Teaching Guides

Research in Practice

Procedures

Community in Focus

BRIEF CONTENTS

MATERNAL-NEWBORN NURSING

Maternal-Newborn Nursing

A Family and Community-Based Approach

SIXTH EDITION

Sally B. Olds, MS, RNC, SANE
Professor Emerita
Beth-El College of Nursing
Colorado Springs, Colorado

Marcia L. London, MSN, RNC, NNP
Associate Professor and Director
Neonatal Nurse Practitioner Program
Beth-El College of Nursing and Health Sciences
University of Colorado at Colorado Springs
Colorado Springs, Colorado

Patricia A. Wieland Ladewig, PhD, RNC, NP
Professor and Academic Dean
School for Health Care Professions
Regis University
Denver, Colorado

PRENTICE HALL HEALTH
Upper Saddle River, New Jersey 07458

ss Cataloging-in-Publication Data

-

orn nursing : a family and community-
lly B. Olds, Marcia L. London, Patricia
5th ed.

..udes bibliographical references and index.
ISBN 0–8053–8070–1
1. Maternity nursing Handbooks, manuals, etc. 2. Community health nursing Handbooks, manuals, etc. I. London, Marcia L. II. Ladewig, Patricia, W. III. Title.
[DNLM: 1. Community Health Nursing. 2. Maternal–Child Nursing.
WY 157.3 044m 1999]
RG951.043 1999
610.73' 678—dc21
DNLM/DLC
for Library of Congress 99-28575
CIP

Manager, Addison Wesley Nursing: Paul Blackburn
Senior Project Editor: Virginia Simione Jutson
Managing Editor: Wendy Earl
Production Supervisor: Bradley Burch
Art and Photo Supervisor: Bradley Burch
Associate Editor: Stephanie Kellogg
Publishing Assistants: Susan Teahan and Peggy Hammett
Text Designer: Cloyce Wall
Cover Designer: Yvo Riezebos
Director of Manufacturing and Production: Bruce Johnson
Manufacturing Buyer: Ilene Sanford

Art and photography credits appear on pages 1052–1054.

Previously published by Addison-Wesley Nursing, A Division of The Benjamin/Cummings Publishing Company, Menlo Park, California 94025.

10 9 8 7 6 5 4 3 2

ISBN 0–8053–8070–3

Prentice-Hall International (UK) Limited, London
Prentice-Hall of Australia Pty. Limited, Sydney
Prentice-Hall Canada Inc., Toronto
Prentice-Hall Hispanoamericana, S.A., Mexico
Prentice-Hall of India Private Limited, New Delhi
Prentice-Hall of Japan, Inc. Tokyo

The authors and publisher would like to thank the agencies that provided settings for many of the photos in this edition, they are: Springs Center for Women, Colorado Springs, Colorado; Alta Bates Hospital, Berkeley, California; and Berkeley Primary Care Access Clinic, Berkeley, California; Eden Medical Center, Castro Valley, California. A special thanks goes to the staff, parents, and newborns associated with these agencies.

Cover image is *I have found My Blue Flower*, quilted by Liesel Niesner and photographed by Charlotte de la Bedoyère. Reproduced with kind permission of Search Press Limited. © Search Press Limited.

Care has been taken to confirm the accuracy of information presented in this book. The authors, editors, and the publisher, however, cannot accept any responsibility for errors or omissions or for the consequences from application of the information in this book and make no warranty, express, or implied, with respect to its contents.

The authors and publisher have exerted every effort to ensure that drug selections and dosages set forth in this text are in accord with current recommendation and practice at time of publication. However, in view of ongoing research, changes in government regulations, and the constant flow of information relating to drug therapy and drug reactions, the reader is urged to check the package inserts of all drugs for any change in indications of dosage and for added warnings and precautions. This is particularly important when the recommended agent is a new and/or infrequently employed drug.

Maternal-Newborn Nursing

A Family and Community-Based Approach

SIXTH EDITION

Sally B. Olds, MS, RNC, SANE
Professor Emerita
Beth-El College of Nursing
Colorado Springs, Colorado

Marcia L. London, MSN, RNC, NNP
Associate Professor and Director
Neonatal Nurse Practitioner Program
Beth-El College of Nursing and Health Sciences
University of Colorado at Colorado Springs
Colorado Springs, Colorado

Patricia A. Wieland Ladewig, PhD, RNC, NP
Professor and Academic Dean
School for Health Care Professions
Regis University
Denver, Colorado

PRENTICE HALL HEALTH
Upper Saddle River, New Jersey 07458

Library of Congress Cataloging-in-Publication Data
Olds, Sally B., 1940–
Maternal-newborn nursing : a family and community-based approach / Sally B. Olds, Marcia L. London, Patricia Wieland Ladewig. — 6th ed.
p. cm
Includes bibliographical references and index.
ISBN 0–8053–8070–1
1. Maternity nursing Handbooks, manuals, etc. 2. Community health nursing Handbooks, manuals, etc. I. London, Marcia L. II. Ladewig, Patricia, W. III. Title.
[DNLM: 1. Community Health Nursing. 2. Maternal–Child Nursing.
WY 157.3 044m 1999]
RG951.043 1999
610.73' 678—dc21
DNLM/DLC
for Library of Congress 99-28575
CIP

Manager, Addison Wesley Nursing: Paul Blackburn
Senior Project Editor: Virginia Simione Jutson
Managing Editor: Wendy Earl
Production Supervisor: Bradley Burch
Art and Photo Supervisor: Bradley Burch
Associate Editor: Stephanie Kellogg
Publishing Assistants: Susan Teahan and Peggy Hammett
Text Designer: Cloyce Wall
Cover Designer: Yvo Riezebos
Director of Manufacturing and Production: Bruce Johnson
Manufacturing Buyer: Ilene Sanford
Art and photography credits appear on pages 1052–1054.

Previously published by Addison-Wesley Nursing, A Division of The Benjamin/Cummings Publishing Company, Menlo Park, California 94025.

Printed in the United States of America.

10 9 8 7 6 5 4 3 2

ISBN 0–8053–8070–3

Prentice-Hall International (UK) Limited, London
Prentice-Hall of Australia Pty. Limited, Sydney
Prentice-Hall Canada Inc., Toronto
Prentice-Hall Hispanoamericana, S.A., Mexico
Prentice-Hall of India Private Limited, New Delhi
Prentice-Hall of Japan, Inc. Tokyo

The authors and publisher would like to thank the agencies that provided settings for many of the photos in this edition, they are: Springs Center for Women, Colorado Springs, Colorado; Alta Bates Hospital, Berkeley, California; and Berkeley Primary Care Access Clinic, Berkeley, California; Eden Medical Center, Castro Valley, California. A special thanks goes to the staff, parents, and newborns associated with these agencies.

Cover image is *I have found My Blue Flower*, quilted by Liesel Niesner and photographed by Charlotte de la Bedoyère. Reproduced with kind permission of Search Press Limited. © Search Press Limited.

Dedication

We have been fortunate to have love in our lives from family, friends, and associates.
As we have interacted with students, clients, and colleagues, our goal has always been to do so in a supportive and loving manner.

And so we dedicate this edition to love . . . to unending support for those who spend their lives providing nursing care to childbearing clients . . . and for those who love and support you.

Know that our love and support is with you always because we are in . . .
a newborn's first cry . . .
the parent's first gaze . . .
a puppy's kiss . . .
the soft breeze that blows . . .
warm sunshine on your face . . .
the creaking of a rocking chair . . .
the smell of rain before it falls . . . .

To our families, with love . . .
Joe Olds, Scott, Roy, Allison, and Dave
David London, Craig, and Matthew
Tim Ladewig, Ryan, and Erik

SBO, MLL, PWL

CONTRIBUTORS

Melody R. Marks Best, RN-C, MS, WHCNP, LCCE
Contributed to Chapter 9
Colorado College
Colorado Springs, Colorado

Deborah A. Bopp, RN, MS
Contributed to Chapters 17 and 19
Memorial Hospital
Colorado Springs, Colorado

Wendy Earl
Contributed to Self-Care Guides
Medical Writer
San Francisco, California

Victoria Flanagan, RN, BSN
Contributed to Chapter 15
Dartmouth-Hitchcock Medical Center
Lebanon, New Hampshire

Kathleen Furniss, RNC, MSN
Contributed to Chapter 5
Asscociates in Woman's Health Care
Wayne, New Jersey

Mary I. Enzman Hagedorn, RN, PhD, CNS, CPNP
Contributed to Chapter 2 and Research in Practice boxes
Beth El College of Nursing and Health Sciences
University of Colorado at Colorado Springs
Colorado Springs, Colorado

Carol Ann Harrigan, RNC, MSN, NNP
Contributed to Chapter 28
Phoenix Childrens' Hospital
Phoenix, Arizona

Mary Ellen Honeyfield, RNC, MS, NNP
Contributed to Chapter 25
Innovative Health Care, Inc.
Denver, Colorado

Virginia Gramzow Kinnick, RN, EdD, CNM
Contributed to Chapter 13
University of Northern Colorado
Greeley, Colorado

Cheryl Pope Kish, RNC, MSN, EdD, WHNP
Contributed to Chapter 33
Georgia College and Georgia State University
Milledgeville, Georgia

Ruth Likler, RNC, BSN
Contributed to Chapter 26
Presbyterian/St. Luke's Medical Center
Denver, Colorado

Deborah Cooper McGee, RNC, MSN
Contributed to Chapter 16
Regis University
St. Luke's Medical Center
Denver, Colorado

Susan Moberly, RN, BSN, ICCE
Contributed to Critical Pathways
Centura Health/Penrose Community Birth Center
Colorado Springs, Colorado

Patricia Moores, RN, PhD, CS
Contributed to Research in Practice boxes
Samuel Merritt College
Oakland, California

Candace Polzella, RD, MSS
Contributed to Chapter 14
The Renfrew Center
Philadelphia, Pennsylvania

Lisa Sams, RN, MSN
Contributed to Chapters 22 and 23
Clinician to Clinician Solutions, Inc.
Arlington, Virginia

Lisa A. Smith-Pedersen, APRN, MSN, CNNP
Contributed to Chapter 30
Northwestern State University of Louisiana
Louisiana State University Medical Center
Shreveport, Louisiana

Monica Taylor, RN, MEd, LCCE
Contributed to Chapter 27
The Toledo Hospital
Toledo, Ohio

Candice Tolve Schoeneberger, RN, PhD, WHCNP
Contributed to Chapter 12
Regis University
Denver, Colorado

Mary E. English Worth, RNC, CRNP
Contributed to Chapter 8
Pennsylvania Reproductive Associates
Philadelphia, Pennsylvania

Sandra Worthington, RNC, MSN, CNM
Contributed to Chapter 3
Planned Parenthood Federation of America, Inc.
New York, New York

REVIEWERS

Kathy Beard, RN, MSN, FNP, ACCE
Covenant Hospital School of Nursing
Lubbock, Texas

Nancy Diane Bingaman, RN, MSN
Monterey Peninsula College
Monterey, California

Janet C. Brookman, RN, DSN
University of Alabama
Huntsville, Alabama

Carol M. Bryant, RN, MSN, EdD
University of Central Oklahoma
Edmond, Oklahoma

Joyceann Fileccia-Walton, RN, BSN, MA
Bayonne Hospital School of Nursing
Bayonne, New Jersey

Evelyn D. French, RN, MSN, PhD
Lourdes College
Sylvania, Ohio

Janice G. Harris, RNC, MSN
Columbus State University
Columbus, Georgia

Carole Kenner, RNC, DNS, FAAN
Consultants with Confidence, Inc.
Milford, Ohio

Betty Lemon, RNC, CNN, MSN, CS
St. Vincent Mercy Medical Center
Toledo, Ohio

Jane McAteer, RN, MN
College of San Mateo
San Mateo, California

Joanette Pete McGadney, RN, PhD
Texas Woman's University
Dallas, Texas

Joan Carley Oliver, RN, BSN, MSNEd, EdD
Mount Hood Community College
Gresham, Oregon

Netha O'Meara, RN, MS, CNS
Wharton County Junior College
Wharton, Texas

Susan A. Orshan, RNC, PhD, FACCE
Woman's Health Consultant
Princeton, New Jersey

Mildred Peters, RN, MSN
Northern Michigan University
Marquette, Michigan

Lenore K. Resick, RN, MSN, CS, CRNP
Duquesne University
Pittsburgh, Pennsylvania

Mimi Sanderlin, ARNP-C, MSN
Valencia Community College
Orlando, Florida

Ida L. Slusher, RN, DSN
Eastern Kentucky University
Richmond, Kentucky

Paula Smith, RNP, MNSc.
Arkansas State University
Jonesboro, Arkansas

Louise Timmer, RN, MSN, EdD
University of California
Sacramento, California

Terry R. Tobin, RN, MSN, MPH
Marquette University
Milwaukee, Wisconsin

Judy E. White, RNC, MA, MSN
Vital Care Home Parenteral Services
Meridian, Mississippi

Marguerite Wright, RN, MSN, RDMS
Gordon College
Barnesville, Georgia

AUTHOR BIOGRAPHIES

Sally B. Olds has provided hands-on maternal-newborn nursing care, and has mentored students and colleagues for more than 30 years. She received her BSN from the University of Kansas and her MS in nursing from the University of Colorado. Completing her Masters degree provided Mrs. Olds with the opportunity to achieve one of her life's goals—teaching nursing students. She began teaching at the Beth-El School of Nursing and Health Science in 1975, eventually becoming the Chair of the Department of Holistic Nursing, and was instrumental in developing the Clinical Nursing Specialist Program in Holistic Health for the Masters program. Her teaching philosophy has been to nurture and support students as they learn, to focus on the positive aspects of learning, and to teach students the importance of respecting the client and family for whom they provide care. Mrs. Olds taught at Beth-El for over 22 years before retiring in 1997, and was named Professor Emerita. She became a Sexual Assault Nurse Examiner (SANE), working one-on-one with sexual assault survivors in 1996, and she continues her involvement with issues affecting women and children. Since her retirement, Mrs. Olds has had more time to spend with her husband and two grown children, and her Old English Sheepdog.

Marcia L. London has been able to combine her two greatest passions—being both a nurse caring for children and families and a teacher for almost 29 years. She received her BSN and School Nurse Certificate from Plattsburgh State University in Plattsburgh, New York. After graduation, she worked as a pediatric nurse at Saint Luke's Hospital in New York City, then moved to Pittsburgh where she began her teaching career. Mrs. London accepted a faculty position at Pittsburgh's Children's Hospital Affiliate program and received her MSN in Pediatrics from University of Pittsburgh in Pennsylvania. Mrs. London began teaching at Beth-El School of Nursing and Health Science in 1974 after opening the first Intensive Care Nursery at Memorial Hospital of Colorado Springs. She has served in many faculty positions at Beth-El, including Assistant Director of the School of Nursing. Mrs. London obtained her post masters Neonatal Nurse Practitioner certificate in 1983, and subsequently developed the Neonatal Nurse Practitioner certificate and the Masters programs at Beth-El. She is active nationally in neonatal nursing and was involved in the development of the Neonatal Nurse Practitioner Educational program guidelines. Mrs. London is currently completing her PhD in Higher Education Administration and Adult Studies at University of Denver in Colorado. She feels fortunate to be involved in the education of her future colleagues and her teaching philosophy is that with support, students can achieve more than they may initially believe they are capable of. Mrs. London and her husband have two sons and two dogs (Samantha and Betsy—daughters by proxy). Her son Matthew is finishing high school and her son Craig is combining college and computers.

Patricia A. Wieland Ladewig received her BSN from the College of Saint Teresa in Winona, Minnesota. After graduation, she worked as pediatric nurse before joining the Air Force. After completing her tour of duty, Dr. Ladewig relocated to Florida where she accepted a faculty position at Florida State University. There she discovered teaching as her calling. Over the years, she taught at several schools of nursing while earning her MSN in Maternal-Newborn Nursing from Catholic University of America in Washington, DC, and her PhD in Higher Education Administration from the University of Denver in Colorado. In addition, she became a Women's Health Nurse Practitioner and maintained a part-time clinical practice. In 1988 Dr. Ladewig became the first director of the nursing program at Regis College in Denver, and in 1991, when the college became Regis University, she became Dean of the School for Health Care Professions. Under her guidance, the Department of Nursing has added a graduate program and the School for Health Care Professions has added two departments: the Department for Physical Therapy and the Department of Health Services Administration and Management. Dr. Ladewig feels that teaching others to be excellent, caring nurses gives her the best of all worlds because it keeps her in touch with the profession she loves and enables her to help shape the future of nursing professionals. When not at work or writing textbooks, Pat and her husband, Tim, enjoy skiing, climbing Colorado's 14'ers (14,000 foot mountains—she has climbed 15 to date), and traveling. They are parents of two college-aged sons, Ryan and Erik.

PREFACE

Caring for childbearing women and their families—in their times of great joy and in their moments of deepest sorrow—is in many ways the essence of nursing. Nurses play a central role in all aspects of the experience, from the earliest days of pregnancy, through the moments of birth, and during the early days of parenthood. Often the quality of the nursing care a family receives profoundly influences their perceptions of the entire experience—for better or for worse. However, the changes occurring in the health care delivery system have staggering implications for nurses everywhere, even nurses caring for childbearing women and their families. Shortened length of stay, the trend toward greater use of home care options, the increasing use of unlicensed assistive personnel, downsizing and mergers of large health care systems, the aging of the population—these and a myriad of other factors are altering the way we practice nursing today and in the future.

Now, more than ever, nurses must be flexible, creative, and open to change. They must be able to think critically and problem solve effectively. They must be able to meet the teaching needs of their clients so that their clients can, in turn, better meet their own health care needs. They must be open to an increasingly multicultural population. They must understand and use the technology available in their chosen area of practice. Most crucially, they must never lose sight of the importance of excellent nursing care in improving the quality of people's lives.

The underlying philosophy of *Maternal-Newborn Nursing: A Family and Community-Based Approach* remains unchanged. We believe that pregnancy and birth are normal life processes and that family members are co-participants in care. We remain committed to providing a text that is accurate and readable; a text that helps students develop the skills and abilities they need now and in the future in an ever-changing health care environment.

Community-Based Nursing Care

By its very nature, maternal-newborn nursing is community-based nursing. Only a brief portion of the entire pregnancy and birth is spent in a birthing center or hospital. Moreover, because of changes in practice, even women with high-risk pregnancies are receiving more care in their homes and in the community and spending less time in hospital settings.

The provision of nursing care in community-based settings is a driving force in health care today and, consequently, is a dominant theme throughout this edition. We have addressed this topic in several ways. *Community-Based Nursing Care* is a heading used throughout the text to assist students in identifying specific aspects of this content. Because we consider *Home Care* to be one form of community-based care, it is often a separate heading under *Community-Based Nursing Care*. Even more importantly, a new chapter, Chapter 32, *Home Care of the Postpartal Family*, provides a thorough explanation of home care as an important aspect of care for childbearing families.

Community in Focus boxes are another exciting new feature in this edition. These boxes describe innovative community nursing programs available in different parts of the United States.

Nursing Care Management

While some books cover the role of the medical community in childbirth as a separate topic, our book gives an overview of all aspects of the childbearing process with a specific emphasis on nursing care throughout pregnancy, labor and birth, and the postpartal period. A new heading, *Nursing Care Management*, delineates the important care management role of the nurse within the organizing framework of the nursing process. Numerous special features reinforce the care management role. The **Assessment Guides** incorporate expected findings, possible alterations, and causes, as well as guidelines for interventions. The **Critical Pathways** help nurses organize care and evaluate its effectiveness. **Procedures** describe interventions specific to maternal-newborn nursing care in illustrated, step-by-step fashion.

Emphasis on Client/Family Teaching

Client and family teaching is a crucial responsibility of the maternal-newborn nurse, one we continue to emphasize strongly and highlight in this sixth edition. Again, our focus is on the teaching that nurses do at all stages of pregnancy and the childbearing process including the important postpartal teaching that is done before and immediately after families are discharged. Thus the chapter on client teaching, Chapter 2, *Community-Based Teaching for Childbearing Families*, has been revised and broadened.

In several places a more detailed discussion of client/family teaching is summarized in the **Teaching Guides**. The perforated **Self-Care Guides** at the back of the book provide students with additional client teaching information and can be removed from the book, photocopied, and handed out to clients. The tear-out **Client/Family Teaching Cards** are also handy tools for the student to use while studying or for quick reference in the clinical setting. Furthermore, a fold-out, full-color **Fetal Development Chart** depicts maternal/fetal development month by month and provides specific teaching guidelines for each stage of pregnancy. Students can use this chart as another tool for study or as a quick clinical reference.

Special Features

In this edition we have streamlined the content to help students focus their study. For example, the Women's Health unit has been reorganized and thoroughly revised, and the content on the pregnant adolescent is now addressed in a new chapter, ***Chapter 13, Adolescent Pregnancy.***

We also provide several features designed to enhance clinical skills and critical thinking abilities:

- **Critical Thinking in Practice** provides brief scenarios that ask students to determine the appropriate response to real-life clinical situations. Suggested answers to the scenarios are provided in Appendix I to give students immediate feedback on their decision-making skills.
- **Critical Thinking Questions** interspersed throughout the text challenge students to think more deeply about the content they are studying and its implications for clinical practice.
- **Critical Pathways** reflect a growing trend in the way nurses manage care and we have included several examples to assist students. These pathways focus on both a normal childbearing experience and on conditions that place a pregnant or postpartum woman or a newborn at high risk.
- **Essential Precautions in Practice** boxes appear throughout the text to help students apply appropriate blood and body fluid precautions in a variety of nursing care situations.
- The **Clinical Tips** are among our favorite features. These tips, or "pearls of wisdom," are gleaned from our own clinical practice or that of colleagues and are addressed directly to the students.
- The **Research in Practice** boxes have been completely updated to reflect the latest research findings, and are redesigned to focus on the applicability of the findings for clinical practice. This helps students grasp the importance of clinical nursing research for effective practice.
- The **Resource Guide** (Appendix J) provides students with the names, telephone numbers, and URLs of various maternal-newborn nursing organizations.

State-of-the-Art Teaching/Learning Tools

Instructors and students alike continue to praise the abundance of in-text learning aids included in our books. With this edition, we have once again created a book that is both easy to learn from and easy to use as a reference. Each chapter begins with learning **Objectives** and a list of **Key Terms,** and ends with a section, **Focus Your Study,** which summarizes important concepts as well as a list of References. Where appropriate, we have included **Drug Guides** for those medications commonly used in maternal-newborn nursing, to guide students in correctly administering medications. Additionally, photographs, quotes, and vignettes from nurses, clients, and students bring a personal perspective to the text by presenting real-life situations. Finally, a **Glossary** of terms (with phonetic pronunciations of those most difficult to pronounce) that are commonly used in the field of maternal-newborn nursing can be found at the back of the book.

Commitment to Diversity

With this edition, we made our text even more inclusive through a commitment to diversity beyond multiculturalism. We realize such an approach is difficult at best, but feel its success cannot be measured simply in terms of specific photos, charts, or tables. Instead, we believe that with its subtle integration of a variety of issues and scenarios affecting maternal-newborn nursing care—beyond an emphasis on ethnicity alone—our approach is more accessible overall.

Complete Teaching/Learning Package

For the Student

- **NEW! Free Companion Web site** for nursing students includes on-line quizzing, chapter outlines, and Internet resources. Visit the Prentice Hall Health Nursing Station at www.prenhall.com/nursing.
- **NEW! Student Tutorial CD-ROM.** This addition to the teaching/learning package is an interactive student program that contains NCLEX-style multiple-

choice and fill-in questions. Students are able to test their knowledge and gain immediate feedback through rationales provided for both right and wrong answers. This CD-ROM is packaged with every copy of the text and is free to students.

- **Clinical Handbook.** Written by the authors, this clinical handbook serves as a portable, succinct quick-reference to guide students in the clinical area.
- **Student Workbook.** Written by the authors, this popular workbook has been revised and updated in keeping with the changes made in this revision. It incorporates strategies for students to focus their study and increase their knowledge.

For the Instructor

- **NEW! Instructor's Presentation CD-ROM.** For lecture presentation purposes, this cross-platform CD-ROM includes illustrations from the text.
- **Instructor's Manual.** Written by Virginia Kinnick, CNM, EdD, this timesaving aid has been thoroughly revised and updated.
- **800-Item Test Bank,** written by Judith M. Wilkinson, PhD, RNC, ARNP, available in printed form or as computer software for IBM-compatible computers, this updated and revised test bank helps faculty quickly and easily create numerous unique examinations.
- **Transparency Acetates.** A set of full-color transparencies provide visual support for lectures.

Acknowledgments

Our goal with every revision is to incorporate the latest research and information from the literature of nursing and related fields to make our text as relevant and useful as possible. This would not be possible without the support and encouragement of our peers. The comments and suggestions we have received from nurse educators and practitioners around the country have helped us keep this text accurate and up-to-date. Whenever a nurse takes the time to write or to speak to one of us at a professional gathering, we recognize again the intense commitment of nurses to excellence in practice. And so we thank our colleagues.

We are grateful, too, to our students, past, present, and future. They stimulate us with their interest; they reinvigorate us with their enthusiasm; they challenge us with their questions to make each edition of this text clear and understandable. We learn so much from them.

In publishing as in health care, quality assurance is an essential part of the process; that is the dimension our reviewers have added. Some reviewers assist us by validating the accuracy of the content, some by their attention to detail, and some by challenging us to examine our ways of thinking and to develop a new awareness about a given topic. Thus we extend our sincere thanks to all those who reviewed the manuscript for this book; their names and affiliations are listed before this preface.

We are also grateful to the contributors to the sixth edition of *Maternal-Newborn Nursing: A Family and Community-Based Approach.* Their knowledge of clinical practice and current literature in their areas of expertise helps make the chapters relevant and accurate. They, too, are listed just before this preface.

The success of a project of this scope requires the skills and dedication of many people. We would personally like to thank the following people:

Ginnie Simione Jutson, our editor, is a very special woman and a long-time friend. Her knowledge and editorial ability are unquestioned. More importantly, from our perspective, she is warm, caring, and compassionate with a great sense of humor and infinite patience. She is also the incredibly lucky mother of a little jewel, Hannah Faith, born during the writing of this edition!

Karen Gulliver stepped in during Ginnie's maternity leave to take over editorial coordination. She was consistently helpful, supportive, and efficient. Thanks, Karen, for the seamless transition.

We are deeply grateful to Stephanie Kellogg for all her behind the scenes efforts. Stephanie coordinated all the reviews and the supplement package. She is a very talented woman.

Sally Peyrefitte, the copy editor, has a remarkable knowledge of grammar and punctuation, a keen eye, and a staggering memory for detail. Her work has improved our manuscript and helped ensure consistency.

What can you say about a man who takes on the responsibilities of a production editor as well as coordination of all art and photos for the manuscript, and who does so with infinite patience, helpfulness, and charm? That man, Bradley Burch, is an exceptional person and a special friend. We would be lost without him.

Kudos to Wendy Earl. She converted many of the Teaching Guides in the text to Self-Care Guides, which students are free to reproduce and share with the childbearing women and families they encounter. This new feature helps students learn to teach clients more effectively.

Many thanks to the in-house staff of Addison Wesley and Wendy Earl Productions for their yeoman's service on behalf of the book, especially Susan Teahan, who prepared and prepped the manuscript, and Peggy Hammett and David Novak for their overall support.

Many thanks as well to Tina Valenzuela of Kwik Kopy Printing in Colorado Springs for her prompt and unfailingly cheerful response to our rush projects. We are grateful to Diane Kern, RN, IBCLE, and Lisa Hoffman, RN, ACCE for providing us with some of the Clinical

Tips included in this text; and thanks, too, to Carol Lawson and Tod Hazlett for updating the Resources Guide, adding URL information, and verifying the 1–800 phone numbers. The Guide is as current as we can make it because of their efforts.

And finally, a warm word of thanks to Paul Blackburn, Manager of AW Nursing. Although we only worked with him for a brief period, we were struck by his warmth, his commitment to excellence, and his wonderful accent!

During these times of uncertainty in the health care environment, we are sustained by our passion for nursing and our vision of what childbirth means. Time and again we have seen the difference a skilled nurse can make in the lives of people in need. We, like you, are committed to helping all nurses recognize and take pride in that fact. Thank you for your letters, your comments, and your suggestions. We are renewed by your support.

SBO, MLL, PWL

Dear Students:

We believe that working with childbearing families gives you the opportunity to experience the essence of nursing at its best. You can play a vital role in helping families learn what they need to know in order to be as independent as possible; you can improve and refine your assessment skills as you work with essentially healthy women and infants, and those with complications; and you can also use the other nursing skills you have learned in a variety of acute and community-based care settings.

We love this field and we know that many of you will as well. Some of you, on the other hand, may find that this area of nursing is not your first interest, and that's OK, too. We would have a real problem if every nurse loved the same area!

We do hope that you will use this opportunity to grow in professional ability and to appreciate the importance of all you do as nurses — not just the technical and organizational tasks, although they are undoubtedly crucial, but also the caring you bring to the role of nurse. When you hold the hand of a laboring woman or help an adolescent plan a way to tell her parents of her pregnancy; when you provide accepting care to a woman with AIDS or gently stroke the skin of a preterm infant; when you rejoice with a delighted father or console a grieving one; you are practicing the heart of nursing.

Caring in an optimal environment is not difficult, but caring in today's practice setting is more of a challenge. Finding a way to maintain a caring environment when you are overworked and stretched by fiscal constraints and a lack of adequate staffing requires great dedication, creativity, and personal resolve. We have attempted to help you translate caring into practice throughout this text through the tone of the book, the photos and art work, the personal quotes, and the content itself with its emphasis on holistic care.

As you work to translate what you learn into practice, please take care of yourselves as well. Providing excellent nursing care is infinitely rewarding and can be energizing, but it is also draining both physically and emotionally. Make time to play, rest, exercise, be with loved ones, and participate in things that rejuvenate you.

We think that nurses are very special people and we are proud to be counted among them. Good luck with your studies! We wish you well.

Sally B. Olds

Marcia L. London

Pat W. Ladewig

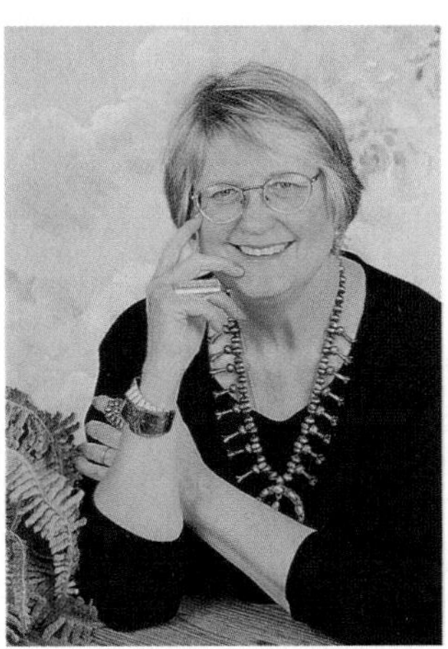

Sally B. Olds

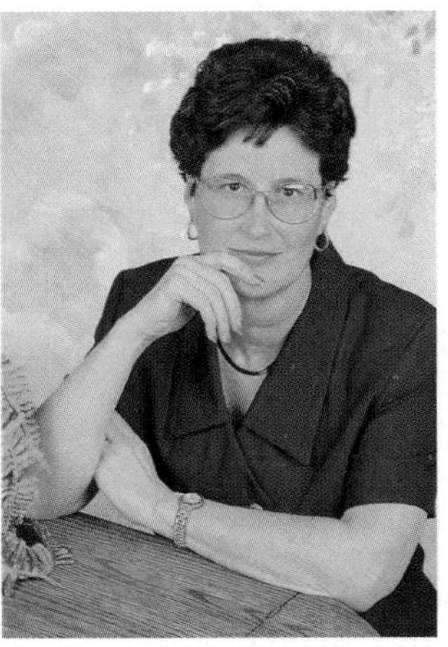

Marcia L. London

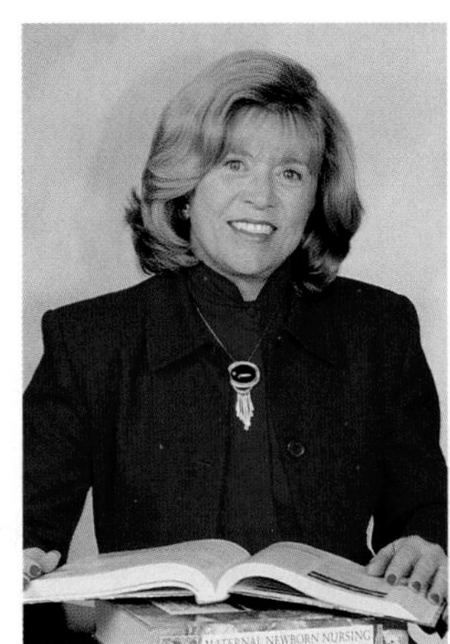

Pat W. Ladewig

To the Student

This textbook contains numerous learning tools to help increase your understanding of key concepts and guide you in applying maternal-newborn nursing care.

CRITICAL THINKING IN PRACTICE boxes use a case study format to further develop effective problem-solving and decision-making skills. Responses are provided in Appendix I.

CRITICAL THINKING IN PRACTICE

A mother calls you to her room. She sounds frightened and says her baby can't breathe. You find the mother cradling her infant in her arms. The infant is mildly cyanotic, waving her arms, and has mucus coming from her nose and mouth. What would you do?

Answer (from Appendix I): Reassure mother that you will help her baby as you carry out the following activities:

- *Position the infant with her head lowered and to the side.*
- *Bulb suction the nares and mouth repeatedly until the airway is cleared.*
- *Hold and comfort the infant when normal respirations are restored.*
- *Reassure the mother, and review this procedure with her.*

NOTE: If bulb suctioning alone does not clear the airway, use DeLee wall suction and administer oxygen as needed to restore normal respirations.

CRITICAL THINKING QUESTIONS are integrated throughout the text to encourage you to select appropriate strategies to support client needs.

CRITICAL THINKING QUESTION

You hear the fetal heart rate just above the expectant woman's navel (umbilicus). You read in the prenatal record that 2 weeks ago, at 35 weeks, the fetal presentation was cephalic. What do you think of your findings? Are they consistent with a cephalic presentation? What might you do to gather additional data?

ESSENTIAL PRECAUTIONS IN PRACTICE boxes, integrated throughout the text, show you how to apply appropriate infection control practices in a variety of situations.

ESSENTIAL PRECAUTIONS IN PRACTICE

During Prenatal Examinations

Examples of times when gloves should be worn include the following:

- When drawing blood for lab work
- When handling urine specimens
- During pelvic examinations (sterile gloves)

In most instances in a clinic or office setting, gowns and goggles are not necessary because splashing of fluids is unlikely.

REMEMBER to wash your hands prior to putting the disposable gloves on and AGAIN immediately after you remove the gloves.

For further information consult OSHA and CDC guidelines.

CRITICAL PATHWAYS provide detailed, time-sequenced guides of anticipated care for women giving birth—whether vaginally or by cesarean section—for healthy newborns and for new mothers.

CRITICAL PATHWAY FOR INTRAPARTAL STAGES

Category	First Stage	Second and Third Stage	Fourth Stage Birth to 1 Hour Past Birth
Referral	**Review prenatal record** **Advise CNM/physician of admission**	**Labor record for first stage**	**Report to recovery room nurse**
Assessments	Admission assessments: Ask about problems since last prenatal visit; labor status (contraction frequency and duration), membrane status (intact or ruptured); coping level; support; woman's desires during labor and birth; ability to verbalize needs; laboratory testing (blood and UA) Intrapartal assessments:Cervical assessment: from 1 to 10 cm dilatation; nullipara (1.2 cm/h), multipara (1.5 cm/h) Cervical effacement: from 0% to 100% Fetal descent: progressive descent from −4 to +4 Membrane assessment: intact or ruptured; when ruptured, Nitrazine positive, fluid clear, no foul odor Comfort level: woman states is able to cope with contractions Behavioral characteristics: facial expressions, tone of voice and verbal expressions are consistent with comfort level and ability to cope Latent Phase: • B/P, P, R q1h if in normal range (B/P 90–140/60–90 or not >30 mm Hg systolic or 15 mm Hg diastolic over baseline; pulse 60–90; respirations 12–20/min, quiet, easy) • Temp q4h unless >37.6C (99.6F) or membranes ruptured then q2h • Uterine contractions q30min (contractions q5–10min, 15–40sec, mild intensity) • FHR q60min (for low-risk women) and q30min (for high-risk women) if reassuring (reassuring FHR has: baseline 120–160, STV present, LTV average, accelerations with fetal movement, no late nor variable decelerations); if nonreassuring, position on side, start O_2, assess for hypotension, monitor continuously, notify CNM/physician Active Phase: • B/P, P, R, q1h if WNL • Temp as above • Uterine contractions q30min: contractions q2–3min, 60 sec, moderate to strong • FHR q30min (for low-risk women) and q15min (for high-risk women) if reassuring; if nonreassuring institute interventions Transition: • B/P, P, R, q30min • Uterine contractions q15–30min: contractions q2min, 60–75 sec, strong • FHR q30min (for low-risk women) and q15min (for high-risk women) if reassuring; if nonreassuring, see above	Second stage assessments: • B/P, P, R q5–15min • Uterine contractions palpated continuously • FHR q15min (for low-risk women) and q5min (for high-risk women) if reassuring; if nonreassuring, monitor continuously Fetal descent: descent continues to birth Comfort level: woman states is able to cope with contractions and pushing Behavioral characteristics: response to pushing, facial expressions, verbalization Third stage assessments: • B/P, P, R q5min • Uterine contractions, palpate occasionally until placenta is delivered, fundus maintains tone and contraction pattern continues to birth of placenta Newborn assessments: • Assess Apgar score of newborn • Respirations: 30–60, irregular • Apical pulse: 120–160 and somewhat irregular • Temperature: Skin temp above 36.5C (97.8F) • Umbilical cord: two arteries, one vein (if one artery, assess for anomalies and urine output) • Gestational age: 38–42 weeks	**Expected Outcomes** Appropriate resources identified and utilized Immediate postbirth assessments of mother q15min for 1h: • B/P: 90–140/60–90; should return to prelabor level • Pulse: slightly lower than in labor; range is 60–90 • Respirations: 12–20/min; easy; quiet • Temperature: 36.2–37.6C (98–99.6F) • Fundus firm, in midline, at the umbilicus • Lochia rubra; moderate amount; <1 pad/h; no free flow or passage of clots with massage • Perineum: sutures intact; no bulging or marked swelling; minimal bruising may be present; no c/o severe pain nor rectal pain • Bladder nondistended; spontaneous void of >100mL clear, straw-colored urine; bladder nondistended following voiding • If hemorrhoids present, no tenseness or marked engorgement; <2 cm diameter Comfort level: <3 on scale of 1 to 10 Energy level: awake and able to hold newborn Newborn assessments if newborn remains with parents: • Respirations: 30–60; irregular • Apical pulse: 120–160 and somewhat irregular • Temperature: skin temp above 36.5C (97.8F); skin feels warm to touch • Skin color noncyanotic • Mucus: small amount, clear, easily suctioned with bulb syringe without skin color change • Behavioral: newborn opens eyes widely if room is slightly darkened • Movements rhythmic; no hand tremors present **Expected Outcomes** Findings indicate normal progression with absence of complications

CONTINUED

Category	First Stage	Second and Third Stage	Fourth Stage Birth to 1 Hour Past Birth
	essments mation athing amily	Orient to expected assessments and procedures Answer questions and provide information Explain comfort measures available Continue advocacy role	Explain immediate assessments and care after this first hour Teach self-massage of fundus and expected findings Instruct to call for assistance if mother desires to get OOB Begin newborn teaching; bulb syringe, positioning; maintaining warmth Assist parents in exploring their newborn Assist with first breastfeeding experience **Expected Outcomes** Client and partner verbalize/demonstrate understanding of teaching
	d or B/P, Perineal clip per woman's request Small enema per woman's request Perform sterile vaginal examination as indicated	Straight cath prn if bladder distended Continue monitoring VS, FHR and sensation if regional block has been given	Straight cath if bladder distended Monitor return of motor ability and sensation if regional block has been given Weigh perineal pads if lochia flow >1 saturated pad in 15 min, presence of boggy uterus and clots; ↓B/P, ↑P **Expected Outcomes** • Maternal/fetal well-being maintained and supported • Mother and newborn experience safe labor and birth • Family participates in process as desired
Activity	Encourage ambulation unless contraindicated Maintain bed rest immediately after administration of IV pain medication, or following regional block Woman rests comfortably between contractions	Position comfortably for birth Woman rests comfortably between pushing efforts & while awaiting birth of placenta	Position of comfort **Expected Outcomes** • Activity maintained as desired unless contraindicated • Comfort enhanced by positioning/movement
Comfort	Institute comfort measures: ambulation, frequent position change, effleurage, focal point, patterned paced breathing, visualization, therapeutic touch, back rub, moist cloths to face, holding hand, words of encouragement, changing underpad, shower, whirlpool, staying with the woman/family, warmed blanket at back, sacral pressure Offer pain medication or administer if requested Assist with administration of regional block	Institute comfort measures: • Second stage: cool cloth to forehead, encouragement, coaching, help support legs while pushing, position of comfort for pushing and birth • Third stage: cool cloth to forehead, assist parents to see newborn, position mother to hold newborn, provide encouragement	Institute comfort measures: • Perineal discomfort: gently cleanse and apply ice pack; position to decrease pressure on perineum • Uterine discomfort: palpate fundus gently • Hemorrhoids: ice pack • General fatigue: position of comfort, encourage rest • Administer pain medication ________ **Expected Outcomes** • Optimal comfort level maintained • Active reductionof pain/discomfort achieved
Nutrition	Ice chips and clear fluids Evaluate for signs of dehydration	Ice chips and clear fluids	Regular diet if assessments are WNL Encourage fluids **Expected Outcomes** Nutritional needs met
Elimination	Voids at least q2h; urine clear, straw-colored, negative for protein Bladder nondistended May have bowel movement Monitor I & O with IVs	May void spontaneously with pushing May pass stool with pushing	Voids spontaneously **Expected Outcomes** Urinary bladder and bowel function unimpaired
Medications	Administer pain medication per woman's request	Local infiltration of anesthetic agent for birth by CNM/physician Pitocin 10 units IM, IVP per IV tubing, or added to IV fluids	Continue Pitocin infusion Administer pain medication ____________ **Expected Outcomes** Comfort enhanced by pain relieving techniques, administration of analgesia agent or an analgesic or anesthetic block

TEACHING GUIDES help you understand how to assess common teaching needs in maternity care situations, create a particular teaching session, and evaluate the session's success.

ASSESSMENT GUIDES summarize assessment findings, alterations and possible causes, and nursing responses to assessment data to help you make distinctions between normal and abnormal clinical findings.

TEACHING GUIDE: WHAT TO EXPECT DURING LABOR

Assessment As the woman is admitted into the birthing area, assess the woman's knowledge regarding the childbirth experience. Her knowledge base will be affected by previous births, attendance at childbirth education classes, and the amount of information she has been able to gather during her pregnancy by asking questions or reading. You may also assess the factors that affect communication and anxiety level. Assess labor progress to determine what to teach and the time available for teaching. If the woman is in early labor and she needs additional information, proceed with teaching.

Nursing Diagnosis The key nursing diagnosis will probably be ***Knowledge Deficit*** related to lack of information about nursing care during labor.

Nursing Plan and Implementation The teaching plan will focus on the assessments and support the woman will receive during labor.

Client Goals At the completion of teaching, the woman will be able to:

- Verbalize the assessments the nurse will complete during labor.
- Discuss the support and comfort measures that are available.

Teaching Plan

Content	*Teaching Method*

• Describe aspects of the admission process, including:
  • Taking an abbreviated history
  • Physical assessment (maternal vital signs [VS], fetal heart rate [FHR], contraction status, status of membranes)
  • Assessment of uterine contractions (frequency, duration, intensity)
  • Orientation to surroundings
  • Introductions to other support staff
  • Determination of woman's and family support person's expectations of the nurse
• Present aspects of ongoing physical care, such as when to expect assessment of maternal VS, FHR, and contractions.
•
	Provide information on the basic assessment and care activities. Allow time for questions and discussion as labor progress permits.

INTRAPARTAL ASSESSMENT GUIDE *CONTINUED*

Nursing Responses to Data†

ess fluid for consistency, amount, odor; ess FHR frequently. Assess fluid at regular rvals for presence of meconium staining. low BSI precautions while assessing amniotic fluid.

h woman that amniotic fluid is continually duced (to allay fear of "dry birth"). h woman that she may feel amniotic fluid kle or gush with contractions. nge Chux pads often.

ess FHR; do vaginal exam to evaluate for lapsed cord; apply fetal monitor for continuous data; report to physician.

e woman's temperature and report to sician.

iate interventions based on particular FHR ern.

ort to physician; after presentation is coned as face, brow, breech, or shoulder, nan may be prepared for cesarean birth.

efully monitor maternal and fetal status.

efully evaluate FHR; apply fetal monitor.

efully evaluate FHR; apply fetal monitor. ort to physician/CNM.

luate woman for problems due to reased oxygen-carrying capacity caused owered hemoglobin.

luate for other signs of infection or for echiae, bruising, or unusual bleeding.

reactive test notify newborn nursery and iatrician.

† column provides guidelines for further assessment nitial nursing intervention.

INTRAPARTAL ASSESSMENT GUIDE *CONTINUED*

Nursing Responses to Data†

Exercise care while doing a perineal prep; note on client record need for follow-up in postpartal period; reassess after birth; refer to physician.

Suspected gonorrhea or chorioamnionitis; report to physician; initiate care to newborn's eyes; notify neonatal nursing staff and pediatrician.

Assess BP and pulse, pallor, diaphoresis; report any marked changes. (Note: Gaping of vagina or anus and bulging of perineum are suggestive signs of second stage of labor.) Universal precautions.

Evaluate whether woman is in true labor; ambulate if in early labor. Evaluate client status and contractile pattern. Obtain a 20-minute EFM monitor strip. Notify physician or CNM.

Evaluate contractions, fetal engagement, position, and cervical dilatation. Inform client of progress.

Evaluate contractions, fetal engagement, and position. Notify physician/CNM if cervix is becoming edematous; work with woman to prevent pushing until cervix is completely dilated. Keep vaginal exams to a minimum.

Evaluate fetal position, presentation, and size. Evaluate maternal pelvic measurements.

Assess for ruptured membranes using Nitrazine test tape before doing vaginal exam. Follow BSI precautions. Instruct woman with ruptured membranes to remain on bed rest if presenting part is not engaged and firmly down against the cervix. Keep vaginal exams to a minimum to prevent infection. When membranes rupture in the birth setting, **immediately assess FHR** to detect changes associated with prolapse of umbilical cord (FHR slows).

†This column provides guidelines for further assessment and initial nursing intervention.

ASSESSMENT GUIDE: INTRAPARTAL—FIRST STAGE OF LABOR

Physical Assessment/ Normal Findings	Alterations and Possible Causes*	Nursing Responses to Data†
Vital Signs		
Blood pressure (BP): < 130 systolic and < 85 diastolic in adult 18 years of age or older or no more than 15–20 mm Hg rise in systolic pressure over baseline BP during early pregnancy (Johannsen, 1993)	High blood pressure (essential hypertension, preeclampsia, renal disease, apprehension or anxiety) Low blood pressure (supine hypotension)	Evaluate history of preexisting disorders and check for presence of other signs of preeclampsia. Do not assess during contractions; implement measures to decrease anxiety and reassess. Turn woman on her side and recheck BP. Provide quiet environment Have O_2 available.
Pulse: 60–90 bpm	Increased pulse rate (excitement or anxiety, cardiac disorders, early shock)	Evaluate cause, reassess to see if rate continues; report to physician.
Respirations: 14–22/min (or pulse rate divided by 4)	Marked tachypnea (respiratory disease), hyperventilation in transition phase	Assess between contractions; if marked tachypnea continues, assess for signs of respiratory disease.
	Hyperventilation (anxiety)	Encourage slow breaths if woman is hyperventilating.
Pulse ox 95% or greater	>90%: hypoxia, hypotension, hemorrhage	Apply O_2; notify physician
Temperature: 36.2–37.6C (98–99.6F)	Elevated temperature (infection, dehydration, prolonged rupture of membranes, epidural regional block)	Assess for other signs of infection or dehydration.
Weight		
25–30 lb greater than prepregnant weight	Weight gain > 30 lb (fluid retention, obesity, large infant, diabetes mellitus, PIH), weight gain < 15 lb (SGA)	Assess for signs of edema. Evaluate pattern from prenatal record.
Lungs		
Normal breath sounds, clear and equal	Rales, rhonchi, friction rub (infection), pulmonary edema, asthma	Reassess; refer to physician.
Fundus		
At 40 weeks' gestation located just below xiphoid process	Uterine size not compatible with estimated date of birth (SGA, large for gestational age [LGA], hydramnios, multiple pregnancy)	Reevaluate history regarding pregnancy dating. Refer to physician for additional assessment.
Edema		
Slight amount of dependent edema	Pitting edema of face, hands, legs, abdomen, sacral area (preeclampsia)	Check deep tendon reflexes for hyperactivity; check for clonus; refer to physician.
Hydration		
Normal skin turgor, elastic	Poor skin turgor (dehydration)	Assess skin turgor; refer to physician for deviations.

*Possible causes of alterations are placed in parentheses.

†This column provides guidelines for further assessment and initial nursing intervention.

Clinical Tips offer practical tips on identifying and coping with clinical situations, much as an experienced mentor would do.

CLINICAL TIP

Doing the pelvic rock on hands and knees may aggravate back strain. Teach women with a history of minor back problems to do the pelvic rock only in the standing position.

Research in Practice boxes report the latest research with a focus on its relevance in clinical practice.

RESEARCH IN PRACTICE

What is this study about? Guatemalan women view pregnancy as a normal physiologic event rather than as an illness. Only 50% of these women seek medical care and the remainder are attended by traditional midwives or comadronas. In order to explore the meaning of the childbirth experience, Lynn Callister and Rosemarie Vega conducted an ethnographic study using the birth stories and perceptions of Guatemalan women.

How was the study done? The principal investigator and a bilingual Latina nursing student interviewed 30 Guatemalan women who had recently given birth to healthy, full-term infants. Interviews took place in a hospital, clinics, homes, and central plazas. Many of the informants lived in small villages, worked in the fields, and wove fabrics to sell. Data analysis included identifying and classifying core concepts from the translated audiotapes.

What were the results of the study? Participants were evenly divided between 15 multiparae and 15 primiparae. Fourteen women gave birth at home with traditional midwives in attendance and 16 gave birth in the hospital, where primarily physicians in training delivered the child. Using midwives allowed the women to give birth in their own homes with more privacy and family support. Midwives would administer herbs to relieve pain and sometimes a small amount of cooking oil to "soften the pain." Some women gave birth in a kneeling or squatting position. Professional care was viewed as safer and less costly than using the services of the traditional midwives. The midwife's fees might consume the family income for an entire month. Because the women viewed birth as a natural, but painful experience, they vocalized their pain. They also used breathing, rhythmic moaning, or rubbing of thighs and abdomen to relieve or cope with pain. Vaginal births in the professional setting were unmedicated. Many women reported being unhappy when they initially learned of their pregnancy due to their concerns about their ability to provide for the child. Paradoxically, children enhance economic security because children can sometimes earn more than their parents and are obligated to care for elderly parents. Predominant themes found by the researchers included a sense of sacredness related to childbearing, a need to rely on God to provide a positive outcome, and the bittersweet paradox of giving birth.

What additional questions might I have? How did the researchers gain access to the participants? Obtaining access is not described. Did the authors conduct any fieldwork or participant observation? Many ethnographic studies include these methods of data collection.

How can I use this study? As the authors state, the study may assist nurses in the provision of culturally competent care if caring for a Central American immigrant from a similar background as the participants of this study. New immigrants may still be tied to the traditions and customs of their country of origin.

SOURCE: Callister, L. C., & Vega, R. (1998). Giving birth: Guatemalan women's voices. *JOGNN, 27,* 289–295.

SELF-CARE GUIDE: SUMMARY OF CONTRACEPTIVE METHODS

Fertility Awareness (also called Natural Family Planning)	***Basal Body Temperature (BBT)*** Methodology: The woman measures and records BBT until ovulation can be predicted according to BBT. Action: Abstain from intercourse for several days before the anticipated time of ovulation and for 3 days after ovulation. ***Rhythm Method (also called Calendar Method)*** Methodology: The woman uses a calendar to calculate the fertile and infertile phases of her menstrual cycle. Action: Abstain from intercourse during the fertile period. ***Cervical Mucus Method (also called Ovulation Method or Billings Method)*** Methodology: The woman assesses cervical mucus for changes in wetness, color, and clearness throughout the menstrual cycle until ovulation can be predicted by the condition of the mucus. Action: Abstain from intercourse when the mucus is wet, clear, and stretchable. ***Symptothermal Method*** Methodology: The woman assesses and records information about primary signs (eg, cycle days, cervical mucus changes) and secondary signs (eg, increased libido, abdominal bloating) until ovulation can be predicted according to the signs. Action: Abstain from intercourse for several days before the anticipated time of ovulation and for 3 days after ovulation.
Situational Contraceptives	***Abstinence*** ***Coitus Interruptus (Withdrawal)*** Methodology/Action: The man withdraws from the vagina when he feels that ejaculation is impending and then ejaculates away from the woman's external genitalia. NOTE: This is one of the least reliable methods of contraception. ***Douching*** Methodology/Action: The woman douches with a saline solution directly after intercourse. NOTE: This is an ineffective method and is not recommended. It may actually facilitate conception by pushing sperm farther up the birth canal.
Spermicides	***Creams, Jellies, Foams, Vaginal Film, Suppositories*** Methodology: The substances destroy or immobilize sperm. Action: The woman inserts one of the substances into the vagina before intercourse. NOTE: Spermicides are minimally effective when used alone, but effectiveness increases when used with a diaphragm, cervical cap, or condom.
Mechanical Contraceptives	***Male Condom*** Methodology: The condom covers the penis and prevents sperm from entering the birth canal. Action: The man applies the condom to the erect penis before vulvar or vaginal contact. ***Female Condom*** Methodology: The condom, which fits over the cervix and also covers a portion of the woman's external genitalia and the base of the man's penis, prevents sperm from entering the birth canal. Action: The woman inserts the condom prior to intercourse. ***Diaphragm*** Methodology: The spermicide-filled diaphragm covers the cervix, preventing sperm from entering the birth canal. Action: The woman fills the diaphragm with spermicidal cream and inserts it into the vagina prior to intercourse. NOTE: The diaphragm must be left in place for 6 hours following intercourse.

Self-Care Guides support client education by providing tear-out, photocopy-ready information sheets to send home with new mothers.

DRUG GUIDES describe the action, use, administration, and nursing considerations for the most important medications used in maternal-newborn nursing.

DRUG GUIDE

Dinoprostone (Cervidil) Vaginal Insert

Pregnancy Risk Category: C

Overview of Maternal-Fetal Action

Dinoprostone is a naturally occurring form of prostaglandin E_2. Dinoprostone can be used at term to ripen the cervix and can stimulate the smooth muscle of the uterus to enhance uterine contractions. A single vaginal insert may be used to ripen the cervix and then oxytocin can be administered 30 minutes later (Zatuchi & Slupik, 1996; Forrest Pharmaceuticals, Inc. Drug Insert, 1995).

Route, Dosage, Frequency

The vaginal insert contains 10 mg of dinoprostone. The insert is placed transversely in the posterior fornix of the vagina, and the client is kept supine for 2 hours but then may ambulate. The dinoprostone is released at approximately 0.3 mg/hour over a 12-hour period. The vaginal insert should be removed by pulling on the retrieval string upon onset of uterine contractions or after 12 hours (Forrest Pharmaceuticals, Inc. Drug Insert, 1995).

Contraindications

- Client with known sensitivity to prostaglandins
- Presence of fetal distress
- Unexplained bleeding during pregnancy
- Strong suspicion of cephalopelvic disproportion
- Client already receiving oxytocin
- Client with 6 or more previous term pregnancies
- Client who is not anticipated to be able to give birth vaginally

Dinoprostone vaginal insert should be used with CAUTION in clients with ruptured membranes, a fetus in breech presentation, presence of glaucoma, or history of asthma (Forrest Pharmaceuticals, Inc., 1995).

Maternal Side Effects

Uterine hyperstimulation with or without fetal distress has occurred in a very small number (2.8–4.7%) of clients. Fewer than 1% of clients have experienced fever, nausea, vomiting, diarrhea, or abdominal pain (Forest Pharmaceuticals, Inc., 1995).

Effects on Fetus/Neonate

Fetal distress (Zatuchi & Slupik, 1996).

Nursing Considerations

- Assess for presence of contraindications.
- Monitor maternal vital signs, cervical dilatation, and effacement carefully.
- Monitor fetal status for presence of reassuring fetal heart rate pattern (baseline 120–160 bpm, presence of short-term variability, average variability, presence of accelerations with fetal movement, absence of late or variable decelerations).
- Remove vaginal insert if uterine hyperstimulation, sustained uterine contractions, fetal distress, or any other maternal adverse actions occur.

COMMUNITY IN FOCUS boxes are informational and inspirational descriptions of community-based care and services.

COMMUNITY IN FOCUS

The Stork's Nest

The Stork's Nest is an innovative educational program co-sponsored by the National March of Dimes Birth Defects Foundation and the Zeta Phi Beta, Inc. sorority, an organization of African-American professional women. Designed primarily for low income women of African-American descent, the program provides incentives for women to attend perinatal educational seminars. In addition to the education provided, women earn points for attending a seminar. These points can then be used to shop for baby clothes at a "store" or Stork's Nest located on site. Individual chapters of the March of Dimes can adopt the basic program as designed or modify it based on their community's needs. The two Stork's Nests sponsored by the Northern Ohio Chapter of the March of Dimes are examples of successful program implementation.

The Stork's Nests located in Cleveland and Akron, which began in 1994 and 1997 respectively, truly represent a community partnership. Each Nest is located in a church that serves a predominantly African-American population. The churches provide space for the seminars and for housing the baby clothes, which are actually arranged as though part of a small store. The Zetas, members of the sorority, staff the Stork's Nests, handle logistics on the day of each seminar, keep track of the points each woman earns, and run the store. Clothing is donated by Gymboree, a nationwide chain of children's clothing stores.

The Northern Ohio Chapter of the March of Dimes has developed the seminars using a nationally developed curriculum, and coordinates the volunteer faculty and clothing donations. Seminars, offered monthly on a Saturday, cover a variety of topics such as "Taking care of oneself during pregnancy," "Caring for a newborn," "Exercise during pregnancy," "Nutrition during pregnancy," and so forth. These seminars cover each topic in depth but in a relaxed atmosphere with time for questions and discussion. Seminar leaders, all volunteers, are often nurses from the prenatal clinics and hospitals that serve this population. These classes are not designed to replace preparation for childbirth classes but to supplement them. On average, 25 women participate in a seminar, although some sessions have had as many as 60 participants. Some women come for one or two seminars, others attend the entire series of classes. Many bring their partners for some sessions. Women can continue to participate for up to one year postpartum. Women learn of the Stork's Nest program from a variety of sources including the clinics where they receive prenatal care, through WIC offices, and from friends. Over 1000 women have participated to date.

Partnerships are an important way of addressing community needs. The Stork's Nests are an example of collaboration at its best and meet an important community need.

SOURCE: Personal communication with John G. Ladd, Director of Program Services, March of Dimes Northern Ohio Chapter.

NURSING CARE MANAGEMENT sections, integrated throughout the text, clearly outline and describe how the nursing process is used to structure effective maternal-newborn care.

NURSING CARE MANAGEMENT

Nursing Assessment and Diagnosis

The nurse should inspect the woman's perineum every 8 to 12 hours for signs of early infection. The REEDA scale helps the nurse remember to consider *r*edness, *e*dema, *e*cchymosis, *d*ischarge, and *a*pproximation. Any degree of induration (hardening) should be immediately reported to the clinician.

Fever, malaise, abdominal pain, foul-smelling lochia, larger than expected uterus, tachycardia, and other signs of infection should be noted and reported immediately so that treatment can begin. The WBC count, a usual objective measure of infection, cannot be used reliably because of the normal increase in white blood cells during the postpartum period; a WBC of 14,000 to 16,000 mm is not an unusual finding. Some clinicians believe that WBC counts of 20,000 plus are not abnormal at this time, likely resulting from the physiologic stress response of labor and also cite a primary increase in neutrophils. An increase in WBC level of more than 30% in a 6-hour period, however, is indicative of infection.

Nursing diagnoses that may apply to the women with a puerperal infection include the following:

- ***Risk for Injury*** related to the spread of infection
- ***Pain*** related to the presence of infection
- ***Knowledge Deficit*** related to lack of information about condition and its treatment
- ***Risk for Altered Parenting*** related to delayed parent-infant attachment secondary to woman's malaise and other symptoms of infection

Nursing Plan and Implementation

Hospital-Based Nursing Care

Careful attention to aseptic technique during labor, birth, and postpartum is essential.

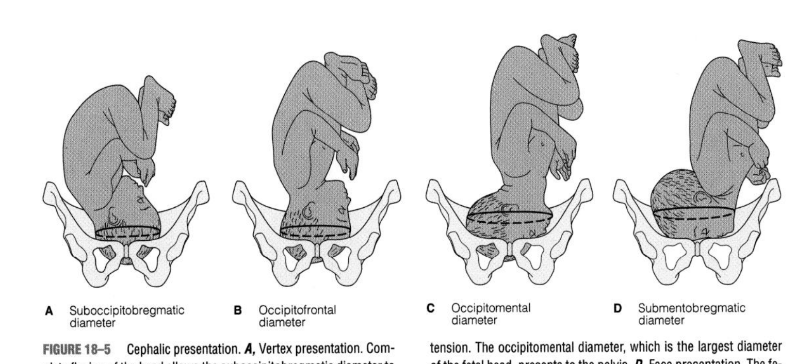

FIGURE 18–5 Cephalic presentation. ***A,*** Vertex presentation. Complete flexion of the head allows the suboccipitobregmatic diameter to present to the pelvis. ***B,*** Military (median vertex) presentation with no flexion or extension. The occipitofrontal diameter presents to the pelvis. ***C,*** Brow presentation. The fetal head is in partial (halfway) extension. The occipitomental diameter, which is the largest diameter of the fetal head, presents to the pelvis. ***D,*** Face presentation. The fetal head is in complete extension, and the submentobregmatic diameter presents to the pelvis.

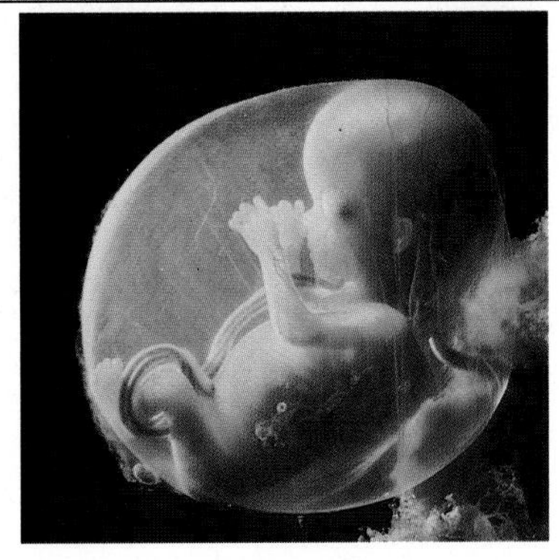

FIGURE 7–23 The fetus at 14 weeks. During this period of rapid growth, the skin is so transparent that blood vessels are visible beneath it. More muscle tissue and body skeleton have developed, which holds the fetus more erect. SOURCE: Nilsson L: *A Child Is Born.* New York: Dell Publishing, 1990.

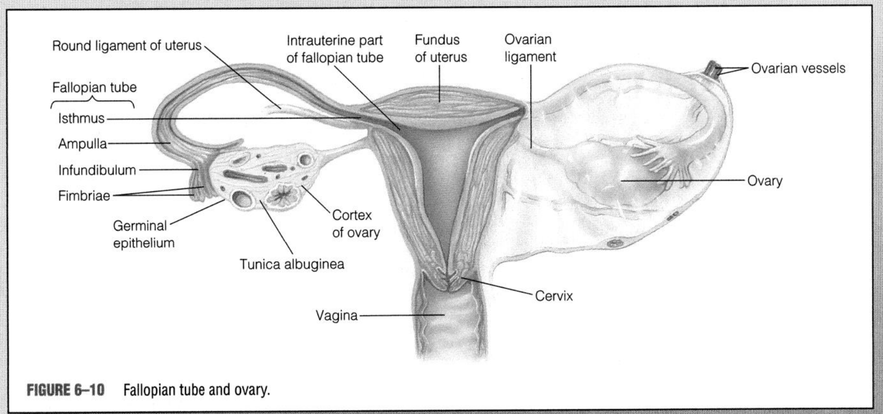

FIGURE 6–10 Fallopian tube and ovary.

FULL-COLOR FORMAT enhances visual learning of anatomy and physiologic processes and highlights key information. Dramatic photographs and personal reflections of childbearing women bring you closer to the childbearing experience.

PROCEDURES breakdown nursing actions and their rationale in an instructional and step-by-step format.

PROCEDURE 19–2 ASSESSING FOR AMNIOTIC FLUID

Nursing Action	*Rationale*
Objective: Assemble equipment.	
• Gather Nitrazine test tape and a pair of disposable gloves.	*Nitrazine test tape reacts to alkaline fluids and confirms presence of amniotic fluid.*
• Have microscope and glass slide available if determining ferning of obtained fluid.	*Microscope is used to detect ferning pattern.*
• Obtain a sterile speculum.	
Objective: Set the stage for the assessment.	
Explain the procedure, indications for the procedure, what the woman will feel, and information that may be obtained. Determine whether she has noted the escape of any clear fluid from the vagina.	*Explanation of the procedure decreases anxiety and increases relaxation.*
Objective: Test fluid.	
• Prior to performing a vaginal examination that uses lubricant, put on gloves. With one gloved hand, spread the labia, and with the other hand place a small section of Nitrazine tape (approx. 2 in long) against the vaginal opening. Take care not to touch tape with bare fingers prior to the test.	*Contamination of the Nitrazine test tape with lubricant can make the test unreliable.* *Enough fluid needs to be placed on the test tape to make it wet. Amniotic fluid is alkaline, and an alkaline fluid turns the Nitrazine test tape a dark blue. If the test tape remains a beige color, the test is negative for amniotic fluid.*
• Compare the color on the test tape to the guide on the back of the Nitrazine test tape container to determine the test results.	
• Amniotic fluid may also be obtained by speculum exam. This is indicated in preterm premature rupture of membranes. If fluid is present in sufficient amount to draw some into a syringe, a small amount of fluid can be placed on a glass slide, allowed to dry, and then examined under a microscope. A ferning pattern confirms the presence of amniotic fluid. See Figure 8–4 for an example of ferning.	*Obtaining a specimen by speculum examination reduces the contamination of the fluid with other substances such as blood and reduces chance of infection for the woman who is not actively laboring.*
Objective: Record information on client's record.	
Record on labor record (eg, SROM, Nitrazine positive).	*Nurse documents status of membranes, intact or ruptured.*

CONTENTS IN DETAIL

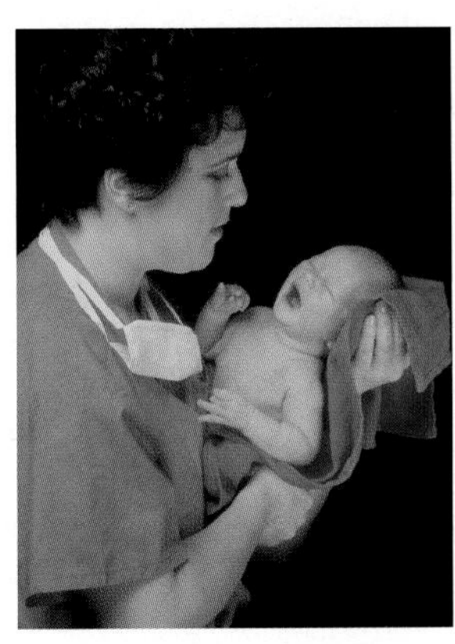

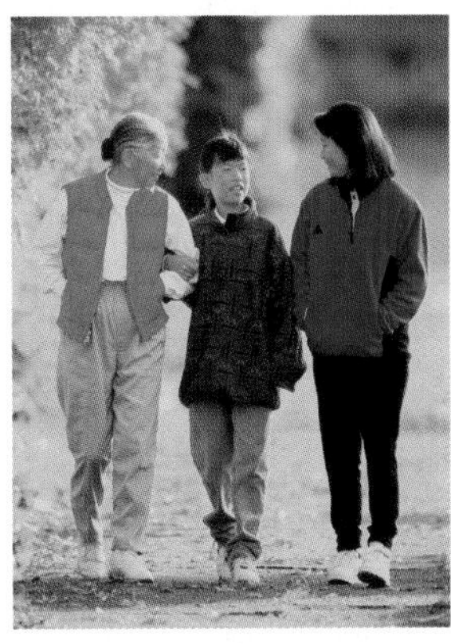

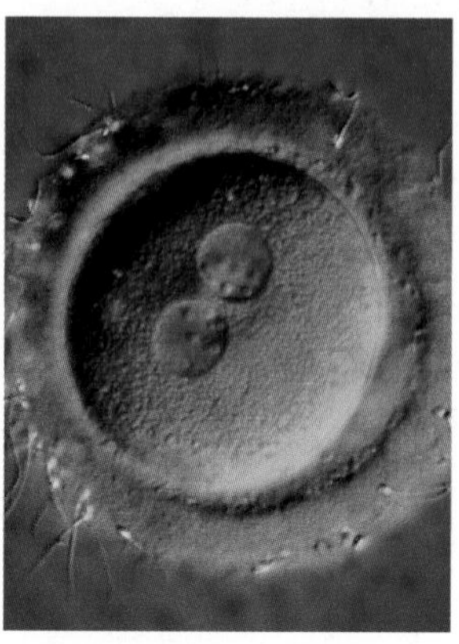

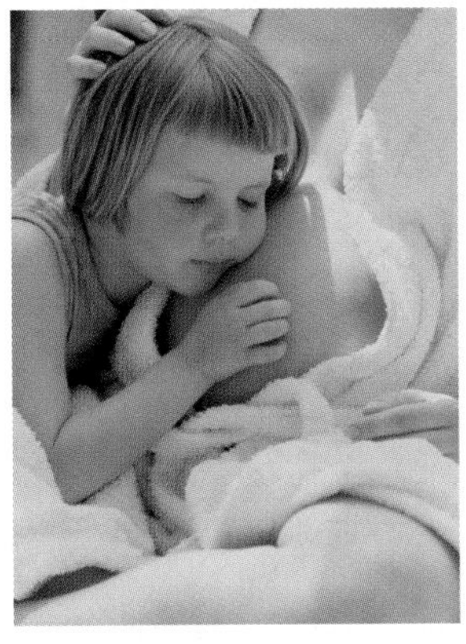

Part Four

Pregnancy 211

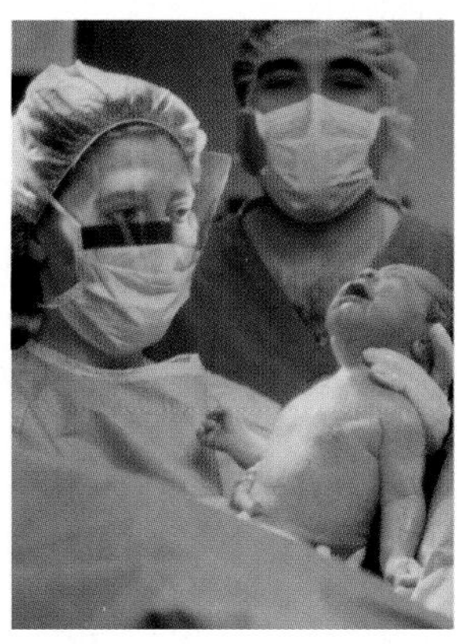

Chapter 21 Pain Management During Birth 581

Chapter 22 Childbirth at Risk 606

Chapter 23 Birth-Related Procedures 651

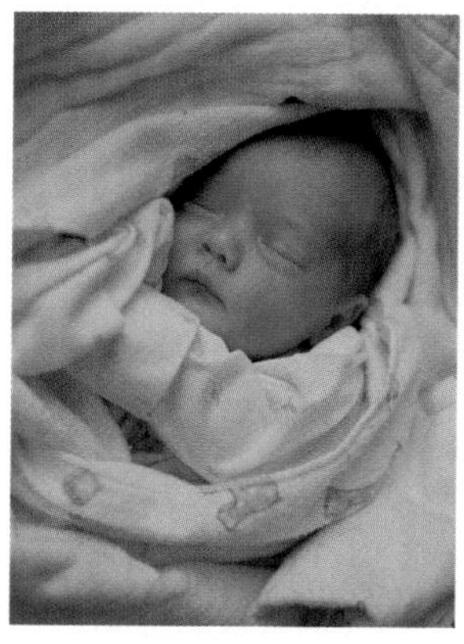

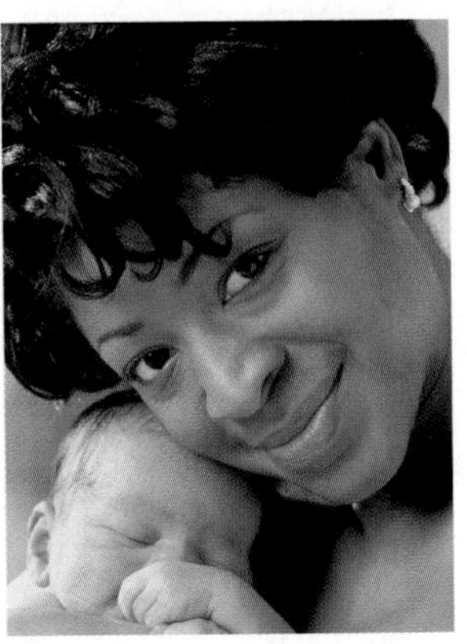

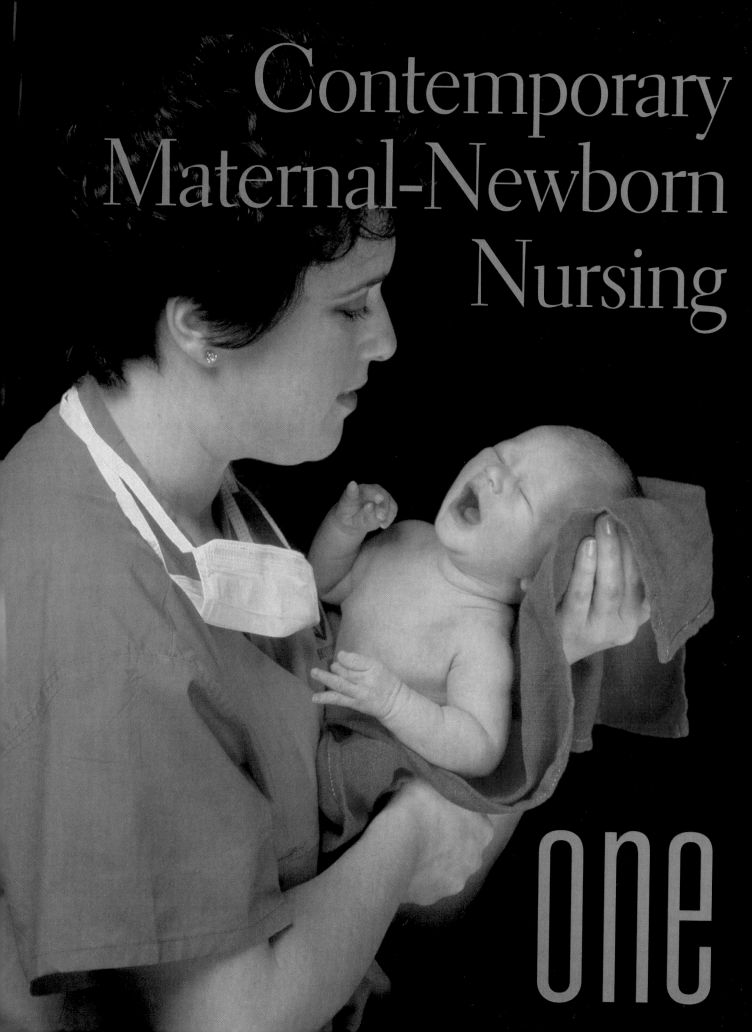

Contemporary Maternal-Newborn Nursing

one

1 Current Issues in Maternal-Newborn Nursing

Key Terms

Artificial insemination (AI)
Assisted reproductive technology (ART)
Certified nurse-midwife (CNM)
Client
Clinical nurse specialist (CNS)
Infant mortality rate
Informed consent
Intrauterine fetal surgery
Maternal mortality rate
Nurse practitioner (NP)
Professional nurse

OUR DAUGHTER JUST TOLD US THAT SHE IS 3 MONTHS pregnant with our first grandchild. As a labor and delivery nurse for 25 years, I've helped with hundreds of births, but it still seems magical to me, especially now. I'm excited for her and a little worried because I know all the risks as well as the joys. She is so happy; when I am with her I just want to laugh out loud. I already know I love being a grandmother, even though I really am too young!

Objectives

- Relate the concept of the expert nurse to nurses caring for childbearing families.
- Discuss the impact of the self-care movement on contemporary childbirth.
- Compare the nursing roles available to the maternal-newborn nurse.
- Delineate significant legal and ethical issues that influence the practice of nursing for childbearing families.
- Evaluate the potential impact of some of the special situations in contemporary maternity care.
- Contrast descriptive and inferential statistics.
- Relate the availability of statistical data to the formulation of further research questions.

THE PRACTICE OF MOST NURSES IS filled with special moments, shared experiences, times in which they know they have practiced the essence of nursing and, in doing so, have touched a life. What is the essence of nursing? Simply stated, nurses care for people, care about people, and use their expertise to help people help themselves.

I like working with students. I enjoy the enthusiasm they bring, the questions they ask, the ways they cause me to examine my practice. I love being a nurse. I am passionate about the importance of what I do, and I feel the need to seize every chance to influence those who will be practicing beside me someday. Last week was a perfect example. I had a nursing student working with me in one of our birthing rooms. It was her first day caring for a laboring woman, and she was scared and excited at the same time. We were taking care of a healthy woman who had two boys at home and really wanted a girl. As labor progressed, the student and I worked closely together monitoring contractions, teaching the woman and her husband, doing what we could to ease her discomfort. Sometimes the student would ask how I knew when to do something, a vaginal exam, for example, and I'd have to think beyond "I just do" to give her some clues. At the birth the student stayed close to the mother, coaching and helping with breathing. The student was excited but felt she had an important role to play, and she handled it beautifully. At the moment of birth the student and the dad were leaning forward watching as the baby just slipped into the world. There wasn't a sound until the student said in a voice filled with awe, "Oh, it's a girl!" Then we all laughed and hugged each other. What a day—using my expertise to help others and helping a future nurse recognize the importance of what we do!

All nurses who provide care and support to childbearing women and their families can make a difference. But how does this happen? How do nurses develop expertise and become skilled, caring practitioners?

In her classic work, Benner (1984) suggested that as nurses develop their skills in making clinical judgments and intervening appropriately, they progress through five levels of competence. Beginning as a novice, the nurse progresses to advanced beginner and then to competent, proficient, and finally, expert nurse.

In the above situation, the student was clearly a novice. Lacking experience, the novice relies on rules to guide actions. As nurses gain experience, they begin to draw on that experience to view situations more holistically, becoming increasingly aware of subtle cues that indicate physiologic and psychologic changes. Expert nurses, like the nurse in the preceding situation, have a clear vision of what is possible in a given situation. This holistic perspective is based on a wealth of knowledge bred of experience and enables nurses to act "intuitively" to provide effective care. In reality nurses' intuition reflects their internalization of information. When faced with a clinical situation, nurses draw almost subconsciously on their stored knowledge and judgment.

This intuitive perception is integral to the "art of nursing," especially in areas such as maternal-newborn nursing, where change occurs quickly and families look to the nurse for help and guidance. Labor nurses become attuned to a woman's progress or lack of progress; nursery nurses detect subtle changes in their infant charges; antepartal and postpartal nurses become adept at assessing and teaching. Similarly, nurses who are cross-trained as LDRP (labor, delivery, recovery, postpartum) nurses become skilled at caring for childbearing families during all phases of childbirth. Thus skilled nursing practice depends on a solid base of knowledge and clinical expertise delivered in a caring, holistic manner.

Empowerment is an important concept for nurses and clients today. Empowerment may be viewed as both a process and an outcome. As an internal process, empowerment results as individuals develop ever-increasing awareness of competence, mastery, and control over their own lives. An empowered self develops as a consequence of five processes—control, competence, credibility, confidence, and comfort. For nurses, these attributes often evolve as they mature in the profession (Moores, 1997).

Control develops as nurses learn to handle their own emotions and to master clinical situations by making and acting on client care decisions. Control issues are often difficult for advanced beginners, who can demonstrate only marginally acceptable performance (Benner, 1984) and they may look to expert nurses for guidance. As nurses provide good nursing care and develop a knowledge base, they gain competence. From this competence flows credibility as others begin to trust and believe in them. Nurses in turn become self-reliant, gaining confidence in their judgment, which is critical to feelings of empowerment. Finally a sense of comfort develops and nurses feel able to predict probable outcomes (Moores, 1997).

Empowered nurses are better able to approach client care situations effectively with full knowledge that they are ethically, legally, and morally accountable for their actions. Empowered nurses are able to interact as equals with other health care providers and collaborate with them to resolve problems and accomplish goals (Moores, 1997). When empowered nurses practice proactively, they anticipate problems before they develop and avoid undesirable client outcomes (Hagedorn, Gardner, Laux, & Gardner, 1997). Empowered nurses share responsibility and accountability with each childbearing family, thereby helping the family become self-determining (Figure 1–1).

My first pregnancy ended in spontaneous abortion at 8 weeks, so this time I decided not to tell anyone I was pregnant until I was 3 months along. We had just told both families the news the preceding day when it happened again. I began bleeding heavily, and we rushed to the ER. Here I was, a maternal-newborn nursing instructor, and I couldn't seem to handle a

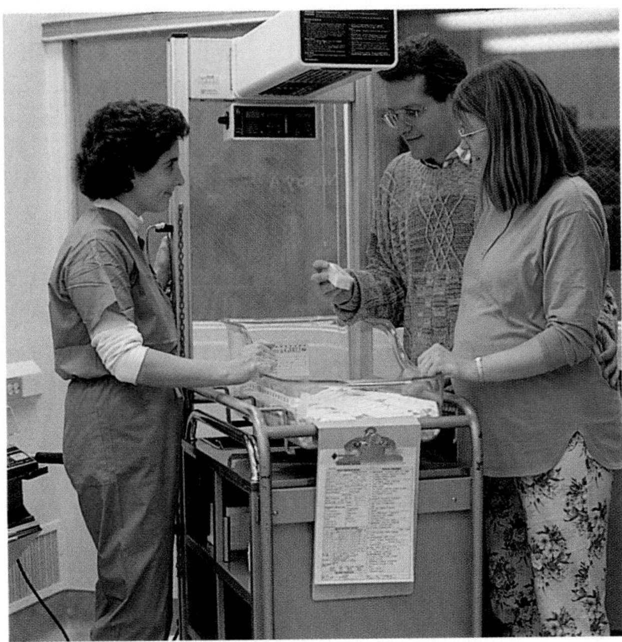

FIGURE 1–1 Individualized education for childbearing couples is one of the prime responsibilities of the maternal-newborn nurse.

pregnancy. I was in the bathroom when I passed the fetus into the Johnny cap. My poor baby—so small, maybe 3 or 4 inches long. I began to sob uncontrollably as I rang for the nurse. I told her what happened, and she helped me to bed. My husband sat with his arm around me as I cried while the nurse took our baby out. A few minutes later, she came back and said, "I saw on your record that you are Catholic. Would you like me to baptize your baby?" I said, "Oh, yes, please," and she left. I've never forgotten how that made me feel. She saw me as a total person. I'm still teaching, and now I have two children. Whenever I teach high-risk pregnancy, I tell that story to the students. I want them to know what a difference a nurse can make.

We believe that many nurses who work with childbearing families are experts: They are sensitive, intuitive, knowledgeable, critical thinkers. They are technically skilled, empowered professionals who can collaborate effectively with others and advocate for those individuals and families who need their support. Such nurses do make a difference in the quality of care that childbearing families receive.

Contemporary Childbirth

The scope of practice of maternal and newborn nurses has changed dramatically in the past 25 years. Today's maternal-newborn nurses have far broader responsibilities and focus more on the specific goals of the individual childbearing woman and her family.

Not only has maternal-newborn nursing changed, so has the whole experience of childbirth. No longer do laboring women leave their partners and family at the labor room door while they work to give birth without the family's loving presence; no longer are newborns routinely whisked away for a prescribed period, to reappear magically for feedings every 4 hours and then return to the safe atmosphere of a central nursery; no longer are young siblings treated like walking sources of infection that threaten every infant. Today fathers are active participants in the birth experience. Families and friends are also often included. Siblings are encouraged to visit and meet their newest family member and may even attend the birth. Today the concept of "family-centered childbirth" is accepted and encouraged.

In addition, new definitions of family are evolving. For example, the family of the single mother may include her mother, sister, another relative, a close friend, or the father of the child. Many cultures also recognize the importance of extended families, where several family members often provide care and support.

The family can generally make choices about many aspects of the childbirth experience, including the place of birth (hospital, free-standing birthing center, or home), the primary caregiver (physician, nurse-midwife, or even lay midwife), and birth-related experiences (methods of childbirth preparation, use of analgesia and anesthesia, and position for labor and birth, for example).

As recently as the early 1990s, women who gave birth vaginally remained in the hospital for approximately 3 days. This provided ample time for nurses to assess the family's knowledge and skill and complete essential teaching. By the mid-1990s, in an effort to control costs, hospitals were routinely discharging new mothers within 12 to 24 hours or less following birth. For women with supportive families, thorough prenatal preparation, and adequate resources for necessary follow-up care, this practice did not necessarily pose a problem. However, because early discharge severely limits the time available for client teaching, women with little knowledge, experience, or support were at greater risk of being inadequately prepared to care for themselves and their newborn infants.

Fortunately, the negative impact of this practice gained recognition nationwide. As a result, Congress passed the Newborns' and Mothers' Health Protection Act of 1996, which took effect in January 1998. This Act provides for a postpartum stay of up to 48 hours following vaginal birth and up to 96 hours following cesarean birth at the discretion of the mother and her health care provider. However, it does not contain a provision for home care follow-up if a new mother chooses to leave the birthing facility earlier than the length of stay mandated by the Act. Some states have developed home care provisions that strengthen the federal legislation, but only slightly more than half require insurance coverage for such care (Carpenter, 1998).

It seems likely that home follow-up nursing care will continue to gain acceptance because it is a cost-effective approach with favorable long-term family outcomes. In addition, families can access a variety of community resources, from local programs focusing on specific topics such as parenting or postpartal exercise to the widely recognized support provided by national organizations such as La Leche League.

For families with access to the Internet, a wealth of information and advice is available. Two examples demonstrate this:

- The National Women's Health Information Center provides information and guidance on a variety of topics related to women's health at their Web site (http://www.4woman.org). They also have a toll-free number, 1-800-994-WOMAN.
- Women seeking information on breastfeeding, breast pumping, and related topics can visit http://www.medela.com, a site created by Medela, a breast pump manufacturer.

Interest in complementary and alternative medicine (CAM) practices is growing nationwide and will have an impact on the care of childbearing families. In response to this trend, the National Institutes of Health now has an Office of Alternative Medicine. Nurses caring for childbearing families need to recognize that approximately one-third of Americans are using some form of unconventional or alternative practice (Wysocki, 1997). Thus it is important for nurses to communicate a willingness to work with the client to recognize and respect these alternative approaches.

The Self-Care Movement

The self-care movement began to emerge in the late 1960s as consumers sought to understand technology and take an interest in their own health and basic self-care skills. More and more people have begun to exercise, control their diet, monitor their psychologic and physiologic status, and in some cases even do their own diagnostic tests. They thus assume many primary care functions. Furthermore, today's health care consumers are requiring greater information and accountability from their health care providers. These consumers recognize that knowledge, indeed, is power.

Practicing self-care—assuming responsibility for one's own health—often requires assertiveness and taking an active role in seeking necessary information. Nurses can foster self-care by providing information readily and by acknowledging people's right to ask questions and become actively involved in their own care.

Maternal-newborn care offers a special opportunity to promote active participation in health care because it is essentially health focused; in most cases, clients are well when they enter the system. The consumer movement that has already influenced childbirth encourages people to speak up for preferences in dealing with health care providers.

Self-care has gained an even broader appeal in recent years because research suggests that it can significantly reduce health care costs. We believe that self-care will be a vital part of health care for years to come. Obviously, self-care is not always realistic or appropriate, especially in acute emergencies, but in many situations it is appropriate. With this in mind, throughout this book we have attempted to suggest ways in which nurses might offer health education that would enable the childbearing family to meet their own health care needs. We see this as one of nursing's most important functions and one that nurses are especially well qualified to perform.

Because of our support of self-care, we have used the term *client* rather than *patient* when referring to the childbearing woman. The term **client** implies an active, rather than a passive, role. The client seeks assistance from professionals who have special skills and knowledge that the client does not. The health care professional offers information and suggestions for a plan of action regarding the client's particular situation. The client can choose not to accept the professional's advice. Furthermore, the health care professional cannot proceed with the plan of action without the client's consent. In this relationship, clients assume responsibility for their decisions.

The nursing profession has been at the forefront in recognizing that people who are able to do so should take an active role in their own health care, and the term *client* best fits this concept. Nurses must understand that it is their professional expertise and skill that the client is seeking. Any attempt to make decisions for the client is inappropriate.

Professional Options in Maternal-Newborn Nursing Practice

As a man, I don't always find it easy to be a labor and delivery nurse. I have three children of my own and attended all their births. It meant a lot to me to be there, and I like helping others to have good childbirth experiences, too. I don't fit some people's image of a nurse; so they refer to me as a "male nurse" as opposed to a real nurse, and they ask why I didn't go into medicine instead. Why can't they understand that I'm a nurse because it's what I really want to be—and I'm darned good at it, too. More men are choosing nursing now, and I think that will help. I hope to see the day when we don't have "female doctors" and "male nurses," but doctors and nurses, period!

Nurses are found in the maternity departments of acute care facilities, in physicians' offices, in clinics, in college health services, in school-based programs dealing with

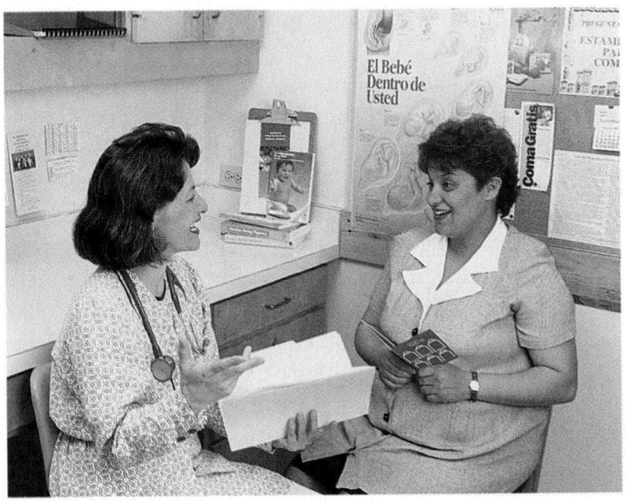

FIGURE 1–2 A certified nurse-midwife confers with her client.

sex education or adolescent pregnancies, in community health services, and in any other setting where a client has a need for maternity care. The depth of nursing involvement in various settings is determined by the qualifications and the role or function of the nurse employed. Many different titles have evolved to describe the professional requirements of the nurse in various maternity care roles. These titles include the following:

- **Professional nurses** are graduates of an accredited basic program in nursing who have successfully completed the nursing examination (NCLEX) and are currently licensed as registered nurses. Professional nurses are usually educated as generalists.
- **Nurse practitioners (NPs)** are professional nurses who have received specialized education in either a master's degree program or a continuing education program and thus can function in an expanded role. Nurse practitioners often provide ambulatory care services to the expectant family (women's health nurse practitioner, family nurse practitioner); some NPs also function in acute care settings (neonatal nurse practitioner, perinatal nurse practitioner). They focus on physical and psychosocial assessment, including health history, physical examination, and certain diagnostic tests and procedures. The nurse practitioner makes clinical judgments and begins appropriate treatments, seeking physician consultation when necessary. The emerging emphasis on community-based care has greatly increased opportunities for NPs.
- **Clinical nurse specialists (CNSs)** are professional nurses with master's degrees who have additional specialized knowledge and competence in a specific clinical area. They assume a leadership role within their specialty and work to improve client care both directly and indirectly.
- **Certified nurse-midwives (CNMs)** are educated in the two disciplines of nursing and midwifery and are certified by the American College of Nurse-Midwives (ACNM). The certified nurse-midwife is prepared to manage independently the care of women at low risk for complications during pregnancy and birth and the care of normal newborns (Figure 1–2).

The term *advanced practice nurse* is used to describe nurses who, by education and practice, function in an expanded nursing role. The term, often used in a legal sense in state nurse practice acts, most frequently applies to NPs, CNSs, CRNAs (certified registered nurse anesthetists), and CNMs. As NPs assume a more prominent role in providing care, the distinctions between the roles of the nurse practitioner and the clinical nurse specialist are beginning to blur and these roles may ultimately merge.

The Health Care Environment

Health care issues are at the top of policy and legislative agendas. Cost, access, and quality of health care have become the "bywords" of the times. In 1960, health care costs in the United States accounted for approximately 5% of the gross domestic product; by 1994 that number had risen to 14% (Dower & O'Neil, 1997). Health care reform is in part a reaction to a cost problem out of control. The real question is whether the United States can develop solutions that are not simply reactive incremental changes, but that truly address the cost issue and other fundamental problems in the system.

In addition to high cost, lack of access to appropriate health care services is a second serious problem in the existing system. Currently about 40 million people in the United States are uninsured; moreover, estimates suggest that another 60 million are underinsured (Shactman & Altman, 1995). The United States spends more per capita than any other country in the world on health care; nevertheless, compared with other industrialized nations, we have higher infant mortality rates, similar life expectancy, and less access to care (Sinclair, 1997). Many people who have insurance fear changing or losing jobs because they may lose health care benefits and access to insurance. They may be denied insurance in the future because of pre-existing conditions. The increase in serious, debilitating illnesses such as AIDS and tuberculosis makes this problem of "job lock" and lack of transferability of insurance benefits even more significant. For some uninsured people, the only access to the health care system is an emergency department. This inappropriate use of expensive services for basic primary care is both an access and a cost problem.

Demographic and environmental changes are increasing the need for services. The number of elderly and chronically ill continues to rise. In the United States, 20.5% of children live in poverty (Lamison-White,

1997). Homelessness, violence, AIDS, and substance abuse are on the increase.

In an effort to curtail costs, many employers have moved from fee-for-service coverage to some form of managed care. Currently almost 75% of Americans covered by employer-provided health insurance are enrolled in some type of managed care organization (Jensen, Morrisey, Gaffney, & Liston, 1997). Thus managed care is now the dominant form of health care delivery in the United States. The move toward managed care has sparked concerns about the quality of health care. Because a fee-for-service model allows the consumer to register dissatisfaction by choosing to seek care elsewhere, quality is a high priority among fee-for-service providers (Langley, 1997). A managed care model, in contrast, limits consumer choice and, in turn, potentially affects quality. Establishing managed care's effects on quality poses a problem because in the US system, quality indicators such as outcomes of care usually have not been well determined. An outcome-based system is essential if there is to be comprehensive health care reform.

Changing the current system requires a new way of thinking and providing services. Primary health care services should be the base on which all other secondary and tertiary services are built. Today in the United States the opposite is still the case. The system emphasizes high-technology care; 75% of third-party payments are for hospital-based acute care. Further, 5% of the population spends 58% of the American health care resources (American Nurses' Association [ANA], 1993). Providing all segments of the population with access to primary health care should be the chief criterion for meaningful reform of the US health care system. This includes a focus on health promotion, prevention, and individual responsibility for one's own health. In this model, secondary health care services would use a smaller proportion of the health care dollar. Such services would include screening, diagnosis, and ongoing treatment and would be provided by clinics or long-term care facilities. Hospitals would concentrate chiefly on providing complex, highly technologic care. In this model, the smallest proportion of the health care dollar and resources would be spent on high-technology tertiary care (ANA, 1993).

The current emphasis on health care reform has yielded an unexpected benefit: Many health care providers and consumers have become more aware of the vitally important role nurses play in providing excellent care to clients and families. The emerging shift in the US health care system presents a significant opportunity for the nursing profession. However, this opportunity for responding to and creating change in nursing and health care delivery requires a new way of thinking. Nurses must clearly articulate their role in the changing environment. They must define and differentiate practice roles and the educational preparation required for those new roles, especially in community-based nursing practice and advanced practice roles such as nurse practitioners and CNMs. Nurses must delineate roles of caregiver and care manager. Nurses must also assume greater roles in promoting health and preventing disease.

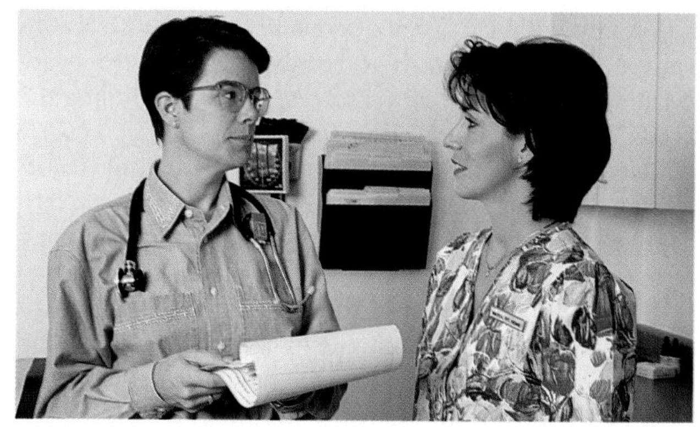

FIGURE 1–3 A collaborative relationship between nurse and physician contributes to excellent client care.

Health care reform will have an impact on women's health and maternal-newborn nursing. Klerman (1994) suggests that several factors, including demographic changes, the need to improve access to care, new research findings, and women's preferences for health care, will contribute to future changes in the field. Changes are predicted in clinical procedures, provider roles, care settings, and financing of care. As access to health care and the need to control costs increase, so will the need for, and utilization of, nurses in advanced practice roles. It is estimated that 80% to 90% of primary and preventive care services can be appropriately and cost-effectively provided by advanced practice nurses. Moreover, process and outcome measures indicate that the care that NPs and CNMs provide is as effective as the care provided by physicians (Sinclair, 1997).

Collaborative Practice

Nursing, if it is to survive, must change education, practice, and research. The uniqueness of nursing practice will become more visible if nursing develops firm partnerships with health professions other than medicine. Nurses should stress coalition building, discipline-specific knowledge and skills, and collaborative advancement (Mundinger, 1994).

Managed care has led to a rethinking of care delivery. One approach that is becoming increasingly popular is collaborative practice. Collaborative practice is a comprehensive model of health care that uses a multidisciplinary team of health professionals to provide cost-effective, high quality care. In maternal-newborn settings, the team generally includes CNMs and nurse practitioners in practice with physicians (often obstetricians or family practice physicians) and may include other health professionals, such as lactation consultants or clinical nurse specialists (Figure 1–3). "All team members are valued for their knowledge and expertise, and each individual has autonomy within a defined scope of practice. Decisions reflect shared responsibility, individual and group accountability, and mutual values and goals—including the commitment to empowering clients and families as partners in their care and members of the collaborative team" (Corry, Williams, & Stapleton, 1997, p 279). In a collaborative approach, no single profession "owns the client." Leadership of the team depends on the issue being addressed and the expertise of the members. All team members must function within their scope of practice, and they must understand the scope of practice of other team members and respect their expertise (Leppert, 1997).

Community-Based Nursing Care

Many advocates of a new direction for health care support the increasing emphasis on primary care. Primary care includes a focus on health promotion, illness prevention, and individual responsibility for one's own health. These services are best provided in community-based settings. Third-party payors and managed care organizations are beginning to recognize the importance of primary care in containing costs and maintaining health. Estimates indicate that by the turn of the century, only 40% of nurses will work in the traditional hospital setting. Community-based health services providing primary care and some secondary care will be available in schools, workplaces, homes, churches, clinics, transitional care programs, and other ambulatory settings.

Weisman (1996) has suggested that the growth and diversity of managed care plans offers both opportunities and challenges for women's health care. The potential exists for managed care organizations to work with consumers to provide a model for coordinated and comprehensive well-woman care that includes improved screening and preventive services. One challenge managed care organizations will face is to determine how to relate to essential community providers of care—organizations such as family planning clinics or women's health centers—that offer a unique service or serve groups of women with special needs (adolescents, disabled women, ethnic or racial minorities). "The extent to which satisfactory contractual relationships are negotiated between managed care plans and community providers may in turn have profound effects on the survival of some of these providers and their future availability to women" (Weisman, 1996, p 3).

Community-based care remains an essential element of health care for uninsured and underinsured individuals as well as for those individuals who benefit from programs such as Medicare or state-sponsored health-related programs. Some of these programs, such as those offered through public health departments, are broad based; others, such as parenting classes for adolescents, are geared to the needs of a specific population.

Community-based care is also part of a trend initiated by consumers, who are asking for a "seamless" system of family-centered, comprehensive, coordinated health care, health education, and social services (Plotnick & Presler, 1996). To effect such a seamless system requires coordination as clients move from primary care services to acute care facilities and then back into the community. The shortened length of hospital stays further mandates the need for coordination of services. Nurses can assume this care management role and perform an important service for individuals and families.

Maternal-newborn nurses are especially sensitive to these changes in health care delivery because the vast majority of health care provided to childbearing families takes place outside hospitals in clinics, offices, and community-based organizations. In addition, maternal-newborn nurses offer specialized services such as childbirth preparation classes or postpartal exercise classes. In essence, we are already expert at providing community-based nursing care. However, it is important that we remain knowledgeable about current practices and trends and open to new approaches to meet the needs of women and children.

Home Care

The provision of health care in the home is emerging as an especially important dimension of community-based nursing care. The shortened length of hospital stays has resulted in the discharge of individuals who still require support, assistance, and teaching. Home care can help fill this gap. Conversely, home care also enables individuals to remain at home with conditions that formerly would have required hospitalization.

Nurses are the major providers of home care services. Home care nurses perform direct nursing care and also supervise unlicensed assistive personnel who provide less skilled levels of service. In a home setting, nurses can use their skills in assessment, therapeutics, communication, teaching, problem solving, and organization to meet the needs of childbearing families. They also play a major role in coordinating services from other providers, such as physical therapists or lactation consultants.

Postpartum and newborn home visits are becoming a recognized way of ensuring that childbearing families make a satisfactory transition from the hospital or birthing center to the home. We see this trend as positive and hope that this method of meeting the needs of childbearing families becomes standard practice. Chapter 32 discusses home care in more detail and provides guidance about making a home visit. In addition, throughout the text we have provided information on how home care can meet the needs of women with health problems such as diabetes or preterm labor, which put them at risk during pregnancy. We believe that home care offers nurses the opportunity to function in an autonomous role and make a significant difference for individuals and families.

Legal Considerations

Professional nursing practice requires full understanding of practice standards, institutional or agency policies, and local, state, and federal laws. Professional practice also requires an understanding of the ethical implications of those standards, policies, and laws that impact care, care providers, and care recipients. Every professional nurse is responsible for obtaining and maintaining current information regarding ethics and laws related to nursing practice and health care.

Scope of Practice

State nurse practice acts protect the public by broadly defining the legal *scope of practice* within which every nurse must function and by excluding untrained or unlicensed individuals from practicing nursing. Although some state practice acts continue to limit nursing practice to the traditional responsibilities of providing client care related to health maintenance and disease prevention, most state practice acts cover expanded practice roles that include collaboration with other professionals in planning and providing care, diagnostic and prescriptive privilege, and the delegation of client care tasks to other specified licensed and unlicensed personnel. Specified care activities for certified nurse-midwives and women's health, perinatal, or neonatal nurse practitioners may include diagnosis and prenatal management of uncomplicated pregnancies, management of births by certified nurse-midwives, and prescribing and dispensing medications using protocols in specified circumstances. A nurse must function within the scope of practice or risk being accused of practicing medicine without a license.

Correctly interpreting and understanding state practice acts enables the nurse to provide safe care within the limits of nursing practice. State boards of nursing may provide official interpretation of practice acts when the limits are not clear. On occasion hospital policy may conflict with a state's nurse practice act. It is important to recognize that hospital or agency policy may restrict the scope of practice specified in a state practice act, but such policy cannot legally expand the scope of practice beyond the limits stated in the practice act.

Nurse practice acts are subject to change. One component of professional nursing practice is the responsibility of each nurse to remain up-to-date regarding scope of practice and even to participate actively in promoting appropriate changes.

CRITICAL THINKING QUESTION

How do changes in nurses' scope of practice come about? Can you describe any efforts by nurses in your region that have resulted in a broadening of their scope of practice?

Nursing Negligence

Negligence is defined as omitting or committing an act that a reasonably prudent person would not omit or commit under the same or similar circumstances. Negligence consists of four elements: (1) there was a duty to provide care; (2) the duty was breached; (3) injury occurred; and (4) the breach of duty caused the injury (proximate cause). Duty may be breached by omission—failing to give a medication, failing to assess properly, failing to notify a physician of a change in a laboring woman's condition, and so on. Duty may also be breached by commission—giving the wrong medication, placing an infant in the wrong crib, and so on. The injury that results may be physical or mental (pain and suffering). In determining whether nursing negligence occurred, the care that was given is compared to the standard of care. If the standard was not met, negligence occurred.

Standards of Nursing Care

Standards of care establish minimum criteria for competent, proficient delivery of nursing care. Such standards are designed to protect the public and are used to judge the quality of care provided. Legal interpretation of actions within standards of care is based on what a reasonably prudent nurse with similar education and experience would do in similar circumstances.

Written standards of care are provided by a number of different sources. The American Nurses Association (ANA) has published standards of professional practice since 1950. In 1973, the ANA Congress for Nursing Practice began to write generic standards for all nurses in all settings. In addition, the ANA Divisions of Practice have published standards that include nursing practice for maternal-child health. The Council of Perinatal Nurses has published standards for perinatal nursing. Other specialty organizations, such as the Association of Women's Health, Obstetric, and Neonatal Nurses (AWHONN), the Association of Operating Room Nurses (AORN), and the National Association of Neonatal Nurses (NANN), have developed standards of specialty practice. Agency policies, procedures, and protocols also provide appropriate guidelines for care standards. The Joint Commission on Accreditation of Healthcare Organizations (JCAHO), a private, nongovernmental agency that audits the operation of hospitals and health care facilities, has also contributed to the development of nursing standards.

Some standards carry the force of law; others, although not legally based, still carry important legal significance. Any nurse who fails to meet appropriate standards of care invites allegations of negligence or malpractice. (*Malpractice* is negligent action of a professional person.) However, any nurse who practices within the guidelines established by agency, local, or national standards is assured that clients are provided with competent nursing care, which, in turn, diminishes the potential for litigation.

Ethical Components of Care Standards

Standards of care are based on a legal model rather than on ethics. However, they incorporate important ethical components that extend the narrow legal interpretation of the term *standard*. Although there is a great deal of interplay between the two disciplines, each has a different perspective.

Law is based primarily on a rights model that establishes rules of conduct to define relationships among individuals. Law may also define relationships to impersonal entities like formal organizations, agencies, or hospitals.

Ethics, in contrast, is based on a responsibility or duty model that considers a wider range of factors than the rights model of law. Ethics incorporates factors such as risks, benefits, other relationships, concerns, and the needs and abilities of persons affected by and affecting decisions.

Law and ethics are interrelated; they share a similar decision process and standards. Both disciplines incorporate fact finding, conflict negotiation, prioritization of related issues and values, and the application of resolutions of particular cases in decision making. Professional nurses must consider the ethical implications of legal decisions and the legal implications of ethical decisions.

Understanding the distinctions among medical or health care decisions, legal decisions, and ethical decisions is important. Consider the case in which parents from a culture unfamiliar to the nurse refuse surgery for their newborn based on a deeply held spiritual belief that intentional cutting of a body will result in spiritual death. Such a decision to forgo surgery may be viewed as negligent in the eyes of the law, unwise and inappropriate from a medical perspective, yet fully justifiable ethically. Similarly, legally sanctioned maintenance of life support for a severely damaged newborn with little hope for meaningful existence may remain a medically viable alternative, but to many it is not ethically justifiable. Recognizing the type of decision to be made often helps measure the worth and outcome of a decision more appropriately.

Clients' Rights

Law and ethics impact all of nursing practice, and several topics have specific implications for maternal-child nursing practice. Clients' rights encompass such topics as informed consent, privacy, and confidentiality.

Informed Consent

Informed consent is designed to allow clients to make intelligent decisions regarding their own health care. Informed consent means that a client, or legally designated decision maker, has granted permission for a specific treatment or procedure based on full information about that specific treatment or procedure as it relates to that client under the specific circumstances of the permission. While this policy is usually enforced for such major procedures as surgery or regional anesthesia, it pertains to any nursing, medical, or surgical intervention. To touch a person without consent (except in an emergency) constitutes battery.

Several elements must be addressed in order to ensure that the client has given informed consent. The information must be clearly and concisely presented in a manner understandable to the client and must include risks and benefits, the probability of success, and significant treatment alternatives. The client also needs to be told the consequences of receiving no treatment or procedure. Finally, the client must be told of the right to refuse a specific treatment or procedure. Each client should be told that refusing the specified treatment or procedure does not result in the withdrawal of all support or care.

Information should be provided by the individual who is ultimately responsible for the treatment or procedure. In most instances, this is a physician. In such cases, the nurse's role may be to witness the client's signature giving consent. A nurse who knows the client and the procedure may certainly help the physician obtain the client's consent by clarifying the information the physician provides. It is also part of the nurse's role to determine that the client understands the information prior to making a decision.

Society grants parents the authority and responsibility to give consent for their minor children. Parents are presumed to possess what a child lacks in maturity, experience, and capacity for judgment in life's difficult decisions. Although the age of majority is 18 years in most states, variations in certain states require that nurses be aware of the law in the state where they practice. Special problems can occur in maternity nursing when a minor gives birth. It is possible, depending upon state law, that a minor may consent to treatment for her infant but not for herself. In some states, however, a pregnant teenager is considered an emancipated minor and may therefore give consent for herself as well.

Additionally, some states require a married woman to obtain the consent of her spouse when a procedure involves sterilization or threatens the life of a fetus. Although childbearing women sign a general consent form on admission to an agency, separate informed consent is often required for surgery, cesarean birth, the administration of anesthesia, tubal ligation, or participation in research.

Refusal of a treatment, medication, or procedure after appropriate information also requires that a client sign a form to release the physician and agency from liability. Jehovah's Witnesses' refusal of blood transfusion or Rh_o(D) immune globulin is an example of such refusal.

Right to Privacy

The right to privacy is the right of a person to keep his or her person and property free from public scrutiny. In the context of health care, the right to privacy dictates that only those responsible for a client's care should examine the client or discuss the client's case. Most states have recognized the right to privacy through statutory or common law, and some states have written that right into their constitution. Professional standards protecting clients' privacy have been adopted by the ANA, National League for Nursing (NLN), and JCAHO. Health care agencies should also have written policies dealing with client privacy.

Laws, standards, and policies about privacy specify that information about clients' treatment, condition, and prognosis can be shared only by the health professionals responsible for their care. Authorization for the release of any client information should be obtained from competent clients or their surrogate decision maker. Although it may be legal to reveal vital statistics such as name, age, occupation, and prognosis, such information is often withheld because of ethical considerations. The client should be consulted regarding what information may be released and to whom. When a client is a celebrity or is considered newsworthy, inquiries may be best handled by the public relations department of the agency.

Confidentiality

Given the highly personal and intimate information requested of clients, the need for maintaining confidentiality is extremely crucial for the development of trust in the relationship between client and provider. Privileged communications exist between client and physician, client and attorney, husband and wife, clergy and those who seek their counsel. In some states nurses are also protected by laws of privilege. Nurses should become well informed regarding privileged communication laws in their state.

A client may waive the right to confidentiality of medical records by action or words. For example, if a childbearing woman sues a physician, hospital, or other care provider, she waives the right to confidentiality of the medical record because the record becomes a source of evidence. Clients commonly consent to disclose information to insurance companies or to their employers. Computerization of medical records has created a greater concern for the integrity of records and the potential invasion of privacy.

In some instances, the public good takes precedence over an individual's right to privacy. For example, state laws require that care providers report gunshot wounds, child abuse, and some communicable diseases.

Special Ethical Situations in Maternity Care

Ethical Decisions

Health care and bioethical literature are filled with examples of ethical decision-making models and frameworks. Decision-making models help nurses and other care providers confront seemingly unresolvable conflicts among the rights, duties, theories, principles, values, and individuals impacted by the ethical dilemmas of practice. There are six critical components of ethical decision making; they are very similar to the components of the nursing process.

1. Establish a means of determining who is involved in the dilemma, who is involved in the decision, and who will be affected by the outcome of the decision. This data-gathering step allows the nurse to identify and define the issue and determine who owns the problem, the information, the decision, and the consequences of it.
2. Establish a mechanism for obtaining all the information relevant to the conflict, including data related to diagnosis, prognosis, treatment options, available health care, and psychosocial, spiritual, financial, and other appropriate resources.
3. Formulate a plan to outline all potential options and the consequences of each option. Be sure that opposing viewpoints are presented and considered. Set individual values aside during this phase in order to encourage divergent views.
4. In the conflict resolution process that follows, review driving and restraining forces, assess risks and benefits, and assess the likelihood of a successful outcome with each option. At this stage, be sure that the moral values of everyone involved are addressed. In addition, review peripheral issues—such as the possible impact on other individuals or systems related to the decision, changes in client condition, pertinent laws, or new information—within the context of general and individual moral principles.
5. Select and act on a plan to resolve the conflict. Before acting on the resolution, determine who is ultimately responsible for the decision, who is most impacted by the outcome, and whether consensus is required.
6. Evaluate the resolution, its consequences, and the decision process itself. This step is critically important to avoid making similar decisions in isolation.

Ethical decisions in maternal-child nursing are often complicated by moral obligations to more than one client. Straightforward solutions to the ethical dilemmas nurses encounter in caring for childbearing families are often, quite simply, not available. By using a formal decision-making structure, nurses may, however, increase the likelihood of addressing multiple needs in complex care situations in an ethically appropriate and legal manner.

Maternal-Fetal Conflict

The status of the fetus as a person has long been debated. Currently the fetus is not viewed as a person by the US Supreme Court even if considered "viable" (Thorp,

Bowes, & Cefalo, 1997). However, advances in technology have enabled physicians to monitor fetal development, to treat fetal problems, and even to provide preembryo diagnosis that may dramatically affect the outcome of the birth of a healthy baby. Increasingly, the fetus is given consideration as a client separate from the mother, although treatment of the fetus necessarily involves the mother. Care providers may confront situations in which two clients assert "possibly contradictory moral claims on . . . [the] fundamental ethical obligation to do good and avoid harm" (J. J. Mitchell, 1994, p 93).

In maternity care the moral assumption is made that the pregnant woman's decisions will be beneficial to both her life and well-being and that of her fetus. In some cases, however, the pregnant woman refuses to consent to a medical intervention that is essential to the well-being of the fetus and of minimal risk to her. Situations also exist in which the pregnant woman engages in high-risk behaviors, such as substance abuse, that jeopardize the health of her fetus. Despite care providers' noble intentions to protect the fetus, coercion of the pregnant woman, even through judicial intervention, is rarely justified.

The American College of Obstetricians and Gynecologists (ACOG) Committee on Ethics 1987 position statement, *Patient Choices: Maternal-Fetal Conflict;* the American Academy of Pediatrics 1988 statement, *Fetal Therapy: Ethical Considerations;* and the American Medical Association Board of Trustees 1990 report, *Legal Interventions During Pregnancy*, all reaffirm the fundamental right of pregnant women to make informed, uncoerced decisions regarding medical interventions. All three major policy statements also recognize that cases of maternal-fetal conflict involve two clients, both of whom deserve respect and treatment. Further, all agree such cases "are best resolved through the use of internal hospital mechanisms including counseling, the intervention of specialists, and the utilization of ethics committees . . . and that a resort to judicial intervention is rarely, if ever, appropriate" (J. J. Mitchell, 1994, p 94).

Abortion

Since the 1973 Supreme Court decision in *Roe v. Wade*, abortion has been legal in the United States. It can be performed until the period of viability, after which abortion is permissible only when the life or health of the mother is threatened. Before viability, the mother's rights are paramount; after viability, the rights of the fetus take precedence.

In the early 1990s individuals and organizations opposed to abortion had worked to limit or abolish abortion by prohibiting Medicaid funding of abortions and putting other restrictions on the procedure. Those favoring abortion were pleased when, in 1993, shortly after taking the oath of office, President Clinton signed executive orders that (1) lifted the gag rule prohibiting most health care providers at federally funded clinics from discussing abortion with pregnant women; (2) permitted the use of fetal tissue in federally funded research, even if the tissue was obtained from an abortion; and (3) permitted overseas US military personnel and their dependents to receive abortions at military hospitals at their own expense. Currently the controversy continues, especially at the state level.

At present the decision for abortion is to be made by a woman and her physician. Nurses (and other care givers) have the right to refuse to assist with the procedure if abortion is contrary to their moral and ethical beliefs. However, if the institution supports abortion, the nurse may be dismissed for refusing. To avoid being placed in a situation contrary to their values and beliefs, nurses should determine the philosophy of an institution before going to work there. A nurse who refuses to participate in an abortion because of moral or ethical beliefs does have a responsibility to ensure that someone with similar qualifications is able to provide appropriate care for the client. Clients may never be abandoned, regardless of the nurse's beliefs.

Fetal Research

Research with fetal tissue has been responsible for remarkable advances in the care and treatment of fetuses with health problems and advances in the treatment of progressive, debilitating adult diseases such as Parkinson's disease, Alzheimer's disease, and DiGeorge's syndrome. Therapeutic research with living fetuses has been instrumental in the treatment of Rh-sensitized infants, the evaluation of lung maturity using the lecithin/sphingomyelin ratio, and the treatment of pulmonary immaturity in the newborn. Because it is aimed at treating a fetal condition, therapeutic fetal research raises fewer ethical questions than does nontherapeutic fetal research (Collins, 1993). To be approved, nontherapeutic research requires that the risk to the fetus be minimal, that the knowledge to be gained be important, and that the information be unobtainable by any other means. Control over research standards and attention to state and federal regulations remain foci of debate regarding fetal research.

Intrauterine fetal surgery, which began in 1981 and developed through therapeutic research, is a therapy for anatomic lesions that can be corrected surgically and are incompatible with life if not treated. Intrauterine fetal surgery involves opening the uterus during the second trimester (prior to viability), treating the fetal lesion, and replacing the fetus in the uterus. The risks to the fetus are substantial, and the mother is committed to cesarean births for this and subsequent pregnancies because the upper, active segment of the uterus is incised during the surgery. The parents must be informed of the experimental nature of the treatment, the risks of the surgery, the commitment to cesarean birth, and alternatives to the treatment.

As with other aspects of maternity care, the pregnant woman's autonomy must be respected. The procedure does involve health risks to the woman, and she retains the right to refuse any surgical procedure. Health care providers must be careful that their zeal for new technology does not lead them to focus unilaterally on the fetus at the expense of the mother ("Fetal Surgery," 1994).

Reproductive Assistance

The number and sophistication of reproductive assistance techniques continue to grow. Infertile couples now have reproductive options that include artificial insemination, intracytoplasmic sperm injection (ICSI), microsurgical epididymal sperm aspiration (MESA), testicular sperm aspiration (TESA), in vitro fertilization, zygote intrafallopian transfer (ZIFT), gamete intrafallopian transfer (GIFT), embryo transfer, oocyte donation, and the possibility for surrogate childbearing.

Artificial insemination (AI) is accomplished by depositing into a woman sperm obtained from her husband, partner, or other donor. Homologous insemination (AIH) involves the husband's or partner's sperm; donor insemination (AID) involves a donor other than the husband or partner. Some women who are single are choosing AID as a childbearing option. No states prohibit AIH, so there is no question of the child's legitimacy. Legal problems may occur with AID, however. Because the child is the biologic child of the mother, legal concerns center around the donor. A donor must sign a form waiving all parental rights. The donor must also furnish accurate health information, particularly regarding genetic traits or diseases. Donor sperm must be tested for HIV. Husbands often are requested to sign a form to agree to the insemination and to assume parental responsibility for the child. Some men legally adopt the child so there is no question of parental rights and responsibilities. Several states have enacted legislation regarding paternity of the child conceived by insemination with donor sperm.

Assisted reproductive technology (ART) is the term used to describe the highly technologic approaches used to produce pregnancy. *Intracytoplasmic sperm injection (ICSI)*, *microsurgical epididymal sperm aspiration (MESA)*, and *testicular sperm aspiration (TESA)* are procedures developed to address severe male factor infertility. ICSI is a microscopic procedure designed to inject a single sperm into the outer layer of an ovum so that fertilization will occur. MESA and TESA involve the retrieval of sperm from the gonadal tissue of men who have azospermia or an ejaculatory disorder (Macklin & White, 1997). While these procedures have been quite promising, they do raise questions about the increased risk of genetic defects related to bypassing of certain aspects of the process of natural selection. In the United States there are no established barriers to the use of these procedures. In the Netherlands, by contrast, a governmental report has recommended that ICSI continue to be available, but not MESA and TESA because they present a greater danger of transmitting genetic defects (Robertson, 1997).

In vitro fertilization and embryo transfer (IVF-ET), a therapy offered to selected infertile couples, is perhaps the best known ART technique. In this process, ovulation is induced, and one or more oocytes are retrieved by transvaginal ultrasound scanning in conjunction with transvaginal aspiration. The oocytes are then fertilized with sperm from the partner or a donor. Three to four embryos are transferred to the woman's uterus when they reach the four- to six-cell stage (Stillman & Gindoff, 1994). *Zygote intrafallopian transfer (ZIFT)* is similar to IVF-ET, except that the developing embryo is implanted in the fallopian tube. The success rates of the procedures are low. Researchers have also begun to use natural cycle IVF (as opposed to the use of medications to stimulate ovulation). This approach eliminates the need to use fertility drugs to stimulate ovulation, with the associated risks of those medications, and results in the implantation of a single oocyte instead of multiple oocytes (Levy & Gindoff, 1994).

Gamete intrafallopian transfer (GIFT) is used in women with at least one functioning tube whose infertility is due to unknown causes or to male factors such as low sperm count. In GIFT, multiple oocytes are retrieved by laparoscopy from the woman or a donor and transferred with sperm directly into the fallopian tubes. The resulting pregnancy is considered in vivo fertilization.

Some effort has been made legislatively to address consumer concerns about ART. In the United States, the Federal Fertility Clinic Success Rate and Certification Act of 1992 (FCSRCA) addresses issues related to laboratory quality and the standardized reporting of pregnancy success rates associated with ART programs. However, it does not contain provisions to deal with the unethical practices that may occur, nor does it address false reporting of success rates (Wilcox & Marks, 1996).

In Canada, the Royal Commission on New Reproductive Technologies was charged with examining the range of technologies related to reproduction. Among its most important recommendations, the Commission advocated legislation to prohibit several aspects of technology, such as selling human eggs, zygotes, sperm, fetuses, or fetal tissue. They also recommended that the government establish a national regulatory body to license and regulate the provision of reproductive technology services in Canada (Baird, 1996).

Surrogate childbearing is another approach to addressing the issue of infertility. Surrogate childbearing occurs when a woman agrees to become pregnant for a childless couple. Depending on the infertile couple's needs, she may be artificially inseminated with the male partner's sperm or a donor's sperm, or she may even receive a gamete transfer. If fertilization occurs, the woman carries the fetus to term and then releases the infant to the couple after birth.

These methods of resolving infertility raise many ethical questions, including the problem of religious objections to artificial conception, the question of who will assume financial and moral responsibility for a child born with a congenital defect, the issue of candidate selection, and the threat of genetic engineering. Other ethical questions include: What should be done with surplus fertilized oocytes? To whom do frozen embryos belong—parents together or separately? The hospital or infertility clinic? Who is liable if a woman or her offspring contracts HIV disease from donated sperm? Should children be told the method of their conception?

Cord Blood Banking

Cord blood, which is taken from a newborn's umbilical cord by the physician or nurse-midwife assisting with the birth, may play a role in combating leukemia, certain other cancers, and other immune and blood system disorders. Cord blood, like bone marrow, contains regenerative stem cells, which are able to replace diseased cells in the affected individual. The value of bone marrow transplants has long been recognized, and a national registry of potential bone marrow donors has been established. The process of collecting bone marrow is expensive and uncomfortable, however, and the National Marrow Donor Registry is able to find a matching bone marrow donor in only 20% to 30% of cases (Randal, 1995).

Cord blood has some advantages over bone marrow: (1) collecting cord blood is less invasive and involves no risk to mother or infant; (2) large-scale cord blood banking would increase the availability of stem cells for minority groups, who are seriously underrepresented in bone marrow registries; (3) cord blood is less likely than bone marrow to trigger a potentially fatal rejection response; (4) cord blood works with a less-than-perfect match; and (5) cord blood is available for use more rapidly than bone marrow. Cord blood also has its limitations. A limited number of cells are available to be transplanted; there is little definitive information about effectiveness based on recipient size; transplantation cannot be repeated; and there is an increased likelihood of leukemic relapse (Crooks, Lill, Feig, & Parkman, 1997).

Cord blood banks that process and store cord blood have now been established in the United States. Families can elect to register their infant's cord blood privately. The blood is collected at birth and the family assumes all costs for analyzing, preparing, and storing the blood. The blood is quickly available for use by the donor, a sibling, or the mother. (During pregnancy, mother and infant seem to become immunologically tolerant of each other.) This option is especially useful in families with a history of cancer or genetic blood disease. Alternatively, families may elect to donate the cord blood to an established registry for use by others.

Sugarman and colleagues (1995) have identified several ethical issues associated with cord blood banking:

- Who owns the blood? The donor? The parents? Private blood banks? Society?
- How can caregivers ensure that informed consent is correctly obtained? It is necessary to ensure that family members understand that, if they choose to donate, the mother will be asked to provide a blood sample and a detailed history about her health and infectious disease status.
- How will obligations to notify the family and donor be addressed if testing of the blood reveals infectious diseases or genetic disorders? Should there be any ongoing assessment of donors so that if health problems develop, recipients can be notified?
- How can the system be set up to maintain privacy and confidentiality?
- How can the harvested blood be distributed fairly, so that it is available to individuals from all races, ethnic groups, and income levels?

The Human Genome Project

The Human Genome Project (HGP) is an international, multidisciplinary effort to explore and map human genetic material. In the United States, the Human Genome Project is a coordinated, 15-year national research program to identify all human genetic material—the genome—by developing a human genetic map of all chromosomes, by improving existing genetic maps, and by determining the complete sequence of human DNA. Jointly sponsored by the US Department of Energy and the National Institutes of Health (NIH), the project is also designed to develop new technologies and techniques to support the effort (Mahowald, 1997). In addition, the HGP is charged with analyzing the legal, ethical, and social implications resulting from the availability of genetic information about individuals; developing public policy options to deal with the complex issues that will arise; and identifying advanced ways of sharing the information that emerges with researchers, scientists, physicians, and others so that the data may quickly be used for the public good (National Center for Human Genome Research, 1996). As part of the effort, the HGP has also established research training programs for pre- and postdoctoral fellows.

The implications of the effort are staggering. For example, in 1989 the gene involved in cystic fibrosis was identified. Subsequently a diagnostic test was developed to identify gene carriers of cystic fibrosis in high-risk individuals and families. Currently the first human gene therapy approaches are being evaluated in federally funded clinical trials. More recently, researchers located two genes implicated in a hereditary form of colon cancer. Once the genes are identified it becomes possible to develop a blood test to detect high-risk individuals (National Center for Human Genome Research, 1996).

As more genetic information becomes available, questions regarding the use and protection of such information arise. Gene manipulation and gene therapy, once limited to science fiction novels, now present a reality that adds to the complex ethical questions of the use and control of technology. Other emerging issues include the question of payment for genetic testing; appropriate counseling following testing; confidentiality; qualifications of individuals engaged in testing, counseling, and interventions; mandated testing; and the right to refuse genetic information.

Implications for Nursing Practice

The complex ethical issues facing maternal-newborn nurses have many social, cultural, legal, and professional ramifications. Nurses, like all health care professionals, need to learn to anticipate ethical dilemmas, clarify their own positions and values related to the issues, understand the legal implications of the issues, and develop appropriate strategies for ethical decision making. To accomplish these tasks, they may read about bioethical issues, participate in discussion groups, or attend courses and workshops on ethical topics pertinent to their areas of practice. Most nurses develop solid skills in logical thinking and critical analysis. These skills, coupled with theoretical knowledge about ethical decision making, can serve nurses well in dealing with the many ethical dilemmas found in health care.

Statistical Data and Maternal-Infant Care

Increasingly nurses are recognizing the value and usefulness of statistics. Health-related statistics provide an objective basis for projecting client needs, planning use of resources, and determining the effectiveness of treatment.

There are two major types of statistics: descriptive and inferential. *Descriptive statistics* describe or summarize a set of data. They report the facts—what is—in a concise and easily retrievable way. How the data are compiled and presented is determined by the question being asked. An example of a descriptive statistic is the birth rate in the United States. Although no conclusion may be drawn from these statistics about *why* some phenomenon has occurred, they can identify certain trends and high-risk "target groups" and generate possible research questions.

Inferential statistics allow the investigator to draw conclusions or inferences about what is happening between two or more variables in a population and to suggest or refute causal relationships between them. For example, descriptive statistics reveal that the infant mortality rate in the United States has declined over the past decade. Exactly why that trend has occurred cannot be answered by simply looking at these data, however. More data and inferential statistics using smaller samples of the population of pregnant women are needed to determine whether this finding is due to earlier prenatal care, improved maternal nutrition, use of electronic fetal monitoring during labor, and/or any number of factors potentially associated with maternal-fetal survival.

Descriptive statistics are the starting point for the formation of research questions. Inferential statistics answer specific questions and generate theories to explain relationships between variables. Theory applied in nursing practice can help change the specific variables that may cause or contribute to certain health problems.

This section discusses descriptive statistics that are particularly important to maternal-newborn health care. Inferences that may be drawn from these descriptive statistics are addressed as possible research questions that may help identify relevant variables.

Birth Rate

Birth rate refers to the number of live births per 1000 people. Table 1–1 provides valuable information about births and birth rates in the United States through 1996. That was the sixth straight year in which the overall birth rate decreased. Birth rates for teens fell 3% to 8% while rates for women in their twenties increased slightly. This is the first increase in that age group since 1990. Concurrently, birth rates rose 2% to 3% for women in their thirties (Ventura, Martin, Curtin, & Mathews, 1998).

In 1990 there were 450,486 live births in Canada, a birth rate of 15.3. In 1992 the birth rate dropped to 14 per 1000 people. Internationally, birth rates vary significantly. Table 1–2 compares the 1994 birth rates of selected countries. Research questions that can be posed about birth rates include the following:

- Is there an association between birth rates and changing societal values?
- Do the differences in birth rates between various age groups reflect education? Changed attitudes toward motherhood?
- Do the differences in birth rates among various countries reflect cultural differences? Do they represent availability of contraceptive information? Are there other factors at work?

Infant Mortality

The **infant mortality rate** is the number of deaths of infants under 1 year of age per 1000 live births in a given population. In 1996 the infant mortality rate was 7.3 (28,487 infant deaths), the lowest rate ever recorded for the United States (Peters, Kochanek, & Murphy, 1998). *Neonatal mortality* is the number of deaths of infants less than 28 days of age per 1000 live births. *Perinatal mortality* includes both neonatal deaths and fetal deaths per 1000 live births. (Fetal death is death in utero at 20 weeks or more gestation.)

The US infant mortality rate has continued to be of concern because the United States has fallen to 22nd place among industrialized nations in infant mortality rankings. Health care professionals, policy makers, and the public have continued to stress the need in the United States for better prenatal care, coordination of health

TABLE 1–1 Births and Birth Rates: 1980 to 1996 (in thousands)

Item	1980	1985	1987	1988	1989	1990	1991	1992	1993	1994	1995	1996
Live births[1] (add 000)	**3,612**	**3,761**	**3,809**	**3,910**	**4,041**	**4,158**	**4,111**	**4,065**	**4,000**	**3,953**	**3,900**	**3,891**
White	2,936	3,038	3,044	3,102	3,192	3,290	3,241	3,202	3,150	3,121	3,099	3,093
Black	568	582	611	639	673	684	683	674	659	636	603	595
American Indian	29	34	35	37	39	39	39	39	39	38	37	38
Asian or Pacific Islander	74	105	117	129	133	142	145	150	153	158	160	166
Age of mother:												
Under 20 years old	562	478	473	489	518	533	532	518	501	518	512	503
20 to 24 years old	1,226	1,141	1,076	1,067	1,078	1,094	1,090	1,070	1,038	1,001	966	945
25 to 29 years old	1,108	1,201	1,216	1,239	1,263	1,277	1,220	1,179	1,129	1,089	1064	1071
30 to 34 years old	550	696	761	804	842	886	885	895	901	906	905	898
35 to 39 years old	141	214	248	270	294	318	331	345	357	372	384	400
40 years old or more	24	29	36	41	46	50	54	58	61	66	70	75
Birth rate per 1,000 population	**15.9**	**15.8**	**15.7**	**16.0**	**16.4**	**16.7**	**16.3**	**15.9**	**15.5**	**15.2**	**14.8**	**14.7**
White	15.1	15.0	14.9	15.0	15.4	15.8	15.4	15.0	14.7	14.4	14.2	14.1
Black	21.3	20.4	20.8	21.5	22.3	22.4	21.9	21.3	20.5	19.5	18.2	17.8
American Indian	20.7	19.8	19.1	19.3	19.7	18.9	18.3	18.4	17.8	17.1	16.6	16.6
Asian or Pacific Islander	19.9	18.7	18.4	19.2	18.7	19.0	18.2	18.0	17.7	17.5	17.3	17.0
Fertility rate per 1,000 women[2]	**68.4**	**66.2**	**65.7**	**67.2**	**69.2**	**70.9**	**69.6**	**68.9**	**67.6**	**66.7**	**65.6**	**65.3**
White[2]	64.8	64.1	63.3	64.5	66.4	68.3	67.0	66.5	65.4	64.9	64.4	64.3
Black[2]	84.7	78.8	80.1	82.6	86.2	86.8	85.2	83.2	80.5	76.9	72.3	70.7
American Indian[2]	82.7	78.6	75.6	76.8	79.0	76.2	75.1	75.4	73.4	70.9	69.1	68.7
Asian or Pacific Islander[2]	73.2	68.4	67.1	70.2	68.2	69.6	67.6	67.2	66.7	66.8	66.4	65.9
Age of mother:												
10 to 14 years old	1.1	1.2	1.3	1.3	1.4	1.4	1.4	1.4	1.4	1.4	1.3	1.2
15 to 19 years old	53.0	51.0	50.6	53.0	57.3	59.9	62.1	60.7	59.6	58.9	56.8	54.4
20 to 24 years old	115.1	108.3	107.9	110.2	113.8	116.5	115.7	114.6	112.6	111.1	109.8	110.4
25 to 29 years old	112.9	111.0	111.6	114.4	117.6	120.2	118.2	117.4	115.5	113.9	112.2	113.0
30 to 34 years old	61.9	69.1	72.1	74.8	77.4	80.8	79.5	80.2	80.8	81.5	82.5	83.9
35 to 39 years old	19.8	24.0	26.3	28.1	29.9	31.7	32.0	32.5	32.9	33.7	34.3	35.3
40 to 44 years old	3.9	4.0	4.4	4.8	5.2	5.5	5.5	5.9	6.1	6.4	6.6	6.8
45 to 49 years old	0.2	0.2	0.2	0.2	0.2	0.2	0.2	0.3	0.3	0.3	0.3	0.3

[1]Excludes births to nonresidents of the United States. Includes other races not shown separately. [2]Per 1,000 women, 15 to 44 years old in specified group. The rate for *age of mother 45 to 49 years old* computed by relating births to mothers 45 years old and over to women 45 to 49 years old.

SOURCE: U.S. National Center for Health Statistics, *Vital Statistics of the United States*, annual; *Monthly Vital Statistics Report;* and unpublished data.

services, and the provision of comprehensive maternal-child services. Recent data do indicate a slow but steady increase in the percentage of US women beginning prenatal care in the first trimester. In 1990, for example, 74.2% of pregnant women began their prenatal care in the first trimester. In 1993 that number was 78.9%; data for 1996 suggest that 81.9% began prenatal care in the first trimester (Ventura et al, 1998). Of course, this number also indicates that one in five women did not begin prenatal care until later, if at all.

Table 1–2 identifies infant mortality rates for selected countries for 1994. As the data indicate, the range is dramatic among the countries listed. Unfortunately, information about birth rates and mortality rates is limited for some countries because of a lack of organized reporting mechanisms.

The information prompts questions about access to health care during pregnancy and following birth, about standards of living, nutrition, sociocultural factors, and more. Additional factors affecting the infant mortality

TABLE 1–2 Live Birth Rates and Infant Mortality Rates in Selected Countries, 1996

Country	Birth Rate	Infant Mortality Rate
Afghanistan	43	147
Argentina	20	19
Australia	14	5
Canada	13	6
China	17	40
Egypt	28	71
Ethiopia	46	122
France	11	6
Iraq	43	58
Japan	10	4
Mexico	26	24
United Kingdom	13	6
United States	14.8	7.2

SOURCE: *1998 World Almanac and Book of Facts.* Newark NJ: World Almanac Books, 1997.

TABLE 1–3 Maternal Mortality Rate per 100,000 Live Births: United States, 1950–1992

Year	Rate
1996[1]	7.6
1995[1]	7.1
1992[1]	7.8
1980[2]	9.2
1970[2]	21.5
1960[2]	37.1
1950[2]	83.3

SOURCES: [1]National Center for Health Statistics: Deaths: Final data for 1996. (November 10, 1998). *National Vital Statistics Reports,* vol 47, no 8. Hyattsville, MD: National Center for Health Statistics, Public Health Services.

[2]National Center for Health Statistics: Births, marriages, divorces, and deaths for August 1994. *Monthly Vital Statistics Report.* vol 42, no 8. Hyattsville, MD: National Center for Health Statistics, Public Health Service, 1995.

[3]National Center for Health Statistics: Advance report of final mortality statistics, 1984. *Monthly Vital Statistics Report.* vol 35, no 6, Suppl (2). DHHS Pub No (PHS) 86–1120. Public Health Service, Hyattsville, MD: September 26, 1986.

rate may be identified by considering the following research questions:

- Does infant mortality correlate with a specific maternal age?
- What are the leading causes of infant mortality in each country?
- Is there a difference in mortality rates among racial groups? If so, is it associated with the availability of prenatal care? With educational level of the mother or father?

Maternal Mortality

Maternal mortality is the number of deaths from any cause during the pregnancy cycle (including the 42-day postpartal period) per 100,000 live births. In 1996, 294 women died of maternal causes as compared to 277 in 1995. As a result, the maternal mortality rate in the US, which had decreased steadily in the last 40 years or more (Table 1–3) rose slightly in 1996. However, the number is not statistically significant (Peters et al, 1998). Factors influencing the decrease in maternal mortality include the increased use of hospitals and specialized health care personnel by antepartal, intrapartal, and postpartal maternity clients; the establishment of care centers for high-risk mothers and infants; the prevention and control of infection with antibiotics and improved techniques; the availability of blood and blood products for transfusions; and the lowered rates of anesthesia-related deaths.

Additional factors to consider may be identified by asking the following research questions:

- Is there a correlation between maternal mortality and age?
- Is there a correlation with availability of health care? Economic status?

Implications for Nursing Practice

Nurses can use statistics in a number of ways. For example, statistical data may be used to

- Determine populations at risk.
- Assess the relationship between specific factors.
- Help establish databases for specific client populations.
- Determine the levels of care needed by particular client populations.
- Evaluate the success of specific nursing interventions.
- Determine priorities in case loads.
- Estimate staffing and equipment needs of hospital units and clinics.

Statistical information is available through many sources, including professional literature; state and city health departments; vital statistics sections of private, county, state, and federal agencies; special programs or agencies (family-planning and similar agencies); and demographic profiles of specific geographic areas. Nurses who use this information will be better prepared to promote the health needs of maternal-newborn clients and their families.

Nursing Research

Research plays a vital role in expanding the science of nursing. It is also a means of improving client care and advancing the profession of nursing.

Nursing research can help clarify the relationships between the health professional and the client. Nursing research also can help determine the psychosocial and physical risks and benefits of nursing and medical interventions.

RESEARCH IN PRACTICE

What is this study about? For decades, high fertility rates among the poor have puzzled clinicians, health care policy makers, and political leaders. A common misconception is that the poor create their own poverty by having children. In this ethnographic study, 15 homeless women were interviewed about their reproductive goals.

How was this study done? Fifteen homeless, pregnant women from five different shelters comprised the sample. Participant observation was the data collection method used to obtain information about these women during their visits to the clinic, emergency room, welfare and housing authorities, during job and apartment hunting, and even during grocery store excursions. General and focused observations occurred at the shelter and the surrounding neighborhood. In-depth interviews were conducted with each of the women surrounding their experience of pregnancy. Data were analyzed for domains and themes.

What were the results of the study? Results revealed one domain, conditions of conceptions, and five themes: 1) the desire for intimacy; 2) victimization and economic survival; 3) lack of access to contraception; 4) uncertain fertility; and 5) hope for the future. All the women revealed that they had little choice in the partner, the timing, the place, or the manner in which conception took place. All became pregnant while they were homeless.

What additional questions might I have? 1)How does homelessness contribute to the desire for intimacy? 2) Are homeless couples increasingly more vulnerable to pregnancy than low-income couples?

How can I use this study? This study revealed that homelessness often diminished women's control over everyday situations. This lack of control was directly related to their vulnerability and pregnancy state. Nurses can play a significant role in education and prevention in this population by providing access to contraception (condoms, cervical caps, and so on) in the shelters. The interplay of individual and situational factors frame the homeless family's ability to manage fertility. This study provides valuable information that can increase professional nurses' sensitivity to this vulnerable population.

SOURCE: Killion, C. (1998). Poverty and procreation among women. *Journal of Nurse Midwifery, 43*(4), 273–279.

The gap between research and practice is being narrowed by the publication of research findings in popular nursing journals, the establishment of departments of nursing research in hospitals, and collaborative research efforts by nurse researchers and clinical practitioners. In addition, nurses can access numerous journal articles giving "how-to" information for translating research into practice.

Critical Thinking: An Example

Each of the tools of critical thinking—knowledge base, nursing process, communication skills, standards of care, statistics, and nursing research—can exist separately, but in practice they overlap and build upon each other. An example of just one possible situation is presented in the following case study.

> Two birthing unit nurses express concerns to each other about the seemingly high number of adolescents who have been giving birth in their unit. At the next staff meeting, they voice their concerns and raise questions about whether the number of teenage mothers seen in their unit is higher than normal. After the discussion, the nurses decide they need to formulate a plan to gather more information. Each nurse volunteers to pursue a particular aspect of the plan of action. Their plan includes contacting the local public health department for local and national statistics on this age group; looking at the availability of health care for adolescents in their community; investigating the particular health problems of pregnant teenagers and risks to their infants; checking the availability of prenatal education groups for adolescents; finding out whether their community has school health programs and what the program content is; looking at national statistics identifying when adolescents seek prenatal care; talking with local certified nurse-midwives, physicians, and prenatal clinic personnel to see if the national statistics apply to their community; collecting information about current legislative issues affecting adolescent health care; seeking further information about the needs of adolescents during pregnancy and birth by doing a library search; and looking for continuing education programs dealing with the pregnant adolescent client.
>
> At subsequent staff meetings, nurses share information and investigate other areas as the need is identified. How they evaluate the data and apply them will depend on the requirements of their maternal-newborn unit and the unique needs of their community.
>
> Possible outcomes may include developing a research study, volunteering in local adolescent clinics, developing and teaching prenatal classes for adolescents, volunteering to teach in community school health programs, organizing a continuing education program on the adolescent mother for community hospitals, and forming a network within their professional nursing organization to stay informed about legislative issues pertaining to adolescents.

As the example illustrates, the application of tools of critical thinking assists the nurse in analyzing data and planning a course of action.

FOCUS YOUR STUDY

- Many nurses working with childbearing families are expert practitioners who are able to serve as role models for nurses who have not yet attained the same level of competence.
- Contemporary childbirth is family centered, offers choices about birth, and recognizes the needs of siblings and other family members.

- The self-care movement, which emerged in the late 1960s, emphasizes personal health goals, a holistic approach, and preventive care.
- A nurse must practice within the scope of practice or be open to the accusation of practicing medicine without a license. The standard of care against which individual nursing practice is compared is that of a reasonably prudent nurse.
- Nursing standards provide information and guidelines for nurses in their own practice, in developing policies and protocols in health care settings, and in directing the development of quality nursing care.
- Informed consent—based on knowledge of a procedure and its benefits, risks, and alternatives—must be secured prior to providing treatment.
- The right to privacy is protected by state constitutions, statutes, and common law.
- Abortion can be performed until the age of viability. Caregivers have the right to refuse to perform an abortion or assist with the procedure.
- Assisted reproductive technology (ART) is the term used to describe highly technologic approaches used to produce pregnancy, including artificial insemination (AI), intracytoplasmic sperm injection (ICSI), in vitro fertilization and embryo transfer (IVF-ET), zygote intrafallopian transfer (ZIFT), and gamete intrafallopian transfer (GIFT).
- Cord blood banking provides the opportunity to make stem cells available to treat a variety of cancers and blood system disorders. Its growing popularity has revealed several ethical issues.
- Descriptive statistics describe or summarize a set of data. Inferential statistics allow the investigator to draw conclusions about what is happening between two or more variables in a population.
- Nursing research plays a vital role in adding to the nursing knowledge base, expanding clinical practice, and expanding nursing theory.

REFERENCES

American Academy of Pediatrics, Committee on Bioethics (1988). Fetal therapy: Ethical considerations. *Pediatrics, 81*(6), 898–899.

American College of Obstetricians and Gynecologists, Committee on Ethics (1987). *Patient choices: Maternal-fetal conflict* (Opinion No. 55). Washington, DC: Author.

American Medical Association, Board of Trustees (1990). Legal interventions during pregnancy. Court-ordered medical treatments and legal penalties for potentially harmful behavior by pregnant women. *Journal of the American Medical Association, 264*(20), 2663–2670.

American Nurses Association (1993). Primary Health care: The nurse solution. In *Nursing facts.* Washington, DC: Author.

Baird, P. A. (1996). New reproductive technologies: The Canadian perspective. *Women's Health Issues, 6*(3), 156–166.

Benner, P. (1984). *From novice to expert.* Menlo Park, CA: Addison-Wesley.

Carpenter, J. A. (1998). Shortening the short stay. AWHONN *Lifelines, 2*(1), 29–34.

Collins, B. A. (1993). Ethical issues in conducting clinical nursing research. *AWHONN's Clinical Issues in Perinatal & Women's Health Nursing, 4*(4), 620–623.

Corry, M. P., Williams, D., & Stapleton, S. R. (1997). Models of collaborative practice: Preparing for maternity care in the 21st century [Meeting report]. *Women's Health Issues,* 7(5), 279–284.

Crooks, G. M., Lill, M., Feig, S., & Parkman, R. (1997). Cord blood—new source of stem cells for transplants. *Contemporary OB/GYN, 42*(8), 114–126.

Department of Commerce (1997). Vital statistics. In *Statistical abstract of the United States, 1997* (117th ed., pp. 70–108). Washington, DC: Author.

Department of Health and Human Services, Secretary's Commission on Nursing (1988). *Final Report* (Vol. 1). Washington, DC: Author.

Donohue, M. (1994). Midwives use advance directive birth plans to build trust. *Medical Ethics Advisor, 10*(3), 43.

Dower, C., & O'Neil, E. (1997). Collaborative practice, regulation, and market forces: A changing health care agenda. *Women's Health Issues,* 7(5), 298–300.

Edwards-Beckett, J. (1990). Nursing research utilization techniques. *Journal of Nursing Administration, 20*(11), 25–30.

Evans, M. I., Johnson, M. P., & Holzgreve, W. (1990). Fetal therapy: The next generation. *Women's Health Issues, 1*(1), 31–33.

Fagin, C. M., & Lynaugh, J. E. (1992). Reaping the rewards of radical change: A new agenda for nursing education. *Nursing Outlook, 40*(5), 213–220.

Fetal surgery: Past, present, and future work in this frontier [Symposium; Special issue]. (1994, April 15). *Contemporary OB/GYN, 39*(S), 59–66.

Gill, S. (1992). The fate of Roe v. Wade. *Hastings Center Report, 22*(5), 24.

Goode, C. J., & Hahn, S. J. (1993). Oocyte donation and in vitro fertilization: The nurse's role with ethical and legal issues. *Journal of Obstetric, Gynecologic, & Neonatal Nursing, 22*(2), 106–111.

Gorman, C. (1994, August). Brave new embryos. *Time, 144*(9), 60–61.

Hagedorn, M. I. E., Gardner, S. L., Laux, M. G., & Gardner, G. L. (1997). A model for professional nursing practice. In S. L. Gardner & M. I. E. Hagedorn (Eds.), *Legal aspects of maternal-child nursing practice* (pp. 67–94). Menlo Park, CA: Addison Wesley Longman.

Heater, B. S., Olson, R. K., & Becker, A. M. (1990). Helping patients recover faster. *American Journal of Nursing, 90*(10), 19–20.

Hurst, B. S., & Schlaff, W. D. (1994, October). Assisted reproduction: What role for ZIFT? [Special issue]. *Contemporary OB/GYN, 39*(S), 9–19.

Jensen, G. A., Morrisey, M. A., Gaffney, S., & Liston, D. K. (1997). The new dominance of managed care: Insurance trends in the 1990s. *Health Affairs, 16*(1), 125–136.

Joint Commission on Accreditation of Healthcare Organizations (1990). *The 1991 Joint Commission accreditation manual for hospitals: Vol. 1. Standards.*

Klerman, L. V. (1994). Perinatal health care policy: How it will affect the family in the 21st century. *Journal of Obstetric, Gynecologic, & Neonatal Nursing, 23*(2), 124–128.

Lamison-White, L. (1997). *Poverty in the United States: 1996* (U.S. Bureau of the Census, Current Population Reports, Series P60-198). Washington, DC: U.S. Government Printing Office.

Leppert, P. C. (1997). The challenges and opportunities of collaborative practice. *Women's Health Issues, 7*(5), 285–288.

Levy, M. J., & Gindoff, P. R. (1994). Who benefits most from natural-cycle IVF? *Contemporary OB/GYN, 39*(2), 11–23.

Loeb, S. (1992). *Nurses handbook of law and ethics.* Springhouse, PA: Springhouse.

Macklin, R., & White, G. B. (1997). Assisted reproductive technologies, ads, and ethics: Philosophical, ethical, and clinical perspectives on the use of advertising in reproductive medicine. A conference held by the National Advisory Board on Ethics in Reproduction [Executive summary]. *Women's Health Issues, 7*(3), 127–131.

Mahowald, M. B. (1997). An overview of the Human Genome Project and its implications for women. *Women's Health Issues, 7*(4), 206–208.

Markowitz, M. S. (1993). Human fetal tissue: Ethical implications for use in research and treatment. *AWHONN's Clinical Issues in Perinatal & Women's Health Nursing, 4*(4), 578–588.

Mathieu, D. (1991). *Preventing fetal harm: Should the State intervene?* Boston, MA: Kluwer Academic.

Mitchell, C. (1990). Ethical dilemmas. *Critical Care Nursing Clinics of North America, 2*(3), 427–430.

Mitchell, J. J. (1994). Maternal-fetal conflict: A role for the healthcare ethics committee. *Healthcare Ethics Committee Forum, 6*(2), 93.

Moore, M. L., & Paul, N. W. (1992). Improving access to prenatal care: Innovative responses to a national dilemma. *Birth Defects: Original Article Series, 28*(4). White Plains, NY: March of Dimes Birth Defects Foundation.

Moores, P. (1997). Empowering women in the practice setting. In S. L. Gardner & M. I. E. Hagedorn (Eds.), *Legal aspects of maternal-child nursing practice* (pp. 9–23). Menlo Park, CA: Addison Wesley Longman.

Mundinger, M. O. (1994). Health care reform: Will nursing respond? *Nursing & Health Care, 15*(1), 28–33.

Peters, K. D., Kochanek, K. D., & Murphy, S. L. (1998, November 10). Deaths: Final data for 1996. *National Vital Statistics Reports, 47*(9), 1–82.

Pettengill, M. M., Gillies, D. A., & Clark, C. C. (1994, Summer). Factors encouraging and discouraging the use of nursing research findings. *Image—the Journal of Nursing Scholarship, 26*(2), 143–147.

Plotnick, J., & Presler, B. (1996). Rugged individualism and compassion: The foundation of public policy. *American Journal of Maternal Child Nursing, 21*(1), 20–33.

Raff, B. S., & Eunpu, D. (1994). The genome project. *Journal of Obstetric, Gynecologic, & Neonatal Nursing, 23*(6), 448–491.

Randal, J. (1995, February). Cord blood offers patients new blood cell source [News]. *Journal of the National Cancer Institute, 87*(3), 164–166.

Robertson, J. A. (1997). Innovations in infertility treatment and the rush to market. *Women's Health Issues, 7*(3), 162–166.

Shactman, D., & Altman, S. (1995). *Market consolidating, antitrust, and public policy in the health care industry: Agenda for future research.* Princeton, NJ: Robert Wood Johnson Foundation.

Sinclair, B. P. (1997). Advanced practice nurses in integrated health care systems. *Journal of Obstetric, Gynecologic, & Neonatal Nursing, 26*(2), 217–223.

Stillman, R. J., & Gindoff, P. R. (1994). Assisted reproductive technology. In J. R. Scott, P. J. DiSaia, C. B. Hammond, & W. N. Spellacy (Eds.), *Danforth's obstetrics and gynecology* (7th ed., pp. 739–756). Philadelphia: Lippincott.

Thorp, J. M., Jr., Bowes, W. A., & Cefalo, R. C. (1997). Medical and legal considerations of court-ordered ob intervention. *Contemporary Obstetrics and Gynecology, 42*(6), 41–48.

Ventura, S. J., Martin, J. A., Curtin, S. C., & Mathews, T. J. (1998, June 30). Report of final natality statistics, 1996. *Monthly Vital Statistics Report, 46*(11S), 1–99.

Weisman, C. S. (1996). Proceedings of women's health and managed care: Balancing cost, access, and quality [Meeting report]. *Women's Health Issues, 6*(1), 1–38.

Wilcox, L. S., & Marks, J. S. (1996). Regulating assisted reproductive technologies: Public health, consumer protection, and public resources. *Women's Health Issues, 6*(3), 175–180.

Wysocki, S. (1997). Unconventional and conventional medicine: Searching for common ground. *Contemporary Nurse Practitioner, 2*(4), 3–15.

2 Community-Based Teaching for Childbearing Families

I CAN REMEMBER MY NURSING INSTRUCTOR STRESSING the need to use every opportunity available to do patient teaching. She told me that, no matter how I felt inside, I was an expert to the patients I cared for unless I acted otherwise. I was afraid to try teaching at first, but I soon realized that people did trust me and believed I knew what I was talking about. I felt good about that, but I felt a tremendous sense of responsibility, too. I had to be sure that I gave only accurate information. Even today, years later, when I don't know something or I'm not sure, I always make it my practice to say, "I don't know the answer, but I will find out for you." And then I do just that!

Objectives

- Delineate the political, sociocultural, and technologic issues that influence client teaching.
- Contrast the behavioral, cognitive field, perceptual-existential, and information-processing theories about learning.
- Compare the key concepts that form the basis of selected theories about the "ways of knowing" or assimilating knowledge.
- Describe the key concepts about adult learners that form the basis of the andragogic model developed by Knowles (1984).
- Summarize the actions an educator needs to take to implement the teaching/learning process effectively.

CLIENT EDUCATION AFFORDS NURSES the opportunity to profoundly influence the health and well-being of those for whom they care. Nurses can appreciate the direct impact of this teaching when a nursing mother recognizes that her baby's refusal to suck results from sleepiness, not rejection of her, or when a new father smiles and cuddles his infant after successfully completing his first "solo" bath at home. In keeping with our philosophy of a shared, mutually respectful relationship between health care provider and the individual, we refer to this teaching as *client teaching* or *health teaching* rather than the more common term *patient teaching.*

Because the nurse is often the primary provider of health teaching, we have attempted to help readers identify key teaching areas and have presented a variety of approaches to help readers identify what and how to teach. This book includes teaching cards, which can be removed and carried in a pocket. These cards contain information about teaching a variety of specific topics, such as exercise during pregnancy, fetal heart monitoring, and breastfeeding. The text also contains a series of detailed teaching guides. Many of the chapters, especially those focusing on normal pregnancy and birth, contain the subheading "Teaching for Self-Care." These sections address areas of teaching about a specific topic. Finally, because we are teachers, too, we have created a special feature entitled "Clinical Tips." This is designed to help the nurse practice more effectively and contains tips we have learned through our own nursing practice or from our nurse colleagues.

This chapter addresses the topic of teaching from both theoretical and practical perspectives. It is designed to provide a framework for the health teaching that is an essential component of the nurse's role in working with the childbearing woman and her family.

Client Teaching in Community-Based Settings

Nursing theorists and educators have long recognized the importance of client teaching and have written about this topic since the middle 1800s (Redman, 1993a; Smith, 1987). In her *Notes on Nursing* (1860/1969), Nightingale spoke of the importance of health and implied that nurses could teach their homebound clients how to achieve efficient drainage and cleanliness and obtain pure air, light, and pure water. In the 1920s, Lavinia Dock praised Margaret Sanger's efforts to provide information to underserved women of that era (Church, 1990). Hildegard Peplau (1952) emphasized that client teaching should be developed around the individual's wants and ability to use the information.

In the 1970s, a rebirth or reemphasis on client education occurred in response to several factors, including a new emphasis on health and self-care; a change in attitude toward physicians; and a trend toward long-term, outpatient, home management of such chronic illnesses as diabetes, hypertension, and sickle cell disease, which required that individuals be knowledgeable about their condition and its treatment (Redman, 1993b). Today this trend toward home management has become a "given" in the health care system, with hospitalization indicated only during crisis periods or to stabilize newly diagnosed conditions.

Childbearing families have traditionally been viewed as important recipients of health teaching to prepare them for the challenges and responsibilities of childrearing. In the late 1980s, health teaching was a major part of the postpartum care provided during a hospitalization that typically lasted 72 hours for a vaginal birth and 4 to 5 days for a cesarean birth. For a time in the mid-1990s, women were being discharged very early—often within 6 to 24 hours following vaginal birth and 24 to 48 hours after cesarean. Outcries from health care providers and concerned individuals about "drive-through deliveries" brought about some changes. Currently, legislation mandates that women have a right to a 48-hour postpartum stay following vaginal births and a 72-hour stay following cesarean births.

Although the time for teaching is still brief, the legislated increase in length of stay does help, and nurses need to use every opportunity to share information creatively with the new family. In planning teaching strategies for the woman and her loved ones, nurses need to recognize that women in the postpartal period often experience transient deficits in cognitive functioning, particularly in memory function. Consequently, verbal instructions may be poorly remembered and should be augmented with written instructions when possible (Eidelman, Hoffman, & Kaitz, 1993).

The traditional model of hospital-based education for the postpartal woman is being replaced by home and community-based health care. Concurrently, the teaching nurses provide during prenatal visits assumes new importance in preparing the pregnant woman for the pregnancy itself and the postpartum period.

Issues Impacting Client Teaching

Political, sociocultural, educational/experience, and technologic issues impact client teaching. Each of these issues creates potential concerns for the client educator.

Political Issues

Political influences affecting client education include the trend toward self-care and taking personal responsibility for health; the current educational climate of empowerment; the changing emphasis on women's health; health

COMMUNITY IN FOCUS

Follow-Up Neonatal Home Care

Home care has played only a limited role in addressing the needs of preterm infants following discharge. Consequently the focus of nursing efforts to date has been on discharge preparation of the family. However, many preterm infants have continuing health needs following discharge. To address these needs and to provide a mechanism for early discharge for qualified infants, one Fort Worth, Texas community has designed an innovative approach using a home care model that represents a partnership between clinical nurse specialists (CNS) and neonatal intensive care unit (NICU) nurses.

The Harris Home Health program is directed by a clinical nurse specialist who works closely with both the Harris Hospital neonatal CNS and perinatal CNS to ensure a seamless system of follow-up care after discharge. Typically home care visits are planned for stable preterm infants who are feeding well and weigh more than 4 lb. The visits are made by specially selected, carefully educated NICU nurses who cared for the infant in the NICU. On average, the infants are visited twice a week until they have attained a weight of 7–8 lb.

Each pattern of visits is planned individually with the family based on their needs and those of their newborn. The initial home visit includes a thorough assessment of the infant including developmental and nutritional status, and of the family's environment, caregiving abilities, and areas of concern. At each subsequent visit the nurse completes a physical assessment of the infant including vital signs, length, and weight.

Parental education is an important aspect of each visit and focuses on a variety of topics such as infection prevention, IV infusion therapy procedures and maintenance, feeding issues, safety, growth and development, and the like. In addition, the home care nurse works with the insurance case manager when necessary to address coverage issues. Referral to community agencies is made as indicated. A home care nurse is available to families round the clock for consultation and guidance about problems or concerns.

The Harris Home Care CNS coordinates the program and orients the NICU nurses who participate. To be eligible, a nurse must have a minimum of one year NICU experience. The orientation program includes both a didactic portion and a home care clinical component under the supervision of the home care CNS or a designated RN preceptor. Ultimately, home care visits will become a part of each NICU nurse's job description.

The Harris Home Care CNS is responsible for modeling nursing expertise, assessing health care needs of the infants in the program, and networking in the community. In addition, the CNS is responsible for collecting outcomes data. These data will focus on three areas: infant outcomes, parent satisfaction and improved caregiving behaviors, and cost effectiveness. Such information should prove invaluable in assessing the effectiveness of this creative new program, which builds on the expertise of nurses in differing roles and is an innovative response to issues of cost containment.

SOURCE: Christian A (1996): Clinical nurse specialists: Creating new programs for neonatal home care. *Journal of Perinatal,* and *Neonatal Nursing 10* (1):54.

care reform; and the issue of jurisdiction over client education, or who decides what, how, and when the client needs to be taught. Politics is potentially present in all social relationships and involves exercising power in any given situation. The novice educator needs to be aware that education is inherently a political process and includes much more than just teaching a circumscribed content to specific individuals. In educating clients, nurses must recognize power behaviors characteristic of any social interaction (Morgan, 1994).

An increased emphasis on health, a trend toward less reliance on health care professionals, and general challenges to authority have all contributed to motivating people to take responsibility for themselves in matters of health (Redman, 1993a; Stanhope & Lancaster, 1992). To practice self-care, the client needs timely, correct health information about how to engage in a healthier lifestyle and to manage or correct problems associated with chronic illness. Nurses, as key members of the health care team, share a responsibility for educating clients in a variety of health care settings on a variety of health-related issues. Nurses play an important role in providing people with the necessary knowledge and skills to promote self-care.

Another client teaching factor with potential political impact is empowerment. The empowered student, whether in a formal educational institution or in a health teaching situation, makes decisions based on knowledge and past experiences. Empowered students and empowered participants in health education seek equality in the educational process. Empowerment becomes a political process when an oppressed group seeks freedom from domination partially through the educational process (Shor & Freire, 1987). As a result of the changing educational process, nurses who participate in health teaching strive to help clients make informed, knowledgeable choices rather than merely comply with instructions. Client and educator negotiate teaching content and share responsibility (Fleming, 1992).

Women's issues have emerged as major factors in health care education. As more people recognize the lack of health information specific to women, more research and new publications have resulted. Knowledge of past and present attitudes toward women as well as current, accurate information based on research with and about women is helpful for anyone who plans health teaching involving mothers, babies, and families.

Even before the recent national movement toward health care reform, the health care industry had responded to political and legislative pressure to reduce costs. This response included shortened hospital stays and increased use of outpatient surgery and community-based facilities. Reduced interaction time with health care professionals intensifies the need for effective, interactive teaching/learning methods that enable the nurse to provide necessary information and ensure that the client has learned the essential material.

Nurses are in a unique position to maximize the health potential of the client. It is imperative that nurses recognize this responsibility as an inherent aspect of professional practice (Morgan, 1994). Many nurses suggest that because client education is a professional expectation and an independent nursing function, nurses have a legal obligation to provide health teaching to their clients (Hagedorn, Gardner, Laux, & Gardner, 1997).

Whatever the circumstance, the nurse must recognize that client education is a dynamic and interactive process that is achieved through a mutual empowerment of nurse and client (Morgan, 1994). The therapeutic benefits of initiating nursing actions that actually empower the client and facilitate equitable nurse–client relationships are gaining recognition in clinical practice. Clients become empowered by applying the knowledge and skill they gain through appropriate education. Indeed, the overriding argument for developing client education as a facet of nursing is based not just on health considerations but on financial constraints (Morgan, 1994). Spellbring (1991) insists that current cost containment in health services will bring client education issues to the forefront of the economic debate.

Sociocultural Issues

Sociocultural issues impact the nurse-educator and the client because both bring their own socioeconomic background, personal values, and cultural beliefs to the situation. If nurses do not recognize their own personal belief system, they will not be aware of how those beliefs impact their approach to client teaching and care.

Many societies are multicultural and contain both a dominant culture and other, smaller cultural groups. The increased frequency of international travel has led to greater mixing of peoples. Nurses increasingly interact with clients of many ethnic backgrounds. However, simply translating educational or health promotional materials from one language to another may create problems. Pictures or illustrations must be appropriate to individuals from the culture. Nevertheless, certain materials, such as informed consent or authorization for specific procedures, need to be translated into other languages. Bilingual health care providers should review any translated materials for accuracy, ease of use, and cultural sensitivity (Poss, Santucci, & Mull, 1993).

The nurse-educator must be aware of cultural norms that are different from the nurse's own belief system. Beliefs and values may vary in terms of time orientation, religious beliefs and practices, folk remedies, cultural healers, and language and communication methods. Sociocultural influences may include folk beliefs about health and illness.

Hispanic folk healers or practitioners may include family members, a curandero or curandera, an espiritualista, a yerbero, or a sabador. Family members who do folk healing are those who possess knowledge of medicine learned from others or through study. Curanderos or curanderas have knowledge about herbs, diet, massage, and rituals. They may have had training or received curative powers as a gift from God. An espiritualista, or spiritualist, is born with the ability to analyze dreams and foretell the future. A yerbero knows about growing and prescribing herbs. A sabador uses massage and manipulation of bones and muscles.

For some people of African descent, a folk practitioner may be a spiritualist, a voodoo priestess, or an "old lady." The spiritualist, usually associated with a fundamentalist Christian church, has been called by God to help others. A voodoo priestess establishes a therapeutic milieu, uses herbs, and can cure illnesses caused by voodoo. An "old lady" gives advice for common illness; her knowledge has been obtained through successful life experiences (Hautman, 1979).

Beliefs about health and illness develop from world views, or how one sees the world. Most cultural groups believe in one of three major world views: magicoreligious, scientific, or holistic (Boyle & Andrews, 1995).

In the magicoreligious worldview, supernatural forces control the world and the people in it. The supernatural forces may be a god, several gods, or other powers. Elements of this belief are found in African, Caribbean, and many Hispanic cultures. Some Western religious groups, such as Christian Scientists, believe in healing through the power of prayer alone (Boyle & Andrews, 1995).

The scientific worldview depends on objective, mechanistic thought processes. In this model, health and health attributes have to be observable and measurable to be real. This biomedical model, ascribed to by most of the dominant American cultural group, places greater importance on physical and chemical interventions than human relationships (Boyle & Andrews, 1995).

The holistic health belief model stresses natural balance and harmony. It is grounded in the belief that natural laws of the universe maintain order; imbalance, disease, and chaos result when these natural laws are violated (Boyle & Andrews, 1995). Holistic worldviews are found in Native American and Asian cultures, for example. Two common metaphors for this belief system include the Chinese concept of yin and yang and the hot/cold theory of disease found in Asian, Hispanic, African, Arabic, Muslim, and Caribbean cultures. Yin, the feminine universal force, encompasses darkness, cold, the negative, inactivity, and emptiness. Opposite qualities—light, warmth,

TABLE 2–1 Cultural Beliefs about Activity and Pregnancy

Prescriptive Beliefs	Restrictive Beliefs	Taboo
Remain active during pregnancy to aid the baby's circulation. (Crow Indian)	Avoid cold air during pregnancy. (Mexican, Haitian, Asian)	Avoid lunar eclipses and moonlight, or the baby may be born with a deformity. (Mexican)
Remain happy to bring the baby joy and good fortune. (Pueblo and Navajo Indian)	Do not reach over your head, or the cord will wrap around the baby's neck. (African American, Hispanic, European American, Asian)	Don't walk on the streets at noon or five o'clock, or the spirits may become angry. (Vietnamese)
Sleep flat on your back to protect the baby. (Mexican)	Avoid weddings and funerals, or you will bring bad fortune to the baby. (Vietnamese)	Don't join in traditional ceremonies like Yei or Squaw dances, or spirits will harm the baby. (Navajo Indian)
Keep active during pregnancy to ensure a small baby and an easy labor. (Mexican)	Do not continue sexual intercourse, or harm will come to you and the baby. (Vietnamese, Filipino, Samoan)	Don't get involved with persons who cast spells, or the baby will be eaten in the womb. (Haitian)
Continue sexual intercourse to lubricate the birth canal and prevent dry labor. (Haitian, Mexican)	Do not tie knots or braid or allow the baby's father to do so, or you will have difficult labor. (Navajo Indian)	Don't say the baby's name before the naming ceremony, or harm might come to the baby. (Orthodox Jewish)
Continue daily baths and frequent shampoos during pregnancy to produce a clean baby. (Filipino)	Do not sew. (Pueblo Indian, Asian)	Don't have your picture taken because it might cause a stillbirth. (African descent)

SOURCE: Adapted from Boyle J. & Andrews M. (1995). *Transcultural concepts in nursing care.* (2nd ed.) Glenview, IL: Scott, Foresman/Little, Brown.

the positive, activity, and fullness—characterize yang, the masculine force (Babcock & Miller, 1994). Certain organs and health conditions are considered to be either yin or yang. Illness results from an imbalance between the two forces. Cancer, menstruation, and wasting are attributed to yin, for example; constipation, infection, and hangovers are characterized as yang conditions.

The hot/cold theory of disease is also based on the idea of balance, in this instance, between hot and cold humors (body fluids). Certain diseases, such as cancer, paralysis, and earache, are cold conditions and need "hot" medicine or food. This can sometimes be confusing because "hot" does not necessarily relate to the temperature or spiciness of food. Examples of "hot" foods include gingerroot, cinnamon, and cod-liver oil.

In addition to health belief models and folk healing beliefs, many cultures have specific beliefs about pregnancy, which may influence client teaching. Some of these beliefs are described in Table 2–1.

In order to obtain pertinent client information, the nurse should always ask cultural assessment questions. Questions similar to those identified in Table 2–2 help both the nurse and the client identify important cultural issues that relate to health teaching. If nurses do not assess and honor cultural differences when teaching, the client will probably follow familiar practices and beliefs rather than attempt new approaches. A comprehensive coverage of cultural concepts is beyond the scope of this chapter; for more in-depth information, see the several excellent texts listed in the references at the end of this chapter.

Education and Experience

Educational and experiential diversity create significant challenges for nurses and other health educators who plan learning activities for childbearing families. For example, nurses in any birthing unit may find themselves concurrently responsible for meeting the postpartum teaching needs of a 15-year-old high school sophomore

TABLE 2–2 Suggested Cultural Questions for a Prenatal Assessment

Do you identify with a particular ethnic group or a specific race?
Tell me about beliefs and practices concerning pregnancy or birth that you learned while you were growing up.
Describe any practices or circumstances that you believe might harm you or your baby.
What foods do you believe to be important during your pregnancy (postpartum or during breastfeeding)?
Do you use or plan to use any type of cultural healer, practitioner, or healing practices as part of your care?

and a business executive with an advanced degree; a woman who teaches English composition and a woman who is functionally illiterate; a woman who has never been inside a hospital or birthing unit and a woman who is a registered nurse. It is essential that nurses be alert to clues about a family's general level of comprehension, experience with the health care system, and reading/language ability.

Most educational programs are planned to meet the needs of the majority of clients using the facility. However, it can be extremely useful to have print materials prepared for different reading levels and interests. In addition, classes focused on the needs of a particular group may be very effective. For example, many nurses offer special classes for pregnant adolescents and have specific print materials available for them.

One of every five adult Americans can be considered functionally illiterate, that is, reading at or below fifth-grade level (Redman, 1993b). Some strategies that can be used with these clients include the following (Salerno, 1997):

- Present survival skills or essential information first.
- Make each point clearly, concisely, and vividly.
- Use simple language and examples in order to help the individual remember verbal information.

- Whenever possible, use visual resources such as line drawings.
- Use large type and a simple format for written materials.
- Have print materials assessed to ensure that they are written at no higher than a fifth grade level.

Technologic Issues

In addition to political and sociocultural issues, technologic concerns also affect health teaching. Nurse-educators have both the ability and technologic access to convey information through many different modalities. Technologic aspects of client education involve issues of literacy as well as the explosion of knowledge and the transmission of information. Today literacy, the ability to read and write, can also be extended to basic knowledge of computers. Therefore, the educator should assess the client's literacy for the medium to be used.

Computer programs and client access to the Internet have added a new dimension to client education. Information on parenting and childbirth techniques is readily available at various Web sites on the Internet. When using any type of technologic tool, such as a computer, to present information, the nurse must ascertain that the client has some comfort with the entire process. Computer literacy is not necessary for the client to use the technology, but clear directions and a basic understanding of program usage are critical.

Technology has transformed health care, but many people are reluctant to reveal how frightening or incomprehensible they find a piece of machinery such as a fetal monitor. The nurse can create a teaching moment by showing the mother that her baby's heart rate varies from minute to minute and then reassuring her that this variability is desirable. Similarly, when the nurse shows the father how the monitor strip measures the contraction that he can feel when he places his hand on the mother's abdomen during labor, teaching takes place. Nurses also incorporate technology into their care on a daily basis and do not always consider how a piece of familiar equipment may appear to the individual for whom it is being used. In many cases, the nurse's teaching about the technology being used puts the client at ease and enhances care.

The movement toward the increased use of technology in the home has created additional challenges for client teaching. Families are being called upon to maintain complicated equipment—from monitors to infusion pumps to suctioning equipment—without the ready access to support found in a hospital. Nurses preparing families to use technologic equipment should establish a formal orientation program, including a skills check list. The client should also have a telephone number to call for immediate assistance in the event of any questions or concerns.

Principles and Assumptions about Teaching and Learning

Client education may be thought of as the process of helping someone learn about specific issues through planned sequences of teaching and supportive activities (Morgan, 1994). Learning implies change, or at least having the information to make a choice about whether or not to change one's thoughts or behavior. Morgan (1994) describes the educational process as a transformative journey; nurses can help clients learn the information needed to decide whether to transform a behavior, belief, or attitude. Most instructional practices are based on learning theory, which has evolved over time. Theory-based teaching helps the nurse make sense of observations, provide a way to examine observations and relationships, organize thinking, and plan actions. Theoretical dimensions of learning include learning theories, ways of knowing, and assumptions about learners.

Theories about Learning

Current learning theories include behavioral theory, Gestalt or cognitive field theory, humanistic or perceptual-existential theory, and information-processing theory. These theories are summarized in Table 2–3.

Early learning theories, probably first conceptualized by Aristotle, focused on associating similar things and remembering them. Centuries later, this idea of associating similar things led to the school of thought known as *behaviorism.* One of the early proponents of behaviorism, Edward Lee Thorndike, found through experimentation that the learner remembered positive responses, acquired behaviors that were rewarded, and rejected behaviors that were not rewarded. Behaviorists believe that learning or behavioral change results from conditioning.

Gestalt or cognitive field theory is based on the premise that the learner is ready to perceive events in a new way. The term *Gestalt* means "totality" or "the whole." This theory suggests that the whole is far more than simply the sum of its parts, so it is not possible to understand a given event or perception by reducing it into parts. This perspective incorporates both the learner and the learning context, which includes all the learner's perceptions and experiences (Babcock & Miller, 1994). Learning eventually becomes the basis for problem solving.

A third type of learning theory, *humanistic* or *perceptual-existential theory*, integrates cognitive and behavioral concepts. According to this theory, learning depends on the learner's actions, thoughts, and feelings. Behavioral change occurs when perceptions are modified. Learning necessitates total involvement by the learner—emotionally, intellectually, and physically. Learning should be self-directed; produce knowledgeable, caring learners; and be valued for its own sake (Babcock & Miller, 1994).

Information processing theory examines how information is encoded and remembered (Babcock & Miller,

TABLE 2–3 Theories of Learning

Theory	Concepts	Application to Teaching in the Clinical Setting
Behavioral	Learning—results from conditioning. Conditioning—occurs when a stimulus and the resultant response lead to a pattern of behavior. Reinforcement—giving a positive or negative reward in response to a behavior; a statement such as, "You're doing great with your breathing" is a positive reinforcement for a laboring client. Shaping—reinforcement becomes intermittent and then fades away and the desired behavior becomes established. Extinction—occurs when no reinforcement occurs; when not rewarded, a behavior gradually decreases, for example, ignoring a child's temper tantrum eventually results in an extinction of the behavior.	A woman in early pregnancy learns that nausea (the stimulus) is reduced when she eats dry crackers before getting out of bed in the morning (response). A change of behavior occurs—with this learned response, the woman now places crackers at her bedside before going to sleep. Teaching the first-time mother to breastfeed, the nurse is initially quite involved with teaching the mother techniques, positioning, hygiene, breast care; as shaping occurs, the nurse gradually withdraws as the new mother gains confidence.
Gestalt or cognitive field	Whole is greater than the sum of its parts; therefore, it is impossible to understand a given event or perception by reducing the phenomenon into parts. Incorporates both learner and the learning context (all the learners' perceptions and experiences). Learning is a process in which the learner progresses in ability from simple recall to combining and synthesizing information to form new ideas. Learning eventually becomes the basis for problem solving.	Parents who have never been in the hospital may consider a skin probe and a cardiac monitor taped to their infant a frightening experience, while the nurse caring for the infant views this technology as simple and noninvasive.
Humanistic, or perceptual existential	Learning depends on the learner's actions, thoughts, and feelings. Behavior changes when perceptions are modified. Learning necessitates total involvement by learner (emotional, intellectual, and physical). Learning should be: • Self-directed. • Produce knowledgeable, caring learners. • Valued. Learning is a transactional process in which individuals gain further understanding, new insights, or more developed cognitive structures.	Clients are allowed to choose what, how, and from whom they will learn. The nurse shares personal stories of childrearing with a new mother who is concerned that she won't be able to care for her new infant.
Information processing	Consists of short-term and long-term memory. Short-term memory—primary and working memory. Primary memory is transient because the contents are constantly displaced by incoming information. Working memory—serves as an entry to long-term memory and has capacity for only few items. Long-term memory—unlimited capacity to store information and includes all the stored information the learner retains for more than a few seconds; provides the basis for learned skills and knowledge. Subsystems of long-term memory include procedural and episodic memory. Procedural memory—stores routines that constitute skills and habits. Episodic memory—contains temporal and situational context of events. Semantic or categorical memory—meanings, facts, and rules independent of context.	In a teaching situation, a woman's episodic memory might help her remember terms like "placenta" and "fetal heart tones" from a prenatal class. Semantic memory would provide more abstract information, such as how nutrients get from the mother to the fetus.

SOURCE: Adapted from Babcock, D. & Miller, M. (1994). *Client education.* St. Louis: Mosby-Year Book.

1994). According to this theory, there are two types of memory: short-term and long-term. Long-term memory provides the basis for learned skills and knowledge.

CRITICAL THINKING QUESTION

Which of the learning theories just presented make the most sense to you? Why?

Ways of Knowing

Learning theories focus on intellectual functions and acquiring information, but several different "ways of knowing" or assimilating knowledge have also been identified. This section describes some of the most widely accepted models of how people use experience and intuition to integrate what they know.

Experiential Learning

Kolb (1984) describes learning as a process in which knowledge is constructed from experience. Colgrove, Schlapman, & Erpelding (1995) describe experiential learning as the process through which the learner transforms knowledge and meaning by reflecting on personal experience, discussing thoughts with others, and reevaluating what the learner knows and understands. The interaction of reflection, discussion, and reevaluation ultimately transforms knowledge into new meanings and ideas (Table 2–4).

TABLE 2–4 Experiential Learning

Concepts	Characteristics	Examples
Reflection	Emphasis lies on the process of learning rather than a focus on outcomes.	Group discusses breastfeeding techniques.
Discussion	Knowledge is continuously derived from experiences.	
Transformation	Learning results from resolving conflicts between concrete experiences and abstract concepts.	The nurse shares a story with client about her or his own fears of being able to parent a child.
Personal knowledge	Learning is a holistic activity.	
	Learning is a process of creating knowledge.	
	Interactions occur between the learner and the environment.	
	Knowledge is the result of perception and interpretation of the learner and is reality based.	
	Teacher and learner share an attitude toward critical thinking and learning.	
	Student and educator are knowledgeable.	
	The nurse is the facilitator and listener.	
	Nurses empower and challenge learners to develop ideas and questions.	

SOURCE: Adapted from Colgrove, S., Schlapman, N., & Erpelding, C. (1995). Experiential learning. In B. Fuszard (Ed.). *Innovative teaching strategies in nursing* (pp. 9–13). Rockville, MD: Aspen Publishers.

Women's Ways of Knowing

To uncover women's ways of knowing, Belenky and her colleagues (1986) interviewed 135 women. They found that these learners progressed through five roles: the silent knower, the received knower, the subjective knower, the procedural knower, and the constructed knower.

Silent knowers perceive words as weapons to separate and diminish people. These women view themselves as seen but never heard and consider authority figures all-powerful. New mothers may feel like silent knowers before they can identify and define their abilities.

Received knowers learn by listening and regard words as central to knowledge. They believe all knowledge originates outside the self, and they listen to and repeat information from authority figures. The received knower can teach others, but only by using the information provided by "experts." A new mother who defers all decision making to her own mother or her husband may be a received knower.

Subjective knowers have found an inner voice and become their own authority. A pervasive theme in the stories of subjective knowers is the loss of trust in male authority due to sexual harassment and abuse. Subjective knowers perceive truth and knowledge as personal, private, and intuitive. The subjective knower needs time to process new information and evaluate it against self-knowledge. This way of knowing may be exemplified by a woman, formerly in an abusive relationship, who begins to seek information about mammograms.

Procedural knowers, usually college students or graduates, have replaced intuition with reason, method, and objectivity. These women have acquired procedures for obtaining and communicating knowledge and may be fascinated by proficient technique or correct sequencing for needed skills. A college student seeking information about contraceptive options exemplifies this way of knowing.

Constructed knowers have integrated all these methods. They construct their own reality by combining known procedure with knowledge they have generated. Constructed knowers have the capacity to empathize with others regardless of their way of knowing. A woman who seeks information about both the role of hormone therapy and the use of herbs and alternative methods such as therapeutic touch in treating symptoms of menopause exemplifies a constructed knower.

Whatever the woman's developmental level of knowing, she needs confirmation of herself as knower. Whereas for men confirmation is important at the end of an educational process, for women "confirmation and community are prerequisites rather than consequences of development" (Belenky et al, 1986, p 194). These authors point out that women do best with "connected teaching" in which the expert explores the learner's needs and abilities and constructs a message that is courteous to her.

Nurses' Ways of Knowing

Carper (1978) and White (1995) identified the patterns of knowing in nursing. These include empiric knowledge, ethical knowledge, personal knowing, aesthetic knowing, and sociopolitical knowing.

Empiric knowledge (the science of nursing) refers to knowledge gained through observation of objective data. *Ethical knowledge* (the moral imperative of nursing) focuses on making ethical judgments based on values, norms, formal codes, and principles. *Personal knowing* (self-understanding) focuses on growth and realization of potential through self-knowledge. *Aesthetic knowing* (the art of nursing) enables the individual to compare new knowledge with prior personal experience, to consider the "possibilities" within a situation. This form of knowing involves intuition, a concept also addressed by Benner (1984) and Noddings and Glaser (1984). *Sociopolitical knowing* focuses on cultural identity because culture influences each person's understanding of health and all that impacts it.

TABLE 2–5 Adult Learning Theory

Concepts	Characteristics	Examples
Climate of mutual respect is most important for learning—trust, support, and caring are essential components.	Learners desire and enact a tendency toward self-direction about learning as they mature.	Readiness of learner depends on previous learning.
		Intrinsic motivation produces more pervasive and permanent learning.
Learning is pleasant and should be emphasized.	Learner's experiences are a rich source for learning.	Positive reinforcement is effective.
Andragogic approaches urge the educator to base teaching on the learner's experiences and interests.	Learners learn more effectively through experiential activities, such as problem solving.	Material should be presented in an organized fashion.
	Learners are aware of specific learning needs generated by real life.	Learning is enhanced by repetition.
	Competency-based learners are learners who wish to apply knowledge to immediate circumstances.	Meaningful tasks and materials are more fully and easily learned.
		Active participation improves retention.
		Lifelong learning is key.

SOURCE: Adapted from Hoff, P. (1995). Adult learning and the nurse. In B. Fuszard (Ed.). *Innovative teaching strategies in nursing* (pp. 3–8). Rockville, MD: Aspen Publishers.

Noddings and Glaser (1984) and Benner (1984) recognize intuition as a way of knowing. Noddings and Glaser indicate that once a person puts aside the urge to control and impose, the person can become intentionally receptive to intuition. This intuitive mode of knowing is oriented toward understanding; the analytic mode, in contrast, is goal oriented.

Benner (1984) describes the expert nurse as having intuitive knowledge about what actions to take in certain situations. This intuitive knowledge arises from years of experience. Intuitive judgment includes six aspects: pattern recognition, similarity recognition, commonsense understanding, skilled know-how, a sense of salience, and deliberative rationality (Leddy & Pepper, 1998). A sense of salience refers to recognizing particularly significant situations, and deliberative rationality involves using analytic interpretation of past experiences to interpret findings. Expert nurses who rely on an intuitive way of knowing may have difficulty describing how they know something, but will often state, "It just feels right."

I've worked in the high-risk nursery for 6 years now, and I really take pride in focusing on families and in helping them understand the purposes of the equipment we use and the procedures we do with the little ones. I want the families to feel that we are a team. Sometimes it is hard, though. I remember trying to explain to one father, a physicist, why his prematurely born son needed to be under an oxygen hood. He kept interrupting me, asking me to tell him the partial pressure of oxygen. I tried to get him to laugh by joking that he probably knew more than I did about the partial pressure of oxygen and then asked him to just let me explain. Still he interrupted. Finally I realized that his reaction was the only way he knew to control what to him was an uncontrollable situation. Once I realized this, I quit trying to explain and turned the conversation to the shock of the preterm birth and the feelings people often have. I could see that talking about his feelings was very hard for him, but finally he did, at least a little.

The nurse just quoted based much of her reaction to the father on aesthetic or intuitive knowing. In doing so she drew on internalized prior experiences. She did not rely on objective data; she sensed the problem.

Assumptions about Adult Learners

Knowles (1984) developed a theory of adult learning, which he termed *andragogy.* As part of his theory, he identified several assumptions about adult learners and how they best learn. Knowles describes five concepts within adult learning patterns: self-concept, experience, readiness to learn, orientation to learning, and motivation (Table 2–5).

Other important assumptions about adult learning and learners relate to repetition, control, active participation, feedback, and organization (Babcock & Miller, 1994). Repetition and practice, especially when applied to tasks, help the learner remember. Having some control over the method or content facilitates learning for adults. Active participation helps the adult form concepts and improves learning. Immediate, positive feedback reinforces behavior. Organization of content can promote or hamper the learning process. By considering all these assumptions about the learner, the nurse can expedite the learning process.

Teaching Guidelines and Strategies

Standards and guidelines for maternal-child nursing and client education have been developed to set forth professional consensus on essential content and responsibilities regarding care and education (Association of Women's Health, Obstetrics, and Neonatal Nurses [AWHONN], 1998; American Academy of Pediatrics [AAP] & Ameri-

RESEARCH IN PRACTICE

What is this study about? Health education is an integral part of maternal-child nursing care. During pregnancy and the postpartum period, nurses educate mothers about health behaviors that enhance positive maternal–infant outcomes, particularly as they relate to self-care and infant care. The purpose of this study was to compare mothers' and nurses' perceptions of postpartum learning needs and effective teaching modalities.

How was the study done? Nurses and mothers in a large urban hospital were asked to complete a questionnaire concerning the mothers' postpartal educational needs. The staff received the questionnaires and an explanation of the study in their employee mailboxes and the women were mailed the questionnaires postpartally. Two hundred thirty-six mothers (26% of the deliveries during the study period at this hospital) and 82 nurses (48% of the nursing personnel) returned their responses to the Davis, Brucher, and MacMullen Postpartum Questionnaire (a Likert scale questionnaire [1 to 4, from very important to not important] that asks 23 questions about infant care and 14 questions about maternal topics that could be taught in the postpartal period).

What were the results of the study? Mothers and nurses were in agreement about the importance of teaching maternal topics. Both mothers and nurses concurred that postpartal complications (eg, stitches/episiotomy/incision and medications) were very important. Help at home, shape-up exercises, and resumption of sexual activities were considered less important by both groups. Several topics were rated differently by mothers and nursing staff. Seventy-four percent of nurses considered breast care a very important learning need, whereas only 49% of the mothers agreed. Likewise, significantly more nurses than mothers reported information on mood changes as very important. The reports on mothers' personal appearance revealed an opposite trend: 19% of the mothers rated shape-up exercises as important, whereas no nurses rated this topic as important. Concerning infant care, 95% of nurses rated infant feeding as very important, whereas only 77% of the mothers rated this item as very important. However, mothers considered the topics of taking infant outside (36% mothers, 15% nurses), spoiling (23% mothers, 10% nurses), and choosing toys (19% mothers, 8% nurses) as very important. Concerning effective teaching methods, most mothers (76%) and nurses (83%) agreed that individual teaching was the most important postpartal teaching strategy. Over one-third (35%) of mothers considered handouts and books very important compared to only 10% of the nursing staff. Audiovisual presentations were rated as very effective by only 28% of mothers and 21% of the nursing staff. Even fewer considered group classes to be important (16% mothers, 13% nurses).

What additional questions might I have? 1) Are individual teaching sessions a more effective way of giving information to mothers postpartally?
2) Why do nurses continue to use audiovisual media and large classroom sessions as the dominant form of postpartal education?

How can I use this study? Nurses cannot realistically teach mothers about every topic related to maternal–infant care during the mother's postpartal stay, particularly with early discharge. It is clear from this study that immediate physical needs of both the mother and infant, as well as signs of illness and complications, need to be addressed. Perhaps less time needs to be spent on infant feeding and breast care. With cost containment as the main objective in most health care institutions, nurses will continue to be challenged to develop new approaches to postpartal education.

SOURCE: Beger, D., & Cook, C. (1998). Postpartal teaching priorities: The viewpoints of nurses and mothers. *JOGNN, 27*(2), 161–168.

can College of Obstetricians and Gynecologists [ACOG], 1997). These guidelines include standards for documentation based on the assessment of learning needs developed with client participation, suggested learning strategies, and the need for evaluation.

Client teaching has been identified as probably the most underdocumented service nurses provide. Often nurses fail to recognize the scope and depth of their teaching. Nurses frequently use an informal and conversational style when teaching the client about care issues without realizing that these teaching moments are based on their professional education and experience (Casey, 1995). Much of the nurse's teaching is incidental and given at a "teachable moment"; therefore, nurses may not document this spontaneous teaching as they would teaching given in a more formal setting (eg, Lamaze, infant care classes).

In caring for childbearing families the nurse frequently addresses the teaching needs of a pregnant woman or new mother, her partner if he is involved, other family members or loved ones, and other children. When feasible, nurses can offer teaching, especially about newborn care, parenting, and postpartum adjustment, to the woman and appropriate family members together. Such group learning tends to be effective because different people remember various aspects of the teaching and ask different questions. Thus the "collective memory" is a strong one. This approach also permits the nurse to emphasize content essential to the woman's well-being, such as the need for adequate rest, good nutrition, and help at home, which she may be hesitant to discuss with her family. However, teaching related to the woman's health history or current status should be done privately (unless the woman requests the presence of others) to permit open discussion and avoid inadvertently causing the woman embarrassment.

Assessing the Situation

When an occasion for teaching arises, the nurse needs to assess the situation, develop and present the teaching session, and examine the outcome to determine what changes, if any, need to be made. Each of these steps is important to the teaching/learning process.

Because individuals have different learning styles, they prefer to give and/or receive information in certain ways. Client educators need to assess the different ways individuals translate experience into knowledge because educators will tend to use their favorite styles, which may or may not be the learner's preferred style.

The nurse should assess several areas prior to beginning a session: the learner, oneself, and the setting. Even if the teaching session is spontaneous, the nurse will have a better outcome by assessing these three areas.

Assessing the learner's readiness to learn consists of appraising the individual's health status, belief system (including cultural background and values), developmental level, and past experiences (Whitman, Graham, Gleit, & Boyd, 1992). To evaluate the learner's health status, the nurse must consider the learner's perception of personal health, degree of physical comfort, extent of anxiety, energy level, and sensory abilities, such as hearing and vision. An uncomfortable individual may have difficulty attending to new information. The learner's belief system encompasses health values, cultural influences, and presumed degree of control over health. The learner's developmental level reflects psychosocial development, ability to comprehend both verbal and written materials, and physical and cognitive maturity. Past experiences, such as prior involvement with a health care environment or interactions with health care professionals, may influence the learner's perceived need for education.

In addition to assessing learners, nurses should also assess their personal abilities, knowledge, and values as they relate to the situation. After examining values and identifying potential strengths and limitations, the nurse-educator must co-create a plan to proceed with a teaching situation. Otherwise the nurse may either allow personal values to shade the presentation or attempt a teaching session without adequate knowledge.

The final step of assessing the situation includes examining the setting. Whether it is a client's room or a more public area, the setting should afford privacy. The individual should be able to ask questions and receive information without feeling embarrassed. The immediate environment should be comfortable and quiet, with potential distractions kept to a minimum. When planning a formal or group presentation, the nurse should ensure that everyone is able to see both the presenter and any audiovisual aids. Prior to planning a group learning session, the nurse should know what resources are available in the intended setting.

Creating the Teaching Session

After assessing the learner, self, and setting, the nurse can develop the teaching session. Elements in creating a teaching session include designing or planning the educational experience, developing the session through the selection of appropriate strategies, and evaluating the effectiveness of the session.

Co-Creating the Educational Experience

The nursing process (a problem-solving approach) and the use of adult education methods, when combined, offer an excellent format for providing client education. Together educators and learners can explore concepts and initiatives that maximize the desired learning outcomes of the clients. This approach allows the client to articulate personal feelings and expectations, and also acknowledges the client's uniqueness and individuality.

Client education takes place in a variety of settings and occurs for a wide number of reasons. The aim of a client teaching moment may be to increase the client's understanding of a specific nursing intervention or to focus on family members to involve them in the care of a new infant. Whatever the circumstances, it is imperative for the nurse to recognize that client education is a dynamic and interactive process that can be achieved through nurse-client empowerment. The enabling factor for client empowerment is the application of knowledge and skills through appropriate nursing action (Hagedorn et al, 1997).

The nurse should select client education strategies on the basis of their potential to enhance individual autonomy and thereby support future decisions concerning desired health behaviors compatible with the client's own lifestyle and perceived health priorities. The key aspect of this collaborative approach to nurse-client encounters is facilitating a dialogue conducive to an effective teaching-learning process. The nurse's actions and strategies should create a climate of exchange in which the client is an active participant rather than a passive receptacle to be filled with knowledge. Dialogue, a two-way process, places joint responsibility for the learning on the nurse and client.

Learners need stability, order, pattern, and predictability. To develop a useful teaching session, nurses need to choose, organize, and present information in a way that helps learning to occur. Useful organizational methods include proceeding from beginning to end, from familiar to unfamiliar, simple to complex, concrete to abstract, specific to general, or general to specific. The method used depends on the desired outcome, the identified subject matter, and the assessed characteristics of the learner.

In a formal or group session, the educator may wish to prepare an advanced organizer—a verbal summary, a written outline, a series of overhead transparencies, or a review of previously learned material and how it correlates to new content. For example, a review of previously learned material might consist of discussing how moss appears to be attached to a rock but can be peeled away with minimal damage to the moss. The nurse can then relate this concept to the way the placenta peels away from the uterine wall, illustrating how it is possible for the mother's and baby's blood not to mix but still allow nutrients to pass across the membrane. An advanced organizer is more abstract and general than the presentation but

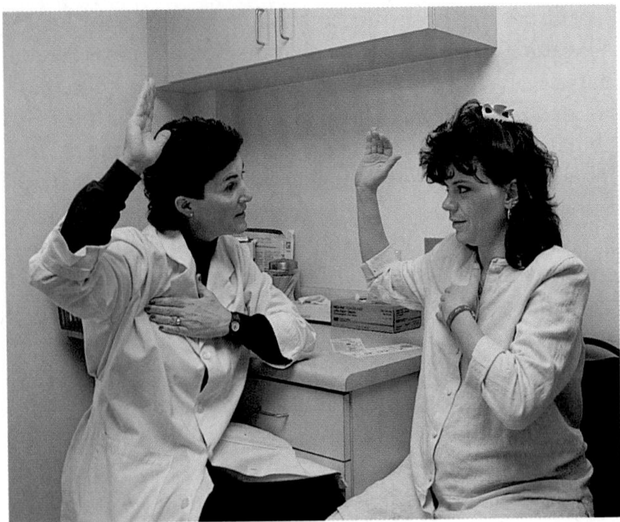

FIGURE 2–1 Teaching strategies that involve multiple forms of sensory input are most effective. In this case, the nurse explains breast self-examination and provides an opportunity for the woman to practice on herself.

inclusive enough to help the learners organize content. Advanced organizers explicate and integrate the information to be presented. Whatever the organizational method, the nurse should arrange the session to help the learner incorporate and retain new information.

Planning and Implementing the Teaching Session

The nurse develops the teaching session in accordance with the client's specific learning needs. The nurse can use a variety of tools and strategies, including activities, materials, events, or techniques, to help learners attain knowledge or skills or develop or modify attitudes. These tools and strategies are used to motivate, stimulate critical thinking and problem solving, provoke a response, or evaluate the transfer of learning. They can be interactional, such as one-to-one instruction; can be a method of conveying information, such as a videotape; or can be an approach, such as using an example to assist with learning.

Teaching strategies can be either direct or indirect. A direct strategy involves face-to-face teacher interaction. Examples include lecture, demonstration, role-playing, and discussion (Figure 2–1). Indirect strategies, such as the use of films, books, or games, provide vicarious or representative experiences, and the teacher's presence may not be required. The nurse selects the strategy based on the needs of the learner, objectives or learning outcomes, teaching content, available resources, and teacher preference (Table 2–6).

Within a teaching session, the teacher's expectations strongly affect the learner's comprehension. Regardless of the teaching strategy, the teacher should establish the environment and accomplish closure within any teaching session. The teacher can provide incentives, such as beverages or gifts, to motivate the learner to attend the session. Closure means more than just a summary of what has been said. It involves combining old and new information, determining appropriateness, formulating associations, and transferring information to new learning experiences.

In preparing print materials or a handout for teaching a specific cultural group, a nurse who is culturally competent must first have developed an awareness of personal biases, assumptions, and prejudices. The nurse should then develop an understanding of the group's subjective culture, specifically their major beliefs, attitudes, roles, and social norms as well as their core cultural values. In developing educational programs or written materials, the nurse should work with a multicultural team composed of colleagues from the culture and community members with an educational and experiential background similar to that of the target audience. They can provide valuable information and help avoid embarrassing or inadvertently insulting mistakes (Freda, 1997).

In general, the nurse should meet three basic criteria when preparing written materials for client teaching (Freda, 1997):

1. Make the material concise, emphasizing the major points without information overload.
2. Use color, graphics, cartoons, varied fonts, and other techniques to make the material interesting.
3. Keep the language simple and free of medical terminology, jargon, and abbreviations.

Evaluating the Teaching Session

After assessing the situation and planning and implementing the teaching session, the nurse should evaluate the process. Evaluation consists of both formative and summative methods.

Formative evaluation assesses the process of the teaching session. It is continuous, allows for change, and provides ongoing feedback. Formative evaluation occurs when teachers ask themselves, "How am I doing? Do they seem to be getting the information?" or checks with the participants about how they feel about the amount of information they have received.

The second type of evaluation, summative evaluation, occurs after the teaching session. It can demonstrate behavioral change based on the teaching objectives or achievement of learning goals or outcomes. Summative evaluation can be accomplished by a variety of methods, including checklists to evaluate and document learning; conversations with clients to discover what they have learned; and observation of participants to ascertain their development of psychomotor skills, alteration of health behaviors, or change in attitudes (Whitman et al, 1992). All teaching sessions, whether impromptu or formal, should entail some type of summative evaluation.

TABLE 2–6 Parental Reactions to Pregnancy

Strategy	Advantages	Limitations
Live, formal lecture with overhead transparencies or slides	Auditory and visual sensory input Same information delivered to large group of learners at one time Straightforward message delivery	Primarily one-way communication Immediate feedback and reinforcement limited or nonexistent
Discussion	Highly interactive Immediate feedback and reinforcement Flexible sequencing of information Branched organization of information	Lack of participation by some learners Message delivered to limited number of learners at one time Message not the same from one group or individual to another from time to time Primarily auditory input
Textbooks, readings	Same information conveyed to large group of learners at one time Flexible or fixed sequencing of information Highly portable Easy to repeat information	Visual input only Reading level may not be appropriate for all learners May lack immediate feedback and reinforcement
Live demonstration with return practice	Personalized role modeling Fixed or flexible sequencing of information Immediate feedback and reinforcement Active, overt, hands-on participation in learning	Not appropriate for large numbers of learners at one time Relatively expensive in terms of teaching time, equipment, and facility needs Scheduling problems
Computer assisted	Saves teaching and learning time Branched sequencing of information Immediate feedback and reinforcement Message easily repeated and manipulated Highly interactive Random access to information	Inadequate programming Scheduling problems Limited to one to three learners at a time Equipment expensive Backup needed in case of equipment failure
Videotape or 16 mm film of interview, lecture, or demonstration	Auditory, visual sensory input Fixed sequencing of information Saves teaching time Overcomes barriers of time, size, space, distance Conveys real action (motion) Message can be repeated Adaptable to group or individual	Learner dependent on equipment Rate and pace controlled by equipment Fixed sequencing of information Difficult to update and revise Equipment expensive; backup needed in case of malfunction Scheduling problems Usually lacks immediate feedback and reinforcement
Audioconferencing	Overcomes barriers of distance Flexible message delivery Highly interactive Immediate feedback and reinforcement Personalized Same information delivered to large group of learners at one time	Primarily auditory input Equipment malfunction Equipment and line time expensive Scheduling problems Message not easily repeated
2 × 2 slides	Easy to rearrange Fixed or flexible sequencing of information Adaptable to group or individual learning Multiple images can be displayed at one time Conveys realism Step-by-step disclosure of information	Still, visual input May lack immediate feedback and reinforcement Learner dependent on hardware May be lost or damaged by learners
Filmstrip	Fixed sequencing of information Step-by-step disclosure of information Adaptable to group or individual learning Message can be repeated Conveys realism	Still, visual input Difficult and expensive to revise Learner dependent on hardware Easily damaged

TABLE 2–6 Teaching Strategies: Advantages and Limitations *continued*

Strategy	Advantages	Limitations
Objects, models, mockups, simulators	Multisensory input Conveys realism Concrete, hands-on, overt participation in learning Immediate feedback and reinforcement	May oversimplify reality Damage, loss of parts Not suitable for large numbers of learners at same time
Teacher-directed clinical practicum	Real experiential learning Multisensory input Hands-on, overt participation in learning Immediate feedback and reinforcement Personalized	Limited to one-on-one or small groups of learners Facilities, scheduling problems Great amount of direct teaching time required
Games, simulations, role play	Can be highly interactive or provide for independent participation in learning Consequences of actions realized Hands-on, overt participation in learning Immediate feedback and reinforcement Flexible sequencing of information Makes learning fun, rewarding Can simulate lifelike experiences	Some learners uncomfortable participating, especially in role playing May oversimplify reality
Modular instruction, learning activity packages	Multisensory input Can accommodate individual learning styles and preferences Facilitates mastery learning Step-by-step disclosure of information Highly organized Linear or branched organization of information Active, overt response Guided practice Easy to repeat information Learner can proceed at own rate and pace Objectives and procedures stated Immediate feedback and reinforcement	Instructor's management and record-keeping time great to track successful completion of modules or activities
Print programmed instruction (as in self-paced books)	Individualized Small, step-by-step disclosure of information Linear or branched organization of information Saves teaching and learning time Active, overt participation in learning Portable Easy to repeat Learner can proceed at own rate and pace Immediate feedback and reinforcement	Visual input only Readability may be a problem May foster boredom Allows learner procrastination

SOURCE: Adapted from Van Hoozer et al. (1987). *The teaching process: Theory and practice in nursing.* Norwalk, CT: Appleton-Century-Crofts.

FOCUS YOUR STUDY

- Although health-related teaching is commonly called *patient teaching*, the term *client teaching* better reflects the notion of an equal partnership between the individual and the health care provider.
- Political factors influencing client education include the trend toward personal responsibility for health and self-care, the current educational climate of empowerment, the changing emphasis on women's health, the issue of jurisdiction over client education, and health care reform.
- Sociocultural values profoundly influence clients' responses to health teaching.
- Technologic tools, such as computers, can effectively enhance learning if the learner is comfortable with the process and not afraid of damaging the equipment.
- Behavioral learning theory is based on concepts of positive responses, reinforced behavior, and rejected behavior, which work together to produce conditioning.

- The information-processing learning theory is based on concepts regarding the ways information is remembered.
- Different "ways of knowing" or assimilating knowledge have been described by theorists. Kolb called learning a process in which knowledge is developed from experience. Belenky and colleagues addressed issues related to women's ways of knowing. Carper identified a framework based on types of knowledge used in nursing. Benner and Noddings and Glaser addressed the concept of intuition as a way of knowing, especially as it relates to the expert nurse.
- The andragogic model explores the characteristics of adult learners and the differences between them and younger learners. These differences involve self-concept, experience, readiness to learn, orientation to learning, and motivation.
- When a teaching moment arises, the nurse-educator needs to assess the situation, develop and present the teaching situation, and examine or evaluate the outcome.

REFERENCES

Ali, N. S. (1993). Preparing student nurses for patient education. *Nurse Educator, 18*(2), 27–29.

American Academy of Pediatrics (AAP) and the American College of Obstetricians and Gynecologists (ACOG). (1997). *Guidelines for perinatal care* (4th ed.). Washington, DC: Authors.

Annand, F. (1993). A challenge for the 1990s: Patient education. *Today's OR Nurse, 15*(1), 31.

Babcock, D. E., & Miller, M. A. (1994). *Client education.* St. Louis, MO: Mosby.

Barnes, L. P. (1992). The illiterate client: Strategies in patient teaching. *MCN: American Journal of Maternal Child Nursing, 17*(3), 127.

Belenky, M. F., Clinchy, B. M., Goldberger, N. R., & Tarule, J. M. (1986). *Women's ways of knowing: The development of self, voice, and mind.* New York: Basic Books.

Benner, P. (1984). *From novice to expert.* Menlo Park, CA: Addison-Wesley.

Bevis, E. O., & Watson, J. (1989). *Toward a caring curriculum: A new pedagogy for nursing.* New York: National League for Nursing.

Boyle, J. S., & Andrews, M. M. (1995). *Transcultural concepts in nursing care* (2nd ed.). Glenview, IL: Scott, Foresman/Little Brown.

Carper, B. (1978). Fundamental patterns of knowing in nursing. *Advances in Nursing Science, 1*(1), 13–23.

Casey, F. S. (1995). Documenting patient education: A literature review. *Journal of Continuing Education in Nursing, 26*(6), 257–260.

Church, O. M. (1990). Nursing's history: What it was and what it was not. In N. L. Chaska (Ed.), *The nursing profession: Turning points* (pp. 3–8). St. Louis, MO: Mosby.

Colgrove, S., Schlapman, N., & Erpelding, C. (1995). Experiential learning. In B. Fuszard (Ed.), *Innovative teaching strategies in nursing* (pp. 9–13). Rockville, MD: Aspen Publishers.

de Tornyay, R., & Thompson, M. (1987). *Strategies for teaching nursing.* New York: Wiley.

Eidelman, A. I., Hoffmann, N. W., & Kaitz, M. (1993). Cognitive deficits in women after childbirth. *Obstetrics & Gynecology, 81*(5 Pt. 1), 764–767.

Fleming, V. E. (1992). Client education: A futuristic outlook. *Journal of Advanced Nursing, 17*(2), 158–163.

Freda, M.C. (1997). Cultural competence in patient education. *Maternal-Child Nursing Journal, 22* (5), 271.

Gilligan, C. (1982). *In a different voice.* Cambridge, MA: Harvard University Press.

Hagedorn, M. I. E., Gardner, S. L., Laux, M. G., & Gardner, G. L. (1997). A model for professional nursing practice. In S. L. Gardner & M. I. E. Hagedorn (Eds.), *Legal aspects of maternal-child nursing practice* (pp. 67–94). Menlo Park, CA: Addison Wesley Longman.

Haggard, A. (1989). *Handbook of patient education.* Rockville, MD: Aspen Publishers.

Hautman, M. A. (1979). Folk health and illness beliefs. *Nurse Practitioner, 4*(4), 23, 26–27, 31.

Hoff, P. (1995). Adult learning and the nurse. In B. Fuszard (Ed.), *Innovative teaching strategies in nursing* (pp. 3–8). Rockville, MD: Aspen Publishers.

Knowles, D. (1984). *Andragogy in action: Applying modern principles of adult learning.* San Francisco: Jossey-Bass.

Kolb, D. (1984). *Experiential learning.* Englewood Cliffs, NJ: Prentice Hall.

Laschinger, H. K. (1990). Review of experimental learning theory research in the nursing profession. *Journal of Advanced Nursing, 15*(8), 985–993.

Leddy, S., & Pepper, J. M. (1998). *Conceptual bases of professional knowledge.* Philadelphia: Lippincott.

Lesgold, A., & Glaser, R. (Eds.). (1989). *Foundations for a psychology of education.* Hillsdale, NJ: Lawrence Erlbaum Associates.

Littlefield, V. (1986). *Health education for women: A guide for nurses and other health professionals.* Norwalk, CT: Appleton-Century-Crofts.

Loreno, P., & Drick, C. A. (1990). Self-care identity formation: A nursing education perspective. *Holistic Nursing Practice, 4*(2), 79–86.

Morgan, A. K. (1994). Client education experiences in professional nursing practice—a phenomenological perspective. *Journal of Advanced Nursing, 19*(4), 792–801.

Nightingale, F. (1969). *Notes on nursing: What it is and what it is not.* New York: Dover. (Original work published 1860)

Noddings, N., & Glaser, R. (1984). *Awakening the inner eye: Intuition in education.* New York: Teachers College Press.

Nurses' Association of the American College of Obstetricians and Gynecologists (1991). *Standards for the nursing care of women and newborns.* Washington, DC: Author.

Peplau, H. (1952). *Interpersonal relations in nursing.* New York: Putnam's.

Poss, R. M., Santucci, M. A., & Mull. C. (1993, February). Education literature for Hispanic patients. *Caring, 12*(2), 104–106.

Rankin, S., & Stallings, K. (1990). *Patient education* (2nd ed.). Philadelphia: Lippincott.

Redman, B. K. (1993a). Patient education at 25 years. Where we have been and where we are going. *Journal of Advanced Nursing, 18*(5), 725–730.

Redman, B. K. (1993b). *The process of patient education* (7th ed.). St. Louis, MO: Mosby Year-Book.

Redman, B., & Thomas, S. (1992). Patient teaching. In G. Bulechek & J. McCloskey (Eds.), *Nursing interventions* (pp. 304–313). Philadelphia: Saunders.

Salerno, S. (1997). *Teaching newborn care to mentally challenged parents.* Paper presented at Beth El College of Nursing, Colorado Springs, CO.

Shor, I., & Freire, P. (1987). *A pedagogy for liberation.* Granby, MA: Bergin & Garvey.

Smith, C. (1987). *Patient education: Nurses in partnership with other health professionals.* Orlando, FL: Grune & Stratton.

Spellbring, A. M. (1991). Nursing's role in health promotion. An overview. *Nursing Clinics of North America, 26*(4), 805–814.

Stanhope, M., & Lancaster, J. (1992). *Community health nursing: Process and practice for promoting health.* St. Louis, MO: Mosby-Year Book.

Van Hoozer, H. L., Bratton, B. D., Ostmoe, P. M., Weinholtz, D., Craft, M. J., Albanese, M. A., & Gjerde, C. L. (1987). *The teaching process: Theory and practice in nursing.* Norwalk, CT: Appleton-Century-Crofts.

White, J. (1995). Patterns of knowing. Review, critique, and update. *Advances in Nursing Science, 17*(4), 73–86.

Whitman, N. I., Graham, B. A., Gleit, C. J., & Boyd, M. D. (1992). *Teaching in nursing practice: A professional model* (2nd ed.). Norwalk, CT: Appleton & Lange.

Wilkins, H. (1993). Transcultural nursing: A selective review of the literature, 1985–1991. *Journal of Advanced Nursing, 18*(4), 602–612.

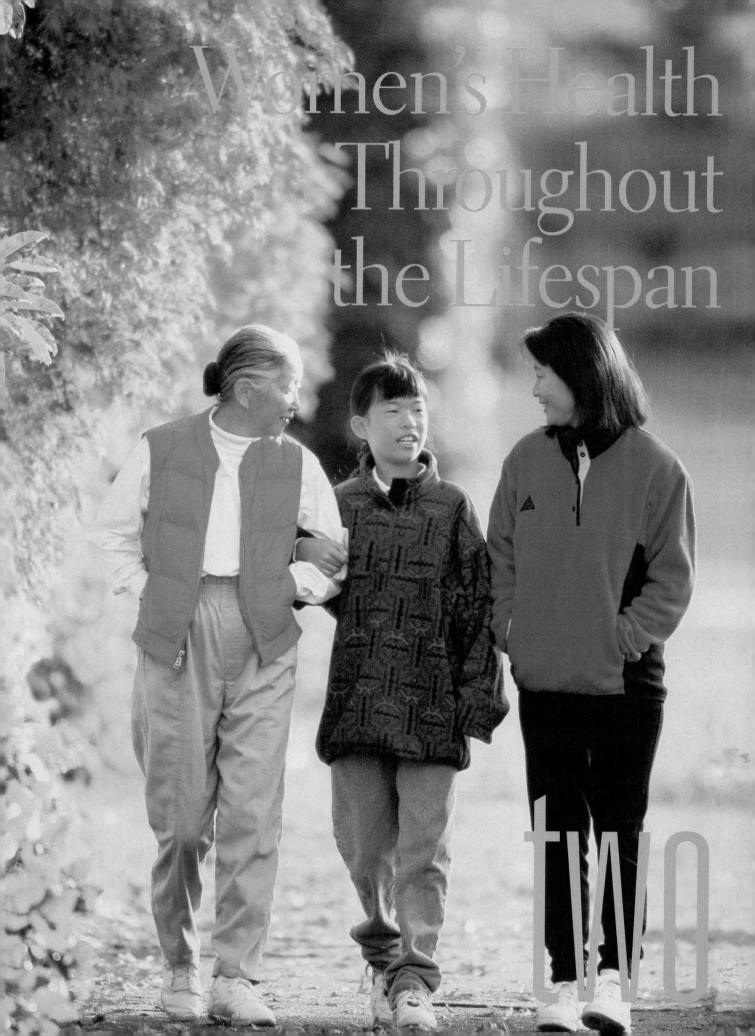
Women's Health
Throughout
the Lifespan
two

3 Women's Health Care

Key Terms

Amenorrhea
Breast self-examination (BSE)
Cervical cap
Climacteric
Coitus interruptus
Colposcopy
Condom
Depo-Provera
Diaphragm
Dysfunctional uterine bleeding
Dysmenorrhea
Dyspareunia
Endometriosis
Fertility awareness methods
Fibrocystic breast disease
Galactorrhea
Hormone replacement therapy (HRT)
Intrauterine device (IUD)
Mammogram
Menopause
Oral contraceptives
Osteoporosis
Pap smear
Pelvic inflammatory disease (PID)
Postcoital contraception
Premenstrual syndrome (PMS)
Sexually transmitted infections (STI)
Spermicides
Subdermal implants (Norplant)
Toxic shock syndrome (TSS)
Tubal ligation
Vasectomy

I WAS 15 WHEN I FELL IN LOVE WITH JOE, A 17-year-old handsome senior on our high school basketball team. My friends were so envious. We didn't plan on becoming sexually involved. It just happened. I knew I should use some method of birth control, but I didn't know where to go. I couldn't talk to my mother. She wouldn't understand. Joe tried condoms, but he didn't like the way they felt. Several months went by and nothing happened, so I ignored the thought of getting pregnant. Then one month my period was late. I was SCARED. My best friend took me to see her nurse practitioner. My pregnancy test was negative. The routine test they took for gonorrhea was positive. Joe refused to believe I got it from him and said we were through. I felt dirty, betrayed, confused, and lonely. My nurse practitioner encouraged me to talk. She taught me about my body and how to protect myself. She helped me build my self-esteem. I realize now that I'm not ready to be in a sexual relationship.

Objectives

- Summarize information that women may need in order to implement appropriate self-care measures for dealing with menstruation.
- Compare the advantages, disadvantages, and effectiveness of the various methods of contraception.
- Delineate basic gynecologic screening procedures indicated for well women.
- Discuss the physical and psychologic aspects of menopause.
- Contrast the common benign and malignant breast disorders.
- Discuss the signs and symptoms, medical therapy, and implications for fertility of endometriosis.
- Discuss abnormal uterine bleeding and abdominal masses.
- Compare vulvovaginal candidiasis and bacterial vaginosis.
- Describe the common sexually transmitted infections (STIs).
- Summarize the health teaching that a nurse needs to provide to a woman with an STI.
- Relate the implications of pelvic inflammatory disease (PID) for future fertility to its pathologic origin, signs and symptoms, and treatment.
- Identify the implications of an abnormal finding during a pelvic examination.
- Contrast cystitis and pyelonephritis.

A WOMAN'S HEALTH CARE NEEDS change throughout her lifetime. As a young girl she requires health teaching about menstruation, sexuality, and personal responsibility. As a teen she needs information about reproductive choices and safe sexual activity. During this time she should also be introduced to the importance of health care practices, such as breast self-examination and regular Pap smears. The mature woman may need to be reminded of these self-care issues and prepared for physical changes that accompany childbirth and aging. By educating women about their bodies, their health care choices, and their right to be knowledgeable consumers, nurses can help women assume responsibility for the health care they receive.

The contemporary woman is likely to encounter various major or minor gynecologic or urinary problems during her lifetime. These problems may provoke a variety of psychologic responses and physical concerns. The nurse can assist a woman in this situation by providing accurate, sensitive, and supportive health education and counseling. To meet the woman's needs, the nurse must have up-to-date information about health care practices and available diagnostic and treatment options.

This chapter provides information about selected aspects of women's health care, with an emphasis on conditions typically addressed in community-based settings. Chapter 4 addresses some of the major social issues women face, while Chapter 5 focuses on violence against women. For more detailed information on any of these subjects or for discussion of gynecologic conditions requiring surgery or extensive therapy, consult more specialized texts.

Community-Based Nursing Care

Women's health refers to a holistic view of women and their health-related needs within the context of their everyday lives. It is based on the awareness that a woman's physical, mental, and social status are interdependent and determine her state of health or illness. The woman's view of her situation, her assessment of her needs, her values, and her beliefs are valid and important factors to be incorporated into any health care intervention. Her views frequently influence the health care of her entire family because women usually coordinate the family's health care needs.

Nurses can work with women to provide health teaching and information about self-care practices in schools, during routine examinations in a clinic or office, at senior centers, at meetings of volunteer organizations, through classes offered by the local health department or community college, or in the home. This community-based focus is the key to providing effective nursing care to women of all ages.

In reality, the vast majority of women's health care is provided outside of acute care settings. Nurses oriented to community-based care are especially effective in recognizing the autonomy of each individual and in dealing with clients holistically. This approach is important in addressing not only physical problems but also major health issues such as violence against women, which may go undetected unless care providers are alert for signs of it.

The Nurse's Role in Addressing Issues of Sexuality

On occasion, most people experience concern and even anxiety about some aspect of sexuality. Societal standards and pressures can cause people to evaluate and compare with others their sexual attractiveness, technical abilities, frequency of sexual interaction, and so on. Appearance and sexual behavior are not the only causes for concern; the reproductive implications of sexual intercourse must also be considered. Some people desire conception; others wish to avoid it. Health factors are another consideration. The increase in the incidence of sexually transmitted infections, especially HIV/AIDS and herpes, has caused many people to modify their sexual practices and activities.

Because sexuality and its reproductive implications are such an intrinsic and emotion-laden part of life, people have many concerns, problems, and questions about sex roles; heterosexual, homosexual, or bisexual orientation; behaviors; education; inhibitions; morality; and related areas such as family planning. Women frequently voice these concerns to the nurse in a clinic or ambulatory setting. Thus the nurse may need to assume the role of counselor on sexual and reproductive matters.

Nurses who assume this role must be secure about their own sexuality. They must also develop an awareness of their own feelings, values, and attitudes about sexuality so that they can be more sensitive and objective when they encounter the values and beliefs of others. Nurses should have accurate, up-to-date information about topics related to sexuality, sexual practices, and common gynecologic problems. They also need to know about the structures and functions of female and male reproductive systems. In some cases women are accompanied by their partners, male or female, so nurses need to be sensitive to the dynamics of the relationship between the partners.

Continuing education for the practicing nurse and appropriate courses in undergraduate and graduate nursing education programs can help nurses achieve this sense of security and the requisite knowledge about aspects of sexuality. These courses can teach nurses about sexual values, attitudes, alternative lifestyles, cultural factors, and misconceptions and myths about sex and reproduction.

Taking a Sexual History

Nurses today are often responsible for taking a woman's initial history, including her gynecologic and sexual history. To be effective in this role, the nurse must have good communication skills and should conduct the interview in a quiet, private place free of distractions. The sexual history is one part of a lengthier health history and covers personal and intimate topics. Nurses should start their interview with less intimate areas, such as medical and surgical history, and proceed to the sexual history toward the end of the history-taking session. This approach helps the woman develop a comfort level with the nurse before disclosing personal information.

Opening the sexual history discussion with a brief explanation of the purpose of such questions is often helpful. For example, the nurse might say, "As your nurse I'm interested in all aspects of your well-being. Often women have concerns or questions about sexual matters, especially when they are pregnant (or starting to be sexually active). I will be asking you some questions about your sexual history as part of your general health history."

It may be helpful to use direct eye contact as much as possible unless the nurse knows it is culturally unacceptable to the woman. The nurse should do little, if any, writing during the interview, especially if the woman seems ill at ease or is discussing very personal issues. Open-ended questions are often useful in eliciting information. For example, "What, if anything, would you change about your sex life?" will elicit more information than "Are you happy with your sex life now?" The nurse should also clarify terminology and proceed from easier topics to those that are more difficult to discuss. Throughout the interview, the nurse should be alert to the client's body language and nonverbal cues. It is essential that the nurse listen, react in a nonjudgmental manner, and use teachable moments to educate women about their bodies. It is also important that the nurse not assume the client is heterosexual. Some clients are open about discussing a lesbian relationship. Others are more reserved until they develop rapport and a sense of trust in the caregiver.

After completing the sexual history, the nurse assesses the information obtained. If there is a problem that requires further medical tests and assessments, the nurse will refer the woman to a nurse practitioner, certified nurse-midwife, physician, or counselor as necessary. In many instances the nurse alone will be able to develop a nursing diagnosis and then plan and implement an appropriate intervention. For example, if the nurse determines that a woman who is interested in conceiving a child does not have a clear understanding of when she ovulates, the nurse may formulate the nursing diagnosis ***Knowledge Deficit*** related to lack of information about the timing of ovulation. The nurse can then evaluate the woman's knowledge through discussion and review and work with the woman to provide necessary knowledge. The nurse might also suggest that the woman keep a menstrual calendar and monitor basal body temperatures to identify the time of ovulation.

The nurse must be realistic in making assessments and planning interventions. It requires insight and skill to recognize when a woman's problem requires interventions that are beyond a nurse's preparation and ability. In such cases, the nurse must make appropriate referrals.

Menstruation

Girls today begin to learn about puberty and menstruation at a surprisingly young age. Unfortunately, the source of their "education" is sometimes their peers and sometimes the media; thus, the information is frequently incomplete, inaccurate, and sensationalized. Nurses who work with young girls and adolescents recognize this and are working hard to provide accurate health teaching and to correct misinformation about menarche (the onset of menses) and the menstrual cycle.

Cultural, religious, and personal attitudes about menstruation are part of the menstrual experience and often reflect negative attitudes toward women. In the past, many myths surrounded menstruation. Women were often isolated or restricted to the company of other women during their monthly flow because they were considered "unclean." Currently there are fewer customs associated with menstruation, although many women hide the fact of menstruation entirely. Sexual intercourse during menstruation is a common practice and is not generally contraindicated. For most couples, the decision is one of personal preference. However, women at high risk for sexually transmitted infections may increase their risk even more if they have intercourse during their periods because the cervix is slightly dilated, permitting easier access of organisms, which may be propelled in the menstrual blood toward the fallopian tubes. (The physiology of menstruation is discussed in Chapter 6.)

Counseling the Premenstrual Girl about Menarche

The average age of menarche is about 12 years for girls in the United States, although many begin their periods at an earlier age. For about 2 years before menarche, a girl experiences a series of physical changes as her body develops. Many girls find it embarrassing or stressful to discuss these changes and the menstrual experience, both because of the many taboos associated with the subject and because of their immaturity. However, the most critical factor in successful adaptation to menarche is the preteen's or adolescent's level of preparedness. Information should be given to premenstrual girls over time, rather than all at once. This allows them to absorb information and develop questions. The following basic information is helpful for young clients:

- *Cycle length.* Cycle length is determined from the first day of one menses to the first day of the next menses. Initially a female's cycle length is about 29 days, but the normal length may vary from 21 to 35 days. As a woman matures, cycle length often shortens to a median of 25+ days just before menopause. Cycle length often varies by a day or two from one cycle to the next, although greater normal variations may also occur.
- *Amount of flow.* The average flow is approximately 30 mL per period. Usually women characterize the amount of flow in terms of the number of pads or tampons used. Flow often is heavier at first and lighter toward the end of the period.
- *Length of menses.* Menses usually lasts from 2 to 8 days, although the length may vary.

The nurse should make it clear that variations in age at menarche, length of cycle, and duration of menses are normal because girls are likely to be concerned if their experience varies from that of their peers. It also is helpful to acknowledge the negative aspects of menstruation (messiness and embarrassment) while stressing its positive role as a symbol of maturity and womanhood.

Educational Topics

The nurse's primary role is to provide accurate information and assist in clarifying misconceptions, so that girls will develop positive self-images and progress smoothly through this phase of maturation.

CRITICAL THINKING QUESTION

How have you been influenced by attitudes and customs about menstruation?

Pads and Tampons

Since early times women have made pads and tampons from cloth or rags, which required washing but were reusable. Some women made them from gauze or cotton balls. Commercial tampons were introduced in the 1930s.

Today adhesive-stripped minipads and maxipads and flushable tampons have made life easier. However, the deodorants and increased absorbency that manufacturers have added to both sanitary napkins and tampons may prove harmful. The chemical used to deodorize can create a rash on the vulva and damage the tender mucous lining of the vagina. Excessive or inappropriate use of tampons can produce dryness or even small sores or ulcers in the vagina.

When taking a menstrual history, the nurse should attempt to determine the amount of bleeding each month. The woman can be asked what type of pad or tampon she uses, how frequently she changes, and how much blood has been absorbed. Women should be advised to change pads frequently, regardless of the amount of blood that is absorbed. If a woman reports she saturates a maxipad every 1 to 2 hours for a couple of days, she may be experiencing a gynecologic problem and subsequent anemia.

CRITICAL THINKING IN PRACTICE

Rita Cooper is a 16-year-old, vivacious teenager who comes to the clinic because of irregular menses. She is captain of the cheerleading squad at the local high school and believes that her periods are "really messed up" and interfering with her cheering activities. She wants to get her periods regulated and asks for birth control pills.

As you take Rita's menstrual history, you find that her menarche was at age 12 and that her periods occur every 24–34 days. She usually has cramps, and the flow, which she describes as heavy, lasts 4–5 days. She uses an average of five tampons per day. What should you advise Rita about her menstrual cycle?

Answers can be found in Appendix I.

Because the use of superabsorbent tampons has been linked to the development of toxic shock syndrome (TSS) (page 64), women should avoid using them. They should use regular-absorbency tampons only for heavy menstrual flow (during the first 2 or 3 days of the period), not during the whole period, and change them every 3 to 6 hours. Because *Staphylococcus aureus*, the causative organism of TSS, is frequently found on the hands, a woman should wash her hands before inserting a fresh tampon and should avoiding touching the tip of the tampon when unwrapping it or before insertion.

In the absence of a heavy menstrual flow, tampons absorb moisture, leaving the vaginal walls dry and subject to injury. The absorbency of regular tampons varies. If the tampon is hard to pull out or shreds when removed, or if the vagina becomes dry, the tampon is probably too absorbent. If a woman is worried about accidental spotting, she can check the diagrams on the packages of regular tampons. Those that expand in width are better able to prevent leakage without being too absorbent.

A woman may want to use tampons only during the day and switch to pads at night to avoid vaginal irritation. She should avoid using tampons on the last spotty days of the period and should never use them for midcycle spotting or leukorrhea. If a woman experiences vaginal irritation, itching, or soreness or notices an unusual odor while using tampons, she should stop using them or change brands or absorbencies.

The choice of sanitary protection must meet the individual's needs and feel comfortable, whether it be pads or tampons.

Vaginal Sprays and Douching

Vaginal sprays are unnecessary and can cause infections, itching, burning, vaginal discharge, rashes, and other problems. They are *not* recommended by health care providers. If a woman chooses to use a spray, she needs to know that these sprays are for external use only and should never be applied to irritated or itching skin or used with sanitary napkins.

Although douching is sometimes used to treat vaginal infections, douching as a hygiene practice is unnecessary because the vagina cleanses itself, and caregivers advise against it. Douching washes away the natural mucus and upsets the vaginal ecology, which can make the vagina more susceptible to infection. Douching with one of the perfumed or flavored douches can cause allergic reactions, and too frequent use of an undiluted or strong douche solution can induce severe irritation, even tissue damage. Propelling water up the vagina may also erode the antibacterial cervical plug and force bacteria and germs from the vagina into the uterus. It is essential that women avoid douching during menstruation because the cervix is dilated to permit the downward flow of menstrual fluids from the uterine lining. Douching may force tissue back up into the uterine cavity, which could contribute to endometriosis. Douching is also contraindicated during pregnancy.

Cleansing the Perineum

The mucous secretions that continually bathe the vagina are completely odor free while they are in the vagina; only when they mingle with perspiration and become exposed to the air does odor develop. Keeping one's skin clean and free of bacteria with plain soap and water is the most effective method of controlling odor. A soapy finger or soft washcloth should be used to wash gently between the labial folds. Bathing is as important (if not more so) during menses as at any other time. A long leisurely soak in a warm tub will promote menstrual blood flow and relieve cramps by relaxing the muscles.

Keeping the vulva fresh throughout the day means keeping it dry and clean. A woman can assure herself of adequate ventilation by wearing cotton panties and clothes loose enough to allow air to circulate. After using the toilet, a woman should always wipe herself from front to back and, if necessary, follow up with a moistened paper towel or toilet paper.

The most important thing to remember is that if an unusual odor persists despite these efforts, a visit to one's health care provider may be indicated. Certain conditions, such as vaginitis, produce a foul-smelling discharge.

Associated Menstrual Conditions

A variety of menstrual irregularities has been identified. An abnormally short duration of menstrual flow is termed *hypomenorrhea;* an abnormally long one is called *hypermenorrhea.* Excessive, profuse flow is called *menorrhagia,* and bleeding between periods is known as *metrorrhagia.* Infrequent and too frequent menses are termed *oligomenorrhea* and *polymenorrhea,* respectively. An *anovulatory cycle* is one in which ovulation does not occur. Such irregularities should be investigated to rule out any disease process.

Amenorrhea

Amenorrhea, the absence of menses, is classified as primary or secondary. Primary amenorrhea is said to occur if menstruation has not been established by 18 years of age. Secondary amenorrhea is said to occur when an established menses (of longer than 3 months) ceases.

Primary amenorrhea necessitates a thorough assessment of the young woman to determine its cause. Possible causes include congenital obstructions, congenital absence of the uterus, testicular feminization (external genitals appear female, but the uterus and ovaries are absent and testes are present), or absence or imbalance of hormones. Success of treatment depends on the causative factors. Many causes are not correctable.

Secondary amenorrhea is caused most frequently by pregnancy. Additional causes include lactation, hormonal imbalances, poor nutrition (anorexia nervosa, obesity, fad dieting), ovarian lesions, strenuous exercise (associated with anorexia nervosa; also with long-distance runners, dancers, and other athletes with low body fat ratios), debilitating systemic diseases, stress of high intensity or long duration, stressful life events, a change in season or climate, use of oral contraceptives, the phenothiazine and chlorpromazine group of tranquilizers, and disorders such as Cushing's syndrome and Sheehan's syndrome. Treatment is dictated by the causative factors. The nurse can explain that once the underlying condition has been corrected—for example, when the client gains sufficient body weight—menses will resume. Female athletes and women who participate in strenuous exercise routines may be advised to increase their caloric intake or reduce their exercise levels for a month or two to see whether a normal cycle resumes. If it does not, medical referral is indicated.

Dysmenorrhea

Dysmenorrhea, or painful menstruation, occurs at, or a day before, the onset of menstruation and disappears by the end of menses. Dysmenorrhea is classified as primary or secondary. Primary dysmenorrhea is defined as cramps without underlying disease. Prostaglandins F_2 and F_{2a}, which are produced by the uterus in higher concentrations during menses, are the primary cause. They increase uterine contractility and decrease uterine artery blood flow, causing ischemia. The end result is the painful sensation of cramps. Dysmenorrhea typically disappears after a first pregnancy and does not occur if cycles are anovulatory. Treatment of primary dysmenorrhea includes oral contraceptives (which block ovulation), prostaglandin inhibitors (such as ibuprofen, aspirin, naproxen), and self-care measures such as regular exercise, rest, heat, and good nutrition. Biofeedback has also been used with some success.

Secondary dysmenorrhea is associated with pathology of the reproductive tract and usually appears after menstruation has been established. Conditions that most frequently cause secondary dysmenorrhea include endometriosis; residual pelvic inflammatory disease (PID); anatomic anomalies, such as cervical stenosis, imperforate hymen, uterine displacement; ovarian cysts; or the presence of an IUD. Because primary and secondary dysmenorrhea may coexist, accurate differential diagnosis is essential for appropriate treatment.

Some nutritionists suggest that vitamins B and E help relieve the discomforts associated with menstruation. Vitamin B_6 may help relieve the premenstrual bloating and irritability some women experience. Vitamin E, a mild prostaglandin inhibitor, may help decrease menstrual discomfort. Avoiding salt can decrease discomfort from fluid retention.

Heat is soothing and promotes increased blood flow. Any source of warmth, from sipping herbal tea to soaking in a hot tub or using a heating pad, may be helpful during painful periods. Massage can also soothe aching back muscles and promote relaxation and blood flow.

Daily exercise can ease existing menstrual discomfort and help prevent cramps and other menstrual complaints. Aerobic exercise—jogging, cycling, aerobic dancing, swimming, and fast-paced walking—is especially helpful. Persistent discomfort should be medically evaluated.

Premenstrual Syndrome

Premenstrual syndrome (PMS) refers to a symptom complex associated with the luteal phase of the menstrual cycle (2 weeks prior to onset of menses). Women over 30 years of age are the most likely to have PMS. The symptoms must, by definition, occur between ovulation and the onset of menses. They repeat at the same stage of each menstrual cycle and include some or all of the following:

- Psychologic: irritability, lethargy, depression, low morale, anxiety, sleep disorders, crying spells, and hostility
- Neurologic: classic migraine, vertigo, syncope
- Respiratory: rhinitis, hoarseness, occasionally asthma
- Gastrointestinal: nausea, vomiting, constipation, abdominal bloating, craving for sweets
- Urinary: retention and oliguria
- Dermatologic: acne
- Mammary: swelling and tenderness

Most women experience only some of these symptoms. The symptoms usually are most pronounced 2 or 3 days before the onset of menstruation and subside as menstrual flow begins, with or without treatment. The exact cause of PMS is unknown, although a variety of theories have been put forth to explain it. These include, for example, hormone imbalance, nutritional deficiency, prostaglandin excess, and endorphin deficiency. Diagnosis is generally made after having the woman keep a menstrual calendar for 2 months on which she carefully records daily symptoms.

NURSING CARE MANAGEMENT

The nurse can help the woman identify specific symptoms and develop healthy behavior. After assessment, the nurse may advise the woman to restrict her intake of foods containing methylxanthines, such as chocolate, cola, and coffee; restrict her intake of alcohol, nicotine, red meat, and foods containing salt and sugar; increase her intake of complex carbohydrates and protein; and increase the frequency of meals. Supplementation with B complex vitamins, especially B_6, may decrease anxiety and depression. When depression is a major symptom, the caregiver may prescribe antidepressants. Vitamin E supplements may help reduce breast tenderness, and a program of aerobic exercises such as fast walking, jogging, or aerobic dancing is generally beneficial. In addition to vitamin supplements, pharmacologic treatments for PMS include progesterone suppositories, diuretics, and prostaglandin inhibitors. All have been effective in some women and not in others. For women who are not planning a pregnancy, low-dose oral contraceptives, which suppress ovulation, are often an effective solution. An empathic relationship with a health care professional to whom the woman feels free to voice concerns is highly beneficial. The nurse can also encourage the woman to keep a journal to help identify life events associated with PMS. Self-care groups and self-help literature both help women gain control over their bodies. ●

Contraception.

The decision to use a method of contraception may be made individually by a woman (or, in the case of vasectomy, by a man) or jointly by a couple. The decision may be motivated by a desire to avoid pregnancy, to gain control over the number of children conceived, or to determine the spacing of future children. In choosing a specific method, consistency of use outweighs the absolute reliability of the given method.

Decisions about contraception should be made voluntarily, with full knowledge of advantages, disadvantages, effectiveness, side effects, contraindications, and long-term effects. Many outside factors influence this choice, including cultural practices, religious beliefs, personality, cost, effectiveness, misinformation, practicality of method, and self-esteem. Different methods of contraception may be appropriate at different times in a couple's life (Table 3–1).

Fertility Awareness Methods

Fertility awareness methods, also known as *natural family planning,* are based on an understanding of the changes that occur throughout a woman's ovulatory cycle. All these methods require periods of abstinence and recording of certain events throughout the cycle; cooperation of the partners is important.

TABLE 3–1 Factors to Consider in Choosing a Method of Contraception

Effectiveness of method in preventing pregnancy	Personal preferences, biases
Safety of the method:	Lifestyle:
Are there inherent risks?	How frequently does client have intercourse?
Does it offer protection against STIs or other conditions?	Does she have multiple partners?
Client's age and future childbearing plans	Does she have ready access to medical care in the event of complications?
Any contraindications in client's health history	Is cost a factor?
Religious or moral factors influencing choice	Partner's support and willingness to cooperate
	Personal motivation to use method

On the one hand, fertility awareness methods are free, safe, and acceptable to many whose religious beliefs prohibit other methods; they provide an increased awareness of the body; they involve no artificial substances or devices; they encourage a couple to communicate about sexual activity and family planning; and they are useful in helping a couple plan a pregnancy.

On the other hand, these methods require extensive initial counseling to be used effectively; they may interfere with sexual spontaneity; they require the couple to maintain records for several cycles before beginning to use them; they may be difficult or impossible for women with irregular cycles to use; and, although theoretically they should be very reliable, in practice they may not be as reliable in preventing pregnancy as other methods.

The *basal body temperature (BBT)* method to detect ovulation requires that a woman take her BBT every morning upon awakening (before any activity) and record the readings on a temperature graph. To do this, she uses a basal body temperature thermometer, which shows tenths of a degree rather than the two-tenths shown on standard thermometers. After 3 to 4 months of recording temperatures, a woman with regular cycles should be able to predict when ovulation will occur. The method is based on the fact that the temperature sometimes drops just before ovulation and almost always rises and remains elevated for several days after. The temperature rise occurs in response to the increased progesterone levels that occur in the second half of the cycle. Figure 3–1 shows a sample BBT chart. To avoid conception, the couple abstains from intercourse on the day of the temperature rise and for 3 days after. Because the temperature rise does not occur until after ovulation, a woman who had intercourse just before the rise is at risk of pregnancy. To decrease this risk, some couples abstain from intercourse for several days before the *anticipated* time of ovulation and then for 3 days after.

The *calendar*, or *rhythm*, *method* is based on the assumptions that ovulation tends to occur 14 days (plus or minus 2 days) before the start of the next menstrual period, that sperm are viable for up to 5 days, and that the ovum is viable for about 24 hours (Hatcher et al, 1998). To use this method, the woman must record her menstrual cycles for 6 to 8 months to identify the shortest and longest cycles. The first day of menstruation is the first day of the cycle. The fertile phase is calculated from 18 days before the end of the shortest recorded cycle through 11 days from the end of the longest recorded cycle (Hatcher et al, 1998). For example, if a woman's cycle lasts from 24 to 28 days, the fertile phase would be calculated as day 6 through day 17. Once this information is obtained, the woman can identify the fertile and infertile phases of her cycle. For effective use of this method, she must abstain from intercourse during the fertile phase. The calendar method is the least reliable of the fertility awareness methods and has largely been replaced by other, more scientific approaches.

The *cervical mucus method*, sometimes called the *ovulation method* or the *Billings method*, involves the assessment of cervical mucus changes that occur during the menstrual cycle. The amount and character of cervical mucus change because of the influence of estrogen and progesterone. At the time of ovulation, the mucus (estrogen-dominant mucus) is clearer, more stretchable (a quality called spinnbarkheit), and more permeable to sperm. It also shows a characteristic fern pattern when placed on a glass slide and allowed to dry.

During the luteal phase, cervical mucus is thick and sticky (progesterone-dominant mucus) and forms a network that traps sperm, making their passage difficult.

To use the cervical mucus method, the woman abstains from intercourse for the first menstrual cycle. She assesses her cervical mucus daily for amount, feeling of slipperiness or wetness, color, clearness, and spinnbarkheit, as the woman becomes familiar with varying characteristics.

The peak day of wetness and clear, stretchable mucus is assumed to be the time of ovulation. To use this method correctly, a woman is advised to abstain from intercourse from the time she first notices that the mucus is becoming clear, more elastic, and slippery until 4 days after the last wet mucus (ovulation) day. Because this method evaluates the effects of hormonal changes, it can be used by women with irregular cycles.

The *symptothermal method* consists of various assessments made and recorded by the couple. These include information regarding cycle days, coitus, cervical mucus changes, and secondary signs such as increased libido, abdominal bloating, mittelschmerz (midcycle abdominal pain), and basal body temperature. Through the various assessments, the couple learns to recognize signs that indicate ovulation. This combined approach tends to improve the effectiveness of fertility awareness as a method of birth control (Berek, Adashi, & Hillard, 1996).

Situational Contraceptives

Abstinence can be considered a method of contraception and, partly because of changing values and the increased risk of infection with intercourse, it is gaining increased

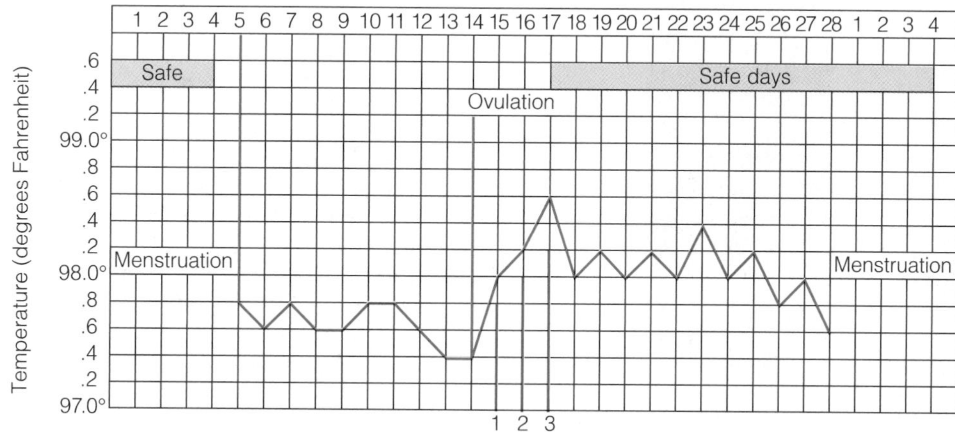

FIGURE 3–1 Sample basal body temperature chart. SOURCE: Crooks R., & Baur K. (1993). *Our sexuality* (5th ed.). Monterey, CA: Brooks/Cole.

acceptance among people of all ages, but especially among adolescents and young adults. In fact, more and more young people are embracing abstinence and making a commitment to delay sexual intercourse until marriage. Some have even signed pledges to that effect.

Coitus interruptus, or withdrawal, is one of the oldest and least reliable methods of contraception. This method requires that the male withdraw from the female's vagina when he feels that ejaculation is impending. He then ejaculates away from the external genitalia of the woman. Failure tends to occur for two reasons:

- This method demands great self-control on the part of the man, who must withdraw just as he feels the urge for deeper penetration with impending orgasm.
- Some preejaculatory fluid, which can contain sperm, may escape from the penis during the excitement phase prior to ejaculation. Because the quantity of sperm in this preejaculatory fluid is increased after a recent ejaculation, this is especially significant for couples who engage in repeated episodes of orgasm within a short period of time.

Couples who use this method should be aware of postcoital contraceptive options should the man fail to withdraw in time.

Douching after intercourse is an ineffective method of contraception and is not recommended. It may actually facilitate conception by pushing sperm farther up the birth canal.

Spermicides

Spermicides, available as creams, jellies, foams, vaginal film, and suppositories, are inserted into the vagina before intercourse. They destroy sperm or neutralize vaginal secretions and thereby immobilize sperm. Spermicides that effervesce in a moist environment offer more rapid protection, and coitus may take place immediately after they are inserted. Suppositories may require up to 30 minutes to dissolve and will not offer protection until they do so. The nurse instructs the woman to insert these spermicide preparations high in the vagina and maintain a supine position.

Spermicides are minimally effective when used alone, but their effectiveness increases in conjunction with a diaphragm, cervical cap, or condom. They provide modest protection from gonorrhea and chlamydia (Hatcher et al, 1998).

The major advantages of spermicides are their wide availability and low toxicity. Although some studies have suggested that the use of spermicides at the time of conception or early in pregnancy may be associated with an increased risk of congenital anomalies, recent studies show no increased incidence (Hatcher et al, 1998).

Mechanical Contraceptives

Mechanical contraceptive methods either prevent the transport of sperm to the ovum or prevent implantation of the ovum/zygote.

The male **condom** offers a viable means of contraception when used consistently and properly (Figure 3–2). Acceptance has been increasing as a growing number of men are assuming responsibility for regulation of fertility. The condom is applied to the erect penis, rolled from the tip to the end of the shaft, before vulvar or vaginal contact. Most condoms have a reservoir tip to allow for collection of ejaculate. When using a condom without a reservoir end, a small space must be left at the end to

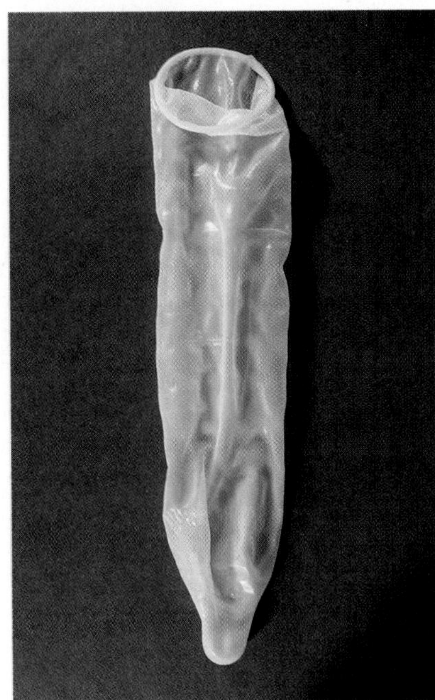

A

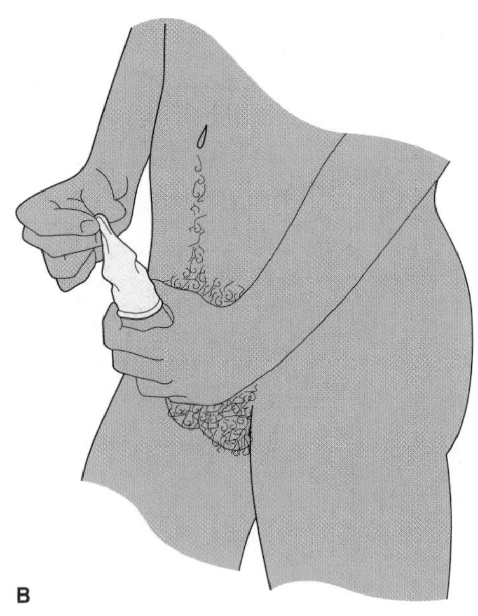

B

FIGURE 3–2 ***A,*** An unrolled condom with reservoir tip. ***B,*** Correct use.

collect the ejaculate, so that the condom will not break at the time of ejaculation. If the condom or vagina is dry, water-soluble lubricants, such as K-Y Jelly, should be used to prevent irritation and possible condom breakage.

Care must be taken in removing the condom after intercourse. For optimal effectiveness, the man should withdraw his penis from the vagina while it is still erect and hold the condom rim to prevent spillage. If after ejaculation the penis becomes flaccid while still in the vagina, the male should hold onto the edge of the condom while withdrawing to avoid spilling the semen and to prevent the condom from slipping off.

The effectiveness of male condoms is largely determined by their use. The condom is small, lightweight, disposable, and inexpensive; it has no side effects, requires no medical examination or supervision, and offers visual evidence of effectiveness. Most condoms are made of latex. Polyurethane and silicone rubber condoms are also manufactured and recommended for individuals allergic to latex. Condoms are available with ribbed or smooth sides, tapered or straight-sided, lubricated or unlubricated, with or without spermicide. "Natural skins" (lambs' intestines) are still available but declining in popularity. All condoms except natural skin condoms offer protection against both pregnancy and sexually transmitted infections (STIs). It has not yet been determined whether condoms lubricated with spermicide are more effective than other lubricated condoms in preventing the transmission of HIV and other STIs (Centers for Disease Control and Prevention [CDC], 1998). However, concurrent use of a vaginal spermicide does increase the overall effectiveness of skin condoms.

The male condom is becoming increasingly popular because of the protection it offers from infections. Significantly, researchers speculate that the recent decrease in the teenage pregnancy rate may be due in part to the increased use of condoms to avoid STIs and HIV infection (Speroff, 1998). For women, sexually transmitted infection increases the risk of pelvic inflammatory disease (PID) and resultant infertility. Many women are beginning to insist that their sexual partners use condoms, and many women carry condoms with them.

Misplacement, perineal or vaginal irritation, and dulled sensation are possible disadvantages of condoms.

The *Reality female condom* (Figure 3–3) is a thin polyurethane sheath with a flexible ring at each end. The inner ring, at the closed end of the condom, serves as the means of insertion and fits over the cervix like a diaphragm. The second ring remains outside the vagina and covers a portion of the woman's perineum. It also covers the base of the man's penis during intercourse. Available over the counter and designed for one-time use, the condom may be inserted up to 8 hours before intercourse. The inner sheath is prelubricated but does not contain spermicide and is not designed to be used with a male condom. Data on its effectiveness against pregnancy are still limited, although the female condom has been compared favorably to other barrier methods. Because it also covers a portion of the vulva it probably provides better protection against some pathogens than other methods. High cost, noisiness during intercourse, and the cumbersome feel of the device make acceptability a problem for some couples.

The **diaphragm** is used with spermicidal cream or jelly and offers a good level of protection from concep-

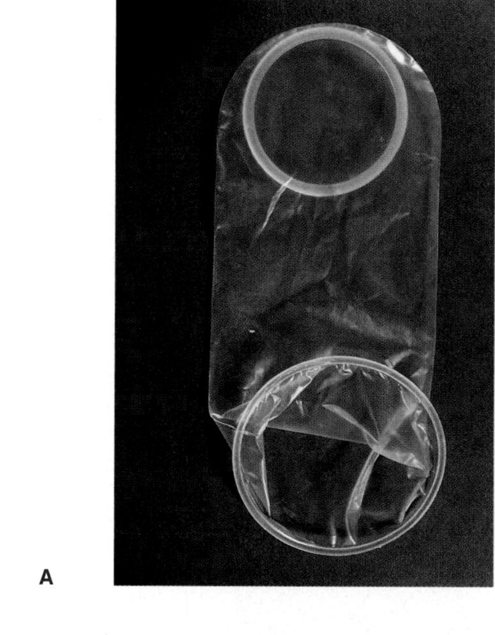

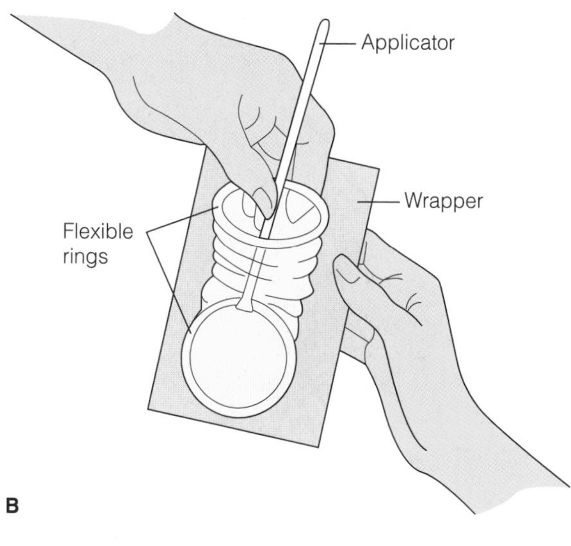

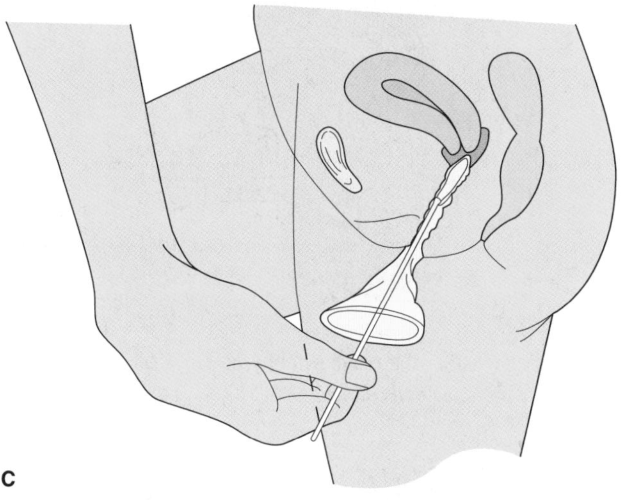

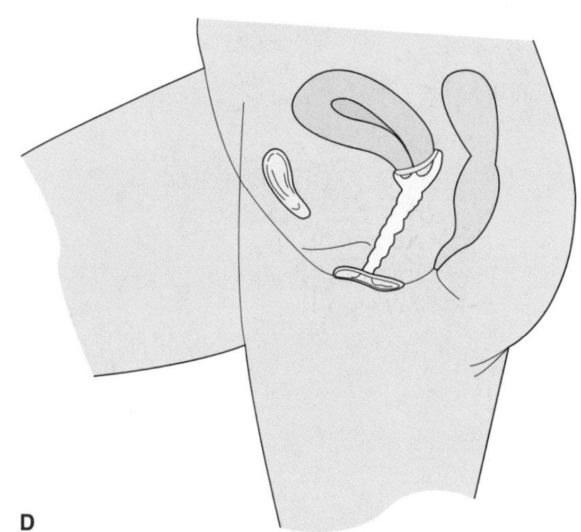

FIGURE 3–3 ***A,*** The female condom. To insert the condom: ***B,*** Remove condom and applicator from wrapper by pulling up on the ring. ***C,*** Insert condom slowly by gently pushing the applicator toward the small of the back. ***D,*** When properly inserted, the outer ring should rest on the folds of skin around the vaginal opening, and the inner ring (closed end) should fit loosely against the cervix. SOURCE: Crooks R., & Baur K. (1993). *Our sexuality* (5th ed.). Monterey, CA: Brooks/Cole.

tion. The woman must be fitted with a diaphragm and given instructions by trained personnel. The diaphragm should be rechecked for correct size after each childbirth and whenever a woman has gained or lost 15 pounds or more.

The diaphragm must be inserted before intercourse, with approximately one teaspoonful (or 1.5 inches from the tube) of spermicidal jelly placed around its rim and in the cup (Figure 3–4). This chemical barrier supplements the mechanical barrier of the diaphragm. The diaphragm is inserted through the vagina and covers the cervix. The last step in insertion is to push the edge of the diaphragm under the pubic symphysis, which may result in a "popping" sensation. When fitted properly and correctly in place, the diaphragm should not cause discomfort to the woman or her partner. Correct placement of the diaphragm can be checked by touching the cervix with a fingertip through the cup. The cervix feels like a small rounded structure and has a consistency similar to that of the tip of the nose. The center of the diaphragm should be over the cervix. If more than 4 hours elapse between insertion of the diaphragm and intercourse, additional spermicidal cream should be used. It is necessary to leave the diaphragm in place for at least 6 hours after coitus. If intercourse is desired again within the 6 hours, another type of contraception must be used or additional spermicidal jelly placed in the vagina with an applicator, taking care not to disturb the placement of the diaphragm. The

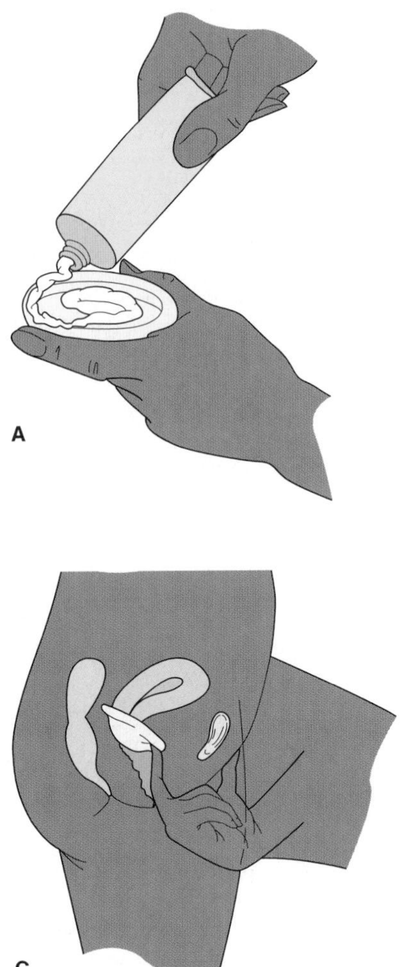

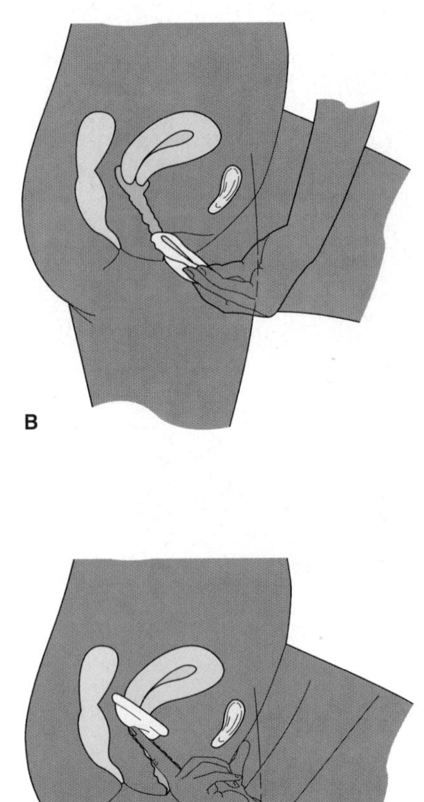

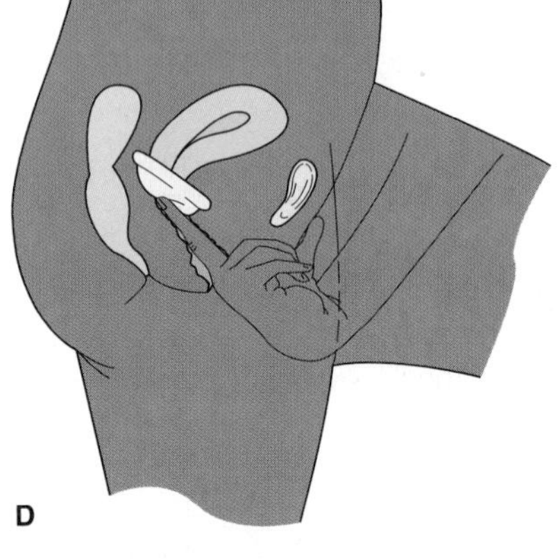

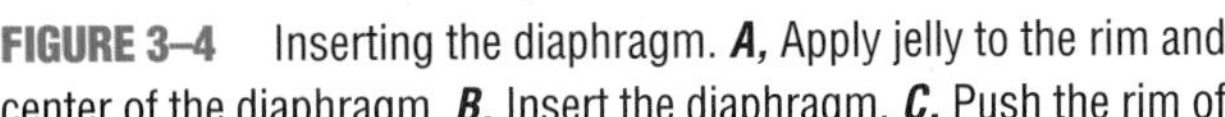

FIGURE 3–4 Inserting the diaphragm. ***A,*** Apply jelly to the rim and center of the diaphragm. ***B,*** Insert the diaphragm. ***C,*** Push the rim of the diaphragm under the pubic symphysis. ***D,*** Check placement of the diaphragm. The cervix should be felt through the diaphragm.

diaphragm should be periodically held up to the light and inspected for tears or holes. It should be cleaned after each use and stored in a clean dry container.

Some couples feel that the use of a diaphragm interferes with the spontaneity of intercourse. The nurse can suggest that the partner insert the diaphragm as part of foreplay.

Diaphragms are an excellent contraceptive method for women who are lactating, who cannot or do not wish to use oral contraceptives, or who wish to avoid the increased risk of PID associated with intrauterine devices. They are also a good choice for older women who can't take oral contraceptives because they smoke but who don't wish to be sterilized. Diaphragm use reduces the incidence of cervical gonorrhea, pelvic inflammatory disease, and tubal infertility. This protection may be due in part to the simultaneous use of a spermicide (Byyny & Speroff, 1996).

Women who object to touching their genitals to insert the diaphragm, check its placement, and remove it may find this method unsatisfactory. It is not recommended for women with a history of urinary tract infection (UTI), because pressure from the diaphragm on the urethra may interfere with complete bladder emptying and lead to recurrent UTIs. Women with a history of toxic shock syndrome should not use diaphragms or any of the barrier methods because they are left in place for prolonged periods. For the same reason, the diaphragm should not be used during a menstrual period or if a woman has abnormal vaginal discharge.

The **cervical cap** (Figure 3–5) is a cup-shaped device, used with spermicidal cream or jelly, that fits snugly over the cervix and is held in place by suction. Effectiveness rates and method of insertion are similar to those for the diaphragm. Unlike the diaphragm, however, the cap may be left in place for up to 48 hours, and it does not require additional spermicide for repeated intercourse. The cervical cap should be inserted at least 20 minutes and not more than 4 hours before intercourse (Hatcher et al, 1998). Advantages, disadvantages, and contraindications are

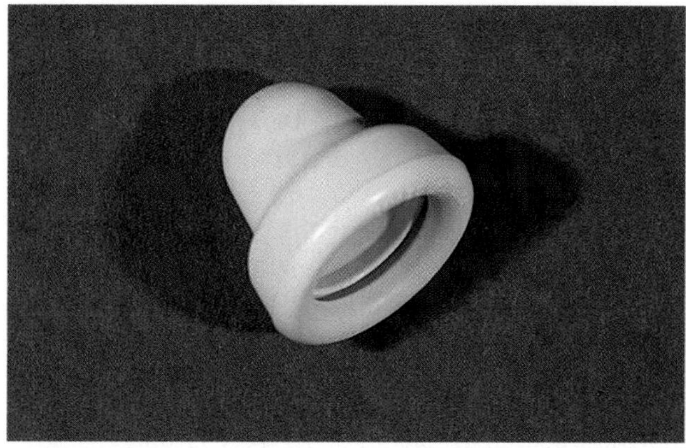

FIGURE 3–5 A cervical cap.

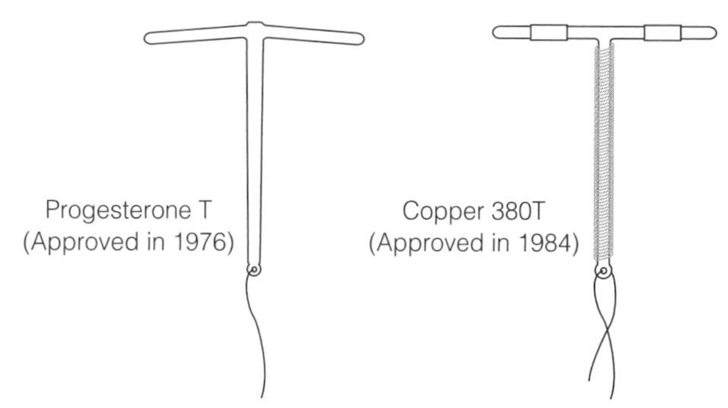

FIGURE 3–6 Two types of IUDs.

similar to those associated with the diaphragm. The cervical cap may be more difficult to fit because of limited size options. It also tends to be more difficult for women to insert and remove.

The **intrauterine device (IUD)** is designed to be inserted into the uterus by a qualified health care provider and left in place for an extended period, providing continuous contraceptive protection. The exact mechanism of IUD action is not clearly understood. Traditionally the IUD was believed to act by preventing the implantation of a fertilized ovum. Thus the IUD was considered an abortifacient or abortion-causing method. This belief is not accurate. IUDs truly are contraceptives; they act by immobilizing sperm in some way and impeding their progress from the cervix through the uterus to the fallopian tubes. The IUD also creates a sterile inflammatory response of the endometrium that is sufficient enough to be spermicidal (Byyny & Speroff, 1996).

The IUDs available today offer excellent contraceptive protection and, contrary to common myth, do not increase the risk of ectopic pregnancy or cause pelvic inflammatory disease (PID). In reality, late development of PID in IUD users probably results from sexually transmitted infection (Kjos, 1997). Unfortunately, although they are widely used throughout the world, IUDs currently account for less than 1% of contraceptive use in the United States (Speroff, 1998). Advantages of the IUD include high rate of effectiveness, continuous contraceptive protection, no coitus-related activity, and relative inexpensiveness over time. Because it is metabolically neutral, the IUD does not interact with medications. Thus it is an excellent form of contraception for women with existing medical problems. Possible adverse reactions to the IUD include discomfort to the wearer, increased bleeding during menses, increased risk of pelvic infection for about 3 weeks following insertion, perforation of the uterus during insertion, intermenstrual bleeding, dysmenorrhea, and expulsion of the device.

Two IUDs are currently available (Figure 3–6). The Progesterone T (Progestasert) must be changed annually and should be used only by women with an allergy to copper. The Copper T380A (ParaGard) is highly effective and can be left in place for up to 10 years. The IUD is recommended only for women who have at least one child and are in a monogamous relationship, because they have the lowest risk of contracting an STI. It is not recommended for women with multiple sexual contacts, because they are at risk for STIs.

The IUD is inserted into the uterus with its string or tail protruding through the cervix into the vagina. It may be inserted during a menstrual period or during the 4- to 6-week postpartum check. After insertion, the clinician instructs the woman to check for the presence of the string once a week for the first month and then after each menses. She does this by inserting her index finger or middle finger into her vagina to feel the string. She is told that she may have some cramping or bleeding intermittently for 2 to 6 weeks and that her first few menses may be irregular. Follow-up examination is suggested 4 to 8 weeks after insertion.

Women with IUDs should contact their health care providers if they are exposed to an STI or if they develop the following warning signs: late period, abnormal spotting or bleeding, **dyspareunia** (pain with intercourse), abdominal pain, abnormal discharge, signs of infection (fever, chills, malaise), or missing string. If a woman becomes pregnant with an IUD in place, the device should be removed.

Oral Contraceptives

The use of hormones, specifically the combination of estrogen and progesterone, is a very successful birth control method. **Oral contraceptives** work by inhibiting the release of an ovum, by creating an atrophic endometrium, and by maintaining cervical mucus that is hostile to sperm. Numerous oral contraceptives are available. The pill is taken daily for 21 days, typically beginning on the Sunday after the first day of the menstrual cycle and ending on a Saturday. In most cases menses will occur 1 to 4 days after the last pill is taken. Seven days after taking her

TABLE 3–2 Side Effects Associated with Oral Contraceptives

Estrogen Effects	Progestin Effects
Alterations in lipid metabolism	Acne, oily skin
Breast tenderness, engorgement; increased breast size	Breast tenderness; increased breast size
Cerebrovascular accident	Decreased libido
Changes in carbohydrate metabolism	Decreased high-density lipoprotein (HDL) cholesterol levels
Chloasma	Depression
Fluid retention; cyclic weight gain	Fatigue
Headache	Hirsutism
Hepatic adenomas	Increased appetite; weight gain
Hypertension	Increased low-density lipoprotein (LDL) cholesterol levels
Leukorrhea, cervical erosion, ectopia	Oligomenorrhea, amenorrhea
Nausea	Pruritus
Nervousness, irritability	Sebaceous cysts
Telangiectasia	
Thromboembolic complications—thrombophlebitis, pulmonary embolism	

last pill, the woman restarts the next cycle of pills. Thus the woman always begins the pill on the same day. Some companies offer a 28-day pack with seven "blank" pills so that the woman never stops taking a pill. The pill should be taken at approximately the same time each day—usually on arising or before retiring in the evening.

Although they are highly effective, oral contraceptives may produce side effects ranging from breakthrough bleeding to thrombus formation. Side effects from oral contraceptives may be either progesterone- or estrogen-related. The use of low-dose (35 μg or less) estrogen preparations has reduced many of the side effects, but the threat of potential risk is sufficient to deter some women from using oral contraceptives.

Absolute contraindications to the use of oral contraceptives include pregnancy, previous history of thrombophlebitis or thromboembolic disease, acute or chronic liver disease of cholestatic type with abnormal function, presence of estrogen-dependent carcinomas, undiagnosed uterine bleeding, heavy smoking, gall bladder disease, hypertension, diabetes, and hyperlipidemia. Women with the following relative contraindications may initiate oral contraceptive use; however, they require close and frequent monitoring. These include women with migraine headaches, epilepsy, depression, oligomenorrhea, and amenorrhea. Women who choose this method of contraception should be fully advised of the potential side effects (Table 3–2).

Oral contraceptives also have some important noncontraceptive benefits. Many women experience relief of uncomfortable menstrual symptoms. Cramps diminish, flow decreases, and the cycle becomes more regular. Mittelschmerz is eliminated, and the incidence of functional ovarian cysts decreases. More importantly, there is a substantial reduction in the incidence of ectopic pregnancy, ovarian cancer, endometrial cancer, iron-deficiency anemia, and benign breast disease. Currently oral contraceptives are considered a wonderful solution to the physiologic problems some women experience during the perimenopause, and their use in nonsmoking women ages 40 to 45 has quadrupled (Speroff, 1998). Because of an increased risk of ischemic heart disease, women over age 35 who smoke should not take oral contraceptives.

The woman using oral contraceptives should contact her health care provider if she becomes depressed, develops a breast lump, becomes jaundiced, or experiences any of the following warning signs: severe abdominal pain, severe chest pain or shortness of breath, severe headaches, dizziness, changes in vision (vision loss or blurring), speech problems, or severe leg pain.

Another oral contraceptive is the seldom-used progesterone-only pill, also called the minipill. It is used primarily by women who have a contraindication to the estrogen component of the combination preparation, such as history of thrombophlebitis, but are strongly motivated to use this form of contraception. The major problems with this preparation are amenorrhea or irregular spotting and bleeding patterns.

Long-Acting Progestin Contraceptives

Subdermal implants (Norplant) consist of silastic capsules containing levonorgestrel, a progestin, which are implanted in the woman's arm. They are effective for up to 5 years (Figure 3–7). Typically, six rods are inserted, although the manufacturer is currently developing Norplant II, which uses only two rods.

Norplant prevents ovulation in most women. It also stimulates the production of thick cervical mucus, which inhibits sperm penetration. Norplant provides effective continuous contraception that is removed from the act of coitus. Possible side effects include spotting, irregular bleeding or amenorrhea, an increased incidence of ovarian cysts, weight gain, headaches, fluid retention, acne, mood changes, and depression. Women should be advised that the implant may be visible, especially in very slender users, and that it requires a minor surgical procedure to insert and remove the implants.

Depot-medroxyprogesterone acetate (DMPA) **(Depo-Provera),** another long-acting progestin, provides highly effective birth control for 3 months when administered as a single intramuscular injection of 150 mg. DMPA, which acts primarily by suppressing ovulation, is safe, convenient, private, and relatively inexpensive. It also separates birth control from the act of coitus. It can safely be given to nursing mothers because it contains no estrogen. DMPA provides levels of progesterone high enough to block the luteinizing hormone (LH) surge, thereby suppressing ovulation. It also thickens the cervical mucus to block sperm penetration. Side effects include menstrual irregularities, headache, weight gain, breast tenderness, and depression. Return of fertility may be delayed for an average of 9 months (Kaunitz & Jordon, 1997).

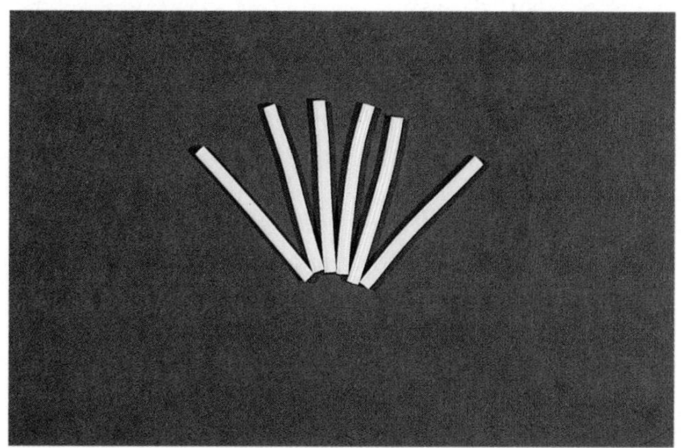

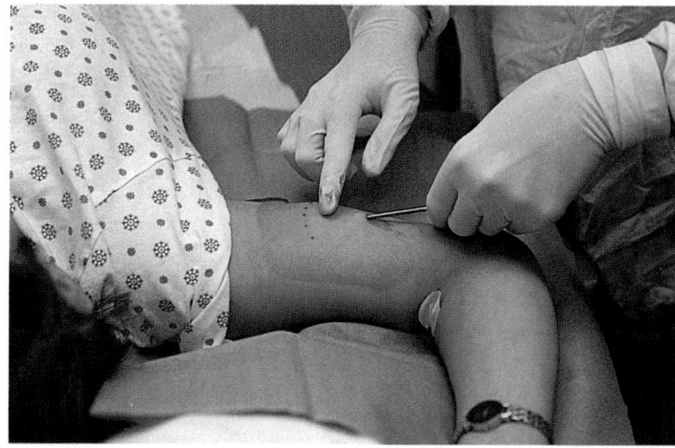

FIGURE 3–7 The Norplant system.

Emergency Postcoital Contraception

Emergency **postcoital contraception** is indicated when a woman is worried about pregnancy because of unprotected intercourse or possible contraceptive failure (eg, broken condom, slipped diaphragm, or too long a time between DMPA injections). The most commonly prescribed emergency postcoital contraceptive is levonorgestrel and ethinyl estradiol (Ovral), a combination oral contraceptive containing 50 μg estrogen. Though sometimes called the "morning-after pill," the phrase is misleading because the woman actually takes two pills as soon after intercourse as possible and two more 12 hours later. This regimen must be initiated within 72 hours after unprotected intercourse. (Lo/Ovral, Levlen, TriLevlin, Nordette, or Triphasil may also be used. When these oral contraceptives are used, the woman takes 4 pills each time.) Other postcoital regimens involve the use of specific doses of levonorgestrel alone without an estrogen and the insertion of a copper IUD (Ellertson, Koenig, Trussell, & Bull, 1997).

Information about postcoital emergency contraception has not been widely disseminated. In 1996, in an effort to increase awareness, an Emergency Contraception Hotline was established (1-888-NOT-2-LATE), and a World Wide Web page was developed (http://opr.princeton.edu/ec/).

Operative Sterilization

Before sterilization is performed on either partner, the clinician provides a thorough explanation of the procedure to both. Each needs to understand that sterilization is not a decision to be taken lightly or entered into at times of psychologic stress, such as separation or divorce. Even though both male and female procedures are theoretically reversible, the permanency of the procedure should be stressed and understood.

Male sterilization is achieved through a relatively minor procedure called a **vasectomy.** This involves surgically severing the vas deferens in both sides of the scrotum. It takes about 4 to 6 weeks and 6 to 36 ejaculations to clear the remaining sperm from the vas deferens. During that period, the couple is advised to use another method of birth control and to bring in two or three semen samples for a sperm count. When the sperm count is negative the couple can safely have unprotected sex. The man is rechecked at 6 and 12 months to ensure that fertility has not been restored by recanalization. Side effects of a vasectomy include pain, infection, hematoma, sperm granulomas, and spontaneous reanastomosis (reconnecting).

Vasectomies can sometimes be reversed by using microsurgery techniques. Restored fertility, as measured by subsequent pregnancy, ranges from 30% to 85%.

Voluntary female sterilization is accomplished by **tubal ligation.** Four procedures are common in the United States:

- Tubal sterilization at the time of laparotomy for a cesarean birth or other abdominal surgery
- Postpartum minilaparotomy soon after a vaginal birth
- Interval sterilization (done at a time unrelated to a pregnancy)
- Laparoscopy

Tubal ligation may be done at any time. However, the postpartal period is an ideal time to perform a tubal ligation because the uterus is enlarged and the tubes are easy to locate. During these procedures the tubes are ligated, clipped, electrocoagulated, banded, or plugged. This interrupts the patency of the fallopian tube, thus preventing the ovum and the sperm from meeting.

Complications of female sterilization procedures include coagulation burns on the bowel, bowel perforation, pain, infection, hemorrhage, and adverse anesthesia effects. Reversal of a tubal ligation depends on the type of procedure performed. The failure rate is 1 to 4 women per 1,000 women sterilized. Reversal is more successful after mechanical occlusion than after electrocoagulation. With microsurgical techniques, a pregnancy rate of up to 75% is possible (Berek et al, 1996).

Male Contraception

The vasectomy and the condom, discussed previously, are currently the only forms of male contraception available in the United States. Hormonal contraception for men has yet to be developed, although studies are under way on testosterone enanthate, which significantly inhibits sperm production in most men. However, it has a long induction period and requires weekly injections. Drug-delivery systems lasting 2 to 3 months are under investigation (Hatcher et al, 1998).

I think I'm like a lot of women. During my life I've used a variety of contraceptive methods. I took the pill back when doses were higher; I used foam alone and had a baby, then used spermicidal cream and condoms more successfully. I never wanted a tubal, and my husband refuses to consider a vasectomy, so the IUD was a perfect alternative for us. I am 47 and I like something I don't have to think about every time we want to make love. Maybe someday there will be more contraceptives for men—it seems only fair—but I'm glad that at least I've had some choices.

NURSING CARE MANAGEMENT

In most cases, the nurse who provides information and guidance about contraceptive methods works with the woman partner, because most contraceptive methods are female oriented. Because a man can purchase condoms without seeing a health care provider, only in the case of vasectomy does a man require counseling and interaction with a nurse. Men should be encouraged to participate in contraceptive services. The nurse can play an important role in helping a woman or couple choose a method of contraception that is acceptable to both partners.

In addition to completing a history and assessing for any contraindications to specific methods, the nurse can spend time with a woman learning about her lifestyle, personal attitudes about particular contraceptive methods, religious and cultural beliefs, personal biases, and plans for future childbearing in order to help the woman select a particular contraceptive method. Once the woman chooses a method, the nurse can help the woman learn to use it effectively. The Teaching Guide: Using a Method of Contraception provides guidelines for helping women use a method of contraception effectively. The Self-Care Guide on contraception methods in the perforated section at the end of this book provides a summary of contraceptive methods for clients. The Guide may be photocopied for use as a handout.

The nurse also reviews any possible side effects and warning signs related to the method chosen and counsels the woman about what action to take if she suspects she is pregnant. In many cases, the nurse is involved in telephone counseling of women who call with questions and concerns about contraception. Thus it is vital that the nurse be knowledgeable about this topic and have resources available to find answers to less common questions. ●

Surgical Interruption of Pregnancy

Although abortion was legalized in the United States in 1973, the associated controversy over moral and legal issues continues. This controversy is as readily apparent in the medical and nursing professions as in other groups.

Many women are strongly opposed to abortion for religious, ethical, or personal reasons. Other women feel that abortion provides a legally available alternative to a pregnancy. A number of physical and psychosocial factors influence a woman's decision to seek an abortion. The presence of a disease or health state that jeopardizes the mother's life and serious, life-threatening fetal problems are frequently suggested as indications for abortion. In other instances, the timing or circumstance of the pregnancy creates an inordinate stress on the woman, prompting her to choose an abortion. Some of these situations may involve contraceptive failure, rape, or incest. Usually the decision is best made by the woman or couple involved. A woman whose life is threatened by the pregnancy may choose to continue the pregnancy, whereas one with no obvious threat may choose abortion.

Abortion in the first trimester is technically easier and safer than abortion in the second trimester. It may be performed by dilatation and curettage (D & C), minisuction, or vacuum curettage. The major risks include perforation of the uterus, laceration of the cervix, systemic reaction to the anesthetic agent, hemorrhage, and infection. Second trimester abortion may be done using dilatation and extraction (D & E), hypertonic saline, systemic prostaglandins, and intrauterine prostaglandins (Berek et al, 1996).

Medical Interruption of Pregnancy

Medical means of interrupting an early pregnancy is becoming available to women in the United States. The antifolate methotrexate can be used alone or in conjunction with misoprostol to terminate a pregnancy up to approximately 50 days from the last menstrual period. Mifepristone (RU 486) blocks progesterone, thereby altering the endometrium and making it unsuitable for implantation. The combination of RU 486 and a prostaglandin has proved to be an effective abortifacient. Currently RU 486 is not manufactured in the United States, although it has gained widespread recognition in Europe and China.

NURSING CARE MANAGEMENT

Important aspects of nursing care for a woman who chooses to have an abortion include providing information about the methods of abortion and associated risks;

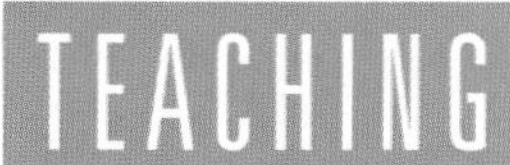

TEACHING GUIDE: USING A METHOD OF CONTRACEPTION

Assessment Determine the woman's general knowledge about contraceptive methods, identify the methods the woman has used previously (if any), identify contraindications or risk factors for any methods, discuss the woman's personal preferences and biases about various methods, and discuss her commitment (and her partner's commitment if appropriate) to a chosen method.

Nursing Diagnosis The key nursing diagnosis will probably be ***Knowledge Deficit*** related to lack of information about the correct use of chosen method of contraception.

Nursing Plan and Implementation The teaching plan will focus on confirming that a chosen method of contraception is a good choice for the woman. You will then help the woman learn the method so that she can use it effectively.

Client Goals At the completion of teaching, the woman will be able to:

- Confirm for herself that the chosen method of contraception is appropriate for her.
- List the advantages, disadvantages, and risks of the chosen method.
- Describe (or demonstrate) the correct procedure for using the chosen method.
- Cite warning signs that should be reported to the caregiver.

Teaching Plan

Content	*Teaching Method*
• Discuss the factors that a woman should consider in choosing a method of contraception (Table 3–1). Stress that the various methods may be appropriate at different times in the woman's life.	*Contraception is a personal decision, so the discussion should take place in a private area free of interruptions. Create a supportive, warm, and comfortable atmosphere by attitude and communication style—both verbal and nonverbal. Use the Self-Care Guide on contraception at the end of this book as a handout to support the discussion.*
• Review the woman's reasons for selecting a particular method and confirm any contraindications to specific methods.	*Recognize that your personal preferences about contraception may be different from those of the woman you are counseling. Your responsibility is to provide accurate information in an open, nonjudgmental way.*
• Discuss the advantages, disadvantages, and risks of the chosen method.	*Focus on open discussion. If a signed permit is required (as with sterilization or IUD insertion), the physician should also discuss the advantages, disadvantages, and risks.*
• Describe the correct procedure for using a method step-by-step. Periodically stop and have the woman review the information for you. If you are teaching a technique (eg, inserting a diaphragm or charting BBT), demonstrate and then have the woman do a return demonstration as appropriate. (Note: If certain aspects are beyond your level of expertise, you can review the content and confirm that the woman has the opportunity to do a return demonstration. For example, an office nurse who does not do cervical cap fittings may describe its use, have the woman try inserting the cap herself, and then have the placement checked by the nurse practitioner or physician.)	*Learning is best accomplished when material is broken down into smaller steps, and it may also be helpful to have a model or chart to enable the woman to visualize what is being described. You may also have a sample of the chosen method available: a package of oral contraceptives, an open IUD, or a symptothermal chart.*
• Provide information on what the woman should do if unusual circumstances arise (she forgets a pill or misses a morning temperature). • Stress warning signs that require immediate action and explain why these signs indicate a risk. Carefully delineate the actions the woman should take: Should she contact her caregiver? Stop the method?	*Provide a written handout identifying the warning signs and the actions a woman should take if an unusual situation develops. For example, what should she do if she vomits or has diarrhea while taking oral contraceptives? What action should she take if she and her partner are using a condom and it breaks?*
• Arrange a follow-up session with the woman, either on the phone or at a return visit, to determine if she has any questions about the method and to ensure that no problems have arisen.	*The woman should know that she is free to call if she has questions or concerns once she starts using the method. This increases her comfort level and enables you to detect potential problems early.*

RESEARCH IN PRACTICE

What is this study about? Breast cancer constitutes a major risk factor for women, especially as they age. Breast screening practices may promote the early detection of breast cancer. Latina women may wait longer to seek treatment for breast cancer symptoms. Programs to encourage breast self-examination have not been successful with older Latina women.

How was the study done? Nilda Peragallo, Patricia Fox, and Melinda Lydia conducted a study about breast care behaviors with 114 Latina women of Mexican or Puerto Rican descent. The researchers wanted to assess general knowledge about breast cancer screening (breast self-examination, clinical breast examination, and mammography), describe screening utilization, and identify barriers that prevent screening practices. Data collection occurred during a 45-to 60-minute interview and included sociodemographic information, acculturation or extent of participation in mainstream US culture, breast cancer knowledge, and breast cancer screening practices. Only 111 women (81 Mexican and 30 Puerto Rican) completed the interview process and these interviews were used in the study.

What were the results of the study? Data analysis showed that acculturation levels were low (2.9% or less) for 70% of the participants (with 76% of the women speaking Spanish only or more than English). Only 40% of Mexican women and 58% of Puerto Rican women had lived a large percentage of their lives in the United States. Forty-nine percent of the women with inconsistent mammogram screening gave all incorrect answers to the questions about breast self-examination.

To analyze breast cancer knowledge, the researchers divided the women into two groups based on consistent or inconsistent breast screening practices. They then completed multiple regression analysis using screening practices as the dependent variables, and sociodemographic characteristics, breast cancer screening knowledge, and acculturation as the independent variables. Significant predictors of consistent breast screening included percentage of time lived in the United States (p=.007) and knowledge of breast self-examination (p=.0103).

What additional questions might I have? Were results of the multiple regression analysis influenced by a nonrandom sample? Does a relationship exist between the dependent variable of inconsistent screening and the independent variable of breast cancer screening knowledge? What were the complete results of the data analysis? Tables illustrating both descriptive and multiple regression results would clarify the report.

How can I use this study? Providing information about breast self-examination and other screening techniques may encourage earlier detection of breast cancer in all women, but it is especially important for women who have lived in the United States for short periods of time.

SOURCE: Peragallo, N. P., Fox, P. G., & Alba, M. L. (1988). Breast care among Latino immigrant women in the U.S. *Health Care for Women International, 19,* 165–172.

counseling regarding available alternatives to abortion and their implications; encouraging the woman to verbalize her feelings; providing support before, during, and after the procedure; monitoring vital signs, intake, and output; providing for physical comfort and privacy throughout the procedure; and teaching the client self-care, the importance of the postabortion checkup, and contraception review. ●

Recommended Gynecologic Screening Procedures

The accepted standard of care for women today involves a variety of screening procedures designed to detect potential problems early to permit the most effective treatment. This section focuses on some of the most commonly used screening procedures: breast self-examination, breast examination by a trained health care provider, mammography, Pap smear, and pelvic examination.

Breast Examination

Like the uterus, the breast undergoes regular cyclical changes in response to hormonal stimulation. Each month, in rhythm with the cycle of ovulation, the breasts become engorged with fluid in anticipation of pregnancy, and the woman may experience sensations of tenderness, lumpiness, or pain. If conception does not occur, the accumulated fluid drains away via the lymphatic network. Mastodynia (premenstrual swelling and tenderness of the breasts) is common. It usually lasts for 3 to 4 days before the onset of menses, but the symptoms may persist throughout the month.

After menopause, adipose breast tissue atrophies and is replaced by connective tissue. The breasts lose elasticity and may droop and become pendulous. The recurring breast engorgement associated with ovulation ceases. If hormone replacement therapy (HRT) is used to counteract other symptoms of menopause, breast engorgement may resume.

Monthly **breast self-examination (BSE)** is a good method for detecting breast masses early. A woman who knows the texture and feel of her own breasts is far more likely to detect changes that develop. Thus it is important for a woman to develop the habit of doing routine BSE as early as possible, preferably as an adolescent. Women at high risk for breast cancer are especially encouraged to be attentive to the importance of early detection through routine BSE.

In the course of a routine physical examination or during an initial visit to the caregiver, the woman should be taught BSE technique and its importance as a monthly practice. The effectiveness of BSE is determined by the woman's ability to perform the procedure correctly.

Breast self-examination should be performed on a regular monthly basis about 1 week after each menstrual period, when the breasts are typically not tender or swollen. See Figures 3–8 and 3–9 and the Self-Care Guide on BSE in the perforated section at the end of this book. The Self-Care Guide may be removed and photocopied for use as a client handout. Breast self-examination is most effective when it uses a dual approach incorporating both inspection and palpation. After menopause, BSE should be performed on the same day each month (chosen by the woman for ease of remembrance).

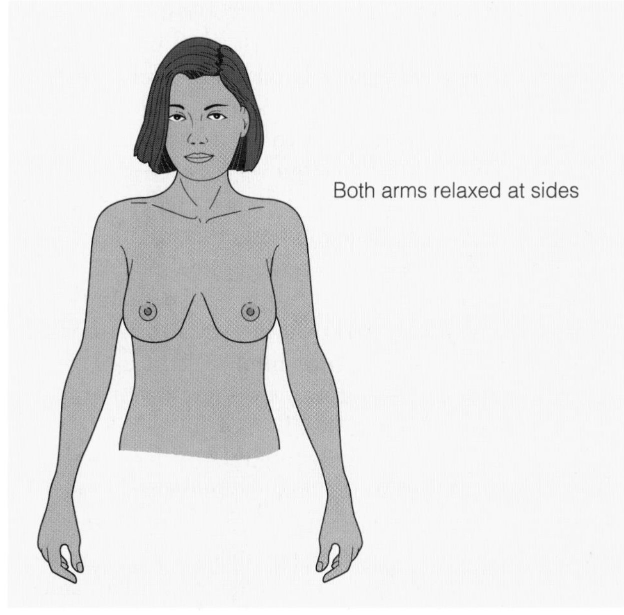

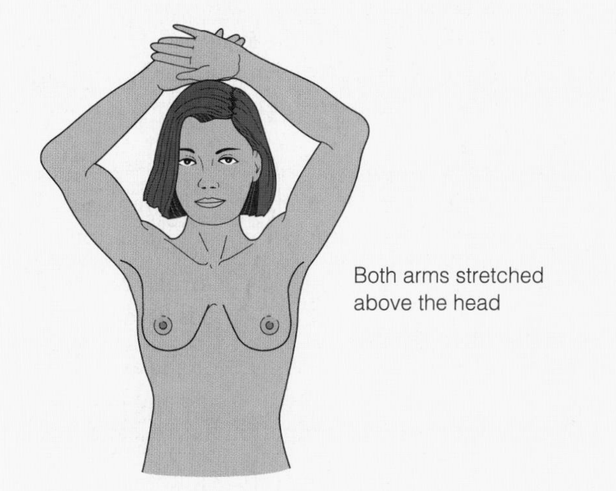

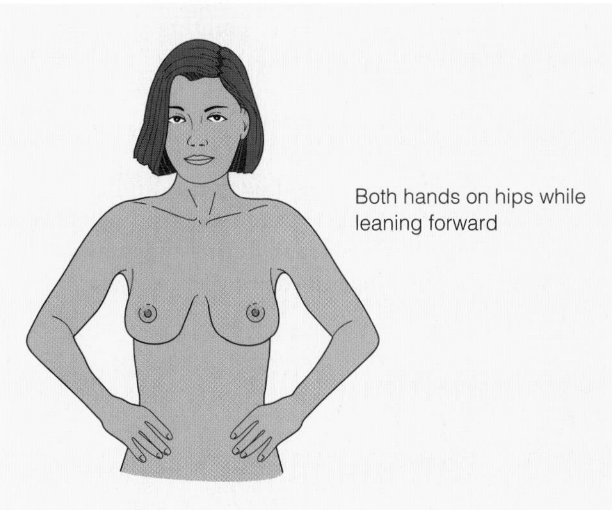

FIGURE 3–8 Positions for inspection of the breasts.

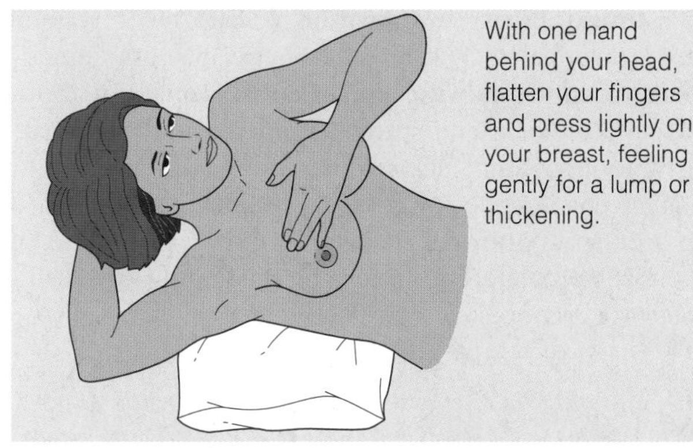

With one hand
behind your head,
flatten your fingers
and press lightly on
your breast, feeling
gently for a lump or
thickening.

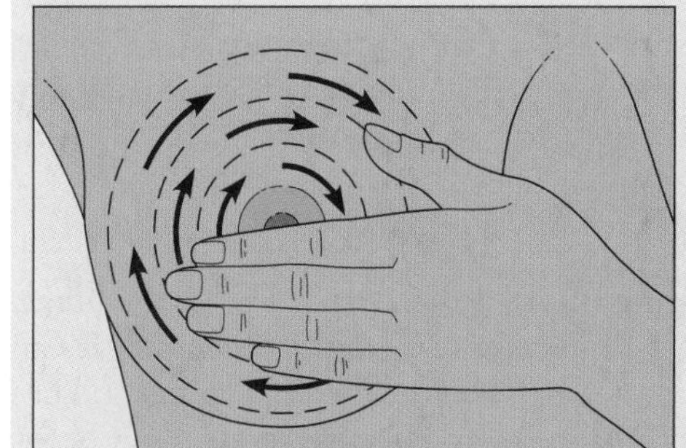

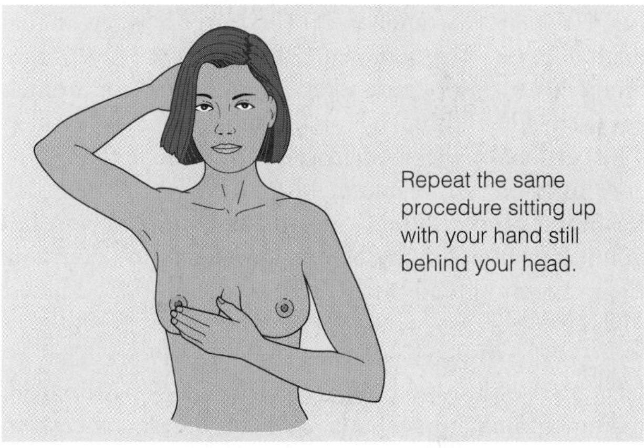

Repeat the same
procedure sitting up
with your hand still
behind your head.

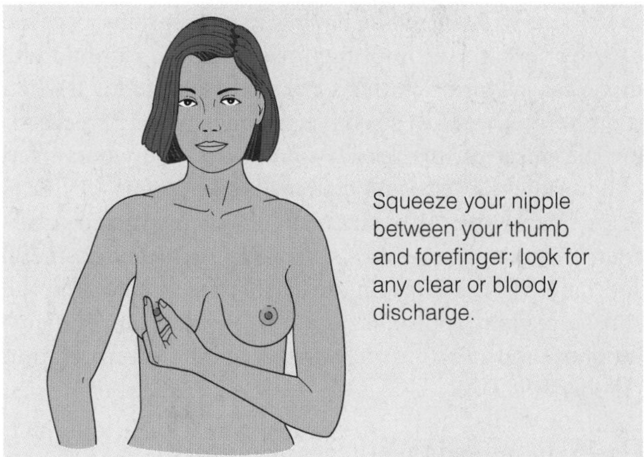

FIGURE 3–9 Procedure for breast self-examination (BSE).

Clinical breast examination (CBE) by a trained health care provider, such as a physician, nurse practitioner, or nurse-midwife, is an essential element of a routine gynecologic examination. Experience in differentiating among benign, suspicious, and worrisome breast changes enables the caregiver to reassure the woman if the findings are normal or move forward with additional diagnostic procedures or referral if the findings are suspicious or worrisome.

CRITICAL THINKING QUESTION

Why do you suppose so many women are unwilling to perform monthly breast self-examination despite its value in detecting cancer early?

Mammography

A **mammogram** is a soft-tissue x-ray image of the breast taken without the injection of a contrast medium. It can detect lesions in the breast before they can be felt and has gained wide acceptance as an effective screening tool for breast cancer. Currently the American Cancer Society suggests that all women age 40 and over have an annual mammogram. The National Cancer Institute (NCI) recommends mammograms every 1 to 2 years for women age 40 to 49 and annually for all women age 50 and older. The National Cancer Advisory Board, which offers guidance to NCI, also recommends that women at high risk for breast cancer should "seek medical advice about beginning mammography before age 40 and to determine their mammography schedule in their 40s" (Taubes, 1997).

Thirty percent of women age 40 to 49 are likely to have a false-positive result requiring biopsy. Moreover, mammograms miss about 25% of breast cancers in women in this age group (Taubes, 1997).

Some women avoid having mammograms because they fear compression of the breasts will be painful. The nurse can suggest that this x-ray study be scheduled when their breasts are least sensitive, which is about 2 weeks after the onset of menses. In some cases, the woman can obtain relief by reducing caffeine intake from 5 to 7 days prior to the test. All women should be instructed to refrain from applying lotions, powders, or other cosmetic substances to the torso on the day of the exam because the substances may appear as questionable areas on the mammogram and may interfere with accurate interpretation (Weber, 1997).

Pap Smear and Pelvic Examination

The purpose of the Papanicolaou smear **(Pap smear)** is to screen for the presence of cellular abnormalities by obtaining a sample containing cells from the cervix and the endocervical canal. Precancerous and cancerous conditions, as well as atypical findings and inflammatory changes, can be identified by microscopic examination. Traditionally the test has been performed by preparing a Pap smear slide. However, the smear was often difficult to read because of obscuring factors such as blood, mucus, overlapping cells, and so forth. More recently, a new test—the ThinPrep™ Pap smear—has been approved by the FDA. In this test, no slide is prepared; instead, the cervical cells are transferred directly to a vial of preservative fluid, thereby preserving the entire specimen. The specimen is sent to a laboratory where a special processor prepares a slide. Research demonstrated that the ThinPrep™ Pap smear significantly improved the detection of abnormal lesions and reduced the number of compromised slides (McPhillips, 1997).

The Pap smear is a screening tool. A definitive diagnosis is made by studying tissue samples obtained by biopsies. Women should be advised to avoid douching, intercourse, female hygiene products, and spermicidal agents for 24 hours prior to a Pap smear. Pap smears should not be obtained during menstruation or when visible cervicitis exists.

Women who have reached the age of 18 and women, regardless of age, who are or have engaged in vaginal/penile intercourse should have a pelvic examination and Pap smear annually.

The pelvic examination consists of three segments: inspection of the vulva; inspection of the vagina and the cervix via a speculum examination; and palpation of the cervix, uterus, and ovaries via a bimanual examination. Some women perceive the pelvic exam as uncomfortable and embarrassing. Any negative feelings can cause women to delay having annual gynecologic examinations. This avoidance may pose a threat to life and health.

To make the pelvic examination less threatening, and thus improve health-seeking behavior, more health care providers are performing what is called an educational pelvic examination. This includes offering the woman a mirror to watch the procedure, pointing out anatomic parts to her and positioning and draping her to allow eye-to-eye contact with the practitioner. The woman is encouraged to participate by asking questions and giving feedback.

Nurse practitioners, certified nurse-midwives, and physicians all perform pelvic examinations. Nurses assist the practitioner and the woman during the examination. Procedure 3–1 provides information on assisting with a pelvic examination.

CLINICAL TIP

Whenever you teach about pelvic examination and Pap smear, be certain that the woman understands that she should not douche for at least 24 hours beforehand. Douching can interfere with the accuracy of the Pap smear. Occasionally a caregiver will specifically request that a woman use a douche before a Pap smear; douching should ONLY be in this circumstance.

PROCEDURE 3–1 ASSISTING WITH A PELVIC EXAMINATION

Nursing Action	*Rationale*
Objective: Provide a warm environment.	
Turn on overhead heat lights, if available, or turn up the thermostat.	
Objective: Assemble and prepare the equipment.	
• Prepare and arrange the following items so that they are easily accessible:	*Equipment organization facilitates the examination.*
a. Vaginal specula of various sizes, warmed with water or on a heating pad prior to insertion.	*A warmed speculum assists in lubrication and facilitates initial insertion when culture and smears are taken.*
b. Gloves.	
c. Water-soluble lubricant.	
d. Materials for Pap smear and cultures.	
e. Good light source.	
• Do not use lubricant on the speculum before insertion.	*Use of lubricant may alter findings or cultures.*
Objective: Prepare the woman.	
• Explain the procedure. If the woman has never had a pelvic examination, show her the equipment and explain the procedure before examination.	*Explanation of the procedure decreases anxiety.*
• Instruct the woman to empty her bladder and to remove clothing below the waist. She may want to leave her shoes on.	*An empty bladder promotes comfort during internal examination. Some women feel more comfortable with shoes on, rather than supporting their weight with bare heels against cold stirrups.*
• Give the woman a disposable drape or sheet to place on her lap. Encourage her to sit on the end of the examining table with the drape across her lap.	
• Position the woman in the lithotomy position with her thighs flexed and adducted. Place her feet in stirrups. Her buttocks should extend slightly beyond the end of the examining table.	
• Drape the woman with the sheet leaving a flap so the perineum can be exposed.	
Objective: Provide support to the woman as the physician or nurse practitioner performs the examination.	
• Explain each part of the examination as it is performed: inspection of external genitals, vagina, and cervix; bimanual examination of internal organs.	*Promotes relaxation.*
• Instruct the woman to relax and breathe slowly.	
• Advise the woman when the speculum is about to be inserted and ask her to bear down.	*When the speculum is inserted, the woman may feel intravaginal pressure. Bearing down helps open vaginal orifice and relaxes perineal muscles.*
• Lubricate the examiner's finger prior to bimanual examination.	*Lubrication decreases friction and eases insertion.*

Nursing Action	*Rationale*
Objective: Provide for the woman's comfort at the end of the examination.	
• Move to the end of the examination table and face the woman's perineum. Cover the woman with the drape. Apply gentle pressure to the woman's knees and encourage her to move toward the head of the table. Offer your hand to the woman, remove her heels from the stirrups, and assist her to a sitting position. Be sure that she is not dizzy and that she is sitting or standing safely before you leave the room.	*The supine position may cause postural hypotension.*
• Provide tissues to wipe lubricant from the perineum.	*Upon assuming a sitting position, vaginal secretions along with lubricant may be discharged.*
• Provide privacy while the woman dresses	

Menopause

Menopause, the time when menses cease, is a time of transition for a woman, marking the end of her reproductive abilities. The years prior to menopause, which mark the change from normal ovulatory cycles to cessation of menses, are known as the perimenopausal or transitional years. The current median age of menopause in the United States is 51.3 years. **Climacteric,** or *change of life* (often used synonymously with menopause), refers to the host of psychologic and physical alterations that occur around the time of menopause.

Psychologic Aspects

An old image of menopausal women as socially irrelevant is undergoing revision, as the average woman will live one-third of her life after menopause. A woman's psychologic adaptation to menopause and the climacteric is multifactorial. She is influenced by her own expectations and knowledge, physical well-being, family views, marital stability, and sociocultural expectations. As the number of women reaching menopause increases, the negative emotional connotations society attaches to menopause are diminishing, enabling menopausal women to cope more effectively and even enabling them to view menopause as a time of personal growth.

My personal response to menopause has surprised me a little. Suddenly 52 doesn't really seem old. I look at pictures of my mother in her early fifties and she seems so much older. I imagine each generation looks back and thinks the same thing. I do wish I had known at 22 what I know now, but I still see myself as learning and growing. Now I am being more selective about my goals for the future—maybe I'll try writing a novel, or I'll take a gourmet cooking class. One thing I am committed to—I intend to do my very best to live each day as it comes and enjoy it to the hilt!

Physical Aspects

The physical characteristics of menopause are linked to the shift from a cyclic to a noncyclic hormonal pattern. Menopause usually occurs between 45 and 52 years of age. The age of onset may be influenced by overall health, nutritional, cultural, lifestyle, or genetic factors. The physiologic mechanisms initiating its onset are not precisely known. The onset of menopause occurs when estrogen levels become so low that menstruation stops.

Beginning 2 to 8 years before menopause, women experience episodes of anovulation, reduced fertility, decreased or increased flow, irregular frequency of menses, and then ultimately, amenorrhea. Generally ovulation ceases 1 to 2 years before menopause, but individual variations exist. FSH levels rise, and ovarian follicles cease to produce estrogen. The uterine endometrium and myometrium atrophy, as do the cervical glands. The uterine cavity constricts. The fallopian tubes and ovaries atrophy extensively. The vaginal mucosa becomes smooth and thin, and the rugae disappear, leading to loss of elasticity. As a result, intercourse can be painful, but this may be overcome by using lubricating gel or saliva. Dryness of the mucous membrane can lead to burning and itching. The vaginal pH level increases as the number of Döderlein's bacilli decreases. This change in the vaginal ecology can lead to an atrophic vaginitis.

Postmenopausal women can remain orgasmic, and some report that sexual interest and activity increase as the need for contraception disappears and personal growth and awareness increase. Other women report a decrease in libido following menopause, which may be related to lowered testosterone levels.

Atrophic changes occur in the ovaries, vagina, vulva, and urethra and in the trigonal area of the bladder. Vulvar atrophy occurs late, and the pubic hair thins, turns gray or white, and may ultimately disappear. The labia shrivel and lose their heightened pigmentation. Pelvic fascia and muscles atrophy, resulting in decreased pelvic support. The breasts become pendulous and decrease in size and firmness.

Many menopausal women experience a vasomotor disturbance commonly known as *hot flashes*, a feeling of heat arising from the chest and spreading to the neck and face. The hot flashes are often accompanied by sweating and sleep disturbances. These episodes may occur as often as 20 to 30 times a day and generally last 3 to 5 minutes. Some women also experience dizzy spells, palpitations, and weakness. Many women find their own most effective ways to deal with the hot flashes. Some report that dressing in layers, using a fan, avoiding alcoholic beverages, or drinking a cool liquid helps relieve distress. Still others seek relief through hormone replacement therapy or herbal therapy.

Long-range physical changes may include **osteoporosis,** a decrease in the bony skeletal mass. This change is thought to be associated with lowered estrogen and androgen levels. Osteoporosis puts an individual at increased risk for fractures of the hip, forearm, and vertebrae. Osteoporosis is more common in women who are middle-aged or older. The following risk factors are also associated with osteoporosis:

- European American or Asian ethnic origin
- Small-boned and thin body type
- Family history of osteoporosis
- Lack of regular weight-bearing exercise
- Nulliparity
- Early onset of menopause
- Consistently low intake of calcium
- Cigarette smoking
- Moderate to heavy alcohol intake

Moreover, the estrogen deprivation that occurs in menopausal women may significantly increase their risk of coronary heart disease. Loss of protein from the skin and supportive tissues causes wrinkling. Postmenopausal women frequently gain weight, which may be due to excessive caloric intake or to lower caloric need with the same level of intake. Another long-range change is a shift in lipid and lipoprotein levels. Estrogen has a protective mechanism that fosters elevated levels of high-density lipoproteins (HDL) and lower low-density lipoprotein (LDL). When estrogen levels fall with menopause, this protective mechanism ceases, potentially placing a woman at increased risk for coronary artery disease, hypertension, and strokes (Westermann, 1997).

Medical Therapy

Hormone Replacement Therapy (HRT)

Hormone replacement therapy (HRT), usually involving estrogen with or without a progestin, was formerly a controversial therapy; currently, however, the American College of Obstetricians and Gynecologists recommends HRT in menopause. Estrogen replacement is helpful in stopping hot flashes and night sweats and in reversing atrophic vaginal changes. Perhaps most significantly, HRT may reduce the incidence of coronary artery disease, the leading cause of death in postmenopausal women (Andrews, 1995). Other benefits of HRT include prevention and treatment of bone loss associated with osteoporosis, improved bladder and vaginal tone, and improved quality of life. It may also improve memory and offer protection against Alzheimer's disease and colon cancer (Rabin, 1998). Possible risks of HRT include increased risk of gallbladder disease; slightly increased risk for venous thrombosis and stroke; possible increased risk of endometrial cancer and systemic lupus erythematosus; and possible increased risk of breast cancer after more than 5 years of use (Rabin, 1998).

When estrogen is given alone, it can produce endometrial hyperplasia and increase the risk of endometrial cancer. Therefore, in women who still have a uterus, estrogen is opposed by giving a progestin for a portion of the cycle. Currently opinion varies on the number of days that progesterone (Provera) should be included. Typically, estrogen is given the first 25 days of the month with 10 mg Provera added during the last 12 days of the estrogen administration (days 14 to 25). With this regimen, 80% to 90% of women will experience monthly withdrawal bleeding. An alternative approach involves the daily administration of 0.625 mg of estrogen with 2.5 mg of Provera, which can be taken as two separate medications or in a combination pill, Prempro™. This regimen is associated with less vaginal bleeding and is sufficient to prevent endometrial hyperplasia and osteoporosis; it also retains most of the cardiovascular beneficial effects of estrogen (Byyny & Speroff, 1996). Although most women prefer to take estrogen orally, some choose the transdermal estrogen skin patch. Estrogen is available in a vaginal cream and is used primarily for urogenital symptoms. For women experiencing decreased libido, combination estrogen-testosterone preparations are available.

Before starting HRT, the woman should undergo a thorough history, physical examination including Pap smear, measurement of cholesterol and liver enzyme levels, and baseline mammogram. An initial endometrial biopsy is no longer routinely recommended for all women beginning HRT; however, biopsy is indicated for women with an increased risk of endometrial cancer and if excessive, unexpected, or prolonged vaginal bleeding occurs (Lichtman, 1996). Women taking estrogen should be advised to stop immediately if they develop headaches, visual changes, signs of thrombophlebitis, or chest pain and to notify their nurse practitioner or physician.

Prevention and Treatment of Osteoporosis

Women with no contraindications to estrogen who are showing evidence of bone loss are good candidates for HRT. Premenopausal or postmenopausal women with four or more risk factors for osteoporosis should have bone mass measurements done. The woman's height should be measured at each visit, because a loss of height is often an early sign that vertebrae are being compressed because of reduced bone mass. A variety of conditions, including malabsorption syndrome, cancer, cirrhosis of the liver, chronic use of cortisone, and rheumatoid arthritis, can cause secondary arthritis, which resembles osteoporosis. If these secondary causes are ruled out, treatment for osteoporosis is instituted.

Prevention of osteoporosis is a primary goal of care. Women are advised to maintain an adequate calcium intake. The Institute of Medicine recommends that women over age 50 have a daily calcium intake of 1200 mg. Most women require supplements to achieve this level. Calcium supplementation is most efficient when single doses do not exceed 500 mg and when taken with a meal. Women are also advised to participate regularly in exercise, consume only modest quantities of alcohol and caffeine, and to stop smoking. This is especially important because alcohol and smoking have a negative effect on the rate of bone resorption.

Alendronate (Fosamax) is a treatment for osteoporosis that acts by inhibiting bone resorption and increasing bone mass. It is recommended for menopausal women with osteoporosis who cannot take estrogen (Barbieri, 1998). Intranasal calcitonin, inhaled once a day, has received FDA approval for the treatment of postmenopausal osteoporosis. However, it produces only limited increases in bone density, and data about its effectiveness in preventing fractures are incomplete (Salvatori & Levine, 1998). Calcium and vitamin D supplements are generally recommended in addition to the alendronate or calcitonin.

Alternative and Complementary Therapies

Many women do not wish to take hormone replacement therapy or have a medical contraindication to it. A variety of therapeutic modalities has been proposed as alternative or complementary treatment or prevention measures for the discomforts and ailments of the perimenopausal and postmenopausal years. These include nutrition and nutrition supplements, such as a diet rich in calcium and vitamins E, D, and B complex. Phytoestrogens, substances with estrogen properties found in a number of foods and herbs, may be helpful. Examples of foods rich in phytoestrogens include carrots, yams, and soy products. Conversely, menopausal women should avoid foods that may trigger symptoms, including caffeine, alcohol, and spicy foods. Weight-bearing exercise, including such activities as walking, jogging, tennis, and running, is a means of increasing bone mass and potentiating the effect of estrogen on bone mass. Pelvic floor, or Kegel's, exercises can help maintain vaginal muscle tone and increase blood circulation to the perineal area. Vaginal lubricants and adequate foreplay can be helpful in maintaining a satisfactory sexual experience. Relaxation techniques, including yoga, meditation, deep breathing, visualization, massage, use of affirmations and biofeedback, may provide a sense of well-being. Herbal remedies—ginseng, for example—can help relieve the symptoms of hot flashes, headaches, fatigue, lack of concentration, decreased libido, and irregular menses. Additional herbal remedies are dong quai, black cohosh, damiana, golden seal, motherwort, licorice root, red raspberry leaves, sarsaparilla, and yerba buena. Other helpful therapies include homeopathy and acupuncture (Lichtman, 1996).

NURSING CARE MANAGEMENT

Menopausal women may need counseling to adjust successfully to this developmental phase of life. Reaction to menopause is determined to a large extent by the kind of life the woman has lived, by the security she has in her feminine identity, and by her feelings of self-worth and self-esteem.

Nurses and other health care professionals can help the menopausal woman achieve high-level functioning at this time in her life. Of paramount importance is the nurse's ability to understand and provide support for the woman's views and feelings. Whether the woman expresses relief and delight or tearfulness and fear, the nurse needs to use an empathetic approach in counseling, health teaching, or providing physical care. Touch and caring, as nursing measures, may enhance the self-actualization of both nurse and client.

Nurses should explore the question of the woman's comfort during sexual intercourse. In counseling, the nurse may say, "After menopause many women notice that their vagina seems drier, and intercourse can be uncomfortable. Have you noticed any changes?" This gives the woman information and may open discussion. The nurse can then go on to explain that the woman can address dryness and shrinking of the vagina by using a water-soluble jelly to help provide relief. Use of estrogen, orally or in vaginal creams, may also be indicated. Increased frequency of intercourse will maintain some elasticity in the vagina. When assessing the menopausal woman, the nurse should address the question of sexual activity openly but tactfully, because the woman may have been socialized to be reticent in discussing sex. Women who do not wish to become pregnant should be counseled to use a method of contraception for one year after her last menstrual period.

The crucial need of women in the perimenopausal period of life is for adequate information about the changes taking place in their bodies and their lives. Supplying that information provides both a challenge and an opportunity for nurses. ●

Care of the Woman with a Disorder of the Breast

Throughout her lifetime, a woman may experience a variety of breast disorders. Some, like mastitis, are acute disorders, whereas others, such as fibrocystic breast disease, are chronic. This section deals with some of the common breast disorders a woman may experience.

Benign Breast Disease

Fibrocystic breast disease, the most common of the benign breast disorders, is most prevalent in women 30 to 50 years of age. It is rare in postmenopausal women who are not taking hormone replacement therapy. Only women with fibrocystic breast disease who show atypical hyperplastic histologic changes (usually found incidentally when a biopsy is done) have an increased risk of developing cancer. Fibrocystic changes may produce an asymptomatic mass but more often are accompanied by pain or tenderness and sometimes nipple discharge. Fluctuation in size and rapid appearance or disappearance of breast masses are common. Cyclic breast pain is the most common symptom. The presence of estrogen seems necessary for the clinical symptoms to occur (Berek et al, 1996).

The woman often reports pain, tenderness, and swelling that occurs just before menses. Physical examination may reveal only mild signs of irregularity, or the breasts may feel dense, with areas of irregularity and nodularity. Women often refer to this as "lumpiness." Some women may also have expressible nipple discharge (Berek et al, 1996).

If the woman has a large, fluid-filled cyst, she may experience a localized painful area as the capsule containing the accumulated fluid distends coincident with her cycle. However, if small cysts form, the woman may experience not a solitary tender lump but a diffuse tenderness. Specific characteristics that differentiate a cyst from a cancerous lesion are mobility, tenderness, and the absence of skin retraction (pulling) in the surrounding tissue.

Mammography, sonography, palpation, and fine-needle aspiration are used to confirm fibrocystic breast disease. Often, fine-needle aspiration provides treatment as well as relief from the tenderness or pain. Treatment of palpable cysts is conservative. Invasive procedures such as biopsy are used only if the diagnosis is questionable.

Women with mild symptoms may benefit from restricting sodium intake and taking a mild diuretic during the week before the onset of menses. This counteracts fluid retention, relieves pressure in the breast, and helps decrease the pain. In other cases, a mild analgesic is necessary. Other treatment approaches include the use of thiamine and vitamin E. In severe cases, the hormone inhibitor danazol is the drug of choice.

Some researchers suggest that methylxanthines (found in caffeine products, such as coffee, tea, colas, chocolate, and some medications) may contribute to the development of fibrocystic breast changes and that limiting intake of these substances will help decrease fibrocystic changes. Other research fails to demonstrate a clear association between methylxanthines and fibrocystic breast changes. Additional medical therapies that are helpful in varying degrees include oral contraceptives, progestins, and bromocriptine. All work on the principle of estrogen suppression and progesterone stimulation or augmentation.

Fibroadenoma is a common benign tumor seen in women in their teens and early twenties. It has not been significantly associated with breast cancer. Fibroadenomas are freely movable, solid tumors that are well defined, sharply delineated, and rounded, with a rubbery texture. They are asymptomatic and nontender.

If there are any disquieting features to the appearance of a lump, fine-needle biopsy or excision of the mass may be indicated. Caution is exercised when deciding upon biopsy because excision of the mass in a young girl may interfere with normal breast development. Watchful observation and possible surgical excision are the only treatments for fibroadenomas. Surgery is often deferred. Surgical removal of the fibroadenoma, when advisable, concludes its treatment.

Intraductal papillomas are tumors growing in the terminal portion of a duct or, sometimes, throughout the duct system within a section of the breast. Symptoms may include a unilateral mass or a spontaneous nipple discharge. They are typically benign but have the potential to become malignant (Berek et al, 1996).

The majority of papillomas present as solitary nodules. These small ball-like lesions may be detected on mammography but often are nonpalpable. The presence of a papilloma is often frightening to the woman, because her primary symptom is a discharge from the nipple that may be serosanguineous or brownish-green due to old blood. The location of the papilloma within the duct system and its pattern of growth determine whether nipple discharge will be present. The lesion must be excised and histologically examined because of the difficulty in differentiating a benign papilloma from a papillary carcinoma. Treatment for benign intraductal papilloma is excision with follow-up care.

Nipple discharge is called **galactorrhea.** It may be physiologic (which is the case with fibrocystic breast disease), drug induced, idiopathic, or pathologic. Clear, milky, straw-colored, or greenish nipple discharge is usually associated with benign conditions, whereas serosanguineous and unilateral discharge is usually associated with malignant conditions. Regardless of its character, all

TABLE 3–3 Summary of Benign Breast Disorders

Condition	Age	Pain	Cancer Risk	Nipple Discharge	Location	Consistency and Mobility	Diagnosis and Treatment
Fibrocystic breast disease	30–50	Yes	Yes with proliferative disease and atypical hyperplasia	Varies: none at all or may be clear, milky, straw-colored, or green	Upper outer quadrant	Multiple lumps occurring bilaterally, influenced by menstrual cycle, nodular	Needle aspiration, Pap smear of nipple discharge, observation, biopsy if unresolved mass exists or mammographic changes, sonography
Fibroadenoma	15–25, median age 20	No	No	No, but milky discharge in pregnancy	Nipple or upper outer quadrant along the lateral side	Solid, well defined, sharply delineated, rounded, rubbery, mobile	Mammography, observation, surgical excision
Intraductal papilloma	Menopausal 50–60	Yes on palpation	Yes with multiple papillomas	Yes: serous, bloody, or brownish-green	No specific location	Nonpalpable or small, ball-like, poorly delineated	Pap smear of nipple discharge, mammography, ductogram, surgical excision
Duct ectasia	45–55	Yes: burning and itching around the nipple	No	Yes in perimenopausal women: thick, sticky, green, greenish-brown, or bloodstained	Mass behind or around the nipple	Poorly circumscribed, inflammation, nipple retraction, axillary lymph adenopathy	Pap smear of breast discharge, mammography, drug therapy for symptoms, surgical excision, observation

breast discharge should have a cytologic evaluation (Berek et al, 1996).

Duct ectasia (comedomastitis), an inflammation of the ducts behind the nipple, commonly occurs during or near the onset of menopause and is not associated with malignancy. The condition typically occurs in women who have borne and nursed children. It is characterized by a thick, sticky nipple discharge and by burning pain, pruritus, and inflammation. Nipple retraction may also be noted, especially in postmenopausal women. Treatment is conservative, with drug therapy aimed at symptomatic relief. The major central ducts of the breast occasionally have to be excised.

Table 3–3 provides a comparison of the most frequently seen benign breast disorders.

Malignant Breast Disease

Cancer of the breast affects one in eight women in the United States. It has a higher mortality rate in women than any other cancer (Spiegel, 1997). Predisposing factors include the following:

- Age—incidence increases steadily with age, especially after 50
- History of previous breast cancer
- Family history of mother or sister with bilateral premenopausal breast cancer
- High-fat diet
- Alcohol consumption (may increase the risk)
- No history of pregnancy
- Longer reproductive phase (early menarche and late menopause)
- Geographic location—high risk areas: North America, northern Europe; in the US, urban North; low-risk areas: Asia, Africa; in the US, rural south.

A malignant neoplasm may originate either in a duct or in the epithelium of the breast lobes. About 50% of breast cancers originate in the upper outer quadrant and spread or metastasize to the axillary lymph nodes. Common sites of distant metastasis are the lymph nodes, lungs, liver, brain, and bone.

As previously discussed, the neoplasm may be discovered by the woman herself or the clinician who palpates or observes an abnormality such as a mass, thickening, nodularity, skin dimpling, nipple retraction, or skin erosion. Routine mammography screening detects masses 2 to 3 years prior to clinical appearance. Other diagnostic modalities include fine-needle biopsy, ultrasonography, thermography, and magnetic resonance imaging (MRI). Biopsy is essential for a diagnosis. Once the diagnosis is made and lymph node involvement evaluated, clinical staging of the disease is determined and a treatment plan that coincides with the stage is initiated.

Surgical treatment used to consist of a mastectomy, which may or may not be followed by reconstructive surgery. More recently, lumpectomy and adjunctive therapy have become a more desirable treatment. Adjunctive therapy includes chemotherapy, radiation, and hormone therapy (Berek et al, 1996). Complementary therapies, such as herbal remedies, therapeutic touch, acupuncture, aromatherapy and massage, combined with the above-mentioned medical treatments are effective additions for many women.

When a woman is confronted with a breast cancer diagnosis, she must decide which therapy is worth what personal risk for her. Although prompt treatment is indicated, a second opinion is encouraged. The emotional feelings a woman experiences can range from fear of the loss of a body part, to fear of the ill effects of treatments, to fear of death. The nurse should encourage the woman to discuss her feelings and concerns, informing her of all procedures, their pros and cons, and alternative options. Family, friends, professionals, and support groups can make significant contributions to a woman's search for information, selection of treatment, and recovery.

For additional information on this important topic, refer to a medical-surgical text. Table 3–4 provides a resource guide about organizations that support cancer research and education.

The physician also felt the lump and thickening and now I'm waiting for my mammogram. In these few days, my thoughts and feelings have been a roller coaster. I'm 46 and I'm wondering if this is it. Am I dying? Now? I am afraid as I have not been afraid since one of our children was very ill. Try as I may to fill my head with other thoughts, it keeps slipping back to this.

NURSING CARE MANAGEMENT

Nursing Assessment and Diagnosis

During the period of diagnosis of any breast disease, the woman may be extremely anxious. The nurse can use therapeutic communication to assess the significance the woman places on her breasts; her current emotional status, coping mechanisms used during periods of stress, and knowledge and beliefs about cancer; and other variables that may influence her coping and adjustment.

Nursing diagnoses that may apply to a woman with a benign disorder of the breast include the following:

- ***Knowledge Deficit*** related to a lack of information about the diagnostic procedures
- ***Anxiety*** related to threat to body image or her life

Nursing Plan and Implementation

During the prediagnosis period, the nurse should clarify misconceptions and encourage the woman to express her anxiety. Once a diagnosis has been made, the nurse should ensure that the woman clearly understands her condition, its association to breast malignancy, and treatment options.

The nurse can also point out that frequent professional breast examinations and regular mammograms are tools that help detect any abnormalities and that the woman who practices monthly BSE, follows her caregiver's advice, and is examined regularly has taken positive action to protect her health.

The nurse can provide psychologic support for the woman with a troublesome diagnosis, supply her with client education materials, and refer her to professional support groups.

TABLE 3–4 Breast Cancer Resources

Organizations	Web Sites
National Cancer Institute (NCI) Cancer Information Service (CIS) 800-4-CAN-CER (800-422-6237)	http://cancernet.nci.nih.gov (produced jointly by the International Cancer Information Center, NCI, and the Office of Cancer Communication)
National Alliance of Breast Cancer Organizations (NABCO) 212-719-0154	http://oncolink.upenn.edu/ (University of Pennsylvania)
American Cancer Society (ACS) 800-227-2345	http://www.access.digex.net/~mkragen/index.html (sponsored by the National Coalition for Cancer Survivorship, a not-for-profit organization)
Susan G. Komen Breast Cancer Foundation 800-I'M AWARE (800-462-9273)	
Y-ME 800-221-2141 (9 to 5 PM CST) or 312-986-8228 (24 hours)	

Evaluation

Expected outcomes of nursing care include the following:

- The woman is able to discuss her fears, concerns, and questions during the period of diagnosis.
- The diagnosis is made quickly and accurately, and treatment initiated, if indicated. ●

Care of the Woman with Endometriosis

Endometriosis is a condition characterized by the presence of endometrial tissue outside the uterine cavity. It is estimated to occur in 7% of women of reproductive age in the United States (Berek et al, 1996). Endometriosis has been found almost everywhere in the body, including the vagina, lungs, cervix, central nervous system, and gastrointestinal tract. The most common location, however, is the pelvis. This tissue responds to the hormonal changes of the menstrual cycle and bleeds in a cyclic fashion. The bleeding results in inflammation, scarring of the peritoneum, and formation of adhesions.

Endometriosis may occur at any age after puberty, although it is most commonly diagnosed in women between ages 20 and 45 and is rare in postmenopausal women. The exact cause of endometriosis is unknown. Proposed causative factors include retrograde menstrual flow of the endometrium, hereditary tendency, and a possible immunologic defect (Corwin, 1997).

The most common symptom of endometriosis is pelvic pain, which is often dull or cramping. Usually the pain is related to menstruation and is thought to be dysmenorrhea by the affected woman. Dyspareunia (painful intercourse) and abnormal uterine bleeding are other common signs. The condition is often diagnosed when the woman seeks evaluation for infertility. Bimanual examination may reveal a fixed, tender, retroverted uterus and palpable nodules in the cul-de-sac. Diagnosis is confirmed by laparoscopy.

Treatment may be medical, surgical, or a combination of the two. During the laparoscopic examination, the physician may surgically resect any visible implants of endometrial tissue, taking care to avoid damaging any organs. Laser vaporization can be used for all but the deepest implants. This allows for more exact removal of tissue, less damage of adjacent tissue, and decreased bleeding. If the woman is experiencing severe dyspareunia or dysmenorrhea, the surgeon may perform a presacral neurectomy. In advanced cases in which childbearing is not an issue, treatment may be a hysterectomy with bilateral salpingo-oophrectomy. If the woman does not desire pregnancy at the present time, she may be started on oral contraceptives. In women with minimal disease and symptoms, treatment includes observation, analgesics, and nonsteroidal anti-inflammatory drugs (NSAIDs). The woman who desires pregnancy and has been unsuccessful in her attempts to conceive is often treated for a designated period of time with a medication that suppresses estrogen synthesis. This causes an atrophy of endometrial implants. Medications commonly used to treat endometriosis include oral contraceptives, progestins, antiprogestins, and gonadotropin-releasing hormones (GnRH).

Combined oral contraceptives (OCs) create a "pseudopregnancy" state that leads to decreased menstrual bleeding and possible amenorrhea. Treatment with OCs is cost effective and can relieve dysmenorrhea and pelvic pain.

Progestins such as medroxyprogesterone acetate (MPA) exert an antiendometriotic effect and ultimate atrophy. The medication is administered intramuscularly every 3 months and the effectiveness of the treatment evaluated every 3 to 6 months. Side effects may include nausea, weight gain, fluid retention, and breakthrough bleeding.

Danazol is an antiprogesterone treatment that is frequently used to treat endometriosis. It suppresses GnRH and has high androgen and low estrogen effects that do not support the growth of the endometrium. It suppresses ovulation and causes amenorrhea. Danazol does have some significant side effects, including hirsutism, vaginal bleeding, acne, oily skin, weight gain, reduced libido, voice changes and hoarseness, clitoral enlargement, and decreased breast size.

GnRH agonists, such as nafarelin acetate (given as a metered nasal spray twice daily) and leuprolide acetate (Lupron), (given once a month as an intramuscular injection), are gaining popularity because many women tolerate them better than danazol and their results in treating endometriosis are comparable. GnRH agonists suppress the menstrual cycle through estrogen antagonism. This may result in the hypoestrogen side effects of hot flashes, vaginal dryness, headache, breast reduction, and loss of bone density (Corwin, 1997).

NURSING CARE MANAGEMENT

Nursing Assessment and Diagnosis

The nurse should be aware of the common symptoms of endometriosis and elicit an accurate history if a woman mentions these symptoms. If a woman is being treated for endometriosis, the nurse should assess the woman's understanding of the condition, its implications, and the treatment alternatives.

Nursing diagnoses that may apply to a woman with endometriosis include the following:

- ***Pain*** related to peritoneal irritation secondary to endometriosis
- ***Ineffective Individual Coping*** related to depression secondary to infertility

Nursing Plan and Implementation

The nurse can be available to explain the condition, its symptoms, treatment alternatives, and prognosis. The nurse can help the woman evaluate treatment options and make appropriate choices. If the woman begins taking medication, the nurse can review the dosage, schedule, possible side effects, and any warning signs. Women are often advised to avoid delaying pregnancy because of the risk of infertility. The woman may wish to discuss the implications of this decision on her life choices, relationship with her partner, and personal preferences. The nurse can be a nonjudgmental listener and help the woman consider her options.

Evaluation

Expected outcomes of nursing care include the following:

- The woman is able to discuss her condition, its implications for fertility, and her treatment options.
- After considering the alternatives, the woman chooses appropriate treatment options. ●

Care of the Woman with Toxic Shock Syndrome (TSS)

Although **toxic shock syndrome (TSS)** has been reported in children, postmenopausal women, and men, it is primarily a disease of women in their reproductive years, especially women at or near menses or during the postpartum period. The causative organism is a strain of *Staphylococcus aureus*. As discussed earlier, the use of superabsorbent tampons has been widely related to an increased incidence of TSS. However, occluding the cervical os with a contraceptive device such as a diaphragm or cervical cap, especially if it is left in place for more than 48 hours, may also increase the risk of TSS (Hatcher et al, 1998).

Early diagnosis and treatment are important in preventing a fatal outcome. The most common signs of TSS include fever (often greater than 38.9 C, or 102 F); desquamation of the skin, especially the palms and soles, which usually occurs 1 to 2 weeks after the onset of symptoms; rash; hypotension; and dizziness. Systemic symptoms often include vomiting, diarrhea, severe myalgia, and inflamed mucous membranes (oropharyngeal, conjunctival, or vaginal). Disorders of the central nervous system, including alterations in consciousness, disorientation, and coma, may also occur.

Laboratory findings reveal elevated blood urea nitrogen (BUN), creatinine, SGOT, SGPT, and total bilirubin, while platelets are often less than 100,000/mm^3.

Women with TSS are generally hospitalized and given supportive therapy, including intravenous fluids to maintain blood pressure. Severe cases may require renal dialysis, administration of vasopressors, and intubation. Penicillinase-resistant antibiotics, while of limited value during the acute phase, do help reduce the risk of recurrence (Sweet & Gibbs, 1995).

NURSING CARE MANAGEMENT

Nurses play a major role in helping to educate women about ways to prevent the development of TSS. Women should understand the importance of avoiding prolonged use of tampons. They should change tampons every 3 to 6 hours and avoid using superabsorbent tampons. Some women may choose to use other products, such as sanitary pads or minipads. The woman who chooses to continue using tampons may reduce her risk by alternating them with pads and avoiding overnight use of tampons.

Postpartal women should avoid the use of tampons for 6 to 8 weeks after childbirth. Women with a history of TSS should never use tampons. Women who use diaphragms or cervical caps should not leave them in place for prolonged periods and should not use them during the postpartum period or when they are menstruating.

Nurses can also help make women aware of the signs and symptoms of TSS so that they can seek treatment promptly if symptoms occur. ●

Care of the Woman with a Vaginal Infection

Vulvovaginal Candidiasis

Vulvovaginal candidiasis (VVC) is also called moniliasis or yeast infection. It is estimated that in their lifetime, 75% of women will have at least one episode of yeast vulvovaginitis, with 40% to 45% having two or more episodes (CDC, 1998). *Candida albicans* is responsible for 85% to 90% of vaginal yeast infections. Other candida species such as *C glabrata* and *C tropicalis*, can cause vulvovaginal symptoms and tend to be resistant to therapy. Predisposing factors to yeast infections include glycosuria, use of oral contraceptives, use of antibiotics, pregnancy, diabetes mellitus, and immunosuppressants.

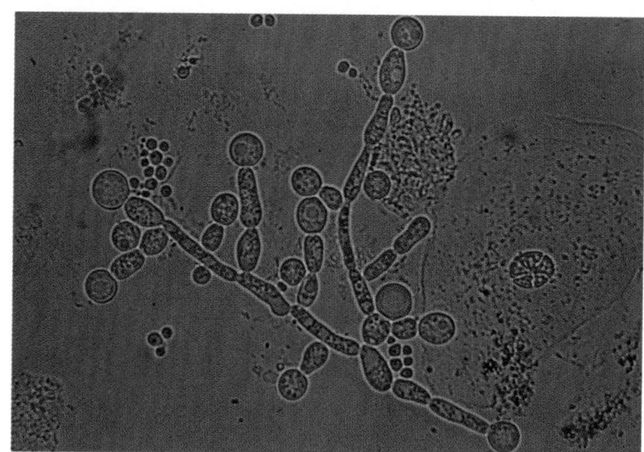

FIGURE 3–10 Hyphae and spores of *Candida albicans.*

The woman often complains of thick, curdy vaginal discharge, severe itching, dysuria, and dyspareunia. A male sexual partner may experience a rash or excoriation of the skin of the penis, and possibly pruritus. The male may be symptomatic and the female asymptomatic.

On physical examination, the woman's labia may be swollen and excoriated if pruritus has been severe. A speculum examination reveals thick, white, tenacious, cheeselike patches adhering to the vaginal mucosa. The diagnosis is made by observing mycelia or pseudohyphae upon direct microscopy in a 10% potassium hydroxide (KOH) preparation (Figure 3–10). A Gram stain or culture positive for the fungus is a more accurate way of diagnosing the causative organism. The pH of the vagina remains 4.5 or less (the normal pH of the vagina is about 4.5).

Medical treatment of VVC includes a single oral dose of 150 mg fluconazole or intravaginal insertion of butoconazole, clotrimazole, miconazole, nystatin, terconazole, or tioconazole suppositories or cream at bedtime for 3 days to 1 week (CDC, 1998). Women with severe symptoms who are treated with oral fluconazole may need a repeat dose in 4 days (Mead, 1998). If the vulva is also infected, the cream is applied topically. Some of these medications are available over the counter. They are indicated for women with a history of yeast infections who clearly recognize the symptoms (Sweet & Gibbs, 1995).

Topical miconazole usually eliminates the yeast infection from the male. However, the CDC states that treatment of the male partner is not necessary unless candidal balanitis (inflammation of the glans penis) is present (CDC, 1998).

If a woman experiences frequent recurrences of monilial vaginitis, she should be tested for an elevated blood glucose level to determine whether a diabetic or prediabetic condition is present. Women at high risk for sexually transmitted infections should also be tested for HIV infection. Pregnant women are treated the same as nonpregnant women (CDC, 1993). Infection at the time of birth may cause thrush (a mouth infection) in the newborn.

NURSING CARE MANAGEMENT

Nursing Assessment and Diagnosis

The nurse caring for the woman should suspect VVC if the woman complains of intense vulvar itching and a curdy, white discharge. Because pregnant women with diabetes mellitus are especially susceptible to this infection, the nurse should be alert for symptoms in these women. In some areas nurses are trained to do speculum examinations and wet-mount preparations and can confirm the diagnosis themselves. In most cases, however, the nurse who suspects a vaginal infection reports it to the woman's health care provider.

Nursing diagnoses that might apply to the woman with VVC include the following:

- ***Risk for Impaired Skin Integrity*** related to scratching secondary to discomfort of the infection
- ***Knowledge Deficit*** related to lack of information about ways of preventing the development of VVC

Nursing Plan and Implementation

If the woman is experiencing discomfort because of pruritus, the nurse can recommend gentle bathing of the vulva with a weak sodium bicarbonate solution. If a topical treatment is being used, the woman will need to bathe the area before applying the medication.

The nurse also discusses with the woman the factors that contribute to the development of VVC and suggests ways to prevent recurrences, such as wearing cotton underwear and avoiding vaginal powders or sprays that may irritate the vulva. Some women report that adding yogurt to the diet or using activated culture of plain yogurt as a vaginal douche helps prevent recurrence by maintaining high levels of lactobacillus.

Evaluation

Expected outcomes of nursing care include the following:

- The woman's symptoms are relieved, and the infection is cured.
- The woman is able to identify self-care measures to prevent further episodes of VVC. ●

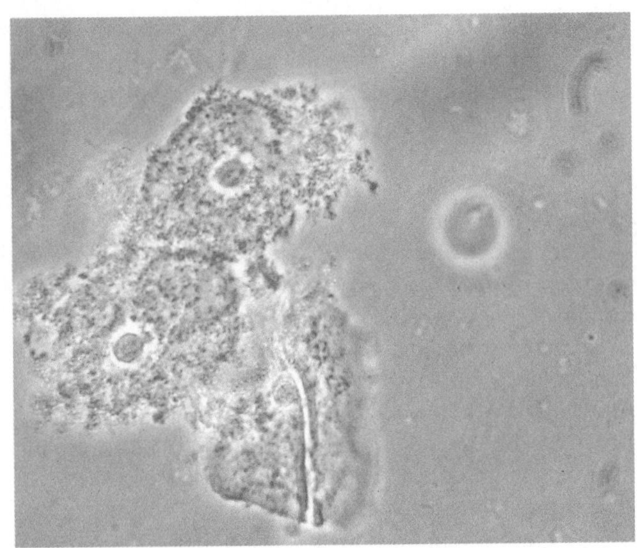

FIGURE 3–11 The characteristic "clue cells" seen in bacterial vaginosis.

Care of the Woman with a Sexually Transmitted Infection

The occurrence of **sexually transmitted infection (STI),** or *sexually transmitted disease (STD),* has increased over the past few decades. In fact, vaginitis and sexually transmitted infections are the most common reasons for outpatient, community-based treatment of women. More than one STI can occur at the same time. All symptomatic women should be tested for other infections.

Bacterial Vaginosis (BV)

Bacterial vaginosis (BV), a sexually associated condition, was formerly referred to as nonspecific vaginitis or *Gardnerella* vaginitis. It is an alteration of normal vaginal bacterial flora that results in the loss of hydrogen-peroxide-producing lactobacilli and an overgrowth of predominantly anaerobic bacteria. Anaerobic bacteria can be found in less than 1% of the flora of normal women. In women with BV, the concentration of anaerobes is 100 to 1000 times higher. Lactobacilli are usually absent (Berek et al, 1996). The cause of this overgrowth is not clear, although sexual intercourse and trauma from douching are sometimes identified as contributing factors. The *Gardnerella vaginalis* and *Mycoplasma hominis* organisms have been found in the vast majority of cases, along with an increased concentration of anaerobic bacteria.

The infected woman often notices an excessive amount of thin, watery, yellow-gray vaginal discharge with a foul odor described as "fishy." The characteristic "clue" cells are seen on a wet-mount preparation, and leukocytes are conspicuously absent (Figure 3–11). The addition of KOH to the vaginal secretions (the "whiff" test) releases a fishy, amine-like odor. The vaginal pH is usually greater than 4.5. Women with BV have an in-

DRUG GUIDE: METRONIDAZOLE (FLAGYL)

Overview of Action

Metronidazole is an antiprotozoal and antibacterial agent. It possesses direct trichomonacidal and amebicidal activity against *T vaginalis* and *E histolytica*. Metronidazole is active in vitro against most obligate anaerobes but does not appear to possess any clinically relevant activity against facultative anaerobes or obligate aerobes. It is used in the treatment of various infections caused by organisms that are sensitive to this drug. It is used predominantly to treat the following infections in women: *T vaginalis,* bacterial vaginosis, endometritis, endomyometritis, tubo-ovarian abscess, and postsurgical vaginal cuff infection.

Route, Dosage, Frequency

Trichomoniasis—1-day treatment: 2 g orally in a single dose; 7-day treatment: 500 mg orally twice a day for 7 consecutive days (CDC, 1998).
Amebiasis—Adults: 750 mg orally three times a day for 5–10 days; children: 35–50 mg/kg/24 hours orally divided into three doses for 10 days.
Bacterial vaginosis—500 mg orally twice a day for 7 consecutive days (CDC, 1998).

Contraindications

First trimester of pregnancy
Breastfeeding women (drug secreted in breast milk)
Impaired kidney or liver function

Side Effects

Convulsive seizures
Peripheral neuropathy
Nausea/Vomiting
Headache
Weakness
Insomnia
Cystitis
Dysuria
Anorexia
Diarrhea
Epigastric distress
Abdominal cramping
Constipation
Metallic taste in mouth
Dizziness
Vertigo
Uncoordination
Ataxia
Confusion
Irritability
Reversible neutropenia and thrombocytopenia
Flattening of the T wave on ECG
Polyuria
Incontinence
Pelvic pressure
Proliferation of *Candida* in the vagina and mouth
Joint pains
Decreased libido
Dryness in the mouth, vulva, and vagina
Dyspareunia
Depression

Nursing Considerations

1. Inform woman about potential side effects.
2. Rule out first trimester pregnancy, and stress the importance of contraceptive compliance during course of treatment.
3. Obtain baseline renal and liver function tests as ordered.
4. Teach woman about the signs, symptoms, and treatment of vulvovaginal candidiasis.
5. Counsel the woman to avoid alcoholic beverages while taking the medication.
6. If the woman is taking oral contraceptives, a backup nonhormonal contraceptive method is recommended during treatment.
7. Take thorough history to rule out the woman's exposure to this medication within the last 6 weeks.
8. Teach woman to monitor the signs and symptoms of her infection.
9. Encourage cooperation with the entire course of treatment.

creased risk of pelvic inflammatory disease (PID), abnormal cervical cytology, postoperative cuff infections after hysterectomy, and postabortion PID. Pregnant women with BV are at risk for premature rupture of membranes, preterm labor, chorioamnionitis and postcesarean endometritis (Berek et al, 1996).

The nonpregnant woman is generally treated with metronidazole (Flagyl) or clindamycin (Cleocin) orally or via vaginal cream (Table 3–5). Because of its potential teratogenic effects, metronidazole is avoided during the first trimester of pregnancy; one full applicator of clindamycin is inserted intravaginally at bedtime instead. Women at high risk for preterm labor should be screened for BV in the second trimester and treated if BV is present. During the second and third trimesters, oral metronidazole or clindamycin or vaginal metronidazole gel can be used (CDC, 1998). Treatment of the male partner has not been shown to improve therapeutic response and therefore is not recommended (Mead, 1998).

Trichomoniasis

Trichomonas vaginalis is a microscopic motile protozoan that thrives in an alkaline environment. The parasite is an anaerobe that has the ability to generate hydrogen, which combines with oxygen to create an anaerobic environment. Most infections are acquired through sexual intimacy. Transmission by shared bath facilities, wet towels, or wet swimsuits may also be possible (CDC, 1998).

Often women with trichomoniasis are asymptomatic or have only mild symptoms. More pronounced symptoms of trichomoniasis may include a yellow-green, frothy, odorous discharge and vulvar itching. The woman may also complain of dysuria and dyspareunia. Occasionally, subepithelial hemorrhages on the cervix (strawberry-like red spots) can be seen with the naked eye; smaller areas of hemorrhage are generally visible with a colposcope. Microscopy visualization of mobile trichomonads and increased leukocytes, a vaginal pH of 4.5 or higher,

TABLE 3–5 Summary of Sexually Transmitted Infections

Disease	Organism	Diagnosis	Treatment: Nonpregnant	Treatment: Pregnant
Vulvovaginal candidiasis	*Candida albicans*	Wet-mount hyphae	Topically applied azole drugs	Topically applied azole drugs
Bacterial vaginosis	*Gardnerella vaginalis* and *Mycoplasma hominis*	Wet-mount clue cells	Metronidazole	Metronidazole after 1st trimester
Trichomoniasis	*Trichomonas vaginalis*	Wet-mount trichomonads	Metronidazole	Metronidazole after 1st trimester
Syphilis	*Treponema pallidum*	Dark-field examination VDRL, RPR, or MHA-TP	Benzathine Penicillin G	Benzathine Penicillin G
Herpes genitalis	Herpes simplex virus	Herpes culture or titre	Acyclovir	None
Chlamydia	*Chlamydia trachomatis*	Chlamydia culture	Doxycycline	Erythromycin base
Gonorrhea	*Neisseria gonorrhoeae*	Gonorrhea culture	Ceftriaxone and doxycycline	Ceftriaxone and erythromycin
Acquired immunodeficiency syndrome	Human immunodeficiency virus	ELISA test and Western blot	Varies	Varies
Genital warts	Human papilloma virus	Virapap, biopsy, Pap smear, colposcopy	Cryotherapy Podophyllum, podofilox	Cryotherapy Trichloracectic acid
Pediculosis pubis	*Phthirus*	Microscopic identification of lice or nits	Permethrin 1% creme rinse or lindane 1% shampoo	Permethrin 1% creme rinse
Scabies	*Sarcoptes scabiei*	Confirmation of symptoms or scraping of furrows	Lindane 1% lotion or permethrin 5% cream	Crotamiton 10% lotion or permethrin 5% cream

and a positive whiff test are diagnostic of *T. vaginitis* (Figure 3–12). Pregnant women with trichomoniasis may be at increased risk for premature rupture of membranes and preterm birth (CDC, 1998).

Treatment for trichomoniasis is metronidazole (Flagyl) administered in a single 2 g dose or 500 mg twice daily for 7 days for both male and female sexual partners. Partners should avoid intercourse until both are cured (CDC, 1998). The woman should be informed that metronidazole is contraindicated in the first trimester of pregnancy because of possible teratogenic effects on the fetus. However, no other adequate treatment exists. For women with severe symptoms after the first trimester, treatment with 2 g metronidazole in a single dose may be considered (CDC, 1998). The woman and her partner should be cautioned to avoid alcohol while taking metronidazole; the combination has an effect similar to that of alcohol and Antabuse—abdominal pain, nausea, flushing, or tremors.

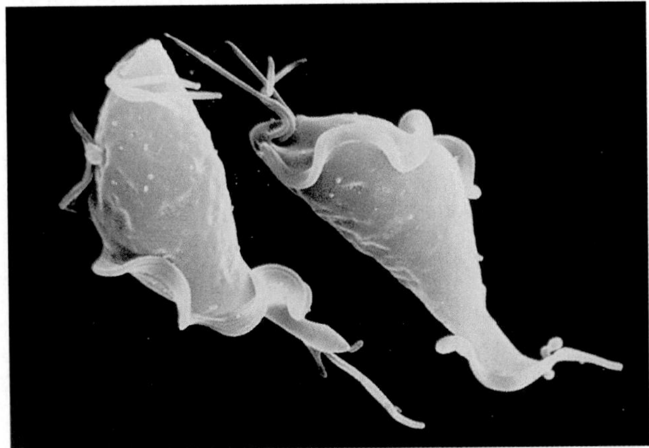

FIGURE 3–12 Microscopic appearance of *Trichomonas vaginalis.*

Chlamydial Infection

Chlamydial infection, caused by *Chlamydia trachomatis*, is the most common STI in the United States. The organism is an intracellular bacterium with several different immunotypes. Immunotypes of chlamydia are responsible for lymphogranuloma venereum and trachoma, which is the world's leading cause of preventable blindness.

Chlamydia is a major cause of nongonococcal urethritis (NGU) in men. In women it can cause infections similar to those that occur with gonorrhea. It can infect the fallopian tubes, cervix, urethra, and Bartholin's glands. Pelvic inflammatory disease, infertility, and ectopic pregnancy are associated with chlamydia. In the United States, newborn exposure to chlamydia in the birth canal of the mother at birth is the most common cause of ophthalmia neonatorum (CDC, 1998). This chlamydial conjunctivitis responds to erythromycin ophthalmic ointment but not to silver nitrate eye prophylaxis. The newborn may also develop chlamydial pneumonia.

Asymptomatic infection is common in both women and men. Symptoms of chlamydia include a thin or mucopurulent discharge, cervical ectopia, friable cervix, burning and frequency of urination, and lower abdominal pain. Women, however, are often asymptomatic. The gold standard diagnostic test for chlamydia has been a culture of cervical cells. More recently, antigen detection, DNA probe assays, and polymerase chain reaction tests have become widely available. Diagnosis is frequently made after treatment of a male partner for NGU or in a symptomatic woman with a negative gonorrhea culture.

The recommended treatment is azithromycin or doxycycline. Sexual partners should also be treated and the couple should abstain from intercourse for 7 days, the course of therapy. Doxycycline and azithromycin are contraindicated during pregnancy. Pregnant women should be treated with erythromycin ethylsuccinate or amoxicillin, although neither is highly effective (CDC, 1998).

Gonorrhea

Gonorrhea is an infection caused by the bacterium *Neisseria gonorrhoeae.* If a nonpregnant woman contracts the disease, she is at risk of developing pelvic inflammatory disease. If a pregnant woman becomes infected after the third month of gestation, the mucous plug in the cervix will prevent the infection from ascending, and it will remain localized in the urethra, cervix, and Bartholin's glands until the membranes rupture. Then it can spread upward. A newborn exposed to a gonococcal-infected birth canal is at risk of developing ophthalmia neonatorum. Eye prophylaxis for all newborns is provided to prevent this complication.

The majority of women with gonorrhea are asymptomatic. Thus it is accepted practice to screen for this infection by doing a cervical culture during the initial prenatal examination. For women at high risk, the culture may be repeated during the last month of pregnancy. Cultures of the urethra, throat, and rectum may also be required for diagnosis, depending on the body orifices used for intercourse.

The most common symptoms of gonorrheal infection include a purulent, greenish-yellow vaginal discharge, dysuria, and urinary frequency. Some women also develop inflammation and swelling of the vulva. The cervix may appear swollen and eroded and may secrete a foul-smelling discharge in which gonococci are present.

Treatment for nonpregnant women consists of antibiotic therapy with ceftriaxone administered intramuscularly and doxycycline or azithromycin administered orally. This combined approach provides dual treatment for gonorrhea and chlamydia because the two infections frequently occur together. Oral doses of ofloxacin, cefixime, and ciprofloxacin are also used to treat *N gonorrhoeae.* Additional treatment may be required if the cultures remain positive 7 to 14 days after completion of treatment. All sexual partners must also be treated, or the woman may become reinfected. Pregnant women should be treated with a recommended cephalosporin, usually ceftriaxone intramuscularly or cefixime orally. This is combined with erythromycin or amoxicillin to address the risk of co-infection with chlamydia (CDC, 1998).

Women should be informed of the need for reculture to verify cure and the need for abstinence or condom use until cure is confirmed. Both sexual partners should be treated if either has a positive test for gonorrhea.

Herpes Genitalis

Herpes infections are caused by the herpes simplex virus (HSV). Two serotypes of HSV cause human infections: HSV-1 and HSV-2. HSV-2 causes most cases of recurrent genital herpes. The clinical symptoms and treatment of both types are the same. At least 45 million people in the United States have been diagnosed with genital HSV-2 infection (CDC, 1998).

The primary episode of herpes genitalis is characterized by the development of single or multiple blisterlike vesicles, which usually occur in the genital area and sometimes affect the vaginal walls, cervix, urethra, and anus. The vesicles may appear within a few hours to 20 days after exposure and rupture spontaneously to form very painful, open, ulcerated lesions. Inflammation and pain secondary to the presence of herpes lesions can cause difficult urination and urinary retention. Enlargement of the inguinal lymph nodes may be present. Flulike symptoms and genital pruritus or tingling also may be noticed. Primary episodes usually last the longest and are the most severe. Lesions heal spontaneously in 2 to 4 weeks.

After the lesions heal, the virus enters a dormant phase, residing in the nerve ganglia of the affected area. Some individuals never have a recurrence, whereas others have regular recurrences. Recurrences are usually less severe than the initial episode and seem to be triggered by emotional stress, menstruation, ovulation, pregnancy, frequent or vigorous intercourse, poor health status or a generally run-down physical condition, tight clothing, or overheating. Diagnosis is made on the basis of the clinical appearance of the lesions, Pap smear or culture of the lesions, and sometimes blood testing for antibodies.

No known cure for herpes exists. Medications are available to provide relief from pain and prevent complications from secondary infection. The recommended treatment of the first clinical episode of genital herpes is oral acyclovir, valacyclovir, or famciclovir. These same medications, in somewhat different dosages, are also recommended for recurrent herpes infection and for daily suppressive therapy for people who have frequent recurrences. Therapy should be started during the prodromal period for the greatest benefit. Acyclovir should not be used during pregnancy because its safety has not been established (CDC, 1998).

Self-care suggestions include cleansing with povidone-iodine (Betadine) solution to prevent secondary infection and with Burow's solution to relieve discomfort. Use of vitamin C or lysine is frequently suggested to prevent recurrence, although studies have not documented the effectiveness of these supplements. Keeping the genital area clean and dry, wearing loose clothing, and wearing cotton underwear or none at all will promote healing. Primary or recurrent lesions will heal without treatment.

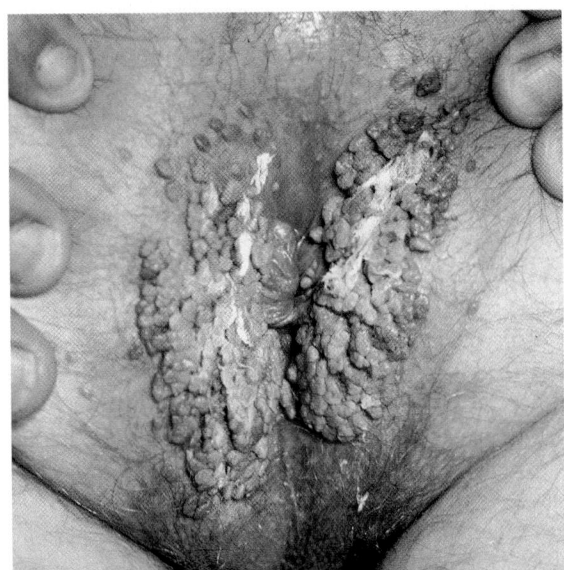

FIGURE 3–13 Condylomata acuminata on the vulva.

If herpes is present in the genital tract of a woman during childbirth, it can have a devastating, even fatal, effect on the newborn. See Chapter 16 for more detail.

> *I've finally come to terms with my herpes. Yes, it's a pain. Yes, I wish I had been more careful. But it's just a virus, an infection. Having herpes doesn't make me a bad person, it doesn't define who I am. I do that by the way I live my life.*

Syphilis

Syphilis is a chronic infection caused by the spirochete *Treponema pallidum*. Syphilis can be acquired congenitally through transplacental inoculation and can result from maternal exposure to infected exudate during sexual contact or from contact with open wounds or infected blood. The incubation period varies from 10 to 90 days, and even though no symptoms or lesions are noted during this time, the woman's blood contains spirochetes and is infectious.

Syphilis is divided into early and late stages. During the early stage (primary), a chancre (painless ulcer) appears at the site where the *Treponema pallidum* organism entered the body. Symptoms include slight fever, loss of weight, and malaise. The chancre persists for about 4 weeks and then disappears. In 6 weeks to 6 months, secondary symptoms appear. Skin eruptions called condylomata lata, which resemble wartlike plaques and are highly infectious, may appear on the vulva. Other secondary symptoms are acute arthritis, enlargement of the liver and spleen, nontender enlarged lymph nodes, iritis, and a chronic sore throat with hoarseness. Transplacentally transmitted syphilis may cause intrauterine growth restriction, preterm birth, and stillbirth.

As a result of the disease's impact on the fetus in utero, serologic testing of every pregnant woman is recommended; some state laws require it. Testing is done at the initial prenatal screening and repeated in the third trimester. Blood studies may be negative if blood is drawn too early in the pregnancy.

During the early primary stage, the diagnosis is made by dark-field microscopic examination of the chancre for spirochetes. Blood tests such as VDRL (Venereal Disease Research Laboratories), RPR (Rapid Plasma Reagin), or the more specific FTA-ABS (fluorescent treponemal antibody absorption test) are commonly done.

For pregnant and nonpregnant women with syphilis of less than a year's duration, the CDC (1998) recommend 2.4 million units of benzathine penicillin G intramuscularly. If syphilis is of long duration (more than 1 year), 2.4 million units of benzathine penicillin G is given intramuscularly once a week for 3 weeks. If a woman is allergic to penicillin, and nonpregnant, doxycycline or tetracycline can be given. The pregnant woman who is allergic to penicillin should be desensitized to penicillin (CDC, 1998). Maternal serologic testing may remain positive for 8 months, and the newborn may have a positive test for 3 months.

Condylomata Acuminata (Venereal Warts)

Condylomata acuminata, also called venereal warts, are a relatively common, sexually transmitted infection caused by the human papilloma virus (HPV). Because of the increasing evidence of a link between HPV and cervical cancer, the condition is receiving increasing attention.

Often a woman seeks medical care after noticing single or multiple soft, grayish-pink, cauliflowerlike lesions in her genital area (Figure 3–13). The moist, warm environment of the genital area is conducive to the growth of the warts, which may be present on the vulva, vagina, cervix, and anus. The incubation period following exposure is 3 weeks to 3 years.

Because condylomata sometimes resemble other lesions and may become cancerous, all atypical, pigmented, and persistent warts should be biopsied and treatment instituted promptly. Diagnosis is usually made by visual appearance. Subclinical diagnosis can be made if characteristic changes are present on a Pap smear.

The CDC does not specify a treatment of choice for genital warts but recommends that treatment be determined based on client preference, available resources, and experience of the health care provider. Client-applied therapies include podofilox solution or gel or imiquimod cream. Provider-administered therapies include cryotherapy with liquid nitrogen or cryoprobe; topical podophyllin; trichloroacetic acid (TCA); bichloroacetic acid (BCA); intralesional interferon; surgical removal by tangential scissor excision, shave excision, or curettage; or laser surgery (CDC, 1998). Imiquimod, podophyllin, and podofilox are not used during pregnancy because they are thought to be teratogenic and in large doses have been associated with fetal death.

Women with HPV infections should have frequent Pap smears to monitor cervical cellular changes. Sex partners are probably infected and do not require treatment unless large exophytic lesions are present. The use of condoms may reduce the risk of transmitting the virus to an uninfected partner.

Pediculosis Pubis (Pubic or Crab Lice)

Pediculosis pubis is caused by *Phthirus*, a grayish, parasitic "crab" louse that lays eggs that attach to the hair shaft. Transmission is primarily by sexual contact, although shared towels and bed linens are also possible sources.

Symptoms include itching, usually in the pubic area. It is treated by applying 1% permethrin creme rinse to the affected area for 10 minutes, plus combing the pubic hair with a fine-toothed comb. Over-the-counter medications can also be used. Retreatment may be necessary. Both partners must be treated and tested for other sexually transmitted infections.

Scabies

Sarcoptes scabiei is an ectoparasitic itch mite. The female mite burrows under the skin to deposit her eggs. Transmission is by intimate sexual contact and contact with household members.

Symptoms include itching that worsens at night or when the individual is warm. Noticeable erythematous, papular lesions or furrows may be present. Prescriptive treatment is 1% lindane (Kwell) lotion applied and then washed off after 8 hours. Permethrin 5% is used in pregnant women. Clothing and bed linens should be washed and dried in a hot dryer or dry cleaned.

Acquired Immunodeficiency Syndrome (AIDS)

Acquired immunodeficiency syndrome (AIDS) is a fatal disorder caused by the human immunodeficiency virus (HIV), which may be transmitted sexually. A medical-surgical text will more fully describe this condition. However, because the diagnosis of HIV/AIDS or the presence of the HIV antibody has implications for a fetus if the woman is pregnant, HIV/AIDS is discussed in greater detail in Chapter 15.

NURSING CARE MANAGEMENT

Nursing Assessment and Diagnosis

The nurse working with women must become adept at taking a thorough history and identifying women at risk for sexually transmitted infections. Risk factors include multiple sexual partners; a partner's involvement with other partners; high-risk sexual behaviors, such as intercourse without barrier contraception or anal intercourse; partners with high-risk behaviors; treatment with antibiotics while taking oral contraceptives; and young age at onset of sexual activity. The nurse should be alert for signs and symptoms of STI and be familiar with diagnostic procedures if it is suspected.

While each STI has certain distinctive characteristics, the following complaints suggest the possibility of infection and warrant further investigation:

- Presence of a "sore" or lesion on the vulva
- Increased vaginal discharge or malodorous vaginal discharge
- Burning with urination
- Dyspareunia
- Bleeding after intercourse
- Pelvic pain

In many instances the woman is asymptomatic but may report symptoms in her partner, especially painful urination or urethral discharge. It is often helpful to ask the woman whether her partner is experiencing any symptoms.

Nursing diagnoses that may apply to a woman with a sexually transmitted infection include the following:

- ***Altered Family Processes*** related to the effects of a diagnosis of sexually transmitted infection on the couple's relationship
- ***Knowledge Deficit*** related to lack of information about the long-term effects of the diagnosis on childbearing status

Nursing Plan and Implementation

In a supportive, nonjudgmental way, the nurse provides the woman who has a sexually transmitted infection with information about the infection, methods of transmission, implications for pregnancy or future fertility, and importance of thorough treatment. If treatment of her partner is indicated, the woman must understand that it is necessary to prevent a cycle of reinfection. She should also understand the need to abstain from sexual activity, if necessary, during treatment.

Some STIs, such as trichomoniasis or chlamydia, may cause a woman concern but, once diagnosed, are rather simply treated. Other STIs may also be fairly simple to treat medically but may carry a stigma and be emotionally devastating for the woman. Thus the nurse should stress prevention with all women and encourage them to require partners, especially new partners, to use a condom.

The sensitive nurse can be especially helpful in encouraging the woman to explore her feelings about the diagnosis. She may experience anger or feel "betrayed" by a partner; she may feel guilt or see her diagnosis as a form of "punishment"; or she may feel concern about the long-term implications for future childbearing or ongoing intimate relationships. She may experience a myriad of emotions that she never expected. Opportunities to discuss her feelings in a nonjudgmental environment can be especially helpful. The nurse can offer suggestions

TABLE 3–6 General Client Teaching About Sexually Transmitted Infections

- The risk of contracting a sexually transmitted infection increases with the number of sexual partners. Because of the extended periods of time between infection with the HIV virus and evidence of infection, intercourse with an individual exposes a woman or man to all the other sex partners of that individual for the past 5 or more years.
- The condom is the best contraceptive method currently available (other than abstinence) for protection from sexually transmitted infections.
- Other contraceptive methods such as the diaphragm, cervical cap, and spermicides also offer some protection against sexually transmitted infections.
- A person diagnosed with a sexually transmitted infection has a responsibility to notify any sexual partners so they can obtain treatment.
- Absence of symptoms or disappearance of symptoms does not mean that treatment is unnecessary if a person suspects a sexually transmitted infection. She or he should be seen for evaluation and treatment. All prescribed medications should be taken completely.
- The presence of a genital infection may lead to an abnormal Pap smear result. Women with certain infections should have more frequent Pap smears according to a schedule recommended by their caregiver.

about support groups, if indicated, and assist the woman in planning for her future with regard to sexual activity.

More subtly, the nurse's attitude of acceptance and matter-of-factness conveys to the woman that she is still an acceptable person who happens to have an infection. Table 3–6 provides a summary of basic information the nurse should share with women who have an STI. STIs that can have an impact on pregnancy or the fetus/neonate are discussed in Chapter 16.

Evaluation

Expected outcomes of nursing care include the following:

- The infection is identified and cured, if possible. If not, supportive therapy is provided.
- The woman and her partner can describe the infection, its method of transmission, its implications, and the therapy.
- The woman copes successfully with the impact of the diagnosis on her self-concept. ●

Care of the Woman with Pelvic Inflammatory Disease

Pelvic inflammatory disease (PID) occurs in approximately 1% of women between ages 15 and 39, although sexually active young women between 15 and 24 have the highest infection rate. The disease is more common in women who have had multiple sexual partners, a history of PID, early onset of sexual activity, a recent gynecologic procedure, or an intrauterine device. It usually produces a tubal infection (salpingitis) that may or may not be accompanied by a pelvic abscess. However, perhaps the greatest problem of PID is postinfection tubal damage, which is closely associated with infertility.

CRITICAL THINKING IN PRACTICE

CW is a 21-year-old, single woman, G0P0, who comes to the office today complaining of excessive, odorous vaginal discharge. She uses an IUD for contraception and has several sex partners. She states that she douches with a medicated douche after intercourse. What should you tell CW about feminine hygiene? What would you tell CW about the relationship between contraceptives and sexually transmitted infections?

Answers can be found in Appendix I.

The organisms most frequently identified with PID include *Chlamydia trachomatis* and *Neisseria gonorrhoeae.* Bacterial vaginosis may facilitate the ascending spread of pathogens. Other aerobic and anaerobic organisms that are often part of the normal vaginal flora have also been found in women with PID (Berek et al, 1996).

Symptoms of PID include bilateral sharp, cramping pain in the lower quadrants, fever, chills, purulent vaginal discharge, irregular bleeding, malaise, nausea, and vomiting. However, it is also possible to be asymptomatic and have normal laboratory values.

Diagnosis consists of a clinical examination to define symptoms, plus blood tests and a gonorrhea culture and test for chlamydia. Physical examination usually reveals direct abdominal tenderness with palpation, adnexal tenderness, and cervical and uterine tenderness with movement (Chandelier sign). A palpable mass is evaluated with ultrasonography. Laparoscopy may be used to confirm the diagnosis and to enable the examiner to obtain cultures from the fimbriated ends of the fallopian tubes.

Except in mild cases, the woman is hospitalized and treated with intravenous administration of cefoxitin sodium, cefotetan disodium, or clindamycin plus gentamicin. Outpatient therapy usually includes antibiotics such as cefoxitin, ceftriaxone, doxycycline, and clindamycin used singly or in combination. A new antibiotic, ofloxacin (Floxin), is now available for women with PID caused by chlamydia or gonorrhea. Ofloxacin, taken twice daily for 10 to 14 days, has a 98% cure rate ("A Simpler Cure," 1997). In addition, supportive therapy is often indicated for severe symptoms. The sexual partner should also be treated. If the woman has an IUD, it is generally removed 24 to 48 hours after antibiotic therapy is started.

NURSING CARE MANAGEMENT

Nursing Assessment and Diagnosis

The nurse is alert to factors in a woman's history that put her at risk for PID. Even though fewer types of IUDs are available, many women still have them, and the nurse

TABLE 3–7 The Bethesda System (TBS) for Classifying Pap Smears

Adequacy of the Specimen

Satisfactory for evaluation

Satisfactory for evaluation but limited by. . .(specify reason)

Unsatisfactory for evaluation

General Categorization (optional)

Within normal limits

Benign cellular changes (See descriptive diagnoses.)

Epithelial cell abnormality (See descriptive diagnoses.)

Descriptive Diagnoses

- Benign cellular changes
  - Infection
    - *Trichomonas vaginalis*
    - Fungal organisms morphologically consistent with *Candida* spp
    - Predominance of coccobacilli consistent with shift in vaginal flora
    - Bacteria morphologically consistent with *Actinomyces* spp
    - Cellular changes associated with herpes simplex virus
    - Other
- Reactive changes
  - Reactive cellular changes associated with:
    - Inflammation (includes typical repair)
    - Atrophy with inflammation ("atrophic vaginitis")
    - Radiation
    - Intrauterine contraceptive device (IUD)
    - Other

Reactive changes *continued*

- Epithelial cell abnormalities
  - Squamous cell
    - Atypical squamous cells of undetermined significance (ASCUS): Qualify*
    - Low-grade squamous intraepithelial lesion (SIL) encompassing HPV[†] mild dysplasia/CIN 1
    - High-grade squamous intraepithelial lesion encompassing: Moderate and severe dysplasia, CIS/CIN 2 and CIN 3
    - Squamous cell carcinoma
  - Glandular cell
    - Endometrial cells, cytologically benign, in a postmenopausal woman
    - Atypical glandular cells of undetermined significance: Qualify*
    - Endocervical adenocarcinoma
    - Endometrial adenocarcinoma
    - Extrauterine adenocarcinoma
    - Adenocarcinoma, not otherwise specified
  - Other malignant neoplasms: Specify
    - Hormonal evaluation (applies to vaginal smears only)
    - Hormonal pattern compatible with age and history
    - Hormonal pattern incompatible with age and history: Specify
    - Hormonal evaluation not possible due to: Specify

*Atypical squamous or glandular cells of undetermined significance should be further qualified as to whether a reactive or a premalignant/malignant process is favored.

[†]Cellular changes of human papillomavirus (HPV)—previously termed koilocytosis, koilocytotic atypia, or condylomatous atypia—are included in the category of low-grade squamous intraepithelial lesion.

should question the woman about possible symptoms, such as aching pain in the lower abdomen, foul-smelling discharge, malaise, and the like. The woman who is acutely ill will have obvious symptoms, but a low-grade infection is more difficult to detect.

Nursing diagnoses that may apply to a woman with PID include the following:

- ***Pain*** related to peritoneal irritation
- ***Knowledge Deficit*** related to a lack of information about the possible effects of PID on fertility

Nursing Plan and Implementation

The nurse plays a vital role in helping to prevent or detect PID. Accordingly, the nurse spends time discussing risk factors related to this infection. The woman who uses an IUD for contraception and has multiple sexual partners needs to understand clearly the risk she faces. The nurse discusses signs and symptoms of PID and stresses the importance of early detection.

The woman who develops PID needs to understand the importance of completing her antibiotic treatment and of returning for follow-up evaluation. She should also understand that one outcome of the infection may be decreased fertility.

Evaluation

Expected outcomes of nursing care include the following:

- The woman describes her condition, her therapy, and the possible long-term implications of PID on her fertility.
- The woman completes her course of therapy and the PID is cured. ●

Care of the Woman with an Abnormal Finding During Pelvic Examination

Abnormal Pap Smear Results

The Bethesda System (TBS) has become the most widely used system in the United States for reporting Pap smear results. The new system was established to provide a uniform format and classification of terminology based on current understanding of cervical disease (Isacson & Kurman, 1995). Early detection of abnormalities allows early changes to be treated before cells reach the precancerous or cancerous stage (Table 3–7).

Notification of an abnormal Pap smear may cause anxiety for the woman, so it is important that she be told in a caring way and then given accurate and complete information about the meaning of the results and about the next steps to be taken. She should also be given time to ask questions and express her concerns.

Diagnostic or therapeutic procedures employed in cases of cellular abnormalities include repetition of Pap smears at shorter intervals, colposcopy and endocervical biopsy, cryotherapy, laser conization, or large loop excision of the transformation zone (LLETZ). Decisions for management are based on the specific report.

Colposcopy has evolved as an appropriate "second step" in many cases of abnormal Pap smear result. The examination, typically done in an office or clinic, permits more detailed visualization of the cervix in bright light, using a microscope with 6 to 40 times magnification. The cervix can be visualized directly and again following application of 3% acetic acid. The acetic acid causes abnormal epithelium to assume a characteristic white appearance. The colposcope can be used to localize and obtain a "directed biopsy." Histologic examination of tissue taken via a biopsy is necessary for a diagnosis.

Women who had first coitus at an early age or have a history of, or a sex partner with a history of, multiple sexual partners, exposure to STIs, immunosuppressive therapy, or antenatal exposure to diethylstilbestrol (DES) have an increased risk of abnormal cell changes and cervical cancer.

Abnormal Uterine Bleeding

During the many years of a woman's reproductive period, she is likely to experience some form of abnormal uterine bleeding. It may occur as spotting between periods, missing several cycles followed by a heavy bleed, or menses that occur every 2 to 3 months. Heavy, unpredictable menstrual periods can cause a woman to experience fatigue, anemia, and embarrassment. Abnormal bleeding may be a symptom that accompanies infertility.

Dysfunctional uterine bleeding (DUB) is characterized by anovulatory cycles with abnormal uterine bleeding that does not have a demonstratable organic cause. Oligomenorrhea, polymenorrhea, menorrhagia, metrorrhagia, menometrorrhagia and intermenstrual bleeding are all forms of DUB. DUB can occur at any age but is most common at either end of the reproductive age span. Adolescents account for 20% of DUB cases due to hypothalmic immaturity after menarche. Perimenopausal women account for 50% of cases due to waning ovarian function. The remaining cases occur among women of reproductive age, generally as a result of polcystic ovary syndrome, hyperprolactinemia, or hypothalmic dysfunction.

The diagnosis is made by excluding organic causes. Laboratory evaluation should include a Pap smear, thyroid function studies, pregnancy test, and possible endometrial biopsy. Additional tests may include ultrasonography, hysteroscopy, adrenal studies, liver function studies, or coagulation studies. The goals of treatment are to control bleeding, prevent or treat anemia, prevent endometrial hyperplasia or cancer, and restore quality of life. Pharmacologic treatment for women who desire a pregnancy such as clomiphene citrate or gonadotropins can be used to induce ovulation. Normal menses should occur after an ovulatory cycle. Conjugated estrogens and synthetic progestins are used in varying doses and regimens to control and regulate the bleeding (Mehring, 1997).

Abnormal bleeding, with or without ovulation, that is caused by organic problems is generally classified as either a systemic or reproductive disorder. Systemic diseases that cause abnormal uterine bleeding include thyroid dysfunction, coagulation disorders, and cirrhosis. Reproductive tract diseases that cause bleeding problems include the following (Mehring, 1997):

- Abnormal pregnancy, such as threatened, missed or incomplete abortion, ectopic pregnancy, or gestational trophoblastic disease
- Endometrial, cervical, or ovarian cancer
- Uterine lesions, such as submucous fibroids, endometrial polyps, or adenomyosis
- Cervical lesions, such as polyps, cervicitis, herpes, or chlamydia

Ovarian Masses

Between 70% and 80% of ovarian masses are benign. More than 50% are functional cysts, occurring most commonly in women 20 to 40 years of age. Functional cysts are rare in women who take oral contraceptives.

Ovarian cysts usually represent physiologic variations in the menstrual cycle. Dermoid cysts (cystic teratomas) comprise 10% of all benign ovarian masses. Cartilage, bone, teeth, skin, or hair can be observed in these cysts. Endometriomas, or "chocolate cysts," are another common type of ovarian mass.

No relationship exists between ovarian masses and ovarian cancer. In reality, ovarian cancer is the most fatal of all cancers in women because it is difficult to diagnose and often has spread throughout the pelvis before it is detected.

A woman with an ovarian mass may be asymptomatic; the mass may be noted on a routine pelvic examination. She may experience a sensation of fullness or cramping in the lower abdomen (often unilateral), dyspareunia, irregular bleeding, or delayed menstruation.

Diagnosis is made on the basis of a palpable mass with or without tenderness and other related symptoms. Radiography or ultrasonography may be used to assist or confirm the diagnosis.

The woman is frequently kept under observation for a month or two because most cysts will resolve on their own and are harmless. Oral contraceptives may be prescribed for 1 to 2 months to suppress ovarian function. If this regimen is effective, a repeat pelvic examination should yield normal findings. If the mass is still present after 60 days of observation and oral contraceptive therapy, a diagnostic laparoscopy or laparotomy may be considered. Tubal or ovarian lesions, ectopic pregnancy, cancer, infection, or appendicitis also must be ruled out before a diagnosis can be confirmed.

Surgery is not always necessary but will be considered if the mass is larger than 6 to 7 cm in circumference; if the woman is over 40 years of age with an adnexal mass, a persistent mass, or continuous pain; or if the woman is taking oral contraceptives. Surgical exploration is also indicated when a palpable mass is found in an infant, a young girl, or a postmenopausal woman. Women may need clear explanations about why the initial therapy is observation. A discussion of the origin and resolution of ovarian cysts may clarify this treatment plan. If a surgical treatment removes or impairs the function of one ovary, the woman needs to be assured that the remaining ovary can be expected to take over ovarian functioning and that pregnancy is still possible.

Women who are taking oral contraceptives should be informed of their preventive effect against ovarian masses.

Uterine Masses

Fibroid tumors, or leiomyomas, are among the most common benign disease entities in women and are the most common reason for gynecologic surgery. Between 20% and 50% of women develop leiomyomas by 40 years of age. The potential for cancer is minimal. Leiomyomas are more common in women of African heritage.

Fibroid tumors develop when smooth muscle cells are present in whorls and arise from uterine muscles and connective tissue. The size varies from 1 to 2 cm to the size of a 10-week fetus. Frequently the woman is asymptomatic. Lower abdominal pain, fullness or pressure, menorrhagia, metrorrhagia, or increased dysmenorrhea may occur, particularly with large leiomyomas. Ultrasonography revealing masses or nodules can assist and confirm the diagnosis. Leiomyoma is also considered a possible diagnosis when masses or nodules involving the uterus are palpated on a pelvic examination.

The majority of these masses require no treatment and will shrink after menopause. Close observation for symptoms or an increase in size of the uterus or the masses may be the only management most women will require. Routine pelvic examinations every 3 to 6 months are recommended unless new symptoms appear.

If a woman notices symptoms, or pelvic examination reveals that the mass is increasing in size, surgery (myomectomy, D & C, or hysterectomy) will be recommended. The route of surgery is typically via an abdominal incision; however, a laparoscopic procedure may be considered. The mass can be excised or ablated. The choice of surgery depends on the age and reproductive status of the woman and the significance of the noted changes. There are no medications or therapies to prevent fibroids. The use of GnRH agonists results in a 40% to 60% decrease in uterine volume. It may be helpful to shrink the fibroid prior to surgery, especially with a laparoscopic procedure (Berek et al, 1996).

Endometrial cancer, most commonly a disease of postmenopausal women, has a high rate of cure if detected early. The hallmark sign is vaginal bleeding in postmenopausal women not treated with hormone replacement therapy. Diagnosis is made by endometrial biopsy or posthysterectomy pathologic examination of the uterus. The treatment is total abdominal hysterectomy (TAH) and bilateral salpingo-oophorectomy. Radiation therapy may also be indicated, depending on the staging of the cancer.

NURSING CARE MANAGEMENT

Only nurses with special training perform pelvic examinations and Pap smears. In most cases, nursing assessment is directed toward evaluating the woman's understanding of the findings and their implications and her psychosocial response.

The woman needs accurate information on the etiology of the disorder, its symptoms, and treatment options. She should be encouraged to report symptoms and keep appointments for follow-up examination and evaluation. The woman needs realistic reassurance if her condition is benign; she may require counseling and effective emotional support if a malignancy is likely. If the management plan includes surgery, she may need the nurse's support in obtaining a second opinion and making her decision. ●

Care of the Woman with a Urinary Tract Infection

A urinary tract infection (UTI) may be life-threatening or a mere inconvenience. Bacteria usually enter the urinary tract by way of the urethra. The organisms are capable of migrating against the downward flow of urine. The shortness of the female urethra facilitates the passage of bacteria into the bladder. Other conditions that are associated with bacterial entry are relative incompetence of the urinary sphincter, frequent enuresis (bedwetting) before adolescence, and urinary catheterization. Wiping from back to front after urination may transfer bacteria from the anorectal area to the urethra.

Voluntarily suppressing the desire to urinate is also a predisposing factor. Retention overdistends the bladder and can lead to an infection. There also seems to be a relationship between recurring UTI and sexual intercourse. General poor health or lowered resistance to infection can increase a woman's susceptibility to UTI.

Asymptomatic bacteriuria (ASB), bacteria in the urine actively multiplying without accompanying clinical symptoms, constitutes about 6% to 8% of UTIs. This becomes especially significant if the woman is pregnant. Between 20% and 30% of pregnant women with untreated ASB will develop cystitis or pyelonephritis. Asymptomatic bacteriuria is almost always caused by one organism.

TABLE 3–8 Measures for Preventing Cystitis

If you use a diaphragm for contraception, try changing methods or using another size diaphragm.
Avoid bladder irritants, such as alcohol, caffeine products, and carbonated beverages.
Increase fluid intake, especially water, to a minimum of six to eight glasses per day.
Make regular urination a habit; avoid long waits.
Practice good genital hygiene, including wiping from front to back after urination and bowel movements.
Be aware that vigorous or frequent sexual activity may contribute to urinary tract infection.
Urinate before and after intercourse to empty the bladder and cleanse the urethra.
Complete medication regimens even if symptoms decrease.
Do not use medication left over from previous infections.
Drink cranberry juice to acidify the urine. This has been found to relieve symptoms in some cases.

If more than one type of bacteria are cultured, the possibility of urine-culture contamination must be considered. The most common cause of ASB is *Escherichia coli.* Other commonly found causative organisms include *Klebsiella* and *Proteus.*

A woman who has had a UTI is susceptible to recurrent infection. If a pregnant woman develops an acute UTI, especially with a high temperature, amniotic fluid may become infected and retard the growth of the placenta (Sweet & Gibbs, 1995).

UTIs are more frequently encountered in pregnant women in part because of dramatic physiologic changes. Muscle tone and activity of the ureter decreases, resulting in reduced passage of urine through the urinary system. The bladder experiences decreased tone, increased capacity, and incomplete emptying. Urinary pH is elevated along with glycogen levels. All of these changes contribute to the increased risk for urinary tract disorders. Pregnant women must be monitored for UTIs throughout the pregnancy in order to prevent ascending renal infections. Treatment in pregnant women includes amoxicillin, nitrofurantoin, cephalexin, trimethoprim-sulfamethoxazole and sulfisoxazole (Sweet & Gibbs, 1995).

Lower Urinary Tract Infection (Cystitis and Urethritis)

Because urinary tract infections ascend, it is important to recognize and diagnose a lower UTI early to avoid the sequelae associated with upper UTI. One common lower UTI is cystitis, or infection of the urinary bladder. Several factors place a woman at increased risk for cystitis, including sexual intercourse, the use of a diaphragm and a spermicide, delayed postcoital micturition, and a history of a recent UTI.

E coli is present in 80% of women with UTIs. *Staphylococcus saprophyticus, Klebsiella, Proteus, Enterobacter,* and *Pseudomonas* are also causative pathogens. Infections without bacteriuria may indicate urethritis and are usually caused by *C trachomatis, N gonorrhoeae* and herpes simplex.

When cystitis develops, the initial symptoms are often acute and include dysuria, specifically at the end of urination. Urgency and frequency along with suprapubic or low back pain also occurs. Cystitis is usually accompanied by a low-grade fever (38.3 C, or 101 F, or lower), and hematuria is occasionally seen. Urine specimens often contain an abnormal number of leukocytes and bacteria. Urethritis symptoms usually have a gradual onset and are associated with a cervicitis or vulvovaginal herpetic lesion.

The diagnosis can be made with a urine culture. Bacteriuria dipstick screening tests are quick office screening tests; however, they have high false-positive and false-negative rates (Sweet & Gibbs, 1995). The treatment depends on the causative pathogen. Oral trimethoprim-sulfamethoxazole, fluoroquinolones, and fomycin tromethamine are frequently used in single-dose, 3-day, and 7-day regimens.

NURSING CARE MANAGEMENT

Nursing Assessment and Diagnosis

During each visit, the nurse notes any complaints from the woman of pain on urination or other urinary difficulties. If any concerns arise, the nurse obtains a clean-catch urine specimen from the woman.

Nursing diagnoses that may apply to a woman with a lower UTI include the following:

- ***Pain*** related to dysuria secondary to the urinary tract infection
- ***Knowledge Deficit*** related to a lack of information about self-care measures to help prevent recurrence of UTI

Nursing Plan and Implementation

Most bacteria enter through the urethra after having spread from the anal area. Therefore, the nurse should make sure the woman is aware of good hygiene practices and provide information on other ways to avoid cystitis (Table 3–8). The nurse should also reinforce instructions or answer questions regarding the prescribed antibiotic, the amount of liquids to take, and the reasons for these treatments. Cystitis usually responds rapidly to treatment, but follow-up urinary cultures are important.

Evaluation

Expected outcomes of nursing care include the following:

- The woman implements self-care measures to help prevent cystitis as part of her personal routine.
- The woman can identify the signs, symptoms, therapy, and possible complications of cystitis.
- The woman's infection is cured. ●

Upper Urinary Tract Infection (Pyelonephritis)

Pyelonephritis (inflammatory disease of the kidneys) is less common but more serious than cystitis and is often preceded by lower UTI. It is more common during the latter part of pregnancy or early postpartum and poses a serious threat to maternal and fetal well-being. Women with symptoms of pyelonephritis during pregnancy have an increased risk of preterm birth and intrauterine growth retardation.

Acute pyelonephritis has a sudden onset with chills, high temperature of 39.6 to 40.6 C (103 to 105 F), and flank pain (either unilateral or bilateral). The right side is almost always involved if the woman is pregnant because the large bulk of intestines to the left pushes the uterus to the right, putting pressure on the right ureter and kidney. Nausea, vomiting, and general malaise may ensue. With accompanying cystitis, the woman may experience frequency, urgency, and burning with urination.

Edema of the renal parenchyma or ureteritis with blockage and swelling of the ureter may lead to temporary suppression of urinary output. This is accompanied by severe colicky (spastic, intense) pain, vomiting, dehydration, and ileus of the large bowel. The woman with acute pyelonephritis will generally have increased diastolic blood pressure, positive fluorescent antibody titer (FA-test), low creatinine clearance, significant bacteremia in urine culture, pyuria, and presence of white blood cell casts.

Often the woman is hospitalized and started on intravenous antibiotics. In the case of obstructive pyelonephritis, a blood culture is necessary. The woman is kept on bed rest. After the sensitivity report is received, the antibiotic is changed as necessary. If signs of urinary obstruction occur or continue, the ureter may be catheterized to establish adequate drainage.

Intravenous treatment options include ampicillin plus gentamicin, ceftriaxone, trimethoprim-sulfamethoxazole, aztreonam, and cefazolin (Sweet & Gibbs, 1995). With appropriate drug therapy, the woman's temperature should return to normal. The pain subsides, and the urine shows no bacteria within 2 to 3 days. Follow-up urinary cultures are needed to determine that the infection has been eliminated completely.

NURSING CARE MANAGEMENT

Nursing Assessment and Diagnosis

During the woman's visit, the nurse obtains a sexual and medical history to identify whether she is at risk for UTI. A clean-catch urine specimen is evaluated for evidence of ASB.

Nursing diagnoses that may apply to a woman with an upper urinary tract infection include the following:

- ***Knowledge Deficit*** related to lack of information about the disease and its treatment
- ***Fear*** related to the possible long-term effects of the disease

Nursing Plan and Implementation

The nurse provides the woman with information to help her recognize the signs of UTI so that she can contact her caregiver as soon as possible. The nurse also discusses hygiene practices, the advantages of wearing cotton underwear, and the need to void frequently to prevent urinary stasis.

The nurse stresses the importance of maintaining a good fluid intake. Drinking cranberry juice daily and taking 500 mg vitamin C help acidify the urine and may help prevent recurrence of infection. Women with a history of UTI find it helpful to drink a glass of fluid before sexual intercourse and to void afterward.

Evaluation

Expected outcomes of nursing care include the following:

- The woman completes her prescribed course of antibiotic therapy.
- The woman's infection is cured.
- The woman incorporates preventive self-care measures into her daily regimen. ●

Pelvic Relaxation

A cystocele is the downward displacement of the bladder, which appears as a bulge in the anterior vaginal wall. Arbitrary classifications of mild to severe are frequently given. Genetic predisposition, childbearing, obesity, and increased age are factors that may contribute to cystocele.

Symptoms of stress incontinence are most common, including loss of urine with coughing, sneezing, laughing, or sudden exertion. Vaginal fullness, a bulging out of the vaginal wall, or a dragging sensation may also be noticeable.

If pelvic relaxation is mild, Kegel exercises are helpful in restoring tone. The exercises involve contracting and relaxing the pubococcygeal muscle. Women have found these exercises helpful before and after childbirth in maintaining vaginal muscle tone. Estrogen may improve the condition of vaginal mucous membranes—especially in menopausal women. Vaginal pessaries or rings may be used if surgery is undesirable or impossible, or until surgery can be scheduled. Surgery may be considered for cystoceles considered moderate to severe.

The nurse may instruct the woman in the use of Kegel exercises. Providing information on causes and contributing factors and discussing possible alternative therapies will greatly assist the woman.

COMMUNITY IN FOCUS

Urinary Incontinence Program

Urinary incontinence is a far more widespread problem than most people realize. Ten percent to 30% of women age 15 to 64 experience it; at least one-third of healthy women over age 65 who dwell in the community are bothered by it; and over 50% of nursing home residents have some form of it. In the US, excluding nursing homes, incontinence costs at least $11.2 billion. In fact, the market for incontinence pads is larger than the market for disposable baby diapers. At this time, no third party payors cover the cost of incontinence pads, so the expense is borne totally by the women themselves. Beyond the expense, however, the figures fail to capture the frustration and embarrassment incontinence can cause and the ways it can negatively impact women who wish to lead active lives.

One nurse practitioner in Chester, Pennsylvania, has established a program to help women overcome the problem. In private practice with two gynecologists, Anne Nichols, MSN, CRNP sees a variety of women, ranging in age from 15 to 102, who are troubled by incontinence. The first step in determining an appropriate treatment regimen for these women is to identify the type of incontinence they are experiencing: stress incontinence, urge incontinence, functional incontinence, or overflow incontinence. Once the type is identified, treatment modalities are discussed with the client, who is an integral part of the decision because she is the one who has to commit to the therapy.

For most women, three simple dietary changes are part of therapy: eliminating caffeine, artificial sweetener, and alcohol. Other interventions may include establishment of a good bowel routine, pelvic floor muscle strengthening exercises (Kegel exercises), biofeedback, urge inhibition techniques, and use of mechanical devices such as a pessary or a reliance device (a form of urethral "plug," which is used during specific activities such as a volleyball game or tennis match, when leakage is most troublesome). For some women, surgery is indicated, and Anne refers them as necessary.

After 3 months of therapy, about 84% of clients report significant improvement in their incontinence. To spread the word about the incontinence treatment program, Anne does community programs on a regular basis, speaking at senior citizen centers and hospitals or to women's groups. She also works with nurses at local clinics, encouraging them to ask every woman about the problem of incontinence.

Incontinence is an invisible problem—seldom spoken of, with little research being done about it. Programs such as this one are greatly needed and are being developed throughout the country. They can make a difference in the quality of life for many women.

SOURCE: Personal communication with Anne Nichols, MSN, CRNP.

FOCUS YOUR STUDY

- Nurses should provide girls and women with clear information about menstrual issues, such as the use of pads and tampons (including warnings regarding deodorant and absorbency); vaginal spray and douching practices; and self-care comfort measures during menstruation, such as maintaining good nutrition, exercising, and applying heat and massage.
- Dysmenorrhea usually begins at, or a day before, the onset of menses and disappears by the end. Hormone therapy (eg, oral contraceptives), nonsteroidal anti-inflammatory drugs, or prostaglandin inhibitors can alleviate dysmenorrhea. Self-care measures include improving nutrition, exercising, applying heat, and getting extra rest.
- Premenstrual syndrome occurs most often in women over 30. Symptoms occur 2 to 3 days before onset of menstruation and subside as menstruation starts, with or without treatment. Medical management usually includes progesterone agonists and prostaglandin inhibitors. Self-care measures include improving nutrition (taking vitamin B complex and E supplements and avoiding methylxanthines, which are found, for example, in chocolate and caffeine), undertaking a program of aerobic exercise, and participating in self-care support groups.
- Fertility awareness methods are "natural," noninvasive methods of contraception often used by people whose religious beliefs prevent their using other methods.
- Mechanical contraceptives such as the diaphragm, cervical cap, and condom act as barriers to prevent the transport of sperm. These methods are used in conjunction with a spermicide.
- The IUD is a mechanical contraceptive. Although its exact method of action is not clearly understood, research suggests it acts by immobilizing sperm or by impeding the progress of sperm from the cervix to the fallopian tubes. In addition, the IUD does have a local inflammatory effect.
- Oral contraceptives (the "pill") are combinations of estrogen and progesterone. When taken correctly, they are the most effective of the reversible methods of fertility control.
- Spermicides are far less effective in preventing pregnancy when they are not used with a barrier method.
- Permanent sterilization is accomplished by tubal ligation for women and vasectomy for men. Although theoretically reversible, clients are advised that the method should be considered irreversible.
- The breasts function in a cyclic process that is regulated by the nervous and hormonal systems. Many women experience breast tenderness and swelling premenstrually.
- Recommendations about the frequency of screening mammograms vary somewhat: the American Cancer Society recommends screening mammograms annually from age 40; the National Cancer Institute recommends mammograms every 1 to 2 years between ages 40 and 49, and annually for all women ages 50 and older.
- Menopause is a physiologic, maturational change in a woman's life. Physiologic changes include the cessation of menses and a decrease in circulating hormones. Hormonal changes sometimes bring unsettling emotional responses. The more common physiologic symptoms are "hot flashes," palpitations, dizziness, and increased perspiration at night.

The woman's anatomy also undergoes changes, such as atrophy of the vagina, reduction in size and pigmentation of the labia, and myometrial atrophy. Osteoporosis becomes an increasing concern.

- Current management of menopause centers around hormone replacement therapy, complementary therapies, and client health care education.
- In fibrocystic breast disease (FBD), the cysts tend to be round, mobile, and well delineated. The woman generally experiences increased discomfort premenstrually. Because of the increased risk of breast cancer, women with FBD should understand the importance of monthly breast self-examination (BSE).
- Galactorrhea should be evaluated with cytologic testing.
- Breast cancer has a higher mortality rate for women than any other cancer. Biopsy is essential for a diagnosis, and prompt treatment is critical.
- Endometriosis is a condition in which endometrial tissue occurs outside the endometrial cavity. This tissue bleeds in a cyclic fashion in response to the menstrual cycle. The bleeding leads to inflammation, scarring, and adhesions. The prime symptoms include dysmenorrhea, dyspareunia, and infertility.
- Treatment of endometriosis may be medical, surgical, or a combination. For the woman not desiring pregnancy at present, oral contraceptives are used. Women desiring pregnancy are treated with danazol.
- Toxic shock syndrome, caused by a toxin of *Staphylococcus aureus*, is most common in women of childbearing age. There is an increased incidence in women who use tampons or barrier methods of contraception, such as the diaphragm and cervical cap, especially if the woman leaves them in place for extended periods of time.
- Abnormal uterine bleeding can occur with or without organic pathology. Treatment is geared toward controlling bleeding, preventing anemia, and detecting pathology.
- Vulvovaginal candidiasis (moniliasis), a vaginal infection caused by *Candida albicans*, is most common in women who use oral contraceptives, are taking antibiotics, are currently pregnant, or have diabetes mellitus. It is generally treated with intravaginal miconazole or clotrimazole suppositories.
- Bacterial vaginosis (*Gardnerella vaginalis* vaginitis), a common vaginal infection, is diagnosed by its characteristic fishy odor and by the presence of "clue" cells on a vaginal smear. It is treated with metronidazole unless the woman is in the first trimester of pregnancy.
- Chlamydial infection is difficult to detect in a woman but may result in PID and infertility. It is treated with antibiotic therapy.
- Herpes genitalis, caused by the herpes simplex virus, is a recurrent infection with no known cure. Acyclovir (Zovirax) may reduce the symptoms.
- Syphilis, caused by *Treponema pallidum*, is a sexually transmitted infection that is treatable if diagnosed. The characteristic lesion is the chancre. Syphilis can also be transmitted in utero to the fetus of an infected woman. The treatment of choice is penicillin.
- Gonorrhea, a common sexually transmitted infection, may be asymptomatic in women initially but may cause PID if not diagnosed early. The treatment of choice is penicillin.
- Condylomata acuminata (venereal warts) are transmitted by the human papilloma virus (HPV). Treatment is indicated, because research suggests a possible link with abnormal cervical changes. The treatment chosen depends on the size and location of the warts.
- Pelvic inflammatory disease may be life threatening and may lead to infertility.
- Women with an abnormal finding on a pelvic examination will need careful explanation of the finding and techniques of diagnosis and emotional support during the diagnostic period.
- The classic symptoms of a lower UTI are dysuria, urgency, frequency, and sometimes hematuria. Oral sulfonamides are the treatment of choice except in middle to late pregnancy.
- An upper UTI is a serious infection that can permanently damage the kidneys if untreated. Generally the woman is acutely ill and may require supportive therapy as well as antibiotics.
- A cystocele is a downward displacement of the bladder into the vagina. Often it is accompanied by stress incontinence. Kegel exercises may help restore tone in mild cases.

REFERENCES

A simpler cure for pelvic infections (1997, April). *Health*, 18.

Andrews, W. C. (1995). Continuous combined estrogen/progestin hormone replacement therapy. *Nurse Practitioner*, (Suppl. 2), 1.

Barbieri, R. L. (1998). Seven steps to the effective treatment of osteoporosis in your practice. *Contemporary OB/GYN*, *43*(2), 30–48.

Berek, J. S. (Ed.), Adashi, E. Y., & Hillard, P. A. (Assoc. Eds.) (1996). *Novak's gynecology* (12th ed.). Baltimore: Williams & Wilkins.

Byyny, R. L., & Speroff, L. (1996). *A clinical guide for the care of older women: Primary and preventive care* (2nd ed.). Baltimore: Williams & Wilkins.

Centers for Disease Control and Prevention (1998). 1998 sexually transmitted disease treatment guidelines. *Morbidity and Mortality Weekly Report*, *47*(RR-1), 1–116.

Corwin, E. J. (1997). Endometriosis: Pathophysiology, diagnosis, and treatment. *The Nurse Practitioner*, *22*(10), 35–51.

Ellertson, C., Koenig, J., Trussell, J., & Bull, J. (1997). How many U.S. women need emergency contraception? *Contemporary OB/GYN*, *42*(10), 103–128.

Hanson, V. (1996). Facing facts on emergency postcoital contraception. *Contemporary OB/GYN*, *41*(6), 31–52.

Hatcher, R. A., Trussell, J., Stewart, F., Cates, W. Jr., Stewart, G. K., Guest, F., & Kowal, D. (1998). *Contraceptive technology*, 17 ed. New York: Ardent Media, Inc.

Isacson, C., & Kurman, R. J. (1995). The Bethesda System: A new classification for managing Pap smears. *Contemporary OB/GYN*, *40*(6), 67–74.

Kaunitz, A., & Jordon, C. (1997). Two long acting hormonal contraceptive options. *Contemporary Nurse Practitioner*, *2*(2), 10.

Kessenich, C. R. (1996). Update on pharmacologic therapies for osteoporosis. *Nurse Practitioner*, *21*(8), 19–24.

Kjos, S. L. (1997). Contraception for women at risk: A case for the intrauterine device. *Contemporary OB/GYN*, *42*(11), 105, 107, 110.

Kupecz, D. (1996). Alendronate for the treatment of osteoporosis. *Nurse Practitioner*, *21*(1), 86.

Lichtman, R. (1996). Perimenopausal and postmenopausal hormone replacement therapy. Part 2. Hormonal regimens and complementary and alternative therapies. *Journal of Nurse-Midwifery, 41*(3), 195–210.

Mead, P. B. (1998). Vaginitis 1998: Update and guidelines. *Contemporary OB/GYN, 43*(1), 116–132.

Mehring, P. (1997). Dysfunctional uterine bleeding. Evaluating this common complaint. *Advance for Nurse Practitioners, 5*(11), 26–28, 31–32.

McPhillips, K. J. (1997). FDA approves more effective Pap test. *Lifelines, 1*(5), 17–18.

Nelson, A. (1995). Patient selection key to IUD success. *Contemporary OB/GYN, 40*(10), 49–62.

Rabin, D. S. (1998). Understanding why women won't take HRT. *Contemporary OB/GYN, 43*(1), 133–137.

Salvatori, R., & Levine, M. (1998). Bisphosphonates for treating and preventing osteoporosis. *Contemporary OB/GYN, 43*(4), 105–120.

Speroff, L. (1998). A quarter century of contraception: Remarkable advances, increasing success. *Contemporary OB/GYN, 43*(5), 13–28.

Spiegel, K. K. (1997). On your markers. Research advances in breast cancer in women. *AWHONN Lifelines, 1*(5), 33–38.

Sweet, R. L., & Gibbs, R. S. (1995). *Infectious diseases of the female genital tract* (3rd ed.). Baltimore: Williams & Wilkins.

Taubes, G. (1997, April). NCI reverses one expert panel, sides with another. *Science, 276*(5309), 27–28.

Weber, E. S. (1997). Questions & answers about breast cancer diagnosis. *American Journal of Nursing, 97*(10), 34–38.

Westermann, C. (1997). Pharmacology and selection of postmenopausal estrogen replacement therapy: The argument for more physiologic agents. *The Female Patient, 22*(6), 15–22.

Wysocki, S. (1997). New options in menstrual protection. A guide for nurse practitioners. *Advance for Nurse Practitioners, 5*(11), 51–54, 81.

Women's Care: Social Issues

4

I DON'T THINK THERE HAS EVER BEEN A MORE exciting time for women. There are many challenges that face us: work, wage and role issues, safety in pregnancy and childbearing, and conflict over women's rights. On the other hand, women have never been more active and involved in the issues that affect them. Moreover, the men who care about us and who recognize the importance of fairness for all are beginning to speak out. I am convinced that together, as people of integrity and vision, we are making a difference.

Key Terms

Child abuse
Child neglect

Objectives

- Describe the concept of feminization of poverty.
- Discuss the current work environment and the factors that affect women's wages.
- Discuss work benefits that affect the childbearing woman.
- Describe environmental hazards present in a childbearing woman's workplace.
- Summarize the philosophical differences in the question of abortion.
- Identify the factors that place parents at risk for child abuse.
- Delineate the short- and long-term effects of child abuse on the child and other members of the family.
- Identify the responsibilities of the nurse who suspects child abuse.
- Cite the community resources available to violence-prone parents.

Women of today have the opportunity to be dynamic, challenging, and challenged individuals. They have opportunities for personal and professional growth that did not exist 30 years ago. Because of political and social changes that have occurred in this country since the early 1970s, women's options have expanded dramatically. Although many women still choose the traditional "women's" careers and become nurses, teachers, and "at-home" mothers, others are entering occupations that until recently were filled almost exclusively by men. More women than ever have joined the ranks of lawyers and judges, managers and corporate heads, scientists, journalists, legislators, construction workers, plumbers, and laborers. Women can be found in almost all occupations and thus are sharing in many of the benefits that come with these positions.

Progress has its costs, however. For example, the woman with a career and a family may have difficulty maintaining both. The woman who would like nothing more than to be an "at-home" wife and mother may be forced by the high cost of living to work outside the home and entrust the care of her children to others. The woman who has devoted her prime childbearing years to establishing a career rather than a family may find herself feeling pressure to find a partner and have children before it is too late.

Nurses must deal with many of the issues facing women, if not personally, then in their clinical practice. To help nurses better understand their clients' concerns and problems, this chapter addresses some of the serious issues facing women today.

Women and Poverty

The harsh economic plight of many women is dramatically reflected in the growing phenomenon referred to as the *feminization of poverty*, a term suggested by Diana Pearce (1993). Simply stated, an increasing number of women live on incomes that fall below the poverty level, which in 1998 was $16,450 for a family of four (Department of Health and Human Services [DHHS], 1998a).

The extent of this problem is enormous and ever-increasing. In 1996, 11% of families lived in poverty. However, only 5.6% of families headed by a married couple lived in poverty, compared to a staggering 32.6% of households headed by single mothers. This disproportion is even more apparent when one considers that although only 18% of families in the United States are headed by a female with no spouse present, 54% of all poor families have a female head (Lamison-White, 1997). With a divorce rate approaching 50% and an out-of-wedlock birth rate of about 25%, the reality is that many children will spend at least a portion of their lives in a single-parent family.

Even more disturbing is the number of children in the United States living in poverty. No other age group, not even the elderly, has a higher rate of poverty. Two risk factors are especially significant in documenting poverty in children: female-headed family and race. Although a disturbing 20.5% of children in the United States live below the poverty level, almost one-third (32.6%) of all children living in female-headed homes fall below the poverty level. The number of children from minority groups who live in female-headed households falling below the poverty level is even more disturbing: 43.7% of African American children and 50.9% of Hispanic children (Lamison-White, 1997). Currently, two-thirds of all poor people in the United States are women and children; it is projected that by the year 2000 they will account for most of the people living in poverty (see Figure 4–1).

The feminization of poverty extends beyond the United States. Since 1975, the number of people living in absolute poverty (earning less than $370 US dollars per year) has more than doubled and is now a shocking 1.3 billion people. Even more disturbingly, 7 out of 10 are women (Intensified Cooperation Organization [ICO], 1998). On a global scale, women must cope with some special problems: They live with the burden of working more than men but are paid less for the same work; they are often expected to bear, raise, and feed many (preferably male) children; they are frequently abused and beaten in their own home; often they have few legal rights. The literacy rate for females is lower than that for males, and education—when available—is more frequently provided for men (Brown et al, 1990).

Although the statistics on poverty may be shocking, they reveal little about what living with poverty is like. It is a day-by-day experience fraught with struggle and hardship.

I never thought this would happen to me. Two months after I became pregnant with our second child, it was over. My husband left us. Suddenly, I am the sole support of myself and my children. Since he left I haven't been able to get a teaching position or any job. So I don't have medical insurance or any benefits to help with this pregnancy. Applying for Medicaid has to be one of the most humiliating experiences I have ever had. I'm an intelligent woman with a college degree, and I couldn't figure out the forms. I'm smart really, surely I am, but I felt so dumb. The lines and the impersonal treatment that I had heard about but never believed were real. I felt like a number, shuttled from one place to the next. I know they don't do it on purpose; they've heard so many awful stories. Still, it hurt. It will take 6 weeks to qualify, and that means I will be more than halfway through my pregnancy. It seems there is no way to win. Only two doctors here accept Medicaid, and they are clear across town. It's all right. I'm thankful that I can get some help now when I need it, but it is so hard. I never dreamed I'd be in this position. I just never dreamed.

Impact of Female-Headed Households

The increase in the number of female-headed families is closely associated with divorce. Almost one out of every two marriages ends in divorce. As a result of divorce the woman's standard of living generally decreases significantly, while the man's increases. This dramatic change in the standard of living is usually associated with the lower earning capacity of women and the fact that women receive custody of the children in over 75% of cases (Clarke, 1995). Only about one-half of divorced women receive full child support payments; about one-fourth receive partial payment, while the remaining one-fourth receive nothing at all (DHHS, 1998b). Moreover, these legally awarded payments are frequently inadequate.

Until recently, society has not really held men accountable for these payments. The status quo is changing, however. Currently society is stepping up efforts to increase child support collection; states are cooperating to help identify noncustodial parents who are delinquent in making their child support payments. The United States Department of Justice is actively investigating and prosecuting individuals who cross state lines to avoid paying child support. In addition, the government now intercepts income tax refunds of delinquent parents. To improve access to information on the subject, the Department of Health and Human Services Office of Child Support Enforcement has an Internet home page that provides information on the enforcement program, explains the process of applying for child support assistance, and provides links to states with similar home pages.

Under the Personal Responsibility and Work Opportunity Act of 1996, a federal case registry and national directory of new hires was established to help address the problem of nonpayment of child support. Employers are required to report all newly hired employees to state agencies, which then transmit the information to the national directory. This makes it easier to track delinquent parents across state lines. Furthermore, states are required to establish central registries of child support orders and centralized collection and disbursement units. The law also permits states to implement tough collection techniques, including garnishing wages, seizing assets, revoking driver's and professional licenses, and, in some cases, requiring mandatory community service of individuals who are delinquent in making child support payments (DHHS, 1998b).

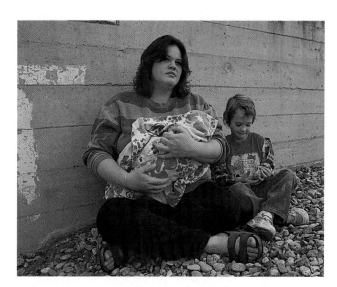

FIGURE 4–1 Two-thirds of Americans living in poverty are women and children.

Impact of the Labor Market

Women have steadily increased their participation in the labor force. In 1970, 43.3% of women were employed; by 1996, that number had increased to 59.3%, and it is predicted that by the year 2005, 61.7% of females over age 16 will be employed (Department of Commerce, 1997). Unfortunately, the average woman employed year-round and full time makes only 74 cents for every dollar earned by a man (US Bureau of the Census, 1998). This disparity is due to a variety of reasons. About one-third of women work in a cluster of occupations—including cashier, child care worker, waitress, nurse, retail sales clerk, elementary school teacher, and secretary—which tend to be poorly paid when compared to male-dominated positions requiring comparable levels of responsibility, skill, and education. Moreover, women comprise two-thirds of part-time workers; as such, their wages typically are lower, and they often have no fringe benefits, such as sick leave and health insurance.

It is true that more women are entering professions previously dominated by men. For example, the percentage of women lawyers increased from 15% in 1983 to 30% in 1996; during the same period, the percentage of women economists increased from 38% to 54%, and the percentage of women physicians increased from 16% to 26% (US Bureau of the Census, 1998). However, the numbers of women in engineering and the hard sciences have not shown comparable increases.

For working divorced or single women with children, the issue of child care is especially difficult. Child care is expensive and may place a burden on the household budget. Moreover, because women face significant responsibilities for ensuring the safety and well-being of their children, employers may view women as unreliable or uncommitted if they miss work when their children become sick. Currently, more enlightened employers are beginning to recognize and accommodate the needs of women in the work force. Like other areas of reform, however, this trend tends to benefit women in better paying, more secure positions far more than it benefits women who are poor and in low-paying positions.

The Welfare System

The welfare system was originally designed to provide assistance to those in need—in many cases, single female heads of households and their children. Unfortunately, the system often failed to provide adequate assistance to raise families above poverty levels and, in many cases, actually provided disincentives for women to work.

In 1996 growing national concern over the failure of the system led to welfare reform via the passage of the Personal Responsibility and Work Opportunity Reconciliation Act. This comprehensive plan no longer offers unlimited support but requires that an individual work in exchange for time-limited assistance. As one of the provisions of the act, the Aid to Families with Dependent Children (AFDC) program is replaced by the Temporary Assistance for Needy Families (TANF) program. Highlights of the new welfare law include the following (DHHS, 1998e):

- States are granted unprecedented flexibility in designing welfare programs to meet the needs of their recipients, but, in turn, they must demonstrate measurable results in moving families toward self-sufficiency and work.
- With few exceptions, recipients must work after 2 years on assistance. By fiscal year 2002, 50% of all families in each state must have left the welfare rolls or be engaged in work activities.
- After 5 cumulative years, families become ineligible for cash aid, although states can exempt up to 20% of their cases from the time limit provision. States can also choose to provide noncash assistance and vouchers for families that have reached the time limit using state funds or Social Security block grant dollars.
- The law provides $14 billion dollars (an increase of $4 billion) in child care funding to enable mothers to have adequate child care as they move into jobs.
- Women on welfare are guaranteed continued health care coverage for their families, including at least 1 year of transitional Medicaid as they leave the welfare rolls for work.
- Welfare recipients must meet state work requirements, which include participation in subsidized or unsubsidized employment, community service, on-the-job training, or 12 months of vocational education. Recipients can also meet the requirement by providing child care services to others who are involved in community service.
- As discussed previously, the act also contains several provisions designed to crack down on noncustodial parents who fail to pay child support.
- For unmarried teenage parents, the law has provisions mandating that they live at home (or in an adult-supervised setting) and stay in school in order to receive assistance.

It is too soon to judge the effectiveness of these reform efforts. In early 1998 Donna Shalala, the secretary of Health and Human Services, announced that for the first time in 25 years, the number of welfare recipients dropped below 10 million (Shalala, 1998). This drop has been attributed to a variety of factors, including strong economic growth nationally; innovative welfare strategies designed to move people from welfare to work, which are being tested by many states; strengthened enforcement of child support laws; and increased funding for child care. As part of the welfare reform law, the Census Bureau has been directed to conduct a Survey of Program Dynamics (SPD) to evaluate the long-term impact of the changes. The SPD will collect data from 1996 to 2001 and compare it to data collected from 1992 to 1995, prior to welfare reform. This will provide 10 years of data to use in assessing short- to medium-term outcomes (Weinberg, Huggins, Kominski, & Nelson, 1997).

CRITICAL THINKING QUESTION

What is involved in acquiring Medicaid? Who would you call if you needed assistance yourself? Where is the office? How long does it take to fill out the form? How long is the form? How much money would you get? Write out a budget for one month based on the money you would receive.

Impact of Aging

In practically all countries worldwide, women comprise the majority of the older population (over age 60). That proportion increases with age so that, globally, 65% of the oldest old (80 years and older) are women. Arber and Ginn (1994) termed this phenomenon *the feminization of later life.* This occurs because women have a longer life expectancy than men, especially in developed countries, where the average difference in life expectancy between the sexes is 7 years. In certain countries, such as Russia, the gap exceeds 10 years. (Researchers attribute this disparity to unusually high levels of current adult male death rates.) In developing countries, the gender gap is narrower (approximately 3 years), which is attributed to high levels of maternal mortality (Gist & Velkoff, 1997). In some developing countries, as Table 4–1 indicates, the life span for both men and women is still less than 60 years.

In the United States, the life expectancy currently is 79 years for women and 73 years for men. Estimates suggest that by 2010, life expectancy will be 81 years and 74 years, respectively (US Bureau of the Census, 1998). Unfortunately, although women tend to live longer than men, they also tend to spend a larger portion of their older years in a disabled state (Colvez, 1996). In reality, older women are more likely than their male counterparts to be widowed, to live alone, to be disabled, and to be poor.

TABLE 4–1 Years of Life Expectancy at Birth by Gender for Selected Countries, 1997

Country	Male Life Expectancy	Female Life Expectancy
Afghanistan	47	46
Argentina	71	78
Australia	77	83
Canada	76	83
China	69	72
Egypt	60	64
Ethiopia	45	48
France	75	83
Japan	77	83
Mexico	70	78
Russia	57	71
Tanzania	40	43
United Kingdom	74	79
United States	73	79

SOURCE: US Bureau of the Census, International Programs Center, International Data Base.

Factors that contribute to the increased economic vulnerability of women include the following (Gist & Velkoff, 1997; Lewis, 1997):

- Women must stretch their financial resources further than men because of their longer life expectancy.
- Older women tend to have less educational preparation than older men.
- Historically women have been economically dependent on men and may have intermittent or nonexistent employment histories.
- Women typically earn less than men and often work in jobs without pension benefits or only limited benefits.
- Women generally have more family caregiving responsibilities than older men.
- Women, more often than men, feel the impact of public policies and programs that place undue financial pressures on them.

Following widowhood, a middle-class woman faces the risk of "cycling into poverty," especially if her husband had a long, costly illness or if his pension shrinks or ceases following his death. However, of all the elderly, women of color have the highest poverty rates (Lewis, 1997). To help keep elderly women from spending their final years in poverty, it is necessary for the nation to develop solutions to the economic concerns caused by a fixed income, to deal with problems of pension inequity, and to address the potentially disastrous effects of staggering health care costs for the uninsured or underinsured.

Homelessness

For many people the thought of a homeless person conjures up a vision of an older man curled in a doorway or making a home under a bridge. However, this vision is less accurate today than in the past; today's homeless people have very different characteristics. In 1985, 27% of the homeless population were families, and 60% were single men. By 1995, those percentages had changed significantly. Homeless families had increased to 36.5% of the homeless population, whereas homeless men had decreased to 46% (Family Impact Seminar, 1996). Many of these families are composed of single mothers and their children.

A major factor contributing to the incidence of homelessness is domestic violence. Research suggests that 50% of homeless women and their children are fleeing from an abusive situation (National Coalition for the Homeless [NCH], 1998). This finding was supported by a survey conducted by the Conference of Mayors, which cited domestic violence as one of the main causes of homelessness (Waxman & Trupin, 1997).

A second factor contributing to homelessness is the high cost of housing. During the past 20 years, housing costs have increased far more than wages or other income sources, especially for women. Single-parent, female-headed households have seen their rent burden increase from an average of 35% of their income in 1974 to over 58% (Wolch & Dear, 1993).

The incidence of homelessness is also related to the extent of a woman's social support system. Because middle-class women typically have relatives and friends with more space and resources, they are able to avoid becoming homeless to a greater extent than poorer women.

Homeless people experience greater health risks and problems than does the general population. Malnutrition predisposes homeless people to a variety of respiratory and nutritional disorders. Moreover, a disproportionately high number of homeless children have not received preventive health care services, such as immunizations.

Homeless women who are pregnant are a special challenge for health care providers. Inadequate prenatal care, limited access to general health care, poor nutrition, and inadequate housing lead to poor birth outcomes, including an increased incidence of low-birth-weight newborns and a higher rate of infant mortality. In addition, as a group they are at risk for many illnesses that could negatively impact their pregnancies, including substance abuse and sexually transmitted infections (Beal & Redlener, 1995).

Effects on Health Care

The effects of poverty on health care are extensive. Since 1981, many funding cuts have directly affected programs that benefited those living in poverty. These cuts have come at a time when the benefits of adequate nutrition and prenatal care have been documented to yield significant health care benefits for every dollar spent.

Medicaid is the major US entitlement program providing health care to low-income people in four categories: children, adults in families, the elderly, and blind and disabled people. Traditionally Medicaid has played an important role in financing maternity care, covering the costs of about 40% of births in the United States. It seems likely that the number of women on Medicaid will decrease in the next few years because welfare reform measures eliminate the automatic connection between TANF and Medicaid and significantly decrease the number of people eligible for Medicaid assistance. In addition, newly established policies requiring that women apply separately for Medicaid may cause a drop in the number of enrollees (Gonen, 1998). These policy changes may have unintended consequences because studies indicate that almost two-thirds of women who leave the Medicaid program become uninsured (Short, 1996).

Lack of health insurance is also a major problem for the poor. Thirty-seven million Americans have no health insurance, and another 7 to 10 million have inadequate coverage. Decreases in health insurance have led to declines in preventive health care that are costing dollars and even lives. For example, children's immunization rates have fallen significantly in recent years, especially among non-whites; as a result, childhood illnesses are on the rise, especially in urban areas. The human and financial costs of the decline in immunization rates are especially devastating in light of the fact that immunizations are not only very effective in preventing illness but also cost-effective; immunizations are estimated to save $10 for every $1 spent (Dutton, 1993).

The issue of universal health care coverage is a significant one, especially for women living in poverty. Statistical data already are beginning to reflect the change in health insurance coverage and funding cuts. Women who do not receive prenatal care are three times more likely to have low-birth-weight babies, and the incidence of low-birth-weight babies is increasing. Moreover, poor areas have shown a marked increase in infant mortality.

Suggestions for Nursing Action

The issue of women and poverty is critical, and the implications for childbearing care are very real. A pregnant woman who is suffering economically may also suffer physically and psychologically. In the end it is often the children who suffer the most, bearing the physical and psychologic scars of their mothers' struggles.

As health care professionals, nurses should be concerned about the issue of women and poverty. The health care system and thus nursing are intricately woven into the political and social structures of society. Nurses often work with women on welfare; they see the effects of poverty on childbearing families and the pain and struggles of these families. The limited resources of these women often frustrates nurses' efforts to provide quality care. What can nurses do about the growing problem of female poverty? The following sections include suggestions for action that nurses can take to ease this crisis.

Personal Action

- Be aware of your own beliefs about poverty and the women who need public assistance.
- Explore your feelings regarding poverty.
- Remain knowledgeable about the impact of poverty on the childbearing woman and her family.
- Speak out to inform others of the facts; correct misconceptions.

Client Action

- Be sensitive in assessing a woman's economic status during intake interviews. Use the knowledge of the current extent of the poverty problem to try to identify women who may be at risk.
- Provide supportive counseling, and determine the woman's ability to follow a treatment plan or accomplish self-care measures, especially when extra expenditure of funds is required.
- Stay knowledgeable about community resources to assist the woman with financial need, and be prepared to offer suggestions and counseling regarding possible resources. It is much more helpful to give a group name and a phone number than to send the woman out to search on her own.

Community Action

- When possible, work with community organizations and planners to identify financial needs of childbearing women in the community.
- Offer your nursing expertise to community groups to help them meet the financial and health needs of childbearing women and their families.

Political Action

- Know your legislators and their views. Be available to discuss issues and act as a resource for them as they become more knowledgeable about issues that affect childbearing women.
- Make your opinions and ideas known to your legislators.
- Support programs that benefit childbearing women and help identify areas that need to be addressed.
- Educate the legislators about the alarming increase in poverty among women.

Research Action

- Investigate the impact of poverty on the health and welfare of childbearing women and their families.

- Document any client's inability to obtain adequate care so that this information will be available for future use.
- Conduct research projects to dispel myths associated with poverty.

Women in the Workplace

The discrepancy between men's and women's wages springs from many factors. In the past, women's wages were purposely set lower than men's simply because it was a woman doing the job. The work of men and women was not valued equally. Unfortunately this belief still lingers, affecting women in the workplace.

Young women traditionally have been socialized in ways that affect their opportunities and expectations, which may also ultimately contribute to wage discrepancy. Boys are encouraged to develop a competitive spirit first in sports and then in other areas of their lives. They learn that "being a winner" and "knowing how to play the game" are valued qualities. Girls are usually not encouraged to develop a competitive spirit; many cultures do not view competitiveness as an important or desirable trait for a girl to have. Girls learn from parents, the media, their peers, and others that physical attractiveness, not intelligence, is the key to popularity and, in turn, to success.

Education is also a significant factor in the socializing of women. Fortunately, parents, educators, and concerned citizens are beginning to recognize that schools must do far more to enhance girls' self-esteem, build their self-confidence, and encourage them to explore a wide range of career options, especially in fields not traditionally seen as welcoming to women. If girls have more positive experiences in academic settings, it seems likely that they will be more eager to pursue higher education and higher-paying jobs, which will lead to a decrease in wage discrepancy.

Currently several factors are exerting a positive force on the issue of wage discrimination.

- The number of women obtaining a college education continues to increase, and these women influence the work environment as they enter the work force. For instance, in 1996, 21% of all women over age 25 had earned a bachelor's degree compared to 26% of all men over 25. However, among 25- to 29-year-olds, women were slightly more likely to have a bachelor's degree (28%) than men (US Bureau of the Census, 1998).
- Many working women are holding their jobs for extended periods and are not as likely to work for short periods. They are gaining more experience in performing their jobs, which has a positive effect on their productivity. As productivity rises, wages generally rise as well.

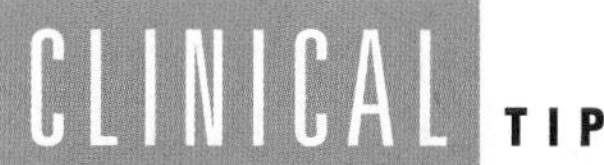

TIP

Speaking out about issues that affect women, children, and families is an integral part of maternal-child nursing. It is difficult for many nurses to do this, so practice with friends and family frequently. Be prepared with accurate information, and try varous techniques for presenting the information. A friendly, supportive audience helps you get started.

- Women have become more involved in the political arena and are raising the issue of comparable worth.

The basic premise of *comparable worth* is that the same wages should be paid for different types of work that require comparable skills, responsibility, education, and experience. This issue is quite controversial. Opponents suggest that, to the extent that job reevaluation results in major increases in women's salaries, comparable worth will increase unemployment and inefficiency, encourage women to remain in female-dominated jobs, decrease US manufacturers' ability to compete with foreign manufacturers, and reallocate limited salary resources away from lower-class, minority men to European American middle-class women. Research suggests, however, that the costs of pay equity adjustments have been overestimated and could be accommodated if phased in gradually and logically (Rhode, 1993). Moreover, in some companies comparable worth is a reality. Major companies such as IBM, AT & T, and Bank of America have instituted some forms of comparable worth. At least 20 states have comparable worth legislation pending or have commissions studying the issue.

Suggestions for Nursing Action

What can women do about wage discrimination? What can nurses do to help clients who are suffering financially because of wage discrimination? The following sections include suggestions for actions nurses can take.

Personal Action

- Seek information regarding the wages for women in your community.
- Share wage information with others so that more people will be informed. When wages are kept secret, disparities are more likely to exist.
- Help women you know maintain their self-esteem and feelings of worth.

Client Action

- Encourage women to push for wage equity.
- Encourage women to talk together about wages so inequities can be identified.

Community Action

- Work with community leaders and groups to identify the lack of adequate jobs and wage inequity in your community.

Political Action

- Educate legislators about the status of women's wages and the impact of low wages on health care for the childbearing woman and her family.
- Support programs that enhance employment opportunities for fair wages for women.

Research Action

- Investigate variables affecting the variations in nurses' salaries across the United States, by sex of the nurse and position.
- Investigate salary-negotiating skills and characteristics of nurses who are able to negotiate.

Maternity Leaves and Child Care Benefits

Maternity Leaves

Combining a career with childbearing can be a challenging task. Moreover, leaving a job to have a child may result at the very least in lost experience, most commonly in lost benefits, perhaps a lost opportunity for promotion, and sometimes loss of the job completely.

Family options improved somewhat in 1993 when the Family and Medical Leave Act (FMLA) was signed into law by President Bill Clinton. This law permits employees to take up to 12 weeks of unpaid leave from work following the birth or adoption of a child or the placement of a foster child. Employees may also take leave if faced with a personal serious illness or the illness of a spouse, child, or parent. During the leave, health insurance benefits must be continued, and employees are entitled to return to their former position or one considered comparable. Coverage is not mandated for employees who work less than 25 hours per week or who have been employed less than 1 year. Under the law, eligible employees are required to provide 30 days' notice when possible and must furnish a physician's statement verifying the need.

Because the Family and Medical Leave Act applies only to companies with 50 or more employees, the vast majority of companies and about 25 million employees are not covered by the law. Those employees still must rely on the policies, if any, that their employers have established.

Discrimination against pregnant women remains an issue in some areas, so women need to be aware of their rights, which were established by the Pregnancy Discrimination Act of 1978. This act guarantees the following:

- A pregnant woman cannot be denied a job if she is able to perform major job functions.
- The same procedure for using sick-leave pay or disability benefits must be used for the pregnant woman as for other employees.
- Employee medical coverage must include pregnancy benefits.
- The mother can use all her maternity benefits without penalty.

When a woman is planning a pregnancy, she should acquire information regarding pregnancy benefits in her work setting. The state in which she lives will also have guidelines or regulations regarding pregnancy. Questions that the woman may need to address include:

- Can I be forced to go on leave because I am pregnant?
- What are my rights to sick leave or disability leave with my pregnancy?
- Can I lose my job for taking disability leave associated with pregnancy?
- Do I have any rights concerning infant care?
- Is my employer required to provide maternity benefits and insurance coverage?

Child Care

Child care has been a working woman's problem for years. Although some fathers are actively involved in meshing work and family responsibilities, child care remains a significant concern because of the high percentage of single-parent households headed by a woman. Access to safe, reliable child care varies. In some areas there is a surplus of child care slots, but in major metropolitan areas availability is an issue. Affordability and quality remain major problems in most areas. A recent study on cost and quality of child care programs in several states revealed that only one in seven programs provides an acceptable level of quality (DHHS, 1998c). In the United States, working women commonly spend 25% of their take-home pay for child care. Typically, a parent pays approximately \$3000 annually, although this cost can reach \$6000 or more in certain areas of the northeast (Ellis, 1993).

Currently some employers provide some form of support for employees' child care needs through referral programs, on-site or near-site centers, or financial assistance. Other creative approaches to handling child care are also gaining in popularity. These include flex-time scheduling, part-time work, job sharing, and telecommuting (working at home).

For many women, however, child care is the most challenging of all the issues they face. At a national level, the first White House Conference on Child Care was held in fall, 1997. In 1998, drawing on information and ideas from the conference, President Clinton declared that the government should lead the way in improving child care and issued an executive directive mandating that by the year 2000 all federally sponsored child care must be nationally accredited with proper background checks performed on all child care workers in federal facilities. That same year the Department of Health and Human Services released a guide for parents to use in selecting child care providers. Among the topics covered, the guide suggests a four-step approach to selecting a quality child care provider (DHHS, 1998c):

- Make the decision to choose quality care.
- Interview potential caregivers carefully.
- Check references.
- Stay involved with the caregiver.

CRITICAL THINKING QUESTION

What benefits will be important for you as you enter your professional career?

Suggestions for Nursing Action

Personal Action

- Examine the maternity and child care benefits in your own work environment. When questions arise or you identify unmet needs, follow the guidelines in your facility to suggest changes or additions in benefit policies.
- Be knowledgeable about the current status of wage inequity and its effect on the childbearing woman's ability to afford adequate child care.
- Once you are prepared with accurate knowledge, speak out at appropriate opportunities to provide information and correct inaccurate information about women's wages.

Client Action

- Talk with women to identify how helpful their benefit packages are.
- Encourage women to investigate the benefits in their own work setting.
- Provide resources that can be used to learn about regulations regarding benefits on the community, state, and national levels.
- Encourage women to pursue their questions regarding benefits until they are answered satisfactorily.

Community Action

- Provide community leaders with information about the need for comprehensive maternal and child care benefits for childbearing women and their families.
- Work within the community to identify benefits for the nursing profession.
- Work with community and professional nursing groups to enhance the status of nursing.
- Work with your professional nursing organizations to improve benefits for nursing.

RESEARCH IN PRACTICE

What is this study about? Female condoms have the potential to protect women against sexually transmitted diseases and to reduce the number of unwanted pregnancies. Additionally, female condoms provide the first barrier method that is controlled by the woman herself. Nabila El-Bassel and her colleagues designed a study to examine the relationships between intention to use female condoms and demographic variables; attitudes toward both male and female condoms; perception of sexual partner's attitude toward female condoms and ability of participant to convince partner to practice safe sex; and social norms related to female condoms.

How was the study done? The researchers recruited 148 women from three methadone clinics. Eligibility criteria included: sexually active; enrolled in a methadone clinic; and inconsistent condom use for 90 days prior to the interview. Because nine participants had already used a female condom, the data analysis incorporated information from the remaining 139 women. Investigators used chi-square and *t*-tests to analyze data collected during structured interviews.

What were the results of the study? The results demonstrated that 56% of the participants had never heard of the female condom, with African American women (66%) and European American women (80%) more likely to have heard about the condom than Latina women (50%) [chi-square=5.7; *df* 2; $p < .05$]. Positive attitudes toward both male and female condoms, perception of sexual partner's attitude toward female condoms, and ability of participant to convince partner to practice safe sex related positively with intent to use female condoms. Other data found during this study included information that in the 90 days prior to the study 35% of the women traded sex for money or drugs; 10% to 50% used some type of drug such as marijuana or freebased cocaine; and male condoms, douching, sterilization, or withdrawal were the most common methods of birth control.

What additional questions might I have? Who was included in the total sample? It is difficult to determine from the report whether the nine participants who had used female condoms were excluded or included in the results. Why were the participants restricted to a methadone clinic? The authors might have incorporated in their research questions the fact that these women are at greater risk for a sexually transmitted disease such as HIV.

How can I use this study? If 56% of the women in this study had never heard of the female condom, then many other women may also be unaware of this method of contraception and protection. Students can discuss the female condom when presenting information to sexually active females.

SOURCE: El-Bassel, N., Krishnan, S. P., Schilling, R. F., Catan, V., & Pollin, S. (1998). Correlates of intention to use the female condom among women taking methadone. *Women's Health Issues, 8,* 112–122.

Political Action

- Write your legislators and support legislation that addresses and corrects wage inequities.
- Let your legislators know if you do not support legislation and why. Educate legislators about the importance of a national policy on parental leave and child care.

Research Action

- Investigate factors currently affecting public view of comparable pay.

Environmental Hazards in the Workplace

As more women enter the work force, they are exposed to an ever-increasing number of chemicals and environmental pollutants. In fact, of the approximately 50,000 chemicals used today in industry, about 500 have been implicated as having potentially hazardous effects on reproduction (Bernhardt, 1990). For example, exposure to volatile organic compounds, dusts, or pesticides increases the risk of female infertility (Smith et al, 1997). Other agents, such as arsenic, formaldehyde, ethylene oxide, and benzene are associated with an increased incidence of spontaneous abortion (Cunningham et al, 1997). Exposure to halogenated hydrocarbons such as polychlorinated biphenyls (PCBs) or anesthetic gases has been linked to both spontaneous abortion and increased incidence of infants born with congenital anomalies.

Other agents have an impact on general health. The incidence of black lung disease in the mining industry and the hazards of exposure to asbestos products are well documented and frightening. Milder chronic respiratory symptoms such as dyspnea, sinusitis, and cough are associated with other industries, including the manufacture of synthetic textiles (Zuskin et al, 1998). Latex allergy is rapidly becoming a significant problem among health care workers, with 2% to 15% demonstrating hypersensitivity symptoms ranging from mild contact dermatitis to severe systemic reactions and anaphylactic shock (Palczynski et al, 1997).

Lead exposure is perhaps the oldest known occupational hazard and has been linked to both reproductive and general health hazards. Increased rates of spontaneous abortion, stillbirths, and prematurity have been documented as well as decreased sperm counts and increased abnormal sperm in men who have been exposed to lead. In addition, lead exposure can cause irreversible health effects, such as central nervous system problems and decreased hearing ability (Staudinger & Roth, 1998).

Questions regarding the safety of exposure to video display terminals (VDTs) have arisen in recent years, and various studies have produced contradictory results. However, at present there is no documented evidence of increased risk of spontaneous abortion or overall fetal loss in women whose work exposed them regularly to VDTs (Cunningham et al, 1997; Schnorr et al, 1991). Until more is known about the possibility of other biologic effects of chronic exposure to the low-frequency electromagnetic fields found with VDTs, women should avoid chronic exposure. Because the strength of the field decreases significantly with distance, women can decrease their exposure by sitting at least 50 cm (20 in.) from the screen and at least 1 m (3.25 feet) from the sides or back of adjacent machines (electromagnetic field strength is typically higher from the back and sides). Exposure is also decreased by turning off VDTs, printers, and other electrical devices when they are not in use (Paul, 1993).

Nurses have an occupational hazard in the exposure inherent in providing care for sick people. Exposure to toxoplasmosis, rubella, cytomegalovirus, herpes simplex, and hepatitis B may affect pregnancy and fetal outcome (Hewitt, Misner, & Levin, 1993). Exposure to HIV infection has also been a concern to health care professionals.

Two governmental agencies have primary responsibility for addressing workplace safety. The Occupational Safety and Health Administration (OSHA), part of the Department of Labor, is responsible for creating and enforcing workplace health and safety regulations. The National Institute for Occupational Safety and Health (NIOSH), which is part of the Department of Health and Human Services, is primarily a research agency. However, it also disseminates information on preventing workplace injury and illness, provides training to occupational safety and health professionals, and investigates potentially hazardous working situations when requested by employers or employees (NIOSH, 1997).

Environmental hazards are increasing with the discovery and development of new products, and these hazards exert their effect on everyone in their environment. Women are at particular risk while they are in the childbearing years. Because no work environment is without risks, it is becoming more important for each woman to become knowledgeable about her own workplace. Information can be obtained from libraries, the public health department, and agencies such as NIOSH and CDC, which collect data regarding environmental hazards. In addition, several teratogen information services are available. Some are sponsored by states for their own residents; some are available for all users; still others are sponsored by major medical centers. Many have e-mail addresses for easy access.

Suggestions for Nursing Action

Environmental hazards are an area of particular interest and importance to maternal-newborn nurses, both personally and professionally. Nurses need to be aware of the risks that they face in their own environment and the risks that childbearing women face in theirs. Nurses can be influential in encouraging more investigation of chemical substances and other hazards so that work environments will be safer for all.

Personal Action

- Be knowledgeable about hazards in your own work environment.
- Collect information regarding the effects of various environmental hazards on the childbearing woman and her family.
- Take time to visit Internet web pages that address the issue, and develop a list of e-mail addresses for teratogen information services.
- Follow guidelines and procedures in the work setting to decrease your risk.

Client Action

- Obtain information about environmental hazards in the woman's work environment.
- Suggest resources to the woman to enhance her knowledge.
- Recommend resource groups to obtain more information.

Community Action

- Work with community leaders and groups to identify environmental hazards in your community.
- Provide education regarding the hazards to childbearing women.

Political Action

- Provide information about environmental hazards in your community to your legislators.
- Educate your legislators regarding the special effects of environmental hazards on the childbearing woman and her family.
- Support legislation that addresses and solves problems involving environmental hazards.

Research Action

- Document problems that are observed during your care of clients.

Abortion

Abortion is a highly charged issue, one that can lead to heated confrontations between supporters and opponents. Even the terms used to refer to those with differing philosophic convictions about abortion are cause for argument. The anti-abortion philosophy is called "pro-life," and the pro-abortion philosophy is dubbed "pro-choice." It is partly this politicizing terminology that works to polarize opposing viewpoints.

The abortion issue is one that different factions have dealt with in one way or another for centuries. For the past 200 years the policies and philosophies in the United States have been directed primarily by the medical community. Through the first half of this century, abortion was not discussed; it was a private matter. As a result, even though people held different opinions about abortion, those adhering to each philosophic position tended to believe their opinions were those of the majority. In the 1960s an effort to clarify laws and philosophies made the issue of abortion an open one, and people came to realize that beliefs about abortion varied greatly.

There are many issues associated with abortion. Four major issues that form the basis of differing feelings about the rightness or wrongness of abortion often arise in public and private discussions. These include the following:

1. *Moral views regarding status of the embryo.* Historically, the status of the embryo has been ambiguous from philosophic, religious, and moral viewpoints. Questions of the legal status of the fetus, the use of medical technology, and the value of children are central to this argument.
2. *The moment that life begins.* Both sides acknowledge that the heartbeat of a developing embryo can be observed by the end of the first month of gestation. However, there is no agreement as to what this fact means. A heartbeat is necessary for life, but the ability to breathe is also critical to maintain life. Does a heartbeat prove that life exists, or does life require a heartbeat and the ability to breathe?
3. *The personhood of the embryo.* Personhood carries with it inalienable rights to due process in our society. The question, then, is whether the embryo is a person with rights to be protected.
4. *Woman's role in society.* The ability to have an abortion gives the woman control over her reproductive life and enables her to function as an autonomous being. This autonomy is perceived by many as essential if women are to enjoy true equality. Others suggest that a pregnant woman has a moral responsibility to humankind to protect and preserve the life she carries regardless of her personal preferences.

Debate about abortion continues as groups speak out and protest publicly against those with opposing views. The Supreme Court continues to consider cases that challenge the 1973 *Roe v Wade* decision. Individual states are also striving to enact abortion policies that address issues such as the following: When can an abortion be done, and under what circumstances? Where can it be done? Is spousal or parental permission required?

The debate extends into the development of new contraceptive techniques. Mifepristone, more commonly known as RU 486, is a drug that has been used to cause abortion. Originally developed in France, RU 486 has met with controversy in the United States.

One question that concerns both pro-abortion and anti-abortion groups is the possible psychologic impact of either choice—having an abortion or carrying an unwanted pregnancy to term. Clearly, on the public scene, in the legislative arena, and in people's private beliefs, abortion is an issue that continues to raise many questions.

The philosophies of nurses mirror those of the society at large. Because it may be difficult for a nurse to provide care for an individual who is participating in a procedure with which the nurse disagrees, nurses who are strongly opposed to abortion are best advised to seek employment in a facility where abortions are not performed. In some settings where abortions are performed, nurses do not have to provide care for women having an abortion if it is against the nurse's own personal philosophy and if another nurse is available to provide care.

Suggestions for Nursing Action

Personal Action

- Explore your own feelings and beliefs regarding abortion.
- Talk with others and gather information about abortion.
- Be knowledgeable about the issues involved.

Client Action

- If your beliefs allow you to care for women considering abortion, provide counseling and support to women as they seek information. If your beliefs do not allow you to care for women who choose abortion, avoid imposing your opinions on them. Provide factual information.
- Be nonjudgmental when working with women, regardless of their personal choices.

Community Action

- Work with community groups that support your views.
- Support adequate health care for all women.

Political Action

- Provide education, support, and assistance to legislators in order to bring about legislation that promotes your philosophy and ensures safe care for women.

Family Violence

Family violence is a major health issue for women worldwide. Violence against women in the form of abuse or sexual assault is covered in detail in Chapter 5. This chapter explores violence against the elderly briefly; violence against children is discussed in more detail.

Elder Abuse

Elder abuse was first recognized publicly in the mid-1980s. Since then the reported incidence has doubled to 241,000 in 1994 (Emery & Laumann-Billings, 1998). Experts anticipate that the problem will continue to grow as the population ages and as illness and financial burdens strain family relationships.

Typically the abuser is a family member or primary caregiver, although the problem of elder abuse by staff in nursing homes and long-term care facilities has been well documented. Four types of elder abuse occur: psychologic abuse, physical abuse, financial abuse, or neglect (by self or caregiver). Multiple forms of abuse often occur simultaneously and tend to intensify with time unless intervention occurs (Lynch, 1997). Factors that increase the risk of elder abuse include shared living arrangements, family history of violence, lack of financial resources, dependence, isolation, poor health, and cognitive impairment. Substance abuse and stressful events in the life of the abuser may also contribute to the risk (Lynch, 1997).

A full discussion of this growing problem, its identification, and treatment is beyond the scope of this textbook. It is imperative, however, that nurses who care for the elderly be alert for signs of abuse and take steps to address the problem when it is identified.

Child Abuse

My daughter looks at me, her eyes brimming with tears and her face strained. We sit across from each other clutching cups of hot chocolate—something to try to bring comfort. She has heard me spill out part of the memories of childhood sexual abuse that I have been reliving and has seen part of the pain inside me. She has listened, and with each word it looks like I have struck her, that the words reach out and lash at her. She is hearing and feeling my pain. I think maybe she shouldn't know; maybe I should protect her; maybe my tormentors were right, I shouldn't tell. But I need her to know. I need her to be able to share this life-changing process with me and know that her mother is all right.

The pain is there, swirling on the red Formica tabletop. It is in her eyes. It is in my fingers clenching the cup. It is in the napkin I twist. It is in my shoulders, which I no longer seem able to hold up. It is in my heart and soul, in every cell of my body. It is in my downward gaze as I consider whether it is all right to look up at her. In that instant before our eyes meet, I fear that I will see doubt and disgust in her eyes. And she looks at me. There is no doubt, no disgust. She says, "I know this happens to people, but, oh no, not you . . . not my mom." And inside I say, "Thank you my daughter, thank you for believing me."

One of the most disastrous results of dysfunctional parenting is **child abuse.** Child abuse arises in part from the cultural sanctioning of physical discipline of children by their parents. Among the many serious effects of child abuse are physical handicaps, poor self-image, inability to love others, antisocial or violent behavior in later life, and death. In 1996 almost 1 million children were confirmed victims of neglect and abuse, and 1077 children died as a result. Of the children who died as a result of abuse or neglect, three-fourths were age 3 or younger (DHHS, 1998d). The problem is far more pervasive than these numbers indicate, however, because of the untold number of cases of abuse or neglect that are never reported.

Child abusers are found among all socioeconomic, religious, and ethnic groups. A small number of abusing parents are mentally ill, but most have less serious problems that respond to intervention. Parents at risk for abusive behavior may manifest one or more of the risk factors identified in Table 4–2.

The parent with a potential for abuse often has low self-esteem, external locus of control, poor impulse control, and heightened response to stress with a less effective personal coping style. The abusive parent may feel isolated and unable to trust others or may be too passive to be able to give. Parents at risk for abuse tend to expect their children to perform for their gratification, and they tend to use severe physical punishment to ensure a child's proper behavior.

Parents who abuse their children are likely to have been abused as children (Coohey & Braun, 1997). In addition, research suggests that single mothers who experienced violent sexual abuse as children were almost six times more likely to physically abuse their children as those who were not sexually abused (Hall, Sachs, & Rayens, 1998). It is important to note, however, that less than half of those who were abused and neglected as children become abusive with their own families (Emery & Laumann-Billings, 1998). This multigenerational pattern of child abuse, although disturbing, does help in identifying families in need of prevention.

Parents with a potential for abuse often expect their children to meet their needs and therefore are most likely to abuse a child who is viewed as "different." Children at risk for abuse may be the result of difficult pregnancies or births or those born at inconvenient times, born out of wedlock, the "wrong" sex, or too active or too passive. Some children are abused because they are the result of a forced pregnancy with an unloved partner or the result of rape or incest. Others have characteristics, such as looks and mannerisms, that evoke negative associations in the abusing parent. Children who have been separated from their families because of prematurity or neonatal disease are more likely to be at risk for abuse. Children with congenital anomalies, mental retardation, hyperactivity, or chronic illness are also at risk. Children with abnormal sleep-wake patterns or feeding difficulties and those who are unresponsive to care might also be at risk if they are living in a family with other risk factors (Mott, James, & Sperhac, 1990). Only a small percentage of premature or difficult children, however, are abused, and for all abused children it is the combination of parental deficiencies and characteristics of the child that create the problems leading to abuse.

TABLE 4–2 Parental Risk Factors for Child Maltreatment

Risk Factor	Assessment Finding
Lack of nurturing experience	Inadequate experience with parenting (eg, multiple foster homes)
	Parent neglected or abused as a child
	Parent expected to meet high demands of own parents as a child
Lack of knowledge of normal growth and development	Inability to read "cues" of child
	Impatience when child does not respond as expected; unreasonable discipline
	Unrealistically high expectations for the child
Isolation	Inadequate use of supports
	Inability to identify resources
	Unknown to others in community
Low self-esteem	Lack of trust, particularly of authority figures
	Expects rejection
High vulnerability to criticism	History of family violence in family of origin or in current family system (eg, female partner abuse)
	Impulsive
Many unmet needs	Feelings of being unloved or having unresponsive partner, unstable marriage, or no relationship at all
	Youthful marriage, forced marriage, unwanted pregnancy
Multiple stressors	Poverty, unemployment, substandard housing, lack of job opportunities
	Inadequate clothing and insufficient food
Substance abuse	Abuse of alcohol or drugs
Role reversal	Emotional immaturity, lack of patience, inability to make judgments
	Preoccupied with self
	Depression
	Dependent on others

SOURCE: Adapted from Mott, S.R., et al (1990). *Nursing care of children and families* (2nd ed). Redwood City, CA: Addison-Wesley Nursing, p 589.

A strong relationship also exists between poverty and child maltreatment. Clearly most poor people do not mistreat their children, and the relationship between poverty and child abuse is not a simple or direct one. Some studies suggest that the difference between poor families who maltreat their children and those who do not lies in the extent of social closeness and mutual caring found in their communities. Conversely, other studies suggest that abusive families are less likely to socialize with their neighbors, seek help from others, or know of community organizations in which they can become involved (Emery & Laumann-Billings, 1998).

Child abuse is most likely to occur during times of crisis. The parent's loss of a job, for example, might be

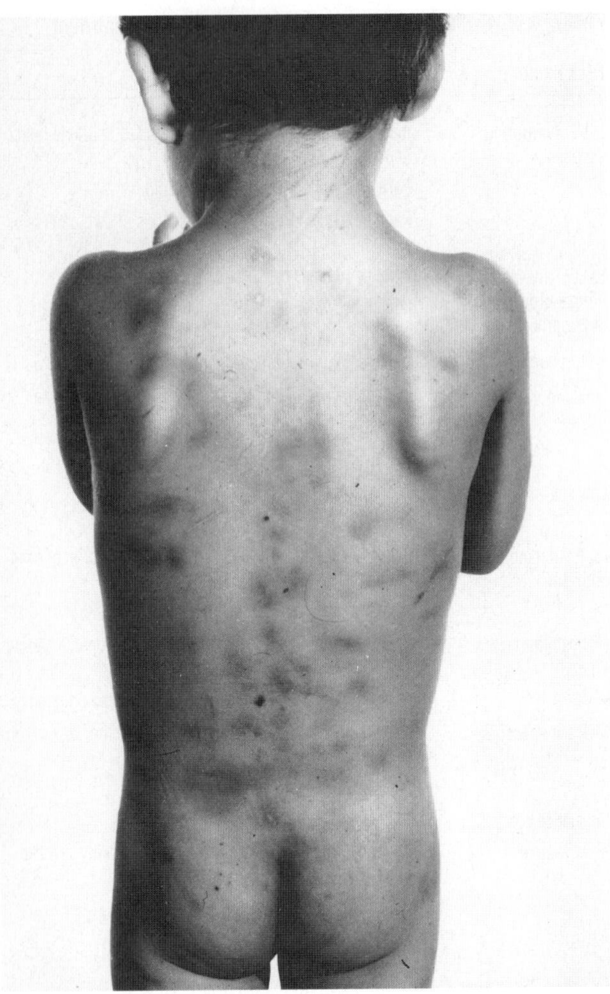

FIGURE 4–2 An abused child may display numerous bruises and scars. SOURCE: Mott, S. R., et al (1990). *Nursing care of children and families* (2nd ed.). Redwood City, CA: Addison-Wesley Nursing, p 603.

just enough to make the crying of a fretful infant unbearable. Some families hover on the brink of perpetual crisis, living with constant changes that contribute to feelings of inadequacy. The magnitude of the crisis is not always in proportion to the abuse. A relatively minor crisis might be viewed as the "last straw" in an unhappy situation.

Solving a crisis for troubled families is not enough if new crises and stressors merely reestablish dysfunctional patterns. Instead, the nurse teaches parents to develop their own coping strategies and to identify when and how to seek help. Parents who learn the problems inherent in isolation, for example, will then seek assistance when under stress and will avoid the patterns of behavior that cause them to abuse their children.

Types of Abuse

Child abuse or maltreatment may be physical, emotional, or sexual. The nurse needs to assess for all forms of abuse (Figure 4–2). The consequences of emotional and sexual abuse are not as obvious as those of physical abuse, but the effects of these types of abuse may last longer and be more damaging to the personal development of the child.

In children less than 1 year old, child abuse is the most common cause of serious head injury, which can result from violent acts such as impact (blows to the head, hitting the head against a wall, and so on), penetrating trauma, asphyxia, and shaking. *Shaken-baby syndrome* is a term used to describe a form of head injury inflicted on younger infants, usually under age 6 months. Caused by vigorous shaking, often in response to frustration, it is characterized by retinal hemorrhages or subdural or subarachnoid bleeding with no external signs of trauma (Kini & Lazoritz, 1998).

Munchausen syndrome by proxy (MSP) is an unusual type of child abuse in which a parent, often the mother, invents or directly induces the child's illness or injury symptoms and then seeks medical assistance, which results in the child's undergoing unnecessary, expensive, potentially harmful medical tests and procedures. The reasons for the perpetrator's need to have the child be ill are not well understood, and MSP remains a difficult problem to diagnose and treat (Smith & Killam, 1994).

Child neglect can be defined as failure by parents or other custodians to meet the medical, emotional, physical, or supervisory needs of a child, whereas child abuse is nonaccidental physical or threatened harm and includes mental and emotional injury, sexual abuse, and sexual exploitation (Allen & Hollowell, 1990). In situations of child abuse and neglect, documentation of evidence is vital.

Documentation

Records provide the legal basis for intervening on behalf of the child. Nursing history and daily notes need to be accurate, timely, and objective. The goal of documentation is to provide a written account of each visit or contact. Because the nursing records may become part of a court proceeding, they need to specify behaviors that indicate progress or failure in providing a safe, nurturing environment for the child. In some neglect cases, much of the evidence is intangible and difficult to prove; therefore, input from many professionals is necessary to convince the court that a child is actually at risk for abuse or neglect. Evidence of risk might include the physician's and nurse's notes on the child, the school nurse's report, and the social worker's impressions during a home visit regarding the child's physical appearance; interactions with parents, peers, and other adults; the child's ability to respond to questions; and the child's general development. Evidence of neglect might include developmental delays, substance abuse, poor medical care, poor school attendance, or lack of supervision. Careful documentation and recorded evidence are essential when presenting a case to the judicial system.

TABLE 4–3 Signs and Symptoms of Physical Abuse

Indication of Abuse	Assessment Findings
Bruises or welts on ears, eyes, mouth, lips, torso, buttocks, genital areas, calves	Injuries in shape of object used to produce them (eg, sticks, belts, hairbrushes, buckles)
	Injuries located on parts of body not usually injured, such as bruising behind the ear, bleeding into the conjunctiva or retina, pinch marks on genitals (normal bruises commonly appear on forehead, shins, knees, elbows)
	Injuries often in various stages of healing
Burns	Shape suggests type of burn
Immersion burns	Immersion burns on feet have "socklike," on hands "glovelike," on buttocks or genitals "donutlike" appearance
Pattern burns	Pattern suggests object used (eg, iron, stove grate, electric burner, heater); small, circular burns on feet, face, hands, chest, or buttocks suggest cigar or cigarette
Friction burns	Friction burns on legs, arms, neck, or torso may be caused by child's having been tied up with rope
Scald burns	Caused by hot liquid poured over trunk or extremities; multiple splash marks may appear on body; depth of burn varies with temperature of liquid, length of contact, and presence of clothing
Fractures of skull, face, nose, orbit, long bones, ribs	Multiple or spiral fractures caused by twisting motion
	Evidence of epiphyseal separations and periosteal shearing
	Shaft fractures from direct blows
	Fractures may be in various stages of healing if earlier fractures went untreated
Lacerations or abrasions on mouth, lips, gums, eyes, genitals	Human bite marks, especially those of adult size, may be evident
	Torn frenulum in infant from forcing object into mouth
	Puncture wounds or deep scratch marks from fingernails around face or genital area
Head trauma	Evidence of increased intracranial pressure in infant (eg, bulging fontanelle)
	Subdural hematomas from being dropped on the head or from receiving blows to the head; if abuse is repetitive, separation of cranial sutures may be evident due to chronic subdural hematoma
	Areas of baldness and swelling from hair being pulled out when dragging the child by the hair
Neck trauma	Limited range of motion from whiplash injury due to being shaken
	Dislocation or subluxation of neck
Somatic	Persistent vomiting or abdominal pain
	Rigid abdomen due to internal bleeding
	Shock
Child's behaviors	Extreme aggressiveness or withdrawal; wariness of adults; fear of going home; apprehension when other children cry
	Appears disinterested or frightened of parents, shows no emotion when parents leave or return
	Indiscriminate friendliness and immediate affection shown toward anyone providing attention
	Vacant stare; no eye contact
	Surveys environment but remains motionless
	Stiffens when approached as if expecting punishment of a physical nature
	Inappropriate response to painful procedures

SOURCE: Adapted from Mott, S.R., et al (1990): *Nursing care of children and families* (2nd ed.), Redwood City, CA: Addison-Wesley Nursing, p 593.

Child Abuse and the Role of the Nurse

By the nature of their work, nurses in a variety of settings are involved in identifying, treating, and preventing child abuse and neglect. In most states, nurses and other health care providers are legally obligated to report any case of suspected child abuse or neglect. The nurse's early detection of child abuse and neglect may lead to the first attempts to intervene and provide services to the child and family.

Family Assessment

Childhood accidents are a common source of injuries; thus every parent who brings a child in for treatment of an injury should not automatically be suspected of abuse. Certain physical and behavioral findings are indicative of abuse, however, and it is important for the nurse to be aware of these clues. Tables 4–3 and 4–4 list the findings indicative of physical and sexual abuse.

In all cases of suspected abuse or neglect, the nurse needs to ask the child and family members present the following questions:

1. How did the accident (or incident) happen?
2. When did the accident happen?
3. Where were the child and other family members at the time?
4. Who was caring for the child at the time?
5. Who saw the accident?
6. What did the child do after the accident?
7. What measures were taken by the parent?

TABLE 4–4 Signs of Sexual Abuse

Physical Signs	Behavioral Signs
Laceration of labia, vagina, or perineum	Advanced knowledge of adult sexual behavior
Irritation, pain, or injury to genital area	Discussion of or implied involvement in sexual activity
Hematomas in genital area	Expression of severe emotional conflict at home with fear of intervention
Vaginal or penile discharge	Reluctance to participate in sports, showers, changing of clothes
Dysuria or urinary frequency	Excessive bathing
Sexually transmitted infection in young child (on eyes, mouth, anus, or genitals)	Sitting carefully because of injuries
Pregnancy	Unusual interest in genital area (eg, fondling of genitals, excessive masturbation, etc)
Itching, bruises, or bleeding in genital area	Sexual acting out with peers
Unexplained vaginal or rectal bleeding	Sleep disturbances (eg, nightmares, fear of sleeping alone)
Enlarged vaginal or rectal orifice	Reluctance to participate in activities with a particular person or at a particular place
Foreign objects in vagina or rectum	Increased number of new fears
Increased rectal pigmentation	Fear of being alone
Gait disturbance	Poor peer relations
Tears in hymen	Depression
	Change in performance at school
	Eating disorders
	Vague somatic complaints
	Extreme shyness
	Increased aggressive or hostile behavior
	Encopresis
	Enuresis
	Self-destructive or suicidal behaviors
	Substance abuse
	Runaway behaviors

SOURCE: Adapted from Mott, S.R., et al (1990). *Nursing care of children and families*, (2nd ed.), Redwood City, CA: Addison-Wesley Nursing, p 597.

Questions to the parents should be phrased in a nonjudgmental way to decrease the likelihood of hostile or defensive responses. For example, it is more effective to ask "How did this burn occur?" than to ask, "How did you do this?" Similarly, open-ended questioning of the child in private ("Would you tell me more about this?") will elicit more information than questions requiring a yes or no response. To protect the child, the nurse should not reveal to the parents information given by the child (Devlin & Reynolds, 1994). After recording answers to these questions, the nurse proceeds with the physical assessment, noting the location, color, and characteristics of all cutaneous lesions. Photographs might be needed as legal evidence.

Orthopedic, surgical, ophthalmologic, and gynecologic examinations also might be needed, depending on the type of injuries. Gynecologic examination includes cultures for gonorrhea and other sexually transmitted infections, microscopic examination for blood and sperm, pregnancy testing, and clothing examination for semen, blood, or pubic hairs. Strict procedures must be followed in collecting evidence and specimens to provide data the courts will accept.

The most important determination to make during the assessment is the risk of reinjury to the victim or injury to other children in the household. Assessment of family functioning, coping strategies, and current state of crisis provides valuable data for such determination. Sometimes, even when the injuries are not severe, hospitalization or foster home placement is necessary. Protection of the child (or children) is always the priority.

In assessing neglected or abused children and their families, the nurse considers the long-term consequences of neglect and their possible effects on family cooperation in meeting goals. Assessment of neglected or abused children and their families includes the following:

- The parents' emotional ability to accept services
- Communication patterns within the family
- The range and availability of services
- The family's use of services
- Supportive counseling for all family members
- The children's growth and developmental patterns
- The parents' attempts to diminish isolation
- The parents' responses to expectations to change behaviors
- The quality of nurturance within the family
- Family dynamics and other risk factors, such as substance abuse or spouse abuse
- Environmental stressors, such as inadequate housing, hygiene, or nutrition

Family Unity and Child Safety

Providing support to marginally functioning parents is generally preferable to removing the child from the home. Removing children is traumatic, and most communities lack adequate foster care homes. Moreover, foster care is more expensive than maintaining the family system.

Without intervention, however, dysfunctional parents tend to continue the cycle of dysfunctional parenting with other children in the family. In some cases, moreover, health care providers' commitment to maintaining the family unit places a child at serious risk of further injury. To decrease this risk, the Adoption and Safe Families Act was enacted in 1997. This new law, while reaffirming the importance of making reasonable efforts to maintain family unity, mandates that a child's safety be the highest priority (DHHS, 1998d).

Support for Dysfunctional Parents

Although both professionals and lay people acknowledge intense feelings concerning child abuse and neglect, they often have little concern for the abusive parents. However, parents as well as children need support in these situations. Working with neglectful and abusive parents is emotionally draining and disturbing for all people involved. Seeing a child victimized calls forth strong emotions, particularly among nurses, who might be required to provide nursing care during the time of the acute injury. A major task for the nurse is helping dysfunctional parents understand the impact of stress and crisis in their lives and the appropriate responses to these crises. In a family that is providing only marginal child care, any stress, however small, might create a crisis. The nurse who identifies stress in dysfunctional families should assess coping strategies and, if indicated, teach appropriate ways to cope with stress.

Most parents need support services as they learn to develop new coping techniques. Group therapy, which provides peer support, might assist abusive parents because finding others with similar problems minimizes isolation. Nurse-therapists can address and help parents verbalize common fears and misconceptions about parenting.

Nurses and other professionals often need to make contracts and establish realistic deadlines in working with families. Dysfunctional families need to be informed that their pattern of child care is inadequate and not acceptable to the community or school system. Facts of legal consequence, including removal of the children, need to be both verbalized and written out. These measures might seem drastic, but if they are handled in too gentle a manner and the family misinterprets the message, valuable time may be lost in mixed messages and conflicts.

Some parents appear to be docile, cooperative, and open but have merely learned responses that please. The nurse therefore must be careful to identify concrete changes that indicate progress; otherwise, the therapeutic contact might end too early for a family that appears to have changed. Periodic evaluation of family dynamics and interagency accomplishments and conflicts should ensure that the family does not manipulate workers or agencies and decrease the effectiveness of the plan. In some instances, a child protective worker is needed to function as coordinator.

Intervention is more effective when multiple resources are available and the family can help choose which resources to use. Most families need to draw on a variety of resources to break the cycle of a dysfunctional lifestyle. Nurses and other health professionals need to be aware of the services available within their communities. They need to help families find those programs most geared to their needs and then coordinate the program goals and the family's progress.

Parents Anonymous, a self-help group for abusive parents, is often an excellent source of information and support for abusive parents seeking to change their behavior. Formerly abusive parents often report increased self-esteem as they assist other parents in distress. Some continue to attend Parents Anonymous meetings long after their initial needs are met, and many parents report pleasurable relationships with their children for the first time in their lives.

Support for the Child

If significant changes in the family are unavoidable, the child needs assistance in working through feelings of having caused the changes. Siblings also need to be included in the treatment plan of an abused or neglected child. If the child is hospitalized, fears of pain or violence are intensified by the unfamiliar surroundings and people. If a parent does visit, the parent is often unsupportive and may be angry with the child. The child is often confused, hurt, and frightened. Nurses and other hospital staff can identify pain, fear, and confusion and help the child discuss those feelings. Nurses need to explain to the child, in developmentally appropriate terms, what will happen and to reassure the child, as much as possible, that the parent will be back. The fewer the number of caregivers, the more likely that the child will establish trusting relationships.

Some children have never heard their names spoken in a gentle voice, and a slow, caring approach is essential to build any degree of trust. Children who withdraw from human contact must be allowed a reasonable period of time in which to grieve and appraise new people. If the child regresses, the regressive behavior needs to be accepted until the child can ease into a more appropriate developmental stage.

Younger children are likely to need nurturing in the form of rocking, cuddling, and soothing. The child initially might appear to reject any comforting, however, or become aggressive in response to overwhelming anxiety. The aggressive behaviors are learned responses to chaotic living and can become a problem if the child manages to manipulate many people. Team members need to set consistent limits in a firm but kindly manner and help the child learn more acceptable behaviors. Aggressive children usually have feelings of deprivation, sadness, and loneliness and may believe themselves to be unworthy and bad. Such children have little faith in their ability to inspire approval and affection.

Individual therapy may help aggressive children discuss family dynamics and the expectations their parents have of them. The therapeutic approach is to face reality honestly and not to arouse expectations in the child that the parent cannot or will not fulfill. Children who have been severely abused or have witnessed severe abuse of a sibling also need support in developing future relationships that are free of fears, guilt, and anxieties. Children facing loss or separation from their parents need therapeutic assistance to handle the loss and time to mourn.

Long-term follow-up of dysfunctional families has no set time for completion. In some instances services are required until the children reach adulthood. Periodic evaluation of parental progress and family growth includes monitoring the behaviors of the children, who might exhibit anger, anxiety, intense loneliness, or apathy. The children's progress in school must also be assessed, together with their response to authority figures. Dysfunctional behaviors suggest that the child needs individual attention.

Suggestions for Nursing Action

Personal Action

- Avoid "rescuer fantasies," which can blind you to the real needs of the child and family.
- Spend time working through your own thoughts and beliefs about child abuse. Identify any stereotypical ideas you may have about abuse and abusers.
- Always bear in mind that the child with whom you are interacting, regardless of the setting, may be in an abusive family environment. Develop skill in identifying these children and in working as a member of an interdisciplinary team.

Client Action

- When possible, advocate for two-nurse teams—one to care for the child and the other to work with the parent. This approach often helps channel negative feelings and maintain lines of communication.
- Be nonjudgmental in working with abusive families.
- Be aware of resources in your community that might assist abusive parents and their children.

Community Action

- Support community programs designed to assist abused children and their parents.
- Be an advocate for educational programs designed to help community members understand the complex factors contributing to child abuse and for effective programs for intervening to break the cycle of abuse.

Political Action

- Provide education, support, and assistance to legislators in enacting laws designed to help abused children and their families break the cycle of violence and dysfunction in which they are caught.

FOCUS YOUR STUDY

- Nurses need to be aware of issues affecting the childbearing woman so that they can better understand the client as she comes to the maternal-newborn health care setting.
- The number of women living in poverty is increasing at a rapid rate. Childbearing women seem to be at particular risk because of current trends in the divorce rate, the frequency with which the mother gains custody of children, and factors in the work environment that make it difficult for women to earn a good wage.
- Women's wages have always been lower than men's because of demand, education, skills, discrimination, and underlying philosophies that deem women's work less valuable. Women are working to change the wage system by pushing for comparable worth legislation.
- Work benefits that affect women include maternity leave and child care. The Family and Medical Leave Act ensures leave for childbirth or adoption but applies only to companies with 50 or more employees. Insurance coverage for childbirth varies by company.
- The belief systems and philosophies regarding abortion are complex. At least four general themes can be identified in arguments for and against abortion: moral views regarding the status of the embryo, the moment that life begins, the personhood of the embryo, and woman's role in society.
- Child abuse is physical, emotional, or sexual violence directed against a child.
- Parents who abuse their children often feel isolated, are unable to trust others, have few supports for coping with stress, or have unrealistic expectations for their children's behavior.
- Indicators of physical abuse include a series of injuries in various stages of healing (especially a series of similar injuries), the family's delay in seeking treatment, use of multiple treatment facilities, and attempts to hide or minimize the abuse, sometimes with special clothing.
- The nurse documents evidence of child abuse by noting and specifically describing parent and child behaviors.
- Nursing actions in cases of child abuse include providing support to the child and parents and providing information about referrals to community resources.

REFERENCES

Allen, J. M., & Hollowell, E. E. (1990). Nurses and child abuse/neglect reporting: Duties, responsibilities, and issues. *Journal of Practical Nursing, 40*(2), 56–59.

Arber, S., & Ginn, J. (1994). Women and aging. *Reviews in Clinical Gerontology, 4*(4), 349–358.

Ashley, B. M., & O'Rourke, K. D. (1994). *Ethics of health care: An introductory textbook.* Washington, DC: Georgetown University Press.

Beal, A. C., & Redlener, I. (1995). Enhancing perinatal outcome in homeless women: The challenge of providing comprehensive health care. *Seminars in Perinatology, 19*(4), 307–313.

Bernhardt, T. H. (1990). Potential workplace hazards to reproductive health: Information for primary prevention. *Journal of Obstetric, Gynecologic, and Neonatal Nursing, 19,* 53.

Brown, L. R., et al. (1990). *State of the World 1990: A Worldwatch Institute report on progress toward a sustainable society.* NY: Norton.

Clarke, S. C. (1995). Advance report on final divorce statistics, 1989 and 1990. *Monthly Vital Statistics Report* (Vol. 43, No. 8, Suppl.). Hyattsville, MD: National Center for Health Statistics.

Collins, J. (1990). Health care of women in the workplace. *Health Care for Women International, 11*(1), 21–32.

Colvez, A. (1996). Disability-free life expectancy. In S. Ebrahim & A. Kalache (Eds.), *Epidemiology in old age.* London: Oxford University Press.

Coohey, C., & Braun, N. (1997). Toward an integrated framework for understanding child physical abuse. *Child Abuse & Neglect, 21*(11), 1081–1094.

Couture, P. D. (1991). *Blessed are the poor?* Nashville, TN: Abingdon Press.

Cunningham, F. G., MacDonald, P. C., Gant, N. F., Leveno, K. J., Gilstrap, L. C., Hankins, G. D. V., Clark, S., L. *Williams obstetrics* (20th ed.). Stamford, CT: Appleton & Lange.

Department of Health and Human Services (1998a, February 24). Annual update of the HHS poverty guidelines. *Federal Register, 63*(36), 9235–9238. On-line via US Government Printing Office access, wais.access.gpo.gov.

Department of Health and Human Services (1998b, March 17). Child support enforcement: A Clinton administration policy (Fact sheet). On-line via http://www.hhs.gov/news/press/1998pres/980317b.html.

Department of Health and Human Services (1998c, April 17). HHS report shows continued record high child abuse and neglect levels (Press release). On-line via http://www.hhs.gov/news/press/1998pres/980417a.html.

Department of Health and Human Services (1998d, May 9). HHS helps parents choose and states better inform parents on quality child care (Press release).

Department of Health and Human Services (1998e, May 27). The Personal Responsibility and Work Opportunity Reconciliation Act of 1996 (Fact sheet). On-line via http://www.hhs.gov/news/press/1998pres/980509.html.

Devlin, B. K., & Reynolds, E. (1994, March). Child abuse: How to recognize it, how to intervene. *American Journal of Nursing, 94*(3), 26.

Dutton, D.B. (1993). Poorer and sicker: Legacies of the 1980s, lessons for the 1990s. In S. Matteo (Ed.), *American Women in the Nineties.* Boston: Northeastern University Press.

Eddins, E. (1993, Spring). Characteristics, health status and service needs of sheltered homeless families. *ABNF Journal, 4*(2), 40–44.

Ellis, J. E. (1993, February 8). What price child care? *Business Week*, 64.

Emery, R. E., & Laumann-Billings, L. (1998). An overview of the nature, causes, and consequences of abusive family relationships: Toward differentiating maltreatment and violence. *American Psychologist, 53*(2), 121–135.

Family Impact Seminar (1996). *Housing is not enough: Helping homeless families achieve self-sufficiency.* Washington, DC.

Gist, Y., & Velkoff, V. (1997, December). *Gender and aging: Demographic dimensions.* Washington, DC: US Bureau of the Census.

Gonen, J. S. (1998, January). Medicaid managed care: The challenge of providing care to low-income women. Briefing paper from the Jacob's Institute of Women's Health, Washington, DC.

Hall, L. A., Sachs, B., & Rayens, M. K. (1998). Mothers' potential for child abuse: The roles of childhood abuse and social resources. *Nursing Research, 47*(2), 87–95.

Hermelin, F. G. (1995). Legislating fair pay. *Working Woman*, 34.

Hewitt, J. B., Misner, S. T., & Levin, P. F. (1993). Health hazards of nursing: Identifying workplace hazards and reducing risks. *AWHONN's Clinical Issues in Perinatal & Women's Health Nursing, 4*(2), 320–327.

Intensified Cooperation Organization (ICO). (1998). *Key issues in health development.* Geneva: World Health Organization: Division of Intensified Cooperation with Countries and Peoples in Greatest Need. Available on-line via http://www.who.ch/ico/key.html.

Karsten, M. F. (1994). *Management and gender.* Westport, CT: Quorum Books.

Kini, N., & Lazoritz, S. (1998). Evaluation for possible physical or sexual abuse. *Pediatric Clinics of North America, 45*(1), 205–219.

Lamison-White, L. (1997). Poverty in the United States: 1996. In US Bureau of the Census, Current Population Reports (Series P60-198). Washington, DC: US Government Printing Office.

Lewis, M. I. (1997, Summer). An economic profile of American older women. *Journal of the American Medical Women's Association, 52*(3), 107–112.

Lynch, S. H. (1997). Elder abuse: What to look for, how to intervene. *American Journal of Nursing, 97*(1), 26–33.

Matteo, S. (1993). *American women in the nineties: Today's critical issues.* Boston: Northeastern University Press.

McAbee, R. R., Gallucci, B. J., & Checkoway, H. (1993). Adverse reproductive outcomes and occupational exposures among nurses: An investigation of multiple hazardous exposures. *AAOHN Journal, 41*(3), 110–119.

Mott, S. R., James, S. R., & Sperhac, A. M. (1990). *Nursing care of children and families* (2nd ed.). Redwood City, CA: Addision-Wesley Nursing.

National Coalition for the Homeless (NCH). (1998, May). *Domestic violence and homelessness.* (NCH Fact sheet no. 8). On-line via http://nch.ari.net/domestic.html.

National Institute for Occupational Safety and Health (NIOSH). (1997, April). NIOSH facts. On-line via http://www.cdc.gov/niosh/nioshfs.html.

Palczynski, C., Walusiak, J., Ruta, U., & Gorski, P. (1997). Occupational allergy to latex: Life threatening reactions in health care workers. Report of three cases. *International Journal of Occupational Medicine & Environmental Health, 10*(3), 297–301.

Paul, M. E. (1993). Physical agents in the workplace. *Seminars in Perinatology, 17*(1), 5–17.

Pearce, D. M. (1993). Something old, something new: Women's poverty in the 1990's. In Matteo, S. (Ed.). *American women in the nineties.* Boston: Northeastern University Press.

Rhode, D. L. (1993). Gender equality and employment policy. In S. Matteo (Ed.), *American women in the nineties.* Boston: Northeastern University Press.

Schnorr, T. M., Grajewski, B. A., Hornung, R. W., Thun, M. J., Egeland, G. M., Murray W. E., Conover, D. L., & Halperin, W. E. (1991, March 14). Video display terminals and the risk of spontaneous abortion. *New England Journal of Medicine, 324*(11), 727–733.

Schumann, D. (1990). Nitrous oxide anesthetic: Risks to healthy personnel. *International Nursing Review, 37*(1), 214–217.

Shalala, D. (1998, February 6). Welfare reform. Remarks presented to the American Enterprise Institute. Washington, DC.

Short, P. F. (1996). *Medicaid's role in insuring low income women.* New York: Commonwealth Fund.

Smith, E. M., Hammonds-Ehlers, M., Clark, M. K., Kirchner, H. L., & Fuortes, L. (1997). Occupational exposures and risk of female infertility. *Journal of Occupational & Environmental Medicine, 39*(2), 138–147.

Smith, K., & Killam, P. (1994). Munchausen syndrome by proxy. *MCN: American Journal of Maternal Child Nursing, 19*(4), 214–221.

Staudinger, K. C., & Roth, V. S. (1998, February 15). Occupational lead poisoning. *American Family Physician, 57*(4), 719–726, 731–732.

US Bureau of the Census (1998, February 24). Women's history month: March 1–31. *Census Bureau facts for features.* Washington, DC: US Census Bureau Public Information Office.

US Bureau of the Census (1997). Labor force, employment, and earnings. In *Statistical abstract of the United States* (117th ed). Washington, DC: US Department of Commerce, Bureau of the Census.

US Department of Commerce (1997). *Statistical abstracts of the United States.* Section 13 Labor Force, Employment, and Earnings. Washington, DC: Author, pp. 393–442.

Waxman, L., & Trupin, R. (1997). A status report on hunger and homelessness in America's cities: 1997. Washington, DC: US Conference of Mayors.

Weinberg, D. H., Huggins, V. J., Kominski, R. A., & Nelson, C. T. (1997, November). A survey of program dynamics for evaluating welfare reform. Paper presented for Statistic Symposium XIV, "New Directions in Surveys and Censuses," Washington, DC: Bureau of the Census.

Wissow, L. (1990). *Child advocacy for the clinician.* Baltimore: Williams & Wilkins.

Wolch J., & Dear, M. (1993). *Malign neglect.* San Francisco: Jossey-Bass.

Zuskin, E., Mustajbegovic, J., Schachter, E. N., Kern, J., Budak, A., & Godnic-Cvar, J. (1998). Respiratory findings in synthetic textile workers. *American Journal of Industrial Medicine, 33*(3), 263–273.

Violence Against Women

5

To my friends I'm living the American dream. My husband is a successful broker; we have a lovely house; we take exotic vacations. Even if I told them about the occasional slap, the shove, the sex when I really didn't want it, they would think it was probably worth putting up with it. Sometimes I do think about leaving, but it would mean admitting I failed. Even as I tell you this, I know it doesn't make sense—he does the hitting, but I feel ashamed. I'm not a battered wife; I can't be. My husband just has a quick temper.

Key Terms

Cycle of violence
Date rape
Domestic violence
Female partner abuse
Rape
Rape trauma syndrome

Objectives

- List the social, psychologic, political, and cultural factors that contribute to the occurrence of female partner abuse and rape.
- Identify the phases of the cycle of violence.
- Describe the myths and facts about female partner abuse.
- Delineate the role of the nurse who cares for battered women.
- Contrast the nonsexual and sexual aspects of rape.
- Compare the types of rape.
- Identify the phases of the rape trauma syndrome.
- Explain the reasons why nurses who care for rape survivors should first explore their personal values and beliefs about rape.
- Discuss the nurse's role as client advocate and counselor with rape survivors.
- Summarize the procedures for collecting and preserving physical evidence of sexual assault.
- Discuss the legal responsibilities of the community to prevent and address violence against women.

VIOLENCE AGAINST WOMEN HAS REACHED epidemic proportions in society today. Experts suggest that as many as one in three women will be the victim of abuse at some time in her life. Violence affects women of all ages, races, and ethnic backgrounds, from all socioeconomic levels, all educational levels, and all walks of life. Two of the most common forms of violence are partner abuse and rape. Society not only accepts these forms of violence against women; it subtly, and sometimes not so subtly, shifts the blame for the violence to the woman herself by asking questions such as, "What did she do to make him so mad?" "Why does she stay?" "What was she doing out so late?"

Violence against women is a major health concern. It costs the health care system millions of dollars and thousands of lives each year. In response to this epidemic, a number of health-related organizations have begun to address the issue. Healthy People 2000 (1992), a national health promotion and disease prevention project, includes in its summary report objectives to decrease violence against women. The Joint Commission on the Accreditation of Healthcare Organizations (JCAHO) has mandated that emergency departments have in place protocols for caring for battered women. The American Nurses Association (1991) advocates education for all nurses in identifying and preventing violence against women as well as routine assessment for abuse in all women.

Historical and Societal Factors Contributing to Violence Against Women

Violence against women is not new. Throughout history, for thousands of years in patriarchal societies, women have been victims of violence. Wives, concubines, sisters, daughters, mothers—none was immune. Female partner abuse (wife battering) is as old as the institution of marriage. Wives were considered the "property" of husbands, subject to their wishes and demands. A husband had the right—even the duty—to "keep her in line," even to kill her. The phrase "rule of thumb" comes from the judicial restriction that when a man beat his wife, the stick he used could be no larger around than the width of his thumb. Outsiders were expected to "keep out of it"; battering was a family matter.

The legal status of women has improved over the years in many cultures. However, many people still hold to the traditional views of male dominance in marriage or any intimate relationship, which can contribute to the occurrence of female partner abuse. Traditionally, rape was viewed not as an act of a man against a woman, but as an act of aggression against another man—the woman's husband or father, that is, her "owner." To rape a man's daughter or wife was the ultimate insult, an act of power. On conclusion of a battle, rape of the wives and daughters of the losers symbolized the triumph of the conquerors and the humiliation of the vanquished.

Violence against women is a means of control by society. Men are generally physically stronger than women and, in a patriarchal society, have greater power and influence. Many women grow up knowing a vague sense of fear that limits their choices and activities because they feel the need always to be on guard. Thus they look to males to serve in the role of "protector," keeping women safe from harm. Unfortunately, these protectors are sometimes the very ones who may perpetrate the acts of violence. But because society often fails to hold men accountable, the violence continues.

Female Partner Abuse

Domestic violence can be defined as collective methods used to exert power and control by one individual over another in an adult domestic or intimate relationship. Gay men, heterosexual women, and lesbian women batter, but by far the majority of abusers are male, and approximately 95% of the victims of this form of violence are women in heterosexual relationships. The partners may be dating, living together, married, separated, or divorced. Because the term *domestic violence* suggests a gender-neutral balance of abuse that is totally inaccurate, the term **female partner abuse** is used in this text.

Female partner abuse is the most common form of violence in the United States but the least reported serious crime. Estimates suggest that a battering incident occurs every 15 seconds in the United States. As many as one in three women will be the victim of assault by her partner in her lifetime. Annually female partner abuse results in 28,700 emergency department visits, 39,000 doctor's office visits, $44 million in total medical costs, and 175,000 lost days of work (Poirier, 1997).

The women's movement and heightened public sensitivity to violence against women have stimulated recognition of the extent of this problem. Forms of abuse may include the following:

- *Physical assault*—pushes, slaps, kicks, punches, knife or gunshot wounds
- *Emotional abuse*—intellectual derision, ridicule, criticism, insults, yelling, coldness, silence, hostility; for example, "You just can't do anything right; what is wrong with you?"
- *Sexual assault*—rape after physical abuse, forced sex while the woman is ill, forced use of objects
- *Economic control*—not allowing the woman to have money of her own, forcing her to ask for everything, and carefully monitoring her, for example, checking gas mileage

- *Social isolation*—not allowing friends and family to visit or making them so uncomfortable that they choose not to visit
- *Destruction of pets and property*—destroying or disposing of treasured objects and killing or maiming pets
- *Threats of violence or harm to the woman or her loved ones*—for example, "If you leave me, I will kill you, your mother, etc."
- *Stalking*—following and watching the woman

Typically these forms of abuse begin slowly and subtly after some form of commitment, such as engagement, onset of a sexual relationship, marriage, first childbirth, or first statement of commitment. The abuse results in a power imbalance, fear, damage to self-esteem, loss of freedom, and, possibly, injury or death.

Contributing Factors

Female partner abuse is a result of the complex and dynamic interaction of social, cultural, political, and psychologic factors.

- *Childhood experiences.* Children who witness or experience abuse and battering are more likely to become batterers (men) or to be abused (women) in their own relationships. Perhaps they view this as normal behavior in intimate relationships.
- *Sex role conditioning.* Some females have been socialized to believe they are inferior, inadequate, and dependent on males for approval. Some males have been socialized to expect these behaviors of females and to expect to be financially successful, aggressive, and independent.
- *Economic insecurity of women.* Women typically receive less pay than men. Those with children are often financially dependent on their partners because their own earning power is limited. When they leave the relationship, they frequently fall into poverty.
- *Ages of children.* Families with young children are subject to more stress and demands; mothers may be more dependent on their husbands for economic and emotional support for themselves and their children.
- *Lack of understanding on the part of professionals.* Law enforcement personnel, clergy, social service agencies, and the judicial system often are unaware of the dynamics of female partner abuse. In addition, they may feel frustrated and impotent when battered women return to their partners.
- *Perception of inequity of power.* Men who feel that they lack power or resources in their homes or jobs may feel the need to prove themselves. As a result, they may assert their superiority by resorting to violence against those they regard as less powerful.
- *Religious traditions.* Some religions support the concept that women are inferior and should be dependent on their husbands. Some religious traditions support patriarchy, which is echoed in some laws and, to an extent, in the economic system.

RESEARCH IN PRACTICE

What is this study about? As part of a larger study concerning reproductive health in Chiapas, Mexico, Namino Glantz, David Halperin, and Linda Hunt explored conjugal physical and sexual violence. Chiapas suffers from lower levels of life expectancy and higher infant and maternal mortality than the remainder of the country. Domestic and sexual violence, a common problem of the area, often encompasses reproductive health issues such as contraception, sterility, sexuality, and pregnancy and birth.

How was the study done? Researchers conducted focused, ethnographic interviews with a convenience sample of 40 mestizo women from 11 municipalities in Chiapas. The interview guide used several techniques to broach sensitive topics, including the introduction of topics through abstract terms, or with hypothetical characters in concrete situations, or with hypothetical narratives such as a couple involved in conjugal violence. Interviewers also asked participants to describe idealized types of individuals such as "good husband" or "bad mother."

What were the results of the study? Participants described 115 events of conjugal violence. Initial descriptive analysis resulted in a typology with four categories: characteristics of event, causes, consequences, and strategies. The characteristics of the 115 events entailed victim (75% hypothetical, 12% informant), perpetrator (98% husband or common-law husband of victim), and nature of violence (physical such as hit [64%], forced sex [31%], and threat [5%]). The primary causes included alcohol (32%), woman committing transgression (32%), and machismo (19%). These women believed that 32% of the time the victim did something to bring about the violent behavior. One example was not having the food ready when the husband got home from work. Another frequent cause of violence—machismo—was attributed to the perpetrator as a male characteristic. The most frequent consequences of the 115 events involved anger (11%), bothered or not at ease (11%), sickness and/or infection (11%), and bruises or lesions (10%). Strategies comprised leaving perpetrator (37%), enduring (32%), and resisting or defending self (31%). The next, or interpretive, phase of the research will focus on understanding the relationships or patterns among the four categories and other variables.

What additional questions might I have? Were there any support systems in place for the study participants if problems resulted from research questions? What did the interviewers do or plan to do if a situation arose in which the participant seemed to be in extreme jeopardy?

How can I use this study? Women in an abusive situation may be reluctant to reveal the violence when confronted directly. An alternative approach might be to employ a technique from this study such as use of a hypothetical situation to introduce the subject of violence.

SOURCE: Glantz, N.M., Halperin, D.C., & Hunt, L.M. (1998, May). Studying domestic violence in Chiapas, Mexico. *Qualitative Health Research 8* (3), 377–92.

Common Myths about Battering and Battered Women

Both professionals and the public believe numerous myths about battering and battered women. These myths often reinforce misunderstanding of battering. Professionals who provide services for battered women need to recognize and counteract these myths. Some commonly accepted myths are discussed here.

- *Battering occurs in a small percentage of the population.* The statistics on reported cases underrepresent the true incidence. As many as one in three women will be the victim of assault by her partner in her lifetime; however, it is estimated that only one in ten women will report battering assaults.
- *Battered women provoke males to beat them; women push men beyond the breaking point and incite physical violence.* It is important to recognize that people are individually responsible for their own behavior. Batterers become violent because of their own internal inadequacies, not because of what the women did or did not do.
- *Alcohol and drug abuse cause battering.* Studies do show a relationship between battering incidents and alcohol or drug use by batterers. In fact, in 1996 over half of those individuals serving prison time for violence against an intimate partner had been using drugs, alcohol, or a combination at the time they committed the incident (US Department of Justice, 1998). However, substance abuse alone cannot be said to cause battering. Some researchers suggest that batterers use alcohol as an excuse to carry out a violent act and shift the blame from themselves to the alcohol. Others suggest that alcohol or drugs reduces the batterer's inhibitions, increasing the likelihood of violent acts. Battered women often blame the violence on the batterer's drunkenness or drug-induced "high" and think the abuse will stop if their partners stop drinking or using drugs. Unfortunately, this usually does not happen.
- *Battered women were battered children.* This myth holds true only in a few cases; the majority did not grow up in violent homes. Most women report that their partners were the first person to beat them.
- *Battered women can easily leave the situation.* Leaving is easier said than done. Women assume they are responsible for their marriages and children; they may still love their partners or husbands, rely on them for financial support, and feel their children need a father. Usually battered women have been psychologically abused and have come to believe that family problems are their fault. They often are isolated by their abuser from family, friends, and agencies that could assist them. Many women with children have no place to go, and shelters sometimes have long waiting lists. Moreover, battered women are at greatest risk for severe battering or murder when they leave the abuser.
- *Batterers and battered women cannot change.* Both batterers and battered women can be resocialized and can learn more effective ways of relating and interacting. Batterers can learn to verbalize their feelings, rechannel their aggressions, and accept the fact that women are not their property to punish or beat. With support, battered women can recognize their own self-worth and develop assertiveness skills.
- *Battered women will be safer when they are pregnant.* Battering may occur for the first time during pregnancy or may escalate in intensity if the woman is already being abused (American College of Obstetricians and Gynecologists [ACOG], 1998). The injury is frequently aimed at the breasts, abdomen, or vagina. Some experts theorize that the partner's low self-esteem is the cause of pregnancy-related abuse. He already views his partner as his personal property and may feel that the fetus is an intruder. He may also resent the extra attention his partner receives from family, friends, and health care providers (Chez, 1994).

Cycle of Violence

Walker (1984), in an effort to better explain the experience of battered women, developed the theory of the **cycle of violence,** which postulates that battering takes place in a cyclic fashion through three phases.

1. In the *tension-building phase,* the batterer demonstrates power and control. This phase is characterized by anger, arguing, blaming the woman for external problems, and possibly minor battering incidents. The woman may blame herself for the battering and believe she can prevent the escalation of the batterer's anger by her own action.
2. The *acute battering incident* is typically triggered by some external event or internal state of the batterer. It is an episode of acute violence distinguished by lack of control, lack of predictability, and major destructiveness. This is generally the briefest of the three phases. Proper interventions can interrupt the cycle of violence before the acute battering incident takes place.
3. The *tranquil, loving phase* is sometimes called the honeymoon period. This phase may be characterized by extremely loving, kind, and contrite behaviors by the batterer as he tries to make up with the woman, or it may simply be manifested by an absence of tension and violence. Without intervention this phase will end at some point, and the cycle of violence will repeat. Over time the cycle of violence increases in severity and frequency.

Characteristics of Battered Women

Battered women may hold traditional views of sex roles. They may have grown up in homes where the woman's role was modeled as submissive, passive, and dependent. These battered women are likely to accept the traditional female role in their marriage or relationship and believe their husbands or partners will love and protect them. They believe in family unity and accept prescribed female sex-role stereotypes, believing it is a woman's responsibility to keep her man happy. Often they believe that they are responsible for the relationship; they have an investment in it and want to make it work. If the relationship fails, they think they have failed as women.

Whereas some battered women were exposed to domestic violence between their parents, others first experience it from their partners.

Battered women typically attribute their beatings to some personal shortcoming or inadequacy because they have been repeatedly accused by their abusers of being "bad" wives or partners and negligent mothers. As these women become more isolated, it becomes harder for them to judge who is right. Convinced that they are to blame, they find it easier to admit their guilt than to confront their partners or husbands. For years the men they love and trust have been telling them how bad or incompetent they are. Eventually they fully believe in their inadequacy, and their low self-esteem reinforces their belief that they deserve to be beaten.

Many battered women are isolated from their families, friends, and neighbors and depend on their partners or husbands for financial and emotional needs. The woman's dependence sets the stage for the partner or husband to exert almost complete control of her environment and finances. The woman ceases to believe that she can be independent or self-sufficient.

After repeated beatings, a woman's self-esteem is virtually nonexistent. She feels embarrassed, depressed, and guilty about a situation over which she has no control. Her sense of hopelessness and helplessness reduces her problem-solving ability. Lack of information of available resources and personal despondency further contributes to her sense of powerlessness. Some women develop a pattern of behavior termed *learned helplessness.* This theory suggests that because experience has taught the woman that she often cannot predict the effects of her actions, she is likely to choose behaviors and responses that have the greatest likelihood of triggering a known response. Learned helplessness often plays a role in a woman's decision to stay in a known situation, even though it is abusive, rather than face the unknown by leaving. More recently, researchers suggest that a *theory of survivorship* better describes the behavior of many women who experience abuse. These women do actively seek help and have found creative ways to survive in abusive relationships when help is not forthcoming (Poirier, 1997; Gondolf, 1988).

Characteristics of Batterers

Batterers come from all racial, ethnic, and religious groups and all professions, occupations, and socioeconomic groups. Batterers often have feelings of insecurity, socioeconomic inferiority, powerlessness, and helplessness that conflict with their assumptions of male supremacy. Emotionally immature or aggressive men may have a tendency to express these overwhelming feelings of inadequacy through violence.

Many batterers feel undeserving of their partners, yet they blame and punish the very person they value. Extreme jealousy and possessiveness are the hallmarks of abusers. They characteristically express their ambivalence by alternating episodes of unmerciful beatings with periods of remorse and loving attention. Extremes in behavior and overreacting are typical patterns.

Some batterers are very calculating and select a partner they feel may be vulnerable. Over a period of time they slowly and purposefully isolate the woman, creating a situation of increased dependence.

Battered women often describe their husbands or partners as lacking respect toward women in general, having come from homes where they have witnessed abuse of their mothers or were themselves abused as children, and having a hidden rage that erupts occasionally. Batterers accept conventional "macho" values, yet when they are not angry or aggressive, they appear childlike, dependent, seductive, manipulative, and in need of nurturing. They may be well respected in the community. This dual personality of batterers reflects the conflict between their belief that they must live up to their macho image and their feelings of inadequacy and insecurity in the role of husband or provider. Combined with low tolerance for frustration and poor impulse control, their pervasive sense of powerlessness leads them to strike out at life's inequities by abusing women.

CRITICAL THINKING QUESTION

Imagine that you have just arrived at a shelter for battered women. You have two children, ages 6 and 8, no cash or credit cards. Because you have been isolated for 10 years, you have no close friends; your parents are living in a nursing home. You haven't held a job since you got married. You will be able to remain at the shelter for 3 weeks. The shelter personnel have helped you find a job as a checker for which you will be paid $6.00/hour. Calculate a budget for 1 month. What problems do you foresee?

NURSING CARE MANAGEMENT

Increased publicity, public sensitivity, and heightened awareness of women's rights are encouraging battered women to leave their homes and seek shelter and community assistance. In the past decade, many communities have developed domestic violence programs, shelters, and resources for battered women. However, the needs of battered women and their children are still insufficiently met.

Battered women enter the health care system in many different settings. Nurses may see them in the physician's office with minor trauma or in the emergency department with multiple severe injuries. Battered women are frequently seen in obstetric services because battering often begins or escalates during pregnancy (ACOG, 1998). Nurses in psychiatric–mental health services frequently counsel women who have been battered, and community health nurses may find battered women during home visits. Unfortunately, emergency departments, hospitals, and social service agencies do not routinely recognize and report battering cases to the legal authorities for action and follow-up, although some states are initiating this policy.

The health care system correctly identifies only 20% of battered women (Moore & Wesa, 1997). Nurses in many different health care settings often come in contact with battered and abused women but fail to recognize them, especially if they have no visible injuries. Nurses who wish to help battered women need advanced knowledge of the dynamics of battered women, assessment skills for recognizing subtle cues of battering, and appropriate intervention skills in counseling and referral.

Working with battered women is sometimes frustrating, and many health care providers feel puzzled when women return to their abusive situations. Nurses must realize that they cannot rescue battered women; these women must decide on their own how to handle the situation, which is often incredibly complex and dangerous. The effective nurse provides battered women with information that empowers them in decision making and supports their decisions.

Nursing Assessment and Diagnosis

Because female partner abuse is so prevalent and so rarely identified by health care providers, many caregivers are now advocating *universal screening of all female clients at every health care encounter.* Screening for female partner abuse should be done privately, with only the nurse and client present, in a safe and quiet place. The woman should be assured that her responses will be kept confidential. Nurses offer a variety of reasons for failing to ask about abuse (Ryan & King, 1998):

- They don't have enough time.
- They believe the question is inappropriate in their health setting (postpartum, general medical unit, etc.).
- Their work setting lacks sufficient privacy.
- They believe the myth that only a certain kind of woman is abused.
- They don't want to hear painful stories of abuse.
- There is a difference in ethnicity or age between the nurse and the client, which makes communication difficult.
- They feel inadequate about intervening if the woman discloses abuse.

Other nurses may be hesitant to ask because they presume that the woman may be offended by the questions. Women are rarely offended by questions about abuse, particularly if prefaced by a statement such as, " Abuse is a major public health problem for women, so we ask all women about it."

McFarlane et al (1997) found that three questions, called the Abuse Assessment Survey, are effective in screening for abuse. These questions are as follows:

1. Have you ever been emotionally or physically abused by your partner or someone important to you?
2. Within the last year, have you been hit, slapped, kicked, or otherwise physically hurt by someone?
3. *(To pregnant women)* Since you've been pregnant, have you been hit, slapped, kicked or otherwise physically hurt by someone?

Signs of possible female partner abuse include:

- Neurologic signs—headaches, including headache following trauma or concussion, tension headache, and migraines; dizziness; paresthesias; unexplained stroke from strangulation; hearing loss; detached retina
- Gynecologic signs—dyspareunia (painful intercourse), sexually transmitted infections, frequent vaginal infections, sexual dysfunction, menstrual disorders, pelvic pain
- Obstetric signs—late onset of prenatal care, premature labor, low-birth-weight infant, excessive concern over fetal well-being, recurrent therapeutic abortion, recurrent spontaneous abortion
- Gastrointestinal signs—dyspepsia, irritable bowel syndrome, globus (sensation of a lump in the throat)
- Musculoskeletal signs—arthralgias (painful joints), chronic pain, osteoarthritis, fibromyalgia
- Psychiatric signs—anxiety, panic, post-traumatic stress disorder, mood disorders, depression, suicide attempts, somatization, eating disorders, substance abuse, child abuse and neglect
- Constitutional signs—fatigue, weight loss, weight gain, multiple somatic complaints, contusions, abrasions, sleep and appetite disturbances, decreased concentration, frequent use of pain medication or tranquilizers
- Trauma—any injury to the female organs, extensive accident history, old fractures, sexual trauma

- Other signs—history of missed appointments or frequently changed appointments; low self-esteem, as seen in the woman's dress, her appearance, and the way she relates to health care providers

When a woman seeks care for an injury, the nurse should be alert to the following cues of abuse:

- Hesitation in providing detailed information about the injury and how it occurred
- Inappropriate affect for the situation
- Delayed reporting of symptoms
- Pattern of injury consistent with abuse, including multiple injury sites involving bruises, abrasions, or contusions to the head (eyes and back of neck), throat, chest, breast, abdomen, or genitals. Nonbattered women's injuries are usually located at one or two sites and on the extremities, such as sprains and strains. Battered women may have scars and evidence of old injuries that have healed.
- Inappropriate explanation for the injuries, such as being "accident prone"
- Lack of eye contact
- Signs of increased anxiety in the presence of the possible batterer, who frequently does most of the talking

The nurse should conduct the assessment interview in a quiet, private place in which the woman can feel safe. When culturally appropriate, it is important to maintain eye contact and avoid excessive note taking. The nurse should assure the woman that her privacy will be respected. It is essential that the nurse remain nonjudgmental, create a warm, caring climate conducive to sharing, and demonstrate a willingness to talk about violence. A battered woman will often interpret the nurse's willingness to discuss violence as permission for her to discuss it as well.

The assessment of the woman who may be experiencing abuse should include information about her strengths and her support system. Strengths may include education, employment history, activities in the home, community involvement, and her ability to cope or handle past problems. The woman's support system may include her family, friends, neighbors, and community agencies or organizations.

During the assessment phase, the nurse begins building a relationship with the woman based on trust, understanding, and advocacy. A woman may feel ashamed and embarrassed about her injuries and situation. It is important to assure her that all information she provides will be kept confidential. Trust begins as the nurse conveys an attitude of unconditional acceptance, empathy, and positive regard for the woman's worth and dignity. Nurses should show that they recognize the woman's feelings and that they accept her right to feel as she does.

In cases where the woman states she has been beaten, kicked, punched, or attacked but does not identify the assailant, the nurse should record the extent of injuries, note the woman's exact words, and describe the incident with a diagnosis of probable battering. Those cases in which the woman states she was beaten by a husband or partner may be diagnosed as battering with all evidence recorded, including the woman's statements.

When abuse or battering is suspected or determined, the nurse should formulate nursing diagnoses based on the assessment findings. Nursing diagnoses related to nonphysical components of abuse or battering may include the following:

- ***Self-Esteem Disturbance*** related to feelings of worthlessness and powerlessness
- ***Knowledge Deficit*** related to lack of information about community resources to assist her

Nursing Plan and Implementation

When a battered woman comes in for treatment, she needs to feel safe physically and safe in talking about her injuries and problems. If a man is with her, the nurse should ask or tell him to remain in the waiting room while the woman is examined. This may reduce her fear, help establish trust, and facilitate her expressions of guilt, shame, and embarrassment, along with pent-up anger, rage, and terror about her battering situation. Anger may be directed toward herself, the batterer, or health professionals.

A battered woman also needs to reestablish a feeling of control over her world. She needs to regain a sense of predictability by knowing what to expect and how she can interact. The nurse should provide sufficient information about what to expect in terms the woman can understand. Simple explanations about how long she will stay, whom she will see, and what will be done are important. Giving the woman control can be accomplished by asking her permission before any activities or procedures and by providing her with choices whenever possible.

The nurse encourages the woman to talk about her injuries and home situation by asking, "How did this happen to you?" or saying, "We often see injuries like yours when a woman has been beaten. Has this happened to you?" Directly confronting the injuries and possible battering may provide an opening for the woman who is trying to cope in private. A woman may continue to deny her battering. The nurse should encourage her to talk but should avoid badgering her.

Supportive counseling and reassurance are professional skills nurses use throughout each phase of the nursing process with a battered woman. The nurse should do the following:

- Let the woman work through her story, problems, and situation at her own pace.

TABLE 5–1 National Domestic Violence Hotline
800-799-SAFE
800-787-3224 (TDD)

- Let the woman know that she is believed and not considered crazy.
- Anticipate her ambivalence in the love-hate relationship with the batterer. She knows he may be loving and contrite after the incident if she has been through the cycle of violence before.
- Respect the woman's capacity to change and grow when she is ready.
- Assist her in identifying specific problems, and support realistic ideas for reducing or eliminating those problems.
- Help clarify the woman's beliefs and myths, and provide information to change her false beliefs.
- Stress that no one should be abused and that the abuse is not her fault.

The appropriate intervention is not to tell an abused woman what to do, but to help her recognize her options and resources and make her own decisions. Even advising or encouraging a woman to leave an abusive situation is not always in the woman's best interest; leaving the home is a major decision with long-lasting consequences. The woman may be economically unable to leave the situation, especially if she has young children. If the woman leaves and then later returns home, both husband and wife may become more frustrated, increasing the possibility of further beatings and even homicide. The most acceptable course of action is one that the woman freely chooses.

Teaching for Self-Care

If the woman returns to an abusive situation, the nurse should encourage her to develop an exit plan for herself and her children, if she has any. As part of the plan, she should pack a change of clothes for herself and the children, including toilet articles and an extra set of car and house keys. She should store these away from the house with a friend or neighbor. If possible, she should have money, identification papers (driver's license, Social Security card), checkbook, savings account information, other financial records (such as mortgage papers, automobile title), and information about the children to help her enroll them in school. She should also plan where she will go, regardless of the day or time. The nurse should ensure that the woman has a planned escape route and emergency telephone numbers she can call, including the local police, a phone hotline, and a women's shelter if one is available in the community.

Community-Based Nursing Care

Besides offering emotional support, medical treatment, and counseling, the nurse should inform any woman who may be in an abusive situation of the services available in the hospital, agency, and community. The nurse can also provide the woman with the phone number of any local resources, as well as the number for the National Domestic Violence Hotline (Table 5–1).

Specifically, a battered woman may need:

- Medical treatment for injuries
- Temporary shelter to provide a safe environment for herself and her children
- Counseling to raise her self-esteem and help her understand the dynamics of family violence
- Legal assistance for protection or prosecution of the batterer
- Financial assistance to provide shelter, food, and clothing
- Job training or employment counseling
- An ongoing support group with counseling on relationships with males and children

A network of community agencies can meet these numerous, varied needs of women, children, and batterers. It is important that employees in these agencies understand the complex dynamics of family violence and female partner abuse as well as how their services and those of other agencies can assist these families. Services that are available to the battered woman are discussed in the following sections.

Emergency Department Services Many battered women are first seen and diagnosed in the emergency departments of their neighborhood hospitals. Emergency department nurses and personnel need to be alert to symptoms of battering, recognize these cues, and encourage women to seek assistance from community agencies. Some states require that suspected cases of abuse and battering be reported to the legal authorities or social service agencies.

Shelter and Housing Since family violence has been recognized as a major social problem, many community agencies have sought federal and state funds to provide needed services and shelters. Shelters differ in the services they provide, depending on the governing body, financial resources and funding agencies, organizational structure, staff qualifications, and range of available community services. Typical shelters provide battered women and their children with a room, beds, food, clothing, and other basic necessities. If professional staff is available, the shelter may offer crisis counseling, individual and group counseling, and information about community agencies such as legal aid, welfare, job training, financial and employment agencies, and women's counseling or support groups.

For safety reasons the location of most shelters is undisclosed, but they can be contacted through a community crisis line. Unfortunately, admission requirements usually state that the woman must have been beaten in the past; this prevents women who are in potentially violent situations from seeking admission until they have been beaten.

Legal Services and Options During incidents of domestic violence, the police are frequently called by the victim or neighbors. Family violence typically occurs on the weekend or in late evening, when most social service agencies are closed; therefore the police department is often the first major agency involved. Most states have laws requiring mandatory arrest if a domestic disturbance report is marked by violence.

Legal options for battered women vary according to state laws and services. In some states a woman may seek a restraining order from the family court or a domestic relations court to protect herself from the batterer. This restraining order specifies that the man may not physically abuse any family members but does not give him a criminal record. Unfortunately, many abusive men violate the restraining order and continue to stalk, harass, intimidate, and abuse their female partner. If the battered woman decides to prosecute, the case is usually heard in criminal court, which handles crimes of assault, harassment, and battery. Criminal court hearings may result in a fine, probation, or a jail sentence if the batterer is convicted, giving the man a criminal record. The prosecution process is often lengthy and may last more than a year. Some state judicial systems are introducing other options, such as mandatory counseling for batterers, in lieu of prosecution. Unfortunately, this counseling does not show great promise for permanent change. Divorce is another legal recourse a woman may choose, but divorce may take several months to a year.

Many battered women are unaware of their legal options. They fear further beatings if they prosecute the batterer. Limited financial resources may also keep them from seeking legal assistance. Some women do not understand the complex judicial process and their options within it. Currently, some communities provide legal advocacy services to help battered women understand the judicial process and its consequences to the woman, children, and batterer.

Financial Services Once battered women leave their homes or seek legal assistance, they usually receive no financial support from the batterer. Without funds battered women and their children are at the mercy of community social service agencies, and it usually takes weeks for papers to be processed before any money is forthcoming. Agencies that may provide financial assistance to battered women include their county

CRITICAL THINKING IN PRACTICE

Marsha Martin, age 23, has come to the emergency department for an injury to her upper left shoulder. She is accompanied by her boyfriend with whom she lives, Fred Schultz. The nurse asks Marsha to tell her the details surrounding the injury to her shoulder. Marsha relates that she is very clumsy and was walking through the house in a hurry when she ran into the door jamb. She said the incident happened 2 hours ago. She complains of discomfort in the shoulder. While relating her story, she often looks at Fred. Fred nods his head in agreement with Marsha's statements. Upon assessment the nurse discovers that Marsha's shoulder is very edematous and bruised. The amount of edema and bruising is not consistent with an injury that happened 2 hours ago. What would you as the nurse do next?

Answers can be found in Appendix I.

welfare department, federal programs (eg, Temporary Assistance for Needy Families), the United Way, women's support groups, religious organizations, and possibly the Salvation Army. There may be other local groups to assist these women in various ways, such as providing food or clothing.

Employment Training or Placement Some battered women are full-time mothers who lack advanced education, training, and job experience. Minimal skills and inadequate transportation often make it difficult for these women to obtain employment with an adequate salary. Women who have children must consider where to place them during working hours as well as the added cost of child care. Often, the woman's choice is restricted to accepting welfare or taking a low-paying job. Either choice usually means lowering the standard of living to mere subsistence.

Some women do seek job training if the opportunities are available, but training provides no guarantee of future job placement. A woman may still have to arrange for financial support and child care while obtaining advanced employment skills or an education.

Counseling Battered women may be offered a variety of counseling services, such as crisis intervention, short-term individual therapy, group therapy, or peer support groups, over an extended period. Counseling and therapy may be provided by specially trained nurses, social workers, psychologists, mental health specialists, or clergy.

Rape

If you really want to help her, the first thing you must do is believe her—even if no weapons were used, she knew the single assailant, she didn't make a police report, and/or there is

no evidence of harm. It is not necessary for you to decide if she was "really raped." She says she was raped, and that's enough. She feels raped, and she needs your support.
~ LINDA E. LEDRAY, *RECOVERING FROM RAPE* ~

In its broadest sense, rape is involuntary sexual contact with another person. The National Crime Victimization Survey defines it as follows: "**Rape** is forced sexual intercourse and includes both psychological coercion as well as physical force. Forced sexual intercourse means vaginal, anal, or oral penetration by the offender(s)." The rapist may be a stranger, acquaintance, spouse or other relative, or an employer. Rape is an act of violence expressed sexually—most commonly, a man's aggression and rage acted out against a woman.

Rape has been reported against females from age 6 months to 93 years, but it remains one of the most underreported violent crimes in the United States. The National Center for Prevention and Control of Rape estimates that one out of three women will be raped at some time in her life. The 1994 Crime Victimization Survey indicated that almost two-thirds of victims of completed rapes did not report the assault to the police (Perkins & Klaus, 1996). Estimates suggest that 1.3 rapes occur every minute in the United States (Haddix-Hill, 1997). Even more disturbing, only 1% of rapists are arrested and convicted (Herman, 1992).

No woman of any age or ethnic background is immune, but statistics indicate that young, unmarried women, women who are unemployed or have a low family income, and students have the highest incidence of rape or attempted rape (Herman, 1992). Adolescent rape survivors are often reluctant to report a rape for several reasons: embarrassment, feelings of guilt, fear of retribution, lack of knowledge of their legal rights, concerns about confidentiality, lack of funds, and limited access to health care. The young adolescent may also avoid disclosing an assault to the authorities because she may be worried about revealing the circumstances, especially if they involved risk-taking behaviors such as underage drinking, drug use, accepting a ride from a stranger, or socializing with older males (Holmes, 1998).

Many people believe the myths that rape commonly occurs at night to provocatively clothed, promiscuous women by unknown assailants. They believe that rapists are sex-starved lunatics who were provoked by the clothing or appearance of the woman. Furthermore, it is a common misconception that no truly virtuous woman can be raped against her will, so that if rape occurs, the woman must have "asked for it." Conversely, the myth continues, there is nothing a woman can do about rape; she should just relax and enjoy it.

The belief in some or all of these myths has shaped people's response to the rape survivor. Research indicates that males in general are more tolerant of rape and people with traditional views of marital roles tend to believe more that women are responsible for causing rape (Caron & Carter, 1997). Culture also plays an important role in people's response to rape. In cultures where virginity is highly valued, a woman may be blamed for damaging the family honor following rape. Similarly, sexually conservative people are more likely to view a rape victim as less desirable.

Like their victims, rapists come from all ethnic backgrounds and walks of life. More than half are under 25 years of age, and three out of five are married and leading "normal" sex lives. Why do these men rape? Of the many theories proposed in answer to this question, none provides a concrete explanation.

Unfortunately, so few rapists are actually caught and convicted that a clear characterization of the assailant has not been developed. Far from being lusty, overly amorous, or perverted, the rapist tends to be emotionally weak and insecure and may have difficulty maintaining interpersonal relationships. Many rapists also have trouble dealing with the stresses of daily life. Such men may become angry and overcome by feelings of powerlessness. They then commit the act of rape as an expression of power or anger (Dupre et al, 1993).

Types of Rape

Rape has been categorized in different ways, which are not mutually exclusive:

- In *blitz rape*, the assailant and victim are strangers, and the rape is sudden and unexpected. The rapist is more likely to use a weapon and threaten violence or murder.
- In *acquaintance rape* (also called *confidence rape*), the assailant is someone with whom the victim had previous nonviolent interaction. The attacker uses deception and trust to gain access to the victim and then betrays that trust.
- In *power rape*, the purpose of the assault is control or mastery. The male uses sexual intercourse to place a woman in a powerless position so that he can feel dominant, potent, and strong. He often believes his victim enjoys the assault, and he exerts only the amount of force necessary to subdue his victim. Often power rape is a planned blitz attack, but most acquaintance rapes are also power rapes.
- In *anger rape*, the sexual assault is used to express feelings of rage. Often the act is characterized by considerable brutality and degradation. Attacks on older women often are a form of anger rape.
- In *sadistic rape*, the assailant has an antisocial personality and delights in torture and mutilation. In this type of rape, the victim and assailant are generally strangers, and the assault is planned. Most rape homicides are sadistic rapes.
- In *gang rape*, the assailants are more commonly younger men responding to peer pressure. Typically, only one or two of the men has a rapist mentality,

TABLE 5–2 Phases of Recovery Following Rape

Phase	Response
Acute Phase (Disorganization)	Fear, shock, disbelief, desire for revenge, anger, anxiety, guilt, denial, embarrassment, humiliation, helplessness, dependence, self-blame, wide variety of physical reactions, lost or distorted coping mechanisms.
Outward Adjustment Phase (Denial)	Survivor appears outwardly composed, denying and repressing feelings; for example, she returns to work, buys a weapon; refuses to discuss the assault; denies need for counseling.
Reorganization	Survivor makes many life adjustments, such as moving to a new residence or changing her phone number; uses emotional distancing; may engage in risky sexual behaviors. May experience sexual dysfunction, phobias, flashbacks, sleep disorders, nightmares, anxiety. Has a strong urge to talk about or resolve feelings; may seek counseling or remain silent.
Integration and Recovery	Time of resolution; survivor begins to feel safe and be comfortable trusting others; places blame on assailant. May become an advocate for others.

but they are able to incite the others to commit acts they would not do individually. Often gang rape can escalate to severe violence as the young men seek to outdo each other.

Date rape is a type of acquaintance rape. This type of rape is commonly found on college campuses and occurs between a dating couple. Estimates indicate that as many as 80% of the rapes that occur on college campuses are date or acquaintance rapes. Unfortunately, only about one out of ten victims of acquaintance rape discloses the assault to police, family, health care providers, or friends (Rickert & Wiemann, 1998). In date rape situations, the male has usually planned to have sex and will do what he feels necessary if denied. Thus in this case the primary motivation of the rapist is sexual gratification (Crooks & Baur, 1998).

In some cases, a rapist uses alcohol or other drugs to sedate his intended victim. Recently flunitrazepam (Rohypnol), a potent sedative-hypnotic that is legal in 80 countries worldwide but illegal in the United States, has received considerable attention as the "date rape drug of choice." Typically Rohypnol, which dissolves easily and is odorless, is slipped into the drink of an unsuspecting woman. Because the drug frequently produces amnesia, the woman may be unable to remember details of her assault; thus prosecution of the rapist is more difficult (Saum & Inciardi, 1997).

Rape Trauma Syndrome

Rape is viewed as a situational crisis, that is, an unanticipated traumatic event that the victim generally is unprepared to handle because it is unforeseen. Following rape, the survivor may experience a cluster of symptoms originally described by Burgess and Holmstrom (1979) as the **rape trauma syndrome.** Burgess and Holmstrom originally described this syndrome as having two phases: the acute phase and the adjustment, or reorganization, phase. Other authors added a third phase: an intermediate, outward adjustment phase. Recently a fourth phase—integration and recovery—has been suggested (Holmes, 1998). The phases of recovery following sexual assault are summarized in Table 5–2. Although the phases of response are discussed individually, they often overlap, as do individual responses and their duration. Other authors have described an alternative "silent reaction."

Acute Phase (Disorganization)

The acute phase of rape trauma syndrome begins during the rape and may last for a few days or up to 3 weeks. The woman may experience fear, shock, disbelief, and sometimes denial. The woman may feel humiliated, guilty, and unclean; her wish to cleanse herself by bathing or douching may be overpowering, even if she knows that by doing so she is destroying evidence. She may feel angry or anxious, powerless or helpless.

The rape survivor may suppress her emotions or may reveal them by crying, sobbing, or acting tense and restless. Survivors who control or mask their emotions may appear calm, composed, or subdued. Many rape survivors also experience alterations in sleep patterns, such as insomnia, nightmares, or crying out at night.

Outward Adjustment Phase (Denial)

Once the acute stage has passed, the survivor may appear adjusted. She returns to work or school and resumes her usual roles. But although she appears composed, she is actually coping by denial and suppression. The survivor needs the outward adjustment phase to cope with the experience of rape; it is a means of regaining control of her life. During this time, she may move to a different residence or may institute security measures, such as installing extra locks or requesting an unlisted telephone number. She may buy a weapon or take a course in self-defense. These activities do not resolve her emotional trauma; they simply push it further into her subconscious. In addition she may get less support from others who perceive her as being "over it."

Reorganization

Denial and suppression cannot sustain the survivor for long. These coping mechanisms, that do not resolve the experience but only mask it, deteriorate; she becomes depressed and anxious and feels a strong urge to talk about the rape. At this point, the woman enters the reorganizational phase of the rape trauma syndrome. She must alter her self-concept and resolve her feelings about the rape.

During this phase, the rape survivor experiences numerous difficulties. Survivors frequently report prolonged menstrual or other gynecologic disorders. The woman may develop phobias. Fears of being indoors or outdoors or of being attacked from behind—depending on how the attack took place—are common. Because of these fears, the woman may alter her lifestyle. If she is afraid of crowds, of being out after dark, or of returning to an empty house, she may become a virtual recluse.

Rape survivors frequently report sexual dysfunction. Some women become totally averse to sexual activity. Those who do try to engage in sex often report a decrease in vaginal lubrication, an inability to be aroused, unusual sensations in the genital area, and an inability to achieve orgasm.

Sleep disorders persist. Survivors report repeated nightmares in which they either relive the rape or thwart the rapist's attempt. In either case the dream contains disturbing violence. The woman repeatedly replays the role of victim until she comes to terms with the experience.

Integration and Recovery

This final phase brings resolution for the woman. She is able to recognize that the blame for her assault lies with her assailant. She begins to be able to trust others again and begins to feel safe in her life and day-to-day activities. She may be filled with a sense of righteous anger and become an advocate for other women (Holmes, 1998).

The Silent Reaction

Women who do not report the rape go through the phases of the rape trauma syndrome without using available support systems. Their reasons for keeping silent vary; a woman may be embarrassed; she may accept society's "temptress view" and blame herself; or she may fear retaliation. Her experience may be discovered much later, perhaps when she seeks professional help in resolving a different crisis.

Some women seek medical help for their physical injuries without disclosing that a rape was the cause. The nurse who suspects that a woman has been raped should seek validation through sympathetic questioning.

Rape as a Cause of Post-Traumatic Stress Disorder

Recent research has demonstrated that rape survivors exhibit high levels of post-traumatic stress disorder (PTSD), the same disorder that developed in many of the veterans of the Vietnam War. To be diagnosed as having PTSD, a person must

- Have been exposed to a traumatic event that triggered feelings of intense fear, horror, or helplessness.
- Reexperience the event in recurrent, intrusive thoughts, images, and perceptions, including, for example, a sense of reliving the experience through, dreams, flashbacks, and hallucinations.
- Persistently avoid stimuli associated with the trauma and demonstrate a generalized "numbing" of responsiveness; demonstrate persistent signs of increased arousal, such as exaggerated startle response, difficulty falling asleep, hyper-vigilance or outbursts of anger, which were not present before the trauma occurred (Clark, 1997).

Post-traumatic stress disorder is marked by varying degrees of intensity. One mitigating factor is individual resiliency. Not surprisingly, the intensity of the post-traumatic disorder is often greatest for women who had psychiatric disorders prior to their assault.

Post-traumatic stress syndrome is difficult to treat. Because the symptoms keep an individual from addressing the problem, she cannot integrate the event into her life, and healing is blocked. Recovery depends on empowering the woman to seek to regain control of her life within the context of healing relationships and professional counseling.

Physical Care of the Rape Survivor

Following rape, repairing tissue damage and preventing complications are primary concerns. As many as 40% of those who are sexually assaulted sustain injuries; of those injured, about 1% require hospitalization and major surgical repair, while 0.1% are fatal (ACOG, 1997). Because rape is a crime as well as a traumatic emergency, however, some aspects of health care are governed by the need to collect and preserve legal evidence for use in prosecuting the assailant. In so doing, health care providers must respect the rights of the rape survivor. To better meet women's needs, many emergency departments use multidisciplinary teams to provide effective care to rape survivors and their families. See the accompanying Community in Focus box on the SANE Program.

Detailed History

Obtaining a detailed history is an essential first step in acquiring necessary medical and forensic data, but it can also be a therapeutic tool if done in a sensitive, caring way. Because a rape survivor may appear relaxed and normal when first seen, caregivers may underestimate her needs, but it is essential that she receive immediate attention. Immediately after the woman has received any necessary emergency care, the nurse takes an explicit history of the event in the woman's own words. Many agencies use a standardized forensic chart containing a history flow sheet to record information obtained. The caregiver should use a nonjudgmental approach and must avoid leading or coaching the woman.

COMMUNITY IN FOCUS

The SANE Program

In many communities, the treatment of a woman immediately following a rape has been almost as traumatic as the rape itself. Often the woman is taken to the local emergency department accompanied by a police officer, and sits in the waiting room while others speculate as to why she requires a police escort. She may have to wait 4–8 hours or more to be seen by the physician, who first has to treat life-threatening emergencies. During this period, she is not allowed to urinate, shower, eat or drink anything, or change her clothes, because these activities might destroy or alter physical evidence. The police officer who accompanies the rape victim is also detained, unable to leave the victim until the examination is completed and specimens obtained, thus preserving the chain of evidence.

In Tulsa, Oklahoma, the Sexual Assault Nurse Examiner (SANE) Program is designed to address this problem. SANE is coordinated by the police department and provides a seamless program of post-rape health care, personal counseling, and prosecution by combining the resources of seven community organizations: the police department, the district attorney's office, Call Rape (rape crisis center), the Victim/Witness Center, the Tulsa City/County Health Department, the University of Oklahoma College of Medicine, and Hillcrest Medical Center (Kauffold, 1996).

Following the report of a rape, provided that the woman's physical injuries are not severe, a police officer brings the rape victim to a special examination suite, away from the busy emergency department. They are met there by a specially trained female sexual assault nurse examiner and a rape crisis counselor. The victim is examined immediately by the SANE nurse, who completes the lengthy examination and gathers all necessary forensic evidence. The hospital ob/gyn resident is available to the nurse if there is a need for further examination and treatment.

Because the evidence collected by the SANE nurses has been of such high quality, the Tulsa District Attorney has designated SANE nurses as expert witnesses in rape trials. Each SANE nurse participates in an extensive training program, agrees to serve as an expert witness if necessary, and takes calls so that nurses are always available to respond when a rape occurs.

Similar programs exist elsewhere. The Sexual Assault Response Team (SART), which started in San Diego, is a multidisciplinary approach that also makes use of SANE nurses. The SART Program is designed to ensure that victims receive necessary health care, emotional support, evidentiary examinations, and referral information. The International Association of Forensic Nurses (the terms *sexual assault nurse examiner* and *forensic nurse* are comparable) estimates that 30–40 new SART programs have started in the United States in the past year (Voelker, 1996).

These programs are highly effective in addressing a real community need. In Tulsa, for example, successful convictions of accused rapists are up significantly (Kauffold, 1996). Equally important, however, the victim of a rape is treated with care and compassion and not victimized a second time.

Collection of Evidence

The collection of evidence may, in itself, be traumatic for the woman. It is valuable to have someone available to provide support and act as an advocate. This person may be a family member or close friend, but often it is a nurse. An interpreter should also be provided as necessary.

The woman should receive a thorough explanation of the procedures to be carried out and should sign a consent form. An important legal concept when dealing with rape survivors is the need to preserve the chain of evidence, meaning that all physical evidence and specimens should remain in the hands of a professional until they are turned over to a police officer. The chain of evidence is preserved to prevent confusion and the possibility of tampering with evidence (Haddix-Hill, 1997). Most agencies have special sexual assault kits that contain all necessary supplies for collecting and labeling evidence.

A careful examination of the entire body is necessary. Vaginal and rectal examinations are performed, along with a complete physical examination for trauma. Any lacerations of the vaginal wall are repaired and noted. A colposcope with photographic capability can be used to document injuries to the genitalia.

Clothing The woman is asked to remove her clothing while standing on a clean paper sheet. The sheet and each piece of clothing are marked, placed in an individual paper bag, sealed, and labeled in a detailed manner.

Swabs of Stains and Secretions Swabs of body stains are analyzed for semen or sperm. Because victims are often forced to commit fellatio, oral swabs are examined for semen. Gonorrhea and chlamydia cultures also are taken from vaginal, rectal, and oral cavities. Specimens of the woman's saliva are examined to determine whether she is a secretor or nonsecretor of certain blood group antigens. If she is a nonsecretor—that is, if these antigens are not present in her saliva—the presence of antigens in her mouth and/or vagina may be evidence of semen from the assailant.

Vaginal, cervical, and rectal swabs are necessary to document the presence of sperm. Because sperm are sensitive to air and do not survive for long periods, a screen for vaginal sperm is performed promptly. A vaginal smear is placed on a wet mount and stained; any sperm that are present will appear light blue. The absence of sperm, however, does not signify that no rape has occurred.

Many rapists suffer from sexual dysfunction during the rape and do not ejaculate, or they may use a condom.

Hair and Scrapings Clippings or scrapings of the woman's fingernails are examined for blood or tissue from the assailant. Approximately 20 to 25 hairs are pulled from her head to analyze the root structure and identify foreign hairs. Her pubic hair is combed to check for loose pubic hair that may have been transferred from the rapist, and 20 to 25 of her pubic hairs are pulled to provide a comparison for forensics. Pulling, although uncomfortable, preserves the root of the hair, the portion needed for forensic comparison.

Blood Samples Blood is drawn to test for syphilis and to determine the woman's blood type. Additional blood may be drawn for a pregnancy test if the woman indicates that she wants to take emergency contraception (Ovral) to prevent pregnancy. She has to have a negative pregnancy test to receive the medication.

Photographs Photographs should be taken of injured areas if possible. Prior to taking any photos, the health care provider should ask the woman to sign an informed consent form.

Prevention of Sexually Transmitted Infections The survivor is offered prophylactic antibiotic treatment for sexually transmitted infections (STIs) and is referred to a clinic specializing in their treatment to evaluate the effectiveness of the therapy. Any identified STIs are treated. If the survivor chooses not to receive prophylactic antibiotic treatment, the nurse should instruct her to be seen by her caregiver in 2 weeks for assessment for any STIs. In addition, because hepatitis B is a risk, the woman who has never been immunized should be given hepatitis B immune globulin immediately if possible but not later than 14 days after exposure; she should also begin the hepatitis B three-dose immunization series immediately (ACOG, 1997). In some states, prophylactic treatment for HIV is also begun.

Prevention of Pregnancy The woman is questioned about her menstrual cycle and contraceptive practices. If she is at risk for pregnancy and a pregnancy test is negative, emergency postcoital contraception is offered. (See Chapter 3 for further discussion.)

NURSING CARE MANAGEMENT

Because rape survivors frequently enter the health care system by way of the emergency department, nurses are often the first to counsel them. Because the caregiver's values, attitudes, and beliefs will necessarily affect the competence and focus of the care, nurses who work with rape survivors must understand their own attitudes and beliefs about rape and rape survivors and resolve any conflicts that may exist.

Nursing Assessment and Diagnosis

Policies for admitting and examining rape survivors vary among institutions. A woman who has been raped is under great stress and needs the sensitive care of professionals who are aware of her special needs. The first priority is creating a safe, secure milieu. Professionals should gather admission information in a quiet, private room and reassure the woman that she is not alone, will not be abandoned, and is safe from a second attack. The survivor's level of emotional distress must be assessed, both for the purpose of planning care and as possible courtroom evidence. Scrupulous documentation is essential because the survivor's medical record is often used in the courtroom to verify her testimony if the rapist is prosecuted. The mental status examination includes the following:

- *General appearance and behavior.* What is the woman's attitude? Her posture? What mannerisms does she display?
- *Consciousness/awareness.* Is the woman oriented to time, place, and identity? Is she able to focus on a subject, theme, or event?
- *Affect and mood.* Is the woman depressed? Anxious? Displaying elation or anxiety? Is she fearful or apathetic? Is she expressing her feelings or controlling them?
- *Motor behavior.* Is the woman inactive, hyperactive, or underactive?
- *Thought control.* How logical is the woman's flow of ideas and associations?
- *Intellectual functioning.* What is her level of general knowledge? How does she express herself? How well does she remember events? How is she coping and solving problems?

Examples of nursing diagnoses that may apply to the rape survivor include the following:

- ***Fear*** related to invasion of personal space secondary to rape
- ***Powerlessness*** related to inability to regain sense of control secondary to rape

Nursing Plan and Implementation

Table 5–3 outlines the general nursing actions that are appropriate during each of the phases of recovery. *It is imperative that control be returned to the woman as quickly as possible.* The nurse can return control by encouraging the woman to make contact. When feasible, the woman should decide on the sequence of forensic events, such as pulling her own hair (head and pubic), having blood drawn after clothes are collected rather than before, and so forth. In this way the nurse helps her deal with her crisis in small, manageable increments. The nurse should encourage the woman to express her feelings and reassure her that anger and fear are normal, appropriate responses. The nurse can also address expressed or unexpressed guilt by assuring the woman that the rape was not her fault.

By explaining the forensic examination and the general sequence of events in the emergency department, the nurse alleviates the client's anxiety related to fear of the unknown. The woman should know what is going to happen and why and how she can assist in each phase of the examination.

Throughout the experience, the nurse acts as the survivor's advocate, providing support without usurping decision making. The nurse need not agree with all the survivor's decisions but should respect and defend her right to make them.

The family members or friends on whom the survivor calls also need nursing care. Like those of the survivor, the reactions of the family will depend on the values to which they ascribe. Many families or mates blame the survivor for the rape and feel angry with her for not having been more careful. They may also incorrectly view the rape as a sexual act rather than as an act of violence. They may feel personally wronged or attacked and see the survivor as being devalued or unclean. Their reactions may compound the survivor's crisis. By spending some time with family members before their first interaction with the survivor, the nurse can reduce their anxiety and absorb their frustrations, sparing the woman further trauma.

Community-Based Nursing Care

A survivor who is in the outward adjustment phase may deny any need for counseling. The nurse, respecting the woman's wishes, does not force counseling on her. The family, however, may still need assistance in coping with anger or guilt. The survivor's behavior may confuse them. By providing information and support, the nurse can help them examine and reconcile their feelings. Many loved ones are able to come to terms with their feelings about the rape by going through a sometimes lengthy process of emotional recovery. To be successful, they must deal with their personal issues and build on their relationship with the woman, who is irreversibly changed. Unfortunately, some loved ones, especially the partners of women who are raped, cannot deal with the reality of the assault and its impact on their lives. Their own personal needs and responses remain more important to them than helping the woman deal with the trauma. Ultimately they may abandon the rape survivor through divorce, by terminating the relationship, or by intense emotional distancing.

TABLE 5–3 Nursing Actions Appropriate to Phases of Recovery Following Rape

Phase	Nursing Action
Acute Phase	Create a safe milieu.
	Explain the sequence of events in the health care facility.
	Allow the woman to grieve and express her feelings.
	Provide care for significant others.
Outward Adjustment Phase	Provide advocacy and support at the level requested by the woman.
	Provide assistance to significant others.
Reorganizational Phase	Establish a trusting relationship.
	Assist the woman to understand her role in the assault.
	Clarify and enhance the woman's feelings.
	Assist the woman in planning for her future.
Integration and Recovery	Acknowledge survivor's success in overcoming trauma; support advocacy efforts.

As the woman enters the reorganizational phase, she usually feels a strong urge to discuss and resolve her feelings about herself and her assailant. During this phase, the survivor may benefit from counseling.

Rape counseling, provided by qualified nurses or other counselors, is a valuable tool in helping the rape survivor come to terms with her assault and its impact on her life. In counseling the woman is encouraged to explore and identify her feelings and determine appropriate actions to resolve her problems and concerns. It is important for the counselor to assist the woman to realize that the rape was not her fault. The fault lies with the rapist. With the counselor, the woman explores her thoughts and feelings about self-care, celebrates her victories, and evaluates her defeats. It is important to emphasize that the loss of control that occurred during the rape was temporary and that the woman does have control over other aspects of her life.

Pregnancy Following Rape

Estimates about the number of pregnancies resulting from rape or coerced sex in an abusive relationship vary. A woman who becomes pregnant as the result of rape needs support and information. In particular, counseling should include information about community resources and all legally available options for dealing with the pregnancy, including keeping the baby, relinquishing it for adoption, or terminating the pregnancy (ACOG, 1997). If the woman carries the pregnancy to term, the nurse should assess the woman carefully for signs of maternal attachment behaviors during the pregnancy and in the postpartal period (Lathrop, 1998). If signs of malattachment develop, counseling may be indicated.

Preventive Education

Community colleges or local rape awareness groups may offer courses in preventive strategies. Some classes focus

TABLE 5–4 Information Resources on Rape

Rape, Abuse, and Incest National Network (RAINN) 800-656-HOPE
National Coalition Against Sexual Assault 912 N. Second Street Harrisburg, PA 17102 717-232-7460 e-mail: ncasa@redrose.net
National Clearinghouse on Marital and Date Rape 2325 Oak Street Berkeley, CA 94708 510-524-1582

on increasing women's awareness of situations in which they are at risk. Others are concerned with changing societal attitudes about rape and rape survivors. Because rape is a considerable risk for any woman, courses in what to do during and after a rape may also be helpful. Nurses who have completed additional education and are thoroughly prepared are well qualified to initiate or participate in preventive instruction.

Rape Crisis Counseling

Most rape crisis counseling centers operate 24 hours a day, 7 days a week. Their services are invaluable. Properly trained telephone counselors can help the woman regain control early in the crisis. Early crisis intervention often encourages the woman to seek professional treatment and assistance. Many rape crisis centers offer free counseling to rape survivors or can refer them to qualified counselors. Information on sexually transmitted infections and pregnancy alternatives may also be obtained from these centers. Table 5–4 provides a brief list of informational resources for survivors of rape.

Prosecution of the Rapist

Legally, rape, like any criminal action, is considered a crime against the state rather than against the victim. Therefore, prosecution of the assailant is a community responsibility in which the district attorney will act on the victim's behalf. The victim, however, must initiate the process by reporting the crime and pressing charges against her assailant. Once authorities have apprehended the alleged rapist, the judicial system is set into motion.

Procedures vary from state to state. A judge or magistrate generally conducts a hearing to determine whether there is sufficient evidence that a crime has in fact been committed and that the accused has committed it. If so, the alleged assailant will be bound over for the grand jury. The grand jury will hear the state's evidence (not that of the defense), again to determine whether the evidence is sufficient for trial. If so, the defendant is indicted; if not, he is acquitted. Once indicted, a defendant must stand trial unless he waives this right. He may elect to have his case heard by a judge rather than a jury. Either a judge or a jury will find the defendant guilty or not guilty, and he will be retained or set free accordingly.

Many rape survivors who have gone through the judicial process refer to it as a second rape—and sometimes a more damaging one. The survivor will be repeatedly asked to identify the assailant and describe the rape in intimate detail. Throughout the pretrial period, the defense attorney may use delaying tactics, obtaining continuances or postponements, further frustrating the survivor and her support system. Publicity may intensify her feelings of humiliation, and if the assailant is released on bail, she may fear retaliation.

During the trial itself, cross-examination by the defense attorney can be a severely degrading experience in which the "victim as temptress" myth is continually evoked. Although some states have altered their laws so that the survivor's sexual history may not be made public, others have not. The defense attorney will try to discredit her testimony, causing her to feel victimized a second time.

The nurse acting as a counselor needs to be aware of the judicial sequence to anticipate rising tension and frustration in the survivor and her support system. They will need consistent, effective support at this crucial time.

FOCUS YOUR STUDY

- Female partner abuse is a common occurrence, but it is the least reported serious crime in the United States.
- Battering occurs in a cyclic pattern called the cycle of violence, which increases in frequency and severity over time.
- Nurses are in an excellent position to intervene and assist battered women by recognizing their cues, diagnosing their problems appropriately, and understanding the complex dynamics of the battering family. The nurse provides information about available community resources, medical attention, and emotional support.
- Estimates suggest that 1.3 rapes occur every minute in the United States, yet a majority of rapes are unreported. Approximately one out of every three women will be raped at some time in her life.
- Why men rape remains a mystery, although it has been established that rape is an act of violence acted out sexually. Most rapes are expressions of anger or power.
- Following rape, the survivor will usually experience an assortment of symptoms known as the rape trauma syndrome. Recent research also links the effects of rape to the post-traumatic stress disorder experienced by many veterans following the Vietnam War. The nursing actions to assist rape survivors are encompassed in the roles of advocate, educator, and counselor.
- Nurses inform the woman of the sequence of events involved in providing her care and developing the chain of evidence and support the survivor's decisions.
- The counseling process used by the nurse follows the crisis intervention model because the survivor is in a situational crisis rather than being ill.
- Widespread education is needed to abolish societal myths surrounding rape.

REFERENCES

American College of Obstetricians and Gynecologists (ACOG) (1998). Mandatory reporting of domestic violence. (ACOG Committee Opinion 200). Washington, DC: Author.

American College of Obstetricians and Gynecologists (ACOG) (1997). *Sexual assault* (ACOG Educational Bulletin 242). Washington, DC: Author.

American Nurses Association (1991). *Position statement on physical violence against women.* Washington, DC: Author.

Bachman, R., & Saltzman, L. E. (1995). Violence against women: Estimates from the redesigned survey. *Bureau of Statistics special report.* Washington, DC: U.S. Department of Justice. (NCJ-154348)

Beckmann, C. R. B., & Groetzinger, L. L. (1989). Treating sexual assault victims: A protocol for health professionals. *Female Patient, 14,* 78.

Bullock, L. F., Sandella, J. A., & McFarlane, J. (1989). Breaking the cycle of abuse: How nurses can intervene. *Journal of Psychosocial Nursing & Mental Health Services, 27*(8), 11–13.

Burge, S. K. (1989). Violence against women as a health care issue. *Family Medicine, 21*(5), 368–373.

Burgess, A. W., & Holmstrom, L. L. (1979). *Rape: Crisis and recovery.* Englewood Cliffs, NJ: Prentice Hall.

Campbell, J. C. (1993). Woman abuse and public policy: Potential for nursing action. *AWHONN's Clinical Issues in Perinatal & Women's Health Nursing, 4*(3), 503–512.

Caron, S. L., & Carter, D. B. (1997). The relationships among sex role orientation, egalitarianism, attitudes toward sexuality, and attitudes toward violence against women. *Journal of Social Psychology, 137*(5), 568–587.

Chez, N. (1994). Helping the victim of domestic violence. *American Journal of Nursing, 94*(7), 32–37.

Clark, C. C. (1997). Posttraumatic stress disorder: How to support healing. *American Journal of Nursing, 97*(8), 26–33.

Crooks, R., & Baur, K. (1998). *Our sexuality* (7th ed.). Monterey, CA: Brooks/Cole.

DeKeseredy, W. S., Schwartz, M. D., & Tait, K. (1993). Sexual assault and stranger aggression on a Canadian university campus. *Sex Roles, 28*(5–6), 263–277.

Dennis, L. I. (1998). Adolescent rape: The role of nursing. *Issues in Comprehensive Pediatric Nursing, 11*(1), 59–70.

Department of Health & Human Services, Public Health Services (1990). *Healthy people 2000* (Publication No. PHS 91-50213). Washington, DC: Author.

Dupre, A. R., Hampton, H. L., Morrison, H., & Meeks, G. R. (1993). Sexual assault. *Obstetrical & Gynecological Survey, 48*(9), 640–648.

Fishwick, N. (1993). Nursing care of rural battered women. *AWHONN's Clinical Issues in Perinatal & Women's Health Nursing, 4*(3), 441–448.

Golan, N. (1978). *Treatment in crisis situations.* New York: Free Press.

Gondolf, E. W. (1988). *Battered women as survivors: An alternative to treating learned helplessness.* Lanham, MA: Lexington Books.

Gordon, M. T., & Riger, S. (1989). *The female fear.* New York: Free Press.

Haddix-Hill, K. (1997). The violence of rape. *Critical Care Nursing Clinics of North America, 9*(2), 167–174.

Herman, J. L. (1992). *Trauma and recovery.* New York: Basic Books.

Holmes, M. M. (1998). The clinical management of rape in adolescents. *Contemporary OB/GYN, 43*(5), 62–78.

Kauffold, M. P. (1996, September). The SANE Solution: Easing the trauma of rape. *Trustee, 49*(8), 6–9.

Kennedy, P. H. (1993). Sexual abuse within adult intimate relationships. *AWHONN's Clinical Issues in Perinatal & Women's Health Nursing, 4*(3), 391–401.

Lathrop, A. (1998). Pregnancy resulting from rape. *Journal of Obstetric, Gynecologic, and Neonatal Nursing, 27*(1), 25–31.

Moore, L., & Wesa, K. (1997). Domestic violence. *Primary Care Update OB/GYNs, 4*(6), 257–260.

Perkins, C., & Klaus, P. (1996). Criminal victimization 1994. *Bureau of Justice statistics bulletin.* Washington, DC: U.S. Department of Justice. (NCJ-158022)

Poirier, L. (1997). The importance of screening for domestic violence in all women. *Nurse Practitioner, 22*(5), 105–108, 111–112, 115 passim.

Renshaw, D. C. (1989). Treatment of sexual exploitation. Rape and incest. *Psychiatric Clinics of North America, 12*(2), 257–277.

Rickert, V. I., & Wiemann, C. M. (1998). Date rape: Office-based solutions. *Contemporary OB/GYN, 43*(3), 133–153.

Ryan, J. & King, M. C. (1998). Scanning for violence: Educational strategies for helping abused women. *AWHONN Lifelines, 2*(3), 36–41.

Saum, C. A., & Inciardi, J. A. (1997, May). Rohypnol misuse in the United States. *Substance Use and Misuse, 32(6),* 723–31.

Stenchever, M. A., & Stenchever, D. H. (1991). Abuse of women: An overview. *Women's Health Issues, 1*(4), 187–192.

US Department of Justice (1998, March). Murder by intimates declined 36% since 1976. Decline greater for male than female victims. *Press release.* Washington, DC: Author.

Voelker, R. (1996, April). Experts hope team approach will improve the quality of rape exams. *Journal of the American Medical Association, 275*(13), 973–974.

Walker, L. (1984). *The battered woman syndrome.* New York: Springer.

Human Reproduction

three

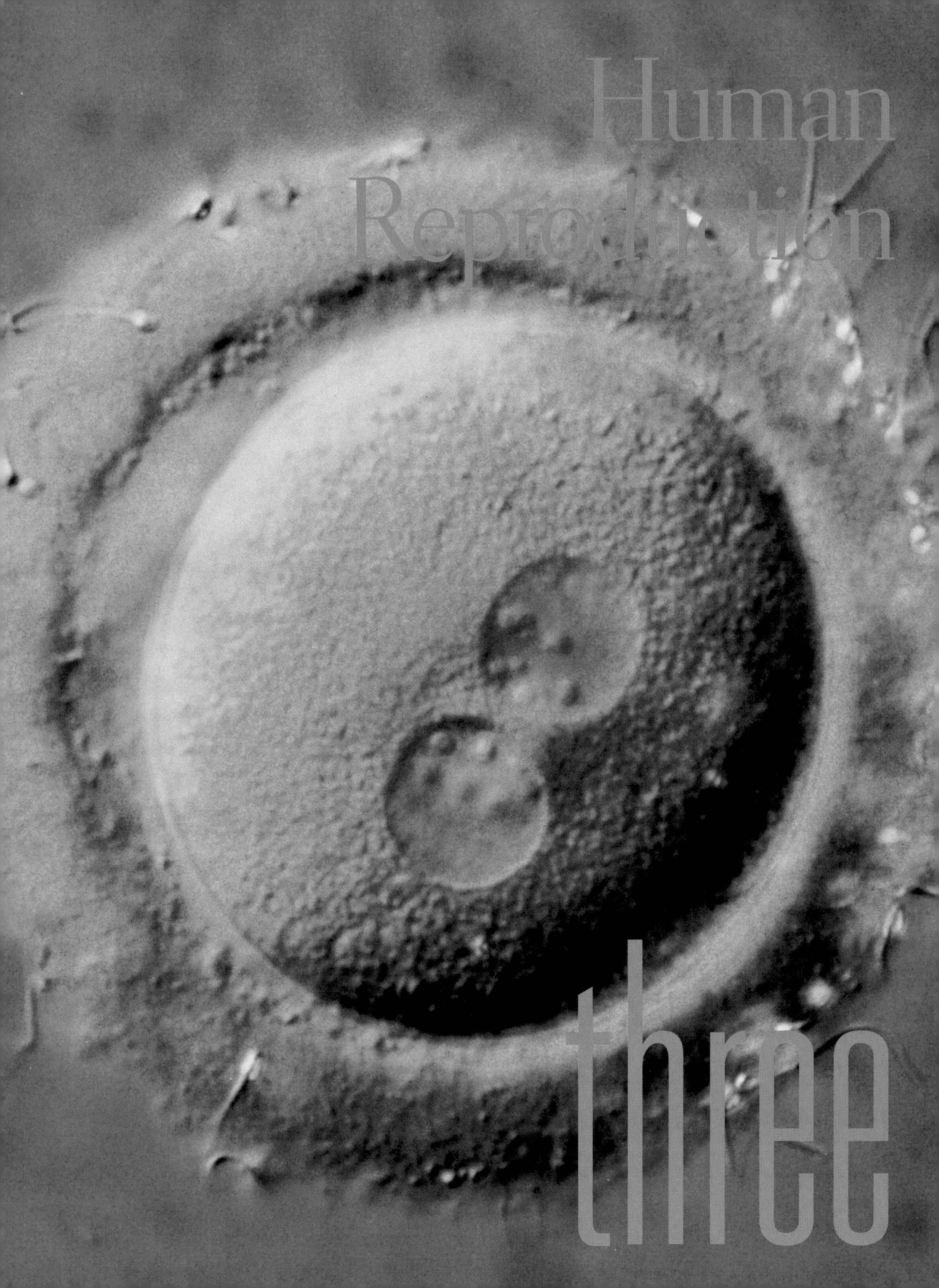

6 The Reproductive System

Key Terms

Ampulla
Areola
Breasts
Cervix
Conjugate vera
Cornua
Corpus
Corpus luteum
Diagonal conjugate
Endometrium
Estrogens
Fallopian tubes
Female reproductive cycle (FRC)
Fimbria
Follicle-stimulating hormone (FSH)
Fundus
Gonadotropin-releasing hormone (GnRH)
Graafian follicle
Human chorionic gonadotropin (hCG)
Ischial spines
Isthmus
Luteinizing hormone (LH)
Myometrium
Nidation
Nipple
Obstetric conjugate
Oocytes
Oogenesis
Ovulation
Ovum
Pelvic diaphragm
Pelvic inlet
Pelvic outlet
Perimetrium
Perineal body
Progesterone
Prostaglandins
Puberty
Pubis
Sacral promontory
Spermatogenesis
Spermatozoa
Testosterone
Transverse diameter
True pelvis
Uterus
Vagina
Vulva

I ALWAYS THOUGHT IT WAS SO BORING TO STUDY anatomy and physiology. Who cares how many bones there are in the pelvis or the muscles involved. But now I'm with mothers having babies, and now it all makes sense.
~ A Nursing Student ~

Objectives

- Summarize the major changes in the reproductive system that occur during puberty.
- Identify key aspects of the female and male reproductive systems that are important to childbearing.
- Summarize the actions of the hormones that affect reproductive functioning.
- Identify the two phases of the ovarian cycle and the changes that occur in each phase.
- Describe the phases of the menstrual cycle, their dominant hormones, and the changes that occur in each phase.
- Discuss the significance of specific female reproductive structures during childbirth.

UNDERSTANDING CHILDBEARING REQUIRES more than understanding sexual intercourse or the process by which the female and male sex cells unite. The nurse must also become familiar with the structures and functions that make childbearing possible and the phenomena that initiate it. This chapter considers the anatomic, physiologic, and sexual aspects of the female and male reproductive systems. It also provides information regarding basic embryologic development in order to increase the understanding of anatomy, physiology, and function. The psychosocial aspects of human sexuality are discussed in Chapter 3.

The female and male reproductive organs are *homologous;* that is, they are fundamentally similar in function and structure. The primary functions of both the female and male reproductive systems are to produce sex cells and to transport the sex cells to locations where their union can occur. The sex cells, called *gametes,* are produced by specialized organs called *gonads.* A series of ducts and glands within both the male and female reproductive systems contributes to the production and transport of the gametes.

Embryonic Development of Reproductive Structures and Processes

Although the genetic sex of an embryo is determined at fertilization, the male and female reproductive systems are undifferentiated for about the first 8 weeks of gestation. This undifferentiated period is followed by a period of rapid, dramatic changes as the reproductive organs differentiate into recognizable structures.

Ovaries and Testes

During the 5th week of gestation, a primitive gonad arises from the intermediate mesoderm tissue known as gonadal ridges. The gonad develops a medulla (inner part of the organ) and cortex (outer part of the organ), which appear in the underlying mesenchyme (embryonic tissue from which connective and muscle tissue arises; see Table 7–1). In genetic males during the 7th and 8th weeks, the medulla develops into a testis, and the cortex regresses. In genetic females by about the 10th week, the cortex develops into an ovary, and the medulla regresses.

Every egg available for maturation in a woman's reproductive life is present at her birth. During fetal life the ovary produces *oogonia,* cells that become primitive eggs called **oocytes,** by the process of **oogenesis** (see Chapter 7). No oocytes are formed after fetal development. About 150,000 oocytes are contained in the ovaries at birth. Each oocyte is contained in a small ovarian cavity called a *primitive follicle.*

Every month during a female's reproductive years, one of the oocytes undergoes a process of cellular division and maturation that transforms it into a fertilizable egg, or **ovum.** At **ovulation,** the ovum is released from its follicle. The remaining follicles and oocytes degenerate over time.

Each testis produces the male gametes, called **spermatozoa** or *sperm,* by a process called **spermatogenesis.** This process is described in Chapter 7. Spermatogenesis of mature sperm does not occur until the onset of puberty (Sanfilippo & Jamieson, 1997).

Figure 6–1 illustrates the embryologic development of the gonads and other internal reproductive organs.

Other Internal Structures

During the undifferentiated period—the first 7 weeks—two pairs of genital ducts develop: the mesonephric and paramesonephric ducts (Malasanos, 1997).

In genetic females the fallopian tubes are formed from the unfused portions of the paramesonephric ducts, and the fused portions give rise to the epithelium and uterine glands. The endometrial stroma and the myometrium (thick layer of smooth muscle in the wall of the uterus) develop from the adjacent mesenchyme.

The vagina is derived from more than one embryologic structure. The vaginal epithelium develops from the endoderm of the urogenital sinus, and the musculature develops from the uterovaginal primordium.

The urethral and paraurethral glands develop from outgrowths of the urethra into the surrounding mesenchyme. Bartholin's glands arise from similar structures.

In genetic males the fetal testes secrete two hormones. The first hormone, testosterone, stimulates the mesonephric ducts to develop into the male genital tract. The other hormone, müllerian regression factor, suppresses the development of the paramesonephric ducts, which would otherwise develop into the female genital tract.

From the mesonephric ducts comes development of the efferent ductule, vas deferens, epididymis, seminal vesicle, and ejaculatory duct. Both the prostate and the bulbourethral glands develop from endodermal outgrowths of the urethra.

External Structures

Genetic males and females possess the same external genitals until the end of the 9th week. By the 12th week differentiation of the external genitals is complete.

If fetal testosterone is not present, the undifferentiated external genitals are feminized. The phallus becomes the clitoris, and the urogenital folds remain open, forming the labia minora. The labioscrotal folds form the labia majora.

If fetal testosterone is present, the undifferentiated external genitals become masculine. The phallus elongates, forming the penis. The fusion of the urogenital

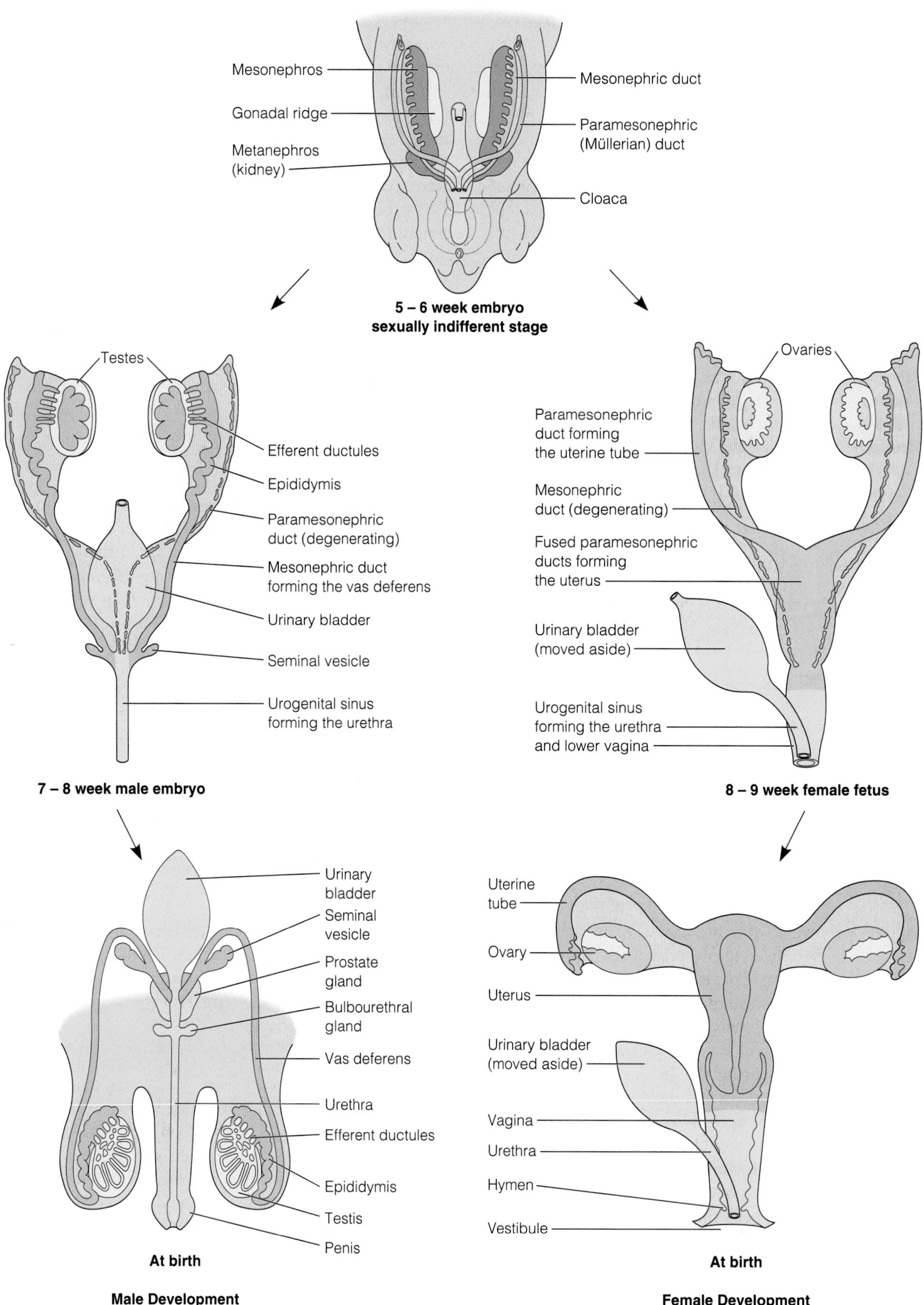
Mesonephros
Gonadal ridge
Metanephros
(kidney)
Mesonephric duct
Paramesonephric
(Müllerian) duct
Cloaca
5 – 6 week embryo
sexually indifferent stage
Testes
Efferent ductules
Epididymis
Paramesonephric
duct (degenerating)
Mesonephric duct
forming the vas deferens
Urinary bladder
Seminal vesicle
Urogenital sinus
forming the urethra
7 – 8 week male embryo
Ovaries
Paramesonephric
duct forming
the uterine tube
Mesonephric
duct (degenerating)
Fused paramesonephric
ducts forming
the uterus
Urinary bladder
(moved aside)
Urogenital sinus
forming the urethra
and lower vagina
8 – 9 week female fetus
Urinary
bladder
Seminal
vesicle
Prostate
gland
Bulbourethral
gland
Vas deferens
Urethra
Efferent ductules
Epididymis
Testis
Penis
At birth
Male Development
Uterine
tube
Ovary
Uterus
Urinary bladder
(moved aside)
Vagina
Urethra
Hymen
Vestibule
At birth
Female Development

FIGURE 6–1 Embryonic differentiation of male and female internal reproductive organs.

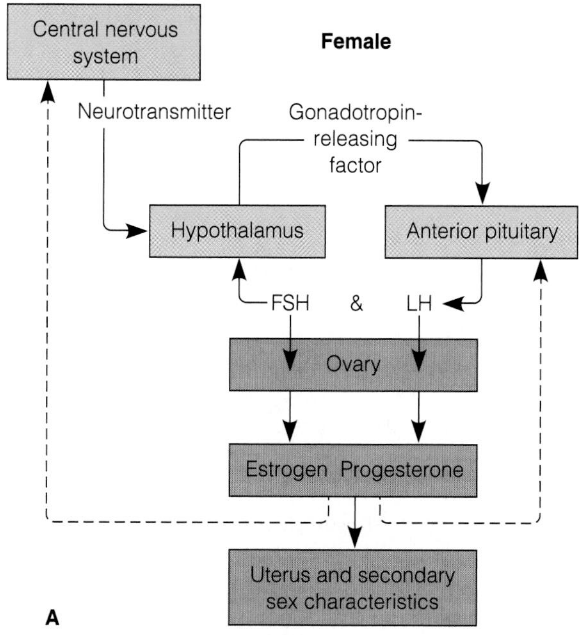

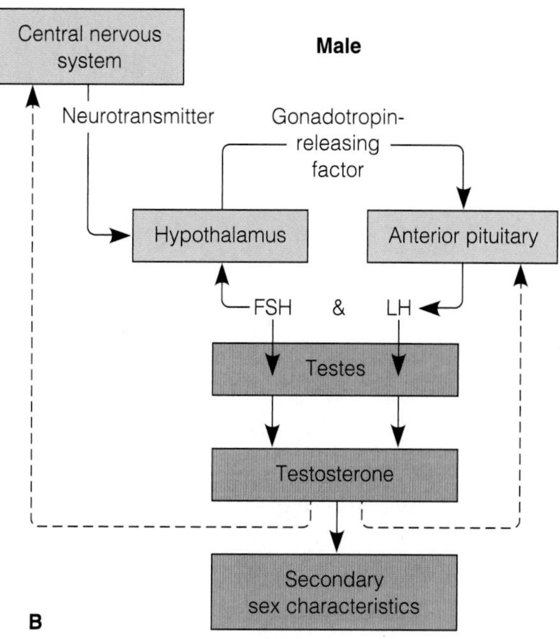

FIGURE 6–2 Physiologic changes leading to onset of puberty. ***A,*** In females; and ***B,*** in males. Solid lines illustrate stimulation of hormone production, and broken lines illustrate inhibition. Through a neurotransmitter the CNS stimulates the hypothalamus, which in turn produces a gonadotropin-releasing factor that causes the anterior pituitary to produce gonadotropins (FSH or LH). These hormones stimulate specific structures in the gonads to secrete steroid hormones (estrogen, progesterone, or testosterone). The rise in pituitary hormone production increases hypothalamus activity. Elevated steroid hormone levels stimulate the CNS and pituitary gland to inhibit hormone production.

folds on the ventral surface of the penis forms the penile urethra, with the urethral meatus moving forward toward the glans penis.

Puberty

The term **puberty** refers to the developmental period between childhood and attainment of adult sexual characteristics and functioning. Generally, boys mature physically about 2 years later than girls. In boys, the age of onset of puberty ranges from 10 to 19 years; 14 years is the average age of onset. In girls, the age of onset ranges from 9 to 17 years; 12 years is the average age of onset. Puberty lasts from 1.5 to 5 years and involves profound physical, psychologic, and emotional changes. These changes include an altered body image, changing roles, and changing societal expectations and responses as the child matures to an adult.

Major Physical Changes

In both girls and boys, puberty is preceded by an accelerated growth rate called adolescent spurt. Widespread body system changes occur, including maturation of the reproductive organs.

Girls experience a broadening of the hips, then budding of the breasts, the appearance of pubic and axillary hair, and the onset of menstruation, called menarche. The average time between breast development and menarche is 2.3 years (Weiss & Goldsmith, 1994).

Boys experience linear growth spurts; an increase in the size of the external genitals; the appearance of pubic, axillary, and facial hair; deepening of the voice; and nocturnal seminal emissions (called wet dreams) without sexual stimulation. These early seminal emissions do not *usually* contain mature sperm (Sanfilippo & Jamieson, 1997).

The physical changes of puberty present themselves differently in each person. The age at onset and progress of puberty vary widely, physical changes overlap, and the sequence of events can vary from person to person. This diversity results from each individual's response to hormonal stimulation.

Physiology of Onset

Puberty is initiated by the maturation of the hypothalamic-pituitary-gonad complex (the *gonadostat*) and input from the central nervous system. The process, which begins during fetal life, is sequential and complex.

The central nervous system releases a neurotransmitter that stimulates the hypothalamus to synthesize and release **gonadotropin-releasing hormone (GnRH)** (Ferin, 1998). GnRH is transmitted to the anterior pituitary, where it causes the synthesis and secretion of the gonadotropins **follicle-stimulating hormone (FSH)** and **luteinizing hormone (LH)** (Figure 6–2).

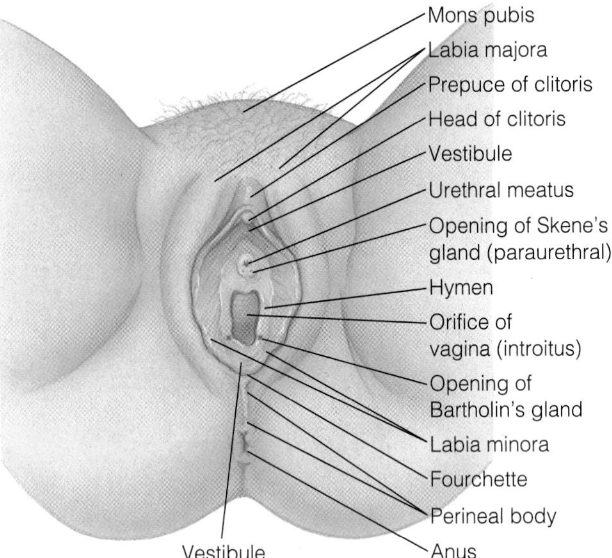

FIGURE 6–3 Female external genitals, longitudinal view.

Although the gonads do produce small amounts of *androgens* (male sex hormones) and *estrogens* (female sex hormones) before the onset of puberty, FSH and LH stimulate increased secretion of these hormones. Androgens and estrogens influence the development of secondary sex characteristics. FSH and LH stimulate the processes of spermatogenesis and maturation of ova.

Other hormones are involved in the onset of puberty. Although less direct, their action is essential. Abnormally high or low levels of adrenocorticotropic hormone (ACTH), thyroid hormone, or growth hormone (GH) can disrupt the onset of normal puberty (Ferin, 1998).

Female Reproductive System

The female reproductive system consists of the external and internal genitals and accessory organs of the breasts. The structure of the bony pelvis is also discussed in this section because of its importance in childbearing.

External Genitals

All the external reproductive organs, except the glandular structures, can be directly inspected. The size, color, and shape of these structures vary extensively among races and individuals.

The female external genitals, called the **vulva** or *pudendum*, include the following structures (Figure 6–3):

- Mons pubis
- Labia majora
- Labia minora
- Clitoris
- Urethral meatus and opening of the paraurethral (Skene's) glands
- Vaginal vestibule (vaginal orifice, vulvovaginal glands, hymen, and fossa navicularis)
- Perineal body

Although they are not actually parts of the female reproductive system, this chapter discusses the urethral meatus and perineal body because of their proximity and relationship to the vulva.

The vulva has a generous supply of blood and nerves. As a woman ages, estrogen secretions decrease, causing gradual atrophy of tissues.

Mons Pubis

The *mons pubis* is a softly rounded mound of subcutaneous fatty tissue beginning at the lowest portion of the anterior abdominal wall. Also known as the *mons veneris*, this structure covers the anterior portion of the symphysis pubis. The mons pubis is covered with pubic hair, typically with the hairline forming a transverse line across the lower abdomen (Figure 6–3). The hair is short and varies from sparse and fine in the Asian woman to heavy, coarse, and curly in the black woman. The mons pubis protects the pelvic bones, especially during coitus.

Labia Majora

The *labia majora* are longitudinal, raised folds of pigmented skin, one on either side of the vulvar cleft (Figure 6–3). As the pair descend, they narrow, enclosing the vulvar cleft, and merge to form the posterior junction of the perineal skin. Their chief function is to protect the structures lying between them. The labia majora are covered by stratified squamous epithelium containing hair follicles and sebaceous glands with underlying adipose and muscle tissue. Immediately under the skin is a sheet of dartos muscle, which is responsible for the wrinkled appearance of the labia majora.

The inner surface of the labia majora in women who have not had children is moist and looks like a mucous membrane, but after many births it is more skinlike (Cunningham et al, 1997). With each pregnancy the labia majora become less prominent.

Because of the extensive venous network in the labia majora, varicosities may occur during pregnancy, and birth trauma or sexual trauma may cause hematomas. The labia majora share an extensive lymphatic supply with the other structures of the vulva, which can facilitate the spread of cancer in the female reproductive organs. Because nerves from the first lumbar and third sacral segment of the spinal cord supply the labia majora, certain regional anesthesia blocks will affect them and cause numbness.

Labia Minora

The *labia minora* are soft folds of skin within the labia majora that converge near the anus, forming the *fourchette*. Each labium minora has the appearance of a shiny mucous membrane, moist and devoid of hair follicles. The labia minora are rich in sebaceous glands, which lubricate and waterproof the vulvar skin and provide bactericidal secretions. Because sebaceous glands do not open into hair follicles but directly onto the surface of the skin, sebaceous cysts commonly occur in this area. The labia minora are composed of erectile tissue and involuntary muscle tissue. Vulvovaginitis in this area is very irritating because of the many tactile nerve endings. The labia minora increase in size at puberty and decrease after menopause due to changes in estrogen levels.

Clitoris

The *clitoris*, located between the labia minora, is about 5 to 6 mm long and 6 to 8 mm across. Its tissue is essentially erectile (Figure 6–3). The glans is partially covered by a fold of skin called the *prepuce*, or clitoral hood. This area often looks like an opening to an orifice and may be confused with the urethral meatus. Accidental attempts to insert a catheter in this area produce extreme discomfort. The clitoris has very rich blood and nerve supplies and is a primary source of female sexual pleasure. In addition, it secretes *smegma*, which along with other vulval secretions has a unique odor that may be sexually stimulating to a man.

Urethral Meatus and Paraurethral Glands

The *urethral meatus* is located 1 to 2.5 cm beneath the clitoris in the midline of the vestibule; it often appears as a puckered, slitlike opening. At times the meatus is difficult to visualize because of the presence of blind dimples, small mucosal folds, or wide variations in location.

The paraurethral glands, or *Skene's glands*, open into the posterior wall of the urethra close to its opening (Figure 6–3). Their secretions help lubricate the vaginal vestibule, facilitating sexual intercourse.

Vaginal Vestibule

The vaginal vestibule is a boat-shaped depression enclosed by the labia majora and visible when they are separated. The vestibule contains the vaginal opening, or *introitus*, which is the border between the external and internal genitals.

The *hymen* is a collar or semi-collar of tissue that surrounds the vaginal opening. The appearance of the hymen changes during the woman's lifetime. From birth to about 3 years of age, the hymen is fluffy and full, and the tissue appears to fold back on itself and to cover the vaginal opening. These characteristics are due to exposure to estrogen in utero. With the loss of exposure to estrogen after birth, the hymen's appearance begins to change to a thin membranous tissue that is still in a collar or semicollar shape. At approximately 3 years of age, the hymen is thin and membranous, with an absence of tissue beneath the urethra (Berenson, 1995). The hymen is without estrogen stimulation and is hypersensitive to touch. At puberty, under the stimulation of the girl's own increasing estrogen levels, the hymen once again becomes more full. For thousands of years, some societies have perpetuated the belief that the hymen covers the vaginal opening and is a sign of virginity. However, modern studies of the female genital anatomy have revealed that the hymen can be broken not only through sexual intercourse, but also through strenuous physical activity, masturbation, menstruation, or the use of tampons, thus dispelling old beliefs.

External to the hymenal tissue at the base of the vestibule are two small papular elevations containing the openings of the ducts of the *vulvovaginal (Bartholin's) glands*. They lie under the constrictor muscle of the vagina. These glands secrete a clear and thick mucus with an alkaline pH that enhances the viability and motility of sperm deposited in the vaginal vestibule.These ducts of the vulvovaginal glands can harbor *Neisseria gonorrhoeae* and other bacteria, which can cause suppuration and abscesses in the Bartholin's glands.

The vestibular area is innervated mainly by the perineal nerve from the sacral plexus. The area is not sensitive to touch generally; however, the hymen contains numerous free nerve endings as receptors to pain.

Perineal Body

The **perineal body** is a wedge-shaped mass of fibromuscular tissue measuring about 4 × 4 × 4 cm, found between the lower part of the vagina and the anal canal (Figure 6–3). The superficial area between the anus and the vagina is referred to as the *perineum*.

The muscles that meet at the perineal body are the external sphincter ani, both levator ani (the superficial and deep transverse perineal), and the bulbocavernosus. These muscles mingle with elastic fibers and connective tissue in an arrangement that allows a remarkable amount of stretching. During the last part of labor, the perineal body thins out until it is just a few centimeters thick. This tissue is the site of the episiotomy or lacerations during childbirth (see Chapter 23).

Female Internal Reproductive Organs

The female internal reproductive organs—the vagina, uterus, fallopian tubes, and ovaries—are target organs for estrogenic hormones. These organs play a unique part in the reproductive cycle (Figure 6–4). The internal reproductive organs can be palpated during vaginal examination and assessed through use of various instruments.

Vagina

The **vagina** is a muscular and membranous tube that connects the external genitals with the uterus (Figure 6–4). It extends from the vulva to the uterus in a position nearly parallel to the plane of the pelvic brim. The vagina is often referred to as the *birth canal* because it forms the lower part of the axis through which the fetus must pass during birth.

Because the cervix of the uterus projects into the upper part of the anterior wall of the vagina, the anterior wall is approximately 2.5 cm shorter than the posterior

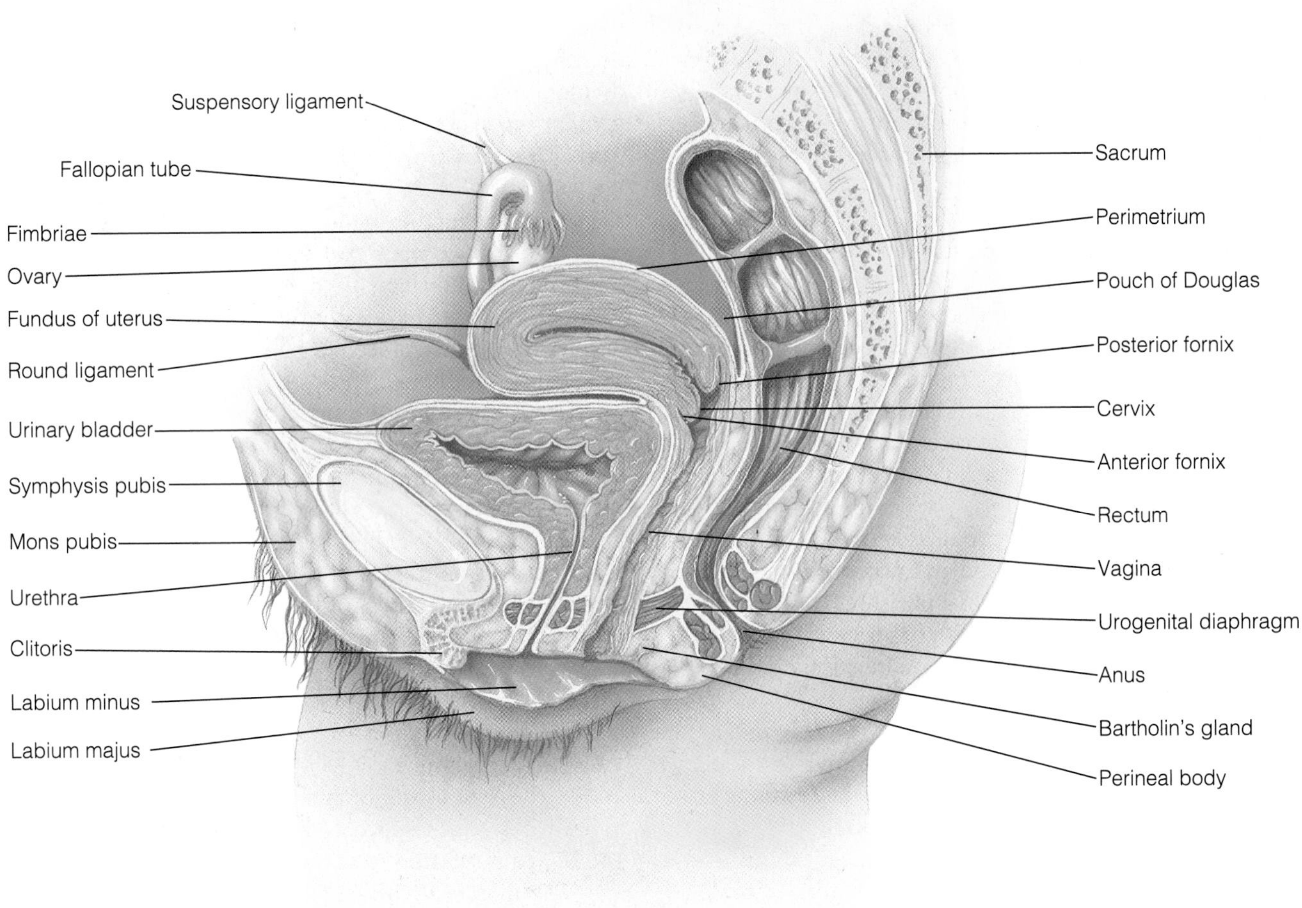

FIGURE 6–4 Female internal reproductive organs.

wall. Measurements range from 6 to 8 cm for the anterior wall and 7 to 10 cm for the posterior wall.

In the upper part of the vagina, which is called the *vaginal vault,* there is a recess or hollow around the cervix called the vaginal *fornix.* Because the walls of the vaginal vault are very thin, various structures can be palpated through the walls and fornix of the vaginal vault, including the uterus, a distended bladder, the ovaries, appendix, cecum, colon, and the ureters.

When a woman lies on her back after intercourse, the space in the fornix permits the pooling of semen. The collection of a large number of sperm near the cervix at or near the time of ovulation in the woman increases the chances of pregnancy.

The walls of the vagina are covered with ridges, or *rugae,* crisscrossing each other. These rugae allow the vaginal tissues to stretch enough for the fetus to pass through during childbirth.

A rich blood supply is needed to maintain a high glycogen content in the epithelial cells as well as to nourish the underlying musculofascial layer, through which the vaginal vault has strong attachments to the cervix. These muscle layers are continuous with the superficial muscle fibers of the uterus. A thin band of striated muscle, the *sphincter vaginae,* is found at the lowest extremity of the vagina. However, the levator ani is the principal muscle that closes the vagina.

During a woman's reproductive life, the vaginal environment is normally acidic (pH 4.0 to 5.0). Secretion from the vaginal epithelium provides a moist environment. The acidic environment is maintained by a symbiotic relationship between lactic acid–producing bacilli (Döderlein's bacillus or lactobacillus) and the vaginal epithelial cells. These cells contain glycogen, which is broken down by the bacilli into lactic acid. The amount of glycogen is regulated by the ovarian hormones. Any interruption of this process can destroy the normal self-cleansing action of the vagina. Such interruption may be caused by antibiotic therapy, douching, or use of vaginal sprays or deodorants. For further discussion, see Chapter 3.

The acidic vaginal environment is normal only during the mature reproductive years and in the first days of life, when maternal hormones are operating in the infant. A relatively neutral pH of 7.5 is normal from infancy until puberty and after menopause.

Each third of the vagina is supplied by a distinct vascular and lymphatic pattern. Although one would expect venous drainage to go directly to the heart and then the lungs, anastomoses of veins are present and make it possible for a pelvic embolism or carcinoma to bypass the heart and lungs and lodge in the brain, spine, or other remote part of the body.

Vaginal lymphatics drain into the external and internal iliac nodes, the hypogastric nodes, and the inguinal glands. The posterior wall drains into nodes lying in the rectovaginal septum. Any vaginal infection follows these routes.

The pudendal nerve supplies what relatively little somatic innervation there is to the lower third of the vagina. Thus vaginal sensation during sexual excitement and coitus is minimal, as is vaginal pain during the second stage of labor.

The vagina has the following functions:

- To serve as the passageway for sperm and for the fetus during birth.
- To provide passage for the menstrual blood flow from the uterine endometrium to the outside of the body.
- To protect against infection from pathogenic organisms.

Uterus

As the core of reproduction and hence continuation of the human race, the uterus, or womb, has been endowed with a mystical aura. Numerous customs, taboos, mores, and values have evolved about women and their reproductive function. Although scientific knowledge has replaced much of this folklore, remnants of old ideas and superstitions persist. To provide effective care, nurses must be cognizant of their own attitudes and beliefs, as well as those of their clients.

The **uterus** is a hollow, muscular, thick-walled, organ shaped like an upside-down pear. It lies in the center of the pelvic cavity between the base of the bladder and the rectum and above the vagina (Figure 6–5). It is level with or slightly below the brim of the pelvis, with the external opening of the cervix (the external os) about the level of the ischial spines. The mature organ weighs about 50 to 70 g and is approximately 7.5 cm long, 5 cm wide, and 1 to 2.5 cm thick.

Many uterine anomalies are thought to be congenital. A normal uterus requires two symmetric, parallel, equal-sized paramesonephric ducts to meet in the midline. Their ultimate fusion gives rises to the fallopian tubes, uterine fundus, cervix, and upper vagina. Anomalies represent the absence of either one or both of the ducts, degrees of failure to fuse, or canalization defects. Uterine malformations such as the uterus bicornuate ("two-horned") and uterus didelphys ("double uterus") are associated with habitual abortion. Because both the urinary and reproductive systems develop from the common urogenital fold in the embryo, anomalies in one system are frequently accompanied by anomalies in the other. Problems of infertility and premature labor and birth are common.

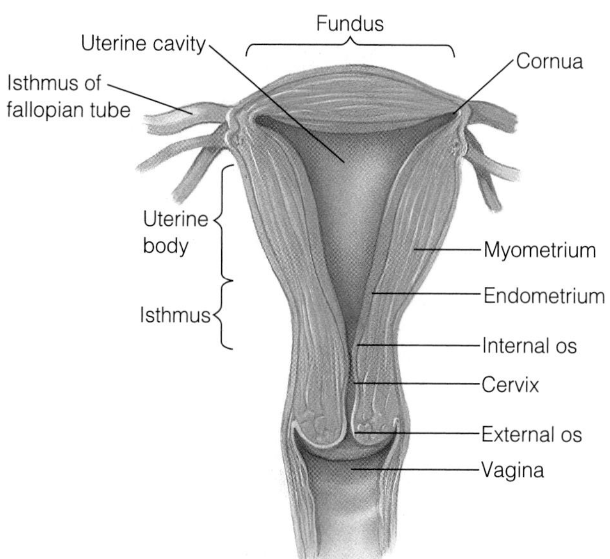

FIGURE 6–5 Structures of the uterus.

The position of the uterus can vary, depending on a woman's posture, number of children borne, bladder and rectal fullness, and even normal respiratory patterns. Only the cervix is anchored laterally. The body of the uterus can move freely forward or backward. The axis also varies. Generally, the uterus bends forward, forming a sharp angle with the vagina. There is a bend in the area of the isthmus of the uterus, and from there the cervix points downward. The uterus is said to be *anteverted* when it is in this position. The anteverted position is considered normal.

The uterus is kept in place by three sets of supports. The upper supports are the broad and round ligaments. The middle supports are the cardinal, pubocervical, and uterosacral ligaments. The lower supports are those structures considered to be the pelvic muscular floor.

The isthmus is a slight constriction in the uterus that divides it into two unequal parts. The upper two-thirds of the uterus is the **corpus,** or *body,* composed mainly of a smooth muscle layer (myometrium). The lower third is the cervix, or neck. The rounded uppermost portion of the corpus that extends above the points of attachment of the fallopian tubes is called the **fundus.** The elongated portion of the uterus where the fallopian tubes enter is called the **cornua.**

The isthmus joins the corpus and the cervix. It is located about 6 mm above the uterine opening of the cervix (the internal os), and it is in this area that the uterine lining changes into the mucous membrane of the cervix; it joins the corpus to the cervix. The isthmus takes on importance in pregnancy because it becomes the lower uterine segment. With the cervix it is a passive segment and

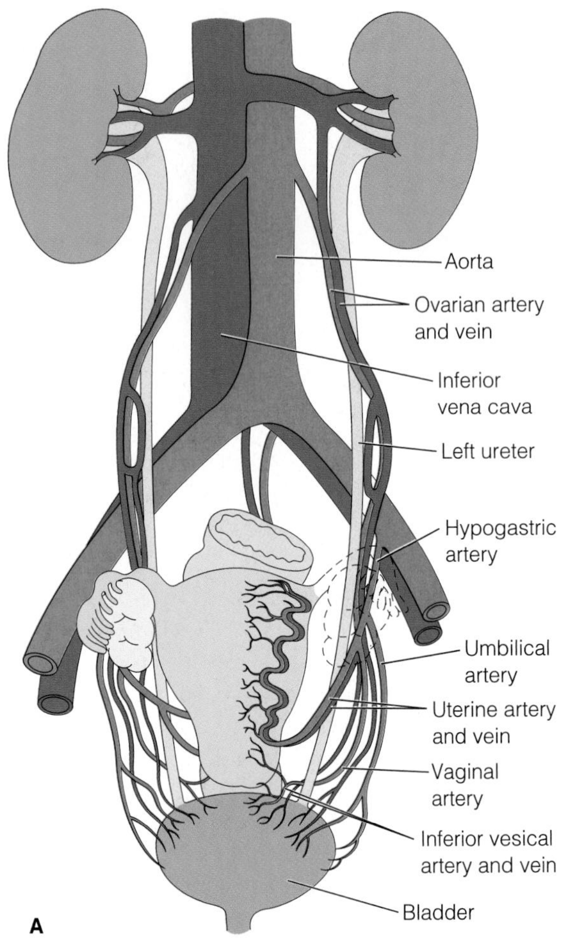

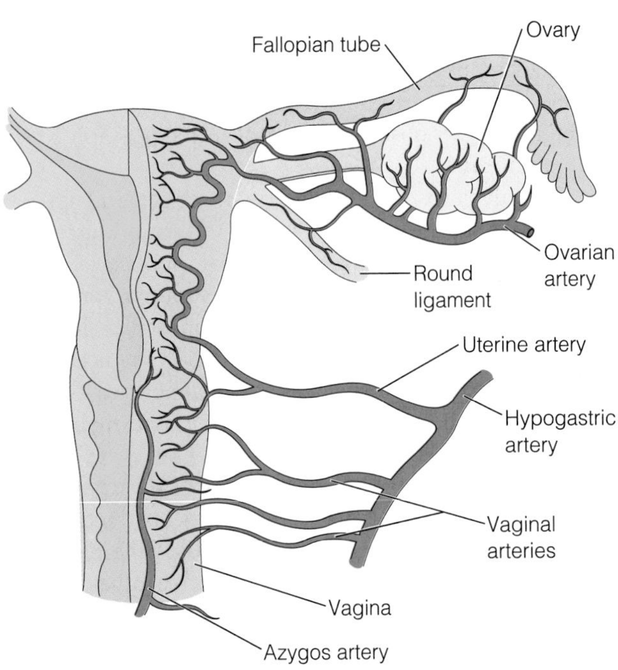

FIGURE 6–6 Blood supply to internal reproductive organs: ***A,*** Pelvic blood supply. ***B,*** Blood supply to vagina, ovary, uterus, and fallopian tube.

not part of the contractile uterus. At birth this thin lower segment, situated behind the bladder, is the site for lower-segment cesarean births (see Chapter 23).

The blood and lymphatic supplies to the uterus are extensive (Figure 6–6). The uterus is innervated entirely by the autonomic nervous system. Even without an intact nerve supply, the uterus can contract adequately for birth. Thus, for example, hemiplegic women have adequate uterine contractions.

Pain of uterine contractions is carried to the central nervous system by the 11th and 12th thoracic nerve roots. Pain from the cervix and upper vagina passes through the ilioinguinal and pudendal nerves. The motor fibers to the uterus arise from the 7th and 8th thoracic vertebrae. Because the sensory and motor levels are separate, epidural anesthesia can be used during labor and birth.

The function of the uterus is to provide a safe environment for fetal development. The uterine lining is cyclically prepared by steroid hormones for implantation of the embryo, a process known as **nidation.** Once the embryo is implanted, the developing fetus is protected until it is expelled.

Both the body of the uterus and the cervix are changed permanently by pregnancy. The body never returns to its prepregnant size, and the external os changes from a circular opening of about 3 mm to a transverse slit with irregular edges.

The Corpus

The uterine corpus is made up of three layers. The outermost layer is the *serosal layer,* or **perimetrium,** which is composed of peritoneum. The middle layer is the *muscular uterine layer,* or **myometrium.** This muscular uterine layer is continuous with the muscle layer of the fallopian tubes and with that of the vagina. This characteristic helps the organs present a unified reaction to various stimuli—ovulation, orgasm, or the deposit of sperm in the vagina. These muscle fibers also extend into the ovarian, round, and cardinal ligaments and minimally into the uterosacral ligaments, which helps explain the vague but disturbing pelvic "aches and pains" reported by many pregnant women.

The myometrium has three distinct layers of uterine (smooth) involuntary muscles (Figure 6–7). The outer layer, found mainly over the fundus, is made up of longitudinal muscles especially suited to expel the fetus during birth. The middle layer is thick and made up of interlacing muscle fibers in figure-eight patterns. These muscle fibers surround large blood vessels, and their contraction produces a hemostatic action (a tourniquetlike action on blood vessels to stop bleeding after birth). The inner muscle layer is made up of circular fibers, which form sphincters at the fallopian tube attachment sites and at the internal os. The internal os sphincter inhibits the expulsion of the uterine contents during pregnancy but stretches in labor as cervical dilatation occurs. An incompetent cervical os can be caused by a torn, weak, or absent sphincter at the internal os. The sphincters at the fallopian tubes prevent menstrual blood from flowing backward into the fallopian tubes from the uterus.

Although each layer of muscle has been discussed as having a unique function, it must be remembered that the uterine musculature works as a whole. The uterine contractions of labor are responsible for the dilatation of the cervix and provide the major force for the passage of the fetus through the pelvic axis and vaginal canal at birth.

The innermost layer of the uterine corpus is the *mucosal layer*, or **endometrium,** which is composed of a single layer of columnar epithelium, glands, and stroma. From menarche to menopause, the endometrium undergoes monthly renewal and degeneration in the absence of pregnancy. As it responds to a governing hormonal cycle and prostaglandin influence as well, the endometrium varies in thickness from 0.5 to 5 mm.

The glands of the endometrium produce a thin, watery, alkaline secretion that keeps the uterine cavity moist. This *endometrial milk* not only assists the sperm as they travel to the fallopian tubes, but also nourishes the developing embryo before it implants in the endometrium (see Chapter 7).

The blood supply to the endometrium is unique. In the myometrium, the radial arteries branch off from the arcuate arteries at right angles. Once inside the endometrium, they become the basal arteries supplying the zona basalis (a layer of the endometrium) and ultimately become the coiled arteries supplying the zona functionalis (also part of the endometrium). The straighter basal arteries are smaller than the coiled arteries and are not sensitive to cyclic hormonal control. Hence the zona basalis portion remains intact and is the site of new endometrial tissue generation. The coiled arteries are extremely sensitive to cyclic hormonal control. Their response is alternate relaxation and constriction during the ischemic, or terminal, phase of the menstrual cycle. This response allows for part of the endometrial tissue to remain intact while other endometrial tissue is shed during menstruation.

When pregnancy occurs and the endometrium is not shed, the reticular stromal cells surrounding the endometrial glands become the decidual cells of pregnancy. The stromal cells are highly vascular, channeling a rich blood supply to the endometrial surface.

The Cervix

The narrow neck of the uterus is the **cervix.** Canal-like, it meets the body of the uterus at the internal os and descends about 2.5 cm to connect with the vagina at the external os (Figure 6–5). Thus it provides a protective portal for the body of the uterus. The cervix is divided by its line of attachment into the vaginal and supravaginal areas. The *vaginal cervix* projects into the vagina at an angle from 45 to 90 degrees. The *supravaginal cervix* is surrounded by the attachments that give the uterus its main

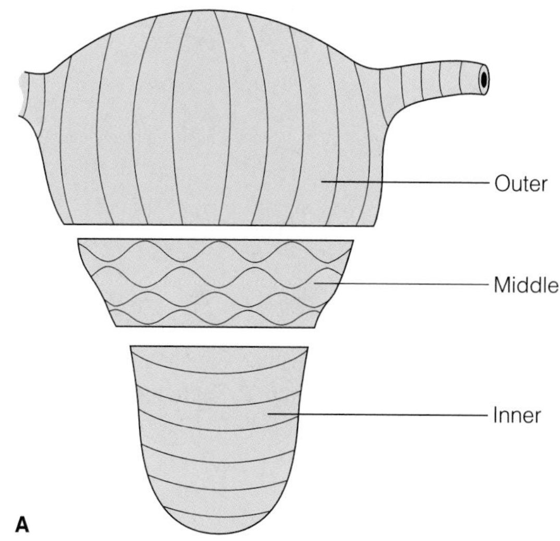

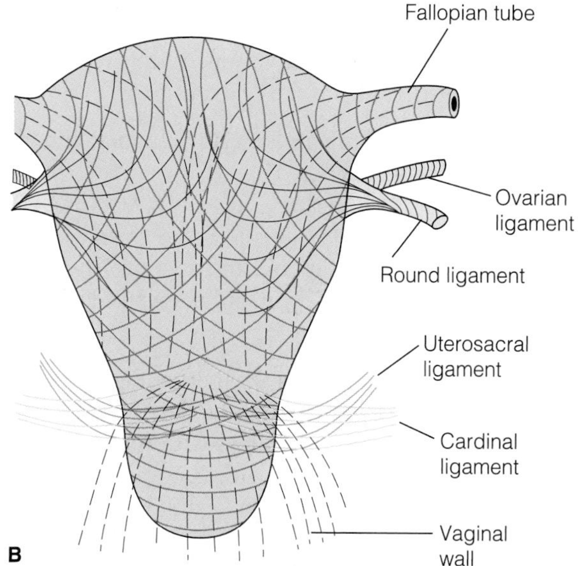

FIGURE 6–7 Uterine muscle layers: ***A,*** Muscle fiber placement. ***B,*** Interlacing of uterine muscle layers.

support: the uterosacral ligaments, the transverse ligaments of the cervix (Mackenrodt's ligaments), and the pubocervical ligaments.

The vaginal cervix appears pink and ends at the external os. The cervical canal appears rosy red and is lined with columnar ciliated epithelium, which contains mucus-secreting glands. Most cervical cancer begins at this *squamocolumnar junction.* The specific location of the junction varies with age and number of pregnancies. Figure 6–8 shows this junction at various stages of a woman's life.

Elasticity is the chief characteristic of the cervix. Its ability to stretch is due to the high fibrous and collagenous content of the supportive tissues and also to the vast number of folds in the cervical lining.

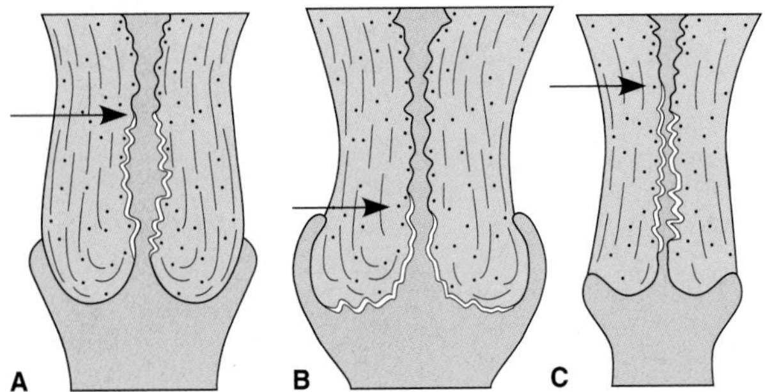

FIGURE 6–8 Changes in squamocolumnar junction (arrows) at various stages of life: ***A,*** Childhood. ***B,*** Reproductive years. ***C,*** Postmenopausal years.

The cervical mucosa has three functions:

- To provide lubrication for the vaginal canal.
- To act as a bacteriostatic agent.
- To provide an alkaline environment to shelter deposited sperm from the acidic vagina.

At ovulation, cervical mucus is clearer, thinner, and more alkaline than at other times.

Uterine Ligaments

The uterine ligaments support and stabilize the various reproductive organs. The ligaments shown in Figure 6–9 are described in this section.

- The *broad ligament* keeps the uterus centrally placed and provides stability within the pelvic cavity. It is a double layer that is continuous with the abdominal peritoneum. The broad ligament covers the uterus anteriorly and posteriorly and extends outward from the uterus to enfold and stabilize the fallopian tubes. The round and ovarian ligaments are at the upper border of the broad ligament. At its lower border, the broad ligament forms the cardinal ligaments. Between the folds of the broad ligament are connective tissue, involuntary muscle, blood and lymph vessels, and nerves.
- The *round ligaments* keep the uterus in place. Each of the round ligaments arises from the sides of the uterus near the fallopian tube insertion. They extend outward between the folds of the broad ligament, passing through the inguinal ring and canals and eventually fusing with the connective tissue of the labia majora. The round ligaments are made up of longitudinal muscle and enlarge during pregnancy. During labor the round ligaments steady the uterus, pulling downward and forward, so that the presenting part of the fetus is forced into the cervix.
- The *ovarian ligaments* anchor the lower pole of the ovary to the cornua of the uterus. They are composed of muscle fibers, which allow the ligaments to contract. This contractile ability influences the position of the ovary to some extent, thus helping the fimbriae of the fallopian tubes to "catch" the ovum as it is released each month.
- The *cardinal ligaments* are the chief uterine supports, suspending the uterus from the side walls of the true pelvis. These ligaments, also known as Mackenrodt's ligaments or transverse cervical ligaments, arise from the sides of the pelvic walls and attach to the cervix in the upper vagina. These ligaments prevent uterine prolapse and also support the upper vagina.
- The *infundibulopelvic ligament* suspends and supports the ovaries. Arising from the outer third of the broad ligament, the infundibulopelvic ligament contains the ovarian vessels and nerves.
- The *uterosacral ligaments* provide support for the uterus and cervix at the level of the ischial spines. Arising on each side of the pelvis from the posterior wall of the uterus, the uterosacral ligaments sweep back around the rectum and insert on the sides of the first and second sacral vertebrae. The uterosacral ligaments contain smooth muscle fibers, connective tissue, blood and lymph vessels, and nerves. Providing support for the uterus and cervix at the level of the ischial spines, they also contain sensory nerve fibers that contribute to dysmenorrhea (painful menstruation; see Chapter 3).

Fallopian Tubes

The two **fallopian tubes,** also known as *oviducts* or *uterine tubes,* arise from each side of the uterus and reach almost to the side of the pelvis, where they turn toward the ovaries (Figure 6–10). Each tube is approximately 8 to 13.5 cm long. A short section of each fallopian tube is inside the uterus; its opening into the uterus is 1 mm in diameter. The fallopian tubes link the peritoneal cavity with the uterus and vagina. This linkage increases a woman's vulnerability to disease processes.

Each fallopian tube may be divided into three parts: the **isthmus,** the ampulla, and the infundibulum or fimbria. The isthmus is straight and narrow, with a thick muscular wall and an opening (lumen) 2 to 3 mm in diameter. It is the site of tubal ligation (a surgical procedure to prevent pregnancy; see Chapter 3).

Next to the isthmus is the curved **ampulla,** which comprises the outer two-thirds of the tube. Fertilization of the secondary oocyte by a spermatozoon usually occurs here. The ampulla ends at the **fimbria,** which is a funnel-like enlargement with many moving fingerlike projections (*fimbriae*) reaching out to the ovary. The longest of these, the *fimbria ovarica,* is attached to the ovary to increase the chances of intercepting the ovum as it is released.

The wall of the fallopian tube is made up of four layers: peritoneal (serous), subserous (adventitial), muscular, and mucous tissues. The peritoneum covers the tubes. The subserous layer contains the blood and nerve supply,

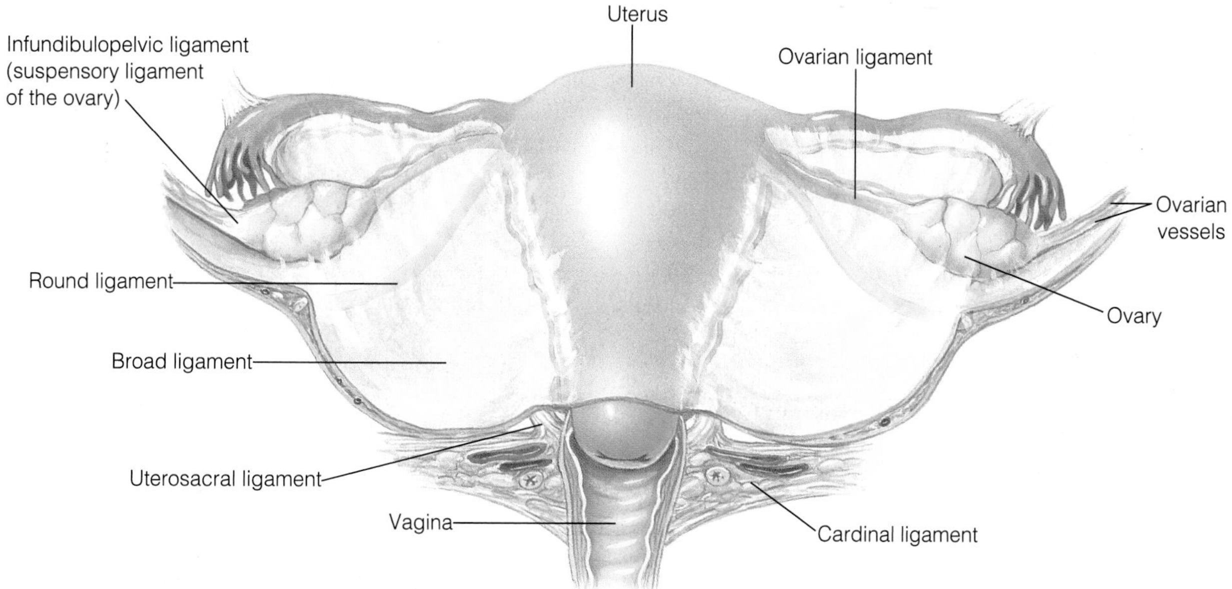

FIGURE 6–9 Uterine ligaments.

and the muscular layer is responsible for the peristaltic movement of the tube. The mucosal layer, immediately next to the muscular layer, is composed of ciliated and nonciliated cells, with the number of ciliated cells more abundant at the fimbria. Nonciliated cells are goblet cells that secrete a protein-rich, serous fluid that nourishes the ovum. The constantly moving tubal cilia propel the ovum toward the uterus. Because the ovum is a large cell, this ciliary action is needed to assist the tube's muscular layer peristalsis. Any malformation or malfunction of the tubes could result in infertility, ectopic pregnancy, or even sterility.

A well-functioning tubal transport system involves active fimbriae close to the ovary, peristalsis of the tube created by the muscular layer, ciliated currents beating toward the uterus, and the proximal contraction and distal relaxation of the tube caused by different types of prostaglandins.

A rich blood and lymph supply serves each fallopian tube. Thus the fallopian tubes have an unusual ability to recover from any inflammatory process. The functions of the fallopian tubes are as follows:

- To provide transport for the ovum from the ovary to the uterus (transport through the fallopian tubes varies from 3 to 4 days).
- To provide a site for fertilization.
- To serve as a warm, moist, nourishing environment for the ovum or zygote (a fertilized egg; see also Chapter 7).

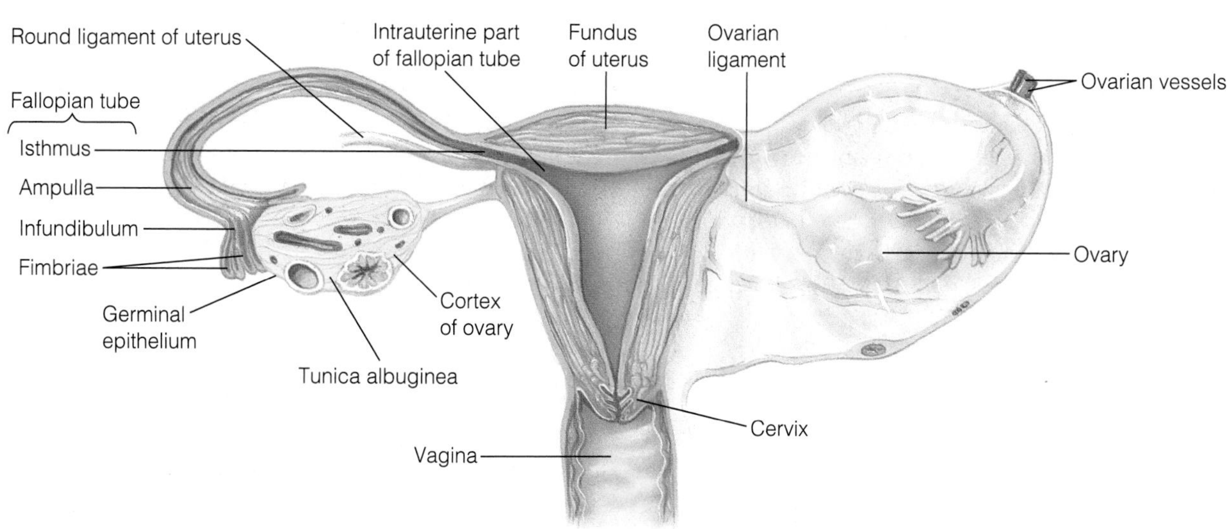

FIGURE 6–10 Fallopian tube and ovary.

Ovaries

The ovaries are two almond-shaped glandular structures just below the pelvic brim. One ovary is located on each side of the pelvic cavity. Their size varies among women and according to the stage of the menstrual cycle. Each ovary weighs 6 to 10 g and is 1.5 to 3 cm wide, 2 to 5 cm long, and 1 to 1.5 cm thick. The ovaries of girls are small but become larger after puberty. They also change in appearance from smooth-surfaced, dull white organs to pitted gray organs. This pitting is caused by scarring due to ovulation. It is rare for both ovaries to be at the same level in the pelvic cavity. The ovary is held in place by the ovarian, broad, and infundibulopelvic ligaments (Figure 6–9), discussed earlier in the chapter.

There is no peritoneal covering for the ovaries. Although this lack of covering assists the mature ovum to erupt, it also allows easier spread of malignant cells from cancer of the ovaries. A single layer of cuboidal epithelial cells, called the germinal epithelium, covers the ovaries. The ovaries are composed of three layers: the tunica albuginea, the cortex, and the medulla. The *tunica albuginea* is dense and dull white and serves as a protective layer. The *cortex* is the main functional part, containing ova, graafian follicles, corpora lutea, degenerated corpora lutea (corpora albicantia), and degenerated follicles. The *medulla* is completely surrounded by the cortex and contains the nerves and the blood and lymphatic vessels.

The ovaries are the primary source of two important hormones: the estrogens and progesterone. *Estrogens* are associated with characteristics contributing to femaleness, including breast alveolar lobule growth and duct development. The ovaries secrete large amounts of estrogens; the adrenal cortex (extraglandular sites) produces minute amounts of estrogens in nonpregnant women.

Progesterone is often called the *hormone of pregnancy* because its effects on the uterus allow pregnancy to be maintained. The placenta is the primary source of progesterone during pregnancy. This hormone also inhibits the action of prolactin in α-lactalbumin synthesis, thereby preventing lactation during pregnancy (Cunningham et al, 1997).

The interplay between the ovarian hormones and other hormones such as FSH and LH is responsible for the cyclic changes that allow pregnancy to occur. The hormonal and physical changes that occur during the female reproductive cycle are discussed later in this chapter. Between the ages of 45 and 55 years, the woman's ovaries secrete decreasing amounts of estrogen. Eventually, ovulatory activity ceases, and menopause occurs.

Bony Pelvis

The female *bony pelvis* has two unique functions:

- To support and protect the pelvic contents.
- To form the relatively fixed axis of the birth passage.

Because the pelvis is so important to childbearing, its structures should be understood clearly.

Bony Structure

The pelvis is made up of four bones: two innominate bones, the sacrum, and the coccyx (or tailbone). The pelvis resembles a bowl or basin; its sides are the innominate bones, and its back is composed of the sacrum and coccyx. Lined with fibrocartilage and held tightly together by ligaments, the four bones join at the symphysis pubis, the two sacroiliac joints, and the sacrococcygeal joints (Figure 6–11).

The *innominate bones*, also known as the *hip bones* or os coxae, are made up of three separate bones: the ilium, the ischium, and the pubis. These bones fuse to form a circular cavity, the *acetabulum*, which articulates with the femur.

The *ilium* is the broad, upper prominence of the hip. The *iliac crest* is the margin of the ilium. The iliac spine, the foremost projection nearest the groin, is the site of attachment for ligaments and muscles.

The *ischium*, the strongest bone, lies under the ilium and below the acetabulum. The L-shaped ischium ends in a marked protuberance, the *ischial tuberosity*, on which the weight of a seated body rests. The **ischial spines** arise near the junction of the ilium and ischium and jut into the pelvic cavity. The shortest diameter of the pelvic cavity is located between the ischial spines. The ischial spines can serve as a reference point during labor to evaluate the descent of the fetal head into the birth canal. (See Chapter 18 and Figure 18–7.)

The **pubis** forms the slightly bowed front portion of the innominate bone. Extending medially from the acetabulum to the midpoint of the bony pelvis, the two pubic bones meet to form a joint, the *symphysis pubis*. The triangular space below this junction is known as the *pubic arch*. The fetal head passes under this arch during birth. The symphysis pubis is formed by heavy fibrocartilage and the superior and inferior pubic ligaments. The mobility of the inferior ligament increases during pregnancy and to a greater extent in subsequent pregnancies than in first pregnancies.

The sacroiliac joints also have a degree of mobility that increases near the end of pregnancy and results in an upward gliding movement. The pelvic outlet may be increased by 1.5 to 2 cm in the squatting, sitting, and dorsal lithotomy positions. These relaxations of the joints are induced by the hormones of pregnancy.

The *sacrum* is a wedge-shaped bone formed by the fusion of five vertebrae. On the anterior upper portion of the sacrum is a projection into the pelvic cavity known as the **sacral promontory**. This projection is another obstetric guide in determining pelvic measurements. (For discussion of pelvic measurements, see Chapter 11.)

The small triangular bone last on the vertebral column is the *coccyx*. It articulates with the sacrum at the sacrococcygeal joint. The coccyx usually moves backward during labor to provide more room for the fetus.

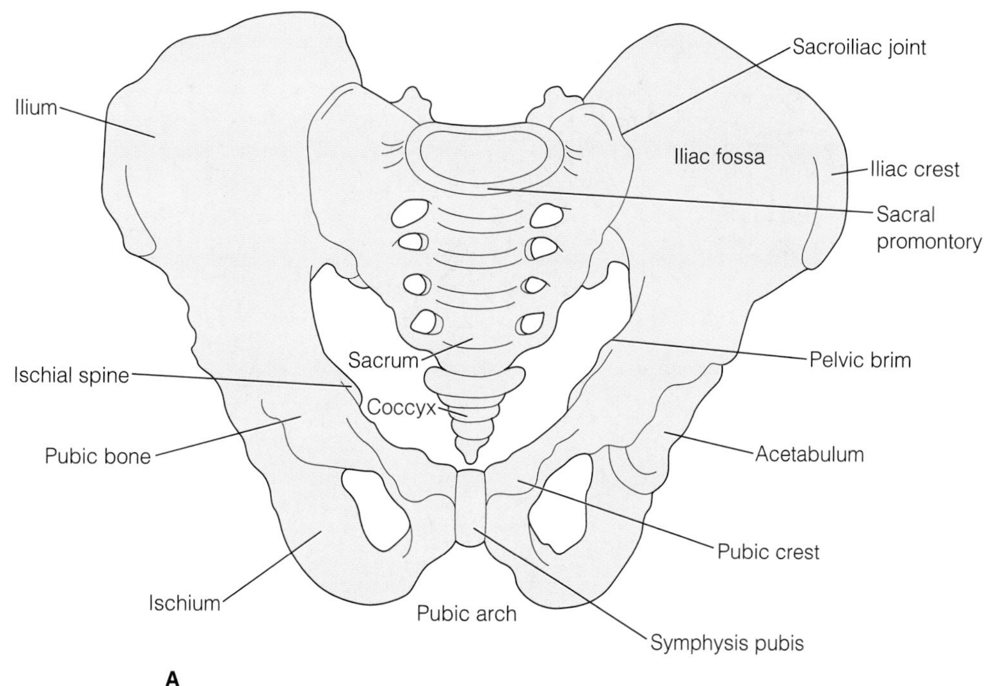

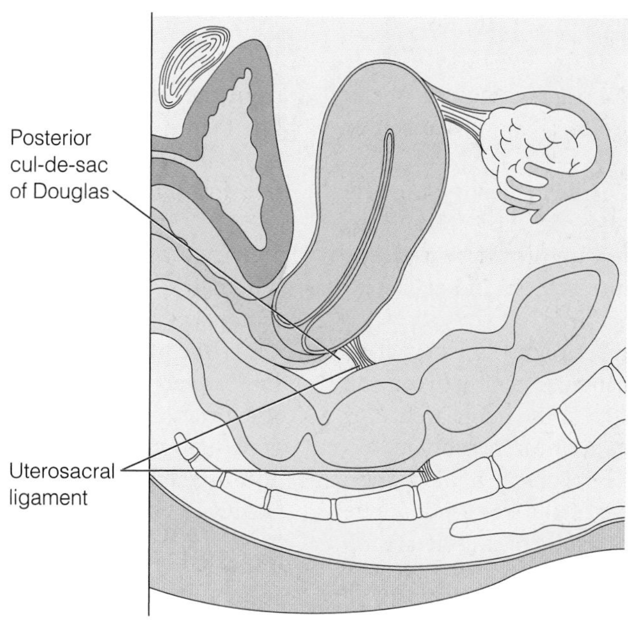

FIGURE 6–11 Pelvis: ***A,*** Pelvic bones. ***B,*** Midsagittal view in supine position with some ligaments.

Pelvic Floor

The muscular *pelvic floor* of the bony pelvis is designed to overcome the force of gravity exerted on the pelvic organs. It acts as a supporting structure to the irregularly shaped pelvic outlet, thereby providing stability and support for surrounding structures.

Deep fascia and the levator ani and coccygeal muscles form the part of the pelvic floor known as the **pelvic diaphragm.** Above it is the pelvic cavity; below and behind it is the perineum. The sacrum is located posteriorly.

The levator ani muscle makes up the major portion of the pelvic diaphragm. It consists of four muscles: the ileococcygeus, pubococcygeus, puborectalis, and pubovaginalis muscles. These muscles form a sling for the pelvic structures. The ileococcygeal muscle, a thin muscular sheet underlying the sacrospinous ligament, helps

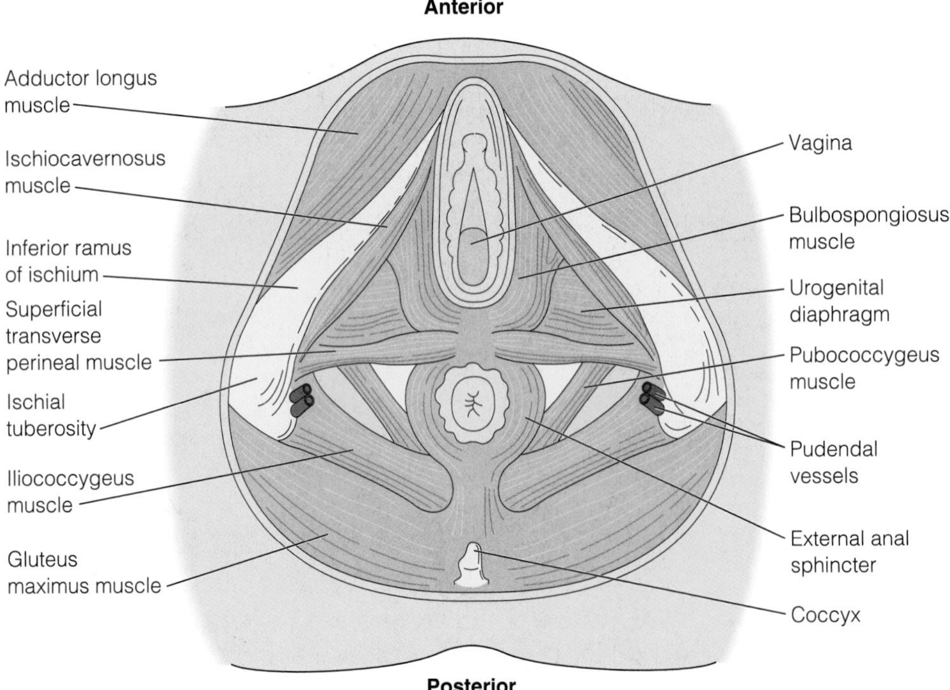

FIGURE 6–12 Muscles of the pelvic floor. (The puborectalis, pubovaginalis, and coccygeal muscles cannot be seen from this view.)

the levator ani support the pelvic organs. Muscles of the pelvic floor are shown in Figure 6–12 and discussed in Table 6–1.

Endopelvic fascia covers the pelvic diaphragm. The components function as a whole, yet they are able to move over one another. This feature provides an exceptional capacity for dilatation during birth and return to prepregnant condition following birth.

The urogenital triangle (diaphragm) is external to the pelvic diaphragm, in the triangular area between the ischial tuberosities and the hollow of the pubic arch. It is made up of superficial and deep perineal membranes extending from the rami of the ischial and pubic bones. Most important in this region are the deep transverse perineal muscles, which are flat bands of muscle arising from the ischiopubic rami and intertwining in the midline to form a seam, or raphe. These muscles are modified to encircle both the urinary meatus and the vaginal orifice, forming the urethral and vaginal sphincters.

Pelvic Division

The pelvic cavity is divided into the false pelvis and the true pelvis (Figure 6–13). The *false pelvis* is the portion above the pelvic brim, or linea terminalis, bounded by the lumbar vertebrae posteriorly, the iliac fossae laterally, and the lower abdominal wall anteriorly. Its primary function is to support the weight of the enlarged pregnant uterus and direct the presenting fetal part into the true pelvis below.

TABLE 6–1 Muscles of the Pelvic Floor

Muscle	Origin	Insertion	Innervation	Action
Levator ani	Pubis, lateral pelvic wall, and ischial spine	Blends with organs in pelvic cavity	Inferior rectal, second and third sacral nerves, plus anterior rami of third and fourth sacral nerves	Supports pelvic viscera; helps form pelvic diaphragm
Iliococcygeus	Pelvic surface of ischial spine and pelvic fascia	Central point of perineum, coccygeal raphe, and coccyx		Assists in supporting abdominal and pelvic viscera
Pubococcygeus	Pubis and pelvic fascia	Coccyx		
Puborectalis	Pubis	Blends with rectum; meets similar fibers from opposite side		Forms sling for rectum, just posterior to it; raises anus
Pubovaginalis	Pubis	Blends into vagina		Supports vagina
Coccygeus	Ischial spine and sacrospinous ligament	Lateral border of lower sacrum and upper coccyx	Third and fourth sacral nerves	Supports pelvic viscera; helps form pelvic diaphragm; flexes and abducts coccyx.

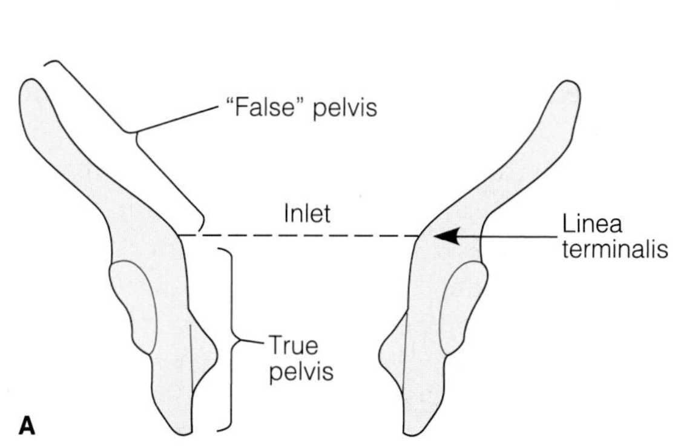

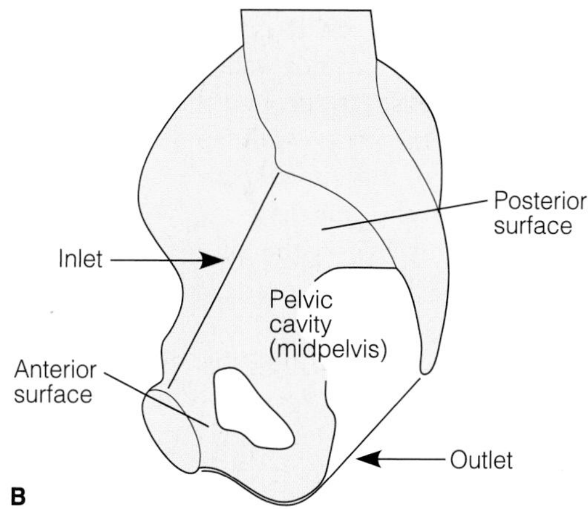

FIGURE 6–13 Female pelvis: ***A,*** The false pelvis is the shallow cavity above the inlet; the true pelvis is the deeper portion of the cavity below the inlet. ***B,*** The true pelvis consists of the inlet, cavity (midpelvis), and outlet.

The **true pelvis** is the portion that lies below the pelvic brim. It is bounded above by the promontory of the sacrum and the upper margins of the pubic bones and below by the pelvic outlet. The true pelvis represents the bony limits of the birth canal. It measures about 5 cm at its anterior wall at the symphysis pubis and about 10 cm at its posterior wall. When a woman is standing upright, the upper portion of the pelvic cavity or canal is directed downward and backward; its lower portion, downward and forward. This forms a curved canal through which the presenting part of the baby must pass during birth (Figure 6–13). The inclination of the pelvis is the angle formed by two planes: a horizontal plane passing through the tip of the coccyx and the superior border of the symphysis pubis, and an inclined plane passing through the sacral promontory and the superior border of the symphysis pubis. This pelvic angle of inclination usually measures 50 to 60 degrees (Figure 6–14).

The true pelvis is extremely important in childbearing because its size and shape must be adequate for normal fetal passage during labor and at birth. The relationship of the fetal head to the true pelvic cavity is of critical importance.

The true pelvis consists of three parts: the inlet, the pelvic cavity, and the outlet. Associated with each part are distinct measurements that aid in evaluating the adequacy of the pelvis for childbirth. The dimensions of the true pelvis and their obstetric implications are described here. Measurement techniques are discussed in Chapter 11. The effects of inadequate or abnormal pelvic diameters on labor and birth are considered in Chapter 19.

The **pelvic inlet** is the upper border of the true pelvis and typically is round in the female. The size and shape of the pelvic inlet are determined by assessing three anteroposterior diameters: the diagonal conjugate, obstetric conjugate, and conjugate vera. (For an in-depth discussion, see Chapter 11.) The **diagonal conjugate** extends from the subpubic angle to the middle of the sacral promontory and is typically 12.5 cm. The diagonal conjugate can be measured manually during a pelvic examination. The **obstetric conjugate** extends from the middle of the sacral promontory to an area approximately 1 cm below the pubic crest. Its length is estimated by subtracting 1.5 cm from the diagonal conjugate. The fetus passes through the obstetric conjugate, and the size of this diameter determines whether the fetus can move down into the birth canal in order for engagement to occur. The true (anatomic) conjugate, or **conjugate vera,** extends from the middle of the sacral promontory to the middle of the pubic crest (superior surface of the symphysis). One additional measurement, the **transverse diameter,** helps determine the shape of the inlet. The transverse diameter is the largest diameter of the inlet.

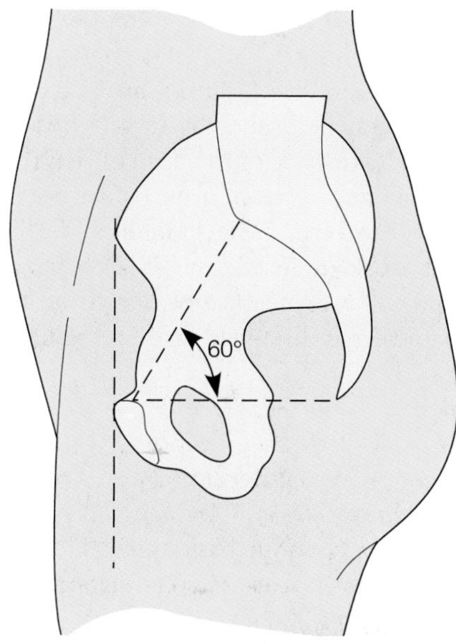

FIGURE 6–14 Pelvic angle of inclination while woman is standing.

The *pelvic cavity* (canal) is a curved canal with a longer posterior than anterior wall. A change in the lumbar curve can increase or decrease the pelvic inclination and can influence the progress of labor because the fetus has to adjust itself to this curved path as well as to the different diameters of the true pelvis.

The **pelvic outlet** is at the lower border of the true pelvis. The size of the pelvic outlet can be determined by assessing the *transverse diameter.* The anteroposterior diameter of the pelvic outlet increases during birth as the presenting part pushes the coccyx posteriorly at the mobile sacrococcygeal joint. Decreased mobility, a large fetal head, and/or a forceful birth can cause the coccyx to break. As the infant's head emerges, the long diameter of the head (occipital frontal) parallels the long diameter of the outlet (anteroposterior).

The transverse diameter (*bi-ischial* or *intertuberous*) extends from the inner surface of one ischial tuberosity to the other. It is the shortest diameter of the pelvic outlet and becomes even shorter if the woman has a narrowed pubic arch. The pubic arch has great importance because the baby must pass under it during birth. If it is narrow, the baby's head may be pushed backward toward the coccyx, making the extension of the head difficult. This situation, known as *outlet dystocia,* may require the use of forceps or a cesarean birth. The shoulders of a large baby may also get stuck under the pubic arch, making birth more difficult. The clinical assessment of each of these obstetric diameters is discussed further in Chapter 11.

Pelvic Types

The Caldwell-Moloy classification of pelves (Figure 6–15) is widely used to differentiate types of bony pelves (Caldwell & Moloy, 1933). *Gynecoid, android, anthropoid,* and *platypelloid* are the four basic types. However, variations in the female pelvis are so great that classic types are not usual.

Each type of pelvis has a characteristic shape, and each shape has implications for labor and birth. The types are described briefly here, and their implications for labor and birth are discussed in detail in Chapter 18.

Gynecoid Pelvis The most common female pelvis is the gynecoid type. The inlet is rounded, with the anteroposterior diameter a little shorter than the transverse diameter. All of the inlet diameters are at least adequate. The posterior segment is broad, deep, and roomy, and the anterior segment is well rounded. The gynecoid midpelvis has nonprominent ischial spines, straight and parallel side walls, and a wide, deep sacral curve. The sacrum is short and slopes backward. All of the midpelvic diameters are at least adequate. The gynecoid pelvic outlet has a wide and round pubic arch; the inferior pubic rami are short and concave. The anteroposterior diameter is long; the transverse diameter, adequate. The capacity of the outlet is adequate. The bones are of medium structure and weight. Approximately 50% of female pelves are classified as gynecoid.

Android Pelvis The normal male pelvis is the android type. The inlet is heart shaped. The anteroposterior and transverse diameters are adequate for birth, but the posterior sagittal diameter is too short, and the anterior sagittal diameter is long. The posterior segment is shallow because the sacral promontory is indented, resulting in a reduced capacity. The anterior segment is narrow, and the forepelvis is sharply angled. The android midpelvis has prominent ischial spines, convergent side walls, and a long, heavy sacrum inclining forward. All of the midpelvic diameters are reduced. The distance from the linea terminalis to the ischial tuberosities is long, yet the overall capacity of the midpelvis is reduced. The android outlet has a narrow, sharp, and deep pubic arch; the inferior pubic rami are straight and long. The anteroposterior diameter is short, and the transverse diameter is narrow. The capacity of the outlet is reduced. The bones are of medium to heavy structure and weight.

Approximately 20% of female pelves are classified as android. The influence of an android pelvis on labor is not favorable. Descent into the pelvis is slow. The fetal head usually engages in the transverse or occipital posterior diameter in asynclitism (oblique presentation) with extreme molding. Arrest of labor is frequent, requiring difficult forceps manipulation (rotation and extraction), and the deep, narrow pubic arch may lead to extensive perineal lacerations. Cesarean birth may be required.

Anthropoid Pelvis The inlet of an anthropoid pelvis is oval, with a long anteroposterior diameter and an adequate but rather short transverse diameter. Both the posterior and anterior segments are deep; the posterior sagittal diameter is extremely long, as is the anterior sagittal diameter. The anthropoid midpelvis has variable ischial spines, straight side walls, and a narrow and long sacrum that inclines backward. The midpelvic diameters are at least adequate, making its capacity adequate. The anthropoid outlet has a normal or moderately narrow pubic arch; the interior pubic rami are long and narrow. The outlet capacity is adequate, and the bones are of medium weight and structure. Approximately 25% of female pelves are classified as anthropoid.

Platypelloid Pelvis The platypelloid type refers to the flat female pelvis. The inlet is distinctly transverse oval, with a short anteroposterior and extremely short transverse diameter. The posterior sagittal and anterior sagittal diameters are short. Both the anterior and posterior segments are shallow. The platypelloid midpelvis has variable ischial spines, parallel side walls, and a wide sacrum with a deep curve inward. Only the transverse diameter is adequate; thus the midpelvic capacity is reduced. The platypelloid outlet has an extremely wide pubic arch; the inferior pubic rami are

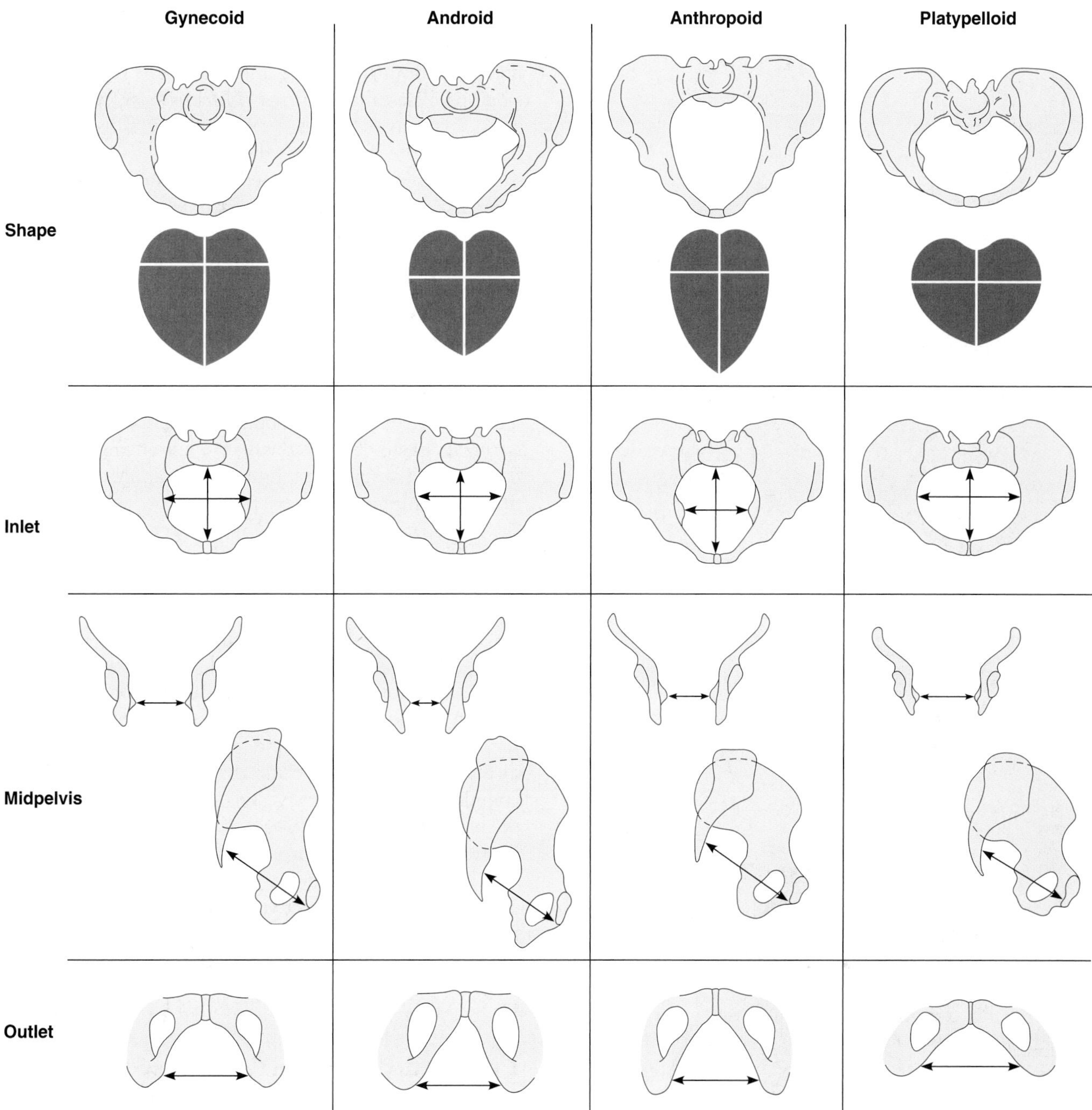

FIGURE 6–15 Comparison of Caldwell-Moloy pelvic types.

straight and short. The transverse diameter is wide, but the anteroposterior diameter is short. The outlet capacity may be inadequate. The platypelloid bones are similar to the gynecoid type. Only 5% of female pelves are classified as platypelloid.

Breasts

The **breasts,** or *mammary glands,* considered accessories of the reproductive system, are specialized sebaceous glands. They are conical and symmetrically placed on the sides of the chest. The greater pectoral and anterior serratus muscles underlie each breast. Suspending the breasts are fibrous tissues, called *Cooper's ligaments,* that extend from the deep fascia in the chest outward to just under the skin covering the breast. The left breast is frequently larger than the right. In different racial groups breasts develop at slightly different levels in the pectoral region of the chest (Rebar, 1999).

In the center of each mature breast is the **nipple,** a protrusion about 0.5 to 1.3 cm in diameter. The nipple is composed mainly of erectile tissue, which becomes more rigid and prominent during the menstrual cycle, sexual

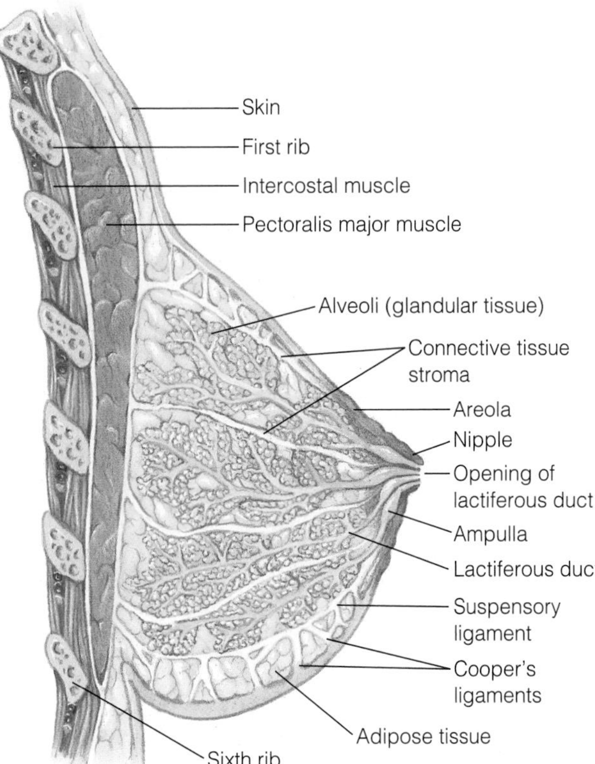

FIGURE 6–16 Anatomy of the breast: The sagittal view of partially dissected left breast.

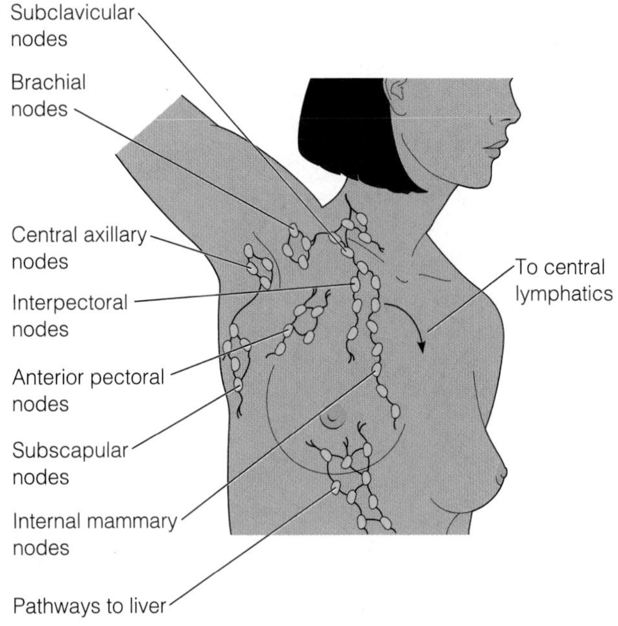

FIGURE 6–17 Lymphatic vessels draining the breast.

excitement, pregnancy, and lactation. The nipple is surrounded by the heavily pigmented **areola,** 2.5 to 10 cm in diameter. Both the nipple and areola are roughened by small papillae called *tubercles of Montgomery.* As an infant suckles, these tubercles secrete a fatty substance that helps lubricate and protect the breasts.

The breasts are composed of glandular, fibrous, and adipose tissue. The glandular tissue consists of acini, or alveoli (Figure 6–16), which are arranged in a series of 15 to 24 lobes separated from each other by adipose and fibrous tissue.

Each lobe is made up of several lobules, which are made up of many grapelike clusters of alveoli around tiny ducts. They are lined with a single layer of cuboidal epithelium, which secretes the various components of milk. The ducts from several lobules combine to form larger *lactiferous ducts,* or *sinuses,* which open on the surface of the nipple. The smooth muscle of the nipple causes erection of the nipple on contraction.

Cyclic hormonal control of the mature breast is complex. Essentially, estrogenic hormones stimulate the growth and development of the ductal epithelium. Progesterone, in association with estrogen, is responsible for the acinar and lobular development during the luteal phase of menstruation. Adrenal corticosteroids, prolactin, somatotropin (growth hormone), and thyroxine are also necessary for estrogen and progesterone to act.

The arterial, venous, and lymphatic systems communicate medially with the internal mammary vessels and laterally with the axillary vessels. Therefore, in cancer of the breast metastasis follows the vascular supply both medially and laterally (Figure 6–17).

The biologic function of the breasts is to provide nourishment and protective maternal antibodies to infants through the lactation process. They are also a source of pleasurable sexual sensation.

Female Reproductive Cycle

The **female reproductive cycle (FRC)** is composed of the ovarian cycle, during which ovulation occurs, and the menstrual cycle, during which menstruation occurs. These two cycles take place simultaneously (see Figure 6–18).

Effects of Female Hormones

After menarche, a woman undergoes a cyclic pattern of ovulation and menstruation (if pregnancy does not occur) for a period of 30 to 40 years. This cycle is an orderly process under neurohormonal control: Each month, one oocyte matures, ruptures from the ovary, and enters the fallopian tube. The ovary, vagina, uterus, and fallopian tubes are major target organs for female hormones.

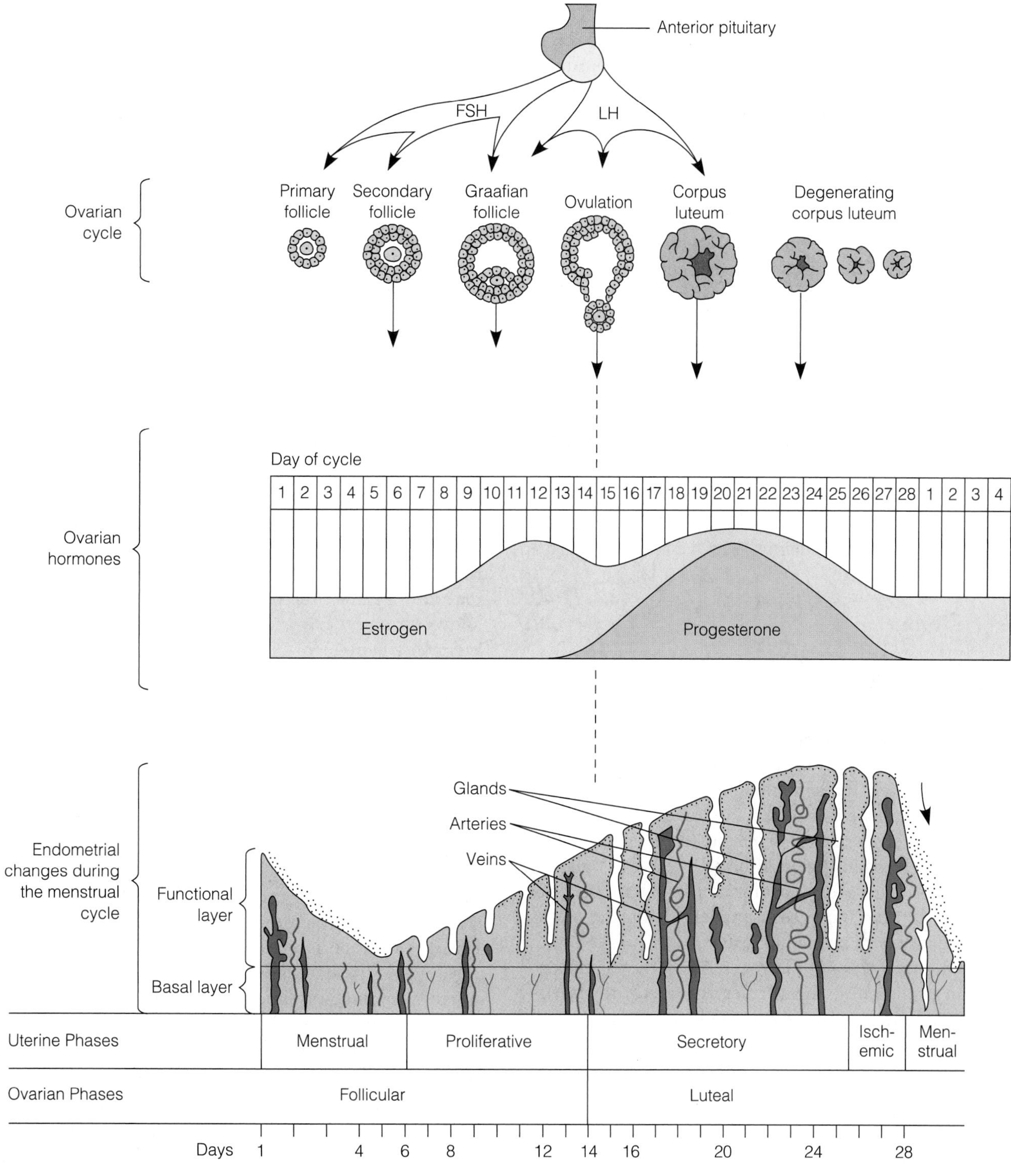

FIGURE 6–18 Female reproductive cycle: Interrelationships of hormones, the four phases of the uterine cycle, and the two phases of the ovarian cycle.

The ovaries not only produce mature gametes, but also secrete hormones. Ovarian hormones include the estrogens, progesterone, and testosterone. The ovary is sensitive to FSH and LH. The uterus is sensitive to estrogen and progesterone. The relative proportions of these hormones control the events of both ovarian and menstrual cycles.

Estrogens

Estrogens are hormones that are associated with those characteristics contributing to "femaleness." The major estrogenic effects are due primarily to three estrogens: estrone, β-estradiol, and estriol. β-estradiol is the major estrogen.

Estrogens control the development of the female secondary sex characteristics: breast development, widening of the hips, and deposits of tissue (fat) in the buttocks and mons pubis. Estrogen also influences the growth of body hair in women. In addition, estrogens assist in the maturation of the ovarian follicles and cause the endometrial mucosa to proliferate following menstruation. The amount of estrogens is greatest during the proliferative (follicular or estrogenic) phase of the menstrual cycle. Estrogens also cause the uterus to increase in size and weight because of increased glycogen, amino acids, electrolytes, and water. Blood supply is expanded as well. Under the influence of estrogens, myometrial contractility increases in both the uterus and the fallopian tubes, and uterine sensitivity to oxytocin increases. Estrogens inhibit FSH production and stimulate LH production.

Estrogens have effects on many hormones and other carrier proteins. This explains the increased amount of protein-bound iodine in pregnant women and in women who use oral contraceptives containing estrogen.

Estrogens may increase libido. They decrease the excitability of the hypothalamus, which may cause an increase in sexual desire.

Progesterone

Progesterone is secreted by the corpus luteum and is found in greatest amounts during the secretory (luteal or progestational) phase of the menstrual cycle. It decreases uterine motility and contractility caused by estrogens, thereby preparing the uterus for implantation after the ovum is fertilized. The endometrial mucosa is in a ready state as a result of estrogenic influence. Progesterone causes the uterine endometrium to increase further its supply of glycogen, arterial blood, secretory glands, amino acids, and water. This hormone is often called the hormone of pregnancy because its effects on the uterus allow pregnancy to be maintained.

Under the influence of progesterone, the vaginal epithelium proliferates, and the cervix secretes thick, viscous mucus. Breast glandular tissue increases in size and complexity. Progesterone also prepares the breasts for lactation.

The temperature rise of about 0.3 to 0.6C (0.5 to 1.0F) that accompanies ovulation and persists throughout the secretory phase of the menstrual cycle is due to progesterone.

Prostaglandins (PGs)

Prostaglandins (PGs) are oxygenated fatty acids that are produced by the cells of the endometrium and are also classified as hormones. Prostaglandins have varied actions in the body. Generally PGE relaxes smooth muscles and is a potent vasodilator; PGF is a potent vasoconstrictor and increases the contractility of muscles and arteries. Although their primary actions seem antagonistic, their basic regulatory functions in cells are achieved through an intricate pattern of reciprocal events. The discussion here sums up their role in ovulation and menstruation.

Prostaglandin production increases during follicular maturation, is dependent on gonadotropins, and is essential to ovulation. Extrusion of the ovum, resulting from the increased contractility of the smooth muscle in the theca layer of the mature follicle, is thought to be caused by PGF_{2a}. Significant amounts of PGs are found in and around the follicle at the time of ovulation.

Although the exact mechanism by which the corpus luteum degenerates in the absence of pregnancy remains obscure, PGF_{2a} is thought to induce progesterone withdrawal, the lowest point of which coincides with the onset of early menses.

During the late secretory phase, the level of PGF_{2a} is higher than that of PGE. This event increases vasoconstriction and contractility of the myometrium, which contributes to the ischemia preceding menstruation. High concentration of PGs may also account for the vasoconstriction of the endometrium venous lacunae allowing for platelet aggregation at vascular rupture points, thereby preventing a rapid blood loss during menstruation. The menstrual flow's high concentration of PGs may also facilitate the process of tissue digestion, which allows for an orderly shedding of the endometrium during menstruation.

Neurohormonal Basis of the Female Reproductive Cycle

The female reproductive cycle is controlled by complex interactions between the nervous and endocrine systems and their target tissues. These interactions involve the hypothalamus, anterior pituitary, and ovaries.

The hypothalamus secretes gonadotropin-releasing hormone (GnRH) to the pituitary gland in response to signals received from the central nervous system. This releasing hormone is often called luteinizing hormone–releasing hormone (LHRH) or follicle-stimulating hormone–releasing hormone (FSHRH) (Ferin, 1998).

In response to GnRH, the anterior pituitary secretes the gonadotropic hormones *follicle-stimulating hormone (FSH)* and *luteinizing hormone (LH)*. FSH is primarily responsible for the maturation of the ovarian follicle. As the follicle matures, it secretes increasing amounts of estrogen, which enhance the development of the follicle (Ferin, 1998). (This estrogen also is responsible for the rebuilding/proliferation phase of the endometrium after it is shed during menstruation.)

Final maturation of the follicle will not come about without the action of LH. The anterior pituitary's production of LH increases sixfold to tenfold as the follicle matures. About 10 to 12 hours after the peak production of LH, ovulation occurs (Speroff, Glass, & Kase, 1994).

The LH is also responsible for the "luteinizing" of the theca and granulosa cells of the ruptured follicle. As a result, estrogen production declines, and progesterone secretion continues. Thus estrogen levels fall a day before ovulation; tiny amounts of progesterone are in evidence. Ovulation takes place following the very rapid growth of the follicle—as the sustained high level of estrogen diminishes and progesterone secretion begins.

The ruptured follicle undergoes rapid change, complete luteinization is accomplished, and the mass of cells becomes the corpus luteum. The lutein cells secrete large amounts of progesterone with smaller amounts of estrogen. (Concurrently, the excessive amounts of progesterone are responsible for the secretory phase of the uterine cycle.) Seven or 8 days following ovulation the corpus luteum begins to involute, losing its secretory function. The production of both progesterone and estrogen is severely diminished. The anterior pituitary responds with increasingly large amounts of FSH; a few days later, LH production begins. As a result, new follicles become responsive to another ovarian cycle and begin maturing.

The Ovarian Cycle

The ovarian cycle has two phases: the *follicular phase* (days 1 to 14) and the *luteal phase* (days 15 to 28 in a 28-day cycle). Figure 6–19 depicts the changes that the follicle undergoes during the ovarian cycle. In women whose menstrual cycles vary, usually it is only the length of the follicular phase that varies, because the luteal phase is of fixed length. During the follicular phase, the immature follicle matures as a result of FSH. Within the follicle, the oocyte grows. A mature **graafian follicle** appears about the 14th day under dual control of FSH and LH. It is a large structure, measuring about 5 to 10 mm. The mature follicle produces increasing amounts of estrogen.

In the mature graafian follicle, the cells surrounding the antral cavity are granulosa cells. The oocyte and follicular fluid are enclosed in the cumulus oophorus. The stromal elements of the ovary are condensed around the follicle in two layers: the theca interna and the theca externa. The theca interna cells resemble the luteal cells of the corpus luteum. In the fully mature graafian follicle, the *zona pellucida* (oolemma), a thick, elastic capsule, develops around the oocyte.

Just before ovulation, the mature oocyte completes its first meiotic division (see Chapter 7 for a description of meiosis). As a result of this division, two cells are formed: a small cell called a *polar body*, and a larger cell called the *secondary oocyte*. The secondary oocyte matures into the ovum. (See Figure 7–4.)

As the graafian follicle matures and enlarges, it comes close to the surface of the ovary. The ovary surface has a blisterlike protrusion 10 to 15 mm in diameter, and the follicle's walls become thin. The secondary oocyte, polar body, and follicular fluid are pushed out. The ovum is discharged near the fimbria of the fallopian tube and is pulled into the tube to begin its journey toward the uterus.

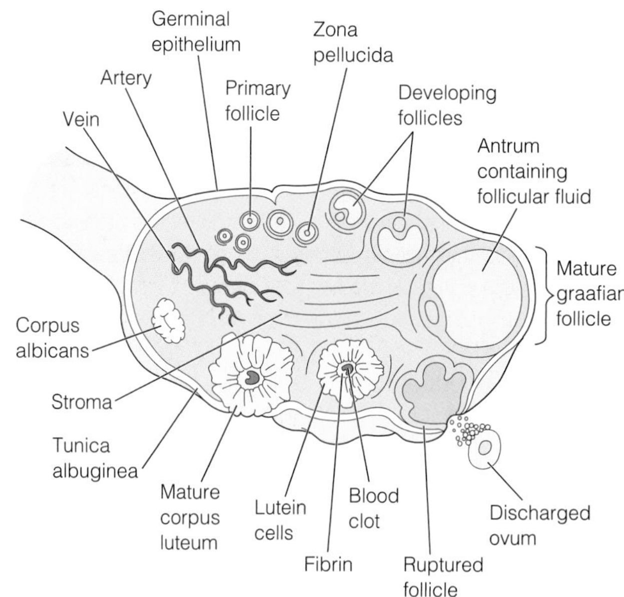

FIGURE 6–19 Various stages of development of the ovarian follicles.

Occasionally ovulation is accompanied by midcycle pain, known as *mittelschmerz*. This pain may be caused by a thick tunica albuginea or by a local peritoneal reaction to the expelling of the follicular contents. Vaginal discharge may increase during ovulation, and a small amount of blood (midcycle spotting) may be discharged as well.

The body temperature increases about 0.3 to 0.6C (0.5 to 1.0F) 24 to 48 hours after the time of ovulation. It remains elevated until the day before menstruation begins. There may be an accompanying sharp basal body temperature drop just before the increase. These temperature changes are useful clinically to determine the approximate time ovulation occurs.

Generally the ovum takes several minutes to travel through the ruptured follicle to the fallopian tube opening. The contractions of the tube's smooth muscle and its ciliary action propel the ovum through the tube. The ovum remains in the ampulla, where it may be fertilized and cleavage can begin. The ovum is thought to be fertile for only 6 to 24 hours. It reaches the uterus 72 to 96 hours after its release from the ovary.

The luteal phase begins when the ovum leaves its follicle. Under the influence of LH the **corpus luteum** develops from the ruptured follicle. Within 2 or 3 days the corpus luteum becomes yellowish and spherical and increases in vascularity. If the ovum is fertilized and implants in the endometrium, the fertilized egg begins to secrete **human chorionic gonadotropin (hCG),** which is needed to maintain the corpus luteum. If fertilization does not occur, within about a week after ovulation the corpus luteum begins to degenerate, eventually becoming

RESEARCH IN PRACTICE

What is this study about? Nancy Fugate Woods and colleagues explored the etiology of perimenstrual symptoms as part of a larger study evaluating the biopsychosocial dimensions of perimenstrual symptom patterns. The researchers examined the relationships among ovarian steroids, stress arousal indicators of cortisol and catecholamines, perceived stress, and symptoms of turmoil and fluid retention when women experienced low symptom severity (LS), premenstrual syndrome (PMS), or premenstrual magnification (PMM).

How was this study done? From an initial sample of 1149 women recruited through local newspapers, 342 women completed an initial 90-day health diary. Of the 118 women who agreed to complete the intensive second portion, only 40 met the criteria for LS pattern, 22 for PMS, and 26 for PMM. Daily urines were assayed for ovarian hormones of estradiol and a progesterone derivative, and cortisol. Due to budget constraints, daily urines for only 49 women were analyzed for epinephrine and norepinephrine. From the daily diary the researchers assessed perceived stress, emotional turmoil, and fluid retention.

What were the results of the study? As noted by the researchers, this study demonstrated a complex interrelationship among ovarian hormones and catecholamines and determined that both are related to emotional turmoil and fluid retention for women experiencing symptoms of PMS and PMM. The pattern of relationship differs for both groups. Women with PMS and PMM perceived higher levels of stress than the LS group. Premenses turmoil and fluid retention were most severe for the PMM group, then PMS, then LS. In comparison of the LS and PMM groups, lower levels of norepinephrine, higher premenses global stress ratings, and estradiol slope predicted premenstrual turmoil. Perceived stress and cortisol correlate with symptoms for women with PMS. For women with PMM, perceived stress, higher epinephrine, lower norepinephrine, and higher estradiol levels in the luteal phase impact emotional turmoil and fluid retention symptoms.

What additional questions might I have? Although the study reported 86 women as the final sample and some explanation is provided, the reported *n* varies from table to table. What was the specific number of subjects evaluated with each variable and why do they change?

How can I use this study? Many women suffer from premenstrual syndrome and believe it to be psychological. Results of this study provide information about the physiologic changes that occur, and may be shared with any woman who desires more knowledge regarding her symptoms.

SOURCE: Woods, N. F., Lentz, M .J., Mitchell, E. S., Shaver, J., & Heitkemper, M. (1998). Luteal phase ovarian steroids, stress arousal, premenses perceived stress, and premenstrual symptoms. *Research in Nursing & Health, 21,* 129–142.

a connective tissue scar called the *corpus albicans.* With degeneration comes a decrease in estrogen and progesterone. This allows for an increase in LH and FSH, which triggers the hypothalamus. Approximately 14 days after ovulation (in a 28-day cycle), in the absence of pregnancy, menstruation begins.

CRITICAL THINKING QUESTION

How would a decrease in FSH affect the proliferation phase of the menstrual cycle?

The Menstrual Cycle

Menstruation is cyclic uterine bleeding in response to cyclic hormonal changes. Menstruation occurs when the ovum is not fertilized and begins about 14 days after ovulation in a 28-day cycle. The menstrual discharge, also referred to as the *menses* or *menstrual flow,* is composed of blood mixed with cervical and vaginal secretions, bacteria, mucus, leukocytes, and other cellular debris. The menstrual discharge is dark red and has a distinctive odor.

A review of the endometrium and its arterial blood supply will provide further understanding of the menstrual process. Blood flow from the spiral arterioles in the superficial endometrium is reduced, leading to a lack of blood and oxygen, which in turn produces tissue death (necrosis) and discharge of the superficial endometrium (menses). At the same time, the straight arterioles provide the basal endometrium with sufficient blood flow to maintain this layer of the endometrium and the endometrial glands (or seeds) that are responsible for the generation of the endometrium in the next female reproductive or menstrual cycle (Figure 6–20). Bleeding is controlled by vasospasm of the straight basal arterioles, resulting in coagulative necrosis at the vessel tips.

Frequently, ovulation does not occur in early menstrual cycles; these are called anovulatory cycles. Early cycles also are often irregular in frequency, amount of flow, and duration. Within several months to 2 to 3 years, a regular cycle becomes established.

Menstrual parameters vary greatly among individuals. Generally, menstruation occurs every 28 days, plus or minus 5 to 10 days. Emotional and physical factors such as illness, excessive fatigue, stress or anxiety, and rigorous exercise programs can alter the cycle interval. Certain environmental factors such as temperature and altitude may also affect the cycle.

The duration of menses is from 2 to 8 days, with the blood loss averaging 30 mL, and the loss of iron averaging 0.5 to 1 mg daily.

The menstrual cycle has four phases: the menstrual phase, proliferative phase, secretory phase, and ischemic phase (Table 6–2). Menstruation occurs during the *menstrual phase.* Some endometrial areas are shed, while others remain. Some of the remaining tips of the endometrial glands begin to regenerate. The endometrium is in a resting state following menstruation. Estrogen levels are low, and the endometrium is 1 to 2 mm deep. During this part of the cycle the cervical mucosa is scanty, viscous, and opaque.

The proliferative phase begins when the endometrial glands enlarge, becoming twisted and longer, in response

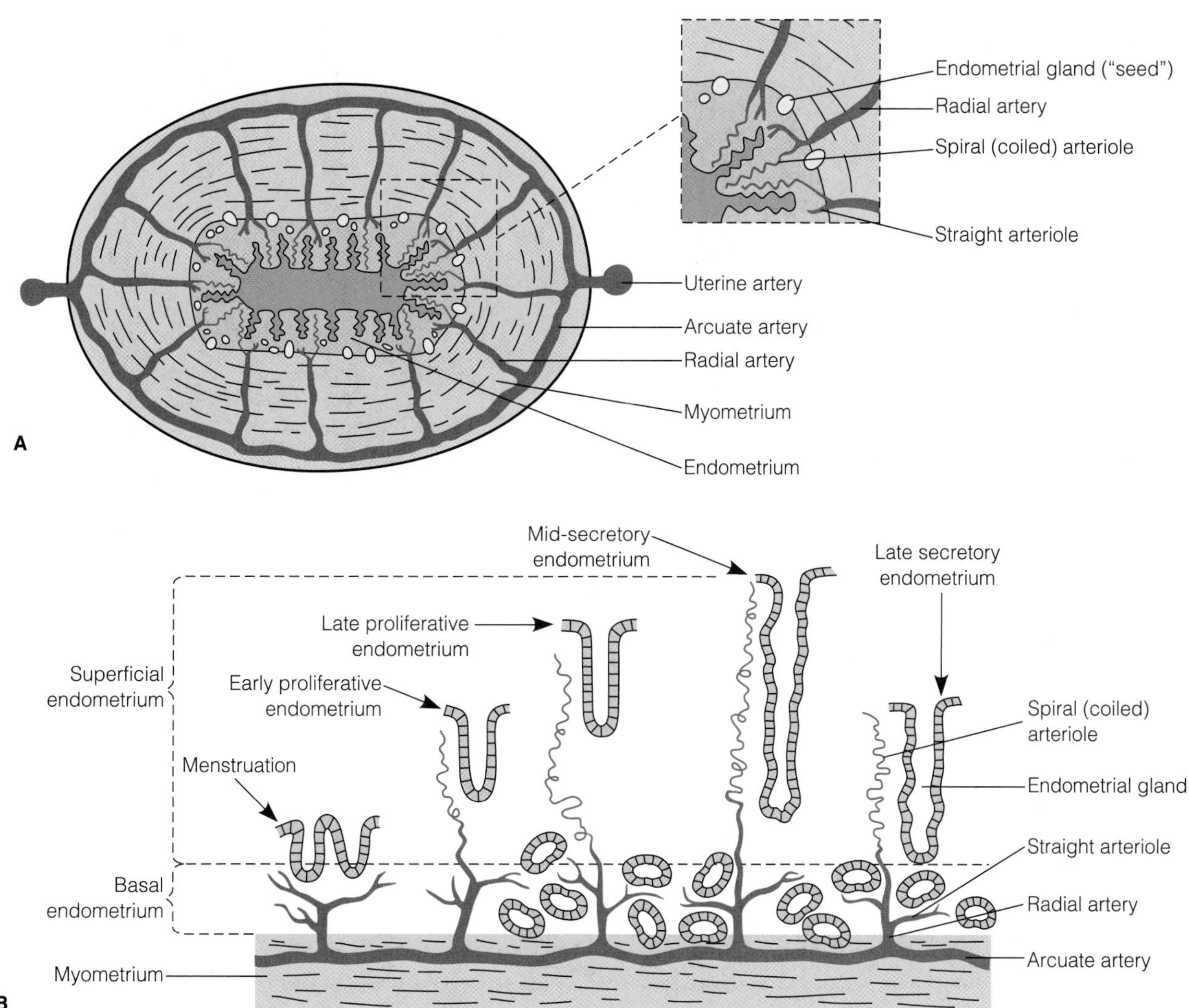

FIGURE 6–20 ***A,*** Blood supply to the endometrium (cross-sectional view of the uterus). ***B,*** Schematic representation of the blood supply during complete menstrual cycle.

TABLE 6–2 Characteristics of Menstrual Cycle and Ovulation

Phase	Characteristics
Menstrual phase (days 1–6)	Estrogen levels are low. Cervical mucus is scanty, viscous, and opaque. Endometrium is shed.
Proliferative phase (days 7–14)	Endometrium and myometrium thickness increases. Estrogen peaks just before ovulation. Cervical mucosa at ovulation: Is clear, thin, watery, and alkaline. Is more favorable to sperm. Has elasticity (*spinnbarkheit*) greater than 5 cm. Shows ferning pattern on microscopic exam. Just prior to ovulation body temperature drops; then at ovulation basal body temperature increases 0.3 to 0.6C, and *mittelschmerz* and/or midcycle spotting may occur.
Secretory phase (days 15–26)	Estrogen drops sharply, and progesterone dominates. Vascularity of entire uterus increases. Tissue glycogen increases, and the uterus is made ready for implantation.
Ischemic phase (days 27–28)	Both estrogen and progesterone levels fall. Spiral arteries undergo vasoconstriction. Endometrium becomes pale. Blood vessels rupture. Blood escapes into uterine stromal cells.

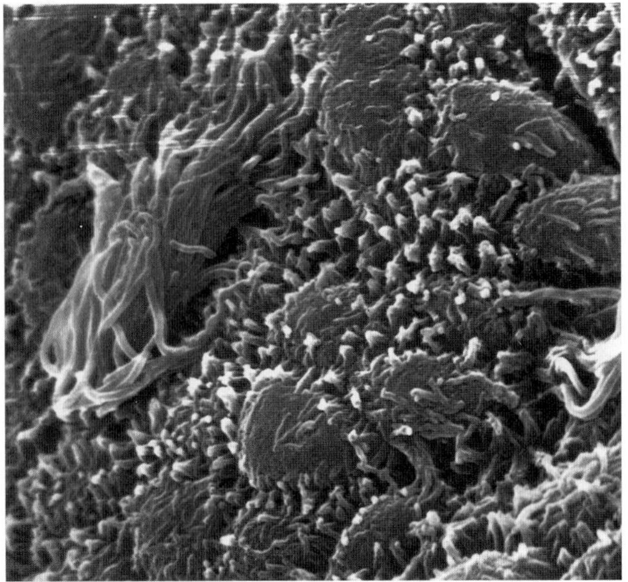

A

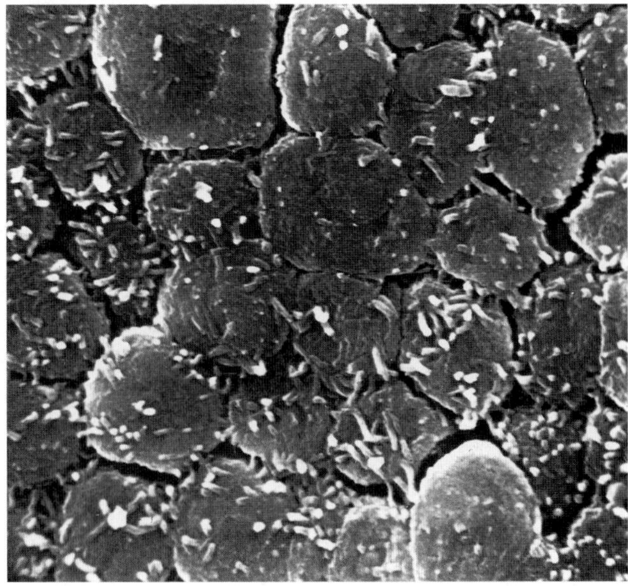

B

FIGURE 6–21 Scanning electron micrographs of the uterine lining during different phases of the uterine cycle. ***A,*** During the luteal phase, some of the cells have cilia, and some are secreting droplets. The secreting cells are covered with microvilli. ***B,*** In the secretory phase, microvilli are still present on the surface of the secreting cells, but the general surface of the lining has a lumpier appearance than during the proliferative phase, and the cilia appear shorter and less numerous. The named phases refer to the uterine condition at the time the photographs were taken.

to increasing amounts of estrogen. The blood vessels become prominent and dilated, and the endometrium increases in thickness sixfold to eightfold. This gradual process reaches its peak just before ovulation. The cervical mucosa becomes thin, clear, watery, and more alkaline, making the mucosa more favorable to spermatozoa. As ovulation nears, the cervical mucous shows increased elasticity, called spinnbarkheit. At ovulation in the *proliferative phase*, the mucus will stretch more than 5 cm. The cervical mucosa pH increases from below 7.0 to 7.5 at the time of ovulation. On microscopic examination, the mucosa shows a characteristic ferning pattern (Figure 8–4 *B*). This ferning pattern is a useful aid in assessment of ovulation time (Table 6–3). For an in-depth discussion, see Chapter 8.

TABLE 6–3 Signs of Ovulation

The cervical mucosa changes in the following ways:

- The amount of mucus increases.
- It appears thin, watery, and clear.
- *Spinnbarkheit* greater than 5 cm is present.
- A ferning pattern appears on microscopic examination.

Basal body temperature increases 0.3 to 0.6C 24 to 48 hours after ovulation.

Mittelschmerz may be present.

Midcycle spotting may occur.

The *secretory phase* follows ovulation. The endometrium, under estrogenic influence, undergoes slight cellular growth. Progesterone, however, causes such marked swelling and growth that the epithelium is warped into folds (Figure 6–21). The amount of tissue glycogen increases. The glandular epithelial cells begin to fill with cellular debris, and the glands become tortuous and dilate. The glands secrete small quantities of endometrial fluid in preparation for a fertilized ovum. The vascularity of the entire uterus increases greatly, providing a nourishing bed for implantation. If implantation occurs, the endometrium, under the influence of progesterone, continues to develop and becomes even thicker (Figure 6–22; see Chapter 7 for an in-depth discussion of implantation).

If fertilization does not occur, the *ischemic phase* begins. The corpus luteum begins to degenerate, and as a result both estrogen and progesterone levels fall. Areas of necrosis appear under the epithelial lining. Extensive vascular changes also occur. Small blood vessels rupture, and the spiral arteries constrict and retract, causing a deficiency of blood in the endometrium, which becomes pale. This ischemic phase is characterized by the escape of blood into the stromal cells of the uterus. The menstrual flow begins, thus beginning the menstrual cycle again. After menstruation, the basal layer remains so that the tips of the glands can regenerate the new functional endometrial layer. See Table 6–4 for a summary of the female reproductive cycle.

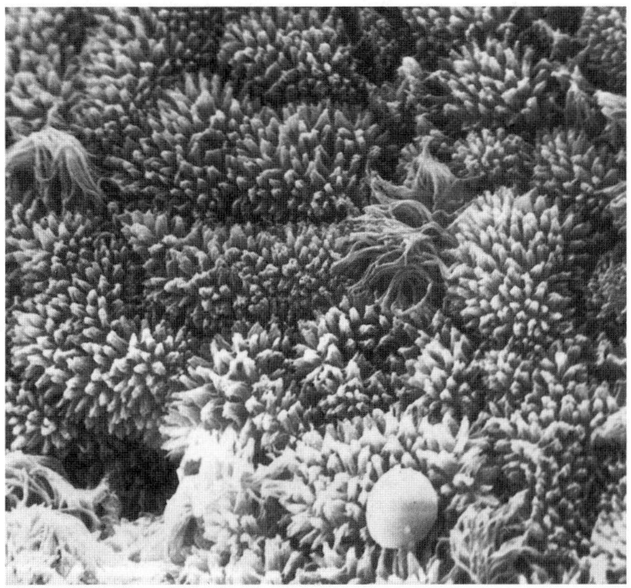

C

FIGURE 6–22 Scanning electron micrograph of the inner lining of the uterus at the time of blastocyst implantation. The blastocyst is an embryo at an early stage of development.

TABLE 6–4 Summary of Female Reproductive Cycle

Ovarian Cycle

Follicular phase (days 1–14): Primordial follicle matures under influence of FSH and LH up to the time of ovulation.

Luteal phase (days 15–28): Ovum leaves follicle; corpus luteum develops under LH influence and produces high levels of progesterone and low levels of estrogen.

Menstrual Cycle

Menstrual phase (days 1–6)

Proliferative phase (days 7–14): Estrogen peaks just prior to ovulation. Cervical mucus at ovulation is clear, thin, watery, alkaline, and more favorable to sperm; shows ferning pattern; and has *spinnbarkheit* greater than 5 cm. At ovulation body temperature drops, then rises sharply and remains elevated.

Secretory phase (days 15–26): Estrogen drops sharply, and progesterone dominates.

Ischemic phase (days 27–28): Both estrogen and progesterone levels drop.

Male Reproductive System

The primary reproductive functions of the male genitals are to produce and transport the male sex cells (sperm) through and eventually out of the genital tract into the female genital tract. The male reproductive system consists of the external and internal genitals (Figure 6–23).

External Genitals

The two external reproductive organs are the penis and the scrotum.

Penis

The *penis* is an elongated, cylindrical structure consisting of a body, termed the *shaft*, and a cone-shaped end called the *glans*. The penis lies in front of the scrotum.

The shaft of the penis is made up of three longitudinal columns of erectile tissue: the paired *corpora cavernosa* and a third, the *corpus spongiosum*. These columns are covered by a dense, fibrous connective tissue and then enclosed by an elastic tissue. The penis is covered by a thin outer layer of skin.

The corpus spongiosum contains the urethra and becomes the glans at the distal end of the penis. The urethra widens within the glans and ends in a slitlike orifice, located in the tip of the glans, called the *urethral meatus*. A circular fold of skin arises just behind the glans and covers it. Known as the *prepuce*, or *foreskin*, it is frequently removed by the surgical procedure of circumcision (Chapter 26). If the corpus spongiosum does not surround the urethra completely, the urethral meatus may occur on the ventral aspect of the penile shaft (hypospadias) or on the dorsal aspect (epispadias).

The penis is innervated by the pudendal nerve. Sexual stimulation causes the penis to elongate, thicken, and stiffen, a process called *erection*. The penis becomes erect when its blood vessels become engorged, a consequence of parasympathetic nerve stimulation. If sexual stimulation is intense enough, the forceful and sudden expulsion of semen occurs through the rhythmic contractions of the penile muscles. This phenomenon is called *ejaculation*.

The penis serves both the urinary and reproductive systems. Urine is expelled through the urethral meatus. The primary reproductive function of the penis is to deposit sperm in the female vagina during sexual intercourse so that fertilization of the ovum can occur.

Scrotum

The *scrotum* is a pouchlike structure that hangs in front of the anus and behind the penis. Composed of skin and the *dartos muscle*, the scrotum shows increased pigmentation and scattered hairs. The sebaceous glands open directly onto the scrotal surface; their secretion has a distinctive odor. Contraction of the dartos and cremasteric muscles shortens the scrotum and draws it closer to the body, thus wrinkling its outer surface. The degree of wrinkling is greatest in young men and at cold temperatures and is least in older men and at warm temperatures.

Inside the scrotum are two lateral compartments. Each compartment contains a testis with its related structures. Because the left spermatic cord grows longer, the left testis and its scrotal sac hang lower than the right. A ridge (raphe) on the external scrotal surface marks the position of the medial septum and continues anteriorly on the urethral surface of the penis but disappears in the perineal area.

The function of the scrotum is to protect the testes and the sperm by maintaining a temperature lower than

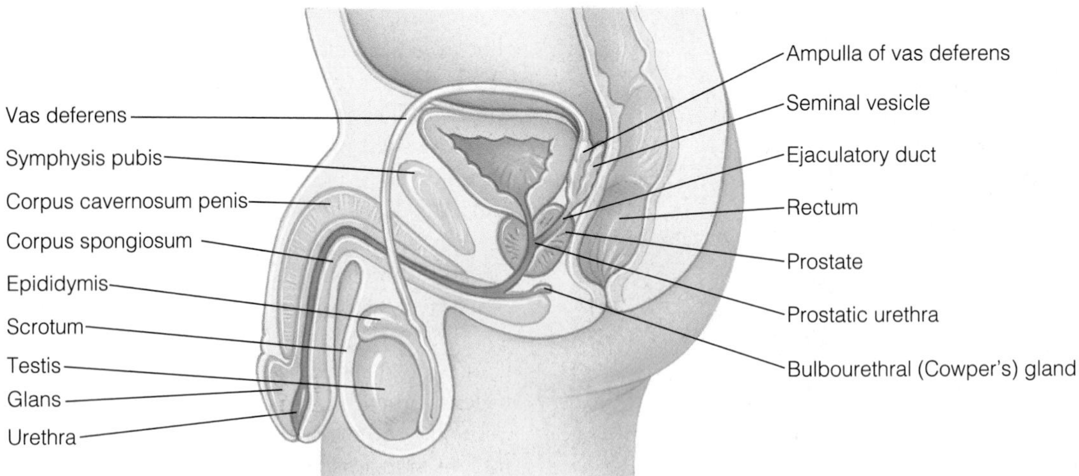

FIGURE 6–23 Male reproductive system, sagittal view.

that of the body. Spermatogenesis will not occur if the testes fail to descend and thus remain at body temperature. Because it is sensitive to touch, pressure, temperature, and pain, the scrotum defends against potential harm to the testes.

Internal Reproductive Organs

The male internal reproductive organs include the gonads (testes or testicles), a system of ducts (epididymis, vas deferens, ejaculatory duct, and urethra), and accessory glands (seminal vesicles, prostate gland, bulbourethral glands, and urethral glands). See Table 6–5 for a summary of male reproductive organ functions.

Testes

The *testes* are a pair of oval, compound glandular organs contained in the scrotum (Figure 6–24). In the sexually mature male, they are the site of spermatozoa production and the secretion of several male sex hormones.

Each testis is 4 to 6 cm long, 2 to 3 cm wide, and 3 to 4 cm deep and weighs 10 to 15 g. Each is covered by a serous membrane and an inner capsule that is tough, white, and fibrous. The connective tissue sends projections inward to form septa, dividing the testis into 250 to 400 lobules. Each lobule contains one to three tightly packed, convoluted *seminiferous tubules* containing sperm cells in all stages of development.

The seminiferous tubules are surrounded by loose connective tissue, which houses abundant blood and lymph vessels and the *interstitial (Leydig's) cells.* The interstitial cells produce testosterone, the primary male sex hormone. The seminiferous tubules come together to form the 20 or 30 straight tubules, which in turn form an anastomosing network of thin-walled spaces, the rete testis. The rete testis forms 10 to 15 efferent ducts that empty into the duct of the epididymis.

Most of the cells lining the seminiferous tubules undergo *spermatogenesis,* a process of maturation in which spermatocytes become spermatozoa. (See Chapter 7 for further discussion of spermatogenesis.) Sperm production varies among and within the tubules, with cells in different areas of the same tubule undergoing different stages of spermatogenesis. The seminiferous tubules also contain *Sertoli's cells,* which nourish and protect the spermatocytes. The sperm are eventually released from the tubules into the epididymis, where they mature further.

Like the female reproductive cycle, the process of spermatogenesis and other functions of the testes are the

TABLE 6–5 Summary of Male Reproductive Organ Functions

The testes house seminiferous tubules and gonads.

- Seminiferous tubules contain sperm cells in various stages of development and undergoing meiosis.
- Sertoli's cells nourish and protect spermatocytes (phase between spermatids and spermatozoa).
- Leydig's cells are the main source of testosterone.
- Epididymides provide an area for maturation of sperm and a reservoir for mature spermatozoa.
- The vas deferens connects the epididymis with the prostate gland, then connects with ducts from the seminal vesicle to become an ejaculatory duct.
- Ejaculatory ducts provide a passageway for semen and seminal fluid into the urethra.
- Seminal vesicles secrete yellowish fluid rich in fructose, prostaglandins, and fibrinogen. This provides nutrition that increases motility and fertilizing ability of sperm. Prostaglandins also aid fertilization by making the cervical mucus more receptive to sperm.
- The prostate gland secretes thin, alkaline fluid containing calcium, citric acid, and other substances. Alkalinity counteracts acidity of ductus and seminal vesicle secretions.
- Bulbourethral (Cowper's) glands secrete alkaline, viscous fluid into semen, aiding in neutralization of acidic vaginal secretions.

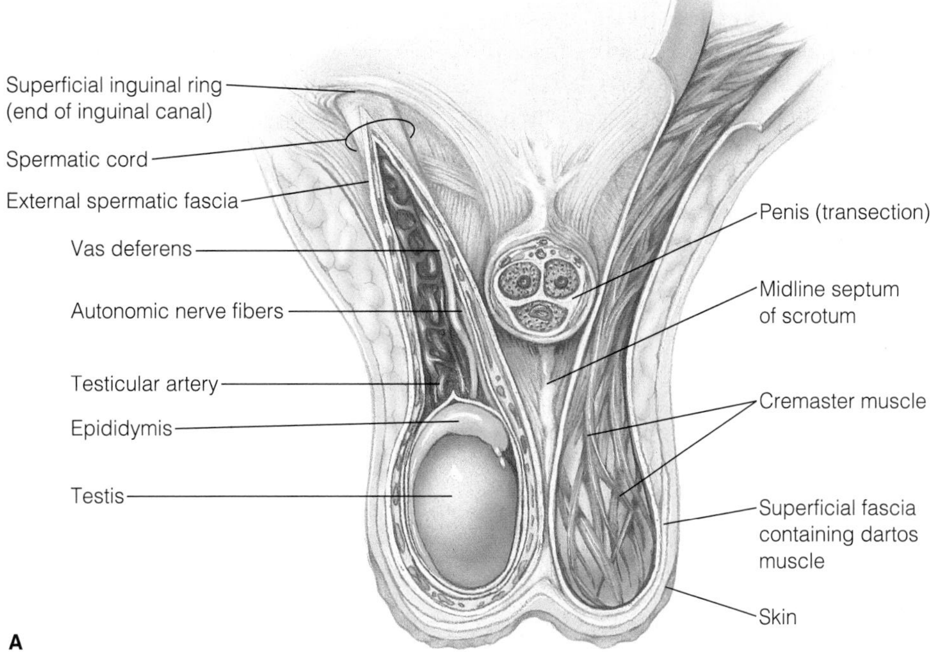

result of complex neural and hormonal controls. The hypothalamus secretes releasing factors, which stimulate the anterior pituitary to release the gonadotropins—FSH and LH. These hormones cause the testes to produce testosterone, which maintains spermatogenesis, increases sperm production by the seminiferous tubules, and stimulates production of seminal fluid.

Testosterone is also responsible for the development of secondary male characteristics and certain behavioral patterns. The effects of testosterone include structural and functional development of the male genital tract, emission and ejaculation of seminal fluid, distribution of body hair, promotion of growth and strength of long bones, increased muscle mass, and enlargement of the vocal cords. The action of testosterone on the central nervous system is thought to produce aggressiveness and sexual drive. The action of testosterone is constant, not cyclic like that of the female hormones. Its production is not limited to a certain number of years, but is thought to decrease with age.

In summary, the primary functions of the testes are to serve as the site of spermatogenesis and to produce testosterone.

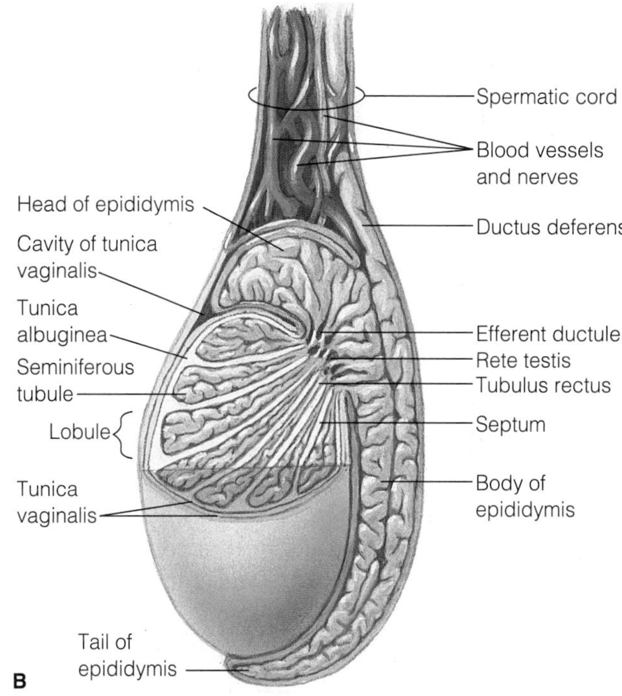

FIGURE 6–24 The testes: ***A,*** External view. ***B,*** Sagittal view showing interior anatomy.

Epididymis

The *epididymis* (plural, *epididymides*) is a duct about 5.6 m long, although it is convoluted into a compact structure about 3.75 cm long. An epididymis lies behind each testis. It arises from the top of the testis, extends downward, and then passes upward, where it becomes the vas deferens.

The epididymis provides a reservoir where spermatozoa can survive for a long period. When discharged from the seminiferous tubules into the epididymis, the sperm are immobile and incapable of fertilizing an ovum. The spermatozoa remain in the epididymis for 2 to 10 days. As the sperm are transported along the tortuous course of the epididymis, they become both motile and fertile.

Vas Deferens and Ejaculatory Ducts

The *vas deferens*, also known as the *ductus deferens*, is about 40 cm long and connects the epididymis with the prostate. One vas deferens arises from the posterior border of each testis. It joins the spermatic cord and weaves over and between several pelvic structures until it meets the vas deferens from the opposite side. Each vas deferens terminus expands to form the *terminal ampulla.* It then unites with the seminal vesicle duct (a gland) to form the ejaculatory duct, which enters the prostate gland and ends in the prostatic urethra. The ejaculatory ducts serve as a passageway for semen and fluid secreted by the seminal vesicles. The main function of the vas deferens is to rapidly squeeze the sperm from their storage sites (the epididymis and distal part of the vas deferens) into the urethra.

Men who choose to take total responsibility for birth control may elect to have a vasectomy. In this procedure, the scrotal portion of the vas deferens is surgically incised or cauterized. Although sperm continues to be produced for the next several years, they can no longer reach the outside of the body. Eventually, the sperm deteriorate and are reabsorbed.

Urethra

The *male urethra* is a passageway for urine and semen. The urethra begins in the bladder and passes through the prostate gland, where it is called the *prostatic urethra.*

The urethra emerges from the prostate gland to become the *membranous urethra.* It terminates in the penis, where it is called the penile urethra. In the penile urethra goblet secretory cells are present, and smooth muscle is replaced by erectile tissue.

Accessory Glands

The male accessory glands are specialized structures under endocrine and neural control. Each secretes a unique and essential component of the total seminal fluid in an ordered sequence.

The *seminal vesicles* are two glands composed of many lobes. Each vesicle is about 7.5 cm long. They are situated between the bladder and rectum and immediately above the base of the prostate. The epithelium lining the seminal vesicles secretes an alkaline, viscous, clear fluid rich in high-energy fructose, prostaglandins, fibrinogen, and amino acids. During ejaculation this fluid mixes with sperm in the ejaculatory ducts. This fluid helps provide an environment favorable to sperm motility and metabolism (Aumüller & Riva, 1992).

The *prostate gland* encircles the upper part of the urethra and lies below the neck of the bladder. Made up of several lobes, it measures about 4 cm in diameter and weighs 20 to 30 g. The prostate is made up of both glandular and muscular tissue. It secretes a thin, milky, alkaline fluid containing high levels of zinc, calcium, citric acid, and acid phosphatase. This fluid protects the sperm from the acidic environment of the vagina and the male urethra, which could be spermicidal.

The *bulbourethral glands (Cowper's glands)* are a pair of small round structures on either side of the membranous urethra. The glands secrete a clear, thick, alkaline fluid rich in mucoproteins that becomes part of the semen. This secretion also lubricates the penile urethra during sexual excitement and neutralizes the acid in the male urethra and the vagina, thereby enhancing sperm mobility.

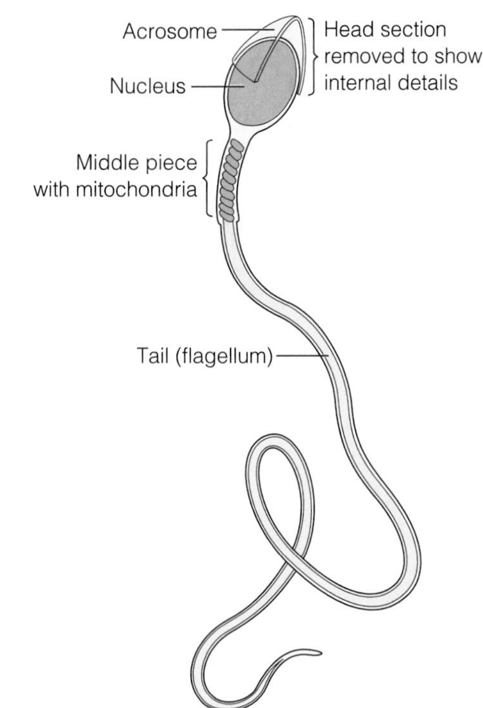

FIGURE 6–25 Schematic illustration of a mature spermatozoon.

The *urethral glands (Littre's glands)* are tiny mucus-secreting glands found throughout the membranous lining of the penile urethra. Their secretions add to those of the bulbourethral glands.

Semen

The male ejaculate, *semen* or *seminal fluid*, is made up of spermatozoa and the secretions of all the accessory glands. The seminal fluid transports viable and motile sperm to the female reproductive tract. Effective transportation of sperm requires adequate nutrients, an adequate pH (about 7.5), a specific concentration of sperm to fluid, and an optimal osmolarity.

A spermatozoon is made up of a head and a tail (Figure 6–25). The head's main components are the *acrosome*, and the *nucleus.* The head carries the male's haploid number of chromosomes (23), and it is the part that enters the ovum at fertilization (Chapter 7). The tail, or *flagellum*, is specialized for motility. The tail is divided into the middle and end piece.

Sperm may be stored in the male genital system up to 42 days, depending primarily on the frequency of ejaculations. The average volume of ejaculate following abstinence for several days is 2 to 5 mL but may vary from 1 to 10 mL. Repeated ejaculation results in decreased volume. Once ejaculated, sperm can live only 2 or 3 days in the female genital tract.

FOCUS YOUR STUDY

- Reproductive activities require complex interactions between the reproductive structures, the central nervous system, and such endocrine glands as the pituitary, hypothalamus, testes, and ovaries.
- At puberty, an alteration in brain sensitivity leads to an increased release of GnRH, which stimulates LH and FSH, leading in the male to an increase in testosterone and in the female to an increase in estrogen and progesterone.
- Estrogen is the principal cause of the events of puberty in females (maturation of ova, enlargement of the uterus and fallopian tubes, deposition of fat in the breasts and hips, and characteristic hair growth).
- Puberty changes for the male (onset of spermatogenesis; enlargement of the penis, scrotum, and testes; voice changes; and characteristic hair growth) occur as a result of increased testosterone production by the testes.
- The female reproductive system consists of the ovaries, where female germ cells and female sex hormones are formed; the fallopian tubes, which capture the ovum and allow transport to the uterus; the uterus, which is the implantation site for the fertilized ovum (blastocyst); the cervix, which is a protective portal for the body of the uterus and the connection between the vagina and the uterus; and the vagina, which is the passageway from the external genitals to the uterus and provides for discharge of menstrual products to the outside of the body.
- The female reproductive cycle may be described in terms of the ovarian cycle, during which ovulation occurs, and the menstrual cycle, during which menstruation occurs. These two cycles take place simultaneously and are under neurohormonal control. The ovarian cycle has two phases: the follicular phase and the luteal phase. During the follicular phase, the primordial follicle matures under the influence of FSH and LH until ovulation occurs. The luteal phase begins when the ovum leaves the follicle and the corpus luteum develops under the influence of LH. The corpus luteum produces high levels of progesterone and low levels of estrogen.
- The menstrual cycle has four phases: menstrual, proliferative, secretory, and ischemic. Menstruation is the actual shedding of the endometrial lining, when estrogen levels are low. The proliferative phase begins when the endometrial glands begin to enlarge under the influence of estrogen and cervical mucosal changes occur; the changes peak at ovulation. The secretory phase follows ovulation, and, influenced primarily by progesterone, the uterus increases its vascularity to make ready for possible implantation. The ischemic phase is characterized by degeneration of the corpus luteum, decreases in both estrogen and progesterone levels, constriction of the spiral arteries, and escape of blood into the stromal cells of the endometrium.
- The male reproductive system consists of the testes, where male germ cells and male sex hormones are formed; a series of continuous ducts through which spermatozoa are transported outside the body; accessory glands that produce secretions important to sperm nutrition, survival, and transport; and the penis, which serves as the reproductive organ of intercourse.

REFERENCES

Aumüller, G., & Riva, A. (1992). Morphology and functions of the human seminal vesicle. *Andrologia, 24*(4), 183–196.

Berenson, A. B. (1995). A longitudinal study of hymenal morphology in the first years of life. *Pediatrics, 95*(4), 490–496.

Caldwell, W. E., & Moloy, H. C. (1933). Anatomical variations in the female pelvis and their effect on labor with a suggested classification [Historical article]. *American Journal of Obstetrics and Gynecology, 26*, 479–505.

Cunningham, F. G., MacDonald, P. C., Gant, N. F., Leveno, K. J., Gilstrap, L. C., Hankins, G. D. V., & Clark, S. L. (1997). *Williams obstetrics* (20th ed.). Stamford, CT: Appleton & Lange.

Ferin, M. (1998). The hypothalamic-hypophyseal-ovarian axis and the menstrual cycle. In J. J. Sciarri & T. J. Watkins (Eds.), *Gynecology and obstetrics* (Vol. 5, Chap. 6, pp 1–15). Hagerstown, MD: Harper and Row.

Malasanos, T. H. (1997). Sexual development of the fetus and pubertal child. *Clinical Obstetrics and Gynecology, 40*(1), 153–167.

Rebar, R. W. (1999). The breast and the physiology of lactation. In R. K. Creasy & R. Resnik (Eds.), *Maternal-fetal medicine: Principles and practice* (4th ed., pp 106–121). Philadelphia: Saunders.

Sanfilippo, J. S., & Jamieson, M. J. (1997). Physiology of puberty. In J. J. Sciarri & T. J. Watkins (Eds.), *Gynecology and obstetrics* (Vol. 5, Chap. 9, pp 1–20). Hagerstown, MD: Harper and Row.

Speroff, L., Glass, R. H., & Kase, N. G. (1994). *Clinical gynecologic endrocrinology and infertility* (5th ed.). Baltimore: Williams & Wilkins.

Weiss, G., & Goldsmith, L. T. (1994). Puberty and pediatric and adolescent gynecology. In J. R. Scott, P. J. DiSaia, C. B. Hammond, & W. N. Spellacy (Eds.), *Danforth's obstetrics and gynecology* (7th ed., pp 611–620). Philadelphia: Lippincott.

7 Conception and Fetal Development

My friends tease me when I say this, but I know the moment my daughter was conceived. My husband and I had both been so busy at work, but we finally went away for a long weekend together. It was wonderful—we got back some of the magic as we took long walks and talked and talked. Until that weekend, whenever we discussed having children it was always "maybe someday." On the second night we decided to skip the diaphragm for the first time ever. Our lovemaking seemed so special that evening, a true reflection of the emotional closeness we had recaptured. I never went back to using the diaphragm after that weekend, but I am convinced that Jennifer is the result of that night together!

Objectives

- Explain the differences between mitotic cellular division and meiotic cellular division.
- Compare the processes by which ova and sperm are produced.
- Describe the process of fertilization.
- Identify the differing processes by which fraternal (dizygotic) and identical (monozygotic) twins are formed.
- Describe in order of increasing complexity the structures that form during the cellular multiplication and differentiation stages of intrauterine development.
- Describe the development, structure, and functions of the placenta and umbilical cord during intrauterine life.
- Summarize the significant changes in growth and development of the fetus in utero at 4, 6, 12, 16, 20, 24, 28, 32, 36, and 40 weeks' gestation.
- Identify the vulnerable periods during which malformations of the various organ systems may occur, and describe the resulting congenital malformations.

Key Terms

Acrosomal reaction
Amnion
Amniotic fluid
Bag of waters (BOW)
Blastocyst
Capacitation
Chorion
Chromosomes
Cleavage
Cotyledon
Decidua basalis
Decidua capsularis
Decidua vera (parietalis)
Diploid number of chromosomes
Ductus arteriosus
Ductus venosus
Ectoderm
Embryo
Embryonic membranes
Endoderm
Fertilization
Fetus
Foramen ovale
Gametes
Gametogenesis
Haploid number of chromosomes
Lanugo
Meiosis
Mesoderm
Mitosis
Morula
Placenta
Postconception age periods
Teratogen
Trophoblast
Umbilical cord
Vernix caseosa
Wharton's jelly
Zygote

EACH PERSON IS UNIQUE. NONETHELESS, everyone has many if not all of the same "parts," which usually function similarly. Even chromosomes, those determinants of the structure and function of organ systems and traits, are made of the same biochemical substances. How does each person become unique, then? The answer lies in the physiologic mechanisms of heredity, the processes of cellular division, and the environmental factors that influence development from the moment a person is conceived. This chapter explores the processes involved in conception and fetal development—the basis of human uniqueness.

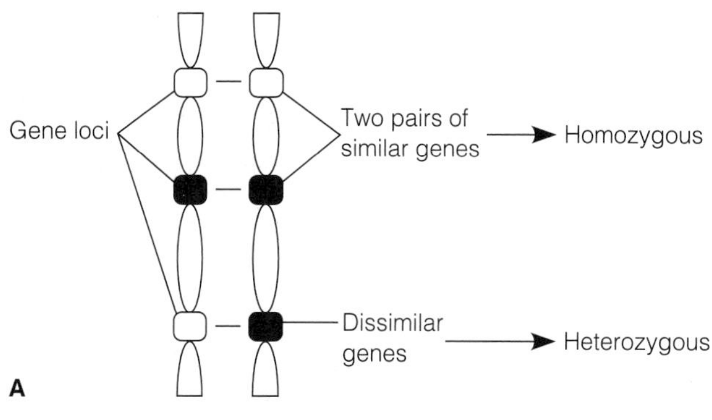

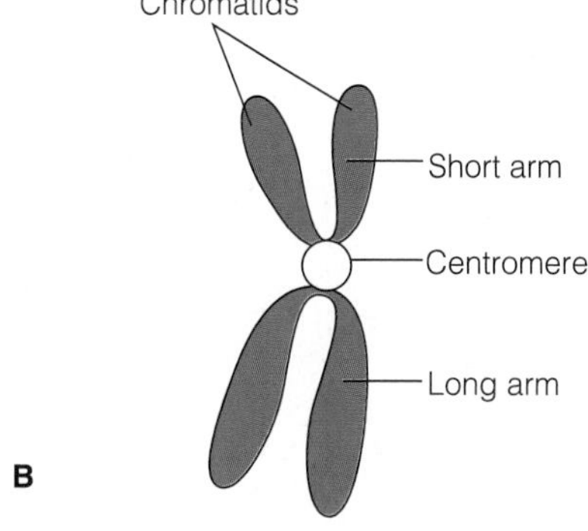

FIGURE 7–1 ***A,*** One pair of homologous chromosomes with similar (homozygous) genes and dissimilar (heterozygous) genes. ***B,*** Classification of chromosomal joining.

Chromosomes

The body (somatic) cells of each individual contain within their nuclei threadlike bodies known as **chromosomes,** which are composed of strands of *deoxyribonucleic acid (DNA)* and protein. Genes are regions in the DNA strands that contain coded information used to determine the unique characteristics of the individual; they are arranged in linear order on the chromosomes.

Each chromosome contains two longitudinal halves called *chromatids,* which are joined together at a point called the centromere. Each member of a chromosome pair carries either similar genes referred to as *homologous* (homozygous) or dissimilar genes referred to as *heterozygous* (Figure 7–1, *A*).

The chromosomes are classified according to their length and to the position of their centromere. When the centromere is centrally located, the longitudinal halves are divided into one short arm region and one long arm region, and the chromosome resembles an X (Figure 7–1, *B*).

Cellular Division

Every human begins life as a single cell (fertilized ovum or zygote). This single cell reproduces itself, and in turn each new cell also reproduces itself in a continuing process. The new cells are similar to the cells from which they came.

Cells are reproduced by either mitosis or meiosis, two different but related processes. **Mitosis** results in the production of diploid body (somatic) cells, which are exact copies of the original cell. Mitosis makes growth and development possible, and in mature individuals it is the process by which our body cells continue to divide and replace themselves. **Meiosis** is the cell division process leading to the development of eggs and sperm needed to produce a new organism.

Mitosis

During mitosis, the cell undergoes several changes, ending in cell division. Although mitosis is a continuous process, it is generally divided into five stages: interphase, prophase, metaphase, anaphase, and telophase (see Figure 7–2).

During interphase, before cell division takes place, the DNA within the chromosomes replicates so that the genes will be doubled. Mitosis begins when the cell enters prophase. The chromosomes condense and form the shape we usually recognize as a chromosome. Next comes the appearance of a mitotic apparatus known as a spindle, in which fine threads extend from the top and bottom poles of the nucleus. At each pole of the spindle, a body known as the centriole is formed, so the threads of the spindle extend from one centriole to the other. Next the nuclear membrane, which separates the nucleus from the cytoplasm, disappears, the nucleus as a separate entity disappears, and the cell enters metaphase.

During metaphase, the chromosomes line up at the equator (midway between the poles) of the spindle. Metaphase is followed by anaphase, in which the two chromatids of each chromosome separate and move to opposite ends of the spindle, where they cluster in masses near the two poles of the cell.

Telophase is essentially the opposite of prophase. A new nuclear membrane forms, separating each newly formed nucleus from the cytoplasm. The spindle disappears, and the centrioles relocate outside of each new nucleus. Within the nucleus the chromosomes lengthen and become threadlike. As telophase nears completion, a furrow develops in the cell cytoplasm and divides it into two

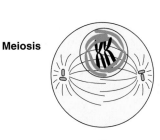

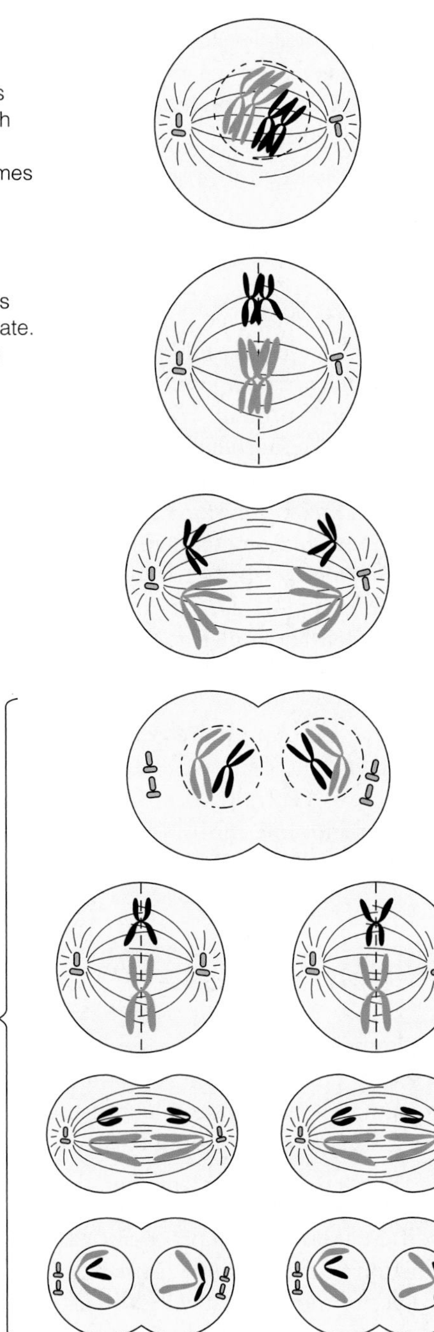

Mitosis
Meiosis
DNA replicates during interphase.
Mitosis or meiosis begins.
Prophase
Each chromosome now has two chromatids. In mitosis, homologous chromosomes do not attach to each other and thus act independently.
In meiosis, homologous chromosomes attach to each other.
Metaphase
In mitosis, each chromosome aligns independently at the metaphase plate.
In the first division of meiosis, each pair of chromosomes aligns at the metaphase plate.
Anaphase
In mitosis, chromatids separate. In meiosis I, chromosomes (not chromatids) separate.
Telophase
Result of mitosis: two identical cells, each with the same number of chromosomes as the original cell
In the second division of meiosis, sister chromatids separate.
Result of meiosis: four haploid cells, each with half as many chromosomes as the original cell

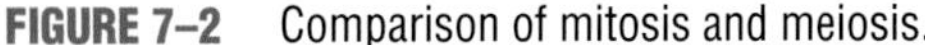

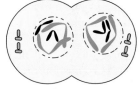

FIGURE 7–2 Comparison of mitosis and meiosis.

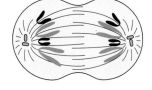

daughter cells, each with its own nucleus. Daughter cells have the same **diploid number of chromosomes** (46) and the same genetic makeup as the cell from which they came. At the end of mitosis, a cell with 46 chromosomes results in two identical cells, each with 46 chromosomes.

Meiosis

Meiosis is a special type of cell division by which diploid cells give rise to haploid gametes (sperm and ova). Meiosis consists of two successive cell divisions (Figure 7–2). In the first division, the chromosomes replicate. Next a pairing takes place between homologous chromosomes (Sadler, 1995). Instead of separating immediately as in mitosis, the similar chromosomes become closely intertwined. At each point of contact, there is a physical exchange of genetic material between the chromatids (arms of the chromosomes). New combinations are provided by the newly formed chromosomes; these combinations account for the wide variation of traits, such as hair or eye color, in people. The chromosome pairs then separate, each member of a pair moving to opposite sides of the cell. (In contrast, during mitosis the chromatids of each chromosome separate and move to opposite poles.) The cell divides, forming two daughter cells, each with 23 double-structured chromosomes—the same amount of DNA as a normal somatic cell. In the second division, the chromatids of each chromosome separate and move to opposite poles of each of the daughter cells. Cell division occurs, resulting in the formation of four cells, each containing 23 single chromosomes, **the haploid number of chromosomes.** These daughter cells contain only half the DNA of a normal somatic cell (Moore & Persaud, 1998).

Mutations may occur during the second meiotic division if two of the chromatids do not move apart rapidly enough when the cell divides. The still-paired chromatids are carried into one of the daughter cells and eventually form an extra chromosome. This condition is referred to as an *autosomal nondisjunction* (chromosomal mutation) and is harmful to the offspring that may result should fertilization occur. The implications of nondisjunction are discussed in Chapter 8.

Another type of chromosomal mutation can occur if chromosomes break during meiosis. If the broken segment is lost, the result is a shorter chromosome; this is known as a deletion. If the broken segment becomes attached to another chromosome, a harmful mutation called a translocation is the result. The effects of translocation are described in Chapter 8.

Gametogenesis

Meiosis occurs during **gametogenesis,** the process by which germ cells, or **gametes,** are produced. The gametes must have a haploid number of chromosomes (23) so that when the female gamete (the egg, or ovum) and the male gamete (sperm, or spermatozoon) unite to form the **zygote,** the normal human diploid number of chromosomes (46) is reestablished.

Oogenesis

Oogenesis is the process by which female gametes or ova are produced. As discussed in Chapter 6, the ovaries begin to develop early in the fetal life of the female. All the ova that the female will produce in her lifetime are present at birth. The ovary gives rise to oogonial cells, which develop into *oocytes.* Meiosis begins in all oocytes before the female infant is born but stops before the first division is complete and remains in this arrested phase until puberty. During puberty the mature primary oocyte continues through the first meiotic division in the graafian follicle of the ovary.

The first meiotic division produces two cells of unequal size with unequal amounts of cytoplasm, but the same number of chromosomes. These two cells are the *secondary oocyte* and a minute *polar body.* Both the secondary oocyte and the first polar body contain 22 double-structured autosomal chromosomes and one double-structured sex chromosome (X). At the time of ovulation, the second meiotic division begins immediately and proceeds as the oocyte moves down the fallopian tube. Again, division is not equal. The secondary oocyte proceeds to metaphase, where its meiotic division is arrested.

When the secondary oocyte completes the second meiotic division after fertilization, the result is a mature ovum with the haploid number of chromosomes and virtually all the cytoplasm. In addition, the second polar body (also haploid) forms at this time (Figure 7–3). The first polar body has now also divided, producing two additional polar bodies. Thus when meiosis is completed, four haploid cells have been produced: three small polar bodies, which eventually disintegrate, and one ovum (Sadler, 1995) (Figure 7–4).

Spermatogenesis

During puberty, the germinal epithelium in the seminiferous tubules of the testes begins the process of spermatogenesis, which produces the male gametes (sperm). As the (diploid number) spermatogonium enters the first meiotic division, it is called the *primary spermatocyte.* During this first meiotic division, the spermatogonium replicates and forms two haploid cells termed *secondary spermatocytes,* each of which contains 22 double-structured autosomal chromosomes and either a double-structured X sex chromosome or a double-structured Y sex chromosome. During the second meiotic division they divide to form four spermatids, each with the haploid number of chromosomes (Figure 7–3). The spermatids undergo a series of changes during which they lose most of their cytoplasm and become sperm (spermatozoa). The nucleus becomes compacted into the head of the sperm, which is covered by a cap called an acrosome. A long tail is produced from one of the centrioles.

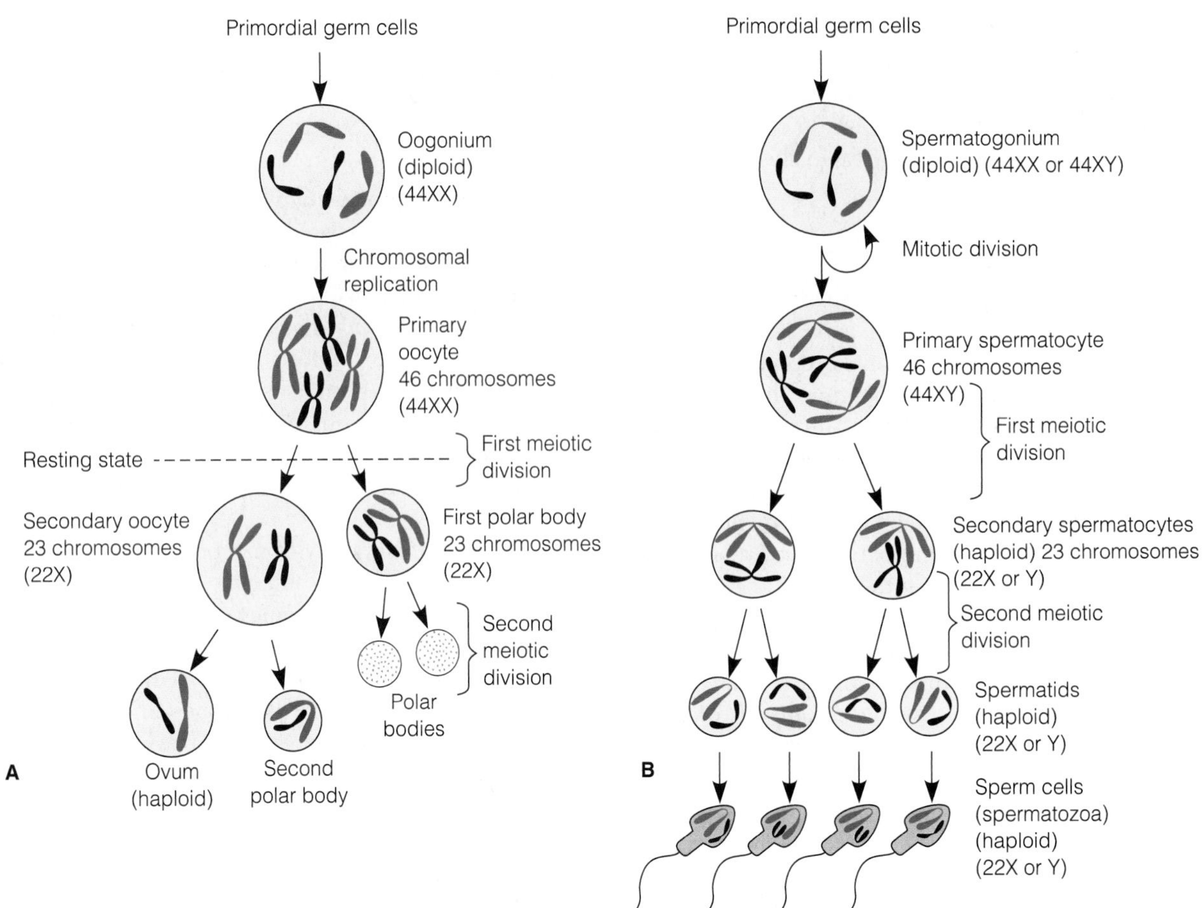

FIGURE 7–3 Gametogenesis involves meiosis within the ovary and testis. ***A,*** During meiosis, each oogonium produces a single haploid ovum once some cytoplasm moves into the polar bodies. ***B,*** Each spermatogonium, in contrast, produces four haploid spermatozoa.

The Process of Fertilization

Fertilization is the process by which a sperm fuses with an ovum to form a new diploid cell, or zygote. Following are the events that lead to fertilization.

Preparation for Fertilization

The process of fertilization usually takes place in the ampulla (outer third) of the fallopian tube. During ovulation, high estrogen levels increase peristalsis within the fallopian tubes, which helps move the ovum through the tube toward the uterus. The ovum has no inherent power of movement. The high estrogen levels also cause a thinning of the cervical mucus, facilitating movement of the sperm through the cervix, into the uterus, and up the fallopian tube.

The ovum's cell membrane is surrounded by two layers of tissue. The layer closest to the cell membrane is called the *zona pellucida*. It is a clear, noncellular layer whose thickness influences the fertilization rate (Bertrand, Van den Bergh, & Englert, 1996). Surrounding the zona pellucida is a ring of elongated cells, called the *corona radiata* because they radiate from the ovum like the gaseous corona around the sun. These cells are held together by hyaluronic acid.

The mature ovum and spermatozoa have only a brief time to unite. Ova are considered fertile for about 24 hours after ovulation. Sperm can survive in the female reproductive tract for 48 to 72 hours but are believed to be healthy and highly fertile for only about the first 24 hours (Moore & Persaud, 1998).

In a single ejaculation, the male deposits approximately 200 to 400 million spermatozoa in the vagina, of which fewer than 200 actually reach the ampulla (Moore & Persaud, 1998). Fructose in the semen, secreted by the seminal vesicles, is the energy source for the sperm. The spermatozoa propel themselves up the female tract by the flagellar movement of their tails. Transit time from the cervix into the fallopian tube can be as short as 5 minutes but usually takes an average of 4 to 6 hours after ejaculation (Cunningham et al, 1997). Prostaglandins in the semen may increase uterine smooth muscle contractions, which help transport the sperm. The fallopian tubes have

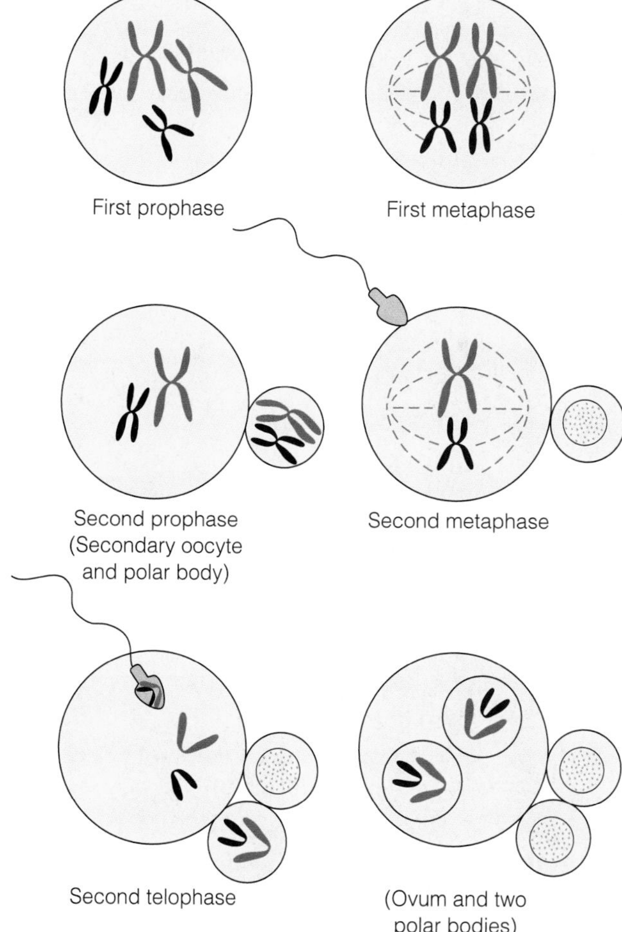

FIGURE 7–4 Human oogenesis and fertilization.

a dual ciliary action that facilitates movement of the ovum toward the uterus and movement of the sperm from the uterus toward the ovary.

The sperm's nucleus, which contains its genetic material, is compacted into the head of the sperm and covered by a protective cap called an acrosome, which is in turn covered by a plasma membrane.

The sperm must undergo two processes before fertilization can occur: capacitation and the acrosomal reaction. **Capacitation** is the removal of the plasma membrane overlying the spermatozoa's acrosomal area and the loss of seminal plasma proteins and the glycoprotein coat. If the glycoprotein coat is not removed, the sperm will not be able to fertilize the ovum (Bar-Ami & Seibel, 1997). Capacitation occurs in the female reproductive tract (aided by uterine enzymes) and is thought to take about 7 hours. Sperm that undergo capacitation take on three characteristics: (1) the ability to undergo the acrosomal reaction, (2) the ability to bind to the zona pellucida, and (3) the acquisition of hypermotility.

The acrosomal reaction follows capacitation. The acrosomes of the millions of sperm surrounding the ovum release their enzymes (hyaluronidase, a protease called acrosin, and corona-dispersing enzymes) and thus break down the hyaluronic acid in the ovum's corona radiata, the outer layer of the ovum (Millette, 1997). This activity is the **acrosomal reaction.** Hundreds of acrosomes must rupture before enough hyaluronic acid in the corona radiata is cleared for a single sperm to penetrate the zona pellucida of the ovum successfully.

At the moment of penetration by a fertilizing sperm, the zona pellucida undergoes a reaction that prevents additional sperm from entering a single ovum. This is known as the block to polyspermy. This cellular change is mediated by release of materials from the cortical granules, organelles found just below the ovum's surface, and is called the *cortical reaction* (Millette, 1997) (Figure 7–5).

The Moment of Fertilization

After the sperm enters the ovum, a chemical signal prompts the secondary oocyte to complete the second meiotic division, forming the nucleus of the ovum and ejecting the second polar body. Then the nuclei of the ovum and sperm swell and approach each other. The true moment of fertilization occurs as the nuclei unite. Their individual nuclear membranes disappear, and their chromosomes pair up to produce the diploid zygote. Since each nucleus contains a haploid number of chromosomes (23), this union restores the diploid number (46). The zygote contains a new combination of genetic material that results in an individual different from either parent and from anyone else.

It is also at the moment of fertilization that the sex of the zygote is determined. The two chromosomes (the sex chromosomes) of the 23rd pair—either XX or XY—determine the sex of an individual. X chromosomes are larger and bear more genes than Y chromosomes. Females have two X chromosomes, and males have an X and a Y chromosome. Whereas the mature ovum produced by oogenesis can have only one type of sex chromosome—an X—spermatogenesis produces two sperm with an X chromosome and two sperm with a Y chromosome. When each gamete contributes an X chromosome, the resulting zygote is female. When the ovum contributes an X chromosome and the sperm contributes a Y, the resulting zygote is male. As discussed in Chapter 8, certain traits are termed sex-linked because they are controlled by the genes on the X sex chromosome. Two examples of sex-linked traits are color blindness and hemophilia.

CRITICAL THINKING QUESTION

How can knowledge of the normal fertilization process assist in helping couples conceive?

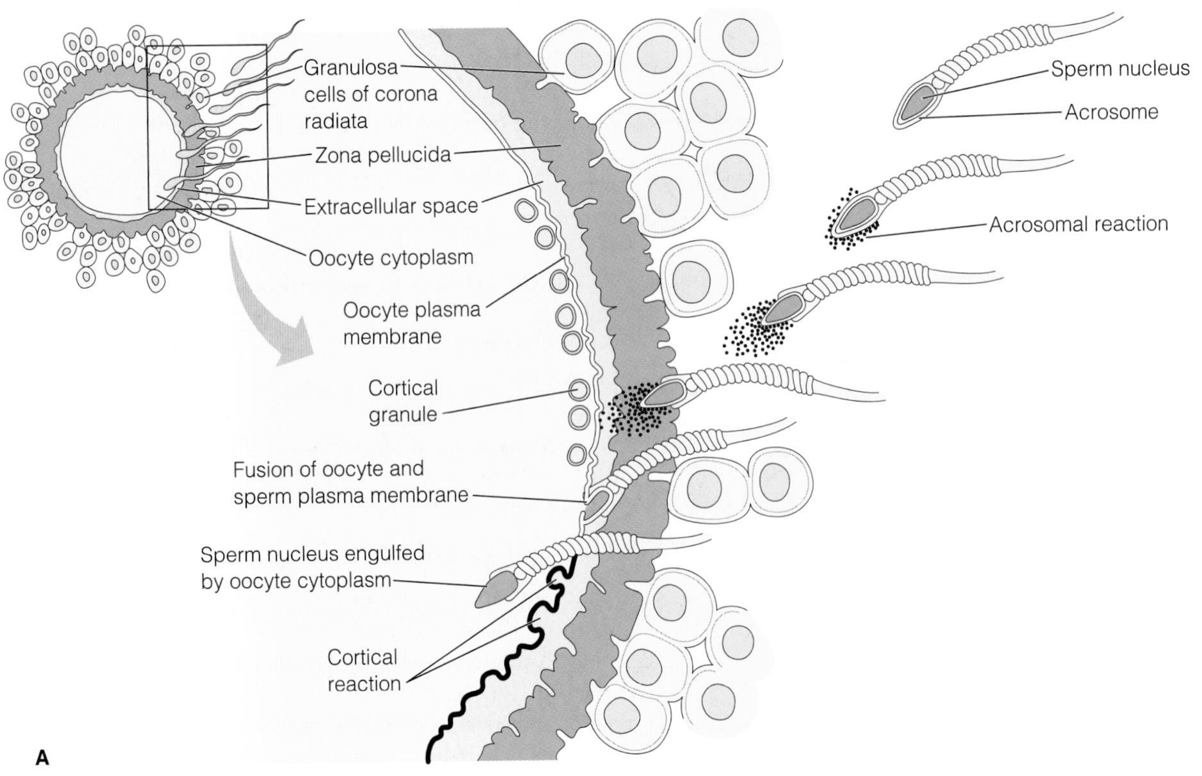

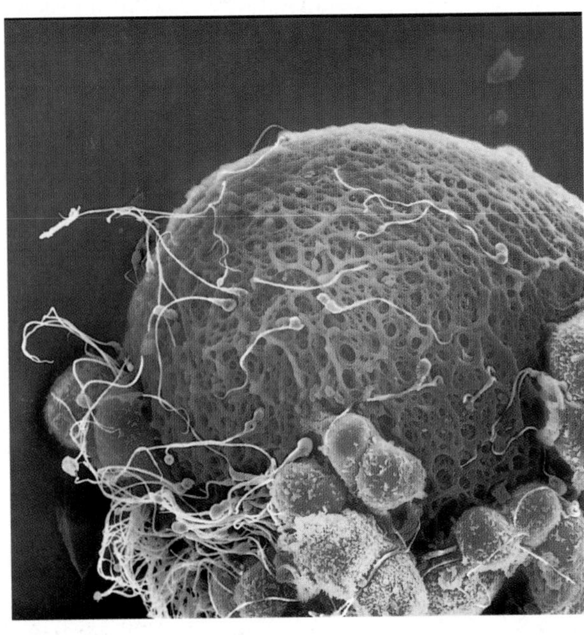

FIGURE 7–5 Sperm penetration of an ovum. ***A,*** The sequential steps of oocyte penetration by a sperm are depicted moving from top to bottom. ***B,*** Scanning electron micrograph of human sperm surrounding a human oocyte (750×). The smaller spherical cells are granulosa cells of the corona radiata. SOURCE: Scanning electron micrograph from Nilsson L: *A Child Is Born.* New York: Dell Publishing, 1990.

Twins

Twinning normally occurs in approximately 1 in 80 pregnancies, and triplets in 1 in 8000 pregnancies (Kochenour, 1997). Twins have been reported to occur more often among black than among white women and more often among white individuals than among women of Asian origin (Benirschke, 1995). Among all groups, as parity (having given birth to a viable infant) increases so does the chance for multiple births.

Twins may be either fraternal or identical (Figure 7–6). If they are fraternal, they are *dizygotic,* which means they arise from two separate ova fertilized by two separate spermatozoa. There are two placentas, two chorions, and two amnions; however, the placentas sometimes fuse and look as if they are one. Despite their birth relationship, fraternal twins are no more similar to each other than they would be to siblings born singly. They may be the same or different sex.

Dizygotic twinning increases with maternal age up to about 35 years of age and then decreases abruptly. The chance of dizygotic twins increases with parity, in conceptions that occur in the first 3 months of a relationship, and with increased coital frequency. The chance of dizygotic twinning decreases during periods of malnutrition and during winter and spring for women living in the northern hemisphere. Studies indicate that dizygotic twins tend to occur in certain families, perhaps because of genetic factors that result in elevated serum gonadotropin levels leading to double ovulation (Benirschke, 1995).

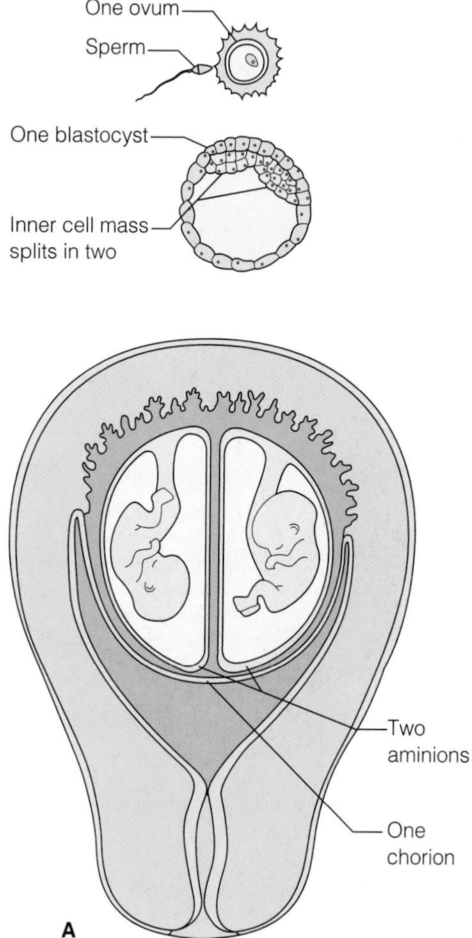

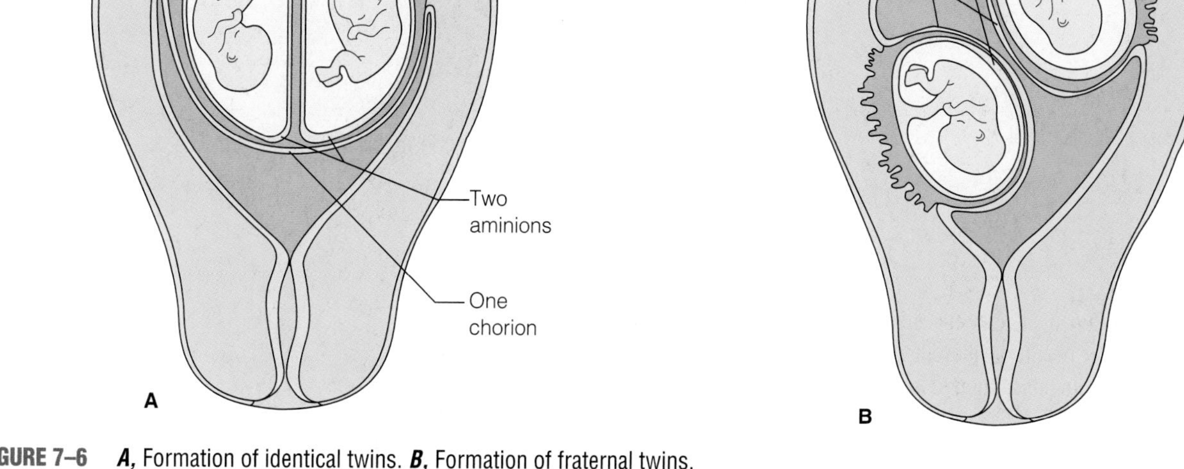

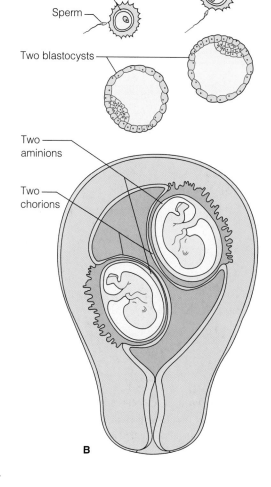

FIGURE 7–6 ***A,*** Formation of identical twins. ***B,*** Formation of fraternal twins.

Identical, or monozygotic, twins develop from a single fertilized ovum. They are of the same sex and have the same genotype (appearance). Identical twins usually have a common placenta (Figure 7–6). Monozygosity is not affected by environment, race, physical characteristics, or fertility. Monozygotic twins originate from division of the fertilized ovum at different stages of early development, after the zygote consists of thousands of cells.

Complete separation of the cellular mass into two parts is necessary for twin formation. The number of amnions and chorions present depends on the timing of the division.

- If division occurs within 3 days of fertilization (before the inner cell mass and chorion are formed), two embryos, two amnions, and two chorions will develop. This dichorionic-diamniotic situation occurs about 20% to 30% of the time, and there may be two distinct placentas or a single fused placenta.
- If division occurs about 5 days after fertilization (when the inner cell mass is formed and the chorion cells have differentiated but those of the amnion have not), two embryos develop with separate amnionic sacs. These sacs will eventually be covered by a common chorion, thus there will be a monochorionic-diamniotic placenta.
- If the amnion has already developed approximately 7 to 13 days after fertilization, division results in two embryos with a common amnionic sac and a common chorion. This type occurs about 1% of the time (Revenis & Johnson, 1994).

Monozygotic twinning is considered a random event and occurs in approximately 3.5 per 1000 live births (Kochenour, 1997). The survival rate of monozygotic twins as a group is 10% lower than that of dizygotic twins, and congenital anomalies are more prevalent. Both twins may have the same malformation.

Intrauterine Development

Development after fertilization can be divided into two phases: cellular multiplication and cellular (embryonic membrane) differentiation. These phases and the process of implantation (nidation), which occurs between them, are discussed next.

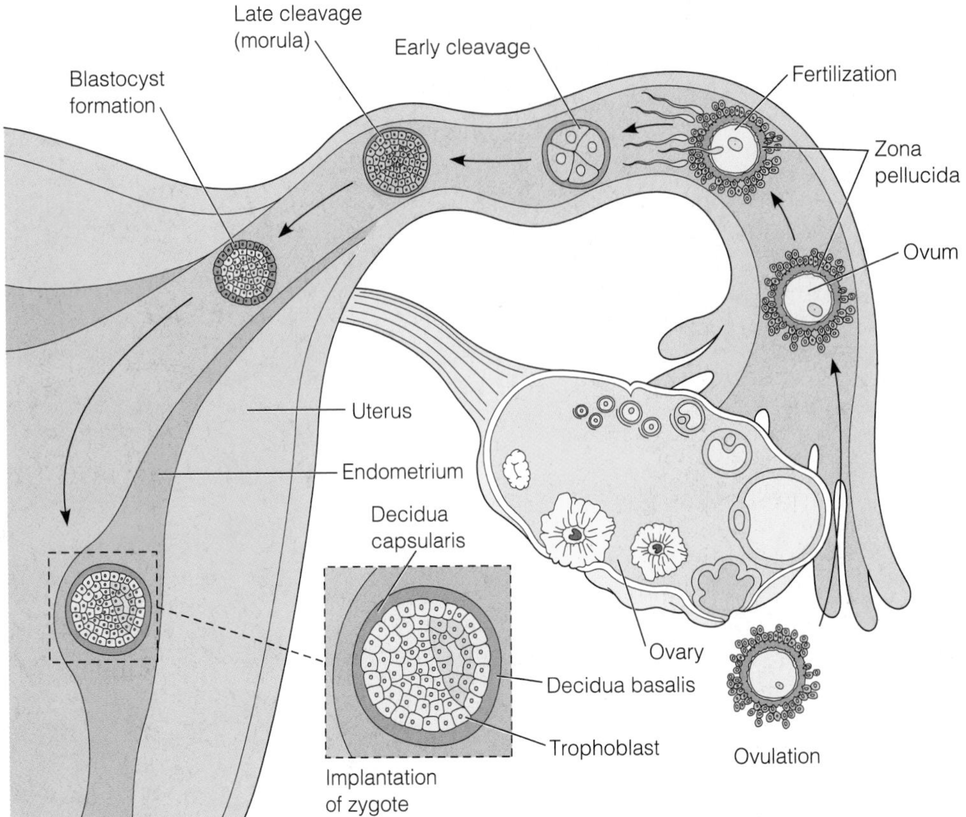

FIGURE 7–7 During ovulation, the ovum leaves the ovary and enters the fallopian tube. Fertilization generally occurs in the outer third of the fallopian tube. Subsequent changes in the fertilized ovum from conception to implantation are depicted.

Cellular Multiplication

Cellular multiplication begins as the zygote moves through the fallopian tube toward the cavity of the uterus. This transportation takes 3 days or more (Cunningham et al, 1997) and is accomplished mainly by a very weak fluid current in the fallopian tube resulting from the beating action of the ciliated epithelium that lines the tube.

The zygote now enters a period of rapid mitotic divisions called **cleavage,** during which it divides into two cells, four cells, eight cells, and so on. These cells, called *blastomeres,* are so small that the developing cell mass is only slightly larger than the original zygote. The blastomeres are held together by the zona pellucida, which is under the corona radiata. The blastomeres will eventually form a solid ball of 12 to 16 cells called the **morula.** As it enters the uterus, the intracellular fluid in the morula increases, and a central cavity forms within the cell mass.

The inner solid mass of cells is called the **blastocyst.** The outer layer of cells that surround the cavity and have replaced the zona pellucida is the **trophoblast.** Eventually, the trophoblast develops into one of the embryonic membranes, called the chorion. The blastocyst develops into a double layer of cells called the embryonic disc, from which the embryo will develop, and the other embryonic membrane, called the amnion. The journey of the fertilized ovum to its destination in the uterus is illustrated in Figure 7–7.

Implantation (Nidation)

While floating in the uterine cavity, the blastocyst is nourished by the uterine glands, which secrete a mixture of lipids, mucopolysaccharides, and glycogen. The trophoblast attaches itself to the surface of the endometrium for further nourishment. The most frequent site of attachment is the upper part of the posterior uterine wall (Figure 7–7). Between days 7 and 9 after fertilization, the zona pellucida disappears, and the blastocyst implants itself by burrowing into the uterine lining and penetrating down toward the maternal capillaries until it is completely covered (Jirasek, 1998). The lining of the uterus thickens below the implanted blastocyst, and the cells of the trophoblast grow down into the thickened lining, forming processes called *villi.*

Under the influence of progesterone, the endometrium increases in thickness and vascularity in preparation for implantation and nourishment of the ovum. After implantation, the endometrium is called the *decidua.* The portion of the decidua that covers the blas-

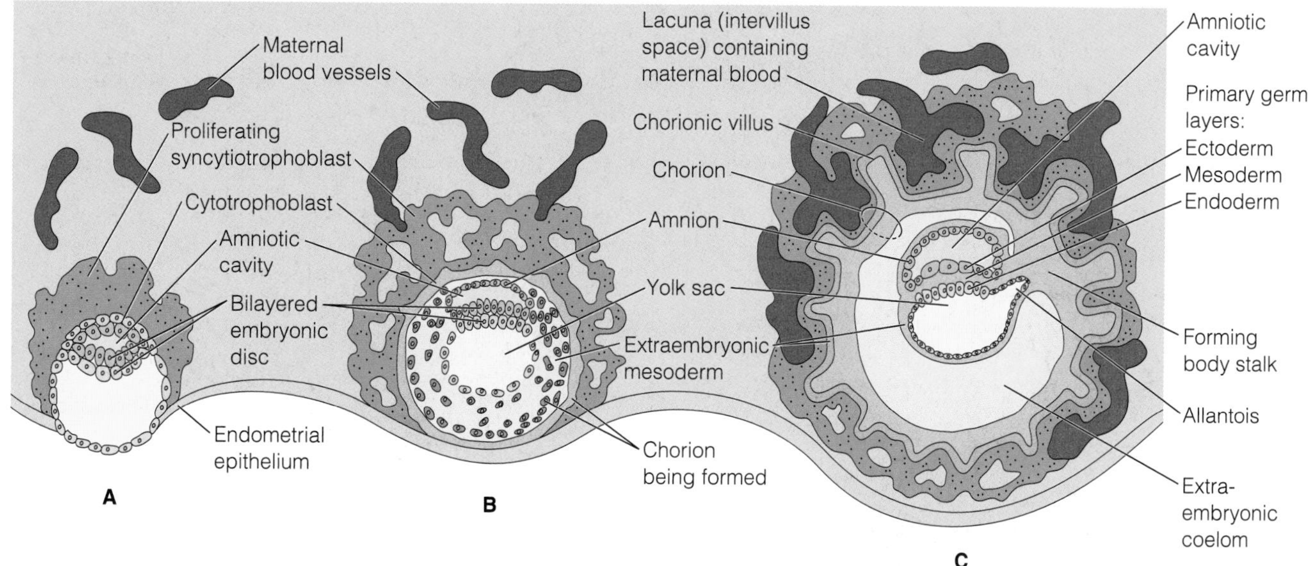

FIGURE 7–8 Formation of primary germ layers. ***A,*** Implantation of a 7½-day blastocyst in which the cells of the embryonic disc are separated from the amnion by a fluid-filled space. The erosion of the endometrium by the syncytiotrophoblast is ongoing. ***B,*** Implantation is completed by day 9, and extraembryonic mesoderm is beginning to form a discrete layer beneath the cytotrophoblast. ***C,*** By day 16, the embryo shows all three germ layers, a yolk sac, and an allantois (an outpouching of the yolk sac that forms the structural basis of the body stalk, or umbilical cord). The cytotrophoblast and associated mesoderm has become the chorion, and chorionic villi are developing. SOURCE: Adapted from Marieb EN: *Human Anatomy and Physiology,* 4th ed. Redwood City, CA: Benjamin/Cummings, 1998, p 1088.

tocyst is called the **decidua capsularis;** the portion directly under the implanted blastocyst is the **decidua basalis;** and the portion that lines the rest of the uterine cavity is the **decidua vera (parietalis)** (Figure 7–7, inset). The maternal part of the placenta develops from the decidua basalis, which contains large numbers of blood vessels. The chorionic villi (described later) in contact with the decidua basalis will form the fetal portion of the placenta.

Cellular Differentiation

Primary Germ Layers

About day 10 to 14 after conception, the homogenous mass of blastocyst cells differentiates into the primary germ layers. These layers, the **ectoderm, mesoderm,** and **endoderm** (Figure 7–8), are formed at the same time as the embryonic membranes. All tissues, organs, and organ systems will develop from these primary germ cell layers (Table 7–1 and Figure 7–9).

TABLE 7–1 Derivation of Body Structures from Primary Cell Layers

Ectoderm	Mesoderm	Endoderm
Epidermis	Dermis	Respiratory tract epithelium
Sweat glands	Wall of digestive tract	Epithelium (except nasal), including pharynx, tongue, tonsils, thyroid, parathyroid, thymus, tympanic cavity
Sebaceous glands	Kidneys and ureter (suprarenal cortex)	Lining of digestive tract
Nails	Reproductive organs (gonads, genital ducts)	Primary tissue of liver and pancreas
Hair follicles	Connective tissue (cartilage, bone, joint cavities)	Urethra and associated glands
Lens of eye	Skeleton	Urinary bladder (except trigone)
Sensory epithelium of internal and external ear, nasal cavity, sinuses, mouth, anal canal	Muscles (all types)	Vagina (parts)
Central and peripheral nervous systems	Cardiovascular system (heart, arteries, veins, blood, bone marrow)	
Nasal cavity	Pleura	
Oral glands and tooth enamel	Lymphatic tissue and cells	
Pituitary gland	Spleen	
Mammary glands		

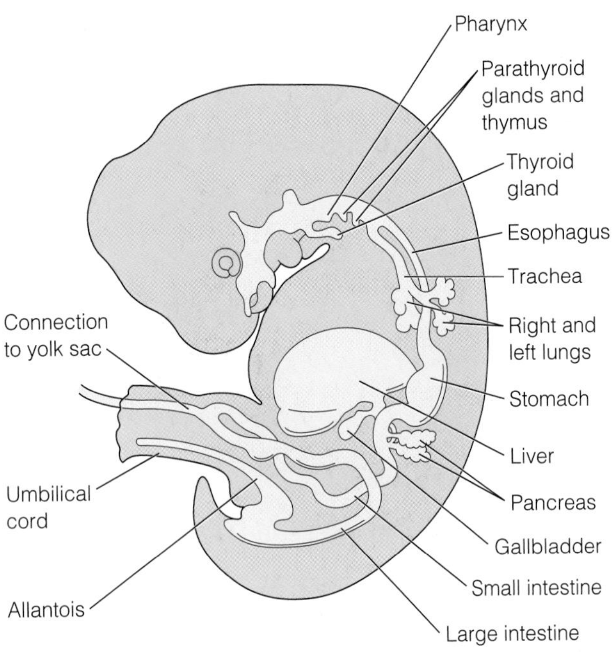

FIGURE 7–9 Endoderm differentiates to form the epithelial lining of the digestive and respiratory tracts and associated glands. SOURCE: Adapted from Marieb EN: *Human Anatomy and Physiology,* 4th ed. Redwood City, CA: Benjamin/Cummings, 1998, p 1092.

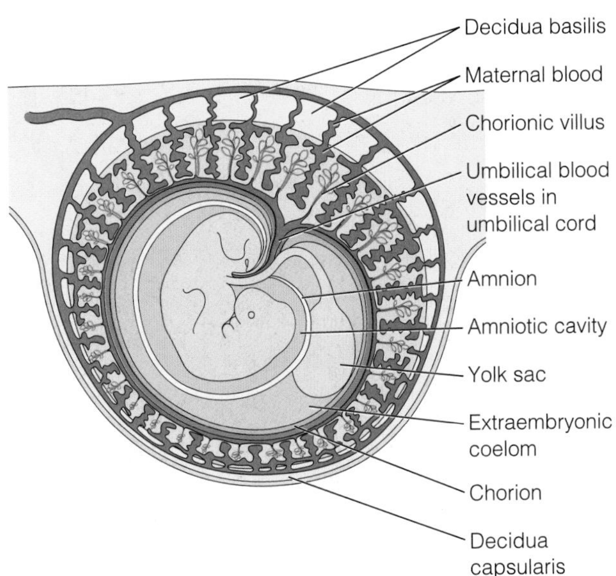

FIGURE 7–10 Early development of primary embryonic membranes. At 4½ weeks, the decidua capsularis (placental portion enclosing the embryo on the uterine surface) and decidua basalis (placental portion encompassing the elaborate chorionic villi and maternal endometrium) are well formed. The chorionic villi lie in blood-filled intervillus spaces within the endometrium. The amnion and yolk sac are well developed. SOURCE: Adapted from Marieb EN: *Human Anatomy and Physiology,* 4th ed. Redwood City, CA: Benjamin/Cummings, 1998, p 1088.

CRITICAL THINKING QUESTION

Why is it important to know which tissues and organs arise from each of the germ layers?

Embryonic Membranes

The **embryonic membranes** begin to form at the time of implantation (Figure 7–10). These membranes protect and support the embryo as it grows and develops inside the uterus. The first membrane to form is the **chorion,** the outermost embryonic membrane that encircles the amnion, embryo, and yolk sac. The chorion is a thick membrane that develops from the trophoblast and has many fingerlike projections, called chorionic villi, on its surface. These chorionic villi can be used for early genetic testing of the embryo at 8 to 10 weeks' gestation by chorionic villi sampling (see Chapter 17). As the pregnancy progresses, the villi begin to degenerate, except for those just under the embryo, which grow and branch into depressions in the uterine wall, forming the fetal portion of the placenta. By the fourth month of pregnancy, the surface of the chorion is smooth except at the place of attachment to the uterine wall.

The second membrane, the **amnion,** originates from the ectoderm, a primary germ layer, during the early stages of embryonic development. The amnion is a thin protective membrane that contains amniotic fluid. The space between the amniotic membrane and the embryo is the *amniotic cavity.* This cavity surrounds the embryo and yolk sac, except where the developing embryo (germ layer disc) attaches to the trophoblast via the umbilical cord. As the embryo grows, the amnion expands until it comes in contact with the chorion. These two slightly adherent membranes form the fluid-filled amniotic sac, also called **bag of waters (BOW),** that protects the floating embryo.

Amniotic Fluid

Amniotic fluid functions as a cushion to protect against injury. It also helps control the embryo's temperature, permits symmetric external growth of the embryo, prevents adherence to the amnion, and allows freedom of movement so that the embryo-fetus can change position freely, thus aiding in musculoskeletal development.

The amount of amniotic fluid is about 30 mL at 10 weeks and increases to 350 mL at 20 weeks. After 20 weeks the volume ranges from 700 to 1000 mL (Moore & Persaud, 1998). The amniotic fluid volume is constantly changing as the fluid moves back and forth across the placental membrane. As the pregnancy continues, the fetus contributes to the volume of amniotic fluid by excreting urine. The fetus also swallows up to 600 mL of the fluid every 24 hours. Approximately 400 mL of amniotic fluid flows out of the fetal lungs each day (Gilbert & Brace,

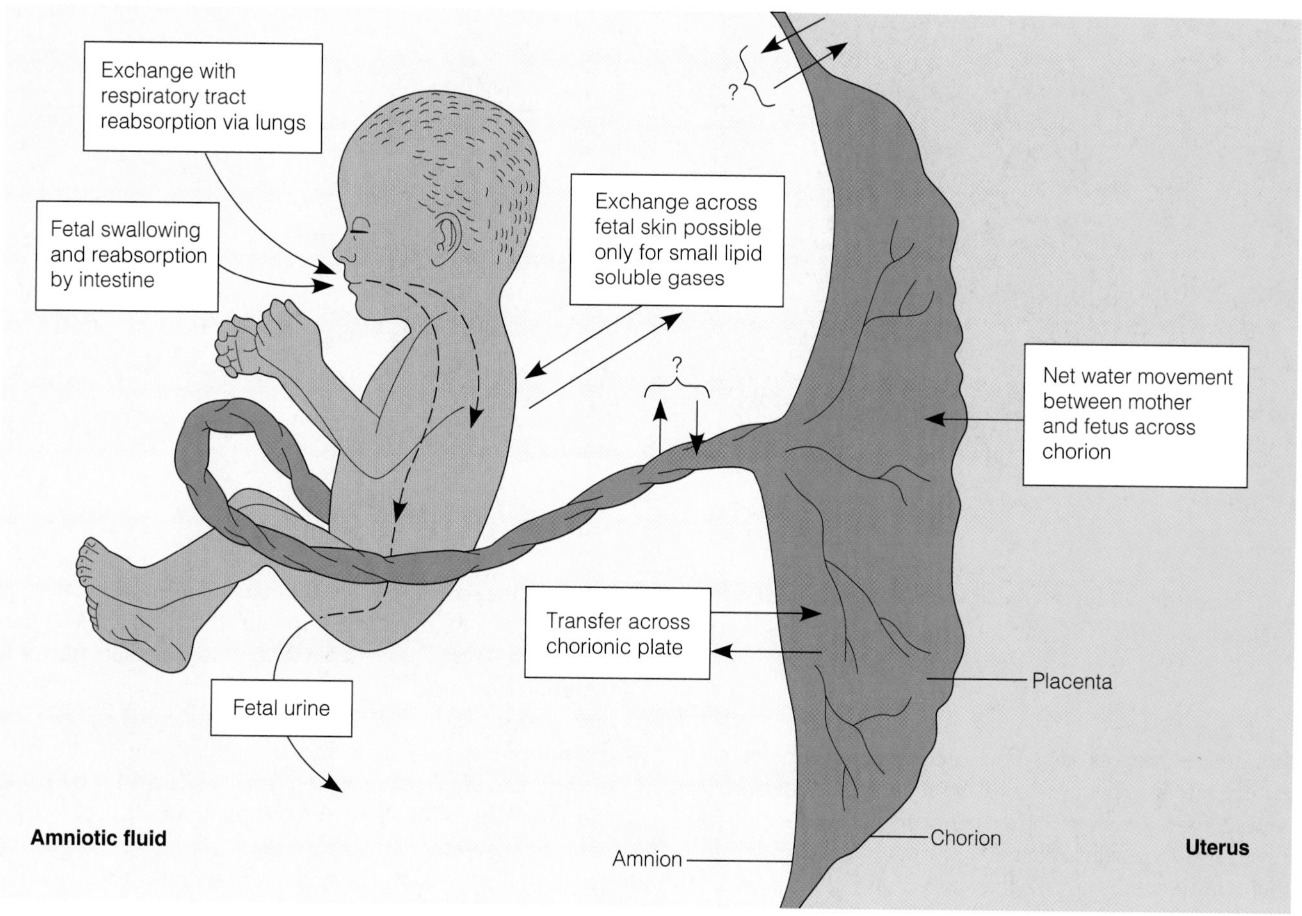

FIGURE 7–11 Summary of the significant pathways of water and solute exchange between the amniotic fluid and fetus. SOURCE: Seeds AE: Current concepts of amniotic fluid dynamics. *Am J Obstet Gynecol* November 1980; 138:575.

1993). Amniotic fluid is slightly alkaline and contains albumin, urea, uric acid, creatinine, lecithin, sphingomyelin, bilirubin, fat, fructose, leukocytes, proteins, epithelial cells, enzymes, and fine hair called **lanugo.** Abnormal variations in amniotic fluid volume are *oligohydramnios* (less than normal amounts of amniotic fluid) and *hydramnios* (higher than normal amounts of amniotic fluid). Hydramnios is also called *polyhydramnios.* Chapter 25 discusses alterations in amniotic fluid volume. Water and solutes must pass between the amniotic fluid and fetus. Figure 7–11 summarizes the major pathways of exchange.

Early in the first trimester of pregnancy, amniotic fluid is iso-osmolar with fetal and maternal plasma and is secreted from the developing trophoblast or embryo. Water and solutes move freely across the fetal skin before the time of skin keratinization. After 23 to 25 weeks, thickening of the fetal skin inhibits this diffusion. During the rest of the pregnancy, the fetal kidneys are the major source of fluid that enters the amniotic sac. Abnormalities of fetal urine production can result in changes in amniotic fluid volume. For example, with obstruction of urine outflow, as in Potter's syndrome, oligohydramnios (less than 400 mL of amniotic fluid) develops. Conversely, Bartter's syndrome results in a fetal diuresis and hydramnios. Hydramnios is amniotic fluid volume of more than 2000 mL or amniotic fluid index (AFI) greater than the 97.5 percentile for the corresponding gestational age. The fetal lungs are also significant contributors to amniotic fluid. Fetal breathing movements are associated with the bidirectional flow of fluid through the trachea. Net outflow from the fetal lungs averages 4.3 mL/kg/hr or 10% of body weight per day (Gilbert & Brace, 1993). This outflow of lung and tracheal fluid is used as the basis for amniotic fluid tests of fetal lung maturity.

The major mechanism by which amniotic fluid is removed in the last half of the pregnancy is fetal swallowing, which occurs mostly during periods of fetal breathing movements. In pregnancy when the fetus does not swallow normal amounts of amniotic fluid (as in esophageal atresia and anencephalus), hydramnios will result. A potential route of amniotic fluid removal is by the transmembranous pathway, that is, the movement of fluid across the amniochorion and into the maternal circulation within the uterine wall. Another major regulator of amniotic fluid volume and composition is the intramembranous pathway. This pathway causes amniotic

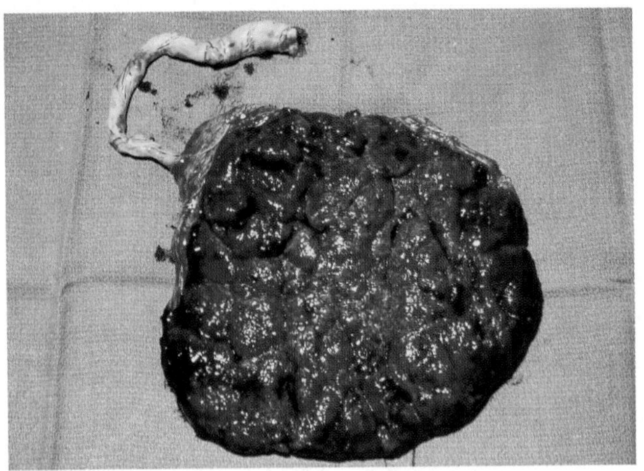

FIGURE 7–12 Maternal side of placenta.

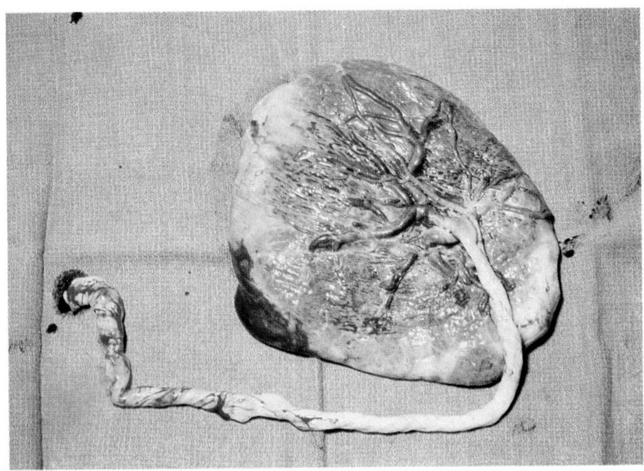

FIGURE 7–13 Fetal side of placenta.

water and/or solutes to be absorbed by the fetal blood that perfuses the fetal surface of the placenta (Gilbert & Brace, 1993).

Yolk Sac

In humans the yolk sac is small and functions only in early embryonic life. It develops as a second cavity in the blastocyst, about day 8 or 9 after conception, and forms primitive red blood cells during the first 6 weeks of development until the embryo's liver takes over the process. As the embryo develops, the yolk sac is incorporated in the umbilical cord, where it can be identified as a degenerate structure after birth.

Placenta

The **placenta** is the means of metabolic and nutrient exchange between the embryonic and maternal circulations. Placental development and circulation does not begin until the third week of embryonic development. The placenta develops at the site where the developing embryo attaches to the uterine wall. Expansion of the placenta continues until about 20 weeks, when it covers about half the inside of the uterus. After 20 weeks' gestation, the placenta becomes thicker but not wider. At 40 weeks' gestation, the placenta is about 15 to 20 cm (5.9 to 7.9 in.) in diameter and 2.5 to 3.0 cm (1.0 to 1.2 in.) in thickness. At that time, it weighs approximately 400 to 600 g (14 to 21 oz).

The placenta has two parts: the maternal portion and the fetal portion. The maternal portion consists of the decidua basalis and its circulation. Its surface is red and fleshlike. The fetal portion consists of the chorionic villi and their circulation. The fetal surface of the placenta is covered by the amnion, which gives it a shiny, gray appearance (Figures 7–12 and 7–13).

Development of the placenta begins with the chorionic villi. The trophoblast cells of the chorionic villi form spaces in the tissue of the decidua basalis. These spaces fill with maternal blood, and the chorionic villi grow into these spaces. As the chorionic villi differentiate, two trophoblastic layers appear: an outer layer called the syncytium (consisting of syncytiotrophoblasts), and an inner layer known as the *cytotrophoblast* (Figure 7–14). The cytotrophoblast thins out and disappears about the fifth month, leaving only a single layer of syncytium covering the chorionic villi. The syncytium is in direct contact with the maternal blood in the intervillous spaces. It is the functional layer of the placenta and secretes the placental hormones of pregnancy.

A third, inner layer of connective mesoderm develops in the chorionic villi, forming *anchoring villi.* These anchoring villi eventually form the *septa* (partitions) of the placenta. These septa divide the mature placenta into 15 to 20 segments called **cotyledons** (subdivisions of the placenta made up of anchoring villi and decidual tissue). In each cotyledon, the *branching villi* form a highly complex vascular system that allows compartmentalization of the uteroplacental circulation. The exchange of gases and nutrients takes place across these vascular systems.

Exchange of substances across the placenta is minimal during the first 3 to 5 months of development because of limited permeability. The villous membrane is initially too thick. As the villous membrane thins, the placental permeability increases until about the last month of pregnancy, when permeability begins to decrease as the placenta ages. In the fully developed placenta, fetal blood in the villi and maternal blood in the intervillous spaces are separated by three to four thin layers of tissue.

Placental Circulation After implantation of the blastocyst, the cells differentiate into fetal cells and trophoblastic cells. The proliferating trophoblast successfully invades the decidua basalis of the endometrium, first opening the uterine capillaries and later opening the larger uterine vessels. The chorionic villi are an outgrowth of the blastocystic tissue. As these

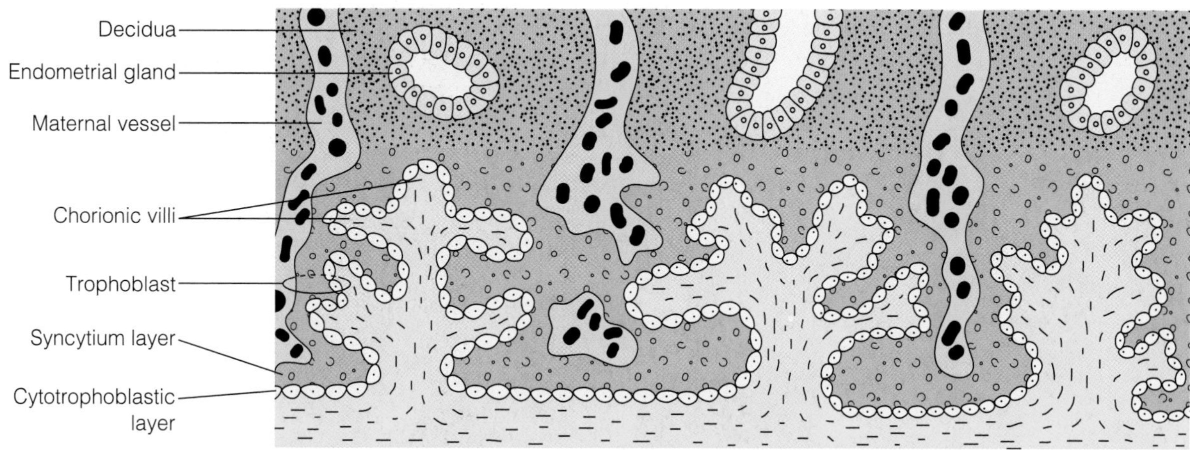

FIGURE 7–14 Longitudinal section of placental villus. Spaces formed in the maternal decidua are filled with maternal blood; chorionic villi proliferate into these maternal blood-filled spaces and differentiate into a syncytium layer and a cytotrophoblast layer.

villi continue to grow and divide, the fetal vessels begin to form. The intervillous spaces in the decidua basalis develop as the endometrial spiral arteries are opened.

By the fourth week the placenta has begun to function as a means of metabolic exchange between embryo and mother. The completion of the maternal-placental-fetal circulation occurs about 17 days after conception, when the embryonic heart begins functioning (Cunningham et al, 1997).

By 14 weeks the placenta is a discrete organ. It has grown in thickness as a result of growth in the length and size of the chorionic villi and accompanying expansion of the intervillous space.

The *cotyledons* of the maternal surface contain branches of a single placental mainstream villus, allowing for some compartmentalization of the uteroplacental circulation. Each cotyledon is a vascular unit containing branching vessels that are distributed throughout a particular lobule and partially separated from other lobules by the cotyledon's thin septal partitions.

The capillaries of the villi are lined with an extremely thin endothelium and are surrounded by a layer of mesenchymal (connective) tissue. This connective tissue is covered by chorionic epithelium consisting of cytotrophoblast and syncytiotrophoblast (Figure 7–14). As previously discussed, the cytotrophoblast thins out and disappears after the fifth month.

In the fully developed placenta's umbilical cord, fetal blood flows through the two umbilical arteries to the capillaries of the villi, and oxygen-enriched blood flows back through the umbilical vein to the fetus (Figure 7–15). Late in pregnancy, a soft blowing sound (*funic souffle*) can be heard over the area of the umbilical cord of the fetus. The sound is synchronous with the fetal heartbeat and the flow of fetal blood through the umbilical arteries.

Maternal blood, rich in oxygen and nutrients, spurts from the spiral uterine arteries into the intervillous spaces. These spurts are produced by the maternal blood pressure. The spurt of blood is directed toward the chorionic plate, and as the blood flow loses pressure, it becomes lateral (spreads out). Fresh blood continually enters and exerts pressure on the contents of the intervillous spaces, pushing blood toward the exits in the basal plate. Blood is then drained through the uterine and other pelvic veins. A *uterine souffle* is also heard in the later months of pregnancy. This uterine souffle, which is timed precisely with the mother's pulse and heard just above the mother's symphysis pubis, is caused by the augmented blood flow entering the dilated uterine arteries.

Circulation within the intervillous spaces depends on maternal blood pressure producing a gradient between arterial and venous channels. The lumen of the spiral uterine artery is narrow when it pierces the chorionic plate and enters the intervillous space, resulting in an increased blood pressure. The pressure in the arteries forces the blood into the intervillous spaces and bathes the numerous small villi in oxygenated blood. As the pressure decreases, the blood flows back from the chorionic plate toward the decidua, where it enters the endometrial veins.

Braxton Hicks contractions (Chapter 10) are believed to facilitate placental circulation by enhancing the movement of blood from the center of the cotyledon through the intervillous space. Placental blood flow is also enhanced when the woman is lying on her left side because the vena cava is not compromised.

Placental Functions Placental exchange functions occur only in those fetal vessels which are in intimate contact with the covering syncytial membrane. The syncytium villi have brush borders containing many microvilli, which greatly increase the exchange rate between maternal and fetal circulation (Sadler, 1995).

The placental functions, many of which begin soon after implantation, include fetal respiration, nutrition,

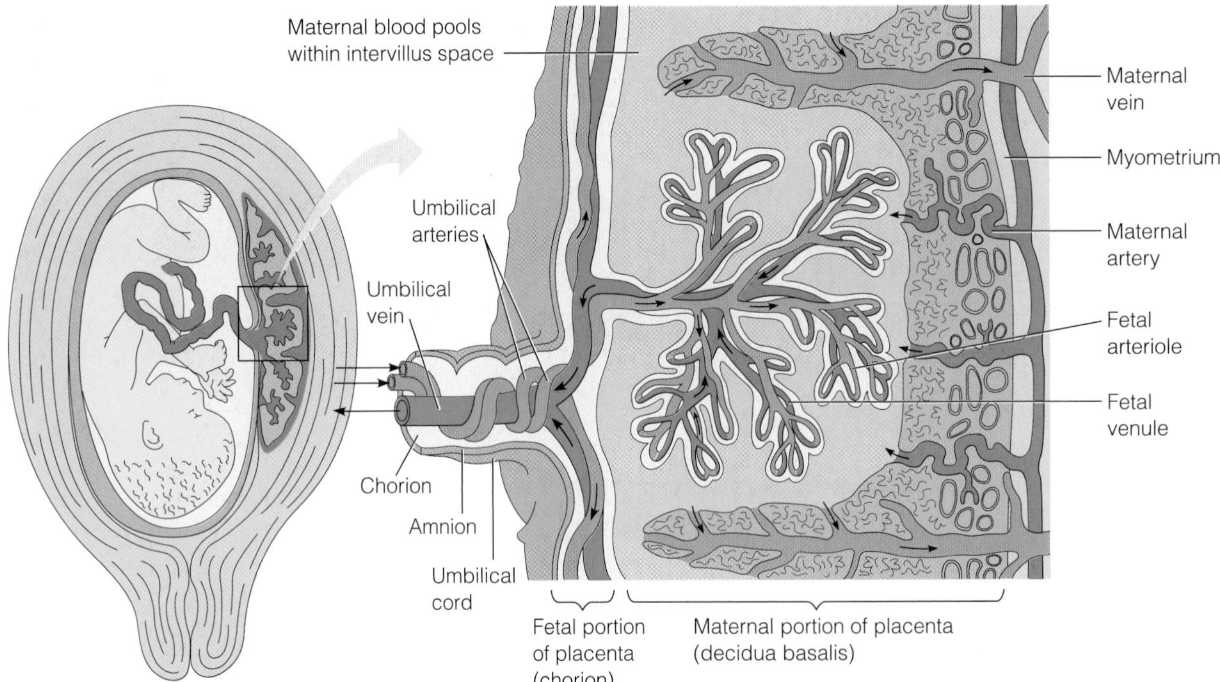

FIGURE 7–15 Vascular arrangement of the placenta. Arrows indicate the direction of blood flow. Maternal blood flows through the uterine arteries to the intervillus spaces of the placenta and returns through the uterine veins to maternal circulation. Fetal blood flows through the umbilical arteries into the villous capillaries of the placenta and returns through the umbilical vein to the fetal circulation.

and excretion. To carry out these functions, the placenta is involved in metabolic and transfer activities. It also has endocrine functions and special immunologic properties.

Metabolic Activities The placenta produces glycogen, cholesterol, and fatty acids continuously for fetal use and hormone production. The placenta also produces numerous enzymes required for fetoplacental transfer, and it breaks down certain substances, such as epinephrine and histamine. In addition it stores glycogen and iron.

Transport Functions The placental membranes actively control the transfer of a wide range of substances by five major mechanisms:

1. *Simple diffusion* moves substances from an area of higher concentration to an area of lower concentration. Substances that move across the placenta by simple diffusion include water, oxygen, carbon dioxide, electrolytes (sodium and chloride), anesthetic gases, and drugs. Insulin and steroid hormones originating from the adrenal glands and thyroid hormones also cross the placenta, but at a very slow rate. The rate of oxygen transfer across the placental membrane is greater than that allowed by simple diffusion, indicating that oxygen is also transferred by facilitated diffusion of some type. Unfortunately many substances of abuse, such as cocaine, cross the placenta via diffusion (Little & Van Beveren, 1996).
2. *Facilitated transport* involves a carrier system to move molecules from an area of greater concentration to an area of lower concentration. Molecules such as glucose, galactose, and some oxygen are transported by this method. The glucose level in the fetal blood ordinarily is approximately 20% to 30% lower than the glucose level in the maternal blood because glucose is being metabolized rapidly by the fetus. This in turn causes rapid transport of additional glucose from the maternal blood into the fetal blood.
3. *Active transport* can work against a concentration gradient, allowing molecules to move from areas of lower concentration to areas of higher concentration. Amino acids, calcium, iron, iodine, water-soluble vitamins, and glucose are transferred across the placenta this way. The measured amino acid content of fetal blood is greater than that of maternal blood, and calcium and inorganic phosphate occur in greater concentration in fetal blood than in maternal blood (McNanley & Woods, 1998).
4. *Pinocytosis* is important for transferring large molecules, such as albumin and gamma globulin. Materials are engulfed by amoebalike cells forming plasma droplets.
5. *Hydrostatic and osmotic pressures* allow the bulk flow of water and some solutes.

Other modes of transfer exist as well. For example, fetal red blood cells pass into the maternal circulation through breaks in the placental membrane, particularly during labor and birth. Certain cells, such as maternal leukocytes, and microorganisms, such as viruses (eg, the human immunodeficiency virus [HIV], which causes acquired immunodeficiency syndrome [AIDS]) and the bacterium *Treponema pallidum* which causes syphilis, can also cross the placental membrane under their own power (Simone, Derewlany, & Koren, 1994). Some bacteria and protozoa infect the placenta by causing lesions and then entering the fetal blood system.

Several factors, including the following, affect transfer rate:

- Molecular size
- Electrical charge
- Lipid solubility
- Placental area
- Diffusion distance
- Maternal-placental-fetal blood flow
- Blood saturation with gases and nutrients
- pK_a of the substance
- Maternal-placental-fetal metabolism of the substance

Substances that have a molecular weight of 1000 daltons or more have difficulty crossing the placenta by simple diffusion. Therefore, heparin, with a molecular weight above 6000, does not cross the placenta, but warfarin sodium (Coumadin), which has a molecular weight in the 300 to 400 range, crosses easily. Electrically charged molecules cross the placenta more slowly. An example is the muscle relaxant succinylcholine. A lipid-soluble substance moves quickly across the placenta into the fetal circulation.

Reduction of the placental surface area, as with abruptio placentae (partial or complete premature separation of a normally implanted placenta) will lessen the area that is functional for exchange. Placental diffusion distance also affects exchange. In conditions such as diabetes and placental infection, edema of the villi increases the diffusion distance, thus increasing the distance the substance has to be transferred.

Changes in blood flow between the fetus and the maternal intervillous space can be influenced by the transfer rate of substances, the ratio of blood on each side of the placenta, and the binding and dissociation abilities of carrier molecules in the blood. Decreased intervillous space blood flow is seen during labor and with certain maternal disease conditions such as hypertension. Mild fetal hypoxia increases the umbilical blood flow, but severe hypoxia results in decreased blood flow.

As the maternal blood picks up fetal waste products and carbon dioxide, it drains back into the maternal circulation through the veins in the basal plate. Fetal blood is hypoxic by comparison; it therefore attracts oxygen from the mother's blood. Affinity for oxygen also increases as the fetal blood gives up its carbon dioxide, which decreases its acidity.

Endocrine Functions The placenta produces hormones that are vital to the survival of the fetus. These include human chorionic gonadotropin (hCG); human placental lactogen (hPL); and two steroid hormones, estrogen and progesterone.

The hormone hCG is similar to LH and prevents the normal involution of the corpus luteum at the end of the menstrual cycle (see Chapter 6). If the corpus luteum stops functioning before the 11th week of pregnancy, spontaneous abortion occurs. The hCG also causes the corpus luteum to secrete increased amounts of estrogen and progesterone.

After the 11th week, the placenta produces enough progesterone and estrogen to maintain pregnancy. In the male fetus, hCG also exerts an interstitial cell–stimulating effect on the testes, resulting in the production of testosterone. This small secretion of testosterone during embryonic development causes male sex organs to grow. Human chorionic gonadotropin may play a role in the trophoblast's immunologic capabilities (ability to exempt the placenta and embryo from rejection by the mother's system). This hormone is used as a basis for pregnancy tests (for discussion of pregnancy tests, see Chapter 10).

Human chorionic gonadotropin is present in maternal blood serum 8 to 10 days after fertilization, just as soon as implantation has occurred, and is detectable in maternal urine at the time of the missed menses. Chorionic gonadotropin reaches its maximum level at 50 to 70 days' gestation and then begins to decrease as placental hormone production increases.

Progesterone is a hormone essential for pregnancy. It increases the secretions of the fallopian tubes and uterus to provide appropriate nutritive matter for the developing morula and blastocyst. It also appears to aid in ovum transport through the fallopian tube (Moore & Persaud, 1998). Progesterone causes decidual cells to develop in the uterine endometrium, and it must be present in high levels for implantation to occur. Progesterone also decreases the contractility of the uterus, thus preventing uterine contractions from causing spontaneous abortion.

Prior to hCG stimulation, the production of progesterone by the corpus luteum reaches a peak about 7 to 10 days after ovulation. Implantation occurs at about the same time as this peak. At 16 days after ovulation, the production of progesterone reaches a level between 25 and 50 mg per day and continues to rise slowly in subsequent weeks (Cunningham et al, 1997). After 10 weeks, the placenta (specifically, the syncytiotrophoblast) takes over the production of progesterone and secretes it in tremendous quantities, reaching levels of more than 250 mg per day late in pregnancy.

By 7 weeks, the placenta produces more than 50% of the estrogens in the maternal circulation. *Estrogens* serve mainly a proliferative function, causing enlargement of the uterus, breasts, and breast glandular tissue. Estrogens also have a significant role in increasing vascularity and vasodilation, particularly in the villous capillaries, near the end of pregnancy. Placental estrogens increase markedly toward the end of pregnancy, to as much as 30 times the daily production in the middle of a normal monthly menstrual cycle. The primary estrogen secreted by the placenta is different from that secreted by the ovaries. The placenta secretes mainly *estriol*, whereas the ovaries secrete primarily *estradiol*. The placenta by itself cannot synthesize estriol. Essential precursors are provided by the adrenal glands of the fetus and are transported to the placenta for the final conversion to estriol.

The hormone *hPL* (human placental lactogen; sometimes referred to as human chorionic somatomammotropin, or hCS) is similar to human pituitary growth hormone; hPL stimulates certain changes in the mother's metabolic processes. These changes ensure that more protein, glucose, and minerals are available for the fetus. Secretion of hPL can be detected by about 4 weeks. New placental proteins have been identified that may have clinical uses. These include SP 1 (Schwangerschaft's protein), and PP 5 (placental protein 5), and others.

Immunologic Properties The placenta and embryo are transplants of living tissue within the same species and are therefore considered *homografts*. Unlike other homografts, the placenta and embryo appear exempt from immunologic reaction by the host. Most recent data suggest that there is a suppression of cellular immunity by the placental hormones (progesterone and hCG) during pregnancy. One theory used to explain this phenomenon suggests that trophoblastic tissue is immunologically inert. It may contain a cell coating that masks transplantation antigens, repels sensitized lymphocytes, and protects against antibody formation.

Umbilical Cord

As the placenta is developing, the **umbilical cord** is also being formed from the amnion. The *body stalk*, which attaches the embryo to the yolk sac, contains blood vessels that extend into the chorionic villi. The body stalk fuses with the embryonic portion of the placenta to provide a circulatory pathway from the chorionic villi to the embryo (Figure 7–13). As the body stalk elongates to become the umbilical cord, the vessels in the cord decrease to one large vein and two smaller arteries. About 1% of umbilical cords have only two vessels, an artery and a vein; this condition may be associated with congenital malformations, primarily of the cardiac and gastrointestinal systems. A specialized connective tissue known as **Wharton's jelly** surrounds the blood vessels in the umbilical cord. This tissue, plus the high blood volume pulsating through the vessels, prevents compression of the umbilical cord in utero. At term, the average cord is 2 cm (0.8 in.) across and about 55 cm (22 in.) long. The cord can attach itself to the placenta at various sites. Central insertion into the placenta is considered normal. (Chapter 22 discusses the various attachment sites.)

Umbilical cords appear twisted or spiraled. This is most likely caused by fetal movement (Benirschke, 1997). A true knot in the umbilical cord rarely occurs; if it does, the cord is usually long. More common are so-called false knots caused by the folding of cord vessels. A *nucbal cord* exists when the umbilical cord encircles the fetal neck.

Development of the Fetal Circulatory System

The circulatory system of the fetus has several unique features that, by maintaining the blood flow to the placenta, provide the fetus with oxygen and nutrients while removing carbon dioxide and other waste products.

Most of the blood supply bypasses the fetal lungs because they do not carry out respiratory gas exchange. The placenta assumes the function of the fetal lungs by supplying oxygen and allowing the fetus to excrete carbon dioxide into the maternal bloodstream. Figure 7–16 shows the fetal circulatory system. The blood from the placenta flows through the umbilical vein, which enters the abdominal wall of the fetus at the site that, after birth, is the umbilicus (belly button). It divides into two branches, one of which circulates a small amount of blood through the fetal liver and empties into the inferior vena cava through the hepatic vein. The second and larger branch, called the **ductus venosus,** empties directly into the fetal vena cava. This blood then enters the right atrium, passes through the **foramen ovale** into the left atrium, and pours into the left ventricle, which pumps it into the aorta. Some blood returning from the head and upper extremities by way of the superior vena cava is emptied into the right atrium and passes through the tricuspid valve into the right ventricle. This blood is pumped into the pulmonary artery, and a small amount passes to the lungs and provides nourishment only. The larger portion of blood passes from the pulmonary artery through the **ductus arteriosus** into the descending aorta, bypassing the lungs. Finally, blood returns to the placenta through the two umbilical arteries, and the process is repeated.

The fetus receives oxygen via diffusion from the maternal circulation because of the gradient difference of Po_2 of 50 mm Hg in maternal blood in the placenta to a 30 mm Hg Po_2 in the fetus. At term the fetus receives oxygen from the mother's circulation at a rate of 20 to 30 mL/min (Sadler, 1995). Fetal hemoglobin facilitates obtaining oxygen from the maternal circulation because it carries as much as 20% to 30% more oxygen than adult hemoglobin. For further discussion, see Chapter 24.

Fetal circulation delivers the highest available oxygen concentration to the head, neck, brain, and heart (coronary circulation) and a lesser amount of oxygenated blood to the abdominal organs and the lower body. This circulatory pattern leads to cephalocaudal (head-to-tail) development in the fetus.

Fetal Heart

The heart of the fetus, as in the adult, is under the control of its own pacemaker. The sinoatrial (S-A) node sets the rate and is supplied by the vagus nerve. Bridging the atrium and the ventricle is the atrioventricular (A-V)

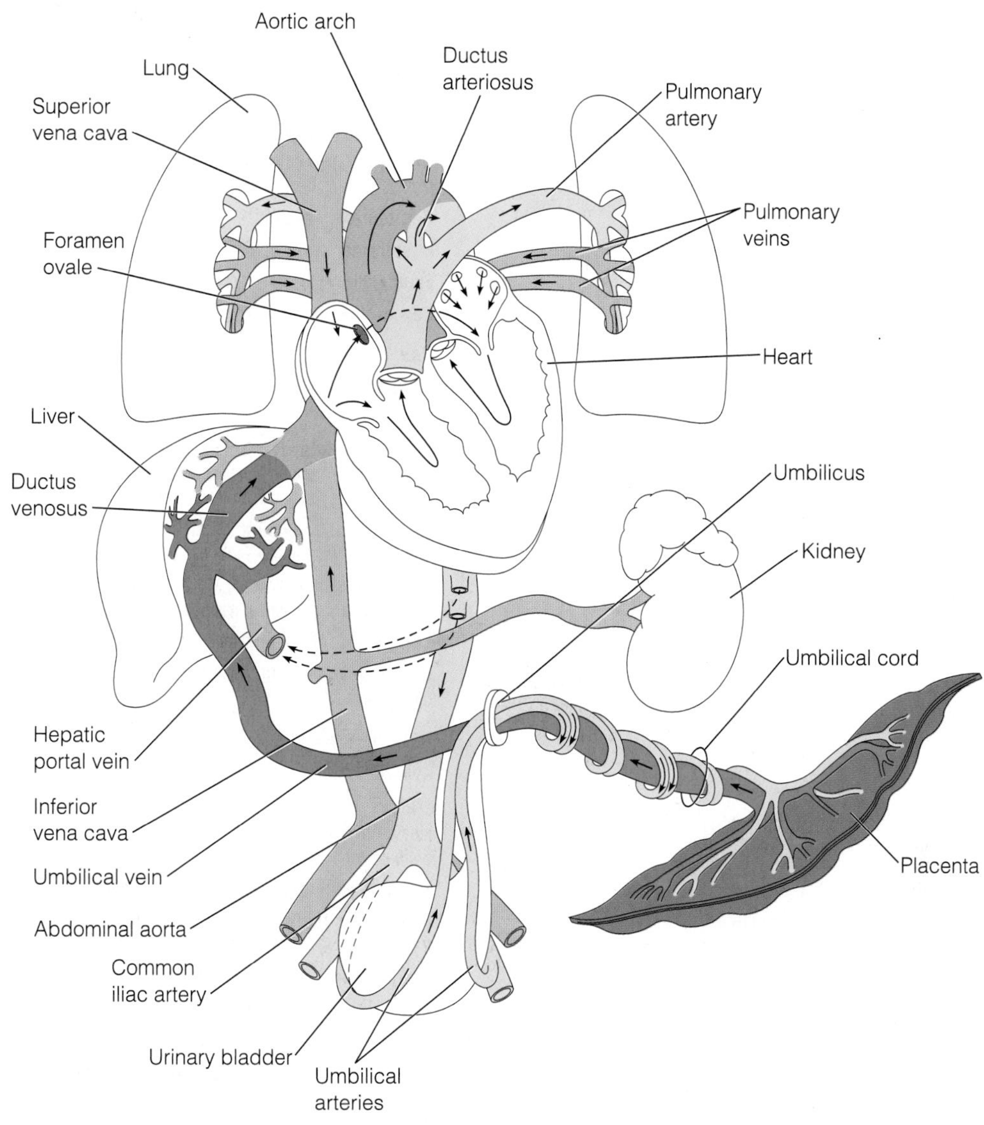

High oxygenation
Moderate oxygenation
Low oxygenation
Very low oxygenation

FIGURE 7–16 Fetal circulation. Blood leaves the placenta and enters the fetus through the umbilical vein. After circulating through the fetus, the blood returns to the placenta through the umbilical arteries. The ductus venosus, the foramen ovale, and the ductus arteriosus allow the blood to bypass the fetal liver and lungs.

node, also supplied by the vagus nerve. Baseline changes in the fetal heartbeat have been shown to be under the influence of this nerve. Atropine will block this effect.

When the fetus is stressed, the sympathetic nervous system causes the release of norepinephrine, which increases the fetal heart rate. To counteract the increase in blood pressure, baroreceptors, which respond to stretch, are present in the vessel walls at the junction of the internal and external carotid arteries. When stimulated, these receptors, under the influence of the vagus and glossopharyngeal nerves, cause the heart rate to slow.

Chemoreceptors in the fetal peripheral and central nervous systems respond to decreased oxygen tensions and to increased carbon dioxide tensions, leading to fetal tachycardia and an increase in blood pressure. The central nervous system (CNS) also has control over heart rate. Increased activity of the fetus in a wakeful period is exhibited in an *increase in the beat-to-beat variability* of the fetal heart baseline. Sleep patterns demonstrate a *decrease in the beat-to-beat baseline variability.* In cases of severe hypoxia, increased levels of epinephrine and norepinephrine act on the fetal heart to produce a faster and stronger rate.

TABLE 7–2 Summary of Organ System Development

Age: 2–3 weeks

Length: 2 mm C–R (Crown-to-Rump)

Nervous system: Groove forms along middle back as cells thicken; neural tube forms from closure of neural groove.

Cardiovascular system: Beginning of blood circulation; tubular heart begins to form during third week.

Gastrointestinal system: Liver begins to function.

Genitourinary system: Formation of kidneys beginning.

Respiratory system: Nasal pits forming.

Endocrine system: Thyroid tissue appears.

Eyes: Optic cup and lens pit have formed; pigment in eyes.

Ear: Auditory pit is now enclosed structure.

Age: 4 weeks

Length: 4–6 mm C–R

Weight: 0.4 g

Nervous system: Anterior portion of neural tube closes to form brain; closure of posterior end forms spinal cord.

Musculoskeletal system: Noticeable limb buds.

Cardiovascular system: Tubular heart beats at 28 days and primitive red blood cells circulate through fetus and chorionic villi.

Gastrointestinal system: Mouth: formation of oral cavity; primitive jaws present; esophagotracheal septum begins division of esophagus and trachea. Digestive tract: stomach forms; esophagus and intestine become tubular; ducts of pancreas and liver forming.

Age: 5 weeks

Length: 8 mm C–R

Weight: Only 0.5% of total body weight is fat (to 20 weeks).

Nervous system: Brain has differentiated and cranial nerves are present.

Musculoskeletal system: Developing muscles have innervation.

Cardiovascular system: Atrial division has occurred.

Age: 6 weeks

Length: 12 mm C–R

Musculoskeletal system: Bone rudiments present; primitive skeletal shape forming; muscle mass begins to develop; ossification of skull and jaws begins.

Cardiovascular system: Chambers present in heart; groups of blood cells can be identified.

Gastrointestinal system: Oral and nasal cavities and upper lip formed; liver begins to form red blood cells.

Respiratory system: Trachea, bronchi, and lung buds present.

Ear: Formation of external, middle, and inner ear continues.

Sexual development: Embryonic sex glands appear.

Age: 7 weeks

Length: 18 mm C–R

Cardiovascular system: Fetal heartbeats can be detected.

Gastrointestinal system: Mouth: tongue separates; palate folds. Digestive tract: stomach attains final form.

Genitourinary system: Separation of bladder and urethra from rectum.

Respiratory system: Diaphragm separates abdominal and thoracic cavities.

Eyes: Optic nerve formed; eyelids appear, thickening of lens.

Sexual development: Differentiation of sex glands into ovaries and testes begins.

Age: 8 weeks

Length: 2.5–3 cm C–R

Weight: 2 g

Musculoskeletal system: Digits formed; further differentiation of cells in primitive skeleton; cartilaginous bones show first signs of ossification; development of muscles in trunk, limbs, and head; some movement of fetus now possible.

Cardiovascular system: Development of heart essentially complete; fetal circulation follows two circuits—four extraembryonic and two intraembryonic.

Gastrointestinal system: Mouth: completion of lip fusion. Digestive tract: rotation in midgut; anal membrane has perforated.

Ear: External, middle, and inner ear assuming final forms.

Sexual development: Male and female external genitals appear similar until end of ninth week.

Age: 10 weeks

Length: 5–6 cm C–H (Crown-to-Heel)

Weight: 14 g

Nervous system: Neurons appear at caudal end of spinal cord; basic divisions of brain present.

Musculoskeletal system: Fingers and toes begin nail growth.

Gastrointestinal system: Mouth: separation of lips from jaw; fusion of palate folds. Digestive tract: developing intestines enclosed in abdomen.

Genitourinary system: Bladder sac formed.

Endocrine system: Islets of Langerhans differentiated.

Eyes: Eyelids fused closed; development of lacrimal duct.

Sexual development: Males: production of testosterone and physical characteristics between 8 and 12 weeks.

Age: 12 weeks

Length: 8 cm C–R; 11.5 cm C–H

Weight: 45 g

Musculoskeletal system: Clear outlining of miniature bones (12–20 weeks); process of ossification is established throughout fetal body; appearance of involuntary muscles in viscera.

NOTE: Age refers to gestational age of fetus/conceptus; fertilization age.

Embryonic and Fetal Development and Organ Formation

Pregnancy is calculated to last an average of 10 lunar months: 40 weeks, or 280 days. This period of 280 days is calculated from the beginning of the last menstrual period to the time of birth. Estimated date of birth (EDB) is usually calculated by this method. The fertilization age or postconception age of the fetus is calculated to be about 2 weeks less, or 266 days (38 weeks). The latter measurement is more accurate because it measures time from the fertilization of the ovum, or conception. The basic events of organ development in the embryo and fetus are outlined in Table 7–2. The time periods used are **postconception age periods.** For detailed discussion of each body system's development, see Chapter 24.

Human development follows three stages. The preembryonic stage consists of the first 14 days of development after the ovum is fertilized; the embryonic stage covers the period from day 15 until approximately the eighth week; and the fetal stage extends from the end of the eighth week until birth.

TABLE 7–2 Summary of Organ System Development *continued*

Age: 12 weeks continued

Gastrointestinal system: Mouth: completion of palate. Digestive tract: appearance of muscles in gut; bile secretion begins; liver is major producer of red blood cells.

Respiratory system: Lungs acquire definitive shape.

Skin: Pink and delicate.

Endocrine system: Hormonal secretion from thyroid; insulin present in pancreas.

Immunologic system: Appearance of lymphoid tissue in fetal thymus gland.

Age: 16 weeks

Length: 13.5 cm C–R; 15 cm C–H

Weight: 200 g

Musculoskeletal system: Teeth beginning to form hard tissue that will become central incisors.

Gastrointestinal system: Mouth: differentiation of hard and soft palate. Digestive tract: development of gastric and intestinal glands; intestines begin to collect meconium.

Genitourinary system: Kidneys assume typical shape and organization.

Skin: Appearance of scalp hair; lanugo present on body; transparent skin with visible blood vessels; sweat glands developing.

Eye, ear, and nose: Formed.

Sexual development: Sex determination possible.

Age: 18 weeks

Musculoskeletal system: Teeth beginning to form hard tissue (enamel and dentine) that will become lateral incisors.

Cardiovascular system: Fetal heart tones audible with fetoscope at 16–20 weeks.

Age: 20 weeks

Length: 19 cm C–R; 25 cm C–H

Weight: 435 g (6% of total body weight is fat)

Nervous system: Myelination of spinal cord begins.

Musculoskeletal system: Teeth beginning to form hard tissue that will become canine and first molar. Lower limbs are of final relative proportions.

Gastrointestinal system: Fetus actively sucks and swallows amniotic fluid; peristaltic movements begin.

Skin: Lanugo covers entire body; brown fat begins to form; vernix caseosa begins to form.

Immunologic system: Detectable levels of fetal antibodies (IgG type).

Blood formation: Iron is stored and bone marrow is increasingly important.

Age: 24 weeks

Length: 23 cm C–R; 28 cm C–H

Weight: 780 g

Nervous system: Brain looks like mature brain.

Musculoskeletal system: Teeth are beginning to form hard tissue that will become the second molar.

Respiratory system: Respiratory movements may occur (24–40 weeks). Nostrils reopen. Alveoli appear in lungs and begin production of surfactant; gas exchange possible.

Skin: Reddish and wrinkled, vernix caseosa present.

Immunologic system: IgG levels reach maternal levels.

Eyes: Structurally complete.

Age: 28 weeks

Length: 27 cm C–R; 35 cm C–H

Weight: 1200–1250 g

Nervous system: Begins regulation of some body functions.

Skin: Adipose tissue accumulates rapidly; nails appear; eyebrows and eyelashes present.

Eyes: Eyelids open (28–32 weeks).

Sexual development: Males: testes descend into inguinal canal and upper scrotum.

Age: 32 weeks

Length: 31 cm C–R; 38–43 cm C–H

Weight: 2000 g

Nervous system: More reflexes present.

Age: 36 weeks

Length: 35 cm C–R; 42–48 cm C–H

Weight: 2500–2750 g

Musculoskeletal system: Distal femoral ossification centers present.

Skin: Pale; body rounded, lanugo disappearing, hair fuzzy or woolly; few sole creases; sebaceous glands active and helping to produce vernix caseosa (36–40 weeks).

Ears: Ear lobes soft with little cartilage.

Sexual development: Males: scrotum small and few rugae present; descent of testes into upper scrotum to stay (36–40 weeks). Females: labia majora and minora equally prominent.

Age: 40 weeks

Length: 40 cm C–R; 48–52 cm C–H

Weight: 3200+ g (16% of total body weight is fat)

Respiratory system: At 38 weeks, lecithin-spingomyelin (L/S) ratio approaches 2:1 (indicates decreased risk of respiratory distress from inadequate surfactant production if born now).

Skin: Smooth and pink; vernix present in skinfolds; moderate to profuse silky hair; lanugo hair on shoulders and upper back; nails extend over tips or digits; creases cover sole.

Ears: Ear lobes firmer due to increased cartilage.

Sexual development: Males: rugous scrotum. Females: labia majora well developed and minora small or completely covered.

SOURCES: Sadler TW: *Langman's Medical Embryology,* 7th ed. Baltimore: Williams & Wilkins, 1995; and Moore KL, Persand TVN: *The Developing Human: Clinically Oriented Embryology,* 6th ed. Philadelphia: Saunders, 1998.

Preembryonic Stage

The first 14 days of human development, starting on the day the ovum is fertilized (conception), are referred to as the *preembryonic stage*, or the *stage of the ovum*. This period is characterized by rapid cellular multiplication and differentiation and the establishment of the embryonic membranes and primary germ layers, discussed earlier.

Embryonic Stage

The stage of the **embryo** starts on day 15 (beginning of the third week after conception or fertilization) and continues until approximately 8 weeks or until the embryo reaches a crown-to-rump (C–R) length of 3 cm (1.2 in.). This length is usually reached about 56 days after fertilization (the end of the eighth gestational week). During the embryonic stage, tissue differentiates into essential organs, and the main external features develop (Figure 7–17). The embryo is most vulnerable to teratogens during this period.

Three Weeks

In the third week, the embryonic disc becomes elongated and pear-shaped, with a broad cephalic end and a narrow

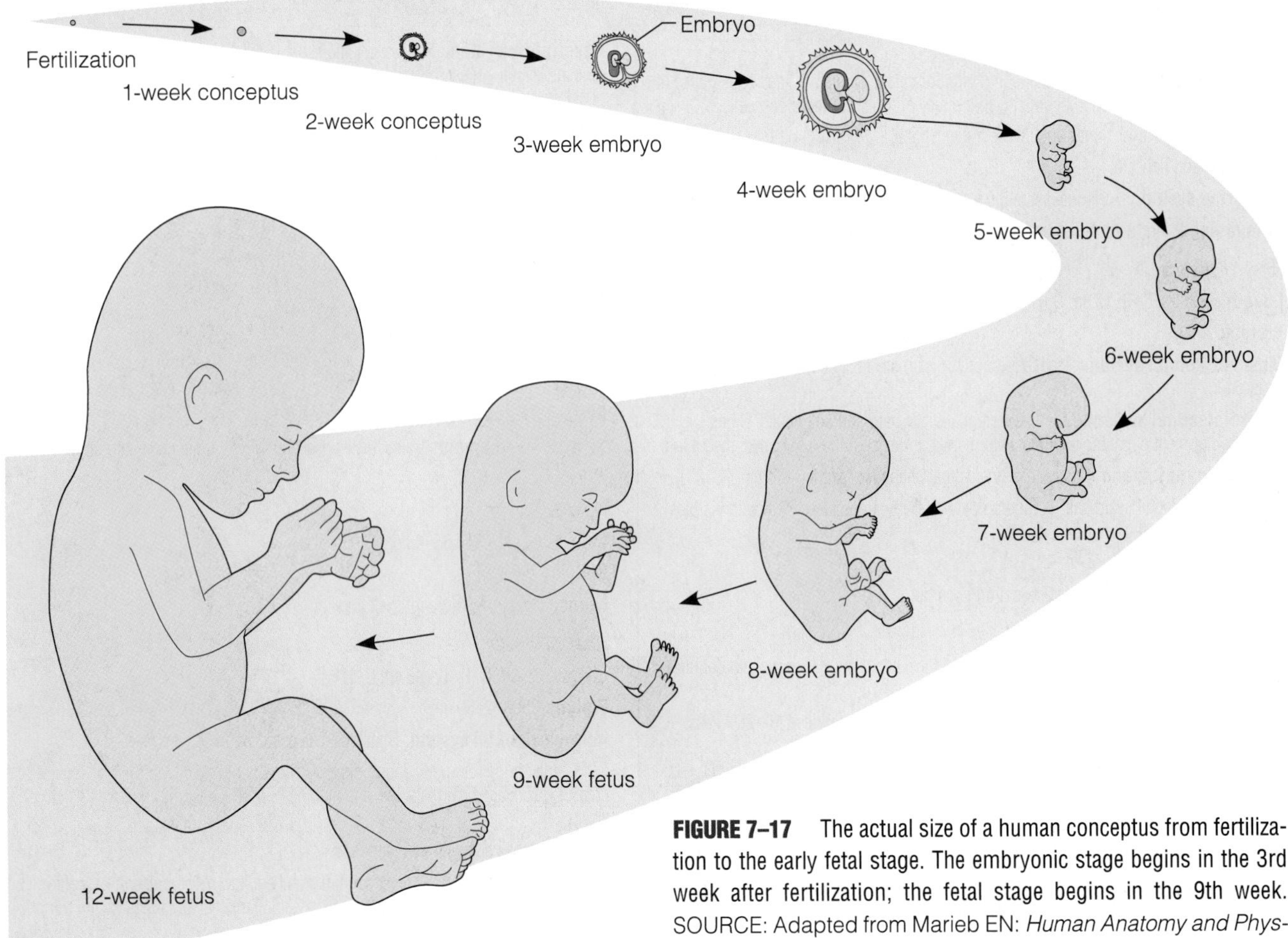

FIGURE 7–17 The actual size of a human conceptus from fertilization to the early fetal stage. The embryonic stage begins in the 3rd week after fertilization; the fetal stage begins in the 9th week. SOURCE: Adapted from Marieb EN: *Human Anatomy and Physiology,* 4th ed. Redwood City, CA: Benjamin/Cummings, 1998, p 1079.

caudal end. The ectoderm has formed a long cylindrical tube called the notochord for brain and spinal cord development. The gastrointestinal tract, created from the endoderm, appears as another tubelike structure communicating with the yolk sac. The most advanced organ is the heart. At 3 weeks, a single tubular heart forms just outside the body cavity of the embryo.

Four to Five Weeks

During days 21 to 32, somites, a series of mesodermal blocks, form on either side of the embryo's midline. The vertebrae that form the spinal column will develop from these somites. Prior to 28 days, arm and leg buds are not visible, but the tail bud is present. The pharyngeal arches—which will form the lower jaw (mandibular arch), hyoid bone, and cartilage of the larynx—develop at this time. The pharyngeal pouches appear now; these pouches will form the eustachian tube and cavity of the middle ear, the tonsils, and the parathyroid and thymus glands. The primordia of the ear and eye are also present (Figure 7–18). By the end of 28 days, the tubular heart is beating at a regular rhythm and pushing its own primitive blood cells through the main blood vessels.

During the fifth week, the optic cups and lens vesicles of the eye form and the nasal pits develop. Partitioning in the heart occurs with the dividing of the atrium. The embryo has a marked C-shaped body, accentuated by the rudimentary tail and the large head folded over a protuberant trunk (Figure 7–19). By day 35, the arm and leg buds are well developed, with paddle-shaped hand and foot plates. The heart, circulatory system, and brain show the most advanced development. The brain has differentiated into five areas, and ten pairs of cranial nerves are recognizable.

Six Weeks

At 6 weeks, the head structures are more highly developed, and the trunk is straighter than in earlier stages. The upper and lower jaws are recognizable, and the external nares are well formed. The trachea has developed, and its caudal end is bifurcated for beginning lung formation. The upper lip has formed, and the palate is developing. The ears are developing rapidly. The arms have begun to extend ventrally across the chest, and both arms and legs have digits, although they may still be webbed. There is a slight elbow bend in the arm, which is more

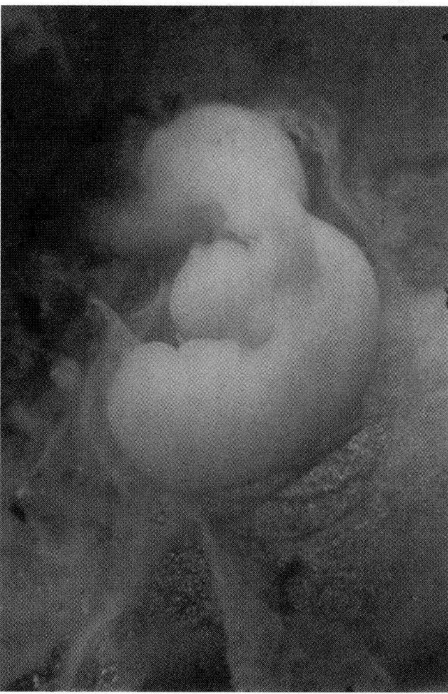

FIGURE 7–18 The embryo at 4 weeks. Pharyngeal arches, pharyngeal pouches, and primordia of the ear and eye are present.

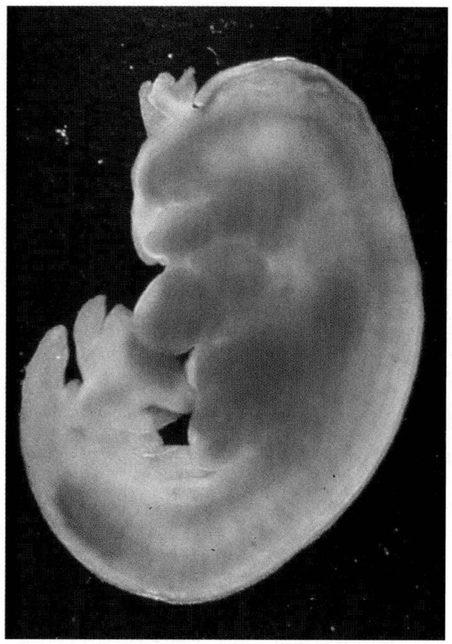

FIGURE 7–19 The embryo at 5 weeks. The embryo has a marked C-shaped body and a rudimentary tail.

advanced in development than the leg. Beginning at this stage the prominent tail will recede. The heart now has most of its definitive characteristics, and fetal circulation begins to be established. The liver begins to produce blood cells.

Seven Weeks

At 7 weeks, the head of the embryo is rounded and nearly erect (Figure 7–20). The eyes have shifted from their original lateral position to a forward location, where they are closer together, and the eyelids are beginning to form. The palate is nearing completion, and the tongue is developing in the formed mouth. The gastrointestinal and genitourinary tracts undergo significant changes during the seventh week. Prior to this time the rectal and urogenital passages formed one tube that ended in a blind pouch; they now separate into two tubular structures. The intestines enter the extraembryonic coelom in the area of the umbilical cord, called umbilical herniation (Moore & Persaud, 1998). At this point the beginnings of all essential external and internal structures are present.

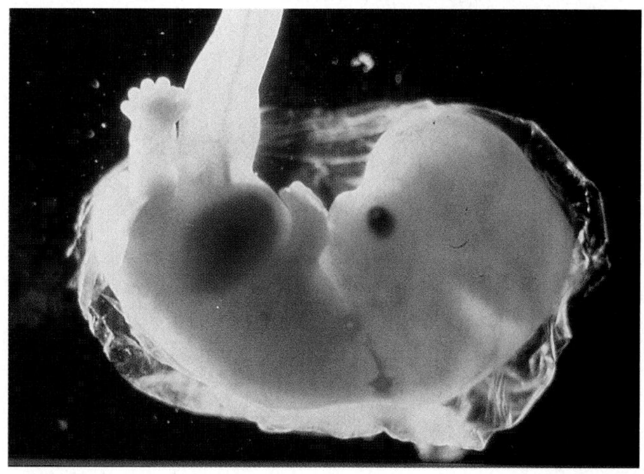

FIGURE 7–20 The embryo at 7 weeks. The head is rounded and nearly erect. The eyes have shifted forward and are closer together, and the eyelids begin to form.

Eight Weeks

At 8 weeks, the embryo is approximately 3 cm (1.2 in.) C–R and clearly resembles a human being (Figure 7–21). Facial features continue to develop. The eyelids begin to fuse. Auricles of the external ears begin to assume their final shape, but they are still set low (Moore & Persaud, 1998). External genitals appear, but the embryo's sex is not clearly identifiable. The rectal passage opens with the perforation of the anal membrane. The circulatory system through the umbilical cord is well established. Long bones are beginning to form, and the large muscles are now capable of contracting.

Fetal Stage

By the end of the eighth week, the embryo is sufficiently developed to be called a **fetus.** Every organ system and external structure that will be found in the full-term newborn is present. The remainder of gestation is devoted to refining structures and perfecting function.

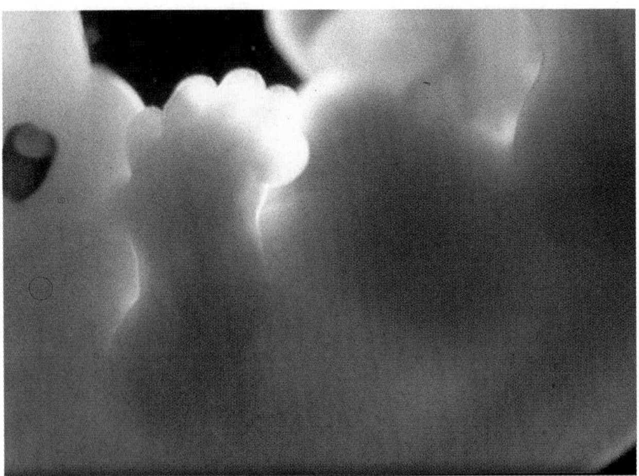

FIGURE 7–21 The embryo at 8 weeks. Although only 3 cm in C–R length, the embryo clearly resembles a human being. Facial features continue to develop.

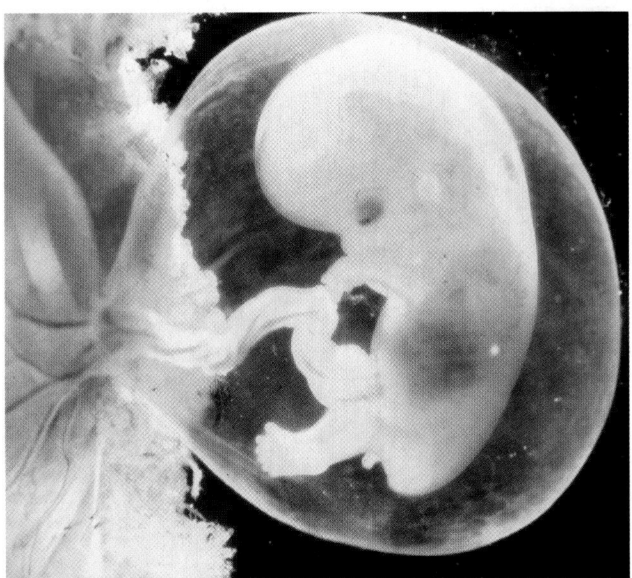

FIGURE 7–22 The fetus at 9 weeks. Every organ system and external structure is present. SOURCE: Nilsson L: *A Child Is Born.* New York: Dell Publishing, 1990.

Nine to Twelve Weeks

By the end of the ninth week, the fetus reaches a C–R length of 5 cm (2 in.) and weighs about 14 g. The head is large and comprises almost half of the fetus's entire size (Figure 7–22). The neck is distinct from the head and body, and both the head and neck are straighter than in previous stages of development.

By 12 weeks, the fetus reaches an 8-cm (3.2-in.) C–R length and weighs about 45 g (1.6 oz). The face is well formed, with the nose protruding, the chin small and receding, and the ear acquiring a more adult shape. The eyelids close at about the tenth week and will not reopen until about 28 weeks. Some reflex movements of the lips suggestive of the sucking reflex have been observed at 3 months. Tooth buds now appear for all 20 of the child's first teeth (baby teeth). The limbs are long and slender, with well-formed digits. The fetus can curl the fingers toward the palm and make a tiny fist. The legs are still shorter and less developed than the arms. The urogenital tract completes its development, well-differentiated genitals appear, and the kidneys begin to produce urine. Red blood cells are produced primarily by the liver. Spontaneous movements of the fetus now occur. Fetal heart tones (the sound of the heart beat) can be ascertained by electronic devices between 8 and 12 weeks. The heart rate is 120 to 160 beats per minute.

Thirteen to Sixteen Weeks

This is a period of rapid growth. At 13 weeks, the fetus weighs 55 to 60 g and is about 9 cm (3.6 in.) in C–R length. Lanugo, or fine hair, begins to develop, especially on the head. The skin is so transparent that blood vessels are clearly visible beneath it. More muscle tissue and body skeleton have developed, which hold the fetus more erect (Figure 7–23). Active movements are present—the fetus stretches and exercises its arms and legs. It makes sucking motions, swallows amniotic fluid, and produces meconium in the intestinal tract. Bronchial tubes are branching out in the primitive lungs, and sweat glands are developing. The liver and pancreas now begin production of their appropriate secretions. By the beginning of week 16, skeletal ossification is clearly identifiable.

Twenty Weeks

The fetus doubles its C–R length and now measures about 19 cm (8 in.). Fetal weight is between 435 and 465 g (15.2 to 16.3 oz). Lanugo covers the entire body and is especially prominent on the shoulders. Subcutaneous deposits of brown fat, which has a rich blood supply, make the skin a little less transparent. Nipples now appear over the mammary glands. The head is covered with fine, "woolly" hair, and the eyebrows and eyelashes are beginning to form. The fetus has nails on both fingers and toes (Figure 7–24). Muscles are well developed, and the fetus is active. Fetal movement, known as *quickening,* is felt by the mother. The heartbeat is audible through the fetoscope. Quickening and fetal heartbeat can help in validating the estimated date of birth.

Twenty-four Weeks

The fetus at 24 weeks reaches a crown-to-heel (C–H) length of 28 cm (11.2 in). It weighs about 780 g (1 lb, 10 oz). The hair on the head is growing long, and eyebrows and eyelashes have formed. The eye is structurally complete and will soon open. The fetus has a reflex hand grip (grasp reflex) and, by the end of 6 months, a startle reflex. Skin covering the body is reddish and wrinkled, with little subcutaneous fat. Skin on the hands and feet has thickened, with skin ridges on palms and soles forming distinct footprints and fingerprints. The skin over the entire body

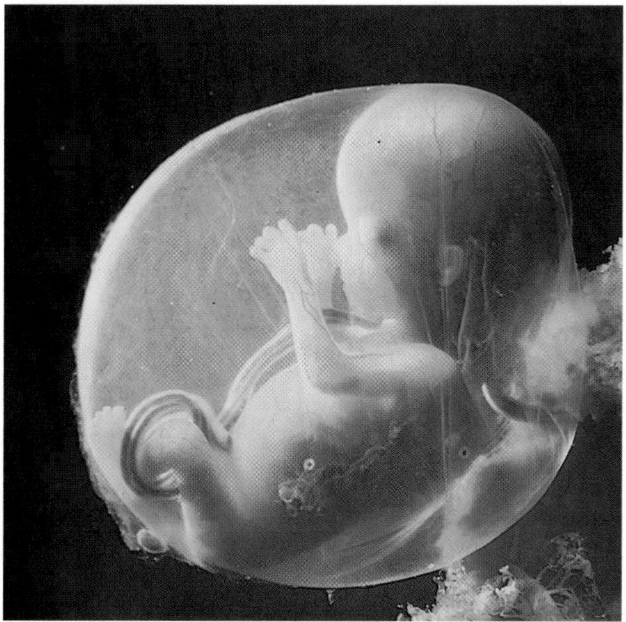

FIGURE 7–23 The fetus at 14 weeks. During this period of rapid growth, the skin is so transparent that blood vessels are visible beneath it. More muscle tissue and body skeleton have developed, which holds the fetus more erect. SOURCE: Nilsson L: *A Child Is Born.* New York: Dell Publishing, 1990.

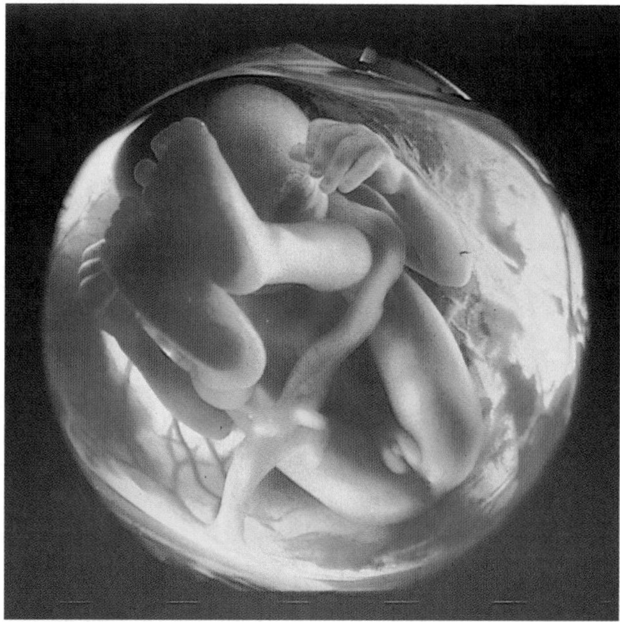

FIGURE 7–24 The fetus at 20 weeks. The fetus weighs approximately 435–465 g and measures about 19 cm. Subcutaneous deposits of brown fat make the skin less transparent. "Woolly" hair covers the head, and nails have developed on the fingers and toes. SOURCE: Nilsson L: *A Child Is Born.* New York: Dell Publishing, 1990.

is covered with a protective cheeselike fatty substance secreted by the sebaceous glands called **vernix caseosa.** The alveoli in the lungs are just beginning to form.

Twenty-five to Twenty-eight Weeks

At 6 calendar months, the fetal skin is still red, wrinkled, and covered with vernix caseosa. During this time the brain is developing rapidly, and the nervous system is complete enough to provide some degree of regulation of body functions. The eyelids open and close under neural control. If the fetus is a male, the testes begin to descend into the scrotal sac. Even though the lungs are still physiologically immature, they are sufficiently developed to provide gas exchange. A fetus born at this time will require immediate and prolonged intensive care in order to survive and to decrease the risk of major handicap. The fetus at 28 weeks is about 35 to 38 cm (14 to 15 in.) long C–H and weighs 1200 to 1250 g (2 lb, 10.5 oz to 2 lb, 12 oz).

Twenty-nine to Thirty-two Weeks

At 30 weeks, the pupillary light reflex is present (Moore & Persaud, 1998). The fetus is gaining weight from an increase in body muscle and fat and weighs about 2000 g (4 lb, 6.5 oz) with a length of about 38 to 43 cm (15 to 17 in.) by 32 weeks of age. The central nervous system (CNS) has matured enough to direct rhythmic breathing movements and partially control body temperature. However, the lungs are not yet fully mature. Bones are now fully developed but are soft and flexible. The fetus begins storing iron, calcium, and phosphorus. In males, the testicles may be located in the scrotal sac but are often still high in the inguinal canal.

Thirty-six Weeks

The fetus is beginning to get plump with less-wrinkled skin covering the deposits of subcutaneous fat. Lanugo hair is beginning to disappear, and the nails reach the edge of the fingertips. By 35 weeks, the fetus has a firm grasp and exhibits spontaneous orientation to light. By 36 weeks of age, the weight is usually 2500 to 2750 g (5 lb, 12 oz to 6 lb, 11.5 oz), and the C–H length of the fetus is about 42 to 48 cm (16 to 19 in.). An infant born at this time has a good chance of surviving but may require some special care, especially if there is intrauterine growth restriction.

Thirty-eight to Forty Weeks

The fetus is considered full term at 38 weeks after conception. The C–H length varies from 48 to 52 cm (18 to 21 in.) with males usually longer than females. Males also usually weigh more than females. The weight at term is about 3000 to 3600 g (6 lb, 10 oz to 7 lb, 15 oz) and varies in different ethnic groups. The skin has a smooth polished look. The only lanugo left is on the upper arms and shoulders. The hair on the head is no longer woolly but coarse and about an inch long. Vernix caseosa is present, with heavier deposits remaining in creases and folds of the skin. The body and extremities are plump, with good skin turgor, and the fingernails extend beyond the fingertips. The chest is prominent but still a little smaller than the head, and mammary glands protrude in both sexes.

TABLE 7–3 Fetal Development: What Parents Want to Know

4 weeks:	The fetal heart begins to beat.
8 weeks:	All body organs are formed.
8–12 weeks:	Fetal heart tones can be heard by Doppler device.
16 weeks:	Baby's sex can be seen. Although thin, the fetus looks like a baby.
20 weeks:	Heartbeat can be heard with fetoscope. Mother feels movement (quickening). Baby develops a regular schedule of sleeping, sucking, and kicking. Hands can grasp. Baby assumes a favorite position in utero. Vernix (lanolinlike covering) protects the body, and lanugo (fine hair) keeps oil on skin. Head hair, eyebrows, and eyelashes present.
24 weeks:	Weighs 1 lb 10 oz. Activity is increasing. Fetal respiratory movements begin.
28 weeks:	Eyes begin to open and close. Baby can breathe at this time. Surfactant needed for breathing at birth is formed. Baby is two-thirds its final size.
32 weeks:	Baby has fingernails and toenails. Subcutaneous fat is being laid down. Baby appears less red and wrinkled.
38–40 weeks:	Baby fills total uterus. Baby gets antibodies from mother.

TABLE 7–4 Developmental Vulnerability Timetable

Weeks Since Conception	Potential Teratogen-Induced Malformation
3	Ectromelia (congenital absence of one or more limbs) Ectopia cordis (heart lies outside thoracic cavity)
4	Omphalocele (herniation of abdominal viscera into the umbilical cord) Tracheoesophageal fistula (abnormal connection between trachea and esophagus) (4–5 weeks) Hemivertebra (4–5* weeks)
5	Nuclear cataract Microphthalmia (abnormally small eyeballs) (5–6* weeks) Facial clefts Carpal or pedal ablation (5–6* weeks)
6	Gross septal or aortic abnormalities Cleft lip, agnathia (absence of the lower jaw)
7	Interventricular septal defects Pulmonary stenosis Cleft palate, micrognathia (smallness of the jaw) Epicanthus Brachycephalism (shortness of the head) (7–8* weeks) Mixed sexual characteristics
8	Persistent ostium primum (persistent opening in atrial septum) Digital stunting (shortening of fingers and toes)

*May occur in several time periods after conception.

SOURCE: Modified from Danforth DN, Scott JR: *Obstetrics and Gynecology,* 5th ed. Philadelphia: Lippincott, 1986, p 319.

The testes are in the scrotum or are palpable in the inguinal canals. As the fetus enlarges, amniotic fluid diminishes to about 500 mL or less, and the fetal body mass fills the uterine cavity. The fetus assumes what is referred to as its *position of comfort,* or lie. The head is generally pointed downward, following the shape of the uterus (and also possibly because the head is heavier than the feet). The extremities and often the head are well flexed. After 5 months, feeding patterns, sleeping patterns, and activity patterns become established, so the fetus at term has its own body rhythms and individual style of response.

Table 7–3 lists some important developmental milestones.

CRITICAL THINKING QUESTION

How can knowing the gestational age of the fetus help us determine the potential effects of a teratogen?

Factors Influencing Embryonic and Fetal Development

Among factors that may affect embryonic development are the quality of the sperm or ovum from which the zygote was formed, the genetic code established at fertilization, and the adequacy of the intrauterine environment. If the environment is unsuitable before cellular differentiation occurs, all the cells of the zygote are affected. The cells may die, which causes spontaneous abortion, or growth may be slowed, depending on the severity of the situation. When differentiation is complete and the fetal membranes have formed, an injurious agent has the greatest effect on those cells undergoing the most rapid growth. Thus the time of injury is critical in the development of anomalies.

Because organs are formed primarily during embryonic development, the growing organism is considered most vulnerable to hazardous agents during the first months of pregnancy. Table 7–4 lists potential malformations related to the time of insult. Any agent, such as a drug, virus, or chemicals, that can cause development of abnormal structures in an embryo is referred to as a **teratogen** (Bishop, Witt, & Sloane, 1997). Chapter 10 discusses the effects of specific teratogenic agents on the developing fetus.

Adequacy of the maternal environment is also important during the periods of rapid embryonic and fetal development. Maternal nutrition can affect brain development. The period of maximum brain growth and myelination begins with the fifth lunar month before birth and continues during the first 6 months after birth. During the first 6 months after birth, there is a twofold increase in myelination; in the second 6 months to 2 years of age, there is a 50% further increase (Volpe, 1995). Amino acids, glucose, and fatty acids are considered to be the primary dietary factors in brain growth. A subtle type of damage that affects the associative capacity of the

RESEARCH IN PRACTICE

What is this study about? Smoking during pregnancy contributes to low birth weight, spontaneous abortion, and diminished infant lung function. Usual advice to smoking pregnant women may be vague and may exclude specifics about how to quit. The National Cancer Institute suggests that clinicians use the "four A's" (Ask, Advise, Assist, and Arrange follow-up) to encourage smoking cessation. Cathy Gebaur, Kwo Chung-Ying, Elaine Haynes, and Mary Ellen Wewers designed a research project and intervention program for pregnant smokers based on the "four A's."

How was the study done? To be eligible for the research project, the women had to be at least 17 years of age, self-reported daily users of tobacco, and pregnant. Participants in the study were informed only that data collection was for the purpose of assessing health behaviors. The researchers assigned 94 women to a control group and 84 to the treatment or intervention group. Advanced practice nurses initially provided individual 15-minute counseling sessions and telephone follow-up 7 to 10 days later.

What were the results of the study? During a clinic visit 6 to 12 weeks after the initial visit, all participants were asked about tobacco use for the previous 7 days. Sixteen (19%) of the treatment group and none of the control group reported abstinence. Thirteen (15.5%) of the self-reported abstainers tested negative on a saliva test. No statistically significant difference between the control and treatment group was reported in number of participants/group, age, race, education, medical information, or rate of smoking at initial visit. The treatment group had more smokers at home, had a longer period of time between the first counseling visit and evaluation visit, and had a statistically lower average of number of cigarettes smoked per day at the evaluation visit.

What additional questions might I have? (1) What was the intervention for the control group? (2) How were participants assigned to their group? (3) If the participants who quit were removed from the results, did the remaining treatment group members still smoke a lower average number of cigarettes per day when compared to the control group?

How can I use this study? With proper training, any nurse (or with supervision, any student nurse) could apply the "four A's," including follow-up with clients who smoke.

SOURCE: Gebaur, C., Chung-Ying, K., Haynes, E. F., & Wewers, M. E. (1998). A nurse-managed cessation intervention during pregnancy. *JOGNN, 27*(1), 47–53.

brain, possibly leading to learning disabilities, may be caused by nutritional deficiency at this stage. Maternal nutrition may also predispose to the development of adult coronary heart disease, hypertension, and diabetes in babies who were small or disproportionate at birth (Godfrey & Barker, 1995; Godfrey et al, 1996). Maternal nutrition is discussed in depth in Chapter 14.

Another prenatal influence on the intrauterine environment is maternal hyperthermia associated with sauna baths or hot tub use. Studies of the effects of maternal hyperthermia during the first trimester have raised concern about possible central nervous system defects and failure of neural tube closure (Jirasek, 1998). The effects of maternal substance abuse on fetal development are discussed in Chapters 15 and 28.

FOCUS YOUR STUDY

- Humans have 46 chromosomes, which are divided into 23 pairs—22 pairs of autosomes and one pair of sex chromosomes.
- Mitosis is the process by which additional somatic (body) cells are formed. It provides growth and development of the organs and replacement of body cells.
- Meiosis is the process by which gametes are formed. It occurs during gametogenesis (oogenesis and spermatogenesis) and consists of two successive cell divisions (reduction division), which produce a gamete with 23 chromosomes (22 chromosomes and 1 sex chromosome)—the haploid number of chromosomes.
- Gametes must have a haploid number (23) of chromosomes so that when the female gamete (ovum) and the male gamete (spermatozoon) unite (fertilization) to form the zygote, the normal human diploid number of chromosomes (46) is reestablished.
- An ovum is considered fertile for about 24 hours after ovulation, and the sperm is believed to be capable of fertilizing the ovum for only about 24 hours after it is deposited in the female reproductive tract.
- Fertilization usually takes place in the ampulla (outer third) of the fallopian tube. Both capacitation and the acrosomal reaction must occur for the sperm to fertilize the ovum. Capacitation is the removal of the plasma membrane, which exposes the acrosomal covering of the sperm head. The acrosomal reaction is the deposit of hyaluronidase in the corona radiata, which allows the sperm head to penetrate the ovum.
- Sex chromosomes are referred to as X and Y. Females have two X chromosomes, and males have an X and a Y chromosome. Y chromosomes are carried only by the sperm. To produce a male child, the mother contributes an X chromosome and the father contributes a Y chromosome.
- Twins are either dizygotic (fraternal) or monozygotic (identical). Dizygotic twins arise from two separate ova fertilized by two separate spermatozoa. Monozygotic twins develop from a single ovum fertilized by a single spermatozoon.
- Intrauterine development first proceeds via cellular multiplication in which the zygote undergoes rapid mitotic division called cleavage. As a result of cleavage, the zygote divides and multiplies into cell groupings called blastomeres, which are held together by the zona pellucida. The blastomeres will eventually become a solid ball of cells called the morula. When a cavity forms in the morula cell mass, the inner solid cell mass is called the blastocyst.
- Implantation usually occurs in the upper part of the posterior uterine wall when the blastocyst burrows into the uterine lining.
- After implantation, the endometrium is called the decidua. Decidua capsularis is the portion that covers the blastocyst. Decidua basalis is the portion that is directly under the blastocyst. Decidua vera is the portion that lines the rest of the uterine cavity.
- Embryonic membranes are called the amnion and the chorion. The amnion is formed from the ectoderm and is a thin protective membrane that contains the amniotic fluid and the embryo. The chorion is a thick membrane that develops from the trophoblast and encloses the amnion, embryo, and yolk sac.
- Amniotic fluid cushions the fetus against mechanical injury, controls the embryo's temperature, allows symmetric external growth, prevents adherence to the amnion, and permits freedom of movement.

- Primary germ layers will give rise to all tissues, organs, and organ systems. The three primary germ cell layers are ectoderm, endoderm, and mesoderm.
- The placenta, which develops from the chorionic villi and the decidua basalis, has two parts. The maternal portion, consisting of the decidua basalis, is red and flesh-looking; the fetal portion, consisting of chorionic villi, is covered by the amnion and appears shiny and gray. The placenta is made up of 15 to 20 segments called cotyledons.
- The placenta serves endocrine functions (production of hPL, hCG, estrogen, and progesterone), metabolic functions, and immunologic functions. It acts as the fetus's respiratory organ, is an organ of excretion, and aids in the exchange of nutrients.
- The umbilical cord contains two umbilical arteries, which carry deoxygenated blood from the fetus to the placenta, and one umbilical vein, which carries oxygenated blood from the placenta to the fetus. The umbilical cord has a central insertion into the placenta.
- Wharton's jelly, a specialized connective tissue, prevents compression of the umbilical cord in utero.
- Fetal circulation is a specially designed circulatory system that provides for oxygenation of the fetus while bypassing the fetal lungs.
- Stages of fetal development include the preembryonic stage (the first 14 days of human development starting at fertilization), the embryonic stage (from day 15 after fertilization, or the beginning of the third week, until approximately 8 weeks after conception), and the fetal stage (from 8 weeks until birth at approximately 40 weeks postconception).
- Significant events that occur during the embryonic stage are that at 4 weeks the fetal heart begins to beat and at 6 weeks fetal circulation is established.
- The fetal stage is devoted to refining structures and perfecting function. The following are some significant developments during the fetal stage:

  At 8 to 12 weeks, all organ systems are formed and now require maturation.

  At 16 weeks, the sex of the fetus can be determined visually.

  At 20 weeks, fetal heartbeat can be auscultated by a fetoscope, and the mother can feel movement (quickening).

  At 24 weeks, vernix caseosa covers the entire body.

  At 26 to 28 weeks, the eyes reopen.

  At 32 weeks, skin appears less wrinkled and red because subcutaneous fat has been laid down.

  At 36 weeks, fingernails reach the ends of fingers.

  At 40 weeks, vernix caseosa is apparent only in creases and folds of skin, and lanugo remains on upper arms and shoulders only.
- The embryo is particularly vulnerable to teratogenesis during the first 8 weeks of cell differentiation and organ system development.

REFERENCES

Bar-Ami, S., & Seibel, M. M. (1997). Oocyte development and meiosis in humans. In M. M. Seibel (Ed.), *Infertility: A comprehensive text* (2nd ed., pp 81–110). Stamford, CT: Appleton & Lange.

Benirschke, K. (1997). Placental casebook. *Journal of Perinatolology, 17*(4), 327–329.

Benirschke, K. (1995). The biology of the twinning process: How placentation influences outcome. *Seminars in Perinatolology, 19*(5), 342–350.

Bertrand, E., Van den Bergh, M., & Englert, Y. (1996). Clinical parameters influencing human zona pellucida thickness. *Fertility and Sterility, 66*(3), 408–411.

Bishop, J. B., Witt, K. L., & Sloane, R. A. (1997). Genetic toxicities of human teratogens. *Mutation Research 396*, 9–43.

Cunningham, F. G., MacDonald, P. C., Gant, N. G., Leveno, K. J., Gilstrap, L. C. III, Hankins, G. D. V., & Clark, S. L. (1997). *Williams obstetrics* (20th ed.). Stamford, CT: Appleton & Lange.

Gilbert, W. M., & Brace, R. A. (1993). Amniotic fluid volume and normal flows to and from the amniotic cavity. *Seminars in Perinatolology* 17(3), 150–157.

Godfrey, K. M., & Barker, D. J. P. (1995). Maternal nutrition in relation to fetal and placental growth. *European Journal of Obstetrics, Gynecology, and Reproductive Biology, 61*, 15–22.

Godfrey, K. M., Robinson, K., Barker, D. J. P., Osmond, C., & Cox, V. (1996). Maternal nutrition in early and late pregnancy in relation to placental and fetal growth. *British Medical Journal, 312*, 410–414.

Jirasek, J. E. (1998). Prenatal development: Growth, differentiation, and their disturbances. In J. J. Sciarri & T. J. Watkins (Eds.), *Gynecology and obstetrics* (Vol 2., Chap. 14, pp 1–14). Hagerstown, MD: Harper and Row.

Kochenour, N. K. (1997). Obstetric management of multiple gestation. In A. A. Fanaroff & R. J. Martin (Eds.), *Neonatal-perinatal medicine: Diseases of the fetus and infant* (6th ed., pp 295–300). St. Louis: Mosby.

Little, B. B., & Van Beveren, T. T. (1996). Placental transfer of selected substances of abuse. *Seminars in Perinatolology 20*(2), 147–153.

McNanley, T., & Woods, J. (1998). Placental physiology. In J. J. Sciarri & T. J. Watkins (Eds.), *Gynecology and obstetrics* (Vol. 3, Chap. 59, pp 1–14). Hagerstown, MD: Harper and Row.

Millette, C. F. (1997). Reproductive physiology of men. In M. M. Seibel (Ed.), *Infertility: A comprehensive text* (2nd ed., pp 221–251). Stamford, CT: Appleton & Lange.

Moore, K. L., & Persaud, T. V. N. (1998). *The developing human: Clinically oriented embryology* (6th ed.). Philadelphia: Saunders.

Revenis, M. E., & Johnson L. A. (1994). Multiple gestations. In G. B. Avery, M. Fletcher, & M. G. MacDonald (Eds.), *Neonatalogy: Pathophysiology and management of the newborn* (4th ed., pp 417–426). Philadelphia: Lippincott.

Sadler, T. W. (1995). *Langman's medical embryology* (7th ed.). Baltimore: Williams & Wilkins.

Simone, C., Derewlany, L. O., & Koren, G. (1994). Drug transfer across the placenta. *Clinics in Perinatology 21*(3), 463–481.

Speroff, L., Glass, R. H., & Kase, N. G. (1994). *Clinical gynecologic endocrinology and infertility* (5th ed.). Baltimore: Williams & Wilkins.

Volpe, J. J. (1995). *Neurology of the newborn* (3rd ed.). Philadelphia: Saunders.

Special Reproductive Concerns

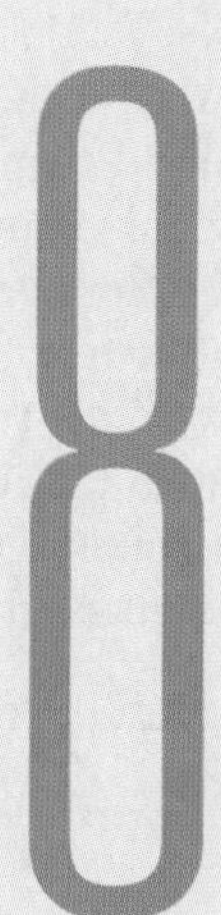

As we sat in the waiting room at the vitro clinic, I felt great apprehension. For 4 years we had been unable to conceive. I'd been through two surgeries, dozens of blood tests, hormone drugs that made me irrational and emotional. It was difficult at times—I blamed myself, felt out of control, and had surprisingly painful reactions to seeing mothers with babies. After many long talks we decided that if in vitro didn't work for us, we would adopt. Still, we felt that we wanted to experience childbirth together.

We were on the brink of the most expensive infertility treatment—the last resort for most infertile couples. Each month's treatment would involve nearly $10,000 of potentially uninsured costs; numerous injections, many of which I would have to administer to myself; egg retrieval; four or five ultrasounds; a dozen blood tests; and only a 30% to 50% chance of conceiving a child. Is this the right thing? Is this the right clinic for us? After so many disappointments did I dare get my hopes up again?

A young nurse burst into the office, excited and out of breath. She'd just come from the lab, having done a blood test, and had discovered that a client was pregnant. Watching the thrill and caring of the nurse's face helped me to decide. Yes, I was in the right place. Yes, it was worth hoping again. Even if in vitro didn't work for us, we had to try.

Objectives

- Identify the components of fertility.
- Describe the elements of the preliminary investigation of infertility.
- Summarize the indications for the tests and associated treatments, including assisted reproductive technologies, that are done in an infertility workup.
- Summarize the physiologic and psychologic effects of infertility.
- Describe the nurse's roles as counselor, educator, and advocate during infertility evaluation and treatment.
- Discuss the indications for preconceptual chromosomal analysis and prenatal testing.
- Identify the characteristics of autosomal dominant, autosomal recessive, and X-linked recessive disorders.
- Compare prenatal and postnatal diagnostic procedures used to determine the presence of genetic disorders.
- Explore the emotional impact on a couple undergoing genetic testing or coping with the birth of a baby with a genetic disorder, and explain the nurse's role in genetic counseling.

Key Terms

Artificial insemination
Autosomes
Basal body temperature (BBT)
Chromosomes
Endometrial biopsy
Ferning capacity
Gamete intrafallopian transfer (GIFT)
Genotype
Huhner test
Hysterosalpingography (HSG)
Infertility
In vitro fertilization (IVF)
Karyotype
Laparoscopy
Mendelian (single-gene) inheritance
Monosomies
Mosaicism
Non-Mendelian (multifactorial) inheritance
Pedigree
Phenotype
Spinnbarkheit
Sterility
Subfertility
Transvaginal ultrasound
Trisomies
Zygote intrafallopian transfer (ZIFT)

MOST COUPLES WHO WANT CHILDREN conceive with little difficulty. Pregnancy and childbirth usually take their normal course, and a healthy baby is born. But some less fortunate couples are unable to fulfill their dream of having a healthy baby because of infertility or genetic problems.

This chapter explores two particularly troubling reproductive problems facing some couples: the inability to conceive, and the risk of bearing babies with genetic abnormalities.

Infertility

Infertility is defined as lack of conception despite unprotected sexual intercourse for at least 12 months (Hatcher et al, 1998). Infertility has a profound emotional, psychologic, and economic impact on both the affected couple and society. Approximately 8% of couples in their reproductive years are infertile (Speroff et al, 1994). **Sterility** is a term applied when there is an absolute factor preventing reproduction. **Subfertility** is used to describe a couple having difficulty conceiving because both partners have reduced fecundity (ability to reproduce). Subfertility may be used interchangeably with the term subfecundity (Hatcher et al, 1998).

Primary infertility identifies those women who have never conceived, whereas *secondary infertility* indicates those who have been pregnant in the past but have not conceived during 1 or more years of unprotected intercourse (Trantham, 1996) or cannot sustain a pregnancy.

Public perception is that the incidence of infertility is increasing, but in fact it may be decreasing. What has changed is the composition of the infertile population; the infertility diagnosis has increased in the age group 25 to 44 because of delayed childbearing and the entry of the baby-boom cohort into this age range.

The perception that infertility is on the rise may be related to the following factors:

- The increase in assisted reproduction techniques
- The increase in availability and use of infertility services
- The increase in insurance coverage of diagnosis of and treatment for infertility
- The increased number of childless women over 35 seeking medical attention for infertility (Speroff et al, 1994)
- Increased incidence of sexually transmitted infections
- The decreasing population of adoptable babies

Essential Components of Fertility

Understanding the elements essential for normal fertility can help the nurse identify the many factors that may cause infertility. The following essential components must be presented for normal fertility.

Female partner:

1. The cervical mucus must be favorable to the survival of spermatozoa and allow passage to the upper genital tract.
2. The fallopian tubes must be patent and have normal fimbria with peristaltic movements toward the uterus to facilitate normal transport and interaction of ovum and sperm.
3. The ovaries must produce and release normal ova in a regular cyclic fashion.
4. There must be no obstruction between the ovaries and the uterus.
5. The endometrium must be in a physiologic state to allow implantation of the blastocyst and to sustain normal growth and development.
6. Adequate reproductive hormones must be present.

Male partner:

1. The testes must produce spermatozoa of normal quality, quantity, and motility.
2. The male genital tract must not be obstructed.
3. The male genital tract secretions must be normal.
4. Ejaculated spermatozoa must be deposited in the female vagina in such a manner that they reach the cervix.

These normal components are correlated with possible causes of deviation in Table 8–1. With the intricacies of the normal male and female reproductive cycle, it is an impressive phenomenon that approximately 92% of the couples in the United States are able to conceive. The remaining 8% of couples suffer infertility due to a male factor (40%), a female factor (40%), or either an unknown cause (unexplained infertility) or a problem with both partners (10% to 20%) (Speroff et al, 1994). In 35% of the infertile couples, multiple causes are present. Professional intervention can help approximately 65% of infertile couples achieve pregnancy (Corson, 1995).

Couples should be referred for infertility evaluation if they have been unable to conceive after at least 1 year of attempting to achieve pregnancy. In women over 35 years of age or couples with a history predisposing them to infertility, it may be appropriate to refer the couple after only 6 months of unprotected intercourse without conception. At 25 years of age, the age at which couples are the most fertile, the average length of time needed to achieve conception is 5.3 months. The average 20- to 30-year-old American couple has intercourse one to three times a week, a frequency that should be sufficient to achieve pregnancy if all other factors are satisfactory. In about 20% of cases, conception occurs within the first month of unprotected intercourse (Speroff et al, 1994). However, age can have a serious impact on the ability to

TABLE 8–1 Possible Causes of Infertility

Necessary Norms	Deviations from Normal
Female	
Favorable cervical mucus	Cervicitis, cervical stenosis, use of coital lubricants, antisperm antibodies (immunologic response)
Clear passage between cervix and tubes	Myomas, adhesions, adenomyosis, polyps, endometritis, cervical stenosis, endometriosis, congenital anomalies (eg, septate uterus, DES exposure)
Patent tubes with normal motility	Pelvic inflammatory disease, peritubal adhesions, endometriosis, IUD, salpingitis (eg, chlamydia, recurrent STIs), neoplasm, ectopic pregnancy, tubal ligation
Ovulation and release of ova	Primary ovarian failure, polycystic ovarian disease, hypothyroidism, pituitary tumor, lactation, periovarian adhesions, endometriosis, premature ovarian failure, hyperprolactinemia, Turner syndrome
No obstruction between ovary and tubes	Adhesions, endometriosis, pelvic inflammatory disease
Endometrial preparation	Anovulation, luteal phase defect, malformation, uterine infection, Asherman's syndrome
Male	
Normal semen analysis	Abnormalities of sperm or semen, polyspermia, congenital defect in testicular development, mumps after adolescence, cryptorchidism, infections, gonadal exposure to x- rays, chemotherapy, smoking, alcohol abuse, malnutrition, chronic or acute metabolic disease, medications (eg, morphine, ASA, ibuprofen), cocaine, marijuana use, constrictive underclothing, heat
Unobstructed genital tract	Infections, tumors, congenital anomalies, vasectomy, strictures, trauma, varicocele
Normal genital tract secretions	Infections, autoimmunity to semen, tumors
Ejaculate deposited at the cervix	Premature ejaculation, impotence, hypospadias, retrograde ejaculation (eg, diabetic), neurologic cord lesions, obesity (inhibiting adequate penetration)

conceive with 1 in 7 women ages 30 to 34, 1 in 5 women ages 35 to 39, and 1 in 4 women in ages 40 to 44 experiencing infertility (Stovall et al, 1991). Finally there continues to be an increase in the number of women who give birth to their first child after the age of 30. It is estimated that by the year 2000, 1 in 2 babies will be born to women over 35 (American College of Obstetrics and Gynecology [ACOG], 1992). The age-related decline in reproductive potential is the principal factor contributing to the increase in the prevalence of infertility in Western society (Sharara & Scott, 1997). Delaying parenthood appears to increase the possibility that one or more of the physiologic processes necessary for conception will be adversely affected (Speroff et al, 1994).

Preliminary Investigation

The easiest and least intrusive infertility testing approach is used first. Extensive testing is avoided until data confirm that the timing of intercourse and the length of coital exposure have been adequate. The nurse informs the couple of the most fertile times to have intercourse during the menstrual cycle. Teaching the couple the signs and timing of ovulation and the most effective times for intercourse within the cycle may solve the problem before extensive testing needs to be initiated (Table 8–1). Primary assessment, including a comprehensive history (with a discussion of genetic conditions) and physical examination for any obvious causes of infertility, is done before a costly, time-consuming, and emotionally trying investigation is initiated. During the first visit for the preliminary investigation, the nurse explains the basic infertility workup. The basic investigation for the couple depends on the individuals' history and usually includes assessment of ovarian function, cervical mucus adequacy and receptivity to sperm, sperm adequacy, tubal patency, and the general condition of the pelvic organs (Bradshaw, 1998). Because approximately 40% of infertility is related to a male factor, a semen analysis should be one of the first diagnostic tests prior to moving on to the more invasive diagnostic procedures involving the woman.

The mutual desire to have children is central to many marriages. A fertility problem is a deeply personal, emotion-laden area in a couple's life. The self-esteem of one or both partners may be threatened if the inability to conceive is seen as a lack of virility or femininity. It is never easy to discuss one's sexual activity, especially when potentially irreversible problems with fertility may exist. The nurse can provide comfort to couples by offering a sympathetic ear, a nonjudgmental approach, and appropriate information and instructions throughout the diagnostic and therapeutic process. Because counseling includes discussion of very personal matters, nurses who are comfortable with their own sexuality are more capable of establishing rapport and eliciting relevant information.

The first interview should include a comprehensive history of both partners and a physical and pelvic exam of the woman. Table 8–2 outlines what a complete infertility physical workup and laboratory evaluation entails for both partners. Figure 8–1 outlines the historical database, diagnostic tests usually performed, and health care interventions in cases of infertility.

Tests for Infertility

After a thorough history and physical examination of both partners, tests may be initiated to identify causes of infertility (Stansberry, 1996). Because of the high incidence of multifactorial infertility, it is important to assess both partners. A thorough evaluation of the woman includes assessment of the hypothalamic/pituitary axis in terms of ovulatory function, as well as structure and

TABLE 8–2 Initial Infertility Physical Workup and Laboratory Evaluations

Female	Male
Physical Examination	**Physical Examination**
Assessment of height, weight, blood pressure, temperature, and general health status	General health (assessment of height, weight, blood pressure)
Endocrine evaluation of thyroid for exophthalmos, lid lag, tremor, or palpable gland	Endocrine evaluation (eg, presence of gynecomastia)
Optic fundi evaluation for presence of increased intracranial pressure, especially in oligomenorrheal or amenorrheal women (possible pituitary tumor)	Visual fields evaluation for bitemporal hemianopia
Reproductive features (including breast and external genital area)	Abnormal hair patterns
Physical ability to tolerate pregnancy	
Pelvic Examination	**Urologic Examination**
Papanicolaou smear	Presence or absence of phimosis
Culture for gonorrhea if indicated and possibly chlamydia or mycoplasma culture (opinions vary)	Location of urethral meatus
Signs of vaginal infections (Chapter 3)	Size and consistency of each testis, vas deferens, and epididymis
Shape of escutcheon (eg, does pubic hair distribution resemble that of a male?)	Presence of varicocele
Size of clitoris (enlargement caused by endocrine disorders)	**Rectal Examination**
Evaluation of cervix: old lacerations, tears, erosion, polyps, condition and shape of os, signs of infections, cervical mucus (evaluate for estrogen effect of spinnbarkheit and cervical ferning)	Size and consistency of the prostate with microscopic evaluation of prostate fluid for signs of infection
Bimanual Examination	Size and consistency of seminal vesicles
Size, shape, position, and motility of uterus	**Laboratory Examination**
Presence of congenital anomalies	Complete blood count
Presence of endometriosis	Sedimentation rate if indicated
Evaluation of adnexa: ovarian size, cysts, fixations, or tumors	Serology
Rectovaginal Examination	Urinalysis
Presence of retroflexed or retroverted uterus	Rh factor and blood grouping
Presence of rectouterine pouch masses	Semen analysis
Presence of possible endometriosis	If indicated, testicular biopsy, buccal smear
Laboratory Examination	Hormonal assays, FSH, LH, prolactin
Complete blood count	
Sedimentation rate if indicated	
Serology	
Urinalysis	
Rh factor and blood grouping	
If indicated, thyroid function tests, prolactin levels, glucose tolerance test, hormonal assays including estradiol, LH, progesterone, FSH, DHEA, androstendione, testosterone, 17-OHP.	

function of the cervix, uterus, fallopian tubes, and ovaries. See Chapter 6 for an in-depth discussion of the fertility cycle. If the man's history indicates, he may be referred to a urologist for a physical exam and further testing. Evaluation of the man may include at least two semen analyses to confirm or rule out a seminal deficiency. More sophisticated tests to evaluate specific sperm function have evolved over the last several years; however, their usefulness or clinical significance is controversial (Kruger & Franken, 1994). These include such tests as the hamster sperm penetration assay (SPA), hemizona (HZA), acrosome reaction assay, sperm density evaluation, and semen immunobead testing for the presence of antisperm antibodies (immunologic infertility).

Assessment of the Woman

Evaluation of Ovulatory Factors Ovulation problems account for approximately 15% of couples' infertility (Speroff et al, 1994). Fertility assessments of the woman are discussed first. For review of the characteristics of the female reproductive cycle, see Table 8–3 and Figure 8–2. A basic test of ovulatory function is the **basal body temperature (BBT)** recording, which aids in identifying follicular and luteal phase abnormalities. At the initial visit, the nurse instructs the woman in the technique of recording basal body temperature, taken only with a BBT thermometer. This special kind of thermometer measures temperature between 35.6C (96F) and 37.8C (100F) and is calibrated by tenths of a degree, making slight temperature changes readily apparent. The woman should take her BBT every morning before rising out of bed (after 6 to 8 hours of uninterrupted sleep) (Moghissi, 1998). Studies have demonstrated that, in addition to the traditional glass/mercury BBT thermometer, tympanic thermometry is a valid method to obtain basal body temperatures. Tympanic thermometry has the advantages of being simple and fast; it takes only a few seconds to get a reading. Several computerized or digitalized BBT devices ("the Rabbit," Fertil-A-Chron) have been developed to identify the fertile period more accurately at home.

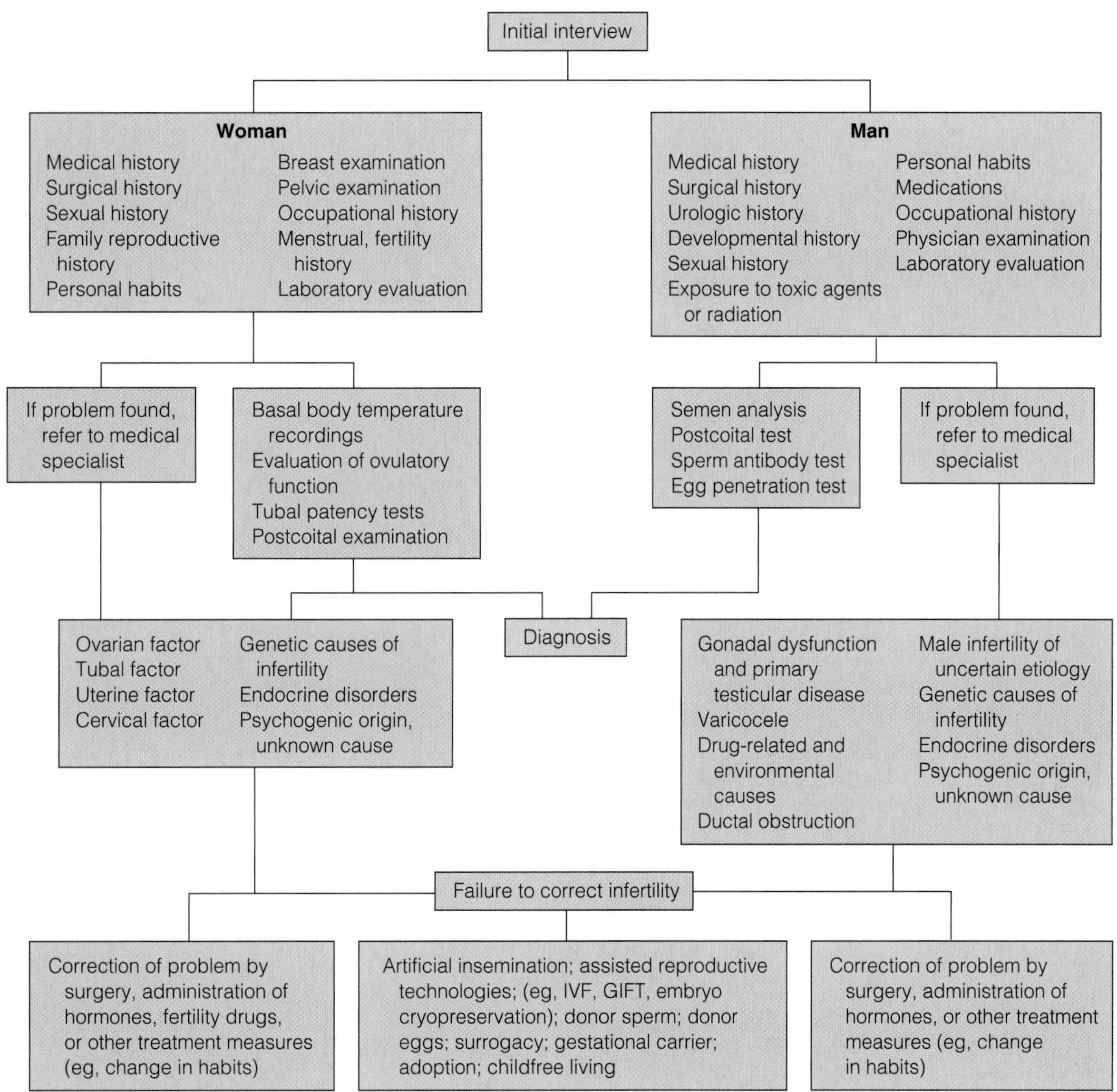

FIGURE 8–1 Flow chart for management of the infertile couple.

The woman should record daily variations on a temperature graph. The temperature graph typically shows a biphasic pattern during ovulatory cycles, whereas in anovulatory cycles it remains monophasic. The woman uses the readings on the temperature graph to detect ovulation and thus to plan the timing of intercourse (Figure 8–3, *A*).

Basal temperature for a woman in the preovulatory phase is usually below 36.7C (98F). As ovulation approaches, production of estrogen increases and at its peak may cause a slight drop, then rise, in the basal temperature. Prior to ovulation, there is a surge of lutenitizing hormone (LH), which stimulates production of progesterone by the corpus luteum, causing a 0.3C to 0.6C (0.5F to 1.0F) rise in basal temperature. These changes in the basal temperature create the typical biphasic pattern. Figure 8–3, *B* shows a biphasic ovulatory BBT chart. Progesterone is thermogenic (produces heat), thereby maintaining the temperature increase during the second half of the menstrual cycle (luteal phase). Temperature elevation does not predict the day of ovulation but provides supportive evidence of ovulation about a day after it has occurred. Actual release of the ovum probably occurs 24 to 36 hours prior to the first temperature elevation (Speroff et al, 1994).

With the additional documentation of coitus, serial BBT charts can be used to indicate retrospectively if, and approximately when, the woman is ovulating and if intercourse is occurring at the proper time to achieve conception. Based on serial BBT charts, the clinician might recommend sexual intercourse *every other day* beginning 3 to 4 days prior to and continuing for 2 to 3 days after the expected time of ovulation.

Hormonal assessments of ovulatory function fall into the following categories:

TABLE 8–3 Female Reproductive Cycle

Ovarian Cycle	Menstrual Cycle
Follicular phase (days 1–14): Primordial follicle matures under influence of FSH and LH up to the time of ovulation. *Luteal phase* (days 15–28): Ovum leaves follicle, corpus luteum develops under LH influence and produces high levels of progesterone and low levels of estrogen.	*Menstrual phase* (days 1–6) *Proliferative phase* (days 7–14): Estrogen peaks just prior to ovulation. Cervical mucus at ovulation is clear, thin, watery, alkaline, and more favorable to sperm; shows ferning pattern; and has spinnbarkheit greater than 8 cm. At ovulation body temperature drops, then rises sharply and remains elevated. *Secretory phase* (days 15–26): Estrogen drops sharply and progesterone dominates. *Ischemic phase* (days 27–28): Both estrogen and progesterone levels drop.

1. *Gonadotropin levels (FSH, LH).* Baseline hormonal assessment of FSH and LH provides valuable information concerning normal ovulatory function. Measured on cycle day 3, FSH is the single most valuable test in assessing ovarian reserve and function and should always be measured, particularly in women over 35, to predict the potential for successful treatment with ovulation induction treatment cycles. High levels predict a very poor outcome for conception and pregnancy (Scott & Hofmann, 1995). LH levels may be measured early in the cycle to rule out disorders associated with androgen excess, causing a disruption in normal follicular development and oocyte maturation. Daily sampling of serum LH at midcycle can detect the LH surge. The day of the LH surge is believed to be the time of maximum fertility. Urine LH ovulation prediction kits are also available for home use to better time postcoital testing, insemination, and coitus (Moghissi, 1998).
2. *Progesterone assays.* Progesterone levels furnish the best evidence of ovulation and corpus luteum function. Serum levels begin to rise with the LH surge and peak about 8 days later. A level of 5 ng/mL 3 days after the LH surge generally confirms ovulation (Moghissi, 1998). On day 21 (7 days postovulation) a level of 10 ng/mL or higher generally indicates an adequate luteal phase.
3. *Prolactin.* Elevated prolactin levels are a frequent cause of ovulatory dysfunction, which may range from a luteal phase defect to anovulation to amenorrhea.
4. *Thyroid stimulating hormone (TSH).* Thyroid hormone is necessary for most body functions, not only metabolism but also specific tissue activities. TSH stimulates prolactin secretion by the pituitary gland (Speroff et al, 1994). Hypothyroidism may have a dramatic effect on ovulatory function and cause menstrual irregularities and bleeding problems.

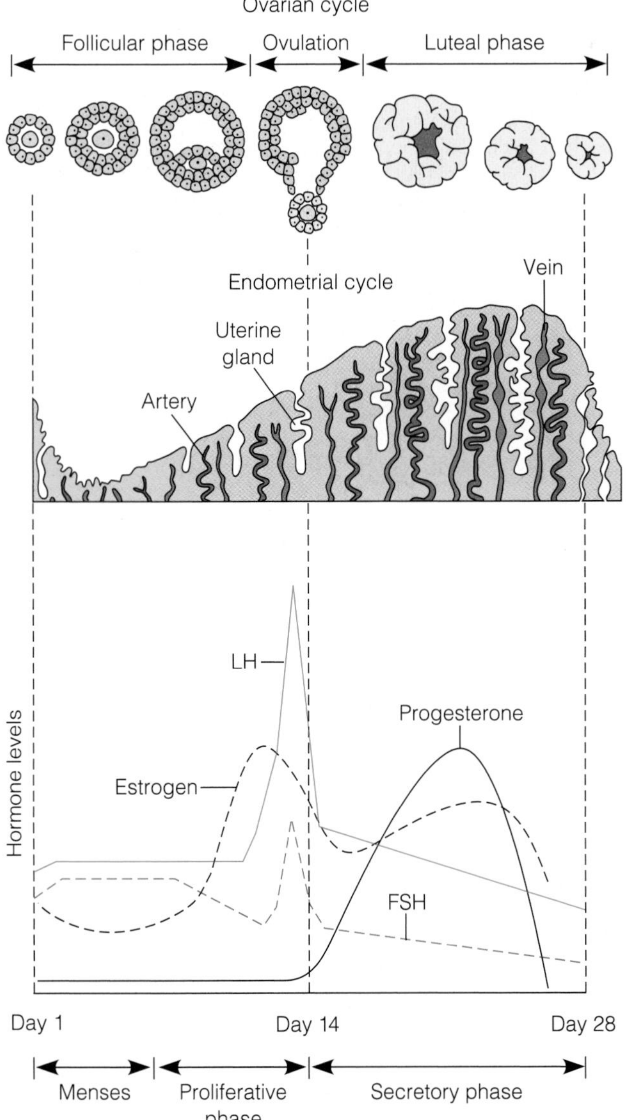

FIGURE 8–2 Sequence of events in a normal reproductive cycle showing the relationship of hormone levels to events in the ovarian and endometrial cycles.

5. *Androgen levels* (testosterone, DHEAS, androstendione). Androgen excess can originate from the adrenal glands, ovaries, or peripheral tissue. Despite the origin, it usually results in specific clinical symptoms such as acne, hirsutism, virilization, and ovulatory dysfunction—which can range from oligomenorrhea to anovulation to amenorrhea.

Endometrial biopsy provides information about the effects of progesterone produced by the corpus luteum after ovulation and endometrial receptivity. The biopsy is performed not earlier than 10 to 12 days after ovulation and involves removing a sample of endometrium with a small pipette attached to suction (Speroff et al, 1994). The woman should be informed that some pelvic discomfort, cramping, and vaginal spotting is normal during and

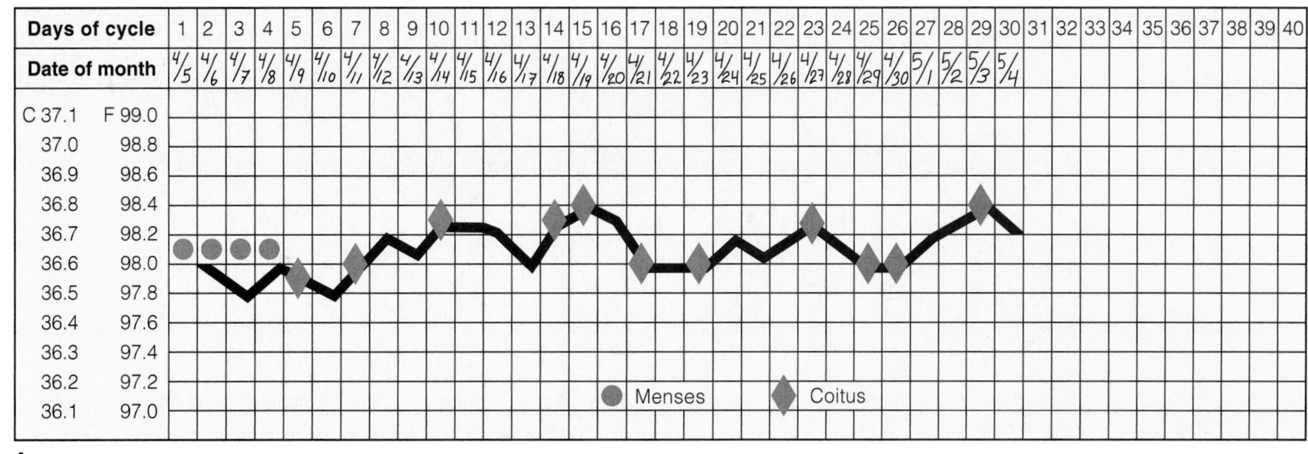

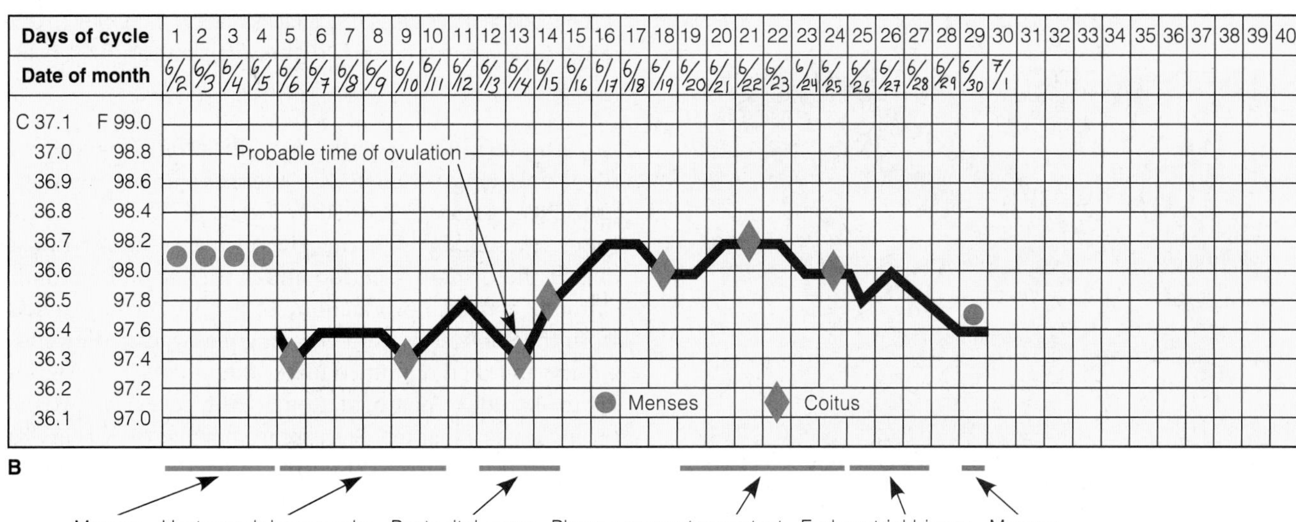

FIGURE 8–3 ***A,*** A monophasic, anovulatory basal body temperature (BBT) chart. ***B,*** A biphasic BBT chart illustrating probable time of ovulation, the different types of testing, and the time in the cycle that each would be performed.

following the procedure. The onset of menses following biopsy should be reported for accurate interpretation of the biopsy report.

A dysfunction may exist if the endometrial lining does not show the expected amount of secretory tissue for that day of the woman's cycle. A repeat biopsy is indicated to confirm luteal phase dysfunction. Serum progesterone levels may also be used in conjunction with endometrial biopsy to confirm adequate luteal phase function.

Transvaginal ultrasound is now an invaluable adjunct in diagnosis and treatment of infertility. Transvaginal ultrasound has rapidly replaced the use of abdominal ultrasounds and is the method of choice for follicular monitoring of women undergoing ovulation induction cycles, for timing ovulation for insemination and intercourse, for retrieving oocytes for in vitro fertilization (IVF), and for monitoring early pregnancy.

The use of transvaginal color flow Doppler to investigate uterine blood flow may in the future help the endocrinologist evaluate the adequacy of the developing follicle, further assessing oocyte maturity and endometrial development and patterns, and improve the diagnosis of luteal phase defect (Moghissi, 1998).

Evaluation of Cervical Factors The cervical mucus cells of the endocervix consist predominately of water. As ovulation approaches, the ovary increases its secretion of estrogen and produces changes in the cervical mucus. The amount of mucus increases tenfold, and the water content rises significantly. At ovulation, mucus elasticity, or **spinnbarkheit,** increases, and the viscosity decreases. Excellent spinnbarkheit exists when the mucus can be stretched 8 to 10 cm or longer (Jewelewicz & Wallach, 1995). This is accomplished by using two glass slides (Figure 8–4, *A*) or by grasping some mucus at the external os and stretching it in the vagina toward the introitus. (See Teaching Guide: Self-Care Methods of Determining Ovulation and the Self-Care Guide: How to Determine Ovulation in the perforated section at the end of this book.)

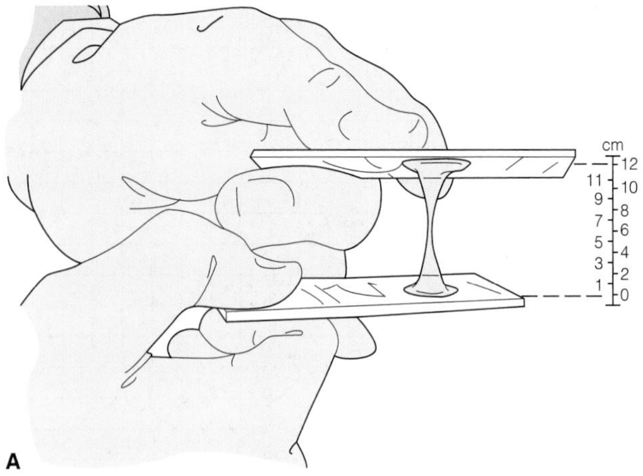

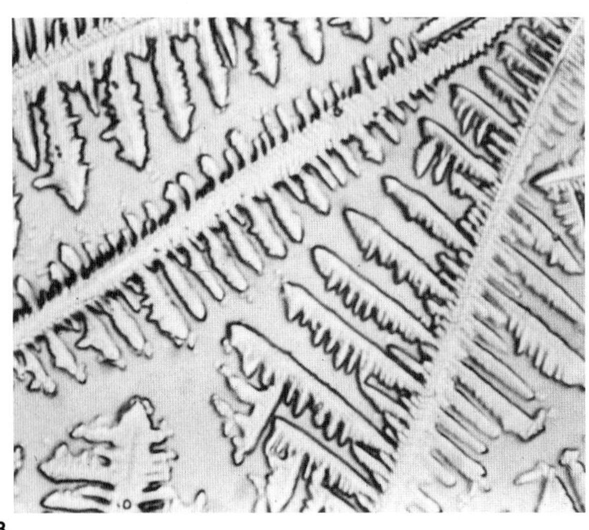
B

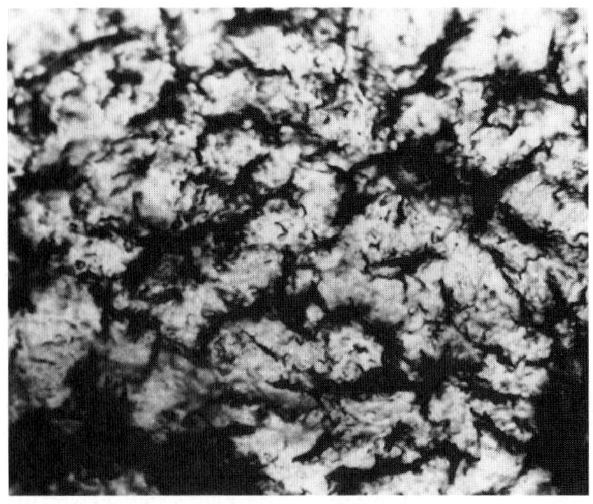
C

FIGURE 8–4 ***A,*** Spinnbarkheit (elasticity). ***B,*** Ferning pattern. ***C,*** Lack of ferning pattern. SOURCE: Speroff L et al: *Clinical Gynecologic Endocrinology and Infertility,* 5th ed. Baltimore: Williams & Wilkins, 1994, p 818.

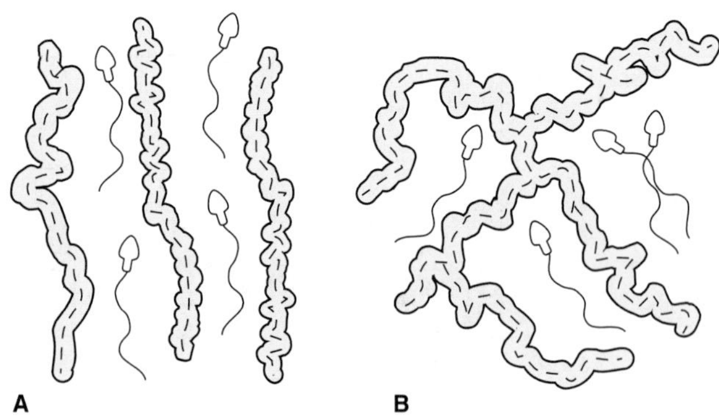

FIGURE 8–5 Sperm passage through cervical mucus. ***A,*** Appearance at the time of ovulation with channels favoring efficient sperm penetration and migration upward. ***B,*** Unfavorable mazelike configuration found at other times of the menstrual cycle. SOURCE: Corson S: *Conquering Infertility.* New York: Prentice Hall, 1990, p 16.

The **ferning capacity** (crystallization) (Figure 8–4, *B*) of the cervical mucus also increases as ovulation approaches. Ferning is caused by *decreased* levels of salt and water interacting with the glycoproteins in the mucus during the ovulatory period and is thus an indirect indication of estrogen production. To test for ferning, mucus from the cervical os is spread on a glass slide, allowed to air dry, and then examined under the microscope. Within 24 to 48 hours postovulation, rising levels of progesterone cause a marked decrease in the quantity of cervical mucus and increase in viscosity and cellularity, resulting in absence of spinnbarkheit and ferning capacity and consequently sperm survival.

To be receptive to sperm, cervical mucus must be thin, clear, watery, profuse, alkaline, and acellular (Geerling, 1995). As shown in Figure 8–5, the mazelike microscopic mucoid strands align in a parallel manner to allow for easy sperm passage. The mucus is termed inhospitable if these changes do not occur.

Cervical mucus inhospitable to sperm survival can have several causes, some of which are treatable. For example, estrogen secretion may be inadequate for the development of receptive mucus. Cervical infection, another cause of mucosal hostility to sperm, can be treated, depending on the type of infection. Cone biopsy, electrocautery, or cryosurgery of the cervix may remove large numbers of mucus-producing glands, creating a "dry cervix" that decreases sperm survival. Finally, treatment with clomiphene citrate may have deleterious effects on cervical mucus due to its antiestrogenic properties. Therapy with supplemental estrogen for approximately 6 days before expected ovulation is sometimes employed to encourage formation of suitable spinnbarkheit (Speroff et al, 1994). However, intrauterine insemination (IUI) is more often the most appropriate therapy to overcome these obstacles. Profuse mucus is necessary for a hospitable sperm environment. The cervix can also be the site of secretory immunologic reactions in which antisperm antibodies are produced, causing agglutination or

Assessment Focus on the woman's knowledge of her own body functions, mucus secretions, and menstrual cycle.

Nursing Diagnoses The essential nursing diagnoses will probably be ***Self-Care Deficit*** related to lack of knowledge of normal body changes occurring with menstruation and ovulation; ***Ineffective Individual Coping*** related to inexperience with self-care measures for determining fertile days.

Nursing Plan and Implementation The teaching plan will include information on expected changes in cervical mucus and body temperature related to menstrual cycle, how to recognize that ovulation has occurred, and self-care methods for determining fertility days.

Client Goals At the completion of teaching, the woman will be able to:

- Accurately identify cervical mucus changes
- Accurately take and record BBT
- Discuss the changes in BBT and cervical mucus that indicate ovulation has occurred
- Summarize physical symptoms that may indicate ovulation has occurred.

Teaching Plan

Content	*Teaching Method*
Basal Body Temperature (BBT) Method	
• Explain that BBT relies on assessing the woman's temperature pattern to determine ovulation.	*Explain why BBT can predict ovulation.*
• Describe the procedure for determining BBT; instruct the woman to record her temperature on a special BBT chart.	*Photocopy the Self-Care Guide at the end of the book that describes the procedure and the findings. Ask the woman to follow along. Demonstrate the BBT thermometer and chart.*
• Describe the expected findings	*Provide pictures of the anovulation cycle and the biphasic cycle.*
• Explain that certain situations can disturb body temperature: excessive alcohol intake, sleeplessness, gastrointestinal or other febrile illness, immunizations, warm or hot climate, jet lag, shift work, or use of electric blanket.	
Cervical Mucus Method	
• Explain that cervical mucus changes throughout the woman's menstrual cycle and that the quality of the mucus can be evaluated to predict ovulation.	*Discuss the rationale for the physical changes. Encourage the woman to ask questions. Use the Self-Care Guide at the end of the book as a handout.*
• Describe the various qualities of cervical mucus throughout the menstrual cycle.	*Show the woman pictures of mucus changes including spinnbarkheit of differing elasticity.*
• Explain that the presence and consistency of the mucus is altered by vaginal infection, vaginal medications such as creams or suppositories, spermicides, lubricants, douching, sexual arousal, or semen.	

➤

Teaching Plan

Content	*Teaching Method*

Other Methods

- Describe other physical findings that may indicate ovulation: slight vaginal spotting, *mittelschmertz,* increased libido.

Evaluation Teaching has been effective if you discussed the BBT and the cervical mucus changes associated with ovulation, demonstrated the BBT procedure and charting of BBT and cervical mucus changes and the woman feels comfortable with BBT and cervical mucus procedure and completion of charting. The woman will be able to describe her body functions, how they change, and how they can be used to identify fertile periods and the time at which ovulation may occur.

---

immobilization of sperm. The most widely used serum sperm bioassay to detect specific classes of antibodies in serum and seminal fluid is immunobead testing by RIA. The treatment for antisperm antibodies may include intrauterine insemination of the male's washed sperm to bypass the cervical factor.

The postcoital test (PCT), also called the **Huhner test,** is performed 1 or 2 days before the expected date of ovulation by previous BBT charts, the length of prior cycles, or urinary LH kit. This examination evaluates the cervical mucus, sperm motility, sperm-mucus interaction, and the sperm's ability to negotiate the cervical mucus barrier (Tredway, 1996).

The couple is asked to have intercourse 8 to 12 hours before examination. The optimal time for the exam is 2 to 3 hours after coitus. A small plastic catheter attached to a 10-mL syringe is placed in the cervix. Mucus is aspirated from the endocervical canal, measured, and examined microscopically for signs of infection, spinnbarkheit, ferning, number of active spermatozoa per high-power field (HPF), and number of sperm with poor or no motility. Because the postcoital exam focuses attention on the timing of intercourse, it has the potential for causing difficulties in the couple's sexual relationship unless the infertile couple has a satisfying sexual relationship (Oei et al, 1996).

Evaluation of Uterine Structures and Tubal Patency Tubal patency tests are usually done after BBT evaluation, semen analysis, and the other less invasive tests have been done and evaluated. Tubal patency and uterine structure are usually evaluated by hysterosalpingography. Other invasive tests of the tubes' function are laparoscopy and hysteroscopy. Hysteroscopy may be performed earlier in the evaluation if the woman's history suggests the potential for tubal or adhesive disease or uterine abnormalities.

Hysterosalpingography (HSG), or hysterogram, involves an instillation of a radiopaque substance into the uterine cavity. As the substance fills the uterus and fallopian tubes and spills into the peritoneal cavity, it is viewed with x-ray techniques. This procedure can reveal tubal patency and any distortions of the uterine cavity. In addition, the water-based dye used in HSG may have a therapeutic effect. This effect may be caused by the flushing of debris, breaking of peritoneal adhesions, stimulation of cilia by the instillation, or improvement of cervical mucus because the iodine may exert a bacteriostatic effect on the mucous membranes and decrease phagocytosis of sperm (Karande et al, 1995).

The hysterosalpingogram should be performed in the follicular phase of the cycle to avoid interrupting an early pregnancy. This timing also avoids the lush secretory changes in the endometrium that occur after ovulation, which may prevent the passage of the dye through the tubes and present a false picture of cornual obstruction. Hysterosalpingography causes moderate discomfort. The pain is referred from the peritoneum (which is irritated by the subdiaphragmatic collection of gas) to the shoulder. The cramping may be decreased if the radiopaque dye is warmed to body temperature before instillation. Women can take an over-the-counter prostaglandin synthesis inhibitor (such as ibuprofen) 30 minutes prior to the procedure to decrease the pain, cramping, and discomfort. HSG can also cause serious recurrence of pelvic inflammatory disease, so prophylactic antibiotics are recommended to prevent infection that could be triggered by the procedure (Corson, 1995).

Hysteroscopy allows the physician to further evaluate any areas of suspicion within the uterine cavity revealed by HSG. It is often done in conjunction with a laparoscopy but can be done independently in the office and does not require general anesthesia. A fiberoptic instrument is placed into the uterus for further evaluation of polyps, myomata (fibroids), or structural variations (Speroff et al, 1994).

Laparoscopy enables direct visualization of the pelvic organs and is usually done 6 to 8 months after HSG unless symptoms or findings suggest the need for earlier evaluation. Diagnostic laporascopy is an outpatient procedure requiring the use of general anesthesia. Generally, a three-puncture approach is used; entry is made through the umbilical area, and supporting instruments are inserted in two suprapubic incisions. The peritoneal cavity is distended with carbon dioxide gas, and the pelvic organs can be directly visualized with a fiberoptic instrument. Tube patency can be assessed by instilling dye into the uterine cavity through the cervix. The pelvis is evaluated for endometriosis, adhesions, organ fixations, pelvic inflammatory disease, tumors, and cysts. The intraperitoneal gas is usually manually expressed at the end of the procedure. In routine preanesthesia instructions, the woman is told that she may have some discomfort from organ displacement and shoulder to chest pain caused by gas in the abdomen. She should be informed that she can resume normal activities as tolerated after 24 hours. Using postoperative pain medication and assuming a supine position may help relieve residual shoulder and chest discomfort caused by any remaining gas.

Assessment of the Man

The semen analysis is the single most important diagnostic study of the man. It should be done early in the couple's evaluation and prior to invasive testing of the woman. Although a postcoital test can provide information about sperm viability, it does not provide sufficient information concerning normal seminal parameters.

To obtain accurate results, the specimen is collected after 2 to 3 days of abstinence and usually by masturbation to avoid contamination or loss of any ejaculate. If the man has difficulty producing sperm by masturbation, special medical grade condoms are available to collect the sperm during intercourse. Regular or nonlatex condoms should not be used because they contain spermicidal agents, and sperm can be lost in the condom. Most lubricants also are spermicidal and should not be used unless approved by the andrology laboratory (Jeyendran, 1998). There may be seasonal as well as incidental variability in count and motility seen in successive semen samples from the same individual. Thus, a repeat semen analysis may be required to assess the man's fertility potential adequately; a minimum of two separate analyses is recommended for confirmation. In the case where a known testicular insult has occurred, such as infection, high fevers, or surgery, a repeat analysis may not be done for at least 2.5 months to allow for new sperm maturation.

Semen analysis provides information about sperm motility and morphology as well as a determination of the absolute number of spermatozoa present (Table 8–4). Debate exists over absolute number and motility of sperm for fertility. Although it is known that low numbers and motility may indicate compromised fertility, other parameters such as morphology, motion patterns, and progression, are important prognostic indicators. Values previously thought to indicate subfertility may in fact be compatible with normal fertility when these factors are considered. An infertile specimen is one that reveals fewer than 20 million sperm per mL, less than 50% motility at 6 hours, or less than 50% normal sperm forms (World Health Organization, 1992). Some studies have indicated that the quality of sperm decreases with increased age. Infants born to 50- to 60-year-old fathers are at risk for trisomy 21 (Speroff et al, 1994).

Treatment of seminal deficiency is directed toward correcting any anatomic or endocrine problems with medical or surgical intervention. In many cases this is not possible, and treatment is directed toward compensating for the seminal deficiency. Treatment options depend on the severity of the seminal problem and may include intrauterine insemination with washed sperm collected from the partner, artificial insemination with donor sperm, or utilization of the assisted reproductive technologies (ARTs).

A variety of environmental factors can affect male fertility. Causes of increased scrotal heat, such as jockey shorts, hot tubs, or occupations requiring long hours of sitting, are thought to decrease fertility potential, but there are no clinical studies to substantiate this belief. Heavy use of marijuana, alcohol, or cocaine within 2 years of testing can depress sperm count and testosterone levels; cigarette smoking may depress sperm motility. Neurologic ejaculatory dysfunction can be caused by alpha blockers, phentolamine, methyldopa, quanethidine,

TABLE 8–4 Normal Semen Analysis

Factor	Value
Volume	>2 mL
pH	7.0 to 8.0
Total sperm count	>20 million/mL
Liquefaction	Complete in 1 hour
Motility	50% or greater
Normal forms	30% or greater

SOURCE: *The WHO Labratory Manual for the Examination of Human Semen and Sperm-Cervical Mucus Interaction,* 3rd ed. Geneva: WHO, 1993.

and reserpine (Speroff et al, 1998). Lead and pesticide exposure can also reduce sperm count (Hatcher et al, 1998).

Spermatozoa have been shown to possess intrinsic antigens that can provoke male immunologic infertility. This is especially apparent following vasectomy reversals or genital trauma, such as testicular torsion, in which autoimmunity to sperm develops (the man produces antibodies to his own sperm). Research now indicates that it is the actual presence of antibodies on the spermatozoal surface, not just the presence of antibodies in the serum, that affects sperm function and thus leads to subfertility. Treatment for antisperm antibodies is directed toward preventing the formation of antibodies or arresting the underlying mechanism that compromises sperm function. Different therapies that have been used, such as immunosuppression with corticosteroids and intrauterine insemination, have not proved effective. The treatment of choice for clinically significant antisperm antibodies is IVF (Jeyendran, 1998).

Methods of Managing Infertility

Pharmacologic Methods

If an ovulatory defect has been identified during fertility testing, the treatment depends on the specific cause of the problem. In the presence of normal ovaries, a normal prolactin level, and an intact pituitary gland, *clomiphene citrate* (Clomid, Serophene) is often used. See Drug Guide: Clomiphene Citrate. Clomiphene citrate acts by competing with estrogen receptor sites at the level of the hypothalamus, the pituitary, and the ovary, thus increasing secretion of FSH and LH, which stimulates follicular growth. This medication induces ovulation in 80% of women by actions at both the hypothalamic and ovarian levels; 40% of these women will become pregnant. Approximately 5% of women develop multiple gestation pregnancies, almost exclusively twins (Speroff et al, 1994).

The woman takes 50 to 250 mg per day orally for 5 days starting from day 3 to 5 after last menses (Hammond, 1996). The woman usually starts with 50 mg per day and, if there is no response, increases the dose by 50 mg per day to a maximum of 200 to 250 mg. The clinician may need to give estrogen simultaneously if cervical mucus decreases.

The woman is informed that if ovulation occurs, it is expected to occur 5 to 10 days after the last dose. The presence of ovulation and evaluation of the response to therapy is assessed by BBT or urinary LH kit monitoring for in-home use, ultrasound evaluation, and possibly progesterone assays in conjunction with an endometrial biopsy.

After the first treatment cycle, a pelvic exam should be done to rule out ovarian enlargement or hyperstimulation. The risk of ovarian hyperstimulation is reported to be 10% but is rarely as severe as that reported with menotropins (gonadotropin therapy). Ovarian enlargement and abdominal discomfort (bloating) may result from follicular growth and the formation of multiple corpus lutea. Persistence of ovarian cysts is a contraindication for subsequent treatment cycle. Other side effects include hot flashes, abdominal distention, bloating, breast discomfort, nausea and vomiting, vision problems, headache, and dryness or loss of hair (Hammond, 1996). Some women experience severe mood swings (Bambi-Hitler syndrome). Supplemental low-dose estrogen may be given to ensure appropriate quality and quantity of cervical mucus, or IUI may be employed to overcome this obstacle.

The nurse determines if the couple has been advised to have sexual intercourse every other day for 1 week beginning 5 days after the last day of medications. The nurse also reminds couples that if the woman doesn't have a period she must be checked for pregnancy before another trial of clomiphene is started.

Self-Care Measures for Clomiphene Citrate (Clomid)

Women can assess the presence of ovulation and possible response to clomiphene therapy by doing BBT and urinary LH tests. The woman should be knowledgeable about side effects and call her health care provider if they occur. When visual disturbances (flashes, blurring, spots) occur, the woman should avoid bright lighting. This side effect disappears within a few days or weeks after discontinuation of therapy (Speroff et al, 1994). The occurrence of hot flashes may be due to the antiestrogenic properties of clomiphene. The woman can obtain some relief through increasing intake of fluids and using fans. Table 8–5 lists some of the drugs commonly used to treat infertility.

Therapy using *human menopausal gonadotropins (hMG),* which include menotropins (Pergonal, Humegon, Repronex) and urofollitropin (Fertinex), is indicated as a first line of therapy for the anovulatory infertile woman with low to normal levels of gonadotropins (FSH and LH) and as a second line of therapy in women who

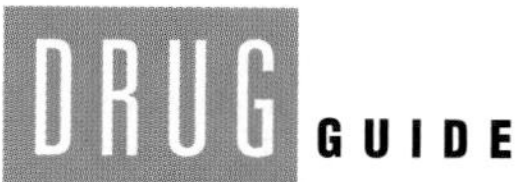

Clomiphene Citrate (Clomid, Serophene)

Overview of Action

Clomid stimulates follicular growth by stimulating the release of FSH and LH. Ovulation is expected to occur 5 to 9 days after last dose. Used when anovulation is caused by hypothalamic dysfunction, luteal phase dysfunction, or oligo-ovulation, and for in vitro fertilization protocols.

Route, Dosage, Frequency

Administered orally. Fifty mg/day to 250 mg/day from day 5 to day 9 (total of 5 days) of the menstrual cycle. Usually start with 50 mg/day and increase dose 50 mg if no response, to a maximum of 250 mg (Speroff et al, 1994). May need to give estrogen simultaneously if decrease in cervical mucus occurs.

Contraindications

Presence of ovarian enlargement, ovarian cysts, hyperstimulation syndrome, liver disease, visual problems, pregnancy.

Side Effects

Antiestrogenic effects may cause decrease in cervical mucus production and endometrial lining development. Other side effects include vasomotor flushes; abdominal distention and ovarian enlargement secondary to follicular growth and development and multiple corpus luteum formation; bloating, pain, soreness, breast discomfort; nausea and vomiting; visual symptoms (spots, flashes); headaches; dryness or loss of hair; multiple pregnancies.

Nursing Considerations

Determine if couple has been advised to have sexual intercourse every other day for 1 week beginning 5 days after the last day of medications.

Instruct couple on use of BBT chart to assess whether ovulation has occurred, or instruct on the use of urinary LH kits to predict the onset of LH surge. Also inform couple that plasma progesterone, cervical mucus, and postcoital test may be done. Remind couples that if the woman doesn't have a period, she must be checked for the possibility of pregnancy before another trial of Clomid is started.

fail to ovulate or conceive with clomiphene citrate therapy and in women undergoing assisted reproduction to induce superovulation. Menotropin is a mixture of FSH and LH in a 1:1 ratio, and urofollitropin is further purified and contains only FSH. Both are natural hormones extracted from the urine of postmenopausal women, purified, and freeze-dried into a powder. HMG is inactive and therefore must be given by intramuscular injection. Immediately prior to injection, the powder is reconstituted with diluent. More recently, however, recombinant FSH has been produced through genetic engineering, giving rise to more consistent preparation. It has been approved by the Food and Drug Administration (FDA) for use where ovulation induction therapy is indicated. Recombinant FSH is homogenous and free of contaminants by proteins (unlike urinary menotropins) and thus allows for subcutaneous administration. It is marketed under the name Gonal-F (follitropin alpha) or Follistim (follitropin beta). Current investigations using recombinant LH are being tested and expected to be FDA approved for clinical use in the near future. It is thought that the use of recombinant gonadotropins will eventually become the preferred preparation and that the use of urinary preparations will be phased out.

Normal functioning of the pituitary is not necessary with menotropins or urofollitropin because their mechanisms of action are direct stimulation of follicular development in the ovary, thus totally bypassing the hypothalamic/pituitary axis. However, normal ovarian reserve and functioning are necessary to ensure that follicles can be stimulated by FSH and LH. As previously described, the single most valuable tests to assess ovarian reserve and function is the FSH level, with elevated levels being a poor prognostic sign for conception and pregnancy.

Menotropins (FSH, LH) are the primary preparations used for therapy. Urofollitropin (FSH only) is indicated for women who have excessive androgen production, such as those with polycystic ovary disease (PCO). Clients with PCO have high endogenous LH levels, and urofollitropin, which is predominantly FSH, is used to equalize the hormonal ratio and induce ovulation.

Gonadotropin therapy requires close observation with serum estradiol levels and ultrasound. Follicle development must be monitored in order to minimize the risk of multiple pregnancy and to avoid ovarian hyperstimulation syndrome. The daily dose of medication given is titrated based on serum estradiol and ultrasound findings. When follicle maturation has occurred, hCG may be administered by intramuscular injection to stimulate ovulation. The couple is advised to have intercourse 24 to 36 hours after hCG administration and for the next 2 days. The multiple birth rate is reported to be about 20%, with less than 1% resulting in multiples greater than triplets. Women who elect to have hMG medication usually have

TABLE 8–5 Drugs Commonly Used to Treat Infertility

Drugs	Indications	
	Women	**Men**
Clomiphene citrate (Clomid, Serophene)	Polycystic ovarian disease (3 days, beginning day 5 of bleeding) Hyperandrogenemia (with no neoplasia) Premature follicular rupture	Low levels of gonadotropins Hypothalamic hypogonadism
Bromocriptine mesylate (Parlodel)	Hyperprolactinemia (functional or pituitary adenoma)	Hyperprolactinemia (functional or pituitary adenoma)
Progesterone	Luteal phase dysfunction	
hMG, menotropins (FSH and LH) (Pergonal) with hCG	Hypothalamic ovulatory dysfunction (after failure of clomiphene) Hypopituitarism Polycystic ovarian disease (rarely) Luteinized unruptured follicle syndrome (after failure of hCG alone) Inadequate cervical mucus In vitro fertilization, GIFT, ZIFT Controlled superovulation	Hypothalamic-pituitary failure due to Kallmann's syndrome or delayed puberty Hypogonadotropic hypogonadism (deficiency of FSH and LH)
hCG	Luteinized unruptured follicle syndrome Induction of ovulation	
FSH, urofollitropin (Metrodin) with hCG	Polycystic ovarian disease	
C_rFSH, follitropin (Gonal F, Follistim) with hCG	In vitro fertilization, GIFT, ZIFT	
GnRH (Factrel)	Hypothalamic ovulatory dysfunction (pulsed infusion)	Hypothalamic-pituitary failure due to Kallmann's syndrome or delayed puberty (pulsed infusion)
GnRH agonist Leuoprolide acetate (Lupron) Nafarelin acetate (Synarel)	Endometriosis Premature follicular rupture In vitro fertilization, GIFT, ZIFT	Hypogonadotropic gonadism

SOURCE: Adapted from Shane J: Evaluation and treatment of infertility. *Clin Symp* 1993; 45:2.

passed through all other forms of management without conceiving. Strong emotional support and thorough education are needed because of the numerous office visits and injections. Often the male partner is instructed, with return demonstration, to administer the daily injections.

When hyperprolactinemia accompanies anovulation, the infertility may be treated with *bromocriptine.* This medication acts directly on the prolactin-secreting cells in the anterior pituitary. It inhibits the pituitary's secretion of prolactin—thus preventing suppression of the pulsatile secretion of FSH and LH. This restores normal menstrual cycles and induces ovulation by allowing FSH and LH production. High prolactin levels may impair production of FSH and LH or block their action on the ovaries. If treatment is successful, the tests of ovulatory function will indicate that ovulation is occurring with a normal luteal phase. Bromocriptine should be discontinued if pregnancy is suspected or at the anticipated time of ovulation because of its possible teratogenic effects. Other side effects include nausea, diarrhea, dizziness, headache, fatigue, and can be attributed to the dopaminergic action of bromocriptine. To mimimize side effects for women who are extremely sensitive, treatment may be initiated with a dose of 2.5 mg, slowly building tolerance toward the usual dose of 2.5 mg bid. Intravaginal administration also has been shown to decrease the occurrence of side effects.

When endometriosis is determined to be the cause of the infertility, *danazol* (Danocrine) may be given to suppress ovulation and menstruation and to effect atrophy of the ectopic endometrial tissue. Temporary suppression has been shown to result in healing of the endometriosis. The treatment regimen may last for 6 to 12 months or longer, depending on the severity of the disease. Other pharmacologic treatments involve use of the oral contraceptives or oral medroxyprogesterone acetate, and gonadotropin-releasing hormone (GnRH) agonists (Brosens, 1997). Medical management of endometriosis and long-term plan for therapy should be based on the individual needs of the woman, including severity of symptoms, the extent of the disease, the woman's age, and desire for fertility. For in-depth discussion of the management and care needed for endometriosis, see Chapter 3.

Gonadotropin-releasing hormone (GnRH) is a therapeutic tool for inducing ovulation, but its use is rare. It is used for women who have insufficient endogenous release of GnRH. Administration is usually by continuous intravenous infusion accomplished by a portable infusion pump with a pulsatile mechanism worn on a belt around the waist. The length of treatment varies from 2 to 4 weeks, and hCG is also given to stimulate ovulation. The risk of multiple gestation and hyperstimulation of the ovaries is less than with hMG therapy, and the treatment is also less expensive (Speroff et al, 1994). Significant client education and support are necessary for effective use of the pump. Some women find the pump cumbersome.

Treatment of luteal phase defects may include the use of progesterone to augment luteal phase progesterone levels or the use of ovulation induction agents, such as clomiphene citrate or menotropins (discussed previously), which will augment proliferative phase FSH production of the developing follicle. Women with luteal phase defects have been found to have decreased FSH production in the proliferative phase. This is associated with a decline in luteal phase progesterone and estrogen production and is manifested by an out-of-phase endometrial biopsy. It is also common to use progesterone supplementation in conjunction with these ovulation induction agents if the drug alone does not correct the luteal phase. Occasionally, hCG therapy may be used in the luteal phase to stimulate corpus luteum production of progesterone.

Artificial Insemination

Artificial insemination with either the partner's semen (*AIH*) or the semen of a donor (*AID*) involves depositing sperm at the cervical os or in the uterus by mechanical means. Therapeutic donor insemination (*TDI*) is the current nomenclature used rather than AID (Speroff et al, 1994).

AIH is generally indicated for such seminal deficiencies as oligospermia (low sperm count), asthenospermia (decreased motility), and teratospermia (low percentage, abnormal morphology); for anatomic defects that are accompanied by inadequate deposition of sperm, such as hypospadias (a congenital abnormal male urethral opening on the underside of the penis); and for ejaculatory dysfunction, such as retrograde ejaculation (Corson, 1995). AIH is also indicated in unexplained infertility and some cases of female factor infertility, specifically infertility due to cervical factors, such as scant or inhospitable mucus, persistent cervicitis, or cervical stenosis. In such cases, intrauterine insemination (IUI) would be indicated in order to bypass the cervical factor. Because the seminal fluid contains high levels of prostaglandins, IUI prevents the violent reaction of nausea, severe cramps, abdominal pain, and diarrhea that can result from the absorption of prostaglandins by the uterine lining (Corson, 1995). Sperm preparation for IUI involves washing sperm from the seminal plasma.

Donor insemination is considered in cases of azoospermia (absence of sperm), severe oligospermia or asthenospermia, inherited male sex-linked disorders, and autosomal dominant disorders (Speroff et al, 1994). In the past several years, indications for donor insemination have expanded to include single women or lesbians desirous of pregnancy. Many states have specified the parental rights of the single woman and the donor, but some continue to remain silent on this issue (Speroff et al, 1994).

Donor insemination has become more complicated and expensive in the last decade because of the need for strict screening and processing procedures to prevent transmission of a genetic defect or sexually transmitted infection to the offspring or recipient. Guidelines established by the American Fertility Society (1994) include mandatory medical and infectious disease screening of both donor and recipient, the need for informed consent from all parties, the need to limit the number of pregnancies per donor, and the need to establish an accurate means of record keeping. Finally, because of the risk of transmitting infectious disease, donated sperm must be frozen and quarantined for 6 months from the time of acquisition and the donor retested at this time before sperm can be released for use. Before AIDS was discovered, fresh semen was used.

With the use of frozen sperm, pregnancy rates with donor insemination are somewhat lower per cycle because the freezing process causes loss of motility in 15% to 20% of the sperm. The usual number of cycles required to initiate pregnancy in a couple with only a male infertility factor is approximately six. Couples who fail to conceive after six to eight cycles of well-timed inseminations require further evaluation and/or aggressive therapy, such as the ARTs.

Numerous factors must be evaluated before AID is performed. Has every possible effort been made to diagnose and treat the cause of the male infertility? Do tests indicate normal ovulation and sperm/ovum transport in the woman? Has the couple had an opportunity to discuss this option with an infertility counselor to explore the issues of secrecy, disclosure, and potential feelings of loss that the couple (particularly the male partner) may feel because of their inability to have a genetic child? After making the decision, the couple should allow themselves time to assess their concerns further and explore their feelings individually and together to ensure that this option is acceptable to both. Couples need to consider how they will feel if the child is born with a congenital anomaly. Congenital anomalies occur in 4% to 5% of all pregnancies, irrespective of whether they result from spontaneous conception or therapeutic insemination.

Intrauterine insemination (IUI), with or without ovulation induction therapy, is an option for many couples before more aggressive treatments, such as in vitro fertilization (IVF) and gamete intrafallopian transfer (GIFT) are employed. Success rates range from 10% to 25%, depending on indications for use and the woman's age.

CRITICAL THINKING QUESTION

Some adult children who were conceived by TDI are now wanting to meet their biological fathers. What issues does this raise for prospective donors, infertility clinics, and TDI conceived children? What would you say to an adolescent who tells you he wants to meet his biological father?

In Vitro Fertilization

In vitro fertilization (IVF) is selectively used in cases in which infertility has resulted from tubal factors, mucus abnormalities, male infertility, unexplained infertility, male and female immunologic infertility, and cervical factors. In IVF, a woman's eggs are collected from her ovaries, fertilized in the laboratory, and placed into her uterus after normal embryo development has begun. If the procedure is successful, the embryo continues to develop in the uterus, and pregnancy proceeds naturally.

The potential for a successful pregnancy with IVF is maximized by replacing three to four embryos rather than only one. For this reason, fertility drugs are used to induce ovulation. Follicular development and oocyte maturity are monitored frequently with ultrasound and hormonal assays. Monitoring usually begins around cycle day 5, and medications are titrated according to individual response. When the follicles appear mature, hCG is given to stimulate final egg maturation and control the induction of ovulation. Egg retrieval is performed approximately 35 hours later.

In the majority of cases, egg retrieval is performed by a transvaginal approach under ultrasound guidance. It is an outpatient procedure performed with intravenous sedation and a cervical block for anesthesia. A needle guide that helps direct the aspirating needle through the posterior vaginal wall into the follicle is attached to the vaginal ultrasound probe. Many follicles can be aspirated with only one puncture, and the procedure generally lasts no more than 30 minutes. The woman usually tolerates the procedure well and is discharged to home within 2 hours with instructions for limited activity for 24 hours.

Once identified, the oocytes are evaluated for maturity and incubated for a period of time prior to insemination. The gametes are incubated in a specially prepared culture medium supplemented with serum to provide nutrients. Fertilization should occur within 18 to 24 hours. Once it is documented, the fertilized eggs are transferred to growth medium and incubated for another 24 to 48 hours, at which time embryo development is assessed.

Embryo replacement is procedurally much like an IUI. After the procedure, the woman is advised to engage in only minimal activity for 12 to 24 hours, and progesterone supplementation is prescribed.

Success with IVF depends on many factors, the two most important of which are the woman's age and the indication. Women with an average of three cycles of IVF have a good chance of achieving pregnancy. Many couples find the emotional, physical, and financial costs of going beyond three cycles too great (Speroff et al, 1994). Clinical delivery rates reported by the Society of Assisted Reproductive Technology (SART) in 1995 were 25.1% per embryo transfer for women regardless of age or indication (Centers for Disease Control and Prevention [CDC], 1997). It should be noted that some centers show increased maternal and neonatal morbidity associated with IVF because of the multiple gestation rates of 15% to 30% (Tallo et al, 1995).

Other Assisted Reproductive Techniques

GIFT and ZIFT **Gamete intrafallopian transfer (GIFT),** developed in 1984, involves the retrieval of oocytes by laparoscopy; immediate placement of the oocytes in a catheter with washed, motile sperm; and placement of the gametes into the fimbriated end of the fallopian tube. Fertilization occurs in the fallopian tube as with normal conception (in vivo), rather than in the laboratory (in vitro). The fertilized egg then travels through the fallopian tube to the uterus for implantation as in normal reproduction. This practice is acceptable to the Catholic church (Robertson, 1995).

GIFT has proven to be a very effective therapy for couples whose infertility results from various seminal deficiencies, unexplained infertility, cervical factors, immunologic factors, and endometriosis when less aggressive means of therapy have failed. In cases of male factor infertility, GIFT offers an opportunity for the egg and an adequate concentration of sperm to meet in the fallopian tube; with coitus, in contrast, sperm with low count or motility may never reach the tube.

The major prerequisite for GIFT is the presence of at least one normal fallopian tube. It is not an appropriate therapy for any woman with a history of PID, tubal disease, or ectopic gestation because the passage of the fertilized ova to the uterus is slowed, thereby increasing the chance of sustaining an ectopic tubal pregnancy.

From the GIFT technology evolved procedures such as **zygote intrafallopian transfer (ZIFT)** and tubal embryo transfer (TET). These procedures involve retrieving oocytes under ultrasound guidance, followed by in vitro fertilization and laparoscopic replacement of the fertilized eggs (ZIFT) or embryos (TET) into the fimbriated end of the fallopian tube. In theory, GIFT, ZIFT, and TET have all been thought to yield higher pregnancy rates because, unlike IVF, these procedures involve placing the conceptus in the fallopian tube, where the environment is more conducive to normal embryo development and implantation than that of a laboratory. However, with refined laboratory culture techniques, IVF success rates approximate those that have been achieved with the GIFT procedure. Moreover, IVF is a much less invasive and costly procedure. For these reasons, GIFT and other tubal procedures have lost some acceptance, and IVF techniques are more often employed.

Embryo Cryopreservation Research has shown that replacing three to four embryos in a treatment cycle offers the best chances for pregnancy. Replacing more than four increases only the chance for a multiple pregnancy (Wolf, 1998). To minimize this risk, excess embryos may be stored using freezing, or cryopreservation. Should a pregnancy not ensue, frozen embryos can be thawed. After they are maintained in culture for a short time to confirm resumption of growth, they are replaced in the woman's uterus at the appropriate time in her menstrual cycle. Thus freezing affords the couple another attempt at pregnancy without having to undergo stimulation and egg retrieval.

Ethical issues to consider in this situation include the following: Who has legal custody of the embryos? How long can they be frozen? What options do the couple have in the event of divorce, death of one or both partners, or if they do not wish to use the embryos at a later date? These issues must be addressed with all couples so that they may make informed decisions when executing their consent forms and legal statements (Robertson, 1995). Perinatal nurses need to be involved in establishing standards and guidelines for assisted reproduction technologies (Jones, 1994). Clinically, the perinatal nurse is instrumental in providing support, education, and counseling to couples considering assisted reproductive methods. The nurse assesses the couple for personal, marital, and parenting difficulties and initiates interventions that help establish family roles and bonds. Follow-up care mechanisms can be set, thereby aiding in individual growth, marital stability, and family development.

In Vitro Fertilization Utilizing Donor Oocytes The use of donor eggs, a natural extension of IVF, is reserved for women who do not produce viable eggs because of premature ovarian failure, surgical removal of the ovaries, advanced maternal age, or inherent oocyte defects but who do have a functional uterus. Women with normal ovarian function may also benefit from egg donation if they have an autosomal dominant or sex-linked genetic disorder such as hemophilia or Duchenne muscular dystrophy.

Oocyte donors may be either known or anonymous. In either case, both donors and recipients undergo extensive psychologic evaluation and counseling to ensure that all parties have explored and discussed potential issues and are comfortable with the process. The nurse functions as a case manager by coordinating the many tests, procedures, and educational and counseling sessions that are involved for the donor and recipient couple.

Once donor eggs are available, they are inseminated with the sperm of the recipient's partner. After fertilization has occurred and embryo development has begun, the embryos are placed in the recipient's uterus. Pregnancies can be achieved and maintained in these women with an estrogen/progesterone replacement protocol. When pregnancy occurs, hormonal support is continued until the placenta is capable of supporting the pregnancy, usually at 10 to 12 weeks.

Micromanipulation and Blastomere Analysis Micromanipulation allows individual eggs and sperm to be handled through the use of very fine, specialized instruments. Using the micromanipulators allows the clinician to handle cells under the microscope with magnification of 200 to 400 times and to inject a sperm cell directly into an egg. This procedure, known as Intracytoplasmic Sperm Injection (ICSI), has revolutionized the treatment of severe male factor infertility. The procedure has achieved fertilization in cases of extremely low sperm concentrations, absence of motility, sperm aspirated directly from the testis, and in cases where previous IVF therapy failed.

Assisted embryo hatching is another micromanipulation procedure that has proved to be an effective adjunct therapy in IVF. It is indicated for women in whom the normal "hatching" process may be impeded because of a hardening or thickening of the zona pellucida. Assisted hatching involves creating a small opening in the zona pellucida of the embryo using micromanipulators. The small opening may facilitate the natural hatching process, allowing the embryo to escape from the zona pellucida and interact with the endometrium for implantation (Smith & Tucker, 1997).

Other recent advances in micromanipulation allow a single cell to be removed from the embryo for genetic study. Couples at risk for having a detectable single gene or chromosomal anomaly may wish to undergo such preimplantation genetic testing, called blastomere analysis (Pickler & Munro, 1994). The single cell is obtained from a six- to eight-cell embryo by a process known as blastomere biopsy (Speroff et al, 1994). The genetic content of the cell is examined using the polymerase chain reaction (PCR) technique. The cell's DNA is amplified 1,000,000 times and examined so that embryos affected with genetic disease are not placed in the mother. Results of genetic testing on the preimplantation embryos are available in 4 to 24 hours, so unaffected embryos may still be placed during the required biologic window of time without the need for cryopreservation.

The diagnosis of genetic disorders before implantation provides couples with the option of forgoing the attempt to establish a pregnancy and thereby avoiding a difficult decision about terminating an affected pregnancy. This technology also raises several issues, including the following:

- Identification of couples at risk. There is a need for criteria that identify couples at risk for diseases that constitute significant hardship and suffering so that "wrongful birth" cases can be avoided.
- Availability of and access to centers providing blastomere analysis. Should society provide access for those at risk for genetic transfer of disease but without the financial resources to pay for the services?

- Analysis of blastomeres for sex gene testing. In X-linked diseases, the only way to prevent the disorder is to select against the Y chromosome.
- Identification of late-onset diseases. The Human Genome Project has aided in the identification of genetic markers for late-onset disease. Couples may wish to choose to implant blastomeres that do not carry these markers.

In Vitro Fertilization Using a Gestational Carrier IVF utilizing a gestational carrier is appropriate for the infertile woman who is genetically sound but unable to carry a pregnancy due to (1) congenital absence or surgical removal of her uterus; (2) a reproductively impaired uterus, myomas, uterine synechiae (adhesion of uterus), or any other congenital abnormalities; or (3) a medical condition that might be life threatening during pregnancy, such as diabetes, immunologic problems, or a severe heart, kidney, or liver disease (Corson et al, 1998).

Use of a gestational carrier allows a couple with any of these conditions to have their own biologic pregnancy (Pergament & Fiddler, 1996). The couple undergoes the IVF procedure, and the resulting embryos are placed in a woman who has contracted with the infertile woman or couple to carry the child. This must be distinguished from surrogate motherhood, wherein the gestational surrogate mother makes a genetic contribution to the child. In the carrier relationship, the carrier has no genetic investment in the child. All participants are required to have medical and psychologic screening as well as legal counsel prior to acceptance into the program.

CRITICAL THINKING QUESTION

What makes a mother? Does motherhood require genetic, gestational, and social contributions to the child?

Community-Based Nursing Care

Infertility therapy taxes a couple's financial, physical, and emotional resources. Treatment can cost over $20,000 a year, and insurance coverage may be limited. Years of effort and numerous evaluations and examinations may take place before a conception occurs, if one occurs at all. In a society that values children and considers them to be the natural result of marriage, infertile couples may face a myriad of tensions and discrimination.

The clinic nurse needs to be constantly aware of the emotional needs of the couple confronting infertility evaluation and treatment. Often an intact marriage will become stressed with the intrusive but necessary infertility procedures and treatments. Constant attention to temperature charts and instructions about their sex life from a person outside the relationship naturally affect the spontaneity of a couple's interactions. Tests and treatments may heighten feelings of frustration or anger between the couple. The need to share this intimate area of a relationship, especially when one or the other is identified as "the cause" of infertility, may precipitate feelings of guilt or shame.

TABLE 8–6 Tasks of the Infertile Couple

Tasks	Nursing Interventions
Recognize how infertility affects their lives and express feelings (may be negative toward self or mate)	Supportive: help to understand and facilitate free expression of feelings
Grieve the loss of potential offspring	Help to recognize feelings
Evaluate reasons for wanting a child	Help to understand motives
Decide about management	Identify alternatives; facilitate partner communication

SOURCE: Sawatzky M: Tasks of the infertile couple. *JOGNN* 1981; 10:132.

The nurse's roles can be summarized as those of counselor, educator, and advocate. Tasks of the infertile couple and appropriate nursing interventions are summarized in Table 8–6. Throughout the evaluation process, nurses can play a key role in lessening the stress these couples must endure by providing them with appropriate resources and accurate information about what treatment entails and what physical, emotional, and financial demands they can anticipate throughout the process (Villaire, 1996). The nurse's ability to assess and respond to emotional and educational needs is essential to give infertile couples control and help them negotiate the treatment process (Johnson, 1996; Boxer, 1996). An assessment tool such as an infertility questionnaire (Table 8–7) may be helpful. Extensive and repeated explanations and written instruction may be necessary because the couple's anxiety often overwhelms their ability to retain all the information given.

Infertility may be perceived as a loss by one or both partners. Affected individuals have described this loss as loss of their relationship with spouse, family, or friends; their health; their status or prestige; their self-esteem and self-confidence; their security; and the potential child. Only one such loss may lead to depression and, in many cases, the crisis of infertility evokes feelings of all these losses (Schoener & Krysa, 1996). Each couple passes through several stages, not unlike those identified by Kübler-Ross: surprise, denial, anger, isolation, guilt, grief, and resolution. The impact of these feelings on the couple and how fast they move into resolution, if ever, may depend on the cause and duration of treatment. Each partner may progress through the stages at different rates (Sandelowski, 1994). Nonjudgmental acceptance and a professional, caring attitude on the nurse's part can go far to dissipate the negative emotions the couple may experience while going through this process.

This is also a time when the nurse may assess the quality of the couple's relationship: Are they able and willing to communicate verbally and share feelings? Are

TABLE 8–7 Infertility Questionnaire

Self-Image

1. I feel bad about my body because of our inability to have a child.
2. Since our infertility, I feel I can do anything as well as I used to.
3. I feel as attractive as before our infertility.
4. I feel less masculine/feminine because of our inability to have a child.
5. Compared with others, I feel I am a worthwhile person.
6. Lately, I feel I am sexually attractive to my wife/husband.
7. I feel I will be incomplete as a man/woman if we cannot have a child.
8. Having an infertility problem makes me feel physically incompetent.

Guilt/Blame

1. I feel guilty about somehow causing our infertility.
2. I wonder if our infertility problem is due to something I did in the past.
3. My spouse makes me feel guilty about our problem.
4. There are times when I blame my spouse for our infertility.
5. I feel I am being punished because of our infertility.

Sexuality

1. Lately I feel I am able to respond to my spouse sexually.
2. I feel sex is a duty, not a pleasure.
3. Since our infertility problem, I enjoy sexual relations with my spouse.
4. We have sexual relations for the purpose of trying to conceive.
5. Sometimes I feel like a "sex machine," programmed to have sex during the fertile period.
6. Impaired fertility has helped our sexual relationship.
7. Our inability to have a child has increased my desire for sexual relations.
8. Our inability to have a child has decreased my desire for sexual relations.

NOTE: The questionnaire is scored on a Likert scale with responses ranging from "strongly agree" to "strongly disagree." Each question is scored separately, and the mean score is determined for each section (Self-Image, Guilt/Blame, Sexuality). The total mean score is then divided by 3. A final mean score of greater than 3 indicates distress.

SOURCE: Bernstein J: Assessment of psychological dysfunction associated with infertility. *JOGNN* 1985; 14(Suppl):63.

they mutually supportive? The answers to these questions may help the nurse identify areas of strength and weakness and construct an appropriate plan of care. Availability of mental health professionals for referral is helpful when the emotional issues become too disruptive in the couple's relationship or life. Couples should be made aware of infertility support and education organizations such as RESOLVE, which may help meet some of these needs and validate their feelings. Finally, individual or group counseling with other infertile couples may help the couple resolve feelings brought about by their own difficult situation.

RESEARCH IN PRACTICE

What is the study about? Approximately 50% of infertile couples will become parents through pregnancy or adoption, and may experience major difficulties during this process. The treatment for infertility is often associated with physical pain and psychologic distress, and fertility workups or adoption procedures may prolong this emotional stress. The effect of these processes on parenting skills of the mother–infant couplet is unknown. The purpose of this study was to examine early parenting interactions in infertile couples who become pregnant through fertility procedures or adoption.

How was this study done? Two groups of infertile couples (30 who achieved pregnancy and 21 who became parents through adoption) and a group of 19 couples without fertility problems were observed interacting with their infants twice, 7 to 21 days after the infant's arrival and 1 week after the first observation at a time when both parents were home. The infants ranged in age from 9 days to 5 months. Exclusion criteria included couples with multiple births who adopted children older than 6 months or whose data collection was delayed until more than 3 weeks after the arrival of the child. Behaviors of the mother, father, and infant were recorded every 10 seconds beginning when the infant was picked up and ending when the infant was put down asleep or after 1 1/2 hours had passed.

What were the results of the study? No differences were found between fertile and infertile biological parents in the interaction behaviors. Adopted infants showed more alertness, less sleeping, more smiles, and more looking around than the biological infants. Adoptive mothers spent less time as the sole interactor with the infant. Adoptive parents spent more time playing with their child, yet held and touched them less than the biological parents. Interestingly, the number of behaviors exhibited by infertile couples was very close to those of fertile couples.

What additional questions do I have? (1) Would parents rate their parenting skills the same as the ratings derived through observation? (2) Were the behaviors noted in adoptive parents due to the older age of their infants when compared to the younger-aged infants of the infertile and fertile couples?

How can I use this study? These findings suggest that neither infertility nor adoption affect parenting interactions with infants. What is unclear is whether the length of time attempting pregnancy or the type of adoption were factors affecting parenting interactions. Specific risk factors regarding infertility (eg, depression, fear of loss of achieved pregnancy) affected parents' perceptions of their ability to parent.

SOURCE: Holditch-Davis, D., Sandelowski, M., & Harris, B. (1998). Infertility and early parent–infant interactions. *Journal of Advanced Nursing, 27*, 992–1001.

Adoption

The adoption of an infant can be a difficult or frustrating experience for all persons involved (Arms, 1990). It is not uncommon for a couple to have to wait for several years before beginning the adoption process. The number of available infants has decreased because many infants are reared by their single mothers instead of being relinquished for adoption, as was customary in the past. In addition, many unwanted pregnancies are being terminated by elective abortion. Some couples seek international adoptions or consider adopting older children, children with handicaps, or children of mixed parentage because the adoption process in such cases is quicker and more children are available. The nurse can assist couples considering adoption by providing information on community resources for adoption as well as by providing support through the adoption process. Couples also need support if they choose to remain childless.

Pregnancy After Infertility

The feeling of being infertile does not necessarily disappear with pregnancy. Although there may be initial ecstasy, the couple may also face a whole new arena of fear and anxieties, and the parents-to-be often do not know where they "fit in." They may feel a great sense of loss and isolation because those who have had no trouble conceiving cannot relate to the physical and emotional pain they endured to achieve the pregnancy. Contact with their past "infertile" support system may vanish when peers learn the couple has resolved their infertility (Braverman & English, 1992).

Although the desperation to become pregnant may have superseded the couple's ability to acknowledge their concerns about undergoing various treatments or procedures, questions about the repeated cycle of fertility drugs or the achievement of pregnancy through IVF technology or cryopreservation may now arise. The expectant couple may be very concerned about the potential of these treatments for adverse effects on the fetus. Couples may need much reassurance throughout the pregnancy to allay these anxieties.

The nurse can assist couples who experience pregnancy after infertility by acknowledging their past experience of infertility treatment; validating their fears and anxieties as they face childbirth classes, birth, and parenting issues; and providing education and support regarding what to anticipate physically and emotionally throughout the pregnancy (Black et al, 1995). These interventions will go a long way toward normalizing the experience for the couple.

Genetic Disorders

Even when conception has been achieved, families can have special reproductive concerns. The desired and expected outcome of any pregnancy is the birth of a healthy, "perfect" baby. Parents experience grief, fear, and anger when they discover that their baby has been born with a defect or a genetic disease. Such an abnormality may be evident at birth or may not appear for some time. The baby may have inherited a disease from one parent, creating guilt and strife within the family.

Regardless of the type or scope of the problem, parents will have many questions: "What did I do?" "What caused it?" "Will it happen again?" The nurse must anticipate the parents' questions and concerns and guide, direct, and support the family (Olsen, 1994). To do so, the nurse must have a basic knowledge of genetics and genetic counseling. Many congenital anomalies and diseases are genetic or have a strong genetic component. Others are not genetic at all. The genetic counselor attempts to categorize the problem and answer the family's questions. Professional nurses can help expedite this process if they understand the principles involved and are able to direct the family to the appropriate resources.

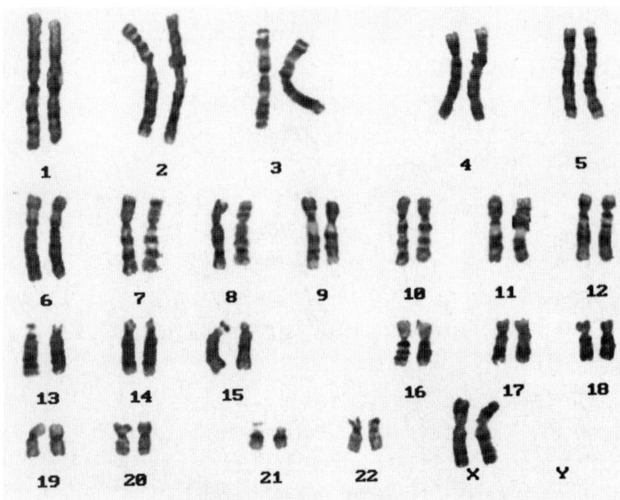

FIGURE 8–6 Normal female karotype. SOURCE: Courtesy David Peakman, Reproductive Genetics Center, Denver, CO.

Chromosomes and Chromosomal Analysis

All hereditary material is carried on tightly coiled strands of DNA known as **chromosomes.** The chromosomes carry the genes, the smallest unit of inheritance, as discussed in greater detail in Chapter 6.

All *somatic (body) cells* contain 46 chromosomes, which is the *diploid number;* the sperm and egg contain half as many (23) chromosomes, or the *haploid number* (see Chapter 7). There are 23 pairs of homologous chromosomes (a matched pair of chromosomes, one inherited from each parent). Twenty-two of the pairs are known as **autosomes** (nonsex chromosomes), and one pair is the sex chromosome, X or Y. A normal female has a 46, XX chromosome constitution, the normal male, 46, XY (Figures 8–6 and 8–7).

The **karyotype,** or pictorial analysis of an individual's chromosomes, is usually obtained from specially treated and stained peripheral blood lymphocytes. Although the use of peripheral blood is an easy, convenient method of obtaining chromosomes, almost any tissue can be examined to get this information. In addition, a piece (1 mm × 1 mm) of placenta taken from a site near the insertion of the cord and deep enough to include chorion may be sent for karyotyping.

Chromosome abnormalities can occur in either the autosomes or the sex chromosomes and can be divided into two categories: abnormalities of number and abnormalities of structure. Even small alterations in chromosomes can cause problems, especially those associated with slow growth and development or with mental retardation. The child does not need to have obvious major

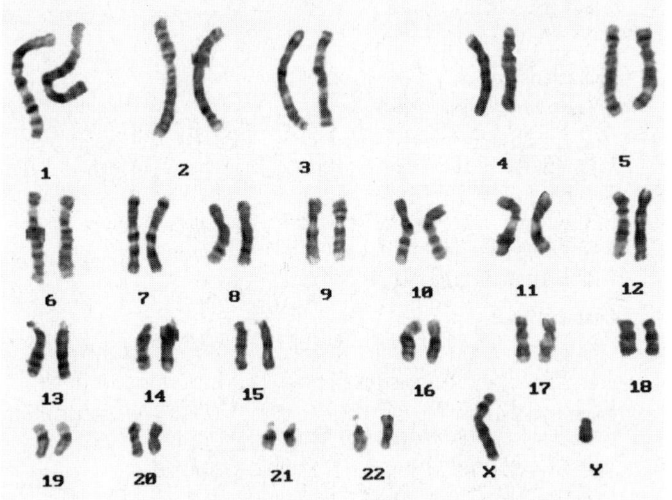

FIGURE 8–7 Normal male karotype. SOURCE: Courtesy David Peakman, Reproductive Genetics Center, Denver, CO.

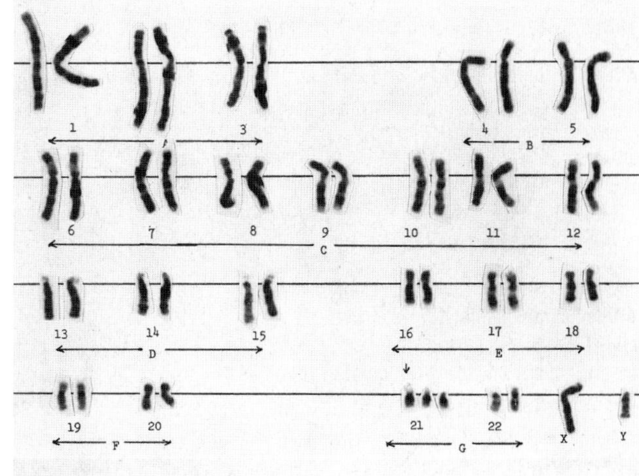

FIGURE 8–8 Karotype of a male who has trisomy 21, Down syndrome. Note the extra chromosome 21. SOURCE: Courtesy Dr Arthur Robinson, National Jewish Hospital and Research Center, Denver, CO.

malformations to be affected. Some of these abnormalities can also be passed on to other offspring; thus in some cases chromosomal analysis is appropriate even if clinical manifestations are mild. Whatever the case, too much or too little genetic material usually produces adverse effects on normal growth and development.

Indications for chromosomal analysis include the following:

- Chromosome syndrome suspected (or clients with a clinical diagnosis of Down syndrome)
- Mental retardation and congenital malformations
- Abnormal sexual development (primary amenorrhea, lack of secondary sex characteristics)
- Ambiguous genitals
- Multiple miscarriages
- Possible balanced translocation carrier (see discussion of abnormalities of chromosome structure in this chapter)

Autosomal Abnormalities

Abnormalities of chromosome number are most commonly seen as trisomies, monosomies, and as mosaicism. In all three cases, the abnormality is most often caused by nondisjunction, which occurs when paired chromosomes fail to separate during cell division. If nondisjunction occurs in either the sperm or the egg before fertilization, the resulting zygote (fertilized egg) will have an abnormal chromosome makeup in all of the cells (trisomy or monosomy).

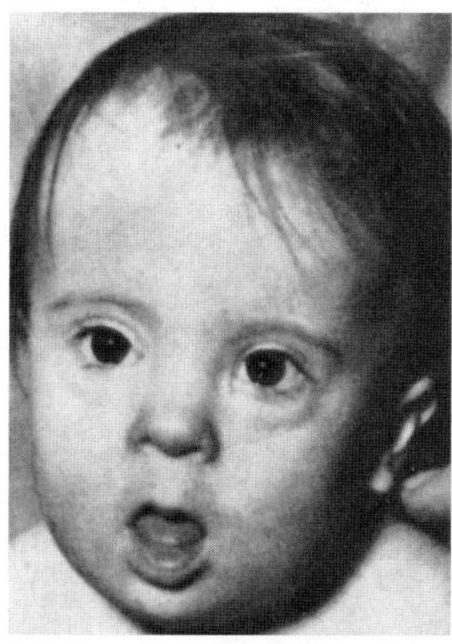

FIGURE 8–9 A child with Down syndrome. SOURCE: Jones KL: *Smith's Recognizable Patterns of Human Malformations,* 4th ed. Philadelphia: Saunders, 1988.

Trisomies are the product of the union of a normal gamete (egg or sperm) with a gamete that contains an extra chromosome. The individual will have 47 chromosomes and be trisomic (have three copies of the same chromosome) for whichever chromosome is extra. Down syndrome (formerly called mongolism) is the most common trisomy abnormality seen in children (Figure 8–8). The presence of the extra chromosome 21 produces distinctive clinical features (Figure 8–9 and Table 8–8).

TABLE 8–8 Chromosomal Syndromes

Altered chromosome	Characteristics
Altered chromosome: 21 Genetic defect: trisomy 21 (Down syndrome) (secondary nondisjunction or 14/21 unbalanced translocation) Incidence: average 1 in 700 live births, incidence variable with age of woman **(Figure 8–9)**	**Characteristics:** CNS: mental retardation; hypotonia at birth Head: flattened occiput; depressed nasal bridge; mongoloid slant of eyes; epicanthal folds; white specking of the iris (Brushfield spots); protrusion of the tongue; high, arched palate; low-set ears Hands: broad, short fingers; abnormalities of finger and foot; dermal ridge patterns (dermatoglyphics); transverse palmar crease (simian line) Other: congenital heart disease
Altered chromosome: 18 Genetic defect: trisomy 18 Incidence: 1 in 3000 live births **(Figure 8–10)**	**Characteristics:** CNS: mental retardation; severe hypotonia Head: prominent occiput; low-set ears; corneal opacities; ptosis (drooping of eyelids) Hands: third and fourth fingers overlapped by second and fifth fingers; abnormal dermatoglyphics; syndactyly (webbing of fingers) Other: congenital heart defects; renal abnormalities; single umbilical artery; gastrointestinal tract abnormalities; rocker-bottom feet; cryptorchidism; various malformations of other organs
Altered chromosome: 13 Genetic defect: trisomy 13 Incidence: 1 in 5000 live births **(Figure 8–11)**	**Characteristics:** CNS: mental retardation; severe hypotonia; seizures Head: microcephaly; microphthalmia and/or coloboma (keyhole-shaped pupil); malformed ears; aplasia of external auditory canal; micrognathia (abnormally small lower jaw); cleft lip and palate Hands: polydactly (extra digits); abnormal posturing of fingers; abnormal dermatoglyphics Other: congenital heart defects; hemangiomas; gastrointestinal tract defects; various malformations of other organs
Altered chromosome: 5p Genetic defect: deletion of short arm of chromosome 5 (cri du chat, or cat cry, syndrome) Incidence: 1 in 20,000 live births **(Figure 8–13)**	**Characteristics:** CNS: severe mental retardation; a catlike cry in infancy Head: microcephaly; hypertelorism (widely spaced eyes); epicanthal folds; low-set ears Other: failure to thrive; various organ malformations
Altered chromosome: XO (sex chromosome) Genetic defect: only one X chromosome in female (Turner syndrome) Incidence: 1 in 300–7000 live female births **(Figure 8–14)**	**Characteristics:** CNS: no intellectual impairment; some perceptual difficulties Head: low hairline; webbed neck Trunk: short stature; cubitus valgus (increased carrying angle of arm); excessive nevi (congenital discoloration of skin due to pigmentation); broad shieldlike chest with widely spaced nipples; puffy feet; no toenails Other: fibrous streaks in ovaries; underdeveloped secondary sex characteristics; primary amenorrhea; usually infertile; renal anomalies; coarctation of the aorta
Altered chromosome: XXY (sex chromosome) Genetic defect: extra X chromosome in male (Klinefelter syndrome) Incidence: 1 in 1000 live male births, approximately 1–2% of institutionalized males	**Characteristics:** CNS: mild mental retardation Trunk: occasional gynecomastia (abnormally large male breasts); eunuchoid body proportions (lack of male muscular and sexual development) Other: small, soft testes; underdeveloped secondary sex characteristics; usually sterile

With the advent of modern surgical techniques and antibiotics, children with Down syndrome are now living into their fifth or sixth decade of life.

The other two common trisomies are trisomy 18 and trisomy 13 (Table 8–8 and Figures 8–10 and 8–11). The prognosis for children with trisomy 13 or 18 is extremely poor. Most children (70%) die within the first 3 months of life as a result of complications related to respiratory and cardiac abnormalities. However, 10% survive the first year of life; therefore, the family needs to plan for the possibility of long-term care of a severely affected infant and for family support.

Monosomies occur when a normal gamete unites with a gamete that is missing a chromosome. In this case, the individual will have only 45 chromosomes and is said to be monosomic. Monosomy of an entire autosomal chromosome is incompatible with life.

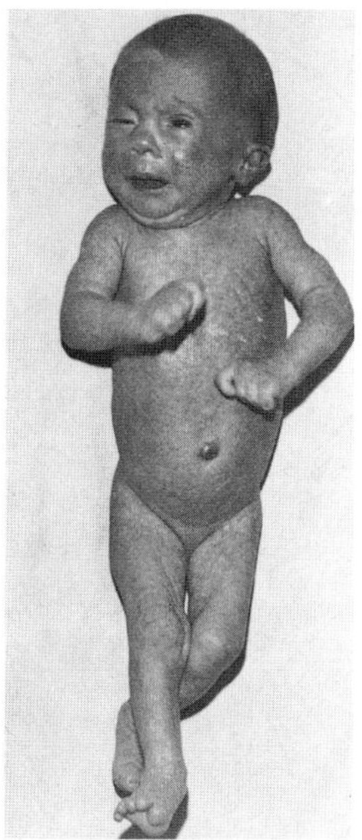

FIGURE 8–10 Infant with trisomy 18. SOURCE: Jones KL: *Smith's Recognizable Patterns of Human Malformations,* 4th ed. Philadelphia: Saunders, 1988.

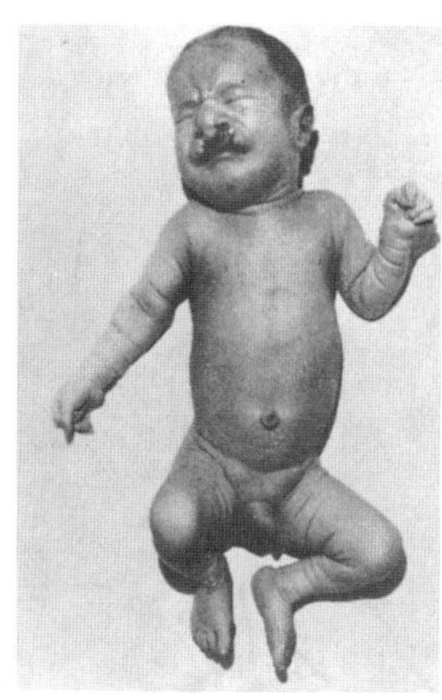

FIGURE 8–11 Infant with trisomy 13. SOURCE: Jones KL: *Smith's Recognizable Patterns of Human Malformations,* 4th ed. Philadelphia: Saunders, 1988.

Mosaicism occurs after fertilization and results in an individual with two different cell lines, each with a different chromosomal number. Mosaicism tends to be more common in the sex chromosomes, but when it does occur in the autosomes, it is most common in Down syndrome. An individual with many of the classic signs of Down syndrome but with normal or near-normal intelligence should be investigated for the possibility of mosaicism.

Abnormalities of chromosome structure involve only parts of the chromosome and generally occur in two forms: translocation, and deletions or additions. As the technology improves, more of these chromosomal structural abnormalities can be detected.

Some children born with Down syndrome have trisomy 21, whereas others have an abnormal rearrangement of chromosomal material known as translocation. Clinically, the two types of Down syndrome are indistinguishable. What is of major importance to the family is that the two different types have significantly different risks of recurrence. The only way to distinguish between the two is to do a chromosome analysis. Risk of trisomy is 1 in 800 live births, in contrast with 1 in 1500 live births with a balanced translocation (Simpson, 1990).

The translocation occurs when the carrier parent has 45 chromosomes, usually with one chromosome fused to another. A common translocation is one in which a particle of chromosome 14 breaks and fuses to chromosome 21. The parent has one normal 14, one normal 21, and one 14/21 chromosome. Since all the chromosomal material is present and functioning normally, the parent is clinically normal. This individual is known as a *balanced translocation carrier.* When a person who is a balanced translocation carrier has a child with a person who has a structurally normal chromosome constitution, the child can have a normal number of chromosomes, be a carrier, or have an extra chromosome 21 (Figure 8–12). Such a child has an *unbalanced translocation* and has Down syndrome.

The other type of structural abnormality seen is caused by *additions or deletions* of chromosomal material. Any portion of a chromosome may be lost or added, generally leading to some adverse effect. Depending on how much chromosomal material is involved, the clinical effects may be mild or severe. Many types of additions and deletions have been described, such as a deletion of the short arm of chromosome 5 (cri du chat, or cat cry, syndrome; Figure 8–13) or the deletion of the long arm of chromosome 18 (Edwards' syndrome). Table 8–8 lists other chromosomal syndromes.

Sex Chromosome Abnormalities

To better understand normal X chromosome function and thus abnormalities of the sex chromosomes, the nurse should know that in females, at an early embryonic stage, one of the two normal X chromosomes becomes inactive. The inactive X chromosome forms a dark-staining area

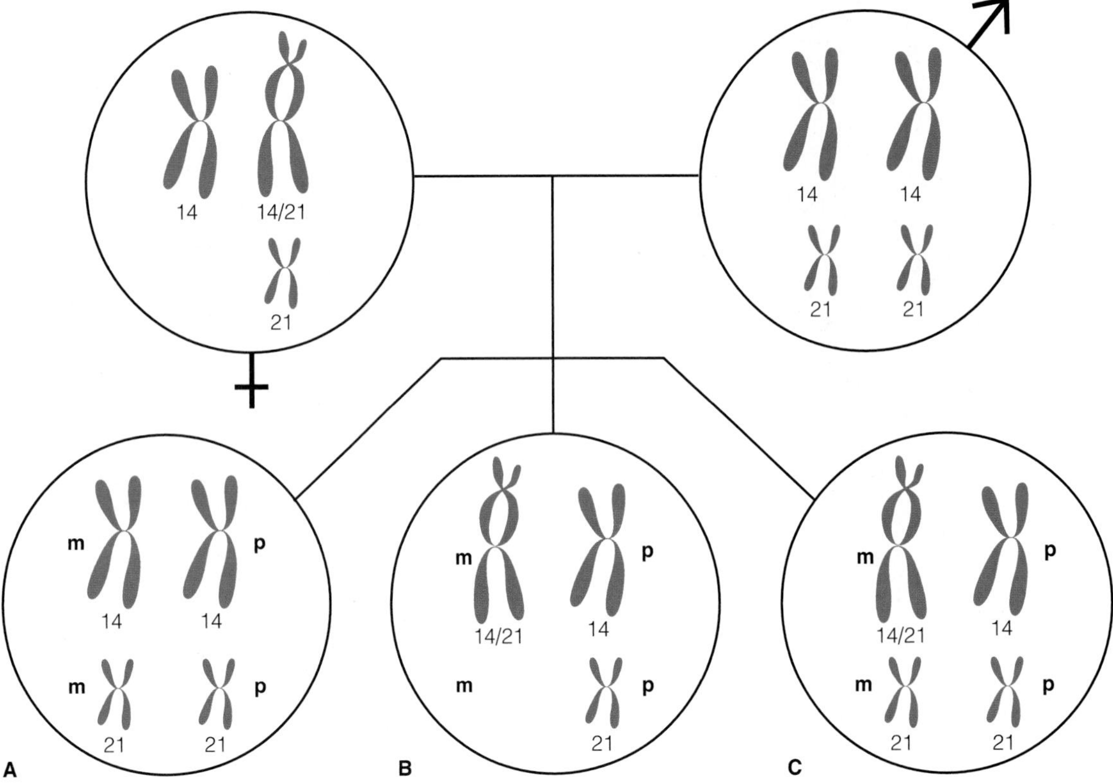

FIGURE 8–12 Diagram of various types of offspring when mother has a balanced translocation between chromosomes 14 and 21 and father has a normal arrangement of chromosomal material. ***A,*** Normal offspring. ***B,*** Balanced translocation carrier. ***C,*** Unbalanced translocation. Child has Down syndrome.

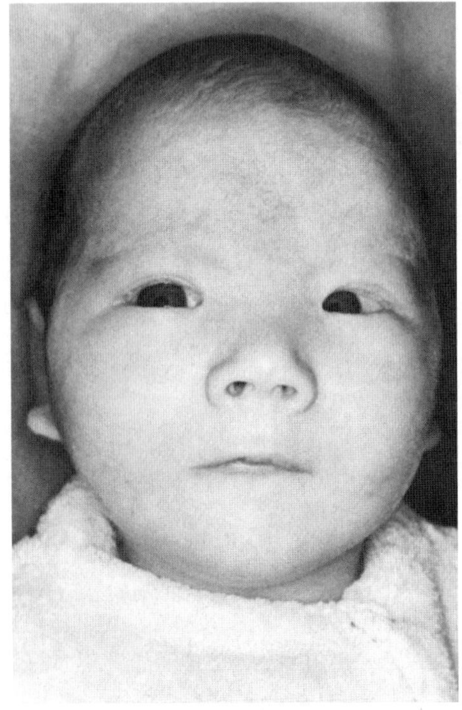

FIGURE 8–13 Infant with cri du chat syndrome resulting from deletion of part of the short arm of chromosome 5. Note characteristic facies with hypertelorism, epicanthus, and retrognathia. SOURCE: Thompson JS, Thompson MW: *Genetics in Medicine,* 5th ed. Philadelphia: Saunders, 1991.

known as the *Barr body*, or sex chromatin body. The normal female has one Barr body because one of her two X chromosomes has been inactivated. The normal male has no Barr bodies because he has only one X chromosome.

The most common sex chromosome abnormalities are Turner syndrome in females (45,X with no Barr bodies present) and Klinefelter syndrome in males (47,XXY with one Barr body present). See Figure 8–14 and Table 8–8 for clinical descriptions of these abnormalities.

The mosaic form of the XO chromosome is associated with daughters of women who took the drug diethylstilbestrol (DES) during pregnancy. The fertility of women with the mosaic form of the XO chromosome

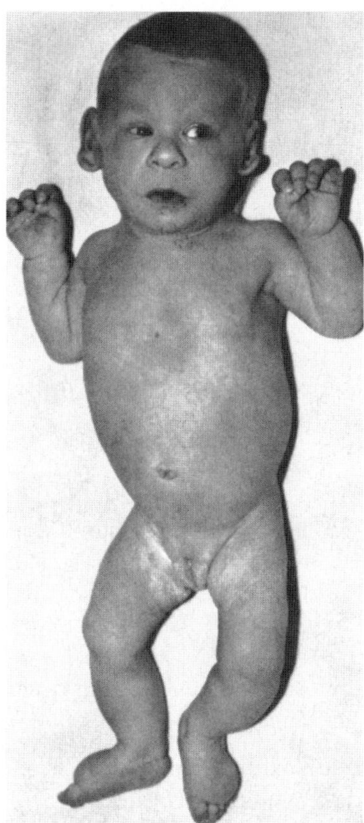

FIGURE 8–14 Infant with Turner syndrome at 1 month of age. Note the prominent ears. SOURCE: Lemli L, Smith DW: The XO syndrome: A study of the differential phenotype in 25 patients. *Journal of Pediatrics* 1963; 63:577.

may not be impaired; however, there is a higher percentage of uterine malformation and hormonal difficulty associated with it, and hence a high degree of miscarriage.

Modes of Inheritance

Many inherited diseases are produced by an abnormality in a single gene or pair of genes. In such instances the chromosomes are grossly normal. The defect is at the gene level. Some of these gene defects can be detected by new technologies, including DNA and other biochemical assays.

There are two major categories of inheritance: **Mendelian, or single-gene, inheritance** and **non-Mendelian, or multifactorial, inheritance.** Each single-gene trait is determined by a pair of genes working together. These genes are responsible for the observable expression of the traits (eg, brown eyes, dark skin), referred to as the **phenotype.** The total genetic makeup of an individual is referred to as the **genotype** (pattern of the genes on the chromosomes). One of the genes for a trait is inherited from the mother; the other, from the father. Individuals who have two identical genes at a given locus are considered to be *homozygous* for that trait. Individuals are considered to be *heterozygous* for a particular trait when they have two different *alleles* (alternate forms

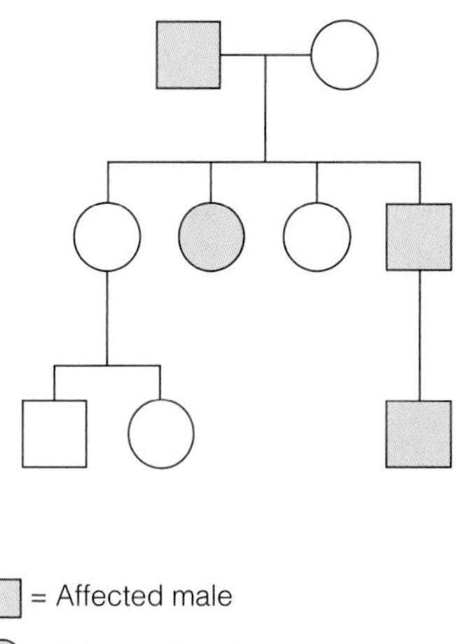

FIGURE 8–15 Autosomal dominant pedigree. One parent is affected. Statistically, 50% of offspring will be affected, regardless of sex.

of the same gene) at a given locus on a pair of homologous chromosomes.

The best known modes of single-gene inheritance are autosomal dominant, autosomal recessive, and X-linked (sex-linked) recessive. There is also a less common, X-linked dominant mode of inheritance and a new identified mode of inheritance, the fragile X syndrome.

Autosomal Dominant Inheritance

An individual is said to have an autosomal dominantly inherited disorder if the disease trait is heterozygous. That is, the abnormal gene overshadows the normal gene of the pair to produce the trait. The following occurs in autosomal dominant inheritance:

- An affected individual generally has an affected parent. The family **pedigree** (graphic representation of a family tree) usually shows multiple generations having the disorder.
- Affected individuals have a 50% chance of passing on the abnormal gene to each of their children (Figure 8–15).
- Males and females are equally affected, and a father can pass the abnormal gene on to his son. This is an important principle when distinguishing autosomal dominant disorders from X-linked disorders.
- Autosomal dominant inherited disorders have varying degrees of presentation. This is an important factor when counseling families concerning autosomal dominant disorders. Although a parent may have a mild form of the disease, the child may have a more severe form.

Some common autosomal dominantly inherited disorders are Huntington's disease, polycystic kidney disease, neurofibromatosis (von Recklinghausen's disease), and achondroplastic dwarfism.

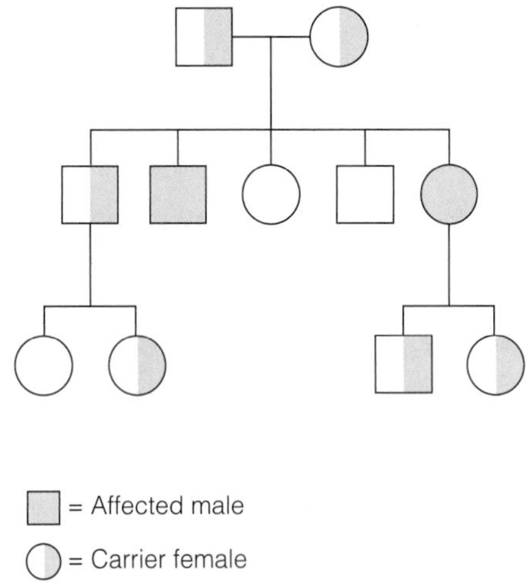

FIGURE 8–16 Autosomal recessive pedigree. Both parents are carriers. Statistically, 25% of offspring will be affected, regardless of sex.

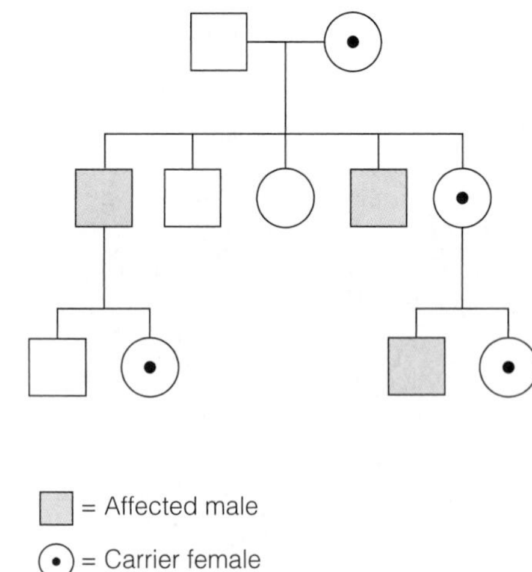

FIGURE 8–17 X-linked recessive pedigree. The mother is the carrier. Statistically, 50% of male offspring will be affected, and 50% of female offspring will be carriers.

Autosomal Recessive Inheritance

In an autosomal recessively inherited disorder, the individual must have two abnormal genes to be affected. The notion of a *carrier state* is appropriate here. A carrier is an individual who is heterozygous for the abnormal gene and clinically normal. It is not until two individuals mate and pass on the same abnormal gene that affected children may appear. It is essential to remember the following facts about autosomal recessive inheritance:

- An affected individual has clinically normal parents, but both parents are carriers of the abnormal gene (Figure 8–16).
- There is a 25% chance of carrier parents passing the abnormal gene on to any of their offspring. Each pregnancy has a 25% chance of resulting in an affected child.
- If the child of two carrier parents is clinically normal, there is a 50% chance that the child is a carrier of the gene.
- Both males and females are equally affected.
- There is an increased history of consanguineous matings.

Some other common autosomal recessive inherited disorders are cystic fibrosis, phenylketonuria (PKU), galactosemia, sickle cell anemia, Tay-Sachs disease, and most metabolic disorders.

X-Linked Recessive Inheritance

X-linked, or sex-linked, disorders are those for which the abnormal gene is carried on the X chromosome. Thus an X-linked disorder is manifested in a male who carries the abnormal gene on his X chromosome. His mother is considered to be a carrier when the normal gene on one X chromosome overshadows the abnormal gene on the other X chromosome. The following occurs in X-linked recessive inheritance:

- There is no male-to-male transmission. Affected males are related through the female line (Figure 8–17).
- There is a 50% chance that a carrier mother will pass the abnormal gene to each of her sons, who will thus be affected. There is a 50% chance that a carrier mother will pass the normal gene to each of her sons, who will thus be unaffected. There is a 50% chance that a carrier mother will pass the abnormal gene to each of her daughters, who become carriers.
- Fathers affected with an X-linked disorder cannot pass the disorder to their sons, but all their daughters become carriers of the disorder.

Common X-linked recessive disorders are hemophilia, Duchenne muscular dystrophy, and some forms of color blindness.

X-Linked Dominant Inheritance

X-linked dominant disorders are extremely rare, the most common being vitamin D–resistant rickets. When X-linked dominance does occur, the pattern is similar to X-linked recessive inheritance except that heterozygous females are affected. It is essential to remember that in X-linked dominant inheritance there is no male-to-male transmission. Affected fathers will have affected daughters, but no affected sons.

Fragile X Syndrome

The fragile X syndrome is a common inherited form of mental retardation second only to Down syndrome among all cases of moderate mental retardation in males (Murray, Cuckle, Taylor & Hewison, 1997). Fragile X syndrome is a CNS disorder linked to a "fragile site" on the X chromosome. Fragile X syndrome is characterized by moderate mental retardation, large protuberant ears, and large testes after puberty. The carrier females are not dysmorphic (having abnormal features), but about one-third are mildly retarded.

Multifactorial Inheritance

Many common congenital malformations, such as cleft palate, heart defects, spina bifida, dislocated hips, clubfoot, and pyloric stenosis, are caused by an interaction of many genes and environmental factors. They are therefore multifactorial in origin. The following occur in multifactorial inheritance:

- The malformations may vary from mild to severe. For example, spina bifida may range in severity from mild, as spina bifida occulta, to more severe, as a myelomeningocele. It is believed that the more severe the defect, the greater the number of genes present for that defect.
- There is often a sex bias. Pyloric stenosis is more common in males, whereas cleft palate is more common among females. When a member of the less commonly affected sex shows the condition, a greater number of genes must usually be present to cause the defect.
- In the presence of environmental influence (such as seasonal changes, altitude, radiation exposure, chemicals in the environment, or exposure to toxic substances), fewer genes may be needed to manifest the disease in the offspring.
- In contrast to single-gene disorders, there is an additive effect in multifactorial inheritance. The more family members who have the defect, the greater the risk that the next pregnancy will also be affected (King & Schimke, 1994).

Although most congenital malformations are multifactorial tracts, a careful family history should always be taken because occasionally cleft lip and palate, certain congenital heart defects, and other malformations can also be inherited as autosomal dominant or recessive traits. Other disorders thought to be within the multifactorial inheritance group are diabetes, hypertension, some heart diseases, and mental illness.

Nongenetic Conditions

Malformations present at birth may be caused by an environmental insult during pregnancy, such as exposure to a drug or an infectious agent (see Chapter 12). Some malformations, however, cannot be explained by genetic mechanisms or teratogens. A referral to a genetic center is warranted with any birth defect. Autosomal dominant conditions such as phocomelia (developmental anomaly characterized by the absence of the upper portion of limbs) can have very minimal expression in a parent but severe effects in a child. False reassurance or information can put any health care professional in jeopardy.

Prenatal Diagnostic Tests

Parent-child and family planning counseling have become a major responsibility of professional nurses. To be effective counselors, nurses need to have the most current knowledge available concerning prenatal diagnosis. It is essential that the couple be completely informed as to the known and potential risks of each of the genetic diagnostic procedures. The nurse needs to recognize the emotional impact on the family of a decision to undergo or not to undergo a genetic diagnostic procedure.

The ability to diagnose certain genetic diseases by various diagnostic tools has enormous implications for the practice of preventive health care. Several methods are available for prenatal diagnosis, although some are still being used on an experimental basis.

Ultrasound may be used to assess the fetus for genetic or congenital problems. With ultrasound, one can visualize the fetal head for abnormalities in size, shape, and structure. (For a detailed discussion of ultrasound technology, see Chapter 17.) Craniospinal defects (anencephaly, microcephaly, hydrocephalus), gastrointestinal malformations (omphalocele, gastroschisis), renal malformations (dysplasia or obstruction), and skeletal malformations (caudal regression, conjoined twins) are only some of the disorders that have been diagnosed in utero by ultrasound.

Screening by ultrasound for congenital anomalies is best done at 18 to 20 weeks, when fetal structures have completed development. There is no information documenting harm to the fetus or long-term effects with exposure to ultrasound. However, there is no guarantee of complete safety; therefore, the practitioner and the parents must evaluate the risks against the benefits on an individual basis (Kuller & Laifer, 1995).

Genetic Amniocentesis

A major method of prenatal diagnosis is genetic amniocentesis (Figure 8–18). The procedure is described in Chapter 17. The indications for genetic amniocentesis include the following:

- *Maternal age 35 or older.* Women 35 or older are at greater risk for having children with chromosome abnormalities. Approximately 95% of trisomy 21 cases occur because of conception after 35 years of age. See Chapter 17 for further discussion. Half of the chromosomal abnormalities due to maternal age are trisomy 21, and half are other abnormalities of chromosome number, such as trisomy 13, 18, XXX, or XXY. The risk of having a live–born infant with a chromosome problem is 1 in 200 for a 35-year-old woman; the risk for trisomy 21 is 1 in 400. At age 45

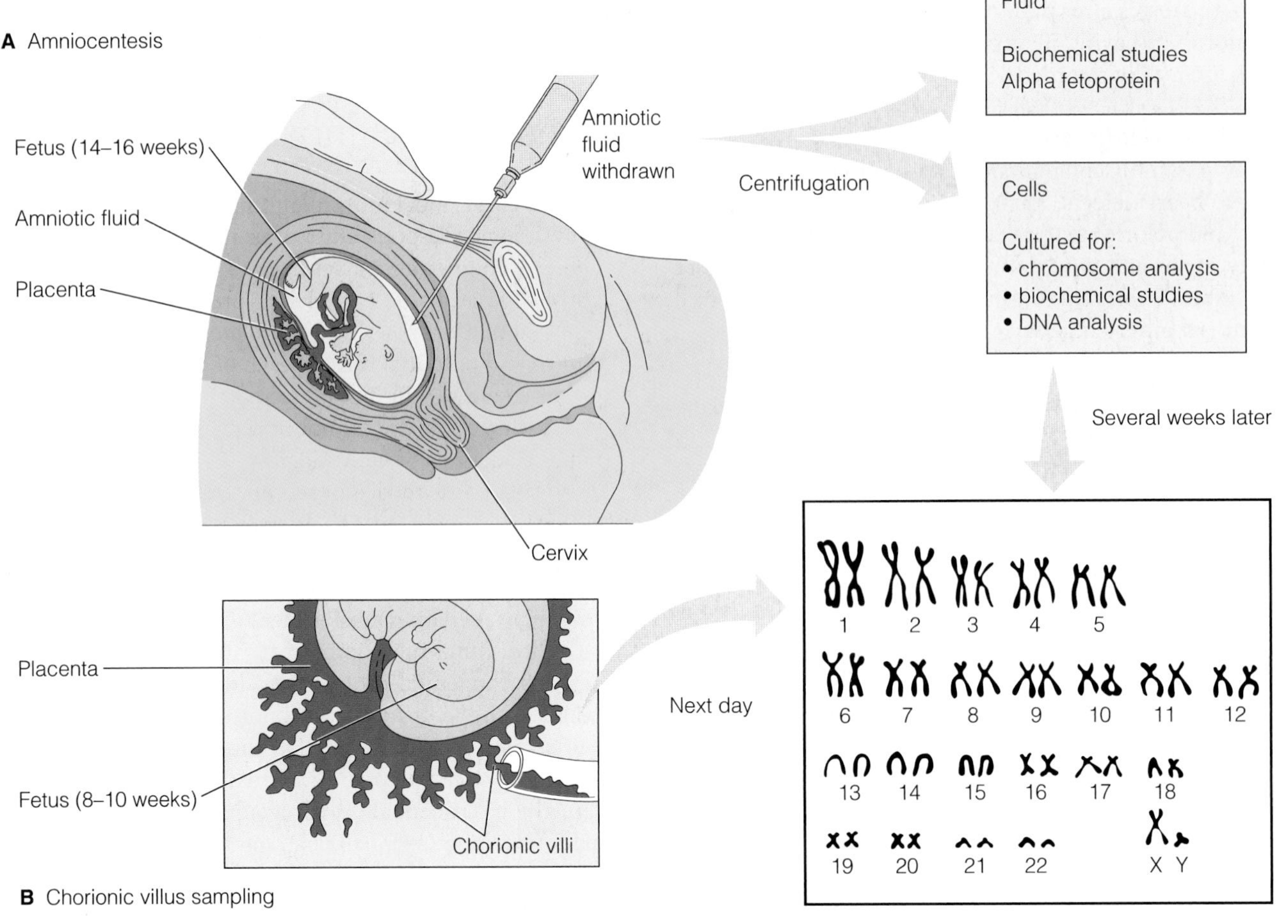

FIGURE 8–18 ***A,*** Genetic amniocentesis for prenatal diagnosis is done at 14 to 16 weeks' gestation. ***B,*** Chorionic villus sampling is done at 8 to 10 weeks, and the cells are karyotyped within 48 to 72 hours.

the risks are 1 in 20 and 1 in 40, respectively (Hook et al, 1988). Table 8–9 presents maternal age-related risks at different gestational ages.

- *Previous child born with a chromosomal abnormality.* Young couples who have had a child with trisomy 21, 18, or 13 have approximately a 1% to 2% risk of a future child having a chromosome abnormality.
- *Parent carrying a chromosomal abnormality (balanced translocation).* For example, a woman who carries a balanced 14/21 translocation has a risk of approximately 10% to 15% that her children will be affected with the unbalanced translocation of Down syndrome; if the father is a carrier, there is a 2% to 5% risk.
- *Mother carrying an X-linked disease.* In families in which the woman is a known or possible carrier of an X-linked disorder, such as Duchenne muscular dystrophy or hemophilia, genetic amniocentesis, chorionic villus sampling (CVS), or percutaneous umbilical cord sampling (PUBS) may be appropriate options. For a known female carrier, the risk of having an affected male fetus is 50%. New technologies such as DNA testing may make it possible to differentiate affected from nonaffected males in some disorders. In disorders where female carriers can be distinguished from noncarriers, only the carrier females would be offered prenatal diagnosis.
- *Parents carrying an inborn error of metabolism that can be diagnosed in utero.* Metabolic disorders detectable in utero include argininosuccinicaciduria, cystinosis, Fabry's disease, galactosemia, Gaucher's disease, homocystinuria, Hunter's syndrome, Hurler's disease, Krabbe's disease, Lesch-Nyhan syndrome, maple syrup urine disease, metachromatic leukodystrophy, methylmalonic aciduria, Niemann-Pick disease, Pompe's disease, Sanfilippo's syndrome, and Tay-Sachs disease.
- *Both parents carrying an autosomal recessive disease.* When both parents are carriers of an autosomal

TABLE 8–9 Risk for Chromosomal Abnormalities at Different Stages of Pregnancy Due to Maternal Age

Maternal Age (Years)	10 Weeks Rates Noted with CVS	17 Weeks Rates Noted with Amniocentesis	Birth: Chromosomal Anomalies	Birth: Down Syndrome*
33		1/200	1/300	1/600
34		1/170	1/250	1/500
35	1/110	1/130	1/200	1/400
36	1/80	1/100	1/170	1/340
37	1/65	1/80	1/130	1/260
38	1/50	1/65	1/100	1/200
39	1/35	1/50	1/80	1/160
40	1/30	1/40	1/65	1/130
41	1/20	1/30	1/50	1/100
42	1/15	1/25	1/40	1/80
43	1/13	1/20	1/30	1/60
44	1/10	1/15	1/25	1/50
45	1/7	1/12	1/20	1/40
46	1/6	1/10	1/16	1/32
47	1/4	1/8	1/12	1/24
48	1/3	1/6	1/10	1/20

*Risk for Down syndrome is approximately half of each number listed above (eg, age 33 risk for live born Down syndrome is 1 in 600).

SOURCES: Approximate (rounded) estimates from Hook EB et al: Maternal age-specific rates of 47, +21 and other cytogenetic abnormalitiesdiagnosed in the first trimester of pregnancy in chorionic villus biopsy specimens: Comparison with rates expected from observations atamniocentesis. *Am J Hum Genet* 1988; 42:797; and Hook EB, Cross PK and Schreimachers DM: Chromosomal abnormality rates at amniocentesis and in live-born infants. *JAMA* 1983; 249:2034. Rates for maternal ages >45 years are based on very small numbers.

recessive disease, there is a 25% risk for each pregnancy that the fetus will be affected. Diagnosis is made by testing the cultured amniotic fluid cells (enzyme level, substrate level, product level, or DNA) or the fluid itself. Autosomal recessive diseases identified by amniocentesis are hemoglobinopathies such as sickle cell anemia, thalassemia, and cystic fibrosis.

- *Family history of neural tube defects.* Genetic amniocentesis is available to those couples who have had a child with neural tube defects or who have a family history of these conditions, which include anencephaly, spina bifida, and myelomeningocele. Neural tube defects are usually multifactorial traits.

Chorionic Villus Sampling (CVS)

Chorionic villus sampling is a technique used in selected regional centers. Its diagnostic capability is similar to that of amniocentesis. Its advantages are that diagnostic information is available at 8 to 10 weeks' gestation and that products of conception are tested directly. (For further discussion, see Chapter 17.)

Percutaneous Umbilical Blood Sampling

Percutaneous umbilical blood sampling (PUBS) is a technique used for obtaining blood that allows for more rapid chromosome diagnosis, for genetic studies, or for transfusion for Rh isoimmunization or hydrops. (For more in-depth discussion, see Chapter 17).

Alpha Fetoprotein (AFP and AFP3)

Alpha fetoprotein tests for AFP in the maternal circulation or amniotic fluid. Maternal serum AFP (MSAFP) is elevated in infants with open neural tube defect, infants with anencephaly, omphalocele, gastroschisis, or multiple gestation (Alteneder, Kenner, Greene, & Pohorecki, 1998). MSAFP is done at 15 to 22 weeks' gestation (Scioscia, 1999). Women with a family history of neural tube defects should consult their prenatal care provider for recommended folic dosages (King & Schimke, 1994). Low MSAFP has been associated with Down syndrome. Ultrasound and amniocentesis are offered with low or high MSAFP. Inaccurate dating is the most common cause for abnormal AFP; therefore, ultrasound dating is very important. With high MSAFP, normal amniotic fluid AFP, and normal ultrasound, there is an increased risk for preterm labor, perinatal death, and intrauterine growth restriction.

Implications of Prenatal Diagnostic Testing

It is imperative that counseling precede any procedure for prenatal diagnosis. Many questions and points must be considered if the family is to reach a satisfactory decision. See Tables 8–10 and 8–11.

With the advent of diagnostic techniques such as amniocentesis, couples at risk, who would not otherwise have additional children, can decide to conceive. Following prenatal diagnosis, a couple can decide not to have a child with a genetic disease. For many couples, prenatal

TABLE 8–10 Couples to Be Offered Prenatal Diagnosis

Couples to Be Offered Prenatal Diagnosis
Women 35 or over at time of birth
Couples having a balanced translocation (chromosomal abnormality)
Mother carrying X-linked disease (eg, hemophilia)
Couples having a previous child with chromosomal abnormality
Couples in which either partner or a previous child is affected with a diagnosable metabolic disorder
Couples in which both partners are carriers for a diagnosable metabolic or autosomal recessive disorder
Family or personal history of neural tube defects
Ethnic groups at increased risk for specific disorders (Table 8–11)
Couples with history of two or more first trimester spontaneous abortions
Women with an abnormal maternal serum alpha fetoprotein (MSAFP or AFP3) test

diagnosis is not a solution because they choose not to prevent the genetic disease by aborting the fetus. The decision whether or not to use prenatal diagnosis can be made only by the family. Even when termination is not an option, prenatal diagnosis can give parents an opportunity to prepare for the birth of a child with special needs, contact other families with a child with similar problems, or contact support services before the birth.

Every pregnancy has a 3% to 4% risk for resulting in an infant with a birth defect. Some birth defects can be diagnosed before birth. When an abnormality is detected or suspected, an attempt is made to determine the diagnosis by assessing the family health history (via the pedigree) and the pregnancy history, and by evaluating the fetal anomaly or anomalies. The parents can then be presented with options. Families with a baby having a lethal anomaly, such as trisomy 13 or 18, may wish to consider nonaggressive intervention.

Prenatal diagnosis cannot guarantee the birth of a normal child. It can only determine the presence or absence of specific disorders (within the limits of laboratory error). Many disorders can be prenatally diagnosed; the list has grown and continues to grow almost daily. Experts on a specific disorder should be consulted before giving information to couples or discussing options.

Treatment of prenatally diagnosed disorders may begin during the pregnancy, thus possibly preventing irreversible damage. For example, a galactose-free diet may be given to a mother carrying a fetus with galactosemia. In light of the philosophy of preventive health care, information on what data can be obtained prenatally should be made available to all couples who are expecting a baby or who are contemplating pregnancy.

CRITICAL THINKING QUESTION

What implications does the Human Genome Project have for families with genetic conditions?

Postnatal Diagnosis

Questions concerning genetic disorders (cause, treatment, and prognosis) are most often first discussed in the newborn nursery or during the infant's first few months of life. When a child is born with anomalies, has a stormy neonatal period, or does not progress as expected, a genetic evaluation may well be warranted. Accurate diagnosis and an optimal treatment plan incorporate:

- Complete and detailed histories to determine whether the problem is prenatal (congenital), postnatal, or familial in origin.
- Thorough physical examination, including dermatoglyphic analysis (Figure 8–19).
- Laboratory analysis, which includes chromosome analysis; enzyme assay for inborn errors of metabo-

TABLE 8–11 Genetic Screening Recommendations for Various Ethnic and Age Groups

Background of Population at Risk	Disorder	Screening Test	Definitive Test
Ashkenazic Jewish	Tay-Sachs disease	Decreased serum hexosaminidase-A	CVS* or amniocentesis for hexosaminidase-A assay
African; Hispanic from Caribbean, Central America, South America	Sickle cell anemia	Presence of sickle cell hemoglobin; confirmatory hemoglobin electrophoresis	CVS or amniocentesis for genotype determination; direct molecular studies
Greek, Italian	β-thalassemia	Mean corpuscular volume <80%; confirmatory hemoglobin electrophoresis	CVS or amniocentesis for genotype determination (direct molecular studies or indirect RFLP† analysis)
Southeast Asian (Vietnamese, Laotian, Cambodian), Philippine	α-thalassemia	Mean corpuscular volume <80%; confirmatory hemoglobin electrophoresis	CVS or amniocentesis for genotype determination (direct molecular studies)
Women over age 35 (EDB) (all ethnic groups)	Chromosomal trisomies	None	CVS or amniocentesis for cytogenetic analysis
Women of any age (all ethnic groups; particularly suggested for women from British Isles, Ireland)	Neural tube defects and selected other anomalies	Maternal serum α-fetoprotein (MSAFP)	Amniocentesis for amniotic fluid, α-fetoprotein, and acetylcholinesterase assays

*Chorionic villus sampling

†Restriction fragment length polymorphism

lism (see Chapter 26 for further discussion on these specific tests); and DNA studies (both direct and by linkage); antibody titers for infectious teratogens, such as toxoplasmosis, rubella, cytomegalovirus, and herpes virus (TORCH syndrome; see Chapter 15).

To make an accurate diagnosis, the geneticist consults with other specialists and reviews the current literature. This lets the geneticist evaluate all the available information before arriving at a diagnosis and plan of action.

Community-Based Nursing Care

Genetic counseling is a communication process in which the genetic counselor tries to provide a family with the most complete and accurate information on the occurrence or the risk of recurrence of a genetic disease in that family (Inati et al, 1994).

In retrospective genetic counseling, time is a crucial factor. One cannot expect a family who has just learned that their child has a birth defect or a genetic abnormality to assimilate any information concerning future risks. However, the couple should never be "put off" from counseling for too long a period, only to find that they have borne another affected child. The perinatal nursing team nurse frequently has the first contact with the family that has a newborn with a congenital abnormality. At the birth of an affected child, the nurse can inform the parents that before they attempt having another child genetic counseling is available. Genetic counseling is an appropriate course of action for any family wondering, "Will it happen again?" The nursery nurse frequently has the first contact with the family that has a newborn with a congenital abnormality. The family nurse practitioner or family-planning nurse is in an excellent position to reach at-risk families before the birth of another baby with a congenital problem. Genetic counseling referral is advised for any of the following categories:

- *Congenital abnormalities, including mental retardation.* Any couple who has a child or a relative with a congenital malformation may be at an increased risk and should be so informed. If mental retardation of unidentified cause has occurred in a family, there may be an increased risk of recurrence. In some cases, the genetic counselor will identify the cause of a malformation as a teratogen (see Chapter 12). The family should be aware of teratogenic substances so they can avoid exposure during any subsequent pregnancy.
- *Familial disorders.* Families should be told that certain diseases may have a genetic component and that the risk of their occurrence in a particular family may be higher than that for the general population. Such disorders as diabetes, heart disease, cancer, and mental illness fall into this category.
- *Known inherited diseases.* Families may know that a disease is inherited but not know the mechanism or the specific risk for them. An important point to remember is that family members who are not at risk for passing on a disorder should be as well informed as family members who are at risk.
- *Metabolic disorders.* Any families at risk for having a child with a metabolic disorder or biochemical defect should be referred for genetic counseling. Because most inborn errors of metabolism are autosomal recessively inherited ones, a family may not be identified as at risk until the birth of an affected child. Carriers of the sickle cell trait can be identified before pregnancy is begun, and the risk of having an affected child can be determined. Prenatal diagnosis of an affected fetus is available on an experimental basis only.
- *Chromosomal abnormalities.* As discussed previously, any couple who has had a child with a chromosomal abnormality may be at an increased risk of having another child similarly affected. This group includes families in which there is concern for a possible translocation.

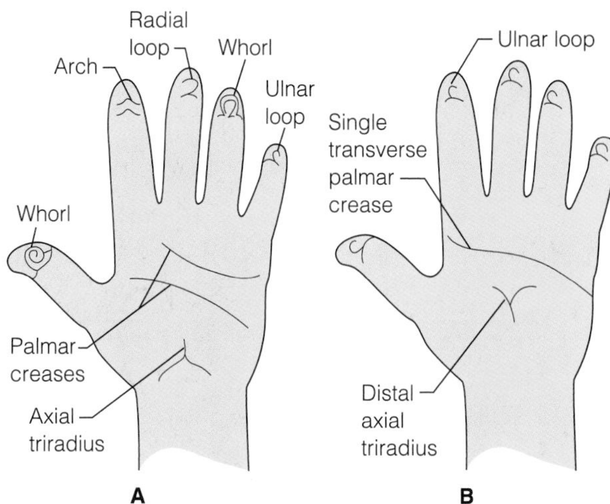

FIGURE 8–19 Dermatoglyphic patterns of the hands in ***A,*** a normal individual and ***B,*** a child with Down syndrome. Note the single transverse palmar crease, distally placed axial triradius, and increased number of ulnar loops.

After the couple have been referred to the genetic clinic, they are sent a form requesting information on the health status of various family members. At this time the nurse can help by discussing the form with the family or clarifying the information needed to complete it.

A pedigree and family health history facilitate identification of other family members who might also be at risk for the same disorder (Figure 8–20). The family being counseled may wish to notify those relatives at risk so that they, too, can be given genetic counseling. When done correctly, the family history and pedigree are two of the most powerful and useful tools for determining a family risk.

The counselor gathers additional information about the pregnancy, the affected child's growth and development, and the family's understanding of the problem.

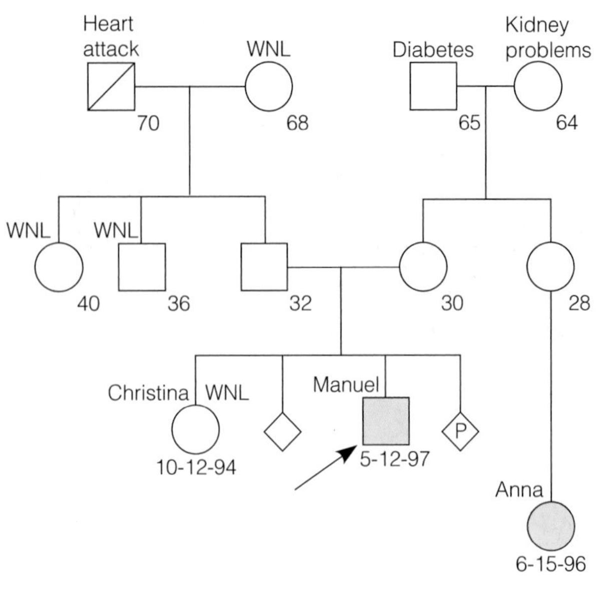

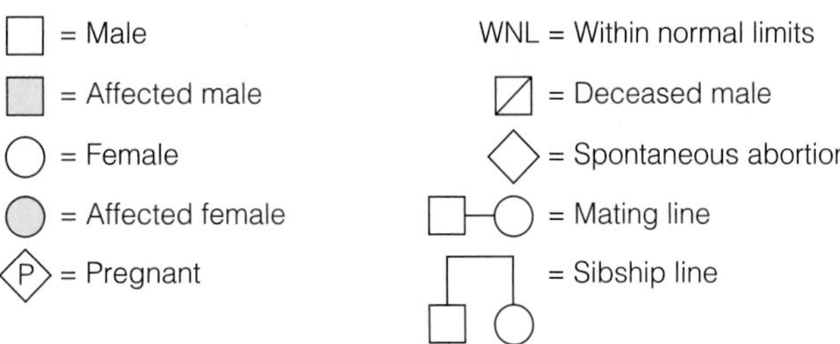

FIGURE 8–20 Screening pedigree. Arrow indicates the nearest family member affected with the disorder being investigated. Numbers refer to the ages of family members.

Generally the child is given a physical examination. Other family members may also be examined. If any laboratory tests, such as chromosomal analysis, metabolic studies, or vital titers, are indicated, they are performed at this time. The genetic counselor may then give the family some preliminary information based on the data at hand.

Finally, the nurse should elicit information concerning ethnic background, family origin, and religion. Many genetic disorders are more common among certain ethnic groups or in particular geographic areas. For example, families from the British Isles are at higher risk of having children with neural tube defects; the Ashkenazi Jews are at higher risk for Tay-Sachs disease; people of African descent for sickle cell anemia; and people of Mediterranean heritage for thalassemias.

Follow-Up Counseling

When all the data have been carefully examined and analyzed, the family returns for a follow-up visit. At this time, the parents are given all the information available, including the medical facts, diagnosis, probable course of the disorder, and any available management; the inheritance pattern for this particular family and their risk of recurrence; and the options or alternatives for dealing with the risk of recurrence. The remainder of the counseling session is spent discussing the course of action that seems appropriate to the family in view of their risk and family goals.

Among those options or alternatives are prenatal diagnosis and early detection and treatment and, in some cases, adoption, artificial insemination, or delayed childbearing.

The family may consider artificial insemination by donor (AID), discussed earlier in this chapter. This alternative is appropriate in several instances; for example, if the man has an autosomal dominant disease, AID would decrease to zero the risk of having an affected child (if the sperm donor is not at risk) because the child would not inherit any genes from the affected parent. If the man is affected with an X-linked disorder and does not wish to continue the gene in the family (all his daughters will be carriers), AID would be an alternative to terminating all pregnancies with a female fetus. If the man is a carrier for a balanced translocation and if termination of pregnancy is against family ethics, AID is the most appropriate alternative. AID is also appropriate if both parents are carriers of an autosomal recessive disease. AID lowers the risk to a very low level or to zero if a carrier test is available. Finally, AID may be appropriate if the family is at high risk for a multifactorial disorder.

Couples who are young and at risk may decide to delay childbearing for a few years. Medical science and medical genetics are continually making breakthroughs in early detection and treatment. These couples may find in a few years that prenatal diagnosis will be available or that a disease can be detected and treated early to prevent irreversible damage.

The family may return to the genetic counselor a number of times to air their questions and concerns. It is desirable for the nurse working with the family to attend many or all of these counseling sessions. Because the nurse has already established a rapport with the family, the nurse can act as a liaison between the family and the genetic counselor. Hearing directly what the genetic counselor says helps the nurse clarify issues for the family, which in turn helps them formulate questions.

When the parents have completed the counseling sessions, the counselor sends them and their physician a letter detailing the contents of the sessions. The family keeps this document for reference. See Table 8–12.

Perhaps one of the most important and crucial aspects of genetic counseling in which the nurse is involved is follow-up counseling. The nurse with the appropriate knowledge of genetics is in an ideal position to help families review what has been discussed during the counseling sessions and to answer any additional questions they might have. As the family returns to the daily aspects of living, the nurse can provide helpful information on the day-to-day aspects of caring for the child, answer questions as they arise, support parents in their decisions, and refer the family to other health and community agencies (Mackta & Weiss, 1994).

TABLE 8–12 Nursing Responsibilities in Genetic Counseling

Identify families at risk for genetic problems.
Assist families in acquiring accurate information about the specific problem.
Act as liaison between family and genetic counselor.
Assist the family in understanding/dealing with information received.
Provide information on support groups.
Aid families in coping with this crisis.
Provide information about known genetic factors.
Assure continuity of nursing care to the family.

If the couple is considering having more children or if siblings want information concerning their affected brother or sister, the nurse should recommend that the family return for another follow-up visit with the genetic counselor. Appropriate options can again be defined and discussed, and any new information available can be given to the family. Many genetic centers have found the public health nurse to be the ideal health professional to provide such follow-up care.

Nurses must be careful not to assume a diagnosis, determine carrier status or recurrence risks, or provide genetic counseling without adequate information and training. Inadequate, inappropriate, or inaccurate information may be misleading or harmful. Health care professionals need to learn the appropriate referral systems and options for care in their region.

FOCUS YOUR STUDY

- A couple is considered infertile when they do not conceive after 1 year of unprotected coitus.
- At least 8% of couples in the United States are infertile.
- A thorough history and physical of both partners is essential as a basis for infertility investigation.
- General fertility investigations include evaluation of ovarian function, cervical mucus adequacy and receptivity to sperm, sperm number and function, tubal patency, general condition of the pelvic organs, and certain laboratory tests.
- Among cases of infertility, 40% involve male factors, 40% involve female factors, 10% to 20% have no identifiable cause, and 35% have multifactorial causes.
- Medications may be prescribed to induce ovulation, facilitate cervical mucus formation, reduce antibody concentration, increase sperm count and motility, and suppress endometriosis.
- The emotional aspect of infertility may be more difficult for the couple than the testing and therapy.
- The nurse needs to be prepared to provide accurate information about infertility and dispel myths.
- The nurse assesses coping responses and initiates counseling referrals as indicated.
- In autosomal dominant disorders, an affected parent has a 50% chance of having an affected child. Such disorders equally affect both males and females. The characteristic presentation will vary in each individual with the gene. Some of the common autosomal dominant inherited disorders are Huntington's disease, polycystic kidney disease, and neurofibromatosis (von Recklinghausen's disease).
- Autosomal recessive disorders are characterized by both parents being carriers; each offspring has a 25% chance of having the disease, a 25% chance of not being affected, and a 50% chance of being a carrier. Males and females are equally affected. Some common autosomal recessive inheritance disorders are cystic fibrosis, phenylketonuria (PKU), galactosemia, sickle cell anemia, Tay-Sachs disease, and most metabolic disorders. X-linked recessive disorders are characterized by no male-to-male transmission; effects limited to males; a 50% chance that a carrier mother will pass the abnormal gene to her sons; a 50% chance that her daughters will be carriers; and a 100% chance that daughters of affected fathers will be carriers. Common X-linked recessive disorders are hemophilia, some forms of color blindness, and Duchenne muscular dystrophy.
- Multifactorial inheritance disorders include cleft lip and palate, spina bifida, dislocated hips, clubfoot, and pyloric stenosis.
- Some genetic conditions that can currently be diagnosed prenatally are neural tube and cranial defects, renal malformations, hemophilia, fragile X syndrome, thalassemia, cystic fibrosis, and many inborn errors of metabolism such as Tay-Sachs disease. This list expands daily as new technology allows more conditions to be detected.
- The chief tools of prenatal diagnosis are ultrasound, maternal serum alpha fetoprotein testing, amniocentesis, chorionic villus sampling, and percutaneous umbilical blood sampling.
- Based on sound knowledge about common genetic problems, the nurse should prepare the family for counseling and act as a resource person during and after the counseling sessions.

REFERENCES

Alteneder, R. R., Kenner, C., Greene, D., & Pohorecki, S. (1998). The lived experience of women who undergo prenatal diagnostic tetsting. *Maternal Child Nursing, 23,* (4), 180–186.

American College of Obstetrics and Gynecology (ACOG). (1992). Later childbearing. ACOG patient education pamphlet APO60. Washington, DC: Author.

American Fertility Society (1994). *Infertility: Questions and answers.* Washington, DC: American Fertility Society, Office of Government Relations.

Arms, S. (1990). *Adoption: A handful of hope.* Berkeley, CA: Celestial Arts.

Black, B. P., Holditch-Davis, D., Sandelowski, M., & Harris, B. G. (1995). Comparison of pregnancy symptoms of infertile and fertile couples. *Journal of Perinatal and Neonatal Nursing, 9*(2), 1–9.

Boxer, A. (1996). Images of infertility. *Nurse Practitioner Forum, 7*(2), 60–63.

Bradshaw, K. D. (1998). Evaluation and management of the infertile couple. In. J. J. Sciarri & T. J. Watkins (Eds.), *Gynecology and obstetrics* (Vol. 5, Chap. 50, pp 1–15). Hagerstown, MD: Harper and Row.

Braverman, A., & English, M. (1992). Creating brave new families with advanced reproductive technologies. *Clinical Issues in Perinatal Women's Health Nursing, 3*(2), 353–363.

Brosens, I. A. (1997). Pathophysiology and medical treatment of endometriosis-associated infertility. In M. M. Seibel (Ed.), *Infertility: A comprehensive text* (2nd ed., pp 189–202). Stamford, CT: Appleton & Lange.

Centers for Disease Control and Prevention (CDC). (1997). *1995 Assisted reproductive technology success rates.* Atlanta: Author.

Corson, S. (1995). *Conquering infertility.* Vancouver: EMIS.

Corson, S. L., Kelly, M., Braverman, A. M., & English, M. E.

(1998). Gestational carrier pregnancy. *Fertility and Sterility, 69*(4), 670–674.

Geerling, J. H. (1995, Nov. 1). Natural family planning. *American Family Physician, 52*(6), 1749–1756, 1759–1760.

Hammond, M. G. (1996). Induction of ovulation with clomiphene citrate. In J. J. Sciarri et al (Eds.), *Gynecology and obstetrics* (Vol. 5). Hagerstown, MD: Harper and Row.

Hatcher, R. A., Stewart, F., Trussell, J., Kowal, D., Guest, F., Stewart, G. K., Gates, W., & Policar, M. (1998). *Contraceptive technology* (17th ed.). New York: Ardent Media, Inc.

Hook, E. B. et al (1988). Maternal age-specific rates of 47, +21 and other cytogenetic abnormalities diagnosed in the first trimester of pregnancy in chorionic villus biopsy specimens: Comparison with rates expected from observations at amniocentesis. *American Journal of Human Genetics, 42*, 797–807.

Inati, M. N, Lazar, E. C., & Haskin-Leahy, L. (1994). The role of the genetic counselor in a perinatal unit. *Seminars in Perinatology, 18*(3), 133–139.

Jeyendran, R. S. (1998). Semen analysis: Method and interpretation. In J. J. Sciarri & T. J. Watkins (Eds.), *Gynecology and obstetrics* (Vol. 5. Chap. 64, pp 1–15). Hagerstown, MD: Harper and Row.

Jewelewicz, R., & Wallach, E. E. (1995). Evaluation of the infertile couple. In E. E. Wallach & H. A. Zacur (Eds.), *Reproductive medicine and surgery*. New York: Mosby.

Johnson, C. L. (1996). Regaining self-esteem: Strategies and interventions for the infertile woman. *Journal of Obstetric, Gynecologic, and Neonatal Nursing, 25*(4), 291–295.

Jones, S. L. (1994). Assisted reproductive technologies: Genetic and nursing implications. *Journal of Obstetric, Gynecologic, and Neonatal Nursing, 23*(6), 492–497.

Karande, V. C., Pratt, D. E., Rabin, D. S., & Gleicher, N. (1995). The limited value of hysterosalpingography in assessing tubal status and fertility potential. *Fertility and Sterility, 63*(6), 1167–1171.

King, C. R., & Schimke, R. N. (1994). Multifactorial inheritance. In J. J. Sciarri & T. J. Watkins (Eds.), *Gynecology and obstetrics* (Vol. 5). Hagerstown, MD: Harper and Row.

Kruger, T. F., & Franken, D. (1994). Evolution of male factor infertility. In S. L. Behram, G. W. Patton, & G. Holtz (Eds.), *Progress in infertility*. Boston: Little, Brown.

Kuller, J. A., & Laifer, S. A. (1995). Contemporary approaches to prenatal diagnosis. *American Family Physician, 52*(8), 2277–2283, 2285–2286.

Mackta, J., & Weiss, J. O. (1994). The role of genetic support groups. *Journal of Obstetric, Gynecologic, and Neonatal Nursing, 23*(6), 519.

Moghissi, K. S. (1998). How to document ovulation. In J. J. Sciarri & T. J. Watkins (Eds.), *Gynecology and obstetrics* (Vol. 5, Chap. 54, pp 1–14). Hagerstown, MD: Harper and Row.

Murray, J., Cuckle, H., Taylor, G., & Hewison, J. (1997). Screening for fragile X syndrome: Information needs for health planners. *Journal of Medical Screening, 4*, 60–94.

Oei, S. G., Helmerhorst, F. M., Bloemenkamp, K. W., & Keirse, M. J. (1996). Effects of the postcoital test on the sexual relationship of infertile couples: A randomized controlled trial. *Fertility and Sterility, 65*(4), 771–775.

Olsen, D. G. (1994). Parental adjustment to a child with a genetic disease: One parent's reflections. *Journal of Obstetric, Gynecologic, and Neonatal Nursing, 23*(6), 516.

Pergament, E., & Fiddler, M. (1996). Current status of preimplantation diagnosis. In J. J. Sciarri & T. J. Watkins (Eds.), *Gynecology and obstetrics* (Vol 5). Hagerstown, MD: Harper and Row.

Pickler, R. H., & Munro, C. L. (1994). Blastomere analysis: Issues for discussion. *Journal of Obstetric, Gynecologic, and Neonatal Nursing, 23*(5), 379–382.

Robertson, J. A. (1995). Ethical and legal issues in human embryo donation. *Fertility and Sterility, 64*(5), 885–894.

Sandelowski, M. (1994). On infertility. *Journal of Obstetric, Gynecologic, and Neonatal Nursing, 23*(9), 749–752.

Sawatzky, M. (1981). Tasks of the infertile couple. *Journal of Obstetric, Gynecologic, and Neonatal Nursing, 10*, 132–133.

Schoener, C. J., & Krysa, L. W. (1996). The comfort and discomfort of infertility. *Journal of Obstetric, Gynecologic, and Neonatal Nursing, 25*(2), 167–172.

Scioscia, A. L. (1999). Preantal genetic diagnosis. In R. K. Creasy & R. Resnik (Eds.), *Maternal-fetal medicine* (4th ed. pp 40–62). Philadelphia: Saunders.

Scott, R. T., & Hofmann, G. E. (1995). Prognostic assessment of ovarian reserve. *Fertility and Sterility, 63* (1) 1.

Shane, J. M. (1993). Evaluation and treatment of infertility. *Clinical Symposia, 45*, 2–32.

Sharara, F. I., & Scott, R. T. (1997). Assessment of ovarian reserve and treatment of low responders. In E. S. Surrey (Ed.), *Reproductive clinics of North America*. Philadelphia: Saunders.

Simpson, J. L. (1990). Genetic factors in obstetrics and gynecology. In J. R. Scott, P. J. DiSaia, C. B. Hammond, & W. N. Spellacy (Eds.), *Danforth's obstetrics and gynecology* (6th ed.). Philadelphia: Lippincott.

Simpson, J. L., & Elias, S. (1993). *Essentials of prenatal diagnosis*. New York: Churchill Livingstone.

Smith, S. E., & Tucker, M. J. (1997). Micromanipulation for assisted reproduction. In J. J. Sciarri & T. J. Watkins (Eds.), *Gynecology and obstetrics* (Vol. 5, Chap. 102, pp 1–19). Hagerstown, MD: Harper and Row.

Speroff, L. Glass, R. H., & Kase, N. G. (1994). *Clinical gynecologic endocrinology and infertility* (5th ed.). Baltimore: Williams & Wilkins.

Stansberry, J. (1996). The infertile couple: An overview of pathophysiology and diagnostic evaluation for the primary care clinician. *Nurse Practitioner Forum*, 7(2), 76–86.

Stovall, D. W., Tomah, S. K., Hammond, L. M., & Talbert, L. M. (1991). The effect of age on female fecundity. *Obstetrics and Gynecology*, 77, 33.

Tallo, C. P., Vohr, B., Oh, W., Rubin, L. P., Seifer, D. B., & Haning, R. V., Jr. (1995). Maternal and neonatal morbidity associated with in vitro fertilization. *Journal of Pediatrics, 127*(5), 794–800.

Thompson, M. W., McInnes, R. R., & Willard, H. F. (1991). *Thompson & Thompson's genetics in medicine* (5th ed.). Philadelphia: Saunders.

Trantham, P. (1996). The infertile couple. *American Family Physician, 54*(3) 1001–1010.

Tredway, A. B. (1996). DR: The postcoital test. In J. J. Sciarri & T. J. Watkins (Eds.), *Gynecology and obstetrics* (Vol. 5). Hagerstown, MD: Harper and Row.

Villaire, M. (1996). Management of genetic information: Professional and ethical challenges in nursing. *Critical Care Nurse, 16*(5), 96–101.

World Health Organization. (1992). *WHO manual for the examination of human semen and sperm–cervical mucus interaction*. Cambridge, England: Cambridge University Press.

Wolf, D. P. (1998). Gamete and embryo cryopreservation. In J. J. Sciarri & T. J. Watkins (Eds.), *Gynecology and obstetrics* (Vol. 5, Chap. 99, pp 1–7). Hagerstown, MD: Harper and Row.

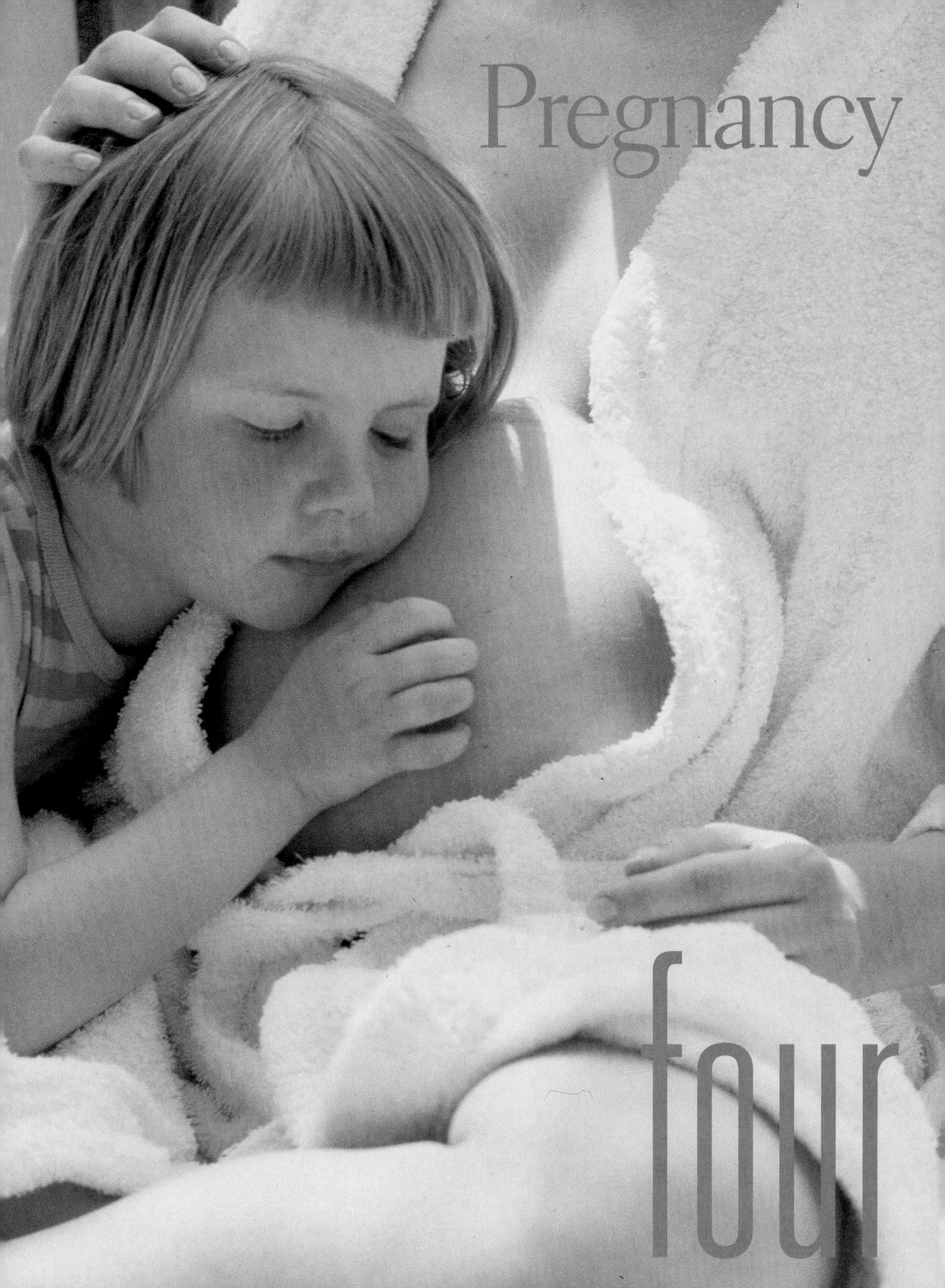

Pregnancy

four

9 Preparation for Parenthood

Key Terms

Birth plan
Disassociation relaxation
Doula
Effleurage
Prenatal education
Progressive relaxation
Psychoprophylactic (Lamaze) method
Touch relaxation

Choices are important. They determine how you experience giving birth and how your baby enters the world. They must be made in the present and lived with in the future.
~ *Pregnant Feelings* ~

Objectives

- Apply the nursing process to help couples prepare for childbirth.
- Identify the various issues related to pregnancy, labor, and birth that require decision making by parents.
- Discuss the basic goals of childbirth education.
- Summarize the role of the doula/labor companion during labor and birth.
- Describe the types of prenatal education programs available to expectant couples and their families.
- Delineate the childbirth educator's role in decreasing anxiety for pregnant women.
- Compare methods of childbirth preparation.

PREPARATION FOR PARENTHOOD BEGINS with one's own birth into a family. Attitudes, feelings, and fears about pregnancy, birth, and parenthood are molded by numerous factors, including relationships within and outside one's own family, cultural conditioning, personal history, and discussions with health care providers.

A person's experiences with parenting or children may have been pleasant or uncomfortable. A person's information about parenthood and related areas may or may not be accurate. Because people bring their beliefs and fears with them to the childbearing period, the nurse can do much to correct misconceptions and calm fears regarding pregnancy, childbirth, and early parenting. One way that a couple can cope with feelings about impending parenthood is to assume an active, participatory role during the preconception, prenatal, intrapartal, and postpartal periods. This involvement enables them to take part in many of the decisions regarding the conduct of the birth. It offers them a degree of control over what could be an overwhelming experience.

Some of the decisions that the childbearing family must consider are presented in this chapter. The chapter addresses issues such as the decision to have a baby, choice of care provider, type of childbirth preparation, place of birth, activities during the birth, method of infant feeding, and choices surrounding the care of the newborn. It also considers the role of the nurse, who provides information that enables the family to make informed decisions.

Throughout this chapter the term "childbearing family" is used. In today's society, the childbearing family may be composed of a man and a woman joined by marriage or simply by mutual personal commitment, a single woman living alone or with another partner or a family member, or a lesbian couple. No matter what the family structure and configuration, the expectant woman and her support person have similar concerns and educational needs during this time. The term "childbearing family" includes all family types.

Today's professional nurse has many opportunities to help the childbearing family make the decisions that are part of pregnancy and birth. The nurse can help families seek preconceptual counseling, select a health care provider, find prenatal classes that meet their needs, and make informed choices. Even more important, as the family works through these decisions, the nurse is able to affirm their decision-making abilities and their ability to take on parenting roles. For first-time parents in particular, the decisions may seem numerous and complicated. The nurse has a unique opportunity to help these families establish a pattern of decision making that will serve them well in their years as parents (Figure 9–1).

Preconception Counseling

One of the first questions a couple should ask before conception is whether they wish to have children. This involves consideration of each person's goals, expectations of their relationship, and desire to be a parent. At times

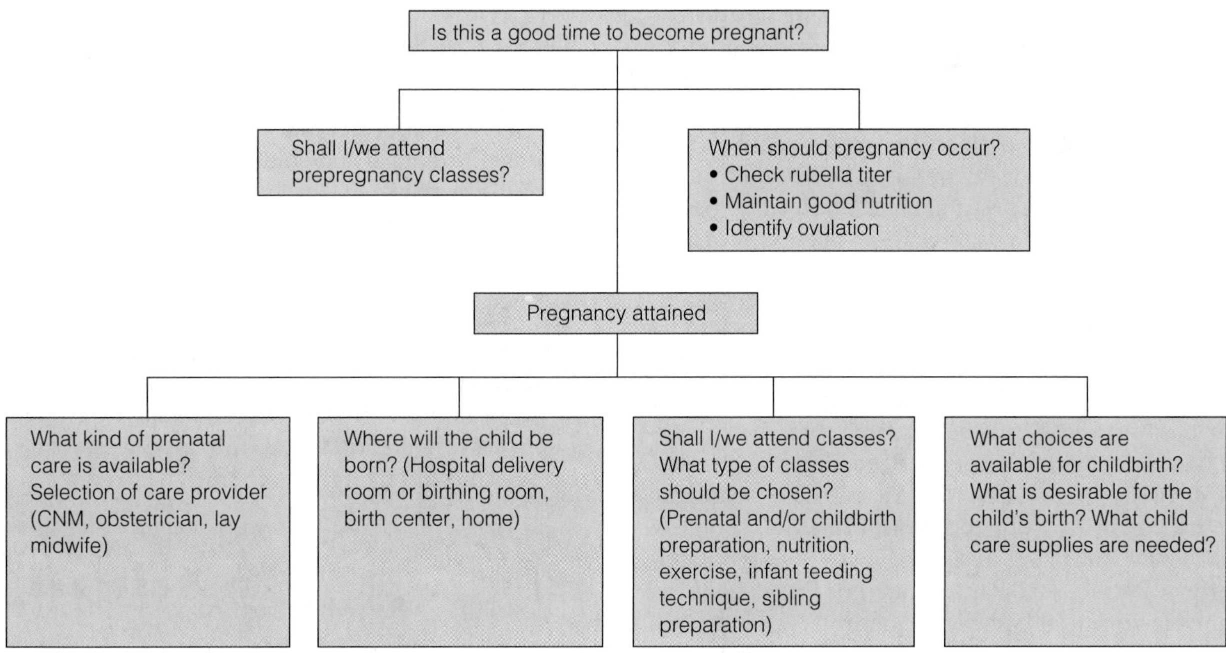

FIGURE 9–1 Pregnancy decision tree.

one individual wishes to have a child while the other does not. In such situations, an open discussion is essential to reach a mutually acceptable decision. In some cases professional counseling for the couple may be necessary.

Couples who wish to have children face a decision about the timing of pregnancy. At what point in their lives do they believe it would be best to become parents? Pregnancy comes as a surprise even when the decision about timing is made, but at least the couple has some control over it.

For couples who have religious beliefs that do not support contraception or who feel that fertility planning is unnatural and wrong, planning the timing of pregnancy is unacceptable and irrelevant. These couples can still take steps to ensure that they are in the best possible physical and mental health when pregnancy occurs.

Preconception Health Measures

The couple is taught about known or suspected health risks. The nurse advises the woman to cease smoking if possible, or to limit her cigarette intake to less than half a pack per day (Tirosh et al, 1996). Because of the hazards of secondhand smoke, it is helpful if her partner refrains from smoking around her. The effects of caffeine are less clearly understood; however, as a precaution the woman is advised to avoid caffeine or limit her intake. Alcohol, social drugs, and street drugs pose a real threat to the fetus. A woman who uses any prescription or over-the-counter medications needs to discuss the implications of their use with her health care provider. It is best to avoid using any medication if possible. Because of the possible teratogenic effects of environmental hazards in the workplace, the nurse urges the couple contemplating pregnancy to determine whether they are exposed to any environmental hazards at work or in their community.

Physical Examination

It is advisable for both partners to have a physical examination to identify any health problems so that they can be corrected if possible. These might include medical conditions such as high blood pressure or obesity; problems that pose a threat to fertility, such as certain sexually transmitted infections; or conditions that keep the individual from achieving optimal health, such as anemia or colitis. If the family history indicates previous genetic disorders, or if the couple is planning pregnancy when the woman is over age 35, the health care provider may suggest that the couple consider genetic counseling. In addition to the history and physical exam, the woman may have the following laboratory tests: urinalysis, complete blood count, Rh factor, Venereal Disease Research Laboratory (VDRL) test, Pap smear, gonorrhea culture, chlamydia screen, and rubella and hepatitis screens (Olds, 1997). Prior to conception the woman is also advised to have a dental examination and any necessary dental work to avoid exposure to x-rays and the risk of infection.

Nutrition

Prior to conception it is advisable for the woman to be at an average weight for her body build and height. The woman is advised to follow a nutritious diet that contains ample quantities of all the essential nutrients. Some nutritionists advocate emphasizing the following nutrients: calcium, protein, iron, B complex vitamins, vitamin C, folic acid, and magnesium. Excessive vitamin intake can cause severe fetal problems and should be avoided.

Exercise

A woman is advised to establish a regular exercise plan beginning at least 3 months before she plans to attempt to become pregnant. The exercise should be one she enjoys and will continue. It needs to provide some aerobic conditioning and some general toning. Exercise improves the woman's circulation and general health and tones her muscles. Once an exercise program is well established, the woman is generally encouraged to continue it during pregnancy.

Contraception

A woman who takes birth control pills is advised to stop the pill and have two or three normal menses before attempting to conceive. This allows the natural hormonal cycle to return and facilitates dating the subsequent pregnancy. A woman using an intrauterine device is advised to have it removed and wait 1 month before attempting to conceive. This allows the endometrium to be resterilized. During the waiting period, she can use barrier methods of contraception (condoms, diaphragm, cervical cap, or spermicides).

Conception

Most preconception recommendations focus on helping the couple attain their best possible health state so that they do not enter pregnancy with unnecessary risks. Conception is a personal and emotional experience, and even if a couple is prepared, they may feel some ambivalence. This is a normal response, but they may require reassurance that the ambivalence will pass. A couple may get so caught up in preparation and in their efforts to "do things right" that they lose sight of the pleasure they derive from each other and their lives together and cease to value the joy of spontaneity in their relationship. It is often helpful for the health care provider to remind an overly zealous couple that moderation is always appropriate and that there is value in "taking time to smell the roses."

CRITICAL THINKING QUESTION

What characteristics would you expect in women or couples who seek preconceptual counseling?

Childbearing Decisions

Care Provider

One of the first decisions facing expectant parents is the selection of a health care provider. The nurse assists them by explaining the various options and outlining what can be expected from each. A thorough understanding of the differences of education preparation, skill level, and general philosophy and characteristics of practice of certified nurse-midwives, obstetricians, family practice physicians, and lay midwives is essential (Harvey et al, 1996). The nurse can encourage expectant parents to investigate the care provider's credentials, basic and special education and training, fee schedule, and availability to new clients; this is often accomplished by telephoning the provider's office. The nurse can also help them develop a list of interview questions for their first visit to a care provider. These could include the following:

- Who is in practice with you, or who covers for you when you are unavailable?
- How do your partners' philosophies compare to yours?
- How do you feel about my partner, other support person, or other children coming to the prenatal visits?
- What weight gain do you recommend and why?
- What are your feelings about (fill in special desires for the birth event, such as different positions assumed during labor, episiotomy, induction of labor, other people present during the birth, breastfeeding immediately after the birth, no separation of infant and parents following birth, and so on)?
- If a cesarean is necessary, can my partner be present?

Choosing a care provider is just one of the decisions pregnant women and couples will make. A method that has assisted many couples in making these choices is called a **birth plan.** In the birth plan, prospective parents identify aspects of the childbearing experience that are most important to them. (A sample birth plan is presented in Figure 9–2.) The birth plan helps identify available options and becomes a tool for communication among the expectant parents, the health care providers, and the health care professionals at the birth setting (Wheeler, 1997).

The plan also helps pregnant women and couples set priorities. Using the plan, they identify areas that they want to incorporate in their own birth experience. Then they can take the birth plan to a visit with their certified nurse-midwife or other care provider and use it in discussing and comparing their wishes with the philosophy and beliefs of the provider. They can also take the birth plan to the birth setting and use it as a basis for communicating their wishes during the childbirth experience.

Sample Birth Plan

Choice	*Choice*
Care provider:	Position during birth:
Certified nurse-midwife	On side
Obstetrician	Hands and knees
Lay midwife	Kneeling
Birth setting	Squatting
Hospital:	Birthing chair
Birthing room	Birthing bed
Delivery room	Other:
Birth center	Family present (sibs)
Home	Filming of birth (videotaping)
Support during labor and birth:	Photography of birth
Partner present	Leboyer
Doula present	Episiotomy
During labor:	No sterile drapes
Ambulate as desired	Partner to cut umbilical cord
Shower if desired	Hold baby immediately after birth
Wear own clothes	Breastfeed immediately after birth
Use hot tub	No separation after birth
Use own rocking chair	Save the placenta
Have perineal prep	Collect cord blood for banking
Have enema	Newborn care:
Water birth	Eye treatment for the baby
Electronic fetal monitor	Vitamin K injection
Membranes:	Heptovac injection
Rupture naturally	Breastfeeding
Amniotomy if needed	Formula feeding
Labor stimulation if needed	Glucose water
Medication:	Circumcision
Identify type desired	Postpartum care:
Fluids or ice as desired	Short stay
Music during labor and birth	48 hour stay after vaginal birth
Massage	Home visits after discharge
Therapeutic touch	Home doula
Healing touch	Other:

FIGURE 9–2 Birth plan for childbirth choices. The column on the left lists various choices that the couple may consider during their childbirth experience. Once the couple has considered each of the choices, they may circle the items they desire.

Expectant parents also need to discuss the qualities they want in a care provider for the newborn, and they may want to visit several before the birth to assure a selection of someone who will meet their needs and those of their child.

There are many more choices that pregnant women and couples will make. Some of these are explored in Table 9–1. Although most birth experiences are very close to the desired experience, at times expectations cannot be met. This may be due to unavailability of some choices in the community or in the presence of unexpected problems during pregnancy or birth. It is important for nurses to help expectant parents keep sight of what is realistic for their situation.

CRITICAL THINKING QUESTION

What forces affect the birth choices available in your community? Does your community have nurse-midwives? Doulas?

TABLE 9–1 Benefits and Risks of Some Consumer Decisions During Pregnancy, Labor, and Birth

Issue	Benefits	Risks
Breastfeeding	No additional expense. Contains maternal antibodies. Decreases incidence of infant otitis media, vomiting, and diarrhea. Easier to digest than formula. Immediately after birth, promotes uterine contractions and decreases incidence of postpartum hemorrhage.	Transmission of pollutants to newborn. Irregular ovulation and menses can cause false sense of security and nonuse of contraceptives. Increased nutritional requirement in mother.
Perineal prep	May decrease risk of infection. Facilitates episiotomy repair.	Nicks can be portal for bacteria. Discomfort as hair grows back.
Enema	May facilitate labor. Increases space for infant in pelvis. May increase strength of contractions. May prevent contamination of sterile field.	Increases discomfort and anxiety.
Ambulation during labor	Comfort for laboring woman. May assist in labor progression by a. Stimulating contractions. b. Allowing gravity to help descent of fetus. c. Giving sense of independence and control.	Cord prolapse will rupture membranes unless engagement has occurred. Birth of infant in undesirable situations.
Electronic fetal monitoring	Helps evaluate fetal well-being. Helps identify fetal stress. Useful in diagnostic testing. Helps evaluate labor progress.	Supine postural hypotension. Intrauterine perforation (with internal uterine pressure device). Infection (with internal monitoring). Decreases personal interaction with mother because of attention paid to the machine. Mother is unable to ambulate or change her position freely.
Whirlpool (jet hydrotherapy)	Increased relaxation. Decreased anxiety. Stimulation of labor. Nonmedicated pain relief. Slight decrease in B/P. Increased diuresis.	May slow contractions if used before active labor is established. Possible risk of infection if membranes are ruptured. Slight increase in maternal temperature and heart rate and fetal heart rate during whirlpool and/or in first 30 min after being in tub (Rogers & Davis, 1995).
Analgesia	Maternal relaxation facilitates labor.	All drugs reach the fetus in varying degrees and with varying effects.
Episiotomy	Decreases irregular tearing of perineum.	Increased pain after birth and for 3 months following birth. Infection. Increased frequency of 3rd- and 4th-degree lacerations (Woolley, 1995).

NOTE: For additional information regarding these issues, refer to Chapter 20.

Choosing the Birth Setting

The nurse can help expectant parents choose a birth setting by suggesting they tour facilities and talk with nurses there, and by talking with friends or acquaintances who are recent parents. Questions that may be asked of new parents include the following:

- What kind of support did you receive during labor? Was it what you wanted?
- If the setting has both labor and delivery rooms and birthing rooms, was a birthing room available when you wanted it?
- Were you encouraged to be mobile during labor or to do what you wanted to do (walking, sitting in a rocking chair, remaining in bed, sitting in a hot tub, standing in a shower, and so on)?
- Was your labor partner or coach treated well?
- Was your birth plan respected? Did you share it with the facility before the birth? If something did not work, why do you think there were problems?
- How were medications handled during labor? Were you comfortable with this?
- Were siblings welcomed in the birth setting? After the birth?
- Was the nursing staff helpful after the baby was born? Did you receive self-care and infant care information? Was it in a usable form? Did you have a choice about what information you got? Did they let you decide what information you needed?

The nurse helps expectant parents understand the array of choices available to them. The nurse can encourage them to consider options early in the pregnancy to allow time for talking with other parents and touring facilities.

What I've seen time and again is that the technology of the hospital overwhelms patients' natural instincts; they are intimidated, afraid of appearing stupid or clumsy or sentimental in a surrounding that seems too efficient and immaculate and intelligent.
~ A MIDWIFE'S STORY ~

The Labor Support Person

Some of the first formal childbirth preparation classes were patterned after a book entitled *Husband Coached Childbirth* by Dr. Robert Bradley, published in 1965. Since that time, husbands and other partners of expectant women have been very involved in acting as "coaches" during childbirth classes, labor, and birth. Recently, however, there has been recognition of the facts that some partners do not want to play an active role during labor and birth, and some pregnant women are not finding the kind of support they desire. Chapman (1991) studied fathers during childbirth and found that they usually take on one of three roles: (1) In the "coach" role, the father actively assists the woman in comfort and breathing techniques and seems to assume responsibility for helping direct the course of her responses during labor. (2) The "teammate" is very willing to help, but waits for direction from the nurse or physician. (3) The "witness" is willing to hold the woman's hand, but for the most part does not seek further involvement and is comfortable simply to observe the process. Chapman's study and other information about partners' comfort levels and their personal and cultural expectations of their role have created awareness that some women need support from another source.

When the partner is not actively involved in supportive, attentive care, most women look to another woman for empathy and help (Robotti & Inman, 1998). Out of this need for companionship and special support in the birthing journey the role of the **doula** has evolved. *Doula* is a Greek word that means "woman's servant." In the birthing environment, doula refers to a companion who provides support but does not perform any clinical tasks. The doula provides emotional, physical, and informational support and acts as an advocate for the woman and her family by verbalizing their wishes to the nurses and physicians or certified nurse-midwives. A doula may also be trained to provide support and care during the postpartum period and in this role is called a home doula (Robotti & Inman, 1998). The doula may accompany the childbearing couple on a volunteer basis or may be paid a fee by the family. Another support person who has been involved in labor and birthing is a *monitrice*. Monitrice is a French word that refers to a specially trained nurse who provides assessment, nursing care, and support. The role of monitrice is not common in the United States.

Siblings at Birth

The couple may decide to have their other children present at the birth. Children who will attend a birth can be prepared through books, audiovisual materials, models, discussion, and sibling classes. Nurses can assist parents with sibling preparation by helping them understand the stresses a child may experience. For example, the child may feel left out when there is a new child to love or disappointed if a brother is born when a sister is expected.

It is highly recommended that the child have his or her own support person or coach whose sole responsibility is tending to the needs of the child. The support person should be well known to the child, warm, sensitive, and flexible, knowledgeable about the birth process, and comfortable with sexuality and birth. This person must be prepared to interpret what is happening to the child and to intervene when necessary. The support person should not be one who would hesitate to leave the birthing room (such as a maternal grandmother) but should be amenable to the child's desire to leave the birthing room.

CLINICAL TIP

Call the birthing facilities in your community and inquire about what choices are available in each facility.

The child should be given the option of relating to the birth in whatever manner she or he chooses as long as it is not disruptive. Children should understand that it is their own choice to be there and that they may stay or leave the room as they choose. To help the child meet her or his goal, the nurse may wish to elicit exactly what the child expects from the experience. The child needs to feel free to ask questions and express feelings.

In general, the presence of siblings at birth engenders feelings of interest and the desire to nurture "our" baby, as opposed to jealousy and rivalry directed at "Mom's" baby. The mother does not disappear mysteriously into the hospital and return with a demanding outsider. Instead, the family attending the birth together finds a new opportunity for closeness and growth by sharing in the birth of a new member.

Classes for Family Members During Pregnancy

Prenatal education programs provide important opportunities to share information about pregnancy and childbirth and to enhance the parents' decision-making skills (Humenick, 1996; Monto, 1996). The content of each class is generally directed by the overall goals of the program. For example, in classes that aim to provide preconceptual information, preparations for becoming pregnant would be the major topics. Other classes may be directed toward childbirth choices available today, preparation of the mother for pregnancy and birth, preparation for cesarean birth, and preparation of specific people such as grandparents or siblings for the birth. The nurse who knows the types of prenatal programs available in the community can direct expectant parents to programs that meet their special needs and learning goals (Walden et al, 1996). Childbirth preparation classes usually contain information about changes in the woman and the developing baby. See Table 9–2.

TABLE 9–2 Possible Content of Classes for Childbirth Preparation

Early Classes (First Trimester)
- Early gestational changes
- Self-care during pregnancy
- Fetal development, environmental dangers for the fetus
- Sexuality in pregnancy
- Birth settings and types of care providers
- Nutrition, rest, and exercise suggestions
- Relief measures for common discomforts of pregnancy
- Psychologic changes in pregnancy
- Information for getting pregnancy off to a good start

Later Classes (Second and Third Trimesters)
- Preparation for birth process
- Postpartum self-care
- Birth choices (episiotomy, medications, fetal monitoring, perineal prep, enema, etc.)
- Relaxation techniques
- Breathing techniques
- Infant stimulation
- Newborn safety issues, such as car seats

Adolescent Preparation Classes
- How to be a good parent
- Newborn care
- Health dangers for the baby
- Healthy diet during pregnancy
- How to recognize when baby is ill
- Baby care: physical and emotional

Breastfeeding Programs
- Advantages and disadvantages
- Techniques of breastfeeding
- Methods of breast preparation
- Involvement of fathers in feeding process

From the expectant parents' point of view, class content is best presented in chronology with the pregnancy (Figure 9–3). Although both parents expect to learn breathing and relaxation techniques and infant care, fathers usually expect facts and mothers expect coping strategies. It is important that the classes begin by finding out what each parent wants to learn and birth alternatives (Humenick, 1996). At times prenatal classes are divided into early and late classes.

Early Classes: First Trimester

Early prenatal classes should include prepregnant women and couples as well as those in early pregnancy. The classes cover early gestational changes; self-care during pregnancy; fetal development and environmental dangers for the fetus; sexuality in pregnancy; birth settings and types of care providers; nutrition, rest, and exercise suggestions; common discomforts of pregnancy and relief measures; psychologic changes in pregnancy for the woman and man; and getting the pregnancy off to a good start by following a healthful lifestyle, learning methods

COMMUNITY IN FOCUS

Healthy Beginnings

More and more communities are acting proactively to improve the parenting skills of their residents and decrease the incidence of child abuse and neglect. One especially successful program is the Healthy Beginnings Program in Hastings, Nebraska. Established in 1990, the program, which is the first mainland replication of the successful Hawaii Healthy Start Program, is a home visitation program designed to help parents be "the best they can be." The program is voluntary and free to participants.

Families enter the program prenatally or up to 3 months following the birth of a child. Approximately 75% of families are referred to the program by a health care professional; the remainder are self-referred or referred by another agency. Once a contact is made, each family is seen by a nurse and a paraprofessional for an interview and initial assessment. The Family Stress Checklist, developed in 1978 by Smith and Carroll of the University of Colorado Health Sciences Center, is used to screen families as low, moderate, or high risk for parenting problems. All moderate and high-risk families are invited to join the program.

The program offers long-term and intensive services. Prenatally, parents participate in a series of nursing home visits to discuss a wide variety of topics related to pregnancy and parenting. Additional nursing visits are scheduled in the home following childbirth and again within the first month. The emphasis of these early visits is on adjustment to the newborn and on learning to read and respond appropriately to the baby's cues. Moreover, six times during the first two years, nurses complete developmental assessments of each child and make appropriate referrals if they identify any concerns or developmental delays. Nurses also regularly assess and educate parents about issues such as age-appropriate developmental expectations and activities, and parent-child interactions and communication.

In addition, the family is visited weekly by a specially trained paraprofessional who helps the family develop parenting skills. To ensure consistency and promote a sense of trust, the family works with the same paraprofessional and nurse throughout the duration of services. These weekly visits last up to a year or more and then progress to biweekly and quarterly visits as the family gains skills and confidence. Visits continue until the child is 5 years old. Throughout the process, families receive case management services including community and professional referrals and networking, health, nutritional and safety assessments, and encouragement to use the health care system appropriately (eg, clinic, ER, phone support). Results to date are impressive. Of the families served by Healthy Beginnings:

- 98% have no child abuse or neglect requiring court involvement.
- 97% of the children are up-to-date on their well child care and immunizations.
- At least 98% of the families have no unintended repeat pregnancies.
- Over 80% of the families are either employed, furthering their education, or both.

SOURCE: Personal communication with Paula Witt, RN, PNP, Director of the Healthy Beginnings Program, and printed program materials.

of coping with stress, and avoiding alcohol and smoking. Early classes should provide information about factors that place the woman at risk for preterm labor and about how to recognize symptoms of preterm labor. Early classes should also present the advantages and disadvantages of bottle or breastfeeding. The majority of women (50% to 80%) have made their infant feeding decision before the sixth month of pregnancy.

Later Classes: Second and Third Trimesters

The later classes focus on preparation for the birth, infant care and feeding, postpartum self-care, birth choices (episiotomy, medications, fetal monitoring, perineal prep, enema, and so forth), and newborn safety issues. Because many parents purchase a car seat before birth, later classes should also include information about the importance of car seats, how they work, and how to select an approved car seat (Baer, 1992).

Broussard and Rich (1990) suggest that infant stimulation concepts be incorporated into childbirth preparation classes. This will aid in the development of parenting skills and enhance prenatal and neonatal bonding. Methods that can be used include tactile, vestibular, auditory, and visual stimulation. Information regarding tactile stimulation can be presented while discussing maternal anatomy and physiology. As the uterine wall thins during the pregnancy, the mother and father are better able to feel the baby, and the fetus can sense the parents' stroking and patting through the abdominal wall. **Effleurage** (a light stroking movement made with the fingertips) can also be used over the abdominal wall to provide tactile stimulation to the fetus.

Vestibular stimulation through movement of the fetus is provided while the expectant woman does the pelvic-tilt exercise. Rocking in a rocking chair is also a comfortable way to provide relaxation for the expectant woman and vestibular stimulation for the fetus. Auditory stimulation can be provided by playing music. Classical music (such as Vivaldi, Mozart, Beethoven, and Bach) is found to be pleasing to the fetus. In the prenatal period, actual visual stimulation for the fetus is not possible. However, the parents can be encouraged to visualize the fetus "as lying calmly inside, all flexed, sucking its thumb, swallowing amniotic fluid, and opening its eyes to look toward the sunlight filtering through the abdominal wall" (Broussard & Rich, 1990, p 384).

Adolescent Parenting Classes

Adolescents have special learning needs during pregnancy. In a study by Roye and Balk (1996), teens identified informational needs during pregnancy. Areas of concern were how to be a good parent, how to care for the new baby, health dangers to the baby, and healthy foods to eat during pregnancy. Teens also identified information needs about how to recognize when the baby is sick, take care of the baby, protect the baby from accidents,

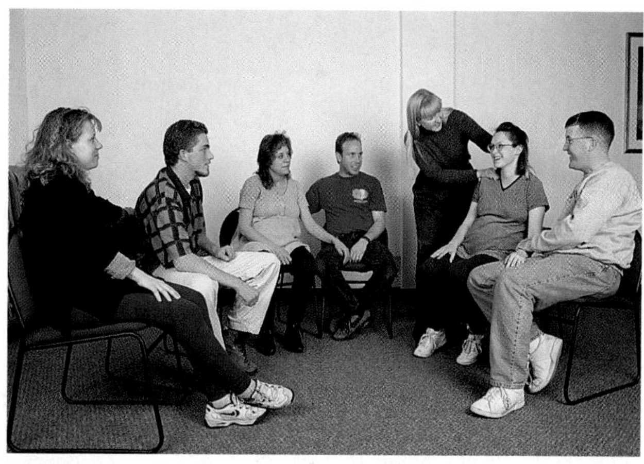

FIGURE 9–3 In a group setting with a nurse-instructor, expectant parents share information about pregnancy and childbirth.

and make the baby feel happy and loved. They were also eager to hear more about the birth process (especially pain during the birth process), the personal health of the mother, the discomforts of pregnancy, changes in life with pregnancy, and sexuality.

Breastfeeding Programs

Programs offering information on breastfeeding are increasing. For many years, a primary source of information has been La Leche League. Information can also be obtained from lactation consultants, birthing centers, hospitals, and health clinics. Content includes advantages and disadvantages, techniques of breastfeeding, and methods of breast preparation. The father's support and encouragement of the mother is vital so it is important to include him in the educational programs decision making. Some fathers may feel negative and resentful about breastfeeding and need opportunities in the prenatal period for discussion and sharing of information.

Sibling Preparation: Adjustment to a Newborn

The birth of a new sibling is a significant event in a child's life. Positive adjustment can be enhanced by attendance at formal sibling preparation classes (Figure 9–4). The classes are usually focused on reducing anxiety in the child, providing opportunities for the child to express feelings and concerns, and encouraging realistic expectations of the newborn. Parents learn strategies to help prepare the child for the birth and to assist the child in coping with a newcomer (Fortier et al, 1991).

Fortier and associates (1991) found that a sibling preparation class made a significant difference in the adjustment of the child to the birth. The child demonstrated fewer behaviors associated with sibling rivalry (crying, whining, clinging, and eating problems). The mothers also felt that they were able to cope more effectively.

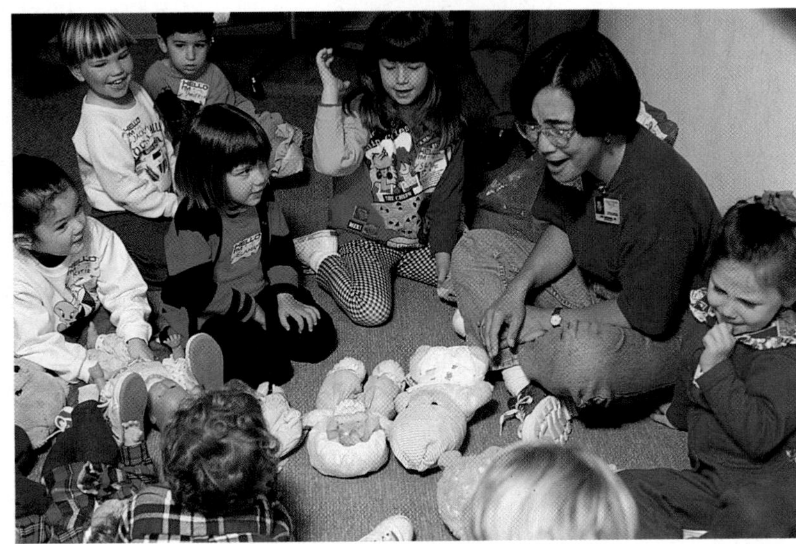

FIGURE 9–4 It is especially important that siblings be well prepared when they are going to be present at the birth. However, even siblings who will not be present at the birth can benefit from information about birth and the new baby ahead of time.

The classes in the study were titled "Siblings Are Special." Parents and their children attended the class together. Many activities were devised to help each child feel special: Children were greeted with badges saying "I'm a big sister" or "I'm a big brother" and "I'm special"; an instant photo was taken of the child so that the picture could be placed in the newborn's hospital crib; and the child decorated a bib for the new baby. Time was allotted at the end of the class for talking with parents about coping skills and providing hints about dealing with sibling jealousy.

Sibling preparation can be addressed through a formal class such as the one just described, or in a less formal way by preparing a booklet for parents that addresses issues affecting both parents and children.

Classes for Grandparents

Grandparents are an important source of support and information for prospective and new parents. They are now being included in the birthing process more frequently. Prenatal programs for grandparents can be an important source of information about current beliefs and practices in childbearing (Roye & Balk, 1996). The most useful content may include changes in birthing and parenting practices and helpful tips for being a supportive grandparent. Grandparents who will be integral members of the labor and birth team need information about being coaches.

Education of the Family Having Cesarean Birth

Preparation for Cesarean Birth

Cesarean birth is an alternative method of birth. Because one out of every four or five births is a cesarean, preparation for this possibility should be an integral part of every childbirth education curriculum. The instructor should treat cesarean birth as a normal event and present factual information that will allow expectant parents to make choices and be full participants in their birth experience. The instructor can emphasize the similarities between cesarean and vaginal births to minimize undertones of "normal" versus "abnormal" birth. This will diminish the feelings of anger, loss, and grief that often accompany cesarean births.

Cesarean birth classes should cover what the parents can expect to happen during a cesarean birth, what they will feel, and what they can do. All pregnant women and couples should be encouraged to discuss with their certified nurse-midwife/physician what the approach would be in the event of a cesarean. They can also discuss their needs and preferences regarding the following:

- Participating in the choice of anesthetic
- Father (or significant other) being present during the birth
- Planning initial contact with their newborn

Preparation for Repeat Cesarean Birth

When expectant parents are anticipating a repeat cesarean birth, they have time to plan and prepare. Many hospitals or local groups (such as C-Sec, Inc.) provide preparation classes for cesarean birth. Parents who have had previous negative experiences need an opportunity to describe what contributed to their feelings. They should be encouraged to identify what they would like to change and to list interventions that would make the experience more positive. Those who have had positive experiences need reassurance that their needs and desires will be met in the same manner. In addition, all parents are encouraged to air any fears or anxieties.

A specific concern of the woman facing a repeat cesarean is anticipation of pain. She needs reassurance that subsequent cesareans are often less painful than the first.

TABLE 9–3 Summary of Selected Childbirth Preparation Methods

Method	Characteristics	Breathing Technique
Lamaze	See narrative discussion.	
Bradley	Frequently referred to as partner- or husband-coached natural childbirth. Uses various exercises and slow controlled abdominal breathing to accomplish relaxation.	Primarily abdominal.
Kitzinger	Uses sensory memory to help the woman understand and work with her body in preparation for birth. Incorporates the Stanislavsky method of acting as a way to teach relaxation.	Uses chest breathing in conjunction with abdominal relaxation.

If her first cesarean was preceded by a long or strenuous labor, she will not experience the same fatigue. Giving this information will help her cope more effectively with all stressful stimuli, including pain. The nurse can remind the client that she has already had experience with how to prevent, cope with, and alleviate painful stimuli.

Preparation for Parents Desiring Vaginal Birth after Cesarean Birth (VBAC)

Parents who have had a cesarean birth and are now anticipating a vaginal birth have unique needs. Because they may have unresolved questions and concerns about the last birth, it is helpful to begin the series of classes with an informational session. During this session, they can ask questions, share experiences, and begin to form bonds with each other. The nurse can supply information regarding the criteria necessary to attempt a trial of labor and identify decisions regarding the birth experience. Some childbirth educators find it helpful to have the parents prepare two birth plans: one for vaginal birth and one for cesarean birth. The preparation of the birth plans seems to help parents take more control of the birth experience and tends to increase the positive aspects of the experience.

After an informational session, the classes may be divided according to the needs of the expectant parents. Those with recent coached childbirth experiences may need only refresher classes, while others may need complete training. Some parents may choose to attend regular classes after participating in the informational session.

Methods of Childbirth Preparation

Overview of Selected Methods

Various methods of childbirth preparation are taught in North America. Some antepartal classes are specifically oriented to preparation for labor and birth, have a name associated with a theory of pain reduction in childbirth, and teach specific exercises to reduce pain. The most common methods of this type are the Lamaze (psychoprophylactic), Kitzinger (sensory-memory), and Bradley (partner-coached childbirth). Each of these methods is designed to provide the woman or couple with self-help measures so that the pregnancy and birth are healthy and happy events. See Table 9–3 for differentiating characteristics of each method.

The programs in prepared childbirth share some similarities. All have an educational component to help eliminate fear. The classes vary in coverage of subjects related to the maternity cycle, but all teach relaxation techniques and all prepare the participants for what to expect during labor and birth. Except for hypnosis, these methods also feature exercises to condition muscles and breathing patterns used in labor. The greatest differences among the methods lie in the theories of why they work and in the relaxation techniques and breathing patterns they teach.

There are several advantages to these methods of childbirth preparation. Most important is that the baby may be healthier because of the reduced need for analgesics and anesthetics. Another is the satisfaction of the parents, for whom childbirth becomes a shared and profound emotional experience. In addition, each method has been shown to shorten labor. All nurses must know how these methods differ, so that they can support each birth experience effectively.

Psychoprophylactic (Lamaze) Method

The **psychoprophylactic method** is the childbirth preparation method generally called "Lamaze classes." *Psychoprophylactic* means "mind prevention." Dr. Fernand Lamaze, a French obstetrician, was the first person to introduce this method of childbirth preparation to the Western world. Proponents of the method formed a nonprofit group called the American Society for Psychoprophylaxis in Obstetrics (ASPO). This organization helped establish many programs throughout the country, and Lamaze has become one of the most popular methods of childbirth education.

The major components of Lamaze classes are education and training. In Lamaze classes, the woman learns about the developing fetus and the changes that occur in the pregnant woman. The woman also learns body-conditioning exercises that can be used during the pregnancy

RESEARCH IN PRACTICE

What is this study about? Prenatal services that do not consider a woman's traditional belief system may unknowingly create barriers to care. Claudia Long and Mary Ann Curry designed a qualitative study to explore the relationship between the use of prenatal care and the traditional beliefs and practices about pregnancy of Native American women.

How was this study done? The study was completed in conjunction with a project to improve birth outcomes for Native American women at two sites in rural Oregon. At one of the sites—a federally recognized reservation—traditional ways and native language were encouraged and maintained. At the other site—a tribal site—only a few elders retained any memory of native language. Researchers conducted focus groups with a total of 32 Native American female elders and 20 young women to explore traditional beliefs and practices about pregnancy and childbirth. Each focus group began with the same question about participants' thoughts about pregnancy and childbirth. Questions for the elder group included past experiences, transmission of cultural beliefs, and role of the family and community during pregnancy and childbirth. Young women were asked what they had been told regarding pregnancy and childbirth, their beliefs about community and family responsibilities, and the differences between the ideal and the reality of health care for pregnant contemporary Native American women.

What were the results of the study? Data analysis of the transcribed focus discussions revealed a central theme concerning the breakdown of transmission of cultural health beliefs. The two major reasons were federal assimilation policies and premature death of elders. Federal assimilation policies incorporated sending young Native Americans to boarding school and forbidding native language and customs. Elders blamed these policies for breaking the family circle and creating problems of substance abuse that impact childrearing. The tribal site participants described very few traditional practices, whereas many from the reservation site identified traditional teaching about pregnancy and childbirth. Elders and young women from both sites identified the passing of the elders as a great loss because although young women could obtain information and support from their mothers, the elders transmitted cultural wisdom. Young women at the tribal site perceived the Western care providers as insensitive and disrespectful. At both sites, the women did not ascribe to the values of Western prenatal care. Young women perceived themselves as living in two worlds in relation to prenatal care.

How can I use this study? In order to provide sensitive care, one must be aware of how one's actions are interpreted based on the care receiver's cultural perspective.

SOURCE: Long, C. R., & Curry, M. A. (1998). Living in two worlds: Native American women and prenatal care. *Health Care for Women International, 19,* 205–215.

and specific relaxation and breathing techniques for labor (Monto, 1996).

Body-Conditioning Exercises

Some body-conditioning exercises, such as the pelvic tilt, pelvic rock, and Kegel exercises, are taught in childbirth preparation classes. Other exercises strengthen the abdominal muscles for the expulsive phase of labor. (See Chapter 10 for a description of recommended exercises.)

Relaxation Exercises

Relaxation during labor allows the woman to conserve energy and allows the uterine muscles to work more efficiently. Without practice it is very difficult to relax the whole body in the midst of intense uterine contractions. However, many people are familiar with **progressive relaxation** exercises such as those taught to induce sleep. One example follows:

- Lie down on your back or side. (The left side position is best for pregnant women.)
- Tighten your muscles in both feet. Hold the tightness for a few seconds, and then relax the muscles completely, letting all the tension drain out.
- Tighten your lower legs, hold for a few seconds, then relax the muscles, letting all the tension drain out.
- Continue tensing and relaxing parts of your body, moving up the body as you do so.

Another type of relaxation exercise, called **touch relaxation,** requires cooperation between the woman and her coach. It is particularly useful in working together during labor (see Table 9–4).

An additional exercise specific to Lamaze is **disassociation relaxation.** This pattern of active relaxation is in contrast to the Read method of passive relaxation (where the woman is taught progressive contraction and relaxation of muscle groups moving from head to toe to promote sleep). The woman is taught to become familiar with the sensation of contracting and relaxing the voluntary muscle groups throughout her body. She then learns to contract a specific muscle group and relax the rest of her body. This process of isolating the action of one group of voluntary muscles from the rest of the body is called neuromuscular disassociation and is basic to the psychoprophylaxis method of prepared childbirth. The exercise conditions the woman to relax uninvolved muscles while the uterus contracts, creating an active relaxation pattern (Table 9–5).

In order to practice the relaxation exercises in a more realistic setting, the coach may use one of three methods to induce some discomfort:

1. The coach places both hands in a grasping position firmly on the upper arm and turns them in opposite directions to create a burning sensation. This is begun slowly and gently and increased at the direction of the woman as she continues to practice relaxation breathing techniques (Figure 9–5).

TABLE 9–4 Touch Relaxation

Practice is vital to the following exercises, which require that the pregnant woman and her partner work very closely together. Tell the woman, "With practice you will train yourself to release not only in response to your partner's touch but also to the touch of doctors or nurses as they examine you. This technique will also help you to be more comfortable with your own body."

Goals

(For her) To recognize and release tension in response to partner's touch; to be able to do this automatically and spontaneously.
(For partner) To recognize her tension in its very early stages; to learn how to touch in a firm yet sensitive way; to concentrate on her problem areas.

Tools

(For her) Conscious relaxation, comfortable positioning, and trust.
(For partner) Sensitivity, patience, and warm hands!

Procedure

She tenses.
Partner touches.
She immediately releases towards touch.
Partner strokes, "drawing" tension from her.
She releases all residual tension.

Sequence

- Contract muscles of the scalp and raise eyebrows. Partner cups hands on either side of the scalp. Immediately release tension in response to the pressure of your partner's touch. Then release any residual tension as your partner strokes your head.
- Frown, wrinkle nose, and squeeze eyes shut. Partner rests hands on brow and then strokes down over temples. Release.
- Grit teeth and clench jaw. Partner rests hands on either side of jaw. Release.
- Press shoulder blades back. Partner rests hands on front of shoulders. Release.
- Pull abdominal wall towards spine. Partner rests hands on sides of abdomen and then strokes down over her hips. Partner might also stroke the lower curve of abdomen across pubic symphysis. Release.
- Press thighs together. Partner touches outside of each leg. Relax and let legs move apart. Partner strokes firmly down outside of leg with light strokes up on inner thigh.
- Press legs outward, still flexed but forcing thighs apart. Partner rests hands with fingers pointing downward, on inner thighs. Firmly strokes down to knees, then lightly strokes upward on outside of leg. Release.
- Tense arm muscles. Partner places hands on the upper arm and shoulder area, one on the inside and one on the outside of the arm. Strokes down to the elbow and then down forearm to wrist, and over fingertips. Release. Repeat with other arm.
- Tighten leg muscles, being careful not to cramp them. Partner touches foot around the instep, firmly without tickling. Release whole leg. Partner moves hands up, placing one on either side of the thigh, stroking down to the knee then down the calf to the foot and over the toes. Release. Repat with other leg.
- Change to the Sims lateral or side-lying position. Raise chin, contracting the muscles at the back of the neck. Partner rests hand on nape of neck and massages. Release.
- Curl into fetal position, crawing shoulders forward. Partner applies pressure to back of shoulders. Strokes upper back. Release.
- Hollow the small of back by arching back. Partner rests hands against either side of spine and follows with stroking down over buttocks. Release.
- Press buttocks together. Partner rests one hand on each buttock. After initial release, strokes down toward thighs.

SOURCE: O'Halloran, S. *Pregnant and Prepared: A Guide to Preparing for Childbirth,* Wayne, NJ.: Avery Publishing Group, 1984, p 45.

TABLE 9–5 Disassociation Relaxation

The uterus, an involuntary muscle over which you have no control, will work most efficiently and effectively when the rest of your body is free from tension. The following exercises will give you further practice in conscious release. They will also give you and your partner a way to evaluate your progress.

Goals

During pregnancy, disassociation relaxation will teach you consciously to release certain sets of muscles, while contracting others, and to disassociate yourself from voluntary tension. During labor, this technique will release all voluntary muscles of your body at will, while the uterus contracts. This conserves energy and fights fatigue.

Tools

Body awareness, touch release, and concentration.

Procedure

Partner gives consistent suggestions.

Partner checks relaxation using touching.

Example

Partner: "Contraction begins."

Mother: Relaxation breath (following with a comfortable rate of breathing).

Partner: [See suggested patterns below.]

Mother: Relaxation breath.

Sequence

"Contract right arm. Hold. Release."

"Contract left arm. Hold. Release."

"Contract right leg. Hold. Release."

"Contract left leg. Hold. Release."

"Contract both arms. Hold. Release."

"Contract both legs. Hold. Release."

"Contract right side (arm and leg). Hold. Release."

"Contract left side (arm and leg). Hold. Release."

"Contract right arm and left leg. Hold. Release."

"Contract left arm and right leg. Hold. Release."

For Variety

"Contract right arm and left leg."

"Release left leg. Contract right leg. Release right arm. Contract left arm."

"Release."

SOURCE: O'Halloran, S. *Pregnant and Prepared: A Guide to Preparing for Childbirth.* Wayne, NJ: Avery Publishing Group,1984, pp 45–46.

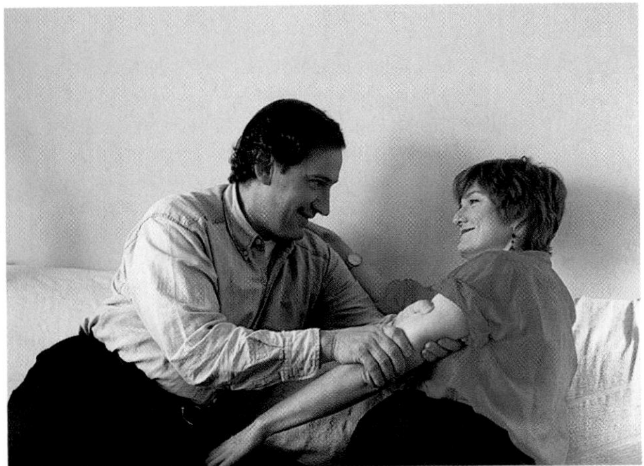

FIGURE 9–5 To help the woman practice relaxing in the presence of discomfort, the coach can induce discomfort by "twisting" the skin of her upper arm or by pinching her inner thigh.

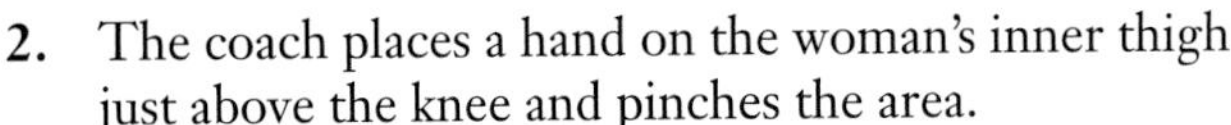

2. The coach places a hand on the woman's inner thigh just above the knee and pinches the area.

While practicing, the coach checks the woman's neck, shoulders, arms, and legs for relaxation. As tense areas are found, the coach encourages the woman to relax those particular body parts. The woman learns to respond to her own perceptions of tense muscles and also to the suggestion from others. The suggestion can come verbally or from touch. The exercises are usually practiced each day so that they become comfortable and easy to do.

A specific type of cutaneous stimulation used prior to the transitional phase of labor is known as abdominal effleurage (Figure 9–6). This light abdominal stroking is used in the Lamaze method of childbirth preparation. It effectively relieves mild to moderate pain, but not intense pain. Deep pressure over the sacrum is more effective for relieving back pain. Additional modalities that may be used to enhance coping in labor include guided imagery, meditation, music, massage, aromatherapy, therapeutic touch, biofeedback, and acupuncture. In addition to the measures just described, the nurse can promote relaxation by encouraging and supporting the client's controlled breathing.

Breathing Techniques

Breathing techniques are a key element of most childbirth preparation programs. They help keep the mother and her unborn baby adequately oxygenated and help the mother relax and focus her attention appropriately. Patterned-paced, breathing techniques are best taught during the final trimester of pregnancy when the expectant mother's attention is focused on the birth experience. The nurse then supports the mother's use of breathing techniques during labor. See Table 9–6. Breathing techniques are described in detail in Chapter 20.

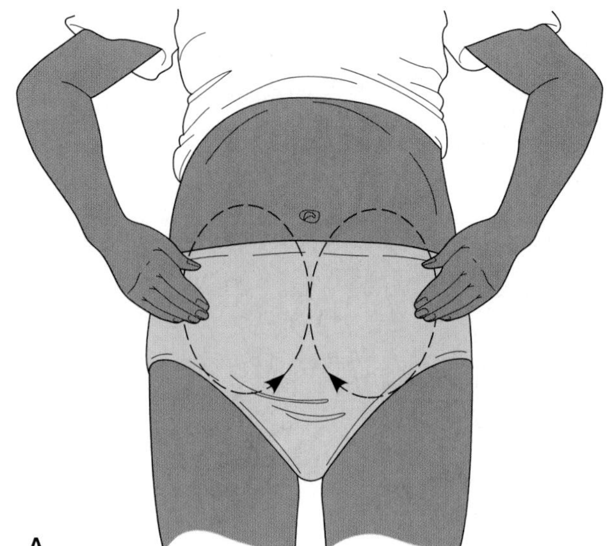

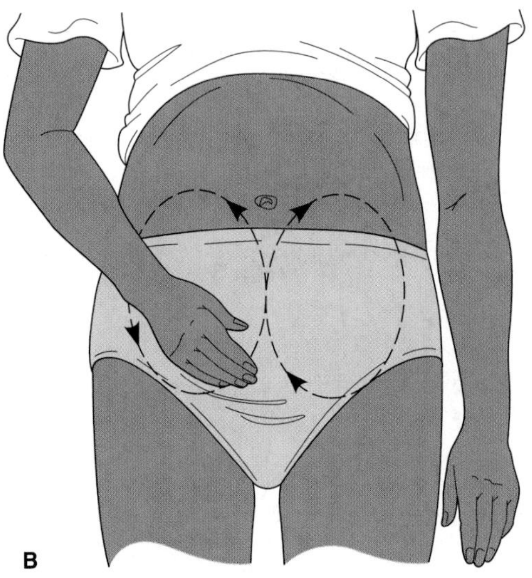

FIGURE 9–6 Effleurage is light stroking of the abdomen with the fingertips. ***A,*** Starting at the symphysis, the woman lightly moves her fingertips up and around in a circular pattern. ***B,*** An alternative approach involves using one hand in a figure-eight pattern. This light stroking can also be done by the support person.

TABLE 9–6 Goals of Breathing Techniques

- Provide adequate oxygenation of mother and baby, open maternal airways, and avoid inefficient use of muscles.
- Increase physical and mental relaxation.
- Decrease pain and anxiety.
- Provide a means of focusing attention.
- Control inadequate ventilation patterns that are related to pain and stress.

Client Education

Nurses involved in childbirth education need to include the concept of individuality when providing information to expectant parents about the process of childbirth and their own pattern of coping. Controversy exists over the use of ritualistic breathing techniques (patterned-paced) in childbirth. The wave of the future in childbirth education is to encourage women to incorporate their natural responses into coping with the pain of labor and birth. Self-care activities that may be used include the following:

- Vocalization or "sounding" to relieve tension in pregnancy and labor.
- Massage (light touch) to facilitate relaxation.
- Breathing in any manner that seems to bring relief. No specific pattern is followed.
- Use of warm water for showers or bathing during labor.
- Visualization (imagery).
- Relaxing music and subdued lighting.

Nurses should encourage expectant women and couples to make the birth a personal experience. The woman might plan, for example, to bring items from home to enhance relaxation and comfort, such as warm socks, slippers, bath powder, lotion, or a favorite blanket. She may wish to bring photographs of parents or friends who cannot be with them in person to share the birth experience. Many expectant parents enjoy listening to tapes of favorite music or watching home videotapes or favorite films. Such personalization of the birth experience may give expectant parents feelings of increased serenity and empowerment.

FOCUS YOUR STUDY

- Prenatal education programs vary in their goals, content, leadership techniques, and method of teaching.
- Prenatal classes may be offered early or late in the pregnancy. The class content varies depending on the type of class and the individual offering it. Expectant parents tend to want information in chronologic sequence with the pregnancy. Adolescents have special learning needs.
- Breastfeeding programs are offered in the prenatal period.
- Siblings are now included in the whole birthing process, and classes for them are available from many sources.
- Grandparents have unique needs for information in grandparents' classes.
- Information regarding cesarean birth is included in antepartal classes to help prepare parents.
- The major types of childbirth preparation methods are Lamaze, Kitzinger, and Bradley.
- Lamaze is a type of psychoprophylactic method. The classes include information on toning exercises, relaxation exercises and techniques, and breathing methods for labor.

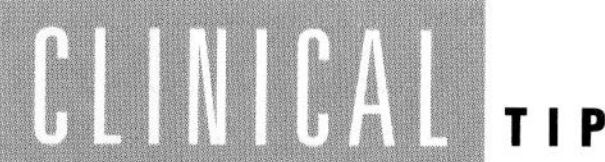

TIP

Practice the techniques for relaxation and patterned-paced breathing. This practice will prepare you for educating expectant parents and laboring women.

REFERENCES

Baer D. (1992). Buckle up! *Lamaze Parent's Magazine*, 95.

Broussard, A. B., & Rich, S. K.(1990). Incorporating infant stimulation concepts into prenatal classes. *Journal of Obstetric, Gynecologic, and Neonatal Nursing, 19*(5), 381.

Chapman, L. (1991). Co-laboring: Expectant fathers' experience during labor and birth. *Maternal-Child Nursing Journal, 5*, 92.

Fortier, J. C. et al. (1991). Adjustment to a newborn: Sibling preparation makes a difference. *Journal of Obstetric, Gynecologic, and Neonatal Nursing, 20*(1), 73.

Harvey, S. et al. (1996). A randomized, controlled trial of nurse-midwifery care. *Birth, 23*, 128.

Kitzinger, S. (1992). Sheila Kitzinger's letter from England: Birth plans. *Birth, 19*(1) 36.

Monto, M. (1996). Lamaze and Bradley childbirth classes: Contrasting perspectives toward the medical model of birth. *Birth, 23*, 193.

Mynaugh, P. A. (1991). A randomized study of two methods of teaching perineal massage: Effects of practice rates, episiotomy rates, and lacerations. *Birth, 18*(3), 153.

Nichols, F. H., & Humenick, S. S. (1988). *Childbirth education: Practice, research and theory.* Philadelphia: Saunders.

Olds, S. B. (1997). Care of the childbearing family. In J. Luckman (Ed.), *Saunders manual of nursing care.* Philadelphia: Saunders.

Robotti, S. B., & Inman M. A. (1998). *Childbirth instructor magazine's guide to careers in birth.*

Rogers, J., & Davis, B. A. (1995). How risky are hot tubs and saunas for pregnant women? *American Journal of Maternal Child Nursing, 20*, 137.

Roye, C., & Balk, S. J. (1997). Evaluation of an intergenerational program for pregnant and parenting adolescents. *American Journal of Maternal Child Nursing, 21*, 32.

Tirosh, F., Libon, D., & Bader, D. (1996). The effect of maternal smoking during pregnancy on sleep respiratory and arousal patterns in neonates. *Journal of Perinatology, 16*, 435.

Walden, C., et al. (1996). Perinatal effects of a pregnancy wellness program in the workplace. *American Journal of Maternal Child Nursing, 21*, 288.

Wheeler, L. (1997). *Nurse-midwifery handbook: A practical guide to prenatal and postpartum care.* Philadelphia: Lippincott.

Woolley, R. J. (1995). Benefits and risks of episiotomy: A review of the English-language literature since Part II. *Obstetrical and Gynecological Survey, 50* (11), 821.

10

Physical and Psychologic Changes of Pregnancy

THE ATMOSPHERE OF APPROVAL IN WHICH I WAS bathed—even by strangers on the street, it seemed—was like an aura I carried with me. . . . This is what women have always done.

~ *Adrienne Rich, Of Woman Born* ~

Objectives

- Identify the anatomic and physiologic changes that occur during pregnancy.
- Relate the physiologic and anatomic changes that occur in the body systems during pregnancy to the signs and symptoms that develop in the woman.
- Compare subjective (presumptive), objective (probable), and diagnostic (positive) changes of pregnancy.
- Contrast the various types of pregnancy tests.
- Discuss the emotional and psychologic changes that commonly occur in a woman, her partner, and her family during pregnancy.
- Summarize cultural factors that may influence a family's response to pregnancy.

Key Terms

Ballottement
Braxton Hicks contractions
Chadwick's sign
Chloasma
Colostrum
Couvade
Goodell's sign
Hegar's sign
Linea nigra
McDonald's sign
Morning sickness
Physiologic anemia of pregnancy
Quickening
Striae
Supine hypotensive syndrome (vena caval syndrome, aortocaval compression)

THROUGH MODERN TECHNOLOGY AND highly evolved research methods, we know a great deal about how pregnancy occurs and what happens to the fetus and the woman's body during gestation. Yet no matter how much we learn about this event, it never ceases to amaze us. First, it is nothing short of a miracle that the union of two microscopic entities—an ovum and a sperm—can produce a living being. Second, the woman's body must undergo extraordinary physical changes to sustain a pregnancy. A pregnant woman's body changes in size and shape, and all her organ systems modify their functions to create an environment that protects and nurtures the growing fetus.

Pregnancy is divided into three trimesters, each a 3-month period. Each trimester has its own predictable developments in both the fetus and the mother. This chapter describes both obvious and subtle physical and psychologic changes caused by pregnancy. It also discusses the various cultural factors that can affect a woman's well-being during pregnancy.

CRITICAL THINKING IN PRACTICE

At 33 weeks' gestation, Elena Martinez, gr 2 p1, who is 5 feet 4 inches tall and who weighs 144 lb (prepregnancy weight = 120), is examined by her certified nurse-midwife. At that time her fundal height is measured as 33 cm. Because of a vacation trip she is not seen again by her midwife until 36 weeks' gestation. At that time her fundus measures 35 cm and she weighs 147 lb. Elena asks you if there is something wrong with her baby's growth. What is your assessment?

Answer may be found in Appendix I.

Anatomy and Physiology of Pregnancy

The changes that occur in the pregnant woman's body are caused by several factors. Many changes are the results of hormonal influences, some are caused by the growth of the fetus inside the uterus, and some are a result of the mother's physical adaptation to the changes that are occurring.

Reproductive System

Uterus

The changes in the uterus during pregnancy are phenomenal. Before pregnancy the uterus is a small, semisolid, pear-shaped organ measuring approximately 7.5 × 5 × 2.5 cm and weighing about 60 g (2 oz). At the end of pregnancy the dimensions are approximately 28 × 24 × 21 cm, with an organ weight of approximately 1000 g (2.2 lb). Its capacity increases from 10 mL to 5000 mL (5 L) or more.

The enlargement of the uterus is primarily a result of an increase in size (hypertrophy) of the preexisting myometrial cells. There is only a limited increase in cell number (hyperplasia). The amount of fibrous tissue between the muscle bands increases markedly, which adds to the strength and elasticity of the muscle wall.

The uterine walls are considerably thicker during the first few months of pregnancy than during the nonpregnant state. The initial changes are stimulated by increased estrogen and progesterone levels and not by mechanical distention (enlargement) by the fetus, placenta, and amniotic fluid. After approximately the third month, the uterine contents begin to exert intrauterine pressure. The myometrial hypertrophy continues during the first few months of pregnancy. Then the musculature begins to distend, resulting in a thinning of the muscle wall to a thickness of about 5 mm or less at term (38 through 41 weeks of gestation). The ease of palpating the fetus through the abdominal wall attests to this thinning.

The circulatory requirements of the uterus increase as the uterus enlarges and the fetus and placenta develop. The size and number of the blood and lymphatic vessels increase greatly. By the end of pregnancy, one-sixth of the total maternal blood volume is contained within the vascular system of the uterus.

Braxton Hicks contractions—irregular contractions of the uterus—occur intermittently throughout pregnancy. They may be palpated bimanually beginning about the fourth month of pregnancy. These contractions help stimulate the movement of blood through the intervillous spaces of the placenta. In late pregnancy as these contractions increase in frequency, they can become uncomfortable and may be confused with true labor contractions.

Cervix

Estrogen stimulates the glandular tissue of the cervix, which increases in cell number and becomes hyperactive. The endocervical glands occupy about half the mass of the cervix at term, as compared to a small fraction in the nonpregnant state. They secrete a thick, tenacious mucus, which accumulates and thickens to form the mucus plug that seals the endocervical canal and prevents the ascent of bacteria or other substances into the uterus. This plug is expelled when cervical dilatation begins. The hyperactive glandular tissue also causes an increase in the normal physiologic mucorrhea, at times resulting in a profuse discharge. Increased vascularization causes both the softening of the cervix **(Goodell's sign)** and a blue-purple discoloration of the cervix **(Chadwick's sign).** Increased vascularization is a result of hypertrophy and engorgement of the vessels below the growing uterus.

Ovaries

The ovaries cease ovum production during pregnancy. Many follicles develop temporarily but never to the point of maturity. The cells lining these follicles, the thecal cells, become active in hormone production and have been called the interstitial glands of pregnancy.

During early pregnancy human chorionic gonadotrophin (hCG) maintains the corpus luteum, which persists and produces hormones until about week 10 to 12 of pregnancy. The corpus luteum engulfs approximately a third of the ovary at its peak of hypertrophy. By the middle of pregnancy it has regressed to almost complete obliteration. The corpus luteum secretes progesterone to maintain the endometrium until the placenta produces enough progesterone to maintain the pregnancy; then the corpus luteum disintegrates slowly.

Vagina

The vaginal epithelium undergoes hypertrophy, increased vascularization, and hyperplasia during pregnancy. As with the cervical changes, these changes are estrogen induced and result in a thickening of mucosa, a loosening of connective tissue, and an increase in vaginal secretions. The secretions are thick, white, and acidic (pH 3.5 to 6.0). The acid pH plays a significant role in preventing infections. However, it also favors the growth of yeast organisms, resulting in moniliasis, a common vaginal infection during pregnancy.

As in the uterus, the smooth muscle cells of the vagina hypertrophy, with an accompanying loosening of the supportive connective tissue. By the end of pregnancy, the vaginal wall and perineal body have become sufficiently relaxed to permit distention of the tissues and passage of the infant.

Because the blood flow to the vagina increases, it may show the same blue-purple color (Chadwick's sign) seen in the cervix.

Breasts

Soon after the woman first misses her menstrual period, estrogen- and progesterone-induced changes occur in the mammary glands. Increases in breast size and nodularity are the result of glandular hyperplasia and hypertrophy in preparation for lactation. By the end of the second month, superficial veins are prominent, nipples are more erectile, and pigmentation of the areola is obvious. Pigmentation tends to be more pronounced in women with dark complexions. Hypertrophy of Montgomery's follicles is noted within the primary areola. **Striae** (purplish stretch marks that slowly turn silver after childbirth) may develop as the pregnancy progresses. Breast changes are often most noticeable in the woman who is pregnant for the first time.

Colostrum, an antibody-rich, yellow secretion, may be expressed manually by the 12th week and may leak from the breasts during the last trimester of pregnancy. Colostrum gradually converts to mature milk during the first few days following childbirth.

Respiratory System

Pulmonary function is modified throughout pregnancy. Pregnancy induces a small degree of hyperventilation as the tidal volume (amount of air breathed with ordinary respiration) increases steadily throughout pregnancy. There is a 30% to 40% rise from nonpregnant values in the volume of air breathed each minute. Between weeks 16 and 40, oxygen consumption increases approximately 15% to 20% to meet the increased needs of the mother as well as those of the fetus and placenta. The vital capacity (maximum amount of air that can be moved in and out of the lungs with forced respiration) increases slightly, while lung compliance (elasticity) and pulmonary diffusion remain constant. Measurements of airway resistance show a marked decrease in pregnancy in response to elevated progesterone levels. This permits increases in oxygen consumption, in carbon dioxide production, and in the respiratory functional reserve.

The diaphragm is elevated and the subcostal angle is increased as a result of pressure from the enlarging uterus. This change causes the rib cage to flare, with a decrease in the vertical diameter and increases in the anteroposterior and transverse diameters. The circumference of the chest may increase by as much as 6 cm. The increase compensates for the elevated diaphragm, and there is no significant loss of intrathoracic volume. Breathing changes from abdominal to thoracic as pregnancy progresses, and descent of the diaphragm on inspiration becomes less possible.

Nasal stuffiness and congestion, referred to as *rhinitis of pregnancy*, are not uncommon. Epistaxis (nose bleeds) may also occur. They are primarily the result of estrogen-induced edema and vascular congestion of the nasal mucosa.

Cardiovascular System

The growing uterus exerts pressure on the diaphragm, pushing the heart upward and to the left and rotating it forward. This lateral displacement makes the heart appear somewhat enlarged on x-ray examination.

Blood volume progressively increases throughout pregnancy, beginning in the first trimester and peaking in the middle of the third trimester at about 45% above nonpregnant levels. This increase is due to increases in both plasma and erythrocytes. No increase occurs in pulmonary capillary wedge pressure or in central venous pressure despite the increase in blood volume. This is due to decreases in both systemic vascular resistance (21%) and pulmonary vascular resistance (34%), which enable the circulation to adapt to higher blood volume while maintaining normal vessel pressures (Cunningham, MacDonald, Gant, Leveno, Gilstrap, Hankins, & Clark, 1997). Cardiac output begins to increase early in pregnancy and peaks at 20 to 24 weeks' gestation at 30% to 50% above prepregnant levels. It then remains elevated for the duration of the pregnancy (Cruikshank, Wigton, & Hays, 1996).

During pregnancy, organ systems receive additional blood flow according to their increased work load. Thus blood flow to the uterus and kidneys increases, whereas hepatic and cerebral flow remains unchanged.

The pulse rate frequently increases during pregnancy, although the amount varies from almost no increase to an increase of 10 to 15 beats per minute. The blood pressure decreases slightly during pregnancy, reaching its lowest point during the second trimester. The blood pressure then gradually increases during the third trimester and is near prepregnant levels at term (when the baby is due).

The femoral venous pressure slowly rises as the uterus exerts increasing pressure on return blood flow. There is an increased tendency toward stagnation of blood in the lower extremities, with a resulting dependent edema and tendency toward varicose vein formation in the legs, vulva, and rectum late in pregnancy. In addition to the effects of increased femoral venous pressure, a reduction of plasma colloid osmotic pressure resulting from a reduction in plasma albumin further maintains the presence of fluid in the extravascular space. The pregnant woman becomes more prone to develop postural hypotension because of the increased blood volume in the lower extremities.

Researchers have long recognized that the enlarging uterus may put pressure on the vena cava when the woman is supine, resulting in **supine hypotensive syndrome,** also called **vena caval syndrome** or **aortocaval compression.** This pressure interferes with returning blood flow and produces a marked decrease in blood pressure with accompanying dizziness, pallor, and clamminess, which can be corrected by having the woman lie on her left side. Research indicates that the enlarging uterus may press on the aorta and its collateral circulation as well (Cunningham et al, 1997) (Figure 10–1).

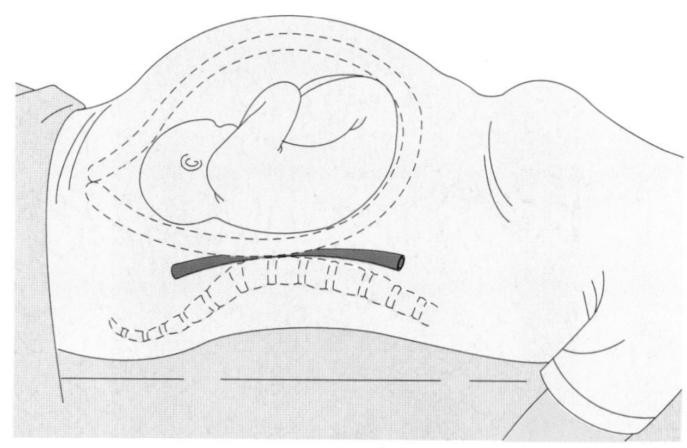

FIGURE 10–1 Vena caval syndrome. The gravid uterus compresses the vena cava when the woman is supine. This reduces the blood flow returning to the heart and may cause maternal hypotension.

The total erythrocyte volume increases by about 30% in women who receive iron supplementation but increases only about 18% without iron supplements (Cruikshank et al, 1996). This increase is necessary to transport the additional oxygen required during pregnancy. The increase in plasma volume averages about 50%. Because the plasma volume increase is greater than the erythrocyte increase, however, the hematocrit, which measures the portion of whole blood that is composed of erythrocytes, decreases slightly. This decrease is sometimes referred to as the **physiologic anemia of pregnancy** (pseudoanemia).

Iron is necessary for hemoglobin formation, and hemoglobin is the oxygen-carrying component of erythrocytes. Thus the increase in erythrocyte levels results in an increased need for iron by the pregnant woman. Even though the gastrointestinal absorption of iron is moderately increased during pregnancy, it is usually necessary to add supplemental iron to the diet to meet the expanded red blood cell and fetal needs.

Leukocyte production equals or is slightly greater than the increase in blood volume. The average cell count is 5000 to 12,000/mm^3, with an occasional woman developing a physiologic leukocytosis of 15,000/mm^3. During labor and the early postpartum period, these levels may reach 25,000/mm^3. The reason for this dramatic increase remains unknown, but similar leukocyte changes occur with physiologic stress such as vigorous exercise. It probably represents the return to the circulation of mature leukocytes that had been shunted out of the circulatory system (Cunningham et al, 1997).

The fibrin level in the blood is increased by as much as 40% at term, and the plasma fibrinogen has been known to increase by as much as 50%. The increased fibrinogen accounts for the nonpathologic rise of the sedimentation rate. Although the clotting time of the pregnant woman does not differ significantly from that of the nonpregnant woman, blood factors VII, VIII, IX, and X are increased so that pregnancy becomes a somewhat hypercoagulable state. These changes, coupled with venous stasis in late pregnancy, place the pregnant woman at increased risk of developing venous thrombosis.

Gastrointestinal System

Many of the discomforts of pregnancy are attributed to changes in the gastrointestinal system. Nausea and vomiting during the first trimester are associated with the hCG secreted by the implanted blastocyst and with a change in carbohydrate metabolism that occurs in early pregnancy. Peculiarities of taste and smell are common and can further aggravate gastrointestinal discomfort. Gum tissue may become hyperemic and softened and may bleed when only mildly traumatized. The secretion of saliva may increase or become excessive (ptyalism).

During the second half of pregnancy, numerous gastrointestinal symptoms are attributable to the pressure of the growing uterus and smooth muscle relaxation due to

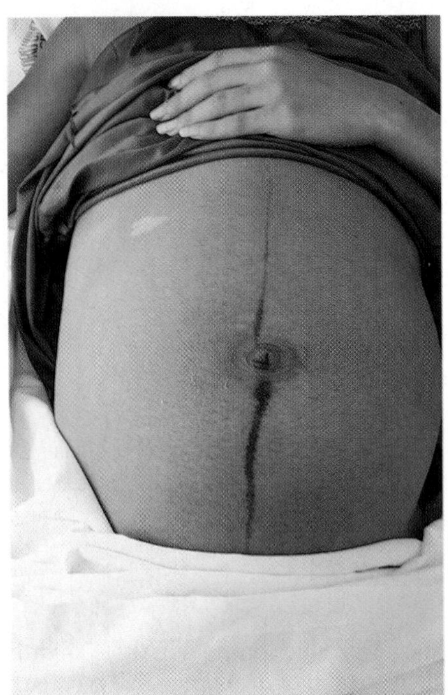

FIGURE 10–2 Linea nigra.

elevated progesterone levels. The intestines are displaced laterally and posteriorly and the stomach superiorly. Heartburn (pyrosis) is caused by the reflux of acidic secretions from the stomach into the lower esophagus as a result of relaxation of the cardiac sphincter. Gastric emptying time and intestinal motility are delayed, leading to frequent complaints of bloating and constipation, which can be aggravated by the smooth muscle relaxation and increased electrolyte and water reabsorption in the large intestine. Hemorrhoids frequently develop if constipation is a problem or, in the second half of pregnancy, from pressure on vessels below the level of the uterus.

Only minor liver changes occur with pregnancy. Plasma albumin concentrations and serum cholinesterase activity decrease with normal pregnancy as with certain liver diseases.

The emptying time of the gallbladder is prolonged during pregnancy as a result of smooth muscle relaxation from progesterone. Hypercholesterolemia may follow, and it can predispose the woman to gallstone formation.

Urinary Tract

During the first trimester, the growing uterus puts pressure on the bladder, producing urinary frequency until the second trimester when the uterus becomes an abdominal organ. Near term, when the presenting part engages in the pelvis, pressure is again exerted on the bladder. This pressure can impair the drainage of blood and lymph from the hyperemic bladder, rendering it more susceptible to infection and trauma. The bladder, normally a convex organ, becomes concave from the external pressure, and its retention capacity is greatly reduced.

Dilation of the kidneys and ureter may occur, most frequently on the right side above the pelvic brim, due to the lie of the uterus. This dilation is accompanied by elongation and curvature of the ureter. There appears to be no single factor accounting for this anatomic variation; instead a combination of ureteral atonia and hypoperistalsis, possibly caused by the placental progesterone and by pressure from the enlarging fetus, seems to be involved. The presence of amino acids and glucose in the urine in conjunction with the tendency toward ureteral atonia and stasis of urine in the ureters may increase the risk of urinary tract infection.

The glomerular filtration rate (GFR) and renal plasma flow (RPF) increase early in pregnancy. The GFR rises by as much as 50% by the beginning of the second trimester and remains elevated until birth. The increase in RPF is slightly less and decreases somewhat during the third trimester (Cunningham et al, 1997). The mechanism for these rises remains unclear, but human placental lactogen (hPL) may play a part.

An increased renal tubular reabsorption rate compensates for the increased glomerular activity. Amino acids and water-soluble vitamins are excreted in greater amounts than in the nonpregnant woman. Glycosuria is not uncommon or necessarily pathogenic during pregnancy but is merely a reflection of the kidneys' inability to reabsorb all of the glucose filtered by the glomeruli. However, pregnancy can be diabetogenic, so the possibility of diabetes mellitus cannot be disregarded.

The increased renal function during pregnancy results in an increased clearance of urea and creatinine and in a lowering of the blood urea and nonprotein nitrogen values. Because of this, measurement of creatinine clearance provides an accurate test of renal functioning during pregnancy.

Skin and Hair

Changes in skin pigmentation commonly occur during pregnancy. These changes are thought to be stimulated by increased estrogen, progesterone, and α-melanocyte-stimulating hormone levels (Cruikshank et al, 1996).

Pigmentation of the skin increases primarily in areas that are already hyperpigmented: the areolae, the nipples, the vulva, the perianal area, and the linea alba. The linea alba refers to the midline of the abdomen from the pubic area to the umbilicus and above. During pregnancy increased pigmentation may cause this area to darken. It is then referred to as the **linea nigra** (Figure 10–2). Some women also develop facial **chloasma,** or the "mask of pregnancy." This is an irregular pigmentation of the cheeks, forehead, and nose that occurs in many women during pregnancy and is accentuated by sun exposure. Similar changes may occur in women who are taking oral contraceptives. Facial chloasma is more prominent in

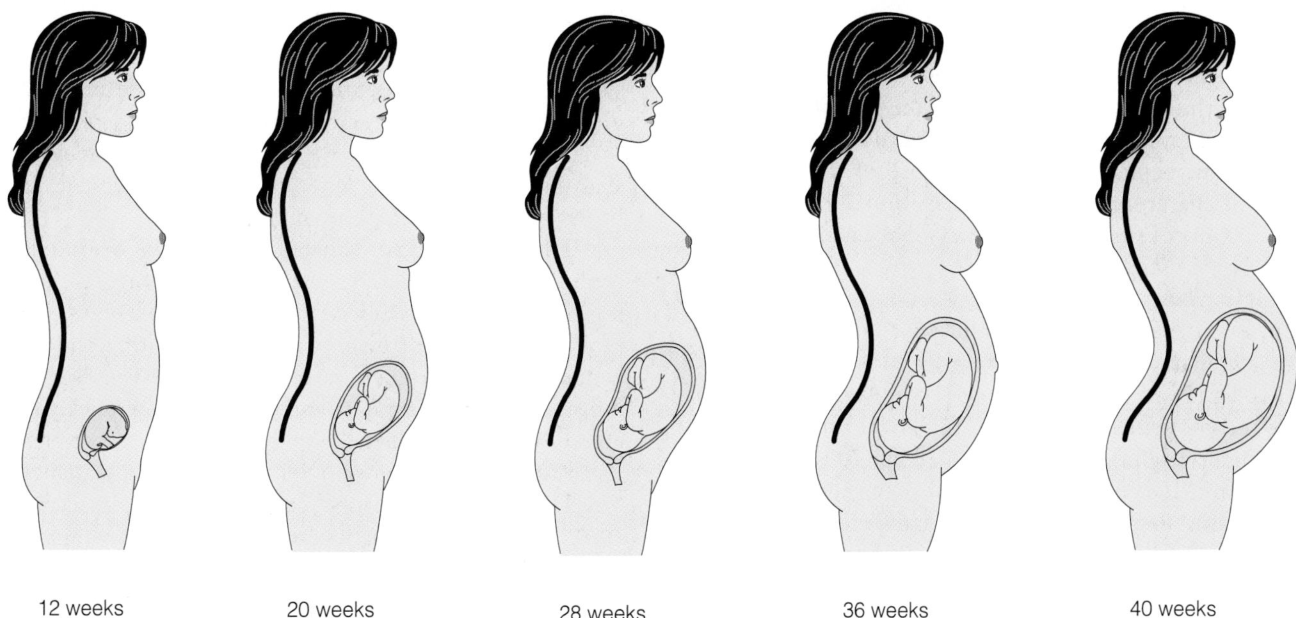

FIGURE 10–3 Postural changes during pregnancy. Note the increasing lordosis of the lumbosacral spine and the increasing curvature of the thoracic area.

dark-haired women and is occasionally disfiguring. Fortunately, it fades or at least regresses soon after birth when the hormonal influence of pregnancy has stopped. In addition the sweat and sebaceous glands are frequently hyperactive during pregnancy.

Striae, or stretch marks, are reddish, wavy, depressed streaks that may occur over the abdomen, breasts, and thighs as pregnancy progresses. They are caused by reduced connective tissue strength due to elevated adrenal steroid levels.

Vascular spider nevi may develop on the chest, neck, face, arms, and legs. They are small, bright-red elevations of the skin radiating from a central body. They may be caused by increased subcutaneous blood flow in response to increased estrogen levels. This condition is of no clinical significance and disappears after pregnancy ends.

The rate of hair growth may decrease during pregnancy, and the number of hair follicles in the resting or dormant phase also decreases. After birth the number of hair follicles in the resting phase increases sharply, and the woman may notice increased shedding of hair for 1 to 4 months. Practically all hair is replaced within 6 to 12 months, however (Cunningham et al, 1997).

Musculoskeletal System

No demonstrable changes occur in the teeth of the pregnant woman. No demineralization takes place. The fairly common occurrence of dental caries during pregnancy has led to the myth "a tooth for every pregnancy." The dental caries that may accompany pregnancy are likely to be caused by inadequate oral hygiene and dental care.

The sacroiliac, sacrococcygeal, and pubic joints of the pelvis relax in the later part of the pregnancy, presumably as a result of relaxin and progesterone. This often causes a waddling gait. A slight separation of the symphysis pubis can often be demonstrated on radiologic examination.

As the pregnant woman's center of gravity gradually changes, the lumbodorsal spinal curve is accentuated, and the woman's posture changes (Figure 10–3). This posture change compensates for the increased weight of the uterus anteriorly and frequently results in low backache. Late in pregnancy, aches in the neck, shoulders, and upper extremities may occur because of shoulder slumping and anterior flexion of the neck accompanying the lumbodorsal lordosis. Paresthesias of the extremities may occur late in pregnancy as a result of pressure on peripheral nerves.

Often pressure of the enlarging uterus on the abdominal muscles causes the rectus abdominis muscle to separate, producing *diastasis recti.* If the separation is severe and muscle tone is not regained postpartally, subsequent pregnancies will not have adequate support, and the woman's abdomen may appear pendulous.

Eyes

Two changes generally occur in the eyes during pregnancy. First, intraocular pressure decreases, probably as a result of increased vitreous outflow. Second, a slight thickening of the cornea occurs, which is generally attributed to fluid retention. Consequently, some pregnant women experience difficulty wearing previously comfortable contact lenses (Cunningham et al, 1997). The change in the corneas generally disappears by 6 weeks postpartum.

Metabolism

Most metabolic functions accelerate during pregnancy to support the additional demands of the growing fetus and its support system. The expectant mother must meet her own tissue replacement needs, those of the fetus, and those preparatory for labor and lactation. No other event in life induces such profound metabolic changes.

Weight Gain

The recommended total weight gain during pregnancy for a woman of normal weight prior to pregnancy is 11.5 to 16 kg (25 to 35 lb); for women who were overweight, the recommended gain is 7 to 11.5 kg (15 to 25 lb); and for underweight women, 12.5 to 18 kg (28 to 40 lb) (Institute of Medicine, 1990). Weight may decrease slightly during the first trimester due to nausea, vomiting, and food intolerances of early pregnancy. The lost weight is soon regained, and an average increase of 1.6 to 2.3 kg (3.5 to 5 lb), 5.5 to 6.8 kg (12 to 15 lb), and 5.5 to 6.8 kg (12 to 15 lb) occurs in the first, second, and third trimesters, respectively.

Adequate nutrition and weight gain are important during pregnancy. Maternal nutrition is discussed in detail in Chapter 14.

Water Metabolism

Increased water retention is a basic chemical alteration of pregnancy. Several interrelated factors cause this phenomenon. The increased level of steroid sex hormones affects sodium and fluid retention. The lowered serum protein also influences the fluid balance, as do the increased intracapillary pressure and permeability. The extra water is needed for the products of conception—the fetus, placenta, and amniotic fluid—and the mother's increased blood volume, interstitial fluids, and enlarged organs.

Nutrient Metabolism

The fetus makes its greatest protein and fat demands during the second half of gestation, doubling in weight in the last 6 to 8 weeks. The increased nitrogen (protein) retention that begins in early pregnancy is initially used for hyperplasia and hypertrophy of maternal tissues, such as the uterus and breasts. Nitrogen must also be stored during pregnancy to maintain a constant level within the breast milk and to avoid depletion of maternal tissues.

Fats are more completely absorbed during pregnancy, resulting in a marked increase in the serum lipids, lipoproteins, and cholesterol and decreased elimination through the bowel. Fat deposits in the fetus increase from about 2% at midpregnancy to almost 12% at term. The excess nitrogen and lipidemia are considered to be a preparation for lactation.

The demand for carbohydrate increases, especially during the last two trimesters. Ketosis can be a problem, especially with the diabetic woman, due to glycosuria, reduced alkaline reserves, and lipidemia. Intermittent glycosuria is not uncommon during pregnancy. When it is not accompanied by a rise in blood sugar levels, glycosuria is a physiologic entity secondary to the increased glomerular filtration rate. Fasting blood sugar levels tend to fall slightly, returning to more normal levels by the sixth postpartal month. The oral glucose tolerance test shows no change with pregnancy.

The possibility of diabetes must not be overlooked during pregnancy. Plasma levels of insulin increase during pregnancy (probably due to hormonal changes), and rapid destruction of insulin takes place within the placenta. Insulin production must be increased by the mother, and any marginal pancreatic function quickly becomes apparent. The diabetic woman often experiences increased exogenous insulin demands during pregnancy.

The demand for iron during pregnancy is accelerated, and the pregnant woman needs to guard against anemia. Iron is necessary for the increase in erythrocytes, hemoglobin, and blood volume, as well as for the increased tissue demands of both woman and fetus.

Iron transfer takes place at the placenta in only one direction—toward the fetus. It has been demonstrated that approximately five-sixths of the iron stored in the fetal liver has been assimilated during the last trimester of pregnancy. This stored iron in the fetal liver compensates in the first 4 months of neonatal life for the normal inadequate amounts of iron available in breast milk and non-iron-fortified formulas.

The progressive absorption and retention of calcium during pregnancy has been noted. The maternal plasma concentration of bound calcium decreases as the levels of bindable plasma proteins fall. Approximately 30 g of calcium is retained in maternal bone for fetal deposition late in pregnancy.

Pregnancy produces little change in the metabolism of most other minerals, other than retention of amounts needed for fetal growth.

Vitamin metabolism does not change appreciably with pregnancy. (See Chapter 14 for the mother's requirements of minerals and vitamins.)

Endocrine System

Thyroid

Pregnancy influences the thyroid gland's size and activity. Often a palpable change is noted, which represents an increase in vascularity and hyperplasia of glandular tissue. Total serum thyroxine (T_4) increases in early pregnancy, and thyroid-stimulating hormone (TSH) decreases. The elevated levels of total T_4 continue until several weeks postpartum, although the level of free serum T_4 returns to normal after the first trimester (Cunningham et al, 1997). Increased thyroxine-binding capacity is evidenced by an increase in serum protein-bound iodine (PBI), probably due to the increased levels of circulating estrogens.

The basal metabolic rate (BMR) increases by as much as 20% to 25% during pregnancy. The increased oxygen consumption is due primarily to fetal metabolic activity.

Parathyroid

The concentration of the parathyroid hormone and the size of the parathyroid glands increase, paralleling the fetal calcium requirements. Parathyroid hormone concentration reaches its highest level of approximately twofold between 15 and 35 weeks of gestation, returning to a normal or even subnormal level before childbirth.

Pituitary

During pregnancy, the pituitary gland enlarges somewhat, but it returns to normal size after birth. There is no significant change in the posterior lobe of the gland, although the anterior lobe increases in weight with each successive pregnancy.

Pregnancy is made possible by the hypothalamic stimulation of the anterior pituitary hormones: FSH, which stimulates follicle growth within the ovary, and LH, which effects ovulation. Pituitary stimulation prolongs the corpus luteal phase of the ovary, which maintains the secretory endometrium for development of the pregnancy. Two additional pituitary hormones, thyrotropin and adrenotropin, alter maternal metabolism to support the pregnancy. Prolactin, also an anterior pituitary secretion, is responsible for initial lactation. (Continued lactation depends on the suckling of the infant.)

The posterior pituitary contains the mechanism for the release of oxytocin and vasopressin, which exert oxytocic, vasopressor, and antidiuretic effects. The main effects of oxytocin are the promotion of uterine contractility and the stimulation of milk ejection from the breasts. Vasopressin causes vasoconstriction, which results in increased blood pressure; it also has an antidiuretic effect and plays an important role in the regulation of water balance. Vasopressin secretion is controlled by changes in plasma osmolarity and blood volume.

Adrenals

Little structural change occurs in the adrenal glands during a normal pregnancy. Estrogen-induced increases in the levels of circulating cortisol result primarily from lowered renal excretion. The circulating cortisol levels regulate carbohydrate and protein metabolism. A normal level resumes 1 to 6 weeks postpartum.

The adrenals secrete increased levels of aldosterone by the early part of the second trimester. The levels of secretion are even more elevated in the woman on a sodium-restricted diet. This increase in aldosterone in a normal pregnancy may be the body's protective response to the increased sodium excretion associated with progesterone (Cunningham et al, 1997).

Pancreas

The pregnant woman has increased insulin needs. The islets of Langerhans are stressed to meet this increased demand, and a latent deficiency may become apparent during pregnancy, producing symptoms of gestational diabetes (Chapter 15).

Hormones in Pregnancy

Several hormones are required to maintain pregnancy. Most of these are produced initially by the corpus luteum; production is then assumed by the placenta. (For an in-depth discussion of placental hormones, see Chapter 7.)

Human Chorionic Gonadotropin (hCG) The trophoblast secretes hCG in early pregnancy. This hormone stimulates progesterone and estrogen production by the corpus luteum to maintain the pregnancy until the placenta is developed sufficiently to assume that function.

Human Placental Lactogen (hPL) Also called human chorionic somatomammotropin (hCS), human placental lactogen (hPL) is produced by the syncytiotrophoblast. This hormone is an antagonist of insulin; it increases the amount of circulating free fatty acids for maternal metabolic needs and decreases maternal metabolism of glucose to favor fetal growth.

Estrogen Secreted originally by the corpus luteum, estrogen is produced primarily by the placenta as early as the seventh week of pregnancy. Estrogen stimulates uterine development to provide a suitable environment for the fetus. It also helps to develop the ductal system of the breasts in preparation for lactation.

Progesterone Progesterone, also produced initially by the corpus luteum and then by the placenta, plays the greatest role in maintaining pregnancy. It maintains the endometrium and also inhibits spontaneous uterine contractility, thus preventing early spontaneous abortion due to uterine activity. In addition, progesterone helps develop the acini and lobules of the breasts in preparation for lactation.

Relaxin Relaxin is detectable in the serum of a pregnant woman by the time of the first missed menstrual period. Relaxin inhibits uterine activity, diminishes the strength of uterine contractions, aids in the softening of the cervix, and has the long-term effect of remodeling collagen. Its primary source is the corpus luteum, but small amounts are believed to be produced by the placenta and uterine decidua throughout pregnancy (Buster & Carson, 1996).

Prostaglandins in Pregnancy

Prostaglandins (PGs) are lipid substances that can arise from most body tissues but occur in high concentrations

TABLE 10–1 Differential Diagnosis of Pregnancy—Subjective Changes

Subjective Changes	Possible Alternative Causes
Amenorrhea	Endocrine factors: early menopause; lactation; thyroid, pituitary, adrenal, ovarian dysfunction
	Metabolic factors: malnutrition, anemia, climatic changes, diabetes mellitus, degenerative disorders, long-distance running
	Psychologic factors: emotional shock, fear of pregnancy or sexually transmitted infection, intense desire for pregnancy (pseudocyesis), stress
	Obliteration of endometrial cavity by infection or curettage
	Systemic disease (acute or chronic), such as tuberculosis or malignancy
Nausea and vomiting	Gastrointestinal disorders
	Acute infections such as encephalitis
	Emotional disorders such as pseudocyesis or anorexia nervosa
Urinary frequency	Urinary tract infection
	Cystocele
	Pelvic tumors
	Urethral diverticula
	Emotional tension
Breast tenderness	Premenstrual tension
	Chronic cystic mastitis
	Pseudocyesis
	Hyperestrinism
Quickening	Increased peristalsis
	Flatus ("gas")
	Abdominal muscle contractions
	Shifting of abdominal contents

in the female reproductive tract and are present in the decidua during pregnancy. The exact functions of PGs during pregnancy are still unknown, although it has been proposed that they are responsible for maintaining reduced placental vascular resistance. The decreased prostaglandin levels may contribute to hypertension and pregnancy-induced hypertension (PIH). Prostaglandins are also believed to play a role in the complex biochemistry that initiates labor, although their specific functions are still being defined (Blackburn & Loper, 1992).

Signs of Pregnancy

Many of the changes women experience during pregnancy are used to diagnose the pregnancy itself. They are called the subjective or presumptive changes, the objective or probable changes, and the diagnostic or positive changes of pregnancy.

Subjective (Presumptive) Changes

The subjective changes of pregnancy are the symptoms the woman experiences and reports. They can be caused by other conditions (Table 10–1) and therefore cannot be considered proof of pregnancy. The following can be diagnostic clues when other signs and symptoms of pregnancy are also present.

Amenorrhea is the earliest symptom of pregnancy. In a healthy woman whose menstrual cycles are regular, missing one or more menstrual periods leads to the consideration of pregnancy.

Nausea and vomiting of pregnancy (NVP) are experienced by almost half of all pregnant women during the first 3 months of pregnancy and result from elevated hCG levels and changed carbohydrate metabolism. The woman may feel merely a distaste for food or may suffer extreme vomiting, which may be accompanied by dehydration and ketosis. Because these symptoms frequently occur in the early part of the day and disappear within a few hours, they are commonly called **morning sickness.** In reality, symptoms may occur at any time. This gastrointestinal disturbance usually appears about 6 weeks after the first day of the last menstrual period and usually disappears spontaneously 6 to 12 weeks later, although it may be prolonged in some instances. Research suggests that women who experience NVP often have a more favorable pregnancy outcome than those who do not (Cruikshank et al, 1996).

Excessive fatigue may be noted within a few weeks after the first missed menstrual period and may persist throughout the first trimester.

Urinary frequency is experienced during the first trimester as the enlarging uterus exerts pressure on the bladder. The increased vascularization and pelvic congestion that occur in each pregnancy can also cause frequent voiding. This symptom decreases during the second trimester, when the uterus is an abdominal organ, but reappears during the third trimester, when the presenting part descends into the pelvis.

Changes in the breasts are frequently noted in early pregnancy. Some women report significant breast changes prior to missing their first menses. Engorgement of the breasts due to the hormone-induced growth of the secretory ductal system results in the subjective symptoms of tenderness and tingling, especially of the nipple area. The veins also become more visible and form a bluish pattern beneath the skin in fair-skinned women.

Quickening, or the mother's perception of fetal movement, occurs about 18 to 20 weeks after the last menstrual period (LMP) in a primigravida (a woman who is pregnant for the first time) but may occur as early as 16 weeks in a multigravida (a woman who has been pregnant more than once). Quickening is a fluttering sensation in the abdomen that gradually increases in intensity and frequency.

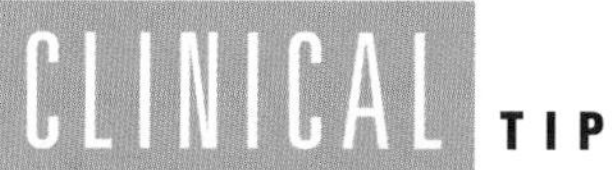

TIP

Some women suggest that it is easiest to imagine the fluttering associated with quickening by letting the outer tips of the eyelashes brush a finger and then imagining that same sensation deep inside the abdomen.

Objective (Probable) Changes

An examiner can perceive the objective changes that occur in pregnancy. They are more diagnostic than the subjective symptoms. However, their presence does not offer a definite diagnosis of pregnancy (Table 10–2).

Changes in the pelvic organs caused by increased vascular congestion are the only physical signs detectable within the first 3 months of pregnancy. These changes are noted on pelvic examination. There is a softening of the cervix, called Goodell's sign. Chadwick's sign is the deep red to purple or bluish coloration of the mucous membranes of the cervix, vagina, and vulva due to increased vasocongestion of the pelvic vessels. (Cunningham et al [1997] consider Chadwick's sign a subjective sign; Scott et al [1994] consider it an objective sign.) **Hegar's sign** is a softening of the isthmus of the uterus, the area between the cervix and the body of the uterus, which occurs at 6 to 8 weeks of pregnancy. This area may become so soft that on a bimanual exam there seems to be nothing between the cervix and the body of the uterus (Figure 10–4). *Ladin's sign* is a soft spot anteriorly in the middle of the uterus near the junction of the body of the uterus and cervix (Figure 10–5, *A*). **McDonald's sign** is an ease in flexing the body of the uterus against the cervix.

The uterus assumes an irregular globular shape during the early months of pregnancy. Irregular softening and enlargement at the site of implantation, known as *Braun von Fernwald's sign*, occurs about the fifth week (Figure 10–5, *B*). Occasionally an almost tumorlike, asymmetric enlargement occurs, called *Piskacek's sign* (Figure 10–5, *C*). Generalized enlargement and softening of the body of the uterus are present after the eighth week of pregnancy. The fundus of the uterus is palpable just above the symphysis pubis at approximately 10 to 12 weeks' gestation and at the level of the umbilicus at 20 to 22 weeks' gestation (Figure 10–6).

Enlargement of the abdomen during the childbearing years is usually regarded as evidence of pregnancy, especially if the enlargement is progressive and is accompanied by a continuing amenorrhea. It is generally more pronounced in a woman whose abdominal musculature has lost some of its tone because of previous childbirth.

As mentioned earlier, Braxton Hicks contractions are irregular, ordinarily painless contractions that occur at irregular intervals throughout pregnancy but are felt with

TABLE 10–2 Differential Diagnosis of Pregnancy—Objective Changes

Objective Changes	Possible Alternative Causes
Changes in pelvic organs	Increased vascular congestion
Goodell's sign	Estrogen-progestin oral contraceptives
Chadwick's sign	Vulvar, vaginal, cervical hyperemia
Hegar's sign	Excessively soft walls of nonpregnant uterus
Uterine enlargement	Uterine tumors
Braun von Fernwald's sign	Uterine tumors
Piskacek's sign	Uterine tumors
Enlargement of abdomen	Obesity, ascites, pelvic tumors
Braxton Hicks contractions	Hematometra, pedunculated, submucous, and soft myomas
Uterine souffle	Large uterine myomas, large ovarian tumors, or any condition with greatly increased uterine blood flow
Pigmentation of skin	Estrogen-progestin oral contraceptives
Chloasma	Melanocyte hormonal stimulation
Linea nigra	
Nipples/areola	
Abdominal striae	Obesity, pelvic tumor
Ballottement	Uterine tumors/polyps, ascites
Pregnancy tests	Increased pituitary gonadotropins at menopause, choriocarcinoma, hydatidiform mole
Palpation for fetal outline	Uterine myomas

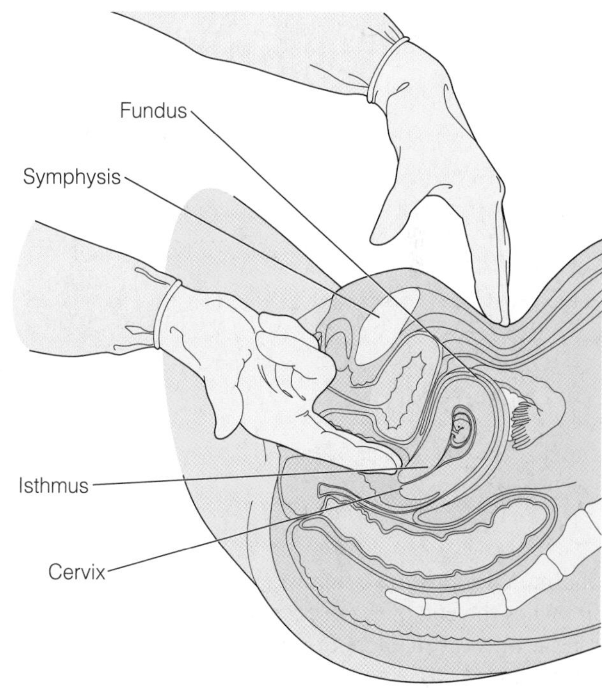

FIGURE 10–4 Hegar's sign, a softening of the isthmus of the uterus, can be determined by the examiner during a vaginal examination.

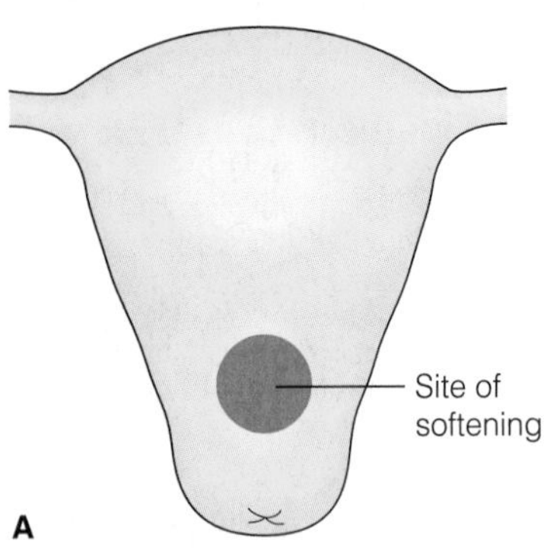

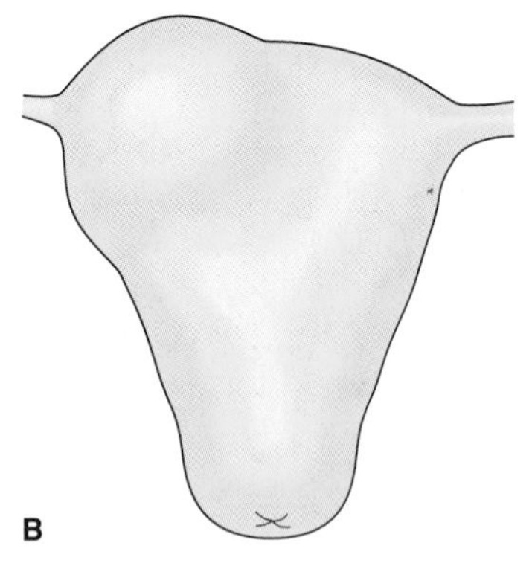

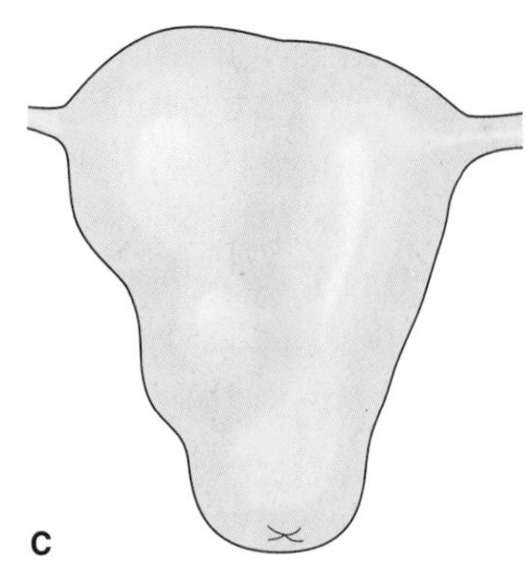

FIGURE 10–5 Early uterine changes of pregnancy. ***A,*** Ladin's sign, a soft spot anteriorly in the middle of the uterus near the junction of the body of the uterus and the cervix. ***B,*** Braun von Fernwald's sign, irregular softening and enlargement at the site of implantation. ***C,*** Piskacek's sign, a tumorlike, asymmetric enlargement.

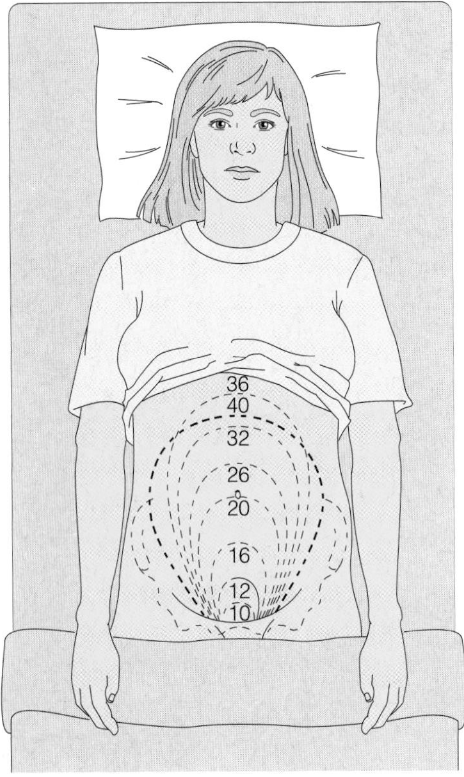

FIGURE 10–6 Approximate height of the fundus at various weeks of pregnancy.

abdominal palpation after week 28. As the woman approaches the end of the pregnancy, these contractions often become more uncomfortable and are then called *false labor*

Uterine souffle may be heard when auscultating the abdomen over the uterus. It is a soft blowing sound at the same rate as the maternal pulse and is due to the increased uterine vascularization and the blood pulsating through the placenta. It is sometimes confused with the *funic souffle*, which is a soft blowing sound of blood pulsating through the umbilical arteries. The funic souffle is at the same rate as the fetal heart rate.

Changes in pigmentation of the skin and the *appearance of abdominal striae* are common manifestations in pregnancy. Facial chloasma occurs in varying degrees after week 16. The pigmentation of the nipple and areola may darken, especially in primigravidas and dark-haired women. The Montgomery glands of the areola may become enlarged. The skin in the midline of the abdomen may develop a pigmented line, the linea nigra. As pregnancy progresses, striae appear on the abdomen and buttocks.

The *fetal outline* may be identified by palpation in many pregnant women after 24 weeks of gestation, becoming easier to distinguish as term approaches. **Ballottement** is the passive fetal movement elicited by pushing up against the cervix with two fingers. This pushes the fetal body up and, as it falls back, the examiner feels a rebound.

Pregnancy tests are based on analysis of maternal blood or urine for the detection of human chorionic gonadotropin, the hormone secreted by the trophoblast. These tests are not considered positive signs of pregnancy because the similarity of hCG and the pituitary-secreted LH occasionally results in cross-reactions. In addition, certain conditions other than pregnancy can cause elevated levels of hCG.

Pregnancy Tests

A variety of assay techniques are available to detect human chorionic gonadotropin during early pregnancy.

- Hemagglutination-inhibition test (Pregnosticon R), an immunoassay, is based on the fact that no clumping of cells occurs when the urine of a pregnant woman is added to the hCG-sensitized red blood cells of sheep.

CLINICAL TIP

Beginning early in pregnancy, have the woman feel her uterus periodically so that she becomes familiar with the size and the way it feels. As her pregnancy progresses she then will be more likely to identify Braxton Hicks contractions and preterm labor, should it occur.

- Latex agglutination test (Gravindex and Pregnosticon slide test), also an immunoassay, is based on the fact that latex particle agglutination is inhibited in the presence of urine containing hCG.

The hemagglutination-inhibition test and the latex agglutination tests are approximately 95% accurate in diagnosing pregnancy and 98% accurate in determining the absence of pregnancy. The tests become positive approximately 10 to 14 days after the first missed menstrual period. The specimen used for the tests is the first early morning midstream urine because it is adequately concentrated for accuracy. The presence of protein substances (such as blood) in the specimen should be avoided because false-positive results may occur.

- *β-subunit radioimmunoassay* or *RIA* uses an antiserum with specificity for the β-subunit of hCG in blood plasma. This is a very accurate pregnancy test that becomes positive a few days after presumed implantation, thereby permitting earlier diagnosis of pregnancy. This test is also used in the diagnosis of ectopic pregnancy or trophoblastic disease. However, because it requires several hours to perform and has only limited sensitivity, it is being replaced by other, simpler, tests such as the immunoradiometric assay (Buster & Carson, 1996).
- *Immunoradiometric assay (IRMA)* (Neocept; Pregnosis) uses a radioactive antibody to identify the presence of hCG in the serum. This test can identify very low concentrations of hCG and requires only about 30 minutes to perform.
- *Enzyme-linked immunosorbent assay (ELISA)* (Model Sensichrome, Quest Confidot) does not use radioisotopes but a substance that results in a color change after binding. A blue color develops, the intensity of which is related to the amount of hCG present. The test is sensitive, quick, and can detect hCG levels as early as 7 to 9 days after ovulation and conception, which is 5 days before the first missed period (Buster & Carson, 1996).
- *Fluoroimmunoassay (FIA)* (Opus hCG; Stratus hCG) uses an antibody tagged with a fluorescent label to detect serum hCG. The test, which takes about 2 to 3 hours to perform, is extremely sensitive and is used primarily to identify and follow hCG concentrations.
- *Radioreceptor assay (RRA)* (Biocept-G) uses the principle of high-affinity receptors to detect pregnancy. It can be performed in about 1 hour, but because it fails to distinguish between hCG and LH, cross-reactions may occur and it has generally been replaced by more effective tests.

Over-the-Counter Pregnancy Tests Home pregnancy tests are available over the counter at a reasonable cost. These enzyme immunoassay tests are quite sensitive and detect even low levels of hCG in urine.

Home pregnancy test instructions are quite explicit and should be followed carefully. Best results are obtained with the first morning-voided urine, although some of the tests can be used on any voided specimen. Furthermore, because the newer kits require only a short wait (usually 3 to 5 minutes), the margin for error is very small.

The false-positive rate of these tests is quite low, but the false-negative results are higher and should be followed up in the presence of pregnancy symptoms. Most of the kits available today can detect a pregnancy as early as the day of a missed period. If the results are negative, the woman should repeat the test in 1 week if she has not started her menstrual period. A false-negative result may lead to delays in beginning prenatal care or the use of drugs that may be harmful to the fetus. It is important that women using the home kits understand that a positive result merely indicates growing trophoblastic tissue and not necessarily a uterine pregnancy. If the woman delays seeking prenatal care after pregnancy is confirmed, an early ectopic pregnancy may be missed.

CRITICAL THINKING QUESTION

What factors might cause a woman to choose a home pregnancy test rather than have a pregnancy test done in a health care facility?

Diagnostic (Positive) Changes

The positive signs of pregnancy are completely objective, cannot be confused with pathologic states, and offer conclusive proof of pregnancy, but they are usually not present until after the fourth month of pregnancy.

The *fetal heartbeat* can be detected with a fetoscope by approximately weeks 17 to 20 of pregnancy. With the electronic Doppler device it is possible to detect the fetal heartbeat as early as weeks 10 to 12. The fetal heart rate is between 120 and 160 beats per minute and must be counted and compared with the maternal pulse for differentiation. Auscultation of the abdomen may reveal sounds other than that of the fetal heart. The maternal pulse, emanating from the abdominal aorta, may be unusually loud, or a uterine souffle may be heard.

Fetal movement is actively palpable by a trained examiner after about 20 weeks' gestation. The movements vary from a faint flutter in the early months to more vigorous movements late in pregnancy.

Visualization of the fetus by ultrasound confirms a pregnancy. The gestational sac can be observed by 4 to 5 weeks' gestation (2 to 3 weeks after conception). Fetal parts and fetal heart movement can be seen as early as 8 weeks. Recently ultrasound using a vaginal probe has been used to detect a gestational sac as early as 10 days after implantation (Cunningham et al, 1997).

Psychologic Response of the Expectant Family to Pregnancy

Pregnancy is a developmental challenge, a turning point, in a family's life and therefore is accompanied by stress and anxiety whether the pregnancy is desired or not. Pregnancy confirms one's biologic capabilities to reproduce. It is evidence of one's participation in sexual activity and as such is an affirmation of one's sexuality. For beginning families, pregnancy is the transition period from childlessness to parenthood. If the pregnancy terminates in the birth of a child, the couple enters a new stage of their life together, one that is irreversible and characterized by awesome responsibilities.

The expectant couple may be unaware of the physical, emotional, and cognitive states peculiar to pregnancy. The couple may anticipate no problem from such a normal event as pregnancy and therefore may be confused and distressed by new feelings and behaviors that are essentially normal.

If the expectant woman is married or has a stable partner, she no longer is only a mate but also must assume the role of mother. Her partner will soon be a father. Career goals and mobility may be altered or thwarted for one or both partners. Each partner begins to see the other in a different light. Their relationship takes on a different meaning to them and within the larger family and community. Their lifestyle changes. With each pregnancy, routines and family dynamics are altered, requiring readjustment and realignment.

If a pregnant woman is without a stable partner, she will still experience changes in role identity and psychobiologic maturation. She must deal alone with the role changes, fears, and adjustments of pregnancy or seek support from family and friends. She also faces the reality of planning for the future as a single parent. Even if the pregnant woman plans to relinquish her infant, she must still deal with the adjustments of pregnancy. She is no longer a separate individual; she must consider the needs of another being who depends on her totally, at least during the pregnancy. This adjustment can be especially difficult without a good support system.

In most pregnancies, whether of a mother with a supportive partner, a single mother, or a relinquishing mother, finances are an important consideration. Traditional lore relegates to the father the role of primary breadwinner, and indeed finances are often a very real concern for fathers. However, in today's society even pregnant women with stable partners recognize the financial impact of a child and may feel concern about financial issues. For the single mother, finances may be a major source of concern.

Decisions about financial matters need to be made at this time. Will the woman work during the pregnancy and return to work after the baby is born? Who will provide child care if she works? Decisions may also need to be made about the division of tasks within the home. Any differences of opinion must be discussed openly and resolved so that the family can meet its members' needs.

The couple must face the realities of labor and birth. Many nonparents have little idea what labor entails. Their information is frequently based on experiences related to them by family members or friends, and these tales are often fraught with myths and exaggerations. Classes in prepared childbirth can help them address this lack of information or misinformation.

Labor is threatening in many respects. Pain, disfigurement, disruption of bodily function, and even death are potential threats for the woman. The man faces the potential disfigurement of his wife, impairment of her health, or her death. Both fear that the baby may be ill or disfigured. The expectant couple is subject to anxiety during this period because no one can provide total reassurance about the outcome.

Pregnancy can be viewed as a developmental stage with its own distinct developmental tasks. It can be a time of support or conflict for a couple, depending on the amount of adjustment each is willing to make to maintain the family's equilibrium. Family dynamics are an important factor in adjusting to pregnancy. Family strengths include the ability of the couple to talk about issues that are important to them, to resolve conflicts and make compromises, and to seek and receive assistance and support from loved ones.

During pregnancy, the couple plans together for the first child's arrival, collecting information on how to be parents. At the same time, each continues to participate in some separate activities with friends or family members. The availability of social support is an important factor in psychosocial well-being during pregnancy. The social network often is a major source of advice for the pregnant woman. However, evidence indicates that both sound and unsound information is given.

Although individual activities are important, some conflict may arise if the couple's activities become too divergent. Thus they may find it necessary to limit their outside associations.

TABLE 10–3 Parental Reactions to Pregnancy

First Trimester	Second Trimester	Third Trimester
Mother's Reactions	**Mother's Reactions**	**Mother's Reactions**
Informs father secretively or openly. Feels ambivalent toward pregnancy, anxious about labor and responsibility of child. Is aware of physical changes, daydreams of possible miscarriage. Develops special feelings for and renewed interest in her own mother, with formation of a personal identity.	Remains regressive and introspective, projects all problems with authority figures onto partner, may become angry as if lack of interest is sign of weakness in him. Continues to deal with feelings as a mother and looks for furniture as something concrete. May have other extreme of anxiety and wait until 9th month to look for furniture and clothes for baby. Feels movement and is aware of fetus and incorporates it into herself. Dreams that partner will be killed, telephones him often for reassurance. Experiences more distinct physical changes; sexual desires may increase or decrease.	Experiences more anxiety and tension, with physical awkwardness. Feels much discomfort and insomnia from physical condition. Prepares for birth, assembles layette, picks out names. Dreams often about misplacing baby or not being able to give birth, fears birth of deformed baby. Feels ecstasy and excitement, has spurt of energy during last month.
Father's Reactions	**Father's Reactions**	**Father's Reactions**
Differ according to age, parity, desire for child, economic stability. Acceptance of pregnant woman's attitude or complete rejection and lack of communication. Is aware of his own sexual feelings, may develop more or less sexual arousal. Accepts, rejects, or resents mother-in-law. May develop new hobby outside of family as sign of stress.	If he can cope, will give her extra attention she needs; if he cannot cope, will develop a new time-consuming interest outside of home. May develop a creative feeling and a "closeness to nature." May become involved in pregnancy and buy or make furniture. Feels for movement of baby, listens to heartbeat, or remains aloof, with no physical contact. May have fears and fantasies about himself being pregnant, may become uneasy with this feminine aspect in himself. May react negatively if partner is too demanding, may become jealous of physician and of physician's importance to partner and her pregnancy.	Adapts to alternative methods of sexual contact. Becomes concerned over financial responsibility. May show new sense of tenderness and concern, treats partner like doll. Daydreams about child as if older and not newborn, dreams of losing partner. Renewed sexual attraction to partner. Feels he is ultimately responsible for whatever happens.

The expectant mother and father both face significant changes during pregnancy and must deal with major psychosocial adjustments (Table 10–3). Other family members, especially other children of the woman or couple, and the grandparents-to-be, must also adjust to the pregnancy.

For some couples, pregnancy is more than a developmental stage; it is a crisis. Crisis can be defined as a disturbance or conflict in which the individual cannot maintain a state of equilibrium. Pregnancy can be considered a *maturational crisis* because it is a common event in the normal growth and development of the family. During such a crisis, the individual or family is in disequilibrium. Egos weaken, usual defense mechanisms lose their effectiveness, unresolved material from the past reappears, and relationships shift. The period of disequilibrium and disorganization is marked by abortive attempts to solve the perceived problems. If the crisis is unresolved, it will result in maladaptive behaviors in one or more family members and possible disintegration of the family. Families who are able to resolve a maturational crisis successfully will return to normal functioning and can even strengthen the bonds in the family relationship.

The Mother

Pregnancy is a condition that alters body image and also necessitates a reordering of social relationships and changes in roles of family members. The way a particular woman meets the stresses of pregnancy is influenced by her emotional makeup, her sociologic and cultural background, and her acceptance or rejection of the pregnancy. However, many women manifest similar psychologic and emotional responses during pregnancy, including ambivalence, acceptance, introversion, mood swings, and changes in body image.

Ambivalence

Initially, even if the pregnancy is planned, there is an element of surprise that conception has occurred. This feeling is generally coupled with a feeling that the timing is wrong, that pregnancy is desirable "some day" but "not now." This ambivalence may be related to feelings that the timing is somehow "wrong;" worries about the need to modify existing relationships or career plans; fears about assuming a new role; unresolved emotional conflicts with the woman's own mother; and fears about pregnancy, labor, and birth. Indirect evidence of ambivalence

RESEARCH IN PRACTICE

What is this study about? Psychologic factors may directly or indirectly impact the outcome of a pregnancy. Use of the Prenatal Psychological Profile (PPP) provides information about pregnant women's perceptions of stress, support from partners, support from others, and feelings of self-esteem. Psychometric properties of convergent validity, internal consistency, and test–retest reliability have been evaluated for this profile with primarily European American women.

How was this study done? Mary Ann Curry, Deborah Burton, and Jonathan Fields compared and evaluated the psychometric properties of the data from five studies that used the PPP with pregnant, culturally diverse women. The Rural Oregon Minority Prenatal Project provided nursing case management to 83 rural Native American and 100 rural Latina women and used the PPP to evaluate the woman's stress before and after intervention. The Low Birthweight Study tested the ability of a biopsychosocial model to predict low birth weight and adverse outcomes of pregnancy for 1223 European American, 406 African American, and 60 Native American women. The North Carolina Birth Prevention study determined if intensive telephone contact with high-risk women could reduce the incidence of preterm delivery for 791 African American and 234 European American women. The Oregon Preterm Birth Prevention study evaluated the effectiveness of three interventions to reduce the incidence of preterm birth among 349 European American women with high-risk pregnancies. The PPP was given before and after the intervention. the San Francisco study used the PPP with 118 African American women to examine the associations of maternal stress, social support, and self-esteem with low birth weight and gestational age.

What were the results of the study? In three of the five studies, women had difficulty with the self-esteem subscale. Difficulties stemmed from both the wording and the cultural implications of the concept, especially for the Native American participants. Internal consistency and test–retest scores denote reliability. Cronbach's alpha scores for support, which measure internal consistency, ranged from 0.92 to 0.96; for self-esteem from 0.76 to 0.89; for stress from 0.67 to 0.78. A scale with a score of 0.70 is considered to be internally consistent. The test–retest scores ranged from 0.52 to 0.76 or moderately stable. The authors evaluated construct validity by determining correlation of the subscales with one another as described in the literature. Exceptions could be culturally based.

What additional questions might I have? What were the psychometric properties from the initial study of the tool? Although the study is cited, the actual findings are not given.

How can I use this study? The scale, which takes only 5 minutes to use, could be used to help initiate discussion, provide important clinical information, or validate current knowledge.

SOURCE: Curry, M. A., Burton, D., & Fields, J. (1998). The prenatal psychosocial profile: A research and clinical tool. *Research in Nursing & Health, 21,* 211–219.

includes complaints about prolonged or frequent depression, considerable physical discomfort, significant dissatisfaction with body shape, excessive mood swings, and difficulty accepting the life changes resulting from the pregnancy (Lederman, 1996).

Such feelings may be even more pronounced if the pregnancy is unintended or unwanted. In fact, research suggests that women with unintended pregnancy experience increased depression, increased stress, decreased support from the father, and decreased overall satisfaction with life (Orr & Miller, 1997).

During the early months, the pregnant woman may consider the possibility of a therapeutic abortion if the pregnancy is unwanted. In the event of religious conflicts about induced abortion, the woman may experience guilt feelings about her thoughts or may tend to focus on the possibility of spontaneous abortion (miscarriage). Even when the pregnancy is planned, thoughts of abortion and miscarriage arise. Concurrently, the pregnant woman may feel guilty for having such negative thoughts and may worry that in some way these thoughts will harm the baby (Robinson & Stewart, 1990).

Acceptance

Acceptance of pregnancy is influenced by many factors. Lower acceptance tends to be related to an unplanned pregnancy and greater evidence of fear and conflict. The woman carrying an unplanned pregnancy tends to experience more physical discomfort and depression. When a pregnancy is well accepted, the woman demonstrates feelings of happiness and pleasure in the pregnancy. She experiences less physical discomfort and shows a high degree of tolerance for the discomforts associated with the third trimester (Lederman, 1996).

Conflicts about adapting to pregnancy are no more pronounced for older pregnant women (age 35 and older) than for younger ones. Moreover, older pregnant women tend to be less concerned about the normal physical changes of pregnancy and are confident about handling issues that arise during pregnancy and parenting. This may be because mature pregnant women have more experience with problem solving. However, mature pregnant women may have fewer pregnant peers and thus may have fewer people with whom to share concerns and expectations (Stark, 1997).

For some women, an unintended pregnancy has more psychologic and social advantages than disadvantages. It provides purpose and direction to life and allows a woman to test the devotion and love of her partner and family (Moos, Peterson, Meadows, Melvin, & Spitz, 1997).

I didn't expect to get pregnant, but my baby seems like a gift from God. Suddenly I feel like I have a purpose in life. I know I have to do the right things so the baby will be okay. Being pregnant made me grow up in a hurry, but I don't regret it—not at all.

During the *first trimester*, evidence of pregnancy is often limited to amenorrhea and to the word of the caregiver that the pregnancy test was positive. Unless she has the opportunity to see the gestational sac during an ultrasound, her baby may not seem real to her. Consequently she may tend to focus on herself and her pregnancy. In an effort to verify her condition, a woman may become minutely conscious of changes in her body that could validate the pregnancy.

The *second trimester* is relatively tranquil. Morning sickness generally passes, the threat of spontaneous abortion diminishes, and the woman begins to accept the reality of her pregnancy. It is not unusual for an enthusiastic primigravida to don maternity clothes at the beginning of this trimester even when it is not truly necessary. The clothing serves as a verification of her pregnant state.

The highlight of the second trimester is quickening, which generally occurs about week 20—midway through the pregnancy. Actual perception of fetal movement frequently produces dramatic changes in the woman. She now perceives her baby as a real person and generally becomes excited about the pregnancy even if she hasn't been prior to this time.

As quickening and her altered physical appearance confirm her pregnant state, the woman adjusts to the idea of change and begins to prepare for her new role and her new set of relationships—with her partner and family, the child-to-be and other children, friends, and loved ones. When the pregnancy is well accepted, the woman takes pleasure in the sensations of pregnancy and attempts to picture her baby in order to know him or her better. She may seek out other women who are pregnant or have recently given birth. She feels well, is excited, and may exhibit the "glow" so often attributed to pregnant women.

The *third trimester* combines a sense of pride with anxiety about what is to come in order for the child to be born. During this time, the special prerogatives of pregnancy may be most marked. As her protruding abdomen proclaims her advanced pregnancy, the woman may find that others become more solicitous, that a chair may be offered in a crowded room, that others may carry her parcels. The woman may actually need this help, she may simply enjoy the attention as a privilege of pregnancy, or she may reject it if she fears that such gestures indicate she is helpless.

During the final trimester, physical discomforts again increase, and adequate rest becomes a necessity. The woman makes final preparation for the baby and may spend long periods considering names for the child. During this time she worries more about the health and safety of her unborn child and may have concerns that she will not behave well during childbirth (Robinson & Stewart, 1990).

The woman may feel vulnerable to rejection, loss, or insult. She may worry about a variety of things and may withdraw into the security and quiet of her home. Toward the end of this period there is often a surge of energy as the woman prepares a "nest" for her infant. Many women report bursts of energy in which they vigorously clean and organize their homes.

Introversion

Introversion, or turning in on oneself, is a common occurrence in pregnancy. An active, outgoing woman may become less interested in previous activities and more concerned with needs for rest and time alone. This concentration of attention permits the woman to plan, adjust, adapt, build, and draw strength in preparation for her child's birth. As she becomes more aware of herself, her partner may feel she is being overly sensitive. He may perceive her introversion and passivity as exclusion of him and may in turn become unable to interact with her, either verbally or physically, or to provide the affection, support, and consideration she requires. This change may result in disequilibrium and stress for the entire family. It is essential that the couple work together to establish new, mutually acceptable patterns of response in order to overcome these blocks to communication.

> *I don't know if this is really considered a problem or not, but at times it seems like a problem. I'm really subject to drastic mood changes. That or I'll be extremely emotional. For no reason at all I'll start crying or just laugh till I can hardly breathe. I don't know why; and if I can't understand it, it's twice as hard for John, especially if I'm bummed out or crying. It don't [sic] seem normal for a person to cry for no reason, and I never did it before.*
>
> ~ QUOTED IN RP LEDERMAN ~
>
> ~ *PSYCHOSOCIAL ADAPTATION IN PREGNANCY, 1996* ~

Mood Swings

Throughout pregnancy, the emotions of many women are characterized by mood swings, from great joy to deep despair. Frequently, the woman will become tearful with little apparent cause. When asked why she is crying, she may find it difficult or impossible to give a reason. The situation may be extremely unsettling for the partner, causing him to feel confused and inadequate. Because the man may feel unable to handle the woman's tears, he often reacts by withdrawing and ignoring the problem. Because the pregnant woman needs increased love and affection, she may perceive his reaction as unloving and nonsupportive. Once the couple understands that this behavior is characteristic of pregnancy, it becomes easier for them to deal with it more effectively—although it will be a source of stress to some extent throughout pregnancy.

Changes in Body Image

Pregnancy produces marked changes in a woman's body within a relatively short period of time. Women perceive that they require more body space as pregnancy progresses (Mercer, 1995). They also experience changes in body image. The degree of this change is related to a certain extent to personality factors, social network responses, and attitudes toward pregnancy. Changes in body image are normal but can be very stressful for the pregnant woman. Explanation and discussion of the changes may help both the woman and her partner deal with the stress associated with this aspect of pregnancy.

Psychologic Tasks of the Mother

Rubin (1984) identified four major tasks that the pregnant woman undertakes to maintain her intactness and that of her family and at the same time incorporate her new child into the family system. These tasks form the basis for a mutually gratifying relationship with her baby:

1. *Ensuring safe passage through pregnancy, labor, and birth.* The pregnant woman feels concern for both her unborn child and herself. She seeks competent maternity care to provide a sense of control. She may also seek knowledge from literature, observation of other pregnant women and new mothers, and discussion with others. The pregnant woman also seeks to ensure safe passage by engaging in self-care activities related to diet, exercise, alcohol consumption, and so forth (Patterson, Freese, & Goldenberg, 1990). In the third trimester, as her movements slow and her body mass increases, she becomes aware of external threats in the environment—a toy on a stair, the awkwardness of an escalator—that pose a threat to her intactness and represent hazards to be overcome. She may worry if her partner is late or she is home alone. Sleep becomes difficult, and she begins to long for the baby's birth, even though it, too, is frightening.
2. *Seeking of acceptance of this child by others.* The birth of a child alters a woman's primary support group, her family, and her secondary affiliative groups. The family generally makes the transition, and the woman slowly and subtly alters her secondary network to meet the needs of her pregnancy. In this adjustment the woman's partner is the most important figure. The partner's support and acceptance influence her completion of her maternal tasks and the formation of her maternal identity. If there are other children in the home, the mother also works to ensure their acceptance of the coming child. Accepting the coming change in exclusive relationships—woman and partner or mother and first child—can be stressful, and the woman will often work to maintain some special time with her partner or older child. Achieving social acceptance of the child and herself as mother may be more difficult for the adolescent mother or single woman. The child to come is not always wanted, and the woman often must direct her energies to changing this situation.
3. *Seeking of commitment and acceptance of self as mother to the infant (binding-in).* During the first trimester, the child remains a rather abstract concept. With quickening, however, the child begins to become a real person, and the mother begins to develop bonds of attachment. The mother experiences the movement of the child within her in an intimate, exclusive way, and out of this experience bonds of love form. The mother develops a fantasy image of her ideal child. This binding-in process, characterized by its strong emotional component, motivates the pregnant woman to become competent in her role and provides satisfaction for her in her role of mother (Mercer, 1995). This possessive love increases her maternal commitment to protect her fetus now and her child after she or he is born.
4. *Learning to give of oneself on behalf of one's child.* Childbirth involves many acts of giving. The man "gives" a child to a woman; she in turn "gives" a child to the man. Life is given to an infant; a sibling is given to older children of the family. The woman begins to develop a capacity for self-denial and learns to delay immediate personal gratification to meet the needs of another. Baby showers and baby gifts are acts of giving that help the mother's self-esteem while also helping her acknowledge the separateness and needs of the coming baby.

Accomplishment of these tasks helps the expectant woman develop her self-concept as mother. The expectant mother who was well nurtured by her own mother may view her mother as a role model and emulate her; the woman who views her own mother a "poor mother" may worry that she will make similar mistakes (Lederman, 1996). A woman's self-concept as mother expands with actual experience and continues to grow through subsequent childbearing and childrearing. Occasionally, a woman never accepts the mother role but plays the role of babysitter or older sister.

The Father

Until fairly recently, the expectant father was often viewed as a "bystander" or observer of his partner's pregnancy. He was necessary for conception, for bill paying, and for providing male guidance as his child matured. This view has changed, and the father of today is expected to fulfill the role of nurturing, caring, involved parent as well as provider. In response to societal pressures, the influence of the feminist movement, and the economic pressures that result in more women employed outside the home, shared parenting and breadwinning have become more commonplace. Then, too, many men have actively sought to be more involved in the experience of childbirth and parenting.

Expectant fathers experience many of the same feelings and conflicts experienced by expectant mothers when the pregnancy has been confirmed. Feelings of ambivalence are prevalent. The extent of ambivalence depends on many factors, such as whether the pregnancy was planned, the man's relationship with his partner, his previous experiences with pregnancy, his age, and his economic stability.

Thus the expectant father must first deal with the reality of the pregnancy and then struggle to gain recognition as a parent from his partner, family, friends, coworkers, society—and from his baby as well. The expectant mother can help her partner be a participant and not merely a helpmate to her if she has a definite sense of the experience as *their* pregnancy and *their* infant and not *her* pregnancy and *her* infant (Jordan, 1990).

The expectant father faces psychologic stress as he makes the transition from nonparent to parent or from parent of one or more to parent of two or more. Sources of stress include financial issues, unexpected events during pregnancy, concern that the baby will not be healthy and normal, worry about the pain the partner will experience in childbirth, and their role during labor and birth. Other sources of stress for expectant fathers include concern over the changing relationship with their partner, diminished sexual responsiveness in their partner or in themselves, change in relationships with their family or male friends, and their ability to parent.

The expectant father must establish a fatherhood role just as the woman develops a motherhood role. Fathers who are most successful at this generally like children, are excited about the prospect of fatherhood, are eager to nurture a child, have confidence in their ability to be a parent, and share the experiences of pregnancy and childbirth with their partners (Lederman, 1996).

First Trimester

After the initial excitement of the announcement of the pregnancy to friends and relatives and their congratulations, an expectant father may begin to feel left out of the pregnancy. He is also often confused by his partner's mood changes and perhaps bewildered by his responses to her changing body. He may resent the attention given to the woman and the need to change their relationship as she experiences fatigue and a decreased interest in sex.

During this time, his child is a "potential baby." Fathers often picture interacting with a child of 5 or 6 rather than a newborn. Even the pregnancy itself may seem unreal until the woman shows more physical signs (Jordan, 1990).

Second Trimester

The father's role in the pregnancy is still vague in the second trimester, but his involvement can be increased by his watching and feeling fetal movement. It is helpful if the father, as well as the mother, has the opportunity to hear the fetal heartbeat. That requires a visit to the nurse-midwife's or physician's office. Involvement of fathers in antepartal care is increasing as fathers become more comfortable with this new role. For many men, seeing the infant on ultrasound is an important experience in accepting the reality of the pregnancy.

Like expectant mothers, expectant fathers need to confront and resolve some of their own conflicts about the fathering they received. A father needs to sort out those behaviors in his own fathering that he wants to imitate and those he wishes to avoid. This process usually occurs gradually as the pregnancy progresses.

Evidence suggests that the father-to-be's anxiety is lessened if both parents agree on the support role the man is to assume during pregnancy and on his projected paternal role. For example, if both see his role as that of breadwinner, the man's stress is low. However, if the man views his role as that of breadwinner and the woman expects him to be actively involved in preparations and child care, his stress increases. Thus the ability of the couple to negotiate a mutually agreeable role for the man may provide a significant coping mechanism for expectant fathers (Diemer, 1997).

The woman's appearance begins to alter at this time too, and men react differently to the physical change. For some it decreases sexual interest; for others it may have the opposite effect. Both partners experience a multitude of emotions, and it continues to be important for them to communicate and accept each other's feelings and concerns. In situations in which the expectant mother's demands dominate the relationship, the expectant father's resentment may increase to the point that he is spending more time at work, involved in a hobby, or with his friends. The behavior is even more likely if the expectant father did not want the pregnancy and/or if the relationship was not a good one prior to the pregnancy.

Third Trimester

If the couple have communicated their concerns and feelings to one another and grown in their relationship, the third trimester is a special and rewarding time. A more clearly defined role evolves at this time for the expectant father, and it becomes more obvious how the couple can prepare together for the coming event. They may become involved in childbirth education classes and make concrete preparations for the arrival of the baby, such as shopping for a crib, car seat, and other equipment. If the expectant father has developed a detached attitude about the pregnancy prior to this time, however, it is unlikely that he will become a willing participant even though his role becomes more obvious.

Concerns and fears may recur. Many men are afraid of hurting the unborn baby during intercourse. The father may also begin to have anxiety and fantasies about what could happen to his partner and the unborn baby during labor and birth and feels a great sense of responsibility. The questions asked earlier in pregnancy emerge again. What kind of parents will he and his partner be? Will he really be able to help his partner in labor? Can they afford to have a baby?

COMMUNITY IN FOCUS

Boot Camp for New Dads

The Boot Camp for New Dads is an innovative program designed to help prospective fathers prepare for parenthood. The program, offered by Exempla Health Care System in Denver, Colorado, is patterned on a model that originated in Irvine, California. The "Boot Camp" is a 3-hour workshop that fathers-to-be typically take during the third trimester of their partner's pregnancy. Each workshop consists of about 15 "rookie" dads and 4 to 5 veterans of the course who have been fathers for 3 to 4 months.

Expectant fathers learn of the course through Exempla or are referred by other hospitals or care providers. A local adoption agency also refers prospective fathers. The cost of the class is $15. Boot Camp workshops are offered three times a month. In addition, once each month the workshop is offered in Spanish. Because of the tremendous success of the program, a workshop for expectant teenage fathers is also available. It includes the basic workshop content but also identifies ways in which the teen father can have a relationship with his child even if he does not have an ongoing relationship with the teen mother.

During the first hour of the Boot Camp workshop, the men gather in a circle and the facilitator asks the fathers-to-be to describe their concerns about becoming fathers. The facilitator records the identified concerns for later use. Typically some common themes emerge from the group. The veteran fathers in the group, who are accompanied by their newborns, are each asked to share three pieces of advice based on their actual experiences as parents.

During the second hour, the men discuss babies. The veteran fathers demonstrate basic baby-care activities such as changing diapers and burping. They also demonstrate calming techniques they have used successfully with their infants. Using a baby model, the facilitator demonstrates basics not covered by the veteran fathers. In addition, the veteran fathers pass their infants to the rookie fathers to hold. This can be an intimidating experience for the expectant fathers.

The third hour of the class addresses specific parenting issues such as forming a parenting team, balancing work and family, the male role in successful breastfeeding, postpartum depression, and shaken baby syndrome. Issues of personal safety such as wearing seat belts and avoiding driving after drinking are also covered. Themes identified during the first hour are addressed at this time as well.

Recently Exempla added a postpartum support element to the fatherhood program called "Huddles." The huddles, which cost $5 and last 2 hours, typically involve about 6 to 8 fathers. In many instances, fathers who join the huddles have not participated in the boot camp and are experiencing difficulty with a specific issue. Fathers may sign up for one or more huddles. At present, each huddle focuses on one of five specific themes:

- *The mechanics of a growing infant,* led by a pediatrician
- *Play time,* which describes ways of playing appropriately with a baby
- *Couples communication AC* (after children), led by a marriage and family counselor
- *Infant brain development*
- *Home alone,* which addresses issues of dads who care for their children for several hours at a time on their own.

Anecdotal support for program success is strong. To identify knowledge change, simple pre- and post-tests are used with the boot camp workshops. The willingness of boot camp graduates to return as veterans also serves as a measure of success. All veterans of the course receive an invitation to return and share their experiences in parenting and, rather surprisingly, approximately 50% do so. Currently Exempla is working to identify more specific outcome measures as well.

The tremendous growth of the program attests to its success and indicates that a real need exists to provide support to expectant fathers. Hopefully programs like Exempla's Boot Camp will proliferate as more and more communities address this need.

SOURCE: Personal communication with Chuck Ault, Coordinator of Fatherhood Programs, Exempla Health Care.

Couvade

The term **couvade** traditionally referred to the observance of certain rituals and taboos by the male to signify the transition to fatherhood. This observance affirms his psychosocial and biophysical relationship to the woman and child. These taboos may have taken specific form—for example, the man may have been forbidden to eat certain foods or carry certain weapons before and immediately after the birth. More recently, the term has been used to describe the unintentional development of physical symptoms, such as fatigue, increased appetite, difficulty sleeping, depression, headache, or backache by the partner of the pregnant woman. Research suggests that those men who demonstrate couvade syndrome tend to have a higher degree of paternal role preparation and be involved in more activities related to this preparation (Longobucco & Freston, 1989).

Siblings

The introduction of a new baby into the family is often the beginning of sibling rivalry. Sibling rivalry results from children's fear of change in the security of their relationships with their parents. Some of the behaviors demonstrating feelings of sibling rivalry may even be directed toward the mother during the pregnancy as she experiences more fatigue and less patience with her toddler, for example. Parents who recognize the situation early in pregnancy and begin constructive actions can help minimize the problems of sibling rivalry.

Preparation of the young child begins several weeks prior to the anticipated birth and is designed according to the age and experience of the child. Because they do not have a clear concept of time, young children should not be told too early about the pregnancy. From the toddler's point of view "several weeks" is an extremely long time. The mother may let the child feel the baby moving in her uterus, explaining that this is "a special place where babies grow." The child can help the parents put the baby clothes in drawers or prepare the nursery.

The concept of consistency is important in dealing with young children. They need reassurance that certain people, special things, and familiar places will continue to exist after the new baby arrives. The crib is an important though transient object in a child's life. If it is to be given to the new baby, the parents should thoughtfully help the child adjust to this change. Any move from crib to bed or from one room to another should precede the baby's birth by at least several weeks. If the new baby must share a room with siblings, the parents must discuss this with the siblings.

If the child is ready for toilet training, it is most effectively done several months before or after the baby's arrival. Parents should know that the older, toilet-trained child may regress to wetting or soiling because he or she sees the new baby getting attention for such behavior. The older, weaned child may want to drink from a bottle again after the new baby comes. If the new mother anticipates these behaviors, they will be less frustrating during her early postpartum days.

During the pregnancy older children should be introduced to a new baby for short periods to get an idea of what a new baby is like. This introduction dispels fantasies that the new arrival will be big enough to be a playmate. Pregnant women may also find it helpful to bring their children to a prenatal visit after they have been told about the expected baby. The children are encouraged to become involved in prenatal care and to ask any questions they may have. They are also given the opportunity to hear the baby's heartbeat, either with a stethoscope or with the Doppler. This helps make the baby more real to them.

If siblings are school-age children, the pregnancy should be viewed as a family affair. Teaching about the pregnancy should be based on the child's level of understanding and interest. Overeager parents may go into lengthier and more in-depth responses than the child is interested in. Some children are more curious than others. Books at their level of understanding can be made available in the home. Involvement in family discussions, attendance at sibling preparation classes, encouragement to feel fetal movement, and an opportunity to listen to the fetal heart supplement the learning process and help make the school-age child feel part of the pregnancy. Sibling preparation classes assist in the transition process for both parents and children. After attending the classes, children often exhibit less anxiety and increased ability to express their feelings.

Older children or adolescents may appear to have a sophisticated knowledge base, but it may be intermingled with many misconceptions. Thus the parents should make opportunities to discuss their concerns and should involve the children in preparation for the new baby.

Even after the birth, siblings need to feel that they are part of a family affair. Changes in hospital regulations allowing siblings to be present at the birth or to visit their mother and the new baby facilitate this process. On arrival at home, siblings can share in "showing off" the new baby.

Sibling preparation for the arrival of a new baby is essential, but other factors are equally important. These include the amount of parental attention focused on the new arrival, amount of parental attention given the older child after the birth of the new arrival, and parental skill in dealing effectively with regressive and/or aggressive behavior.

Grandparents

The first relatives told about a pregnancy are usually the grandparents. Although relationships with parents can be very complex, this period in a family's life most often promotes a closer relationship between the expectant couple and their parents. Usually the expectant grandparents become increasingly supportive of the expectant couple, even if conflicts previously existed.

Grandparents may be unsure about the amount of involvement they are "allowed" during the pregnancy and childbearing process. Most want to be helpful; some may bestow advice and/or gifts unsparingly. Because grandparenting can occur over a wide span of years, people's response to this role can vary considerably. For some, this new role may occur at a relatively young age, and the connotation of aging that accompanies the role may affect their response to the pregnancy. The younger grandparent may also be involved in work and other activities and may not demonstrate as much interest as the young couple would like.

It can be difficult for even sensitive grandparents to know how much involvement the couple wants. Expectant couples want to feel in control of their new situation, which may be initially difficult in their changing roles. Grandparents find that this factor, as well as changing roles in their own life (eg, retirement, financial concerns, menopause of the expectant grandmother, death of a friend), may contribute to conflicts in the changing family structure. Some parents of expectant couples may already be grandparents and have already developed their own style of grandparenting, which will be an important factor in how they respond to the pregnancy.

Childbearing and childrearing practices are very different for today's childbearing couple. It helps family cohesiveness for young couples to share with interested grandparents what today's practices are and why they feel they are effective. At the same time, it is important for young couples to listen to any differences expectant grandparents want to explain. When grandparents give advice, it helps to remember that they care. When their recommendations seem effective, it is significant to grandparents that young couples do listen and follow their advice.

Occasionally young couples feel they are receiving more advice than they can tolerate. Too often they perceive parents' suggestions as criticizing their ability to prepare adequately for the childbearing process—and later as criticizing their care of the newborn. It is useful for the young couple to discuss the problem and agree on a plan of action. The role of the helping grandparents when the new baby is brought home needs to be clarified before the event to ensure a comfortable situation for all.

In some areas, classes for grandparents provide information about changes in birthing and parenting practices. These classes help familiarize grandparents with new parents' needs and may offer suggestions for ways in which the grandparents can supporting the childbearing woman or couple.

Cultural Diversity and Pregnancy

CRITICAL THINKING QUESTION

How might nurses become more aware of their own cultural beliefs and biases about pregnancy and childbirth? How can they distinguish their own personal biases from essential, factual information?

A universal tendency exists to create ceremonial rituals and rites around important life events. Thus pregnancy, childbirth, marriage, and death are often tied to ritual. Many of these rituals have their origins in the practices of ancient human beings (Spector, 1996). The rituals, customs, and practices of a group are a reflection of the group's values. Thus the identification of cultural values is useful in planning and providing culturally sensitive care. An understanding of male and female roles, family lifestyles, or the meaning of children in a culture may explain reactions of joy or shame. Pregnancy is a joyful event in a culture that values children. In some cultures, however, pregnancy is a shameful event if it occurs outside of marriage.

Health values and beliefs are also important in understanding reactions and behavior. Certain behaviors can be expected if a culture views pregnancy as a sickness, whereas other behaviors can be expected if pregnancy is viewed as a natural occurrence. Prenatal care may not be a priority for women who view pregnancy as a natural occurrence. For example, in India pregnancy is not considered an illness but a normal physiologic event, so a traditional Indian woman may seek health care only in the event of a problem (Choudhry, 1997). On the other hand, health care in southeast Asia is crisis oriented, with symptom relief as the goal (D'Avanzo, 1992).

Generalizations about cultural characteristics or cultural values are difficult because not every individual in a culture may display these characteristics. Just as variations are seen *among* cultures, variations are also seen *within* cultures. These variations are often related to social and economic factors such as class, income, and education. For example, because of their exposure to the American culture, a third-generation Chinese American family might have very different values and beliefs from those of a traditional Chinese family who has recently immigrated to America. For this reason, the nurse needs to supplement a general knowledge of cultural values and practices with a complete assessment of the individual's values and practices.

Attitudes about pregnancy may vary somewhat among cultures. Americans of African descent, for example, usually consider pregnancy as a state of wellness. Mexican Americans generally view pregnancy as a natural and desirable condition, and most Native American groups consider pregnancy a normal process. In all these cultures, children are desired. Children ensure continuation of the family and cultural values. A woman who gives birth to a child, especially a son, often achieves higher status. This is true in traditional Chinese families, for example. Similarly, in the western United States, people of the Mormon faith view motherhood as the most important aspect of a woman's life, comparable with the male role of priesthood (Conley, 1990). In Mexican American society and among many Hispanic groups, having children is evidence of the male's virility and is a sign of manliness, or machismo, a desired trait.

Health Beliefs

Although pregnancy is perceived as a natural occurrence in many cultures, it may also be viewed as a time of increased vulnerability. Individuals with European/Western ideas might expect the woman to be away from work before and right after childbirth. Individuals of many cultures take certain protective precautions based on their beliefs. For example, many women of Malawi, Africa avoid preparing clothes for the infant during the prenatal period because they believe that this action will lead to the birth of a stillborn infant (Gennaro, Kamwendo, Mbweza, Kershbaumer, 1998). Similarly, many southeast Asian women fear that they will have a complicated labor and birth if they sit in a doorway or on a step. Thus they tend to avoid areas near doors in waiting rooms and examining rooms. Some Hmong women fear that sharp instruments may cause cleft lip or abortion. Consequently they avoid contact with scissors or knives during pregnancy (Mattson, 1995).

In the Mexican American culture, the concept of *mal aire*, or bad air, is sometimes related to evil spirits. It is thought that air, especially night air, may enter the body and cause harm. Preventive measures, such as keeping the windows closed or covering the head, are used. For many southeast Asians, "wind" represents a bad external influence that may enter a person when the body is vulnerable, such as during and after childbirth or during surgery (Mattson, 1995).

Most of the taboos stemming from the belief in evil spirits relate to fears of injuring the unborn child. Taboos also emanate from the fear that a pregnant woman has evil powers. For this reason, pregnant women are sometimes prohibited from taking part in certain activities with other people.

The equilibrium model of health is based on the concept of balance between light and dark, heat and cold. Eastern philosophical belief focuses on the notion of yin and yang. Yin represents the female, passive principle—darkness, cold, wetness—and yang is the masculine, active part—light, heat, and dryness. When the two are combined, they are all that can be.

The hot-cold classification is seen in cultures in Latin America, the Near East, and Asia. The dimensions and meanings of this classification vary, however, and require further investigation. Spanish priests brought the concept of "hot" and "cold" to Mexico, where it was combined with ancient Aztec beliefs. Consequently, some Mexican Americans may consider illness to be an excess of either hot or cold (Spector, 1996). To restore health, imbalances are often corrected by the proper use of foods, medications, or herbs. These substances are also classified as hot or cold. For example, an illness attributed to an excess of coldness will be treated only with hot foods or medications. The classification of foods is not always consistent, but it does conform to a general structure of traditional knowledge. Certain foods, spices, herbs, and medications are perceived to cool or heat the body. These perceptions do not necessarily correspond to the actual temperature; some hot dishes are said to have a cooling quality.

Southeast Asians believe it is important to keep the woman "warm" after the birth because blood, which is considered "hot," has been lost, and the woman is at risk of becoming "cold." Therefore, they avoid cold drinks and foods following birth (Mattson & Lew, 1992). In contrast, many women in India consider pregnancy a "hot" period and eat "cool" foods to counterbalance the hot state (Choudhry, 1997).

The concepts of hot and cold are not as important in Native American or African American beliefs. There are some similarities, however, in all of these groups because of the emphasis on a balance in nature.

Health Practices

Health care practices during pregnancy are influenced by numerous factors, such as the prevalence of traditional home remedies and folk beliefs, the importance of indigenous healers, and the influence of professional health care workers. In an urban setting the age, length of time in the city, marital status, and strength of the family may affect these patterns. Socioeconomic status is also important because modern medical services are more accessible to those who can afford them.

An awareness of alternative health sources is crucial for health professionals because these practices affect health outcomes. For example, many members of the Mexican American community utilize the *partera*, a lay midwife, as a healer who gives advice and treats illnesses during pregnancy as well as being in attendance during labor and birth (Spector, 1996).

Indigenous healers are also important in some cultures. In the Mexican American culture the healer is called a *curandero* or *curandera.* In some Native American tribes the medicine man may fulfill the healing role. Herbalists are often found in Asian cultures; and faith healers, root doctors, and spiritualists are sometimes consulted in the African American culture.

Cultural Factors and Nursing Care

In recent years people from a variety of cultures have immigrated to North America. This influx of people has had a significant impact on the health care system. Numerous differences often exist in beliefs, values, health care practices and expectations, language, world views, and etiquette between these newly arrived people and the majority of health care providers.

Health care providers are often unaware of the cultural characteristics they themselves demonstrate. Without cultural awareness, caregivers tend to project their own cultural responses onto foreign-born clients; clients from different socioeconomic, religious, or educational groups; or clients from different regions of the country. This leads caregivers to assume that clients are demonstrating a specific behavior for the same reason that they themselves would. Moreover, health care providers frequently fail to recognize that medicine has its own culture, which has been dominated historically by traditional, middle-class values and beliefs (American College of Obstetrics and Gynecology [ACOG], 1998).

Ethnocentrism "refers to an individual's belief that his or her own cultural group's beliefs and values are the best or the only acceptable beliefs. It includes an inability to understand the world view or beliefs of another culture" (Eliason, 1993). To a certain extent, most people are guilty of ethnocentrism, at least some of the time. Thus the nurse who values stoicism during labor may be uncomfortable with the more vocal response of a Latin American woman. Another nurse may be disconcerted by the southeast Asian woman who believes that pain is something to be endured rather than alleviated and is very intent on maintaining self-control in labor (Mattson & Lew, 1992).

Health care providers sometimes believe that if members of other cultures do not share Western values, they should adopt them. This is especially difficult for some nurses caring for childbearing families if the nurse is a firm believer in the equality of the sexes and feminism. The nurse may find it difficult to remain silent if a woman from a Middle Eastern culture defers to her husband in decision making. It is important to remember that pressure to defy cultural values and beliefs can be stressful and anxiety provoking for these women.

TABLE 10–4 Providing Effective Prenatal Care to Families of Different Cultures

Nurses who are interacting with expectant families from a different culture or ethnic group can provide more effective, culturally sensitive nursing care by

- Critically examining their own cultural beliefs.
- Identifying personal biases, attitudes, stereotypes, and prejudices.
- Making a conscious commitment to respect the values and beliefs of others.
- Using sensitive, current language when describing their culture.
- Learning the rituals, customs, and practices of the major cultural and ethnic groups with whom they have contact.
- Including cultural assessment and assessment of the family's expectations of the health care system as a routine part of prenatal nursing care.
- Incorporating the family's cultural practices into prenatal care as much as possible.
- Fostering an attitude of respect for and cooperating with alternative healers and caregivers whenever possible.
- Providing for the services of an interpreter if language barriers exist.
- Learning the language (or at least several key phrases) of at least one of the cultural groups with whom they interact.
- Recognizing that ultimately it is the woman's right to make her own health care choices.
- Evaluating whether client's health care beliefs have any potential negative consequences for the client's health.

To address issues of cultural diversity in the provision of health care, emphasis is being placed on developing *cultural competency*, that is, the skills and knowledge necessary to appreciate, understand, and work with individuals from different cultures. It requires self-awareness, awareness and understanding of cultural differences, and the ability to adapt clinical skills and practices as necessary (ACOG, 1998).

Members of minority culture groups are often found living in a certain area of a community. The nurse can begin developing cultural competence by becoming knowledgeable about the cultural practices of local groups. For example, is it considered courteous to avoid eye contact? Should last names be used in conversation as a sign of respect? Is a female health care provider necessary? Do communication and language barriers exist? If so, how can they be addressed?

Cultural assessment is an important aspect of prenatal care. Health care professionals are becoming increasingly aware of the importance of addressing cultural, physiologic, and psychologic needs in the prenatal assessment in order to provide culture-specific health care during pregnancy (Pritham & Sammons, 1993). The nurse should identify the main beliefs, values, and behaviors that relate to pregnancy and childbearing. This includes information about ethnic background, amount of affiliation with the ethnic group, patterns of decision making, religious preferences, language, communication style, and common etiquette practices. The nurse can also explore the woman's (or family's) expectations of the health care system.

In planning care, the nurse considers the extent to which the woman's personal values, beliefs, and customs are in accord with those of the woman's identified cultural group, the nurse providing care, and the health care agency. If discrepancies exist, the nurse then considers whether the woman's system is supportive, neutral, or harmful in relation to possible interventions. If the woman's system is supportive or neutral, it can be incorporated into the plan. For example, individual food practices or methods of pain expression may differ from those of the nurse or agency but would not necessarily interfere with the nursing plan. However, certain cultural practices might pose a threat to the health of the childbearing woman. For example, some Filipino women will not take any medication during pregnancy. The health care provider may consider a certain medication essential to the woman's well-being. In this case, the woman's cultural belief may be detrimental to her own health. The nurse and client must carefully discuss the reasons for her refusal. After discussing and understanding the reasons, the nurse faces three possible outcomes: (a) identifying ways to persuade the woman to accept the proposed medication; (b) accepting the woman's decision to refuse the medication if she is not willing to adapt her belief system; or (c) explaining alternative therapies that might be acceptable to the woman in light of her cultural beliefs. Table 10–4 summarizes the key actions a nurse can take to become more culturally aware.

FOCUS YOUR STUDY

- Virtually all systems of a woman's body are altered in some way during pregnancy. Blood pressure decreases slightly during pregnancy. It reaches its lowest point in the second trimester and gradually increases to near normal levels in the third trimester. The enlarging uterus may exert pressure on the vena cava when the woman lies supine. This is called the vena caval syndrome.
- A physiologic anemia may occur during pregnancy because the total plasma volume increases more than the total number of erythrocytes. This produces a drop in the hematocrit.
- The glomerular filtration rate increases during pregnancy. Glycosuria may be caused by the body's inability to reabsorb all the glucose filtered by the glomeruli.
- Changes in the skin include the development of chloasma; linea nigra; darkened nipples, areolae, and vulva; striae; and spider nevi.
- Insulin needs increase during pregnancy. A woman with a latent deficiency state may respond to the increased stress on the islets of Langerhans by developing gestational diabetes.
- The subjective (presumptive) signs of pregnancy are those symptoms experienced and reported by the woman, such as amenorrhea, nausea and vomiting, fatigue, urinary frequency, breast changes, and quickening.
- The objective (probable) signs of pregnancy can be perceived by the examiner but may be caused by conditions other than pregnancy.
- The diagnostic (positive) signs of pregnancy can be perceived by the examiner and can be caused only by pregnancy.
- During pregnancy the expectant woman may experience ambivalence, acceptance, introversion, emotional lability, and changes in body image.

- Rubin (1984) has identified four developmental tasks for the pregnant woman: (1) ensuring safe passage through pregnancy, labor, and birth; (2) seeking acceptance of this child by others; (3) seeking commitment and acceptance of self as mother to the infant; and (4) learning to give of oneself on behalf of one's child.
- Fathers also face a series of adjustments as they accept their new role.
- Siblings of all ages require assistance in dealing with the birth of a new baby.
- Cultural values, beliefs, and behaviors influence a couple's response to childbearing and the health care system.
- Ethnocentrism is the belief that one's own cultural beliefs, values, and practices are the best ones, indeed the only ones worth considering.
- A cultural assessment should focus on factors that will influence the practices of the childbearing family with regard to their health needs.

REFERENCES

American College of Obstetricians and Gynecologists (ACOG) (1998). Cultural competency in health care. (ACOG Committee Opinion 201). Washington, DC: Author.

Biasella, S. A. (1993). A comprehensive perinatal education program. *AWHONN's Clinical Issues in Perinatal & Women's Health Nursing, 4*(1), 5–19.

Blackburn, S. T., & Loper, D. L. (1992). *Maternal, fetal, and neonatal physiology: A clinical perspective.* Philadelphia: Saunders.

Buster, J. E., & Carson, S. A. (1996). Endocrinology and diagnosis of pregnancy. In S. G. Gabbe, J. R. Niebyl, & J. L. Simpson (Eds.), *Obstetrics: Normal and problem pregnancies* (3rd ed.). New York: Churchill Livingstone.

Camann, W. R., & Ostheimer, G. W. (1990). Physiological adaptations during pregnancy. *International Anesthesiology Clinics, 28*(1), 2–10.

Choudhry, U. K. (1997). Traditional practices of women from India: Pregnancy, childbirth, and newborn care. *Journal of Obstetric, Gynecologic, & Neonatal Nursing, 26*(5), 533–539.

Clark, S. L., Cotton, D. B., Lee, W., Bishop, C., Hill, T., Southwick, J., Pivarnik, J., Spillman, T., DeVore, G. R., Phelan, J., Hankins, G. D. V., Benedetti, T. J., & Tolley, D. (1989). Central hemodynamic assessment of normal term pregnancy. *American Journal of Obstetrics & Gynecology, 161*(6, Pt. 1), 1439–1442.

Conley, L. J. (1990). Childbearing and childrearing practices in Mormonism. *Neonatal Network, 9*(3), 41–48.

Conner, G. K., & Denson, V. (1990). Expectant fathers' response to pregnancy: Review of literature and implications for research in high-risk pregnancy. *Journal of Perinatal & Neonatal Nursing, 4*(2), 33–42.

Cruikshank, D. P., Wigton, T. R., & Hays, P. M. (1996). Maternal physiology in pregnancy. In S. G. Gabbe, J. R. Niebyl, & J. L. Simpson (Eds.), *Obstetrics: Normal & problem pregnancies* (3rd ed.). New York: Churchill Livingstone.

Cunningham, F. G., MacDonald, P. C., Gant, N. F., Leveno, K. J., Gilstrap, L. C., III, Hankins, G. D. V., & Clark, S. L. (1997). *Williams obstetrics* (20th ed.). Stamford, CT: Appleton & Lange.

D'Avanzo, C. E. (1992). Bridging the cultural gap with Southeast Asians. *MCN, American Journal of Maternal Child Nursing, 17*(4), 204–208.

Demystifying ovulation and pregnancy kits for your patients [Special issue]. (1993, April 15). *Contemporary OB/GYN, 38*(S), 67–69.

Diemer, G. A. (1997). Expectant fathers: Influence of perinatal education on stress, coping, and spousal relations. *Research in Nursing & Health, 20*(4), 281–293.

Eliason, M. J. (1993). Ethics and transcultural nursing care. *Nursing Outlook, 41*(5), 225–228.

Gennaro, S., Kamwendo, L. A., Mbweza, E., Kershbaumer, R. (1998). Childbearing in Malawi, Africa. *Journal of Obstetric, Gynecologic, and Neonatal Nursing, 27*(2), 191–196.

Hofmeyr, G. J., Marcos, E. F., & Butchart, A. M. (1990). Pregnant women's perceptions of themselves: A survey. *Birth, 17*(4), 205–206.

Hollingsworth, A. O., Brown, L. P., & Brooten, D. A. (1980). Indochina moves to Main Street. The refugees and childbearing: What to expect. *RN, 43*(11), 45–48.

Hytten, F. E. (1991). Weight gain in pregnancy. In F. E. Hytten & G. Chamberlain (Eds.), *Clinical physiology in obstetrics* (2nd ed.). Oxford, England: Blackwell Scientific Publications.

Institute of Medicine (1990). *Nutrition during pregnancy: I. Weight gain.* Washington, DC: National Academy Press.

Jordan, P. L. (1990). Laboring for relevance: Expectant and new fatherhood. *Nursing Research, 39*(1), 11–16.

Khanobdee, C., Sukratanachaiyakul, V., & Gay, J. T. (1993). Couvade syndrome in expectant Thai fathers. *International Journal of Nursing Studies, 30*(2), 125–131.

Kimura, M., Amino, N., Tamaki, H., Mitsuda, N., Miyai, K., & Tanizawa, O. (1990). Physiologic thyroid activation in normal early pregnancy is induced by circulating hCG. *Obstetrics & Gynecology, 75*(5), 775–778.

Lederman, R. P. (1996). *Psychosocial adaptation in pregnancy* (2nd ed.). New York: Springer.

Lee, R. V., D'Alauro, F., White, L. M., & Cardinal, J. (1988). Southeast Asian folklore about pregnancy and parturition. *Obstetrics & Gynecology, 71*(4), 643–646.

Longobucco, D. C., & Freston, M. S. (1989). Relation of somatic symptoms to degree of paternal-role preparation of first-time expectant fathers. *Journal of Obstetric, Gynecologic, and Neonatal Nursing, 18*(6), 482–488.

Mattson, S. (1995). Culturally sensitive perinatal care for Southeast Asians. *Journal of Obstetric, Gynecologic, and Neonatal Nursing, 24*(4), 335–341.

Mattson, S., & Lew, L. (1992). Culturally sensitive prenatal care for Southeast Asians. *Journal of Obstetric, Gynecologic, and Neonatal Nursing, 21*(1), 48–54.

Mercer, R. T. (1995). *Becoming a mother.* New York: Springer.

Moos, M. K., Petersen, R., Meadows, K., Melvin, C. L., & Spitz, A. M. (1997). Pregnant women's perspectives on intendedness of pregnancy. *Women's Health Issues, 7*(6), 385–392.

Oakley, A., Rajan, L., & Gant, A. (1990). Social support and pregnancy outcome. *British Journal of Obstetrics & Gynaecology, 97*(2), 155–162.

Orr, S. T., & Miller, C. A. (1997). Unintended pregnancy and the psychosocial well-being of pregnant women. *Women's Health Issues, 7*(1), 38–46.

Patterson, E. T., Freese, M. P., & Goldenberg, R. L. (1990). Seeking safe passage: Utilizing health care during pregnancy. *Image, 22*(1), 27–31.

Pritham, U. A., & Sammons, L. N. (1993). Korean women's attitudes toward pregnancy and prenatal care. *Health Care for Women International, 14*(2), 145–153.

Robinson, G. E., & Stewart, D. E. (1990). Motivation for motherhood and the experience of pregnancy. *Canadian Journal of Psychiatry–Revue Canadienne de Psychiatrie, 34*(9), 861–865.

Rubin, R. (1975). Maternal tasks in pregnancy. *Maternal-Child Nursing Journal, 4*(3), 143–153.

Rubin, R. (1984). *Maternal identity and the maternal experience.* New York: Springer.

Scott, J. R., DiSaia, P. J., Hammond, C. B., & Spellacy, W. N. (1994). *Danforth's obstetrics and gynecology* (7th ed.). Philadelphia: Lippincott.

Spector, R. E. (1996). *Cultural diversity in health and illness.* (2nd ed.). Norwalk, CT: Appleton & Lange.

Spero, D. (1993). Sibling preparation classes. *AWHONN's Clinical Issues in Perinatal & Women's Health Nursing, 4*(1), 122–131.

Stark, M. A. (1997). Psychosocial adjustment during pregnancy: The experience of mature gravidas. *Journal of Obstetric, Gynecologic, and Neonatal Nursing, 26*(2), 206–211.

St. Clair, P. A., & Anderson, N. A. (1989, September). Social network advice during pregnancy: Myths, misinformation, and sound counsel. *Birth, 16*(3), 103–108.

Stern, P. N., Tilden, V. P., & Maxwell, E. K. (1985). Culturally induced stress during childbearing: The Filipino-American experience. *Health Care for Women International, 6*(1–3), 105–121.

Tomilson, B., White, M. A., & Wilson, M. E. (1990). Family dynamics during pregnancy. *Journal of Advanced Nursing, 15* (6), 683–688.

Antepartal Nursing Assessment

11

OUR DAUGHTER, ONE OF THE AUTHORS OF THIS book, invited me to write a few paragraphs. What would I write about? How about comparing the father's role at childbirth when she was born to the role of today's father? The father of the 1940s. . . . Main objective: Get your wife to the hospital on time. No delays. Don't wait too long. You're not schooled in delivering babies. Next, check her in and find the father's waiting lounge. You won't be needed until the baby is born. Fathers are really useless at this time. Try not to be nervous. Smoking is in fashion so you're well equipped with a fresh pack. Coffee is available. Lots and lots of coffee. This hospital is very considerate. The delivery may take a long time. It's always at night.

It seems babies are never born in the daytime. You're tired. Maybe you can pace. It's hard to pace in a room 10 feet square. Delivery may take anywhere from 20 minutes to 20 hours. Hope it's not 20 hours.

More coffee, more cigarettes, no sleep. What a drain on the father. . . . The baby finally comes. Two hours later the doctor remembers the father is waiting. "It's a beautiful, healthy baby girl. Mother and baby are doing fine. You can see them now, but only for 5 minutes." What a relief. The pressure is finally off. Isn't nature wonderful? . . . Today's father, my son. Schooled in Lamaze. Drives his wife to the hospital. Coaches her through her labor. Helps her find a comfortable position to birth their baby. His camera is ready. The baby is born. He cuts the cord. What a relief. The pressure is finally off. Isn't nature wonderful?

Objectives

- Summarize the essential components of a prenatal history.
- Define common obstetric terminology found in the history of maternity clients.
- Identify factors related to the father's health that should be recorded on the prenatal record.
- Describe the normal physiologic changes one would expect to find when performing a physical assessment on a pregnant woman.
- Explain the use of Nägele's rule to determine the estimated date of birth.
- Develop an outline of the essential measurements that can be determined by clinical pelvimetry.
- Describe areas that should be evaluated as part of the initial assessment of psychosocial factors related to a woman's pregnancy.
- Relate the danger signs of pregnancy to their possible causes.

Key Terms

Abortion
Antepartum
Diagonal conjugate
Estimated date of birth (EDB)
Gestation
Gravida
Intrapartum
Multigravida
Multipara
Nägele's rule
Nulligravida
Nullipara
Obstetric conjugate
Para
Postpartum
Postterm labor
Prenatal
Preterm or premature labor
Primigravida
Primipara
Risk factors
Stillbirth
Term

TODAY NURSES ARE ASSUMING A MORE important role in prenatal care, particularly in the area of assessment. The certified nurse-midwife has the education and skill to perform in-depth prenatal assessments. The nurse practitioner may share the assessment responsibilities with a physician. An office nurse, whose primary role may be to counsel and meet the psychologic needs of the expectant family, performs assessments in those areas.

The nurse should establish an environment of comfort and open communication with each prenatal visit, conveying concern for the woman as an individual and being available to listen and discuss the woman's concerns and desires. A supportive atmosphere coupled with the information found in the prenatal assessment guides in this chapter will enable the nurse to identify needed areas of education and counseling.

Initial Client History

The course of a pregnancy depends on a number of factors, including the prepregnancy health of the woman, presence of disease states, emotional status, and past health care. Ideally, health care before the advent of pregnancy has been adequate, and antenatal care will be a continuation of that established care. One important method of determining the adequacy of a woman's prepregnancy care is a thorough history.

Definition of Terms

The following terms are used in recording the obstetric history of maternity clients:

- **Antepartum:** Time between conception and onset of labor, usually used to describe the period during which a woman is pregnant; used interchangeably with **prenatal.**
- **Intrapartum:** Time from onset of labor until the birth of the infant and placenta.
- **Postpartum:** Time from birth until the woman's body returns to an essentially prepregnant condition.
- **Gestation:** The number of weeks since the first day of the last menstrual period (LMP).
- **Abortion:** Birth that occurs before the end of 20 weeks' gestation.
- **Term:** The normal duration of pregnancy (38 to 42 weeks' gestation).
- **Preterm** or **premature labor:** Labor that occurs after 20 weeks but before the completion of 37 weeks of gestation.
- **Postterm labor:** Labor that occurs after 42 weeks of gestation.
- **Gravida:** Any pregnancy, regardless of duration, including present pregnancy.
- **Nulligravida:** A woman who has never been pregnant.
- **Primigravida:** A woman who is pregnant for the first time.
- **Multigravida:** A woman who is in her second or any subsequent pregnancy.
- **Para:** Birth after 20 weeks' gestation, regardless of whether the infant is born alive or dead.
- **Nullipara:** A woman who has not given birth at more than 20 weeks' gestation.
- **Primipara:** A woman who has had one birth at more than 20 weeks' gestation, regardless of whether the infant is born alive or dead.
- **Multipara:** A woman who has had two or more births at more than 20 weeks' gestation.
- **Stillbirth:** A fetus born dead after 20 weeks' gestation.

The terms *gravida* and *para* refer to pregnancies, not to the fetus. Thus twins, triplets, and other multiple fetuses count as one pregnancy and one birth.

The following examples illustrate how these terms are applied in clinical situations:

1. Jean Sanchez has one child born at 38 weeks and is pregnant for the second time. At Jean's initial prenatal visit, the nurse indicates her obstetric history as "gravida 2 para 1 ab 0." Jean Sanchez's present pregnancy terminates at 16 weeks' gestation. She is now "gravida 2 para 1 ab 1."
2. Liz Buehl is pregnant for the fourth time. She has a child born at 35 weeks at home. She lost one pregnancy at 10 weeks' gestation and gave birth to another infant stillborn at term. At her prenatal assessment the nurse records Liz Buehl's obstetric history as "gravida 4 para 2 ab 1."

To provide more comprehensive data, a more detailed approach is used in some settings. Using the detailed system, *gravida* keeps the same meaning, but that of *para* is altered somewhat to focus on the number of infants born rather than the number of deliveries. A useful acronym for remembering the system is TPAL.

T: number of *term* infants born; that is, the number of infants born at the completion of 37 weeks' gestation or beyond.

P: number of *preterm* infants born, that is, the number of infants born after 20 weeks' but before the completion of 37 weeks' gestation.

A: number of pregnancies ending in either spontaneous or therapeutic *abortion.*

L: number of currently *living* children to whom the woman has given birth.

Using this approach, the nurse would have initially classified Jean Sanchez (described in the first example) as "gravida 2 para 1001." Following her spontaneous abortion, she would be "gravida 2 para 1011." Liz Buehl would be described as "gravida 4 para 1111" (Figure 11–1).

Client Profile

The history is essentially a screening tool that identifies the factors that may detrimentally affect the course of a pregnancy. For optimal prenatal care, the nurse should obtain the following information for each maternity client at the first prenatal assessment:

1. Current pregnancy
   - First day of last normal menstrual period (LMP)
   - Presence of cramping, bleeding, or spotting since LMP
   - Woman's opinion about when conception occurred and when infant is due
   - Woman's attitude toward pregnancy (Is pregnancy planned? Wanted?)
   - Results of pregnancy test, if completed
   - Any discomforts since LMP, such as nausea, vomiting, urinary frequency, fatigue, breast tenderness
2. Past pregnancies
   - Number of pregnancies
   - Number of abortions, spontaneous or induced
   - Number of living children
   - History of previous pregnancies: length of pregnancy, length of labor and birth, type of birth (vaginal, forceps or vacuum extraction, cesarean), type of anesthesia used, if any, woman's perception of the experience, complications (antepartal, intrapartal, postpartal)
   - Neonatal status of previous children: Apgar scores, birth weights, general development, complications, feeding patterns (breast/bottle)
   - Loss of a child (miscarriage, elective or medically indicated abortion, stillbirth, neonatal death, relinquishment, death after the neonatal period). What was the experience like for her? What coping skills helped? How did her partner, if involved, respond?
   - Blood type and Rh factor (If negative, ask about medication prescribed after birth to prevent sensitization.)
   - Prenatal education classes, resources (books)
3. Gynecologic history
   - Previous infections: vaginal, cervical, tubal, sexually transmitted
   - Previous surgery
   - Age of menarche

Name	Gravida	**T**erm	**P**reterm	**A**bort	**L**iving Child
Jean Sanchez	2	1	0	0	1
Liz Buehl	4	1	1	1	1

FIGURE 11–1 The TPAL approach provides more detailed information about the woman's pregnancy history.

   - Regularity, frequency, and duration of menstrual flow
   - History of dysmenorrhea
   - Sexual history
   - Contraceptive history (If birth control pills were used, did pregnancy immediately follow cessation of pills? If not, how long after?)
   - Date of last Pap smear, any history of abnormal Pap smear
4. Current medical history
   - Weight
   - Blood type and Rh factor, if known
   - General health, including nutrition, regular exercise program (type, frequency, duration)
   - Any medications being taken currently (including nonprescription medications) or since the onset of pregnancy
   - Previous or present use of alcohol, tobacco, or caffeine (Ask specifically about the amounts of alcohol, cigarettes, and caffeine [specify coffee, tea, colas, chocolate] consumed each day.)
   - Illicit drug use or abuse (Ask about specific drugs such as cocaine, crack, marijuana.)
   - Drug and other allergies
   - Potential teratogenic insults to this pregnancy, such as viral infections, medications, x-ray examinations, surgery, cats in home (possible source of toxoplasmosis)
   - Presence of disease conditions, such as diabetes, hypertension, cardiovascular disease, renal problems
   - Record of immunizations (especially rubella)
   - Presence of any abnormal symptoms
5. Past medical history
   - Childhood diseases
   - Past treatment for any disease condition: Any hospitalizations? History of hepatitis? Rheumatic fever? Pyelonephritis?
   - Surgical procedures
   - Presence of bleeding disorders or tendencies (Has she received blood transfusions?)

CRITICAL THINKING IN PRACTICE

Karen Blade, a 23-year-old, G1P0, is 10 weeks pregnant when she sees the certified nurse-midwife (CNM) for her first prenatal exam. She has been experiencing some mild nausea and fatigue but otherwise is feeling well. She asks the CNM about continuing with her routine exercises (walking 3 miles a day and lifting light weights). She also asks about using the heated pool and a hot tub. What should she be told?

Answers can be found in Appendix I.

6. Family medical history
   - Presence of diabetes, cardiovascular disease, hypertension, hematologic disorders, tuberculosis, preeclampsia-eclampsia (pregnancy-induced hypertension [PIH])
   - Occurrence of multiple births
   - History of congenital diseases or deformities
   - History of mental illness
   - Occurrence of cesarean births
   - Cause of death of deceased parents or siblings
7. Religious/cultural history
   - Does the woman wish to specify a religious preference on her chart? Does she have any religious beliefs or practices that might influence her health care or that of her child, such as prohibition against receiving blood products, dietary considerations, circumcision rites, or other practices?
   - Are there practices in her culture or that of her partner that might influence her care or that of her child?
8. Occupational history
   - Occupation
   - Physical activities (Does she stand all day, or are there opportunities to sit and elevate her legs? Does she do any heavy lifting?)
   - Exposure to chemicals or other harmful substances
   - Opportunity for regular lunch and breaks for nutritious snacks
   - Provision for maternity leave
9. Partner's history
   - Presence of genetic conditions or diseases
   - Age
   - Significant health problems
   - Previous or present alcohol intake, drug use, tobacco use
   - Blood type and Rh factor
   - Occupation
   - Educational level
   - Attitude toward the pregnancy
10. Personal information
    - Age
    - Educational level
    - Race or ethnic group (to identify need for prenatal genetic screening or counseling)
    - Stability of living conditions
    - Economic level
    - Housing
    - Any history of emotional or physical deprivation or abuse of herself or children (Does she experience any abuse in her current relationship? Ask specifically whether she has been hit, slapped, kicked, or hurt within the past year or since she has been pregnant. Ask whether she is afraid of her partner or anyone else. If yes, who?)
    - History of emotional problems
    - Support systems
    - Overuse or underuse of health care system
    - Acceptance of pregnancy
    - Personal preferences about the birth (expectations of both the woman and her partner, presence of others, and so on)
    - Plans for care of child following birth

Obtaining Data

In many instances, nurses use a questionnaire like the one shown in Figure 11–2 to obtain information. The woman should complete the questionnaire in a quiet place with a minimum of distractions.

The nurse can obtain further information in a direct interview, which allows the pregnant woman to expand or clarify her responses to questions and gives the nurse and client the opportunity to begin developing a good relationship. The expectant father should be encouraged to attend the initial and subsequent prenatal assessments. He is often able to contribute information to the history and may use the opportunity to ask questions and express concerns that may be of particular importance to him.

I didn't know what to expect when I went for my first prenatal visit. I'm clean now and wanted to be honest, but I was afraid they would yell if I told them about some of the really dumb things I did in high school—the drinking and marijuana and sex and stuff. I really liked the nurse-midwife who was taking care of me, so I decided to be straight with her—for the baby's sake, you know. She was great about everything and really made me feel okay.

Name ____ Age __________

Address ____ Home Phone __________

What was the last year of schooling completed? __________

How old were you when your menstrual periods started? __________

How many days does a normal period last? __________

How many days are there between periods? __________

Do you have cramping with your periods? yes ___ no ___

Is the pain: minimal ______

moderate ______

severe ______

What was the date of your last normal menstrual period? ______

Have you had bleeding or spotting

since your last menstrual period? yes ___ no ___

Have you been on birth control pills? yes ___ no ___

If yes, when did you stop taking them? __________

How many previous pregnancies have you had? __________

How many living children do you have? __________

Have you had any abortions or stillbirths? yes ___ no ___

If yes, how many? __________

Were any of your previous babies born prematurely?

yes ___ no ___

List the birth weight of all previous children.

1. __________ 3. __________

2. __________ 4. __________

Did any of your children have problems immediately after birth?

yes ___ no ___

If yes, check the problems that occurred:

___ Respiratory ___ Feeding

___ Jaundice ___ Heart

___ Bleeding

Did you have any problems with:

previous pregnancies? yes ___ no ___

If yes, what was the problem? __________

previous labors? yes ___ no ___

If yes, what was the problem? __________

previous postpartal periods: yes ___ no ___

if yes, what was the problem? __________

Are you Rh negative: yes ___ no ___

Did you receive RhoGAM after each pregnancy? yes ___ no ___

What is your present weight? __________

Are you presently taking any prescription or nonprescription drugs?

yes ___ no ___

If yes, please list the medications:

1. __________ 3. __________

2. __________ 4. __________

Do you smoke? yes ___ no ___

If yes, how many cigarettes per day? __________

How much alcohol do you consume each day? __________

each week? __________

How much caffeine do you consume each day? __________

If you have had any of the following diseases, place a check beside it.

___ Chickenpox ___ High blood pressure

___ Mumps ___ Heart disease

___ Measles (3 day) ___ Respiratory disease

___ Measles (2 week) ___ Kidney disease

___ Asthma ___ Frequent bladder infections

___ Hepatitis

If any of the following diseases is present in your family, place a check beside the item.

___ Diabetes ___ Preeclampsia-eclampsia

___ Cardiovascular disease ___ Multiple pregnancies

___ High blood pressure ___ Congenital disorder

___ Breast cancer

The following questions pertain to the father of this child.

What is the father's age? __________

Does he take prescription or nonprescription drugs?

yes ___ no ___

If yes, please list the medications:

1. __________ 3. __________

2. __________ 4. __________

What is his alcohol intake each day? __________

each week? __________

FIGURE 11–2 Sample prenatal questionnaire.

Prenatal High-Risk Screening

A highly significant part of the prenatal assessment is the screening for high-risk factors. **Risk factors** are any findings that have been shown to have a negative effect on pregnancy outcome, either for the woman or her unborn child. Many risk factors can be identified during the initial prenatal assessment; others may be detected during subsequent prenatal visits. It is important that high-risk pregnancies be identified early so that appropriate interventions can be instituted immediately.

All risk factors do not threaten the pregnancy to the same degree. Thus many agencies use a risk-scoring sheet to determine the degree of risk. The sheet is initiated at

TABLE 11–1 System for Determining Risk of Spontaneous Preterm Birth

Points Assigned	Socioeconomic Factors	Previous Medical History	Daily Habits	Aspects of Current Pregnancy
1	Two children at home Low socioeconomic status	Abortion × 1 Less than 1 year since last birth	Works outside home	Unusual fatigue
2	Maternal age 18–20 years or > 40 years Single parent	Abortion × 2	Smokes more than 10 cigarettes per day	Gain of less than 5 kg by 32 weeks
3	Very low socioeconomic status Height < 150 cm Weight < 45 kg	Abortion × 3	Heavy or stressful work Long, tiring trip	Breech at 32 weeks Weight loss of 2 kg Head engaged at 32 weeks Febrile illness
4	Maternal age < 18 years	Pyelonephritis		Bleeding after 12 weeks Effacement Dilatation Uterine irritability
5		Uterine anomaly Second trimester abortion DES exposure Cone biopsy		Placenta previa Hydramnios
10		Preterm birth Repeated second trimester abortion		Twins Abdominal surgery

NOTE: The score is computed by adding the number of points given any item. The score is computed at the first visit and again at 22 to 26 weeks' gestation. A total score of 10 or more places the woman at high risk of spontaneous preterm birth.

SOURCE: Adapted from Creasy RK, Gummer BA, and Liggins GC: A system for predicting spontaneous preterm birth. *Obstet Gynecol* 1980; 55:692.

the first visit and becomes a permanent part of the woman's record. Information may be updated throughout the pregnancy as necessary. It is always possible that a pregnancy may begin as low risk and change to high risk because of complications. Risk is also assessed intrapartally and postpartally.

Table 11–1 is an example of one risk-scoring protocol that evaluates the woman for factors that increase her risk of spontaneous preterm birth. Table 11–2 identifies the major risk factors currently recognized. The table describes maternal and fetal/neonatal implications should the risk be present in the pregnancy. In addition to the factors listed, the perinatal health team also needs to evaluate such psychosocial factors as ethnic background; occupation and education; financial status; environment, including living arrangements and location; and the woman's and her family's or significant other's concept of health, which might influence her attitude toward seeking health care.

Initial Antepartal Assessment

CRITICAL THINKING QUESTION

What approaches might the nurse use to assess the woman's psychosocial status effectively at the initial visit? What behavioral cues in the woman might be helpful?

The antepartal assessment focuses on the woman holistically by considering physical, cultural, and psychosocial factors that influence her health. At the initial visit the woman may be concerned with the diagnosis of pregnancy. However, during this visit she and her primary support person are also evaluating the health team that she has chosen. The establishment of the nurse-client relationship will help the woman evaluate the health team and also provide the nurse with a basis for developing an atmosphere that is conducive to interviewing, support, and education. Because many women are excited and anxious at the first antepartal visit, the initial psychosocial-cultural assessment is general.

As part of the initial psychosocial-cultural assessment the nurse discusses with the woman any religious, cultural, or socioeconomic factors that influence the woman's expectations of the childbearing experience. It is especially helpful if the nurse is familiar with common practices of various religious and cultural groups who reside in the community. If the nurse gathers this data in a tactful, caring way, it can help make the childbearing woman's experience a positive one.

After the history is obtained, the woman is prepared for the physical examination. The physical examination begins with assessment of vital signs; then the woman's body is examined. The pelvic examination is performed last.

Before the examination, the woman should provide a clean urine specimen. When the bladder is empty, the woman is more comfortable during the pelvic examination, and the examiner can palpate the pelvic organs more

TABLE 11–2 Prenatal High-Risk Factors

Factor	Maternal Implications	Fetal/Neonatal Implications
Social-Personal		
Low income level and/or low educational level	Poor antenatal care Poor nutrition ↑ risk of preeclampsia	Low birth weight Intrauterine growth retardation (IUGR)
Poor diet	Inadequate nutrition ↑ risk anemia ↑ risk preeclampsia	Fetal malnutrition Prematurity
Living at high altitude	↑ hemoglobin	Prematurity IUGR
Multiparity > 3	↑ risk antepartum/postpartum hemorrhage	Anemia Fetal death
Weight < 45.5 kg (100 lb)	Poor nutrition Cephalopelvic disproportion Prolonged labor	IUGR Hypoxia associated with difficult labor and birth
Weight > 91 kg (200 lb)	↑ risk hypertension ↑ risk cephalopelvic disproportion	↓ fetal nutrition
Age < 16	Poor nutrition Poor antenatal care ↑ risk preeclampsia ↑ risk cephalopelvic disproportion	Low birth weight ↑ fetal demise
Age > 35	↑ risk preeclampsia ↑ risk cesarean birth	↑ risk congenital anomalies ↑ chromosomal aberrations
Smoking one pack/day or more	↑ risk hypertension ↑ risk cancer	↓ placental perfusion → ↓ O_2 and nutrients available Low birth weight IUGR Preterm birth
Use of addicting drugs	↑ risk poor nutrition ↑ risk of infection with IV drugs	↑ risk congenital anomalies ↑ risk low birth weight Neonatal withdrawal Lower serum bilirubin
Excessive alcohol consumption	↑ risk poor nutrition Possible hepatic effects with long-term consumption	↑ risk fetal alcohol syndrome
Preexisting Medical Disorders		
Diabetes mellitus	↑ risk preeclampsia, hypertension Episodes of hypoglycemia and hyperglycemia ↑ risk cesarean birth	Low birth weight Macrosomia Neonatal hypoglycemia ↑ risk congenital anomalies ↑ risk respiratory distress syndrome
Cardiac disease	Cardiac decompensation Further strain on mother's body ↑ maternal death rate	↑ risk fetal demise ↑ perinatal mortality
Anemia: hemoglobin < 9 g/dL (white) < 29% hematocrit (white) < 8.2 g/dL hemoglobin (black) < 26% hematocrit (black)	Iron deficiency anemia Low energy level Decreased oxygen-carrying capacity	Fetal death Prematurity Low birth weight
Hypertension	↑ vasospasm ↑ risk CNS irritability → convulsions ↑ risk CVA ↑ risk renal damage	↓ placental perfusion → low birth weight Preterm birth
Thyroid disorder Hypothyroidism	↑ infertility ↓ BMR, goiter, myxedema	↑ spontaneous abortion ↑ risk congenital goiter Mental retardation → cretinism
Hyperthyroidism	↑ risk postpartum hemorrhage ↑ risk preeclampsia Danger of thyroid storm	↑ incidence congenital anomalies ↑ incidence preterm birth ↑ tendency to thyrotoxicosis
Renal disease (moderate to severe)	↑ risk renal failure	↑ risk IUGR ↑ risk preterm birth
DES exposure	↑ infertility, spontaneous abortion ↑ cervical incompetence	↑ spontaneous abortion ↑ risk preterm birth

➤

TABLE 11–2 Prenatal High-Risk Factors *continued*

Factor	Maternal Implications	Fetal/Neonatal Implications
Obstetric Considerations		
Previous Pregnancy		
Stillborn	↑ emotional/psychologic distress	↑ risk IUGR ↑ risk preterm birth
Habitual abortion	↑ emotional/psychologic distress ↑ possibility diagnostic workup	↑ risk abortion
Cesarean birth	↑ possibility repeat cesarean birth	↑ risk preterm birth ↑ risk respiratory distress
Rh or blood group sensitization	↑ financial expenditure for testing	Hydrops fetalis Icterus gravis Neonatal anemia Kernicterus Hypoglycemia
Large baby	↑ risk cesarean birth ↑ risk gestational diabetes	Birth injury Hypoglycemia
Current Pregnancy		
Rubella (first trimester)		Congenital heart disease Cataracts Nerve deafness Bone lesions Prolonged virus shedding
Rubella (second trimester)		Hepatitis Thrombocytopenia
Cytomegalovirus		IUGR Encephalopathy
Herpesvirus type 2	Severe discomfort Concern about possibility of cesarean birth, fetal infection	Neonatal herpesvirus type 2 2° hepatitis with jaundice Neurologic abnormalities
Syphilis	↑ incidence abortion	↑ fetal demise Congenital syphilis
Abruptio placenta and placenta previa	↑ risk hemorrhage Bed rest Extended hospitalization	Fetal/neonatal anemia Intrauterine hemorrhage ↑ fetal demise
Preeclampsia/eclampsia (PIH)	See hypertension	↓ placental perfusion → low birth weight
Multiple gestation	↑ risk postpartum hemorrhage	↑ risk preterm birth ↑ risk fetal demise
Elevated hematocrit > 41% (white) > 38% (black)	Increased viscosity of blood	Fetal death rate 5 times normal rate
Spontaneous premature rupture of membranes	↑ uterine infection	↑ risk preterm birth ↑ fetal demise

easily. After emptying her bladder, the woman is asked to disrobe and is given a gown and sheet or some other protective covering.

Increasing numbers of nurses, such as certified nurse-midwives and other nurses in advanced practice, are prepared to perform physical examinations. The nurse who has not yet fully developed these specific assessment skills assesses the woman's vital signs, explains the procedures to allay apprehension, positions her for examination, and assists the examiner as necessary. Each nurse is responsible for operating at the expected standard for a professional with that individual nurse's skill and knowledge base.

Thoroughness and a systematic procedure are the most important considerations when performing the physical portion of an antepartal examination (see the Initial Prenatal Assessment Guide on page 259). To promote completeness, the Initial Prenatal Assessment Guide is organized into three columns that address the areas to be assessed, the variations or alterations that may be observed, and nursing responses to the data. The nurse should be aware that certain organs and systems are assessed concurrently with other systems during the physical portion of the examination. Essential Precautions in Practice: During Prenatal Examinations provides basic information on appropriate body fluid precautions.

Text continues on page 268.

ASSESSMENT GUIDE: INITIAL PRENATAL ASSESSMENT

Physical Assessment/ Normal Findings	Alterations and Possible Causes*	Nursing Responses to Data†
Vital Signs		
Blood pressure (BP): 90–140/60–90 mm Hg	High BP (essential hypertension; renal disease; pregestational hypertension; apprehension or anxiety associated with pregnancy diagnosis, exam, or other crises; PIH if initial assessment not done until after 20 weeks' gestation)	BP > 140/90 requires immediate consideration; establish woman's BP; refer to physician if necessary. Assess woman's knowledge about high BP; counsel on self-care and medical management.
Pulse: 60–90 beats/min. Rate may increase 10 beats/min during pregnancy	Increased pulse rate (excitement or anxiety, cardiac disorders)	Count for 1 full minute; note irregularities.
Respiration: 16–24 breaths/min (or pulse rate divided by four). Pregnancy may induce a degree of hyperventilation; thoracic breathing predominant	Marked tachypnea or abnormal patterns	Assess for respiratory disease.
Temperature: 36.2–37.6C (98–99.6F)	Elevated temperature (infection)	Assess for infection process or disease state if temperature is elevated; refer to physician/CNM.
Weight		
Depends on body build	Weight < 45 kg (100 lb) or > 91 kg (200 lb); rapid, sudden weight gain (PIH)	Evaluate need for nutritional counseling; obtain information on eating habits, cooking practices, foods regularly eaten, income limitations, need for food supplements, pica and other abnormal food habits. Note initial weight to establish baseline for weight gain throughout pregnancy.
Skin		
Color: Consistent with racial background; pink nail beds	Pallor (anemia); bronze, yellow (hepatic disease, other causes of jaundice)	The following tests should be performed: complete blood count (CBC), bilirubin level, urinalysis, and blood urea nitrogen (BUN).
	Bluish, reddish, mottled; dusky appearance or pallor of palms and nail beds in dark-skinned women (anemia)	If abnormal, refer to physician.
Condition: Absence of edema (slight edema of lower extremities is normal during pregnancy)	Edema (PIH); rashes, dermatitis (allergic response)	Counsel on relief measures for slight edema. Initiate PIH assessment; refer to physician.
Lesions: Absence of lesions	Ulceration (varicose veins, decreased circulation)	Further assess circulatory status; refer to physician if lesion severe.
Spider nevi common in pregnancy	Petechiae, multiple bruises, ecchymosis (hemorrhagic disorders; abuse)	Evaluate for bleeding or clotting disorder. Provide oportunities to discuss abuse if suspected.

*Possible causes of alterations are placed in parentheses.

†This column provides guidelines for further assessment and initial nursing intervention.

Physical Assessment/ Normal Findings	Alterations and Possible Causes*	Nursing Responses to Data†
Moles	Change in size or color (carcinoma)	Refer to physician.
Pigmentation: Pigmentation changes of pregnancy include linea nigra, striae gravidarum, chloasma		Assure woman that these are normal manifestations of pregnancy and explain the physiologic basis for the changes.
Café-au-lait spots	Six or more (Albright's syndrome or neurofibromatosis)	Consult with physician.
Nose		
Character of mucosa: Redder than oral mucosa; in pregnancy nasal mucosa is edematous in response to increased estrogen, resulting in nasal stuffiness (rhinitis of pregnancy) and nosebleeds	Olfactory loss (first cranial nerve deficit)	Counsel woman about possible relief measures for nasal stuffiness and nosebleeds (epistaxis); refer to physician for olfactory loss.
Mouth		
May note hypertrophy of gingival tissue because of estrogen	Edema, inflammation (infection); pale in color (anemia)	Assess hematocrit for anemia; counsel regarding dental hygiene habits. Refer to physician or dentist if necessary. Routine dental care appropriate during pregnancy (no x-ray studies, no gas).
Neck		
Nodes: Small, mobile, nontender nodes	Tender, hard, fixed or prominent nodes (infection, carcinoma)	Examine for local infection; refer to physician.
Thyroid: Small, smooth, lateral lobes palpable on either side of trachea; slight hyperplasia by third month of pregnancy	Enlargement or nodule tenderness (hyperthyroidism)	Listen over thyroid for bruits, which may indicate hyperthyroidism. Question woman about dietary habits (iodine intake). Ascertain history of thyroid problems; refer to physician.
Chest and Lungs		
Chest: Symmetric, elliptical, smaller anteroposterior (A-P) than transverse diameter	Increased A-P diameter, funnel chest, pigeon chest (emphysema, asthma, chronic obstructive pulmonary disease [COPD])	Evaluate for emphysema, asthma, pulmonary disease (COPD).
Ribs: Slope downward from nipple line	More horizontal (COPD) Angular bumps Rachitic rosary (vitamin C deficiency)	Evaluate for COPD. Evaluate for fractures. Consult physician. Consult nutritionist.
Inspection and palpation: No retraction or bulging of intercostal spaces (ICS) during inspiration or expiration; symmetrical expansion	ICS retractions with inspiration, bulging with expiration; unequal expansion (respiratory disease)	Do thorough initial assessment. Refer to physician.

*Possible causes of alterations are placed in parentheses.

†This column provides guidelines for further assessment and initial nursing intervention.

Physical Assessment/ Normal Findings	Alterations and Possible Causes*	Nursing Responses to Data†
Tactile fremitus	Tachypnea, hyperpnea, Cheyne-Stokes respirations (respiratory disease)	Refer to physician.
Percussion: Bilateral symmetry in tone	Flatness of percussion, which may be affected by chest wall thickness	Evaluate for pleural effusions, consolidations, or tumor.
Low-pitched resonance of moderate intensity	High diaphragm (atelectasis or paralysis), pleural effusion	Refer to physician.
Auscultation: Upper lobes: bronchovesicular sounds above sternum and scapulas; equal expiratory and inspiratory phases	Abnormal if heard over any other area of chest	Refer to physician.
Remainder of chest: vesicular breath sounds heard; inspiratory phase longer (3:1)	Rales, rhonchi, wheezes; pleural friction rub; absence of breath sounds; bronchophony, egophony, whispered pectoriloquy	Refer to physician.
Breasts		
Supple; symmetric in size and contour; darker pigmentation of nipple and areola; may have supernumerary nipples, usually 5–6 cm below normal nipple line	"Pigskin" or orange-peel appearance, nipple retractions, swelling, hardness (carcinoma); redness, heat, tenderness, cracked or fissured nipple (infection)	Encourage monthly self-breast checks; instruct woman how to examine own breasts.
Axillary nodes unpalpable or pellet sized	Tenderness, enlargement, hard node (carcinoma); may be visible bump (infection)	Refer to physician if evidence of inflammation.
Pregnancy changes: **1.** Size increase noted primarily in first 20 weeks. **2.** Become nodular. **3.** Tingling sensation may be felt during first and third trimester; woman may report feeling of heaviness. **4.** Pigmentation of nipples and areolas darkens. **5.** Superficial veins dilate and become more prominent. **6.** Striae seen in multiparas. **7.** Tubercles of Montgomery enlarge. **8.** Colostrum may be present after 12th week. **9.** Secondary areola appears at 20 weeks, characterized by series of washed-out spots surrounding primary areola. **10.** Breasts less firm, old striae may be present in multiparas.		Discuss normalcy of changes and their meaning with the woman. Teach and/or institute appropriate relief measures. Encourage use of supportive, well-fitting brassiere.

*Possible causes of alterations are placed in parentheses.

†This column provides guidelines for further assessment and initial nursing intervention.

Physical Assessment/ Normal Findings	Alterations and Possible Causes*	Nursing Responses to Data†
Heart		
Normal rate, rhythm, and heart sounds *Pregnancy changes:* **1.** Palpitations may occur due to sympathetic nervous system disturbance. **2.** Short systolic murmurs that ↑ in held expiration are normal due to increased volume.	Enlargement, thrills, thrusts, gross irregularity or skipped beats, gallop rhythm or extra sounds (cardiac disease)	Complete an initial assessment. Explain normalcy of pregnancy-induced changes. Refer to physician if indicated.
Abdomen		
Normal appearance, skin texture, and hair distribution; liver nonpalpable; abdomen nontender *Pregnancy changes:* **1.** Purple striae may be present (or silver striae on a multipara) as well as linea nigra. **2.** Diastasis of the rectus muscles late in pregnancy.	Muscle guarding (anxiety, acute tenderness); tenderness, mass (ectopic pregnancy, inflammation, carcinoma)	Assure client of normalcy of diastasis. Provide initial information about appropriate postpartum exercises. Evaluate client anxiety level. Refer to physician if indicated.
3. Size: Flat or rotund abdomen; progressive enlargement of uterus due to pregnancy. 10–12 weeks: Fundus slightly above symphysis pubis. 16 weeks: Fundus halfway between symphysis and umbilicus. *20–22 weeks:* Fundus at umbilicus. *28 weeks:* Fundus three finger breadths above umbilicus. *36 weeks:* Fundus just below ensiform cartilage.	Size of uterus inconsistent with length of gestation (intrauterine growth retardation [IUGR] multiple pregnancy, fetal demise, hydatidiform mole)	Reassess menstrual history regarding pregnancy dating. Evaluate increase in size using McDonald's method. Use ultrasound to establish diagnosis.
4. Fetal heartbeats: 120–160 beats/min may be heard with Doppler at 10–12 weeks' gestation; may be heard with fetoscope at 17–20 weeks.	Failure to hear fetal heartbeat with Doppler (fetal demise, hydatidiform mole)	Refer to physician. Administer pregnancy tests. Use ultrasound to establish diagnosis.
5. Fetal movement palpable by a trained examiner after the 18th week.	Failure to feel fetal movements after 20 weeks' gestation (fetal demise, hydatidiform mole)	Refer to physician for evaluation of fetal status.
6. Ballottement: During fourth to fifth month fetus rises and then rebounds to original position when uterus is tapped sharply.	No ballottement (oligohydramnios)	Refer to physician for evaluation of fetal status.

*Possible causes of alterations are placed in parentheses.

†This column provides guidelines for further assessment and initial nursing intervention.

Physical Assessment/ Normal Findings	Alterations and Possible Causes*	Nursing Responses to Data†
Extremities		
Skin warm, pulses palpable, full range of motion; may be some edema of hands and ankles in late pregnancy; varicose veins may become more pronounced; palmar erythema may be present	Unpalpable or diminished pulses (arterial insufficiency); marked edema (PIH)	Evaluate for other symptoms of heart disease; initiate follow-up if woman mentions that her rings feel tight. Discuss prevention and self-treatment measures for varicose veins; refer to physician if indicated.
Spine		
Normal spinal curves: Concave cervical, convex thoracic, concave lumbar	Abnormal spinal curves: flatness, kyphosis, lordosis	Refer to physician for assessment of cephalopelvic disproportion (CPD).
In pregnancy lumbar spinal curve may be accentuated	Backache	May have implications for administration of spinal anesthetics; see Chapter 12 for relief measures.
Shoulders and iliac crests should be even	Uneven shoulders and iliac crests (scoliosis)	Refer very young women to a physician; discuss back-stretching exercises with older women.
Reflexes		
Normal and symmetrical	Hyperactivity, clonus (PIH)	Evaluate for other symptoms of PIH.
Pelvic Area		
External female genitals: Normally formed with female hair distribution; in multiparas, labia majora loose and pigmented; urinary and vaginal orifices visible and appropriately located	Lesions, hematomas, varicosities, inflammation of Bartholin's glands; clitoral hypertrophy (masculinization)	Explain pelvic examination procedure (Procedure 3–1). Encourage woman to minimize her discomfort by relaxing her hips. Provide privacy.
Vagina: Pink or dark pink; vaginal discharge odorless, nonirritating; in multiparas, vaginal folds smooth and flattened; may have episiotomy scar	Abnormal discharge associated with vaginal infections	Obtain vaginal smear. Provide understandable verbal and written instructions about treatment for woman and partner, if indicated.
Cervix: Pink color; os closed except in multiparas, in whom os admits fingertip	Eversion, reddish erosion, Nabothian or retention cysts, cervical polyp; granular area that bleeds (carcinoma of cervix); lesions (herpes, human papilloma virus [HPV]) Presence of string or plastic tip from cervix (intrauterine device [IUD] in uterus)	Provide woman with a hand mirror and identify genital structures for her; encourage her to view her cervix if she wishes. Refer to physician if indicated. Advise woman of potential serious risks of leaving an IUD in place during pregnancy; refer to physician for removal.
Pregnancy changes: 1–4 weeks' gestation: Enlargement in anteroposterior diameter	Absence of Goodell's sign (inflammatory conditions, carcinoma)	Refer to physician.

*Possible causes of alterations are placed in parentheses.

†This column provides guidelines for further assessment and initial nursing intervention.

Physical Assessment/ Normal Findings	Alterations and Possible Causes*	Nursing Responses to Data†
4–6 weeks' gestation: Softening of cervix (Goodell's sign), softening of isthmus of uterus (Hegar's sign); cervix takes on bluish coloring (Chadwick's sign) 8–12 weeks' gestation: Vagina and cervix appear bluish-violet in color (Chadwick's sign)		
Uterus: Pear-shaped, mobile; smooth surface	Fixed (pelvic inflammatory disease [PID]); nodular surface (fibromas)	Refer to physician.
Ovaries: Small, walnut-shaped, nontender (ovaries and fallopian tubes are located in the adnexal areas)	Pain on movement of cervix (PID); enlarged or nodular ovaries (cyst, tumor, tubal pregnancy, corpus luteum of pregnancy)	Evaluate adnexal areas; refer to physician.
Pelvic Measurements		
Internal measurements:	Measurement below normal	Vaginal birth may not be possible if deviations are present.
1. Diagonal conjugate at least 11.5 cm (Figure 11–7)		
2. Obstetric conjugate estimated by subtracting 1.5–2 cm from diagonal conjugate	Disproportion of pubic arch	
3. Inclination of sacrum	Abnormal curvature of sacrum	
4. Motility of coccyx; external intertuberosity diameter > 8 cm	Fixed or malposition of coccyx	
Anus and Rectum		
No lumps, rashes, excoriation, tenderness; cervix may be felt through rectal wall	Hemorrhoids, rectal prolapse; nodular lesion (carcinoma)	Counsel about appropriate prevention and relief measures; refer to physician for further evaluation.
Laboratory Evaluation		
Hemoglobin: 12–16 g/dL; women residing in high altitudes may have higher levels of hemoglobin	< 12 g/dL (anemia)	Note: Wear gloves when drawing blood. Hemoglobin < 12 g/dL requires nutritional counseling. < 11 g/dL requires iron supplementation.
ABO and Rh typing: Normal distribution of blood types	Rh negative	If Rh negative, check for presence of anti-Rh antibodies. Check partner's blood type; if partner is Rh positive, discuss with woman the need for antibody titers during pregnancy, management during the intrapartal period, and possible candidacy for RhIgG.

*Possible causes of alterations are placed in parentheses.

†This column provides guidelines for further assessment and initial nursing intervention.

Physical Assessment/ Normal Findings	Alterations and Possible Causes*	Nursing Responses to Data†
Complete blood count (CBC)		
Hematocrit: 38%–47%; physiologic anemia (pseudoanemia) may occur	Marked anemia or blood dyscrasias	Perform CBC and Schilling differential cell count.
Red blood cells (RBC): 4.2–5.4 million/μL		
White blood cells (WBC): 5000–12,000/μL	Presence of infection; may be elevated in pregnancy and with labor	Evaluate for other signs of infection.
Differential		
Neutrophils: 40%–60%		
Bands: up to 5%		
Eosinophils: 1%–3%		
Basophils: up to 1%		
Lymphocytes: 20%–40%		
Monocytes: 4%–8%		
Syphilis tests: serologic test for syphilis (STS), complement fixation test, Venereal Disease Research Laboratory (VDRL) test—nonreactive	Positive reaction STS—tests may have 25%–45% incidence of biologic false-positive results; false results may occur in individuals who have acute viral or bacterial infections, hypersensitivity reactions, recent vaccinations, collagen disease, malaria, or tuberculosis.	Positive results may be confirmed with the fluorescent treponemal antibody absorption (FTA-ABS) tests; all tests for syphilis give positive results in the secondary stage of the disease; antibiotic tests may cause negative test results.
Gonorrhea culture: Negative	Positive	Refer for treatment.
Urinalysis (u/a): Normal color, specific gravity; pH 4.6–8.0	Abnormal color (porphyria, hemoglobinuria, bilirubinemia); alkaline urine (metabolic alkalemia, *Proteus* infection, old specimen)	Repeat u/a; refer to physician.
Negative for protein, red blood cells, white blood cells, casts	Positive findings (contaminated specimen, kidney disease)	Repeat u/a; refer to physician.
Glucose: Negative (small degree of glycosuria may occur in pregnancy)	Glycosuria (low renal threshold for glucose, diabetes mellitus)	Assess blood glucose; test urine for ketones.
Rubella titer: Hemagglutination-inhibition test (HAI) > 1:10 indicates woman is immune	HAI titer < 1:10	Immunization will be given on postpartum or within 6 weeks after childbirth. Instruct woman whose titers are , >1:10 to avoid children who have rubella.
Hepatitis B screen for hepatitis B surface antigen (HBsAg); negative	Positive	If negative, consider referral for hepatitis B vaccine. If positive, refer to physician. Infants born to women who test positive are given hepatitis B immune globulin soon after birth followed by first dose of hepatitis B vaccine.

*Possible causes of alterations are placed in parentheses.

†This column provides guidelines for further assessment and initial nursing intervention.

Physical Assessment/ Normal Findings	Alterations and Possible Causes*	Nursing Responses to Data†
HIV screen: Offered to all women; encouraged for those at risk; negative	Positive	Refer to physician.
Illicit drug screen: Offered to all women; negative	Positive	Refer to physician.
Sickle cell screen for clients of African descent: Negative	Positive; test results would include a description of cells	Refer to physician.
Pap smear: Negative	Test results that show atypical cells	Refer to physician. Discuss the meaning of the findings with the woman and importance of follow-up.

Cultural Assessment	Variations to Consider*	Nursing Responses to Data†
Determine the woman's fluency in English	Woman may be fluent in a language other than English.	Work with a knowledgeable translator to provide information and answer questions.
Ask the woman how she prefers to be addressed.	Some women prefer informality; others prefer to use titles.	Address the woman according to her preference. Maintain formality in introducing oneself if that seems preferred.
Determine customs and practices regarding prenatal care:	Practices are influenced by individual preference, cultural expectations, or religious beliefs.	Honor a woman's practices and provide for specific preferences unless they are contraindicated because of safety.
• Ask the woman if there are certain practices she expects to follow when she is pregnant.	Some women believe that they should perform certain acts related to sleep, activity, or clothing.	Have information printed in the language of different cultural groups that live in the area.
• Ask the woman if there are any activities she cannot do while she is pregnant.	Some women have restrictions or taboos they follow related to work, activity, sexual, environmental, or emotional factors.	
• Ask the woman whether there are certain foods she is expected to eat or avoid while she is pregnant. Determine whether she has lactose intolerance.	Foods are an important cultural factor. Some women may have certain foods they must eat or avoid; many women have lactose intolerance and have difficulty consuming sufficient calcium.	Respect the woman's food preferences, help her plan an adequate prenatal diet within the framework of her preferences, and refer to a dietician if necessary.
• Ask the woman whether the gender of her caregiver is of concern.	Some women are comfortable only with a female caregiver.	Arrange for a female caregiver if it is the woman's preference.
• Ask the woman about the degree of involvement in her pregnancy that she expects or wants from her support person, mother, and other significant people.	If the woman does have a partner, she may not want this person involved in the pregnancy. For some the role falls to the woman's mother or a female relative or friend.	Respect the woman's preferences about her partner/husband's involvement; avoid imposing personal values or expectations.
• Ask the woman about her sources of support/counseling during pregnancy	Some women seek advice from a family member, *curandera,* tribal healer, and so forth.	Respect and honor the woman's sources of support.

*Possible causes of alterations are placed in parentheses.

†This column provides guidelines for further assessment and initial nursing intervention.

Psychosocial Assessment	Variations to Consider*	Nursing Responses to Data†
Psychologic Status		
Excitement and/or apprehension; ambivalence	Marked anxiety (fear of pregnancy diagnosis, fear of medical facility)	Establish lines of communication. Active listening is useful. Establish trusting relationship. Encourage woman to take active part in her care.
	Apathy Display of anger with pregnancy diagnosis	Establish communication and begin counseling. Use active listening techniques.
Educational Needs		
May have questions about pregnancy or may need time to adjust to reality of pregnancy		Establish educational, supporting environment that can be expanded throughout pregnancy.
Support Systems		
Can identify at least two or three individuals with whom woman is emotionally intimate (partner, parent, sibling, friend)	Isolated (no telephone, unlisted number); cannot name a neighbor or friend whom she can call upon in an emergency; does not perceive parents as part of her support system	Institute support system through community groups. Help woman to develop trusting relationship with health care professionals.
Family Functioning		
Emotionally supportive Communications adequate Mutually satisfying Cohesiveness in times of trouble	Long-term problems or specific problems related to this pregnancy, potential stressors within the family, pessimistic attitudes, unilateral decision making, unrealistic expectations of this pregnancy and/or child	Help identify the problems and stressors, encourage communication, discuss role changes and adaptations.
Economic Status		
Source of income is stable and sufficient to meet basic needs of daily living and medical needs	Limited prenatal care Poor physical health Limited use of health care system Unstable economic status	Discuss available resources for health maintenance and the birth. Institute appropriate referral for meeting expanding family's needs—food stamps and so forth.
Stability of Living Conditions		
Adequate, stable housing for expanding family's needs	Crowded living conditions Questionable supportive environment for newborn	Refer to appropriate community agency. Work with family on self-help ways to improve situation.

*Possible causes of alterations are placed in parentheses.

†This column provides guidelines for further assessment and initial nursing intervention.

ESSENTIAL PRECAUTIONS IN PRACTICE

During Prenatal Examinations

Examples of times when gloves should be worn include the following:

- When drawing blood for lab work
- When handling urine specimens
- During pelvic examinations (sterile gloves)

In most instances in a clinic or office setting, gowns and goggles are not necessary because splashing of fluids is unlikely.

REMEMBER to wash your hands prior to putting the disposable gloves on and AGAIN immediately after you remove the gloves.

For further information consult OSHA and CDC guidelines.

Nursing interventions based on assessment of the normal physical and psychosocial changes, as well as the cultural influences associated with pregnancy and client teaching and counseling needs that have been mutually defined, are discussed further in Chapter 12.

Determination of Due Date

Childbearing families generally want to know the "due date," or the date around which childbirth will occur. Historically, the due date has been called the *estimated date of confinement (EDC).* The concept of confinement is, however, rather negative, and there is a trend in the literature to avoid it by referring to the birth date as the *EDD,* or *estimated date of delivery.* However, childbirth educators often stress that babies are not "delivered" like a package; they are born. In keeping with a view that emphasizes the normality of the process, we have chosen to refer to the due date as the **EDB (estimated date of birth)** throughout this text.

To calculate the EDB, it is helpful to know the first day of the woman's last menstrual period (LMP). However, some women have episodes of irregular bleeding or fail to keep track of menstrual cycles. Thus other techniques also help determine how far along a woman is in her pregnancy, that is, at how many weeks' gestation she is. Other techniques that can be used include evaluating uterine size, determining when quickening occurs, using ultrasound to visualize the gestational sac and obtain regular measurements of the embryo/fetus, auscultating fetal heart rate initially with a Doppler device and later a fetoscope (special type of stethoscope designed to auscultate fetal heart rate).

Nägele's Rule

The most common method of determining the EDB is **Nägele's rule.** To use this method, begin with the first

CLINICAL TIP

When assessing blood pressure, have the pregnant woman sit up with her arm resting on a table so that her arm is at the level of her heart.

Expect a decrease in her blood pressure from baseline during the second trimester because of normal physiologic changes. If this decrease doesn't occur, evaluate further for signs of pregnancy-induced hypertension (PIH).

day of the last menstrual period, subtract 3 months, and add 7 days. For example,

First day of LMP	November 21
Subtract 3 months	− 3 months
	August 21
Add 7 days	+ 7 days
EDB	August 28 (of the next year)

It is simpler to change the months to numeric terms:

November 21 becomes	11–21
Subtract 3 months	− 3
	8–21
Add 7 days	+ 7
EDB	August 28 (of the next year)

A gestation calculator or "wheel" permits the caregiver to calculate the EDB even more quickly (Figure 11–3).

If a woman with a history of menses every 28 days remembers her LMP and was not taking oral contraceptives prior to becoming pregnant, Nägele's rule may be a fairly accurate determiner of her predicted birth date. However, if her cycle is irregular or 35 to 40 days in length, the time of ovulation may be delayed by several days. *Ovulation usually occurs 14 days before the onset of the next menses, not 14 days after the previous menses.* Thus Nägele's rule, while helpful, is not foolproof. Nägele's rule is of no use in calculating EDB for (1) women with markedly irregular periods that include one or more months of amenorrhea; (2) women who are amenorrheic but ovulating and conceive while breastfeeding; or (3) women who conceive before regular menstruation is established following discontinuation of oral contraceptives or termination of a pregnancy (Varney, 1997).

Uterine Assessment

Physical Examination

When a woman is examined in the first 10 to 12 weeks of her pregnancy and the nurse practitioner, certified nurse-midwife, or physician thinks that her uterine size is compatible with her menstrual history, uterine size may be the single most important clinical method for dating her pregnancy. In many cases, however, women do not seek obstetric care until well into their second trimester, when

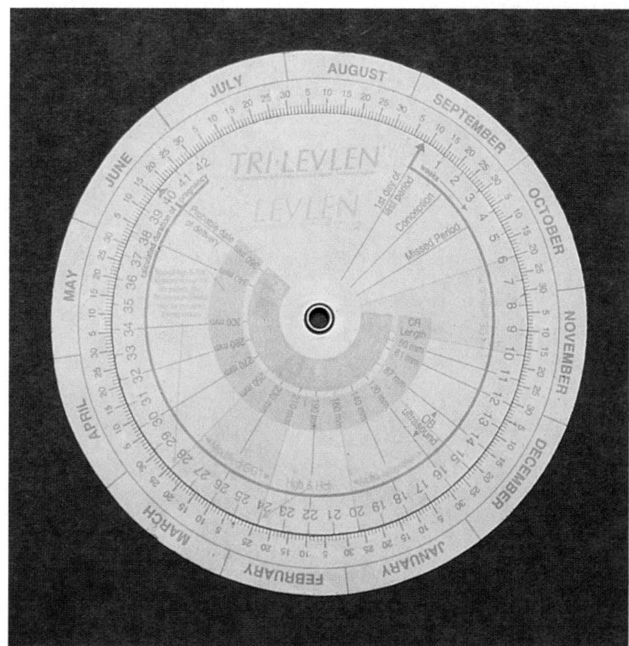

FIGURE 11–3 The EDB wheel can be used to calculate the due date. To use it, place the "last menses began" arrow on the date of the woman's LMP. Then read the EDB at the arrow labeled 40. In this case the LMP is April 30 and the EDB is February 4.

it becomes much more difficult to evaluate specific uterine size. In the case of the obese woman, it is most difficult to determine uterine size early in pregnancy because the uterus is more difficult to palpate.

Fundal Height

Fundal height may be used as an indicator of uterine size, although this cannot be used late in pregnancy. A centimeter tape measure is used to measure the distance from the top of the symphysis pubis over the curve of the abdomen to the top of the uterine fundus (McDonald's method) (Figure 11–4). Fundal height in centimeters correlates well with weeks of gestation between 22 to 24 weeks and 34 weeks. At 26 weeks' gestation, for example, fundal height is probably about 26 cm. To be most accurate, fundal height should be measured by the same examiner each time. The woman should empty her bladder before the examiner takes the measurement (Cunningham et al, 1997). Maternal position (trunk elevation, knee flexion) also influences fundal height measurement (Engstrom et al, 1993). If the woman is very tall or very short, fundal height will differ. In the third trimester, variations in fetal weight decrease the accuracy of fundal height measurements. Unfortunately, this method of dating a pregnancy can be quite inaccurate in the following situations:

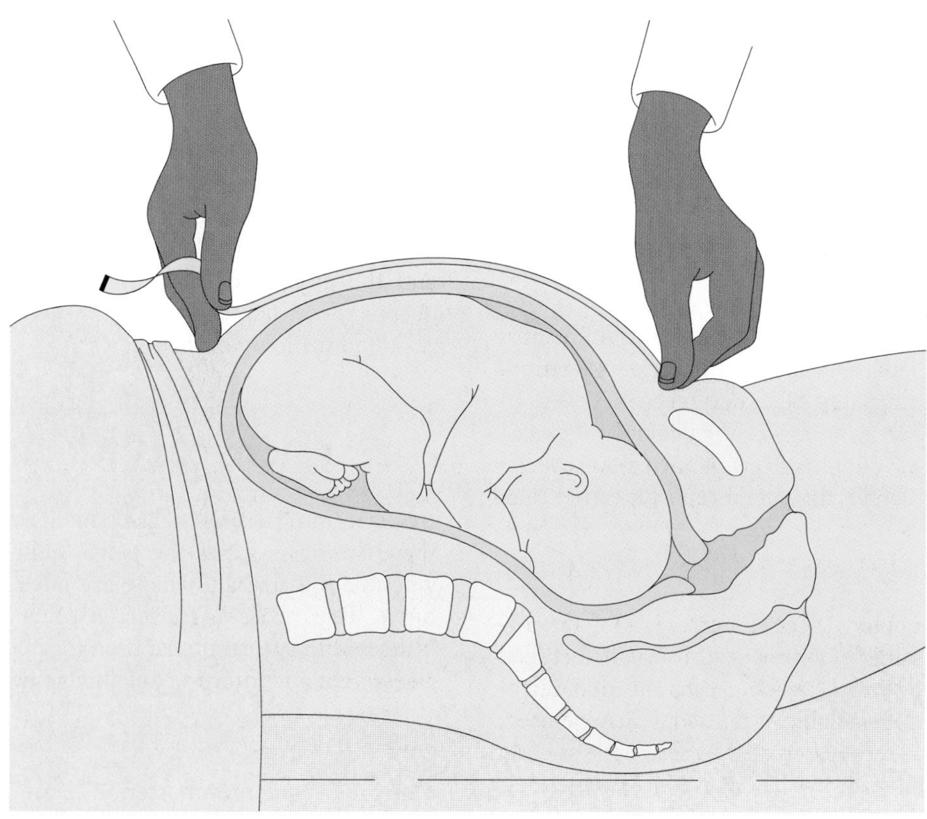

FIGURE 11–4 A cross-sectional view of fetal position when McDonald's method is used to assess fundal height.

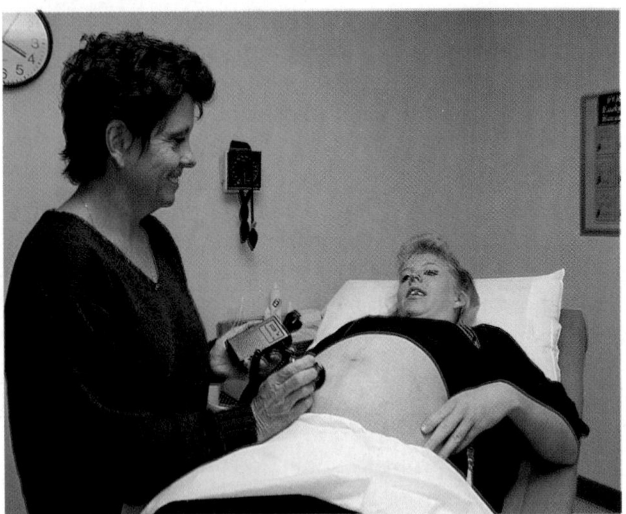

FIGURE 11–5 Listening to the fetal heartbeat with a Doppler device.

- obese women (because of difficulty palpating the fundus accurately)
- women with uterine fibroids (because uterine size may be distorted)
- in women who develop hydramnios (because the excess fluid increases uterine size, leading the examiner to conclude the fetus is larger than it is)

Measurements of fundal height from month to month and week to week may yield other information, as well. For example, a lag in the progression of fundal height may indicate intrauterine growth restriction (IUGR); a sudden increase in height may indicate the presence of twins or hydramnios.

Fetal Development

Quickening

Fetal movements felt by the mother may give some indications that the fetus is nearing 20 weeks' gestation. However, quickening may be experienced between 16 and 22 weeks' gestation, so this is not a completely accurate method. Because multiparous women have experienced quickening before, they often report it earlier than a primigravida does.

Fetal Heartbeat

The ultrasonic Doppler device (Figure 11–5) is the primary tool for assessing fetal heartbeat. It may detect fetal heartbeat at about 10 to 12 weeks' gestation. If an ultrasonic Doppler is not available, a fetoscope may be used. The fetal heartbeat can be detected by fetoscope as early as week 16 and almost always by 19 or 20 weeks of gestation. In the case of twins or the obese woman, it may be later before the fetal heartbeat can be detected.

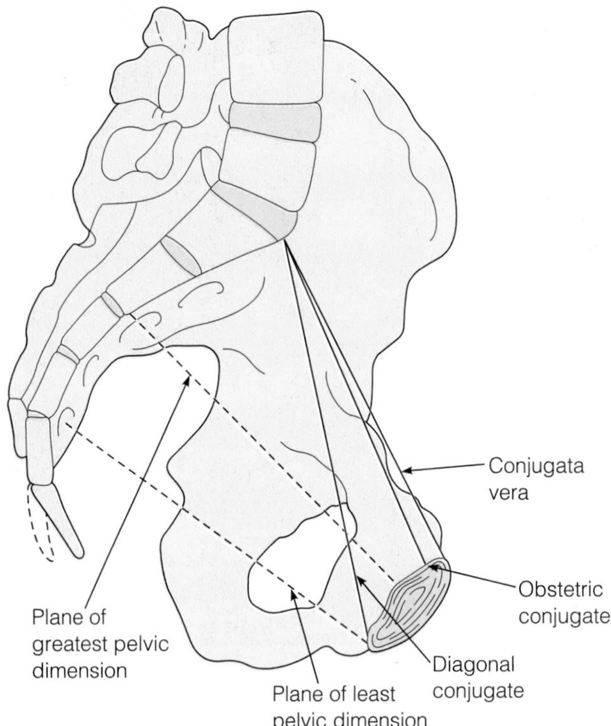

FIGURE 11–6 Anteroposterior diameters of the pelvic inlet and their relationship to the pelvic planes.

Ultrasound

In the first trimester, ultrasound scanning can detect a gestational sac as early as 5 to 6 weeks after the LMP, fetal heart activity by 9 to 10 weeks and occasionally earlier, and fetal breathing movement by 11 weeks of pregnancy. Crown-to-rump measurements can be made for assessment of fetal age until the fetal head can be defined. Biparietal diameter measurements can be made by approximately 12 to 13 weeks and are most accurate between 20 and 30 weeks, when rapid growth in biparietal diameter occurs. (See Chapter 17 for an in-depth discussion of ultrasound scanning of the fetus.)

Assessment of Pelvic Adequacy

By performing a series of assessments and measurements, the examiner assesses the pelvis vaginally to determine whether the size and shape are adequate for a vaginal birth. This process is referred to as *clinical pelvimetry.* Nurses with special preparation may perform the vaginal assessment and interpret pelvimetry findings.

Pelvic Inlet

The important anteroposterior diameters of the inlet for childbearing are the diagonal conjugate, the obstetric conjugate, and the conjugata vera, or true conjugate (Figure 11–6). Other diameters are the transverse (approximately 13.5 cm) and the oblique (averages 12.75 cm).

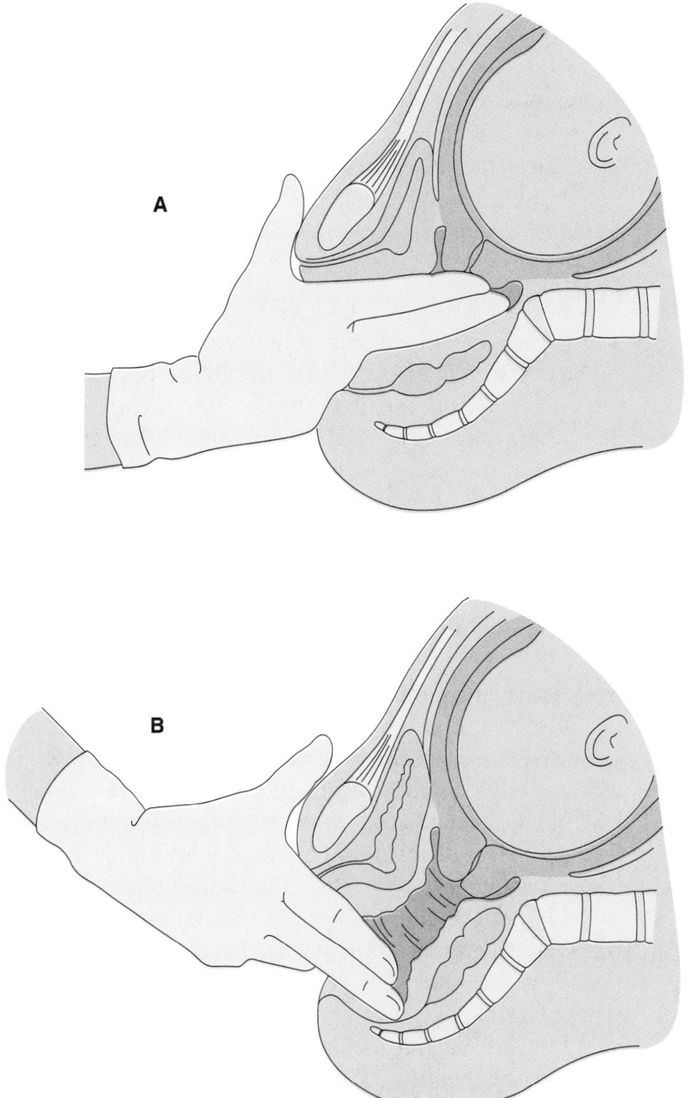

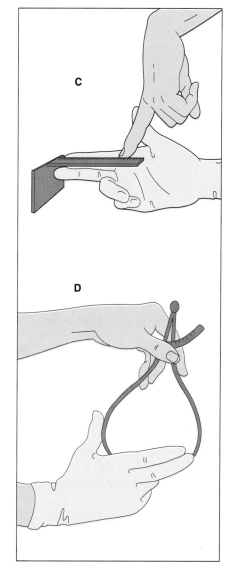

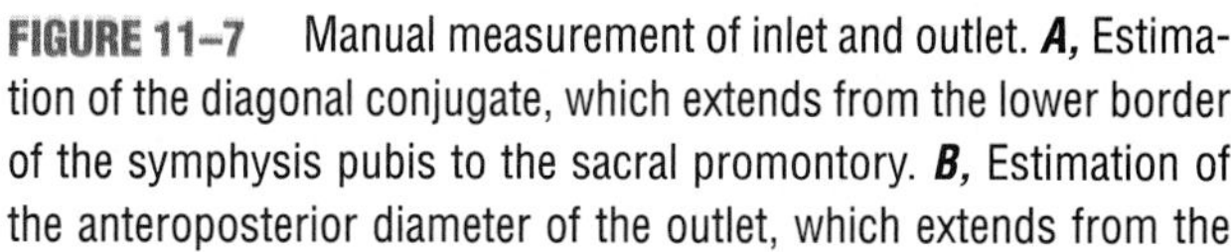

FIGURE 11–7 Manual measurement of inlet and outlet. ***A,*** Estimation of the diagonal conjugate, which extends from the lower border of the symphysis pubis to the sacral promontory. ***B,*** Estimation of the anteroposterior diameter of the outlet, which extends from the lower border of the symphysis pubis to the tip of the sacrum. ***C*** and ***D,*** Methods that may be used to check the manual estimation of anteroposterior measurements.

The anteroposterior diameters of the pelvic inlet may be assessed by attempting to reach from the lower border of the symphysis pubis to the sacral promontory with the middle finger. The clinician should determine the length of the finger before attempting this. The **diagonal conjugate** can then be measured by marking the place where the proximal part of the hand makes contact with the pubis (Figure 11–7). Then the examiner measures the distance (which normally measures at least 11.5 cm). The **obstetric conjugate** is the smallest and thus the most important anteroposterior diameter through which the fetus must pass. It extends from the middle of the sacral promontory to the upper inner point on the symphysis. Because it cannot be measured manually (but only by x-ray examination), it is estimated by subtracting 1.5 to 2 cm from the length of the diagonal conjugate. It should measure 10 cm or more in order for an average size baby (7.5 to 8 lb) to pass through without difficulty. The *true conjugate* extends from the upper border of the symphysis pubis to the middle of the sacral promontory. It can be determined by subtracting 1 cm from the diagonal conjugate.

Pelvic Cavity (Midpelvis)

Important midpelvic measurements include the plane of least dimension, or midplane (anteroposterior diameter, normally 11.5 to 12 cm; posterior sagittal diameter, 4.5 to 5 cm; and transverse diameter [interspinous], 10 cm). The planes of the midpelvis cannot be accurately measured by clinical examination. An evaluation of adequacy

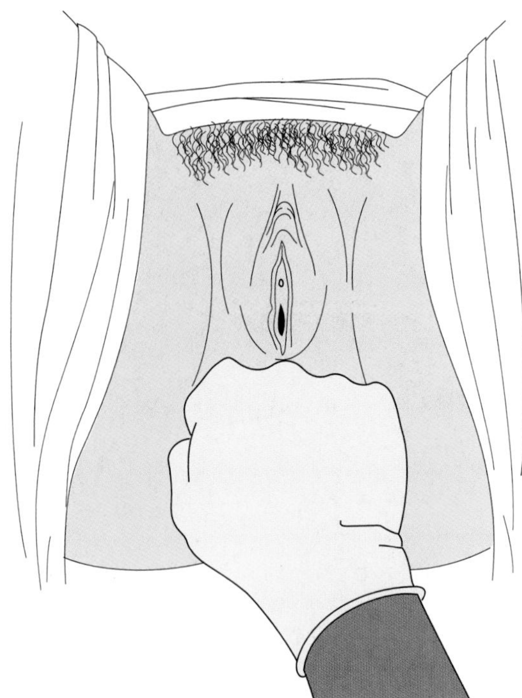

FIGURE 11–8 Use of a closed fist to measure the outlet. Most examiners know the distance between their first and last proximal knuckles. If they don't, they can use a measuring device.

is made based on the prominence of the ischial spines and degree of convergence of the side walls.

Location of the sacrospinous ligament, a firm ridge of tissue, makes location of the ischial spines easier. When this ligament is located, the examiner should run the fingers along it laterally toward the anterior portion of the pelvis. The spines may range from a small, firm bump like the knuckle of a finger (termed *not encroaching*) to a very prominent bone (called *encroaching*).

The sacrosciatic notch should admit two fingers. A wide notch means that the sacrum curves posteriorly, giving the anteroposterior diameter of the midpelvis a greater length. A narrow notch indicates a decreased diameter. The width of the sacrosciatic notch is more accurately evaluated through x-ray examination but can be estimated through vaginal examination.

The length of the sacrospinous ligament is measured by tracing the ligament from its origin on the ischial spines to its insertion on the sacrum. It is usually 4 cm or two to three finger breadths long.

The capacity of the cavity can be assessed by sweeping the fingers down the side walls bilaterally to evaluate the shape of the pelvic side walls. They may be termed *convergent* (closer together at the outlet than the inlet, like a funnel), *divergent* (side walls farther apart at the outlet, which typically means the pubic arch will have a wide angle), or *straight* (normal finding). The curvature, inclination, and hollowness of the sacrum help indicate the capacity of the posterior pelvis. It is estimated digitally by palpating the sacrococcygeal junction and by inching up toward the promontory. The examiner then estimates the hollowness of the sacrum. A flat or shallow sacrum has less room; a hollow sacrum is considered normal.

The plane of greatest pelvic dimensions represents the largest portion of the pelvic cavity and has no obstetric significance.

Pelvic Outlet

The anteroposterior diameter of the pelvic outlet (9.5 to 11.5 cm), which extends from the lower border of the symphysis pubis to the tip of the sacrum, can be measured digitally (Figure 11–7). The transverse diameter of the outlet is measured by placing the fist between the ischial tuberosities. It usually measures 8 to 10 cm (Figure 11–8). The posterior sagittal diameter, the third important outlet diameter, normally measures at least 7.5 cm.

The mobility of the coccyx is determined by pressing down on it with the forefinger and middle finger during the initial vaginal examination. An immobile coccyx can decrease the diameter of the outlet.

The subpubic angle is estimated by palpating the bony structure externally. It should be 85 to 90 degrees. The subpubic angle is estimated by placing two fingers side by side at the border of the symphysis (Figure 11–9). The angle is probably less if the examiner cannot separate his or her fingers.

The length and shape of the pubic rami affect the transverse diameter of the outlet. The pubic ramus is expected to be short and concave inward, as opposed to straight and long.

The height and inclination of the symphysis pubis are measured, and the contour of the pubic arch is estimated. Excessively long or angulated bone structure shortens the diameter of the obstetric conjugate. Height can be determined by placing the index finger of the gloved hand up to the superior border of the symphysis. The examiner should measure the length of the first phalanx of the index finger (normally about 2.5 cm). Inclination can be determined by externally placing one finger on the top of the symphysis while the internal finger palpates the internal margin. An imaginary line is drawn between the fingers, and the angle is estimated.

A posterior inclination with the lower border of the pubis slanting inward decreases the anteroposterior diameter. *The anteroposterior sagittal diameter is the most significant diameter of the outlet because it is the shortest diameter through which the infant must pass.* Estimating the contour of the pubic arch provides information on the width of the angle at which these bones come together. The pubic arch has obstetric importance; if it is narrow, the infant's head may be pushed backward toward the coccyx, making extension of the fetal head difficult, which may lengthen the second stage of labor.

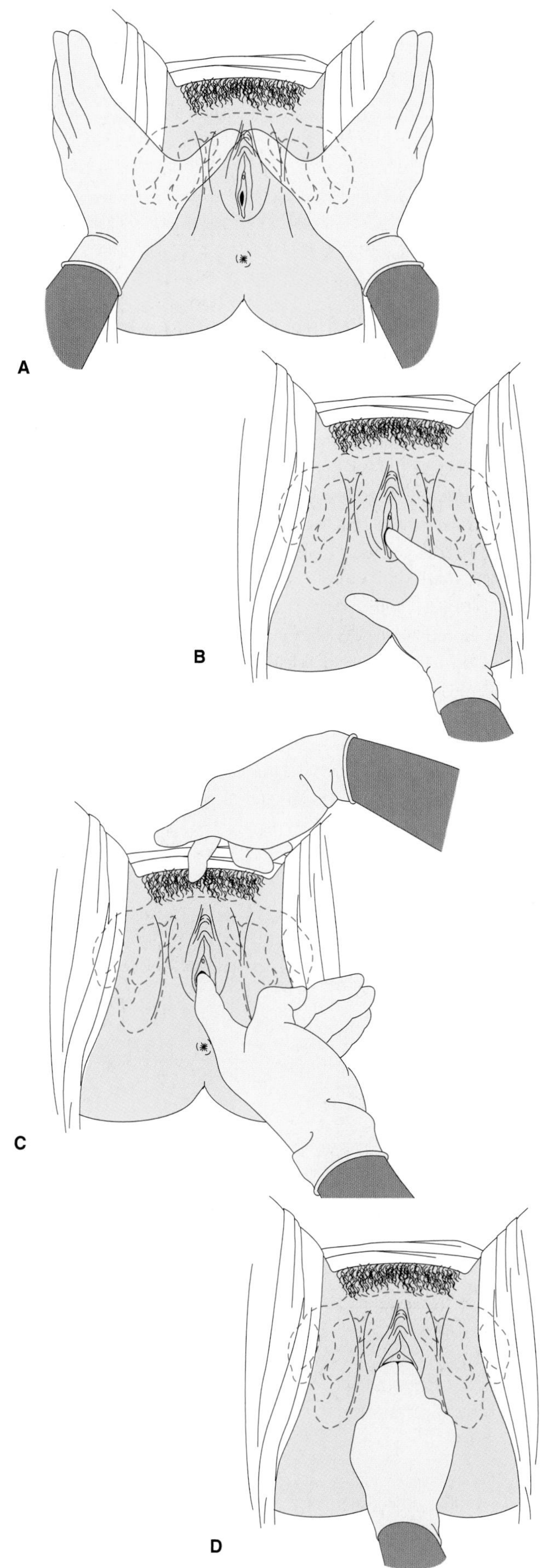

Subsequent Client History

At subsequent prenatal visits, the nurse continues to gather data about the family's adjustment to the pregnancy and the course of the pregnancy to date. The nurse asks the pregnant woman how she thinks the pregnancy is progressing. In what ways is it the same as her expectations, and how is it different? The nurse also asks about the adjustment of the support person and expectations of the support person and other children, if any, in the family. As the pregnancy progresses, the nurse asks about preparations the family has made for the new baby. Taking time to address psychosocial issues is necessary in helping the nurse assess the family's success in meeting their developmental tasks.

The nurse also asks specifically whether the woman has experienced any discomfort, especially the kinds of discomfort that are often seen at specific times during a pregnancy. The nurse inquires about physical changes that relate directly to the pregnancy, such as the woman's perception of fetal movement. Other pertinent information includes any exposure to contagious illnesses, medical treatment and therapy prescribed for nonpregnancy problems since the last visit, and any prescription or over-the-counter medications that were not prescribed as part of the woman's prenatal care.

The danger signs that a woman should report immediately are generally discussed during the initial prenatal visit and reviewed when she comes for her second prenatal visit. Many caregivers also provide printed information on the subject written in lay terms. Table 11–3 identifies the danger signs of pregnancy and possible causes for each.

Periodic prenatal examinations offer the nurse an opportunity to assess the childbearing woman's psychologic needs and emotional status. If the woman's partner attends the prenatal visits, his needs and concerns can also be identified.

The interchange between the nurse and woman will be facilitated if it takes place in a friendly, trusting environment. The nurse should give the woman sufficient time to ask questions and to air concerns. If the nurse provides the time and demonstrates genuine interest, the

Text continues on page 276.

FIGURE 11–9 Evaluation of the outlet. ***A,*** Estimation of the subpubic angle. ***B,*** Estimation of the length of the pubic ramus. ***C,*** Estimation of the depth and inclination of the pubis. ***D,*** Estimation of the contour of the subpubic angle.

COMMUNITY IN FOCUS

Baby Network

The Baby Network in Clarement, New Hampshire, is an example of the success that can result when a multidisciplinary group of health care and human service professionals works together to address a community need. Although Clarement is a small community, it has many resources available to address the health needs of pregnant women and their families. However, before Baby Network began, there was no established method for coordinating services for all women.

In 1994 representatives from Valley Regional Hospital, Planned Parenthood, several physician offices, Connecticut Valley Home Care, University of New Hampshire Cooperative Extensi-1on, WIC, and support programs such as Early Interventions and Good Beginnings met to plan an approach that would provide comprehensive, fully integrated care for the childbearing family including prenatal care and education, inpatient services, post-birth care, and parenting support. The outcomes included a common mission and goal setting among the various providers and a commitment to monthly meetings for ongoing collaboration. The Baby Network supports a case management model of care delivery to coordinate all resources.

When a pregnancy is diagnosed, either in a physician's office or the prenatal clinic, a care manager from Valley Regional Hospital or Planned Parenthood's Prenatal Program is assigned to the woman. The care manager, an experienced, specially trained maternal-child health nurse, conducts an initial assessment interview, usually at the woman's second prenatal visit, and assigns the woman to one of four categories:

1. No need for further care management because of very low risk, adequate support and knowledge
2. 4–8 visit plan will be started
3. Multiple high-risk parameters warrant an extended visit plan as the need presents
4. Future consultations are refused by the woman

The majority of primigravidas fall into category 2.

The care manager follows a standard protocol of nutritional guidance, general health maintenance, education, psychosocial interventions, and community referrals throughout the pregnancy, tailoring the care plan as necessary when unique concerns or problems arise. The care manager works closely with the woman and her family as well as the physicians and clinic staff to address needs. Community referrals and connections to parent support agencies such as Good Beginnings or WIC are part of the philosophy of continuity of care and "wrapping" of services around the family.

Because of the integration of Connecticut Valley Home Care, the care managers can offer skilled nursing home visits as part of the service they provide, thereby decreasing the need for more expensive inpatient care for needs such as mild pregnancy-induced hypertension monitoring, glucose control for diabetics, and IV hydration therapy. The care managers make daily rounds in the LDRP unit, have case conferences as needed, and complete a summary for the acute care team so that they are also familiar with the woman and her family prior to admission. When the woman is admitted for labor, the acute care team notifies the care manager so that postpartum plans can be finalized. The care manager completes maternal-newborn home assessments and provides skilled, in-home nursing care if necessary. In addition, for the three months following birth, a Good Beginnings volunteer is available to provide additional family support.

Baby Network continues to develop as the members explore new, creative ways of enhancing the provision of health services to improve pregnancy outcomes and ensure a consistent high quality of care for childbearing families. The program is making a difference to the people it serves and to the care providers working within it.

SOURCE: Personal communication with Becky Gentes, RN, Maternal/Child Services Director for Valley Regional Healthcare, and printed materials.

TABLE 11–3 Danger Signs in Pregnancy

The woman should report the following danger signs in pregnancy immediately:

Danger Sign	Possible Cause
Sudden gush of fluid from vagina	Premature rupture of membranes
Vaginal bleeding	Abruptio placentae, placenta previa Lesions of cervix or vagina "Bloody show"
Abdominal pain	Premature labor, abruptio placentae
Temperature above 38.3C (101F) and chills	Infection
Dizziness, blurring of vision, double vision, spots before eyes	Hypertension, preeclampsia
Persistent vomiting	Hyperemesis gravidarum
Severe headache	Hypertension, preeclampsia
Edema of hands, face, legs, and feet	Preeclampsia
Muscular irritability, convulsions	Preeclampsia, eclampsia
Epigastric pain	Preeclampsia–ischemia in major abdominal vessel
Oliguria	Renal impairment, decreased fluid intake
Dysuria	Urinary tract infection
Absence of fetal movement	Maternal medication, obesity, fetal death

TABLE 11–4 Guide to Prenatal Assessment of Parenting

Areas Assessed	Sample Questions
I. Perception of complexities of mothering A. Desires baby for itself Positive: 1. Feels positive about pregnancy Negative: 1. Wants baby to meet own needs such as someone to love her, someone to get her out of unhappy home	1. Did you plan on getting pregnant? 2. How do you feel about being pregnant? 3. Why do you want this baby?
B. Expresses concern about impact of mothering role on other roles (wife, career, school) Positive: 1. Realistic expectations of how baby will affect job, career, school, and personal goals 2. Interested in learning about child care Negative: 1. Feels pregnancy and baby will make no emotional, physical, or social demands on self 2. Has no insight that mothering role will affect other roles or lifestyle	1. What do you think it will be like to take care of a baby? 2. How do you think your life will be different after you have your baby? 3. How do you feel this baby will affect your job, career, school, and personal goals? 4. How will the baby affect your relationship with your boyfriend or husband? 5. Have you done any reading, babysitting, or made any things for a baby?
C. Gives up routine habits because "not good for baby" (eg, quits smoking, adjusts time schedule) Positive: 1. Gives up routines not good for baby (quits smoking, adjusts eating habits)	
II. Attachment A. Strong feelings regarding sex of baby. Why? Positive: 1. Verbalizes positive thoughts about the baby Negative: 1. Baby will be like negative aspects of self and partner	1. Why do you prefer a certain sex? (Is reason inappropriate for a baby?) 2. Note comments client makes about baby not being normal and why client feels this way.
B. Interested in data regarding fetus (eg, growth and development, heart tones) Positive: 1. As above Negative: 1. Shows no interest in fetal growth and development, quickening, and fetal heart tones 2. Expresses negative feelings about fetus by rejecting counseling regarding nutrition, rest, hygiene	
C. Fantasies about baby Positive: 1. Follows cultural norms regarding preparation 2. Time of attachment behaviors appropriate to her history of pregnancy loss Negative: 1. Bonding conditional depending on sex, age of baby, and/or labor and birth experience 2. Woman considers only own needs when making plans for baby 3. Exhibits no attachment behaviors after critical period of previous pregnancy 4. Failure to follow cultural norms regarding preparation	1. What did you think or feel when you first felt the baby move? 2. Have you started preparing for the baby? 3. What do you think your baby will look like—what age do you see your baby at? 4. How would you like your new baby to look?
III. Acceptance of child by significant others A. Acknowledges acceptance by significant other of the new responsibility inherent in child Positive: 1. Acknowledges unconditional acceptance of pregnancy and baby by significant others 2. Partner accepts new responsibility inherent with child 3. Timely sharing of experience of pregnancy with significant others	1. How does your partner feel about this pregnancy? 2. How do your parents feel? 3. What do your friends think? 4. Does your partner have a preference regarding the baby's sex? Why? 5. How does your partner feel about being a father? 6. What do you think he'll be like as a father?

Areas Assessed	Sample Questions
Negative:	7. What do you think he'll do to help you with child care?
1. Significant others not supportively involved with pregnancy	8. Have you and your partner talked about how the baby might change your lives?
2. Conditional acceptance of pregnancy depending on sex, race, age of baby	9. Who have you told about your pregnancy?
3. Decision making does not take in needs of fetus (eg, spends food money on new car)	
4. Takes no/little responsibility for needs of pregnancy, woman/fetus	
B. Concrete demonstration of acceptance of pregnancy/baby by significant others (eg, baby shower, significant other involved in prenatal education)	1. Note if partner attends clinic with client (degree of interest; eg, listens to heart tones). Significant other plans to be with client during labor and birth.
Positive:	2. Is your partner contributing financially?
1. Baby shower	
2. Significant other attends prenatal class with client	
IV. Ensures physical well-being	
A. Concerns about having normal pregnancy, labor and birth, and baby	1. What have you heard about labor and birth?
1. Preparing for labor and birth, attends prenatal classes, interested in labor and birth	2. Note data about client's reaction to prenatal class.
2. Aware of danger signs of pregnancy	
3. Seeks and uses appropriate health care (eg, time of initial visit, keeps appointments, follows through on recommendations)	
Negative:	
1. Denies signs and symptoms that might suggest complications of pregnancy	
2. Verbalizes extreme fear of labor and birth—refuses to talk about labor and birth	
3. Fails appointments, fails to follow instructions, refuses to attend prenatal classes	
B. Family/client decisions reflect concern for health of mother and baby (eg, use of finances, time)	
Positive:	
1. As above	

NOTE: When "Negative" is not listed in a section, the reader may assume that negative is the absence of positive responses.

SOURCE: Modified and used with permission of the Minneapolis Health Dept, Minneapolis, MN.

woman will feel more at ease bringing up questions that she may believe are silly or concerns that she has been afraid to verbalize. The nurse who has an accurate understanding of all the changes of pregnancy is most able to answer questions and provide information. See the foldout color chart, "Maternal-Fetal Development," for vivid illustrations of some of this information.

The nurse should also be sensitive to religious, spiritual, cultural, and socioeconomic factors that may influence a family's response to pregnancy, as well as to the woman's expectations of the health care system. The nurse can avoid stereotyping clients simply by asking each woman about her expectations for the antepartal period. Although many women's responses may reflect what are thought to be traditional norms, other women will have decidedly different views or may have expectations that represent a blending of beliefs or cultures.

During the prenatal period, it is essential that the nurse begin assessing the developing readiness of the woman (and her partner, if possible) to take on the responsibilities of parenthood successfully. Table 11–4 identifies areas for assessment and provides some sample questions the nurse might use to obtain necessary information. If the woman's responses are primarily negative, the nurse can plan interventions for the prenatal and postpartal periods.

Subsequent Antepartal Assessment

The Subsequent Prenatal Assessment Guide, which begins on page 277, provides a systematic approach to the regular physical examinations the pregnant woman

Text continues on page 280.

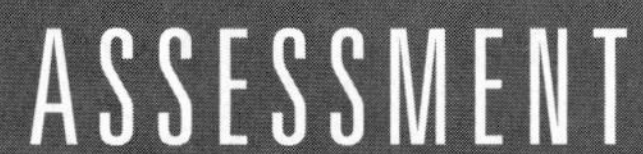

GUIDE: SUBSEQUENT PRENATAL ASSESSMENT

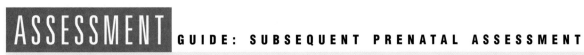

Physical Assessment/ Normal Findings	Alterations and Possible Causes*	Nursing Responses to Data†
Vital Signs		
Temperature: 36.2–37.6C (98–99.6F)	Elevated temperature (infection)	Evaluate for signs of infection. Refer to physician.
Pulse: 60–90/min Rate may increase 10 beats/min during pregnancy	Increased pulse rate (anxiety, cardiac disorders)	Note irregularities. Assess for anxiety and stress.
Respiration: 16–24/min	Marked tachypnea or abnormal patterns (respiratory disease)	Refer to physician.
Blood pressure: 90–140/60–90 (falls in second trimester)	> 140/90 or increase of 30 mm systolic and 15 mm diastolic (PIH)	Assess for edema, proteinuria, hyperreflexia. Refer to physician. Schedule appointments more frequently.
Weight Gain		
First trimester: 1.6–2.3 kg (3.5–5 lb) *Second trimester:* 5.5–6.8 kg (12–15 lb) *Third trimester:* 5.5–6.8 kg (12–15 lb)	Inadequate weight gain (poor nutrition, nausea, IUGR) Excessive weight gain (excessive caloric intake, edema, PIH)	Discuss appropriate weight gain. Provide nutritional counseling. Assess for presence of edema or anemia.
Edema		
Small amount of dependent edema, especially in last weeks of pregnancy	Edema in hands, face, legs, feet (PIH)	Identify any correlation between edema and activities, blood pressure, or proteinuria. Refer to physician if indicated.
Uterine Size		
See Initial Prenatal Assessment Guide for normal changes during pregnancy	Unusually rapid growth (multiple gestation, hydatidiform mole, hydramnios, miscalculation of EDB)	Evaluate fetal status. Determine height of fundus (p 269). Use diagnostic ultrasound.
Fetal Heartbeat		
120–160/min Funic souffle	Absence of fetal heartbeat after 20 weeks' gestation (maternal obesity, fetal demise)	Evaluate fetal status.
Laboratory Evaluation		
Hemoglobin: 12–16 g/dL Pseudoanemia of pregnancy	< 12 g/dL (anemia)	Provide nutritional counseling. Hemoglobin is repeated at 7 months' gestation. Women of Mediterranean heritage need a close check on hemoglobin because of possibility of thalassemia.
Maternal serum α-fetoprotein (MSAFP): normal levels (done at 16–18 weeks' gestation)	Elevated (neural tube defect, underestimated gestational age, multiple gestation, fetal demise, Rh disease)	Refer to physician.

*Possible causes of alterations are placed in parentheses.

†This column provides guidelines for further assessment and initial nursing intervention.

Physical Assessment/ Normal Findings	Alterations and Possible Causes*	Nursing Responses to Data†
Indirect Coombs Test done on Rh− women: negative (done at 28 weeks' gestation)	Rh antibodies present (maternal sensitization has occurred)	If Rh− and unsensitized, RhIgG prophylaxis given (see Chapter 16). If Rh antibodies present, RhIgG *not* given; fetus monitored closely for isommune hemolytic disease.
50 g, 1-hour glucose screen (done between 24 and 28 weeks' gestation)	Plasma glucose level > 140 mg/dL (gestational diabetes mellitus [GDM])	Discuss implications of GDM. Refer for a diagnostic glucose tolerance test.
Urinalysis: See Initial Prenatal Assessment Guide for normal findings	See Initial Prenatal Assessment Guide for deviations	Repeat urinalysis at 7 months' gestation. Dipstick test at each visit.
Protein: Negative	Proteinuria, albuminuria (contamination by vaginal discharge, urinary tract infection, PIH)	Obtain dipstick urine sample. Refer to physician if deviations are present.
Glucose: Negative	Persistent glycosuria (diabetes mellitus)	Refer to physician.
Note: Glycosuria may be present due to physiologic alterations in glomerular filtration rate and renal threshold		

Cultural Assessment	Variations to Consider*	Nursing Responses to Data†
Determine the mother's (and family's) attitudes about the sex of the unborn child.	Some women have no preference about the sex of the child; others do. In many cultures boys are especially valued as firstborn children.	Provide opportunities to discuss preferences and expectations; avoid a judgmental attitude to the response.
Ask about the woman's expectations of childbirth. Will she want someone with her for the birth? Whom does she choose? What is the role of her partner?	Some women want their partner present for labor and birth; others prefer a female relative or friend. Some women expect to be separated from their partner once cervical dilatation has occurred (Andrews & Boyle, 1998).	Provide information on birth options, but accept the woman's decision about who will attend.
Ask about preparations for the baby. Determine what is customary for the woman.	Some women may have a fully prepared nursery; others may not have a separate room for the baby.	Explore reasons for not preparing for the baby. Support the mother's preferences, and provide information about possible sources of assistance if the decision is related to a lack of resources.

Psychosocial Assessment	Variations to Consider*	Nursing Responses to Data†
Expectant Mother		
Psychologic status:		
First trimester: Incorporates idea of pregnancy; may feel ambivalent, especially if she must give up desired role; usually looks for signs of verification of pregnancy, such as increase in abdominal size or fetal movement	Increasing stress and anxiety Inability to establish communication; inability to accept pregnancy; inappropriate response or actions; denial of pregnancy; inability to cope	Encourage woman to take an active part in her care. Establish lines of communication. Establish a trusting relationship. Counsel as necessary. Refer to appropriate professional as needed.

*Possible causes of alterations are placed in parentheses.

†This column provides guidelines for further assessment and initial nursing intervention.

Psychosocial Assessment	Variations to Consider*	Nursing Responses to Data†
Expectant Mother *continued*		
Second trimester: Baby becomes more real to woman as abdominal size increases and she feels movement; she begins to turn inward, becoming more introspective		
Third trimester: Begins to think of baby as separate being; may feel restless and may feel that time of labor will never come; remains self-centered and concentrates on preparing place for baby	Inadequate information	Teach and/or institute appropriate relief measures (Chapter 12).
Educational needs: *Self-care measures and knowledge about the following:* Health promotion Breast care Hygiene Rest Exercise Nutrition Relief measures for common discomforts of pregnancy Danger signs in pregnancy (Table 11–3)		
Sexual activity: Woman knows how pregnancy affects sexual activity	Lack of information about effects of pregnancy and/or alternative positions during sexual intercourse	Provide counseling.
Preparation for parenting: Appropriate preparation (Table 11–4)	Lack of preparation (denial, failure to adjust to baby, unwanted child) (Table 11–4)	Counsel. If lack of preparation is due to inadequacy of information, provide information (Chapter 12).
Preparation for childbirth: *Client aware of following:* **1.** Prepared childbirth techniques **2.** Normal processes and changes during childbirth		If couple chooses particular technique, refer to classes (see Chapter 9 for description of childbirth preparation techniques). Encourage prenatal class attendance. Educate woman during visits based on current physical status. Provide reading list for more specific information.
3. Problems that may occur as a result of drug and alcohol use and of smoking	Continued abuse of drugs and alcohol; denial of possible effect on self and baby	Review danger signs that were presented on initial visit.
Woman has met other physician and/or nurse-midwife who may be attending her birth in the absence of primary caregiver	Introduction of new individual at birth may increase stress and anxiety for woman and partner	Introduce woman to all members of group practice.

*Possible causes of alterations are placed in parentheses.

†This column provides guidelines for further assessment and initial nursing intervention.

Psychosocial Assessment	Variations to Consider*	Nursing Responses to Data†
Impending labor: *Client knows signs of impending labor:* **1.** Uterine contractions that increase in frequency, duration, intensity **2.** Bloody show **3.** Expulsion of mucous plug **4.** Rupture of membranes	Lack of information	Provide appropriate teaching, stressing importance of seeking appropriate medical assistance.
Expectant Father		
Psychologic status: *First trimester:* May express excitement over confirmation of pregnancy and of his virility; concerns move toward providing for financial needs; energetic; may identify with some discomforts of pregnancy and may even exhibit symptoms	Increasing stress and anxiety Inability to establish communication Inability to accept pregnancy diagnosis Withdrawal of support Abandonment of the mother	Encourage expectant father to come to prenatal visits. Establish lines of communication. Establish trusting relationship.
Second trimester: May feel more confident and be less concerned with financial matters; may have concerns about wife's changing size and shape, her increasing introspection		Counsel. Let expectant father know that it is normal for him to experience these feelings.
Third trimester: May have feelings of rivalry with fetus, especially during sexual activity; may make changes in his physical appearance and exhibit more interest in himself; may become more energetic; fantasizes about child but usually imagines older child; fears of mutilation and death of woman and child		Include expectant father in pregnancy activities as he desires. Provide education, information, and support. Increasing numbers of expectant fathers are demonstrating desire to be involved in many or all aspects of prenatal care, education, and preparation.

*Possible causes of alterations are placed in parentheses.

†This column provides guidelines for further assessment and initial nursing intervention.

should undergo for optimal prenatal care, and a model for evaluating both the pregnant woman and the expectant father, if he is involved in the pregnancy.

The frequency of subsequent visits should be determined by the woman's individual needs and the assessment of her risks. Generally, the recommended frequency of prenatal visits is as follows:

- Every 4 weeks for the first 28 weeks of gestation
- Every 2 weeks until 36 weeks' gestation
- After week 36, every week until childbirth

During the subsequent antepartal assessments, most women demonstrate ongoing psychologic adjustment to pregnancy and ever-improving coping skills. However, some women may exhibit signs of psychologic problems. These signs may include one or more of the following:

- Increasing anxiety
- Inability to establish communication
- Inappropriate responses or actions
- Denial of pregnancy
- Inability to cope with stress
- Intense preoccupation with the sex of the baby
- Failure to acknowledge quickening
- Failure to plan and prepare for the baby (for example, living arrangements, clothing, feeding methods)
- Indications of substance abuse

If the woman's behavior indicates possible psychologic problems, the nurse should provide ongoing support and counseling and also refer the woman to appropriate professionals.

FOCUS YOUR STUDY

- A complete history forms the basis of prenatal care and is reevaluated and updated as necessary throughout the pregnancy.
- The initial prenatal assessment is a careful and thorough physical examination and cultural and psychosocial assessment designed to identify variations and potential risk factors.
- Laboratory tests completed at the initial visit, such as a complete blood count, ABO and Rh typing, urinalysis, Pap smear, gonorrhea culture, rubella titer, and various blood screens, provide information about the woman's health during early pregnancy and also help detect potential problems.
- The estimated date of birth can be calculated using Nägele's rule. Using this approach, one begins with the first day of the last menstrual period, subtracts 3 months, and adds 7 days. A "wheel" may also be used to calculate the EDB.
- Accuracy of the EDB may be evaluated by physical examination to assess uterine size, measurement of fundal height, and ultrasound. Perception of quickening and auscultation of fetal heartbeat are also useful tools in confirming the gestation of a pregnancy.
- The diagonal conjugate is the distance from the lower posterior border of the symphysis pubis to the sacral promontory. The obstetric conjugate is estimated by subtracting 1.5 to 2.0 cm from the length of the diagonal conjugate.
- As part of the assessment of the pelvic cavity (midpelvis), the prominence of the ischial spines is assessed, the sacrosciatic notch and the length of the sacrospinous ligament are measured, and the shape of the pelvic side walls is evaluated. Finally, the hollowness of the sacrum is determined.
- The anteroposterior diameter of the pelvic outlet is determined, the mobility of the coccyx is assessed, the suprapubic angle is estimated, and the contour of the pubic arch is evaluated to assess the adequacy of the pelvic outlet.
- The nurse begins evaluating the woman psychosocially during the initial prenatal assessment. This assessment continues and is modified throughout the pregnancy.
- Cultural and ethnic beliefs may strongly influence the woman's attitudes and apparent cooperation with care during pregnancy

REFERENCES

Andrews, M. M., & Boyle, J. S. (1998). *Transcultural concepts in nursing care* (2nd ed.). Glenview, IL: Scott, Foresman/Little, Brown.

Cunningham, F. G., MacDonald, P. C., Gant, N. F., Leveno, K. J., Gilstrap, L. C., III, Hankins, G. D. V., & Clark, S. L. (1997). *Williams obstetrics* (20th ed.). Stamford, CT: Appleton & Lange.

Engstrom, J. L., Piscioneri, L. A., Low, L. K., McShane, H., & McFarlin, B. (1993). Fundal height measurement. Part 3. The effect of maternal position on fundal height measurements. *Journal of Nurse-Midwifery, 38*(1), 23–27.

Milunsky, A., Ulcickas, M., Rothman, K. J., Willett, W., Jick, S. S., & Jick, H. (1992, Aug. 19). Maternal heat exposure and neural tube defects. *Journal of the American Medical Association, 268*(7), 882–885.

Varney, H. (1997). *Varney's midwifery* (3rd ed.). Sudbury, MA: Jones and Bartlett.

12 The Expectant Family: Needs and Care

Key Terms

Fetal alcohol syndrome (FAS)
Fetal movement record (FMR)
Kegel exercises
Leukorrhea
Lightening
Nipple preparation
Pelvic tilt
Ptyalism
Teratogens

I DON'T KNOW HOW I TIMED IT, BUT MY NURSING program OB rotation finishes up right about my due date. Watching all the births during my rotation has been really exciting. The labor and delivery nurses laugh and say my hormones should be hopping now, but I think this baby is subliminally telling me that we won't "hatch" until I take my last final exam!

Objectives

- Summarize communication skills that nurses can use to enhance effectiveness in making nursing assessments and implementing care.
- Explain the causes of the common discomforts of pregnancy and appropriate measures to alleviate these discomforts.
- Develop a plan of care incorporating anticipatory guidance of the pregnant woman and her family to maintain and promote well-being for each trimester of pregnancy.
- Discuss the significance of cultural considerations in managing nursing care during pregnancy.
- Describe the significance of using the nursing process to promote health in the woman and her family during pregnancy.
- Describe factors that have contributed to the increased incidence of pregnancy in women over age 35.
- Compare similarities and differences in the needs of expectant women in various age groups.

FROM THE MOMENT A WOMAN FINDS out that she is pregnant, she faces a future marked by dramatic changes. Her appearance will be altered. Her relationships will change. She will experience a variety of unique physical changes throughout the pregnancy. Even her psychologic state will be affected.

Her family must also adjust to the pregnancy. Roles and responsibilities of family members will change as the woman's ability to perform certain activities changes. They too must adapt psychologically to the situation.

The expectant woman and her family will probably have many questions about the pregnancy and its impact on her and the other members of the family. In addition, the daily activities and health care practices of the woman become of concern when she and her family realize that what she does can affect the well-being of the unborn child.

Nurses caring for pregnant women need a clear understanding of pregnancy and the changes it brings if they are to be effective in managing nursing care. With this in mind, Chapter 10 provided a database for the nurse by presenting material related to the normal physical and psychologic, social, and cultural changes of pregnancy. Chapter 11 then used that database to begin a discussion of nursing care management by focusing on client assessment. This chapter further addresses nursing care management as it relates to the needs of the expectant woman and her loved ones.

NURSING CARE MANAGEMENT

Nursing Diagnosis

The nurse may see a pregnant woman only once every 3 to 4 weeks during the first several months of her pregnancy. To ensure continuity of care, therefore, a written care plan that incorporates assessment data, nursing diagnoses, and client goals is essential.

The nurse can anticipate that, for many women with a low-risk pregnancy, certain nursing diagnoses will be made more frequently than others. Nursing diagnoses will, of course, vary from woman to woman and according to the time in the pregnancy. Examples of common nursing diagnoses include the following:

- ***Constipation*** related to the physiologic effects of pregnancy
- ***Altered Sexuality Patterns*** related to discomfort during late pregnancy

After formulating an appropriate diagnosis, the nurse establishes related goals to guide the nursing plan and interventions.

Nursing Plan and Implementation

Once nursing diagnoses have been identified, the next step is to establish priorities of nursing care. Sometimes priorities of care are based on the most immediate needs or concerns perceived by the woman. For example, during the first trimester, a woman is probably not ready to hear about labor and birth because she is likely to have more immediate concerns, such as nausea or concerns about sexual intimacy with her partner.

The woman's priorities may not always be the same as the nurse's. If the safety of the woman or her fetus is at issue, however, that takes priority over other concerns of the woman or her family. It is the responsibility of medical and nursing professionals to help the woman and her family understand the significance of a problem and to plan appropriate interventions to deal with it.

The intervention methods most used by nurses in caring for the expectant woman and her family are communication techniques and teaching-learning strategies. These intervention methods are often used in groups, such as early pregnancy classes and childbirth education classes, but the nurse in the prenatal setting also applies these techniques with individuals.

Community-Based Nursing Care

Prenatal care, especially for women with low-risk pregnancies, is community based, typically in a clinic or private office. The health care community recognizes the value of providing a primary care nurse in these settings to coordinate care for each childbearing family. The nurse in a clinic or health maintenance organization (HMO) may be the only source of continuity for the woman, who may see a different physician or certified nurse-midwife at each visit. The nurse can be extremely effective in working with the expectant family by providing them with necessary and complete information about pregnancy, self-care measures, and community resources or referral agencies. Communities often have a wealth of services and educational opportunities available for pregnant women and their families, and the knowledgeable nurse can help the woman access these services. This allows the family to assume equal responsibility with health care providers in working toward their common goal of a positive childbearing experience.

Relieving the expectant woman's discomforts, maintaining her physical health, and providing anticipatory guidance are important parts of nursing care management. In addition, the nurse helps meet the needs of the woman's family to better maintain the harmony and integrity of the family unit. The nurse does this by providing support and prenatal education. If the nurse is effective, family members may gain greater problem-solving ability, self-esteem, self-confidence, and ability to participate in health care.

Although the father of the baby is present in most cases, his presence cannot be assumed. If he is not a part of the family structure, it is important to assess the woman's support system to determine what significant persons in her life will play a major role during this childbearing experience.

When the father is part of the family or support system, providing anticipatory guidance to him is a necessary part of any plan of care. He may need information about the anatomic, physiologic, and emotional changes that occur during pregnancy and postpartum, the couple's sexuality and sexual response, and the reactions that he may experience. He may wish to express his feelings about breastfeeding versus bottle feeding, the sex of the child, and other topics. If it is culturally acceptable to the couple and personally acceptable to him, the nurse refers the couple to expectant parents' classes for further information and support from other couples.

The nurse assesses the father's intended degree of participation during labor and birth and his knowledge of what to expect. If the couple prefers that his participation be minimal or restricted, the nurse supports their decision. With this type of consideration and collaboration, the father is less apt to develop feelings of alienation, helplessness, and guilt during the pregnancy. The relationship between the couple may be strengthened and his self-esteem raised. He is then better able to provide physical and emotional support to his partner during labor and birth.

In the plan for prenatal care, the nurse incorporates a discussion about the negative feelings that older children may have. Parents may be distressed to see an older child become aggressive toward the newborn. Parents who are unprepared for the older child's feeling of anger, jealousy, and rejection may respond inappropriately in their confusion and surprise. The nurse emphasizes that open communication between parents and children (or acting out feelings with a doll if the child is too young to verbalize) helps children master their feelings and may prevent them from hurting the baby when they are unsupervised. Children may feel less neglected and more secure if they know that their parents are willing to help with their anger and aggressiveness.

Parents may be encouraged to bring their children to antepartal visits. Seeing what is involved and listening to the fetal heartbeat may make the pregnancy more real to siblings. Many agencies also provide sibling classes geared to different ages and levels of understanding.

Home Care Home care can be of benefit to any pregnant woman, but it is especially effective in removing barriers for women who have difficulty accessing health care. These barriers may include lack of locally available health care facilities, problems with transportation to the facility, or schedule conflicts with available appointment times because of employment hours or family responsibilities.

In-home nursing assessments vary according to the scope of practice of the nurse and include current history and those screening procedures typically completed in an office or clinic: vital signs, weight, urine screen, physical activity, dietary intake. Advanced practice nurses can also assess reflexes, perform tests of fetal well-being, and even do cervical examinations. Once the assessments are completed, the nurse can determine the level of follow-up home care or telephone contact (Springer, Spatz, & Donahue, 1994).

A prenatal home care visit or phone contact can also be useful for women who anticipate a short inpatient stay after childbirth. At the prenatal contact, the nurse explains the postpartum program and answers any questions the woman or her family have.

Although the use of home care for women with uncomplicated pregnancies is growing, it is most often used for women with prenatal complications that can be managed without hospitalization if effective nursing assessment and care are provided in the home (see Chapters 15 and 16).

Teaching for Self-Care

Throughout the prenatal period the nurse provides informal and formal teaching to the childbearing family designed to help the family carry out self-care when appropriate and to report changes that may indicate a possible health problem. The teaching is most effective if timed to coincide with the woman's (couple's) readiness and needs (Table 12–1). The nurse also provides anticipatory guidance to help the family plan for changes that will occur following childbirth. Issues that could be possible sources of postpartal stress should be discussed by the expectant couple. Issues to be resolved beforehand may include the sharing of infant and household chores, help in the first few days, reapportionment of family finances, options for babysitting to allow the mother (and couple) some free time, the mother's return to work after the baby's birth, and sibling rivalry.

Relationship changes with in-laws should be addressed as well as the woman's or couple's expectations of the grandparents. Although some grandparents are eager to assist with child care by babysitting, others are not. The parents should also give some thought to the best ways of dealing with possible conflicts with the grandparents over childraising approaches. Couples resolve these issues in different ways; however, postpartal adjustment is easier for a couple who agrees on the issues beforehand than for a couple who does not confront and resolve these issues.

Cultural Considerations in Pregnancy

As discussed in Chapter 10, specific actions during pregnancy are often determined by cultural beliefs. Some beliefs, which have been passed down from generation to generation, may be called "old wives' tales." These beliefs had meaning at one time, but the meanings have often been lost with the passing of time. Other beliefs have definite meanings that are retained. Table 12–2 describes activities that are encouraged or forbidden by specific cultures. The table is not meant to be all-inclusive; it offers

TABLE 12–1 Topics for Client Teaching During Pregnancy

All Three Trimesters
Discomforts of pregnancy (see Table 12–3)
Nutrition and weight gain
Sexual activity
Sibling preparation
First Trimester
Attitude toward pregnancy
Exercise and rest
Smoking; use of alcohol and other drugs
Traveling
Fetal growth and development
Danger signals associated with spontaneous abortion
Employment
Early pregnancy classes
Second Trimester
Concerns related to changes in body
Fetal growth and development
Fetal movement
Clothing
Care of skin and breasts
Beginning preparation for care of the infant (equipment and room)
Decisions about infant feeding
Third Trimester
Exercise and rest
Traveling
Danger signals
Preparation for labor and birth
Completion of preparation in home for new baby
Decisions about the infant (circumcision, method of feeding, and so forth)
Decision making for the early postpartum period
Education about psychologic and physical expectations in the early postpartum period

a few examples of cultural activities that may be important to some clients during the prenatal period.

In working with clients of another culture, the health care professional should be as open as possible to other beliefs. If certain activities are not harmful, there is no need to impose one's beliefs and practices upon a person of another culture. If the activities are proving to be harmful, the nurse can consult or work with someone within the culture or someone aware of cultural beliefs and values to see whether the client's behavior can be modified.

Relief of the Common Discomforts of Pregnancy

Common discomforts of pregnancy are often referred to as minor discomforts by health care professionals. These discomforts, however, are not minor to the pregnant woman.

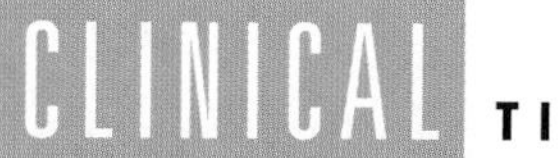

TIP

At each prenatal visit, focus your teaching on changes or possible discomforts the woman might encounter during the coming month and the next trimester. If the pregnancy is progressing normally, spend a few minutes describing her baby at this stage of development.

Most of the discomforts of pregnancy are a result of physiologic and anatomic changes and are fairly specific to each of the three trimesters. Table 12–3 identifies the common discomforts of pregnancy, their possible causes, and the self-care measures that might relieve the discomfort.

First Trimester

Nausea and Vomiting

Nausea and vomiting are early symptoms in pregnancy. These symptoms appear sometime after the first missed menstrual period and usually cease by the fourth missed menstrual period. Approximately 70% to 90% of pregnant women experience some degree of nausea, and 50% experience at least one episode of vomiting (O'Brien & Zhou, 1995). Some women develop an aversion only to specific foods; many experience nausea on arising in the morning; and others experience nausea throughout the day or in the evening.

The exact cause of nausea and vomiting of pregnancy is unknown but is believed to be multifactorial. Research has identified possible hormonal, metabolic, neurologic, and psychosomatic factors contributing to its development. Human chorionic gonadotropin (hCG) is often cited as a major factor because it begins to be present in the body at about the time symptoms of morning sickness usually begin and hCG levels are subsiding when the discomfort of nausea and vomiting usually ends. Research has not yet confirmed this theory, however (Cunningham et al, 1997). Changes in carbohydrate metabolism, fatigue, and emotional factors may also play a role in the development of nausea and vomiting of pregnancy.

Teaching for Self-Care Treatment of nausea and vomiting is not always successful, but the symptoms can be reduced. The nurse must assess the onset, frequency, and duration of symptoms and actual nutritional intake to be helpful in suggesting methods of relief. Physical assessment of the woman should include particular attention to skin color, texture, and turgor as well as vital signs and bowel sounds (Davis, 1996). For some women, nausea may be relieved simply by avoiding the odor of certain foods or other conditions that precipitate the problem. If nausea occurs most frequently during early morning, the woman may find it helpful to eat dry crackers or toast before arising and to rise from bed slowly. Rising slowly and avoiding sudden position

TABLE 12–2 Cultural Beliefs and Practices During Pregnancy

Here are a few examples of cultural beliefs and practices related to pregnancy. It is important not to make assumptions about a client's beliefs, because cultural norms vary greatly within a culture and from generation to generation. The nurse should observe the client carefully and take the time to ask questions. Clients will benefit greatly from the nurse's increased awareness of their cultural beliefs and practices.

Belief or Practice	Nursing Consideration
Home Remedies	
Pregnant women of Native American background may use herbal remedies. An example is the dandelion, which contains a milky juice in its stem believed to increase breast milk flow in mothers who choose to breastfeed (Spector, 1996). Clients of Chinese descent may drink ginseng tea for faintness after childbirth or as a sedative when mixed with bamboo leaves. Some people of African heritage may use self-medication for pregnancy discomforts—for example, laxatives to prevent or treat constipation (Spector, 1996).	Find out what medications and home remedies your client is using, and counsel your client regarding overall effects. It is common for individuals to avoid telling health care workers about home remedies; the client may feel this will be judged unfavorably. Phrase your questions in a sensitive, accepting way.
Nutrition	
Some women of Italian background may believe that it is necessary to satisfy desires for certain foods in order to prevent congenital anomalies. Also, they may believe that they must eat food that they smell, or else the fetus will move "inside," which will result in a miscarriage. Pregnant women of African descent may continue the tradition of eating clay, dirt, or starch, which they believe will benefit the mother and fetus (Spector, 1996). In order to practice Tae Kyo, a set of rules for safe childbirth, pregnant women of Korean descent may practice food taboos by eating particular high-quality foods and avoiding other foods believed to cause an unhealthy fetus (Choi, 1995).	Discuss the client's beliefs and practices in regard to nutrition during pregnancy. Obtain a diet history from the client. Discuss the importance of a well-balanced diet during pregnancy, with consideration of the client's cultural beliefs and practices. In some cases, you might want to suggest remedies that may be more effective—for example, eating high-fiber foods to reduce constipation. If the home remedy is not harmful, there is no reason to ask a client to discontinue this practice.
Alternative Health Care Providers	
Pregnant women of Mexican background may choose to seek out the care of a *partera* (midwife) for prenatal and intrapartal care. A *partera* speaks their language, shares a similar culture, and can deliver pregnant women at home or in a birthing center instead of a hospital. Some people in Hispanic-American communities may use the *curandero,* the folk healer. The *curandero* frequently uses herbs, massage, and religious artifacts for treatment (Spector, 1996).	Discuss the variety of choices of health care providers available to the pregnant woman. Contrast the benefits and risks of different settings for prenatal care and birth. Provide reassurance that the goal of health care during pregnancy and birth is a healthy outcome for mother and baby, with respect for the specific cultural beliefs and practices of the client.
Exercise	
Pregnant women of Italian descent may fear changing their body position in certain ways because they believe this may cause the fetus to develop abnormally (Spector, 1996). Some people of Southeast Asian background believe that inactivity during pregnancy will result in a difficult labor (Mattson, 1995). Some people of European, African, and Mexican descent believe that reaching over the head during pregnancy can harm the baby.	Ask your client whether there are any activities she is afraid to do because of the pregnancy. Assure her that reaching over her head will not harm the baby, and evaluate other activities related to their effect on the pregnancy.
Spirituality	
Native Americans of the Navajo tribe may meet with the medicine man 2 months prior to birth, feeling that the prayers will ensure a safe birth and healthy baby. Some people of European background may tend to pay more attention to spirituality in their life to alleviate fears and ensure a safe birth.	Encourage the use of support systems and spiritual aids that provide comfort for the mother.

changes throughout the day may also help prevent nausea due to hypotensive episodes. In addition, the woman can be advised to avoid brushing her teeth right after eating, because this, too, may trigger vomiting.

Generally, it is helpful to eat small meals every 2 to 3 hours during the day and to avoid greasy or highly seasoned foods. Food may be salted to taste. The salt increases the palatability of the food and replaces any chloride lost when the woman vomits hydrochloric acid from the stomach. Eating dry meals and taking all liquids, including soups, between meals may help some women by avoiding overdistention of the stomach. Sudden changes in blood sugar levels can be avoided if the small meals are high in low-fat protein or complex carbohydrates. Some women find that slowly sipping herbal tea (peppermint, chamomile, raspberry leaf, spearmint) or a carbonated beverage helps reduce nausea.

More recently, some women have obtained relief from acupressure wrist bands. As an alternative to the wrist bands, women can be taught to use acupressure to the pressure point located proximal to the wrist crease. Research suggests that women who do this procedure for 10 minutes four times each day experience significantly less nausea (Belluomini, Litt, Lee, & Katz, 1994). Although health care providers are reluctant to prescribe any medication during pregnancy, some women find 10 to 25 mg pyridoxine (vitamin B_6) helpful in reducing symptoms (Peleg & Niebyl, 1997).

Although some nausea is common, the woman who suffers from extreme nausea coupled with vomiting requires further assessment. She should be advised to contact her care provider if she vomits more than once per day or shows signs of dehydration, such as dry mouth, decreased amounts of highly concentrated urine, and the like. In such cases, the physician or CNM may order antiemetics. However, antiemetics should be avoided if at all possible during the first trimester because of the danger of teratogenic effects on embryo development.

TABLE 12–3 Self-Care Measures for Common Discomforts of Pregnancy

Discomfort	Influencing Factors	Self-Care Measures
First Trimester		
Nausea and vomiting	Increased levels of hCG Changes in carbohydrate metabolism Emotional factors Fatigue	Avoid odors or causative factors. Eat dry crackers or toast before arising in morning. Have small but frequent meals. Avoid greasy or highly seasoned foods. Take dry meals with fluids between meals. Drink carbonated beverages.
Urinary frequency	Pressure of uterus on bladder in both first and third trimesters	Void when urge is felt. Increase fluid intake during the day. Decrease fluid intake *only* in the evening to decrease nocturia.
Fatigue	Specific causative factors unknown May be aggravated by nocturia due to urinary frequency	Plan time for a nap or rest period daily. Go to bed earlier. Seek family support and assistance with responsibilities so that more time is available to rest.
Breast tenderness	Increased levels of estrogen and progesterone	Wear well-fitting, supportive bra.
Increased vaginal discharge	Hyperplasia of vaginal mucosa and increased production of mucus by the endocervical glands due to the increase in estrogen levels	Promote cleanliness by daily bathing. Avoid douching, nylon underpants, and pantyhose; cotton underpants are more absorbent; powder can be used to maintain dryness if not allowed to cake.
Nasal stuffiness and nosebleed (epistaxis)	Elevated estrogen levels	May be unresponsive, but cool air vaporizer may help; avoid use of nasal sprays and decongestants.
Ptyalism (excessive, often bitter salivation)	Specific causative factors unknown	Use astringent mouthwashes, chew gum, or suck hard candy.
Second and Third Trimesters		
Heartburn (pyrosis)	Increased production of progesterone, decreasing gastrointestinal motility and increasing relaxation of cardiac sphincter, displacement of stomach by enlarging uterus, thus regurgitation of acidic gastric contents into the esophagus	Eat small and more frequent meals. Use low-sodium antacids. Avoid overeating, fatty and fried foods, lying down after eating, and sodium bicarbonate.
Ankle edema	Prolonged standing or sitting Increased levels of sodium due to hormonal influences Circulatory congestion of lower extremities Increased capillary permeability Varicose veins	Practice frequent dorsiflexion of feet when prolonged sitting or standing is necessary. Elevate legs when sitting or resting. Avoid tight garters or restrictive bands around legs.
Varicose veins	Venous congestion in the lower veins that increases with pregnancy Hereditary factors (weakening of walls of veins, faulty valves) Increased age and weight gain	Elevate legs frequently. Wear supportive hose. Avoid crossing legs at the knees, standing for long periods, garters, and hosiery with constrictive bands.
Hemorrhoids	Constipation (see following discussion) Increased pressure from gravid uterus on hemorrhoidal veins	Avoid constipation. Apply ice packs, topical ointments, anesthetic agents, warm soaks, or sitz baths; gently reinsert into rectum as necessary.
Constipation	Increased levels of progesterone, which cause general bowel sluggishness Pressure of enlarging uterus on intestine Iron supplements Diet, lack of exercise, and decreased fluids	Increase fluid intake, fiber in the diet, and exercise. Develop regular bowel habits. Use stool softeners as recommended by physician.
Backache	Increased curvature of the lumbosacral vertebrae as the uterus enlarges Increased levels of hormones, which cause softening of cartilage in body joints Fatigue Poor body mechanics	Use proper body mechanics. Practice the pelvic tilt exercise. Avoid uncomfortable working heights, high-heeled shoes, lifting heavy loads, and fatigue.
Leg cramps	Imbalance of calcium/phosphorus ratio Increased pressure of uterus on nerves Fatigue Poor circulation to lower extremities Pointing the toes	Practice dorsiflexion of feet in order to stretch affected muscle. Evaluate diet. Apply heat to affected muscles.

TABLE 12–3 Self-Care Measures *continued*

Discomfort	Influencing Factors	Self-Care Measures
Second and Third Trimesters		
Faintness	Postural hypotension Sudden change of position causing venous pooling in dependent veins Standing for long periods in warm area Anemia	Arise slowly from resting position. Avoid prolonged standing in warm or stuffy environments. Evaluate hematocrit/hemoglobin.
Dyspnea	Decreased vital capacity from pressure of enlarging uterus on the diaphragm	Use proper posture when sitting and standing. Sleep propped up with pillows for relief if problem occurs at night.
Flatulence	Decreased gastrointestinal motility leading to delayed emptying time Pressure of growing uterus on large intestine Air swallowing	Avoid gas-forming foods. Chew food thoroughly. Get regular daily exercise. Maintain normal bowel habits.
Carpal tunnel syndrome	Compression of median nerve in carpal tunnel of wrist Aggravated by repetitive hand movements	Avoid aggravating hand movements. Use splint as prescribed. Elevate affected arm.

Nausea and vomiting generally cease by the fourth month of pregnancy. If they do not, hyperemesis gravidarum (a complication of pregnancy discussed in Chapter 16) must be considered.

Urinary Frequency

Urinary frequency is a common discomfort of pregnancy. It occurs early in pregnancy and again during the third trimester because of the pressure of the enlarging uterus on the bladder. Coughing or sneezing in the last month may even cause leakage of urine. Although the glomerular filtration rate increases in pregnancy, it does not cause a significant increase in urine output. As long as other symptoms of urinary tract infection do not appear, frequency of urination is considered normal during the first and third trimesters.

Teaching for Self-Care There are no methods of decreasing the frequency of urination in pregnancy. Fluid intake should never be decreased to prevent frequency. The woman should be encouraged to maintain an adequate fluid intake: at least 2000 mL/day. She should also be encouraged to empty her bladder frequently (approximately every 2 hours while awake).

Frequent bladder emptying helps decrease the incidence of leakage of urine. Because frequency often results in several trips to the bathroom each night, it is important to remind the woman to consider safety factors in the home, such as a clear path to the bathroom, the use of a night light, and the like. The woman who leaks urine may choose to wear pantyliners during the day. If she does, she should change them as soon as they become damp to avoid perineal excoriation and to avoid contamination of the perineum from the rectal area if the pads move back and forth as she walks. Tightening of the pubococcygeus muscle, which supports internal organs and controls voiding, can help maintain good perineal tone. This procedure, known as Kegel exercise, is discussed in Perineal Exercises, later in this chapter.

Although frequency is considered normal during the first and third trimesters, signs of bladder infection, such as painful urination, burning with voiding, or blood in the urine, should be reported to the woman's health care provider.

Fatigue

Marked fatigue, often out of proportion to the woman's normal pattern, is so common in early pregnancy that it is considered a presumptive sign of pregnancy. It is aggravated if the woman has to arise several times each night because of urinary frequency. Typically, it resolves soon after the end of the first trimester.

Teaching for Self-Care Scheduling activities to allow for napping is helpful. Women should be encouraged to use every opportunity available to rest, including going to bed earlier in the evening. The woman's partner, if he is involved in the pregnancy, needs to understand that the fatigue is normal and will subside. He can be encouraged to assume more home responsibilities to support the woman and enable her to rest.

Breast Tenderness

Sensitivity of the breasts occurs early and continues throughout the pregnancy. Increased levels of estrogen and progesterone contribute to the soreness and tingling felt in the breasts and to the increased sensitivity of the nipples.

Teaching for Self-Care A well-fitting, supportive brassiere gives the most relief for this discomfort. The qualities of a properly supportive brassiere are discussed in Breast Care, later in this chapter.

Increased Vaginal Discharge

Increased whitish vaginal discharge, called **leukorrhea,** is common in pregnancy. It occurs as the result of hyperplasia of vaginal mucosa and increased production of mucus

COMMUNITY IN FOCUS

The M.O.M. Center

Women with physical disabilities or chronic illnesses often have difficulty finding a caregiver who is knowledgeable about the impact of a pregnancy on their disability as well as their needs during pregnancy and the postpartum period. The M.O.M. (Making Options for Motherhood) Center at Thomas Jefferson University (TJU) Hospital in Philadelphia, Pennsylvania was established to help address this issue.

The program began at the request of a pregnant woman with spina bifida. She wanted advice about dealing with parenting, and she sought a support group of people who could relate to her needs and concerns. Two perinatologists, a project coordinator, and a nurse practitioner from a high-risk maternity practice at TJU held a community meeting to get input from other women with physical disabilities about their experiences. The response was remarkable. Many women reported that they had been told they should never have babies and received little or no support when they became pregnant. Moreover, few offices have equipment designed to accommodate the needs of women with disabilities.

The M.O.M. Center uses an interdisciplinary approach to identify and meet specific needs. Women with a variety of disabilities such as sensory deficits, spinal cord injury, cerebral palsy, spina bifida, multiple sclerosis, and limb abnormalities are seen at the Center. The coordinator of the Center, nurse practitioner Toba Spector, and the perinatologist work closely with other health care providers such as social services, physical therapists, and occupational therapists to identify concerns and provide accommodations for women during their pregnancies and postpartally, when parenting issues arise. The Center has special equipment to accommodate women with physical needs, including an adjustable examination table and a scale that weighs a woman in a wheelchair. Specialists such as urologists, neurologists, endocrinologists, and internists who are involved in a woman's ongoing treatment also become part of the interdisciplinary team.

The M.O.M. Center offers preconception counseling as well. During these sessions, the woman is given the information necessary to make an informed choice. This may include data about the impact and risks of pregnancy on her condition; necessary accommodations for medications, activities, and so on; potential risks to a fetus or newborn associated with the mother's disability or her medications; and the challenges she will face in mothering her infant. If a woman has a less common condition such as Wilson's Disease (an autosomal recessive abnormality characterized by a copper deficiency in the plasma), the Center staff will extensively research the literature and help the woman plan accordingly.

Initially the M.O.M. Center tried to establish a support group for these women. However, they found that because of the variety of disabilities there were few common needs. Now the Center uses a "buddy" system when possible, pairing women considering pregnancy or in early pregnancy with a woman who has a similar condition and has completed a pregnancy. This approach has worked well.

Postpartal women are followed for up to 6 months. Certain conditions are exacerbated by pregnancy, so coordination with the appropriate specialist is essential. Part of the follow-up includes home visits by a nurse, physical therapist, or occupational therapist as needed. Women are given information about adaptive equipment and purchasing advice. Ms. Spector reports that babies are remarkable in their ability to adapt and the mothers find ways to meet their infants' needs.

The Center staff have participated in training sessions to increase their sensitivity to the needs of women with physical disabilities. The staff has found that most women are knowledgeable about their condition, abilities, and limitations; thus an approach that acknowledges the woman's expertise and experience tends to be most effective.

The M.O.M. Center has made a difference in the lives of many women. As word of its work has spread, referrals have increased. This innovative program is meeting a significant community need.

SOURCE: Personal communication with Toba L. Spector, CRNP, MSN, Coordinator of the M.O.M. Center, Thomas Jefferson University.

by the endocervical glands. In addition, the increased acidity of the secretions encourages the growth of *Candida albicans*, and the woman is thus more susceptible to monilial vaginitis.

Teaching for Self-Care Cleanliness is important in preventing excoriation and vaginal infections. Daily bathing is adequate; douching should be avoided during pregnancy. The woman should avoid nylon underpants and pantyhose because they retain heat and moisture in the genital area; absorbent cotton underpants should be worn to help prevent problems. The pregnant woman should be encouraged to report any change in vaginal discharge, any irritation in the perineal area, and intense vaginal itching. These changes frequently indicate vaginal infections.

Nasal Stuffiness and Epistaxis

Once pregnancy is well established, elevated estrogen levels may produce edema of the nasal mucosa, resulting in nasal stuffiness, nasal discharge, and obstruction (rhinitis of pregnancy). Epistaxis (nosebleed) may also result.

Teaching for Self-Care Cool air vaporizers and normal saline nose drops may be helpful. However, the problem is often unresponsive to treatment. Women experiencing these problems find it difficult to sleep and may resort to medicated nasal sprays and decongestants to relieve the problem. Such interventions can exaggerate the nasal stuffiness and create other discomforts. The use of any medication in pregnancy should be avoided if possible.

Ptyalism

Ptyalism is a rare discomfort of pregnancy in which excessive, often bitter, saliva is produced. Its cause has not been established, although stimulation of the salivary glands by the ingestion of starch has been suggested as a possible cause (Cunningham et al, 1997). Effective treatments are limited.

Teaching for Self-Care Using astringent mouthwashes, chewing gum, or sucking on hard candy may minimize the problem of ptyalism. It may also be helpful to reduce or limit starch intake.

Second and Third Trimesters

It is difficult to classify discomforts as specifically occurring in the second or third trimester because many problems are due to individual variations in women. The symptoms discussed in this section usually do not appear until the third trimester in primigravidas but occur earlier with each succeeding pregnancy.

Heartburn (Pyrosis)

Heartburn is the regurgitation of acidic gastric contents into the esophagus. It creates a burning or irritating sensation in the esophagus and radiates upward, sometimes leaving a bad taste in the mouth. Heartburn appears to be primarily a result of the displacement of the stomach by the enlarging uterus. The increased production of progesterone in pregnancy, decreases in gastrointestinal motility, and relaxation of the cardiac sphincter also contribute to heartburn.

Teaching for Self-Care Heartburn is aggravated by overeating, ingesting fatty and fried foods, and lying down soon after eating. The woman should therefore avoid these situations. The woman should be encouraged to drink an adequate amount of fluid (8 to 10 8-ounce glasses) each day and to eat smaller, more frequent meals to accommodate the decreased size of her stomach. Good posture is important because it allows more room for the stomach to function. The caregiver may recommend a low-sodium antacid, such as aluminum hydroxide (Amphojel) or a combination of aluminum hydroxide and magnesium hydroxide (Maalox). Because aluminum alone tends to cause constipation and magnesium alone is associated with diarrhea, the combined approach is more desirable. Sodium bicarbonate (baking soda) and Alka-Seltzer should be avoided because of the potential for electrolyte imbalance.

Ankle Edema

Most women experience ankle edema in the last part of pregnancy because of the increasing difficulty of venous return from the lower extremities. Prolonged standing or sitting and warm weather increase the edema. It is also associated with varicose veins. Ankle edema becomes a concern only when accompanied by hypertension or proteinuria or when the edema is not postural in origin.

Teaching for Self-Care The aggravating conditions just mentioned should be avoided. If the woman has to sit or stand for long periods, frequent dorsiflexion of her feet will help contract muscles, thereby squeezing the fluid back into circulation. The pregnant woman should not wear tight garters or other restrictive bands around her legs. During rest periods, the woman should elevate her legs and hips as described in the following section on varicose veins.

Varicose Veins

Varicose veins are a result of weakening of the walls of veins or faulty functioning of the valves. Poor circulation in the lower extremities predisposes the woman to varicose veins in the legs and thighs, as does prolonged standing or sitting. The weight of the gravid uterus in the pelvis aggravates the development of varicosities in the legs and pelvic area by preventing good venous return. Increased maternal age, excessive weight gain, a large fetus, heredity, and multiple pregnancy can all contribute to the problem.

Vulvar varicosities may also be a problem in pregnancy, although they are less common. Varicosities in the vulva and perineum cause aching and a sense of heaviness.

Treatment of varicose veins by surgery or the injection method is not recommended during pregnancy. The woman should be aware that treatment may be needed after pregnancy because the problem will be aggravated by a succeeding pregnancy.

Teaching for Self-Care Regular exercise, such as swimming, cycling, or walking, promotes venous return, which helps prevent varicosities. Avoiding factors that contribute to venous stasis is also helpful. The pregnant woman should avoid standing or sitting for prolonged periods. She should also avoid crossing her legs at the knees because of the pressure on her veins. She should not wear garters or hosiery with constricting bands, such as knee-high hose. However, supportive hose or elastic stockings may be extremely helpful. Supportive hose should be put on in the morning and should be washed daily with soap and warm water to help retain elasticity.

The pregnant woman should be encouraged to elevate her legs level with her hips when she sits. She can enhance comfort by supporting the entire leg rather than simply propping her feet up on a stool, which may lead to hyperextension of the knees. The woman who sits or stands for long periods should walk around frequently to promote venous return to the heart. She can also be encouraged to dorsiflex her feet, hold the position for 3 seconds, then release, with 8 to 10 repetitions several times each day. Venous return is most effectively promoted if the woman lies down with her feet elevated several times a day. To avoid difficulty related to pressure of the uterus on the vena cava, the woman can lie with her legs elevated on pillows and a pillow placed under one hip to displace the uterus to one side (Figure 12–1).

Support for vulvar varicosities can be provided by wearing two sanitary pads inside the underpants. Elevation of only the legs aggravates vulvar varicosities by creating stasis of blood in the pelvic area. Therefore it is important that the pelvic area also be elevated to promote venous drainage into the trunk of the body. More than one firm pillow under the hips may be needed to accomplish this elevation. Near the end of pregnancy, this position may be extremely awkward; the woman may best relieve uterine pressure on the pelvic veins by resting on her side. Blocks may also be placed under the foot of her bed to elevate it slightly.

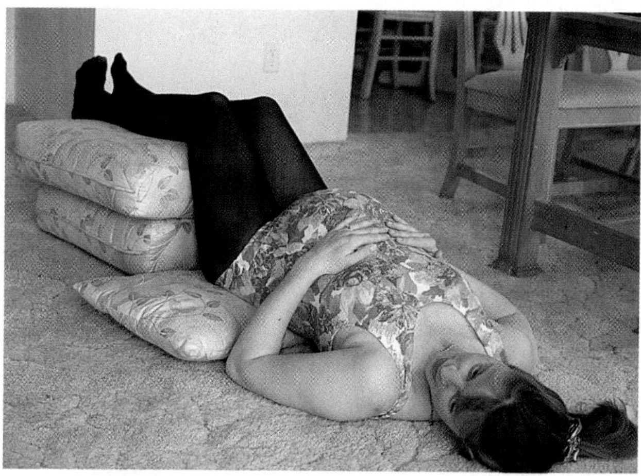

FIGURE 12–1 Swelling and discomfort from varicosities can be decreased by lying down with the legs and one hip elevated (to avoid compression of the vena cava).

Flatulence

Flatulence results from decreased gastrointestinal motility, leading to delayed emptying, and from pressure upon the large intestine by the growing uterus. Air swallowing may also contribute to the problem.

Teaching for Self-Care The woman should be advised to avoid gas-forming foods and to chew her food thoroughly. Regular bowel habits and exercise can also decrease flatulence.

Hemorrhoids

Hemorrhoids are varicosities of the veins around the lower end of the rectum and anus. In the nonpregnant state, hemorrhoids are usually caused by the straining that occurs with constipation. During pregnancy, the gravid uterus presses on the veins and interferes with venous circulation. As the pregnancy progresses, the straining that accompanies constipation can contribute to the development of hemorrhoids.

Some women may not be bothered by hemorrhoids until the second stage of labor, when the hemorrhoids appear as they push just before birth. Hemorrhoids that occur in pregnancy or at birth usually become asymptomatic after the early postpartal period.

Symptoms of hemorrhoids include itching, swelling, pain, and bleeding. Internal hemorrhoids are located above the anal sphincter and are responsible for bleeding, usually with defecation. They are not usually painful unless they protrude from the anus. External hemorrhoids are located outside the anal sphincter. They are not usually the source of bleeding or pain; however, thrombosis of the hemorrhoids can occur, and in that case they become extremely painful. The thrombosis may resolve itself in 24 hours, or it can be treated in the physician's office by incising and evacuating the blood clot. Women who have hemorrhoids prior to pregnancy probably experience more difficulties with them during pregnancy.

Teaching for Self-Care Relief can be achieved by gently and carefully reinserting the hemorrhoids. The woman lies on her side or in the knee to chest position. She places some lubricant on her finger and presses against the hemorrhoids, pushing them inside. She holds them in place for 1 to 2 minutes and then gently withdraws her finger. The anal sphincter should then hold them inside the rectum. The woman will find it especially helpful if she can then maintain a side-lying (Sims') position for a time, so this procedure is best done before bed or prior to a daily rest period.

Avoiding constipation is important in preventing or relieving the discomfort of hemorrhoids. Relief measures for existing hemorrhoid symptoms include ice packs, use of topical ointments and anesthetic agents, and warm soaks.

The woman should contact her health care provider if the hemorrhoids become hardened and noticeably tender to touch. Rectal bleeding that is more than spotting following defecation should also be reported.

Constipation

Conditions in pregnancy that predispose the woman to constipation include general bowel sluggishness caused by increased progesterone and steroid metabolism; displacement of the intestines, which increases with the growth of the fetus; and oral iron supplements, which most pregnant women need.

Teaching for Self-Care Increased fluid intake (at least 2000 mL/day), adequate roughage or bulk in the diet, regular bowel habits, and adequate daily exercise can often maintain good bowel function in women who have not had previous problems. Some women find it helpful to drink a warm beverage or glass of prune juice in the morning. Women should leave sufficient time following breakfast so that the natural action of the body will produce defecation.

In severe or preexisting cases of constipation, the woman may need a mild laxative, stool softeners, or suppositories as recommended by her caregiver.

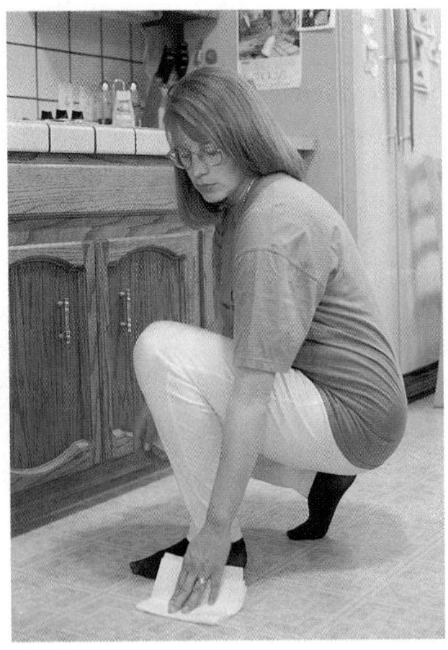

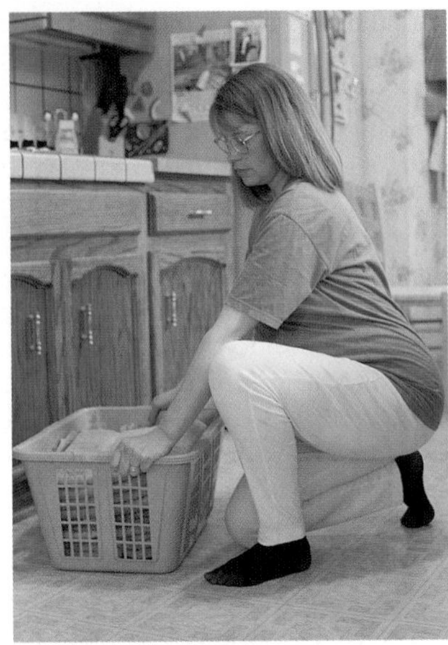

FIGURE 12–2 When picking up objects from floor level or lifting objects, the pregnant woman must use proper body mechanics.

Backache

Many pregnant women experience backache due primarily to the increased curvature of the lumbosacral vertebrae that occurs as the uterus enlarges and becomes heavier. Circulating steroid hormones cause a softening and relaxation of pelvic joints, contributing to the problem. If the woman does not learn how to correct this curvature, the strain on the muscles and ligaments will cause backache.

Teaching for Self-Care An exercise called the pelvic tilt (discussed later in this chapter) can help restore proper body alignment. As the anterior pelvis is tilted upward, the curvature of the back is automatically decreased, relieving much of the discomfort. If proper body alignment is maintained throughout pregnancy, backaches can be relieved or even prevented. See Exercises to Prepare for Childbirth, later in this chapter.

The use of proper posture and good body mechanics throughout pregnancy is important. The pregnant woman should avoid bending over to lift or pick up items from the floor. The strain is felt in the muscles of the back. Leg muscles should be used to do the work instead. The woman can keep her back straight by bending her knees to lower her body into the squatting position (Figure 12–2). She should place her feet 12 to 18 inches apart to maintain body balance. When lifting a heavy object, such as a child, she should place one foot flat on the floor, slightly in front of the other foot, and lower herself to the other knee. The object is held close to her body for lifting. This same principle of keeping the back straight and bending the knees applies when the woman sits down or gets out of a chair. Work heights that require constant bending can contribute to backache and should be adjusted as necessary.

A pendulous abdomen contributes to backache by increasing the curvature of the spine. The use of a supportive maternity girdle is discussed in Clothing, later in this chapter, as is the role of high-heeled shoes in increasing the lumbosacral curvature.

Leg Cramps

Leg cramps are painful muscle spasms in the gastrocnemius muscles. They occur most frequently at night after the woman has gone to bed but may occur at other times. Extension of the foot can often cause leg cramps. The nurse should warn the pregnant woman not to extend the foot during childbirth preparation exercises or during rest periods.

The exact cause of leg cramps is not known. Proposed contributing factors include an inadequate calcium intake, an imbalance in the calcium/phosphorus ratio, pressure of the enlarged uterus on the pelvic nerves leading to the legs, or pressure on the pelvic vessels causing impaired circulation.

Leg cramps are more common in the third trimester because of increased weight of the uterus on the nerves supplying the lower extremities. Fatigue and poor circulation in the lower extremities contribute to this problem.

Teaching for Self-Care The woman can achieve immediate relief of the muscle spasm by stretching the muscle. With the woman lying on her back, another person can press the woman's knee down to straighten her leg while pushing her foot toward her leg (Figure 12–3). The woman may also stand and put her foot flat on the floor. Massage and warm packs can be used to alleviate discomfort from leg cramps. Stretching exercises before bedtime may help prevent leg cramps. The caregiver may recommend that the woman drink no more than a pint of milk daily and take calcium carbonate or that she drink a quart of milk daily and take aluminum hydroxide gel. The gel absorbs phosphorus and eliminates it directly through the intestinal tract. The treatment recommendations depend on the frequency of the leg cramps.

Faintness

Many pregnant women occasionally feel faint, especially in warm, crowded areas. Faintness is caused by a combination of changes in the blood volume and postural hypotension due to venous pooling of blood in the dependent veins. Sudden change of position or standing for prolonged periods can cause this sensation, and fainting can occur.

Teaching for Self-Care The nurse should first be certain that the pregnant woman understands the symptoms of faintness. These include slight dizziness, a "swirling" or "floating" sensation, and a decreased ability to hear or focus attention. If a woman feels faint from prolonged standing or being in a warm, crowded room, she should sit down and lower her head between her knees. If this procedure does not help, the woman should be assisted to an area where she can lie down and get fresh air. When arising from a resting position, she should move slowly. Women whose jobs require standing in one place for long periods should march in place regularly to increase venous return from the legs.

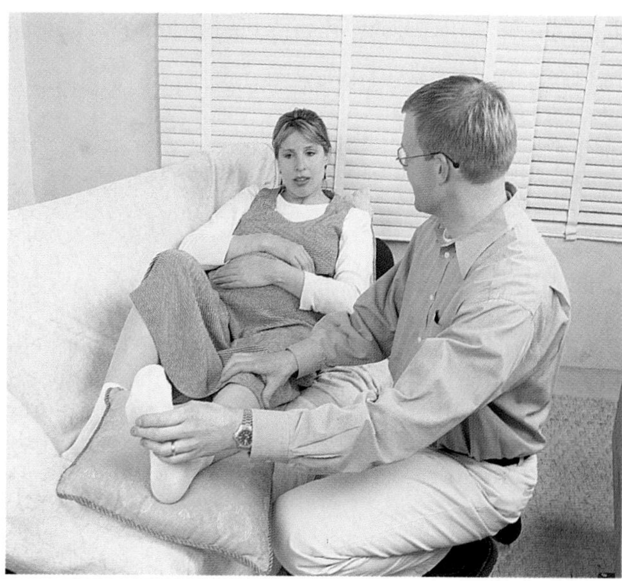

FIGURE 12–3 The expectant father can help relieve the woman's painful leg cramps by flexing her foot and straightening her leg.

Shortness of Breath

Shortness of breath occurs as the uterus rises into the abdomen and causes pressure on the diaphragm. This problem worsens in the last trimester as the enlarged uterus presses directly on the diaphragm, decreasing vital capacity. The primigravida experiences considerable relief from shortness of breath in the last few weeks of pregnancy, when **lightening** occurs, and the fetus and uterus move down in the pelvis. Because the multigravida does not usually experience lightening until labor, shortness of breath will continue throughout her pregnancy.

Teaching for Self-Care During the day, sitting straight in a chair and using proper posture when standing help provide relief. If distress is great at night, the woman can sleep propped up in bed with several pillows behind her head and shoulders.

Difficulty Sleeping

Although the pregnant woman may experience difficulty sleeping for many of the same psychologic reasons as the nonpregnant woman, many physical factors also contribute to this problem. The enlarged uterus may make it difficult to find a comfortable position for sleep, and an active fetus may aggravate the problem. The other discomforts of pregnancy such as urinary frequency, shortness of breath, and leg cramps may also be contributing factors.

Teaching for Self-Care The pregnant woman may find it helpful to drink a warm (caffeine-free) beverage before bed and may benefit from a soothing backrub given by her partner or a family member. Pillows may be used to provide support for her back, between her legs, or for her upper arm when she lies on her side. Relaxation techniques may also help. The woman should avoid caffeine products, stimulating activity, and sleeping medication.

Round Ligament Pain

As the uterus enlarges during pregnancy, the round ligaments stretch, hypertrophy, and lengthen as the uterus rises up in the abdomen. Round ligament pain is attributed to this stretching.

Teaching for Self-Care The woman may feel concern when she first experiences round ligament pain because it is often intense and causes a "grabbing" sensation in the lower abdomen and inguinal area. The nurse should warn women of this possible discomfort. Few treatment measures really alleviate this discomfort, but understanding the cause will help decrease anxiety. Once the caregiver has ascertained that the cause of the discomfort is not related to a medical complication such as appendicitis or gallbladder disease, the woman may find that a heating pad applied to the abdomen brings some relief. She may also benefit from bringing her knees up on her abdomen.

Carpal Tunnel Syndrome

Carpal tunnel syndrome (CTS) results from compression of the median nerve in the carpal tunnel of the wrist. The syndrome is commonly bilateral but may be more pronounced in the dominant hand and is characterized by numbness, tingling, or burning in the fleshy part of the

TABLE 12–4 The National Women's Health Information Center
For information on issues of importance to women's health:
Telephone: 1-800-994-WOMAN
Internet address: http://www.4woman.org
Sponsor: US Public Health Service Office on Women's Health

palm near the thumb. During pregnancy, weight gain and edema may contribute to the development of CTS (Samuels, 1996). The syndrome is aggravated by repetitive hand movements, such as typing, and may disappear following birth. Treatment involves splinting, avoiding aggravating movements, and in some cases injecting steroids into the carpal tunnel. Surgery is indicated in severe cases.

Teaching for Self-Care Although the condition is not preventable, the woman should be advised to avoid aggravating activities and use her splint as directed.

Promotion of Self-Care During Pregnancy

The pregnant woman is faced with the important responsibility of maintaining her health not only for her sake but also for the sake of her fetus. Nurses can help promote maternal and fetal well-being by providing expectant couples with accurate and complete information about health behaviors that can affect pregnancy and childbirth. Some women prefer to gather their own information. The nurse can refer these women to a variety of sources, including the National Women's Health Information Center, which is sponsored by the US Public Health Service's Office on Women's Health (Table 12–4).

Fetal Activity Monitoring

Many caregivers encourage pregnant women to monitor their unborn child's well-being by regularly assessing fetal activity. Vigorous fetal activity generally provides reassurance of fetal well-being, whereas a marked decrease in activity or cessation of movement may indicate possible fetal compromise requiring immediate evaluation. Fetal activity is affected by sound, drugs, cigarette smoking, fetal sleep state, blood glucose levels, and time of day. At times, a healthy fetus may be minimally active or inactive.

Fetal activity monitoring, beginning at 28 weeks' gestation, is recommended for all pregnant women because of the clearly established relationship between decreased fetal activity and fetal death (Druzin & Gabbe, 1996). A variety of methods for assessing fetal activity has been developed. They focus on having the woman keep a **fetal movement record (FMR),** such as the Cardiff Count-to-Ten Method (Figure 12–4). A FMR is a noninvasive technique that enables the pregnant woman to monitor and record fetal well-being easily and without expense. The woman's perceptions of fetal movements and her commitment to completing a movement record may vary. Ideally, when the woman understands the purpose of the assessment, how to complete the form, whom to call with questions, and what to report and has the opportunity for follow-up during each visit, she will see this as an important activity. The Self-Care Guide, Assessing Fetal Activity, at the end of this book describes the Cardiff Count-to-Ten Method and provides guidelines for using the scoring card (see Figure 12–4).

Breast Care

Whether the pregnant woman plans to bottle feed or breastfeed her infant, proper support of the breasts is important to promote comfort, retain breast shape, and prevent back strain, particularly if the breasts become large and pendulous. The sensitivity of the breasts in pregnancy is also relieved by good support.

A well-fitting, supportive brassiere has the following qualities:

- The straps are wide and do not stretch (elastic straps soon lose their tautness due to the weight of the breasts and frequent washing).
- The cup holds all breast tissue comfortably.
- The brassiere has tucks or other devices that allow it to expand, thus accommodating the enlarging chest circumference.
- The brassiere supports the nipple line approximately midway between the elbow and shoulder. At the same time, the brassiere is not pulled up in the back by the weight of the breasts.

Cleanliness of the breasts is important, especially as the woman begins producing colostrum. Colostrum that crusts on the nipples should be removed with warm water. The woman planning to breastfeed should not use soap on her nipples because of its drying effect.

Nipple preparation, begun during the third trimester, helps prevent soreness during the early days of breastfeeding. Nipple preparation promotes the distribution of the natural lubricants produced by Montgomery's tubercles and helps develop the protective layer of skin over the nipple. Women who are planning to nurse can begin by going braless when possible and by exposing their nipples to sunlight and air. Rubbing the nipples removes protective lubrication and should be avoided, but rolling the nipple may be beneficial. This is done by grasping the nipple between thumb and forefinger and gently rolling and pulling on it. A woman with a history of preterm labor is advised not to do this because nipple stimulation triggers the release of oxytocin. (See Chapter 17 for further discussion.)

Nipple rolling is more difficult for women with flat or inverted nipples, but it is still a useful preparation for

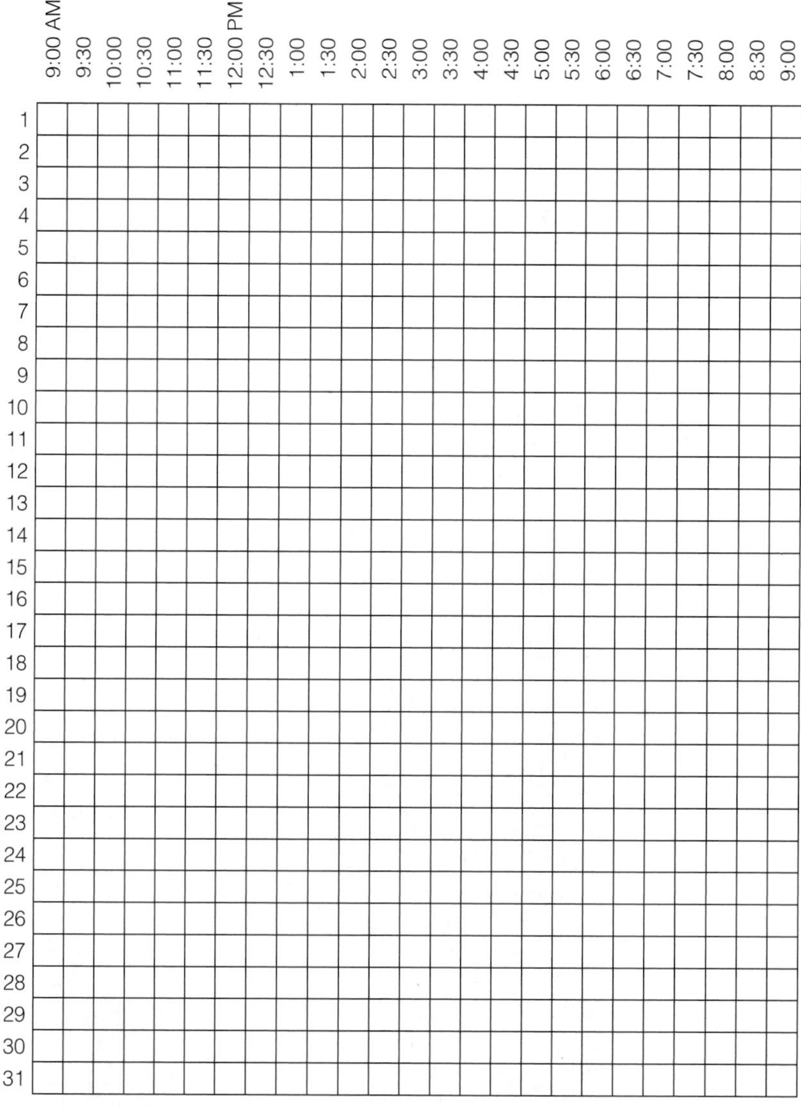

FIGURE 12–4 An adaptation of the Cardiff Count-to-Ten scoring card for fetal movement assessment.

breastfeeding. Nipple inversion is usually diagnosed during the initial antepartal assessment. Occasionally, a nipple appears inverted at all times. In other cases, the nipple appears normal initially, but pressure on the alveoli with the examiner's thumb and finger causes the nipple to retract. The normal or flat nipple protrudes when this is done (Figure 12–5).

The woman with nipple inversion can increase nipple protractility by performing Hoffman's exercises (Figure 12–6) (Hoffman, 1953). If the nipple is truly inverted, she can wear special breast shields (such as Woolrich or Eschmann shields) for the last 3 or 4 months of pregnancy (Figure 12–7). These shields tend to absorb moisture, so they should not be worn more than a few hours at a time. Breast shields appear to be the only measure that really helps women with inverted nipples.

Oral stimulation of the nipple by the woman's partner during sex play is also an excellent technique for toughening the nipple in preparation for breastfeeding. The couple who enjoy this stimulation should be encouraged to continue it throughout the pregnancy, except when the woman has a history of preterm labor, as discussed earlier.

Clothing

Maternity clothes are constructed with fuller lines to allow for the increase in abdominal size during pregnancy. Skirts and slacks have soft elastic waistbands and a stretchable panel over the abdominal area. Maternity clothing is expensive, however, and is worn for a relatively short time. Women can economize by sharing clothes with friends, sewing their own garments, or buying used maternity clothing.

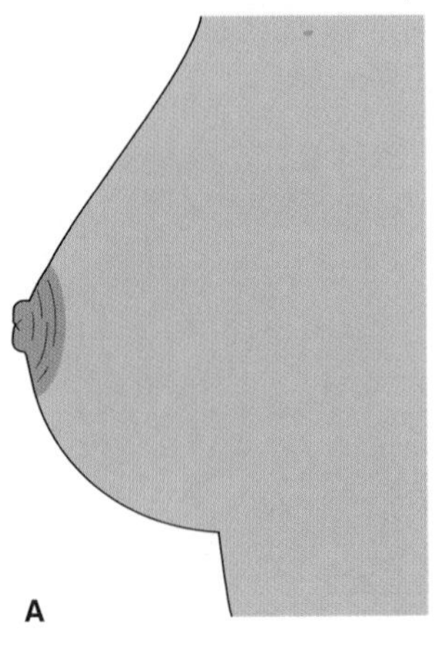

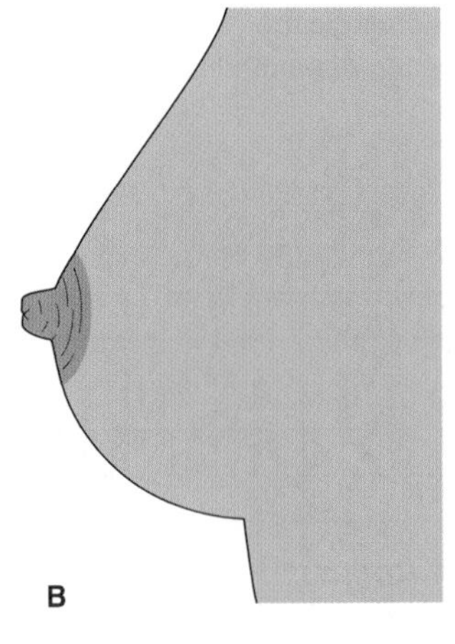

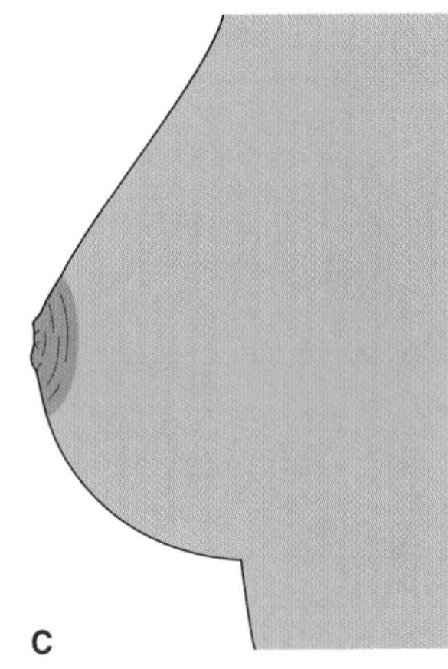

FIGURE 12–5 ***A,*** When not stimulated, normal and inverted nipples often look alike. ***B,*** When stimulated, the normal nipple protrudes. ***C,*** When stimulated, the inverted nipple retracts. However, great variation exists; in some women, for example, one or both nipples always appear inverted, even when not stimulated.

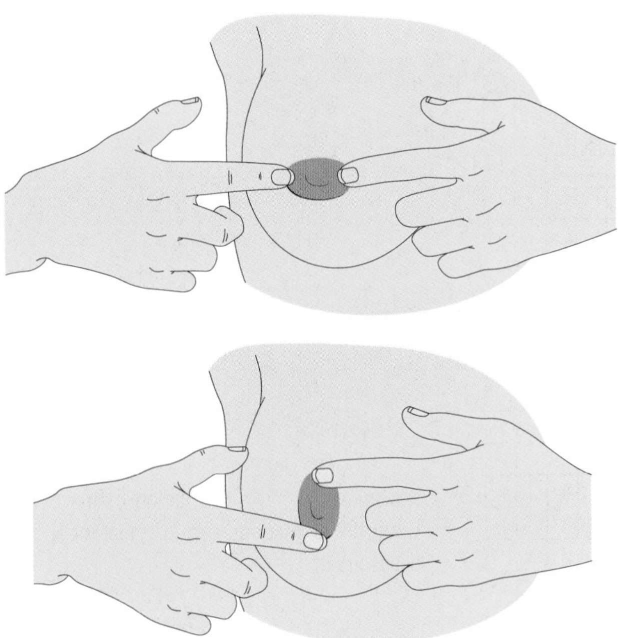

FIGURE 12–6 Hoffman's exercises are designed to increase nipple protractility. The woman is instructed to place her thumbs or index fingers opposite each other near the edge of the areola. She then presses into the breast and stretches outward to break any adhesions. This is done both horizontally and vertically.

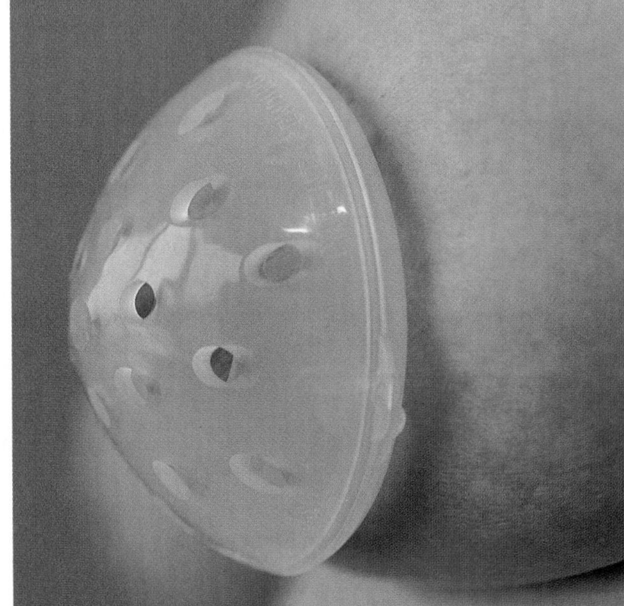

FIGURE 12–7 This breast shield is designed to increase the protractility of inverted nipples. Worn the last 3 to 4 months of pregnancy, they exert gentle pulling pressure at the edge of the areola, gradually forcing the nipple through the center of the shield. They may be used after birth if necessary.

Clothing should be loose and nonconstricting. Maternity girdles are seldom worn today and are not necessary for most women. They are sometimes used by women athletes, such as runners, dancers, or gymnasts, who maintain a light workout schedule during pregnancy. Women with large, pendulous abdomens may also benefit from a well-fitting, supportive girdle. Without this support, the pendulous abdomen increases the curvature of the spine and is a source of backache and general discomfort. Tight leg bands on girdles should be avoided.

High-heeled shoes aggravate back discomfort by increasing the curvature of the spine. They should not be worn if the woman experiences backache or problems with her balance. Shoes should fit properly and feel comfortable.

Bathing

Daily bathing is important because of the increased perspiration and mucoid vaginal discharge that occurs during pregnancy. The woman may take either a shower or a tub bath, according to her preference. Caution is needed during tub baths because balance becomes a problem as pregnancy advances. Rubber tub mats and hand grips are valuable safety devices. Moreover, vasodilation due to the warm water may cause the woman to experience some faintness when she attempts to get out of the tub. Thus she may require assistance, especially in the third trimester. *To avoid introducing infection, tub baths are contraindicated in the presence of vaginal bleeding or when the membranes are ruptured.*

Employment

Although research suggests no differences in perinatal outcomes between pregnant women who are employed and those who are not, these data may be influenced by the "healthy worker effect." This effect suggests that more healthy women continue to work during their pregnancies. Thus when these women are compared with nonworking pregnant women, the groups may not actually be comparable in terms of health, economic status, or educational level (DeJoseph, 1993). Pregnant women who are employed in jobs that require prolonged standing do have a higher incidence of preterm birth (Cunningham et al, 1997).

Major deterrents to employment during pregnancy include fetotoxic hazards in the environment, excessive physical strain, overfatigue, and medical or pregnancy-related complications. In the last half of pregnancy, occupations involving balance should be adjusted to protect the mother.

Fetotoxic hazards in the environment are always a concern to the expectant couple. If the pregnant woman or the woman contemplating pregnancy is working in industry, she should contact her company physician or nurse about possible hazards in her work environment and should do her own reading and research on environmental hazards as well.

Travel

If medical or pregnancy complications are not present, there are no restrictions on travel. Pregnant women should avoid travel if there is a history of bleeding or pregnancy-induced hypertension or if multiple births are anticipated.

Travel by automobile can be especially fatiguing, aggravating many of the discomforts of pregnancy. The pregnant woman needs frequent opportunities to get out of the car and walk. (A good pattern to follow is to stop every 2 hours and walk around for approximately 10 minutes.) She should wear both lap and shoulder belts. The lap belt should fit snugly and be positioned under the abdomen and across the upper thighs. Seat belts play an important role in preventing maternal mortality with subsequent fetal loss (Cunningham et al, 1997). Fetal loss in car accidents is also caused by placental separation as a result of uterine distortion. Use of the shoulder belt decreases the risk of traumatic flexion of the woman's body, thus decreasing the risk of placental separation.

As pregnancy progresses, travel by airplane or train is recommended for long distances. To avoid the development of phlebitis, pregnant women should be advised to request an aisle seat and walk about the plane at regular intervals. The availability of medical care at her destination is an important consideration for the near-term woman who travels.

Activity and Rest

CRITICAL THINKING QUESTION

What factors should be considered in advising a woman about exercise during pregnancy?

Exercise during pregnancy helps maintain maternal fitness and muscle tone, leads to improved self-image, increases energy, improves sleep, relieves tension, helps control weight gain, promotes regular bowel function, and is associated with improved postpartum recovery. Normal participation in regular exercise can continue and in fact is encouraged throughout an uncomplicated pregnancy. Physically fit women who run or do aerobic exercise regularly during pregnancy have been found to have less fetal distress during labor, shorter active labors, fewer cesarean births, and less meconium-stained amniotic fluid (Cunningham et al, 1997).

Before beginning an exercise program, a pregnant woman should be examined by her certified nurse-midwife or physician. A pregnant woman who is already in an exercise program can discuss her degree of participation with her caregiver. Women should also seek the opinion of their health care provider about taking part in strenuous sports, such as skiing and horseback riding. In general, the skilled sportswoman is no longer discouraged from participating in these activities if her pregnancy is uncomplicated. Pregnancy is not the time, however, to learn a new or strenuous sport.

High-risk activities requiring balance and coordination, such as sky diving, mountain climbing, ice skating, surfing, and racquetball should be avoided. In addition, women who are or may become pregnant should be advised not to scuba dive. Reports suggest that the fetus may be at greater risk during a dive than the mother. Risks include hyperoxia, hypoxia, hypercapnia, asphyxia, and decompression sickness (Speroff, 1997).

Certain conditions do contraindicate exercise. These include preterm rupture of the membranes, pregnancy-induced hypertension, incompetent cervix (cerclage), persistent second or third trimester bleeding, a history of

CRITICAL THINKING IN PRACTICE

Constance Petrowski, a 24-year-old, G1P0, world-class marathon runner, is 11 weeks pregnant when she sees the nurse-midwife for her first prenatal exam. Because of her low body fat, her menses have always been irregular, and it had not occurred to Constance that she might be pregnant. Constance tells the certified nurse-midwife that she has just begun serious training for a marathon that is to take place when Constance is about 22 weeks pregnant. Constance says she has been told that it is fine to continue any physical activity at which one is proficient and says that she would like to compete in the marathon because she believes she has a chance to come in as one of the top three women runners. What should the nurse tell Constance about competing in the marathon?

Answers can be found in Appendix I.

preterm labor in the prior or current pregnancy, or intrauterine growth retardation. Women with other obstetric conditions or preexisting medical conditions, such as chronic hypertension or cardiac or pulmonary disease, should be evaluated carefully to determine whether any form of exercise is appropriate (American College of Obstetricians and Gynecologists [ACOG], 1994).

Research related to the effects of maternal exercise on the fetus is varied and contradictory. Exercise can lead to increased maternal core temperature and hyperthermia. However, research suggests that the incidence of neural tube defects or other birth defects is not increased in the pregnancies of women who continue to exercise, even vigorously, during early pregnancy (ACOG, 1994).

Uterine blood flow is reduced during exercise as blood is shunted from visceral organs to muscles. The fetus does seem able to withstand this stress, however, without developing hypoxia. For most healthy pregnant women with no additional risk factors for preterm labor, exercise does not increase the incidence of preterm labor and birth or baseline uterine activity (ACOG, 1994).

The American College of Obstetricians and Gynecologists (ACOG) has formulated guidelines about exercise during pregnancy (ACOG, 1994). These include:

- Even mild to moderate exercise is beneficial during pregnancy. Regular exercise—that is, at least three times a week—is preferred.
- After the first trimester, women should avoid exercising in the supine position. In most pregnant women, the supine position is associated with decreased cardiac output. Because uterine blood flow is reduced during exercise as blood is shunted from the visceral organs to the muscles, the remaining cardiac output is further decreased. Similarly, women should avoid standing motionless for prolonged periods.
- Because decreased oxygen is available for aerobic exercise during pregnancy, women should modify the intensity of their exercise based on their symptoms, should stop when they become fatigued, and should avoid exercising to the point of exhaustion. Non-weight-bearing exercises, such as swimming or cycling, are recommended because they decrease the risk of injury and provide fitness with comfort.
- As pregnancy progresses and the center of gravity changes, especially in the third trimester, exercises in which the loss of balance could pose a risk to mother or fetus should be avoided. Similarly, the woman should avoid any type of exercise that might result in even mild abdominal trauma.
- A normal pregnancy requires an additional 300 kcal per day. Women who exercise regularly during pregnancy should be careful to ensure that they consume an adequate diet.
- To augment heat dissipation, especially during the first trimester, pregnant women who exercise should wear appropriate clothing, ensure adequate hydration, and avoid the prolonged overheating associated with vigorous exercise in hot, humid weather. By the same token, they should avoid hot tubs and saunas. Research suggests that maternal exposure to heat (hot tubs, sauna, or fever) in the first trimester is associated with an increased risk of neural tube defects, mental deficiencies, seizures, facial abnormalities, and external ear anomalies in the fetus/newborn (Rogers & Davis, 1995).

The woman should avoid reaching her maximum physical effort during pregnancy. Two tips help her exercise in the safe range (Speroff, 1997):

1. While exercising, the pregnant woman should be able to carry on a conversation.
2. The upper limit of the woman's pulse rate should not exceed 70% of 220 minus her age. For example, a 28-year-old pregnant woman should not let her pulse rate increase above 126 bpm.

In addition to the previously discussed recommendations, the nurse may suggest that the woman wear a supportive bra and appropriate shoes when exercising. She should be advised to warm up and stretch to help prepare the joints for activity and cool down with a period of mild activity to help restore circulation and avoid pooling of blood. A moderate, rhythmic exercise routine involving large muscle groups such as swimming, cycling, walking, or cross-country skiing is best. Jogging or running is acceptable for women already conditioned to these activities as long as they avoid exercising at maximum effort and overheating.

Warning signs of overexertion include the following: back pain, absent fetal movement, difficulty walking, dizziness or faintness, pain, palpitations, pubic pain, shortness of breath, tachycardia, uterine contractions, vaginal bleeding, or fluid loss (Artal & Buckenmeyer, 1995). The woman should stop exercising if these occur and modify her exercise program. If the symptoms persist, the woman should contact her caregiver.

Adequate rest in pregnancy is important for both physical and emotional health. Women need more sleep throughout pregnancy, particularly in the first and last trimesters, when they tire easily. Without adequate rest, pregnant women have less resilience.

Finding time to rest during the day may be difficult for women who work or have small children. The nurse can help the expectant mother examine her daily schedule to develop a realistic plan for short periods of rest and relaxation.

Sleeping becomes more difficult during the last trimester because of the enlarged abdomen, increased frequency of urination, and greater activity of the fetus. Finding a comfortable position becomes difficult for the pregnant woman. Figure 12–8 shows a position most pregnant women find comfortable. Progressive relaxation techniques similar to those taught in prepared childbirth classes can help prepare the woman for sleep.

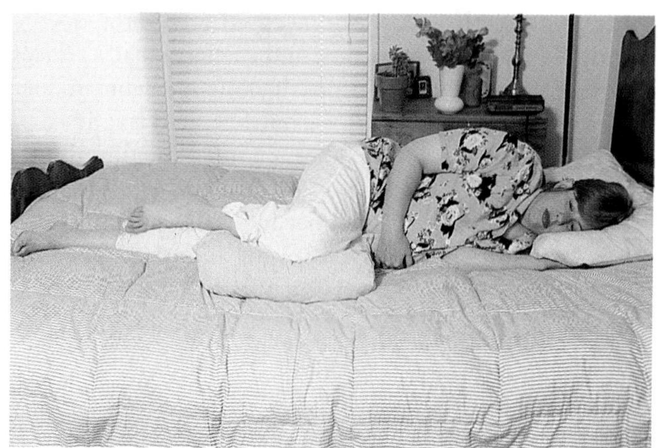

FIGURE 12–8 Position for relaxation and rest as pregnancy progresses.

Exercises to Prepare for Childbirth

Certain exercises help strengthen muscle tone in preparation for birth and promote more rapid restoration of muscle tone after birth. The woman can reduce some physical changes of pregnancy considerably by faithfully practicing prescribed body-conditioning exercises. Many body-conditioning exercises for pregnancy are taught; a few of the more common ones are discussed here.

The **pelvic tilt,** or pelvic rocking, helps prevent or reduce back strain and strengthens abdominal muscle tone. To do the pelvic tilt, the pregnant woman lies on her back and puts her feet flat on the floor. This bent position of the knees helps prevent strain and discomfort. She decreases the curvature in her back by pressing her spine toward the floor. With her back pressed to the floor, the woman tightens her buttocks and abdominal muscles as she tucks in her buttocks. The pelvic tilt can also be performed on hands and knees (Figure 12–9), while sitting in a chair, or while standing with the back against a wall. The body alignment achieved when the pelvic tilt is correctly done should be maintained as much as possible throughout the day.

CLINICAL TIP

Doing the pelvic rock on hands and knees may aggravate back strain. Teach women with a history of minor back problems to do the pelvic rock only in the standing position.

Abdominal Exercises

A basic exercise to increase abdominal muscle tone is tightening abdominal muscles in synchronization with respirations. It can be done in any position, but it is best learned while the woman lies supine. With knees flexed and feet flat on the floor, the woman expands her abdomen and slowly takes a deep breath. As she slowly exhales, she gradually pulls in her abdominal muscles until they are fully contracted. She relaxes for a few seconds and then repeats the exercise.

Partial sit-ups strengthen abdominal muscle tone and are done according to individual comfort levels. When doing a partial sit-up, the woman lies on the floor as described above (Figure 12–10). This exercise is done with the knees bent and the feet flat on the floor to avoid undue strain on the lower back. She stretches her arms toward her knees as she slowly pulls her head and shoulders off the floor to a comfortable level. (If she has poor abdominal muscle tone, she may not be able to pull up very far.) She then slowly returns to the starting position, takes a deep breath, and repeats the exercise. To strengthen the oblique abdominal muscles, she repeats the process, but stretches the left arm to the side of her right knee, returns to the floor, takes a deep breath, and then reaches with the right arm to the left knee.

These exercises can be done approximately five times in a sequence, and the sequence can be repeated several times during the day as desired. It is important that the woman do the exercises slowly to prevent muscle strain and overtiring.

Perineal Exercises

Perineal muscle tightening, also referred to as **Kegel exercises,** strengthens the pubococcygeus muscle and increases its elasticity (Figure 12–11). The woman can feel the specific muscle group to be exercised by stopping urination midstream. However, doing Kegel exercises while urinating is discouraged because this practice has been associated with urinary stasis and urinary tract infection.

Childbirth educators sometimes use the following technique to teach Kegel exercises. They tell the woman to think of her perineal muscles as an elevator. When she relaxes, the elevator is on the first floor. To do the exercises, she contracts, bringing the elevator to the second, third, and fourth floors. She keeps the elevator on the fourth floor for a few seconds, and then gradually relaxes the area. If the exercise is properly done, the woman does not contract the muscles of the buttocks and thighs.

Kegel exercises can be done at almost any time. Some women use ordinary events—for instance, stopping at a red light—as a cue to remember to do the exercise. Others do Kegel exercises while waiting in a checkout line, talking on the telephone, or watching television.

Inner Thigh Exercises

The pregnant woman should assume a cross-legged sitting position whenever possible. This "tailor sit" stretches the muscles of the inner thighs in preparation for labor and birth.

Sexual Activity

As a result of the physiologic, anatomic, and emotional changes of pregnancy, the couple usually have many

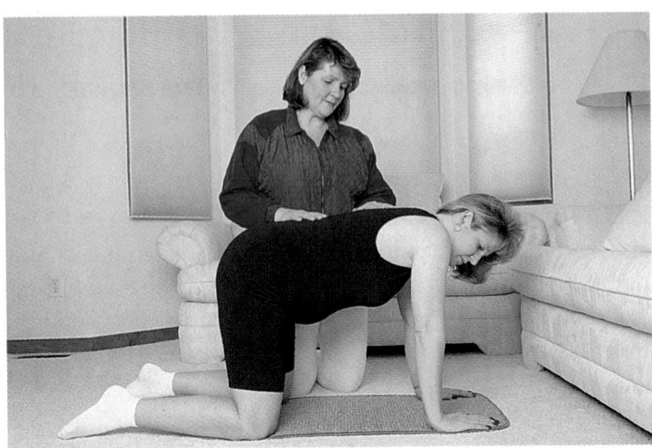

A

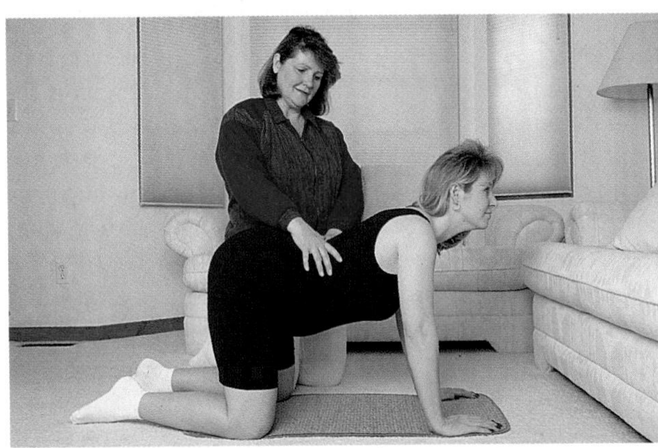

B

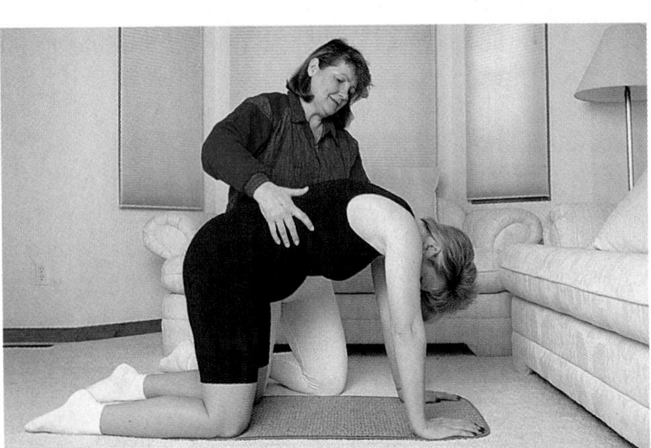

C

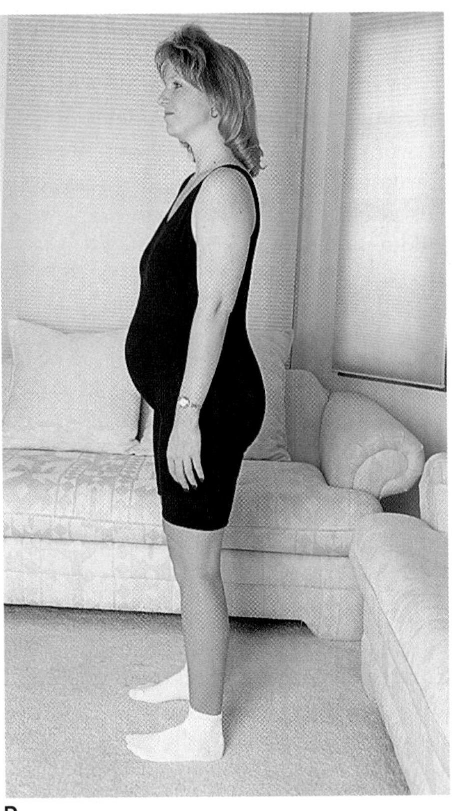

D

FIGURE 12–9 ***A,*** Starting position when the pelvic tilt is done on hands and knees. The back is flat and parallel to the floor, the hands are under the head, and the knees are directly under the buttocks. ***B,*** A prenatal yoga instructor offers pointers for proper positioning for the first part of the tilt: head up, neck long and separated from the shoulders, buttocks up, and pelvis thrust back, allowing the back to drop and release on an inhaled breath. ***C,*** The instructor helps the woman assume the correct position for the next part of the tilt. It is done on a long exhalation, allowing the pregnant woman to arch her back, drop her head loosely, push away from her hands, and draw in the muscles of her abdomen to strengthen them. Note that in this position the pelvis and buttocks are tucked under, and the buttock muscles are tightened. ***D,*** Proper posture. The knees are slightly bent but not locked, the pelvis and buttocks are tucked under, thereby lengthening the spine and helping support the weighty abdomen. With her chin tucked in, this woman's neck, shoulders, hips, knees, and feet are all in a straight line perpendicular to the floor. Her feet are parallel. This is also the starting position for doing the pelvic tilt while standing.

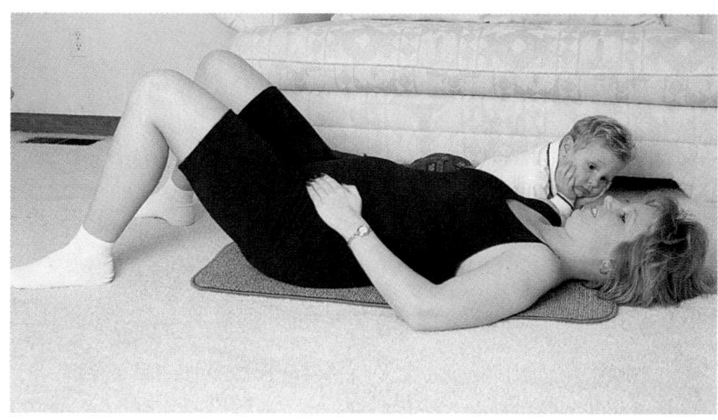

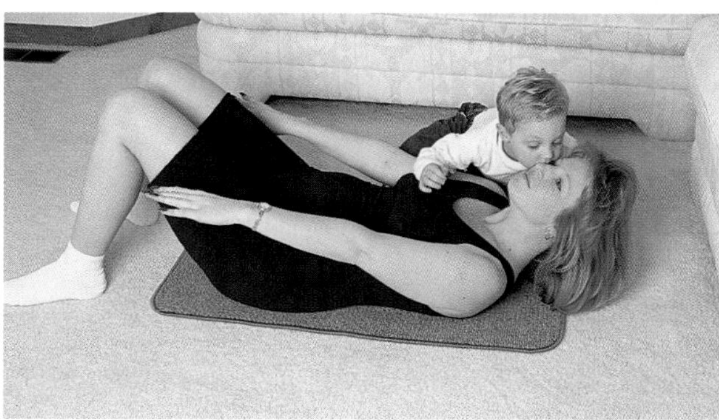

FIGURE 12–10 The pregnant woman can strengthen her abdominal muscles by doing partial sit-ups.

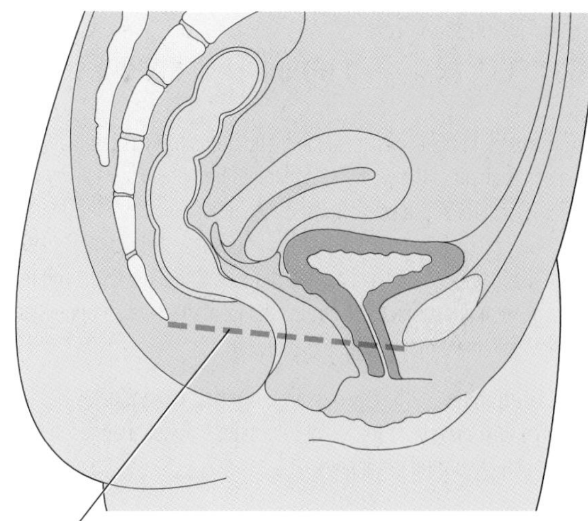

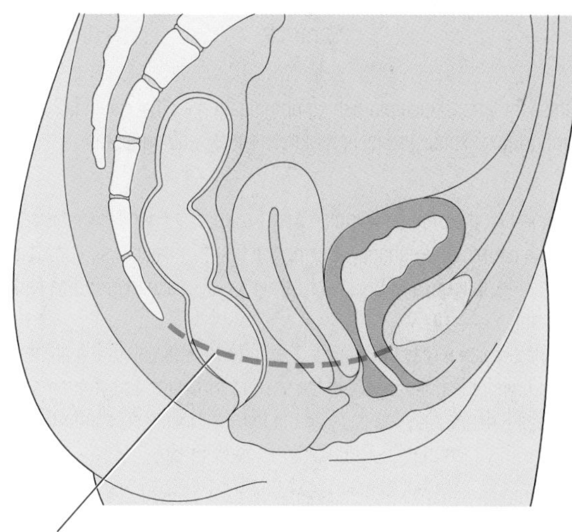

FIGURE 12–11 Kegel exercises. The woman tightens the pubococcygeus muscle to improve support to the pelvic organs.

questions and concerns about sexual activity during pregnancy. Often these questions are about possible injury to the baby or the woman during intercourse and about changes in the desire each partner feels for the other.

In the past, couples were frequently warned to avoid sexual intercourse during the last 6 to 8 weeks of pregnancy to prevent complications such as infection or premature rupture of the membranes. However, these fears seem to be unfounded. In a healthy pregnancy, there is no valid reason to limit sexual activity. Intercourse is contraindicated when bleeding is present or the membranes are ruptured. Women with a history of preterm labor or premature rupture of the membranes and those who experience strong uterine contractions following intercourse should be advised to use a condom or avoid sexual activity because increased uterine activity may be due to breast stimulation, female orgasm, or prostaglandins in the male ejaculate (Johnson, Walker, & Niebyl, 1996).

The expectant mother may experience changes in sexual desire and response. Often these are related to the various discomforts that occur throughout pregnancy. For instance, during the first trimester, fatigue or nausea and vomiting may decrease desire, and breast tenderness may make the woman less responsive to fondling of her breasts. During the second trimester, many of the discomforts have lessened, and with the vascular congestion of the pelvis the woman may experience even greater sexual satisfaction than she experienced prior to pregnancy.

During the third trimester, interest in coitus may again decrease as the woman becomes more uncomfortable and fatigued. In addition, shortness of breath, painful pelvic ligaments, urinary frequency, and decreased mobility may lessen sexual desire and activity. If they are not already using them, the couple should consider coital positions other than male superior, such as side-by-side, female superior, and vaginal rear entry.

Sexual activity does not have to include intercourse. Many of the nurturing and sexual needs of the pregnant

TEACHING GUIDE: SEXUAL ACTIVITY DURING PREGNANCY

Assessment In many cases teaching about this topic is coupled with ongoing assessment of the woman's understanding of sexual activity during pregnancy. Occasionally, a woman will indicate her beliefs about sexual activity during pregnancy by asking a direct question. This is most likely to occur if you and your client have a good rapport. Often, however, you must ask some general questions to determine the woman's level of understanding, or a general statement may trigger a discussion.

Nursing Diagnosis The key nursing diagnosis will probably be ***Knowledge deficit*** related to lack of information about changes in sexuality and sexual activity during pregnancy.

Nursing Plan and Implementation The teaching plan will focus on discussion or you may use a "question-and-answer" format. The presence of both partners may be beneficial in fostering communication between them and is acceptable unless personal or cultural factors indicate otherwise.

Client Goals At the completion of teaching the woman will be able to:

- Relate the changes in sexuality and sexual response that may occur during pregnancy to changes in technique, frequency, and response.
- Explore personal attitudes, beliefs, and expectations about sexual activity during pregnancy.
- Cite maternal factors that would contraindicate sexual intercourse.

Teaching Plan

Content	*Teaching Method*
• Stress the importance of open communication so that the couple feels comfortable expressing feelings, preferences, and concerns.	*Some couples are skilled at expressing their feelings about sexual activity. Others find it difficult and can benefit from specific suggestions. Provide opportunities for discussion throughout the teaching session.*
• Explain that the pregnant woman may experience changes in desire during the course of pregnancy. During the first trimester, discomforts such as nausea, fatigue, and breast tenderness may make intercourse less desirable. Some women may have fewer discomforts and may find that their sexual desire is unchanged. In the second trimester, as symptoms decrease, desire may increase. In the third trimester, discomfort and fatigue may lead to decreased desire in the woman.	*Universal statements that give permission, such as "Many couples experience changes in sexual desire during pregnancy. What kind of changes have you experienced?" are often effective in starting discussion. Depending on the woman's (or couple's) level of knowledge and sophistication, part or all of this discussion may be necessary.*
• Explain that men may notice changes in their level of desire, too. Among other things, this phemomenon may be related to feelings about their partner's changing appearance, their belief about the acceptability of sexual activity with a pregnant woman, or concern about hurting the woman or fetus. Some men find the changes of pregnancy erotic; others must adjust to the notion of their partner as a mother.	*If the partner is present, approach him in the same nonjudgmental way used above. If not, ask the woman if she has noticed any changes in her partner or if he has expressed any concerns.*
• Explain that the woman may notice that orgasms are much more intense during the last weeks of pregnancy and may be followed by cramping. Because of the presence of the enlarging uterus on the vena cava, the woman should not lie flat on her back for intercourse after about the fourth month. If the couple prefer that position, a pillow should be placed under her right hip to displace the uterus. Alternate positions such as side-lying, female superior, or vaginal rear entry may become necessary as her uterus enlarges.	*Deal with any specific questions about the physical and psychologic changes that the couple may have.*
• Stress that the sexual activities that both partners enjoy are generally acceptable. It is not advisable, however, for couples who favor anal sex to go from anal penetration to vaginal penetration because of the risk of introducing *E coli* into the vagina.	*Discussion about various sexual activities requires that you be comfortable with your sexuality and that you be tactful. Often you may find it advisable to volunteer information about yourself to show that discussion of sexual variations is acceptable.*

TEACHING GUIDE *CONTINUED*

Teaching Plan

Content	*Teaching Method*
• Suggest that alternative methods of expressing intimacy and affection such as cuddling, holding and stroking each other, and kissing may help maintain the couple's feelings of warmth and closeness. If the man feels desire for further sexual release, his partner may help him masturbate to ejaculation, or he may prefer to masturbate in private. Advise the woman who is interested in masturbation as a form of gratification that the orgasmic contractions may be especially intense in later pregnancy.	*The couple may be content with these approaches to meeting their sexual needs, or they may require assurance that such approaches are indeed "normal."*
• Stress that sexual intercourse is contraindicated once the membranes are ruptured or if bleeding is present. Women with a history of preterm labor may be advised to avoid intercourse because the oxytocin that is released with orgasm stimulates uterine contractions and may trigger preterm labor. Because oxytocin is also released with nipple stimulation, fondling the breasts may be contraindicated as well.	*An explanation of the contraindications accompanied by their rationale provides specific guidelines that most couples find helpful.*

Evaluation Determine the effectiveness of teaching by evaluating the woman's (or couple's) response to information throughout the discussion. You may also ask the woman to express information—such as the contraindications to intercourse—in her own words. Follow-up sessions and questions from the woman also provide information about teaching effectiveness.

woman can be satisfied by cuddling, kissing, and being held. The warm, sensual feelings that accompany these activities can be an end in themselves. Her partner, however, may need to masturbate more frequently than before.

The sexual desires of men are also affected by many factors in pregnancy. These include the previous relationship with the partner, acceptance of the pregnancy, attitudes toward the partner's change of appearance, and concern about hurting the expectant mother or baby. Some men may withdraw from sexual contact because of a belief that sex with a pregnant woman is immoral. This may be especially true for the couple whose religious beliefs teach that sexual intercourse is only for procreation. Some men find it difficult to view their partners as sexually appealing while they are adjusting to the concept of her as a mother. Other men feel their partner's pregnancy is arousing and experience feelings of increased happiness, intimacy, and closeness.

The expectant couple should be aware of their changing sexual desires, the normality of these changes, and the importance of communicating these changes to each other so that they can make nurturing adaptations. The nurse has an important role in addressing the sexuality concerns of the expectant couple in order to enhance the mother's self-image and promote a healthy, caring relationship for the couple (Alteneder & Hartzell, 1997). The couple must feel free to express concerns about sexual activity, and the nurse must be able to respond and give anticipatory guidance in a comfortable manner. See the accompanying Teaching Guide.

Dental Care

Proper dental hygiene is important in pregnancy. In spite of such discomforts as nausea and vomiting, gum hypertrophy and tenderness, possible ptyalism, and heartburn, regular oral hygiene must not be neglected.

The pregnant woman is encouraged to have a dental checkup early in her pregnancy. General dental repair and extractions can be done during pregnancy, preferably under local anesthetic. The woman should inform her dentist of her pregnancy so that she is not exposed to teratogenic substances. Dental x-ray examinations and extensive dental work should be delayed when possible until after birth. Extensive dental care during pregnancy requires consultation between the dentist and the woman's health care professional.

Immunizations

All women of childbearing age need to be fully aware of the risks of receiving specific immunizations if pregnancy

TABLE 12–5 Summary of Recommendations for Immunization During Pregnancy

Live Virus Vaccines	Inactive Bacterial Vaccines	Hyperimmune Globulins
Measles–contraindicated	Cholera–to meet international travel requirements	Hepatitis B–potexposure prophylaxis; given along with hepatitis B vaccine initially, then vaccine alone at 1 and 6 months
Mumps–contraindicated	Pneumoccoccus–same as nonpregnant	Rabies–postexposure prophylaxis
Poliomyelitis–not routine; increased risk exposure	Plague–selective vaccination of exposed persons	Tetanus–postexposure prophylaxis
Yellow fever–travel to high-risk areas only	Typhoid–travel to endemic areas	Varicella–consider for postexposure (within 96 months)
Inactive Virus Vaccines	**Toxoids**	**Pooled Immune Serum Globulins**
Influenza–underlying diseases; client request	Tetanus-diptheria–same as nonpregnant	Hepatitis A–postexposure prophylaxis
Rabies–same as nonpregnant		Measles–postexposure prophylaxis
Hepatitis B–at high risk and negative for B antigen		

SOURCE: Cunningham FG et al: *Williams Obstetrics*, 20th ed. Stamford, CT: Appleton & Lange, 1997, p 243.

is possible. Expectant women, especially those who intend to travel internationally, should be aware of the immunizations that are contraindicated during pregnancy. Immunizations with attenuated live viruses, such as rubella vaccine, should not be given in pregnancy because of the possible harmful effect of the live viruses on the developing embryo. Vaccinations using killed viruses can be used. Recommendations for immunizations during pregnancy are summarized in Table 12–5.

Teratogenic Substances

Substances that adversely affect the normal growth and development of the fetus are called **teratogens.** Many of these effects are readily apparent at birth, but others may not be identified for years. A well-known example is the development of cervical cancer in adolescent females whose mothers took diethylstilbestrol (DES) during pregnancy.

Many substances are suspected teratogens. Substances that have documented teratogenic effects include some pesticides and exposure to radiation (x-rays, radioactive iodine, and atomic fallout) in the first trimester of pregnancy.

Some environmental factors are also suspected to be teratogenic; however, the complexities of the interrelationships among them make causal relationships difficult to demonstrate. For example, expectant women who live in high-altitude areas have been found to have an increased incidence of small-for-gestational-age (SGA) babies.

Medications are perhaps the most likely documented teratogens, but other factors can also harm the fetus, including certain infections such as rubella, syphilis, herpesvirus type 2, toxoplasmosis, and cytomegalovirus (CMV). Hyperthermia, especially if it occurs in the critical period of organ development, may account for the increased incidence of congenital anomalies that has been associated with the use of hot tubs and saunas early in pregnancy (Rogers & Davis, 1995).

During pregnancy, women need to have adequate information available and a realistic perspective on potential environmental hazards. Factors that are suspected to be hazardous to the general population should obviously be avoided if possible.

Medications

The use of medication in pregnancy is of great concern. Studies have demonstrated that the average pregnant woman takes many more medications than commonly believed, including over-the-counter (OTC) drugs as well as prescription drugs. Medications sold over the counter can be as dangerous as prescription drugs. For example, aspirin is known to inhibit prostaglandin synthesis. This may result in prolonged pregnancy or labor if the woman has used aspirin regularly. Aspirin also interferes with platelet functioning, which may increase the risk of bleeding antepartally or at birth (Niebyl, 1996).

Many pregnant women need medication for therapeutic purposes, such as the treatment of infections, allergies, or other pathologic processes. In these situations, the problem can be extremely complex. Known teratogenic agents are not prescribed and usually can be replaced by medications considered safe. Even when a woman is highly motivated to avoid taking any medications, she may have taken potentially teratogenic medications before her pregnancy was diagnosed, especially if she had an irregular menstrual cycle.

The greatest potential for gross abnormalities in the fetus occurs during the first trimester of pregnancy, when fetal organs are first developing. The classic period of teratogenesis in a woman with a 28-day cycle extends from day 31 after the LMP (17 days after fertilization) to day 71 (54 days after fertilization) (Niebyl, 1996). Many factors influence teratogenic effects, including the specific identity and dose of the teratogen, the state of embryo development, and the genetic sensitivity of the mother and fetus (ACOG, 1997c). For example, the commonly prescribed acne medication isotretinoin (Accutane) is associated with a high incidence of spontaneous abortion and congenital malformations if taken early in pregnancy. Valproic acid, an anticonvulsant, is associated with an increased risk of spina bifida.

To provide information for caregivers and clients, the Food and Drug Administration has developed the follow-

RESEARCH IN PRACTICE

What is the study about? Each year between 500,000 and 700,000 infants are exposed annually to illicit drugs in utero. According to the National Institute on Drug Abuse, of the 60 million women of childbearing age (15 to 44 years) residing in the United States, 50.8% use alcohol, 29% smoke cigarettes, 8% use illicit drugs, 6.5% use marijuana, and 3.5% use cocaine. Surveys from the National Institute on Drug Abuse indicate that a general decline in the use of illicit drugs has occurred over the last 20 years. When the mother and/or infant are exposed to stressors (eg, substance abuse and its concomitant medical problems), their interactions are at risk. The purpose of this study was to determine whether teaching comforting and interacting techniques to substance-abusing mothers within 24 hours of childbirth would improve mother–infant interactions 48 to 72 hours after hospital discharge.

How was the study done? This study used an intervention (experimental), control, and comparison group pretest, posttest design. The study was conducted in a 550-bed, inner city, private hospital that predominately serves indigent mothers and has 1800 births a year. Eighty-three women whose urine was positive for drugs during their prenatal visits at a high-indigent populated clinic were invited to participate in the study. Sixty mother–infant couplets completed the study. Inclusion criteria were: (a) a newborn weighing a minimum of 2500 gms and 37 to 42 weeks gestation; (b) mothers and newborns without serious or life-threatening problems at birth; (c) both mother and newborn having positive drug tests at birth. Three groups (experimental, control, and comparison groups) each containing 20 participants (10 first-time mothers and 10 mothers with more than one child) served as the sample for this study. Two observers, blinded to the population and the mother's drug history, completed the Nursing Child Assessment Feeding Scale (NCAFS) on all couplets within 24 hours of birth. Mothers in the experimental group were shown a culturally sensitive video demonstrating techniques on comforting and interacting with a high-risk newborn. The researchers showed the mothers how to recognize the newborn's cues, and demonstrated methods of comforting. Mothers in the control group were given a booklet based on the concepts in the video. Forty-eight to seventy-two hours after discharge, each mother was observed feeding the infant in her home setting. Control and comparison groups were given a booklet on infant interactions in the home setting.

What were the results of the study? At the home visit, couplets in the experimental group showed significant improvement in their total NCAFS score. The mean home NCAFS increased 8.5 points and the NCAFS score of the control group decreased by 2.6 points.

What additional questions might I have? (1) What effects might the home setting have on the mother's ability to respond to the infant's cues (eg, increased stress, more responsibilities, increased people interacting with the infant); and (2) Do drug-addicted infants show different cues overall than nonaddicted infants?

How can I use this study? The study poses interesting nursing interventions that can impact couplet interactions in drug-addicted mothers. The nursing assessments and counseling during the feeding experience may be important factors for improving couplet interactions. A video and educational program stressing the effects of substance use on pregnancy, the developing fetus, and couplet interaction could be presented at the first prenatal visit. Continued discussion of interaction skills and teaching at subsequent visits could better prepare these mothers for optimal parenting. After childbirth, early assessment of couplet interactions could provide information to aid nurses in designing interventions to assist mothers in developing more sensitive responses to their infants' behavioral cues.

SOURCE: French, E., Pituch, M., Brandt, J., & Pohorecki, S. (1998). Improving interactions between substance abusing mothers and their substance exposed newborns. *JOGNN, 27*(3), 262–269.

ing classification system for medications administered during pregnancy:

Category A. Controlled studies in women have demonstrated no associated fetal risk. Few drugs fall into this category. Vitamin C is cited as a category A drug as long as its use does not exceed the recommended dietary allowance.

Category B. Either animal studies show no risk, but there are no controlled studies in women; or animal studies indicate a risk, but controlled human studies fail to demonstrate a risk. The penicillins fall into this category.

Category C. Either (1) no adequate studies, either in animals or women, are available; or (2) animal studies show teratogenic effects, but no controlled studies in women are available. Many drugs fall into this category, and the lack of information poses a problem for caregivers. Zidovudine, a drug used to decrease perinatal transmission of human immunodeficiency virus (HIV), falls into this category.

Category D. Evidence of human fetal risk does exist, but the benefits of the drug in certain situations are thought to outweigh the risks. Examples in this category include tetracycline, vincristine, lithium, and hydrochlorothiazide.

Category X. The demonstrated fetal risks clearly outweigh any possible benefit. An example of a drug in this category is isotretinoin (Accutane), the acne medication, which can cause multiple central nervous system (CNS), facial, and cardiovascular anomalies.

If a woman has taken a drug in category D or X, she should be informed of the risks associated with that drug and of her alternatives. Similarly, a woman who has taken a drug in the safer categories can be reassured (Cunningham et al, 1997).

This system, while useful, has been criticized because the letter system suggests a risk grading that is not necessarily accurate. More importantly, not all drugs in a category have the same risk level. Currently the FDA is working to develop a new labeling system (Whitney, 1999).

Although the first trimester is the critical period for teratogenesis, some medications are known to have teratogenic effect when taken in the second and third trimesters. For example, tetracycline taken in late pregnancy is commonly associated with staining of teeth in children and has been shown to depress skeletal growth, especially in preterm infants. Sulfonamides taken in the last weeks of pregnancy are known to compete with bilirubin attachment of protein-binding sites, increasing the risk of jaundice in the newborn (Niebyl, 1996). Warfarin (Coumadin), a commonly prescribed anticoagulant, is associated with CNS defects following fetal exposure during the second and third trimesters (Cunningham et al, 1997). Because heparin does not cross the placenta, it is safer for the fetus than warfarin and other anticoagulants.

Pregnant women should avoid all medication if possible. If no alternative exists, it is wisest to select a well-known medication rather than a newer drug whose potential teratogenic effects may not be known. When possible, the oral form of the drug should be used, and it should be prescribed in the lowest possible therapeutic dose for the shortest time possible. Finally, the caregiver should carefully consider the multiple components of the medication.

A woman clearly has a right to the most comprehensive information available concerning medications. The nurse can assist her by suggesting appropriate references and helping her research information. Some excellent reference books on drugs and pregnancy are currently available and should be part of the library of every office and clinic that provides prenatal care. In addition, several on-line databases that provide information on teratogens are available for convenient reference.

The nurse should remind the woman of the need to check with her caregiver about medications she was taking when pregnancy occurred and about any nonprescription drugs she is contemplating using. Any medication with possible teratogenic effects must be avoided.

Tobacco

Smoking has been linked to higher infertility rates in both men and women. In women, smoking has been identified as a factor in ovulatory, tubal function, and implantation disorders, as well as oocyte depletion and early pregnancy loss. In men, smoking has been linked to impaired sperm concentration and changes in sperm motility and morphology (ACOG, 1997b).

Infants of mothers who smoke tend to have a lower birth weight and a higher incidence of perinatal deaths than infants of mothers who do not smoke (Cunningham et al, 1997). In addition, mothers who smoke have an increased risk of spontaneous abortion, preterm birth, placenta previa, abruptio placentae, and premature rupture of the membranes. This risk is related to the number of cigarettes smoked (ACOG, 1997b). Research also links maternal smoking, both during pregnancy and afterward, with an increased risk of sudden infant death syndrome (SIDS), as well as with an increased risk of acute respiratory illnesses and chronic respiratory symptoms for infants (ACOG, 1997b).

The specific mechanism by which smoking affects the fetus is not known. However, the main ingredients in cigarette smoke that account for adverse effects in the fetus are carbon monoxide and nicotine because they decrease the availability of oxygen to maternal and fetal tissues (ACOG, 1997b). Cigarette smoking can also cause adverse fetal effects by decreasing maternal appetite, which can negatively impact maternal nutrition (Bottoms, 1996).

Although fewer women smoke today than 20 years ago, research indicates that approximately 23% of women in the United States smoke (Kendrick & Merritt, 1996). At the time of conception, approximately one-third of women smoke; by the first prenatal visit, 20% of these smokers will have quit (ACOG, 1997b). Unfortunately, a majority of women who quit smoking during pregnancy resume after birth; this percentage is lower for women who quit early in pregnancy. This finding suggests that although women are aware of the potential impact of smoking on the fetus, they may be less knowledgeable about the effects of passive smoke on the baby.

Studies demonstrate that any decrease in smoking during pregnancy improves fetal outcome, and researchers continue to explore approaches designed to help women quit smoking. Pregnancy may be a difficult time for a woman to stop smoking, but the nurse should encourage her to reduce the number of cigarettes she smokes daily. The need to protect her unborn child may dramatically increase her motivation.

Alcohol

Alcohol is now considered one of the primary teratogens in the Western world. Fetuses of women who are heavy drinkers are at increased risk for developing **fetal alcohol syndrome (FAS).**

The effects of moderate consumption of alcohol during pregnancy are not clearly known, but research suggests there is an increased incidence of lower birth weight and of some neurologic effects, such as attention deficit disorder. Evidence suggests that the risk of teratogenic effects increases proportionately with increased average daily intake of alcohol. Although studies of light drinkers demonstrate a degree of risk for adverse pregnancy effects similar to that of nondrinkers, no safe level of drinking during pregnancy has been identified, and caregivers recommend that pregnant women be advised to abstain from all alcohol during pregnancy (Niebyl, 1996).

Alcohol passes the placental barrier within minutes after consumption, with fetal blood alcohol levels becoming equivalent to maternal blood alcohol levels. The effects of alcohol consumption vary according to the stage of fetal development. During the first trimester, alcohol probably alters embryonic development; throughout pregnancy, alcohol may interfere with cell division and growth; in the third trimester, the time of most rapid brain growth, alcohol may alter CNS development and contribute to growth retardation (Cunningham et al,

1997). The risk of neurologic damage is lessened if heavy drinking ceases in the third trimester. Decreased consumption of alcohol in midpregnancy is associated with a lower incidence of growth retardation.

Assessment of a woman's alcohol intake should be a chief part of each woman's medical history, with questions asked in a direct, nonjudgmental manner. All women should be counseled about the role of alcohol in pregnancy. When pregnant women become aware of the risk of alcohol to the fetus, most usually attempt to modify their alcohol consumption. If heavy consumption is involved, these women should be referred early to an alcoholic treatment program. Because the drug disulfiram (Antabuse), which is often used in the treatment of alcoholism, is suspected teratogen, a woman in such a program should inform her counselor if she becomes pregnant.

Counseling about the effects of alcohol during pregnancy has been effective and should, of course, continue. Because the most profound impact of alcohol occurs in the first weeks after conception, nurses and other health care providers will see the most dramatic decrease in the effects of alcohol during pregnancy by increasing their teaching efforts in the period prior to conception.

Caffeine

Current research reveals no evidence that caffeine increases reproductive or teratogenic risk in humans. However, maternal coffee consumption does decrease iron absorption and may increase the risk of anemia (Niebyl, 1996). Until more definitive data are available, nurses should advise women of common sources of caffeine, including coffee, tea, colas, and chocolate, and suggest they use good judgment in moderating their caffeine intake.

Marijuana

The prevalence of marijuana use in our society raises concerns about its effect on the fetus, but to date no teratogenic effects of marijuana use during pregnancy have been documented (Cunningham et al, 1997). Research on marijuana use in pregnancy is difficult, however, because it is an illegal drug. Unreliability of reporting, lack of a representative population, inability to determine strength or composition of the marijuana used, presence of herbicides, and use of other drugs at the same time are major factors complicating the research being done.

Cocaine

A woman who uses cocaine is at increased risk for acute myocardial infarction, cardiac arrhythmias, ruptured ascending aorta, seizures, cerebrovascular accidents, hyperthermia, bowel ischemia, and sudden death (Cunningham et al, 1997). During pregnancy, cocaine use has been related to abruptio placentae, preterm birth, fetal distress, low birth weight, neonatal withdrawal, SIDS, and spontaneous pneumothorax (Chan, Pham, & Reece, 1997). Several congenital anomalies in the neonate have also been linked to maternal cocaine use, including genitourinary anomalies, congenital heart defects, limb reduction defects, CNS anomalies, prune belly syndrome, and segmental intestinal atresia (Cunningham et al, 1997). (See also Chapter 15.)

As cocaine becomes more widely used by women of childbearing age, health care providers must become alert to early signs of cocaine use. Hutchins and Dipietro (1997) found that six psychosocial factors are predictive of cocaine use during pregnancy: (1) family history of alcohol or drug problems, (2) introduction to drugs by a male partner, (3) depression, (4) lack of social support, (5) current partner who is a substance abuser, and (6) an unstable living situation. It is often difficult for a nurse or physician to face the fact that a client may be using cocaine, but ongoing alertness and an open, nonjudgmental approach are important in early detection. Urine screening for cocaine is valuable, but because cocaine is metabolized rapidly, the drug screen is negative within 24 to 48 hours after cocaine use. Thus it is probable that many abusers are missed.

Evaluation

Throughout the antepartal period, evaluation is an essential part of effective nursing care. As nurses ask questions of the pregnant woman and her family or make observations of physical changes, they are evaluating the results of previous interventions. In evaluating the effectiveness of the interventions, the nurse should not be afraid to try creative solutions if they are logical and carefully thought out. This is especially important in dealing with families from other cultures. If a practice is important to a woman and not harmful, the culturally competent nurse will not discourage it.

In completing an evaluation, the nurse must also recognize situations that require referral for further evaluation. For example, a woman who has gained 4 lb in 1 week probably does not require counseling about nutrition; she needs further assessment for pregnancy-induced hypertension. The nurse who has a sound knowledge of theory will recognize this and act immediately.

The ongoing and cyclic nature of the nursing process is especially evident in the prenatal setting. However, throughout the course of pregnancy nurses can use certain criteria to determine the quality of care provided. In essence, nursing care has been effective if the following have been met:

- The common discomforts of pregnancy are quickly identified and are relieved or lessened effectively.
- The woman is able to discuss the physiologic and psychologic changes of pregnancy.
- The woman implements appropriate self-care measures, if they are indicated, during pregnancy.
- The woman avoids substances and situations that pose a risk to her well-being or that of her child.
- The woman seeks regular prenatal care.

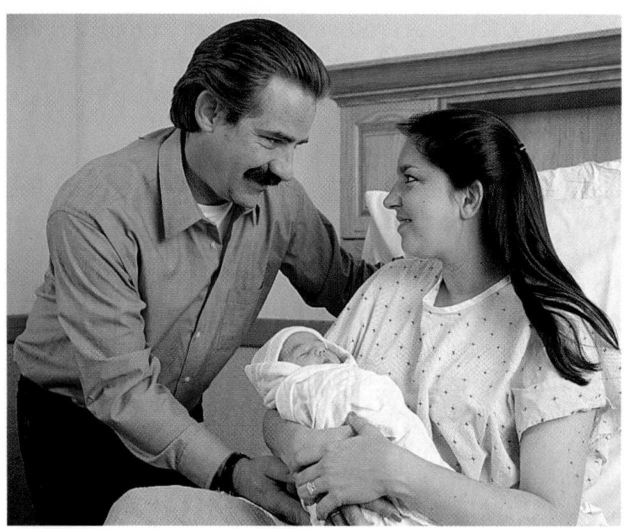

FIGURE 12–12 For many older couples, the decision to have a child may be a very rewarding one.

Care of the Expectant Couple Over 35

Today an increasing number of women are choosing to have their first baby after age 35. In fact, the rate of first births to women between the ages of 35 and 39 more than doubled between 1980 and 1992 in the United States. For women between the ages of 40 and 44, the birth rate increased by 40% during the same period (US Bureau of the Census, 1993). Many factors contribute to this trend, including the following:

- The availability of effective birth control methods
- The expanded roles and career options available for women
- The increased number of women obtaining advanced education, pursuing careers, and delaying parenthood until they are established professionally
- The increased incidence of later marriage and second marriage
- The high cost of living, which causes some young couples to delay childbearing until they are more secure financially
- The increased number of women in this older reproductive age group due to the "baby boom" between 1946 and 1964 (Dildy, Jackson, Fowers, Oshiro, Varner, & Clark, 1996).
- The increased availability of specialized fertilization procedures, which offers opportunities for women who had previously been considered infertile

There are advantages to having a first baby after the age of 35. Single women or couples who delay childbearing until they are older tend to be well educated and financially secure. Usually their decision to have a baby was deliberately and thoughtfully made. Women over age 35 tend to be more emotionally stable, obtain early prenatal care, and demonstrate healthy behaviors during their pregnancy (Catanzarite, Deutchman, Johnson, & Scherger, 1995). Moreover, research indicates that pregnant women over age 35 have less fear of helplessness and loss of control during labor than younger pregnant women (Stark, 1997). Given their greater life experiences, they also are much more aware of the realities of having a child and what it means to have a baby at their age (Figure 12–12). Many of the women have experienced fulfillment in their careers and feel secure enough to take on the added responsibility of a child. Some women are ready to make a change in their lives, desiring to stay home with a new baby. Those who plan to continue working tend to be more able to afford good child care.

Medical Risks

Historically, medical professionals considered women who were over 30 at the time of their first pregnancy, and especially those who were 35 or older, at higher risk for maternal or fetal complications. This age-related concern began to change during the 1980s, when studies comparing healthy pregnant women over 35 years of age with healthy younger women did not confirm these beliefs. However, the current medical literature does report some adverse pregnancy outcomes associated with advanced maternal age.

In the United States and Canada over the past 30 years, the risk of fetal death has declined dramatically for women of all ages as a result of advances in maternal health and obstetric practice. However, the risk for fetal death remains highest among women age 35 and older. Research indicates that women age 35 and older, with a fetal loss of 6 deaths per 1000 live births, are approximately twice as likely to have a stillbirth as women under age 35 (3 deaths per 1000 live births) (Fretts, Schmittdiel, McLean, Usher, & Goldman, 1995). This may be due in part to the decreased ability of the uterine blood vessels of the older women to accommodate to the needs of pregnancy. It may also be related to the fact that older women may experience multiple gestation (a risk factor for fetal death) after fertility-enhancing treatments (Fretts et al, 1995).

Women over 35 are more likely to have chronic medical conditions (Catanzarite et al, 1995). Preexisting medical conditions, such as hypertension or diabetes, probably play a more significant role than age in maternal well-being and the outcome of pregnancy. The frequency of medical complications in pregnant women over 35 increases in the cardiovascular, neurologic, connective tissue, renal, and pulmonary systems. Also, placenta previa, abruptio placentae, preterm birth, spontaneous abortion, low-birth-weight infants, macrosomia, and congenital malformations occur more frequently (Cunningham et al, 1997).

The cesarean birth rate is also increased in pregnant women over 35. This practice may be related to increased concern by the woman and physician about the pregnancy outcome (Cunningham et al, 1997).

The risk of conceiving a child with Down syndrome does increase with age, especially over 35. The use of amniocentesis or chorionic villus sampling (CVS) is routinely offered to all women over age 35 to permit the early detection of several chromosomal abnormalities, including Down syndrome. Routine genetic testing has not been offered to couples in which the only risk is advanced paternal age, because there is not sufficient evidence to determine a specific paternal age at which to start genetic testing. However, advanced paternal age does affect autosomal dominant diseases, such as neurofibromatosis, achondroplasia, and Marfan syndrome (ACOG, 1997a). Research has also focused on the use of multiple marker screening to detect Down syndrome and trisomy 18. This involves a blood test to detect levels of specific serum markers, namely alpha-fetoprotein (AFP), human chorionic gonadotropin (hCG), and unconjugated estriol. When these tests in combination show certain patterns of increase or decrease, they are considered positive, and the woman is advised to consider amniocentesis. Although these tests are not as definite as amniocentesis or chorionic villus sampling in detecting abnormalities, they are safer and less expensive (Rose & Mennuti, 1995).

Special Concerns of the Expectant Couple Over 35

No matter what their age, most expectant couples have concerns regarding the well-being of the fetus and their ability to parent. The older couple has additional concerns related to their age, especially the closer they are to 40 or more. Some couples are concerned about whether they will have enough energy to care for a new baby. Of greater concern is their ability to deal with the needs of the older child when they too are older.

The financial concerns of an older couple are usually different from those of a younger couple. The older couple is generally more financially secure than the younger couple. However, when their "baby" is ready for college, the older couple may be near retirement and might not have the means to provide for their child.

While considering their financial future and future retirement, the older couple may be forced to face their own mortality. Certainly this is not uncommon in midlife, but instead of confronting this issue at 40 to 45 years of age or later, the older expectant couple may confront the issue several years earlier as they consider what will happen as their child grows.

The older couple facing pregnancy following a late or second marriage or after therapy for infertility may find themselves somewhat isolated socially. They may feel "different" because they are often the only couple in their peer group expecting their first baby. In fact, many of their peers are likely to be parents of adolescents or young adults and may be grandparents as well.

The response of older couples who already have children to learning that the woman is pregnant may vary greatly depending on whether the pregnancy was planned or unexpected. Other factors influencing their response include the attitudes of their children, family, and friends to the pregnancy; the impact on their lifestyle; and the financial implications of having another child. Sometimes couples who had previously been married to other mates will choose to have a child together. The concept of blended family applies to situations in which "her" children, "his" children, and "their" children come together as a new family group.

Health care professionals may treat the older expectant couple differently from the way they would a younger couple. Older women may be asked to submit to more medical procedures, such as amniocentesis and ultrasound, than younger women. An older woman may be prevented from using a birthing room or birthing center even if she is healthy because her age is considered to put her at risk.

The woman who has delayed pregnancy may be concerned about the limited amount of time that she has to bear children. When pregnancy does not occur as quickly as she hoped, the older woman may become increasingly anxious as time slips away on her "biological clock." When an older woman becomes pregnant but experiences a spontaneous abortion, her grief for the loss of her unborn child is exacerbated by her anxiety about her ability to conceive again in the time remaining to her.

NURSING CARE MANAGEMENT

Nursing Assessment and Diagnosis

In working with a woman in her 30s or 40s who is pregnant, the nurse makes the same assessments as are appropriate in caring for any woman who is pregnant. These include assessing physical status, the woman's understanding of pregnancy and the changes that accompany it, any health teaching needs that exist, the degree of support the woman has available to her, and her knowledge of infant care. In addition, the nurse explores the woman's and her partner's attitudes about the pregnancy and their expectations of the impact a baby will have on their lives.

The nursing diagnoses that are applicable to any pregnant woman apply to the pregnant woman who is over the age of 35. Examples of other nursing diagnoses that may apply include the following:

- ***Decisional Conflict*** related to unexpected pregnancy
- ***Impaired Social Interaction*** related to changes associated with pregnancy

Nursing Plan and Implementation

Once an older couple has decided to have a child, it is the nurse's responsibility to respect and support them in this decision. As with any client, the nurse needs to discuss risks, identify concerns, and promote strengths. The woman's age should not be made an issue. To promote a sense of well-being, the nurse should treat the pregnancy as "normal" unless specific health risks are identified.

As the pregnancy continues, the nurse should identify and discuss concerns the woman may have related to her age or to specific health problems. The older woman who has made a conscious decision to become pregnant often has carefully thought through potential problems and may actually have fewer concerns than a younger woman or one with an unplanned pregnancy.

Childbirth education classes are important in promoting adaptation to the event of childbirth for expectant couples of any age. However, older expectant couples, who are still in the minority, often feel uncomfortable in classes where the majority of participants are much younger. Because of the differences in age and life experiences, many of the needs of the older couple may not be met in the class. The nurse teaching a childbirth education class should try to anticipate the informational needs of the older couple. At the same time, the nurse should not make the couple feel uncomfortable by drawing attention to their age. As the number of expectant older couples increases, the nurse may find it useful to offer an "over 35" childbirth education class to accommodate the specific needs of older couples. Such classes are being developed in some larger urban areas.

Women who are over 35 years of age and having their first baby tend to be better educated than other health care consumers. These clients frequently know the kind of care and services they want and are assertive in their interactions with the health care system. The nurse should neither be intimidated by these individuals nor assume that they do not need anticipatory guidance and support. Instead, the nurse should support the couple's strengths and be sensitive to their individual needs.

In working with older expectant couples, the nurse needs to be sensitive to their special needs. A particularly difficult issue these couples face is the possibility of bearing an unhealthy child. Because of the risk of Down syndrome in these families, amniocentesis is encouraged. Chorionic villus sampling may also be suggested if available in the area. The decision to have amniocentesis can be difficult to make merely on the basis of its possible risks to the fetus. But that becomes almost a minor concern when the couple thinks of the implications of the possible findings of Down syndrome or other chromosomal abnormalities. The finding of abnormalities means that the couple may be faced with an even more difficult decision about continuing the pregnancy.

A couple's decision to have amniocentesis is usually related to their beliefs and attitudes about abortion. Generally, amniocentesis is not even considered by couples who are strongly opposed to abortion for any reason. Health professionals must respect the couple's decision, take a nonjudgmental approach , and provide them with emotional support throughout the pregnancy.

The decision to have an abortion is a painful one even when couples are not opposed to abortion on political or philosophic grounds. Even though the couple may believe that terminating a high-risk pregnancy is right for their family, they may feel a great deal of ambivalence about amniocentesis. If the results are such that the couple elects to have an abortion, they will usually feel much grief for their loss.

Many health professionals assume that the couple who agrees to amniocentesis will also elect to have an abortion if Down syndrome or another condition is diagnosed. This is not necessarily the case. Some couples choose not to have an abortion after being informed that their unborn child has genetic abnormalities.

For the couple who agrees to amniocentesis, the first few months of pregnancy are a difficult time. Amniocentesis cannot be done until 14 weeks of pregnancy, and the chromosomal studies take roughly 2 weeks to complete. Their fear that the fetus is at risk may delay the successful completion of the psychologic tasks of early pregnancy.

The nurse can support couples who decide to have amniocentesis in several ways:

- The nurse should make sure that the couple is aware of the risks of amniocentesis and why it is being performed.
- The nurse who is present during the amniocentesis procedure can offer comfort and emotional support to the expectant woman. The nurse can also provide information about the procedure as it is being performed.
- The nurse can facilitate a support group for women during the difficult waiting period between the procedure and the results.
- If the results indicate that the fetus has Down syndrome or another genetic abnormality, the nurse can ensure that the couple has complete information about the condition, its range of possible manifestations, and its developmental implications.
- The nurse can support the couple in their decision about continuing or terminating the pregnancy. It is essential that the nurse and other health professionals involved with the couple not impose their philosophic or political beliefs about abortion on the couple. The decision is the couple's, and it should be based on their belief system and a nonbiased presentation of risks and choices from caregivers.

Amniocentesis is discussed further in Chapter 17.

Evaluation

Expected outcomes of nursing care include the following:

- The woman and her partner are knowledgeable about the pregnancy and make appropriate health care choices.
- The expectant couple (and their children) are able to cope successfully with the pregnancy and its implications for the future.
- The woman receives effective health care throughout her pregnancy and during birth and the postpartum period.
- The woman and her partner develop skills in child care and parenting as necessary. ●

FOCUS YOUR STUDY

- Providing anticipatory guidance about childbirth, the postpartum period, and childrearing is a primary responsibility of the nurse caring for women in an antepartal setting.
- The nurse assesses the expectant father's knowledge level and intended degree of participation and then works with the couple to help ensure a satisfying experience.
- Culturally based practices and forbidden activities may have a major impact on the childbearing family.
- The common discomforts of pregnancy occur as a result of physiologic and anatomic changes. The nurse provides the woman with information about self-care activities aimed at reducing or relieving discomfort.
- To make appropriate self-care choices and ensure healthful habits, a pregnant woman requires accurate information about a range of subjects from exercise to sexual activity, from bathing to immunization.
- Teratogenic substances are substances that adversely affect the normal growth and development of the fetus.
- A pregnant woman should avoid taking medications or using over-the-counter preparations during pregnancy.
- Evidence exists that smoking, consuming alcohol, or using social drugs during pregnancy may be harmful to the fetus.
- Maternal assessment of fetal activity keeps the woman "in touch" with her fetus and provides ongoing assessment of fetal status.
- Childbirth among women over 35 is becoming increasingly common. It poses fewer health risks than previously believed and offers advantages for the woman or couple who makes the choice.
- A major risk for the older expectant couple relates to the increased incidence of Down syndrome in children born to women over age 35. Amniocentesis can provide information as to whether the fetus has Down syndrome. The couple can then decide whether they wish to continue the pregnancy.

REFERENCES

Alteneder, R. R., & Hartzell, D. (1997). Addressing couples' sexuality concerns during the childbearing period: Use of the PLISSIT model. *Journal of Obstetric, Gynecologic, & Neonatal Nursing, 26*(6), 651–658.

American College of Obstetricians and Gynecologists (ACOG). (1994). *Exercise during pregnancy and the postpartum period.* (ACOG Technical Bulletin No. 189). Washington, DC: Author.

American College of Obstetricians and Gynecologists (ACOG). (1997a). *Advanced paternal age.* (ACOG Committee Opinion No. 189). Washington, DC: Author.

American College of Obstetricians and Gynecologists (ACOG). (1997b). *Smoking and women's health.* (ACOG Educational Bulletin No. 240). Washington, DC: Author.

American College of Obstetricians and Gynecologists (ACOG). (1997c). *Teratology* (ACOG Educational Bulletin No. 236). Washington, DC: Author.

Artal, R., & Buckenmeyer, P. J. (1995). Exercise during pregnancy and postpartum. *Contemporary OB/GYN, 40*(5), 62–90.

Belluomini, J., Litt, R. C., Lee, K. A., & Katz, M. (1994). Acupressure for nausea and vomiting of pregnancy: A randomized, blinded study. *Obstetrics & Gynecology, 84*(2), 245–248.

Bottoms, S. F. (1996). High-risk pregnancy: Smoking. *Contemporary OB/GYN, 41*(12), 13–16.

Catanzarite, V., Deutchman, M., Johnson, C. A., & Scherger, J. E. (1995, Jan. 15). Pregnancy after 35: What's the real risk? *Patient Care, 29*(1), 41–48, 51.

Chan, L., Pham, H., & Reece, E. A. (1997). Pneumothorax in pregnancy associated with cocaine use. *American Journal of Perinatology, 14*(7), 385–388.

Choi, E. C. (1995). A contrast of mothering behaviors in women from Korea and the United States. *Journal of Obstetric, Gynecologic, & Neonatal Nursing, 24*(4), 363–369.

Clapp, J. F. (1996). The effect of continuing regular endurance exercise on the physiologic adaptations to pregnancy and pregnancy outcome. *American Journal of Sports Medicine, 24*(Suppl. 2), S28–S29.

Cunningham, F. G., MacDonald, P. C., Gant, N. F., Leveno, K. J., Gilstrap, L. C., III, Hankins, G. D. V., & Clark, S. L. (1997). *Williams obstetrics* (20th ed.). Stamford, CT: Appleton & Lange.

Davis, D. C. (1996). The discomforts of pregnancy. *Journal of Obstetric, Gynecologic, & Neonatal Nursing, 25*(1), 73–81.

DeJoseph, J. F. (1993). Redefining women's work during pregnancy: Toward a more comprehensive approach. *Birth, 20*(2), 86–93.

Dildy, G. A., Jackson, G. M., Fowers, G. K., Oshiro, B. T., Varner, M. W., & Clark, S. L. (1996). Very advanced maternal age: Pregnancy after age 35. *American Journal of Obstetrics & Gynecology, 175*(3 Pt. 1), 668–674.

Druzin, M. L., & Gabbe, S. G. (1996). Antepartum fetal evaluation. In S. G. Gabbe, J. R. Niebyl, & J. L. Simpson (Eds.), *Obstetrics: Normal & problem pregnancies* (3rd ed.). New York: Churchill Livingstone.

Freda, M. C., Mikhail, M., Mazloom, E., Polizzotto, R., Damus, K., & Merkatz, I. (1993). Fetal movement counting: Which method? *American Journal of Maternal Child Nursing, 18*(6), 314–321.

Fretts, R. C., Schmittdiel, J., McLean, F. H., Usher, R. H., & Goldman, M. B. (1995, Oct. 12). Increased maternal age and the risk of fetal death. *New England Journal of Medicine, 333*(15), 953–957.

Hoffman, J. B. (1953). A suggested treatment for inverted nipples. *American Journal of Obstetrics and Gynecology, 66*, 346.

Hutchins, E., & DiPietro, J. (1997). Psychosocial risk factors associated with cocaine use during pregnancy: A case-control study. *Obstetrics and Gynecology, 90*(1), 142–147.

Johnson, T. R. B., Walker, M. A., & Niebyl, J. R. (1996). Preconception and prenatal care. In S. G. Gabbe, J. R. Niebyl, & J. L. Simpson (Eds.), *Obstetrics: Normal and problem pregnancies* (3rd ed.). New York: Churchill Livingstone.

Kendrick, J. S., & Merritt, R. K. (1996). Women and smoking: An update for the 1990s. *American Journal of Obstetrics and Gynecology, 175*(3 Pt. 1), 528–535.

Larson, J. D., & Rayburn, W. F. (1996). Gestational heartburn: What role for medications? *Contemporary OB/GYN, 41*(8), 95–117.

Mattson, S. (1995). Culturally sensitive perinatal care for Southeast Asians. *Journal of Obstetric, Gynecologic, and Neonatal Nursing, 24*(4), 335–341.

Niebyl, J. R. (1996). Drugs in pregnancy and lactation. In S. G. Gabbe, J. R. Niebyl, & J. L. Simpson (Eds.), *Obstetrics: Normal and problem pregnancies* (3rd ed.). New York: Churchill Livingstone.

O'Brien, B., & Zhou, Q. (1995). Variables related to nausea and vomiting during pregnancy. *Birth, 22*(2), 93–100.

Peleg, D., & Niebyl, J. R. (1997). Prescribing antiemetic therapy during pregnancy. *Contemporary OB/GYN, 42*(6), 164–171.

Rogers, J., & Davis, B. A. (1995). How risky are hot tubs and saunas for pregnant women? *American Journal of Maternal Child Nursing, 20*(3), 137–140.

Rose, N. C., & Mennuti, M. T. (1995). Multiple marker screening for women 35 and older. *Contemporary OB/GYN, 40*(9), 55–68.

Samuels, P. (1996). Neurological disorders. In S. G. Gabbe, J. R. Niebyl, & J. L. Simpson (Eds.), *Obstetrics: Normal and problem pregnancies* (3rd ed.). New York: Churchill Livingstone.

Soltes, B. A., Anderson, R., & Radwanska, E. (1996). Morphologic changes in offspring of female mice exposed to ethanol before conception. *American Journal of Obstetrics and Gynecology, 175*(5), 1158–1162.

Spector, R. E. (1996). *Cultural diversity in health and illness* (4th ed.). Stamford, CT: Appleton & Lange.

Speroff, L. (1997). Protocols for high risk pregnancy: Exercise. *Contemporary OB/GYN, 42*(9), 11–25.

Springer, M., Spatz, D., & Donahue, D. (1994). Maternal-fetal physical assessment in the home setting: Role of the advanced practice nurse. *Journal of Obstetric, Gynecologic, & Neonatal Nursing, 23*(8), 720–725.

Stark, M. A. (1997). Psychosocial adjustment during pregnancy: The experience of mature gravidas. *Journal of Obstetric, Gynecologic, & Neonatal Nursing, 26*(2), 206–211.

US Bureau of the Census. (1993). *Statistical abstract of the United States* (113th ed.). Washington, DC: Author.

Whitney, J. L. (1999). Drug labeling and pregnancy update: What has the FDA done lately? *Contemporary OB/GYN, 44*(1), 85–95.

Adolescent Pregnancy

13

I AM A FRESHMAN IN COLLEGE, AND SO IS MY daughter. I had her when I was 15, and that forced me to grow up in a hurry. For years I've thought about being a nurse, and now is my chance. Please understand, my daughter is very precious to me, but a part of me knows that if I had it to do over, I would change so much of my life—if only I had known!

Objectives

- Describe different reasons for teenage pregnancy and their implications for nursing care.
- Summarize the developmental tasks of adolescence and the impact that pregnancy superimposes on these tasks.
- Identify the physical, psychologic, and sociologic risks faced by an adolescent who is pregnant.
- Describe successful community approaches to adolescent pregnancy prevention.
- Delineate characteristics of the fathers of children of adolescent mothers.
- Discuss the reactions of the adolescent's family and social support groups to her pregnancy.
- Formulate a plan of care to meet the needs of a pregnant adolescent.

Key Terms

Birth rate
Early adolescence
Emancipated minors
Late adolescence
Middle adolescence

ADOLESCENT PREGNANCY IS A MULTIFACETED issue with no single cause or cure. For a teen, pregnancy comes at a time when her physical development and the developmental tasks of adolescence are incomplete. She is not prepared psychologically or economically for parenthood. Thus both she and her child are at high risk. The negative socioeconomic impact on society is also significant. This chapter explores the incidence, risk factors, and consequences of adolescent pregnancy. It then presents the role of the nurse in meeting the special needs and concerns of pregnant adolescents and their families and concludes with a discussion of efforts to prevent adolescent pregnancy.

Overview of Adolescence

Physical Changes

Puberty, that period during which an individual becomes capable of reproduction, is a maturational process that can last from 1.5 to 6 years and generally coincides with adolescence. The major physical changes of puberty include a growth spurt, weight change, and the appearance of secondary sexual characteristics. Menarche, or the time of the first menstrual period, usually occurs in the last half of this maturational process, with the average age between 12 and 13.

The initial menstrual cycles are usually irregular and often anovulatory for the first 12 to 18 months; however, this is not true for all females. Some adolescents do not use contraception during this time because they falsely assume that they cannot get pregnant. Even if their initial menstrual cycles are anovulatory, there is no certainty about when the first ovulatory cycle will occur; thus contraception is important during this time for all adolescents who are sexually active.

Psychosocial Development

Although it is well documented that the onset of puberty now occurs at a younger age, there are no data to indicate that psychosocial development, particularly cognitive development, occurs at an earlier age. Developmental tasks of adolescence have been described by many writers and are based on a variety of classic theories. These tasks are issues that individuals may struggle with at other times in their lives, but they are especially significant during adolescence to help ensure a successful transition from childhood to adulthood. The following are major developmental tasks of this period (Steinberg, 1993):

- Developing an identity
- Gaining autonomy and independence
- Developing intimacy in a relationship
- Developing comfort with one's own sexuality
- Developing a sense of achievement

Resolving these tasks is a developmental process that occurs over time. This developmental process is reflected in the behaviors of youths during early, middle, and late adolescence. Although average ages for the completion of tasks have been identified, these ages are somewhat arbitrary and are affected by many factors such as culture, religion, and socioeconomic status.

In **early adolescence** (age 14 and under), the teen still sees authority in the parents. However, she begins the process of "leaving the family" by spending more time with friends, especially friends of the same sex. Conformity to peer group standards is reflected in her behavior and in the clothes she wears. During this phase, the adolescent has a rich fantasy life. In addition, she is struggling to become comfortable with her changing body and body image and to fit this image with her fantasy life. Much time is spent in front of the mirror. The adolescent in this phase is very egocentric and is a concrete thinker. She has only minimal ability to see herself in the future or foresee the consequences of her behavior. She perceives her locus of control as external; that is, her destiny is controlled by others, such as parents and school authorities.

Middle adolescence (15 to 17 years) is the time for challenging. Experimenting with drugs, alcohol, and sex is a common avenue for rebellion. The middle adolescent seeks independence and turns increasingly to her peer group. Peer group identification is obvious in her choice of dress, makeup, hair style, and music. During this phase, the adolescent may believe that she is invincible and will not suffer negative consequences from risk-taking behaviors. These years are often a time of great turmoil for the family as the adolescent struggles for independence and challenges the family's values and expectations.

The middle adolescent wants to be treated as an adult. However, fear of adult responsibility may cause fluctuation in behavior. At times she seems like a child; at other times she is surprisingly mature. She is beginning to move from concrete thinking to formal operational thought but is not yet able to anticipate the long-term implications of all her actions.

In **late adolescence** (18 to 19 years), the young woman is more at ease with her individuality and decision-making ability. She can think abstractly and anticipate consequences. During this time, she becomes more confident of her personal identity. The late adolescent is capable of formal operational thought. She is learning to solve problems, to conceptualize, and to make decisions. These abilities help her see herself as having control, which leads to the ability to understand and accept the consequences of her behavior.

Table 13–1 describes successful resolution of each of the developmental tasks of adolescence and identifies high risk factors for adolescent pregnancy.

TABLE 13–1 Developmental Tasks of Adolescence

Tasks	Description of Successful Resolution	High-Risk Factors for Teen Pregnancy
Developing an identity	As individuals enter puberty, their physical appearance begins to change, and others begin to respond differently to them. The media present idealized images of the teenage female. Self-esteem may fluctuate, and hormonal changes create awareness of sexual desire. Adolescents experience confusion about their self-image. This is a time of experimentation until they become comfortable with who they are.	If the young adolescent feels she cannot live up to parents' expectations or is in a dysfunctional family situation, she may adopt a negative identity. She may become rebellious and actively involved in risk-taking behaviors, such as substance abuse and early sexual activity.
Gaining independence	Adolescents gradually move away from parental control and are influenced by peers. Eventually, they develop values that help govern their behavior responsibly without extrinsic control of peers or parents.	Peer pressure is highest during early and middle adolescence. If peers are involved in antisocial behavior, this influences their behavior and all other developmental tasks. Substance abuse and sexual activity are common in these groups.
Developing emotional intimacy in relationships	Adolescents begin to develop a close emotional attachment with another individual. They can share innermost feelings and have empathy for the other. This usually begins with a friend of the same sex and eventually develops into a trusting and loving relationship with someone of the opposite sex.	Sexual activity may be an attempt to meet needs for intimacy. This is a problem for victims of neglect or abuse. Although sexual intercourse has become a common adolescent experience, emotional intimacy is not associated with the majority of dating relationships, and most teenage marriages end in divorce.
Developing comfort with their sexuality	Puberty causes a new awareness of sexual desire and new meaning about physical contact with others. Adolescents learn to express sexual feelings appropriately and comfortably in a relationship.	Many young adolescent females who become sexually involved at an early age do so for a variety of reasons that do not lead to comfort with their own sexuality: peer pressure, pressure from an older male partner, rebellion against parents, sexual abuse and its consequences.
Gaining a sense of achievement	Adolescents begin to look toward the future and compare talents, work skills, and/or academic achievement with reality in preparing for adult working roles.	Those who drop out of school prematurely tend to be from economically disadvantaged backgrounds. Data show that early sexual experimentation by adolescents correlates with poor school performance whatever their background (Stevens-Simon, Kelly, Singer, & Cox, 1996). Use of contraception is more likely among adolescent females who are high academic achievers and have a future orientation (Alan Guttmacher Institute, 1994).

SOURCE: Adapted from Steinberg L: *Adolescence,* 5th ed. New York: McGraw Hill, 1999.

Incidence of Adolescent Pregnancy

Over one million teenage girls in the United States become pregnant each year, and most of these pregnancies are unplanned (US Dept of Health and Human Services, 1995). Of these pregnancies, approximately one-third are terminated by therapeutic abortion, and about 14% end in miscarriage. More than half the teens who become pregnant give birth and keep their babies. Very few adolescents give up their babies for adoption (National Campaign to Prevent Teen Pregnancy, 1997b).

The **birth rate** (number of births per 1000 women) for adolescents has dropped steadily in the US from 1991 (62.1) to 1996 (54.7) (Ventura, Curtin, & Mathews, 1998). However, the United States continues to have one of the highest levels of adolescent childbearing among industrialized nations—almost three times as high as France, and nine times the level in Japan (Alan Guttmacher Institute, 1998). The incidence of sexual activity among teens in other countries is as high as in the United States. Researchers suggest that these countries may have lower adolescent pregnancy rates because of family influences, a greater openness about sexuality, better access to contraceptives, and a more comprehensive approach to sex education (Peckham, 1993).

Factors Contributing to Adolescent Pregnancy

Among American adolescents, there is tremendous peer pressure to become sexually active during their teen years. Premarital sexual activity is commonplace. Sexual innuendo permeates every aspect of the popular media, including music, music videos, television, and movies, but issues of sexual responsibility are commonly ignored. Sexual activity among adolescents has increased significantly. In 1994, 56% of adolescent females and 73% of adolescent males had had sexual intercourse by age 18, as compared to 35% of females and 55% of males in 1970 (Alan Guttmacher Institute, 1994). Figure 13–1 identifies reasons teens cite for having sex.

Adolescent males tend to have their first experience of sexual intercourse at an earlier age than females, and they have more sexual partners in their teenage years. Most teens have their first experience of sexual intercourse during middle or late adolescence. Those who become sexually active at an earlier age tend to have behavioral problems including drug use and delinquency (Seidman & Rieder, 1994; Huizinga, Loeber, & Thornberry, 1993). They may also have been sexually abused at a young age (Esparza & Esperat, 1996).

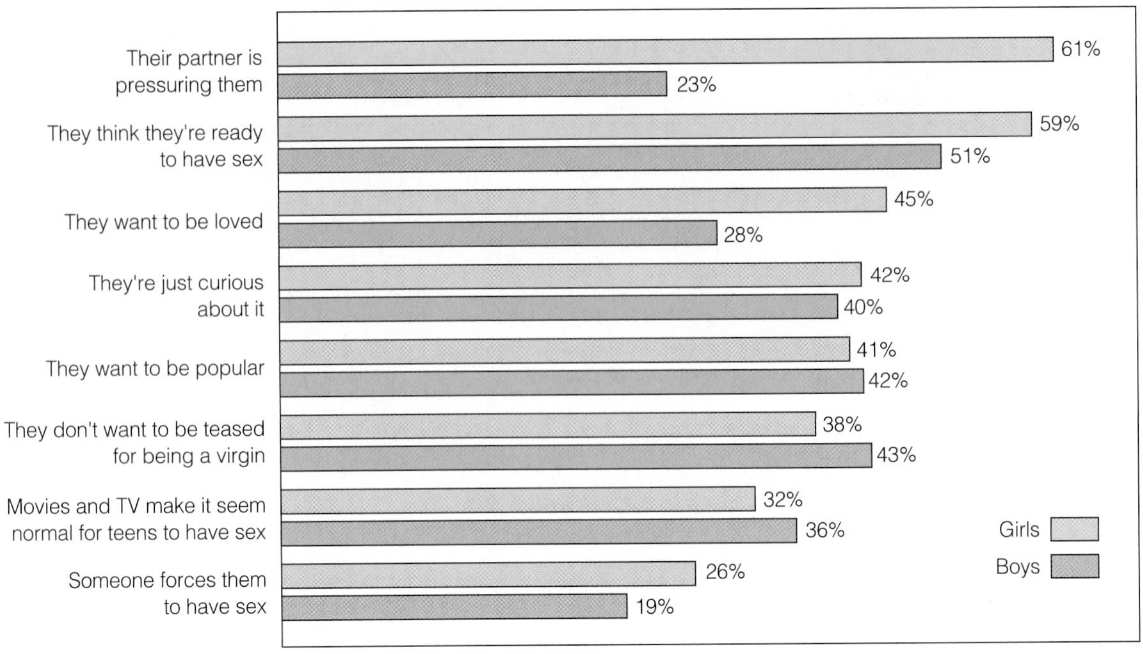

FIGURE 13–1 Why teens have sex. SOURCE: The Kaiser Family Foundation Survey on Teens and Sex: What They Say. *Teens Today Need to Know, and Who They Listen To.* June 1996. Menlo Park, CA: The Harry J. Kaiser Family Foundation.

About three-fourths of adolescents use some form of contraception (often a condom) the first time they have sexual intercourse (Alan Guttmacher Institute, 1994). Statistics have demonstrated an increased use of condoms among the adolescent population, probably because of the tremendous educational efforts related to the human immunodeficiency virus (HIV) (National Campaign to Prevent Teen Pregnancy, 1997b). Once adolescents have their first sexual experience, however, subsequent sexual experiences may occur infrequently. As a result, they do not consistently use contraceptives nor protect themselves from sexually transmitted infections (Seidman & Rieder, 1994). The most common responses by teens when asked why they didn't use birth control is that they did not plan or expect to have sex (National Campaign to Prevent Teen Pregnancy, 1997b).

Pregnancy risk taking (sexual activity without use of pregnancy prevention measures) is believed to stem from a variety of factors. For many adolescents, no conscious decision is made about being sexually active, and the initial experience of sexual intercourse often is not planned. As part of their growth and development, young adolescents do not tend to anticipate the consequences of their behavior and depend more on an external locus of control, such as a parent or other authority figure; so, it is not surprising that they would not use contraception. In addition, accurate sex education may not have been part of their learning experiences, and pregnancy risk taking has been linked to lack of knowledge about contraception. Because of teens' lack of knowledge about sexuality, many health care providers advocate sex education in schools, and at a younger age than previously provided. Others feel that sex education is the responsibility of the parents and are concerned that sex education in the schools will promote sexual activity. Review of research on sex education, however, demonstrates that it does not increase initiation of sexual activity at an earlier age (Kirby et al, 1994). Other factors affecting the use of contraception include access or availability, cost of supplies, and concern regarding confidentiality.

Teenage pregnancy is more socially acceptable today than in the past. In research about pregnant adolescents, many of those who did not use contraception stated that they were ambivalent about getting pregnant or wanted to get pregnant (Kirby, 1997). One study also found that these teenagers were more likely to have dropped out of school and to have known the father for at least 6 months prior to conception (Stevens-Simon, Kelly, Singer, & Cox, 1996).

The adolescent girl may use pregnancy for various subconscious or conscious reasons: to punish her father or mother, to escape from an undesirable home situation, to gain attention, or to feel that she has someone to love and to love her. As a result, some young teenagers may deliberately plan to get pregnant. Pregnancy may also be a young woman's form of delinquency. Pregnant adolescents often have troubled family relationships, poor school achievement, and exposure to drug abuse.

Teens with future goals (ie, college or job) tend to use birth control more consistently. If they do become pregnant, they are more likely to have an abortion. Adolescents who do not have such goals or who lack access to middle-class opportunities, in contrast, tend to maintain their pregnancies. Some consider pregnancy their only way to attain adult status. Eighty-five percent of births to unmarried teens occur to those from families who are poor or near poor (Alan Guttmacher Institute, 1994). Recent revisions of welfare policies (see Chapter 4) are expected to have significant impact, although it may not be on pregnancy rates but on the welfare of children of adolescent mothers.

The adolescent birth rate is higher among African American and Hispanic teens than white. This discrepancy may reflect the fact that a greater percentage of African American and Hispanic teens are sexually active (Clark, Cohall, & Joffe, 1998). The discrepancy probably also reflects the impact of poverty—a disproportionately higher number of African American and Hispanic youths live in poverty—and the influence of ethnic or cultural norms.

Studies with Hispanic teens have demonstrated significant intracultural variations in attitudes toward teen pregnancy. The Hispanic population is the most rapidly growing minority population in the United States and is expected to be the largest minority group, and with the youngest population, in the new century. Those teens who speak only Spanish tend to be part of a growing migrant population, with a majority being of Mexican descent (Smith & Weinman, 1995). This group tends to have the more traditional values of the Mexican culture, with strong family values. If the adolescent is married, early and subsequent childbearing is encouraged (Erickson, 1994; Smith & Weinman, 1995). Second-generation Hispanic adolescents are more likely to be bilingual and strive to succeed in this new culture, so teen pregnancy may be more of a disappointment if pregnancy interrupts educational aspirations. Acculturated Hispanic teens who are involved in high-risk behaviors appear to have characteristics similar to non-Hispanic teens, with socioeconomic influences being a significant factor contributing to teen pregnancy (Smith & Weinman, 1995).

A large number of teens who become pregnant, compared to teens who have not been pregnant, had been sexually abused as children. Some studies have reported that anywhere from 40% to 60% of pregnant teens have experienced sexual abuse early in their lives (Esparza & Esperat, 1996; Smith, 1996). The association between early childhood sexual abuse and teen pregnancy appears to be related to higher-risk behaviors in adolescents who have been abused. In fact, maltreatment of any kind is a high-risk contributor to early teen pregnancy (Becker-Lausen & Rickel, 1995; Stock, Bell, Boyer, & Connell, 1997).

Teenage pregnancy can result from an incestuous relationship. The psychologic turmoil experienced by the incest victim may obliterate thought of the risk of pregnancy, especially for the early adolescent. Late adolescents may fear the possibility of pregnancy, but for a variety of psychologic reasons may deny the reality. In the very young adolescent, incest or sexual abuse should be suspected as a possible cause of pregnancy. Teenage pregnancy could also be caused by other nonvoluntary sexual experiences, such as acquaintance rape.

In addition to the high-risk factors already discussed, the younger the teen when she first gets pregnant, the more likely she will have another pregnancy in her teens (East & Felice, 1996). Moreover, the likelihood of repeat pregnancies increases when the teen is living with her sexual partner and has dropped out of school. Daughters of women who had a baby in their early teens are also at higher risk for teen pregnancy (Jones & Mondy, 1994). Similarly, siblings of adolescent parents have been found to be at higher risk for earlier sexual activity and adolescent pregnancy.

In the United States, the results of teenage childbearing cost taxpayers $6.9 billion each year (Maynard, 1997). Simply delaying these births could result in significant savings because of the improvement in both education and occupational status of these young women (Long, Marquis, & Harrison, 1994). In addition, children of adolescent parents are at a disadvantage in many ways because teens are not developmentally or economically prepared to be parents. Consequently, their children tend to have behavioral problems, do not do as well in school, and are less likely to complete high school. There are also higher rates of abuse and neglect than among those who delay childbearing, resulting in significantly higher rates of foster care placement (National Campaign to Prevent Teen Pregnancy, 1997b).

International Perspective

Currently more than 15 million births—slightly more than 10% of all births worldwide—are to women under age 20. In many parts of North Africa, Asia, and the Middle East, early childbearing is, fortunately, declining; however, little has changed in sub-Saharan Africa and Latin America (Alan Guttmacher Institute, 1998). Cultural factors often play a significant role in the desirability of early pregnancy. Specifically, adolescent women are more likely to welcome a pregnancy in a country where Islam is the predominant religion, where large families are desired, where social change is slow in coming, and where most childbearing occurs within marriage. Early pregnancy is less desired in countries where the reverse is true. Moreover, throughout the world, the higher a woman's educational level, the more likely she is to delay marriage and childbirth (Alan Guttmacher Institute, 1998).

TABLE 13–2 Initial Reaction to Awareness of Pregnancy

Age	Adolescent Behavior	Nursing Implications
Early adolescent (14 and under)	Fears rejection by family and peers. Enters health care system with an adult, most likely mother (parents still seen as locus of control). Value system still closely reflects that of parents, so still turns to parents for decision or approval of decision. Pregnancy probably not result of intimate relationship. Is self-conscious about normal adolescent changes in body. Self-consciousness and low self-esteem likely to increase with rapid breast enlargement and abdominal enlargement of pregnancy.	Be nonjudgmental in approach to care. Focus on needs and concerns of adolescent, but if parent accompanies daughter, include parent in plan of care. Encourage both to express concerns and feelings regarding pregnancy and options: abortion, maintaining pregnancy, adoption. Be realistic and concrete in discussing implications of each option. During physical exam of adolescent, respect increased sense of modesty. Explain in simple and concrete terms physical changes that are produced by pregnancy versus puberty. Explain each step of physical exam in simple and concrete terms.
Middle adolescent (15–17 years)	Fears rejection by peers and parents. Unsure in whom to confide. May seek confirmation of pregnancy on own with increased awareness of options and services, such as over-the-counter pregnancy kits and Planned Parenthood. If in an ongoing, caring relationship with partner (peer), may choose him as confidant. Economic dependence on parents may determine if and when parents are told. Future educational plans and perception of parental support or lack of support are significant factors in decision regarding termination or maintenance of the pregnancy. Possible conflict in parental and own developing value system.	Be nonjudgmental in approach to care. Reassure the adolescent that confidentiality will be maintained. Help adolescent identify significant individuals in whom she can confide to help make a decision about the pregnancy. Be aware of state laws regarding requirement of parental notification if abortion intended. Also be aware of state laws regarding requirements for marriage: usually, minimum age for both parties is 18; 16- and 17-year-olds are, in most states, allowed to marry only with consent of parents. Encourage adolescent to be realistic about parental response to pregnancy.
Older adolescent (18–19 years)	Most likely to confirm pregnancy on own and at an earlier date due to increased acceptance and awareness of consequences of behavior. Likely to use pregnancy kit for confirmation. Relationship with father of baby, future educational plans, own value system are among significant determinants of decision about pregnancy.	Be nonjudgmental in approach to care. Reassure the adolescent that confidentiality will be maintained. Encourage adolescent to identify significant individuals in whom she can confide. Refer to counseling as appropriate. Encourage adolescent to be realistic about parental response to pregnancy.

The Adolescent Mother

Physiologic Risks

Adolescents over age 15 who receive early, thorough prenatal care are at no greater risk during pregnancy than women over 20 years. Unfortunately, many adolescents fail to seek early prenatal care. Those who do seek care may fail to cooperate with recommendations. In addition, teenage mothers are more likely to smoke than older pregnant women and less likely to gain sufficient weight during their pregnancy (Ventura et al, 1998). Thus risks for pregnant adolescents include preterm births, low-birth-weight (LBW) infants, pregnancy-induced hypertension (PIH) and its sequelae, iron deficiency anemia, and cephalopelvic disproportion. In the adolescent age group, prenatal care is the critical factor that most influences pregnancy outcome.

Iron deficiency anemia is a problem in all pregnant women. The adolescent who begins her pregnancy already anemic, however, is at increased risk and must be followed closely and counseled carefully regarding nutrition during pregnancy. The increased risk of cephalopelvic disproportion (CPD) is a concern in adolescent pregnancy, especially with the early adolescent, because of a lack of pelvic maturity.

Teenagers 15 to 19 years old have a high incidence of sexually transmitted infections, including herpesvirus, syphilis, and gonorrhea. The incidence of chlamydial infection is also increased in this age group. The presence of such infections during a pregnancy greatly increases the risk to the fetus (refer to Chapter 16). Other problems seen in adolescents are alcohol and drug use. By the time pregnancy is confirmed in young women, the fetus may already be harmed by these substances.

Psychologic Risks

The most profound psychologic risk to the adolescent who maintains her pregnancy is the interruption of progress in her developmental tasks. Although adolescents have become sexually active at an earlier age and the incidence of adolescent pregnancy has increased, the developmental tasks of this age group remain the same. Add to this the tasks of pregnancy, and the young woman has an overwhelming amount of psychologic work to do, the success of which will affect her own and her newborn's future.

Table 13–2 identifies typical behaviors of the early, middle, and late adolescent when she becomes aware of her pregnancy. In reviewing these behaviors, the nurse should realize that other factors may influence the age at which the behaviors are seen.

Sociologic Risks

A substantial body of research indicates that the adolescent mother is at higher risk for social and economic disadvantages than her teenage counterpart who is not pregnant and lives in the same social environment. Being forced into adult roles before completing adolescent de-

CRITICAL THINKING IN PRACTICE

Cindy Lenz, a 15-year-old Gr1PO, is 16 weeks pregnant when she arrives for her second prenatal visit. She is drinking diet soda and eating potato chips as she waits for her appointment. Her 18-year-old boyfriend is with her. While reviewing her history the nurse remembers that Cindy had tried to get pregnant for several months. Her boyfriend, a high school dropout, has a part-time job. Cindy is still living at home, although she does not get along with her mother or sister. She does plan to stay in school until her baby is born because she has two other friends at school who are also pregnant. As the nurse weighs Cindy, she asks a few questions about her nutritional habits and finds that Cindy eats a lot of junk food and very few vegetables or fruits. How should the nurse discuss Cindy's nutritional needs with her?

Answers can be found in Appendix I.

velopmental tasks causes a series of events that affects the adolescent's entire life. These events may result in a prolonged dependence on parents, lack of stable relationships with the opposite sex, and lack of economic and social stability.

Many teen mothers drop out of school during their pregnancy. This tendency may have as much to do with low academic achievement and low academic commitment as it does with the pregnancy. Many never complete their education. Lack of education reduces the quality of jobs available to these women. Childbearing at an early age is a strong predictor for need for public assistance, especially in lower socioeconomic groups and when the pregnant adolescent's family will not support her (National Campaign to Prevent Teen Pregnancy, 1997b).

Adolescent mothers frequently fail to establish a stable family, especially if they have a second child while still an adolescent. Their family structure tends to be a single-parent, matriarchal family structure, often the same type in which the adolescent herself was raised.

Some pregnant adolescents choose to marry the father of the baby, who may also be a teen. Unfortunately, the majority of adolescent marriages end in divorce (Roye & Balk, 1996). This fact is not surprising because pregnancy and marriage interrupt their "childhood" and basic education. Failure to be self-supporting logically follows lack of education and lost career goals. Lack of maturity in dealing with an intimate relationship also contributes to marital breakdown in this age group.

In general, children of teenage mothers are found to be at a developmental disadvantage compared to children whose mothers were older at the time of their birth. Many factors contribute to these differences, but the strongest evidence indicates that the adverse social and economic conditions facing teenage mothers are significant factors. These factors result in high rates of family instability, disadvantaged neighborhoods, poor academic performance, and higher rates of behavior problems.

RESEARCH IN PRACTICE

What is this study about? Women who are abused during pregnancy experience higher rates of biophysical complications (eg, spontaneous abortion or preterm deliveries) and psychosocial problems (eg, depression or anxiety). Adolescents who become pregnant may be at risk for abuse. Mary Ann Curry, Beth Doyle, and Jennifer Gilhooley developed a study to describe the incidence of abuse among pregnant adolescents and to determine if abuse impacted high school participation, substance abuse, complications of pregnancy, and infant birth weight.

How was the study done? From a larger study to test a model for predicting adverse pregnancy outcomes, the researchers collected data from 559 adolescents regarding incidence of abuse. The researchers used the three developmental stages of adolescence as a framework for assessing the abuse: early adolescence from ages 10 to 13, middle adolescence from 14 to 17, and late adolescence from 18 to 21. Data collection tools included a questionnaire soliciting demographic information, current high school participation and whether or not the present pregnancy was planned. Additional tools included an abuse assessment screen and a confidential self-report of current cigarette, marijuana, alcohol, and other drug use. Information about pregnancy complications was obtained from the prenatal record. After each interview, participants were asked if they wanted to discuss information disclosed in the interview with their provider and offered assistance in making contact.

What were the results of the study? Thirty-seven percent of the pregnant teens reported abuse. Middle adolescents reported the highest percentage (over 50%). Late adolescents reported the least; however, 30% of this age group still reported being abused. When broken down by type of abuse and specific age, the 17-year-old group reported the most overall abuse (54%), with 52% affirming that they had been hit, slapped, kicked, or otherwise physically abused within the last year. Thirty-eight percent of the 13 to 14-year-old group reported an occurrence of abuse during pregnancy. The teenagers who reported abuse had a higher incidence of low-birth-weight babies, although the difference was not statistically significant. Statistically significant differences did exist with high school participation (55% drop-out rate for abused teens as compared to 42% for nonabused teens), substance abused (higher rate of smoking) and pregnancy complications (more reports of second trimester bleeding among abused subjects). The investigators found no difference between the groups regarding planned pregnancies.

What additional questions might I have? Although not a focus of this study, one might ask what a comparative study of nonpregnant teens would reveal regarding incidence of abuse.

How can I use this study? Nurses need to be aware of the potential for abuse and to assess for abuse, especially during pregnancy. The researchers in this study used three questions to assess for abuse. If students ask these questions, they must have a plan for response to positive replies.

SOURCE: Curry, M. A., Doyle, B. A., & Gilhooley, J. (1998). Abuse among pregnant adolescents: Differences by developmental age. *Maternal Child Nursing, 23*(3), 144–150.

TABLE 13–3 The Early Adolescent's Response to the Developmental Tasks of Pregnancy

Stage	Developmental Tasks of Pregnancy	Early Adolescent's Response to Pregnancy	Nursing Implications
First trimester	Pregnancy confirmation. Seeking early prenatal care as a confirmation tool. Begins to evaluate her diet and general health habits. Initial ambivalence common. Usually supportive partner.	May delay confirmation of pregnancy until late part of first trimester or later. Reasons for delay may include lack of awareness that she is pregnant, fear of confiding in anyone, or denial. Rapid enlargement and sensitivity of breasts are embarrassing and frightening to early adolescent–may be perceived as changes of puberty. If confiding in mother, may be experiencing family turmoil in response to pregnancy.	Explain physiologic changes of pregnancy versus those associated with puberty. Explain that ambivalence is normal with any pregnancy, but recognize it as a much greater concern with adolescent pregnancy. Emphasize need for good nutrition as important for her well-being as much as infant's (prevention of PIH and anemia). Use simple explanations and lots of audiovisuals. Have adolescent listen to fetal heart rate (FHR) with Doppler.
Second trimester	Changes in physical appearance begin, and fetal movement is experienced, causing pregnancy to be experienced as a reality. Begins wearing maternity clothes to accommodate the physical changes. As a result of quickening she perceives her fetus as a real baby and begins preparing for the maternal role and new relationships with her partner and members of her family.	Some teenagers may delay validation of pregnancy until now, with family turmoil occurring at this time. Abdominal enlargement and quickening may be perceived as loss of control over body image. May try to maintain prepregnant weight and wear restrictive clothing to control and conceal changing body. Becomes dependent on her own mother for support. Egocentric; unable to develop a maternal role at this time.	Continue to discuss importance of good nutrition and adequate weight gain as noted above. Discuss ways of utilizing common teenage clothing (large sweatshirts, blouses) to promote comfort but preserve adolescent image to some degree. Discuss plans being made for baby, continued educational plans, and role of teen's parents.
Third trimester	At end of second trimester begins to view fetus as separate from self. Buys baby clothes and supplies. Prepares a place for the baby. Realistic about what baby is like. Prepares to give birth to infant. Anxiety increases as labor and birth approach and has concerns about well-being of fetus.	May focus on "wanting it to be over." May have trouble individuating fetus. May have fantasies, dreams, or nightmares about childbirth. Natural fears of labor and birth greater than with older primigravida. Probably has not been in a hospital, and may associate this with negative experiences.	Assess whether adolescent is preparing for baby by buying supplies and preparing a place in the home. Childbirth education important. Provide hospital tour. Assess for discomforts of pregnancy, such as heartburn and constipation. Adolescent may be uncomfortable mentioning these and other problems.

There is also an increased incidence of abuse and neglect (National Campaign to Prevent Teen Pregnancy, 1997b).

The increased incidence of maternal complications, premature birth, and low-birth-weight babies among adolescent mothers also has an impact on society because many of these mothers are on welfare. The need for increased financial support for good prenatal care and nutritional programs remains critical.

Table 13–3 identifies the early adolescent's response to the developmental tasks of pregnancy. The early adolescent's response reflects her level of development, with pregnancy as an interruption of the normal process of development. The middle and late adolescents respond differently, reflecting their maturational progress through the developmental tasks. In addition to her maturational level, the amount of nurturing the pregnant adolescent receives is also a critical factor in the way in which she handles pregnancy and motherhood.

Partners of Adolescent Mothers

Almost half of the fathers of infants of adolescent mothers are not teens themselves, but are 20 years of age or older (Landry & Forest, 1995; East & Felice, 1996). Of these men, approximately one-fifth are 6 years or more older than the adolescent mother (Taylor, Chavez, Chabra, & Boggess, 1997). The poorer the adult father's education, the greater the risk of his paternity, possibly because these men are seeking intellectual and emotional equals. Often the older partners of pregnant adolescents are similar to adolescent fathers socioeconomically. They have experienced early school failure, are unemployed, and no more likely to support the mother than adolescent fathers (Roye & Balk, 1996). Psychosocial development of these adult fathers is also more similar to that of an adolescent father than to that of adult men who have not fathered a child. Adult paternity also tends to be higher when the teenage mother is born outside the United States, which may reflect cultural norms (Taylor et al, 1997).

When the father is an adolescent, he, too, generally has not yet completed the developmental tasks of his age group and is no better prepared psychologically to deal with the consequences of pregnancy than the adolescent mother. Consequently, the adolescent who attempts to assume his responsibility as a father faces many of the same psychologic and sociologic risks as the adolescent mother. The mother and father are generally from similar socioeconomic backgrounds and have similar educational levels.

Although not married, many adolescent couples are involved in meaningful relationships. These men may be very involved in the pregnancy and may be present for the birth. Unfortunately, research indicates that there is decreasing contact with the mother and infant over time, even when fathers are involved in the birth (Roye & Balk, 1996).

Some adolescent fathers face negative reactions from people, including their own family and the family of the young woman. Feelings of anger, shame, and disappointment may be aimed at them. Even at the time of childbirth, the mother of the pregnant adolescent may discourage the presence of the adolescent father.

The lack of responsibility shown by some unwed fathers has caused a shift in cultural and community attitudes. Fathers are being included on birth certificates far more frequently today than in the past. This helps ensure the father's rights and encourages him to meet his responsibilities to his child. In addition, legal paternity gives children access to military and social security benefits and to medical information about their fathers.

In some situations, the pregnant adolescent may not want to identify or contact the father of the baby, and the father may not readily acknowledge paternity. Those situations include rape, exploitative sexual relations, incest, and casual sexual relations. If health care providers suspect any of the first three causes, further investigation into the situation is important for the well-being of the pregnant adolescent, and referral to other resources should be made as appropriate.

In situations in which the adolescent father wants to assume some responsibility, health care providers should support him in his decision. It is important, however, that the pregnant adolescent have the opportunity to decide whether she wants the father to participate in her health care.

If the adolescents perceive that they have a caring relationship, the adolescent father may want to be supportive and protective but probably does not understand the physical and psychologic changes that his partner is experiencing. The young man will need education regarding pregnancy, childbirth, child care, and parenting.

Although the adolescent father may have been included in the health care of the young woman throughout the pregnancy, it is not unusual for her to want her mother as her primary support person during labor and birth. This is especially true with younger adolescents. It is important both to support her wishes and also to acknowledge and support the adolescent father's wishes as appropriate.

As a part of counseling, the nurse should assess the young man's stressors, his support systems, his plans for involvement in the pregnancy and childbearing, and his future plans. He should be referred to social services for an opportunity to be counseled regarding his educational and vocational future. When the father is involved in the pregnancy, the young mother feels less deserted, more confident in her decision making, and better able to discuss her future.

Reactions of Family and Social Supports to Adolescent Pregnancy

The reactions of family members and support groups to adolescent pregnancy are as varied as the motivation and cause of the pregnancy. In families who foster educational and career goals for their children, adolescent pregnancy is often a shock. Anger, shame, and sorrow are common reactions. The majority of pregnant adolescents from these families are most likely to use contraception or choose abortion, with the exception of those teens whose cultural and religious beliefs prevent them from seeking an abortion.

In populations in which adolescent pregnancy is more prevalent and more socially acceptable, family and friends may be more supportive of the adolescent parents. In many cases, friends as well as the teen's mother are present at the birth. The expectant couple may also have friends who are already teen parents. For some male partners of these adolescent mothers, pregnancy and the birth of a baby are seen as a sign of adult status and increased sexual prowess—a sense of pride.

The mother of the pregnant adolescent is usually among the first to be told about the pregnancy. She typically becomes involved with decision making, especially with the younger adolescent, about issues such as maintaining the pregnancy, abortion, and dealing with the father-to-be and his family. As discussed previously, the pregnant adolescent may not want to identify or contact the father of the baby, especially in situations where rape or other exploitative sex was involved, or with casual sexual relationships. Family input in these matters is important in the adolescent's decision making.

Once the decision about the pregnancy has been made, it is usually the mother who helps the teen access health care and accompanies her to her first visit. If the pregnancy is maintained, the mother may participate in prenatal care classes and can be an excellent support system for her daughter. She should be encouraged to participate if the mother-daughter relationship is positive. If the baby's father is involved in the pregnancy, he and the pregnant teen's mother may be able to work together to support the teenage mother. The mother should be updated on obstetric practice to clarify any misconceptions she might have. During labor and birth, the mother may be a key figure for her daughter. Drawing on her own experience, she can offer reassurance and instill confidence in the adolescent.

It is commonly believed that after the baby is born, the adolescent and her infant will fare better if they live in the same household as the teen's mother, now the grandmother. Increasingly, however, research suggests that the best outcomes for the adolescent and her infant occur when the grandmother provides regular assistance but they do not live together (Spieker & Bensley, 1994).

COMMUNITY IN FOCUS

The School/Community Sexual Risk Reduction Model

The high incidence of adolescent pregnancy is of great concern nationwide, and communities have employed a variety of approaches to address the issue. The School/Community Sexual Risk Reduction Model is a comprehensive, multidisciplinary, communitywide model that has achieved significant success in reducing the incidence of unintended pregnancy among never-married teenagers and pre-teens. The model is designed to provide regular doses of multiple interventions directed at the adolescent population in general with higher levels of intervention for at-risk adolescents. The Model was originally developed and implemented in two South Carolina counties–Bamberg County and Hampton County. Evaluation of the success of the effort revealed a 54% decrease in the estimated pregnancy rate for teens aged 14 to 17 (Vincent et al, 1987).

The Model is designed to address issues related to adolescent pregnancy through a variety of interventions, including training and workshops about sexuality for parents, community members, and other professionals; graduate-level course work about sexuality education for teachers; age-appropriate, comprehensive, school-based sexuality education for students in grades K to 12; student access to contraceptives and health services; use of mass media approaches to increase community awareness and involvement; close cooperation with school officials to plan school-based interventions; peer support and education programs; and student activities focused on awareness of alternatives and skill development.

When teen pregnancy became a focus of concern in Kansas, the Kansas Health Foundation, an organization committed to improving the quality of health in Kansas, decided to support initiatives to reduce adolescent pregnancy rates. The Foundation reviewed the literature and sought out "success stories" of models that used community-based approaches, stressed primary prevention, and were sustainable long term. The Foundation was impressed with the results achieved by the South Carolina School/Community Model and decided to support a replication project in selected Kansas counties. To ensure fidelity to the major components of the model, the Model's co-director and originator was employed as a co-director for the Kansas project.

Following a Request for Proposal (RFP) process, three counties were selected for implementation: a rural county, an urban county, and a county with a major military facility and resultant transient population. To promote feelings of ownership, each county selected its own name for the project and minor modifications were made to address the specific issues unique to each site. The Kansas-based co-director of the project works closely with the three sites to provide technical assistance, guidance, and support.

The School/Community Model is an exciting, dynamic approach to addressing an important problem. Equally exciting, however, is the Kansas approach—one of respect for success, a willingness to learn from others, and a commitment to implementing faithfully the South Carolina model. This type of sharing forms the basis for the spread of successful models and is a credit to both states.

SOURCES: Personal communication with Dr. Adrienne Paine-Andrews, Program Co-Director and Courtesy Assistant Professor, Department of Human Development, University of Kansas, Lawrence, Kansas. Also adapted from information found in: Paine-Andrews, A. et al: Replicating a community initiative for preventing adolescent pregnancy: From South Carolina to Kansas. *Family Community Health* April, 1996; 19(1);14; and Vincent, M. et al: Reducing adolescent pregnancy through school and community-based education. *JAMA*, 1987; 257, 3382.

The adolescent period can be a turbulent one between the adolescent and her parents without the superimposed stress of adolescent parenting. One of the developmental tasks of this time is the need to gain autonomy and independence; therefore, conflicts between mother and daughter are no surprise, especially with the struggle between the teen's need for independence and the increased dependence that results from her need for financial and psychologic support in caring for the new infant. Children of adolescent parents experience more negative outcomes, including more aggressive behavior at a young age, when the adolescent is in constant conflict with her mother and becomes less involved in parenting.

The younger the adolescent when she gives birth, however, the more she needs support from her mother. East and Felice (1996) found that younger mothers across all socioeconomic levels had little commitment to the mothering role or to their infants. The researchers suggest that because of their young age, these very young mothers are not psychologically able to make the needed commitment.

NURSING CARE MANAGEMENT

In working with adolescents, the nurse should remember that they often think differently than adults. Adolescents, especially younger adolescents, tend to be more concrete thinkers and may not plan ahead for more than a few days. As a result, nurses need to recognize that missed appointments are not unusual. Missed appointments may also be caused by other factors such as a lack of transportation, especially for those teens who are not old enough to drive. Then, too, many adolescents have never before accessed health care without a parent. If they are unable to share their concerns with a parent, they must be highly motivated to seek health care independently for purposes of contraception, treatment of sexually transmitted infections, or for diagnosis of pregnancy.

Nursing Assessment and Diagnosis

The nurse needs to establish a database to plan interventions for the adolescent mother and family. Areas of assessment include history of family health and personal physical health, developmental level and impact of pregnancy, and emotional and financial support. The nurse also assesses the family and social support network and the father's degree of involvement in the pregnancy.

As with all pregnant women, it is important that the caregiver have information on the teen's general physical health. This may be the first time many adolescents have ever provided a health history. The nurse may find it helpful to ask very specific questions and give examples if the young woman appears confused about a question. The nurse may find that the teen's mother is best able to answer questions about family history because the adolescent is often unaware of this information.

The following areas should be assessed:

- Family and personal health history
- Medical history
- Menstrual history
- Obstetric and gynecologic history
- Substance abuse history

It is important to assess the maturational level of each individual. The adolescent's development level and the impact of pregnancy is reflected in the degree to which the teen recognizes the realities and responsibilities involved in pregnancy and parenting. The mother's self-concept (including body image), her relationship with the significant adults in her life, her attitude toward her pregnancy, and her coping methods in the situation are just a few of the significant factors that need to be assessed.

The socioeconomic status of the pregnant teen often places the baby at risk throughout life, beginning with conception. It is essential that the nurse assess family and social support as well as the extent of financial support.

Adolescent lifestyles and support systems vary greatly. It is imperative that the interdisciplinary health team have information about the expectant adolescents' feelings and perceptions about themselves, their sexuality, and the coming baby; their knowledge of, attitude toward, and anticipated ability to care for and support the infant; and their maturational level and needs.

The nursing diagnoses that are applicable to any pregnant woman apply to the pregnant adolescent. Other nursing diagnoses are influenced by the adolescent's age, support systems, socioeconomic situation, health, and maturity. Examples of nursing diagnoses more specific to the pregnant adolescent may include the following:

- ***Altered Nutrition: Less than Body Requirements*** related to poor eating habits
- ***Self-Esteem Disturbance*** related to unanticipated pregnancy

Nursing Plan and Implementation

Community-Based Nursing Care

Early, thorough prenatal care is the strongest and most critical determinant for reducing risk for the adolescent mother and her newborn. The nurse needs to understand the special needs of the adolescent mother to meet this challenge successfully. Many new and innovative community-based agencies have evolved to provide care for high-risk clients throughout the childbearing experience and beyond. For example, an Early Intervention Program in California provides a planned program that includes preparation for motherhood classes and a series of focused prenatal and postpartum home visits made by specially educated public health nurses as well as monthly home visits for the infant's first year of life. Early results demonstrate a reduced rate of preterm births and fewer days of infant hospitalization (Koniak-Griffin, Mathenge, Anderson, & Verzemnieks, 1999).

Nurses in all community-based agencies can help adolescents access the health care system as well as social services and other support services (ie, food banks and WIC). These nurses are also involved extensively in counseling and client teaching.

Issue of Confidentiality Most states in the US have passed legislation that confirms the right of some minors to assume the rights of adults. These adolescents are referred to as **emancipated minors.** An adolescent may be considered emancipated if he or she is self-supporting and living away from home, married, pregnant, a parent, or in the military. The pregnant adolescent, even if very young, is considered emancipated and has the right and responsibility to consent to health care for herself and later for her child. She is entitled to respect and confidentiality in her dealings with health care providers. Only with her consent can other adults, including her parents, be included in communication.

Development of a Trusting Relationship with the Pregnant Adolescent The nurse needs to be attentive to the special problems of adolescents. The first visit to the clinic or office may be fraught with anxiety on the part of the young woman. She may be nervous not only because of her situation, but also because this may well be her first exposure to the health care system since early childhood. Making this experience as positive as possible for the young woman will encourage her cooperation in returning for follow-up care and ensure a favorable attitude toward the importance of health care, whether she chooses to terminate or maintain the pregnancy.

Depending on how young the adolescent is, this may be her first pelvic examination, an anxiety-provoking experience for any woman. The nurse can help provide a thorough explanation of the procedure. A gentle and thoughtful examination technique will help the young woman to relax. A mirror is helpful in allowing the client to see her cervix, educating her about her anatomy, and giving her a part in the exam.

Developing a trusting relationship with the pregnant adolescent is essential. Honesty and respect for the individual and a caring attitude promote self-esteem. As the

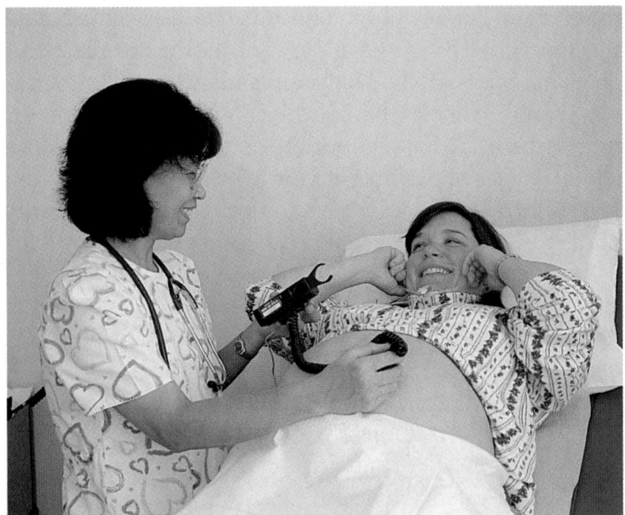

FIGURE 13–2 The nurse gives a young mother an opportunity to listen to her baby's heartbeat.

nurse develops a trusting relationship with the young woman, the nurse's attitudes about self-care and responsibility affect the adolescent's maturation process.

CRITICAL THINKING QUESTION

Imagine that you are a nurse in a clinic caring for a young adolescent who recently learned that she is pregnant and is trying to decide what to do. What are your own beliefs about adolescent pregnancy, abortion, relinquishment, and single parenting? How would you approach your discussion of choices with the adolescent?

Promotion of Self-Esteem and Problem-Solving Skills The nurse assists the adolescent in her decision-making and problem-solving skills so that she can proceed with her developmental tasks and begin to assume responsibility for her life as well as her newborn's life. An overview of what the young woman will experience over the prenatal course, along with thorough explanations and rationale for each procedure as it occurs, will foster the adolescent's understanding and give her some measure of control. Actively involving the young woman in her care will give her a sense of participation and responsibility (Figure 13–2).

Adolescents tend to be egocentric, and even the realization that their health and habits affect the fetus may not be regarded as important by them. It is often helpful to emphasize the effects of these practices on the client herself. Because of their immature cognitive development, adolescents need help in problem solving, in visualizing themselves in the future, and in imagining what the consequences of their actions might be. Moreover, the nurse needs to understand that the adolescent must meet the developmental tasks of pregnancy in addition to the stage-related developmental tasks she is already coping with. Table 13–3 identifies the developmental tasks of pregnancy and the early adolescent's response to pregnancy, with implications for nursing care.

Promotion of Physical Well-Being Baseline weight and blood pressure measurements will be valuable in assessing weight gain and predisposition to pregnancy-induced hypertension. The adolescent may be encouraged to take part in her care by measuring and recording her weight. The nurse may use this time as an opportunity for assisting the young woman in problem solving: "Have I gained too much or too little weight?" "What influence does my diet have on my weight?" "How can I change my eating habits?"

The nurse can also introduce the subject of nutrition during measurement of baseline and subsequent hemoglobin and hematocrit values. Because the adolescent is at risk for anemia, she will need education regarding the importance of iron in her diet. Indeed, basic education about nutrition is a critical component of care for pregnant teens.

Pregnancy-induced hypertension represents the most prevalent medical complication of pregnant adolescents. Blood pressure readings of 140/90 mm Hg are not acceptable as the determinant of PIH in adolescents. Women aged 14 to 20 years without evidence of high blood pressure usually have diastolic readings between 50 and 66 mm Hg. Gradual increases from the prepregnant diastolic readings, along with excessive weight gain, must be evaluated as precursors to PIH. This is one reason why early prenatal care is vital to the effective management of the adolescent.

Adolescents have an increased incidence of sexually transmitted infections (STIs). The initial prenatal examination should include gonococcal and chlamydial cultures and wet prep for *Candida*, *Trichomonas*, and *Gardnerella*. Tests for syphilis should also be done. Education about STIs is important, as is careful observation of herpetic lesions or other symptoms throughout the young woman's pregnancy. Although today's teens are knowledgeable about AIDS, they know much less about other STIs, especially with regard to symptoms and risk reduction. If the adolescent's history indicates that she is at increased risk for HIV, she should be given information about it and offered HIV screening.

The nurse should also discuss substance abuse with adolescents. It is important to review the risks associated with the use of tobacco, caffeine, drugs, and alcohol. The young woman should be aware of the effects of these substances on her development as well as on the development of the fetus.

Ongoing care should include the same assessments that the older woman receives. Special attention should be paid to evaluating fetal growth by determining when quickening occurs and by measuring fundal height, fetal heart tones, and fetal movement. The corresponding dates of auscultating fetal heart tones with the date of last menstrual period and quickening can be helpful in determining correct estimates of time of birth. If there is a question of size-date discrepancy by 2 cm either way, an ultrasound is warranted to establish fetal age so that instances of intrauterine growth restriction (IUGR) may be diagnosed and treated early.

Promotion of Family Adaptation The nurse assesses the family situation during the first prenatal visit and ascertains the level of involvement the adolescent desires from each of her family members and the father of the child, as well as her perception of their present support. A sensitive approach to daughter-mother relationships helps motivate their communication. If the mother and daughter agree, the mother should be included in the client's care.

The nurse should also help the mother assess her daughter's needs and assist her in meeting them. Some adolescents become more dependent during pregnancy, and some become more independent. The mother can ease and encourage her daughter's self-growth by understanding how best to respond and support the adolescent.

Finally, the father of the adolescent's infant should not be forgotten in promoting the family's successful adaptation to the pregnancy. He should be included in prenatal visits, classes, health teaching, and in the birth itself to the extent that he wishes and that is acceptable to the teenage mother. He should also have the opportunity to express his feelings and concerns and to have his questions answered.

Facilitation of Prenatal Education Some school systems are currently attempting to meet prenatal education needs in a variety of ways. The most effective method appears to be mainstreaming the pregnant adolescent in academic classes with her peers and adding classes appropriate to her needs during pregnancy and initial parenting experiences. Classes about growth and development, beginning with the newborn and early infancy, can help teenage parents have more realistic expectations of their infants and may help decrease child abuse. Mainstreaming pregnant adolescents in school is also an ideal way to help them complete their education while learning the skills they need to cope with childbearing and parenting. Vocational guidance in this setting is also most beneficial to their future.

Regardless of the setting for teaching, the developmental tasks of the pregnant teenagers are an important consideration. As stated previously, early adolescents especially tend to be oriented to the present and to be concrete thinkers. As a result, teaching needs to be simple, direct, and responsive to their more immediate needs. For example, teaching about preparation for birth is most effective in the last weeks of pregnancy when this topic is of greater concern and teens are more motivated to practice breathing and relaxation techniques for labor.

Although some childbirth educators believe that older couples can be role models for pregnant adolescents, most believe that prenatal classes with other teens

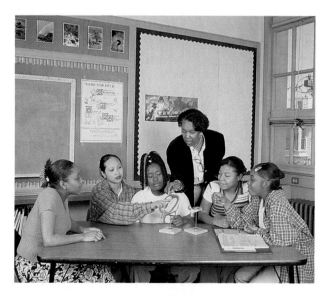

FIGURE 13–3 Young adolescents may benefit from prenatal classes designed specifically for them.

is generally preferable even though these classes can be challenging to teach (Figure 13–3). Attendance may be sporadic. The pregnant teen may be accompanied by her mother, her boyfriend, or her girlfriends. Those who bring girlfriends may bring a different one each time. In such cases, giggling and side conversations may occur. Such activity reflects the short attention span of the teen and is fairly typical. Thus, to keep the attention of the participants it is important to use a variety of teaching strategies, including age-appropriate audiovisual aids, demonstrations, and games.

Goals for prenatal classes may include some or all of the following:

- Providing anticipatory guidance about pregnancy
- Preparing the participants for labor and birth
- Helping participants identify the problems and conflicts of teenage pregnancy and parenting
- Increasing self-esteem
- Providing information about available community resources
- Helping participants develop more adaptive coping skills

Topics on parenting, although sometimes included in prenatal classes for adolescents, tend to be less effective, again because adolescents tend to be oriented to the present. Parenting skills are crucial, but adolescents generally are not ready to learn about these skills until birth makes the newborn a reality.

Hospital-Based Nursing Care

The adolescent's mother is often present during the teen's labor and birth. The sexual partner of the adolescent may also be present, although he may or may not be the father of the baby. Close girlfriends may also arrive soon after the teen is admitted. It is important on admission for the nurse to ask the pregnant adolescent who will be her primary support person in labor and who she wants involved in her labor and birth. This information may also be included on her prenatal record.

The adolescent in labor has the same care needs as any pregnant woman. However, the importance of a sustained presence for her cannot be overemphasized. The nurse must be readily available and should answer questions simply and honestly, using lay terminology. The nurse can also help the adolescent's support people understand their roles in assisting the teen. If the father is involved, the nurse can encourage him to work within his own level of comfort to play an active role in all phases of the birth process, perhaps by feeding ice chips to the mother, timing her contractions, and coaching her with her breathing. The nurse can also let the couple know that holding hands, back rubs, and supportive touching is acceptable and therapeutic (Mills, 1997).

During the postpartum period, most teens do not foresee that they will become sexually active in the near future and are often adamant about the fact that they will not become pregnant again for an extended period. However, the statistics demonstrate a different reality. Prior to discharge, therefore, the nurse's teaching should include information about the resumption of ovulation and the importance of contraception. It is especially helpful to do this teaching with the sexual partner present. The nurse can encourage the couple to use condoms and spermicide until another method is started.

As part of discharge planning, the nurse should ensure that the teen is aware of community resources available to assist her and her family. Postpartum classes, especially with peers, can be extremely beneficial. Such classes address a variety of topics, including postpartum adaptation, infant and child development, parenting skills, and the like.

Prevention of Adolescent Pregnancy

Beginning in the 1980s, the federal government allocated millions of dollars for abstinence-only sex education programs because of the belief of some legislators that abstinence was the only method of prevention that would work or would be accepted by the general public. They believed that funding adolescent contraceptive services would appear to condone sexual activity (Wilcox, Limber, O'Bierne, & Bartels, 1996). Unfortunately, there is little evidence published in the professional literature to support the effectiveness of the abstinence-only programs. Even in the best programs, the results have been disappointing (Wilcox et al, 1996). Abstinence-plus programs are slightly more encouraging in delaying sexual activity (Frost & Forrest, 1995). Although research on the effectiveness of abstinence-only programs had been discouraging, congressional support increased dramatically when the Personal Responsibility and Work Opportunity Act of 1996 was passed. This legislation provided $50 million annually to states for abstinence-only programs.

National Campaign to Prevent Teen Pregnancy

A new national effort to prevent teen pregnancy was initiated in 1996 with the establishment of the National Campaign to Prevent Teen Pregnancy. Its purpose is to reduce teenage pregnancy by one-third by the year 2005 (National Campaign to Prevent Teen Pregnancy, 1997b). The Campaign is a private, nonprofit organization made up of a broad spectrum of religious, political, social, human services, health, and academic organizations. The Association of Women's Health, Obstetric, and Neonatal Nurses (AWHONN) is one of the professional organizations that joined this group and made a commitment to focus on adolescent pregnancy prevention.

Accomplishments in the National Campaign's first year included legislative proposals from bipartisan groups in Congress to allocate money to fund better evaluation of adolescent pregnancy prevention programs and for one-time incentive grants for communities (Cockey, 1997). The National Campaign also has commitments to adolescent pregnancy prevention from such media groups as MTV and ABC Daytime (National Campaign to Prevent Teen Pregnancy, 1997b).

One of the first actions of the National Campaign was to commission a task force to do a comprehensive review of the incidence of adolescent pregnancy and its impact on the nation. At the same time, another task force was commissioned to review the research on the effectiveness of pregnancy prevention programs. The purpose of these task forces was to provide accurate information based on fact and research. In the first year, the National Campaign summarized the results in several publications. Not surprisingly, they have found that adolescent pregnancy is a multifaceted problem with no easy answers. The best approach in local areas needs to be based on strong, communitywide involvement with a variety of programs directed at multiple causes of the problem. No one program can be effective by itself in changing the rate of teenage pregnancy (Kirby, 1997).

Current Community Challenges

One of the major problems in local communities continues to be intense conflict among different groups about how to approach adolescent pregnancy prevention. Some groups feel that abstinence is the only answer, whereas others feel that abstinence programs will not work with the many teens who are already sexually active. The latter groups feel that sex education and easy availability of contraception are the answers. Ironically, a comprehensive review of research suggests that neither of the proposed solutions, individually or together, is as effective in reducing the teen pregnancy rate as many believe. The risk fac-

TABLE 13–4 Community Approaches to Preventing Adolescent Pregnancy

I. Planning

- Involve all sectors of the community (eg, business groups, religious groups, civic organizations, health and human service providers, schools, media).
- Commit to adequate, long-term funding.
- Include teens in planning effective programs.
- Target high-risk populations within the community.
- Target males as well as females.
- Plan programs that are culturally appropriate and age appropriate as well as locally relevant.

II. Sample Components of a Community Program

- Youth development activities, such as tutoring, mentoring, after-school activities, community volunteer work.
- Community-based adolescent health clinics.
- School drop-out prevention.
- Opportunities for career counseling and job training.
- Comprehensive sexuality education, which not only includes accurate information about sexually transmitted infections and contraception, but also teaches adolescents skills to avoid peer pressure and promote responsible relationships.
- Educational programs for teachers and religious leaders who teach sexuality education.
- Educational program for parents on communication skills and increasing knowledge.
- Training peers to be educators and to give support.

III. Evaluation

- Evaluation of the process is essential and should include reports about services that are being delivered plus basic demographics (ie, who attends the program over time).
- Knowledge, attitudes, and intent should also be evaluated; however, these factors have not been found to be well related to the adolescents' actual behaviors (Philliber & Namerow, 1995).
- Evaluation of the impact of specific programs may be too expensive for most communities because it involves experimental research that is difficult to implement (ie, large sample size, control groups, random assignment into groups, and long-term follow-up).
- Pregnancy rates and birth rates are not likely to change rapidly (Kirby, 1997; Moore & Sugland, 1996).

tors most closely associated with teen birth rates appear to be poverty, low educational achievement, poor self-esteem, family dysfunction, and high-risk behaviors in general. Thus research suggests that programs to address these societal problems and give teens hope for a different future are more effective than programs narrowly focused on teen sexual activity (Moore & Sugland, 1996; Stevens-Simon et al, 1996). In teen populations who have job accessibility and education, easy and confidential access to sex education and contraception is also important in reducing the teen pregnancy rates (see Table 13–4).

As a result of site visits to communities that have launched programs for adolescent pregnancy prevention, members of the National Campaign concluded that adults must "agree to disagree" and individual groups must be encouraged to move ahead with their different programs because a variety of approaches is needed.

The cause or motivation for pregnancy varies from one community to another. In inner-city areas where there are higher rates of poverty, low self-esteem, school failure, early behavioral problems, and delinquent behaviors, emphasis on programs that promote self-esteem, deal with these social ills, and provide hope for these youth will be critical. However, similar characteristics have been identified by the National Campaign's Task Forces in successful programs, no matter what type of offering or community. Some of the critical characteristics include the following:

- Involvement of adolescents in planning programs
- The need for good role models from the same cultural and racial backgrounds
- The need for long-term and intensive programs
- The need to focus on the adolescent males

FOCUS YOUR STUDY

- Many factors contribute to the increase in the teenage pregnancy rate, including earlier age of first sexual intercourse, lack of knowledge about conception, lack of easy access to contraception, lessened stigma associated with adolescent pregnancy in some populations, poverty, early school failure, and early childhood sexual abuse.
- Adolescent pregnancy prevention programs should be multifaceted, target males as well as females, and involve community-wide approaches.
- Almost half of the fathers of infants of adolescent mothers are age 20 or older, but they are often similar to adolescent fathers psychosocially and are no more likely to be able to support the mother.
- Factors affecting an adolescent's response to pregnancy include her degree of achievement of the developmental tasks of adolescence (which can be closely associated with age), as well as cultural, religious, and socioeconomic factors.
- Often the adolescent has little understanding of pregnancy, childbirth, or parenting. Consequently, education is a primary responsibility of the nurse.

REFERENCES

Acgs, G. (1996). The impact of welfare on young mothers' subsequent childbearing decisions. *Journal of Human Resources, 31*(4), 898–907.

Alan Guttmacher Institute. (1994). *Sex and America's teenagers.* New York: Author.

Alan Guttmacher Institute. (1996). Issues in brief: Risks and realities of early childbearing. Washington, DC: Author.

Alan Guttmacher Institute. (1998). Facts in brief: Teen sex and pregnancy. http://www.agi-usa.org/pubs/fb_teensex.html#ab

Bachman, J. A. (1993). Self-described learning needs of pregnant teen participants in an innovative university/community partnership. *Maternal-Child Nursing Journal, 21*(2), 65–71.

Barton, J. R., Stanziano, G. J., Jacques, D. L., Bergauer, N. K., & Sibai, B. M. (1995). Monitored outpatient management of mild gestational hypertension remote from term in teenage pregnancies. *American Journal of Obstetrics and Gynecology, 173*(6), 1865–1868.

Becker-Lausen, E., & Rickel, A. U. (1995). Integration of teen pregnancy and child abuse research: Identifying mediator variables for pregnancy outcome. *Journal of Primary Prevention, 16*(8) 39–53.

Chase-Lansdale, P. L., Brooks-Gunn, J., & Zamsky, E. S. (1994). Young African-American multigenerational families in poverty: Quality of mothering and grandmothering. [Special issue]. *Child Development, 65*(2), 373–393.

Clark, L. R., Cohall, A. T., & Joffe, A. (1998). Beyond the birds and the bees: Talking to teens about sex. *Contemporary OB/GYN, 43*(4), 35–61.

Cockey, C. D. (1997). Preventing teen pregnancy: It's time to stop kidding around. *AWHONN Lifelines, 1*(3), 32–40.

East, P. L. (1996). Do adolescent pregnancy and childbearing affect younger siblings? *Family Planning Perspectives, 28*(4), 148–153.

East, P. L., & Felice, M. E. (1996). *Adolescent pregnancy and parenting: Findings from a racially diverse sample.* New Jersey: Lawrence Erlbaum Assoc.

Erickson, P. I. (1994). Lessons from a repeat pregnancy prevention program for Hispanic teenage mothers in east Los Angeles. *Family Planning Perspectives, 26*(4), 174–178.

Esparza, D. V., & Esperat, M. C. R. (1996). The effects of childhood sexual abuse on minority adolescent mothers. *Journal of Obstetric, Gynecologic, & Neonatal Nursing, 25*(4), 321–328.

Frost, J. J., & Forrest, J. D. (1995). Understanding the impact of effective teenage pregnancy prevention programs. *Family Planning Perspectives, 27*(5), 188–195.

Jones, M. E., & Mondy, L. W. (1994). Lessons for prevention and intervention in adolescent pregnancy: A five-year comparison of outcomes of two programs for school-aged pregnant adolescents. *Journal of Pediatric Health Care, 8*(4), 152–159.

Kaunitz, A. M. (1997). Contraception for the adolescent patient. *International Journal of Fertility and Women's Medicine, 42*(1), 30–38.

Kirby, D. (1997). *No easy answers: Research findings on programs to reduce teen pregnancy (summary).* Washington, DC: National Campaign to Prevent Teen Pregnancy.

Kirby, D., Short, L., Collins, J., Rugg, D., Kolbe, L., Howard, M., Miller, B., Sonenstein, F., & Zabin, L. S. (1994). School-based programs to reduce sexual risk behaviors: A review of effectiveness. *Public Health Reports, 109*(3), 339–360.

Koniak-Griffin, D., Mathenge, C., Anderson, N.L.R. & Verzemnieks, I. (1999). An early intervention program for adolescent mothers: A nursing demonstration project. *Journal of Obstetric, Gynecologic, & Neonatal Nursing, 28*(1):51–59.

Landry, D. J., & Forrest, J. D. (1995). How old are US fathers? *Family Planning Perspectives, 27*(4), 159–161, 165.

Long, S. H., Marquis, M. S., & Harrison, E. R. (1994). The costs and financing of perinatal care in the United States. *American Journal of Public Health, 84*(9), 1473–1478.

Maynard, R. A. (Ed.). (1996). *Kids having kids: A Robin Hood Foundation special report on costs of adolescent childbearing.* New York: Robin Hood Foundation.

Maynard, R. A. (Ed.). (1997). *Kids having kids: Economic costs and social consequences of teen pregnancy.* Washington, DC: Urban Institute Press.

Mills, C. B. (1997). Taking time to care: Making ways to help teen parents. *AWHONN Lifelines, 1*(5), 70–72.

Moore, K., Miller, B., Glei, D., & Morrison, D. R. (1995). *Adolescent sex, contraception and childbearing: A review of recent research.* Washington, DC: Child Trends, Inc.

Moore, K., & Sugland, B. (1996). *Next steps and best bets: Approaches to preventing adolescent childbearing.* Washington, DC: Child Trends, Inc.

National Campaign to Prevent Teen Pregnancy. (1997a). *Snapshots from the front line: Lessons about teen pregnancy prevention from states and communities.* Washington, DC: Author.

National Campaign to Prevent Teen Pregnancy. (1997b). *Whatever happened to childhood? The problem of teen pregnancy in the United States.* Washington, DC: Author.

Peckham, S. (1993). Preventing unintended teenage pregnancies. *Public Health, 107,* 125.

Philliber, S., & Namerow, P. (1995). Trying to maximize the odds: Using what we know to prevent teen pregnancy. Paper presented at technical assistance workshop to support the Teen Pregnancy Prevention Program. Division of Reproductive Health, Centers for Disease Control and Prevention, Atlanta, GA, December 13–15, 1995.

Rosenberg, H. M., Ventura, S. J., Maurer, J. D., Heuser, R. L., & Freedman, M. A. (1996, Oct. 4). Births and deaths: United States, 1995. *Monthly Vital Statistics Report, 45*(3 Suppl. 2).

Roye, C. F., & Balk, S. J. (1996). The relationship of partner support to outcomes for teenage mothers and their children: A review. *Journal of Adolescent Health, 19*(2), 86–93.

Seidman, S. N., & Rieder, R. O. (1994). A review of sexual behavior in the United States. *American Journal of Psychiatry, 151*(3), 330–341.

Sells, C. W., & Blum, R. W. (1996). Morbidity and mortality among US adolescents: An overview of data and trends. *American Journal of Public Health, 86*(4), 513–519.

Smith, C. (1996). The link between childhood maltreatment and teenage pregnancy. *Social Work Research, 20*(3) 131–141.

Smith, P. B., & Weinman, M. L. (1995). Cultural implications for public health policy for pregnant Hispanic adolescents. *Health Values: The Journal of Health Behavior, Education, & Promotion, 19*(1), 3–9.

Spieker, S. J., & Bensley, L. (1994). Roles of living arrangements and grandmother social support in adolescent mothering and infant attachment. *Developmental Psychology, 30*(1), 102–111.

Steinberg, L. (1993). *Adolescence* (3rd ed.). New York: McGraw-Hill.

Stevens-Simon, C., Kelly, L., Singer, D., & Cox, A. (1996). Why pregnant adolescents say they did not use contraceptives prior to conception. *Journal of Adolescent Health, 19*(1), 48–53.

Stock, J. L., Bell, M. A., Boyer, D. K., & Connell, F. A. (1997). Adolescent pregnancy and sexual risk-taking among sexually abused girls. *Family Planning Perspectives, 29*(5), 200–203, 227.

Taylor, D., Chavez, G., Chabra, A., & Boggess, J. (1997). Risk factors for adult paternity in births to adolescents. *Obstetrics & Gynecology, 89*(2), 199–205.

US Department of Health and Human Services. (1995, Sept.). *Report to Congress on out-of-wedlock childbearing.* Washington, DC: Author.

Ventura, S. J., Curtin, S. C., & Mathews, T. J. (1998). Teenage births in the United States: National and state trends, 1990–96. National Vital Statistics System. Hyattsville, MD, National Center for Health Statistics.

Wilcox, B. L., Limber, S. P., O'Bierne, H., & Bartels, C. L. (1996, Nov. 18). *Adolescent abstinence promotion programs: An evaluation of evaluations.* Paper presented at the biennial meeting of the American Public Health Association, New York, NY.

Maternal Nutrition

14

I'M TRYING TO BE VERY CAREFUL ABOUT WHAT I EAT. I've had more salads and fresh fruit than I can remember. Sometimes, though, I get a "cookie attack" and indulge myself. My husband says I should eat oatmeal cookies so I could feel that my cravings were nutritionally sound!

Objectives

- Identify the role of specific nutrients in the diet of the pregnant woman.
- Compare nutritional needs during pregnancy, postpartum, and lactation with nonpregnant requirements.
- Discuss effects of maternal nutrition on fetal outcomes.
- Evaluate adequacy and pattern of weight gain during different stages of pregnancy.
- Plan adequate prenatal vegetarian diets based on nutritional requirements of pregnancy.
- Describe ways in which various physical, psychosocial, and cultural factors can affect nutritional intake and status.
- Compare recommendations for weight gain and nutrient intakes in the pregnant adolescent with those for the mature pregnant adult.
- Describe basic factors a nurse should consider when offering nutritional counseling to a pregnant adolescent.
- Compare nutritional counseling issues for nursing and nonnursing mothers.
- Formulate a nutritional care plan for pregnant women based on a diagnosis of nutritional problems.

Key Terms

Calorie

Folic acid

Kilocalorie

Lactase deficiency (lactose intolerance)

Lacto-ovovegetarians

Lactovegetarians

Pica

Recommended Dietary Allowance (RDA)

Vegans

A WOMAN'S NUTRITIONAL STATUS PRIOR to and during pregnancy can significantly influence her health and that of her unborn child. In most prenatal clinics and offices, nurses provide nutritional counseling directly or work closely with dietitians in providing any necessary nutritional assessment and teaching.

This chapter focuses on the nutritional needs of a normal pregnant woman. Special sections consider the nutritional needs of the pregnant adolescent and the woman after birth.

Good prenatal nutrition is the result of proper eating throughout life, not just during pregnancy, although pregnancy may motivate a woman to improve poor eating habits. Many factors influence a woman's ability to achieve good prenatal nutrition, including the following:

- *General nutritional status prior to pregnancy.* Nutritional deficits at conception and the early prenatal period may influence the outcome of the pregnancy.
- *Maternal age.* An expectant adolescent must meet the nutritional needs for her own growth in addition to the nutritional needs of pregnancy.
- *Maternal parity.* A mother's nutritional needs and the outcome of her pregnancy are influenced by the number of pregnancies she has had and the intervals between them.

A mother's nutritional status does affect her fetus. Factors influencing fetal well-being are interrelated, but nutrient deficiencies alone can produce measurable effects on cell and organ growth of the developing fetus.

Fetal growth occurs in three overlapping stages: (1) growth by increase in cell number, (2) growth by increase in cell number and cell size, and (3) growth by increase in cell size alone. The nutritional problems that interfere with cell division may have permanent consequences. If the nutritional insult occurs when cells are mainly enlarging, the changes are usually reversible when normal nutrition resumes.

Growth of fetal and maternal tissues requires increased quantities of nutrients. These are listed in the **recommended dietary allowances (RDAs)** as specific allowances for pregnant and lactating women (Table 14–1). The RDAs distinguish between the first and second 6-month periods of lactation to reflect the differences in the amount of milk produced (750 mL and 600 mL, respectively) as the baby begins to consume solid foods (National Research Council, 1989).

The pregnant woman can obtain most of the recommended nutrients by eating a well-balanced diet each day. The basic food groups and recommended amounts during pregnancy and lactation are presented in Table 14–2.

TABLE 14–1 Recommended Dietary Allowances (RDAs) for Nonpregnant, Pregnant, and Lactating Females, revised 1989*

						Fat-Soluble Vitamins				Water-Soluble Vitamins							Minerals						
Age (years) and Sex Group	Weight[†] kg	Weight[†] lb	Height[†] cm	Height[†] in	Protein	Vitamin A	Vitamin D	Vitamin E	Vitamin K	Vitamin C	Thiamine	Riboflavin	Niacin	Vitamin B_6	Folate	Vitamin B_{12}	Calcium	Phosphorus	Magnesium	Iron	Zinc	Iodine	Selenium
					g	μgR[‡]	μg[§]	mg α TE[‖]	μg	← mg	mg	mg →	mg NE[¶]	mg	← μg	μg →	← mg	mg	mg	mg	mg →	← μg	μg →
Females																							
11–14	46	101	157	62	46	800	10	8	45	50	1.1	1.3	15	1.4	150	2.0	1200	1200	280	15	12	150	45
15–18	55	120	163	64	44	800	10	8	55	60	1.1	1.3	15	1.5	180	2.0	1200	1200	300	15	12	150	50
19–24	58	128	164	65	46	800	10	8	60	60	1.1	1.3	15	1.6	180	2.0	1200	1200	280	15	12	150	55
25–50	63	138	163	64	50	800	5	8	65	60	1.1	1.3	15	1.6	180	2.0	800	800	280	15	12	150	55
51+	65	143	160	63	50	800	5	8	65	60	1.0	1.2	13	1.6	180	2.0	800	800	280	10	12	150	55
Pregnant					60	800	10	10	65	70	1.5	1.6	17	2.2	400	2.2	1200	1200	320	30	15	175	65
Lactating																							
1st 6 months					65	1300	10	12	65	95	1.6	1.8	20	2.1	280	2.6	1200	1200	355	15	19	200	75
2nd 6 months					62	1200	10	11	65	90	1.6	1.7	20	2.1	260	2.6	1200	1200	340	15	16	200	75

*The allowances, expressed as average daily intakes over time, are intended to provide for individual variations among most normal persons as they live in the United States under usual environmental stresses. Diets should be based on a variety of common foods in order to provide other nutrients for which human requirements have been less well defined.

[†]Weights and heights of reference adults are actual medians for the US population of the designated age, as reported by NHANES II. The median weights and heights of those under 19 years of age were taken from Hamill PVV et al: Physical growth. National Center for Health Statistics Percentiles. *Am J Clin Nutr* 1979; 32:607. The use of these figures does not imply that the height-to-weight ratios are ideal.

[‡]Retinol equivalents. 1 retinol equivalent = 1 μg retinol or 6 μg β-carotene.

[§]As cholecalciferol. 10 μg cholecalciferol = 400 IU of vitamin D.

[‖]α-Tocopherol equivalents. 1 mg d-α tocopherol = 1 α-TE.

[¶]1 NE (niacin equivalent) is equal to 1 mg of niacin or 60 mg of dietary tryptophan.

SOURCE: *Recommended Dietary Allowances,* 10th ed. 1989 National Academy of Sciences, National Research Council, Food and Nutrition Board. Washington, DC.

TABLE 14–2 Daily Food Plan for Pregnancy and Lactation

Food Group	Nutrients Provided	Food Source	Recommended Daily Amount During Pregnancy	Recommended Daily Amount During Lactation
Dairy products	Protein; riboflavin; vitamins A, D, and others; calcium; phosphorus; zinc; magnesium	Milk—whole, 2%, skim, dry, buttermilk Cheeses—hard, semisoft, cottage Yogurt—plain, low-fat Soybean milk—canned, dry	Four (8 oz) cups (five for teenagers) used plain or with flavoring, in shakes, soups, puddings, custards, cocoa Calcium in 1 cup milk equivalent to 1½ cups cottage cheese, 1½ oz hard or semisoft cheese, 1 cup yogurt, 1½ cups ice cream (high in fat and sugar)	Four (8 oz) cups (five for teenagers); equivalent amount of cheese, yogurt and so forth
Meat and meat alternatives	Protein; iron; thiamine, niacin, and other vitamins; minerals	Beef, pork, veal, lamb, poultry, animal organ meats, fish, eggs; legumes; nuts, seeds, peanut butter, grains in proper vegetarian combination (vitamin B_{12} supplement needed)	Three servings (one serving = 2 oz), combination in amounts necessary for same nutrient equivalent (varies greatly)	Two servings
Grain products, whole grain or enriched	B vitamins; iron; whole grain also has zinc, magnesium, and other trace elements; provides fiber	Breads and bread products such as cornbread, muffins, waffles, hotcakes, biscuits, dumplings, cereals, pastas, rice	Six to 11 servings daily: one serving = one slice bread, ¾ cup or 1 oz dry cereal ½ cup rice or pasta	Same as for pregnancy
Fruits and fruit juices	Vitamins A and C; minerals; raw fruits for roughage	Citrus fruits and juices, melons, berries, all other fruits and juices	Two to four servings (one serving for vitamin C): one serving = one medium fruit, ½–1 cup fruit, 4 oz orange or grapefruit juice	Same as for pregnancy
Vegetables and vegetable juices	Vitamins A and C; minerals; provides roughage	Leafy green vegetables; deep yellow or orange vegetables such as carrots, sweet potatoes, squash, tomatoes; green vegetables such as peas, green beans, broccoli; other vegetables such as beets, cabbage, potatoes, corn, lima beans	Three to five servings (one serving of dark green or deep yellow vegetable for vitamin A): one serving = ½–1 cup vegetable, two tomatoes, one medium potato	Same as for pregnancy
Fats	Vitamins A and D; linoleic acid	Butter, cream cheese, fortified table spreads; cream, whipped cream, whipped toppings; avocado, mayonnaise, oil, nuts	As desired in moderation (high in calories): one serving = 1 tbsp butter or enriched margarine	Same as for pregnancy
Sugar and sweets		Sugar, brown sugar, honey, molasses	Occasionally, if desired	Same as for pregnancy
Desserts		Nutritious desserts such as puddings, custards, fruit whips, and crisps; other rich, sweet desserts and pastries	Occasionally, if desired	Same as for pregnancy
Beverages		Coffee, decaffeinated beverages, tea, bouillon, carbonated drinks	As desired, in moderation	Same as for pregnancy
Miscellaneous		Iodized salt, herbs, spices, condiments	As desired	Same as for pregnancy

NOTE: The pregnant woman should eat regularly, three meals a day, with nutritious snacks of fruit, cheese, milk, or other foods between meals if desired. (More frequent but smaller meals are also recommended.) Four to 6 (8 oz) glasses of water and a total of 8 to 10 (8 oz) cups total fluid intake should be consumed daily. Water is an essential nutrient.

RESEARCH IN PRACTICE

What is this study about? Optimal maternal weight gain may reduce the risk of maternal obesity while optimizing fetal growth. Anne Paxton and her colleagues developed a four-compartment model to estimate maternal body fat by measuring weight, total water, bone mineral mass, and body density of pregnant women.

How was the study done? The researchers obtained data from 200 pregnant African American, Latina, and European American women at 14 and 37 weeks' gestation. Data collection included measuring height, weight, total body water (with deuterium isotopes), body density (through underwater weighing), 11 skinfold thicknesses, and 12 circumferences. Bone mineral mass determination occurred postpartum because the testing used radiation.

What were the results of the study? The researchers compared estimates of body fat derived from their model to the estimates generated from existing anthropometric formulas for nonpregnant women. At week 14, mean body fat estimates of 17.7 to 23.5 kg were found using the traditional formulas, with an estimate of 21.4 kg with the four-compartment model. These values were all statistically different from one another. At week 37, the estimate of change in body fat ranged from 3.3 to 5.2 kg, with the lowest estimate coming from the multicompartment formula. The investigators also developed new anthropometric equations to determine change in body fat during pregnancy and to determine body fat mass at term. The equation, which determined change in body fat, explained 73% of the variance and consisted of the following: Fat change, kg = 0.77 (weight change, kg) + 0.07 (change in thigh skinfold thickness, mm) − 6.13. The equation for body fat mass at term explained 89% of the variance and incorporated the following: fat mass at term, kg = 0.40 (weight, week 37, kg) + 0.16 (biceps skinfold thickness, week 37, mm) + 0.15 (thigh skinfold thickness, week 37, mm) − 0.09 (wrist circumference, week 37, mm) + 0.10 (prepregnancy weight) − 6.56. The researchers validated the findings by using a repeated measure ANOVA to compare results of the new anthropometric equations to the multicompartment findings and across strata of gestational weight gain, prepregnancy body mass index, ethnicity, and socioeconomic status.

What additional questions might I have? Were all of the assumptions of ANOVA met? No table of results was provided, so it is difficult to evaluate whether there were adequate numbers of subjects within each group.

How can I use this study? The anthropometric equations to determine change in maternal body fat or fat mass at term are simple to calculate given prepregnancy weight, weight at 37 weeks, and correct skinfold thickness measurements at weeks 14 and 37.

SOURCE: Paxton, A., Lederman, S. A., Heymsfield, S. B., Wang, J., Thornton, J. C., & Pierson, R. N. (1998). Anthropometric equations for studying body fat in pregnant women. *American Journal of Clinical Nutrition, 67,* 104–110.

TABLE 14–3 Recommended Total Weight Gain Ranges for Pregnant Women

Prepregnancy Weight-for-Height Category	Recommended Total Gain lb	kg
Low (BMI <19.8)	28–40	12.5–18
Normal (BMI 19.8–26)	25–35	11.5–16
High (BMI >26.0–29.0)	15–25	7.0–11.5
Obese (BMI >29.0)	≥15	≥7.0

NOTE: For singleton pregnancies. The range for women carrying twins is 16–20 kg (35–45 lb). Young adolescents (<2 years after menarche) and African American women should strive for gains at the upper end of the range. Short women (<157 cm or <62 in) should strive for gains at the lower end of the range.

SOURCE: Institute of Medicine Subcommittee for a Clinical Application Guide. *Nutrition During Pregnancy and Lactation: An Implementation Guide.* Washington, DC: National Academy Press, 1992, p 44.

Maternal Weight Gain

Maternal weight gain is an important factor in fetal growth and infant birth weight. An adequate weight gain over time indicates an adequate caloric intake. It does not, however, ensure that the woman has a sufficient nutrient intake. The diet may not be of high enough nutritional quality even though its caloric content supports the recommended weight gain. The pregnant woman must maintain the nutritional quality of her diet as her weight gain progresses.

Weight gain, even in women with a healthy pregnancy outcome, tends to be quite variable. Optimal weight gain depends on the woman's weight for height (body mass index [BMI]) and her prepregnant nutritional state. The Institute of Medicine (1992) recommends weight gain in terms of optimum ranges based on prepregnant BMI (Table 14–3). Adequate maternal weight gain contributes to the tissue expansion and growth of both the mother and the developing fetus.

The pattern of weight gain during pregnancy is also important. Inadequate prenatal weight gain, particularly during the second trimester, is associated with reduced birth weight in the newborn (Hickey, Cliver, McNeal, Hoffman, & Goldberg, 1996). For women of normal weight, the recommended pattern consists of a gain of 1.6 to 2.3 kg (3.5 to 5 lb) during the first trimester, followed by an average gain of 0.5 kg (1 lb) per week during the last two trimesters. The rate of weight gain in the second and third trimesters needs to be slightly higher for underweight women and slightly lower (0.7 lb per week) for overweight women (Institute of Medicine, 1990). A maternal weight gain of 1.5 lb per week has been suggested for normal weight women during the second half of a twin pregnancy. Underweight women should strive for a gain of 1.75 lb/week after 20 weeks' gestation (Lantz, Chez, Rodriguez, & Porter, 1996).

The average maternal weight gain is distributed as follows:

5.0 kg (11 lb)	Fetus, placenta, amniotic fluid
0.9 kg (2 lb)	Uterus
1.8 kg (4 lb)	Increased blood volume
1.4 kg (3 lb)	Breast tissue
2.3 to 4.5 kg (5–10 lb)	Maternal stores

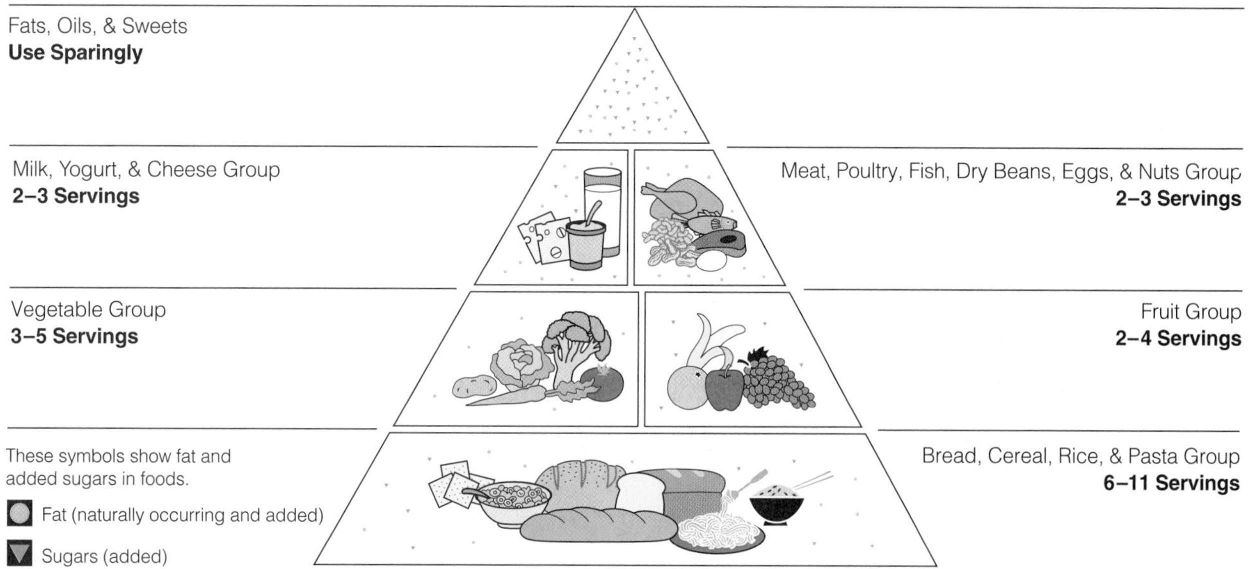

FIGURE 14–1 The Food Guide Pyramid provides a quick reference for people interested in healthy eating. The largest portion of the pyramid is devoted to grains, rice, bread, and pasta, whereas the smallest portion is devoted to fats, oils, and sweets, which should be used sparingly. SOURCE: US Dept of Agriculture; US Dept of Health and Human Services.

Low maternal weight gain has been associated with preterm births (Siega-Riz, Adair, & Hobel, 1994), low-birth-weight infants, and fetal growth retardation. A high maternal weight gain can result in a large-for-gestational-age infant, complications during birth (Abrams, 1994), and possibly even an increased risk of congenital malformations, particularly of the central nervous system (Prentice & Goldberg, 1996).

Because of this association between maternal weight gain and pregnancy outcome, most caregivers pay particular attention to weight gain during pregnancy. Weight gain charts can be useful in monitoring the rate of weight gain over time. If a significant deviation from the anticipated pattern occurs, the cause should be determined and appropriate interventions planned with the woman.

As mentioned above, weight gain alone does not guarantee adequate nutrition. A diet may be high in energy (calories) but low in vitamins, minerals, or complex carbohydrates and protein. Pregnancy is not a time to diet, and severe caloric restriction during pregnancy can result in maternal ketosis. Counseling the pregnant woman to eat according to the Food Guide Pyramid (Figure 14–1) places less emphasis on the amount of her weight gain and more on the quality of her intake.

CLINICAL TIP

Weight varies with time of day, variations in clothing, inaccurate scale adjustment, or weighing error. Do not overemphasize a single weight. Notice the pattern of weight gain.

Nutritional Requirements

The RDA for calories and almost all nutrients increases during pregnancy, although the amount of increase varies with each nutrient. These increases reflect the additional requirements of both the mother and the developing fetus (Table 14–1).

CRITICAL THINKING QUESTION

In counseling a pregnant woman about nutrition, what would you tell her about the role that the RDAs play?

Calories

The term **calorie** (cal) stands for the amount of heat required to raise the temperature of 1 gram of water 1 degree centigrade. The **kilocalorie** (kcal) is equivalent to 1000 cal and is the unit used to express the energy value of food.

The RDA for energy is no caloric increase during the first trimester and a daily increase of 300 kcal during the second and third trimesters. Women with a twin pregnancy should add an additional 300 kcal, for a total of 600

CRITICAL THINKING IN PRACTICE

Diane Fernandez is 14 weeks pregnant. The rate and total amount of her weight gain during the first trimester have been consistent with recommendations. She has gained an average of 0.5 kg (1 lb) per week during both of the past 2 weeks. Her appetite is good, and she consumes three meals per day and snacks between meals on occasion.

Diane has altered her diet because she is concerned about excessive weight gain. She told the nurse that she has decreased her intake from the bread and dairy groups in order to limit her calorie intake. Because she has omitted most dairy products, she has increased her consumption of salads and broccoli to provide calcium sources.

A diet history revealed the following:

Grain	3–4 servings, mainly cereal and rice
Fruit	2–4 servings, fresh fruit
Vegetables	3–5 servings, salads, peas, corn, broccoli
Meat	4–5 servings, beef, pork, chicken
Dairy	occasionally cheese, ice cream, pudding
Fats, oils, sweets	occasionally salad dressings, margarine, desserts
Beverages	8–10 servings, soda, juices, water

After assessing her diet history, what is your evaluation of Diane's diet? How could you counsel her?

Answers can be found in Appendix I.

kcal above nonpregnant levels (American College of Obstetricians and Gynecologists [ACOG], 1998a). Weight gains should be monitored regularly, and dietary recommendations should be individualized to help the pregnant woman meet her caloric needs. Prepregnant weight, height, maternal age, activity, and health status all affect caloric requirements.

The Self-Care Guide, "How to Add 300 kcal to Your Diet," provides basic nutritional information to pregnant women and offers suggestions for increasing caloric intake. It may be copied for use as a handout.

Carbohydrates

Carbohydrates provide the body's primary source of energy as well as fiber necessary for proper bowel functioning. If the total caloric intake is not adequate, the body uses protein for energy. Protein then becomes unavailable for growth needs. In addition, protein breakdown leads to ketosis. Ketosis can be a problem, especially in diabetic women, because of glycosuria, reduced alkaline reserves, and lipidemia.

The carbohydrate and caloric needs of the pregnant woman increase, especially during the last two trimesters. Carbohydrate intake promotes weight gain and growth of the fetus, placenta, and other maternal tissues. Dairy products, fruits, vegetables, and whole-grain cereals and breads all contain carbohydrates.

Protein

During pregnancy, the woman needs increased amounts of protein to provide amino acids for fetal development, blood volume expansion, and growth of other maternal tissues, such as breasts and uterus. Protein also contributes to the body's overall energy metabolism. The RDA for protein during pregnancy is 60 g, an increase of about 14 g (Table 14–1).

The quality of dietary protein is as important as the total amount consumed. The quality is determined by the complex of amino acids that makes up the protein. Proteins are said to be complete when they are made up of all the amino acids necessary to sustain growth and are considered incomplete when they lack some of the necessary amino acids. Proteins of animal origin are generally complete, and proteins of plant origin are incomplete.

To obtain high-quality protein in the diet, it is best to eat a variety of foods. Animal products, such as lean meats, fish, poultry, and eggs, are sources of high-quality, complete protein. Dairy products are also important protein sources. A quart of milk supplies 32 g of protein, more than half the average daily protein requirement. Milk can be incorporated into the diet in a variety of dishes, including soups, puddings, custards, sauces, yogurt, and beverages such as hot chocolate and fruited milk drinks. Various kinds of hard and soft cheeses and cottage cheese are also excellent protein sources, although cream cheese is categorized as a fat source only. Table 14–4 provides information on the protein content of common foods.

TABLE 14–4 Amount of Protein in Common Foods

Food	Protein (g)
Dairy Products	
Milk, 8 oz	8
Cheese: cheddar, Swiss, and so forth, 1 oz	7
Cottage cheese ¼ cup	7
Meat and Meat Alternatives	
Meat, fish, poultry, 1 oz	7
Egg, 1	7
Cooked dry beans & peas, ½ cup	7
Cooked soybeans, ½ cup	11
Peanut butter, 2 tbsp	7
Peanuts (3 tbsp), cashews/almonds (5 tbsp)	7
Breads and Cereals	
Bread, 1 slice	2
Buns, biscuits, muffins, 1	2
Cooked cereals and grains, ½ cup	2
Breakfast cereal, 1 oz	2
Vegetables and Fruits	
Vegetables, ½ cup	0.5–1
Fruits & juices, ½ cup	0.5

Women who have allergies to milk, who have lactose intolerance, or who practice vegetarianism may find dried or canned soy milk acceptable. It can be used in cooked dishes or as a beverage. Tofu, or soybean curd, can replace cottage cheese.

If the woman consumes little or no protein from animal sources, it will be necessary to combine foods of plant origin to obtain the amino acids necessary for a complete protein. Examples of combined proteins are beans and rice, peanut butter on whole-grain bread, and whole-grain cereal and milk. Adequate dietary protein can be obtained by consuming a varied diet; protein and amino acid supplements are not recommended (Institute of Medicine, 1990).

Fat

Fats are valuable sources of energy for the body. Fats are more completely absorbed during pregnancy, resulting in a marked increase in serum lipids, lipoproteins, and cholesterol and decreased elimination of fat through the bowel. Fat deposits in the fetus increase from about 2% at midpregnancy to almost 12% at term. US dietary guidelines recommend that fat calories should not exceed 30% of the total daily caloric intake and that less than 10% should be saturated fat (US Department of Agriculture & US Department of Health and Human Services [USDA/USDHHS], 1990).

When dairy products are used as a regular part of the diet, it may be helpful to select items that have a reduced fat content. Selecting lean cuts of meats, fish, and poultry will also help decrease dietary fat.

Minerals

The woman can increase minerals needed for the growth of new tissue during pregnancy by improving mineral absorption and increasing mineral intake.

Calcium and Phosphorus

Calcium and phosphorus are involved in the mineralization of fetal bones and teeth, energy and cell production, and acid-base buffering. Calcium is absorbed and used more efficiently during pregnancy. Some calcium and phosphorus are required early in pregnancy, but most of the fetus's bone calcification occurs during the last 2 or 3 months. Teeth begin to form at about 8 weeks' gestation and are formed by birth. The 6-year molars begin to calcify just before birth. This means that calcium is particularly important as a structural element. Additional calcium is stored in the maternal skeleton as a reserve for lactation. For the mother, calcium supplementation during pregnancy has been shown to reduce the risk of preeclampsia (DeCherney & Koos, 1997).

The RDA for calcium for the pregnant or lactating woman, regardless of age, is 1200 mg/day. If calcium intake is not adequate, fetal needs will be met at the mother's expense by demineralization of maternal bone.

TABLE 14–5 Foods that Provide Comaprable Amounts of Calcium

Food	Amount
Dairy Products	
Milk	8 oz
Cheese, cheddar	1½ oz
Pudding, vanilla	1 cup
Fruits	
Figs	10
Raisins	2 cups
Vegetables	
Broccoli	2½ cups
Collards	1 cup
Kale	3 cups
Mustard greens	3½ cups
Turnip greens	1½ cups
Fish	
Salmon, canned, with bones	⅔ cup
Sardines	6
Nuts	
Almonds	4 oz
Brazil nuts	½ cup
Miscellaneous	
Molasses, blackstrap	2 tbsp

SOURCE: Data from Pennington JAT: *Bowes and Church's Food Values of Portions Commonly Used,* 15th ed. Philadelphia: Lippincott, 1989.

A diet that includes 4 cups of milk or an equivalent dairy alternate (Table 14–2) will provide sufficient calcium. Smaller amounts of calcium are supplied by legumes, nuts, dried fruits, and dark green leafy vegetables (such as kale, broccoli, collard greens, and beet greens). It is important to remember that some of the calcium in beet greens, spinach, and Swiss chard is bound with oxalic acid, which makes it less available to the body. Larger amounts of these foods need to be consumed if they are substituted for dairy sources of calcium (Table 14–5).

The RDA for phosphorus is the same as the RDA for calcium: 1200 mg/day for the pregnant or lactating woman. Phosphorus is readily supplied through calcium- and protein-rich foods, especially milk, eggs, and meat.

Iodine

Iodine is an essential part of the thyroid hormone, thyroxine. Inorganic iodine is excreted in the urine during pregnancy. Enlargement of the thyroid gland may occur if iodine is not replaced by adequate dietary intake or additional supplement. Iodine deficiency is the most widespread nutritional cause of impaired brain development. This can result in cretinism and lesser degrees of retardation (Wada & King, 1994).

A woman can meet the iodine requirement of 175 mg/day by using iodized salt. Seafood is also a good source of iodine. Plant sources vary because they reflect the iodine content of the soil in which they grow. When sodium is restricted, the physician may prescribe an iodine supplement.

Sodium

The sodium ion is essential for proper metabolism and the regulation of fluid balance. Sodium intake in the form of salt is never entirely curtailed during pregnancy, even when hypertension or PIH is present. The woman can obtain moderate sodium intake (2 to 3 g) by using fresh food lightly seasoned to taste during cooking. The use of extra salt at the table should be avoided. Salty foods, such as potato chips, ham, sausages, and sodium-based seasonings, can be eliminated to avoid excessive intake.

Zinc

Zinc is a part of numerous enzymes and is involved in protein metabolism and the synthesis of DNA and RNA. It is essential for normal fetal growth and development as well as milk production during lactation. Even a mild zinc deficiency may be associated with maternal and fetal morbidity (Prasad, 1996). Fortunately, zinc absorption increases during pregnancy (Fung, Ritchie, Woodhouse, Roehl, & King, 1997). The RDA during pregnancy is 15 mg. Best sources of zinc are meats, shellfish, and poultry. Good sources include whole grains and legumes.

Magnesium

Magnesium is essential for cellular metabolism and structural growth. The RDA for pregnancy is 320 mg. Good sources include milk, whole grains, dark green vegetables, nuts, and legumes.

Iron

Iron requirements increase during pregnancy because of the growth of the fetus and placenta and the expansion of maternal blood volume (Allen, 1997). Anemia in pregnancy is mainly caused by low iron stores, although it may also result from inadequate intake of other nutrients, such as vitamins B_6 and B_{12}, folic acid, ascorbic acid, copper, and zinc. Women with poor diet histories, frequent conceptions, or records of prior iron depletion are particularly at risk.

Iron deficiency anemia may be associated with preterm birth and higher maternal mortality (Allen, 1997). Iron deficiency anemia is generally defined as a decrease in the oxygen-carrying capacity of the blood. This significantly reduces the hemoglobin per decaliter of blood, the volume of packed red cells per decaliter of blood (hematocrit), or the number of erythrocytes.

The normal hematocrit in the nonpregnant woman is 38% to 47%. In the pregnant woman, the level may drop to as low as 34%, even when nutrition is adequate. This condition is called the *physiologic anemia of pregnancy* (see Chapter 10).

Fetal demands for iron further contribute to symptoms of anemia in the pregnant woman. The fetal liver stores iron, especially during the third trimester. The infant needs this stored iron during the first 4 months of life to compensate for the normally inadequate levels of iron in breast milk and non-iron-fortified formulas.

To prevent anemia, the woman must balance iron requirements and intake. Doing so is a problem for nonpregnant women and a greater one for pregnant women. By carefully selecting foods high in iron, the woman can increase her daily iron intake considerably. Lean meats, dark green leafy vegetables, eggs, and whole-grain and enriched breads and cereals are the foods usually depended on for their iron content. Other iron sources include dried fruits, legumes, shellfish, and molasses.

Iron absorption is generally higher for animal products than for vegetable products. However, the woman may enhance absorption of iron from nonmeat sources by combining them with meat or a food rich in vitamin C.

The most iron that can reasonably be obtained from the average diet is about 15 to 18 mg/day. However, the RDA for iron during pregnancy is 30 mg. Thus during pregnancy a supplement of simple iron salt, such as ferrous gluconate, ferrous fumarate, or ferrous sulfate is needed. The CDC recommends a daily supplement of 30 mg elemental iron beginning at the first prenatal visit. Iron deficiency anemia is treated with a daily ferrous iron supplement of 60 to 120 mg. When the hematocrit becomes normal for the stage of pregnancy, the dose of iron should be decreased to 30 mg/day (CDC, 1998b). Unfortunately, iron supplements often cause gastrointestinal discomfort, especially if taken on an empty stomach. Once the woman begins taking an iron supplement, taking it after a meal may help reduce gastrointestinal discomfort.

Vitamins

Vitamins are organic substances necessary for life and growth. They are found in small amounts in specific foods and generally cannot be synthesized by the body in adequate amounts.

Vitamins are grouped according to their solubility. Those that dissolve in fat are A, D, E, and K; those soluble in water include vitamin C and the B complex vitamins. An adequate intake of all vitamins is essential during pregnancy; however, several are required in larger than normal amounts to fulfill specific needs.

A balanced diet generally provides necessary vitamins without the need for supplementation. Despite this, many people who are concerned about nutrition have become involved in the practice of taking exceptionally large doses—megadoses—of vitamins. However, in vitamin therapy, more is not necessarily better. Megadoses of vitamins, especially vitamins A, D, C, and B_6, have been documented to have a negative effect on the fetus. Furthermore, excessive intake of one vitamin may interfere with the body's use of another vitamin. For example, excessive intake of vitamin C may block the body's use of vitamin B_{12}. Consequently, although it is important to meet the RDA of vitamins during pregnancy, megadoses are best avoided.

Fat-Soluble Vitamins

The fat-soluble vitamins A, D, E, and K are stored in the liver and thus are available should the dietary intake become inadequate. They are not excreted in the urine, so excessive consumption of these vitamins, particularly vitamins A and D, can lead to toxicity (Oakley & Erickson, 1995). Symptoms of fat-soluble vitamin toxicity include nausea, gastrointestinal upset, dryness and cracking of the skin, and loss of hair.

Vitamin A is involved in the growth of epithelial cells, which line the entire gastrointestinal tract and compose the skin. Vitamin A plays a role in the metabolism of carbohydrates and fats. The body cannot synthesize glycogen in the absence of vitamin A, and the body's ability to handle cholesterol is also affected. In addition, the protective layer of tissue surrounding nerve fibers does not form properly if vitamin A is lacking.

Probably the best-known function of vitamin A is its effect on vision in dim light. A person's ability to see in the dark depends on the eye's supply of retinol, a form of vitamin A. In this manner, vitamin A prevents night blindness. Vitamin A is associated with the formation and development of healthy eyes in the fetus.

If maternal stores of vitamin A are adequate, the overall effects of pregnancy on the woman's vitamin A requirements are not remarkable. The blood serum level of vitamin A decreases slightly in early pregnancy, rises in late pregnancy, and falls before the onset of labor. Thus the RDA for vitamin A (800 mg) does not increase during pregnancy.

Deficiencies of vitamin A are not common. However, an inadequate maternal intake has been associated with preterm birth, intrauterine growth restriction, and decreased birth weight (Institute of Medicine, 1990). Although routine supplementation with vitamin A is not recommended, supplementation with 5000 IU is indicated for women whose dietary intake may be inadequate, specifically strict vegetarians and recent emigrants from countries where deficiency of vitamin A is endemic (ACOG, 1998b).

Excessive intake of preformed vitamin A is toxic to both children and adults. Research suggests that excessive intake of vitamin A in the fetus can cause birth defects (Oakley & Erickson, 1995).

Rich plant sources of vitamin A include deep green and yellow or deep orange vegetables and some fruits; animal sources include liver, egg yolk, cream, butter, fortified margarine, and milk.

Vitamin D is best known for its role in the absorption and utilization of calcium and phosphorus in skeletal development. To supply the needs of the developing fetus, the pregnant woman should have a vitamin D intake of 10 mg/day.

Main food sources of vitamin D include fortified milk, margarine, butter, liver, and egg yolks. Drinking a quart of vitamin D-fortified milk daily provides the vitamin D needed during pregnancy.

Excessive intake of vitamin D is not usually a result of eating but of taking high-potency vitamin preparations. Overdoses during pregnancy can cause hypercalcemia or high blood calcium levels due to withdrawal of calcium from the skeletal tissue. Symptoms of toxicity are excessive thirst, loss of appetite, vomiting, weight loss, irritability, and high blood calcium levels.

The major function of vitamin E, or tocopherol, is as an antioxidant. Vitamin E takes on oxygen, thus preventing another substance from undergoing chemical change. For example, vitamin E helps spare vitamin A by preventing its oxidation in the intestinal tract and the tissues. It decreases the oxidation of polyunsaturated fats, thus helping to retain the flexibility and health of the cell membrane. In protecting the cell membrane, vitamin E affects the health of all cells in the body.

Vitamin E is also involved in certain enzymatic and metabolic reactions. It is an essential nutrient for the synthesis of nucleic acids required in the formation of red blood cells in the bone marrow. Vitamin E is beneficial in treating certain types of muscular pain and intermittent claudication, in surface healing of wounds and burns, and in protecting lung tissue from the damaging effects of smog. These functions may help explain the abundant claims and cures attributed to vitamin E, many of which have not been scientifically proved.

The newborn's need for vitamin E has been widely recognized. Human milk provides adequate vitamin E, whereas cow's milk is lower in vitamin E content. Deficiency symptoms of vitamin E are related to long-term inability to absorb fats. In humans, malabsorption problems exist in cases of cystic fibrosis, liver cirrhosis, postgastrectomy, obstructive jaundice, pancreatic problems, and sprue.

The recommended intake of vitamin E increases from 8 IU for nonpregnant females to 10 IU for pregnant women. The vitamin E requirement varies with the polyunsaturated fat content of the diet. Vitamin E is widely distributed in foodstuffs, especially vegetable fats and oils, whole grains, greens, and eggs.

Some pregnant women massage vitamin E oil on the abdominal skin to make it supple and possibly prevent permanent stretch marks. It is questionable whether taking high doses orally will accomplish this goal or satisfy any other claims related to vitamin E's role in reproduction or virility. In addition, excessive intake of vitamin E has been associated with abnormal coagulation in the newborn.

Vitamin K, or menadione as used synthetically in medicine, is an essential factor for the synthesis of prothrombin; its function is thus related to normal blood clotting. Synthesis occurs in the intestinal tract by the *Escherichia coli* normally inhabiting the large intestine. However, the body's need for vitamin K is not totally met through synthesis. Green leafy vegetables and liver are excellent sources. The RDA for vitamin K does not increase during pregnancy.

Intake of vitamin K is usually adequate in a well-balanced prenatal diet. Secondary problems may arise if an illness results in malabsorption of fats or if antibiotics are used for an extended period. Antibiotics inhibit vitamin K synthesis by destroying intestinal *E coli.*

Water-Soluble Vitamins

Water-soluble vitamins are excreted in the urine. Only small amounts are stored, so there is little protection from dietary inadequacies. Thus adequate amounts must be ingested daily. During pregnancy, the concentration of water-soluble vitamins in the maternal serum falls, whereas high concentrations are found in the fetus.

The requirement for vitamin C (ascorbic acid) is increased in pregnancy from 60 to 70 mg. The major function of vitamin C is to aid the formation and development of connective tissue and the vascular system. Ascorbic acid is essential to the formation of collagen. Collagen is like a cement that binds cells together, just as mortar holds bricks together. If the collagen begins to disintegrate due to lack of ascorbic acid, cell functioning is disturbed, and cell structure breaks down, causing muscular weakness, capillary hemorrhage, and eventual death. These are symptoms of scurvy, the disease caused by vitamin C deficiency. Newborns of women who have taken megadoses of vitamin C may experience a rebound form of scurvy.

Maternal plasma levels of vitamin C progressively decline throughout pregnancy, with values at term being about half those at midpregnancy. It appears that ascorbic acid concentrates in the placenta; levels in the fetus are 50% or more above maternal levels.

A nutritious diet should meet the pregnant woman's needs for vitamin C without additional supplementation. Common food sources of vitamin C include citrus fruit, tomatoes, cantaloupe, strawberries, potatoes, broccoli, and other leafy green vegetables. Ascorbic acid is readily destroyed by water and oxidation. Therefore foods containing vitamin C should have limited exposure to air, heat, and water during storage and cooking.

The B vitamins include thiamine (B_1), riboflavin (B_2), niacin, folic acid, pantothenic acid, vitamin B_6, and vitamin B_{12}. These vitamins serve as vital coenzyme factors in many reactions, such as cell respiration, glucose oxidation, and energy metabolism. Consequently, the quantities needed invariably increase as caloric intake increases to meet the metabolic and growth needs of the pregnant woman.

The thiamine requirement increases from the prepregnant level of 1.1 mg/day to 1.5 mg/day. Sources include pork, liver, milk, potatoes, enriched breads, and cereals.

Riboflavin deficiency is manifested by cheilosis (fissures and cracks of the lips and the corners of the mouth) and other skin lesions. During pregnancy women may excrete less riboflavin and still require more because of increased energy and protein needs. An additional 0.3 mg/day is recommended. Sources include milk, liver, eggs, enriched breads, and cereals.

Niacin requirements increase by 2 mg/day during pregnancy and 5 mg/day during lactation. Sources of niacin include meat, fish, poultry, liver, whole grains, enriched breads, cereals, and peanuts.

Folic acid, or folate, is required for normal growth, reproduction, and lactation and prevents the macrocytic, megaloblastic anemia of pregnancy. An inadequate intake of folic acid has been associated with neural tube defects (NTD) (spina bifida, anencephaly). Research indicates that up to 70% of spina bifida and anencephaly could be prevented by adequate intake of folic acid (Berry, 1998; Centers for Disease Control and Prevention [CDC], 1992). Consequently, all women of childbearing age should consume 0.4 mg of folic acid daily to reduce the risk of a pregnancy affected by neural tube defects (CDC, 1992). Large-dose supplementation (4.0 mg/day) is recommended only for women who have had a previous NTD-affected pregnancy and are planning another pregnancy (ACOG, 1996). Large-dose supplementation should begin, if possible, 1 month before conception and should continue for the first 3 months of pregnancy ("Folic Acid for Prevention of Neural Tube Defects," 1993). This level of folic acid should be taken only by prescription and under the supervision of a qualified health care provider.

Megaloblastic anemia due to folate deficiency is seldom found in the United States, but those caring for pregnant women must be aware that it does occur. Folate deficiency can also be present in the absence of overt anemia.

Folate cannot be synthesized by the human body. It must be acquired from dietary sources. The best food sources are fresh green leafy vegetables, liver, peanuts, and whole-grain breads and cereals.

Folic acid can be made inactive by oxidation, ultraviolet light, and heating. It can be easily lost during improper storage and cooking. To prevent unnecessary loss, foods should be stored covered to protect them from light, cooked with only a small amount of water, and not be overcooked.

No allowance has been set for pantothenic acid in pregnancy, but 5 mg/day is considered a safe, adequate intake. Sources include meats, egg yolk, legumes, and whole grain cereals and breads.

Vitamin B_6 (pyridoxine) has long been associated biochemically with pregnancy. The RDA for vitamin B_6 during pregnancy is 2.2 mg, an increase of 0.6 mg over the allowance for nonpregnant women. Because pyridoxine is associated with amino acid metabolism, a higher than average protein intake requires an increased pyridoxine intake.

Vitamin B_{12}, or cobalamin, is the cobalt-containing vitamin found only in animal sources. Rarely is B_{12} deficiency found in women of reproductive age. Vegans can develop a deficiency, however, so it is essential that their dietary intake be supplemented with this vitamin. Occasionally, vitamin B_{12} levels decrease during pregnancy but increase again after birth. The RDA during pregnancy is 2.2 mg/day, an increase of 0.2 mg.

A deficiency may also be due to a congenital inability to absorb vitamin B_{12} resulting in pernicious anemia; infertility is a complication of this type of anemia.

Folic acid and iron are the only nutritional supplements generally recommended during pregnancy. The increased need for other vitamins and minerals can usually be met with an adequate diet. To avoid possible deficiencies, however, many health care professionals still recommend a daily vitamin supplement.

Fluid

The nutrient water is essential for life and is found in all body tissues. It is necessary for many biochemical reactions. It also serves as a lubricant, acts as a medium of transport for carrying substances in and out of the body, and aids in the regulation of body temperature. A pregnant woman should consume at least 8 to 10 (8 oz) glasses of fluid each day, of which 4 to 6 glasses should be water. Other beverages such as juices and milk can contribute water as well as other nutrients to the diet. Sodas and diet sodas should be used in moderation because they do not contribute to the nutritional value of the diet.

Caffeine is found in beverages, foods, and medications. It is a central nervous system stimulant and passes readily to the fetus, who is unable to metabolize it effectively (Institute of Medicine, 1990). Caffeinated beverages have a diuretic effect, which may be counterproductive to increasing fluid intake.

Caffeine use during pregnancy remains controversial. However, no significant evidence has been found linking caffeine consumption to birth defects; heavy consumption (> 300 mg/day) has been linked to lowered birth weight (Hinds, West, Knight, & Harland, 1996). Two (8 oz) glasses of caffeinated beverages per day is considered a safe level of consumption (Narod, De Sanjose, & Victora, 1991).

Vegetarianism

Vegetarianism is the dietary choice of many people, for religious, health, or moral reasons. There are several types of vegetarians. **Lacto-ovovegetarians** include milk, dairy products, and eggs in their diet. **Lactovegetarians** include dairy products but no eggs in their diet. **Vegans** are strict vegetarians who will not eat any food from animal sources.

In their position statement on vegetarian diets, the American Dietetic Association stated that "vegetarian diets are healthful and nutritionally adequate when appropriately planned" (ADA, 1988a). People following vegetarian diets tend to have lower blood pressure; a lower incidence of coronary artery disease, osteoporosis, gallstones, kidney stones, and diverticulitis; and weights closer to desirable levels than do nonvegetarians (ADA, 1988b).

The expectant woman who is vegetarian must eat the proper combination of foods to obtain adequate nutrients. If her diet allows, she can obtain ample and complete proteins from dairy products and eggs. Plant protein quality may be improved if consumed with these animal proteins. If the diet contains less than four servings of milk and dairy products, calcium supplementation may be necessary.

If the woman follows a vegan diet, careful planning is necessary to obtain sufficient calories and complete proteins. Obtaining sufficient calories to achieve adequate weight gains can be difficult because vegan diets tend to be higher in fiber and therefore filling. Low prepregnancy weight and optimum pregnancy weight gains are often a problem. Supplementation with energy-dense foods helps provide increased energy intake to prevent the body from using protein for caloric needs.

If energy intake is adequate, the woman can usually meet protein needs by combining complementing proteins. Complete protein may be obtained by eating different types of complementary proteins, such as legumes and whole-grain cereals, nuts and whole grain cereals, or nuts and legumes, over the course of a day (ADA, 1988b).

Because vegans use no animal products, a daily supplement of 4 mg of vitamin B_{12} is necessary. If soy milk is used, only partial supplementation may be needed. If no soy milk is taken, daily supplements of 1200 mg of calcium and 10 mg of vitamin D are needed.

A vegan diet may be low in iron and zinc because the best sources of these minerals are found in animal products. In addition, a high-fiber intake may reduce mineral (calcium, iron, and zinc) bioavailability (Wada & King, 1994). The nurse should emphasize the use of foods containing these nutrients.

Figure 14–2 depicts the vegetarian food pyramid. A guide to vegetarian food groups is provided in Table 14–6.

Factors Influencing Nutrition

Besides having knowledge of nutritional needs and food sources, the nurse needs to be aware of other factors that affect a client's nutrition. What are the age, lifestyle, dietary practices, and culture of the pregnant woman? What food beliefs and habits does she have? What a person eats is determined by availability, economics, and

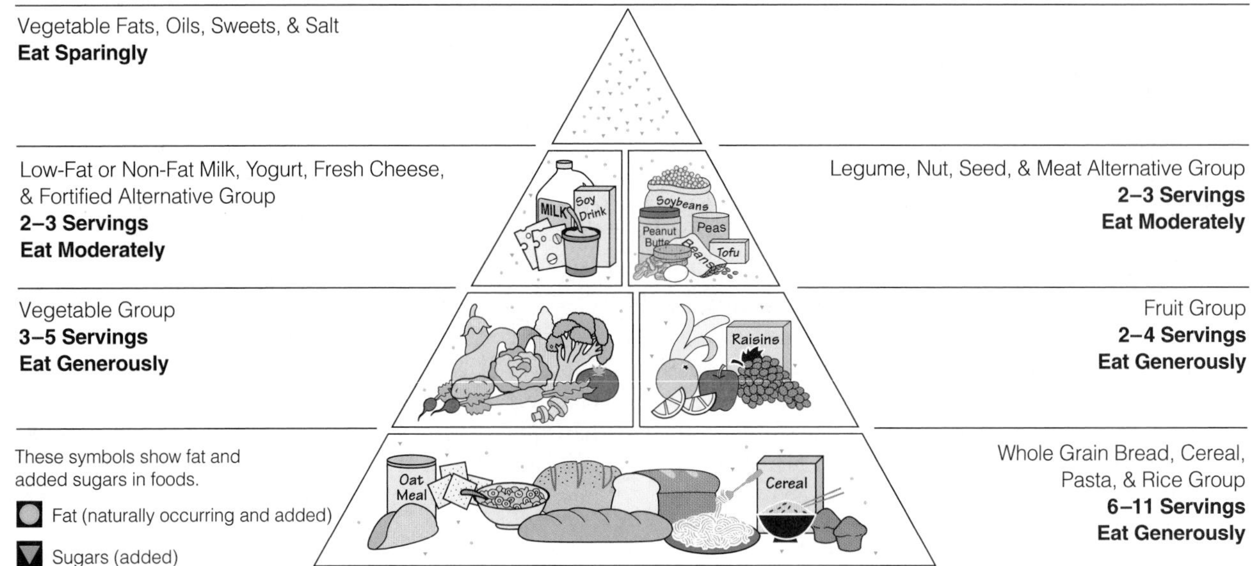

FIGURE 14–2 **The vegetarian food pyramid.** SOURCE: Adapted from The Health Connection, 55 West Oak Ridge Drive, Hagerstown, MD 21740-7390.

symbolism. These and other factors influence the expectant mother's acceptance of the nurse's intervention.

Eating Disorders

Eating disorders are most common in adolescent girls and young women. They are psychologic disorders that can have a major impact on physiologic well-being.

Anorexia nervosa is an eating disorder characterized by an extreme fear of weight gain and fat. People with this disorder have distorted body images and perceive themselves as fat even though they are extremely underweight. Their dietary intake is very restricted in both variety and quantity. In addition to their restrictive eating, they may engage in excessive exercise or purging behaviors to prevent weight gain.

The eating disorder bulimia is characterized by binge eating (secretly consuming large amounts of food in a short time) and purging. Self-induced vomiting is the most common method of purging; laxatives or diuretics may also be used. Individuals with bulimia often maintain a normal or close to normal weight for their height, so their eating disorder may not be apparent.

Pregnancy is likely to exacerbate the symptoms and consequences of an eating disorder. The treatment needs of a woman with an eating disorder can best be met by a team approach that includes medical, dietetic, and psychiatric practitioners. The pregnant adolescent or young woman with an eating disorder needs to be closely monitored and supported throughout her pregnancy.

Lactase Deficiency (Lactose Intolerance)

Some individuals have difficulty digesting milk and dairy products. This condition, known as **lactase deficiency,** or **lactose intolerance,** results from an inadequate amount of the enzyme lactase, which breaks down the milk sugar lactose into smaller digestible substances.

Lactase deficiency is found in many people of African, Mexican, Native American, Ashkenazic Jewish, and Asian descent (Institute of Medicine, 1990). People who are not affected are mainly of Northern European heritage. Symptoms may include abdominal distention, discomfort, nausea, vomiting, loose stools, and cramps. When counseling pregnant women who might be intolerant of milk and milk products, the nurse should be

TABLE 14–6 Vegetarian Food Groups

Food Group	Mixed Diet	Lacto-ovovegetarian	Lacto-vegetarian	Vegan
Grain	Bread, cereal, rice, pasta	Bread, cereal, rice, pasta	Bread, cereal, rice, pasta	Bread, cereal, rice, pasta
Fruit	Fruit, fruit juices	Fruit, fruit juices	Fruit, fruit juices	Fruit, fruit juices
Vegetable	Vegetables, vegetable juices	Vegetables, vegetable juices	Vegetables, vegetable juices	Vegetables, vegetable juices
Dairy and dairy alternatives	Milk, yogurt, cheese	Milk, yogurt, cheese	Milk, yogurt, cheese	Fortified soy milk, rice milk
Meat and meat alternatives	Meat, fish, poultry, eggs legumes, tofu, nuts, nut butters	Eggs, legumes, tofu, nuts, nut butters	Legumes, tofu, nuts, nut butters	Legumes, tofu, nuts, nut butters

TABLE 14–7 Suggestions to Improve Lactose Tolerance in Lactase-Deficient Clients

- Decrease the portion size of milk or dairy products.
- Use cultured or fermented dairy products (buttermilk, cheese, yogurt).
- Use lactase-treated dairy products.
- Add a lactase enzyme to milk.
- Take a lactase tablet at meals.

aware that tolerances vary between individuals and even a partial serving of milk or dairy products can produce symptoms. Suggestions to improve a person's tolerance to lactose are presented in Table 14–7.

Pica

Pica is the persistent eating of substances such as ice, freezer frost, cornstarch, laundry starch, baby powder, clay, dirt, and other nonnutritive substances. Most women who eat such substances do so only during pregnancy.

Iron deficiency anemia is the most common concern with pica. The ingestion of laundry starch or certain types of clay may contribute to iron deficiency by replacing iron-containing foods from the diet or by interfering with iron absorption. In fact, research indicates that women with pica, regardless of substance, tend to have lower hemoglobin levels at birth than women who do not have pica (Rainville, 1998). The ingestion of large quantities of clay could fill the intestine and cause fecal impaction. The ingestion of starch may be associated with excessive weight gain.

Nurses should be aware of pica and its implications for the woman and her fetus. Assessment for pica is an important part of the nutritional history. However, women may be embarrassed about their cravings or reluctant to discuss them for fear of criticism. It is helpful if the nurse uses a nonjudgmental approach. Reeducation of the expectant woman is important in helping her to decrease or eliminate this practice.

Common Discomforts of Pregnancy

Gastrointestinal functioning can be altered at various times throughout pregnancy, resulting in nausea, vomiting, heartburn, and constipation. Although these changes can be uncomfortable for the woman, they are seldom a major problem. Minor dietary modifications may provide relief for some individuals (see Chapter 12, Table 12–3).

Cultural, Ethnic, and Religious Influences

Cultural, ethnic, and, occasionally, religious backgrounds determine one's experiences with food and influence food preferences and habits (Figure 14–3). People of different nationalities are accustomed to eating foodstuffs available in their country of origin and prepared in a manner consistent with the customs and traditions of their ethnic and cultural group. In addition, the laws of certain religions allow particular foods, prohibit others, and direct the preparation and serving of meals.

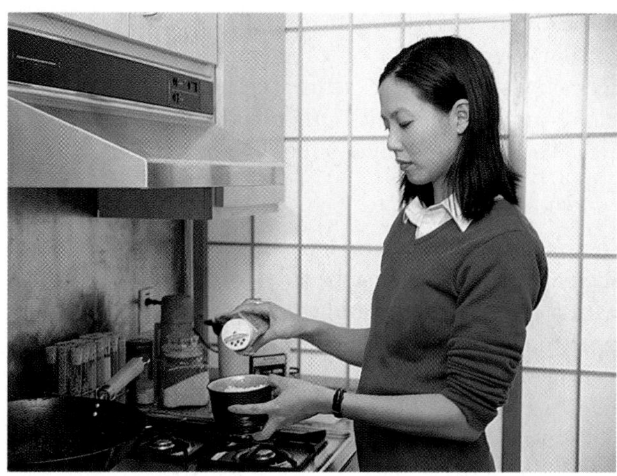

FIGURE 14–3 Cultural factors affect food preferences and habits.

In each culture, certain foods have symbolic significance. Generally, these symbolic foods are related to major life experiences such as birth, death, or developmental milestones. Although generalizations have been made about the food practices of ethnic and religious groups, there are many variations. Food customs will differ among groups in various regions of the same country, among families within local regions, and among individuals within the same family. The extent to which the use of traditional ethnic foods and customs are continued is affected by the recency of immigration, the extent of exposure to other cultures, and the availability, quality, and cost of the traditional foods.

The relationship of food to pregnancy is reflected in beliefs or sayings. Nurses frequently hear that the pregnant woman must "eat for two" or that the fetus takes from the mother all the nutrients it needs. Less frequently, nurses may learn that women believe that food cravings are determining nutrient needs.

When working with a pregnant woman from any ethnic background, the nurse needs to understand the cultural influences on the woman's eating habits and to identify beliefs she may have about foods and pregnancy. Talking with the client can enable the nurse to determine the level of influence that traditional food customs exert. Only then can the nurse provide dietary advice in a manner that is meaningful to the client.

Psychosocial Factors

The sharing of food has long been a symbol of friendliness, warmth, and social acceptance in many cultures. Food is also symbolic of motherliness; that is, taking care of the family and feeding them well is a part of the traditional mothering role. Some foods and food-related practices are associated with status. Certain items may be prepared "just for company." Other foods are served only on special occasions—holidays such as Thanksgiving, for example.

Socioeconomic Factors

Socioeconomic level may be a determinant of nutritional status. Poverty-level families are unable to afford the same foods that higher-income families can. Thus pregnant women with low incomes are frequently at risk for inadequate intake of nutrients, especially iron, calcium, zinc, folate, vitamin B_6, and pantothenic acid (Wunderlich, Hongu, Courter, & Bendixen, 1996).

Education

Knowledge about the basic components of a balanced diet is essential. The nurse must present written and oral communication in a manner consistent with a client's level of comprehension. Often educational level is related to economic status, but even people on very limited incomes can prepare well-balanced meals if their knowledge of nutrition is adequate.

Psychologic Factors

Emotions directly affect nutritional well-being. For example, food may be used as a substitute for the expression of emotions such as anger or frustration, or as a way of expressing feelings of joy. The expectant woman's attitudes and feelings about her pregnancy may influence her food consumption. The woman who is depressed or who does not wish to be pregnant may manifest these feelings by loss of appetite or by an overindulgence of certain foods.

The Pregnant Adolescent

Nutritional care of the pregnant adolescent is of particular concern to health care professionals. Many adolescents are nutritionally at risk due to a variety of complex and interrelated emotional, social, and economic factors that may adversely affect dietary intake. The increased energy and nutrient demands of pregnancy place the pregnant adolescent at even greater risk (Story & Alton, 1996).

Nutritional Concerns

General Concerns

In their position statement, the ADA states that "pregnant adolescents as a group are nutritionally at risk and require nutritional intervention early and throughout the duration of their pregnancies" (ADA, 1989a, p 104). Nutritional status is an important, modifiable variable in any pregnancy, but especially in adolescent pregnancy because teens are more likely than older women to be underweight at the onset of pregnancy and to gain less weight during pregnancy. Good maternal weight gain during adolescent pregnancy significantly improves fetal growth and reduces mortality.

Important nutrition-related factors to assess in pregnant adolescents include low prepregnant weight, low weight gain during pregnancy, younger age with regard to menarche, smoking, excessive prepregnant weight, anemia, unhealthy lifestyle (drugs, alcohol use), chronic disease, and history of an eating disorder (ADA, 1989b). Each of these factors can independently affect the adolescent's nutrient intake and, consequently, the status of the pregnancy.

The psychosocial development of adolescents often results in a compromised nutritional intake. As adolescents become more independent, they make more of their own food choices; these may be influenced, either positively or negatively, by peer acceptance.

Physiologic maturation plays a role in the development of a body image and self-concept. Weight gain and changes in body appearance occur as growth and development progress. This may be difficult for some adolescent girls to accept and can lead to a negative self-concept and possible restrictive food choices. In some cases, a negative body image can be a contributing factor in the development of eating disorders.

The weight gain of pregnancy can be affected by the adolescent's attitudes. She may have trouble consuming a diet that will support the desired weight increase. Negative attitudes about gaining weight during pregnancy are most common among heavier or depressed adolescents and those who do not perceive their families as supportive (Stevens-Simon et al, 1993).

In determining nutrient needs for pregnant adolescents, the nurse needs to consider the number of years that have passed since menstruation began. Adolescent women generally are considered physiologically mature about 4 years after menarche because linear growth is usually completed by this time. Their nutritional needs would be similar to those of other "adult" women.

Adolescents who become pregnant fewer than 4 years after menarche, however, are at a high biologic risk because of their physiologic and anatomic immaturity. They are most likely to be growing, which can impact the fetus's development. Growing adolescents have infants who weigh less than those of nongrowing adolescents and adults 19 to 29 years of age (Scholl & Hediger, 1993). Nutritional needs for these young women will be higher than for those whose growth has been completed.

Very little information is currently available on the nutritional needs of pregnant adolescents. Estimates are usually obtained by using the RDA for nonpregnant teenagers (ages 11 to 14 or 15 to 18) and adding nutrient amounts recommended for all pregnant women (Table 14–1). Although the RDAs are based on chronologic age, they are probably the best available figures to use if the pregnant female is still growing. If mature, the pregnant adolescent has nutritional needs approaching those reported for pregnant adults. However, young adolescents (13 to 15 years) need to gain more weight than older adolescents (16 years or older) to produce babies of equal size. Thus in determining the optimum weight gain for a pregnant adolescent, the nurse needs to consider the following:

- Recommended weight gain for a normal pregnancy
- Amount of weight gain expected during the post-menarcheal year during which the pregnancy occurs

The recommended weight gain during pregnancy was addressed earlier in this chapter. Weight gain needs to be higher for adolescents than for adults to reduce the risk of low birth weight.

The weight gain for a normal pregnancy and the expected weight gain due to growth would be added together to obtain a recommended weight gain for the pregnant adolescent. Young adolescents (2 years after menarche) should strive for a weight gain at the upper end of the range of weight gain for adults (Table 14–3).

Specific Nutrient Concerns

Caloric needs of pregnant adolescents vary widely. Major factors in determining caloric needs include whether growth has been completed and the physical activity level of the individual. Figures as high as 50 kcal/kg have been suggested for young, growing teens who are very active physically. A satisfactory weight gain will confirm adequacy of caloric intake in most cases.

An inadequate iron intake is a major concern with the adolescent diet. Iron needs are high for the pregnant teen due to the requirement for iron by the enlarging maternal muscle mass and blood volume. Iron supplements—providing 30 to 60 mg of elemental iron—are definitely indicated.

Calcium is another nutrient that demands special attention from pregnant adolescents. Inadequate intake of calcium is frequently a problem in this age group. Adequate calcium intake is needed to support normal growth and development of the fetus as well as growth and maintenance of calcium stores in the adolescent. Calcium supplementation is indicated for teens with an aversion to or intolerance of milk unless other dairy products or significant calcium sources are consumed in sufficient amounts.

Because folic acid plays a role in cell reproduction, it is also an important nutrient for pregnant teens. As previously indicated, a supplement is often suggested for pregnant females, whether adult or teenager.

Other nutrients and vitamins must be considered when evaluating the overall nutritional quality of the teenager's diet. Nutrients that have frequently been found to be deficient in this age group include zinc and vitamins A, D, and B_6. Inclusion of a wide variety of foods—especially fresh and lightly processed foods—is helpful in obtaining adequate amounts of trace minerals, fiber, and other vitamins. A low-dose vitamin and mineral supplement may be necessary when the diet is not adequate (Institute of Medicine, 1990).

Dietary Patterns

Healthy adolescents often have irregular eating patterns. Many skip breakfast, and most tend to be frequent snackers. Teens rarely follow the traditional three-meals-a-day pattern; their day-to-day intake often varies drastically; and they eat food combinations that may seem bizarre to adults. Despite this, adolescents usually achieve a better nutritional balance than most adults would expect.

In assessing the diet of the pregnant adolescent, the nurse should consider the eating pattern over time, not simply a single day's intake. This pattern is critical because of the irregularity of most adolescent eating patterns. Once the pattern is identified, counseling can be directed toward correcting deficiencies.

Counseling Issues

CRITICAL THINKING QUESTION

What approaches might be most effective in helping the pregnant teenager develop a more nutritionally sound eating pattern?

A positive approach to nutritional counseling for the pregnant adolescent is more effective than a negative one. The nurse must be ready to suggest nutrient-dense foods that pregnant teens can choose in many places and at any time. If an adolescent's family member does most of the meal preparation, it may be useful to include that person in the discussion if the adolescent agrees. Involving the expectant father in counseling may be beneficial. If the teen is remaining in school, cooperation can also be sought from school lunch personnel.

The pregnant teenager will soon become a parent, and her understanding of nutrition will influence not only her well-being but also that of her child. However, teens tend to live in the present, and counseling that stresses long-term changes may be less effective than more concrete approaches. Messages should emphasize the following (Skinner, Carruth, Ezell, & Shaw, 1996):

- eating for the mother's health
- eating for the baby's health
- eating for the mother's physical comfort
- food rather than nutrients

In many cases, classes with other teens are effective. In a group atmosphere, adolescents often work together to plan adequate meals including foods that are their special favorites.

Postpartum Nutrition

Nutritional needs will change following the birth. Nutrient requirements will vary depending on whether the mother decides to breastfeed. An assessment of postpartal nutritional status is necessary before the nurse provides nutritional guidance.

Postpartal Nutritional Status

Postpartal nutritional status is determined primarily by assessing the new mother's weight, hemoglobin and hematocrit levels, clinical signs, and dietary history.

As previously discussed, an ideal weight gain for the normal-weight woman during pregnancy is between 11.5 and 16 kg (25 and 35 lb). After birth, there is a weight loss of approximately 10 to 12 lb. Additional weight loss will be most rapid during the first few weeks after birth as the uterus returns to normal size, tissue fluids are released, and maternal blood volume returns to normal. The mother's weight will then begin to stabilize. Weight loss may also be affected by lactation. Individual weight loss of women who breastfeed will vary but tends to be greater than that of those who do not if breastfeeding continues for at least 6 months (Dewey, Heinig, & Nommsen, 1993).

The rate of postpartum weight loss is influenced by many factors. Some women approach their prepregnancy weight several weeks after birth; most approach this weight about 6 months later. The amount of weight gained during pregnancy is a major determinant of weight loss after childbirth. Generally, the more weight gained during pregnancy, the more is lost postpartum.

It is important to evaluate the mother's current weight, ideal weight for her height, weight before pregnancy, and weight before the birth. Women who are interested in weight reduction should be referred to a dietitian. Different guidelines for weight loss are used for nursing mothers and nonnursing mothers.

Hemoglobin and erythrocyte values vary after birth, but they should return to normal levels within 2 to 6 weeks. Hematocrit levels should rise gradually due to hemoconcentration as extracellular fluid is excreted. The hematocrit is usually checked at the postpartum visit to detect any anemia. Mothers can be encouraged to eat a diet high in iron. Iron supplements are generally prescribed for 2 to 3 months following birth to replenish supplies depleted by pregnancy.

The nurse assesses any clinical symptoms the new mother may be experiencing. Food cravings and aversions typically drop significantly during the postpartal period and do not usually pose a problem. However, constipation is a common problem following birth. The nurse can encourage the woman to maintain a high fluid intake to keep the stool soft. Dietary sources of fiber and physical exercise are also helpful in preventing constipation.

The nurse obtains specific information on diet and eating habits directly from the woman. Visiting the mother during mealtimes provides an opportunity for unobtrusive nutritional assessment. Which foods has a woman selected? Has she avoided fruits and vegetables? Is her diet nutritionally sound? A comment focusing on a positive aspect of her meal selection may initiate a discussion of nutrition.

The dietitian should be informed about any woman whose cultural or religious beliefs require specific foods. Appropriate meals can then be prepared for her. The nurse may also refer women with unusual eating habits or numerous questions about food or nutrition to a dietitian. In all cases, the nurse should provide literature on nutrition so that the woman will have a source of appropriate information at home.

Nutritional Care of Nonnursing Mothers

After birth, the nonnursing mother's dietary requirements return to prepregnancy levels (Table 14–1). If the mother has a good understanding of nutritional principles, it is sufficient to advise her to reduce her daily caloric intake by about 300 kcal and to return to prepregnancy levels for other nutrients.

If the mother has a poor understanding of nutrition, this is an opportunity to teach her the basic principles and the importance of a well-balanced diet. Her eating habits and dietary practices will eventually be reflected in the diet of her child.

If the mother has gained excessive weight during pregnancy (or perhaps was overweight before pregnancy), referral to a dietitian is appropriate. The dietitian can design weight-reduction diets to meet nutritional needs and food preferences. Weight loss goals of 1 to 2 lb per week are usually suggested.

In addition to learning how to meet her own nutritional needs, the new mother will usually be interested in learning how to provide for her infant's nutritional needs. A discussion of infant feeding, which includes topics such as selecting infant formulas, formula preparation, and vitamin and mineral supplementation, is appropriate and generally well received.

Nutritional Care of Nursing Mothers

Nutrient Needs

Nutrient needs increase during breastfeeding. Table 14–1 lists the RDAs during breastfeeding for specific nutrients. Table 14–2 provides a sample daily food guide for lactating women. A few key nutrients need further discussion.

Calories One of the most important factors in the breastfeeding woman's diet is calories. An inadequate caloric intake can reduce milk volume. However, milk quality generally remains unaffected. The nursing mother should increase her caloric intake by 200 kcal over the pregnancy requirements (that is, a 500 kcal increase from her prepregnancy requirement). This results in a total of about 2500 to 2700 kcal/day for most women.

Depending on her own dietary preferences, the nursing mother can use the general food guide pyramid or the vegetarian food pyramid to assess her dietary intake. She should strive to include a variety of foods from each food group. Her caloric intake needs to provide enough energy to sustain lactation. After her weight stabilizes several weeks following childbirth, weight loss should not exceed more than 1 lb/week for nursing mothers.

Protein An adequate protein intake is essential while breastfeeding because protein is an important component of breast milk. An intake of 65 g/day during the first 6 months of breastfeeding and 62 g/day during the second 6 months is recommended. As in pregnancy, it is important that the woman consume adequate nonprotein calories in order to prevent the use of protein as an energy source.

Calcium Calcium is also an important nutrient in milk production, and increases over nonpregnancy needs are expected. Requirements during breastfeeding remain the same as requirements during pregnancy: 1200 mg/day. An inadequate intake of calcium from food sources necessitates the use of calcium supplements.

Iron Iron needs during lactation are not substantially different from those of nonpregnant women because iron is not a principal component of breast milk. However, as previously mentioned, continued supplementation of the mother for 2 to 3 months after parturition is advisable in order to replenish maternal stores depleted by pregnancy.

Fluids Liquids are especially important during lactation because inadequate fluid intake may decrease milk volume. The recommended fluid intake of 8 to 10 (8 oz) glasses daily can be met by the consumption of water, juices, milk, and soups.

Counseling Issues

In addition to counseling nursing mothers on how to meet their increased nutrient needs during breastfeeding, nurses should discuss a few issues related to infant feeding. For example, many mothers are concerned about how specific foods they eat will affect their babies during breastfeeding. Generally, there are no foods the nursing mother must avoid except those to which she might be allergic. Occasionally, however, some nursing mothers find that their babies are affected by certain foods. Onions, turnips, cabbage, chocolate, spices, and seasonings are commonly listed as offenders. The best advice to give the nursing mother is to avoid those foods she suspects cause distress in her infant. For the most part, however, she should be able to eat any nourishing food she wants without fear that her baby will be affected. For further discussion of successful infant feeding, see Chapter 27.

NURSING CARE MANAGEMENT

Nursing Assessment and Diagnosis

The nurse needs to assess nutritional status in order to plan an optimal diet with each woman. The nurse may gather data by consulting the woman's chart and by interviewing her. Information is obtained about (1) the woman's height and weight and her weight gain during pregnancy; (2) pertinent laboratory values, especially hemoglobin and hematocrit; (3) clinical signs that have possible nutritional implications, such as constipation, anorexia, or heartburn; and (4) diet history to determine the woman's views on nutrition as well as her specific nutrient intake.

The nurse can obtain a diet history by asking the woman to complete a 24-hour diet recall, in which she lists everything consumed in the previous 24 hours, including foods, fluids, and any supplements. At least 3 days of diet recalls should be done to compensate for daily variations. Diet may also be evaluated using a food frequency questionnaire. The questionnaire lists common categories of foods and asks the woman how frequently in a day (or week) she consumes foods from the list. Common categories include vegetables, fruits, milk or cheese, meat or poultry, fish, desserts or sweets, coffee or tea, and alcoholic beverages. This method may be less reliable because it requires the individual to be accurate in generalizing about her intake.

In some instances, the nurse will ask the woman to keep a food record or diary of everything she eats for a specified period of time (such as a week). This provides a clearer picture of nutritional patterns and may prompt the woman to make changes if the diary reveals areas of deficiency or excess.

During the data-gathering process, the nurse has an opportunity to discuss important aspects of nutrition in the context of the family's needs and lifestyle. The nurse also seeks information about psychologic, cultural, and socioeconomic factors that may influence food intake.

The nurse can use a nutritional questionnaire to gather and record important facts. This information provides a database the nurse can use to develop an intervention plan to fit the woman's individual needs. The sample questionnaire shown in Figure 14–4 has been filled in to demonstrate this process.

Once the data are obtained, the nurse begins to analyze the information, formulate appropriate nursing diagnoses, and develop client goals. For a woman during the first trimester, for example, the diagnosis may be ***Altered Nutrition: Less than Body Requirements*** related to nausea and vomiting. In many cases the diagnosis may be related to excessive weight gain. In such cases the diagnosis might be ***Altered Nutrition: More than Body Requirements*** related to excessive calorie intake. Although these diagnoses are broad, the nurse must be specific in addressing issues such as inadequate intake of nutrients such as iron, calcium, or folic acid; problems with nutrition

NUTRITIONAL QUESTIONNAIRE

Name Susan Longmont Date 8-15-01

Age 20

Ethnic group Caucasian

Religion Protestant

Gravida 1 Para 0 EDB 4-7-02

Age of youngest child? NA

Birth weights of previous children? NA

Usual nonpregnant weight 115 Present weight 125

Weight gain during last pregnancy? NA

Vitamin supplements? none

Current medications? aspirin for headache

Do you smoke? yes How much per day? 1-1½ packs

Eating patterns:

1. How many meals per day? 2 when 12:30 pm 6:30 pm
2. How many snacks per day? 3 when 10:30 am 4:00 pm 10:00 pm
3. What other foods are important to your usual diet? chocolate and candy bars
4. Amount per day 4 bars/week
5. Do you have any different food preferences now? no
6. Do you eat nonfoods such as:

		Amount
laundry starch	no	NA
ice	yes	10 cubes/day
other (name)	no	NA

7. What foods do you dislike or do not eat? spinach and dried beans
8. For added information complete a typical daily intake (24 hour recall is suggested).

Do you have special problems in food preparation such as:

1. Physical disability yes ___ no ✓ Explain ___
2. Cooking appliances yes ___ no ✓ Explain ___
3. Refrigeration of food yes ___ no ✓ Explain ___

Who does the meal planning? I do. shopping? We both do.

cooking? I do most of the time but my husband likes to help.

Are there transportation problems? We have only one car but we go in the evening.

Financial situation: My husband is working and going to school.

I am not working. Foodstamps yes w/c no

Do you have any previous nutritional problems? No. I have never paid much attention to food before, but now I have lots of questions.

Are there any problems with this pregnancy? Nausea Yes, in the morning.

Constipation No Other NA

Assessment by the nurse following the completion of the questionnaire.

Basic estimated nutrient and caloric value of typical daily intake.

Please circle one of the following:

Protein intake was	low	**(adequate)**	high
Caloric intake was	low	adequate	**(high)**
Calcium intake was	**(low)**	adequate	high
Iron intake was	**(low)**	adequate	high
Vitamin C intake was	low	**(adequate)**	high

FIGURE 14–4 Sample nutritional questionnaire used in nursing management of a pregnant woman.

due to a limited food budget; problems related to physiologic alterations, such as anorexia, heartburn, or nausea; and behavioral problems related to excessive dieting, anorexia nervosa, or bulimia. In some instances, the diagnosis ***Knowledge Deficit*** may seem most appropriate.

Nursing Plan and Implementation

After the nursing diagnosis is made, the nurse can plan an approach to correct any nutritional deficiencies or improve the overall quality of the diet.

Teaching for Self-Care

In counseling the pregnant woman, the nurse needs to avoid "talking down" to her or "preaching" to her. The nurse should present information in a clear, logical way, using appropriate language but avoiding jargon. Examples are often helpful in clarifying material. The nurse should also answer all questions appropriately and clearly.

When a person requires nutritional counseling, a dietary change usually is necessary. Change is often difficult, however. Counseling will be more effective if the nurse understands the client's values and explains the needed change in a way that is meaningful to the client. Because the pregnant woman must follow the plan, it should be developed in cooperation with her, be suitable for her financial level and background, and be based on reasonable, achievable goals.

The following example demonstrates one way a nurse can implement a plan with a client based on the nursing diagnosis.

Diagnosis: ***Altered Nutrition: Less than Body Requirements*** related to low intake of calcium

Client goal: The woman will increase her intake of calcium to the RDA level.

Implementation:

1. Plan with the woman additional milk or dairy products that she can reasonably add to the diet (specify amounts).
2. Encourage the use of other calcium sources, such as leafy green vegetables and legumes.
3. Plan for the addition of powdered milk in cooking and baking.
4. If none of the above are realistic or acceptable, consider the use of calcium supplements.

Most families can benefit from guidance about food purchasing and preparation. The nurse should advise women to plan food purchases thoughtfully by preparing menus and a grocery list before shopping. It is also helpful to advise clients to monitor sales, compare brands, and be selective when purchasing "convenience" foods, which tend to be expensive. Other techniques for keeping food costs down without jeopardizing quality include buying food in season, using bulk foods when appropriate, using whole-grain or enriched products, buying lower-grade eggs (grading has no relation to the egg's nutritional value but indicates color of the shell and delicacy of flavor), and avoiding fancy grades of food and foods in elaborate packaging.

Community-Based Nursing Care

Food is a significant portion of a family's budget, and meeting nutritional needs may be a challenge for families on limited incomes. Community-based services offered through clinics, local agencies, schools, and volunteer organizations are effective in addressing these needs. Increasingly nurses play an important role in managing such community-based services, especially those services focusing on client education. In addition, most communities offer special assistance to qualifying families to meet their nutritional needs. The Food Stamp Program provides stamps or coupons for participating households whose net monthly income is below a specified level. These stamps can be used to purchase food for the household each month.

The Special Supplemental Food Program for Women, Infants, and Children (WIC) is designed to assist pregnant or breastfeeding women with low incomes and their children under 5 years of age. The program provides food assistance, nutrition education, and referrals to health care providers. The food distributed, including dried beans and peas, peanut butter, eggs, cheese, milk, fortified adult and infant cereals, juice, and iron-fortified infant formula, is designed to provide good sources of iron, protein, and certain vitamins for individuals with an inadequate diet. Research indicates that participation in the WIC program during pregnancy and infancy is associated with a reduced risk of infant death (Moss & Carver, 1998). In addition, the WIC program is credited with helping reduce the incidence of low birth weight in infants and in decreasing the incidence of anemia in the infants and young children of low-income families (Owen & Owen, 1997).

Evaluation

Once a plan has been developed and implemented, the nurse and client may wish to identify ways of evaluating its effectiveness. Evaluation may involve keeping a food journal, writing out weekly menus, returning weekly for weighing, and the like. If anemia is a special problem, periodic hematocrit assessments are also indicated.

Women with serious nutritional deficiencies are referred to a dietitian. The nurse can then work closely with the dietitian and the client to improve the pregnant woman's health by modifying her diet. ●

FOCUS YOUR STUDY

- Maternal weight gains averaging 11.5 to 16 kg (25 to 35 lb) for a normal-weight woman are associated with the best reproductive outcomes.
- If the diet is adequate, folic acid and iron are the only supplements generally recommended during pregnancy.

- Women should not restrict caloric intake to reduce weight during pregnancy.
- Pregnant women should be encouraged to eat regularly and to eat a wide variety of foods, especially fresh and lightly processed foods.
- Taking megadoses of vitamins during pregnancy is unnecessary and potentially dangerous.
- Pregnant women who eat vegetarian diets should place special emphasis on obtaining ample complete proteins, calories, calcium, iron, vitamin D, vitamin B_{12}, and zinc through food sources or supplementation if necessary.
- Evaluation of physical, psychosocial, and cultural factors that affect food intake is essential before the nurse can determine nutritional status and plan nutritional counseling.
- Adolescents who become pregnant less than 4 years after menarche have higher nutritional needs and are considered to be at high biologic risk.
- Weight gains during adolescent pregnancy must accommodate recommended gains for a normal pregnancy plus necessary gains due to growth.
- After childbirth, the nonnursing mother's dietary requirements return to prepregnancy levels.
- Nursing mothers require an adequate caloric and fluid intake to maintain ample milk volume.

REFERENCES

Abrams, B. (1994). Weight gain and energy intake during pregnancy. *Clinical Obstetrics & Gynecology, 37*(3), 515–527.

Allen, L. H. (1997). Pregnancy and iron deficiency: Unresolved issues. *Nutrition Reviews, 55*(4), 91–101.

American College of Obstetricians and Gynecologists (ACOG). (1993). *Folic acid for the prevention of neural tube defects.* (ACOG Committee Opinion No. 120). Washington, DC: Author.

American College of Obstetricians and Gynecologists (ACOG). (1996). *Nutrition and women.* (ACOG Educational Bulletin No. 229). Washington, DC: Author.

American College of Obstetricians and Gynecologists (ACOG). (1998a, November). *Special problems of multiple gestation.* (ACOG, Educational Bulletin No. 253). Washington, DC: Author.

American College of Obstetricians and Gynecologists (ACOG). (1998b). *Vitamin A supplementation during pregnancy.* (ACOG Committee Opinion No. 196). Washington, DC: Author.

American Dietetic Association. (1988a, March). Position of the American Dietetic Association: Vegetarian diets. *Journal of the American Dietetic Association, 88,* 351.

American Dietetic Association. (1988b, March). Position of the American Dietetic Association: Vegetarian diets—Technical support paper. *Journal of the American Dietetic Association, 88,* 352–355.

American Dietetic Association. (1989a, January). Position of the American Dietetic Association: Nutrition management of adolescent pregnancy. *Journal of the American Dietetic Association, 89,* 104.

American Dietetic Association. (1989b, January). Position of the American Dietetic Association: Nutrition management of adolescent pregnancy—Technical support paper. *Journal of the American Dietetic Association, 89,* 105–109.

Berry, A. (1998). Focusing on folic acid. *AWHONN Lifelines, 2* (4), 19–20.

Bower, C. (1995). Folate and neural tube defects. *Nutrition Reviews, 53*(9 Pt. 2), S33–S38.

Centers for Disease Control and Prevention (CDC). (1992, Sept. 11). Recommendations for the use of folic acid to reduce the number of cases of spina bifida and other neural tube defects. *Morbidity & Mortality Weekly Report, 41*(RR-14), 1–7.

Centers for Disease Control and Prevention (CDC). (1998, April 3). Recommendations to prevent and control iron deficiency in the United States. *Morbidity and Mortality Weekly Report, 47* (No. RR-3), 1–36.

Crane, N. T., Wilson, D. B., Cook, D. A., Lewis, C. J., Yetley, E. A., & Rader, J. I. (1995). Evaluating food fortification options: General principles revisited with folic acid. *American Journal of Public Health, 85*(5), 660–666.

DeCherney, A. H., & Koos, B. (1997, June 19). Obstetrics and gynecology: Encouraging results with cord blood stem cell transplantation. Updated analysis shows effectiveness of zidovudine in preventing maternal HIV transmission. Calcium supplementation decreases the incidence of preeclampsia. *JAMA, 277*(23), 1878–1879.

DeLong, G. R. (1993). Effects of nutrition on brain development in humans. *American Journal of Clinical Nutrition, 57*(2 Suppl.), 286S–290S.

Dewey, K. G., Heinig, M. J., & Nommsen, L. A. (1993). Maternal weight-loss patterns during prolonged lactation. *American Journal of Clinical Nutrition, 58*(2), 162–166.

Folic acid for prevention of neural tube defects. (1993, July). *Contraception, 4*(3), 11.

Freda, M. C., Andersen, H. F., Damus, K., & Merkatz, I. R. (1993). What pregnant women want to know: A comparison of client and provider perceptions. *Journal of Obstetric, Gynecologic, & Neonatal Nursing, 22*(3), 237–144.

Fung, E. B., Ritchie, L. D., Woodhouse, L. R., Roehl, R., & King, J. C. (1997). Zinc absorption in women during pregnancy and lactation: A longitudinal study. *American Journal of Clinical Nutrition, 66*(1), 80–88.

General Accounting Office. (1992, May). *Early intervention: Federal investments like WIC can produce savings* (Document HRD 92–19). Washington, DC: Author.

Hickey, C. A., Cliver, S. P., McNeal, S. F., Hoffman, H. J., & Goldenberg, R. L. (1996). Prenatal weight gain patterns and birth weight among nonobese black and white women. *Obstetrics & Gynecology, 88*(4 Pt. 1), 490–496.

Hinds, T. S., West, W. L., Knight, E. M., & Harland, B. F. (1996). The effect of caffeine on pregnancy outcome variables. *Nutrition Reviews, 54*(7), 203–207.

Hine, R. J. (1996). What practitioners need to know about folic acid. *Journal of the American Dietetic Association, 96*(5), 451–452.

Institute of Medicine, Subcommittee for a Clinical Application Guide. (1992). *Nutrition during pregnancy and lactation: An implementation guide.* Washington, DC: National Academy Press.

Institute of Medicine, Subcommittee on Dietary Intake and Nutrient Supplements During Pregnancy, Committee on Nutrition Status During Pregnancy and Lactation, Food and Nutrition Board. (1990). *Nutrition during pregnancy: Weight gain and nutrient supplements.* Washington, DC: National Academy Press.

Lantz, M. E., Chez, R. A., Rodriguez, A., & Porter, K. B. (1996). Maternal weight gain patterns and birth weight outcome in twin gestation. *Obstetrics & Gynecology, 87*(4), 551–556.

López-Jaramillo, P., Delgado, F., Jacome, P., Teran, E., Ruano, C., & Rivera, J. (1997). Calcium supplementation and the risk of preeclampsia in Ecuadorian pregnant teenagers. *Obstetrics & Gynecology, 90*(2), 162–167.

Moss, N., & Carver, K. (1998). The effect of WIC and Medicaid on infant mortality in the United States. *American Journal of Public Health, 88* (9): 1354–1361.

Narod, S. A., De Sanjose, S., & Victora, C. (1991). Coffee during pregnancy: A reproductive hazard? *American Journal of Obstetrics and Gynecology, 164*,(4), 1109–1114.

National Research Council, Food and Nutrition Board. (1989). *Recommended dietary allowances* (10th ed.). Washington, DC: National Academy Press.

Nordentoft, M., Lou, H. C., Hansen, D., Nim, J., Pryds, O., Rubin, P., & Hemmingsen, R. (1996). Intrauterine growth retardation and premature delivery: The influence of maternal smoking and psychosocial factors. *American Journal of Public Health, 86*(3), 347–354.

Oakley, G. P, Jr., & Erickson, J. D. (1995, Nov. 23). Vitamin A and birth defects. Continuing caution is needed. [Editorial]. *New England Journal of Medicine, 333*(21), 1414–1415.

Owen, A. L., & Owen, G. M. (1997). Twenty years of WIC: A review of some effects of the program. *Journal of the American Dietetic Association, 97*(7), 777–782.

Prasad, A. S. (1996). Zinc deficiency in women, infants and children. *Journal of the American College of Nutrition, 15*(2), 113–120.

Prentice, A., & Goldberg, G. (1996). Maternal obesity increases congenital malformations. *Nutrition Reviews, 54*(5), 146–150.

Rainville, A. J. (1998). Pica practices of pregnant women are associated with lower maternal hemoglobin levels at delivery. *Journal of the American Diabetic Association, 98* (3), 293–296.

Repke, J. T. (1994). Calcium and vitamin D. *Clinical Obstetrics & Gynecology, 37*(3), 550–557.

Rose, N. C., & Mennuti, M. T. (1994). Periconceptional folate supplementation and neural tube defects. *Clinical Obstetrics & Gynecology, 37*(3), 605–620.

Schauberger, C. W., Rooney, B. L., & Brimer, L. M. (1992). Factors that influence weight loss in the puerperium. *Obstetrics & Gynecology, 79*(3), 424–429.

Scholl, T. O., & Hediger, M. L. (1993). A review of the epidemiology of nutrition and adolescent pregnancy: Maternal growth during pregnancy and its effect on the fetus. *Journal of the American College of Nutrition, 12*(2), 101–107.

Siega-Riz, A. M., Adair, L. S., & Hobel, C. J. (1994). Maternal underweight status and inadequate rate of weight gain during the third trimester of pregnancy increases the risk of preterm delivery. *Journal of Nutrition, 126*(1), 146–153.

Skinner, J. D., Carruth, B. R., Ezell, J. M., & Shaw, A. (1996). How and what do pregnant adolescents want to learn about nutrition? *Journal of Nutritional Education, 28*(5), 266–271.

Stevens-Simon, C., Nakashima, I., & Andrews, D. (1993). Weight gain attitudes among pregnant adolescents. *Journal of Adolescent Healthcare, 14*(5), 369–372.

Story, M., & Alton, I. (1996). Adolescent nutrition: Current trends and critical issues. *Topics in Clinical Nutrition, 11*(3), 56–69.

Sullivan, C. A., & Martin, J. N., Jr. (1994). Sodium and pregnancy. *Clinical Obstetrics & Gynecology, 37*(3), 558–573.

US Department of Agriculture & US Department of Health and Human Services. (1990). *Nutrition and your health: Dietary guidelines for Americans* (3rd ed.). (Home and Garden Bulletin No. 232). Washington, DC: Authors.

Wada, L., & King, J. C. (1994). Trace element nutrition during pregnancy. *Clinical Obstetrics & Gynecology, 37*(3), 574–586.

Wunderlich, S. M., Hongu, N. K., Courter, A., & Bendixen, C. A. (1996). Nutrient intake and nutritional status of low-income pregnant women. *Topics in Clinical Nutrition, 12*(1), 66–73.

Yu, S. M., Keppel, K. G., Singh, G. K., & Kessel, W. (1996). Preconceptional and prenatal multivitamin-mineral supplement use in the 1988 National Maternal and Infant Health Survey. *American Journal of Public Health, 86*(2), 240–242.

15 Pregnancy at Risk: Pregestational Problems

Key Terms

Acquired immunodeficiency syndrome (AIDS)

Crack

Gestational diabetes mellitus

Macrosomia

I'VE BEEN A NURSE FOR 25 YEARS NOW, AND I'VE never seen anything change nursing practice more than HIV/AIDS has. Nursing students today will take universal precautions for granted because they won't know any other way, but I can remember when we could touch more freely. I remember drying a newly born infant and stroking him—my hands warm against his skin. I remember a time when people didn't think twice before trying to stop bleeding or give other first aid at an accident scene. I know this way is safer, but a part of me mourns what we have lost.

Objectives

- Summarize the effects of alcohol and illicit drugs on the childbearing woman and her fetus/newborn.
- Discuss the pathology, treatment, and nursing care of pregnant women with diabetes.
- Discriminate among the four major types of anemia associated with pregnancy with regard to signs, treatment, and implications for pregnancy.
- Discuss acquired immunodeficiency syndrome (AIDS), including care of the pregnant woman with HIV/AIDS, neonatal implications, and ramifications for the childbearing family.
- Describe the effects of various heart disorders on pregnancy, including their implications for nursing care.
- Compare the effects of selected gestational medical conditions on pregnancy.

EVEN THOUGH IT IS A NORMAL PROCESS, pregnancy is biologically, physiologically, and psychologically stressful. Pregnancy may even be life-threatening, especially for those with pregestational conditions such as substance abuse, diabetes, anemia, HIV infection, and cardiac disease. For these women, pregestational counseling is especially important in order to identify early interventions designed to diminish the adverse effects of pregnancy on both the mother and fetus. In some cases, interventions prior to conception may be critical (American Academy of Pediatrics [AAP] & American College of Obstetricians and Gynecologists [ACOG], 1997).

Disruptive conditions that arise during pregnancy are the result of many high-risk factors, such as maternal age, blood type, socioeconomic status, parity, psychologic well-being, and predisposing chronic illnesses. Prenatal care is aimed toward identification, assessment, and care management of women whose pregnancies are at risk because of potential or existing complications.

This chapter focuses on women with pregestational medical disorders and their possible effects on the outcome of pregnancy.

CLINICAL TIP

Keep in mind that at least 1 of 10 women in the United States, regardless of socioeconomic status or ethnic background, is currently abusing a substance. If you consider that possibility with every woman, you will ask the important questions about drug use and be alert for signs of substance abuse.

Care of the Woman Practicing Substance Abuse

Substance abuse occurs when an individual experiences difficulties with work, family, social relations, and health as a result of alcohol or drug use. The American College of Obstetricians and Gynecologists (1994b) estimates that, at a minimum, 10% of women in the childbearing years are substance abusers. Moreover, approximately 5.5% of pregnant women use an illicit drug during pregnancy (National Pregnancy and Health Survey, 1996). Because illicit drug users seldom use only one drug, it is necessary to complete a thorough drug and alcohol abuse history with each client (Jessup, 1997).

Because women of childbearing age (15 to 44 years) make up a substantial proportion of the drug-using population, the problem has major significance for women and children. In testimony to these statistics is the increasing number of drug-exposed infants being born throughout the United States. Indiscriminate use of drugs during pregnancy, particularly in the first trimester, may adversely affect the health of the woman and the growth and development of her fetus. Drugs that are commonly misused include alcohol, cocaine, marijuana, amphetamines, barbiturates, hallucinogens, heroin, and other narcotics. Table 15–1 identifies common addictive drugs and their effects on the fetus and newborn.

Drug use during pregnancy may be the most frequently missed diagnosis in all of maternity care. Substance-abusing women typically do not seek prenatal care until late in their pregnancy, may be noncompliant, or may present in labor with no prenatal care. Even when they do seek care early, physicians and nurses may fail to ask the woman about drug and alcohol use because of their own lack of knowledge, discomfort, or biases.

Providing prenatal care to chemically dependent women presents multiple dilemmas and challenges to clinicians. However, pregnancy represents a period in most women's lives when they recognize the need for and are receptive to caring and responsive interventions. By optimizing the prenatal experience of chemically dependent women, maternal-fetal outcomes will be improved and the groundwork laid for the ongoing therapeutic services that are needed to maintain the health and well-being of the mother and child (Kenner & D'Apolito, 1997).

The substance-abusing woman who seeks prenatal care may not voluntarily reveal her addiction, so caregivers should be alert for a history or physical signs that suggest substance abuse (Table 15–2). Because substance abuse has increased rapidly in the past decade, it is helpful to discuss the specific substances that are abused to increase understanding of this serious problem.

Substances Commonly Abused During Pregnancy

Alcohol

Alcohol abuse has increased dramatically among women in the United States. The incidence is highest among women 20 to 40 years old; alcoholism is also seen in teenagers. Chronic abuse of alcohol can undermine maternal health by causing malnutrition (especially folic acid and thiamine deficiencies), bone marrow suppression, increased incidence of infections, and liver disease. As a result of alcohol dependence, the woman may have withdrawal seizures in the intrapartal period as early as 12 to 48 hours after she stops drinking. Delirium tremens may occur in the postpartal period, and the newborn may suffer a withdrawal syndrome.

The effects of alcohol on the fetus may result in a group of signs referred to as fetal alcohol syndrome (FAS). The syndrome has characteristic physical and mental abnormalities that vary in severity and combination. (See discussion in Chapter 28.) There is no definitive answer to how much alcohol a woman can safely consume during pregnancy. The expectant woman should "play it safe" by avoiding alcohol completely during the

TABLE 15–1 Possible Effects of Selected Drugs of Abuse/Addiction on Fetus and Neonate

Maternal Drug	Effect on Fetus/Neonate
Depressants	
Alcohol	Mental retardation, microcephaly, midfacial hypoplasia, cardiac anomalies, intrauterine growth restriction (IUGR), potential teratogenic effects, fetal alcohol syndrome (FAS), fetal alcohol effects (FAE)
Narcotics	
Heroin	Withdrawal symptoms, convulsions, death, IUGR, respiratory alkalosis, hyperbilirubinemia
Methadone	Fetal distress, meconium aspiration; with abrupt termination of the drug, severe withdrawal symptoms, neonatal death
Barbiturates	Neonatal depression, increased anomalies; teratogenic effect(?); withdrawal symptoms, convulsions, hyperactivity, hyperreflexia, vasomotor instability Bleeding (with excessive doses)
Phenobarbital	
"T's and Blues" (combination of the following)	
Talwin (narcotic)	Safe for use in pregnancy; depresses respiration if taken close to time of birth
Amytal (barbiturate)	See barbiturates
Tranquilizers	
Phenothiazine derivatives	Withdrawal, extrapyramidal dysfunction, delayed respiratory onset, hyperbilirubinemia, hypotonia or hyperactivity, decreased platelet count
Diazepam (Valium)	Hypotonia, hypothermia, low Apgar score, respiratory depression, poor sucking reflex, possible cleft lip
Antianxiety drugs	
Lithium	Congenital anomalies, especially Ebstein anomaly; lethargy and cyanosis in the newborn
Stimulants	
Amphetamines	
Amphetamine sulfate (Benzedrine)	Generalized arthritis, learning disabilities, poor motor coordination, transposition of the great vessels, cleft palate
Dextroamphetamine sulfate (dexedrine sulfate)	Congenital heart defects, hyperbilirubinemia
Cocaine	Cerebral infarctions, microcephaly, learning disabilities, poor state organization, decreased interactive behavior, CNS anomalies, cardiac anomalies, genitourinary anomalies, sudden infant death syndrome (SIDS)
Caffeine (more than 600 mg/day)	Spontaneous abortion, IUGR, increased incidence of cleft palate; other anomalies suspected
Nicotine (half to one pack cigarettes/day)	Increased rate of spontaneous abortion, increased incidence of placental abruption, SGA, small head circumference, decreased length, SIDS
Psychotropics	
PCP ("angel dust")	Flaccid appearance, poor head control, impaired neurologic development
LSD	Chromosomal breakage?
Marijuana	IUGR, potential impaired immunologic mechanisms

early weeks of pregnancy, when organogenesis is occurring. During the remainder of the pregnancy, she may have an occasional drink, although none at all is safest.

The nursing staff in the maternal-newborn unit must be aware of the manifestations of alcohol abuse so that they can prepare for the client's special needs. The care regimen includes sedation to decrease irritability and tremors, seizure precautions, intravenous fluid therapy for hydration, and preparation for an addicted neonate. Although high doses of sedatives and analgesics may be necessary for the woman, caution is advised because these can cause fetal depression.

Breastfeeding generally is not contraindicated, although alcohol is excreted in breast milk. Excessive alcohol consumption may intoxicate the infant and inhibit maternal let-down reflex. Discharge planning for the alcohol-addicted mother and newborn should be correlated with the social service department of the hospital.

Cocaine/Crack

Cocaine use is one of the most serious epidemics affecting the childbearing family. Approximately 1 in 10 pregnant women is believed to use cocaine, with even higher rates reported in urban areas (Kenner & D'Apolito, 1997). Cocaine acts at the nerve terminals to prevent the reuptake of dopamine and norepinephrine, which in turn results in vasoconstriction, tachycardia, and hypertension. Placental vasoconstriction decreases blood flow to the fetus.

Cocaine is usually taken in three ways: snorting, smoking, and intravenous injection. **Crack** is a form of free-base cocaine that is made up of baking soda, water, and cocaine mixed into a paste and microwaved to form a rock. The rock can then be smoked. Many women, especially those in low-income areas, favor this form of the drug over other forms because it is cheaper and readily available. In addition, smoking crack leads to a quicker, more intense high because the drug is absorbed through the large surface area of the lungs.

The onset of effects of cocaine occurs rapidly, but the euphoria lasts only about 30 minutes. This profound euphoria and excitement are usually followed by irritability, depression, pessimism, fatigue, and a strong desire for more cocaine. This pattern often leads the user to take repeated doses to sustain the effect. Cocaine metabolites may be present in the urine of a pregnant woman for up to 4 to 7 days following use.

The cocaine user is difficult to identify prenatally. Because cocaine is an illegal substance, many women are reluctant to volunteer information about their drug use. The nurse who is familiar with the woman may recognize subtle signs of cocaine use, including mood swings and appetite changes, and withdrawal symptoms such as de-

TABLE 15–2 Factors Associated with the Substance Abuser

Behavioral	Medical	Historical
Vague history regarding personal or medical problems	Liver disease, hepatomegaly	Alcohol- or drug-abusing partner
Conflicts with significant others or domestic violence	Pancreatitis	Many emergency department contacts
History of child abuse or neglect	Hypertension	Many physician contacts
Decreased job performance or chronic unemployment	Gastritis, esophagitis	Child with neonatal narcotic abstinence syndrome
Suicidal gestures, thoughts or attempts	Neurologic disorders	Child with alcohol-related birth defects
Car accidents	Poor nutritional status	Placement of other children outside the home
Citation for driving while intoxicated	Hematologic disorders	Complex perinatal histories and outcomes
Depression	Seropositivity for HIV	Psychiatric treatment or hospital admissions
Irritability or agitation	Bacteremia	Affective disorders
Difficulty concentrating	Alcoholic myopathy	Infants with low birth weight
Mood swings, outbursts of anger	Sensory impairment	Frequent physician prescriptions for mood-altering drugs
Inappropriate behavior	Problems of sepsis	Family history of alcoholism or other drug dependency
Memory lapses and losses or blackouts	Cellulitis	Sudden infant death syndrome
Intoxicated behavior	Hepatitis	Family dissolution
Smell of alcohol on breath	Abscesses	
Unreliability or unpredictable behavior	Mitral valve disease	
Missed appointments	Septicemia	
Intense daily drama, family chaos	Swelling and redness of hands	
Slurred speech	Overdose	
Staggering gait	Withdrawal effects	
	Pulmonary infections	
	Hair loss	
	Erratic menses	
	Loss of appetite	
	Poor dental hygiene	
	Anemia	
	Tuberculosis	
	Sexually transmitted infection	
	Obstetric complications, including spontaneous abortion, abruptio placentae, breech presentations, previous cesarean section, eclampsia, intrauterine growth retardation, premature labor and delivery and premature rupture of membranes, intrauterine fetal death, postpartum hemorrhage	

SOURCE: Adapted from Weiner SM: Nursing care of the drug-dependent pregnant woman during withdrawal treatment. In Jessup M (Ed), *Drug dependency in pregnancy: Managing withdrawal.* Sacramento, CA: Maternal and Child Health Department of Health Services, State of California, 1977, p 222

pression, irritability, nausea, lack of motivation, and psychomotor changes.

Major adverse maternal effects of cocaine use include seizures and hallucinations, pulmonary edema, respiratory failure, and cardiac problems. Women who use cocaine have an increased incidence of spontaneous first-trimester abortion, abruptio placentae, intrauterine growth restriction (IUGR), preterm birth, and stillbirth.

Exposure of the fetus to cocaine in utero increases the risk of IUGR, small head circumference, cerebral infarctions, shorter body length, altered brain development, malformations of the genitourinary tract, and lower Apgar scores at birth. Newborns who were exposed to cocaine in utero may have neurobehavioral disturbances, marked irritability, an exaggerated startle reflex, labile emotions, and an increased risk of sudden infant death syndrome (SIDS). These newborns have poor interactive behaviors, have difficulty responding appropriately to voices, and fail to respond well to consoling behaviors. These complications may interfere with maternal-infant attachment and increase the infant's risk of abuse and neglect (Kenner & D'Apolito, 1997).

Cocaine does cross into the breast milk and may cause such symptoms in the breastfeeding infant as extreme irritability, vomiting, diarrhea, dilated pupils, and apnea. Thus women who continue to use cocaine following childbirth should avoid nursing.

Marijuana

Approximately 15% of pregnant women use marijuana, often in conjunction with alcohol and tobacco. Men who smoke marijuana may have decreased sperm counts and may develop gynecomastia (enlarged breasts); women may experience menstrual cycle irregularities. To date, however, there is no evidence that marijuana has any teratogenic effects on the fetus. One study has reported an increase in precipitous labors (less than 3 hours) in heavy marijuana users, but these results have not been confirmed (Niebyl, 1996). The impact of heavy marijuana use on pregnancy is difficult to evaluate because of the variety of social factors that may influence the results.

Infants exposed to marijuana in utero have been reported to have increased fine tremors, prolonged startles, irritability, and poor habituation to visual stimuli, but these symptoms were not present in follow-up at 12 and 24 months of age (Fanaroff & Martin, 1997).

Phencyclidine (PCP)

Phencyclidine (PCP) is a popular hallucinogen that can be smoked, taken orally, or injected intravenously. The onset of effects occurs in 2 to 4 minutes and lasts about 4 to 6 hours, with no withdrawal state. The drug causes confusion, delirium, and hallucinations and may produce feelings of euphoria. Signs of PCP use include constricted pupils, ataxia, nystagmus, double vision (diplopia), dizziness, and diaphoresis. The greatest risk for the pregnant woman is overdose or a psychotic response. Signs of overdose include hypertension, hyperthermia, diaphoresis, and possible coma, which may jeopardize fetal well-being.

PCP has been associated with neurobehavioral problems including wild behavior states, flaccid appearance, and poor head control (Fanaroff & Martin, 1997).

Heroin

Heroin is an illicit central nervous system (CNS) depressant narcotic that alters perception and produces euphoria. It is an addictive drug that is generally administered intravenously, although a snortable form of heroin called Karachi is available. Pregnancy in women who use heroin is considered high risk because of the associated increased incidence of poor nutrition, iron deficiency anemia, and pregnancy-induced hypertension (PIH). There is also an increased rate of breech position, abnormal placental implantation, abruptio placentae, preterm labor, premature rupture of the membranes (PROM), and meconium staining. Heroin users also have a higher incidence of sexually transmitted infection because many must rely on prostitution to support their drug habit.

The fetus of a heroin-addicted woman is at increased risk for IUGR, meconium aspiration, and hypoxia. The newborn frequently shows signs of heroin addiction, such as restlessness; lack of habituation; shrill, high-pitched cry; irritability; fist sucking; vomiting; and seizures. Signs of withdrawal usually appear within 72 hours and may last for several days. The newborn may exhibit poor consolability for 3 months or more. These behaviors may interfere with successful maternal-infant attachment and increase the potential for parenting problems in an already high-risk mother.

Today is the anniversary of my Julie's death. She died of a heroin overdose. During the years before her death, we tried everything to help her, but nothing worked. She would disappear, sometimes for weeks, and then reappear filled with good intentions to kick her habit—but she never could. She was 29 when I lost her, and 3 months pregnant with our grandchild. I miss her so. I don't know if my heart will ever mend.

Methadone

Methadone is the most commonly used drug in the treatment of women who are dependent on opioids such as heroin. Methadone blocks withdrawal symptoms and the craving for street drugs. Dosage should be individualized at the lowest possible therapeutic level. Methadone does cross the placenta and has been associated with complications such as PIH, hepatitis, placental problems, and abnormal fetal presentation (Kearney, 1997).

Prenatal exposure to methadone may result in reduced head circumference, poor motor coordination, increased body tension, and delayed achievement of motor skills. The neonate may experience withdrawal symptoms that are more severe than those associated with heroin.

Clinical Therapy

Antepartal care of the pregnant addict involves medical, socioeconomic, and legal considerations. The use of a team approach allows for the comprehensive management necessary to provide safe labor and childbirth for the woman and her fetus.

The management of drug addiction may include hospitalization as necessary to initiate detoxification. "Cold turkey" withdrawal is not advisable during pregnancy because of potential risk to the fetus. Maintenance and support therapy are given during weekly prenatal visits.

Urine screening is also done regularly throughout pregnancy if the woman is a known or suspected substance abuser. This testing is helpful in identifying the type and amount of drug being abused.

CRITICAL THINKING QUESTION

What psychosocial factors contribute to the onset of substance abuse?

NURSING CARE MANAGEMENT

Nursing Assessment and Diagnosis

Nurses and other health care providers should make it a practice to screen all pregnant women for substance abuse. Several simple screening tools are available. In addition, the nurse should be alert for clues in the history or appearance of the woman that suggest substance abuse (refer to Table 15–2). If abuse is suspected, the nurse needs to ask direct questions, beginning with less threatening questions about use of tobacco, caffeine, and over-the-counter medications. The nurse can then progress to questions about alcohol consumption and finally ques-

COMMUNITY IN FOCUS

Pregnant and Addicted Women's Program

The Pregnant and Addicted Women's Program in Spokane, Washington, is an exciting example of how a community can succeed in tackling a major health problem when its members use a creative, multidisciplinary approach. In 1995, two nurses at Deaconess Medical Center—Maureen Shogan, RNC, MN, a neonatal clinical nurse specialist, and Ann Seaburg, RNC, MHA, a neonatal intensive care unit (NICU) nurse manager—became concerned about the number of addicted infants they were treating. Although a state program was in place at Deaconess Medical Center to provide voluntary, 26-day inpatient therapy for pregnant and addicted women, it was not well utilized. The nurses rallied support for a study to determine the scope of the problem in their community.

All four medical centers in the city came together to fund the study, and the Inland Northwest Regional Perinatal Center provided a staff person to track the demographics, handle the specimens, and so forth. For the study, meconium samples were obtained from 820 newborns and analyzed for opiates, marijuana, and cocaine. (At that time, methamphetamines were not a problem in the community.) Nurses in all four hospitals responded enthusiastically, obtaining the needed specimens according to the study protocol. The results indicated that 7.8% of the women who gave birth had used at least one of these substances; 8% of women admitted for birth reported alcohol use before birth.

Once the seriousness of the problem had been documented, it was easier to take action. In the year following the study, admissions for inpatient therapy doubled as more physicians and care providers became attuned to signs of substance abuse in the pregnant women they treated. Because of the high costs of inpatient treatment and the difficulties many women have arranging care for other children when they are hospitalized, inpatient stays have been shortened somewhat and are often followed by intensive, long-term residential care at a site such as Isabella House. At Isabella House, women and their children are residents. During the day, the mothers participate in treatment while their children attend a therapeutic day-care center across the street.

The community also established a special Child Protection Team, which deals exclusively with pregnant and addicted women and their children. The team is interdisciplinary in nature, composed of public health nurses, NICU nurses, social workers, child psychologists, drug counselors, and occupational therapists. Under this approach, infants of addicted mothers are automatically considered high risk. Child Protective Services caseworkers present the cases of all such infants to the special team, which meets weekly. The team members review each case and make decisions about appropriate referral, treatment, and follow-up. In addition, under the auspices of Inland Northwest Regional Perinatal Center, outreach programs on substance abuse among pregnant women are presented to health care workers in rural parts of Washington and Idaho, both in person and via telemedicine conferencing.

The state of Washington is also taking the problem of substance abuse during pregnancy very seriously. House Bill 3103, which was passed in 1998, mandates that assessment criteria to identify substance abuse be developed and followed by any care provider who comes into contact with pregnant or lactating women. This will probably take the form of a brief series of screening questions similar to those used to identify victims of abuse. A curriculum will also be developed to educate care providers about the problem itself, the screening tools, and appropriate "next steps" when substance abuse is suspected.

This important effort began because two nurses identified a need and took action. It is a tribute to them and to the community they serve.

SOURCE: Personal communication with Maureen Shogan, RNC, MN, neonatal clinical nurse specialist, Deaconess Medical Center and Valley Medical Center.

tions focusing on past and current use of illicit drugs. The nurse who is matter-of-fact and nonjudgmental in approach is more likely to elicit honest responses.

Nursing assessment of the woman who is a known substance abuser focuses on her general health status, with specific attention to nutritional status, susceptibility to infections, and evaluation of all body systems. The nurse also assesses the woman's understanding of the impact of substance abuse on herself and her pregnancy. Some women are reluctant to discuss their substance abuse; others are quite open about it. Once the nurse establishes a relationship of trust, the nurse can gain information to use in planning the woman's ongoing care.

Nursing diagnoses that may apply to abuse include the following:

- ***Altered Nutrition: Less than Body Requirements*** related to inadequate food intake secondary to substance abuse
- ***Risk for Infection*** related to use of inadequately cleaned syringes and needles secondary to IV drug use
- ***Knowledge Deficit*** related to lack of information about the impact of substance abuse on the fetus

Nursing Plan and Implementation

Preventing substance abuse during pregnancy is the ideal nursing goal and is best accomplished through education. Unfortunately, many women who are substance abusers do not receive regular health care and may not seek care until far along in their pregnancy.

The nurse's role in providing prenatal care for the woman who is a substance abuser focuses on ongoing assessment and client teaching. Research indicates, however, that some maternal-newborn nurses have only limited knowledge about substance abuse and that these same nurses have attitudes that may be more negative and punitive than positive and supportive toward women who abuse substances during pregnancy (Selleck & Redding, 1998). It is essential that nurses caring for childbearing families develop the knowledge and skill necessary to identify pregnant women who abuse substances. To provide care that is truly effective, it is equally important that nurses develop and maintain a nonjudgmental, nonpunitive, positive attitude when caring for women who are substance abusers.

When the nurse encounters a pregnant woman who screens positive for substance abuse, the nurse should review for the woman what she has reported and express concern for the health of the mother and infant. The nurse can then go on to state the belief that the mother is concerned about the baby's health and stress the need for the woman to stop using drugs or alcohol during pregnancy. The nurse can then discuss possible strategies to help the woman quit (addiction treatment programs, 12-step programs, individual counseling) and suggest a referral for more in-depth assessment by a specialist. If feasible, the nurse can make an appointment while the woman is in the office or clinic. Finally the nurse should make a follow-up appointment to see the woman again after her drug or alcohol assessment. The knowledgeable nurse can provide information about the relationship between substance abuse and existing health problems and the implications for the woman's unborn child. By establishing a relationship of trust and support, the nurse may foster the woman's cooperation.

Preparation for labor and birth should be part of the prenatal planning. Fear, tension, or discomfort may be relieved through nonnarcotic psychologic support and careful explanation of the labor process. If pain medication is necessary, it should not be withheld, however, because the notion that it will contribute to further addiction is not correct. Preferred methods of pain relief include the use of psychoprophylaxis and regional or local anesthetics, such as pudendal block and local infiltration. These techniques decrease risk of additional fetal respiratory depression. Immediate intensive care should be available for the newborn, who will probably be depressed, small for gestational age (SGA), and premature. For care of the addicted newborn, see Chapter 28.

Evaluation

Expected outcomes of nursing care include the following:

- The woman is able to describe the impact of substance abuse on herself and her unborn child.
- The woman successfully gives birth to a healthy infant.
- The woman agrees to cooperate with referral to social services (or other appropriate community agency) for follow-up care after discharge. ●

Care of the Woman with Diabetes Mellitus

Diabetes mellitus, an endocrine disorder of carbohydrate metabolism, results from inadequate production or utilization of insulin. Insulin, produced by the beta cells of the islets of Langerhans in the pancreas, lowers blood glucose levels by enabling the glucose to move from the blood into muscle and adipose tissue cells.

Carbohydrate Metabolism in Normal Pregnancy

Carbohydrate metabolism is affected early in pregnancy by a rise in serum levels of estrogen, progesterone, and other hormones. These hormones stimulate insulin production by the maternal pancreatic beta cells and increase tissue response to insulin early in pregnancy. Therefore an anabolic (building up) state exists during the first half of pregnancy with storage of glycogen in the liver and other tissues.

In the second half of pregnancy, placental secretion of human placental lactogen (hPL) and prolactin (from the decidua), as well as elevated cortisol and glycogen, cause increased resistance to insulin and decreased glucose tolerance. This diminished effectiveness of insulin results in a catabolic (destructive) state during fasting periods (eg, during the night and after meal absorption). Because increasing amounts of circulating maternal glucose and amino acids are being diverted to the fetus, maternal fat is metabolized during fasting periods much more readily than in a nonpregnant person. This process is called accelerated starvation. Ketones may be present in the urine as a result of lipolysis (maternal metabolism of fat).

The delicate system of checks and balances that exists between glucose production and glucose use is stressed by the growing fetus, who derives energy from glucose taken solely from maternal stores. This stress is referred to as the diabetogenic effect of pregnancy. Thus any preexisting disruption in carbohydrate metabolism is augmented by pregnancy, and any diabetic potential may precipitate gestational diabetes mellitus.

Pathophysiology of Diabetes Mellitus

In diabetes mellitus, the pancreas does not produce sufficient amounts of insulin to allow necessary carbohydrate metabolism. With inadequate amounts of insulin, glucose cannot enter the cells but remains outside in the blood. The body cells become energy depleted while the blood glucose level remains elevated. Fats and proteins in the body tissues are then oxidized by the cells as a source of energy. This results in wasting of fat and muscle tissue of the body, negative nitrogen balance due to protein breakdown, and ketosis due to fat metabolism. The strong osmotic force of the glucose concentration in the blood

TABLE 15–3 Classification of Diabetes Mellitus (DM) and Other Categories of Glucose Intolerance

Diabetes mellitus
- Type I, insulin-dependent (IDDM)
- Type II, noninsulin-dependent (NIDDM)
  - Nonobese NIDDM
  - Obese NIDDM
- Secondary diabetes

Impaired glucose tolerance (IGT)

Gestational diabetes mellitus (GDM)

SOURCE: National Diabetes Data Group of National Institutes of Health, *Diabetes* 1979; 28:1039. Adapted with permission from the American Diabetes Association Inc.

TABLE 15–4 White's Classification of Diabetes in Pregnancy

Class	Criterion
A	Chemical diabetes
B	Maturity onset (age over 20 years), duration under 10 years, no vascular lesions
C_1	Age 10 to 19 years at onset
C_2	10 to 19 years' duration
D_1	Under 10 years at onset
D_2	Over 20 years' duration
D_3	Benign retinopathy
D_4	Calcified vessels of legs
D_5	Hypertension
E	No longer sought
F	Nephropathy
G	Many failures
H	Cardiopathy
R	Proliferating retinopathy
T	Renal transplant (added by Tagatz and colleagues of the University of Minnesota)

SOURCE: White P: Classification of obstetric diabetes. *Am J Obstet Gynecol* 1978; 130:228. Used with permission.

pulls water from the cells into the blood, which results in cellular dehydration. The high level of glucose in the blood eventually spills over into the urine, producing glycosuria. Osmotic pressure of the glucose in the urine prevents reabsorption of water into the kidney tubules, causing extracellular dehydration.

These pathologic developments cause the four cardinal signs and symptoms of diabetes mellitus: polyuria, polydipsia, weight loss, and polyphagia. Polyuria (frequent urination) results because water is not reabsorbed by the renal tubules because of the osmotic activity of glucose. Polydipsia (excessive thirst) is caused by dehydration from polyuria. Weight loss (seen in insulin-dependent diabetes, also called type I diabetes) is due to the use of fat and muscle tissue for energy. Polyphagia (excessive hunger) is caused by tissue loss and a state of starvation, which results from the inability of the cells to utilize the blood glucose. Diagnosis of diabetes is based on the presence of clinical symptoms and laboratory tests showing elevated glucose levels in the blood.

Classification of Diabetes Mellitus

States of altered carbohydrate metabolism have been classified several different ways. Table 15–3 shows the current accepted classification, a result of the 1979 report of a special committee of the National Institutes of Health (National Diabetes Data Group, 1979). This classification contains three main categories: diabetes mellitus (DM), impaired glucose tolerance (IGT), and gestational diabetes mellitus (GDM).

Table 15–4 shows White's classification of diabetes in pregnancy. This classification is useful for describing the extent of the disease.

Gestational diabetes mellitus is defined as carbohydrate intolerance of variable severity with onset or first recognition during pregnancy. It results from (1) an unidentified preexistent disease, (2) the unmasking of a compensated metabolic abnormality by the added stress of pregnancy, or (3) a direct consequence of the altered maternal metabolism stemming from changing hormonal levels. Diet therapy is the cornerstone of intervention for GDM, but insulin therapy is indicated when dietary management is inadequate (Owen, Phelan, Landon, & Gabbe, 1995).

In most instances, the overt diabetic manifestation disappears postpartum, though subtle manifestations of impaired insulin secretory capacity may remain. Although gestational diabetes mellitus incidence rates vary, many of these individuals progress to overt type II diabetes mellitus with time (Peters, Kjos, Xiang, & Buchanan, 1996).

Influence of Pregnancy on Diabetes

Pregnancy can affect diabetes significantly. First, the physiologic changes of pregnancy can drastically alter insulin requirements. Second, pregnancy may accelerate the progress of vascular disease secondary to diabetes.

The disease may be more difficult to control during pregnancy because insulin requirements are changeable. Insulin need frequently decreases early in the first trimester. Levels of hPL, an insulin antagonist, are low; energy demands of the embryo are minimal; and the woman may be consuming less food due to nausea and vomiting. Nausea and vomiting may also cause dietary fluctuations, which can increase the risk of hypoglycemia or insulin shock. Insulin requirements usually begin to rise late in the first trimester as glucose use and glycogen storage by the woman and fetus increase. As a result of placental maturation and production of hPL and other hormones, insulin requirements may double or quadruple by the end of pregnancy.

Increased energy needs during labor may require more insulin to balance intravenous glucose. After delivery of the placenta, insulin requirements usually decrease abruptly with loss of hPL in the maternal circulation.

Other factors contribute to the difficulty in controlling the disease. As pregnancy progresses, the renal

RESEARCH IN PRACTICE

What is this study about? Women with established diabetes and elevated blood sugar levels early in pregnancy may give birth to a child with a major congenital defect. Emily Holing, Carla Beyer, Zane Brown, and Fredrick Connell designed a study to determine what conditions promote or discourage effective pregnancy planning for diabetic woman, including the maintenance of optimal blood sugars before conception and during the early weeks of pregnancy.

How was the study done? The investigators collected data from 85 English-speaking postpartum women over the age of 16 with established diabetes. At the request of the Institutional Review board, data collectors excluded women with adverse pregnancy outcomes such as stillbirth. Researchers obtained data from a self-administered questionnaire, medical record reviews, and an interview. The questionnaire incorporated demographics, access to health care, type of diabetic provider, frequency of visits, and diabetic complications. Interview questions covered eight themes: contraceptive use, pregnancy planning behavior, desire for motherhood, partner relationships, health locus of control, knowledge about diabetes and pregnancy, medical advice received, and relationship with health care provider.

What were the results of the study? Of the 85 women interviewed, only 34 (41%) had planned their pregnancy. Seventy percent of the women with unplanned pregnancies used contraception less than half of the time. When compared with women who planned their pregnancy, women with unplanned pregnancies had significantly higher glycohemoglobin levels at the first prenatal visit and in the 3rd trimester, were more likely to attribute their health outcomes to powerful others, were less satisfied with their partner relationships, and were less likely to know that they needed to be in good diabetic control to help prevent birth defects. Thirty-five (70%) of the women with unplanned pregnancies stated that being pregnant made them very happy. A majority of this group of women (70%) also related that their health care providers either gave them no sense of encouragement or actually discouraged them from becoming pregnant. Only 28% of this group described a positive relationship with their provider as opposed to 71% for the women with a planned pregnancy. Researchers concluded that discouraging pregnancy by a health care provider may sever communication and encourage unplanned pregnancies when women subconsciously want to become pregnant.

What additional questions might I have? did all of the women seek prenatal care? Were the first glycohemoglobin levels obtained at approximately the same week of gestation?

How can I use this study? Rather than discourage a woman with established diabetes from becoming pregnant, health care providers can initiate discussions about the importance of optimal blood sugar control and the relationship between hyperglycemia and congenital defects.

SOURCE: Holing, E. V., Beyer, C. S., Brown, Z. A., & Connell, F. A. (1998). Why don't women with diabetes plan their pregnancies? *Diabetes Care, 21*(6), 889–895.

threshold for glucose decreases. There is an increased risk of ketoacidosis, which may occur at lower serum glucose levels in the pregnant woman with diabetes than in the nonpregnant diabetic. The vascular disease that accompanies diabetes may progress during pregnancy. Hypertension may occur. Nephropathy may result from renal impairment, and retinopathy may develop.

The primary concern for the pregnant woman who has diabetes is control of circulating blood glucose levels. If control can be achieved and maintained, diabetes generally does not worsen during pregnancy. The woman's health status may even improve because of close medical supervision.

Influence of Diabetes on Pregnancy Outcome

The pregnancy of a woman who has diabetes carries a higher risk of complications, especially perinatal mortality and congenital anomalies. The risk has been reduced by the recent recognition of the importance of tight metabolic control (blood glucose between 70 mg/dL and 120 mg/dL). New techniques for monitoring blood glucose, delivering insulin, and monitoring the fetus have also reduced perinatal mortality.

Maternal Risks

Maternal health problems in diabetic pregnancy have been greatly reduced by the team approach to early prenatal care and emphasis on maintaining control of blood glucose levels. The prognosis for the pregnant woman with gestational, type I, or type II diabetes that has not resulted in significant vascular damage is positive. However, diabetic pregnancy still carries higher risks for complications than normal pregnancy.

Hydramnios, or an increase in the volume of amniotic fluid, occurs in 10% to 20% of pregnant diabetics. It is thought to be a result of excessive fetal urination because of fetal hyperglycemia (Golan, Wolman, Saller, & David, 1993). Premature rupture of membranes and onset of labor may result, but only occasionally does this pose a threat.

Pregnancy-induced hypertension (PIH) occurs more often in diabetic pregnancies, especially when diabetes-related vascular changes already exist.

Hyperglycemia due to insufficient amounts of insulin can lead to *ketoacidosis* as a result of the increase in ketone bodies (which are acidic) in the blood released when fatty acids are metabolized. Ketoacidosis usually develops slowly, but it may develop more rapidly in the pregnant woman because of the hyperketonemia associated with accelerated starvation in the nonfed state. The tendency for higher postprandial glucose levels because of decreased gastric motility and the contrainsulin effects of hPL also predispose the woman to ketoacidosis. If the ketoacidosis is not treated, it can lead to coma and death of both mother and fetus.

Another risk to the pregnant woman with diabetes is a difficult labor *(dystocia)*, caused by fetopelvic disproportion if fetal macrosomia exists. The pregnant woman with diabetes is also at increased risk for monilial vaginitis and urinary tract infections because of increased glycosuria, which contributes to a favorable environment for bacterial growth. If untreated, asymptomatic bacteriuria can lead to pyelonephritis, a serious kidney infection.

During pregnancy, about 15% of diabetic women will have some increase in *retinopathy*. Severe proliferative retinopathy can lead to blindness if not treated with laser coagulation (Puza & Malee, 1996).

Fetal-Neonatal Risks

It is now clear that many of the problems of the neonate result directly from high maternal plasma glucose levels. In the presence of severe maternal ketoacidosis, the risk of fetal death increases to 50% (Garner, 1995). Fetal enzyme systems cease functioning in an acidic environment.

The incidence of *congenital anomalies* in diabetic pregnancies is 5% to 10% and is the major cause of death for infants of diabetic mothers. Research suggests that this increased incidence of congenital anomalies is related to multiple factors including high glucose levels in early pregnancy (Landon, 1996). The anomalies often involve the heart, central nervous system, and skeletal system. Septal defects, coarctation of the aorta, and transposition of the great vessels are the most common heart lesions seen. Central nervous system anomalies include hydrocephalus, meningomyelocele, and anencephaly. One anomaly, sacral agenesis, appears only in infants of diabetic mothers. In sacral agenesis, the sacrum and lumbar spine fail to develop and the lower extremities develop incompletely. To reduce the incidence of congenital anomalies, preconception counseling and strict diabetes control before conception and in the early weeks of pregnancy are indicated.

Characteristically, infants of type I diabetic mothers (or classes A, B, and C; see Table 15–4) are large for gestational age (LGA) as a result of high levels of fetal insulin production stimulated by the high levels of glucose crossing the placenta from the mother. Sustained fetal hyperinsulinism and hyperglycemia ultimately lead to excessive growth, called **macrosomia,** and deposition of fat. If born vaginally, the macrosomic infant is at increased risk for birth trauma such as fractured clavicle or brachial plexus injuries due to shoulder dystocia. To prevent such injuries, cesarean birth may be indicated if birth weight is expected to exceed 4500 g (ACOG, 1994a).

After birth, the umbilical cord is severed, and thus the generous maternal blood glucose supply is eliminated. However, continued islet cell hyperactivity leads to excessive insulin levels and depleted blood glucose (hypoglycemia) in 2 to 4 hours. Macrosomia can be significantly reduced by tight maternal blood glucose control.

Infants of diabetic mothers with vascular involvement may demonstrate *intrauterine growth restriction (IUGR)*. This occurs because vascular changes in the mother decrease the efficiency of placental perfusion, and the fetus is not as well sustained in utero.

Respiratory distress syndrome appears to result from inhibition, by high levels of fetal insulin, of some fetal enzymes necessary for surfactant production. *Polycythemia* in the neonate is due primarily to the diminished ability of glycosylated hemoglobin in the mother's blood to release oxygen. *Hyperbilirubinemia* is a result of the inability of immature liver enzymes to metabolize the increased bilirubin resulting from the polycythemia. *Hypocalcemia*, characterized by signs of irritability or even tetany, may occur. The cause of these low calcium levels in infants of diabetic mothers is not known (Spellacy, 1994).

Clinical Therapy

Detection and Diagnosis of Gestational Diabetes

Gestational diabetes is more common than pregestational diabetes. It is estimated to occur in 3% to 6% of pregnancies. Therefore screening for its detection is a standard part of prenatal care. If diabetes is suspected, further testing is undertaken for diagnosis.

Two screening tests are commonly administered to pregnant women:

1. *Urine testing.* Tes-Tape and Diastix are generally used to test the pregnant woman's urine for glucose at her first prenatal visit and again on subsequent visits. Glycosuria is not diagnostic of diabetes mellitus, but the presence of glycosuria is an indication for glucose tolerance testing. In the nonpregnant adult, glucose is not generally spilled into the urine until the blood sugar level is 180 mg/dL or greater. During pregnancy, the renal threshold is lower, and glucose may spill into the urine when blood glucose levels are 130 mg/dL. Urine is also tested for ketones using Ketostix or Acetest. Both are simple tests for detecting ketones in the urine and are usually done routinely for type I (ketosis-prone) diabetes.
2. *50 g oral glucose tolerance test.* All pregnant women, regardless of risk factors, should be screened for diabetes toward the end of the second trimester (24 to 28 weeks). Women with risk factors (age over 30; family history of diabetes; a prior macrosomic, malformed, or stillborn infant; obesity; hypertension; or glucosuria) should be screened when first seen for prenatal care (ACOG, 1994a). The oral glucose load is administered without regard to time of day or time of last meal, and venous plasma glucose is measured 1 hour later. A plasma level that exceeds 140 mg/dL indicates a need for further diagnostic testing.

During pregnancy, gestational diabetes is diagnosed using a 3-hour, 100 g oral glucose tolerance test (OGTT). To do this test, the woman eats a high-carbohydrate (greater than 200 g carbohydrate daily) diet for 3 days before her scheduled test. She then ingests 100 g oral glucose solution in the morning after an overnight fast for at least 8 hours but not more than 14 hours. Plasma glucose is measured fasting and at 1, 2, and 3 hours. The woman should remain seated and not smoke throughout the test. Gestational diabetes is diagnosed if two or more of the following values are met or exceeded:

CRITICAL THINKING IN PRACTICE

Patti Chang is a 35-year-old, gravida 3, para 2, well-educated, active Chinese American woman with no history of glucose intolerance. Her two children were born healthy at 36 weeks' gestation. She receives the usual 50 g glucose tolerance test at 26 weeks' gestation, and her plasma level is 160 mg/dL. She seems irritated and frustrated when her obstetrician tells her that it would be best to perform a 3-hour fasting glucose tolerance test. After the physician leaves the room, Patti asks the nurse the following questions: Will the glucose hurt my baby? What will the treatment be? How will the nurse answer the questions? Why does Patti seem so upset?

Answers can be found in Appendix I.

Fasting	105 mg/dL
1 hour	190 mg/dL
2 hour	165 mg/dL
3 hour	145 mg/dL

The result is considered borderline abnormal if only one value is elevated, and the OGTT is repeated in 1 month.

Laboratory Assessment of Long-Term Glucose Control

Glycosylated hemoglobin (HbA_{1c}) is a laboratory test that loosely reflects glucose control over the previous 4 to 8 weeks. It measures the percentage of glycohemoglobin in the blood. Glycohemoglobin, or HbA_{1c}, is the hemoglobin to which a glucose molecule is attached. The test is not reliable for screening for gestational diabetes or for close daily control, but it is useful as an indicator of overall blood glucose control. Women with abnormal HbA_{1c} values greater than 10% are at most significant risk for having a fetus with malformations (ACOG, 1994a).

Antepartal Management of Diabetes

The major goals of medical care for a pregnant woman with diabetes—whether gestational or pregestational—are (1) to maintain a physiologic equilibrium of insulin availability and glucose utilization during pregnancy and (2) to deliver an optimally healthy mother and newborn. To achieve these goals, good prenatal care using a team approach is a top priority. The team consists of an obstetrician, an endocrinologist, a perinatologist, a diabetes nurse-educator, a perinatal nurse, a nutritionist, a social worker, and, most importantly, the diabetic woman and her partner if he is involved in the pregnancy. Education of the couple and their active involvement in managing her care are essential for a good outcome.

For the woman with gestational diabetes, the diagnosis may be a shock, leaving her frightened and anxious (Brown & Hare, 1995). She needs clear explanation and teaching to enlist her participation in ensuring a good outcome. The diabetes nurse-educator plays a major role in this counseling.

The woman with pregestational diabetes needs to understand changes she can expect during pregnancy; thus she should receive such teaching in preconception counseling. At the initial prenatal visit, height, weight, and vital signs are assessed along with a thorough assessment of thyroid and cardiac function. Special attention is given to dating the pregnancy. Laboratory data are obtained, and the diabetes is classified using White's criteria. Women should be screened for diabetic neuropathy, and a fundoscopic examination is done to detect any retinopathy. In some cases, the woman may be referred to an ophthalmologist for further evaluation.

Dietary Regulation The pregnant woman requires about 300 calories per day more than she does when she is not pregnant to meet increased metabolic demands. In general, women need approximately 30 kcal/kg of ideal body weight (IBW) during the first trimester and 35 to 36 kcal/kg IBW during the second and third trimesters. If ketonuria develops or the woman complains of hunger, the number of calories may be increased. Dietary guidelines are similar for women with gestational and pregestational diabetes. Approximately 50% to 60% of the calories should come from complex carbohydrates, 12% to 20% from protein, and 20% to 30% from fats (Cunningham et al, 1997). This caloric intake is divided among three meals and three snacks. The prebedtime snack is the most important and must include both protein and complex carbohydrates to prevent hypoglycemia at night. Because it is so important that the pregnant woman follow these guidelines, a nutritionist works out meal plans based on the woman's life-style, culture, and food preferences and teaches her food exchanges so she can vary and plan her own meals. Cookbooks for people with diabetes are available and can be a great help.

Glucose Monitoring Glucose monitoring is an essential part of diabetes management for determining the need for insulin and assessing glucose control. Many physicians have the woman come in for a weekly assessment of her fasting glucose levels and one or two postprandial levels. In addition, frequent self-monitoring of glucose levels is paramount in maintaining good glucose control. Self-monitoring is discussed on page 363.

Insulin Administration Whether the woman with gestational diabetes needs additional insulin (over her own body production) depends on how well her blood glucose levels can be maintained by diet alone. Individuals with pregestational diabetes usually have type I diabetes, requiring insulin administration. Whether the client has gestational or pregestational diabetes, human insulin should be used because it is the least likely to cause an allergic response. If the woman has previously used bovine or porcine insulin, she may require smaller doses of human insulin to achieve the same pharmacologic effect. She is instructed to take an initial glucose reading at 2 AM to avoid nocturnal or early morning hypoglycemic episodes.

Insulin is given either in multiple injections or by continuous subcutaneous infusion. Multiple injections are used more commonly and with excellent results. Most women will need a mixture of intermediate and regular insulin twice daily. Often two-thirds of the total insulin dose is taken with breakfast in a 2:1 ratio of intermediate to regular. The remaining third is taken with the evening meal in a 1:1 ratio. Some centers now use a three-dose or four-dose approach. With the three-dose approach, two thirds of the insulin dose is taken before breakfast in a 2:1 ratio of NPH to regular insulin; the remaining regular insulin dose is then taken before dinner, and the remaining NPH dose is taken at bedtime. With the four-dose approach, regular insulin is taken before each meal and NPH is taken at bedtime. The three- and four-dose approaches are used to stabilize blood glucose levels and avoid episodes of nocturnal hypoglycemia (Idrogo & Mazze, 1998). It is important to remember that the amount of insulin needed usually increases during each trimester of pregnancy.

Oral hypoglycemics are never used during pregnancy because they cross the placenta, may be teratogenic, and stimulate fetal insulin production (ACOG, 1994a).

Evaluation of Fetal Status Information about the well-being, maturation, and size of the fetus is important for planning the course of the pregnancy and the timing of birth. Because pregnancies complicated by diabetes are at increased risk of neural tube defects, *maternal serum α-fetoprotein (AFP)* screening is done during weeks 16 to 20 of gestation (see Chapter 17).

Daily maternal evaluation of *fetal activity*, begun at about 28 weeks, is effective and simple to do. The woman is taught a particular method for counting fetal movements (see Chapter 12). She records the results on a special card, and brings the card to each subsequent office visit.

Nonstress testing (NST) is usually begun weekly at about 28 weeks. If evidence of IUGR, PIH, oligohydramnios, or poorly controlled blood glucose exists, testing may begin as early as 26 weeks and may be done more often. NSTs are increased to twice weekly at 32 weeks' gestation. If the NST is nonreactive, a fetal biophysical profile or *contraction stress test* is performed (Gabbe, 1996). If the woman requires hospitalization (for example, to control glycemia or for complications), NSTs may be done daily.

Ultrasound at 18 weeks establishes gestational age and diagnoses multiple pregnancy or congenital anomalies. It is repeated at 28 weeks to monitor fetal growth for IUGR or macrosomia. Some physicians order *fetal biophysical profiles* (ultrasound evaluation of fetal well-being in which fetal breathing movements, fetal activity, reactivity, muscle tone, and amniotic fluid volume are assessed) as part of an ongoing evaluation of fetal status.

Intrapartal Management of Diabetes Mellitus

During the intrapartal period, medical therapy includes the following:

- *Timing of birth.* Most diabetic pregnancies are allowed to go to term, with spontaneous labor, thereby decreasing the risk of respiratory distress in the neonate. In pregnancies in which there is evidence of fetal macrosomia, fetal compromise, or elevated maternal HbA_{1c}, amniocentesis is done for lecithin/sphingomyelin (L/S) ratio and the presence of phosphatidylglycerol (PG). Whereas levels of 2:1 for the L/S ratio indicate fetal lung maturity in the nondiabetic pregnancy, levels of up to 3.5:1 L/S ratio have been found necessary at some centers before low risk of respiratory distress syndrome (RDS) is achieved. The presence of phosphatidylglycerol (PG) seems to enhance lecithin activity, and its presence is considered favorable for lung maturity. Fetal lung maturity must be weighed against other considerations when deciding time of childbirth. If preterm labor occurs, tocolytic therapy and β-sympathomimetic drugs should *not* be administered because they may worsen maternal glucose control (Cunningham et al, 1997).
- *Labor management.* The degree of prenatal maintenance of normal maternal glucose levels (euglycemia) and the maintenance of maternal euglycemia during labor are important in preventing neonatal hypoglycemia. Maternal insulin requirements often decrease dramatically during labor. Consequently, maternal glucose levels are measured hourly to determine insulin need. Often two intravenous lines are used, one with a 5% dextrose solution and one with a saline solution. The saline solution is then available if a bolus is needed or for piggybacking insulin. Insulin clings to the plastic intravenous bag and tubing. To ensure that the woman receives the desired dose, the intravenous tubing must be flushed with insulin before the prescribed amount is added. During the second stage of labor and the immediate postpartum period, the woman may not need additional insulin. The intravenous insulin is discontinued with the completion of the third stage of labor.

Postpartal Management of Diabetes Mellitus

Maternal insulin requirements fall significantly postpartally because the levels of hPL, progesterone, and estrogen fall after placental separation, and their anti-insulin effect ceases, resulting in decreased blood glucose levels. The diabetic mother may require no insulin for the first 24 hours or only one-fourth to one-half her previous dose. Then, reestablishment of insulin needs based on blood glucose testing is necessary. Diet and exercise levels must also be redetermined.

Diabetic control and the establishment of parent-child relationships in light of neonatal needs are the priorities of this period. If her newborn must be cared for in a special care nursery, the mother needs support and information about the baby's condition. Every effort must be made to provide as much contact as possible between the parents and their newborn.

Breastfeeding is encouraged as beneficial to both mother and baby. The composition of breast milk is not altered by diabetes, and infants of mothers with diabetes gain weight appropriately. The lactating mother with diabetes often has a sense of well-being and diminished insulin needs even while increasing caloric intake. Blood glucose levels may be lower because glucose is transferred from serum to breast to be converted to lactose, and energy is expended in milk production. Caloric needs increase during lactation to 500 to 800 kcal above prepregnant requirements. Insulin must be adjusted according to individual needs. Home blood glucose monitoring should continue for the insulin-dependent diabetic.

The woman and her partner, if he is involved, should receive information on family planning. Barrier methods of contraception (diaphragm and condom) used with spermicide are safe, effective, and inexpensive and are the method of choice for insulin-dependent diabetic women. The use of oral contraceptives (OCs) by diabetic women is controversial. Some evidence suggests that women with diabetes may be at greater risk for OC complications such as myocardial infarction and thrombophlebitis (Landon, 1996). Many physicians who prescribe low-dose OCs to women with diabetes restrict them to women who have no vascular disease and who do not smoke. The progesterone-only pill has a higher failure rate but is otherwise safer. Elective sterilization is chosen by many couples who have completed their families.

It's hard to realize that I have gestational diabetes and to know that it increases my chances of getting diabetes later. My grandmother had diabetes, so I always thought of it as an old person's disease. All the finger sticks, watching my diet, keeping track has taken some getting used to. I'll be glad when our baby is born and I can put this behind me, at least for now.

NURSING CARE MANAGEMENT

The Critical Pathway on page 365 for a woman with diabetes mellitus summarizes nursing management during the antepartum, intrapartum, and postpartum periods.

Nursing Assessment and Diagnosis

Whether diabetes (usually type I) has been diagnosed before pregnancy occurs or the diagnosis is made during pregnancy (GDM), careful assessment of the disease process and the woman's understanding of diabetes is important. Thorough physical examination, including assessment for vascular complications, any signs of infectious conditions, and urine and blood testing for glucose, is essential on the first prenatal visit. Follow-up visits are usually scheduled twice a month during the first two trimesters and weekly during the last trimester.

Assessment also yields vital information about the woman's ability to cope with the combined stress of pregnancy and diabetes and her ability to follow a recommended regimen of care. It is necessary to determine the woman's knowledge about diabetes and self-care before formulating a teaching plan.

Nursing diagnoses that may apply to the pregnant woman with diabetes mellitus include the following:

- ***Risk for Altered Nutrition: More than Body Requirements*** related to imbalance between intake and available insulin
- ***Risk for Injury*** related to possible complications secondary to hypoglycemia or hyperglycemia
- ***Altered Family*** *Processes* related to the need for hospitalization secondary to DM.

Nursing Plan and Implementation

Prepregnancy counseling may be provided by a nurse and a physician, using a team approach. Ideally, the couple is seen prior to pregnancy so that the diabetes can be assessed by ophthalmologic evaluation, electrocardiographic study, and a 24-hour urine collection for creatinine clearance and protein excretion. Prepregnancy counseling about the importance of tight glucose control is cost-effective in preventing congenital anomalies. If the diabetes is of recent onset without vascular complications, the outcome of pregnancy should be good, provided that glucose levels are controlled.

Community-Based Nursing Care

In many cases, women with gestational diabetes mellitus are stabilized in the hospital, and necessary teaching for self-care is begun. Women with preexisting diabetes may also require hospitalization for stabilization of their diabetes. In either case, the majority of ongoing teaching and supervision of pregnant women with diabetes is then carried out by nurses in clinics, community agencies, and the women's homes.

Effective Insulin Use The nurse ensures that the couple understands the purpose of the insulin, the types of insulin the woman is to use, the number of doses she is to receive daily, and the correct procedure for its administration. The woman's partner is also instructed about insulin administration in case it should be necessary for him to give it. For some highly motivated women whose glucose levels are not well controlled with multiple injections, the continuous insulin infusion pump may improve glucose control.

The nurse teaches the client how and when to monitor her blood sugar, the desired range of blood sugar levels, and the importance of good control (Figure 15–1). Most women use a glucose meter because it provides a more accurate reading; some women use a visual method of blood testing instead. With either method, the nurse teaches the client to follow the manufacturer's directions exactly, to wash hands thoroughly before puncturing her finger, and to touch the blood droplet, not her finger, to the test pad on the strip.

With a blood glucose meter, an electronic eye measures the blood sugar, and a digital reading is given. The blood droplet should cover the test pad because uncovered portions are read as low sugar. The glucose meter is a portable pocket-sized device that is more accurate than the visual, color comparison method. Some meters are able to store and recall a specified number of readings, which helps ensure the accuracy of recorded results.

With the visual method, the woman waits the prescribed time and then compares the color on the strip with a color chart provided on the strip bottle. The test strips must be stored as directed, and unused strips should be discarded after their expiration date.

The nurse may offer the client the following tips regarding finger puncture: (1) Various spring-loaded devices are available that make puncturing easier. (2) Hanging the arm down for 30 seconds increases blood flow to the fingers. (3) The sides of fingers should be punctured instead of the ends because the ends contain more pain-sensitive nerves.

Diabetic clients need to keep a record of each blood sugar reading as a guide for management. Specific record sheets are available for this purpose.

Planned Exercise Program Exercise is encouraged for the woman's overall well-being. If she is used to a regular exercise program, she is encouraged to continue. She is advised to exercise after meals, when blood sugar levels are high, to wear diabetic identification, to carry a simple sugar such as hard candy, to monitor her blood glucose levels regularly, and to avoid injecting insulin into an extremity that will soon be used during exercise.

If she has not been following a regular exercise plan, she is encouraged to begin gradually. Because exercise can alter metabolism, the woman's blood glucose should be well controlled before she begins an exercise program. Women with GDM should *not* use unusual, strenuous, and excessive exercise in an attempt to reduce glucose levels (Idrogo & Mazze, 1998).

Teaching for Self-Care

Using the information gained during the nursing assessment of the pregnant woman with diabetes, the nurse provides appropriate teaching to the woman and her family so that the woman can meet her own health care needs as much as possible.

- *Glucose monitoring.* Home blood glucose monitoring is the most accurate and convenient way to determine insulin dose and assess control. It should be taught at the first visit after the diagnosis of gestational diabetes has been established. The woman with pregestational diabetes may already be monitoring her own blood sugar. Women are taught to perform the procedure four to six times per day—generally at least a fasting blood sugar before breakfast, then a postprandial test 2 hours after each meal. Women are encouraged to maintain blood sugars in the normal ranges as follows: fasting (before eating or taking insulin), 60 to 90 mg/dL; before other meals, 60 to 105 mg/dL; 2 hours after each meal, less than 120 mg/dL (Landon, 1996).

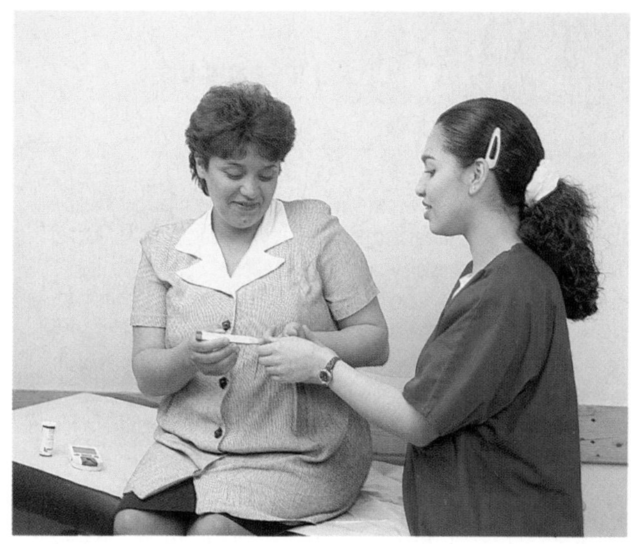

FIGURE 15–1 The nurse teaches the pregnant woman with gestational diabetes mellitus how to do home glucose monitoring.

- *Symptoms of hypoglycemia and ketoacidosis.* The pregnant diabetic woman must recognize symptoms of changing glucose levels and take appropriate action by immediately checking her capillary blood glucose level. If it is less than 60 mg/dL, she is advised to take 20 g of carbohydrate, wait 20 minutes, and then retest her glucose level. She can obtain the necessary carbohydrate by drinking 14.5 oz whole milk, 12 oz orange or apple juice, or 13.3 oz cola (Mandeville, 1992). Many people overtreat their symptoms by continuing to eat. This can cause a rebound hyperglycemia. The woman should carry a snack at all times and should have other fast sources of glucose (simple carbohydrates such as hard candy) at hand so that she can treat an insulin reaction when milk is not available. Family members are also taught how to inject glucagon in the event that food does not work or is not feasible, for instance, in the presence of severe morning sickness.
- *Smoking.* Smoking has harmful effects on the maternal vascular system and the developing fetus and is contraindicated for both pregnancy and diabetes.
- *Travel.* Insulin can be kept at room temperature while traveling. Insulin supplies should be kept with the traveler and not packed in the baggage. Most airlines can supply special meals if notified a few days before departure. The woman should wear a diabetic identification bracelet or necklace. In

COMMUNITY IN FOCUS

Gestational Diabetes Program

The Memorial HealthCare System (MHCS) is a 10-hospital, community-based, not-for-profit, integrated health care system located in Houston, Texas. A large system, each year MHCS has about 12,000 births; it also serves approximately 400 women with gestational diabetes mellitus. To address the special health care needs of women with gestational diabetes, the System established the Gestational Diabetes Program, which is managed by diabetes nurse educators.

Pregnant women with gestational diabetes are referred directly to the program by their caregiver. Each woman is seen individually by a diabetes nurse educator for assessment and one-on-one education. The educational services provided include blood sugar testing; use of the glucometer; documentation of blood sugars; pathophysiology of diabetes in pregnancy; pharmacology of insulin; administration of insulin; signs and symptoms of hypo- and hyperglycemia; danger signs of pregnancy; fetal assessment; and explanation of the medical and nursing care of women with gestational diabetes. The diabetes nurse educators coordinate services with the dietitians, who perform nutritional assessments and dietary planning and counseling. Educational protocols are standardized throughout the System. In addition, group classes are offered on selected topics.

Diabetes educators also provide 24-hour on-call services so that a knowledgeable educator is always available to answer questions or address concerns. During the postpartum period, a diabetes nurse educator visits each woman with gestational diabetes in the hospital and continues to work with her until her blood glucose levels are normalized and she no longer requires insulin therapy.

The multidisciplinary team members involved in the care of women with gestational diabetes mellitus include diabetes nurse educators, dietitians, physicians and their staff, home health nurses, social workers, pharmacists, perinatologists, neonatologists, ultrasonographers, and chaplains. The Gestational Diabetes Program was recently credentialed by the American Diabetic Association. Evaluation data to date reveal overwhelmingly positive maternal and fetal outcomes for women who participate in the program.

SOURCE: Personal communication with Vicki Lucas, PhD, RNC, former Director of Women's and Children's Services, Memorial HealthCare System, Houston, Texas.

addition, the woman should check with her physician for any instructions or advice before leaving.

- *Support groups.* Many communities have diabetes support groups or education classes, which can be helpful to women with newly diagnosed diabetes.
- *Cesarean birth.* Chances for a cesarean birth increase if the pregnant woman is diabetic. This possibility should be anticipated—enrollment in cesarean birth preparation classes may be suggested. Many hospitals offer classes, and information is available through organizations such as Cesarean/Support Education and Concern (C/Sec, Inc); Cesarean Birth Council; or the Cesarean Association for Research, Education, Support and Satisfaction in Birthing (Caress). The couple may prefer simply to discuss cesarean birth with the nurse and their obstetrician and read some books on the topic.

ESSENTIAL PRECAUTIONS IN PRACTICE

A Pregnant Woman with Diabetes Mellitus

In caring for a pregnant woman with diabetes mellitus, follow all precautions that are established for any hospitalized pregnant, laboring, or postpartal woman. In addition, remember the following specifics:

- Wear gloves when doing finger sticks for glucose levels, when starting IVs, when testing urine for ketones, or when drawing blood for other laboratory tests.
- When teaching a woman to do her own blood glucose testing, have gloves available and put them on if it becomes necessary to help the woman obtain a blood sample. The woman does not need to wear gloves during the procedure.
- Dispose of needles, syringes, lancets, and other sharp objects in appropriately labeled containers.

REMEMBER to wash your hands prior to putting the disposable gloves on and AGAIN immediately after you remove the gloves.

For further information, consult OSHA and CDC guidelines.

Hospital-Based Nursing Care

Hospitalization may become necessary during the pregnancy to evaluate blood glucose levels and adjust insulin dosages. In such cases, nurses monitor the woman's status and continue to provide teaching so that the woman is knowledgeable about her condition and its management. Essential Precautions in Practice: A Pregnant Woman with Diabetes highlights key safety measures the nurse should remember.

During the intrapartal period, the nurse must have a clear understanding about the impact of labor on the condition. The nurse carefully monitors the woman's status, maintains her intravenous fluids, is alert for signs of hypoglycemia, and provides the care indicated for any woman in labor. If a cesarean birth is indicated, the nurse provides appropriate care as described in Chapter 23.

Evaluation

Expected outcomes of nursing care include the following:

- The woman is able to discuss her condition and its possible impact on her pregnancy, labor and birth, and postpartal period.
- The woman participates in developing a health care regimen to meet her needs and follows it throughout her pregnancy.
- The woman avoids developing hypoglycemia or hyperglycemia.

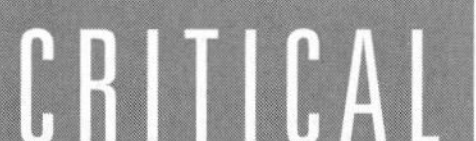

CRITICAL PATHWAY FOR A WOMAN WITH DIABETES MELLITUS

Category	Antepartal Management	Intrapartal Management*	Postpartal Management*
Referral	• Perinatologist • Endocrinologist • Neonatologist • Social worker • Psych clinical nurse practitioner • Diabetes nurse educator • Dietary/nutritionist • Physical therapy, occupational therapy	• Obtain prenatal record	• Home nursing referral if indicated • Diabetes nurse educator **Expected Outcomes** Appropriate resources identified and utilized
Assessment	• Electronic fetal monitoring as indicated • Nonstress test as indicated • Ultrasound as indicated • Amniocentesis for lung maturity at 34–36 weeks • α-fetoprotein (done usually at 16 weeks)	• Assess for signs and symptoms (s/sx) of hypoglycemia (sweating, periodic tingling, disorientation, shakiness, pallor, clammy skin, irritability, hunger, headache and blurred vision) during labor • Continuous electronic fetal monitoring • Assess glucose levels with glucometer as ordered or if s/sx of hypoglycemia occur	• Assess glucose levels with glucometer—generally insulin requirements fall significantly in the postpartum phase • Continue normal postpartum assessment q8h • Feeding technique with newborn: should be progressing • Vital signs assessment: q8h; all WNL; report temperature > 38C (100.4F) • Continue assessment of comfort level **Expected Outcomes** Assessment findings indicate control of blood sugar levels with related complications minimized. Fetal growth and development unimpaired
Teaching/ psychosocial	• Room orientation • Notify RN of s/sx of hyper/hypoglycemia, uterine contractions, decreased fetal movement, vaginal leaking and/or bleeding, dysuria • Assess family status and/or additional psychosocial needs • Evaluation of client learning needs • Importance of following diet • Tour of ICN • Prebirth teaching for vaginal and/or cesarean (CS) • Evaluation of teaching effectiveness	• Evaluation of teaching effectiveness • Continuing evaluation of ongoing learning needs	• Complete normal postpartum teaching **Expected Outcomes** Client verbalizes/demonstrates understanding of diabetic and health care education
Nursing care management and reports	• CBC • UA/dipstick for protein and ketones • Biochemistry profile • Glycosylated hemoglobin level (Hb_{A1C}) daily • 24-hour urine for protein and creatinine clearance • Fingerstick blood sugar (BS), every am, before meals, and 2 hours after meals • Vital signs q4h • Fundal height weekly • Daily weight	• Glucose levels monitored as directed	• Continue sitz bath prn • May shower if ambulating without difficulty • DC buffalo cap if present **Expected Outcomes** Labs/reports reflect stable, controlled blood sugar Maternal/fetal well-being maintained. Active involvement of client in plan of care for diabetic management
Activity	• Bed rest with bathroom privileges • Diversional activity	• Bed rest as tolerated	• Up ad lib **Expected Outcomes** Level of activity has not exacerbated condition
Comfort	• Assess for discomfort • Provide comfort measures as needed	• Assess for discomfort • Provide comfort measures as needed	• Continue with pain management techniques **Expected Outcomes** Optimal comfort maintained

*Interventions for a woman with a normal labor and birth and during the early postpartum period may be found in those appropriate critical pathways.

CRITICAL PATHWAY FOR A WOMAN WITH DIABETES MELLITUS *CONTINUED*

Category	Antepartal Management	Intrapartal Management*	Postpartal Management*
Nutrition	• American Dietetic Association (ADA) per order • Encourage fluids	• Ice chips Hard candy, PRN	• Encourage breastfeeding • Increase calorie needs 500–800 kcal • Continue diet and fluids **Expected Outcomes** Nutritional needs met, with emphasis on diabetic control
Elimination	• Review measures to prevent UTI	**Expected Outcomes** Monitor and record intake and output	**Expected Outcomes** Intake and output WNL
Medications	• IV ____ @ ____ mL/h/buffalo cap • Insulin as ordered →__________ • Prenatal vitamins and iron	• Two IV lines are usually used, one with 5% dextrose solution and one with a saline solution (saline line is used for insulin if needed) • The IV insulin is usually discontinued with completion of 3rd stage of labor	• May take own prenatal vitamins • RhoGAM and rubella vaccine administered if indicated **Expected Outcomes** BS levels within acceptable medical parameters
Discharge planning/ home care	• Explain purpose of scheduled tests and procedures • Include family in diabetic teaching • Assess family support	• Assess family support	• Review discharge instruction sheet and check list • Describe postpartum warning signs and when to call CNM/physician • Provide prescriptions • Gift pack given to woman • Arrangements made for baby pictures if desired • Postpartum visit scheduled • Newborn check scheduled **Expected Outcomes** Discharge teaching completed with emphasis on follow-up health care needs and adequate support network
Family involvement	• Identify available support persons • Assess family perceptions of situation	• Involve support persons in care	• Evidence of parental bonding behaviors apparent • Involve support persons in care: teaching • Plans being made for providing support to mother following discharge **Expected Outcomes** Family utilizes resources
Date			

*Interventions for a woman with a normal labor and birth and during the early postpartum period may be found in those appropriate critical pathways.

- The woman gives birth to a healthy newborn.
- The woman is able to care for her newborn.

Care of the Woman with Anemia

Anemia indicates inadequate levels of hemoglobin (Hb) in the blood. Anemia is defined as hemoglobin less than 12 g/dL in nonpregnant women and less than 10g/dL in pregnant women (Cunningham et al, 1997). Race, altitude, smoking, and medications can affect the normal limits of hemoglobin. Regardless of socioeconomic status, blacks normally have hemoglobin levels about 1 g/dL lower than those of whites (Payton & White, 1995). The lower limit of normal tends to be higher for women who smoke and those who live at higher altitudes because their bodies require a greater quantity of red blood cells to maintain their tissue oxygen levels. For example, a pregnant woman who lives in Denver, Colorado (elevation 5280 feet), would be considered anemic if her hemoglobin dropped below 10.5 g/dL. Similarly, the lower limit of normal for a pregnant woman who smokes ½ to 1 pack of cigarettes per day would increase by 0.3 g/dL to 10.3 g/dL (Varney, 1997). Reference tables are available that indicate these adjustments in the lower level of normal hemoglobin.

The common anemias of pregnancy are due either to insufficient hemoglobin production related to nutritional deficiency in iron or folic acid during pregnancy, or to hemoglobin destruction in inherited disorders, specifically sickle cell anemia and thalassemia.

Iron Deficiency Anemia

Dietary iron is needed to synthesize hemoglobin. Because hemoglobin is necessary to transport oxygen, a deficiency of iron may affect the body's transport of oxygen.

Iron deficiency anemia is the most common medical complication of pregnancy, primarily as a consequence of expansion of plasma volume without normal expansion of maternal hemoglobin mass (Cunningham et al, 1997; Varney, 1997). About 50% of pregnant women have hematocrits less than 32% and are anemic (Samuels, 1996). Approximately 200 mg of iron will be conserved due to the functional amenorrhea of pregnancy, but a pregnant woman needs approximately 1000 mg more iron intake during the pregnancy. Between 300 and 400 mg of iron is transferred to the fetus; 500 mg is needed for the increased red blood cell mass in the woman's own increased circulating blood volume; another 100 mg is needed for the placenta; and about 280 mg is needed to replace the 1 mg of iron lost daily through feces, urine, and sweat.

The greatest need for increased iron intake occurs in the second half of pregnancy. When the iron needs of pregnancy are not met, maternal hemoglobin falls below 11 g/dL. Serum ferritin levels, indicating iron stores, are below 12 mg/L.

Many women begin pregnancy in a slightly anemic state. In pregnancy, mild anemia can rapidly become more severe; therefore, it needs immediate treatment.

Maternal Risks

The woman with iron deficiency anemia may be asymptomatic, but she is more susceptible to infection, may tire easily, has an increased chance of PIH and postpartal hemorrhage, and tolerates poorly even minimal blood loss during birth. Healing of an episiotomy or an incision may be delayed. If the anemia is severe (Hb less than 6 g/dL), cardiac failure may ensue.

Fetal-Neonatal Risks

There is evidence of increased risk of low birth weight, prematurity, stillbirth, and neonatal death in infants of women with severe iron deficiency (maternal Hb less than 6 g/dL). The infant is not iron deficient at birth due to active transport of iron across the placenta, even when maternal iron stores are low. However, these babies do have lower iron stores and are at increased risk for developing iron deficiency during infancy.

Clinical Therapy

The first goal of health care is to prevent iron deficiency anemia. If it occurs, the goal is to return low iron and hemoglobin levels to normal. To prevent anemia, the CDC (1998) recommends starting low-dose (30 mg/day) supplements of iron at the first prenatal visit. If anemia is diagnosed, the dosage should be increased to 60 to 120 mg/day of iron. If the woman remains anemic after one month of therapy, further evaluation is indicated. With a twin pregnancy, a larger dose is needed. If a large dose of oral iron causes vomiting, diarrhea, or constipation, or if the anemia is discovered late in pregnancy, parenteral iron may be needed.

NURSING CARE MANAGEMENT

Nursing Assessment and Diagnosis

The main presenting symptom of iron deficiency anemia may be fatigue. Nutritional history usually gives evidence of poor dietary intake of iron. Physical examination reveals pallor of skin and conjunctiva. Laboratory studies show Hb values below 11 g/dL, serum ferritin levels below 12 μg/L, and possibly microcytic and hypochromic red blood cells (a late finding).

Nursing diagnoses that may apply to a pregnant woman with iron deficiency anemia include the following:

- ***Altered Nutrition: Less than Body Requirements*** related to inadequate intake of iron-containing foods
- ***Constipation*** related to daily intake of iron supplements

CRITICAL THINKING QUESTION

In addition to iron supplements, what other sources of iron can the nurse recommend to a pregnant woman with iron deficiency anemia?

Nursing Plan and Implementation

Community-Based Nursing Care

The nurse stresses the importance of iron supplements during pregnancy. Supplements are indicated because dietary sources cannot meet the extra requirements. The woman is taught to take iron tablets with vitamin C (eg, orange juice) to increase absorption. Iron absorption is reduced by 40% to 50% if the tablets are taken with meals. However, gastrointestinal upset is more likely if they are taken on an empty stomach. The client may tolerate the iron better if she starts with small doses and gradually increases the dosage over several days. She is informed that her stool will turn black and may be more formed. She is also advised to keep the tablets out of the reach of children because ingestion may be fatal to a young child.

Evaluation

Expected outcomes of nursing care include the following:

- The woman is able to identify the risks associated with iron deficiency anemia during pregnancy.

- The woman takes her iron supplements as recommended.
- The woman's hemoglobin levels remain normal or return to normal during her pregnancy. ●

Folic Acid Deficiency Anemia

Folate deficiency is the most common cause of megaloblastic anemia during pregnancy, affecting between 1% and 4% of pregnant women in the United States. It is more prevalent with twin pregnancies.

Folic acid is needed for DNA and RNA synthesis and cell duplication. In its absence, immature red blood cells fail to divide, become enlarged (megaloblastic), and are fewer in number. With the tremendous cell multiplication that occurs in pregnancy, an adequate amount of folic acid is crucial. However, increased urinary excretion of folic acid and fetal uptake can rapidly result in folic acid deficiency. It is usually diagnosed late in pregnancy or the early puerperium. Hemoglobin levels as low as 3 to 5 g/dL may be found.

Clinical Therapy

Diagnosis of folic acid deficiency anemia may be difficult. Women with this anemia often present with nausea, vomiting, and anorexia. Serum folate levels typically fall as pregnancy progresses. Even though folate levels are lower with deficiency, they will fluctuate with diet. Measurement of erythrocyte folate status is more reliable but indicates folate status of several weeks previously. Typically the blood smear reveals that the newly formed erythrocytes are macrocytic. Bone marrow biopsy is diagnostic but rarely used due to the discomfort it causes.

Folic acid deficiency during pregnancy is prevented by a daily supplement of 0.4 mg of folate. Treatment of deficiency consists of 1 mg folic acid supplement. Because iron deficiency anemia almost always coexists with folic acid deficiency, the woman also needs iron supplements.

NURSING CARE MANAGEMENT

The nurse can help the pregnant woman avoid folate deficiency by teaching her food sources of folic acid and cooking methods for preserving folic acid. The best sources are fresh leafy green vegetables, red meats, fish, poultry, and legumes. As much as 50% to 90% of folic acid can be lost by cooking in large volumes of water. Microwave cooking destroys more folic acid than conventional cooking.

Sickle Cell Anemia

Sickle cell anemia (HbSS) is a recessive autosomal disorder in which the normal adult hemoglobin, hemoglobin A (HbA), is abnormally formed. It occurs primarily in people of African descent and occasionally in people of Mediterranean origin (ie, Greeks, Italians, Arabs, and Turks) (Cruikshank, 1994). The anemia is characterized by acute, recurring, painful episodes. Individuals with the disorder are homozygous for the sickle cell gene. They inherit from each parent an allele causing an amino acid substitution in the two beta protein chains in the hemoglobin molecule. This abnormal hemoglobin is called hemoglobin S (HbS). Heterozygous individuals are carriers for sickle cell anemia but are usually asymptomatic. This condition is called sickle cell trait (HbSA). One of the beta protein chains formed in their hemoglobin is normal; the other has the amino acid substitution. Sickle cell trait occurs in 1 out of 12 African Americans; sickle cell anemia is found in 1 out of 576 (Cunningham et al, 1997).

Hemoglobin S causes the red blood cells to be sickle or crescent shaped. In conditions of low oxygenation, normal hemoglobin is soluble, but HbS becomes semisolid and distorts the red blood cell shape. These erythrocytes easily interlock and clog capillaries, particularly in organs characterized by slow flow and high oxygen extraction, such as the spleen, bone marrow, and placenta. This phenomenon, called sickling, varies in frequency depending on the amount of the S hemoglobin in the red blood cells (there is seldom a crisis with levels below 40%) and other hemoglobin factors. Diagnosis is confirmed by hemoglobin electrophoresis or a test to induce sickling in a blood sample.

Maternal Risks

Women with sickle cell trait have a good prognosis for pregnancy if they have adequate nutrition and prenatal care. They are, however, at increased risk for nephritis, bacteriuria, and hematuria, and tend to become anemic.

Women with sickle cell anemia have considerably more risk during pregnancy. Low oxygen pressure—caused by high temperature, dehydration, infection, or acidosis, for example—may precipitate a vaso-occlusive crisis. The crisis produces sudden attacks of pain that may be general or localized in bones or joints, lungs, abdominal organs, or the spinal cord. The pain is due to ischemia in the tissues from occluded capillaries. Vaso-occlusive crises occur more often in the second half of pregnancy.

Maternal mortality due to sickle cell anemia is rare. However, 50% to 67% of pregnant woman with sickle cell anemia develop infections, often urinary tract infections or pulmonary infections, because of impaired immune functioning (Samuels, 1996). Congestive heart failure or acute renal failure may also occur.

Fetal-Neonatal Risks

The incidence of fetal death during and immediately following an attack has decreased greatly in recent years but is still high. Perinatal mortality is estimated to be 15% (Samuels, 1996). Prematurity and IUGR are also associated with sickle cell anemia. Fetal death is believed to be due to sickling attacks in the placenta.

Clinical Therapy

Folic acid supplements are indicated for women with sickle cell anemia. Maternal infection should be treated promptly because dehydration and fever can trigger sickling and crisis. Vaso-occlusive crisis is best treated by a perinatal team in a medical center. Proper management requires close observation and evaluation of all symptoms. The term *sickle cell crisis* should be applied only after all other possible causes for the pain are excluded (Cunningham et al, 1997).

Rehydration with intravenous fluids, administration of oxygen, antibiotics and analgesics, and monitoring of fetal heart rate are important aspects of therapy. Antiembolism stockings are used postpartally.

If vaso-occlusive crisis occurs during labor, the previous therapies are instituted and the woman is kept in a left lateral position. Oxytocics may be used if needed. Episiotomy and outlet forceps are recommended to shorten the second stage of labor.

Several antisickling agents are being researched, and in the future sickle cell crisis may be prevented.

NURSING CARE MANAGEMENT

Nursing Assessment and Diagnosis

The woman with sickle cell anemia usually relates a history of frequent illnesses and recurrent abdominal and joint pains and is found to be extremely anemic. The woman may appear undernourished and have long, thin extremities. Ulcers are often present on her ankles. Anemia may be severe.

A diagnosis of sickle cell anemia is confirmed by hemoglobin electrophoresis or a test to induce sickling in a blood sample. The woman is assessed for infection, which is associated with one-third of sickle cell crises in adults. Infections most often seen during pregnancy or postpartum are pneumonia, urinary tract infections, puerperal endomyometritis, and osteomyelitis.

Fetal status is assessed during a crisis by electronic fetal monitoring. During labor, the woman's vital signs and the fetal heart rate (FHR) are assessed frequently. Compatible blood should be available for transfusion. Oxygen is administered if necessary. The woman is assessed for joint pains and other signs of sickle cell crisis.

Nursing diagnoses that might apply to the pregnant woman with sickle cell anemia include the following:

- ***Pain*** related to the effects of sickle cell crisis
- ***Knowledge Deficit*** related to lack of understanding of the need to avoid exposure to infection secondary to the risk of a sickle cell crisis

Nursing Plan and Implementation

Teaching for Self-Care

The nursing goal for a pregnant woman with sickle cell disease is to provide effective health teaching to help prevent a sickle cell attack (crisis), improve the anemia, and prevent infection. The nurse teaches the woman to increase hydration, use good hygiene, avoid people with infections, seek immediate treatment for infection, and take folic acid supplements. Folic acid is important because of its role in red blood cell production. The woman with sickle cell anemia maintains her hemoglobin levels by intense erythropoiesis and thus requires folic acid supplements. Bed rest is sometimes recommended to decrease the chance of preterm labor. Other nursing interventions are aimed at facilitating the medical therapy and alleviating anxiety through support and education.

Genetic counseling is recommended when both parents have the disease or are known carriers.

Evaluation

Expected outcomes of nursing care include the following:

- The woman is able to describe her condition and identify its possible impact on her pregnancy, labor and childbirth, and postpartal period.
- The woman takes appropriate health care measures to avoid a sickle cell crisis.
- The woman gives birth to a healthy infant.
- The woman and her caregivers quickly identify and successfully manage any complications that arise. ●

Thalassemia

The thalassemias are a group of autosomal recessive disorders characterized by a defect in the synthesis of the alpha or beta chains in the hemoglobin molecule. The one most frequently encountered in the United States is β-thalassemia. Symptoms are caused by the shortened life span of the red blood cells, which result in active erythropoiesis in the liver, spleen, and bones. This produces hepatosplenomegaly and sometimes bony malformations. The thalassemias are seen most often in persons from Greece, Italy, or southern China and are also known as Mediterranean anemia and Cooley's anemia. Early identification and of thalassemia and preventive management avoids unnecessary treatment of anemia (ACOG, 1996).

If the woman is heterozygous for β-thalassemia, half of the beta chains are formed normally. This is β-thalassemia minor, or β-thalassemia trait. Mild anemia is usually the only symptom.

Persons born homozygous for the disease have β-thalassemia major. Because newborns have fetal hemoglobin (HbF), which does not have beta chains, no symptoms are present for several months. Once infants with β-thalessemia major start producing adult type hemoglobin (HbA), they develop severe anemia and are dependent on transfusions, from which they eventually develop iron overload. Iron chelation therapy must be instituted soon after chronic transfusions are begun because excess iron damages the liver and heart. Without chelation therapy, these infants do not live past the second or third decade, and those who reach puberty are often amenorrheic and infertile (Bergan, Kliegman, & Arvin, 1996).

Maternal-Fetal-Neonatal Risks

The woman with β-thalassemia minor has mild anemia with small (microcytic) red cells. This mild anemia must be distinguished from iron deficiency anemia because a woman with β-thalassemia minor should not receive iron therapy. (A woman with iron deficiency anemia typically has low serum iron and serum ferritin levels, whereas the woman with β-thalessemia minor has normal levels.) Beta-thalessemia minor varies in degree of severity from extremely mild (minima) anemia, which results in a relatively smooth pregnancy, to a more symptomatic form (intermedia). Pregnancy is rare in women with β-thalessemia major. If it does occur, the woman generally has severe anemia, needs transfusion therapy, and is at risk for congestive heart failure (Samuels, 1996).

Clinical Therapy

Folic acid supplements are indicated for women with thalassemia, but iron supplements are not given. Those with thalassemia intermedia and thalessemia major may need transfusion and chelation therapy. They should avoid exposure to infections and seek treatment promptly if an infection develops. Their care is similar to that of women with sickle cell anemia (Samuels, 1996).

NURSING CARE MANAGEMENT

The woman with thalassemia needs to understand her disease and the possibility of transmitting it to her offspring. These clients have lived with thalassemia since childhood but may have questions regarding its effect on pregnancy outcome and their own prognosis.

Care of the Woman with Acquired Immunodeficiency Syndrome (AIDS)

Acquired immunodeficiency syndrome (AIDS), caused by the human immunodeficiency virus (HIV), is one of today's major health concerns. As of December 1997, a total of 641,086 cases of AIDS was reported in the United States (CDC, 1997). Homosexual and bisexual males are still the largest group of infected individuals. Women accounted for 16% of the cases. Rates among black women are significantly higher than in white women. HIV infection is now the fourth leading cause of death for all women ages 25 to 44, but it is the *leading cause* of death for black women of the same age (Peters, Kochenek, & Murphy, 1998). In 1997, 473 new pediatric cases were reported for a cumulative pediatric total of 8086 (1.2%), including both males and females under the age of 13. Of these pediatric cases, 91% were infants born to mothers who were infected with HIV during the prenatal or intrapartum period or while breastfeeding.

Homosexual intercourse is the primary method of transmission in men (45% of cases), whereas intravenous drug use is the means of transmission for 15% of cases. In HIV-infected women, 41% acquired the disease through heterosexual sex, while 26% acquired it through intravenous drug use (CDC, 1997). Because HIV/AIDS is increasing more rapidly among women than men, experts believe that HIV/AIDS in the US is beginning to reflect the more gender-equal patterns of infection seen in developing countries (Eyler, 1996).

Pathophysiology of HIV/AIDS

HIV found in blood, semen, vaginal fluid, and breast milk has been implicated in disease transmission, although the virus has been isolated in urine, tears, cerebrospinal fluid, lymph nodes, brain tissue, and bone marrow. HIV shedding has also been detected in the genital tract of women.

Once infected with the virus, the individual develops antibodies that can be detected with enzyme-linked immunosorbent assay (ELISA) and confirmed with the Western blot test. Antibodies can be detected in most individuals 6 to 12 weeks after exposure, but in rare circumstances the latent period is longer. An asymptomatic period of approximately 5 to 10 years follows seroconversion (Duff, 1996). The majority of pregnant women fall into this category.

The diagnosis of AIDS is made when an individual is HIV positive and is identified as having one of several specific opportunistic infections. AIDS can also be diagnosed without laboratory evidence of HIV infection when one of the opportunistic infections is definitively diagnosed and there is no other known cause for the immune deficiency.

Maternal Risks

AIDS-defining diseases that are more common in women than men include wasting syndrome, esophageal candidiasis, and herpes simplex virus disease. Kaposi's sarcoma is rare in women. Non-AIDS-defining gynecologic conditions, such as vaginal *Candida* infections and cervical pathology, are prevalent among women at all stages of HIV infection.

Many women who are HIV positive choose to avoid pregnancy because of the risk of infecting the fetus and the likelihood of dying before the child is raised. Women who do become pregnant should be advised that pregnancy is not believed to accelerate the progression of HIV/AIDS, that the use of zidovudine (ZDV), formally called azidothymidine (AZT), during pregnancy significantly reduces the risk of transmitting HIV to the fetus, and that most medications used to treat HIV can be taken during pregnancy (Eyler, 1996).

Fetal-Neonatal Risks

HIV transmission can occur during pregnancy and through breast milk; however, it is believed that at least 50% of all infection occurs during labor and birth (Landesman et al, 1996). Beginning in the early 1990s, rates of mother-to-child transmission of HIV began to decrease in Europe and the United States, possibly because of changes in clinical management. For HIV-infected pregnant women who received no prophylactic medication, the rate of transmission to the newborn is now about 17%. However, for HIV-infected pregnant women who receive prophylactic therapy with zidovudine (ZDV) and give birth vaginally, this rate drops to 6.6% (Mandelbrot et al, 1998). Moreover, for HIV-infected women who receive zidovudine prophylaxis and give birth by elective cesarean (prior to rupture of membranes), the rate of transmission drops to less than 1% (0.8%) (Mandelbrot et al, 1998). These decreases in transmission are dramatic ones. It is now necessary to determine whether the benefits of cesarean birth outweigh the risks.

Following birth, infants will often have a positive antibody titer, which reflects the passive transfer of maternal antibodies. Infected infants are usually asymptomatic at birth. More than half the children born antibody-positive lose maternal antibody by 15 months of age and remain asymptomatic (Bergan et al, 1996).

Infected newborns are likely to be small for gestational age (SGA) at birth. Facial characteristics that may indicate the newborn had been infected with HIV early in gestation include microcephaly; patulous lips; a prominent, boxlike forehead; increased distance between the inner canthus of the eyes; a flattened nasal bridge; and a mild obliquity of the eyes. The mortality rate for these infants is especially high.

The signs of AIDS in infants may include failure to thrive, hepatosplenomegaly, interstitial lymphocytic pneumonia, recurrent infections, cell-mediated immunodeficiency, evidence of Epstein-Barr virus, and neurologic abnormalities. Recurrent bacterial infections are common in children with AIDS; Kaposi's sarcoma is rare. The prognosis for an infected child remains poor.

Encephalopathy, characterized by delayed developmental milestones or the loss of acquired skills, including cognitive abilities, is found in 50% to 90% of children with AIDS. Treatments that prevent the central nervous system effects of HIV have yet to be identified. Well-controlled developmental studies are needed to clarify the relationship between HIV and child development to help professionals design appropriate, school-based educational plans (Guralnick, 1997).

Clinical Therapy

The goal for antenatal care is to offer HIV testing and counseling to all pregnant women. Initial testing is done using ELISA, followed by a confirmatory Western blot assay. Women who test positive should be counseled about the implications of the diagnosis for themselves and their fetus in order to ensure an informed reproductive choice. The care of the woman who chooses to continue her pregnancy should focus on stabilizing the disease, preventing opportunistic infections and transmission of the virus from mother to fetus, and providing psychosocial and educational support. ZDV therapy should be recommended to all infected pregnant women to reduce the rate of perinatal transmission. This 3-part therapy includes oral administration of the drug on a daily basis beginning at 14 weeks' gestation, intravenous administration during labor and birth, and oral administration to the newborn for the first 6 weeks of life (ACOG, 1997).

To minimize the risk that the mother will develop resistance to suboptimal therapy during pregnancy, many physicians use a combination of potent antiretroviral medications. Based on current data, zidovudine should be part of any combination regimen to prevent perinatal transmission (Carpenter et al, 1998). The decision about which regimen is most appropriate should be determined following discussion with the woman about the risks and benefits based on her individual HIV status.

HIV-infected women should be evaluated and treated for other sexually transmitted infections and for conditions occurring more commonly in women with HIV, such as tuberculosis, cytomegalovirus, toxoplasmosis, and cervical dysplasia. HIV-infected women with no history of hepatitis B should receive the hepatitis vaccine, which is not contraindicated prenatally, as well as the pneumococcal vaccine and an annual flu shot. In addition to routine prenatal laboratory tests, a platelet count and a complete blood count with differential should be obtained at the first prenatal visit and repeated each trimester to identify anemia, thrombocytopenia, and leukopenia, which are associated both with HIV infection and with antiviral therapy.

The woman with HIV also should be assessed regularly for serologic changes that indicate the disease is progressing. This is determined by the absolute CD4+ T-lymphocyte count, which provides the number of helper T4 cells. When CD4+ counts fall to $200/mm^3$ or lower, opportunistic infections such as *Pneumocystis carinii* pneumonia are more likely to develop, and prophylaxis should be instituted using oral trimethoprim-sulfamethoxazole (TMP-SMX) (ACOG, 1997).

At each prenatal visit, asymptomatic HIV-infected women are monitored for early signs of complications, such as weight loss in the second or third trimesters or fever. The mouth is inspected for signs of infections such as thrush (candidiasis) or hairy leukoplakia; the lungs are auscultated for signs of pneumonia; and the lymph nodes, liver, and spleen are palpated for signs of enlargement. Each trimester the woman should have a visual examination and a fundoscopic examination to detect such complications as toxoplasmosis retinitis. Further discussion of therapy for the pregnant woman who is HIV positive or who has AIDS may be found in journal articles and specialty texts.

A pregnancy complicated by HIV infection, even if asymptomatic, is considered high risk, and the fetus is monitored closely. Weekly nonstress testing is begun at 32 weeks' gestation, and serial ultrasounds are done to detect intrauterine growth restriction. Biophysical profiles are also indicated (see Chapter 17). Invasive procedures such as amniocentesis are avoided when possible to prevent the contamination of a noninfected infant.

Intrapartal care is similar to that for all pregnant women, although strict adherence to universal precautions is crucial to avoid nosocomial infection. To prevent exposure of an uninfected infant to HIV during labor and birth, invasive procedures such as vaginal examinations following rupture of the membranes, fetal scalp electrode monitoring, fetal scalp sampling, and vacuum extraction should be done only after carefully evaluating the risks and benefits (ACOG, 1997).

Women who are HIV positive are at increased risk for complications such as intrapartal or postpartal hemorrhage, postpartal infection, poor wound healing, and infections of the genitourinary tract. Thus they need careful monitoring and appropriate therapy as indicated.

Following childbirth, the HIV-positive woman should be referred to a physician knowledgeable about treating individuals with HIV infection (ACOG, 1997). Because of the profound implications of HIV infection for the woman, her family, the fetus/newborn, and her health care providers, screening is recommended for all pregnant women, but especially those at increased risk, including the following: prostitutes; women whose current or previous sex partners have been bisexual, have abused IV drugs, had hemophilia, or tested positive for HIV; women who are or have been intravenous drug users; and women from countries where heterosexual transmission is common. In addition, clinics located in areas with a large HIV-positive population may require routine HIV screening of all prenatal clients.

NURSING CARE MANAGEMENT

Nursing Assessment and Diagnosis

A woman who tests positive for HIV may be asymptomatic or may present with any of the following signs or symptoms: fatigue, anemia, malaise, progressive weight loss, lymphadenopathy, diarrhea, fever, neurologic dysfunction, cell-mediated immunodeficiency, or evidence of Kaposi's sarcoma (purplish, reddish-brown lesions, either externally or internally).

If a woman tests HIV positive or is involved in a relationship that places her at high risk, the nurse should assess the woman's knowledge level about the disease, its implications for her and her fetus, and self-care measures the woman can take.

Examples of nursing diagnoses that might apply for an HIV-positive pregnant woman include the following:

- ***Knowledge Deficit*** related to lack of information about HIV/AIDS and its long-term implications for the woman and her unborn child
- ***Risk for Infection*** related to altered immunity secondary to HIV/AIDS
- ***Ineffective Family Coping*** related to the implications of a positive HIV test in one of the family members

Nursing Plan and Implementation

Community-Based Nursing Care

Nurses need to help women understand that HIV/AIDS is a fatal disease. HIV infection can be avoided if women avoid sharing intravenous drug needles and practice safe sex, including insisting that their sex partners wear a latex condom for each act of intercourse.

Women at risk for AIDS should be offered premarital and prepregnancy screening for HIV antibodies (ACOG, 1997). They should be given clear information about the implications of a diagnosis of HIV, including societal attitudes. Access to information about the disease and about the test results empowers women by enabling them to make informed decisions about their sexual activities and about becoming pregnant.

A detailed drug and sexual history of each prenatal client is the first step in perinatal HIV/AIDS prevention. All women should be offered HIV counseling. The following are counseling guidelines for HIV testing:

- The nurse should discuss HIV testing during the normal prenatal assessment.
- The nurse should assure the woman of confidentiality, explaining the difference between anonymity and confidentiality.
- The nurse should provide an environment that is private, comfortable, and nonjudgmental.
- The nurse should provide the woman information about AIDS, including pathophysiology, mode of transmission of HIV, high-risk behaviors, and methods of decreasing transmission, such as practicing safe sex and not sharing needles.
- If the woman chooses to have an antibody test for HIV (ELISA, Western blot), written consent should be obtained.
- Posttest counseling should be provided. A negative test means that no HIV antibodies were found; it does not ensure that the woman has not been infected with the virus, because antibodies may not be detected for 6 weeks to 6 months after exposure.
- If test results are positive, supportive follow-up is necessary. This includes an explanation of the implications for the woman and her unborn child as well as the value of ZDV therapy, recommended medical therapy, follow-up of sex partners, transmission prevention, discussion of immediate posttest plans, and

referral to appropriate psychologic and educational services. The nurse should tell the woman not to donate blood or blood products and not to share toothbrushes, razors, and other implements that could be contaminated with blood.

This information can be overwhelming to the woman who is HIV positive and should be provided orally and in writing. She will need more than one counseling session to absorb the information. The initial reaction may be one of shock or denial, so it is important that the nurse allow her a little time to think and to give her empathy and support. The nurse needs to stress that being HIV positive does not mean that the woman has AIDS but that she can transmit the virus to others (by sexual contact, sharing IV drug needles, and donating blood) and to her fetus during pregnancy. Most people do develop AIDS within 10 years. It is currently impossible to prevent AIDS from developing in people who are HIV positive or to predict when they will develop the disease.

In monitoring the asymptomatic HIV-positive pregnant woman, the nurse should be alert for nonspecific symptoms such as fever, weight loss, fatigue, persistent candidiasis, diarrhea, cough, skin lesions, and behavior changes. Laboratory findings—such as decreased hemoglobin, hematocrit, and T4 lymphocytes; elevated erythrocyte sedimentation rate (ESR); and abnormal complete blood count, differential, and platelets—may indicate complications or progression of the disease.

Education about optimal nutrition and maintenance of wellness are important and should be reviewed frequently with the woman.

Hospital-Based Nursing Care

The Critical Pathway for a Woman with HIV/AIDS beginning on page 374 summarizes essential nursing management during the antepartum, intrapartum, and postpartum periods.

In both community and hospital settings, the nurse faces the important task of taking the precautions necessary to protect staff, other clients, and families from exposure to HIV while meeting the needs of the childbearing woman with this infection.

In 1987, the CDC stated that the prevalence of AIDS and the risk of exposure faced by health care workers is significant enough that precautions should be taken with all clients (not only those with known HIV infection), especially in dealing with blood and body fluids. These are now called *universal precautions*.

Nurses who deal with childbearing families are exposed to blood and body fluids and should pay careful attention to the CDC guidelines, including the following:

1. Caregivers should wear disposable latex gloves when having contact with a client's mucous membranes, nonintact skin, body fluids, or blood. Contact includes, for example, changing chux pads, peripads, diapers, or dressings; starting or discontinuing intravenous fluids; and drawing blood.
2. After giving care to a client, the caregiver should remove gloves and wash hands before caring for another client.
3. In addition to gloves, caregivers should wear protective coverings, such as a plastic apron, gown, mask, and eye or face shield during any procedures that frequently result in contamination from splashing of body fluids. These include amniotomy, vaginal examination, vaginal or cesarean birth, suctioning, and care of the newborn until after the initial bath has been done. (Note: Full-sized glasses are considered sufficient eye protection. Although agencies are required to provide eye shields, nurses may choose to purchase their own eye goggles and clean them with soap and water before and after each use.)
4. At birth, the newborn should be suctioned with a disposable bulb syringe or mucus extractor attached to wall suction at a low setting. DeLee mucus traps with mouth suction are not used because of the risk of inadvertently ingesting secretions.
5. Similar care should be taken during any resuscitation procedures. To avoid the need for mouth-to-mouth resuscitation, sufficient mouthpieces and ventilation equipment should be available. Disposable resuscitation masks are recommended.
6. Syringes and needles are disposed of in a special puncture-resistant container. Needles are *never* recapped using two hands; a one-handed scoop technique is acceptable. Needles should never be twisted or broken by hand.
7. In the event that a glove is torn, it should be removed, the hands should be cleansed, and new gloves should be applied. It is critical to remember that gloves are *not* a substitute for handwashing.
8. Gloves and protective coverings should also be worn during any cleaning procedures.

Teaching for Self-Care

The psychologic implications of HIV/AIDS for the childbearing family are staggering. The woman is faced with the knowledge that she and her newborn, if infected, have a decreased life expectancy. If her infant is not infected, she must face the probability that others will raise her child. She may have feelings of fear, helplessness, anger, and isolation. If she shares her diagnosis with others, she may face rejection and condemnation. The couple must deal with the impact of the illness on the partner, who may or may not be infected, and on other children. Dealing with the tasks and responsibilities of a newborn may be especially difficult if the woman is physically depleted or if she is trying to come to grips with the long-term implications of her condition.

The nonjudgmental, supportive nurse plays an essential role in preserving confidentiality and the client's right to privacy. In addition, the nurse can help ensure that the

Text continues on page 376.

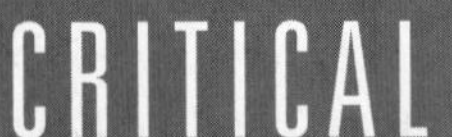

PATHWAY FOR A WOMAN WITH HIV/AIDS

Category	Antepartal Management	Intrapartal Management*	Postpartal Management*
Referral	• Perinatologist • Internist • Social worker • Psych clinical nurse practitioner • Dietary/nutritionist • Infectious disease consult	• Obtain prenatal record	• Home nursing referral if indicated **Expected Outcomes** Appropriate resources identified and utilized

Assessment	• Obtain course of present pregnancy
	• Assess estimated gestational age
	• Assess any sensitivity to medications
	• Obtain history of any infections
	• Obtain complete physical examination to include:
	  • Fetal size, fetal status (FHR), and fetal maturity
	  • Signs of fatigue, weakness, recurrent diarrhea, pallor, night sweats
	  • Lymphadenopathy
	  • Present weight and amount of weight gain or weight loss
	  • Presence of nonproductive cough, fever, sore throat, chills, shortness of breath (*Pneumocystis carinii* pneumonia)
	  • Dark purplish marks or lesions, especially on the lower extremities (Kaposi's sarcoma)
	  • Oral, gingival lesions
	• Obtain diagnostic studies:
	  • Ultrasound
	  • Fetal maturity studies (L/S ratio, PG creatinine)
	  • Hemoglobin and hematocrit
	  • WBC
	  • HIV-I
	  • CD4+ T lymphocyte count
	  • ESR
	  • Differential
	  • Platelet count
		• Assess for signs of infection	• Monitor daily Hct
			• Continue normal postpartum assessment q8h
			• Feeding technique with newborn: should be progressing
			• TPR assessment: q8h; all WNL; report temperature > 38C (100.4F)
			• Continue assessment of comfort level
			Expected Outcomes
			Potential/actual health problems and complications identified and minimized

Teaching/ psychosocial	• Room orientation • Explain signs and symptoms (s/sx) of worsening disease and importance of notifying RN • Explain s/sx of labor • Increase pt awareness of fetal monitoring • Evaluation of client teaching	• Tour of ICN • Discuss with woman: a. Mode of childbirth b. Postpartum expectation	• Implement normal postpartum teaching and psychosocial support **Expected Outcomes** Client verbalizes/demonstrates understanding and incorporation of teaching
Nursing care management and reports	• Assess emotional response so that support and teaching can be planned accordingly • Weigh woman • Obtain food history • Establish rapport • Provide opportunities to talk without interruption • Monitor for signs of infection • Maintain appropriate isolation precautions	• Ongoing monitoring of blood pressure • Electronic fetal monitoring in place • Try to have same nurses caring for woman during her hospitalization • Maintain appropriate BSI precautions • Monitor for signs of infection Provide supportive care	• Continue sitz baths prn • May shower if ambulating without difficulty • DC buffalo cap (saline lock) if present • Maintain appropriate isolation precautions • Monitor for signs of infection **Expected Outcomes** Maternal/fetal well-being maximized Active involvement of client in plan of care to include physical, emotional, and spiritual needs
Activity	• Decreased stimulation in room • Limit visitors	Encourage position change and activity as tolerated	• Up ad lib **Expected Outcome** Level of activity has not exacerbated condition

*Interventions for a woman with a normal labor and birth and during the early postpartum period may be found in those appropriate critical pathways.

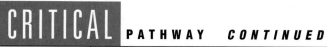

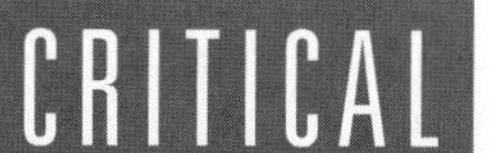

PATHWAY *CONTINUED*

Category	Antepartal Management*	Intrapartal Management*	Postpartal Management*
Comfort	• Assess for discomfort • Provide comfort measures as needed	• Assess for discomfort • Provide comfort measures as needed	• Continue with pain management techniques **Expected Outcome** Optimal comfort maintained
Nutrition	• Plan high-protein, high-calorie diet	• Ice chips; popsicles	• Continue diet and fluids **Expected Outcome** Nutritional needs met with emphasis on appetite enhancement and reduction of deficiencies
Elimination			**Expected Outcome** Intake and output WNL
Medications		• Continuous IV infusion	• May take own prenatal vitamins • RhoGAM administered if indicated • Rubella vaccine administered if indicated **Expected Outcomes** Perfusion and hydration supported Ongoing treatments maintained

Discharge planning/ home care	• Assess home care needs
	• If the client is asymptomatic, the primary nursing activity is client teaching regarding
	  • Disease process
	  • Screening and health care for sex partners as appropriate
	  • Impact of disease on pregnancy
	  • Methods of HIV transmission
	  • Precautions to take in preventing the spread of infection
	  • Options in regard to pregnancy
	  • Available community resources
	  • Signs and symptoms to report to health care provider including common discomforts of pregnancy such as nausea and fatigue and complications such as premature rupture of membranes, vaginal bleeding, and preterm labor
	  • Importance of regular prenatal visits
	• Provide teaching regarding nutritional needs
	• Refer to community resources
	• Discuss disease process, impact on pregnancy, and pregnancy options
	• Provide support and counseling
			• Review discharge instruction sheet and check list
			• Describe postpartum warning signs and when to call CNM/physician
			• Provide prescriptions and gift pack
			• Arrangements made for baby pictures
			• Postpartum visit scheduled
			• Newborn check scheduled
			• Discuss the implications of breastfeeding (current information suggests that the virus may be spread in breast milk)
			• Provide information on transmission of HIV and measures to prevent infection. Discuss household safety issues (eg, it is acceptable to use same dishes, safe to sleep in same bed, safe to use same bathroom, can hold and hug children, should avoid using razors and tooth-brushes and should wear gloves and use 10% bleach solution to clean spills of body fluids or disinfect bathroom). Inform the woman that sexual abstinence is safest; otherwise latex condoms should be used.
			Expected Outcomes
			Discharge teaching completed with emphasis on follow-up continuing health care needs, adequate support network

Family Involvement	• Assess woman's major concerns re: losing fetus, relationship with other children, relationship with partner • Assess support systems	• Encourage family member to stay with the woman as long as possible throughout labor and childbirth	• Family members urged to visit • Continue to involve support persons in teaching • Shows parental bonding behaviors • Plans made for providing support to mother following discharge. Support persons verbalize understanding of need for woman to rest, eat nutritionally, recover. **Expected Outcomes** Family demonstrates resource utilization, integration of newborn into family, helpful coping skills
Date			

*Interventions for a woman with a normal labor and birth and during the early postpartum period may be found in those appropriate critical pathways.

woman receives complete, accurate information about her condition and ways she might cope. This usually involves a referral to social services for follow-up care.

Evaluation

Expected outcomes of nursing care include the following:

- The woman discusses the implications of her positive HIV antibody screen (or diagnosis of AIDS), its implications for herself and her unborn child, the method of transmission, and treatment options.
- The woman uses information regarding referral to social services (or other agency) for follow-up assistance and counseling.
- The woman begins to verbalize her feelings about her condition and its implications in an atmosphere she finds supportive. ●

Care of the Woman with Heart Disease

A healthy woman with a normal heart has adequate cardiac reserve to adjust easily to the demands of pregnancy. The woman with heart disease, however, has decreased cardiac reserve, making it more difficult for her heart to accommodate the higher work load of pregnancy.

Approximately 1% of pregnant women are at risk because of pregestational heart disease. Heart disease ranks fourth after hypertension, hemorrhage, and infection as a cause of maternal mortality. Although rheumatic heart disease used to predominate, at least half of all cases of heart disease currently encountered during pregnancy are caused by congenital heart defects (Cunningham et al, 1997). Other less common causes of heart disease in pregnancy include Marfan syndrome, peripartum cardiomyopathy, and Eisenmenger syndrome. All can cause significant maternal mortality. Mitral valve prolapse is usually asymptomatic but is addressed here because of its frequent occurrence during pregnancy.

Congenital heart defects have become a more common finding in pregnant women as improved surgical techniques enable females born with heart defects to live to childbearing age. The exact pathology depends on the specific defect. Congenital defects most often seen in pregnant women include tetralogy of Fallot, atrial septal defect, ventricular septal defect, patent ductus arteriosus, and coarctation of the aorta. When surgical repair can be accomplished with no remaining evidence of organic heart disease, pregnancy may be undertaken with confidence. In such cases, antibiotic prophylaxis is recommended to prevent subacute bacterial endocarditis at the time of birth. When congenital heart disease is associated with cyanosis, whether the defect was originally uncorrected or the correction failed to relieve the cyanosis, the woman should be counseled to avoid pregnancy because the risk to both her and the fetus would be high. She also needs to know that there is about 2% to 4% chance that the baby will inherit the disorder because most congenital heart defects are believed to be polygenetic and multifactorial in origin (Ward, 1994).

Rheumatic heart disease has declined rapidly in the last four decades, because of prompt identification of pharyngeal infections caused by group A β-hemolytic streptococcus and the availability of penicillin for treatment. Rheumatic fever, which may develop in untreated streptococcal infections, is an inflammatory connective tissue disease that can involve the heart, joints, central nervous system, skin, and subcutaneous tissue. When the heart is affected, mitral valve stenosis is the most common and serious lesion. Aortic valve involvement, manifested by aortic insufficiency, is the second most common problem. The tricuspid and pulmonic valves are rarely affected.

Recurrent acute inflammation from bouts of rheumatic fever causes scar tissue to form on the valves. The scarring results in stenosis (narrowing) of the mitral valve, which may be accompanied by mitral regurgitation. Obstructed blood flow across the narrow valve from the left atrium to the left ventricle can lead to elevated left atrial pressure and elevated pulmonary venous and capillary pressures.

The increased blood volume of pregnancy, coupled with the pregnant woman's need for increased cardiac output, stresses the heart of a woman with mitral valve stenosis. She may develop dyspnea, orthopnea, and pulmonary edema and is at increased risk for congestive heart failure (CHF). Even the woman who has no symptoms at the onset of pregnancy is at risk for CHF.

When the aortic valve is involved, the scarring usually leaves the valve unable to close completely (aortic incompetence or insufficiency) during diastole. Blood then regurgitates back into the left ventricle, leading to volume overload of the left ventricle and inadequate perfusion of the coronary arteries. Occasionally there is both aortic stenosis and regurgitation.

With mild aortic insufficiency, the woman may be asymptomatic. But if the valve dysfunction worsens, she may experience dyspnea and even chest pain (due to inadequate blood flow to the heart muscle) with exertion.

Marfan syndrome is an autosomal dominant disorder of connective tissue in which there may be serious cardiovascular involvement—usually dissection or rupture of the aorta. Because maternal mortality rate may be as high as 25% to 50%, a pregnant woman with Marfan syndrome needs very careful cardiovascular assessment and counseling regarding her prognosis for pregnancy (Rossiter, Repke, Morales, Murphy, & Pyeritz, 1995). Because of its inheritance pattern, there is a 50% chance that the disease will be passed on to offspring.

Mitral valve prolapse (MVP) is usually an asymptomatic condition that is found in as many as 15% of women of childbearing age (Cunningham et al, 1997). The condition is more common in women than in men and seems to be inherited. In MVP, the mitral valve leaflets tend to prolapse into the left atrium during ventricular systole because the chordae tendineae that support them are long and thin. As a result, some mitral regurgitation may occur. On auscultation a midsystolic click and a late systolic murmur are heard.

Women with MVP usually tolerate pregnancy well, and the prognosis is excellent. Most women require assurance that they can continue with normal activities. A few women experience symptoms such as palpitations, chest pain, and dyspnea, which are usually due to arrhythmias. They are often treated with propranolol hydrochloride (Inderal). Limiting caffeine intake also helps decrease palpitations. Women should be given antibiotic prophylaxis if there is mitral valve regurgitation, valvular damage, or other risk factors (Cunningham et al, 1997).

Peripartum cardiomyopathy is a dysfunction of the left ventricle that occurs in the last month of pregnancy or the first 5 months postpartum in a woman with no previous history of heart disease. The symptoms are related to congestive heart failure: dyspnea, orthopnea, chest pain, palpitations, weakness, and edema. The cause is unknown, although symptoms are often attributable to chronic hypertension, mitral stenosis, obesity, or viral myocarditis. The condition usually presents with anemia and infection; consequently, treatment focuses on underlying abnormalities. Digitalis, diuretics, anticoagulants, sodium restriction, and bed rest are often part of the treatment. Peripartum cardiomyopathy may resolve with bed rest as the heart gradually returns to normal size. Counseling about future pregnancies is based on the extent of the heart enlargement (Cunningham et al, 1997).

Eisenmenger syndrome is not a congenital defect, but a complication that can develop with cardiac lesions characterized by left-to-right shunting (as with atrial septal defects or ventricular septal defects). This shunting can result in progressive pulmonary hypertension. As pulmonary vascular resistance increases the shunting becomes bidirectional or reverses to right-to-left shunting. This condition cannot be corrected surgically and is associated with maternal mortality rates approaching 50% (Eisenmenger Syndrome, 1998).

Clinical Therapy

Women with congenital heart disease should be managed by a maternal-fetal specialist (AAP & ACOG, 1997). The primary goal of medical management is early diagnosis and ongoing treatment of the woman with cardiac disease. Echocardiogram, chest x-ray, electrocardiogram, auscultation of heart sounds, and sometimes cardiac catheterization are essential for establishing the type and severity of the heart disease. The severity of heart disease can also be determined by the individual's ability to perform ordinary physical activity. The following classification of functional capacity for those with cardiac disease has been standardized by the Criteria Committee of the New York Heart Association (1979):

- *Class I. Uncompromised.* No limitation of physical activity and no symptoms of cardiac insufficiency. Ordinary physical activity causes no discomfort; anginal pain is not present.
- *Class II. Slightly compromised.* Slight limitation of physical activity. Ordinary physical activity causes fatigue, dyspnea, palpitation, or anginal pain.
- *Class III. Markedly compromised.* Marked limitation of physical activity. During less than ordinary physical activity, the person experiences excessive fatigue, dyspnea, palpitation, or anginal pain.
- *Class IV. Severely compromised.* Unable to carry on any physical activity without experiencing discomfort. Even at rest, the person experiences symptoms of cardiac insufficiency or anginal pain; discomfort increases with any physical activity.

Women in classes I and II usually experience a normal pregnancy and have few complications, whereas those in classes III and IV are at risk for more severe complications, which may affect both maternal and fetal outcomes. Preconception counseling is important for these women in order to optimize maternal and fetal outcomes.

Because anemia increases the work of the heart, it should be diagnosed early and treated. Infection also increases the cardiac work load, so even minor infections should be treated thoroughly. To reduce the risk of pyelonephritis, monthly screening for asymptomatic bacteriuria is indicated, with antibiotic therapy as needed.

As pregnancy progresses, it is important to minimize cardiac workload and promote tissue perfusion. Consequently, the woman's activity should be limited. Weight gain may also be limited to about 15 lb and a daily sodium intake of only 2 to 4 g is recommended (Mason & Bobrowski, 1998).

Drug Therapy

Besides the iron and vitamin supplements prescribed during pregnancy, the pregnant woman with heart disease may need additional drug therapy to maintain health. Antibiotics, usually penicillin if not contraindicated by allergy, are used to prevent recurrent bouts of rheumatic fever and subsequent heart valve damage. Antibiotics are also recommended during labor and the early postpartum period for either acquired or congenital disease to prevent bacterial endocarditis. If the woman develops coagulation problems, the anticoagulant heparin may be used. Heparin offers the greatest safety to the fetus because it does not cross the placenta. The thiazide diuretics and furosemide (Lasix) may be used to treat congestive heart failure if it develops. Digitalis glycosides and common antiarrhythmic drugs may be used to treat cardiac failure and arrhythmias. These agents do cross the placenta but have no reported teratogenic effect; however, they have not been adequately studied to establish their safety in pregnancy (Cunningham et al, 1997).

Labor Spontaneous natural labor with adequate pain relief is usually recommended for clients in classes I and II. Special attention should be given to the prompt recognition and treatment of any signs of heart failure. Those in classes III and IV may need to be hospitalized prior to onset of labor for cardiovascular stabilization. They may also require invasive cardiac monitoring during labor.

Childbirth Use of low forceps provides the safest method of birth, with lumbar epidural anesthesia to reduce the stress of pushing. Cesarean is used only if fetal or maternal indications exist, not on the basis of heart disease alone.

CRITICAL THINKING QUESTION

What specific information does the nurse need to help the pregnant woman with heart disease plan her schedule to avoid stress and allow sufficient time for rest?

NURSING CARE MANAGEMENT

Nursing Assessment and Diagnosis

The nurse assesses the stress of pregnancy on the functional capacity of the heart during every antepartal visit. The nurse notes the category of functional capacity assigned to the woman, takes the woman's pulse, respirations, and blood pressure and compares them to the normal values expected during pregnancy and to the woman's previous values. The nurse then determines the woman's activity level, including rest, and any changes in the pulse and respirations that have occurred since previous visits. The nurse also identifies and evaluates other factors that would increase strain on the heart. These might include anemia, infection, anxiety, lack of support system, and household and career demands.

The following symptoms, if they are progressive, are indicative of congestive heart failure, the heart's signal of its decreased ability to meet the demands of pregnancy:

- Cough (frequent, with or without hemoptysis)
- Dyspnea (progressive, upon exertion)
- Edema (progressive, generalized, including extremities, face, eyelids)
- Heart murmurs (heard on auscultation)
- Palpitations
- Rales (auscultated in lung bases)

Progressiveness of the cycle is the critical factor, because some of these same symptoms are seen to a minor degree in a pregnancy without cardiac problems.

Nursing diagnoses that might apply to the pregnant woman with heart disease include the following:

- ***Decreased Cardiac Output:*** easy fatigability
- ***Impaired Gas Exchange*** related to pulmonary edema secondary to cardiac decompensation
- ***Fear*** related to the effects of the maternal cardiac condition on fetal well-being

Nursing Plan and Implementation

Nursing care is directed toward maintaining a balance between cardiac reserve and cardiac work load.

Community-Based Nursing Care

Antepartum Period Nursing actions are designed to meet the physiologic and psychosocial needs of the pregnant woman with heart disease. The priority of nursing actions varies according to the severity of the disease process and the individual needs of the woman as determined by nursing assessment.

The woman and her family should thoroughly understand her condition and its management and should recognize signs of potential complications. This will increase their understanding and decrease anxiety. When the nurse provides explanations, uses printed material, and offers frequent opportunities to ask questions and discuss concerns, the woman is better able to meet her own health care needs and seek assistance appropriately.

As part of health teaching, the nurse explains the purposes of the dietary and activity changes that are required. A diet is instituted that is high in iron, protein, and essential nutrients but low in sodium, with adequate calories to ensure normal weight gain. Such a diet best meets the nutrition needs of the client with cardiac disease. Excessive weight gain is avoided because it taxes the heart. To help preserve her cardiac reserves, the woman may need to restrict her activities. In addition, 8 to 10 hours of sleep and frequent daily rest periods, are essential. The nurse can encourage the woman to rest in the side-lying position to promote optimal placental perfusion. Because upper respiratory infections may tax the heart and lead to decompensation, the woman must avoid contact with sources of infection.

During the first half of pregnancy, the woman is seen approximately every 2 weeks to assess cardiac status. During the second half of pregnancy, the woman is seen weekly. These assessments are especially important between weeks 28 and 30, when the blood volume reaches maximum amounts. If symptoms of cardiac decompensation occur, prompt medical intervention is indicated to correct the cardiac problem.

Hospital-Based Nursing Care

Intrapartum Period Labor and birth exert tremendous stress on the woman and her fetus. This stress could be fatal to the fetus of a woman with cardiac disease because the fetus may be receiving an inadequate oxygen and blood supply. Thus the intrapartal care of a woman with cardiac disease is aimed at reducing the amount of physical exertion and accompanying fatigue.

The nurse evaluates maternal vital signs frequently to determine the woman's response to labor. A pulse rate greater than 100 beats per minute or respirations greater than 24 per minute may indicate beginning cardiac decompensation, especially if accompanied by dyspnea, and require further evaluation. The nurse also auscultates the woman's lungs frequently for rales and carefully observes for other signs of developing decompensation.

To ensure cardiac emptying and adequate oxygenation, the nurse encourages the laboring woman to assume either a semi-Fowler's position with lateral tilt or side-lying position with her head and shoulders elevated. Oxygen by mask, diuretics to reduce fluid retention, sedatives and analgesics, prophylactic antibiotics, and digitalis may also be used as indicated by the woman's status.

The nurse remains with the woman to support her. It is essential that the nurse keep the woman and her family informed of labor progress and management plans, collaborating with them to fulfill their wishes for the birth experience as much as possible. The nurse needs to maintain an atmosphere of calm to lessen the anxiety of the woman and her family.

Continuous electronic fetal monitoring is used to provide ongoing assessment of the fetus's response to labor. To prevent overexertion and the accompanying fatigue, the nurse encourages the woman to sleep and relax between contractions and provides her with emotional support and encouragement. During pushing, the nurse encourages the woman to use shorter, more moderate open glottis pushing (see Chapter 23), with complete relaxation between pushes. The nurse monitors vital signs closely during the second stage.

Postpartum Period The postpartal period is a significant time for the woman with cardiac disease. After birth, the intra-abdominal pressure and the venous pressure are reduced, the splanchnic vessels engorge, and blood flow to the heart increases. As extravascular fluid returns to the bloodstream for excretion, cardiac output and blood volume increase. This physiologic adaptation places great strain on the heart and may lead to decompensation, especially in the first 48 hours postpartum.

So that the health care team can detect any possible problems, the woman may remain in the hospital longer than the low-risk woman postpartally. Her vital signs are monitored frequently, and she is assessed for signs of decompensation. She stays in the semi-Fowler's or side-lying position, with her head and shoulders elevated, and begins a gradual, progressive activity program. Appropriate diet and stool softeners facilitate bowel movement without undue strain.

The postpartum nurse gives the woman opportunities to discuss her birth experience and helps her deal with any feelings or concerns that cause her distress. The nurse also encourages maternal-infant attachment by providing frequent opportunities for the mother to interact with her child.

Because there is no evidence that cardiac output is compromised during lactation, the only concern about breastfeeding for women with cardiovascular disease is related to medications that the mother may be taking (Friedman & Polifka, 1996). These must be evaluated for their ability to pass into the milk and for any effect of the drug on lactation. The nurse can assist the breastfeeding mother to a comfortable side-lying position with her head moderately elevated or to a semi-Fowler's position. To conserve the mother's energy, the nurse should position the newborn at the breast and be available to burp the baby and reposition him or her at the other breast.

In addition to providing the normal postpartum discharge teaching, the nurse should ensure that the woman and her family understand the signs of possible problems resulting from her heart disease or from other postpartal complications. For women with heart disease, postpartum complications such as hemorrhage, thromboembolism, anemia, and infection pose a real threat and may even precipitate heart failure.

The nurse plans with the woman an activity schedule that is gradual, progressive, and appropriate to her needs and home environment. The nurse provides appropriate health teaching, including information about resumption of sexual activity and contraception. Visiting nurse or homemaker assistance referrals may be necessary, depending on the woman's status.

Evaluation

Expected outcomes of nursing care include the following:

- The woman is able to discuss her condition and its possible impact on her pregnancy, labor and birth, and the postpartal period.
- The woman participates in developing an appropriate health care regimen and follows it throughout her pregnancy.
- The woman gives birth to a healthy infant.
- The woman avoids congestive heart failure, thromboembolism, and infection.
- The woman is able to identify signs and symptoms of possible postpartum complications.
- The woman is able to care effectively for her newborn infant. ●

Other Medical Conditions and Pregnancy

A woman with a preexisting medical condition should be aware of the possible impact of pregnancy on her condition, as well as the impact of her condition on the outcome of her pregnancy. Table 15–5 discusses some of the less common medical conditions vis-à-vis pregnancy.

TABLE 15–5 Less Common Medical Conditions and Pregnancy

Condition	Brief Description	Maternal Implications	Fetal/Neonatal Implications
Rheumatoid arthritis	Chronic inflammatory disease believed to be caused by a genetically influenced antigen-antibody reaction. Symptoms include fatigue, low-grade fever, pain and swelling of joints, morning stiffness, pain on movement. Treated with salicylates, physical therapy, and rest. Corticosteroids used cautiously if not responsive to above.	Usually there is remission of rheumatoid arthritis symptoms during pregnancy, often with a relapse postpartum. Anemia may be present due to blood loss from salicylate therapy. Mother needs extra rest, particularly to relieve weight-bearing joints, but needs to continue range-of-motion exercises. If in remission, may stop medication during pregnancy.	Possibility of prolonged gestation and longer labor with heavy salicylate use. Possible teratogenic effects of salicylates.
Epilepsy	Chronic disorder characterized by seizures; may be idiopathic or secondary to other conditions, such as head injury, metabolic and nutritional disorders such as PKU or vitamin B_6 deficiency, encephalitis, neoplasms, or circulatory interferences. Treated with anticonvulsants.	Vast majority of pregnancies in women with seizure disorders are uneventful and have an excellent outcome. Women with more frequent seizures before pregnancy may have exacerbations during pregnancy, but this may be related to lack of cooperation with drug regimen or sleep deprivation. During pregnancy the woman should continue to be treated with the medication that best controls her seizures. Folic acid therapy should be started prior to conception if possible. Folic acid and vitamin D are indicated throughout pregnancy (Samuels 1996c).	There is an increased incidence of stillbirth in women with epilepsy. Also, anticonvulsant medications are associated with increased incidence of congenital anomalies, especially cleft lip and heart defects, although the incidence has decreased in recent years. This may be due to the fact that the current ability to determine blood levels of medications has led to more accurate dosages and the resultant use of a single medication; consequently multiple medications are used less often (Samuels 1996c).
Hepatitis B	Hepatitis B, caused by the hepatitis B virus (HBV), is a major, growing health problem. Groups at risk include those from areas with a high incidence (primarily developing countries), illegal IV drug users, prostitutes, homosexuals, those with multiple sex partners, or occupational exposure to blood, although many infected people have no identifiable source of infection. HBV transmission is blood borne, primarily sexually and perinatally transmitted. Because of the dramatic increase and the difficulty of vaccinating high-risk individuals before they become infected, the CDC now recommends (1) testing all pregnant women for the presence of hepatitis B surface antigen (HBsAG); (2) routine vaccination of all newborns; (3) vaccination of older children at high risk for hepatitis B; (4) vaccination of children age 11–12 years who have not previously received the vaccine; (5) vaccination of adolescents and adults at high risk for infection (CDC, 1998).	Hepatitis B does not usually affect the course of pregnancy. However, chronic HBV carriers have a great potential for infecting others when exposure to blood and bodily fluids occurs. In addition, chronic carriers may develop long-term sequelae, such as chronic liver disease and liver cancer. Approximately 4000 to 5000 deaths are caused annually by liver disease associated with chronic HBV infection. It is now recommended that all pregnant women be tested for the presence of hepatitis B surface antigen (HBsAg). A woman who is negative may be given the hepatitis vaccine.	Perinatal transmission most often occurs at or near the time of childbirth. More important, the risk of becoming a chronic carrier of the HBV is inversely related to the age of the individual at the time of initial infection (Crawford & Pruss, 1993). Therefore infants infected perinatally have the highest risk of becoming chronically infected if not treated. Recommendations now include routine vaccination of all neonates born to HBsAg-negative women and immunoprophylaxis to all newborns of HBsAg-positive women.
Hyperthyroidism (thyrotoxicosis)	Enlarged, overactive thyroid gland; increased T_4:TBG ratio and increased BMR. Symptoms include muscle wasting, tachycardia, excessive sweating, and exophthalmos. Treatment by antithyroid drug propylthiouracil (PTU) while monitoring free T_4 levels. Surgery used only if drug intolerance exists.	Mild hyperthyroidism is not dangerous. Increased incidence of PIH and postpartum hemorrhage if not well controlled. Serious risk related to thyroid storm characterized by high fever, tachycardia, sweating, and congestive heart failure. Now occurs rarely. When diagnosed during pregnancy, may be transient or permanent.	Neonatal thyrotoxicosis is rare. Even low doses of antithyroid drug in mother may produce a mild fetal/neonatal hypothyroidism; higher dose may produce a goiter or mental deficiencies. Fetal loss not increased in euthyroid women. If untreated, rates of abortion, intrauterine death, and stillbirth increase. Breastfeeding contraindicated for women on antithyroid medication because it is excreted in the milk (may be tried by woman on low dose if neonatal T_4 levels are monitored).
Hypothyroidism	Characterized by inadequate thyroid secretions (decreased T_4:TBG ratio), elevated TSH, lowered BMR, and enlarged thyroid gland (goiter). Symptoms include lack of energy, excessive weight gain, cold intolerance, dry skin, and constipation. Treated by thyroxine replacement therapy.	Long-term replacement therapy usually continues at same dosage during pregnancy as before. Weekly nonstress test (NST) after 35 weeks' gestation.	If mother untreated, fetal loss 50%; high risk of congenital goiter or true cretinism. Therefore newborns are screened for T_4 level. Mild TSH elevations present little risk because TSH does not cross the placenta.

TABLE 15–5 Less Common Medical Conditions and Pregnancy *continued*

Condition	Brief Description	Maternal Implications	Fetal/Neonatal Implications
Maternal phenylketonuria (PKU) (hyperphenylalaninemia)	Inherited recessive single gene anomaly causing a deficiency of the liver enzyme needed to convert the amino acid phenylalanine to tyrosine, resulting in high serum levels of phenylalanine. Brain damage and mental retardation occur if not treated early.	Low phenylalanine diet is mandatory before conception and during pregnancy. The woman should be counseled that her children will either inherit the disease or be carriers, depending on the zygosity of the father for the disease. Treatment at a PKU center is recommended.	Risk to fetus if maternal treatment not begun preconception. In untreated women increased incidence of fetal mental retardation, microcephaly, congenital heart defects, and growth retardation. Fetal phenylalanine levels are approximately 50% higher than maternal levels.
Multiple sclerosis	Neurologic disorder characterized by destruction of the myelin sheath of nerve fibers. The condition occurs primarily in young adults, more commonly in females, and is marked by periods of remission; progresses to marked physical disability in 10 to 20 years.	Associated with remission during pregnancy, but with slighly increased relapse rate postpartum (Confavreux, Hutchinson, Hours, Cortinovis-Tourniaire, & Moreau, 1998). Rest is important; help with child care should be planned. Uterine contraction strength is not diminished, but because sensation is frequently lessened, labor may be almost painless.	Increased evidence of a genetic predisposition. Therefore reproductive counseling is recommended.
Systemic lupus erythematosus (SLE)	Chronic autoimmune collagen disease, characterized by exacerbations and remissions; symptoms range from characteristic rash to inflammation and pain in joints, fever, nephritis, depression, cranial nerve disorders, and peripheral neuropathies.	Women are generally advised that SLE should be in remission for at least 5–7 months before conceiving. Pregnancy does not appear to alter the long-term prognosis of women with SLE, but maternal morbidity and mortality increase. They also face an increased risk of permanent renal or CNS deterioration after pregnancy (Classen, Paulson & Zacharias, 1998). Most maternal deaths occur in the postpartal period and are caused by pulmonary hemorrhage or lupus pneumonitis (Samuels, 1996a).	Increased incidence of spontaneous abortion, stillbirth, prematurity, and IUGR. Infants born to women with SLE may have characteristic skin rash, which usually disappears by 12 months. Infants are at increased risk for complete congenital heart block, a condition that can be diagnosed prenatally. Fetal echocardiography is then performed to rule out other cardiac defects (Samuels, 1996a).
Tuberculosis (TB)	Infection caused by *Mycobacterium tuberculosis;* inflammatory process causes destruction of lung tissue, increased sputum, and coughing. Associated primarily with poverty and malnutrition and may be found among refugees from countries where TB is prevalent. Treated with isoniazid and either ethambutol or rifampin or both.	The incidence of tuberculosis has begun to increase significantly since the late 1980s, and it is increasingly associated with HIV infection (Simpkins et al, 1996). If TB inactive due to prior treatment, relapse rate no greater than for nonpregnant women. When isoniazid is used during pregnancy, the woman should take supplemental pyridoxine (vitamin B_6). Extra rest and limited contact with others is required until disease becomes inactive.	If maternal TB is inactive, mother may breastfeed and care for her infant. If TB is active, neonate should not have direct contact with mother until she is noninfectious. Isoniazid crosses the placenta, but most studies show no teratogenic effects. Rifampin crosses the placenta. Possibility of harmful effects still being studied.

FOCUS YOUR STUDY

- Almost any health problem that a person can have when not pregnant can coexist with pregnancy. Some problems, such as anemias, may be exacerbated by pregnancy. Others, such as collagen disease, may go into temporary remission with pregnancy. Regardless of the health problem, careful health care is needed throughout pregnancy to improve the outcome for mother and fetus.
- The diagnosis of high-risk pregnancy can shock an expectant couple. Providing emotional support, teaching about the condition and prognosis, and educating for self-care are important nursing measures that help the client cope.
- Substance abuse (either drugs or alcohol) not only is detrimental to the mother's health but also may have profound lasting effects on the fetus.
- The key point in the care of the pregnant woman with diabetes is scrupulous maternal plasma glucose control. This is best achieved by home blood glucose monitoring, multiple daily insulin injections, and a careful diet. To reduce incidence of congenital anomalies and other problems in the neonate, the woman should be euglycemic (have a normal blood glucose) throughout the pregnancy. Diabetics, even more than most other clients, need to be educated about their conditions and involved with their own care.
- HIV infection, which is transmitted via blood and body fluids, may also be transmitted transplacentally to the fetus. Currently there is no definitive therapy for HIV/AIDS. Nurses should employ blood and body fluid precautions (universal precautions) in caring for all women to avoid potential spread of infection.
- Cardiac disease during pregnancy requires careful assessment, limitation of activity, and knowing and reporting signs of impending cardiac decompensation by both client and nurse.

REFERENCES

American Academy of Pediatrics (AAP) & American College of Obstetricians and Gynecologists (ACOG). (1997). *Guidelines for perinatal care* (4th ed.). Elk Grove Village, IL: Author.

American College of Obstetricians and Gynecologists (ACOG). (1994a). *Diabetes and pregnancy* (ACOG Technical Bulletin No. 200). Washington, DC: Author.

American College of Obstetricians and Gynecologists (ACOG). (1994b). *Substance abuse in pregnancy* (ACOG Technical Bulletin No. 195). Washington, DC: Author.

American College of Obstetricians and Gynecologists (ACOG). (1995). *Preconceptional care* (ACOG Technical Bulletin No. 205). Washington, DC: Author.

American College of Obstetricians and Gynecologists (ACOG). (1996). *Hemoglobinopathies in pregnancies* (ACOG Technical Bulletin No. 220). Washington, DC: Author.

American College of Obstetricians and Gynecologists (ACOG). (1997). *Human immunodeficiency virus infections in pregnancy* (ACOG Technical Bulletin No. 232). Washington, DC: Author.

Bergan, R., Kliegman, R., & Arvin, A. (Eds.). (1996). *Textbook of pediatrics*. Philadelphia: Saunders.

Brown, F., & Hare, J. (1995). *Diabetes complicating pregnancy*. New York: Wiley-Liss.

Carpenter, C. C. J., Fischl, M. A., Hammer, S. M., Hirsch, M. S., Jacobsen, D. M., Katzenstein, D. A. et al. (1998). Antiretroviral therapy for HIV infection in 1998. *Journal of the American Medical Association, 280*(1), 78–85.

Centers for Disease Control and Prevention (CDC). HIV/AIDS Surveillance Report, 1997. Vol 9, no 2.

Centers for Disease Control and Prevention (CDC). (1998). 1998 guidelines for the treatment of sexually transmitted diseases. *Morbidity & Mortality Weekly Report, 47*(No. RR-1).

Centers for Disease Control and Prevention (CDC) (1998, April 3). Recommendations to prevent and control iron deficiency in the United States. *Morbidity & Mortality Weekly Report, 47*(No. RR-3), 1–36.

Classen, S. R., Paulson, P. R., & Zacharias, S. R. (1998). Systemic lupus erythematosus: Perinatal and neonatal implications. *Journal of Obstetric, Gynecologic, & Neonatal Nursing, 27*(5), 493–500.

Confavreux, C., Hutchinson, M., Hours, M. M., Cortinovis-Tourniaire, P., & Moreau, T. (1998). Rate of pregnancy-related relapse in multiple sclerosis. *New England Journal of Medicine, 339*(5), 339–340.

Crawford, N., & Pruss, A. (1993). Preventing neonatal hepatitis B infection during the perinatal period. *Journal of Obstetric, Gynecologic, & Neonatal Nursing, 22*(6), 491.

Criteria Committee of the New York Heart Association. (1979). *Nomenclature and criteria for diagnosis of diseases of the heart and blood vessels* (8th ed.). New York: Heart Association.

Cruikshank, D. P. (1994). Cardiovascular, pulmonary, renal, and hematologic disorders in pregnancy. In J. R. Scott, P. J. DiSaia, C. B. Hammond, & W. N. Spellacy (Eds.), *Danforth's obstetrics and gynecology* (7th ed.). Philadelphia: Lippincott.

Cunningham, F. G., MacDonald, P. C., Gant, N. F., Leveno, K. J., Gilstrap, L. C., III., Hankins, G. D. V., & Clark, S. L. (1997). *Williams obstetrics* (20th ed.). Stamford, CT: Appleton & Lange.

Duff, P. (1996). Maternal and perinatal infections. In S. G. Gabbe, J. R. Niebyl, & J. L. Simpson (Eds.), *Obstetrics: Normal & problem pregnancies* (3rd ed.). New York: Churchill-Livingstone.

Eisenmenger Syndrome. (1998). http://www.cachnet.org/consensus/eisen.htm#PartI

Eyler, A. E. (1996). Current issues in the primary care of women with HIV. *The Female Patient, 21*, 15–29.

Fanaroff, A., & Martin, R. (Eds.). (1997). *Neonatal-perinatal medicine: Diseases of the fetus and infant*. St. Louis: Mosby.

Friedman, J. M., & Polifka, J. E. (1996). *The effects of drugs on the fetus and nursing infant*. Baltimore: Johns Hopkins University Press.

Gabbe, S. G. (1996). High risk pregnancy: Diabetes mellitus. *Contemporary OB/GYN, 41*(7), 13–15.

Garner, P. (1995, July 15). Type I diabetes mellitus and pregnancy. *Lancet, 346*(8968), 157–161.

Golan, A., Wolman, I., Saller, Y., & David, M. P. (1993). Hydramnios in singleton pregnancy: Sonographic prevalence and etiology. *Gynecologic & Obstetric Investigation, 35*(2), 91–93.

Guralnick, M. J. (1997). *The effectiveness of early intervention*. Baltimore: Paul Brookes.

Hsu, H. W., Moye, J., Jr., Kunches, L., Ng, P., Shea, B., Caldwell, B., Demaria, A., Mofenson, L., & Grady, G. F. (1992). Perinatally acquired human immunodeficiency virus infection: Extent of clinical recognition in a population-based cohort [Massachusetts Pediatric HIV Surveillance Working Group]. *Pediatric Infectious Disease Journal, 11*(11), 941–945.

Idrogo, M. A., & Mazze, R. S. (1998). Gestational diabetes: Implications for women's health. *The Female Patient, 23*(5), 19–34.

Jensen, C. E., Tuck, S. M., & Wonke, B. (1995). Fertility in beta thalassaemia major: A report of 16 pregnancies, preconceptual evaluation and a review of the literature. *British Journal of Obstetrics & Gynaecology, 102*(8), 625–629.

Jessup, M. (1997). Addiction in women: Prevalence, profiles, and meaning. *Journal of Obstetric, Gynecologic, & Neonatal Nursing, 26*(4), 449–458.

Kearney, M. H. (1997). Drug treatment for women: Traditional models and new directions. *Journal of Obstetric, Gynecologic, & Neonatal Nursing. 26*(4), 459–468.

Kenner, C., & D'Apolito, K. (1997). Outcomes for children exposed to drugs in utero. *Journal of Obstetric, Gynecologic, & Neonatal Nursing, 26*(5), 595–603.

Keohane, N. S., & Lacey, L. A. (1991). Preparing the woman with gestational diabetes for self-care. Use of a structured teaching plan by nursing staff. *Journal of Obstetric, Gynecologic, & Neonatal Nursing, 20*(3), 189–193.

Landesman, S. H., Kalish, L. A., Burns, D. N., Minkoff, H., Fox, H. E., Zorrilla, C., Garcia, P., Fowler, M. G., Mofenson, L., & Tuomala, R. (1996, June 20). Obstetrical factors and the transmission of human immunodeficiency virus type 1 from mother to child: The Women and Infants Transmission Study. *New England Journal of Medicine, 334*(25), 1617–1623.

Landon, M. B. (1996). Diabetes mellitus and other endocrine diseases. In S. G. Gabbe, J. R. Niebyl, & J. L. Simpson (Eds.), *Obstetrics: Normal & problem pregnancies* (3rd ed.). New York: Churchill-Livingstone.

Lowdermilk, L., Perry, S., & Bobak, S. (1997). *Maternity and women's health care*. St. Louis: Mosby.

Mandelbrot, L., Le Chenadec, J., Berribi, A., Bongain, A., Benifla, J. L., Delfraissey, J. F., Blanche, S., & Mayaux, M. J. (1998 July 1). Perinatal HIV-1 transmission: Interaction between zidovudine prophylaxis and mode of delivery in the French Perinatal Cohort. *Journal of the American Medical Association, 280*(1), 55–60.

Mandeville, L. (1992). Diabetes mellitus in pregnancy. In L. Mandeville & N. Troiano (Eds.), *High-risk intrapartum nursing*. Philadelphia: Lippincott.

Margono, F., Mroueh, J., Garely, A., White, D., Duerr, A., & Minkoff, H. L. (1994). Resurgence of active tuberculosis among pregnant women. *Obstetrics & Gynecology, 83*(6), 911–914.

Mason, B. A., & Bobrowski, R. A. (1998). Cardiac disease. *Contemporary OB/GYN, 43*(8), 15–26.

McCain, G. C., & Deatrick, J. A. (1994). The experience of high-risk pregnancy. *Journal of Obstetric, Gynecologic, & Neonatal Nursing, 23*(5), 421–427.

National Diabetes Data Group. (1979). *Classification of diabetes mellitus and other categories of glucose intolerance.* Washington, DC: National Institutes of Health (NIH).

National Institute on Drug Abuse. (1991). *National household survey on drug abuse: Population estimates of 1990.* Rockville, MD: Author.

Niebyl, J. R. (1996). Drugs in pregnancy and lactation. In S. G. Gabbe, J. R. Niebyl, & J. L. Simpson (Eds.), *Obstetrics: Normal & problem pregnancies* (3rd ed.). New York: Churchill-Livingstone.

Owen, J., Phelan, S. T., Landon, M. B., & Gabbe, S. G. (1995). Gestational diabetes survey. *American Journal of Obstetrics & Gynecology, 172*(2 Pt. 1), 615–620.

Payton, R. G., & White, P. J. (1995). Primary care for women: Assessment of hematologic disorders. *Journal of Nurse-Midwifery, 40*(2), 120–136.

Peters, K. D., Kochenek, M. A., and Murphy, S. L. Deaths: Final data for 1996. *National Vital Statistics Reports, 47*(9), 1–44.

Peters, R. K., Kjos, S. L., Xiang, A., & Buchanan, T. A. (1996, Jan. 27). Long-term diabetogenic effect of single pregnancy in women with previous gestational diabetes mellitus. *Lancet, 347*(8996), 227–230.

Pollack, C. V., Jr. (1993). Emergencies in sickle cell disease. *Emergency Medicine Clinics of North America, 11*(2), 365–378.

Puza, S. W., & Malee, M. P. (1996). Utilization of routine ophthalmologic examinations in pregnant diabetic patients. *Journal of Maternal-Fetal Medicine, 5*(1), 7–10.

Rossiter, J. P., Repke, J. T., Morales, A. J., Murphy, E. A., & Pyeritz, R. E. (1995). A prospective longitudinal evaluation of pregnancy in the Marfan syndrome. *American Journal of Obstetrics & Gynecology, 173*(5), 1599–1606.

Samuels, P. (1996a). Collagen vascular diseases. In S. G. Gabbe, J. R. Niebyl, & J. L. Simpson (Eds.), *Obstetrics: Normal & problem pregnancies* (3rd ed.). New York: Churchill-Livingstone.

Samuels, P. (1996b). Hematologic complications of pregnancy. In S. G. Gabbe, J. R. Niebyl, & J. L. Simpson (Eds.), *Obstetrics: Normal & problem pregnancies* (3rd ed.) (pp 1083–1100). New York: Churchill-Livingstone.

Samuels, P. (1996c). Neurologic disorders. In S. G. Gabbe, J. R. Niebyl, & J. L. Simpson (Eds.), *Obstetrics: Normal & problem pregnancies* (3rd ed.). New York: Churchill-Livingstone.

Selleck, C. S., & Redding, B. A. (1998). Knowledge and attitudes of registered nurses toward perinatal substance abuse. *Journal of Obstetric, Gynecologic, & Neonatal Nursing, 27*(1), 70–77.

Shields, L. E., Gan, E. A., Murphy, H. F., Sahn, D. J., & Moore, T. R. (1993). The prognostic value of hemoglobin A1c in predicting fetal heart disease in diabetic pregnancies. *Obstetrics & Gynecology, 81*(6), 954–957.

Simpkins, S. M., Hench, C. P., & Bhatia, G. (1996). Management of the obstetric patient with tuberculosis. *Journal of Obstretric, Gynecologic, & Neonatal Nursing, 25*(5): 305–312.

Smith, J. A., Espeland, M., Bellevue, R., Bonds, D., Brown, A. K., & Koshy, M. (1996). Pregnancy in sickle cell disease: Experience of the cooperative study of sickle cell disease. *Obstetrics & Gynecology, 87*(2), 199–204.

Spellacy, W. N. (1994). Diabetes mellitus and pregnancy. In J. R. Scott, P. J. DiSaia, C. B. Hammond, & W. N. Spellacy (Eds.), *Danforth's obstetrics and gynecology* (7th ed.). Philadelphia: Lippincott.

Temmerman, M., Chomba, E. N., Ndinya-Achola, J., Plummer, F. A., Coppens, M., & Piot, P. (1994). Maternal human immunodeficiency virus-1 infection and pregnancy outcome. *Obstetrics & Gynecology, 83*(4), 495–501.

Varney, H. (1997). *Varney's midwifery.* Boston: Jones and Bartlett.

Ward, K. (1994). Genetics and prenatal diagnosis. In J. R. Scott, P. J. DiSaia, C. B. Hammond, & W. N. Spellacy (Eds.), *Danforth's obstetrics and gynecology* (7th ed.) (pp 201–224). Philadelphia: Lippincott.

16

Pregnancy at Risk: Gestational Onset

Key Terms

Abortion
Eclampsia
Ectopic pregnancy
Erythroblastosis fetalis
Gestational trophoblastic disease (GTD)
HELLP syndrome
Hydatidiform mole
Hydrops fetalis
Hyperemesis gravidarum
Incompetent cervix
Miscarriage
Preeclampsia
Pregnancy-induced hypertension (PIH)
Premature rupture of membranes (PROM)
Preterm labor
Rh immune globulin (RhoGAM)
Tocolysis

NOT LONG AGO, MY HUSBAND AND I HAPPILY FOUND out that we were expecting our second child, and although we had experienced it before, we anxiously looked forward to each exciting step along the way. On my second routine prenatal visit, however, we were told that no heartbeat was evident and that I appeared to be nowhere near my then estimated 14 weeks. An ultrasound verified what my doctor had suspected: There was no viable pregnancy—I had miscarried. I was suddenly overwhelmed with a feeling of great loss. But after my D & C, that feeling of loss turned to one of fear and uncertainty as my doctor informed me that no fetal development had existed; I had had a molar pregnancy.

As my doctor told me about the disease and explained the potential risks, it occurred to me that the possibility existed that I might never have another child. Suddenly, my healthy, happy toddler became the most important element in my life—how blessed I was to have her!

Although some anxiety still exists, I now approach my weekly follow-up visits with a renewed sense of being. It will be at least another year before my husband and I might again rejoice in the anticipation of a second child; but for now we rejoice more fully in the precious one we have.

Objectives

- Discuss the medical therapy and nursing care of a woman with hyperemesis gravidarum.
- Contrast the etiology, medical therapy, and nursing interventions for the various bleeding problems associated with pregnancy.
- Identify the medical therapy and nursing interventions indicated in caring for a woman with an incompetent cervix.
- Discuss the nursing care for a woman experiencing premature rupture of the membranes or preterm labor.
- Describe the development and course of hypertensive disorders associated with pregnancy.
- Explain the cause and prevention of hemolytic disease of the newborn secondary to Rh incompatibility.
- Compare Rh incompatibility to ABO incompatibility with regard to occurrence, treatment, and implications for the fetus/newborn.
- Summarize the effects of surgical procedures on pregnancy, and explain ways in which pregnancy may complicate diagnosis of conditions that require surgery.
- Discuss the implications of trauma due to accidents or battering for the pregnant woman and her fetus.
- Describe the effects of infections on the woman and her unborn child.

PREGNANCY IS USUALLY A NORMAL, uncomplicated experience. In some cases, however, problems arise during the pregnancy that place the woman and her unborn child at risk. Regular prenatal care serves to detect these potential complications quickly so that effective care can be provided. This chapter focuses on problems that primarily occur during pregnancy, those with a gestational onset.

Care of the Woman with Hyperemesis Gravidarum

Nausea and vomiting of mild to moderate intensity are common during early pregnancy, affecting at least 75% of pregnant women (Scialli, 1998). Symptoms typically subside early in the second trimester. **Hyperemesis gravidarum,** a relatively rare condition, is excessive vomiting during pregnancy. Hyperemesis can progress to a point at which the woman not only vomits everything she swallows but retches between meals. Dehydration, electrolyte imbalances, acidosis, weight loss, ketonuria, and possibly hepatic and renal damage are attributable to hyperemesis (Cruikshank, Wigtin, & Hays, 1996).

Hyperemesis occurs more frequently in women under age 25 who are primigravidas or multiparous with a history of previous hyperemesis. An association exists with women who are overweight or have a multiple gestation (Wolf, 1996). The cause of hyperemesis during pregnancy is still unclear, but human chorionic gonadotropin (hCG) plays a role. A temporary suppression of thyroid-stimulating hormone occurs in normal pregnancy and is correlated with the rise in hCG. Other mechanisms that may relate to hyperemesis are displacement of the gastrointestinal tract, hypofunction of the anterior pituitary gland and adrenal cortex, abnormalities of the corpus luteum, and psychologic factors (Nageotte, Briggs, Towers, & Astrat, 1996). Interestingly, hyperemesis is rare in populations of developing countries (Williams, 1996).

In severe cases, the pathology of hyperemesis begins with dehydration. This leads to fluid-electrolyte imbalance and alkalosis from the loss of hydrochloric acid. More prolonged vomiting can result in loss of predominantly alkaline intestinal juices and the occurrence of acidosis. Hypovolemia from dehydration leads to hypotension and increased pulse rate, with increased hematocrit and blood urea nitrogen levels and decreased urine output. Severe potassium loss (hypokalemia) interferes with the ability of the kidneys to concentrate urine and disrupts cardiac functioning. Starvation causes muscle wasting and severe protein and vitamin deficiencies. Jaundice, hyperpyrexia, and peripheral neuritis may develop.

The diagnostic criteria for hyperemesis include a history of intractable vomiting in the first half of pregnancy, dehydration, ketonuria, and a weight loss of 5% of prepregnancy weight.

Clinical Therapy

The goals of treatment include controlling vomiting, correcting dehydration, restoring electrolyte balance, and maintaining adequate nutrition. If the woman with intractable nausea and vomiting does not respond to frequent small meals of simple carbohydrates and the occasional use of antiemetics, she may require intravenous fluids on an outpatient basis. Typically 1 to 3 liters of lactated Ringer's solution will provide temporary relief (Rayburn & Carey, 1996). Pyridoxine 100 mg added to each liter of IV fluid may help in reducing symptoms (Reece, Hobbins, Mahoney, & Petrie, 1996). If the woman's symptoms do not improve, hospitalization may be necessary.

When hospitalization is required, the initial workup should include an ultrasound to exclude the possibility of molar pregnancy (see page 392). Initially the woman is given nothing by mouth; intravenous fluids are administered to correct dehydration. Potassium chloride is typically added to the IV infusion to prevent hypokalemia (Scialli, 1998). If significant starvation has occurred, supplementation with thiamine, folic acid, and other B vitamins is indicated. Desired urine output is a minimum of 1000 mL/24 hours. Agents commonly used to control nausea and vomiting of hyperemesis gravidarum are phenothiazines (prochlorperazine, chlorpromazine, promethazine) and antihistamines (meclizine, dimenhydrinate, diphenhydramine). The dopamine antagonist metoclopramide or the apomorphine antagonist droperidol may also be helpful (Williams, 1996). If the woman does not respond to this management, total parenteral nutrition may be used to meet the caloric and nutritional needs of the woman and her fetus.

When the woman's condition has improved, oral feedings are started. Six small dry feedings followed by clear liquids is one suggested treatment. Another method is 1 oz of water offered each hour, followed as tolerated by clear, then nourishing liquids, progressing on succeeding days to low-fat soft and regular diets. Outpatient or home care is available to help the woman maintain enteral and parenteral nutritional therapies while staying at home. This option has the added benefit of giving the home care nurse the opportunity to observe family interactions and assess the home environment.

NURSING CARE MANAGEMENT

Nursing Assessment and Diagnosis

When a woman is hospitalized for control of vomiting, the nurse must regularly assess the amount and character of further emesis, intake and output, fetal heart rate, maternal vital signs, initial weight, evidence of jaundice or bleeding, and the woman's emotional state.

Nursing diagnoses that may apply to the woman with hyperemesis gravidarum include the following:

- ***Altered Nutrition: Less than Body Requirements*** related to persistent vomiting secondary to hyperemesis
- ***Fear*** related to the effects of hyperemesis on fetal well-being

Nursing Plan and Implementation

Community-Based Nursing Care

The initial evaluation of the woman is designed to distinguish between morning sickness, which is amenable to self-care, and real nutritional risk. The nurse should take this opportunity to evaluate possible family and lifestyle stressors. It is wise to include both the woman and her family in the discussion of strategies to reduce nausea and vomiting she can try at home, including such tactics as resting with her feet up and head elevated or slowly sipping carbonated beverages when nauseated. Herbal tea, such as spearmint, peppermint, raspberry, chamomile, or ginger root, may be helpful. Odors, exposure to fresh air, very hot or cold liquids, ice, and straws should be avoided. If the nausea and vomiting progress to a point where oral intake is not tolerated and dehydration is evident, medical intervention is required.

Home Care Parenteral therapy provided at home in collaboration with a physician and registered dietitian is sometimes used to allow the woman to remain in her home and help decrease health care costs. It also gives the nurse an opportunity to observe family interactions and evaluate the home environment. This assessment is often useful in determining the pregnant woman's level of support, any significant stressors in her life, her understanding of nutrition and self-care measures, and so forth.

Hospital-Based Care

Nursing care should be supportive and directed at maintaining a relaxed, quiet environment away from food odors or offensive smells. Once oral feedings are started, food should be attractively served. Oral hygiene is important because the mouth is dry and may be irritated from vomitus. Weight gain or loss should be monitored regularly. Because emotional factors have been found to play a major role in this condition, psychotherapy may be recommended. With proper treatment, the prognosis is favorable.

Teaching for Self-Care

As part of client teaching, the nurse should review actions the woman can take to prevent or decrease nausea. These are discussed in Chapter 12.

Evaluation

Expected outcomes of nursing care include the following:

- The woman is able to explain hyperemesis gravidarum, its therapy, and its possible effects on her pregnancy.
- The woman's condition is corrected, and possible complications are avoided. ●

Care of the Woman with a Bleeding Disorder

During the first and second trimesters of pregnancy the major cause of bleeding is **abortion.** This is the expulsion of the fetus prior to viability, which is considered 20 weeks' gestation or weight of less than 500 g (Cunningham et al, 1997). Abortions are either spontaneous, occurring naturally, or induced, occurring as a result of artificial or mechanical interruption. **Miscarriage** is a lay term applied to spontaneous abortion.

Other complications that can cause bleeding in the first half of pregnancy are ectopic pregnancy and gestational trophoblastic disease. In the second half of pregnancy, particularly in the third trimester, the two major causes of bleeding are placenta previa and abruptio placentae.

General Principles of Nursing Intervention

Spotting is relatively common during pregnancy and can occur following sexual intercourse or exercise as a result of trauma to the highly vascular cervix. However, the woman is advised to report any spotting or bleeding that occurs during pregnancy so that it can be evaluated.

It is often the nurse's responsibility to make the initial assessment of bleeding. In general, the following nursing measures should be implemented for pregnant women being treated for bleeding disorders:

- Monitor blood pressure and pulse frequently.
- Observe woman for behaviors indicative of shock, such as pallor, clammy skin, perspiration, dyspnea, or restlessness.
- Count pads and weigh pads to assess amount of bleeding over a given time period; save any tissue or clots expelled.
- If pregnancy is of 12 weeks' gestation or beyond, assess fetal heart tones with a Doppler.
- Prepare for intravenous therapy. There may be standing orders to start IV therapy on bleeding clients.
- Prepare equipment for examination.
- Have oxygen therapy available.

- Collect and organize all data, including antepartal history, onset of bleeding episode, laboratory studies (hemoglobin, hematocrit, and hormonal assays).
- Obtain an order to type and cross-match for blood if there is evidence of significant blood loss.
- Assess coping mechanisms and support system of woman in crisis. Give emotional support to enhance her coping abilities by continuous, sustained presence, by clear explanation of procedures, and by communicating her status to her family. Most importantly, prepare the woman for possible fetal loss. Assess her expressions of anger, denial, guilt, depression, or self-blame.
- Assess the family's response to the situation.

Spontaneous Abortion

Many pregnancies end in the first trimester as a result of spontaneous abortion. Statistics are inaccurate because some women may have aborted without being aware that they were pregnant during the early weeks of gestation, when the bleeding may be seen as a heavy menstrual period. If these very early abortions are included, the actual incidence of spontaneous abortion may be as high as 50% to 78% (Coddington, 1996). However, when only clinically recognized pregnancies are considered, the incidence falls to 10% to 15% (Simpson, 1996). Up to 5% of childbearing couples experience two consecutive miscarriages; about 1% experience three or more (Scott & Branch, 1998).

When a spontaneous abortion occurs, the woman and her family may search for a cause so that they can plan knowledgeably for future family expansion. However, even with current technology and medical advances, a direct cause cannot always be determined.

A majority of first trimester spontaneous abortions are related to chromosomal abnormalities. Other causes include teratogenic drugs, faulty implantation due to abnormalities of the female reproductive tract, a weakened cervix, placental abnormalities, chronic maternal diseases, endocrine imbalances, and maternal infections. Some people believe that psychic trauma, alcohol consumption, and accidents are primary causes of abortion, but statistics do not support this belief.

The pathophysiology of spontaneous abortion differs according to the cause. In most cases, embryonic death occurs, which results in loss of hCG and decreased progesterone and estrogen levels. The uterine decidua is then sloughed off (vaginal bleeding), and the uterus becomes irritable, contracts, and usually expels the embryo/fetus. In late spontaneous abortion, the cause is usually a maternal factor, for example, incompetent cervix or maternal disease, and fetal death may not precede the onset of abortion.

Spontaneous abortion can be extremely distressing to the couple desiring a child. Chances for carrying the next pregnancy to term after one spontaneous abortion are as good as they are for the general population. Thereafter, however, chances of successful pregnancy decrease with each succeeding abortion. Following two to three consecutive losses, a woman and her partner should be evaluated and are candidates for genetic counseling (Coddington, 1996).

Classification

Spontaneous abortions are subdivided into the following categories so that they can be differentiated clinically:

1. *Threatened abortion.* Unexplained bleeding, cramping, or backache indicate that the fetus may be in jeopardy. Bleeding may persist for days. The cervix is closed. It may be followed by partial or complete expulsion of pregnancy (Figure 16–1). Evaluation for hydatidiform mole or ectopic pregnancy is advisable.
2. *Imminent abortion.* Bleeding and cramping increase. The internal cervical os dilates. Membranes may rupture. The term *inevitable abortion* also applies.
3. *Complete abortion.* All the products of conception are expelled. The uterus is contracted and the cervical os may be closed.
4. *Incomplete abortion.* Part of the products of conception are retained, most often the placenta. The internal cervical os is dilated.
5. *Missed abortion.* The fetus dies in utero but is not expelled. Uterine growth ceases, breast changes regress, and the woman may report a brownish vaginal discharge. The cervix is closed. Diagnosis is made based on history, pelvic examination, and a negative pregnancy test and may be confirmed by ultrasound if necessary. If the fetus is retained beyond 4 weeks, fetal autolysis (breakdown of cells or tissue) results in the release of thromboplastin, and disseminated intravascular coagulation (DIC) may develop.
6. *Habitual abortion.* Abortion occurs consecutively in three or more pregnancies.
7. *Septic abortion.* Presence of infection. Septic abortion is less common since the availability of legal abortion. May occur with prolonged, unrecognized rupture of the membranes, pregnancy with intrauterine device (IUD) in utero, or criminal attempts to terminate a pregnancy.

Clinical Therapy

One of the more reliable indicators of potential spontaneous abortion is the presence of pelvic cramping and backache. These symptoms are usually absent in bleeding caused by polyps, ruptured cervical blood vessels, or cervical erosion.

Evaluations to help determine the cause of vaginal bleeding include ultrasound scanning for the presence

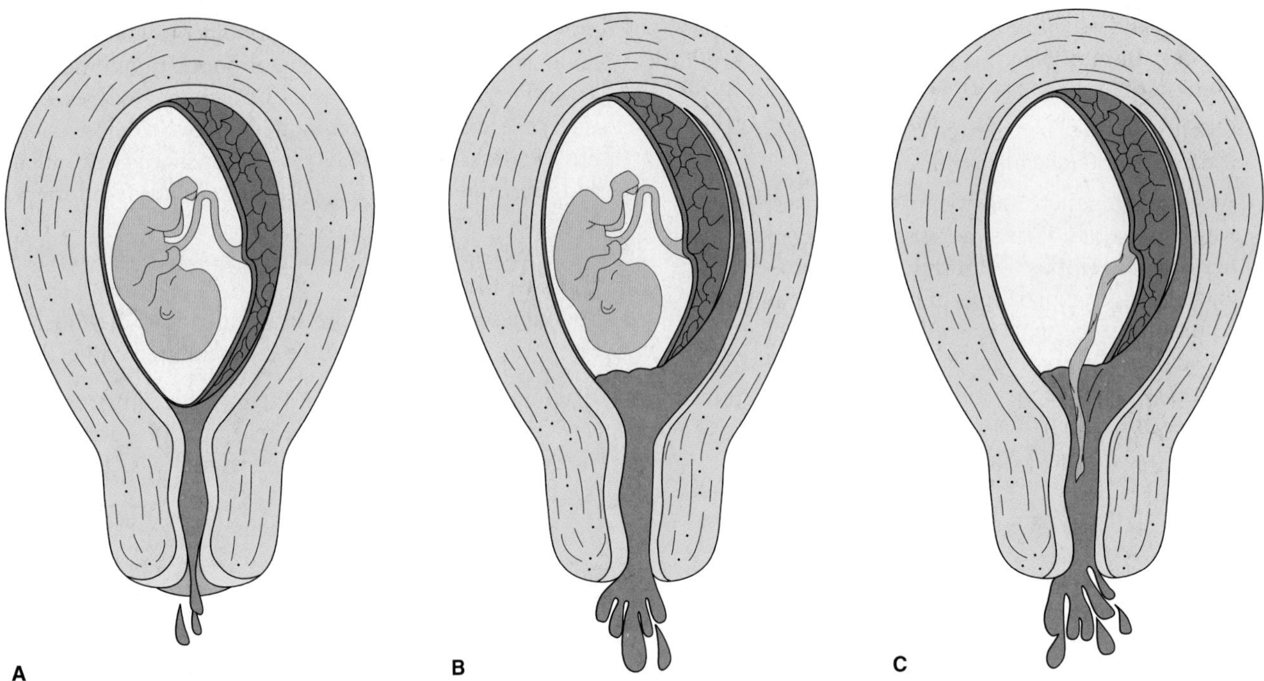

FIGURE 16–1 Types of spontaneous abortion. ***A,*** Threatened. The cervix is not dilated, and the placenta is still attached to the uterine wall, but some bleeding occurs. ***B,*** Imminent. The placenta has separated from the uterine wall, the cervix has dilated, and the amount of bleeding has increased. ***C,*** Incomplete. The embryo/fetus has passed out of the uterus; however, the placenta remains.

of cardiac activity or a gestational sac and laboratory determination of hCG level. The latter can confirm a pregnancy, but because the hCG level falls slowly after fetal death, it cannot confirm a live embryo/fetus. Hemoglobin and hematocrit levels are obtained to assess blood loss. Blood is typed and cross-matched for possible replacement needs.

The therapy prescribed for the pregnant woman with bleeding is bed rest, abstinence from coitus, and perhaps sedation. If bleeding persists and abortion is imminent or incomplete, the woman may be hospitalized, intravenous therapy or blood transfusions may be started to replace fluid, and dilation and curettage or suction evacuation is performed to remove the remainder of the products of conception. If the woman is Rh negative and not sensitized, Rh immune globulin (RhoGAM) is given within 72 hours. (See discussion on Rh sensitization later in this chapter.)

In missed abortions, the products of conception eventually are expelled spontaneously. If this does not occur within 1 month to 6 weeks after fetal death, hospitalization is necessary. Suction evacuation, or dilation and curettage, is done if the pregnancy is in the first trimester. Beyond 12 weeks' gestation, induction of labor by intravenous oxytocin and intra-amniotic prostaglandin $F_{2\alpha}$, intravaginal prostaglandin E_2, or intravaginal misoprostol (a synthetic prostaglandin E_1 analog) may be used to expel the dead fetus.

Currently major research is underway to determine the effectiveness of a variety of treatment approaches for repeat early pregnancy loss, such as administration of intravenous immune globulin (IVIG) alone or in conjunction with progesterone suppositories, heparin administration, and administration of the partner's leukocytes to the pregnant woman, but results are not yet available (Scott & Branch, 1998).

CRITICAL THINKING QUESTION

What questions would you ask a woman who is 8 weeks pregnant and calls to report that she is having a small amount of vaginal bleeding? What recommendations would you make to this woman?

NURSING CARE MANAGEMENT

Nursing Assessment and Diagnosis

The nurse assesses the amount and appearance of any vaginal bleeding and monitors the woman's vital signs and degree of discomfort. The woman's blood type and antibody status should be identified to determine the need for RhoGAM (see page 424). If the pregnancy is 10 to 12 weeks or more, fetal heart rate should be assessed by

Doppler. The nurse also assesses the responses of the woman and her family to this crisis and evaluates their coping mechanisms and ability to comfort each other.

Nursing diagnoses that may apply include the following:

- ***Fear*** related to possible pregnancy loss
- ***Pain*** related to abdominal cramping secondary to threatened abortion
- ***Anticipatory Grieving*** related to expected loss of unborn child

Nursing Plan and Implementation

Community-Based Nursing Care

If a woman in her first trimester of pregnancy begins cramping or spotting, she may be evaluated on an outpatient basis if the bleeding is not heavy. Providing emotional support is an important task for nurses caring for women who have spontaneously aborted. Couples who approached the pregnancy with feelings of joy and a sense of expectancy now feel grief, sadness, and possibly anger.

Because many women, even with planned pregnancies, feel some ambivalence initially, guilt is a common emotion. The woman may harbor negative feelings about herself, ranging from lowered self-esteem resulting from a belief that she is lacking or abnormal in some way, to a notion that the abortion may be a punishment for some wrongdoing.

The nurse can offer invaluable psychologic support to the woman and her family by encouraging them to verbalize their feelings, allowing them the privacy to grieve, and listening sympathetically to their concerns about this pregnancy and future ones. The nurse can aid in decreasing any feelings of guilt or blame by supplying the woman and her family with information regarding the causes of spontaneous abortion and possibly referring them to clergy or other health care professionals for additional help, such as a genetic counselor if there is a history of habitual abortions.

The grieving period following a spontaneous abortion usually lasts 6 to 24 months. Many couples can be helped during this period by an organization or support group established for parents who have lost a fetus or newborn.

We lost our baby together. I know, you could say I never really had a baby, except during those few hours when it was already over and done with, but I guess these things aren't entirely logical. I loved my baby. . . . Absorbed in pain and self-pity, still I was flooded with adoration for this tiny, not yet shaped baby who had lived in me.
~ A Midwife's Story ~

The physical pain of the cramps and the amount of bleeding may be more severe than a couple anticipates, even when they are prepared for the possibility of an abortion. Nurses need to be aware that couples feel unprepared for their first experience of spontaneous abortion. Nurses should offer support in dealing with the physical experience by explaining why the discomfort is occurring and by offering analgesics for pain relief.

Hospital-Based Nursing Care

A suction dilation and curettage (D & C) is performed if the woman experiences an incomplete or missed abortion. This can be performed on an outpatient basis, and, barring any complications, the woman can return home a few hours after the procedure with instructions for self-care. An Rh negative woman with a negative antibody screen should be given RhoGAM prior to discharge.

Teaching for Self-Care

If the woman had a D & C, a competent adult should remain with her for the first 12 to 24 hours. The pregnant woman is instructed to report all episodes of heavy bleeding, fever, foul-smelling vaginal discharge, or abdominal tenderness to her health care provider. The woman who experiences a pregnancy loss requires information about possible causes of the loss and the chances of recurrence with a future pregnancy. She may also require information about the grief process so she is prepared for it when she goes home. In addition, she should receive information about available resources, including support groups to help her cope with her feelings related to the loss of the pregnancy. The woman's partner or a family member should be included in the educational process when possible to assist him or her in personal grief work as well as to provide tools to help support the woman through the loss.

Evaluation

Expected outcomes of nursing care include the following:

- The woman is able to explain spontaneous abortion, the treatment measures employed in her care, and long-term implications for future pregnancies.
- The woman suffers no complications.
- The woman and her partner are able to begin verbalizing their grief and recognize that the grieving process usually lasts several months. ●

Ectopic Pregnancy

Ectopic pregnancy is an implantation of a fertilized ovum in a site other than the endometrial lining of the uterus. It may result from a number of different causes, including tubal damage caused by pelvic inflammatory disease; previous pelvic or tubal surgery; endometriosis; previous ectopic pregnancy; presence of an IUD; high

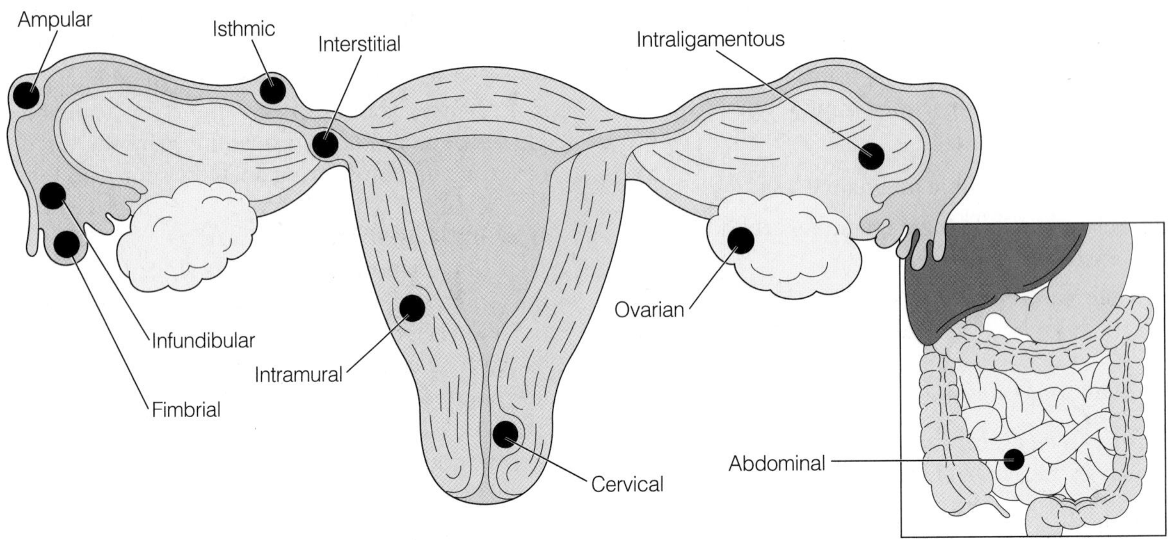

FIGURE 16–2 Various implantation sites in ectopic pregnancy. The most common site is within the fallopian tube, hence the name "tubal pregnancy."

levels of progesterone, which can alter the motility of the egg in the fallopian tube; congenital anomalies of the tube; in vitro fertilization; advanced maternal age; and douching (Reece et al, 1995).

The incidence of ectopic pregnancy in the US has risen dramatically from 4.5 per 1000 pregnancies in 1970 to 19.7 in 1992 (Mortality and Morbidity Weekly Report [MMWR], 1995). Because maternal mortality from other causes is declining, ectopic pregnancy is now the primary cause of maternal mortality in the first trimester of pregnancy.

The actual pathogenesis of ectopic pregnancy occurs when the fertilized ovum is prevented or slowed in its progress down the tube. The fertilized ovum implants in either the fallopian tube or the ovary, peritoneal cavity, cervix, or uterine cornua (Figure 16–2). The most common location for implantation of an ectopic pregnancy is the ampulla of the tube.

Initially, the normal symptoms of pregnancy may be present, specifically, amenorrhea, breast tenderness, and nausea. The hormone hCG is present in the blood and urine. With an ectopic implantation, the trophoblastic cells grow into the adjacent tissue, often the tubal wall, and arterial vessels. This results in internal hemorrhage. The faulty implantation of the placenta causes fluctuation of hormone levels. Hormones first stimulate the endometrial lining of the uterus to grow, but fluctuation in levels cannot support the endometrium, and vaginal bleeding ensues. The implanted ovum quickly begins to rupture the fallopian tube if it is implanted there. The woman may experience one-sided lower abdominal pain or diffuse lower abdominal pain and vasomotor disturbances such as fainting or dizziness. In about 50% of cases, referred right shoulder pain occurs from blood irritating the subdiaphragmatic phrenic nerve.

In many instances, the symptoms are not obvious. One-fourth of ectopic pregnancies may involve uterine enlargement. Physical examination usually reveals adnexal tenderness; an adnexal mass is palpable in approximately one-half of the cases.

If internal hemorrhage is profuse, the woman rapidly develops signs of hypovolemic shock. More commonly, the bleeding is slow (chronic), and the abdomen gradually becomes rigid and very tender. If bleeding into the pelvic cavity has been extensive, vaginal examination causes extreme pain, and a mass of blood may be palpated in the cul-de-sac of Douglas.

Laboratory tests may reveal low hemoglobin and hematocrit levels and rising leukocyte levels. In a normal pregnancy β-hCG titers double every 48 hours from 3 to 6 weeks gestation. Ectopic pregnancies are associated with β-hCG titers that increase more slowly.

Clinical Therapy

It is important to differentiate an ectopic pregnancy from other disorders with similar clinical presenting pictures. Consideration must be given to possible spontaneous abortion, ruptured corpus luteum cyst, appendicitis, salpingitis, torsion of the ovary, ovarian cysts, and urinary tract infection.

The measures below are used to establish the diagnosis of ectopic pregnancy and assess the woman's status:

- A careful assessment of menstrual history, particularly the LMP.
- Careful pelvic exam to identify any abnormal pelvic masses and tenderness.
- Laboratory testing as described previously.
- Ultrasonography. In a normal pregnancy, transvaginal ultrasound should detect an intrauterine gesta-

tional sac when the β-hCG is greater than 1500 mIU/mL. By transabdominal scan, an intrauterine sac may not be identified until the β-hCG levels reach 6500 mIU/mL. Confirming an intrauterine pregnancy nearly eliminates the diagnosis of ectopic pregnancy.

- Laporoscopy. If the presence or absence of an ectopic pregnancy cannot be confirmed by other measures, laporoscopic intervention may be necessary for both diagnosis and treatment.

Once an ectopic pregnancy is confirmed, therapy options are reviewed with the woman. Medical management using methotrexate is indicated for the woman who desires future pregnancy if her ectopic pregnancy is unruptured and of 3.5 cm size or less and if her condition is stable. In addition, there must be no fetal cardiac motion, the woman must have no evidence of thrombocytopenia or leukopenia and must be free of kidney or liver disease. The medication is administered intramuscularly. As an outpatient, the woman is monitored for increasing abdominal pain. β-hCG titers are monitored regularly. β-hCG titers increase for 1 to 4 days and then decrease. As many as one-fourth of women require a second dose of methotrexate (ACOG, 1998).

If surgery is indicated and the woman desires future pregnancies, a laparoscopic linear salpingostomy will be performed to evacuate the ectopic pregnancy gently and preserve the tube. If the tube is ruptured or if future childbearing is not an issue, laparoscopic salpingectomy (removal of the tube) is performed. If the woman is in shock and unstable, an abdominal incision will be made. During surgery, the most important risk to be considered is potential hemorrhage. Bleeding must be controlled, and replacement therapy should be on hand. The Rh negative nonsensitized woman is given Rh_o(D) immune globulin to prevent sensitization.

NURSING CARE MANAGEMENT

Nursing Assessment and Diagnosis

When the woman with a suspected ectopic pregnancy is admitted to the hospital, the nurse assesses the appearance and amount of vaginal bleeding. The nurse monitors vital signs, particularly blood pressure and pulse, for evidence of developing shock.

It is also the nurse's responsibility to assess the woman's emotional status and coping abilities and to evaluate the couple's informational needs. If surgery is necessary, the nurse performs the ongoing assessments appropriate for any client postoperatively.

Nursing diagnoses that may apply for a woman with an ectopic pregnancy include the following:

- ***Anticipatory Grieving*** related to the loss of the pregnancy
- ***Pain*** related to abdominal bleeding secondary to tubal rupture
- ***Knowledge Deficit*** related to lack of information about treatment of ectopic pregnancy and its long-term implications

Nursing Plan and Implementation

Community-Based Nursing Care

Women with ectopic pregnancy are often seen initially in a clinic or office setting. Nurses need to be alert to the possibility of ectopic pregnancy if a woman presents with complaints of abdominal pain and lack of menses for 1 to 2 months. Once an initial evaluation is complete, if no ultrasound is available, the woman should be referred to another facility where ultrasound is available. The nurse plays an important role in monitoring the woman's condition and in providing her with information.

A woman with a confirmed ectopic pregnancy who meets the criteria for methotrexate administration is followed as an outpatient. The nurse should advise the woman that some abdominal pain is common following the injection but it is generally mild and lasts only 24 to 48 hours. More severe pain might indicate treatment failure and should be evaluated. The woman should also report heavy vaginal bleeding, dizziness, or tachycardia (ACOG, 1998). In addition, the nurse should stress the need to return for follow-up hCG testing.

For all women treated for ectopic pregnancy, a follow-up phone call by the nurse may be especially welcome. It gives the woman the opportunity to ask any questions she may have. In addition, the nurse can use the opportunity to assist the woman in dealing with her grief.

Hospital-Based Nursing Care

Once a diagnosis of ectopic pregnancy is made and surgery is scheduled, the nurse starts an IV as ordered and begins preoperative teaching. The nurse should report signs of developing shock to the physician immediately and initiate interventions. If the woman is experiencing severe abdominal pain, the nurse can administer appropriate analgesics and evaluate their effectiveness.

Teaching for Self-Care

Teaching is an important part of nursing care. The woman may want her condition and various procedures explained. She may need instruction regarding measures to prevent infection, symptoms to report (pain, bleeding, fever), and her follow-up visit.

The woman and her family will need emotional support during this difficult time. Their feelings and responses to this crisis will probably be similar to those that occur in cases of spontaneous abortion. As a result, similar nursing actions are required.

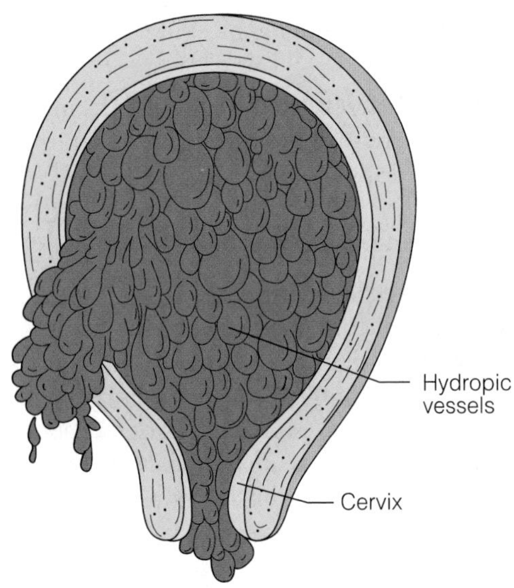

FIGURE 16–3 Hydatidiform mole. A common sign is vaginal bleeding, often brownish (the characteristic "prune juice" appearance) but sometimes bright red. In this figure, some of the hydropic vessels are being passed. This occurrence is diagnostic for hydatidiform mole.

Evaluation

Expected outcomes of nursing care include the following:

- The woman is able to explain ectopic pregnancy, treatment alternatives, and implications for future childbearing.
- The woman and her caregivers detect possible complications early and manage them appropriately.
- The woman and her partner are able to begin verbalizing their loss and recognize that the grieving process usually lasts several months. ●

Gestational Trophoblastic Disease

Gestational trophoblastic disease (GTD) includes partial or complete hydatidiform mole, invasive mole (chorioadenoma destruens), and choriocarcinoma.

Hydatidiform mole (molar pregnancy) is a disease in which (1) abnormal development of the placenta occurs, resulting in fluid-filled, grapelike clusters; and (2) the trophoblastic tissue proliferates. The significance of this disease for the woman who has it is the loss of the pregnancy and the possibility, though remote, of developing choriocarcinoma, a form of cancer, from the trophoblastic tissue.

Molar pregnancies are classified into two types, complete and partial, both of which meet the above criteria. Little is known about the cause of either type, but some of the pathophysiology has been clarified. The *complete mole* develops from an anuclear ovum that contains no maternal genetic material, an "empty" egg. In most cases, a haploid sperm, 23X, fertilizes the egg and duplicates before the first cell division. The conceptus then contains in its cells a 46XX chromosomal set of totally paternal origin (Berkowitz, Goldstein, & Bernstein, 1996). The embryo dies very early, when just a few millimeters long and before embryo-placental circulation has been established. Therefore, the hydropic (fluid-filled) vesicles that form from the chorionic villi are avascular in the complete mole. No embryonic or fetal tissue or membranes are found. Choriocarcinoma seems to be associated primarily with the complete mole.

The *partial mole* usually has a triploid karyotype, that is, 69 chromosomes. Most often, a normal ovum with 23 chromosomes is fertilized by two sperm (dispermy) or by a sperm that has failed to undergo the first meiosis and therefore contains 46 chromosomes. In about one-fifth of the cases, the ovum did not undergo reduction division, so it contains 46 chromosomes and is fertilized by a normal sperm (Berkowitz et al, 1996).

In partial molar pregnancy, the villi are often vascularized and may be hydropic only in sections of the placenta rather than universally as with a complete mole. Often partial moles are recognized only after spontaneous abortion, or they may go unnoticed. Unlike the complete mole, the fetus usually survives to 8 or 9 weeks' gestation and occasionally longer. Twin pregnancies in which a normal fetus coexists with a molar pregnancy have been reported (Copeland & Landon, 1996).

The incidence of GTD varies significantly worldwide. In the United States, hydatidiform mole occurs in about 1 in 1000 to 1500 pregnancies. In Japan, however, the incidence may be as high as 2 in 500 pregnancies (Copeland & Landon, 1996). The incidence of molar pregnancy increases with extremes in maternal age and has a familial tendency. The risk of repeat molar pregnancy has been reported as 1% after one molar pregnancy. After two molar pregnancies, the risk of developing a mole in subsequent pregnancy is about 20% (Berkowitz et al, 1996).

Invasive mole (chorioadenoma destruens) is similar to a complete mole but involves the uterine myometrium. Treatment is the same as for a complete mole.

Clinical Therapy

Diagnosis of hydatidiform mole is often suspected in the presence of the following signs:

- Vaginal bleeding is almost universal with molar pregnancies and may occur as early as the fourth week or as late as the second trimester. It is often brownish, "like prune juice," due to liquefaction of the uterine clot, but it may be bright red.
- Anemia occurs frequently due to the loss of blood.

- Hydropic vesicles may be passed and, if so, are diagnostic (Figure 16–3). With a partial mole, the vesicles are often smaller and may not be noticed by the woman.
- Uterine enlargement greater than expected for gestational age is a classic sign, present in about 50% of cases. In the remainder of cases, the uterus is appropriate or small for the gestational stage. Enlargement is due to the proliferating trophoblastic tissue and to a large amount of clotted blood.
- Absence of fetal heart sounds in the presence of other signs of pregnancy is a classic sign of molar pregnancy. (Only rarely has a viable fetus been born in a partial molar pregnancy.)
- Markedly elevated serum hCG may be present due to continued secretion by the proliferating trophoblastic tissue.
- Very low maternal serum α-fetoprotein level (MSAFP)
- Hyperemesis gravidarum may occur, probably as a result of the high levels of hCG.
- Pregnancy-induced hypertension (PIH) may be seen, especially if the molar pregnancy continues into the second trimester. Because PIH is a disease of late pregnancy, if symptoms occur in the first half of pregnancy, molar pregnancy must be considered as the first diagnosis.

Ultrasound is the primary means of diagnosing a molar pregnancy, usually after 6 to 8 weeks, when the vesicular enlargement of the villi can be identified.

Therapy begins with suction evacuation of the mole and curettage of the uterus to remove all fragments of the placenta. Early evacuation decreases the possibility of other complications. If the woman is older and has completed her childbearing, or if there is excessive bleeding, hysterectomy may be the treatment of choice to reduce the incidence of malignant sequelae.

Complications associated with hydatidiform mole that require medical recognition and therapy include the following:

- Anemia
- Hyperthyroidism
- Infection, usually seen with late diagnosis and spontaneous abortion of the mole
- Disseminated intravascular coagulation (DIC)
- Trophoblastic embolization of the lung, usually seen after molar evacuation of a significantly enlarged uterus (this creates a cardiorespiratory emergency)
- Theca-lutein ovarian cysts, which may be small or large enough to displace the uterus

Malignant GTD, usually choriocarcinoma, develops following evacuation of a mole in 20% of women. To detect this serious problem early and initiate treatment, follow-up care is essential. Follow-up consists of baseline chest x-ray examination to detect metastasis; physical examination, including pelvic exam; and regular measurements of serum hCG levels. Initially, hCG levels are monitored weekly until a normal level is obtained for 3 consecutive weeks; hCG levels are rechecked 2 to 4 weeks after the first normal level to confirm the finding; hCG levels are then monitored every month for 6 months, then every 2 months for 6 months (Oi, 1996).

Effective contraception is needed during this time to prevent pregnancy and the resulting confusion about the cause of changes in hCG levels. In addition, pregnancy could mask an hCG rise associated with malignant GTD.

Continued high or rising hCG levels in women who have had molar pregnancy but are not currently pregnant indicate malignant GTD (choriocarcinoma). Treatment at a center specializing in GTD is advised. Once pregnancy has been ruled out, full physical examination, chest x-ray exam, abdominopelvic CT scan, and brain CT scan are done to rule out metastatic spread. Chemotherapy is then begun using methotrexate alone or in combination with other chemotherapy agents.

After treatment, careful follow-up monitoring of hCG levels is important. Malignant GTD is curable if diagnosed early and treated appropriately. Malignant sequelae appear to be increased with repetitive moles (Oi, 1996).

NURSING CARE MANAGEMENT

Nursing Assessment and Diagnosis

It is important for nurses involved in antepartal care to be aware of symptoms of hydatidiform mole and observe for them at each antepartal visit. The classic symptoms used to diagnose molar pregnancy are found more frequently with the complete than with the partial mole. The partial mole may be difficult to distinguish from a missed abortion prior to evacuation.

When the woman is hospitalized for evacuation of the mole, the nurse should monitor vital signs and vaginal bleeding for evidence of hemorrhage. In addition, the nurse determines whether abdominal pain is present and assesses the woman's emotional state and coping ability.

Nursing diagnoses that may apply to a woman with a hydatidiform mole include the following:

- ***Fear*** related to the possible development of choriocarcinoma
- ***Knowledge Deficit*** related to a lack of understanding of the need for regular monitoring of hCG levels
- ***Anticipatory Grieving*** related to the loss of the pregnancy

CRITICAL THINKING IN PRACTICE

Your friend Rachel Glassman is 6 months pregnant and mentions to you that she is developing symptoms of a bladder infection. She has had several bladder infections over the past few years and feels she has warded off others by increasing her fluid intake and drinking acidic juices. She tells you she plans to use the same approach this time because she just had her prenatal appointment last week. She assures you that if symptoms persist, she will discuss it with her caregiver at her next prenatal visit. What advice would you give her?

Answers can be found in Appendix I.

Nursing Plan and Implementation

Community-Based Nursing Care

When molar pregnancy is suspected, the woman needs emotional support. The nurse can relieve some of the woman's anxiety by answering questions about the disease process and explaining what ultrasound and other diagnostic procedures will entail. If a molar pregnancy is diagnosed, the nurse supports the childbearing family as they deal with their grief about the lost pregnancy. Health care counselors, the hospital chaplain, or their own clergy may be of assistance in helping them deal with this loss.

Hospital-Based Nursing Care

When the woman is hospitalized for evacuation of the mole, explanation of the curettage procedure is necessary. Although the physician is responsible for providing this explanation, the woman and her partner may have many questions and concerns that the nurse can discuss with them. The nurse may also clarify areas of confusion or misunderstanding.

Typed and cross-matched blood must be available for surgery because of previous blood loss and the potential for hemorrhage. Oxytocin is administered to keep the uterus contracted and prevent hemorrhage. In addition, acute renal failure, a syndrome of rapid onset, may occur when significant hemorrhage results in absolute loss of fluid volume. Following surgery, the nurse carefully observes the woman's urinary output, watches for further signs of bleeding, and assesses for any signs of infection.

If the woman is Rh negative and not sensitized, she is given $Rh_o(D)$ immune globulin to prevent antibody formation. (See discussion on Rh sensitization later in this chapter.)

Teaching for Self-Care

The woman needs to know the importance of the follow-up visits. She is advised to use contraception to delay becoming pregnant again until after the follow-up program is completed.

Evaluation

Expected outcomes of nursing care include the following:

- The woman has a smooth recovery following successful evacuation of the mole.
- The woman is able to explain GTD, its treatment, follow up, and long-term implications for pregnancy.
- The woman and her partner are able to begin verbalizing their grief at the loss of their anticipated child.
- The woman is able to discuss the importance of follow-up assessment and indicates her willingness to cooperate with the regimen. ●

Placenta Previa

In placenta previa, the placenta is improperly implanted in the lower uterine segment, sometimes over the internal os. As the lower uterine segment contracts and the cervix dilates in the later weeks of pregnancy, the placental villi are torn from the uterine wall, thus exposing the uterine sinuses at the placental site. Bleeding begins, but because its amount depends on the number of sinuses exposed, it may initially be either scanty or profuse. The classic symptom is painless vaginal bleeding usually occurring after 20 weeks' gestation. See Chapter 22 for an in-depth discussion of placenta previa.

Abruptio Placentae

Abruptio placentae is the premature separation of a normally implanted placenta from the uterine wall. It occurs prior to birth, usually during the labor process. See Chapter 22 for an in-depth description of abruptio placentae.

Care of the Woman with an Incompetent Cervix

Many questions remain unanswered about **incompetent cervix.** The classic definition presents cervical incompetence as painless dilatation of the cervix without contractions. The woman is usually unaware of contractions and presents with advanced effacement and dilatation and, possibly, bulging membranes. The emerging view is that cervical incompetence and *cervical resistance* to labor occur as a continuum from complete incompetence through, perhaps, excessive *competence* demonstrated by those women who have prolonged labors (Iams, 1997).

Factors that may contribute to the tendency for the cervix to dilate prematurely can be divided into two categories: congenital incompetence and acquired incompetence. Congenitally incompetent cervix may be found in women exposed to diethylstilbestrol (DES) or those with a bicornuate uterus. Acquired cervical incompetence may be related to inflammation, infection, subclinical uterine activity, cervical trauma, or increased uterine volume (as with a multiple gestation).

Incompetent cervix occurs in 0.1 to 1.0% of all pregnancies and is responsible for up to 20% of all midtrimester fetal losses (Niebyl, 1996). A woman's obstetric history may give her health care provider an indication of increased risk for incompetent cervix. Factors include repetitive second trimester losses, previous preterm birth, progressively earlier births with each subsequent pregnancy, short labors, previous elective abortion or cervical manipulation, DES exposure, or other uterine anomaly. These women will benefit from close surveillance of cervical length with transvaginal ultrasound beginning at about 18 weeks' gestation. Cervical effacement occurs from the internal os out and can be seen on ultrasound as "funneling." Alteration is apparent in transvaginal scan when fundal pressure is applied or the woman assumes a standing position. Fully 100% give birth prematurely. In addition, women at risk for incompetent cervix need to be informed early in pregnancy of warning signs of impending birth, such as lower back pain, pelvic pressure, and changes in vaginal discharge.

Incompetent cervix has been managed by a variety of methods. Women who are at risk and have cervical lengths of 25 to 30 mm may be managed conservatively with bed rest, avoidance of heavy lifting, and no coitus. For those who have had previous losses, an elective cervical cerclage may be placed late in the first trimester or early in the second trimester. A cervical cerclage involves using a heavy suture to reinforce the cervix at the level of the internal os. The McDonald cerclage utilizes a purse-string technique high up on the cervix to tie it closed. The Shirodkar method uses a submucosal band placed at the level of the internal os (Iams, 1996a). An emergency cerclage may be performed for women who have advanced effacement or dilatation with or without prolapsing fetal membranes. In this situation, tocolytics (drugs that stop labor) and broad-spectrum antibiotics are given preoperatively and for 24 to 48 hours postoperatively.

The woman assumes the Trendelenburg position to help reduce pressure on the cervix. Cerclage should not be placed if intra-amniotic infection, fetal death, fetal anomaly, vaginal bleeding, or premature rupture of the membranes exists. Vaginal cultures should be done to identify bacterial vaginosis, group B streptococcus, or sexually transmitted infections.

Following an uncomplicated elective cerclage, the woman is discharged after 24 to 48 hours. An emergency cerclage, however, requires hospitalization for 5 to 7 days or longer. After 37 completed weeks' gestation, the suture may be cut and vaginal birth permitted, or the suture may be left in place and a cesarean birth performed to avoid repeating the procedure in subsequent pregnancies.

Care of the Woman with Premature Rupture of Membranes

Spontaneous rupture of the membranes prior to the onset of labor is known as **premature rupture of membranes (PROM).** Some authorities define PROM as the rupture of the bag of waters any time before the onset of labor; others require that a specific period elapse without labor, generally between 1 and 12 hours. Preterm PROM has been described as rupture before 37 weeks' gestation. Prolonged rupture of the membranes is rupture more than 24 hours before birth (Haeyl & Williams, 1996; Reece et al, 1996).

Although the cause of PROM is unknown, a variety of factors correlate with its occurrence. An incompetent cervix may be the cause of second trimester PROM. Cervicitis, urinary tract infection (UTI), amniocentesis, placenta previa, abruptio placentae, hydramnios, trauma, multiple pregnancy, and maternal genital tract anomalies may also result in PROM. Other risk factors include smoking, substance abuse, connective tissue disorders, fetal anomalies, and lower socioeconomic status (Reece et al, 1996).

A clinical diagnosis of chorioamnionitis occurs in approximately 10% of cases of PROM (Iams, 1996a). Preterm labor occurs in most circumstances in which intrauterine infection is present, contributing to neonatal morbidity and mortality.

Preterm PROM occurs in about 1% of all pregnancies but accounts for one-third of all preterm births, making it the leading cause of these births (Lovett, Weiss, Diogo, Williams, & Garite, 1997). The onset of labor occurs within 24 hours in 60% to 80% of women with preterm PROM, which means that 20% to 40% may have a latency period of 7 days or more (Haeyl & Williams, 1996).

Maternal Risks

Maternal risk is related to infection, specifically chorioamnionitis (intra-amniotic infection resulting from bacterial invasion and inflammation of the membranes before birth) and endometritis (infection of the endometrium postpartally that may be related to chorioamnionitis or may occur independently) (Garite & Spellacy, 1994).

Abruptio placentae occurs more frequently in women with PROM. It is not clear whether infection causes inflammation of the decidua, which facilitates

TABLE 16–1 Currently Used Plans for Women with Premature Rupture of Membranes

Preterm
Expectant management (observation); birth when labor or clinical infection develops
Fetal pulmonary status determined by amniotic fluid testing; birth if fetus is mature
Risk of infection determined by amniotic fluid Gram stain, white cell count, glucose and culture; maternal white cell count and C-reactive protein, assessment for maternal fever or uterine tenderness; assessment for fetal well-being through electronic fetal monitoring or ultrasound for biophysical profile scoring; birth if infection develops
Administration of corticosteroids, with or without birth in 48 hours after first dose; tocolytics as needed
Birth after an arbitrary latent period (eg, 16–72 hours)
Assess for group B streptococci (or *Neisseria gonorrhoeae*); treatment indicated if positive
Combinations of the above
Term
Induction if spontaneous labor does not begin in approximately 12 hours, or if cervix is ripe, or if there are other complications (eg, PIH)
Expectant management for women with uncomplicated pregnancies and cervix unfavorable for induction

premature separation, or whether the bleeding episode contributes to a weakening of the membranes, which eventually leads to rupture (Reece et al, 1996).

Fetal-Neonatal Risks

The most common neonatal complication in pregnancies involving PROM before 37 weeks' gestation is respiratory distress syndrome (RDS) (see Chapter 29), which occurs in 10% to 40% of newborns. Infection is documented in less than 10% of newborns. The preterm fetus is further jeopardized by the associated risks of malpresentation (especially breech) and prolapse of the umbilical cord (see Chapter 25). Perinatal mortality largely depends on gestational age (Kappy et al, 1993).

Umbilical cord compression may occur related to decreased amniotic fluid volume and may result in fetal asphyxia and, in severe cases, death. When membranes rupture very early in gestation, marked oligohydramnios may result in intrauterine growth restriction, hypoplastic lungs, and limb deformities due to compression. There are conflicting opinions as to whether PROM accelerates pulmonary maturation of fetuses.

Clinical Therapy

Any time a woman complains of watery vaginal discharge or a sudden gush of fluid, rupture of the membranes must be considered. The woman should be questioned regarding the time of initial loss of fluid, the color, consistency, amount, and any odor noted. These questions not only help to determine whether there is blood, meconium, or vernix present, but also may help to differentiate PROM from increased vaginal secretions associated with infection or preterm labor, urinary incontinence, normal leukorrhea of pregnancy, or the passage of the mucus plug.

During the initial physical inspection, any fluid leaking from the vaginal introitus can be checked with nitrazine paper. This test relies on the fact that amniotic fluid is more alkaline (pH 7.0 to 7.5) than normal vaginal secretions (pH 4.5 to 5.5). A color change in the paper to blue-green or blue is highly suggestive of ruptured membranes. Factors that can yield a false positive result are contamination of the fluid with blood, semen, urine, or antiseptic cleansers (Heyl & Williams, 1996). The elevated pH associated with the bacterial vaginosis can also lead to misleading results. If there is copious fluid leaking from the vaginal introitus, the diagnosis of PROM is considered confirmed.

If further evaluation is required, a sterile speculum exam is done. Unless the woman is in active labor, direct digital exam of the cervix or vagina is avoided until a management plan has been determined. Speculum exam relies on gross pooling of amniotic fluid in the vaginal vault. The woman can be asked to "bear down," performing a Valsalva maneuver, if fluid is not visualized in the vagina. The woman may also remain in a supine position for several hours to allow collection of fluid to occur; the exam is then repeated. In addition to performing a nitrazine test on the fluid, a fern test can be performed by applying a thin sample of secretions onto a clean slide and looking for microscopic evidence of a fernlike pattern (see Chapter 19). Vaginal cultures for group B streptococcus, *Chlamydia*, and *Gonorrhea* may be obtained at this time. Ultrasound can be used to look for reduced amniotic fluid.

In situations in which the diagnosis of PROM cannot be made with any certainty, an amniocentesis may be performed to instill either indigo carmine or Evan's blue dye. A tampon is inserted in the vagina for several hours and then is inspected for blue tinged fluid. The woman should be warned that as the dye is absorbed, it will temporarily change her urine to a green color.

Concurrently, fetal well-being should be assessed through a fetal heart rate tracing or biophysical profile. In addition, the gestational age of the fetus must be calculated in order to decide on a management plan (see Table 16–1). At greater than 36 weeks' gestation, labor will begin in 50% of women within 12 hours (Ghidini & Romero, 1996). Labor induction may be delayed for 12 to 24 hours unless a situation exists that would preclude expectant management.

Management of PROM in the absence of infection and gestation of less than 37 weeks is usually conservative. Amniocentesis may be done to evaluate for intra-amniotic infection. Fetal lung maturity studies will also be done if the fetus is nearing 34 weeks' gestation (American Academy of Pediatrics [AAP] & American College of Obstetricians and Gynecologists [ACOG], 1997). The woman is hospitalized on bed rest. An admission complete blood count (CBC), C-reactive protein (CRP), and urinalysis are obtained. Regular nonstress tests (NSTs) or biophysical profiles are used to monitor fetal well-being. Maternal blood pressure, pulse, and temperature are assessed every 4 hours. Regular laboratory evaluations should be performed to detect maternal infection. After initial treatment and observation, if leaking of fluid ceases, some women may be followed at home (Heyl & Williams, 1996). The woman is advised to continue bed rest (with bathroom privileges), monitor her temperature four times a day, and avoid intercourse, douches, and tampons. The woman is advised to contact her physician and return to the hospital if she has fever, uterine tenderness or contractions, increased leakage of fluid, decreased fetal movement, or a foul vaginal discharge. Weekly NSTs should be continued.

Authorities disagree regarding the ideal management of preterm PROM. Prophylactic antibiotics are often administered for the first 48 hours while awaiting culture results. If vaginal cultures are positive, antibiotics will be continued for at least 7 days. If amniotic fluid studies indicate a low glucose level, high white blood cell (WBC) count, a positive Gram stain, or organisms in the fluid, immediate birth is indicated. When a cervical cerclage is in place, it should be removed promptly (Queenan & Hobbins, 1996; Iams, 1996a).

Corticosteroid administration remains somewhat controversial. The 1994 National Institutes of Health Consensus Conference concluded that antenatal steroid administration is effective in reducing respiratory distress syndrome. Antenatal steroid treatment is associated with a significant decrease in the incidence of neonatal intraventricular hemorrhage and a reduction of necrotizing enterocolitis (Iams, 1996b). Because of concern regarding immunosuppression related to steroid administration, the debate centers on the risks and benefits for glucocorticoid administration in the presence of PROM. It is common practice to use antenatal steroid between 24 and 32 to 34 weeks' gestation unless fetal pulmonary maturity can be documented. (See Drug Guide: Betamethasone.)

Use of tocolytics is generally not indicated in the woman who has ruptured membranes. Short-term use of tocolytics may be considered, however, to allow a course of steroids to be delivered.

NURSING CARE MANAGEMENT

Nursing Assessment and Diagnosis

Determining the duration of the rupture of membranes is a significant component of the antepartal assessment. The nurse asks the woman when her membranes ruptured and when contractions began because the risk of infection may be directly related to the time involved. Gestational age is determined to prepare for the possibility of a preterm birth. The nurse observes the mother for signs and symptoms of infection, especially by reviewing her WBC, CRP, temperature, and pulse rate, and the character of her amniotic fluid. If the mother has a fever, the nurse checks hydration status. Fetal heart rate tracings should be watched for tachycardia, loss of variability, or decelerations. When a preterm or cesarean birth is anticipated, the nurse evaluates the childbirth preparation and coping abilities of the woman and her partner.

Nursing diagnoses that may be used with PROM include the following:

- ***Risk for Infection*** related to premature rupture of membranes
- ***Impaired Gas Exchange*** in the fetus related to compression of the umbilical cord secondary to prolapse of the cord
- ***Risk for Ineffective Individual Coping*** related to unknown outcome of the pregnancy

Nursing Plan and Implementation

Nursing actions should focus on the woman, her partner, and the fetus. Uterine activity and fetal response to the labor are evaluated, but vaginal exams are not done unless absolutely necessary. The woman is encouraged to rest on her right or left side to promote optimal uteroplacental perfusion. Comfort measures may help promote rest and relaxation. The nurse must also ensure that hydration is maintained, particularly if the woman's temperature is elevated.

Teaching for Self-Care

Education is another important aspect of nursing care. The couple needs to understand the implications of PROM and all treatment methods. It is important to address side effects and alternative treatments. The couple needs to know that although the membranes are ruptured, amniotic fluid continues to be produced.

Providing psychologic support for the couple is critical. The nurse may reduce anxiety by listening empathetically, relaying accurate information, and providing explanations of procedures. It may be necessary to prepare the couple for a cesarean birth, a preterm newborn, and the possibility of fetal or neonatal demise.

Evaluation

Expected outcomes of nursing care include the following:

- The woman's risk of infection and cord prolapse are decreased.
- The couple is able to discuss the implications of PROM and all treatment options.
- The pregnancy is maintained without trauma to the mother or fetus. ●

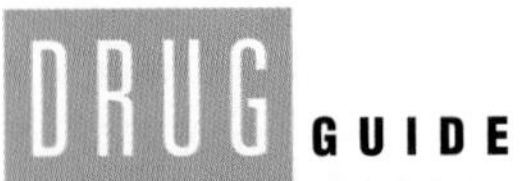

Betamethasone (Celestone Solupan)

Overview of Maternal-Fetal Action

Studies have provided ample evidence that glucocorticoids such as betamethasone are capable of inducing pulmonary maturation and decreasing the incidence of respiratory distress syndrome in preterm infants. The mechanism by which corticosteroids accelerate fetal lung maturity is unclear, but it is related to the stimulation of enzyme activity by the drug. The enzyme is required for biosynthesis of surfactant by the type II pneumocytes. Surfactant is of major importance to the proper functioning of the lung in that it decreases the surface tension of the alveoli. Glucocorticoids also increase the rate of glycogen depletion, which leads to thinning of the interalveolar septa and increases the size of the alveoli. The thinning of the epithelium brings the capillaries into closer proximity with the air spaces and improves oxygen exchange.

Route, Dosage, Frequency

Prenatal maternal intramuscular injections of 12 mg of betamethasone are given once a day for 2 days. Dexamethasone may also be given in doses of 6 mg every 12 hours for four doses (NIH Consensus Development Conference, 1994). To obtain maximum results, birth should be delayed for at least 24 hours after completing the first round of treatment. The effect of corticosteroids may be transient. Currently, it is suggested that the treatment regimen be repeated every week up to 34 weeks' gestation for the undelivered fetus with an immature lung profile.

Contraindications

Inability to delay birth
Adequate L/S ratio
Presence of a condition that necessitates immediate birth (eg, maternal bleeding)
Presence of maternal infection, diabetes mellitus, hypertension
Gestational age greater than 34 completed weeks

Maternal Side Effects

Increased risk for infection has not been supported in large studies. There may, however, be some increase in the incidence of infection in women with premature rupture of the membranes. Maternal hyperglycemia may occur during corticosteroid administration. Insulin-dependent diabetics may require insulin infusions for several days to prevent ketoacidosis. Corticosteroids possibly may increase the risk of pulmonary edema, especially when used concurrently with tocolytics (Iams, 1996a; NIH Consensus Development Conference, 1994).

Effects on Fetus/Neonate

Lowered cortisol levels at birth, but rebound occurs by 2 hours of age
Hypoglycemia
Increased risk of neonatal sepsis
Animal studies have shown serious fetal side effects such as reduced head circumference, reduced weight of the fetal adrenal and thymus glands, and decreased placental weight. Human studies have not shown these effects, however.

Nursing Considerations

Assess for presence of contraindications.
Provide education regarding possible side effects.
Administer betamethasone deep into gluteal muscle, avoiding injection into deltoid (high incidence of local atrophy). (Dexamethasone may be administered IM or IV.)
Periodically evaluate BP, pulse, weight, and edema.
Assess lab data for electrolytes and blood glucose.
Although concomitant use of betamethasone and tocolytic agents has been implicated in increased risk of pulmonary edema, the betamethasone has little mineral corticoid activity; therefore, it probably doesn't add significantly to the salt and water retention effects of beta-adrenergic agonists. Other causes of noncardiogenic pulmonary edema should also be investigated if pulmonary edema develops during administration of betamethasone to a woman in preterm labor.

Care of the Woman at Risk Due to Preterm Labor

Labor that occurs between 20 and 37 completed weeks of pregnancy is referred to as **preterm labor.** Prematurity continues to be the number one perinatal and neonatal problem in the United States today—it is estimated that 8% of all births in the United States and 15% of births from socioeconomically underprivileged populations occur prior to 37 weeks' gestation (AAP & ACOG, 1997). Risk factors that play a role in the development of preterm labor can be categorized as obstetric, medical, or sociodemographic (Iams, 1996a). Despite the use of risk scoring systems for the identification of women at risk, the use of tocolytic therapy, and home uterine activity monitoring, the rate of preterm births in the United States has not changed significantly in the past 40 years (Heyl & Williams, 1996).

Table 16–2 presents a list of risk factors for spontaneous preterm birth.

Maternal Risks

The major risks for the woman involve psychologic stress factors related to her concern for her unborn child. Physiologic maternal risks are related to possible medical treatments for preterm labor, such as tocolysis and prolonged bed rest, or are related to the cause of preterm labor, such as hemorrhage from placental abruption or placenta previa.

RESEARCH IN PRACTICE

What is this study about? Many neonatal deaths occur as a result of preterm birth or birth occurring before 37 weeks' gestation. Preterm babies often have very low birth weights, and if they survive, they contribute to morbidity, mortality, and health care costs for children. The most common method of managing preterm birth is through the management of preterm labor. Often, following an in-hospital stabilization period, the woman will self-manage her preterm labor at home with periodic visits to her health care provider. In spite of potential adverse consequences related to prolonged bed rest and stressed family relationships, little has been documented about the experience of self-managed preterm labor. Roberta Durham designed a grounded theory study to explore the process of managing preterm labor at home.

How was the study done? The investigator's convenience sample of 25 women managing preterm labor at home met the following criteria: pregnancies of less than 36 weeks' gestation, minimum 21 years of age, English-speaking, and able to give consent. From audiotaped, transcribed participant interviews, the researcher used grounded theory methodology to identify codes, develop categories and themes, and explicate theory. Ongoing discussion with a group of substantive experts and affirmation of analysis from research participants strengthened the credibility and validity of the emerging theory.

What were the results of the study? Three temporal phases of managing preterm labor emerged from the data, with the first being the diagnostic phase or the period of gathering information and settling in at home. The negotiation phase included balancing family, career, and household needs with the prescription for bed rest (the common method of managing preterm labor). The third, or preparation, phase focused on preparing for the impending birth. The negotiation phase placed the woman in multiple situations where the needs generated by her roles conflicted with the activity restrictions used to manage preterm labor at home. The women used three major strategies to resolve these conflicts: testing, cheating, and piggybacking. With testing, the woman would extend the limits of the activity restriction and monitor the consequences. Cheating occurred when the woman performed activities restricted by their medical providers. Piggybacking resulted from adding a prohibited activity to a medically sanctioned activity.

How can I use this study? Students can discuss the phases and strategies used by these women for managing activity restrictions at home when caring for women with preterm labor. If the woman recognizes utilization of the same strategies, the student and the woman may be able to problem-solve together to resolve demands that may result in cheating or piggybacking.

SOURCE: Durham, R. F. (1998). Strategies women engage in when managing preterm labor at home. *Journal of Perinatology, 18*(1), 61–64.

Fetal-Neonatal Risks

Mortality increases for neonates born before 37 weeks' gestation. Although the preterm infant is faced with many maturational deficiencies (fat storage, heat regulation, immaturity of organ systems), the most critical factor is the lack of development of the respiratory system—to the extent that life cannot be supported. In some instances, such as severe maternal diabetes or serious isoimmunization, continuation of the pregnancy may be more life-threatening to the fetus than the hazards of prematurity. See Chapter 29 for in-depth consideration of the preterm newborn.

TABLE 16–2 Risk Factors for Spontaneous Preterm Labor

Multiple gestation	Cervical shortening < 1 cm
DES exposure	Uterine irritability
Known cervical incompetence	Age (<18 or >35)
Polyhydramnios	Low socioeconomic status
Uterine anomaly	Cigarettes—more than 10/day
Cervix dilated > 1 cm at 32 weeks	Substance abuse
Second trimester abortion	Poor weight gain
Fetal abnormality	More than 2 first trimester abortions
Febrile illness	Non-white race
Bleeding after 12 weeks	Cervical cerclage in situ
History of pyelonephritis or other maternal infection	In vitro fertilization (singleton or multiple gestation)
Maternal medical disease	STI (trichomoniasis, chlamydia, bacterial vaginosis)
Previous preterm birth	
Previous preterm labor with term birth	Anemia
Abdominal surgery during 2nd or 3rd trimester	Abdominal trauma
	Foreign body (IUD)
History of cone biopsy	

Clinical Therapy

Prompt diagnosis of preterm labor is difficult because many symptoms that are common in normal pregnancy may herald the onset of preterm labor. These include the following:

- Abdominal pain
- Back pain
- Pelvic pain
- Menstrual-like cramps
- Vaginal bleeding
- Increased vaginal discharge (may be pinkish stained)
- Pelvic pressure
- Urinary frequency
- Diarrhea

Some women have frequent contractions without change in the cervix. In these women, a clinical assay for fetal fibronectin (fFN) may aid in diagnosis. Fetal fibronectin is an extracellular matrix protein that is normally found in the fetal membranes and the decidua. The presence of fFN after 20 weeks' gestation is abnormal until near term, when it appears again. Fetal fibronectin testing has been found to be valuable in predicting spontaneous preterm birth within 7 days of testing (Iams, 1996a; Escher-Davis, 1996).

Assessing cervical length by transvaginal ultrasonography is another diagnostic tool. A cervical length of at

TABLE 16–3 Criteria for Diagnosis of Preterm Labor

Gestation 20–37 weeks

and

Documented uterine contractions
(4/20 minute, 8/60 minute)

and

Documented cervical change

or

Cervical effacement of 80%

or

Cervical dilatation 1 cm

SOURCE: American Academy of Pediatrics & American College of Obstericians and Gynecologists: *Guidelines for Perinatal Care,* 4th ed. Washington, DC: Author, 1997 p 128.

least 30 mm is good evidence that the woman is not in preterm labor.

A woman suspected of being in preterm labor should have a digital cervical examination and be observed for a minimum of 1 to 2 hours to determine uterine activity. At the end of this time, the cervix should be reexamined, preferably by the same person, to determine whether there has been any change in effacement or dilatation. Preterm labor is often associated with urinary tract infections, so it is prudent to obtain a clean catch or catheterized urine specimen in order to identify and treat infection. Table 16–3 summarizes common criteria for diagnosing preterm labor.

No attempt is made to stop labor if any of the following conditions exist (Reece et al, 1995):

- Fetal demise
- Lethal fetal anomaly
- Severe preeclampsia/eclampsia
- Hemorrhage/abruptio placentae
- Chorioamnionitis
- Maternal cardiac disease
- Poorly controlled diabetes mellitus, hypertension, or thyrotoxicosis
- Fetal maturity
- Acute fetal distress

The initial management of preterm labor is directed toward maintaining good uterine profusion, detecting uterine contractions, and assessing fetal well-being. Maternal laboratory studies include CBC, CRP, vaginal cultures, and uterine cultures. Amniotic fluid cultures are sometimes done to rule out intra-amniotic infection as a cause of preterm labor.

The goal of clinical therapy is to prevent preterm labor from advancing to a point that no longer responds to medical treatment. Hydration has long been used to decrease the frequency of uterine contractions, but there has been no scientific support for the practice. IV hydration with large quantities of hypertonic fluids increases the risk of pulmonary edema and should be used with caution (Urbanski, 1997).

Tocolysis is the use of medications in an attempt to stop labor. If the cervix is dilated more than 3 to 4 cm and more than 50% effaced, the effect of tocolytics on labor is reduced. If labor cannot be arrested, the priority becomes successful preterm birth and management of its psychologic effect on the woman and her partner.

Drugs currently used for tocolysis include beta-adrenergic agonists (also called β-mimetics), magnesium sulfate ($MgSO_4$), prostaglandin synthetase inhibitors, and calcium channel blockers. The β-mimetics (ritodrine [Yutopar] and terbutaline sulfate [Brethine]) and magnesium sulfate are the most widely used tocolytics. Although ritodrine is FDA approved for use in preterm labor, it is much less frequently employed than terbutaline, which is not FDA approved for this use. Terbutaline and magnesium sulfate are preferred for treating preterm labor because they are effective and significantly less expensive than ritodrine (Heyl & Williams, 1996).

Although tocolytic drugs do suppress contractions and allow prolongation of pregnancy, they may cause significant side effects, the most serious of which is maternal pulmonary edema. Reducing the dose and duration of therapy sometimes decreases side effects.

Currently, preterm labor is initially treated with IV tocolytics, typically magnesium sulfate. Therapy with $MgSO_4$ is indicated in women with cardiopulmonary disease, diabetes, or infection; in all other cases, the selection of $MgSO_4$ or β-mimetics depends on the experience of the health care providers. Once uterine activity is stopped, the woman can be weaned to subcutaneous terbutaline for a short time and then is placed on oral tocolysis.

Although preventing preterm labor is the primary goal of tocolysis, delaying birth can significantly reduce neonatal morbidity and mortality by providing time for fetal therapy and transfer to a tertiary care center if necessary. The ACOG Committee on Obstetric Practice (1994) recommends that corticosteroids (typically betamethasone or dexamethasone) be administered antenatally to women at risk of preterm birth because of their beneficial effect on fetal lung maturation. Any women who are candidates for tocolysis are candidates for antenatal corticosteroids, regardless of fetal gender, race, or availability of surfactant therapy for the newborn, especially between 24 and 34 weeks' gestation (ACOG, 1994).

Magnesium sulfate, long used in the treatment of PIH, has been gaining favor in the treatment of preterm labor because it is effective and has fewer side effects than beta-adrenergic agonists. The usual recommended loading dose is 4 to 6 g IV over 20 to 30 minutes. The maintenance dose is then 2 to 4 g/hour titrated to deep tendon reflexes and serum magnesium levels. The therapy is maintained for 12 to 24 hours at the lowest rate to significantly diminish contractions. The maternal serum level that is usually necessary for tocolysis seems to be 5.5 to 7.5 mg/dL (Heyl & Williams, 1996).

Side effects with the loading dose may include flushing, a feeling of warmth, headache, nystagmus, nausea, dry mouth, and dizziness. Other side effects include lethargy and sluggishness and a risk of pulmonary edema if the woman has predisposing conditions such as multiple gestation, infection, or hydramnios; has had excessive IV fluid administration; or concurrent β-sympathomimetic therapy. See Drug Guide: Magnesium Sulfate on page 402 for other side effects. Fetal side effects may include hypotonia and lethargy that persist for 1 or 2 days following birth.

Of the calcium channel blockers approved for use in the United States, nifedipine appears to have the most clinical promise as a tocolytic. Nifedipine acts by reducing the flow of extracellular calcium ions into the intracellular space of the myometrial smooth muscle cells, thereby inhibiting contractile activity (Elliott, 1997). Nifedipine is well absorbed either orally or sublingually. The most common side effects are related to arterial vasodilation, that is, hypotension, tachycardia, facial flushing, and headache. Because the mechanism of action of nifedipine is different from the beta-adrenergic drugs, co-administration of nifedipine and terbutaline or ritodrine may prove beneficial in the treatment of preterm labor. Because both magnesium sulfate and nifedipine block calcium, however, co-administration of them has been implicated in serious maternal side effects related to low calcium levels.

Prostaglandins enhance the formation of myometrial gap junctions and stimulate the influx of intracellular calcium ions needed for muscle contraction. Prostaglandin synthetase inhibitors, therefore, are a logical choice for tocolysis. Indomethacin or sulindac are the prostaglandin synthetase inhibitors most often used to suppress labor. Maternal side effects are few. Dyspepsia, nausea, vomiting, depression, and dizzy spells may occur. On rare occasions, psychosis or renal failure may result. These drugs are best administered with an antacid to reduce the chance of gastrointestinal (GI) upset (Viamontes, 1996).

Indomethacin crosses the placenta readily, and oligohydramnios and premature closure of the fetal ductus arteriosus may occur with long-term use. Consequently the drug is not recommended after 32 weeks' gestation for a course of therapy longer than 48 hours.

Atosiban, a drug with selective effects on the uterus and breast, has been approved for use in a study of preterm labor in humans. Preliminary results show a significant decrease in uterine contraction frequency compared with a control group (Viamontes, 1996).

NURSING CARE MANAGEMENT

Nursing Assessment and Diagnosis

During the antepartal period, the nurse identifies the woman at risk for preterm labor by noting the presence of predisposing factors. The primary areas for ongoing assessment are change in risk status for preterm labor, educational needs of the woman and her loved ones, and the woman's responses to medical and nursing interventions.

Nursing diagnoses that may apply to the woman with preterm labor include the following:

- ***Knowledge Deficit*** related to lack of information about causes, identification, and treatment of preterm labor
- ***Fear*** related to early labor and birth
- ***Ineffective Individual Coping*** related to need for constant attention to pregnancy

Nursing Plan and Implementation

Community-Based Nursing Care

Once uterine activity stops, the woman is sometimes placed on oral tocolysis. She may then be discharged and followed by home care nurses or as part of a specialized prematurity prevention program.

Home Care

Home care frequently involves programs that combine home monitoring of uterine activity with daily contact between the woman and a nurse. The monitor consists of a contraction sensor belt the woman wears around her abdomen. A small electronic recorder worn at the waist collects and transmits uterine activity data via the telephone to be interpreted by a nurse at a receiving center. The woman also receives in-depth education about the signs and symptoms of preterm labor and how to palpate for contractions. If uterine activity is excessive or if symptoms are reported, the woman is referred to her certified nurse-midwife or physician for prompt evaluation.

Although the combination of the electronic monitor and nursing care seems to be effective, it is not clear at this point whether the value lies in the electronic monitor or in the education and follow-up by a nurse (Devoe, 1996). In spite of this controversy, home uterine activity monitoring continues to be widely used.

Once at home, the woman usually receives weekly or biweekly visits from the home care nurse. During visits from the home care nurse, physical assessments similar to those done in the hospital are completed. Weekly cervical exams may be performed to enhance detection of preterm labor. Consideration of the woman's ability to care for herself, the impact of the changes in relationships that will occur, and care of any young children in the home are among the issues that affect the woman's ability to cope effectively with this situation. The home care nurse needs to be alert to any signs that the woman is failing to achieve the emotional and developmental tasks of pregnancy, such as lack of maternal attachment. An individualized nursing management plan helps focus on each woman's specific needs.

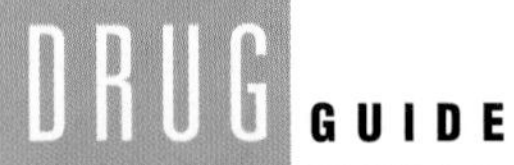

Magnesium Sulfate ($MgSO_4$)

Pregnancy Risk Category: B

Overview of Obstetric Action

$MgSO_4$ acts as a CNS depressant by decreasing the quantity of acetylcholine released by motor nerve impulses and thereby blocking neuromuscular transmission. This action reduces the possibility of convulsion, which is why $MgSO_4$ is used in the treatment of preeclampsia. Because magnesium sulfate secondarily relaxes smooth muscle, it may decrease the blood pressure, although it is not considered an antihypertensive. $MgSO_4$ may also decrease the frequency and intensity of uterine contractions; as a result it is also used as a tocolytic in the treatment of preterm labor.

Route, Dosage, Frequency

$MgSO_4$ is generally given intravenously to control dosage more accurately and prevent overdosage. An occasional physician still prescribes intramuscular administration. However, it is painful and irritating to the tissues and does not permit the close control that IV administration does. The intravenous route allows for immediate onset of action. It must be given by infusion pump for accurate dosage.

For Treatment of Preterm Labor

Loading dose: 4–6 g $MgSO_4$ in 250 mL solution administered over a 30-minute period.
Maintenance dose: 2–4 g/hour via infusion pump (Iams, 1996).

For Treatment of Preeclampsia

Loading dose: 6 g $MgSO_4$ is administered over a 15–20-minute period.
Maintenance dose: 2 g/hour via infusion pump (Usta & Sibai, 1996).
Note: $MgSO_4$ is excreted via the kidneys. Because women in preterm labor typically have normal renal function, they generally require higher levels of magnesium to achieve a therapeutic range than women who have preeclampsia and may have compromised renal function. Maintenance dose may need to be adjusted based on serum magnesium levels.

Maternal Contraindications

Diagnosed maternal myasthenia gravis is the only absolute contraindication to the administration of $MgSO_4$. A history of myocardial damage or heart block is a relative contraindication to use of the drug because of the effects on nerve transmission and muscle contractility. Extreme care is necessary in administration to women with impaired renal function because the drug is eliminated by the kidneys, and toxic magnesium levels may develop quickly.

Maternal Side Effects

Most maternal side effects are dose related. Lethargy and weakness related to neuromuscular blockade are common. Sweating, a feeling of warmth, flushing, and nasal congestion may be related to peripheral vasodilation. Other common side effects include nausea and vomiting, constipation, visual blurring, headache, and slurred speech. Signs of developing toxicity include depression or absence of reflexes, oliguria, confusion, respiratory depression, circulatory collapse, and respiratory paralysis. Rapid administration of large doses may cause cardiac arrest.

Effects on Fetus/Neonate

The drug readily crosses the placenta. Some authorities suggest that transient decrease in FHR variability may occur; others report that no change occurred. In general $MgSO_4$ therapy does not pose a risk to the fetus. Occasionally, the newborn may demonstrate neurologic depression or respiratory depression, loss of reflexes, and muscle weakness. Ill effects in the newborn may actually be related to fetal growth retardation, prematurity, or perinatal asphyxia.

Nursing Considerations

1. Monitor the blood pressure closely during administration.
2. Monitor maternal serum magnesium levels as ordered (usually every 6–8 hours). Therapeutic levels are in the range of 4.8–9.6 mg/dL. Reflexes often disappear at serum magnesium levels of 8–12 mg/dL; respiratory depression occurs at levels of 15–17 mg/dL; cardiac arrest occurs at levels above 30 mg/dL (Sibai, 1996; Silver, 1996).
3. Monitor respirations closely. If the rate is less than 12/minute, magnesium toxicity may be developing, and further assessments are indicated. Many protocols require stopping the medication if the respiratory rate falls below 12/minute.
4. Assess knee jerk (patellar tendon reflex) for evidence of diminished or absent reflexes. Loss of reflexes is often the first sign of developing toxicity. Also note marked lethargy or decreased level of consciousness and hypotension.
5. Determine urinary output. Output less than 30 mL/hour may result in the accumulation of toxic levels of magnesium.
6. If the respirations or urinary output fall below specified levels or if the reflexes are diminished or absent, no further magnesium should be administered until these factors return to normal.
7. The antagonist of magnesium sulfate is calcium. Consequently, an ampule of calcium gluconate should be available at the bedside. The usual dose is 1 g given IV over a period of about 3 minutes.
8. Monitor fetal heart tones continuously with IV administration.
9. Continue $MgSO_4$ infusion for approximately 24 hours after birth as prophylaxis against postpartum seizures if given for PIH.
10. If the mother has received $MgSO_4$ close to birth, the newborn should be closely observed for signs of magnesium toxicity for 24–48 hours.

NOTE: Protocols for magnesium sulfate administration may vary somewhat according to agency policy. Consequently, individuals are referred to their own agency protocols for specific guidelines.

TEACHING GUIDE: PRETERM LABOR

Assessment During the antepartal period, the woman is usually screened for factors that place her at risk for preterm labor. You may then assess the woman's understanding of the danger of preterm labor, the signs of preterm labor, and the actions she can take to prevent it. If she is on a home monitoring program, assess the woman's understanding of the purpose and rationale for the program.

Nursing Diagnosis The key nursing diagnosis will probably be ***Knowledge Deficit*** related to lack of information about the risks of preterm labor and the self-care measures to prevent it.

Nursing Plan and Implementation Your teaching will focus on the risks of preterm labor, the functions of and procedures for home monitoring, and self-care activities to decrease the risk of preterm labor.

Client Goals At the completion of teaching the woman will be able to:

- Discuss the risks of preterm labor.
- Describe the purpose of home monitoring.
- Demonstrate the correct procedures for doing home monitoring.
- Explain self-care measures that help decrease the risk of preterm labor.

Teaching Plan

Content	*Teaching Method*
• Describe the dangers of preterm labor, especially the risk of prematurity in the infant, and all the potential problems.	*Discuss the risks specifically. Many people understand in a general way that prematurity can be dangerous, but they fail to understand how the baby is affected.*
• Stress the value of home monitoring in evaluating uterine activity on a regular basis. Emphasize that many of the early symptoms of labor, such as backache and increased bloody show, may be subtle initially. Home monitoring can often detect increased uterine activity in the early stages before cervical changes progress to the point where it is impossible to stop labor. Studies have demonstrated that home uterine monitoring programs offer little or no significant difference in preterm delivery compared with clients followed by daily contact with the nurse and no home uterine monitoring (Iams, 1996b).	*Use handouts during the discussion. Help the woman clearly understand the value of the program because, to be successful, it requires a real commitment on her part.*
If the woman is to be part of a home monitoring program, the monitoring nurse will usually do the initial teaching. Be prepared to reinforce the information provided and answer questions that may arise.	*Teach the woman how to palpate for uterine contractions. Do a demonstration and ask for a return demonstration.*
• Summarize self-care measures, such as maintaining generous fluid intake (2 to 3 quarts daily), voiding every 2 hours, avoiding lifting and overexertion, avoiding nipple stimulation or orgasm, limiting sexual activity, and cooperating with activity restrictions and bed rest requirements.	*Use a handout during the discussion. Provide opportunities for discussion. If the woman has concerns about certain recommendations, try to modify the approach to best meet her needs.*

Evaluation At the end of the teaching session the woman will be able to discuss the risks of preterm labor, demonstrate home monitoring techniques and explain their rationale, and implement self-care activities to decrease the risks of preterm labor.

Teaching for Self-Care

Once the woman at risk for preterm labor has been identified, she needs to be taught about the importance of recognizing the onset of labor. Increasing the woman's awareness of the subtle symptoms of preterm labor is one of the most important teaching objectives of the nurse (see Teaching Guide: Preterm Labor). Signs and symptoms of preterm labor include the following:

- Uterine contractions that occur every 10 minutes or less with or without pain
- Mild menstrual-like cramps felt low in the abdomen

TABLE 16–4 Self-Care Measures to Prevent Preterm Labor

Rest two or three times a day lying on your left side.

Drink 2 to 3 quarts of water or fruit juice each day. Avoid caffeine drinks. Filling a quart container and drinking from it will eliminate the need to keep track of numerous glasses of fluid.

Empty your bladder at least every 2 hours during waking hours.

Avoid lifting heavy objects. If small children are in the home, work out alternatives for picking them up, such as sitting on a chair and having them climb on your lap.

Avoid prenatal breast preparation such as nipple rolling or rubbing nipples with a towel. This is not meant to discourage breastfeeding but to avoid the potential increase in uterine irritability.

Pace necessary activities to avoid overexertion.

Sexual activity may need to be curtailed or eliminated.

Find pleasurable ways to help compensate for limitations of activities and boost the spirits.

Try to focus on 1 day or 1 week at a time rather than on longer periods of time.

If on bed rest, get dressed each day and rest on a couch rather than becoming isolated in the bedroom.

SOURCE: Prepared in consultation with Susan Bennett, RN, ACCE, Coordinator of the Prematurity Prevention Program.

- Constant or intermittent feelings of pelvic pressure that may feel like the baby pressing down
- Rupture of membranes
- Low, dull backache, which may be constant or intermittent
- A change in the vaginal discharge (an increase in amount, a change to more clear and watery, or a pinkish tinge)
- Abdominal cramping with or without diarrhea

The woman is also taught to evaluate contraction activity once or twice a day. She does so by lying down tilted to one side with a pillow behind her back for support. The woman places her fingertips on the fundus of the uterus (which is above the umbilicus after 20 weeks' gestation). She checks for contractions (hardening or tightening in the uterus) for about 1 hour. It is important for the pregnant woman to know that uterine contractions occur occasionally throughout the pregnancy. If they occur every 10 minutes for 1 hour, however, the cervix could begin to dilate, and labor could continue.

The nurse ensures that the woman knows when to report signs and symptoms. If contractions occur every 10 minutes (or less) for 1 hour, if any of the other signs and symptoms are present for 1 hour, or if clear fluid begins leaking from the vagina, she should telephone her physician/nurse-midwife, clinic, or hospital birthing unit and make arrangements to be checked for ongoing labor.

If the woman experiences any preterm labor symptoms for more than 15 minutes while physically active, she should be instructed to do the following:

- Empty her bladder.
- Lie down tilted toward her side.
- Drink 3 to 4 (8 oz) cups of fluid.
- Palpate for uterine contractions, and if contractions occur 10 minutes apart or less for 1 hour, notify the health care provider.
- Rest for 30 minutes after the symptoms have subsided, and gradually resume activity.
- Call her health care provider if symptoms persist, even if uterine contractions are not palpable.

Caregivers need to be aware that the woman is knowledgeable and attuned to changes in her body and to take her call seriously. When a woman is at risk for preterm labor, she may have many episodes of contractions and other signs or symptoms. If she is treated positively, she will feel freer to report problems as they arise. Other preventive measures the woman could follow are presented in Table 16–4.

Hospital-Based Nursing Care

Providing supportive nursing care to the woman in preterm labor is important during hospitalization. This care consists of promoting bed rest, monitoring vital signs (especially blood pressure and respirations), measuring intake and output, and continuous monitoring of FHR and uterine contractions. Placing the woman on her left side facilitates maternal-fetal circulation. Vaginal examinations are kept to a minimum. If tocolytic agents are being administered, the mother and fetus are monitored closely for any adverse effects.

Whether preterm labor is arrested or proceeds, the woman and her partner, if he is involved, experience intense psychologic stress. Decreasing the anxiety associated with the unknown and the risk of a preterm newborn is a primary aim of the nurse. The nurse also recognizes the stress of prolonged bed rest and of lack of sexual contact and helps the couple find satisfactory ways of dealing with these stresses. With empathetic communication, the nurse can facilitate the couple's expression of their feelings, which commonly include guilt and anxiety, thereby helping the couple identify and implement coping mechanisms. The nurse also keeps the couple informed about the labor progress, the treatment regimen, and the status of the fetus so that their full cooperation can be elicited. In the event of imminent vaginal or cesarean birth, the couple should be offered brief but ongoing explanations to prepare them for the actual birth process and the events following the birth.

Evaluation

Expected outcomes of nursing care include the following:

- The woman can discuss the cause, identification, and treatment of preterm labor.
- The woman affirms that her fears about early labor are decreased.

- The woman states that she feels comfortable in her ability to cope with her situation and has resources to call on if needed.
- The woman can identify signs and symptoms of preterm labor that need to be reported to her caregiver.
- The woman can describe appropriate self-care measures to initiate in the event that she experiences any preterm labor.
- The woman successfully gives birth to a healthy infant. ●

Care of the Woman with a Hypertensive Disorder

Hypertension is the most common medical disorder in pregnancy, complicating 7% to 10% of all pregnancies. Various attempts have been made to classify these disorders. The following classification is recommended by the American College of Obstetricians and Gynecologists (Sibai, 1996):

- Preeclampsia-eclampsia
- Chronic hypertension
- Chronic hypertension with superimposed preeclampsia
- Late or transient hypertension

Preeclampsia and Eclampsia

Preeclampsia is the most common hypertensive disorder in pregnancy. It is characterized by the development of hypertension, proteinuria, and edema. Because hypertension alone may be present early in the disease process, that finding is the basis for diagnosis.

The definition of preeclampsia is an increase in systolic blood pressure of 30 mm Hg or an increase of diastolic pressure of 15 mm Hg over baseline. These blood pressure changes must be noted on at least two occasions 6 hours or more apart for the diagnosis to be made. Ideally, the blood pressures should be compared with a baseline established in the first trimester. In the absence of baseline values, a blood pressure of 140/90 has been accepted as hypertension.

Preeclampsia and eclampsia are two categories of **pregnancy-induced hypertension (PIH).** The term *preeclampsia* indicates that this is a progressive disease unless there is intervention to control it. **Eclampsia** means "convulsion." If a woman has a convulsion, she is considered "eclamptic." Most often, preeclampsia is seen in the last 10 weeks of gestation, during labor, or in the first 48 hours after childbirth. Although birth of the fetus is the only known cure for preeclampsia, it can be controlled with early diagnosis and careful management.

The cause of PIH remains unknown, despite much research over many decades. The condition's former name, "toxemia of pregnancy," was based on a theory that a toxin produced in a pregnant woman's body caused the disease. The term is no longer applicable, however, because the theory has not been substantiated.

PIH occurs in 10% to 14% of all primigravidas and 5.7% to 7.3% of multiparas. Among black primigravidas, the incidence is 15% to 20%, and in young primigravidas with twin pregnancies it is 30% (Sibai, 1996). It is seen more often in primigravidas, teenagers younger than 18, and women over 35. Women with a family history of PIH are at higher risk for it, as are women with a large placental mass associated with multiple gestation, hydatidiform mole, Rh incompatibility, and diabetes mellitus.

Pathophysiology of PIH

Preeclampsia is a multisystemic disorder characterized by reduced perfusion to maternal organs. Although the etiology of preeclampsia is still unclear, some of the pathophysiologic mechanisms in operation have been uncovered. Two of these mechanisms, vasospasm and early hemodynamic alterations (Figure 16–4), are based on research examining the response of pregnant women to the infusion of pressor agents. Women who develop PIH become more sensitive to pressor agents rather than less sensitive to them, as in normal pregnancy. This response has been linked to the ratio between the prostaglandins prostacyclin and thromboxane. Prostacyclin, a vasodilator produced by endothelial cells, decreases blood pressure, prevents platelet aggregation, and promotes uterine blood flow. Thromboxane, produced by platelets, causes vessels to constrict and platelets to clump together (Brennecke et al, 1995). Prostacyclin is decreased in preeclampsia, allowing the potent vasoconstrictor and platelet-aggregating effects of thromboxane to dominate. These hormones are produced partially by the placenta, which would help explain the reversal of the condition when the placenta is removed and why the incidence is increased when there is a larger than normal placental mass, such as in hydrops, multiple pregnancy, or hydatidiform mole (Sibai, 1996). There also seems to be an increased risk of pregnancy-induced hypertension in women with preexisting vascular disease.

The underlying pathology in preeclampsia seems to be related to maternal vasospasm or vascular endothelial damage. The constricted and dilated areas occur throughout the arterial system as well as in major organs, the uterus, and placenta. Women who develop preeclampsia have been found to have an elevated cardiac output and an associated hyperdynamic vasodilation in the first trimester that causes endothelial damage. The vasodilation acts as a compensatory mechanism, allowing

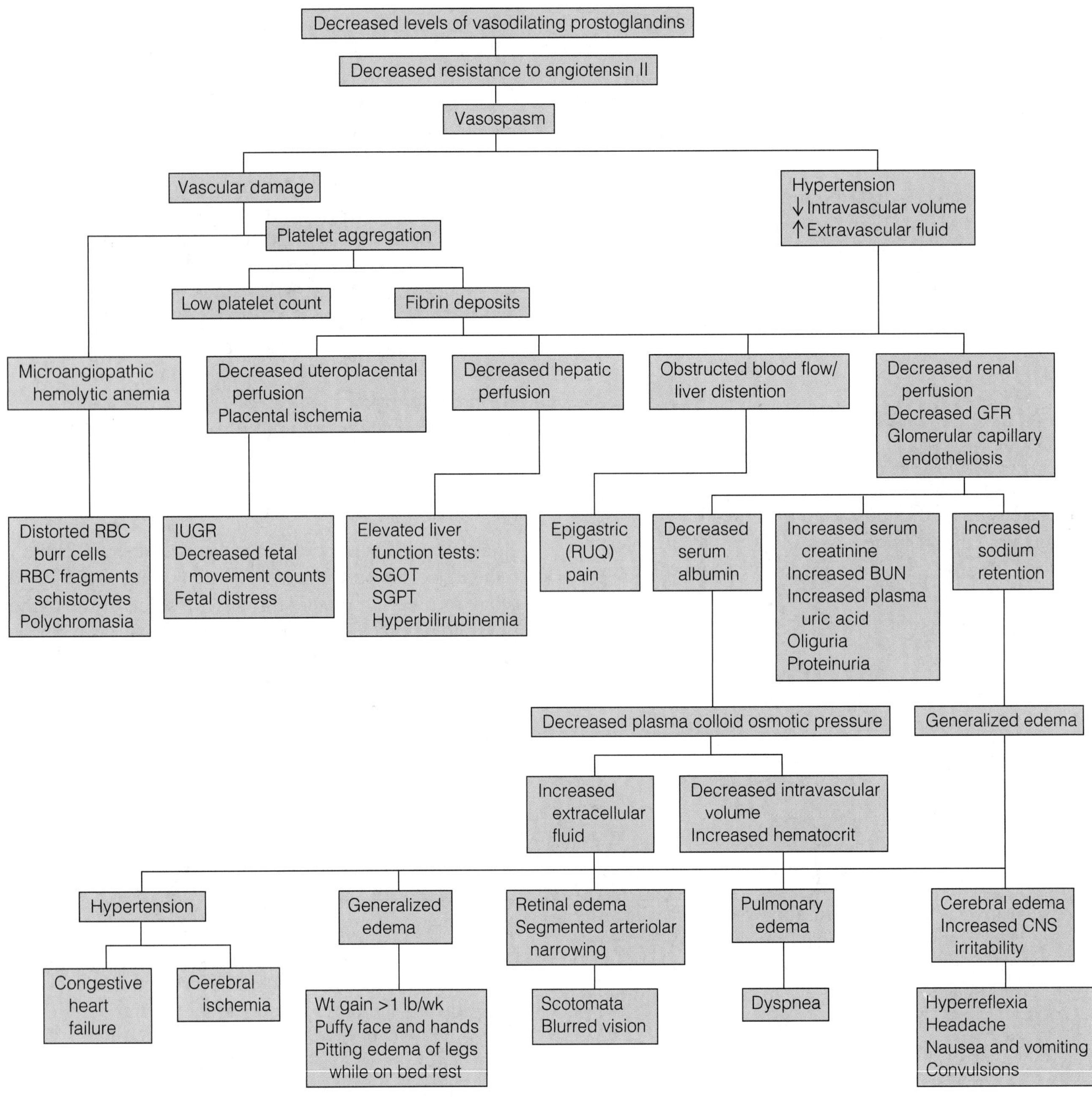

FIGURE 16–4 Clinical manifestations and possible pathophysiology of PIH.

maintenance of a normal blood pressure in spite of the high cardiac output. The vascular endothelium is damaged by the high flow rate and the pressure of the blood rushing through the vessels. The body responds to the endothelial damage with platelet aggregation and adherence to the damaged sites. Platelet aggregation may influence the prostacyclin:thromboxane ratio, affecting the course of the disease. As the disease progresses, the compensatory vasodilation begins to fail. The blood pressure starts to increase, and the systemic vascular resistance (SVR) may increase in an effort to protect end organs from damage. The elevated SVR reduces cardiac output, leading to a low-output, high-resistance state.

Recently, attention has been directed to another theory, which postulates that uteroplacental ischemia acts as a trigger for preeclampsia, with other factors playing contributory roles. Although the prostacyclin-thromboxane imbalance may provide an explanation for the clinical features of preeclampsia, this theory is now being challenged as the primary cause. In the woman with preeclampsia, in addition to a reduced production of the vasoactive substance prostacyclin, there is also a decreased production of nitric oxide. Nitric oxide is a potent vasodilator and important regulator of maternal blood pressure. Nitric oxide synthesis in the placenta may play a meaningful role in maintaining a low-pressure, high-flow placental system and also may prevent intervillous thrombosis. The loss of normal vasodilatation of uterine arterioles results in decreased placental perfusion (Figure 16–5), potentially leading to fetal growth restriction and chronic hypoxia or distress.

Evidence is mounting to suggest that in preeclampsia a hypoxic fetoplacental unit stimulates secretion of factors into maternal circulation that cause a dysfunction of vascular endothelial cells. The resulting dysfunction is demonstrated by the typical maternal changes in preeclampsia, such as the characteristic glomerular changes, increased capillary permeability, elevation of serum endothelin levels—known to induce vasoconstriction—and cellular fibronectin (cFN) (Davidge, Signorella, Lykins, Gilmour, & Roberts, 1996). Fibronectin is an extracellular matrix protein that is thought to play a role in the normal adherence of the placenta to the decidua of the uterus. The question remains unanswered as to whether endothelial dysfunction is the cause or the result of preeclampsia.

Decreased renal perfusion is associated with PIH. With a reduction in glomerular filtration rate (GFR), serum levels of creatinine, blood urea nitrogen (BUN), and uric acid begin to rise from normal pregnant levels, while urine output diminishes. For each 50% decrease in GFR, serum creatinine and BUN plasma levels double, while sodium is retained in increased amounts. Sodium retention results in increased extracellular volume and increased sensitivity to angiotensin II. The typical kidney lesion of preeclampsia involves swollen glomerular capillary endothelial cells containing fibrin deposits. Stretching of the capillary walls allows the large protein molecules, primarily albumin, to escape into the urine, decreasing serum albumin.

Edema is usually more profound in preeclampsia than in normal pregnancy. Its pathologic basis is twofold:

1. The higher salt retention draws out intravascular fluid.
2. Plasma colloid osmotic pressure decreases due to serum albumin loss through edematous renal glomeruli and damaged vascular endothelium. This causes fluid movement to extracellular spaces.

The decreased intravascular volume causes increased viscosity of the blood and a corresponding rise in hematocrit.

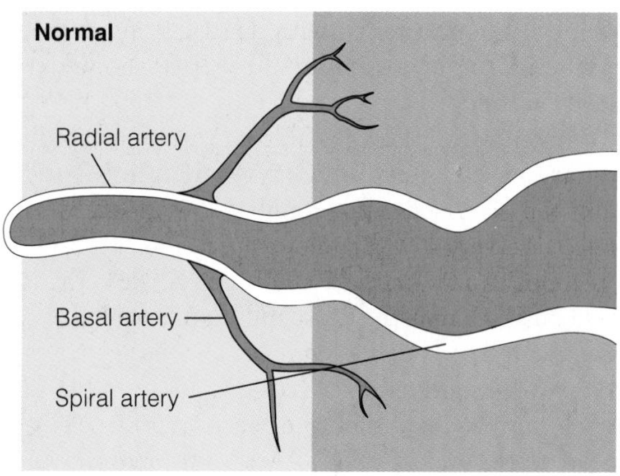

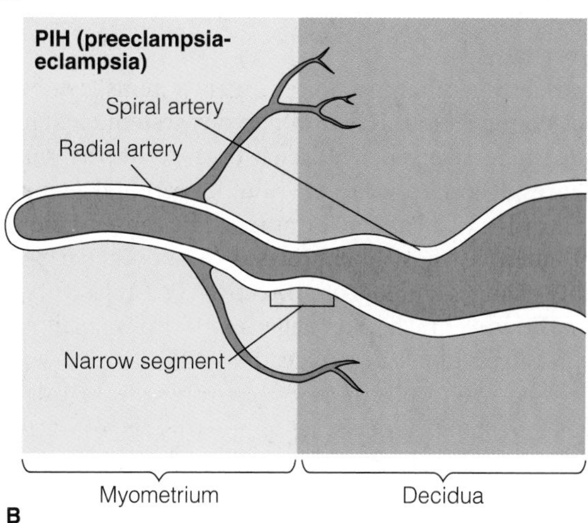

FIGURE 16–5 ***A,*** In a normal pregnancy, the passive quality of the spiral arteries permits increased blood flow to the placenta. ***B,*** In PIH vasoconstriction of the myometrial segment of the spiral arteries occurs.

HELLP Syndrome **HELLP syndrome** (**h**emolysis, **el**evated **l**iver enzymes, and **l**ow **p**latelet count) is sometimes associated with severe preeclampsia, although it may occur before the signs and symptoms of preeclampsia develop. Ninety percent of women with HELLP syndrome present with symptoms before 36 weeks' gestation.

The hemolysis that occurs is termed *microangiopathic hemolytic anemia.* It is thought that red blood cells are distorted or fragmented during passage through small, damaged blood vessels. Elevated liver enzymes occur from blood flow that is obstructed due to fibrin deposits. Hyperbilirubinemia and jaundice may also be seen. Liver distention causes epigastric pain. Thrombocytopenia is a frequent finding in PIH. Vascular damage is associated with vasospasm, and platelets aggregate at sites of damage, resulting in low platelet count (less than 100,000/mm^3).

Symptoms may include nausea, vomiting, malaise, flulike symptoms, or epigastric pain (Sibai, 1996). This may lead to misdiagnoses of gastroenteritis, hepatitis, gallbladder disease, pyelonephritis, renal disease, or thrombocytopenia purpura. Regardless of their blood pressure or the presence of protein in their urine, women presenting with the above symptoms should have a CBC with platelet count and liver enzymes drawn. Perinatal morbidity and mortality with HELLP syndrome are high; therefore the possibility of HELLP should be considered carefully.

Women with HELLP syndrome are best cared for in a tertiary care center. Initially, the mother's condition should be assessed and stabilized, especially if her platelets are very low. Platelet transfusions are indicated for platelet counts below 20,000/mm^3. The fetus is also assessed using a nonstress test and biophysical profile. All women with true HELLP syndrome should give birth regardless of gestational age. Labor may be induced with oxytocin in women with a ripe cervix at 30 weeks' gestation or more. At less than 30 weeks' gestation cesarean birth is indicated (Sibai, 1996).

Maternal Risks

Preeclampsia can impact most organ systems, causing serious complications. Central nervous system changes include hyperreflexia, headache, and eclamptic seizure. Seizures of eclampsia are the result of cerebral edema and occur in 1% of all affected women. The cause of the cerebral edema is most likely related to endothelial permeability changes and loss of protective cerebral autoregulation. Intracerebral hemorrhage is a rare complication, but the most common cause of death in preeclamptic women. Increased intraocular pressure can cause retinal detachment, but spontaneous reattachment usually occurs with reduction in blood pressure and diuresis.

Acute tubular necrosis may result from underperfusion of the kidneys. This is associated with hypovolemia and renal vasoconstriction. Although many women with preeclampsia will have oliguria, most do not develop acute tubular necrosis. One of the more common problems related to preeclampsia is pulmonary edema due to increased capillary permeability.

Thrombocytopenia complicates severe preeclampsia in about 10% of women. The exact mechanism is not fully understood, but platelet consumption is believed to be related to endothelial damage and activation of thrombin. Abruptio placentae is a risk associated with preeclampsia. The release of procoagulants, such as thromboplastin, can result in acute disseminated intravascular coagulation (DIC).

Subcapsular hematoma of the liver is a rare but important occurrence in women with preeclampsia and HELLP syndrome. In addition to the signs of preeclampsia, the physical examination may reveal hepatomegaly and peritoneal irritation. Rupture of a subcapsular hematoma is a life-threatening event. The woman may complain of right shoulder pain or severe epigastric pain persisting for several hours before circulatory collapse is evident. This is a surgical emergency requiring a multidisciplinary approach to management. Maternal and fetal mortality is over 50%, and women who survive are at risk for adult pulmonary distress syndrome, pulmonary edema, and acute renal failure in the postoperative period (Silver, 1996).

Women who have preeclampsia complicated by HELLP syndrome do tend to have a somewhat longer clinical and hematologic recovery time than those who do not develop HELLP.

Fetal-Neonatal Risks

Infants of women with hypertension during pregnancy tend to be small for gestational age (SGA) because of intrauterine growth retardation. The cause is related specifically to maternal vasospasm and hypovolemia, which result in fetal hypoxia and malnutrition. In addition, the newborn may be premature because of the necessity for early birth.

Perinatal mortality associated with preeclampsia is approximately 10%, and that associated with eclampsia is 20%. When preeclampsia is superimposed on chronic hypertension, perinatal mortality may be higher.

At birth, the newborn may be oversedated because of medications administered to the woman. The newborn may also have hypermagnesemia due to treatment of the woman with large doses of magnesium sulfate.

Clinical Therapy

The goals of medical management are prompt diagnosis of the disease; prevention of cerebral hemorrhage, convulsion, hematologic complications, and renal and hepatic diseases; and birth of an uncompromised newborn as close to term as possible. Reduction of elevated blood pressure is essential in accomplishing these goals.

Clinical Manifestations and Diagnosis The most commonly occuring clinical manifestations and diagnoses are related to eclampsia.

Mild Preeclampsia The diagnosis of mild preeclampsia is made based on the following blood pressure findings: a rise in systolic blood pressure of 30 mm Hg or more or a rise in diastolic blood pressure of 15 mm Hg or more above the baseline on two occasions at least 6 hours apart. If an early first trimester blood pressure reading is not available for a baseline parameter, 140/90 is used to designate mild preeclampsia.

Generalized edema, seen as puffy face, hands, and dependent areas such as the ankles and lower legs, may be present. Edema is identified by a weight gain of more than 1.5 kg/month (3.3 lb) in the second trimester or more than 0.5 kg/week (1.1 lb) in the third trimester. Edema is assessed on a 1+ to 4+ scale. Proteinuria is often a late sign of preeclampsia. It may not be present until the disease has progressed to the severe or eclamptic stage. If proteinuria is present with mild preeclampsia, protein is generally between 300 mg/L (1+ dipstick) and 1 g/L (2+ dipstick). This is measured in a midstream clean-catch or catheter-derived urine specimen. Over a 24-hour period, less than 5 g of protein would be lost in the urine.

Severe Preeclampsia Severe preeclampsia may develop suddenly. The following clinical signs are often present (AAP & ACOG, 1997):

- Blood pressure of 160/110 or higher on two occasions at least 6 hours apart while the woman is on bed rest
- Proteinuria ≥5 g/L in 24 hours or 3+ or greater on two random urine samples collected at least 4 hours apart
- Oliguria: urine output ≤500 mL in 24 hours
- Cerebral or visual disturbances
- Pulmonary edema or cyanosis
- Epigastric or right upper quadrant pain
- Impaired liver function
- Thrombocytopenia
- Fetal growth restriction

Other signs or symptoms that may be present include headache, blurred vision or scotomata (spots before the eyes), narrowed segments on the retinal arterioles when examined with an ophthalmoscope, retinal edema (retinas appear wet and glistening) on funduscopy, dyspnea due to pulmonary edema, moist breath sounds on auscultation, pitting edema of lower extremities while on bed rest, epigastric pain, hyperreflexia, nausea and vomiting, irritability, and emotional tension.

Eclampsia Eclampsia, characterized by convulsion or coma, may occur before the onset of labor, during labor, or early in the postpartal period. Late postpartal eclampsia (convulsions occurring more than 48 hours following birth) occurs rarely but has been documented (Sibai, 1996). Some women experience only one convulsion, especially if it occurs late in labor or during the postpartal period. Others may have from 2 to 20 or more. Unless they occur extremely frequently, the woman often regains consciousness between convulsions.

Antepartal Management The only known cure for PIH is birth of the infant. Recent research has focused on preventing PIH in at-risk women through the use of low-dose (50 to 150 mg daily) aspirin. Aspirin is known to block the action of an enzyme, cyclooxygenase, essential to the production of prostaglandins. This results in lowered levels of thromboxane, the vasoconstrictor. At the same time, levels of the vasodilator prostacyclin are not significantly affected. Widespread prophylactic use of aspirin is not yet indicated on the basis of current studies. However, it is reasonable to use low-dose aspirin in women with a history of fetal loss after the first trimester, a previous episode of severe fetal growth restriction in a previous pregnancy, or a history of severe early onset preeclampsia. Treatment should begin between 12 and 18 weeks' gestation (Brennecke et al, 1995).

TABLE 16–5 Signs and Symptoms of Worsening Preeclampsia
Increasing edema, especially of hands and face (If on bed rest, observe for sacral edema.)
Worsening headache
Epigastric pain
Visual disturbances
Decreasing urinary output
Nausea/vomiting
Bleeding gums
Disorientation
Generalized complaints of not feeling well

Home Care of Mild Preeclampsia In general, women with proteinuric preeclampsia should be admitted to the hospital. However, with changes in health care, more attention has been given to decreasing inpatient hospital days for women whose symptoms allow.

A woman should be considered for management at home if she meets the following criteria: Blood pressure ≤ 150/100, proteinuria less than 1 g/24 hours or < 3+ dipstick, platelet count greater than 120,000 mm^3, and normal fetal growth if not at term or showing signs of complicating factors such as vaginal bleeding. She must have a basic understanding of her condition, be able to recognize the signs and symptoms of worsening preeclampsia (Table 16–5), be able to accurately count fetal movements, be cooperative, and know when to call the doctor. She is not restricted to bed rest (Frangieh & Sibai, 1996).

The woman monitors her blood pressure, weight, and urine protein daily. Weight gains of 1.4 kg (3 lb) in 24 hours or 1.8 kg (4 lb) in a 3-day period are generally cause for concern. Remote NSTs are performed on a daily to biweekly basis. Companies that provide this service have equipment that allows phone transmission of blood pressure readings as well as fetal monitor tracings. This eliminates concerns about inaccurate reporting on the part of the woman. Nursing contact varies from daily to weekly, depending on physician request. Laboratory testing regularly evaluates platelet counts, uric acid and BUN, liver enzymes, and 24-hour urine specimens for creatinine clearance and total protein. Any woman with worsening symptoms or severe preeclampsia should be hospitalized.

Hospital Care of Mild Preeclampsia The woman is placed on bed rest, primarily in the left lateral recumbent position, to decrease pressure on the vena cava, thereby increasing venous return, circulatory volume, and placental and renal perfusion. Improved renal blood flow helps decrease angiotensin II levels, promotes diuresis, and lowers blood pressure.

Diet should be well balanced and moderate to high in protein (80 to 100 g/day, or 1.5 g/kg/day) to replace protein lost in the urine. Sodium intake should be moderate, not to exceed 6 g/day. Excessively salty foods should be avoided, but strict sodium restriction and diuretics are no longer used in treating preeclampsia.

Tests to evaluate fetal status are done more frequently as a pregnant woman's preeclampsia progresses. These tests are described in detail in Chapter 17. Monitoring fetal well-being is essential to achieving a safe outcome for the fetus. The following tests are used:

- Fetal movement record
- Nonstress test
- Ultrasonography every 3 to 4 weeks for serial determination of growth
- Biophysical profile
- Serum creatinine determinations
- Amniocentesis to determine fetal lung maturity
- Doppler velocimetry beginning at 30 to 32 weeks to screen for fetal compromise

Maternal well-being is monitored by the following:

- Blood pressure four times daily
- Daily weight and daily evaluation for worsening edema, persistent headache, visual changes, or epigastric pain
- Daily urine dipstick for protein; 24-hour urine for total protein and creatinine
- CBC with platelet count every 2 days
- Serum creatinine, uric acid, and liver function tests (AST, ALT, LDH, bilirubin) one to two times per week

Severe Preeclampsia If the uterine environment is considered detrimental to fetal growth and maturation, birth may be the treatment of choice for both mother and fetus even if the fetus is immature. Other medical therapies for preeclampsia include the following:

- *Bed rest.* Bed rest must be complete. Stimuli that may bring on a convulsion should be reduced.
- *Diet.* A high-protein, moderate-sodium diet is given as long as the woman is alert and has no nausea or indication of impending convulsion.
- *Anticonvulsants.* Magnesium sulfate is the treatment of choice for convulsions. Its CNS-depressant action reduces the possibility of convulsion. Blood levels of $MgSO_4$ should be maintained at therapeutic levels (levels vary according to laboratory). Excessive blood levels may produce respiratory paralysis or cardiac arrest. (See Drug Guide: Magnesium Sulfate on page 402.)
- *Corticosteroids.* Although the use of corticosteroids remains controversial, betamethasone or dexamethasone is often administered to the woman whose fetus has an immature lung profile. Therapy must be administered 24 to 48 hours prior to birth to maximize the beneficial effect (Clewell, 1997).
- *Fluid and electrolyte replacement.* The goal of fluid intake is to achieve a balance between correcting hypovolemia and preventing circulatory overload. Fluid intake may be oral or supplemented with intravenous therapy. Intravenous fluids may be started "to keep lines open" in case they are needed for drug therapy, even when oral intake is adequate. Criteria vary for determining appropriate fluid intake. Electrolytes are replaced as indicated by daily serum electrolyte levels.
- *Sedatives.* A sedative, such as diazepam (Valium) or phenobarbital, is sometimes given to encourage quiet bed rest.
- *Antihypertensives.* Aldomet (Methyldopa), normodyne (Labetalol), and nifedipine (Procardia) are antihypertensives that may be administered orally for the acute treatment of severe preeclampsia. In general, antihypertensive therapy is given for diastolic blood pressures of 110 or above. The therapeutic goal is to maintain the diastolic blood pressure between 90 and 100 mm Hg. Decreasing the diastolic below 90 mm Hg may decrease uterine blood flow, causing fetal compromise. Intravenous antihypertensives are used for hypertension unresponsive to oral medication or for hypertensive crises.

Eclampsia Approximately 19% of women with preeclampsia develop eclampsia (Silver, 1996). Eclampsia includes the occurrence of either seizure or coma. Seizures may be focal, multifocal, or generalized. The etiology of the seizure is most likely related to cerebral vasospasm, edema, hemorrhage, ischemia, and hypertensive or metabolic encephalopathy. Many women experience an increase in deep tendon reflexes (DTRs) before seizure, but seizures may also occur without hyperreflexia. The woman with preeclampsia should be monitored for signs and symptoms of impending eclampsia: scotomata, which can appear as dark spots or flashing lights in the field of vision; blurred vision; epigastric pain; vomiting; persistent or severe headache, generally frontal in location; neurologic hyperactivity; pulmonary edema; or cyanosis.

If a seizure occurs, nursing assessment should include time of onset, progress of the seizure, body involvement, duration, presence of incontinence, status of the fetus, and signs of placental abruption. The airway should be maintained and oxygen administered during the seizure. The woman is positioned on her side to avoid aspiration. Suctioning may be necessary to keep the airway clear; a tongue blade should not be inserted into the back of the throat because it may stimulate the gag reflex. To prevent injury, side rails should be up and padded, but the woman should not be restrained.

A bolus of 4 to 6 g magnesium sulfate is administered intravenously over 5 minutes in an attempt to break the seizure. Magnesium failures require the addition of a second agent, such as 10 mg of diazepam administered intravenously up to a maximum of 30 mg. Dilantin may be used for seizure prevention: A bolus of 10 mg/kg of body weight is piggybacked to a main line and infused at a rate no greater than 50 mg/minute. A second bolus of 5 mg/kg of dilantin is given 2 hours later with maintenance doses beginning 12 hours later and repeated every 8 to 12 hours based on serum levels of the drug. The therapeutic range of dilantin is 10 to 20 μg/mL (Sisson & Sauer, 1996).

During a seizure fetal bradycardia may occur. If possible, the fetus is allowed to recover before birth. The seizure increases uterine irritability and may cause a precipitous birth. Therefore a minimum ratio of one nurse to one client is imperative to assess fetal and maternal status. While she is still unconscious, the woman should be observed for onset of labor. The woman is also observed for signs of placental separation (see Chapter 25). She should be checked every 15 minutes for vaginal bleeding, which may or may not be present with abruptio placentae. The abdomen is palpated for uterine rigidity.

Following a seizure, frequent auscultation of maternal lungs is required to assess for complications from aspiration and to rule out pulmonary edema, which is common in eclamptic clients. The woman is watched for circulatory and renal failure and for signs of cerebral hemorrhage. Furosemide (Lasix) may be given in low doses for pulmonary edema; digitalis may be given for circulatory failure. Intake and output are monitored hourly.

A woman may have a single convulsion or many convulsions, usually followed by a period of coma. She may be combative and confused as she wakens, but having a family member at her side helps to reduce her agitation. Also, it is important to avoid bright light, noises, and frequent disturbances.

The most serious complication, cerebral hemorrhage, arises from uncontrolled hypertension. Loss of vision, which is usually temporary, is a sign of impending hemorrhage. Blood pressure control with intravenous hydralazine has been the preferred treatment until after birth because of extensive experience with its use and rare reports of adverse fetal affects. Intravenous options are Labetalol, diazoxide, or nitroprusside. Nitroprusside has been restricted to hypertensive crises when childbirth is imminent and other medications have not worked. Fetal cyanide poisoning may occur if the drug is continued and birth is delayed. Use of nitroprusside requires an arterial line because of its quick action and profound effects on blood pressure.

Intrapartal Management Labor may be induced by intravenous oxytocin when there is evidence of fetal maturity and cervical readiness. In very severe cases, cesarean birth may be necessary regardless of fetal maturity.

The woman may receive both intravenous oxytocin and $MgSO_4$ simultaneously. Because $MgSO_4$ has depressant action on smooth muscle, uterine contractions may diminish, and labor may be augmented with oxytocin. Equipment and intravenous lines for both fluids must be checked frequently to ensure that they are being administered at the proper rate. Infusion pumps should be used to guarantee accuracy. Bags and tubings must be labeled carefully.

Meperidine (Demerol) or fentanyl may be given intravenously for pain relief in labor. A pudendal block is often used for childbirth. An epidural block may be used if it is administered by a skilled anesthesiologist who is knowledgeable about preeclampsia.

Childbirth in the Sims' position should be considered. If the lithotomy position is used, a wedge should be placed under the right buttock to displace the uterus. The wedge should also be used if birth is by cesarean. Oxygen is administered to the woman during labor if need is indicated by fetal response to the contractions.

Eclampsia Often the woman with eclampsia is cared for in an intensive care unit until labor begins or is induced. Invasive hemodynamic monitoring of either central venous pressure (CVP) or pulmonary artery wedge pressure (PAWP) may be instituted using a Swan-Ganz catheter. Both these procedures carry risk to the woman, and the decision to use them should be made judiciously. Invasive hemodynamic monitoring is indicated for the woman with the following (Fox, Troiano, & Graves, 1996):

- Urine output less than 30 mL/hr for 3 hours with lack of response to an intravenous fluid bolus
- Pulmonary edema resulting in impaired maternal oxygenation
- Administration of a vasoactive drug, such as nitroprusside or dopamine

When the woman's vital signs have stabilized, urinary output is good, and the maternal and fetal hypoxic and acidotic states are alleviated, birth of the fetus should be considered. Birth is the only known cure for PIH. If the newborn will be preterm, it may be necessary to transfer the woman to a tertiary center for childbirth. The woman and her partner deserve careful explanation about the status of the fetus and woman and the treatment they are receiving. Plans for childbirth and further treatment must be discussed with them.

A pediatrician or neonatal nurse practitioner must be available to care for the newborn at birth. This caregiver must be aware of all amounts and times of medication the woman has received during labor.

Postpartum Management The woman with preeclampsia usually improves rapidly after childbirth, although seizures can still occur during the first 48 hours postpartum. A woman who has required $MgSO_4$ antepartally will continue to receive the infusion for about 24 hours postpartum. Antihypertensive medication

CLINICAL TIP

Common errors in measuring blood pressure include the following:

1. Incorrect cuff size—a cuff that is too small results in a falsely elevated blood pressure, whereas one that is too large falsely lowers blood pressure.
2. Elevating the arm above the level of the heart, such as occurs when a woman lies on her left side using her right arm for a blood pressure measurement, will falsely lower the blood pressure 10 to 20 mm Hg.
3. Korotkoff's phase—when blood pressure is checked during pregnancy, the disappearance of sound (phase V) may be unusually low. To standardize measurements, the muffling of sound, (phase IV) is the preferred indicator.
4. Anxiety and exercise can elevate blood pressure. Wait 10 minutes after the woman's arrival to check a resting blood pressure.

may also be required for a time. Postpartum nurses should be acutely aware of the possibility of a worsening of the maternal condition in the immediate postpartum period. The potential for HELLP syndrome, liver rupture, or seizure continues, and one should not be lulled into a false sense of security once birth has occurred.

Women with PIH are not at greater risk for developing chronic hypertension later in life, but if blood pressure fails to return to normal parameters during the postpartum period, further evaluation is indicated to rule out underlying causes for hypertension. Young women are generally healthy and may not have sought regular health care before pregnancy, increasing the likelihood of a preexisting problem becoming evident during pregnancy or in the postpartum period.

NURSING CARE MANAGEMENT

Nursing Assessment and Diagnosis

An essential part of nursing assessment is to obtain a baseline blood pressure early in pregnancy. Arterial blood pressure varies with position and is highest when the woman is sitting, intermediate when she is supine, and lowest when she is in the left lateral recumbent position. Therefore it is important that the woman be in the same position when the blood pressure is measured each visit.

Blood pressure is taken and recorded at each antepartal visit. If the blood pressure rises or if the normal slight decrease in blood pressure expected between 8 and 28 weeks of pregnancy does not occur, the woman should be followed closely.

When blood pressure and other signs indicate that the preeclampsia is worsening, hospitalization is necessary to monitor the woman's condition closely. The nurse then assesses the following:

TABLE 16–6 Deep Tendon Reflex Rating Scale

Rating	Assessment
4+	Hyperactive; very brisk, jerky, or clonic response; abnormal
3+	Brisker than average; may not be abnormal
2+	Average response; normal
1+	Diminished response; low normal
0	No response; abnormal

- *Blood pressure.* Blood pressure should be determined every 1 to 4 hours, more frequently if indicated by medication or other changes in the woman's status.
- *Temperature.* Temperature should be determined every 4 hours, every 2 hours if elevated or if PROM has occurred.
- *Pulse and respirations.* Pulse rate and respiration should be determined along with blood pressure.
- *Fetal heart rate.* The fetal heart rate should be determined with the blood pressure or monitored continuously with the electronic fetal monitor if the situation indicates.
- *Urinary output.* Every voiding should be measured. Frequently, the woman will have an indwelling catheter. In this case, hourly urine output can be assessed. Output should be 700 mL or greater in 24 hours or at least 30 mL per hour.
- *Urine protein.* Urinary protein is determined hourly if an indwelling catheter is in place or with each voiding. Readings of 3+ or 4+ indicate loss of 5 g or more protein in 24 hours.
- *Urine specific gravity.* Specific gravity of the urine should be determined hourly or with each voiding. Readings over 1.040 correlate with oliguria and proteinuria.
- *Edema.* The face (especially eyelids and cheekbone area), fingers, hands, arms (ulnar surface and wrist), legs (tibial surface), ankles, feet, and sacral area are inspected and palpated for edema. The degree of pitting is determined by pressing over bony areas.
- *Weight.* The woman is weighed daily at the same time, wearing the same robe or gown and slippers. Weighing may be omitted if the woman is to maintain strict bed rest, or a bed scale may be used.
- *Pulmonary edema.* The woman is observed for coughing. The lungs are auscultated for moist respirations.
- *Deep tendon reflexes.* The woman is assessed for evidence of hyperreflexia in the brachial, wrist, patellar, or Achilles tendons (Table 16–6). The patellar reflex is the easiest to assess (Procedure 16–1: Assessing Deep Tendon Reflexes and Clonus). Clonus should also be assessed by vigorously dorsiflexing the

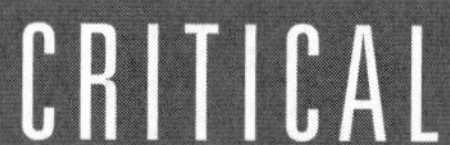

PATHWAY FOR A WOMAN WITH PREGNANCY-INDUCED HYPERTENSION

Category	Antepartal Management	Intrapartal Management*	Postpartal Management*
Referral	• Perinatologist • Internist • Social worker • Psych clinical nurse practitioner • Dietary/nutritionist	• Obtain prenatal record	• Home nursing referral if indicated **Expected Outcomes** Appropriate resources identified and utilized
Assessment	• Electronic fetal monitoring (EFM) ___ q4h ___ q8h ___ Continuous • NST: ___ qd • Ultrasound as indicated • Assess for headache, visual disturbances, epigastric pain, edema, DTRs, clonus, and protein in urine	• Assess prenatal BP readings and compare to baseline reading • Assess for headache, visual disturbances, epigastric pain, edema, DTRs, clonus, and protein in urine	• BP q4h for first 48h then q8h until discharge • Monitor daily Hct • Continue normal postpartum assessment q8h • Feeding technique with newborn: should be progressing • TPR assessment: q8h; all WNL: report temperature >38C (100.4F) • Continue assessment of comfort level • Assess for headache, visual disturbances, epigastric pain, edema, DTRs, clonus, and protein in urine **Expected Outcomes** Findings indicate hypertension reduced or stabilized Unstable/escalating hypertension identified in timely manner
Teaching/ psychosocial	• Room orientation • Explain signs and symptoms (s/sx) of worsening disease and importance of notifying RN • Explain s/sx of labor • Increase pt awareness of fetal monitoring, importance of bed rest and lying on left side • Evaluation of client teaching	• Tour of ICN • Discuss with woman: a. Mode of childbirth b. Progression of disease and possible use of $MgSO_4$ prior to birth c. Postpartum expectation	• Implement normal postpartum teaching and psychosocial support (see Chapter 28) **Expected Outcomes** Verbalizes/demonstrates understanding of teaching Incorporates teaching of BP management into Self-care

Nursing care management and reports	• CBC daily
	• Biochemical profile
	• U/A/Dipstick for protein and ketones with each void as well as specific gravity
	• 24 hour urine for total protein and creatinine clearance
	• VS q4h or more frequently if indicated
	• I&O q8h; fluid restriction ___ mL as ordered
	• DTR and clonus q4h; report 3+ or 4+ results
	• Daily weight
	• Seizure precautions
	  • Headache, visual distress, epigastric pain → report abnormal findings
	  • Edema (ongoing)
	  • Auscultate lungs for moist respirations and report
	  • Assess hourly for vaginal bleeding and/or uterine irritability or contractions
	• Observe for alertness, mood changes, and signs of impending convulsion or coma
	• Assess emotional response so that support and teaching can be planned accordingly
		• Ongoing monitoring of blood pressure
		• Ongoing monitoring of edema
		• Assess urine for proteinuria every shift
		• Electronic fetal monitoring in place
		• Assess woman for worsening signs of PIH (placental separation, pulmonary edema, renal failure, and fetal distress)
		• Try to have same nurses caring for woman during her hospitalization
			• Continue sitz bath prn
			• May shower if ambulating without difficulty
			• DC buffalo cap (heparin lock) if present
			• Continue to monitor VS, breath sounds, edema, epigastric pain, DTRs, clonus, and protein in urine until return to normal limits
			Expected Outcomes
			Hypertension reduced or controlled
			Maternal/fetal complications quickly identified and minimized
			Feels safe in environment and remains injury free

Comfort	• Assess for discomfort • Provide comfort measures as needed	• Assess for discomfort • Provide comfort measures as needed	• Continue with pain management techniques **Expected Outcomes** Comfort level is maintained

➤

CRITICAL PATHWAY FOR A WOMAN WITH PREGNANCY-INDUCED HYPERTENSION *CONTINUED*

Category	Antepartal Management	Intrapartal Management*	Postpartal Management*
Activity	• BR with BRP • Decreased stimulation in room • Limit visitors • Encourage left lateral recumbent position	• Positioned on side • Encouraged to push while lying on side • Birth is in a side-lying position if possible	• Up ad lib when VS have stabilized **Expected Outcomes** Level of activity has not exacerbated condition
Nutrition	• Reg diet	• Ice chips	• Continue diet and fluids **Expected Outcomes** Nutritional needs met
Elimination	• Report urine output <30 mL/hr or urine specific gravity >1.040	• Monitor urine output	• Monitor urine output • I/O recorded for 48h after birth **Expected Outcomes** Intake and output WNL

Medications	• Buffalo cap or IV
	• If gestational age indicates:
	  • Celestone Soluspan
	  • TRH
	• $MgSO_4$ per infusion pump if indicated
	• Assess home care needs
		• Continuous IV infusion
		• $MgSO_4$ infusion pump if indicated
			• Continue $MgSO_4$ as indicated
			• May take own prenatal vitamins
			• RhoGAM and rubella vaccine administered if indicated
			Expected Outcomes
			Hypertensive crisis prevented
			Pain level controlled
			Perfusion of tissues supported

Discharge planning/ home care			• Review discharge instruction and checklist • Describe postpartum warning signs and when to call CNM/physician • Provide prescriptions. Gift pack given to woman. • Arrangements made for baby pictures if desired • Postpartum visit scheduled • Newborn check scheduled **Expected Outcomes** Discharged with plan for follow-up health care and blood pressure monitoring Support network identified
Family involvement	• Assess woman's major concerns: eg, fear for fetus, relationship with other children, relationship with partner	• Encourage family member to stay with the woman as long as possible throughout labor and childbirth	• Family members urged to visit • Continue to involve support persons in teaching • Evidence of parental bonding behaviors apparent • Plans being made for providing support to mother following discharge. Support persons verbalize understanding of need for woman to rest, eat nutritionally, recover. **Expected Outcomes** Family able to participate as desired
Date			

*Interventions for a woman with a normal labor and birth and during the early postpartum period may be found in those appropriate critical pathways.

woman's foot while her knee is held in a flexed position. Normally no clonus is present. If it is present, it is measured as one to four beats, or sustained, and is recorded as such.

- *Placental separation.* The woman should be assessed hourly for vaginal bleeding and/or uterine rigidity.
- *Headache.* The woman should be questioned about the existence and location of any headache.
- *Visual disturbance.* The woman should be questioned about any visual blurring or changes, including scotomata. The results of the daily funduscopic exam should be recorded on the chart.

- *Epigastric pain.* The woman should be asked about any epigastric pain. It is important to differentiate it from simple heartburn, which tends to be familiar and less intense. Nausea and vomiting or right upper quadrant pain, occasionally radiating to the back are also of concern.
- *Laboratory blood tests.* Daily tests of hematocrit to measure hemoconcentration; BUN, creatinine, and uric acid levels to assess kidney function; clotting studies for any indication of thrombocytopenia or DIC; liver enzymes; and electrolyte levels for deficiencies are all indicated.
- *Level of consciousness.* The woman is observed for alertness, mood changes, and any signs of impending convulsion or coma.
- *Emotional response and level of understanding.* The woman's emotional response should be carefully assessed so that support and teaching can be planned accordingly.

In addition, the nurse continues to assess the effects of any medications administered. Because the administration of prescribed medications is an important aspect of care, the nurse is, of course, familiar with the more commonly used medications, their purpose, implications, and associated untoward or toxic effects.

Examples of nursing diagnoses that may apply for the pregnant woman with preeclampsia/eclampsia include the following:

- ***Fluid Volume** Deficit* related to fluid shift from the intravascular to extravascular space secondary to vasospasm and endothelial injury.
- ***Risk of Injury*** to the woman related to convulsion secondary to cerebral edema.

Nursing Plan and Implementation

Community-Based Nursing Care

A woman with PIH has several major concerns. She may fear losing the fetus. She may worry about her personal relationship with her other children and her personal and sexual relationship with her partner. She may be concerned about finances—health insurance does not always cover all the tests, prolonged hospitalization, and so on, that may be associated with complications during pregnancy. Finally, the woman may be depressed or resentful about being left alone or may feel bored. If she has small children, she may have difficulty providing for their care. The woman who does not have children may worry that she never will.

The nurse should identify and discuss each of these areas with the woman and her partner. It is necessary to explain to them the reasons for bed rest. A woman with mild preeclampsia may feel very well and be unable to see the need for resting even a few hours a day. The nurse can refer the couple to many community resources, such as homemaking services, a support group for the partner, or a hot-line. Arrangements may be made for the partner to attend childbirth classes if both are not able to, or a nurse may be found to teach the classes privately.

The woman needs to know which symptoms are significant and should be reported at once. Usually, the woman with mild preeclampsia is seen once or twice a week, but she may need to come in earlier if symptoms indicate the condition is progressing. She must understand her diet plan, which must match her culture, finances, and lifestyle.

CLINICAL TIP

When caring for a woman with PIH who is receiving IV magnesium sulfate, it is imperative that you follow protocols for monitoring blood levels of magnesium. You are probably already aware of the common signs of increasing magnesium levels, such as diminished reflexes and decreased respiratory rate. However, there are some subtle clues you can also watch for that may suggest either the therapeutic or toxic range. When a woman's magnesium level is in the therapeutic range, she usually has some slurring of speech, awkwardness of movement, and decreased appetite. If the woman begins to have difficulty swallowing and begins to drool, she may be approaching the toxic range.

Hospital-Based Nursing Care

The development of worsening preeclampsia is a cause for increased concern to the woman and her family. The most immediate concerns of the woman and her partner usually are about the prognosis for herself and the fetus. The nurse can offer honest and hopeful information. She can explain the plan of therapy and the reasons for procedures to the extent that the woman or her partner are interested. The nurse should keep the couple informed of the fetal status and should also take the time to discuss other concerns the couple may express. The nurse provides as much information as possible and seeks other sources of information or aid for the family as needed. Nurses can offer to contact a member of the clergy or counselor for additional support if the couple so chooses.

The nurse should maintain a quiet, low-stimulus environment for the woman. The woman should be placed in a private room in a quiet location where she can be watched closely. Visitors are limited to close family or main support persons. The woman should maintain the left lateral recumbent position most of the time, with side rails up for her protection. Unlimited phone calls are avoided because the phone ringing unexpectedly may be too jarring. To avoid a sense of isolation, however, some women find it preferable to limit calls to a certain time of the day rather than refusing all calls.

Nursing Management of Eclampsia The occurrence of a convulsion is frightening to any family members who

PROCEDURE 16–1 ASSESSING DEEP TENDON REFLEXES AND CLONUS

Nursing Action	*Rationale*
Objective: Assemble and prepare equipment.	
Obtain a percussion hammer. If one is not available, the side of the hand is also useful in assessing deep tendon reflexes (DTRs).	*A percussion hammer permits accurate delivery of a brisk tap.*
Objective: Prepare woman.	
Explain the procedure, indications for it, and information that will be obtained. At a minimum, check the patellar reflex. Most nurses check a second reflex, such as the biceps, triceps, or brachioradialis.	*Explanation decreases anxiety and increases cooperation. DTRs are assessed to gain information about CNS status and to assess the effects of $MgSO_4$ if the woman is receiving it.*
Objective: Elicit reflexes.	
Patellar reflex. The woman is positioned with her legs hanging over the edge of the bed (feet should not be touching the floor) (Figure 16–6). She may also lie supine with her knees slightly flexed and supported by the nurse. The nurse briskly strikes the patellar tendon, which is located just below the patella. Normal response is extension or a thrusting forward of the foot. Biceps reflex. The woman's arm is flexed at the elbow with the nurse's thumb placed on the biceps tendon. The nurse's thumb is struck in a slightly downward motion and response is assessed. Normal response is flexion of the arm.	*Correct positioning and technique are essential to elicit the reflex. The correct position causes the muscle to be slightly stretched. Then when the tendon is stretched with the tap, the muscle should contract.*

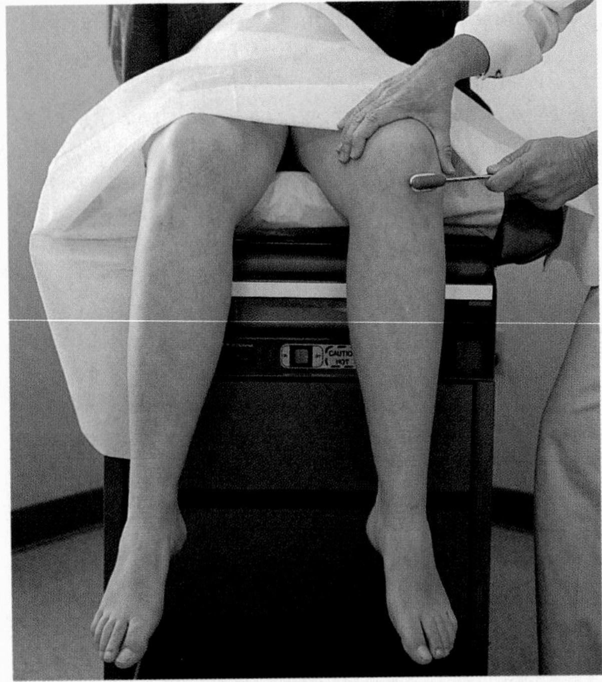

FIGURE 16–6 Correct position for eliciting patellar reflex: sitting.

Objective: Grade reflexes.	
Reflexes are graded on a scale of 0 to 4+. See Table 16–6 on page 412.	*Normally reflexes are 1+ or 2+. With CNS irritation, hyperreflexia may be present; with high magnesium levels reflexes may be diminished or absent.*

PROCEDURE 16–1 *CONTINUED*

Nursing Action	*Rationale*
Objective: Assess for clonus.	
With the knee flexed and the leg supported, vigorously dorsiflex the foot, maintain the dorsiflexion momentarily, and then release (Figure 16–7).	*Clonus indicates more pronounced hyperreflexia and is indicative of CNS irritability.*
Normal response: The foot returns to its normal position of plantar flexion. Clonus is present if the foot "jerks" or taps against the examiner's hand. If so, the number of taps or beats of clonus is recorded.	

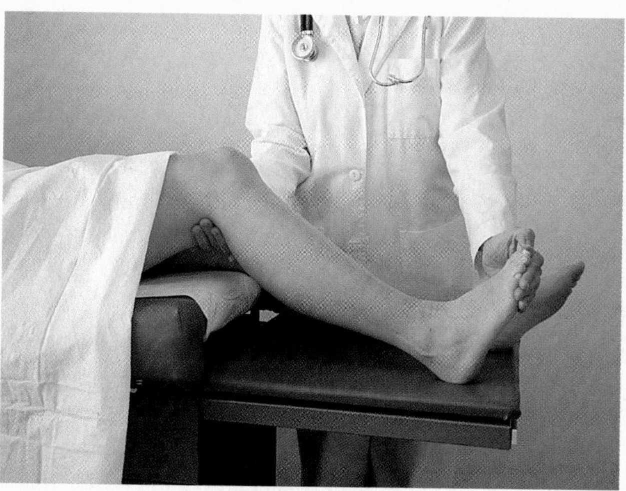

FIGURE 16–7 To elicit clonus, sharply dorsiflex the foot.

Nursing Action	*Rationale*
Objective: Report and record findings.	
For example: DTRs 2+, no clonus or DTRs 4+, 2 beats clonus.	*Provides a permanent record.*

may be present, although the woman will not be able to recall it when she becomes conscious. Therefore, offering explanations to family members, and to the woman herself later, is essential.

When the tonic phase of the convulsion begins, the woman should be turned to her side (if she is not already in that position) to aid circulation to the placenta. Her head should be turned face down to allow saliva to drain from her mouth. Attempting to insert a padded tongue blade has been questioned, and in many facilities it is no longer advocated. In others, it is used if it can be done without force because it may prevent injury to the woman's mouth. The side rails should be padded or a pillow put between the woman and each side rail.

After 15 to 20 seconds, the clonic phase starts. When the thrashing subsides, intensive monitoring and therapy begin. An oral airway is inserted, the woman's nasopharynx is suctioned, and oxygen administration is begun by nasal catheter. Fetal heart tones are monitored continuously. Maternal vital signs are monitored every 5 minutes until they are stable, then every 15 minutes. Essential Precautions in Practice: A Woman with PIH summarizes the specific precautions a nurse should take in caring for a woman with PIH in addition to the normal precautions indicated for all laboring women.

Nursing Management During Labor and Birth The plan of care for the woman with PIH in labor depends on both maternal and fetal condition. The woman may have mild or severe preeclampsia, may become eclamptic during labor, or may have been eclamptic before the onset of labor. Therefore, careful monitoring of blood pressure and checking for edema and proteinuria are necessary for all women in labor. The prenatal record should be obtained so that current blood pressure readings may be compared with the baseline reading.

The woman with preeclampsia in labor is kept positioned on her side as much as possible. Both woman and fetus are monitored carefully throughout labor. Signs of progressing labor are noted. In addition, the nurse must

ESSENTIAL PRECAUTIONS IN PRACTICE

A Woman with PIH

In caring for a woman with PIH, follow all precautions established for any hospitalized pregnant, laboring, or postpartal woman. In addition, remember the following specifics.

- Wear gloves when testing urine for proteinuria, when starting IV for $MgSO_4$ therapy, when doing finger sticks to test hematocrit, or when drawing blood for other laboratory tests.
- If eclampsia occurs and the woman convulses, wear gloves when removing the airway.
- If incontinence occurs during the convulsion, wear a protective gown and gloves when cleansing the woman and while changing the bedding.
- Dispose of needles, syringes, lancets, and other sharp objects in appropriately labeled containers.

REMEMBER to wash your hands prior to putting disposable gloves on and AGAIN immediately after you remove the gloves.

For further information, consult OSHA and CDC guidelines.

be alert for indications of worsening preeclampsia, placental separation, pulmonary edema, circulatory renal failure, and fetal distress.

During the second stage of labor the woman is encouraged to push while lying on her side. If she is unable to do so comfortably or effectively, she can be helped to a semisitting position for pushing and resume the lateral position between each contraction. Birth is in the side-lying position if possible. If the lithotomy position is used, a wedge is placed under the woman's hip.

A family member is encouraged to stay with the woman as long as possible throughout labor and childbirth. This is especially needed if the woman has been transferred to a high-risk center from another facility. The woman in labor and the family member or support person should be oriented to the new surroundings and kept informed of progress and plan of care. The woman should be cared for by the same nurses throughout her hospital stay.

Nursing Management During the Postpartal Period

The amount of postpartal vaginal bleeding should be noted carefully. Because the woman with preeclampsia is hypovolemic, even normal blood loss can be serious. Rising pulse rate and falling urine output are indications of excessive blood loss. The uterus should be palpated frequently and massaged when needed to keep it contracted.

Blood pressure and pulse are checked every 4 hours for 48 hours. Hematocrit may be measured daily. The woman is instructed to report any headache or visual disturbance. *No ergot preparations, such as methergine, are given because they have a hypertensive effect.* Intake and output recordings are continued for 48 hours postpartum. Increased urinary output within 48 hours after birth is a highly favorable sign. With the diuresis, edema recedes and blood pressure returns to normal.

Postpartal depression can develop after the long ordeal of the difficult pregnancy. Family members are urged to visit, and as much mother-infant contact as possible should be allowed. There may be fears about a future pregnancy. The couple needs information about the chance of preeclampsia occurring again. They also should be given family planning information. Oral contraceptives may be used if the woman's blood pressure has returned to normal by the time they are prescribed (usually 4 to 6 weeks postpartum).

Evaluation

Expected outcomes of nursing care include the following:

- The woman is able to explain PIH, its implications for her pregnancy, the treatment regimen, and possible complications.
- The woman suffers no eclamptic seizures.
- The woman and her caregivers detect signs of increasing severity of the PIH or possible complications early so that appropriate treatment measures can be instituted.
- The woman gives birth to a healthy newborn. ●

Chronic Hypertensive Disease

Chronic hypertension exists when the blood pressure is 140/90 or higher before pregnancy or before the 20th week of gestation or persists 42 days following childbirth. If the diastolic blood pressure is greater than 80 mm Hg during the second trimester, chronic hypertension should be suspected. For the majority of chronic hypertensive women, the disease is mild. One of the challenges the health care team faces is differentiating chronic hypertension from preeclampsia. This is even more difficult if a woman arrives for her first prenatal visit during the second trimester when blood pressure is generally lower and preexisting hypertension is more difficult to recognize.

Early prenatal care is important to determine accurately the gestational age and the severity of hypertension. At the time of the first visit, the woman should be counseled on several aspects of her pregnancy (Sibai, 1996; Zuspan, 1996):

- *Nutrition.* Sodium is limited to about 2 g per day; the woman is advised about recommended weight gain.
- *Bed rest.* Frequent rest periods are advisable. At a minimum, the woman should rest twice a day for 1-hour periods of time.
- *Medication.* Studies have shown that women with mild chronic hypertension have outcomes similar to

the general maternity population. Therefore, unless the blood pressure is over 160/110, antihypertensive medications are not used during pregnancy. Methyldopa is generally the first choice for use in pregnancy when medication is required.

- *Prenatal visits.* Counseling regarding the importance of frequent prenatal visits to reduce the incidence of adverse outcomes for mother or fetus is stressed.
- *Blood pressure monitoring.* The woman and her partner can be taught how to monitor blood pressure at home and maintain a record to be brought to each prenatal visit. Home monitoring is often more accurate because the woman is in a familiar environment and relaxed.
- *Fetal movement.* Starting at about 24 weeks, the woman should begin to keep fetal movement records and notify her care provider of any significant decrease in fetal movement.

During the first prenatal visit, the woman should have a thorough physical examination, which includes a funduscopic examination, blood pressure and pulses in all four extremities, and auscultation of chest and flanks. Laboratory work includes a urinalysis and culture; 24-hour urine for protein, creatinine clearance, sodium, and potassium; CBC; serum electrolytes; and a glucose tolerance test. The usual prenatal laboratory assessments and an ultrasound for confirming gestational age are also done if the woman is currently pregnant.

A woman with chronic hypertension generally has more frequent prenatal visits. She should be seen every 2 to 3 weeks in the first two trimesters and then more frequently in the third trimester, depending on how she and the fetus are progressing. Twenty-four hour urines, serum creatinine, uric acid, hematocrit, and ultrasound examinations are repeated at least once in the second and third trimesters.

Chronic Hypertension with Superimposed PIH

Preeclampsia develops in approximately 10% to 40% of women previously found to have chronic hypertension. When elevations of systolic blood pressure 30 mm Hg above the baseline or of diastolic blood pressure 15 mm Hg above the baseline are discovered on two occasions at least 6 hours apart, when proteinuria develops, or when edema occurs in the upper half of the body, the woman needs close monitoring and careful management. If the woman has underlying renal disease, it may be very difficult to confirm the diagnosis of superimposed preeclampsia. A rise in serum uric acid is helpful in identifying preeclampsia, which frequently occurs late in the second trimester or early in the third.

Late or Transient Hypertension

Late hypertension exists when transient elevation of blood pressure occurs during labor or in the early postpartal period, returning to normal within 10 days postpartum.

Care of the Woman at Risk for Rh Sensitization

Rh sensitization results from an antigen-antibody immunologic reaction within the body. Sensitization most commonly occurs when an Rh negative woman carries an Rh positive fetus, either to term or terminated by spontaneous or induced abortion. It can also occur if an Rh negative nonpregnant woman receives an Rh positive blood transfusion, experiences an Rh positive tubal pregnancy, has an amniocentesis, or any other traumatic event that might allow Rh positive fetal cells to enter the circulation of an Rh negative woman.

A number of known red blood cell (RBC) antigens are involved in the Rh system, all of which are controlled by three pairs of genes: Cc, Dd, and Ee. Antigens in the D group are usually involved in incompatibility between the mother and fetus, although other RBC antigens can also cause isoimmunization. The factors implicated in pathogenesis, in order of antigenic potential, are D, C, E, c, e, and, hypothetically, d (no antisera for the d antigen has been found, so the d nomenclature is used to identify the absence of D). There are many genetic combinations (genotypes) possible, such as CDE, cDe, Cde, and so forth. Individuals who are homozygous for the D antigen (DD) or heterozygous (Dd) are Rh positive because the D antigen is dominant; those whose genotype is dd, homozygous for the recessive antigen, are Rh negative.

During a normal pregnancy, small amounts of fetal blood (< 0.5 mL) may cross the placenta. An Rh negative mother whose fetus is Rh positive may develop anti-D antibodies in response to this exposure. During delivery of the placenta or as a result of trauma, even larger quantities of fetal blood can enter maternal circulation. After exposure to the Rh positive antigen, the primary response is development of gamma M immunoglobin (IgM). This primary response develops slowly over several weeks or months (Slotnick, 1996). IgM antibodies are large and do not cross the placenta. Once a woman is isoimmunized, she is immunized for life.

Following the primary response, the production of immune globulin G (IgG) anti-D antibody develops rapidly. IgG is capable of crossing the placenta and coating the fetal Rh (D) positive red cells, causing hemolysis. A second exposure to a very small amount of Rh (D) positive cells produces a rapid secondary immune response, developing in a few days and stronger than the primary response (Figure 16–8). Thus although hemolysis is not generally a problem for the fetus during a first pregnancy, it may create problems during subsequent pregnancies.

The hemolysis caused by the IgG antibody in the fetus creates fetal anemia. The fetus responds by increasing

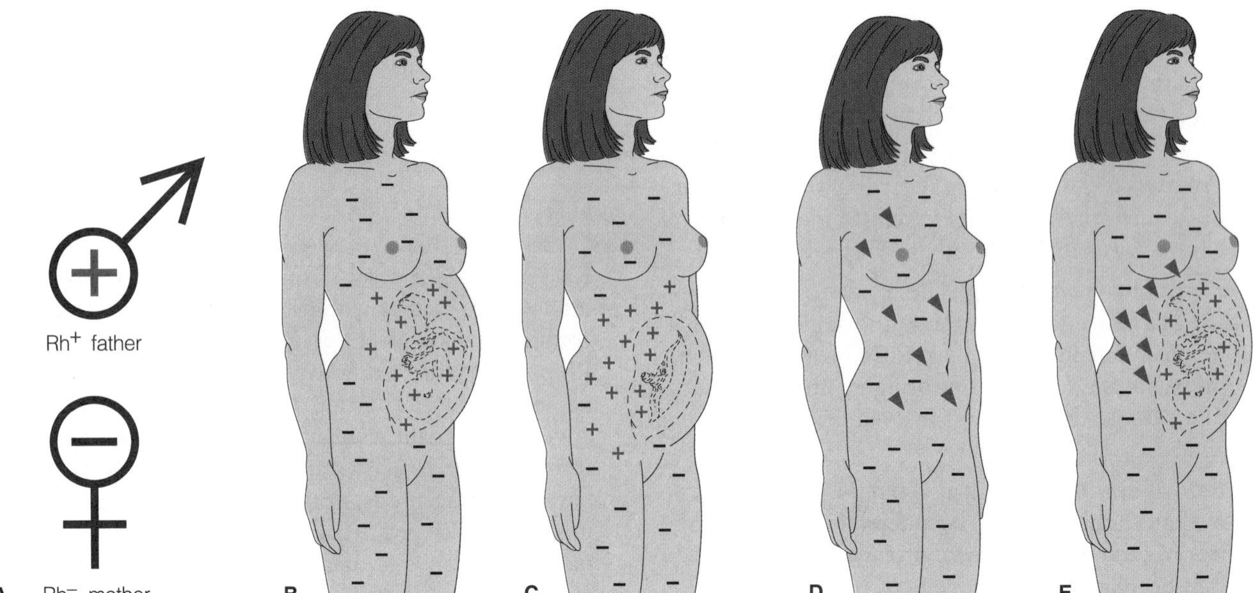

FIGURE 16–8 Rh isoimmunization sequence. ***A,*** Rh positive father and Rh negative mother. ***B,*** Pregnancy with Rh positive fetus. Some Rh positive blood enters the mother's blood. ***C,*** As the placenta separates, the mother is further exposed to the Rh positive blood. ***D,*** The mother is sensitized to the Rh positive blood; anti–Rh positive antibodies (triangles) are formed. ***E,*** In subsequent pregnancies with an Rh positive fetus, Rh positive red blood cells are attacked by the anti–Rh positive maternal antibodies, causing hemolysis of red blood cells in the fetus.

red cell production. The presence of nucleated RBCs (erythroblasts) is why the term **erythroblastosis fetalis** was coined for this severe hemolytic disease of the fetus and newborn. Immune suppression with Rh immune globulin (RhoGAM) appears to be effective as long as it occurs before the development of IgG antibodies.

Approximately 87% of white Americans, 92% to 93% of African Americans, and 99% of Asian populations are Rh positive (Jackson & Branch, 1996). An Rh negative woman who gives birth to an Rh positive, ABO compatible infant has a 16% risk of becoming sensitized as a result of her pregnancy.

CRITICAL THINKING QUESTION

What problems arise for the fetus if the mother is Rh positive and the father is Rh negative?

Fetal-Neonatal Risks

Although maternal sensitization can now be prevented by appropriate administration of **Rh immune globulin (RhoGAM,** or RhIgG), infants still die of hemolytic disease secondary to Rh incompatibility. In the fetus, red blood cell destruction leads to hyperbilirubinemia and anemia. If treatment is not initiated, this anemia can cause marked fetal edema, called **hydrops fetalis.** Congestive heart failure may result, as well as marked jaundice (called *icterus gravis*), which can lead to neurologic damage (*kernicterus*).

The possibility also exists that an Rh negative female fetus carried by an Rh positive mother may become sensitized in utero. This female would not demonstrate signs of hemolytic disease, but because she would be sensitized before even becoming pregnant, she would have a positive antibody screen when receiving prenatal care with her first Rh positive fetus.

Rh sensitization and the resultant hemolytic disease of the newborn are less common today because of the development of RhIgG. See Chapter 29 for treatment of the newborn affected by Rh sensitization.

Screening for Rh Incompatibility and Sensitization

At the first prenatal visit, (1) a history is taken of previous sensitization, abortions, blood transfusions, or children who developed jaundice or anemia during the neonatal period; (2) maternal blood type (ABO) and Rh factor are determined, and a routine Rh antibody screen is done; and (3) other medical complications, such as diabetes, infections, or hypertension are identified. An antibody screen (indirect Coombs' test) is done to determine whether an Rh negative woman is sensitized (has developed isoimmunity) to the Rh antigen. The indirect Coombs' test measures the number of antibodies in the maternal blood. If the Rh negative woman is not D-isoimmunized, a repeat D antibody determination should be made at 28 weeks' gestation, and the expectant woman should receive 300 μg Rh immune globulin (Queenan, 1996). Rh immune globulin is also administered after any amniocentesis, regardless of gestational age, after chorionic villi sampling, if there is an episode of bleeding during pregnancy, or if there has been maternal trauma. In addition, Rh immune globulin must be administered to any Rh negative woman who experiences a first trimester spontaneous or induced abortion, or an ectopic pregnancy.

If the woman is Rh negative (dd), the father of the unborn child is asked to come into the clinic or physician's office to be assessed for his Rh factor and blood type. If he is homozygous for Rh positive (DD), all his offspring will be Rh positive. If he is heterozygous (Dd), 50% of his offspring will be Rh negative and 50% heterozygous for Rh positive. If the father is Rh negative, all their children will be Rh negative, and no Rh incompatibility with the mother will occur. If the father is Rh positive or the mother is known to have previously carried an Rh positive fetus, further testing and careful management are needed.

Anti-D antibody titers should be determined every 2 to 4 weeks beginning at 16 to 18 weeks, biweekly during the third trimester, and the week before the due date. If the test shows a maternal antibody titer of 1:16 or greater, a delta optical density (ΔOD) analysis of the amniotic fluid is performed. If the titer is 1:16 or less late in pregnancy, birth at 38 weeks or spontaneous labor at term can be anticipated.

Negative antibody titers can consistently identify the fetus not at risk. However, the titers cannot reliably point out the fetus in danger because the level of the titer does not correlate with the severity of the disease. For instance, in a severely sensitized woman antibody titers may be moderately high and remain at the same level although the fetus is being more and more severely affected. Conversely, a woman sensitized by previous Rh positive fetuses may show a high fixed antibody titer during a pregnancy in which the fetus is Rh negative. Fetal assessment includes percutaneous umbilical cord blood sampling (PUBS), amniocentesis, amniotic fluid analysis, and ultrasound. Previously, PUBS was the only direct method of assessing the Rh status of a fetus. This procedure requires a highly skilled physician and places the fetus at greater risk than does amniocentesis. It is now possible, however, to determine fetal Rh status from an amniotic fluid specimen using polymerase chain reaction (PCR).

Ultrasound should be done at 14 to 16 weeks to determine gestational age. Thereafter serial ultrasounds and amniotic fluid analysis should be done to follow fetal progress. The presence of ascites and subcutaneous edema are signs of severe fetal involvement (fetal hydrops). Other indicators of the fetal condition include an increase in fetal heart size, hydramnios, and placental thickness and texture (Queenan, 1996). Ultrasound evaluation cannot distinguish mild from severe fetal anemia unless hydropic changes are present.

The concentration of bilirubin pigments in the amniotic fluid declines during normal pregnancy. Hemolysis would result in a higher ΔOD level. Amniotic fluid, obtained by transabdominal amniocentesis, is separated from its cellular components by centrifuge. The amount of pigment from the degradation of red blood cells can be measured in the amniotic fluid. The fluid is subjected to spectrophotometric studies to determine the severity of the fetal hemolytic process. The ΔOD value and gestational age determine the plan of obstetric-pediatric management.

If the spectrophotometric readings are in zone I (the lowest zone) ΔOD at 450 nm, a normal or mildly anemic neonate may be anticipated, and birth at term may be permitted. Prognosis for this newborn is good, but phototherapy or exchange transfusion may be necessary. A reading in zone II (the middle zone) ΔOD at 450 nm indicates a moderately anemic fetus who may be hydropic or stillborn if born at term. Fetuses with a ΔOD in the upper zone II need to be followed with a PUBS or repeat amniocentesis within the week. Once the fetus reaches viability, induced vaginal or cesarean birth is indicated. The exact timing of birth needs to be determined individually based on factors such as fetal well-being, lung maturity, and previous obstetric history. A fair prognosis and possible need for exchange transfusion are anticipated. Readings within zone III (the highest zone) ΔOD at 450 nm indicate a severely affected fetus who may require intrauterine transfusion every 1 to 2 weeks between weeks 26 and 32 until viability is reached, followed by birth, usually by cesarean. Neonatal exchange transfusion is anticipated. Prognosis is guarded.

Fetal monitoring may identify the very ill fetus by documenting less movement or lack of movement. The appearance of sinusoidal pattern suggests fetal anemia and a deteriorating fetal condition (see Chapter 19).

Clinical Therapy

The goal of medical management is the birth of a mature fetus who has not developed severe hemolysis in utero. This requires early identification and treatment of maternal conditions that predispose the infant to hemolytic disease, coordinated obstetric-pediatric treatment for the seriously affected newborn, and prevention of Rh sensitization if none is present.

Antepartal Management

Two primary interventions are used by the physician to aid the fetus whose blood cells are being destroyed by maternal antibodies: early birth of the fetus and intrauterine transfusion, both of which carry risks. Ideally, birth should be delayed until fetal pulmonary maturity is confirmed at about 36 to 37 weeks. This is possible for most pregnancies with spectrophotometric readings in zones I and II. Severely sensitized fetuses may require birth at 32 to 34 weeks.

Intrauterine transfusion is done to correct the anemia produced by the red blood cell hemolysis and thereby improve fetal oxygenation. This may be done either intravascularly through PUBS or intraperitoneally as early as 18 weeks. Intravascular transfusion has greatly improved the outcome for severely affected fetuses. Under ultrasound visualization, the umbilical vein is entered, and the fetus is temporarily paralyzed with 0.1 mg/kg estimated fetal weight of pancuronium bromide. A fetal hematocrit is obtained; then leukocyte-poor Rh negative packed red blood cells (PRBCs) are transfused. The volume of PRBCs is determined by a formula based on estimated normal blood volume, the pretransfusion hematocrit, the hematocrit of the blood to be transfused, and the desired hematocrit (Jackson & Branch, 1996). Repeat transfusions can be scheduled as necessary until the fetus is sufficiently mature to tolerate birth. Prior to this technology, transfusions were done by introducing the needle into the fetal abdomen and peritoneal cavity. Blood was transfused through a catheter into the peritoneal cavity, where diaphragmatic lymphatics absorbed the RBCs into fetal circulation.

About 80% to 90% of transfused fetuses survive. The procedure is hazardous to the fetus, however. Complications include fetal distress, fetal hematoma, fetal-maternal hemorrhage, fetal death, and chorioamnionitis. Birth is delayed until at least 32 weeks' gestation if possible. Premature newborns are generally more susceptible to damage from hemolytic disease. They often require exchange transfusion and usually require intensive nursery care.

Postpartal Management

The goals of postpartal care are to prevent sensitization in the as-yet-unsensitized pregnant woman and to treat the isoimmune hemolytic disease in the newborn.

The Rh negative mother who has no titer (indirect Coombs' negative, nonsensitized) and who has given birth to an Rh positive fetus (direct Coombs' negative) is given an intramuscular injection of 300 μg RhIgG globulin (RhoGAM, HypRho-D) within 72 hours so that she does not have time to produce antibodies to fetal cells that entered her bloodstream when the placenta separated. This protocol reduces the incidence of antenatal sensitization by 93%. RhIgG works to destroy the fetal cells in the maternal circulation before sensitization occurs, thereby blocking maternal antibody production. This provides temporary passive immunity for the mother, which prevents the development of permanent active immunity (antibody formation).

The normal dose of RhIgG should suppress the immune response to approximately 30 mL Rh positive whole blood. However, if a larger fetomaternal bleed may have occurred, a Kleihauer-Betke test can be performed. This test is used to obtain an estimate of the size of a fetomaternal bleed. Based on the findings, an additional 300 μg of RhIgG is given for every 30 mL of fetal whole blood in the woman's circulation at a rate of 300 μg every 12 hours until the total necessary dose is given (Jackson & Branch, 1996).

When the woman is Rh negative and not sensitized and the father is Rh positive or unknown, RhIgG is also given after each abortion, ectopic pregnancy, amniocentesis, PUBS, or external version. After any maternal trauma, a Kleihauer-Betke test can be performed to identify the need for RhIgG administration. If abortion or ectopic pregnancy occurs in the first trimester, a smaller (50 μg) dose of RhIgG (MICRhoGAM or Mini-Gamulin Rh) is used. A full dose is used following second trimester amniocentesis. Occasionally, sensitization can occur antepartally due to small transplacental bleeds. To prevent this from occurring, an antibody screen is performed on an Rh negative woman at 28 weeks' gestation. If it is negative, 300 μg RhIgG is administered prophylactically (Slotnick, 1996). RhIgG is not given to the newborn or the father. It is not effective for and should not be given to a previously sensitized woman. However, sometimes after childbirth or an abortion, the results of the blood test do not clearly show whether the mother is already sensitized to the Rh antigen. In such cases, RhIgG should be given because it will cause no harm. Table 16–7 summarizes the major considerations in caring for an Rh negative woman. The treatment of the newborn with isoimmune hemolytic disease is discussed in Chapter 29.

NURSING CARE MANAGEMENT

Nursing Assessment and Diagnosis

As part of the initial prenatal history the nurse asks the mother whether she knows her blood type and Rh factor. Many women are aware that they are Rh negative and that this status has implications for pregnancy. If the woman knows she is Rh negative, the nurse can assess the woman's knowledge of what that means. The nurse can also ask the woman whether she ever received RhIgG, whether she has had any previous pregnancies and their outcome, and whether she knows her partner's Rh factor. Should the partner be Rh negative, there is no risk to the fetus, who will also be Rh negative.

If the woman does not know what Rh type she is, intervention cannot begin until the initial laboratory data are obtained. If the woman is Rh negative, the father's blood type and zygosity, if he is Rh positive, are obtained. Once that is complete, the nurse plans intervention based on the findings.

If the woman becomes sensitized during her pregnancy, nursing assessment focuses on the knowledge level and coping skills of the woman and her family. The nurse also provides ongoing assessment during procedures to evaluate fetal well-being, such as ultrasound and amniocentesis.

Postpartally, the nurse reviews data about the Rh type of the fetus. If the fetus is Rh positive, the mother is Rh negative, and no sensitization has occurred, nursing assessment reveals the need to administer RhIgG within 72 hours of birth.

TABLE 16–7 Rh Sensitization

When trying to work through Rh problems, the nurse should remember the following:

- A potential problem exists when an Rh negative mother and an Rh positive father conceive a child who is Rh positive.
- In this situation, the mother may become sensitized or produce antibodies to her fetus' Rh positive blood.

The following tests are used to detect sensitization:

- Indirect Coombs' tests—done on the mother's blood to measure the number of Rh positive antibodies
- Direct Coombs' test—done on the infant's blood to detect antibody-coated Rh positive RBCs.

Based on the results of these tests, the following may be done:

- If the mother's indirect Coombs' test is negative and the infant's direct Coomb's test is negative (confirming that sensitization has not occurred), the mother is given RhIgG within 72 hours of birth.
- If the mother's indirect Coomb's test is positive and her Rh positive infant has a positive direct Coomb's test, RhIgG is *not* given; in this case, the infant is carefully monitored for hemolytic disease.
- It is recommended that RhIgG be given at 28 weeks antenatally to decrease possible transplacental bleeding concerns.
- RhIgG is also administered after each abortion (spontaneous or therapeutic), ectopic pregnancy, amniocentesis, chorionic villi sampling (CVS), percutaneous umbilical blood sampling (PUBS), fetal cephalic version, or maternal trauma.

Nursing diagnoses that might apply to the pregnant woman at risk for Rh sensitization include the following:

- ***Knowledge Deficit*** related to a lack of understanding of the need to receive RhIgG and when it should be administered
- ***Ineffective Individual Coping*** related to depression secondary to the development of indications of the need for fetal exchange transfusion

I've been a nurse for over 32 years now. I remember when RhoGAM first started to be used—what a difference it made in the lives of so many women. Young women who are Rh negative today will hopefully never know the pain and tragedy the simple absence of a blood factor can mean. It is nothing short of miraculous!

Nursing Plan and Implementation

During the antepartal period, the nurse explains the mechanisms involved in isoimmunization and answers any questions the woman and her partner may have. It is imperative that the woman understand the importance of receiving RhIgG after every spontaneous or therapeutic abortion or ectopic pregnancy if she is not already sensitized. The nurse also explains the purpose of the RhIgG administered at 28 weeks if the woman is not sensitized.

If the woman is sensitized to the Rh factor, it poses a threat to any Rh positive fetus she carries. The nurse provides emotional support to the family to help them deal with their grief and any feelings of guilt about the infant's condition. Should an intrauterine transfusion become necessary, the nurse continues to provide emotional support while also assuming responsibilities as part of the health care team.

During labor, the nurse caring for an Rh negative woman who has not been sensitized ensures that the woman's blood is assessed for any antibodies and also has been cross-matched for RhIgG. On the postpartum unit, the nurse generally is responsible for administering the RhIgG (see Procedure 16–2: Administration of Rh Immune Globulin [RhIgG] on page 424).

Evaluation

Expected outcomes of nursing care include the following:

- The woman is able to explain the process of Rh sensitization and its implications for her unborn child and for subsequent pregnancies.
- If the woman has not been sensitized, she is able to explain the importance of receiving RhIgG when necessary and cooperates with the recommended dosage schedule.
- The woman gives birth to a healthy newborn.
- If complications develop for the fetus (or newborn), they are detected quickly, and therapy is instituted.

Care of the Woman at Risk Due to ABO Incompatibility

ABO incompatibility is rather common (occurring in 20% to 25% of pregnancies) but rarely causes significant hemolysis. In most cases, ABO incompatibility is limited to type O mothers with a type A or B fetus. The group B fetus of an A mother and the group A fetus of a B mother are only occasionally affected. Group O infants, because they have no antigenic sites on the red blood cells, are never affected regardless of the mother's blood type. The incompatibility occurs as a result of the maternal antibodies present in her serum and interaction between the antigen sites on the fetal red blood cells.

Anti-A and anti-B antibodies are naturally occurring; that is, women are naturally exposed to the A and B antigens through the foods they eat and through exposure to infection by gram-negative bacteria. As a result, some women have high serum anti-A and anti-B titers before they become pregnant. Once the woman becomes pregnant, the maternal serum anti-A and anti-B antibodies cross the placenta and produce hemolysis of the fetal red blood cells. With ABO incompatibility, the first infant is frequently involved, and no relationship exists between the appearance of the disease and repeated sensitization from one pregnancy to the next.

Unlike the case of Rh incompatibility, treatment is never warranted antepartally. As part of the initial assessment, however, the nurse should note whether the potential for an ABO incompatibility exists. This alerts caregivers so that following birth the newborn can be

PROCEDURE 16–2 ADMINISTRATION OF Rh IMMUNE GLOBULIN (RhIgG) (RhoGAM, HypRho-D)

Nursing Action	*Rationale*
Objective: Confirm that Rh immune globulin is indicated.	
Confirm that mother is Rh negative by checking her prenatal or intrapartal record. Then confirm that sensitization has not occurred—maternal indirect Coombs' negative. Confirm that infant is Rh positive. (A sample of the infant's cord blood is generally sent to the lab immediately after birth for typing and cross-matching.) If infant is Rh positive, confirm that sensitization has not occurred—direct Coombs' negative.	*Sensitization occurs when an Rh negative woman is exposed to Rh positive blood. She develops antibodies to the Rh positive blood. These antibodies can attack the fetal red blood cells, causing profound anemia. If both the direct and indirect Coombs' tests are negative, sensitization has not occurred, and Rh immune globulin is indicated.*
Objective: Confirm that the woman does not have a history of allergy to immune globulin preparations.	
Review entries on medication allergies in client chart, and ask woman specifically whether she has had any allergic reactions to medications, globulins, or blood products.	*Rh immune globulin is made from the plasma portion of blood. Allergic reactions are possible.*
Objective: Explain purpose and procedure. Have consent signed.	
Many agencies require informed consent before administering Rh immune globulin.	*The woman should clearly understand the purpose of the procedure, its rationale, and the procedure itself, including any risks. Generally, the primary side effects are erythema and tenderness at the injection site and allergic responses.*
Objective: Obtain correct medication.	
Rh immune globulin is available from the blood bank or pharmacy according to agency policy. Lot numbers for the drug and the cross-match should be the same.	*Because blood products are involved in the preparation, careful verification is essential.*
Objective: Confirm client identity, and administer medication in deltoid muscle.	
Medication is administered intramuscularly within 72 hours of childbirth. The normal dose of 300 μg provides passive immunity following exposure of up to 15 mL of transfused RBCs or 30 mL of fetal blood. If a larger bleed is suspected (as in cases of severe abruptio placentae), additional doses may be administered at one time using multiple sites or at regular intervals as long as all doses are given within 72 hours of childbirth.	*The medication causes passive immunity to occur and "tricks" the body into believing that it is not necessary to develop antibodies. Immunization is indicated any time there is a potential for maternal exposure to Rh positive blood. It is given prophylactically at 28 weeks' gestation, within 72 hours after the birth of an Rh positive Coombs' negative child, and following any spontaneous or therapeutic abortion, ectopic pregnancy, or amniocentesis.*
Objective: Complete education for self-care.	
Provide opportunities for the woman to ask questions and express concerns.	*Many women, especially primigravidas, are not aware of the risks for an Rh positive fetus of a sensitized Rh negative mother. They must understand the importance of receiving medication for each pregnancy to ensure continued protection.*
Objective: Complete client record.	
Chart according to agency procedure. Most agencies chart lot number, route, dose, client education.	*Provides a permanent record.*

assessed carefully for the development of hyperbilirubinemia (Chapter 29). Fewer than 1% of affected fetuses require an exchange transfusion after birth (Jackson & Branch, 1996).

Care of the Woman Requiring Surgery During Pregnancy

Although elective surgery should be delayed until the postpartal period, essential surgery can generally be undertaken during pregnancy. Surgery does pose some risks. The incidence of spontaneous abortion is increased for women who have surgery in the first trimester. There is also an increased incidence of fetal mortality and of low-birth-weight (less than 2500 g) infants. When surgery is necessary, the incidence of premature labor and intrauterine growth restriction increases (Reedy, Källen, & Kuehl, 1997).

Clinical Therapy

The most common reason for surgery during pregnancy (not related to trauma or obstetric conditions) is acute appendicitis followed by cholecystectomy (Reedy, Uy, Thompson, & Rayburn, 1998). Although general preoperative and postoperative care is similar for pregnant and nonpregnant women, special considerations must be kept in mind whenever the surgical client is pregnant. The early second trimester is the best time to operate because there is less risk of causing spontaneous abortion or early labor, and the uterus is not so large as to impinge on the abdominal field.

The preoperative chest radiograph and electrocardiogram, which are routine for persons over age 40, should be done on the same basis for the pregnant woman. If a chest radiograph is done, the fetus should be shielded from the radiation. Because of decreased intestinal motility and decreased free gastric acid secretion during pregnancy, stomach emptying time is delayed, which increases risk of vomiting during induction of anesthesia and during the postoperative period. Therefore, a nasogastric tube is recommended prior to major surgery. An indwelling urinary catheter prevents bladder distention, decreases risk of injury to the bladder, and promotes ease of monitoring output. Support stockings during and after surgery help prevent venous stasis and the development of thrombophlebitis. Fetal heart tones must be monitored before, during, and after surgery.

Pregnancy causes increased secretions of the respiratory tract and engorgement of the nasal mucous membrane, often making breathing through the nose difficult. Because of this, pregnant women often need an endotracheal tube for respiratory support during surgery. Caregivers must guard against maternal hypoxia during surgery because uterine circulation will be decreased and fetal oxygenation can decline very quickly. During surgery and the recovery period, the woman is positioned to allow optimal uteroplacental–fetal circulation. A wedge is placed under her hip to tip the uterus and thereby avoid pressure by the fetus on the maternal vena cava.

Spinal or epidural anesthesia is preferred because local anesthetics are not associated with birth defects. Caution must be exercised because this type of anesthesia may produce hypotension and respiratory apnea in the pregnant woman. The frequency and degree of the hypotension increase with higher anesthetic levels. This can be prevented in many cases with a preanesthetic infusion of 900 to 1000 mL of fluid.

Blood loss during surgery is monitored carefully. Measurement of fetal heart tones gives the best indication of blood loss. Because of the normal increased blood volume of pregnancy, uterine blood flow may be reduced significantly before the maternal blood pressure begins to fall. Fluid replacement should be done with balanced electrolyte solution and, if needed, with whole blood.

NURSING CARE MANAGEMENT

Nursing Assessment and Diagnosis

During the preoperative period, the nurse assesses the pregnant woman's health status in the same way that any preoperative client is assessed. Is there any sign of respiratory infection, fever, urinary tract infection, or anemia? Are laboratory values all within normal limits for surgery (except in the case of emergency surgery, which may, of necessity, be done even with abnormal laboratory values)? Do the woman and her family understand the surgical procedure? Do they know what to expect postoperatively? Do they have any questions or concerns?

The nurse also considers the impact of surgery on the woman's pregnancy. Is the fetal heart rate normal? Does the woman understand the implications of surgery with regard to her pregnancy? How is she coping?

Intraoperatively, fetal heart rate is assessed if at all possible. Postoperatively, the nurse completes all necessary postoperative assessments and also continues to assess fetal status, primarily by monitoring the fetal heart rate.

Nursing diagnoses that might apply to the pregnant woman who requires surgery include the following:

- ***Altered Tissue Perfusion*** (fetal) related to the effects of general anesthesia on fetal oxygenation
- ***Anxiety*** related to lack of knowledge of preoperative and postoperative procedures
- ***Fear*** related to the possible effect of surgery on fetal outcome

Nursing Plan and Implementation

Much of the nurse's care during the preoperative period is directed toward the educational needs of the woman and her family. The nurse plans time to review the procedure and answer any questions the family may have. The nurse recognizes that the need for surgery during the woman's pregnancy is probably very distressing for the family. The nurse works to help decrease their anxiety by providing information and emotional support.

Postoperatively, the nurse is caring for two clients: the mother and her unborn child. In addition to monitoring the status of both, the nurse considers both in providing care. If surgery is done in the first trimester, the nurse should be aware of the potential teratogenic effect of any medications prescribed and should discuss the implications with the surgeon and obstetrician. During the third trimester, the nurse, recognizing the potential for vena caval syndrome if the woman lies flat on her back, helps the woman maintain a side-lying position. To avoid inadequate oxygenation, the nurse encourages the woman to turn, breathe deeply, and cough regularly and also to use any ventilation therapy, such as incentive spirometry, to avoid developing pneumonia. The pregnant woman is also at increased risk for thrombophlebitis, so the nurse applies antiembolism stockings, encourages leg exercises while the woman is confined to bed, and begins ambulation as soon as possible. In addition, the nurse encourages the woman to maintain or resume an adequate diet as soon as possible. If cultural factors influence the woman's dietary practices, the nurse and dietitian should work together to meet the woman's needs.

Discharge teaching is especially important. The woman and her family should have a clear understanding of what to expect regarding activity level, discomfort, diet, medications, and any special considerations. In addition, they ought to know any warning signs that they should report to their physician immediately.

Evaluation

Expected outcomes of nursing care include the following:

- The woman is able to explain the surgical procedure, its risks and benefits, and its implications for her pregnancy.
- Caregivers maintain adequate maternal oxygenation throughout surgery and postoperatively.
- Potential complications are avoided or detected early and treated successfully.
- The woman is able to describe any necessary post-discharge activities, limitations, and follow-up and agrees to cooperate with the recommended regimen.
- The woman maintains her pregnancy successfully. ●

Care of the Woman Suffering Trauma from an Accident

Accidents and injury are the leading causes of death in women of reproductive age. Accidental injury has been estimated to complicate approximately 7% of all pregnancies and account for 200,000 injuries to pregnant women each year (Leiserowitz, 1996; Coleman, Trianfo, & Rund, 1997). Domestic abuse may be the etiology of trauma and is discussed in the next section.

In early pregnancy, body changes increase the potential for injury through fatigue, fainting spells, and hyperventilation. Late in pregnancy, the woman has less balance and coordination and may fall. Her protruding abdomen is vulnerable to a variety of minor injuries. The fetus is usually well protected by the amniotic fluid, which distributes the force of a blow equally in all directions, and by the muscle layers of the uterus and abdominal wall. In early pregnancy, while the uterus is still in the pelvis, it is shielded from blows by the surrounding pelvic organs, muscles, and bony structures. Trauma that causes concern includes blunt trauma, from an automobile accident, for example; penetrating abdominal injuries, such as knife or gunshot wounds; and the complications of maternal shock, premature labor, and spontaneous abortion.

Maternal mortality most often occurs from head trauma or hemorrhage. Uterine rupture results from strong deceleration forces in an automobile accident in fewer than 1% of pregnant women (Leiserowitz, 1996). All automobile passengers should wear seat belts. The small risk of uterine or placental injury from seat belt use is far outweighed by the fact that maternal death is the most common cause of fetal death. Traumatic separation of the placenta can occur even if the site of injury is remote from the abdomen. It results in a high rate of fetal mortality. Premature labor is another serious hazard to the fetus, often following rupture of membranes during an accident. Premature labor can ensue even if the woman is not injured.

Maternal fractures, even of the pelvis, are tolerated well. However, ruptured bladder, retroperitoneal hemorrhage, and shock are complications to watch for with a fractured pelvis.

Complications caused by trauma are more common after assault than after motor vehicle accidents. Fetal or placental injury occurs in 60% to 90% of gunshot wounds to the abdomen, with a 40% to 70% chance of fetal mortality (Leiserowitz, 1996). Stab wounds tend to cause less damage than bullet wounds.

Clinical Therapy

The goals of clinical therapy are to stabilize the injury and promote well-being for both mother and fetus. Thus clinical therapy initially focuses on ensuring airway adequacy, maintaining ventilation and adequate circulatory volume, controlling acute bleeding, and splinting fractures to prevent vascular or tissue injury. The Glasgow Coma Scale is useful in evaluating for neurologic deficit. Once the mother is stabilized, fetal status is assessed.

Care must be taken at the scene of the injury to avoid the development of supine hypotensive syndrome. A wedge is generally placed under the woman's right hip. A neck brace is used if a neck injury is suspected, or the woman is placed on a backboard and the entire board is tilted to displace the uterus. Prompt treatment of maternal hypotension or hypovolemia also averts poor fetal oxygenation. Obstetric consultation is necessary to ensure that the needs of both mother and fetus are met.

In cases of noncatastrophic trauma, that is, where the mother's life is not directly threatened, fetal monitoring for 4 hours should be sufficient if there is no vaginal bleeding, uterine tenderness, contractions, or leaking amniotic fluid. Abruptio placentae may occur following a blow to the abdomen as the flexible myometrium of the uterus sustains a contour-changing impact that the relatively inelastic placenta cannot match. The increased intrauterine pressure during the blow further shears the placenta from the underlying decidua basalis. Abruptio placentae may occur in up to 5% of women who sustain minor injuries and in up to 66% of women who sustain major abdominal trauma (Leiserowitz, 1996). Increased uterine irritability in the first few hours following trauma helps identify women who may be at high risk for this potentially catastrophic complication. If the woman is bleeding, contracting, or has uterine tenderness or a nonreassuring fetal heart rate tracing, a 24- to 48-hour observation is recommended.

Fetomaternal hemorrhage occurs four to five times more often in pregnant women who have experienced trauma. A Kleihauer-Betke test may be useful in helping identify unsensitized Rh negative women who have experienced fetal-maternal bleeds due to trauma. RhIgG should be given to any unsensitized Rh negative woman to be certain she is covered for small fetal hemorrhages that may be below the sensitivity of the Kleihauer-Betke test.

There has been controversy regarding the use of beta-adrenergic tocolytics in pregnant women following trauma because of the concerns regarding hemodynamic instability and the potential for masking uterine irritability or contractions that forewarn of abruptio placentae. Radiographic studies should be performed as needed to evaluate injuries regardless of fetal exposure.

When cardiopulmonary resuscitation (CPR) is performed on the pregnant woman late in gestation, perimortem cesarean birth is advocated if CPR is unsuccessful in the first 4 minutes. Chest compressions are less effective in the third trimester due to compression of the inferior vena cava by the gravid uterus. Cesarean birth alleviates this compression and improves resuscitation efforts in both the fetus and the mother.

NURSING CARE MANAGEMENT

Nursing Assessment and Diagnosis

Each individual must be assessed according to the type and extent of her injuries. As with all trauma victims, initial assessments focus on adequacy of the airway, evidence of breathing, existence of cardiovascular stability, and extent of injury. When an injured woman is pregnant, it is necessary to assess fetal status as well in order to avoid fetal hypoxia. Frequent maternal blood gas determinations are indicated if respiratory function is compromised.

Assessment should include a review of the specific history of past and present pregnancies to avoid incorrect interpretation of vital signs. Caregivers do diagnostic tests as necessary, avoiding radiology in favor of ultrasonography whenever possible.

Ongoing assessments include evaluation of intake and output and other indicators of shock, normal postoperative evaluation in those women requiring surgery, determination of neurologic status, and assessment of mental outlook and anxiety level.

Nursing diagnoses that might apply to the pregnant woman suffering trauma include the following:

- ***Pain*** related to the effects of the trauma experienced
- ***Constipation*** related to immobility secondary to the effects of the accident
- ***Fear*** related to the effects of the trauma on fetal well-being

Nursing Plan and Implementation

As a member of the health care team the nurse is actively involved in the ongoing assessment of the status of the woman and fetus. The nurse also has a primary responsibility to assess the childbearing woman's emotional state. The trauma victim must be oriented to her situation and receive explanation and reinforcement as necessary to help her understand any interventions. Family members should be involved as appropriate. The nurse also gives the pregnant woman an opportunity to discuss her feelings and concerns.

Evaluation

Expected outcomes of nursing care include the following:

- The woman and her family are able to understand the effects of the trauma on her and on her unborn child.
- Adequate maternal oxygenation is maintained to ensure fetal well-being.
- The woman's pain is adequately relieved, and her trauma is treated.
- Potential complications are quickly identified, and appropriate interventions are instituted.
- The woman gives birth to a healthy newborn.
- If the trauma results in fetal demise, the woman is able to verbalize her feelings and begin working through the grief process. ●

COMMUNITY IN FOCUS

Healthy Beginnings

More and more communities are acting proactively to improve the parenting skills of their residents and decrease the incidence of child abuse and neglect. One especially successful program is the Healthy Beginnings Program in Hastings, Nebraska. Established in 1990, the program, which is the first mainland replication of the successful Hawaii Healthy Start Program, is a home visitation program designed to help parents be "the best they can be." The program is voluntary and free to participants.

Families enter the program prenatally or up to three months following the birth of a child. Approximately 75% of families are referred to the program by a health care professional; the remainder are self-referred or referred by another agency. Once a contact is made, each family is seen by a nurse and paraprofessional for an interview and initial assessment. The Family Stress Checklist, developed in 1978 by Smith and Carroll of the University of Colorado Health Sciences Center, is used to screen families as low, moderate, or high risk for parenting problems. All moderate and high-risk families are invited to join the program.

The program offers long-term and intensive services. Prenatally, parents participate in a series of nursing home visits to discuss a wide variety of topics related to pregnancy and parenting. Additional nursing visits are scheduled in the home following childbirth and again within the first month. The emphasis of these early visits is on adjustment to the newborn and on learning to read and respond appropriately to the baby's cues. Moreover, six times during the first 2 years, nurses complete developmental assessments of each child and make appropriate referrals if they identify any concerns or developmental delays. Nurses also regularly assess and educate parents about issues such as age-appropriate developmental expectations and activities, and parent-child interactions and communication.

In addition, the family is visited weekly by a specially trained paraprofessional who helps the family develop skill in parenting. To ensure consistency and promote a sense of trust, the family works with the same paraprofessional and nurse throughout the duration of services. These weekly visits last up to a year or more and then progress to biweekly and quarterly visits as the family gains skills and confidence. Visits continue until the child is 5 years old. Throughout the process, families receive case management services, including community and professional referrals and networking; health, nutritional, and safety assessments; and encouragement to use the health care system appropriately (clinic, emergency department, phone support). Results to date are impressive. Of the families served by Healthy Beginnings:

- 98% have no child abuse or neglect requiring court involvement.
- 97% of the children are up-to-date on their well child care and immunizations.
- At least 98% of the families have no unintended repeat pregnancies.
- Over 80% of the families are either employed, furthering their education, or both.

SOURCE: Personal communication with Paula Witt, RN, PNP, director of the Healthy Beginnings Program, and printed program materials.

Care of the Battered Pregnant Woman

Female partner abuse often begins or increases during pregnancy. In fact, abuse during pregnancy affects one in six women (McFarlane & Parker, 1996). Physical abuse may result in loss of pregnancy, preterm labor, low-birth-weight infants, injury to the fetus, and fetal death. The first step toward helping the battered woman is to identify her. She needs support, confidence in her decision making, and the recognition that she can help herself.

Chronic psychosomatic symptoms can be an indicator of abuse. The woman may have nonspecific or vague complaints. It is important to assess old scars around the head, chest, arms, abdomen, and genitalia. Any bruising or evidence of pain is also evaluated. The nurse should be especially alert for signs of bruising or injury to the woman's breasts, abdomen, or genitals because these areas are common targets of violence during pregnancy. Other indicators include a decrease in eye contact, silence when the partner is in the room, and a history of nervousness, insomnia, drug overdose, or alcohol problems. Frequent visits to the emergency department and a history of accidents without understandable causes are possible indicators of abuse.

The goals of treatment are to identify the woman at risk, increase her decision-making abilities to decrease the potential for further abuse, and provide a safe environment for the pregnant woman and her unborn child. It is important to provide an environment that is private, accepting, and nonjudgmental so that the woman can express her concerns. She needs to be aware of community resources available to her, such as emergency shelters; police, legal, and social services; and counseling. Nurses need to recognize that, ultimately, it is the woman's decision either to seek assistance or to return to old patterns.

Because abuse often begins during pregnancy, it may be a new and unexpected experience for the woman. She may believe that it is an isolated incident that will occur only during the pregnancy. She needs to know that battering may well occur following childbirth and may extend to the child as well. This is an important time for the nurse to provide information and establish a trusted link for the woman with a health care professional. Although the nurse may feel unsuccessful if the woman chooses to return to her partner, in the long term the information the nurse provides may help the woman make choices that end the violence. For further discussion of female partner abuse, see Chapter 5.

Care of the Woman with a TORCH Infection

Infectious diseases in the TORCH group are those identified as causing serious harm to the embryo/fetus. These are **to**xoplasmosis, **r**ubella, **c**ytomegalovirus, and **h**erpes simplex virus. (Some sources identify the O as "other infections.") The TORCH identification assists health team members to assess quickly the potential risk to each woman in pregnancy.

The importance of understanding what these infections are and identifying risk factors cannot be overemphasized. Exposure of the woman during the first 12 weeks of gestation may cause developmental anomalies. The three major viral infections are rubella, cytomegalovirus, and herpes simplex virus. Toxoplasmosis is a protozoal infection.

Toxoplasmosis

Toxoplasmosis is caused by the protozoan *Toxoplasma gondii.* It is innocuous in most adults but can be devastating to the immunosuppressed person. When contracted in pregnancy, it can profoundly affect the fetus. The pregnant woman may contract the organism by eating raw or poorly cooked meat, by drinking unpasteurized goat's milk, or by contact with the feces of infected cats, either through the cat litter box or by gardening in areas frequented by cats (Sever, 1998). The percentage of childbearing women in North America who are seropositive for toxoplasmosis varies. In the United States, approximately 40% to 50% of adults have antibodies to this organism. Toxoplasmosis is more common in Western Europe. In Paris, more than 80% of women of childbearing age have antibodies to this organism (Duff, 1996).

Fetal-Neonatal Risks

Maternal infection during the first trimester is associated with the lowest incidence of fetal infection but often results in a spontaneous abortion if the fetus contracts the infection. The highest rate of fetal infection (65%) occurs when the mother contracts the infection in the third trimester, but almost 90% of infants are born without clinical signs of infection. In very mild cases, retinochoroiditis may be the only recognizable damage, and it and other manifestations may not appear until adolescence or young adulthood. Severe neonatal disorders associated with congenital infection include convulsions, coma, microcephaly, and hydrocephalus. The infant with a severe infection may die soon after birth. Survivors are often blind, deaf, and severely retarded. Treatment of the mother can reduce the incidence of fetal infection by 60% (Cohen & Goldstein, 1996).

Clinical Therapy

The goal of medical treatment is to identify the woman at risk for toxoplasmosis and to treat the disease promptly if diagnosed. Diagnosis can be made by serologic testing, including the IgM and IgG fluorescent antibody tests. Elevated IgM titers are detectable 5 days after infection and may remain elevated for one year or more (Dugoff, 1996). The indirect florescent Ab test (IFAT), the indirect hemagglutination test (IHAT), or the Sabin-Feldman dye test are also used to establish the diagnosis.

If diagnosis can be established by physical findings, history, and positive serologic results, the woman may be treated with sulfadiazine, pyrimethamine, and spiramycin. If toxoplasmosis is diagnosed before 20 weeks' gestation, pyrimethamine should be avoided unless a therapeutic abortion is planned. Sulfadiazine and erythromycin may be used during the first half of pregnancy.

NURSING CARE MANAGEMENT

Nursing Assessment and Diagnosis

The incubation period for the disease is 10 days. The woman with acute toxoplasmosis may be asymptomatic, or she may develop myalgia, malaise, rash, splenomegaly, fever, headache, and enlarged posterior cervical lymph nodes. Symptoms usually disappear in a few days or weeks.

Nursing diagnoses that might apply to the pregnant woman with toxoplasmosis include the following:

- ***Risk for Altered Health Maintenance*** related to lack of knowledge about ways in which a pregnant woman can contract toxoplasmosis
- ***Anticipatory Grieving*** related to potential effects on infant of maternal toxoplasmosis

Nursing Plan and Implementation

The nurse caring for women during the antepartal period has the primary opportunity to discuss methods of prevention of toxoplasmosis with the childbearing woman. The woman must understand the importance of avoiding poorly cooked or raw meat, especially pork, beef, lamb, and, in the arctic region, caribou. Fruits and vegetables should be washed. She should avoid contact with the cat litter box by having someone else clean it. In addition, because it takes approximately 48 hours for a cat's feces to become infectious, the litter should be cleaned frequently. The nurse should also discuss the importance of the woman's wearing gloves when gardening and of avoiding garden areas frequented by cats.

Evaluation

Expected outcomes of nursing care include the following:

- The woman is able to discuss toxoplasmosis, its method of transmission, the implications for her fetus, and measures she can take to avoid contracting it.
- The woman implements health measures to avoid contracting toxoplasmosis.
- The woman gives birth to a healthy newborn. ●

Rubella

The effects of rubella (German measles) are no more severe for pregnant women, nor are there greater complications in pregnant women, than in nonpregnant women of comparable age. However, the effects of this infection on the fetus and newborn are great if maternal infection occurs during the first 5 months of pregnancy (Sever, 1996).

Despite the availability of a rubella vaccine, up to 20% of women of childbearing age are not rubella immune (Cohen & Goldstein, 1996). These figures emphasize the need for routine immunization programs. Prepubertal and nonpregnant women of childbearing age who do not have antirubella antibodies should be immunized with the live attenuated rubella vaccine. Although no fetal infection has resulted from immunization of a pregnant woman, pregnancy should be avoided for 3 months after immunization (Cohen & Goldstein, 1996). Nurses need to be aware of the importance of postpartum immunization of the nonimmune woman to decrease unnecessary perinatal transmission.

Fetal-Neonatal Risks

The period of greatest risk for the teratogenic effects of rubella on the fetus is during the first trimester, when 80% to 90% of the fetuses exposed will be affected, resulting in spontaneous abortion or serious abnormalities, such as heart damage, cataracts, and mental retardation. If infection occurs early in the second trimester, the resultant fetal effect is most often permanent hearing impairment, microcephaly, or psychomotor retardation.

Clinical signs of congenital infection are congenital heart disease, IUGR, and cataracts. Cardiac involvements most often seen are patent ductus arteriosus and narrowing of peripheral pulmonary arteries. Cataracts may be unilateral or bilateral and may be present at birth or develop in the neonatal period. A petechial rash is seen in some infants, and hepatosplenomegaly and hyperbilirubinemia are frequently seen. Other abnormalities, such as mental retardation or cerebral palsy, may become evident in infancy. Diagnosis in the newborn can be conclusively made in the presence of these conditions and with an elevated rubella IgM antibody titer at birth.

Infants born with congenital rubella syndrome are infectious and should be isolated. These infants may continue to shed the virus for months.

The expanded rubella syndrome relates to effects that may develop for years after the infection. These include an increased incidence of insulin-dependent diabetes mellitus; sudden hearing loss; glaucoma; and a slow, progressive form of encephalitis.

Clinical Therapy

The best therapy for rubella is prevention. Live attenuated vaccine is available and should be given to all children. Women of childbearing age should be tested for immunity and vaccinated if susceptible and if it is established that they are not pregnant. Health counseling in high school and in premarital clinic visits can stress the importance of screening prior to planning a pregnancy.

As part of the prenatal laboratory screen the woman is evaluated for rubella using hemagglutination inhibition (HAI), a serology test. The presence of a 1:16 titer or greater is evidence of immunity. A titer less than 1:8 indicates susceptibility to rubella.

Because the vaccine is made with attenuated virus, pregnant women are not vaccinated. However, it is considered safe for newly vaccinated children to have contact with pregnant women.

If a woman who is pregnant becomes infected during the first trimester, therapeutic abortion is an alternative.

NURSING CARE MANAGEMENT

Nursing Assessment and Diagnosis

A woman who develops rubella during pregnancy may be asymptomatic or may show signs of a mild infection, including a maculopapular rash, lymphadenopathy, muscular achiness, and joint pain. The presence of IgM antirubella antibody is diagnostic of a recent infection. These titers remain elevated for approximately 1 month following infection.

Nursing diagnoses that may apply to the woman who develops rubella early in her pregnancy include:

- ***Ineffective Family Coping*** due to an inability to accept the possibility of fetal anomalies secondary to maternal rubella exposure
- ***Risk for Altered Health Maintenance*** related to lack of knowledge about the importance of rubella immunization prior to becoming pregnant

Nursing Plan and Implementation

Nursing support and understanding are vital for the couple contemplating abortion due to a diagnosis of rubella. Such a decision may initiate a crisis for the couple who have planned their pregnancy. They need objective data to understand the possible effects on their fetus and the prognosis for the offspring.

Evaluation
Expected outcomes of nursing care include the following:

- The woman is able to describe the implications of rubella exposure during the first trimester of pregnancy.
- If exposure occurs in a woman who is not immune, she is able to identify her options and make a decision about continuing her pregnancy that is acceptable to her and her partner.
- The nonimmune woman receives the rubella vaccine during the early postpartal period.
- The woman gives birth to a healthy infant. ●

Cytomegalovirus

Cytomegalovirus (CMV) belongs to the herpes simplex virus group and causes both congenital and acquired disorders. The significance of this virus in pregnancy is related to its ability to be transmitted by asymptomatic women across the placenta to the fetus or by the cervical route during birth.

CMV is the most common viral cause of intrauterine infection (Scott, Hollier, & Dias, 1997). Nearly half of adults have antibodies for the virus. The virus can be found in urine, saliva, cervical mucus, semen, and breast milk. It can be passed between humans by any close contact such as kissing, breastfeeding, and sexual intercourse. Asymptomatic CMV infection is particularly common in children and gravid women. It is a chronic, persistent infection in that the individual may shed the virus continually over many years. The cervix can harbor the virus, and an ascending infection can develop after birth. Although the virus is usually innocuous in adults and children, it may be fatal to the fetus.

Accurate diagnosis in the pregnant woman depends on the presence of CMV in the urine, a rise in IgM levels, and identification of the CMV antibodies within the serum IgM fraction. At present no treatment exists for maternal CMV or for the congenital disease in the newborn.

Fetal-Neonatal Risks

The cytomegalovirus is the most frequent agent of viral infection in the human fetus. It infects 0.5% to 2.5% of newborns. Ninety percent of infected fetuses will be asymptomatic at birth, the remaining 10% will have abnormalities of varying severity. There is a 20% to 30% mortality rate among the symptomatic infants, and 90% of the survivors have significant neurologic complications (Cohen & Goldstein, 1996; Scott et al, 1997). Subclinical infections in the newborn are capable of producing mental retardation and auditory deficits, sometimes not recognized for several months, or learning disabilities not seen until childhood. CMV may be the most common cause of mental retardation.

For the fetus, this infection can result in extensive intrauterine tissue damage that leads to fetal death; in survival with microcephaly, hydrocephaly, cerebral palsy, or mental retardation; or in survival with no damage at all.

The infected neonate is often SGA. The principal tissues and organs affected are the blood, brain, and liver. However, virtually all organs are potentially at risk. Hemolysis leads to anemia and hyperbilirubinemia. Thrombocytopenia and hepatosplenomegaly may also develop.

Herpes Simplex Virus

It has been estimated that more than 30 million people are infected with genital herpes and that more than 500,000 new cases are diagnosed in the United States each year (Scott et al, 1997). Herpes simplex virus (HSV-I or HSV-II) infection can cause painful lesions in the genital area. Lesions may also develop on the cervix. This condition and its implications for nonpregnant women are discussed in Chapter 3. However, because the presence of herpes lesions in the genital tract may profoundly affect the fetus, herpes infection as it relates to a pregnant woman is discussed here as part of the TORCH complex of infections.

Fetal-Neonatal Risks

Hormonal changes in pregnancy may make a woman more susceptible to infection and cause a primary herpes infection to be more severe than in a nonpregnant woman. A primary infection can also increase the risk of spontaneous abortion when infection occurs in the first trimester. Preterm labor, intrauterine growth restriction, and neonatal infection are greater risks if the primary infection occurs late in the second trimester or early in the third trimester. The single most predictive factor for recurrence frequencies of HSV is the severity of the initial outbreak. The more severe the initial outbreak, the more likely it is to have frequent outbreaks. Recurrence rates seem higher in pregnant women, and the likelihood of recurrence increases with advancing gestational age. Another important point is that asymptomatic viral shedding occurs on approximately 5% of the days in the first several months after initial infection (lasting 24 to 36 hours), then falls to about 1% of the days after that. A woman who has a primary outbreak of herpes during her current pregnancy has a 36% chance of an outbreak at the time of childbirth. Those with recurrent herpes have a 25% chance of outbreak during the last month of pregnancy, and 11% to 14% will have an outbreak at the time of birth (Scott et al, 1997).

The risk to the fetus varies with the route of birth and whether the lesion that is present at the time of birth is primary or recurrent. If the woman has a primary, asymptomatic lesion at the time of birth, the risk of transmission is 33% for a vaginal birth. If a symptomatic primary lesion is present, the risk of transmission jumps to 50% for a vaginal birth. Exposure of the neonate to a recurrent lesion drops the risk of transmission to 4% for a symptomatic lesion and 0.04% (1/10,000) for an asymptomatic lesion. Cesarean birth is not a fail-safe measure for preventing neonatal herpes infection. Moreover, 20% to 30% of infants who are diagnosed with herpes infections in the neonatal period are born by cesarean (Scott et al, 1997).

The infected infant is often asymptomatic at birth but after an incubation period of 2 to 12 days develops symptoms of fever (or hypothermia), jaundice, seizures, and poor feeding. Approximately one-half of infected infants develop the characteristic vesicular skin lesions. Vidarabine has been useful in decreasing serious effects from neonatal herpes, but no definitive treatment exists as yet. Some experts treat asymptomatic infants who were exposed to herpes simplex virus during birth with acyclovir. Positive herpes cultures taken 24 to 48 hours after birth should be obtained before treatment (CDC, 1998).

Clinical Therapy

In the past, serial cultures were done on a woman with a history of herpes. If the most recent culture prior to labor was negative, she was allowed to give birth vaginally. Because that practice was not based on any scientific evidence, in 1988 serial HSV cultures were abandoned. The current practice is to examine the woman for any evidence of lesions and question her regarding the existence of prodromal symptoms. If either is present, a cesarean is performed. If there is no evidence of infection, the woman is allowed to give birth vaginally.

Oral antiviral therapies are available, including acyclovir (Zovirax), famciclovir and valacyclovir. At this time, acyclovir is the only drug for herpes that has been studied during pregnancy (Brown, 1999). Currently, there is no evidence that there are any adverse fetal effects related to exposure to any of these drugs during any trimester. Use of acyclovir beginning several weeks prior to anticipated childbirth for the purpose of suppressing the herpes virus is controversial. Some researchers feel it decreases the incidence of herpes outbreak; others (Brown, 1999) feel that prophylactic use to suppress recurrent HSV infection is not appropriate until the clinical trials currently underway are completed.

Vaccines against herpes have not yet been developed that are superior to acyclovir suppression. Researchers remain optimistic that an adequate vaccine will be developed, but currently acyclovir remains the antiviral agent of choice in pregnancy (Scott et al, 1997).

NURSING CARE MANAGEMENT

Nursing Assessment and Diagnosis

During the initial prenatal visit, it is important to learn whether the woman or her partner have had previous herpes infections. If so, ongoing assessment is indicated as pregnancy progresses.

Nursing diagnoses that may apply to the pregnant woman with HSV include the following:

- ***Pain*** related to the presence of lesions secondary to herpes infection
- ***Sexual Dysfunction*** related to unwillingness to engage in sexual intercourse secondary to the presence of active herpes lesions
- ***Ineffective Individual Coping*** related to depression secondary to the risk to the fetus if herpes lesions are present at birth

Nursing Plan and Implementation

Nurses need to be particularly concerned with client education about this fast-spreading disease. Women should be informed about what herpes is, how it is spread, and preventive measures. Women should also receive information about the association of genital herpes with spontaneous abortion, neonatal mortality and morbidity, and the possibility of cesarean birth. A woman needs to inform her future health care providers of her infection. She also should know of the possible association of genital herpes with cervical cancer and the importance of a yearly Pap smear.

The woman who acquired HSV as an adolescent may be devastated as a mature young adult who wants to have a family. Clients may be helped by counseling that allows expression of the anger, shame, and depression so often experienced by women with herpes. Literature may be helpful and is available from Planned Parenthood and many public health agencies. The American Social Health Association has established the HELP program to provide information and the latest research results on genital herpes. The association has a quarterly journal, *The Helper*, for nurses and herpes clients.

Evaluation

Expected outcomes of nursing care include the following:

- The woman is able to describe her infection with regard to its method of spread, expected medical therapy, comfort measures, implications for her pregnancy, and long-term implications.
- The woman has appropriate cultures done as recommended throughout her pregnancy.
- The woman gives birth to a healthy infant. ●

Other Infections in Pregnancy

In addition to the TORCH infections, other infections contribute to risk during pregnancy (Table 16–8). Spontaneous abortion is frequently the result of a severe maternal infection. Evidence exists that links infection and prematurity. In addition, if the pregnancy is carried to term in the presence of infection, the risk of maternal and fetal morbidity and mortality increases. Thus it is essential to maternal and fetal health that infection be diagnosed and treated promptly.

TABLE 16–8 Infections That Put Pregnancy at Risk

Condition and Causative Organism	Signs and Symptoms	Treatment	Implications for Pregnancy
Urinary Tract Infections			
Asymptomatic bacteriuria (ASB): *E coli, Klebsiella, Proteus* most common	Bacteria present in urine on culture with no accompanying symptoms.	Oral sulfonamides early in pregnancy, ampicillin and nitrofurantoin (Furadantin) in late pregnancy.	Women with ASB in early pregnancy may go on to develop cystitis or acute pyelonephritis by third trimester if not treated. Oral sulfonamides taken in the last few weeks of pregnancy may lead to neonatal hyperbilirubinemia and kernicterus.
Cystitis (lower UTI): Causative organisms same as ASB	Dysuria, urgency, frequency; low-grade fever and hematuria may occur. Urine culture (clean catch) show ↑ leukocytes. Presence of 10^5 (100,000) or more colonies bacteria per mL urine.	Same.	If not treated, infection may ascend and lead to acute pyelonephritis.
Acute pyelonephritis: Causative organisms same as ASB	Sudden onset. Chills, high fever, flank pain. Nausea, vomiting, malaise. May have decreased urine output, severe colicky pain, dehydration. Increased diastolic BP, positive FA test, low creatinine clearance. Marked bacteremia in urine culture, pyuria, WBC casts.	Hospitalization; IV antibiotic therapy. Other antibiotics safe during pregnancy include carbenicillin, methenamine, cephalosporins. Catheterization if output is ↓. Supportive therapy for comfort. Follow-up urine cultures are necessary.	Increased risk of premature birth and intrauterine growth restriction (IUGR). These antibiotics interfere with urinary estriol levels and can cause false interpretations of estriol levels during pregnancy.
Vaginal Infections			
Vulvovaginal candidiasis (yeast infection): *Candida albicans*	Often thick, white, curdy discharge, severe itching, dysuria, dyspareunia. Diagnosis based on presence of hyphae and spores in a wet mount preparation of vaginal secretions.	Intravaginal insertion of miconazole or clotrimazole suppositories at bedtime for 1 week. Cream may be prescribed for topical application to the vulva if necessary.	If the infection is present at birth and the fetus is born vaginally, the fetus may contract thrush.
Bacterial vaginosis: *Gardnerella vaginalis*	Thin, watery, yellow-gray discharge with foul odor often described as "fishy." Wet mount preparation reveals "clue cells." Application of KOH (potassium hydroxide) to a specimen of vaginal secretions produces a pronounced fishy odor.	Nonpregnant women treated with oral metronidazole (Flagyl). In second and third trimesters, oral metronidazole administered in a lower dose; clindamycin orally or metronidazole vaginal gel are alternatives (CDC, 1998).	Metronidazole has potential teratogenic effects when used in the 1st trimester. Possible ↑ risk of PROM and preterm birth. Confirmatory studies needed (CDC, 1998).
Trichomoniasis: *Trichomonas vaginalis*	Occasionally asymptomatic. May have frothy greenish-gray vaginal discharge, pruritus, urinary symptoms. Strawberry patches may be visible on vaginal walls or cervix. Wet mount preparation of vaginal secretions shows motile flagellated trichomonads.	During early pregnancy symptoms may be controlled with clotrimazole vaginal suppositories. Both partners are treated, but no adequate treatment exists. After first trimester, a single 2 g dose of metronidazole may be used (CDC, 1998).	Metromidazole has potential teratogenic effects. Associated with ↑ risk of PROM and preterm birth (CDC, 1998).
Sexually Transmitted Infections			
Chlamydial infection: *Chlamydia trachomatis*	Women are often asymptomatic. Symptoms may include thin or purulent discharge, urinary burning and frequency, or lower abdominal pain. Lab test available to detect monoclonal antibodies specific for *Chlamydia.*	Although nonpregnant women are treated with tetracycline, it may permanently discolor fetal teeth. Thus pregnant women are treated with erythromycin ethyl succinate.	Infant of woman with untreated chlamydial infection may develop newborn conjunctivitis, which can be treated with erythromycin eye ointment (but not silver nitrate). Infant may also develop chlamydial pneumonia. May be responsible for premature labor and fetal death.

➤

TABLE 16–8 Infections That Put Pregnancy at Risk *continued*

Condition and Causative Organism	Signs and Symptoms	Treatment	Implications for Pregnancy
Sexually Transmitted Infections *continued*			
Syphilis: *Treponema pallidum,* a spirochete	Primary stage: chancre, slight fever, malaise. Chancre lasts about 4 weeks, then disappears. Secondary stage: occurs 6 weeks to 6 months after infection. Skin eruptions (condyloma lata); also symptoms of acute arthritis, liver enlargement, iritis, chronic sore throat with hoarseness. Diagnosed by blood tests such as VDRL, RPR, FTA-ABS. Dark-field examination for spirochetes may also be done.	For syphilis less than 1 year in duration: 2.4 million U benzathine penicillin G IM. For syphilis of more than 1 year's duration: 2.4 million U benzathine penicillin G once a week for 3 weeks. Sexual partners should also be screened and treated.	Syphilis can be passed transplacentally to the fetus. If untreated, one of the following can occur: second trimester abortion, stillborn infant at term, congenitally infected infant, uninfected live infant.
Gonorrhea: *Neisseria gonorrhoeae*	Majority of women asymptomatic; disease often diagnosed during routine prenatal cervical culture. If symptoms are present they may include purulent vaginal discharge, dysuria, urinary frequency, inflammation and swelling of the vulva. Cervix may appear eroded.	Nonpregnant women are treated with cefixime orally or ceftriaxone IM plus doxycycline. Pregnant woman are treated with ceftriaxone plus erythromycin (CDC, 1998). If the woman is allergic to ceftriaxone, spectinomycin is used. All sexual partners are also treated.	Infection at time of birth may cause ophthalmia neonatorum in the newborn.
Condyloma acuminata: caused by a papovavirus	Soft, grayish-pink lesions on the vulva, vagina, cervix, or anus.	Podophyllin not used during pregnancy. Trichloroacetic acid, liquid nitrogen, or cryotherapy CO_2 laser therapy done under colposcopy is also successful (CDC, 1998).	Possible teratogenic effect of podophyllin. Large doses have been associated with fetal death.

Urinary tract, vaginal, and sexually transmitted infections are discussed in detail in Chapter 3. Table 16–8 provides a summary of these infections and their implications for pregnancy.

FOCUS YOUR STUDY

- Hyperemesis gravidarum, excessive vomiting during pregnancy, may cause fluid and electrolyte imbalance, dehydration, and signs of starvation in the mother and, if severe enough, death of the fetus. Treatment is aimed at controlling the vomiting, correcting fluid and electrolyte imbalance, correcting dehydration, and improving nutritional status.
- Several health problems associated with bleeding arise from the pregnancy itself, such as spontaneous abortion, ectopic pregnancy, and gestational trophoblastic disease. The nurse needs to be alert to early signs of these situations, to guard the woman against heavy bleeding and shock, to facilitate the medical treatment, and to provide educational and emotional support.
- Incompetent cervix, the premature dilatation of the cervix, is the most common cause of second trimester abortion. It is treated surgically with a Shirodkar or McDonald cerclage, which involves placing a suture in the cervix to keep it closed.
- Premature rupture of the membranes and preterm labor both place the fetus at risk. Women with PROM and no signs of infection are managed conservatively with bed rest and careful monitoring of fetal well-being. Women with a history of preterm labor may be placed on home fetal monitoring programs. If preterm labor develops, tocolytics are often effective in stopping labor but do have associated side effects.
- Hypertension may exist prior to pregnancy or, more often, may develop during pregnancy. Pregnancy-induced hypertension can lead to growth retardation for the fetus and, if untreated, may lead to convulsions (eclampsia) and even death for the mother and fetus. A woman's understanding of the disease process helps motivate her to maintain the required rest periods in the left lateral position. Antihypertensive or anticonvulsive drugs may be part of the therapy.
- Rh incompatibility can exist when an Rh negative woman and an Rh positive partner conceive a child who is Rh positive. The use of RhIgG has greatly decreased the incidence of severe sequelae due to Rh incompatibility because the drug "tricks" the body into thinking antibodies have been produced in response to the Rh antigen.
- The impact of surgery or trauma on the pregnant woman and her fetus is related to timing in the pregnancy, seriousness of the situation, and other factors influencing the situation.

- Physical violence often begins or continues during pregnancy. The nurse needs to be alert for signs of abuse, including bruising or injury to the breasts, abdomen, and genitals. The nurse should provide the woman information about violence and about community resources available to assist her.
- Urinary tract infections are a common problem in pregnancy. If untreated, the infection may ascend, causing more serious illness for the mother. Urinary tract infections are also associated with an increased risk of premature labor.
- TORCH is an acronym standing for toxoplasmosis, rubella, cytomegalovirus, and herpes, all of which pose a grave threat to the fetus.
- Sexually transmitted infections pose less of a threat to the fetus if detected and treated as soon as possible.

REFERENCES

Abi-Said, D. (1997). A case-control evaluation of treatment efficacy: The example of magnesium sulfate prophylaxis against eclampsia in patients with preeclampsia. *Journal of Clinical Epidemiology 50*(4), 419–423.

American Academy of Pediatrics (AAP) & American College of Obstetricians and Gynecologists (ACOG). (1997). Obstetric complications. In *Guidelines for perinatal care* (4th ed.)(pp 127–146). Elk Grove Village, IL: Author.

American College of Obstetricians and Gynecologists (ACOG). (1989, Jan. 3). Doctors announce campaign to combat domestic violence. (ACOG news release). Washington, DC: Author.

American College of Obstetricians and Gynecologists (ACOG). (1994). *Antenatal corticosteroid therapy for fetal maturation.* (ACOG Committee Opinion No. 147). Washington, DC: Author.

American College of Obstetricians and Gynecologists (ACOG). (1998, December). *Medical management of tubal pregnancy.* (ACOG Practice Bulletin No. 3). Washington, DC: Author.

Berkowitz, R. S., Goldstein, D. P., & Bernstein, M. R. (1996). Update on gestational trophoblastic disease. *Contemporary OB/GYN, 41*(4), 21–29.

Brennecke, S. P, Brown, M. A., Crowther, C. A., Hague, W. M., King, J., McCowan, L., Morris, J., North, R., Pattison, N., Tippett, C., & Wilson, D. (1995). Aspirin and prevention of preeclampsia. *Australian and New Zealand Journal of Obstetrics and Gynaecology, 35*(1), 37–42.

Brown, Z. A. (1999, January). Herpes simplex virus infection in pregnancy. *Contemporary OB/GYN, 44*(1), 27–34.

Centers for Disease Control and Prevention (CDC). (1998). 1998 sexually transmitted disease treatment guidelines. *Mortality and Morbidity Weekly Report, 47*(RR-1), 1–116.

Clewell, W. H. (1997). Hypertensive emergencies in pregnancy. In M. R. Foley & T. H. Strong (Eds.), *Obstetric intensive care: A practical manual* (pp 63–76). Philadelphia: Saunders.

Coddington, C. C. (1996). Spontaneous abortion. In K. R. Niswander & A. T. Evans (Eds.), *Manual of obstetrics* (pp 261–271). Boston: Little, Brown.

Coleman, M. T., Trianfo, A., & Rund, D. A. (1997). Nonobstetric emergencies in pregnancy: Trauma and surgical conditions. *American Journal of Obstetrics and Gynecology, 177*(3), 497–502.

Cohen, S. H., & Goldstein, E. (1996). Infectious disease complications. In K. R. Niswander & A. T. Evans (Eds.), *Manual of obstetrics* (pp 153–184). Boston: Little, Brown.

Copeland, L. J., & Landon, M. B. (1996). Malignant diseases and pregnancy. In S. G. Gabbe, J. R. Niebyl, & J. L. Simpson (Eds.), *Obstetrics: Normal & problem pregnancies* (3rd ed.). New York: Churchill Livingstone.

Cruikshank, D. P, Wigton, T. R., & Hays, P. M. (1996). Maternal physiology in pregnancy. In S. G. Gabbe, J. R. Niebyl, & J. L. Simpson (Eds.), *Obstetrics: Normal & problem pregnancies* (3rd ed.). New York: Churchill-Livingstone.

Cunningham, F. G., MacDonald, P. C., Gant, N. F., Leveno, K. J., Gilstrap, L. C., III, Hankins, G. D. V., & Clark, S. L. (1997). *Williams obstetrics* (20th ed.). Stamford, CT: Appleton & Lange.

Current trends in ectopic pregnancy—United States, 1990–1992. (1995, June 27). *Mortality and Morbidity Weekly Report, 44*(3), 46–48.

Davidge, S. T., Signorella, A. P., Lykins, D. L., Gilmour, C. H., & Roberts, J. M. (1996). Evidence of endothelial activation and endothelial activators in cord blood of infants of preeclamptic women. *American Journal of Obstetrics and Gynecology, 175*(5), 1301–1307.

Dekker, G. A., de Vries, J. I. P., Doelitzsch, P. M., Huijgens, P. C., von Blomberg, B. M. E., Jakobs, C., & van Geijn, H. L. P. (1995). Underlying disorders associated with severe early-onset preeclampsia. *American Journal of Obstetrics and Gynecology, 173*(4), 1042–1048.

Depp, R. (1996). Cesarean delivery. In S. G. Gabbe, J. R. Niebyl, & J. L. Simpson (Eds.), *Obstetrics: Normal & problem pregnancies* (3rd ed.). New York: Churchill-Livingstone.

Dizon-Townson, D. S., Nelson, L. M., Easton, K., & Ward, K. (1996). The factor V Leiden mutation may predispose women to severe preeclampsia. *American Journal of Obstetrics and Gynecology, 175*(4), 902–906.

Dugoff, L. (1996). Toxoplasmosis. In J. T. Queenan & J. C. Hobbins (Eds.), *Protocols for high-risk pregnancies* (pp 382–386). Cambridge, MA: Blackwell.

Elliott, J. P. (1997). Management of complications associated with administration of tocolytic therapy. In M. R. Foley & T. H. Strong (Eds.), *Obstetric intensive care: A practical manual* (pp 336–346). Philadelphia: Saunders.

Escher-Davis, L. (1996). Fetal fibronectin: A biochemical marker for preterm labor. *AWHONN Voice, 4*(3), 1, 6.

Fox, D. B., Troiano, N. H., & Graves, C. R. (1996). Use of the pulmonary artery catheter in severe preeclampsia: A review. *Obstetrical and Gynecological Survey, 51*(11), 684–695.

Friedman, S. A., Schiff, E., Emeis, J. J., Dekker, G. A., & Sibai, B. M. (1995). Biochemical corroboration of endothelial involvement in severe preeclampsia. *American Journal of Obstetrics and Gynecology, 172*(1), 202–203.

Garite, T. J., & Spellacy, W. N. (1994). Premature rupture of membranes. In J. R. Scott, P. J. DiSaia, C. B. Hammond, & W. N. Spellacy (Eds.), *Danforth's obstetrics and gynecology* (7th ed.). Philadelphia: Lippincott.

Gilstrap, L., Phelan, J., & Iams, J. (1996, April). Controversies and management of preterm labor. *OB/GYN Management,* 71–84.

Ghidini, A., & Romero, R. (1996). Prelabor rupture of membranes. In J. T. Queenan & J. C. Hobbins (Eds.), *Protocols for high-risk pregnancies* (pp 547–557). Cambridge, MA: Blackwell.

Graczykowski, J. W., & Seifer, D. B. (1997). Successful treatment of persistent ectopic pregnancy. *Contemporary OB/GYN, 42*(10), 53–64.

Hagay, Z. J., Biran, G., Ornoy, A., & Reece, E. A. (1996). Infectious cytomegalovirus infection: A long standing problem still seeking a solution. *American Journal of Obstetrics and Gynecology, 174*(1), 241–247.

Heyl, P. S., & Williams, M. C. (1996). Preterm delivery. In K. R. Niswander & A. T. Evans (Eds.), *Manual of obstetrics* (pp 431–450). Boston: Little, Brown.

Iams, J. (1996a). Preterm birth. In S. G. Gabbe, J. R. Niebyl, & J. L. Simpson (Eds.), *Obstetrics: Normal & problem pregnancies* (3rd ed.) (pp 743–820). New York: Churchill-Livingstone.

Iams, J. (1996b). Tocolysis. In J. T. Queenan & J. C. Hobbins (Eds.), *Protocols for high-risk pregnancies* (pp 539–546). Cambridge, MA: Blackwell.

Iams, J. (1997). ACOG Annual Clinical Meeting. Las Vegas, Nevada.

Jackson, M., & Branch, D. W. (1996). Isoimmunization in pregnancy. In S. G. Gabbe, J. R. Niebyl, & J. L. Simpson (Eds.), *Obstetrics: Normal & problem pregnancies* (3rd ed.) (pp 899–932). New York: Churchill-Livingstone.

Jones, D. P. (1996). The nursing management of women experiencing preterm labor: Clinical guidelines and why they are needed. *Journal of Obstetric, Gynecologic, and Neonatal Nursing, 25*(7), 569–592.

Kappy, K. A., McTigue, M., & Guzman, E. R. (1993). Premature rupture of the membranes. In R. A. Knuppel & J. E. Drucker (Eds.), *High-risk pregnancy: A team approach* (2nd ed.). Philadelphia: Saunders.

Kupfermine, M. J., Peaceman, A. M., Wigton, T. R., Rehnberg, K. A., & Socol, M. L. (1995). Fetal fibronectin levels are elevated in maternal plasma and amniotic fluid of patients with severe preeclampsia. *American Journal of Obstetrics and Gynecology, 172*(2), 649–654.

Leiserowitz, G. S. (1996). Surgical and gynecologic complications. In K. R. Niswander & A. T. Evans (Eds.), *Manual of obstetrics* (pp 239–260). Boston: Little, Brown.

Leylek, O. A., Cetin, A., Toyaksi, M., & Erselcan, T. (1996). Hyperthyroidism in hyperemesis gravidarum. *International Journal of Gynecology & Obstetrics, 55*, 33–37.

Lindoff, C., Ingemarsson, I., Martinsson, G., Segelmark, M., Tysell, H., & Astedt, B. (1997). Preeclampsia is associated with a reduced response to activated protein C. *American Journal of Obstetrics and Gynecology, 176*(2), 457–461.

Lovett, S. M., Weiss, J. D., Diogo, M. J., Williams, P. T., & Garite, T. J. (1997). A prospective, double-blind, randomized, controlled clinical trial of ampicillin-sulbactam for preterm premature rupture of membranes in women receiving antenatal corticosteroid therapy. *American Journal of Obstetrics and Gynecology, 176*(5), 1030–1038.

Lucas, L. S., & Jordan, E. T. (1997). Phenytoin as an alternative treatment for preeclampsia. *Journal of Obstetric, Gynecologic, and Neonatal Nursing, 26*(3), 263–269.

McFarlane, J., & Parker, B. (1996). Physical abuse, smoking and substance use during pregnancy: Prevalence, interrelationships, and effects on birth weight. *Journal of Obstetric, Gynecologic, and Neonatal Nursing, 25*(4), 313–319.

McIntyre-Seltman, K., & Andrews-Detrich, L. J. (1996). Ectopic pregnancy. In K. R. Niswander and A. T. Evans (Eds.), *Manual of obstetrics* (pp 273–282). Boston: Little, Brown.

Morris, N. H., Eaton, B. M., & Dekker, G. (1996). Nitric oxide, the endothelium, pregnancy and preeclampsia. *British Journal of Obstetrics and Gynaecology, 103*(1), 4–15.

Nageotte, M. D., Briggs, G. G., Towers, C. V., & Astrat, T. (1996). Droperidol and diphenhydraminek in the management of hyperemesis gravidarum. *American Journal of Obstetrics and Gynecology, 174*(6), 1801–1806.

National Institutes of Health (NIH) Consensus Development Conference. (1994). Effect of corticosteroids for fetal maturation on perinatal outcomes. *National Institutes of Health Consensus Development Conference Statement.* Washington, DC.

Niebyl, J. R. (1996). Incompetent cervix. In J. T. Queenan & J. C. Hobbins (Eds.), *Protocols for high-risk pregnancies* (pp 446–451). Cambridge, MA: Blackwell.

Oi, R. H. (1996). Diseases of the placenta. In K. R. Niswander & A. T. Evans (Eds.), *Manual of obstetrics* (pp 451–468). Boston: Little, Brown.

Queenan, J. T. (1996). Rh and other blood group immunizations. In J. T. Queenan & J.C. Hobbins (Eds.), *Protocols for high-risk pregnancies* (pp 523–534). Cambridge, MA: Blackwell.

Rayburn, V. F., & Carey, J. C. (1996). Prenatal care. In *Obstetrics and Gynecology.* Baltimore: Williams & Wilkins.

Reece, E. A., Hobbins, J. C., Mahoney, M. J., & Petrie, R. H. (1996). *Handbook of medicine of the fetus and mother.* Philadelphia: J. B. Lippincott Company.

Reedy, M. B., Källen, B., & Kuehl, T. J. (1997). Laparoscopy during pregnancy: A study of five fetal outcome parameters with use of the Swedish Health Registry. *American Journal of Obstetrics and Gynecology, 177*(3), 673–679.

Reedy, M., Uy, K., Thompson, E., & Rayburn, W. L. (1998, April 15). Laparoscopy during pregnancy: A safe alternative to laparotomy? *Contemporary OB/GYN, 43*, 75–91.

Scialli, A. R. (1998). Protocols for high-risk pregnancy: Nausea and vomiting. *Contemporary OB/GYN, 43*(5), 13–16.

Scott, J. R., & Branch, W. (1998). Immunology of early pregnancy loss. *Contemporary OB/GYN, 43*(6), 40–53.

Scott, L. L., Hollier, L. M., & Dias, K. (1997). Perinatal herpesvirus infections: herpes simplex, varicella, and cytomegalovirus. *Infectious Disease Clinics of North America, 11*(1), 27–51.

Sever, J. L. (1996). Rubella. In J. T. Queenan & J. C. Hobbins (Eds.), *Protocols for high-risk pregnancies* (pp 27–52). Cambridge, MA: Blackwell.

Sever, J. L. (1998). Toxoplasmosis in pregnancy. *Contemporary OB/GYN, 43*, 12, 21–24.

Sibai, B. M. (1996). Hypertension in pregnancy. In S. G. Gabbe, J. R. Niebyl, & J. L. Simpson (Eds.), *Obstetrics: Normal & problem pregnancies* (3rd ed.) (pp 935–996). New York: Churchill Livingstone.

Silver, H. (1996). Hypertensive disorders. In K. R. Niswander & A. T. Evans (Eds.), *Manual of obstetrics* (pp 283–295). Boston: Little, Brown.

Sisson, M. C., & Sauer, P. M. (1996). Pharmacologic therapy for pregnancy-induced hypertension. *The Journal of Perinatal and Neonatal Nursing, 9*(4), 1–12.

Slotnick, R.N. (1996). Isoimmunization. In K. R. Niswander & A. T. Evans (Eds.), *Manual of obstetrics* (pp 329–335). Boston: Little, Brown.

Tincello, D. G., & Johnstone, M. J. (1996). Treatment of hyperemesis gravidarum with the 5-HT3 antagonist ondansetron (Zofran). *Postgraduate Medical Journal, 72*(853), 688–689.

Urbanski, P. K. (1997). How does hydration affect preterm labor? *AWHONN Lifelines, 1*(3), 25.

Usta, I. M., & Sibai, B. M. (1996). Preeclampsia. In J. T. Queenan & J. C. Hobbins (Eds.). *Protocols for high-risk pregnancies* (pp 505–516). Cambridge, MA: Blackwell.

Viamontes, C. M. (1996). Pharmacologic intervention in the management of preterm labor: An update. *Journal of Perinatal and Neonatal Nursing, 9* (4), 13–30.

Williams, M. C. (1996). Hepatic, biliary, and gastrointestinal complications. In K. R. Niswander & A. T. Evans (Eds.). *Manual of obstetrics*, Boston: Little, Brown.

Wolf, J. L. (1996). *Liver disease in pregnancy. Medical Clinics of North America, 80*(5), 1167–1187.

Wong, G. (1997). Maternal postural challenge as a functional test for cervical incompetence. *Journal of Ultrasound Medicine, 16*(3), 169–175.

Zuspan, F. P. (1996). Chronic hypertension. In J. T. Queenan & J. C. Hobbins (Eds.), *Protocols for high-risk pregnancies* (pp 292–300). Cambridge, MA: Blackwell.

17 Assessment of Fetal Well-Being

Key Terms

Amniocentesis

Biophysical profile (BPP)

Chorionic villus sampling (CVS)

Contraction stress test (CST)

Fetal acoustic stimulation test (FAST)

Fetoscopy

Lecithin/sphingomyelin (L/S) ratio

Nonstress test (NST)

Percutaneous umbilical blood sampling (PUBS)

Phosphatidylglycerol (PG)

Surfactant

Ultrasound

My first pregnancy was so tenuous that I didn't know from one moment to the next how it would end. I hoped for our baby's safety, but in the end the baby died. When I became pregnant the next time, I was very nervous. Being able to see the baby on ultrasound helped me so much. I knew then that our baby was alive and growing.

Objectives

- Identify indications for antenatal fetal surveillance.
- Relate indications for ultrasound examination to the information that can be obtained from this procedure.
- Outline pertinent information regarding assessment of fetal activity to be discussed with the woman.
- Compare the procedures for the nonstress test, contraction stress test, and biophysical profile, including the indications, contraindications, and predictive value of each.
- Describe components of a biophysical profile used to evaluate fetal well-being.
- Discuss the nipple stimulation contraction stress test.
- Contrast genetic amniocentesis and chorionic villus sampling in evaluation of chromosomes.
- Summarize counseling regarding triple screen testing and the implications of abnormal values.
- Discuss the nurse's role in antenatal surveillance with regard to high-risk pregnancy management.

DURING THE PAST TWO DECADES, increasing interest has been focused on the problems of the at-risk pregnant woman, both for her health management and for conditions that may affect her unborn child. High-risk women and infants have a significantly greater chance of morbidity (illness) and mortality (death), both before and after childbirth. However, perinatal morbidity and mortality can be considerably reduced by early, skillful diagnosis and highly intensive antepartum care of the pregnant woman.

Several tests can be used to assess fetal well-being during the pregnancy. These tests include diagnostic ultrasound, fetal stress tests, and amniocentesis for lung maturity studies. In addition, after the seventh month of pregnancy the expectant woman can assess fetal movements each day. The tests and assessment methods provide information about fetal well-being, including normal growth of the fetus, the presence of congenital anomalies, the location of the placenta, and fetal lung maturity (Table 17–1). At times just one test will be done; in other circumstances, a combination of the tests is beneficial.

Each pregnancy must be considered individually in terms of what diagnostic and antenatal surveillance tests would provide information for the best outcome for the woman and her fetus. One must be certain the advantages outweigh the potential risks and expense. Each of these tests has its limitations in terms of screening, diagnostic accuracy, and applicability. Combining information obtained from various diagnostic and antenatal surveillance tests can provide an overall assessment of fetal well-being during the management of the high-risk pregnancy.

Indications for Antenatal Testing

Women who are considered to be at risk and who may require assessment of fetal well-being include women with the following complications:

- Decreased fetal movement
- Elevated maternal serum α-fetoprotein (MSAFP) or triple screen (alphafetoprotein, human chorionic gonadotrophin [hCG] and unconjugated estriol [UE3])
- Fetal heart rate arrhythmias
- Hemoglobinopathies
- History of preterm labor or birth, risk of preterm labor with current pregnancy, chromosomal or inherited biochemical disorders, and unexplained stillborn or intrapartal fetal death
- Hydramnios or oligohydramnios
- Infections, immunodeficiencies
- Maternal systemic disease, such as anemia, antiphospholipid syndrome, chronic hypertension, cyanotic heart disease, gestational or insulin-dependent diabetes, hyperthyroidism, or lupus
- Multiple gestation
- Pregnancy past 41 completed weeks of gestation (postdate)
- Pregnancy-induced hypertension
- Preterm premature rupture of membranes (prior to 37 completed weeks of gestation)

TABLE 17–1 Summary of Screening and Diagnostic Tests

Goal	Test	Timing
To validate the pregnancy	Ultrasound: gestational sac volume	5 and 6 weeks after last menstrual period (LMP) by endovaginal ultrasound
To determine how advanced the pregnancy is	Ultrasound: crown–rump length Ultrasound: biparietal diameter, femur length, abdomen circumference	6 to 10 weeks' gestation 13 to 40 weeks' gestation
To identify normal growth of the fetus	Ultrasound: biparietal diameter Ultrasound: head:abdomen ratio Ultrasound: estimated fetal weight	Most useful from 20 to 30 weeks' gestation 13 to 40 weeks' gestation About 24 to 40 weeks' gestation
To detect congenital anomalies and problems	Ultrasound Chorionic villus sampling Amniocentesis Fetoscopy Percutaneous blood sampling Triple test	18 to 40 weeks' gestation 8 to 12 weeks' gestation 16 to 18 weeks' gestation 18 weeks' gestation Second and third trimesters About 10 weeks' gestation
To localize the placenta	Ultrasound	Usually in third trimester or before amniocentesis
To assess fetal status	Biophysical profile Maternal assessment of fetal activity Nonstress test Contraction stress test	Approximately 28 weeks to birth About 28 weeks to birth Approximately 28 weeks to birth After 28 weeks
To diagnose cardiac problems	Fetal echocardiography	Second and third trimesters
To assess fetal lung maturity	Amniocentesis L/S ratio Phosphatidylglycerol Phosphatidylcholine	33 to 40 weeks 33 weeks to birth 33 weeks to birth 33 weeks to birth
To obtain more information about breech presentation	Ultrasound	Just before labor is anticipated or during labor

TABLE 17–2 Sample Nursing Approaches to Pretest Teaching

Assess whether the woman knows the reason the screening or diagnostic test is being recommended.
Examples:
"Has your doctor/nurse-midwife told you why this test is necessary?"
"Sometimes tests are done for many different reasons. Can you tell me why you are having this test?"
"What is your understanding about what the test will show?"

Provide an opportunity for questions.
Examples:
"Do you have any questions about the test?"
"Is there anything that is not clear to you?"

Explain the test procedure, paying particular attention to any preparation the woman needs to do prior to the test.
Example:
"The test that has been ordered for you is designed to . . ." (Add specific information about the particular test. Give the explanation in simple language.)

Validate the woman's understanding of the preparation.
Example:
"Tell me what you will have to do to get ready for this test."

Give permission for the woman to continue to ask questions if needed.
Example:
"I'll be with you during the test. If you have any questions at any time, please don't hesitate to ask."

- Suspected intrauterine growth restriction
- Vaginal bleeding

Each of these complications may increase the risk to the expectant woman and her fetus. The list is not complete; other preexisting medical diseases may place the woman at risk and call for the physician or certified nurse-midwife to recommend diagnostic assessment of the fetus. See Chapter 11 for prenatal high-risk factors and Chapters 15 and 16 for discussion of various conditions that may threaten the mother or fetus during pregnancy.

CRITICAL THINKING QUESTION

Many women who undergo fetal surveillance testing are at high risk. What techniques can you use to make sure the woman and her fetus are treated as a complete unit, rather than treating the woman as a "vessel" for the baby? Watch for and listen to the language that is used during the testing situations that you participate in. How would you reword some of the comments that the examiners make to the woman to help her feel more of a part of the process?

NURSING CARE MANAGEMENT

A variety of nurses in many settings will have an opportunity to interact and provide care. Nurses who perform antenatal assessment tests are perinatal nurse practitioners, and/or nurses who have received additional specialized perinatal education and practice. The nurse, whatever the role, is a vital link between the woman and the physician or certified nurse-midwife.

Nursing Assessment and Diagnosis

Nursing assessment begins with a history of the present prenatal course and possible indications for the particular diagnostic test. The nurse assesses the woman and her partner's knowledge regarding the reason the test is being advised, the information that the woman and her support person have regarding the test, their questions and concerns, and the presence of any psychosociocultural factors that may influence the teaching or learning process (see Table 17–2). During the test and ongoing care, the nurse completes needed assessments to monitor the status of the woman and her fetus.

The primary nursing diagnoses are directed toward providing information regarding the diagnostic test and minimizing any risks to the woman and her unborn child. The woman may also be fearful of the outcome of the test, and the nurse can play an important role in providing education, support, and counseling. Examples of nursing diagnoses that may be applicable include:

- ***Knowledge Deficit*** related to insufficient information about the fetal assessment test and its purpose, benefits, risks, and alternatives
- ***Fear*** related to the specific test or possible unfavorable test results
- ***Disruption in Bonding*** due to high-risk label

Nursing Plan and Implementation

The nursing plan of care will be directed toward each specific nursing diagnosis. The nurse generally plays a vital role in providing needed and desired information regarding the diagnostic test. The nurse also functions as an advocate for the expectant woman by helping her clarify question areas and obtain needed information. The nurse frequently knows the areas about which most women have questions and can anticipate many of their fears. When the woman is not able to verbalize questions, the nurse can assist by bringing up questions that other women have had.

In any interaction with the expectant woman, it is important to remember that carrying a high-risk label is frequently a heavy burden. Some women seem to appear to take the complicated pregnancy in course, whereas others may use denial to get through each day and attempt to keep up all former activities to the best of their ability. Other women may exhibit great anxiety regarding their baby, whereas others seem to be rather disconnected and do not seem to be in touch with the reality of the baby. Such a woman may know she is pregnant and that the pregnancy is complicated, but she seems to hold back on prenatal bonding with her baby in case something goes wrong and the baby has problems or does not live. She may defer thinking about names or getting supplies and clothes for the baby. In some instances, these characteristics parallel risk factors for possible bonding difficulties after birth. However, in the case of the high-risk mother, it is more of a day-by-day process of self-protection and a coping strategy. In all instances, the nurse assesses the situation for each pregnant woman and provides nonjudgmental, supportive, caring nursing care. Establishing a trusting relationship will hopefully open the possibilities for the woman to talk with the nurse and perhaps share her concerns and fears and receive support.

Community-Based Nursing Care

Nurses within the office of the physician or certified nurse-midwife or in community clinics will have the first contact with the pregnant woman. Nurses in perinatal community clinics or in perinatal centers within hospital settings may subsequently perform some of the fetal surveillance tests.

Home Care

Nurses provide a variety of services in the home. Because the home care nurse frequently sees the woman over a period of time, the home care nurse may be the most likely person to develop a comprehensive assessment of the woman and her family. The home care nurse has many advantages, including the ability to visit the family in their own setting, reiterate teaching, complete needed assessments, and assist the family in connecting with appropriate resources in the community. The nurse participates in overall management of care and conducting other assessment tests, such as tests for preterm labor and nonstress tests, and in helping the woman complete daily fetal movement counts ("kick counts").

Maternal Assessment of Fetal Movement

Fetal movement counting is used as a screening procedure in the evaluation of fetal well-being. Clinicians generally agree that vigorous fetal movement (activity) provides reassurance of fetal well-being and that marked reduction in fetal movement or disappearance of fetal movement may occur shortly before fetal death (Richardson & Gagnon, 1999).

Although there is considerable variation among individuals, the average number of daily fetal movements during the third trimester is approximately 720 (or 30 gross fetal body movements per hour) (Druzin & Gabbe, 1996). In women with a multiple gestation daily fetal movements are significantly higher. During the last few weeks of gestation, the fetus spends 60% to 70% of its time in an active sleep state. Abrupt movement of the limbs, trunk, and head are characteristic (Druzin & Gabbe, 1996).

The woman can perform daily counting of fetal movement in a variety of ways. One tool is the Cardiff Count-to-Ten method. The woman begins counting fetal movements at the same time each day and continues counting until she has noted ten movements. She records the movements on a special graph. If there are ten movements in 10 hours or less, the test is completed for that day. If there are fewer than 10 movements in a period of 10 hours for 2 consecutive days or no fetal movement in 10 hours, the woman should immediately contact her certified nurse-midwife or physician (Simpson & Creehan, 1996). See the Self-Care Guide: How to Assess Fetal Activity, in the perforated section at the end of the book.

Although maternal assessment of fetal movement is a subjective means of evaluating fetal status, it has been found to be an excellent screening test. Furthermore, it is simple for the woman to perform, does not interfere with normal daily routines, costs nothing, provides reassurance, and may enhance maternal attachment as the expectant woman spends time each day focusing on feeling her baby move. Pregnant women need to understand that fetal movements are significant and that they change during pregnancy, both in number and strength. The expectant woman should be reassured that there are fetal rest-sleep states during which minimal or no movement may occur for an hour or so as the fetus rests.

Community-Based Nursing Care

The caregiver's responsibility is to teach the expectant woman how to do the fetal movement counts and to provide additional information so that she understands the importance and pertinence of the assessment. Because the kick counts are important, it is the responsibility of the caregivers to ask about the fetal movements and to look at the Cardiff Count-to-Ten record. The nurse must also take calls regarding the woman's questions and concerns seriously and provide additional information as needed.

In 1981, I visited the First International Peace Hospital in Shanghai. At the prenatal clinic, the mothers and fathers were given a small jar that contained many small black stones. The couple was instructed to complete a fetal kick count each day by starting at a similar time and then placing a stone in the jar with each fetal movement. Toward the end of the pregnancy, the father was encouraged to place his hand on the expectant mother's abdomen and feel the movements. Then he was responsible for placing the stones in the jar. The mothers and fathers seemed so proud when they brought their recording of the movements back to the clinic for review.

I have always wondered what it would have been like to hold my baby in my arms after birth and look at the jar of stones. A simple jar but so special.

~ Sally ~

Ultrasound

Ultrasonography is the use of intermittent high-frequency sound waves to create a image of the fetus (Figure 17–1). **Ultrasound** is the most common diagnostic procedure; approximately 70% of pregnant women in the United States receive at least one ultrasound examination during their pregnancy (Simpson & Creehan, 1996).

Ultrasound images are obtained by placing a transducer to the woman's abdomen or labia majora, or by inserting an endovaginal transducer into the woman's

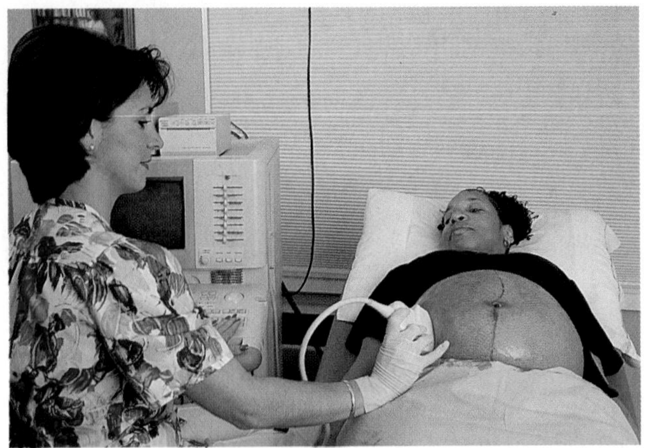

FIGURE 17–1 Ultrasound scanning permits visualization of the fetus in utero.

vagina (Figure 17–2). Ultrasound may be used to evaluate both structural and functional characteristics, including eye movements, fetal breathing movements, cardiac activity, limb movement, tone, and urination (Figure 17–3). Because ultrasound is used for many purposes during pregnancy, the American College of Obstetricians and Gynecologists (ACOG) (1994) standardized the content for ultrasound exam and created guidelines for basic screening, limited screening, and comprehensive ultrasound examinations (ACOG, 1993).

A *basic screening ultrasound* examination is adequate for the majority of pregnant women. The exam may be done by a nurse, certified nurse-midwife, obstetrician, or ultrasound technician who has had specialized education and training in performing the examination. The basic screening ultrasound is intended to provide the following information:

- Documentation of a gestational sac early in the pregnancy
- Fetal number
- Assessment of gestational age
- Survey of fetal anatomy for major malformations
- Fetal presentation
- Placental location
- Assessment of amniotic fluid volume
- Evaluation for maternal pelvic masses

A *limited ultrasound* examination is more involved than the basic screening examination and may be done in antepartum or intrapartum settings. It may include the following:

- More detailed assessment of amniotic fluid volume
- Fetal biophysical profile testing
- Ultrasonography-guided amniocentesis
- Ultrasound used with external cephalic version

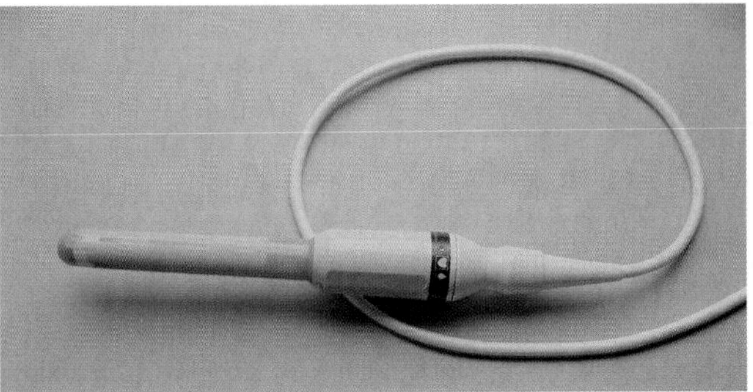

FIGURE 17–2 Endovaginal ultrasound transducer.

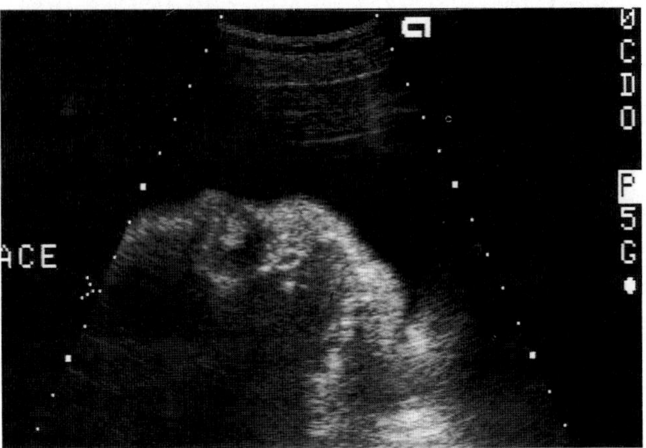

FIGURE 17–3 Ultrasound of fetal face.

- Examination to determine fetal life or death in the presence of complications or cessation of fetal movement
- Localization of placenta in the presence of antepartum hemorrhage
- Confirmation of fetal presentation near term or in the intrapartal area

CRITICAL THINKING QUESTION

Take a few moments and think about how you would react to seeing your fetus by ultrasound. Would it make you feel anxious or more comfortable? Why would you want or not want to know the sex of the fetus? What if you didn't want to know and the ultrasonographer told you? What reactions have you seen in the clinical setting? What differences are there between the expectant woman or couple who wants to know the sex of the fetus and those who don't? If the couple does not want to know the sex, how is that request complied with?

AWHONN (Association of Women's Health, Obstetric, and Neonatal Nurses) (1993) set educational guidelines and nursing practice competencies (expectations) for experienced obstetric nurses to perform limited ultrasound examinations. The guidelines indicate that the nurse must complete an educational program that includes didactic presentations and a clinical practicum. Limited ultrasound exams may also be performed by obstetricians and certified nurse-midwives.

A *comprehensive ultrasound* examination may be indicated for a woman who, from previous ultrasound examination or clinical evaluation, is suspected of carrying a fetus with a physiologic or anatomic defect. The comprehensive examination should be conducted by a professional (usually an obstetrician) with extensive training and experience in performing this examination and interpreting findings. Serial ultrasound (more than one ultrasound done over a period of time) may be used to assess and compare structural abnormalities or masses.

Ultrasound safety has been investigated over the course of 25 years in clinical, in vitro, and animal studies. A safe level of ultrasound has been set by the Food and Drug Administration to less than 94 mW/cm^2 during fetal imaging (Cunningham et al, 1997a). Most instruments used in diagnostic ultrasonography produce energies no greater than 10 to 20 mW/cm^2. Ultrasound exposure at this intensity has not been found to cause any harmful biologic effects on ultrasound operators (the person who does the exam), pregnant women, fetuses, or other clients. Infants exposed in utero have shown no significant differences in fetal risks (Cunningham et al, 1997a).

Procedures

There are three methods of ultrasound scanning: transabdominal, endovaginal, and translabial scanning.

Transabdominal Ultrasound

In the transabdominal approach, a transducer is moved across the abdomen. The woman is usually scanned with a full bladder, except when ultrasound is used to localize the placenta before amniocentesis. When the bladder is full, the examiner can assess other structures, especially the vagina and cervix, in relation to the bladder. This is particularly important when vaginal bleeding is noted and placenta previa is the suspected cause. The woman is advised to drink 1 to 1.5 quarts of water approximately 2 hours before the examination, and she is asked to refrain from emptying her bladder. If the bladder is not sufficiently filled, she is asked to drink 3 to 4 (8 oz) glasses of water and is rescanned 30 to 45 minutes later. Mineral oil or a transmission gel is generously spread over the woman's abdomen, and the sonographer slowly moves a transducer over the abdomen to obtain a picture of the contents of the uterus. Ultrasound testing takes 20 to 30 minutes. The woman may feel discomfort due to pressure applied over a full bladder. In addition, if the woman lies on her back during the test, shortness of breath can develop. this may be relieved by elevating her upper body during the test.

Endovaginal Ultrasound

The endovaginal approach uses a probe inserted into the vagina. Once inserted, the endovaginal probe is close to the structures being imaged and so produces a better, clearer image. The improved images obtained by endovaginal ultrasound have enabled sonographers to identify structures and fetal characteristics earlier in pregnancy than was possible with the transabdominal approach (Chervenak & Gabbe, 1996).

After the procedure is fully explained to the woman, she is prepared in the same manner as for a pelvic examination: in lithotomy position, with appropriate drapes to provide privacy and a female attendant in the room. It is important that her buttocks are at the end of the table so that, once inserted, the probe can be moved in various directions. The small, lightweight vaginal transducer is covered with a specially fitted sterile sheath, a condom, or one finger of a glove. Ultrasound coupling gel is then applied to the covering, making insertion into the vagina easier and providing a medium for enhancing the ultrasound image. In addition to providing a clearer image than the transabdominal method, the endovaginal procedure can be accomplished with an empty bladder. Most women do not feel discomfort during the ultrasound exam. The probe is smaller than a speculum, so insertion is usually completed with ease. The woman may feel some movement of the probe during the exam as various structures are imaged. Some women may want to insert the probe themselves to enhance their comfort; others may feel embarrassed even to be asked. The certified nurse-midwife, physician or ultrasonographer offers the choice based on the clinician's comfort level and the rapport the clinician has established with the woman.

A less common scanning method, translabial ultrasound, may be used in combination with transabdominal ultrasound. The transducer is placed on the woman's labia but is not inserted into the vaginal vault.

Clinical Application

ACOG (1993) has established guidelines regarding the information that should be obtained by ultrasound in each trimester, including biometry (fetal measurements) and a survey of fetal anatomy.

CRITICAL THINKING QUESTION

Think of the implications of knowing the first day of the last menstrual period when calculating the estimated date of birth. If you were leading a preconceptual class, how would you focus on this information so that women would be able to understand the implications? What type of tool or graph might you develop to help the women keep track of their cycles? What could make it fun?

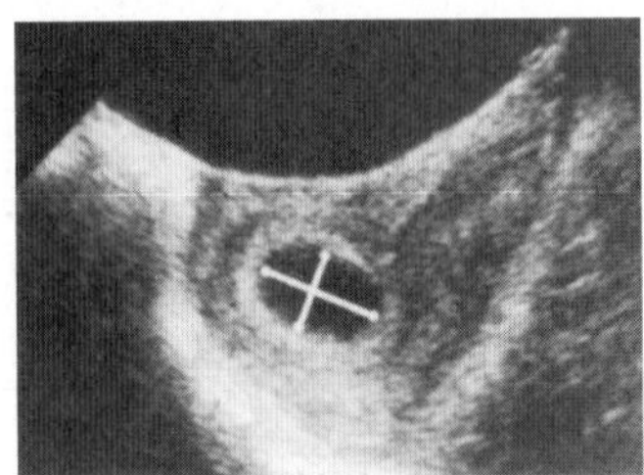

FIGURE 17–4 Measurement of the gestational sac. The ultrasound shows the uterus; the blackened oval area is the gestational sac. The fluid in the gestational sac does not generate echoes from the ultrasound and thus appears dark in contrast to the uterine tissue sur-rounding it. The lines through the gestational sac represent measurements that are taken. SOURCE: Callen PW: *Ultrasonography in Obstetrics and Gynecology,* 2nd ed. Philadelphia: Saunders, 1988, p 49.

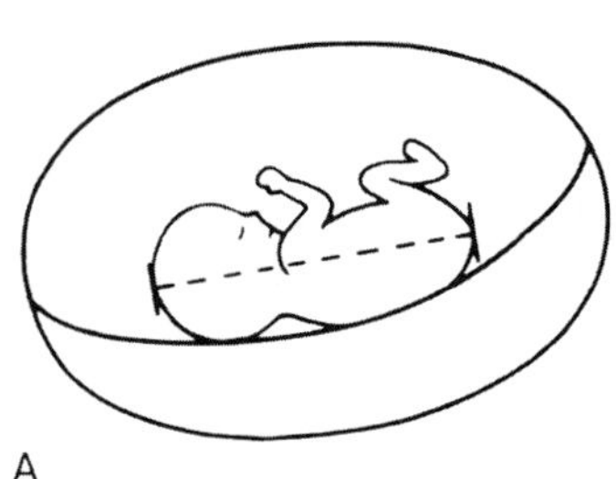

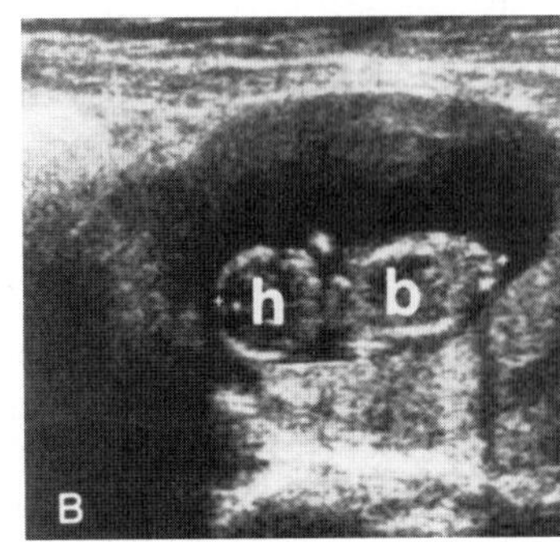

FIGURE 17–5 Measurement of the crown–rump length. ***A,*** Schematic diagram. Dotted line shows the measurement from the top of the crown (head) to the bottom of the rump. ***B,*** Ultrasound scan of the pregnant uterus, showing the longest length of a 9-weekfetus. The head (h) can be differentiated from the body (b), but the internal anatomy cannot be clearly distinguished. SOURCE: Callen PW: *Ultrasonography in Obstetrics and Gynecology,* 2nd ed. Philadelphia: Saunders, 1988, p 50.

First Trimester Pregnancy

Transvaginal ultrasound often provides better and earlier first trimester assessment of pregnancy. With either abdominal or transvaginal methods, the following information should be obtained:

- Presence or absence of the intrauterine gestational sac (Figure 17–4)
- Identification of the embryo or fetus
- Fetal number
- Presence or absence of fetal cardiac activity
- Crown–rump length (Figure 17–5)
- Evaluation of the uterus and adnexal structures

With abdominal ultrasound, the gestational sac is visible at 6 weeks' gestation by menstrual dates. Transvaginal ultrasound allows the gestational sac to be identified by 5 menstrual weeks' gestation. Similarly, fetal heart activity can be detected with abdominal scanning at 7 weeks' gestation by menstrual dating and at 6 weeks' gestation with transvaginal scanning.

First trimester bleeding is the most common indication for early ultrasonography. Blighted ovum or an embryonic pregnancy can be diagnosed by the failure to detect a fetus within a normal gestational sac after 6 weeks' gestation by menstrual dating. Missed abortion is diagnosed by the absence of cardiac activity in an embryo after 7 weeks' gestation. In women with suspected ectopic pregnancy, the main contribution of ultrasonography is demonstration of a gestational sac within the uterus, thereby confirming intrauterine pregnancy. Multiple pregnancy can be diagnosed only when multiple fetuses have documented cardiac activity. Variability in the fusion of the amnion and chorion in early pregnancy may give the appearance of more than one gestational sac.

During the first trimester, measurement of the crown–rump length (CRL) of the fetus is most useful for accurate dating of a pregnancy. The correlation between fetal length and age is excellent because pathologic disorders will minimally affect fetal growth in the first trimester. The measurement should be taken from the top of the fetal head to the outer rump, excluding limbs or yolk sac. A general formula is CRL in cm + 6.5 equals gestational age in weeks. CRL is no longer accurate after 12 weeks due to the extension and flexion of the active fetus (Callen, 1994).

Second Trimester Pregnancy

In the second trimester, the ultrasound measurements of the fetal biparietal diameter, femur length, and abdominal and head circumferences are used to estimate gestational age and fetal weight. The average of the gestational age predictions generated by each of these measurements provides the best estimate of fetal age. However, utilizing the averaging method may adversely affect the gestational age estimate if one of the measurements is grossly incompatible with the others. For example, measurements may show a small biparietal diameter secondary to compression of the fetal head in oligohydramnios or breech presentation. When this occurs, the abnormal value is deleted from the calculation of the mean gestational age.

Biparietal Diameter In the second trimester, the biparietal diameter (BPD) is the most accepted means of measuring the fetal head and is the single most common measurement for estimating gestational age. Between 17 and 24 weeks' gestation is the optimal time for this measurement; at this point it has a predictive value of ± 5 to 7 days. The BPD should be measured at the level of the thalamus and the cavum septi pelludidi (Figure 17–6).

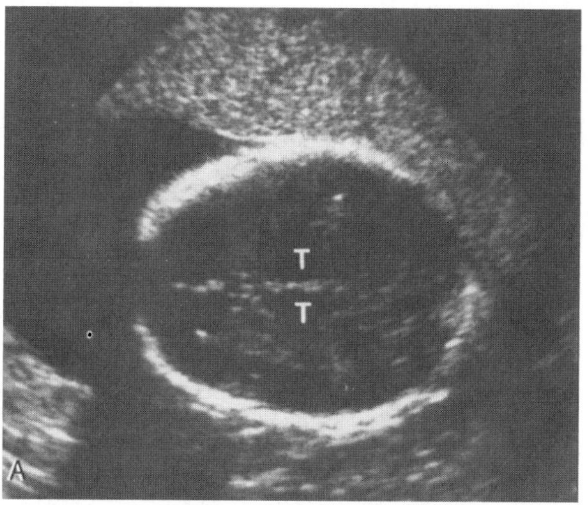

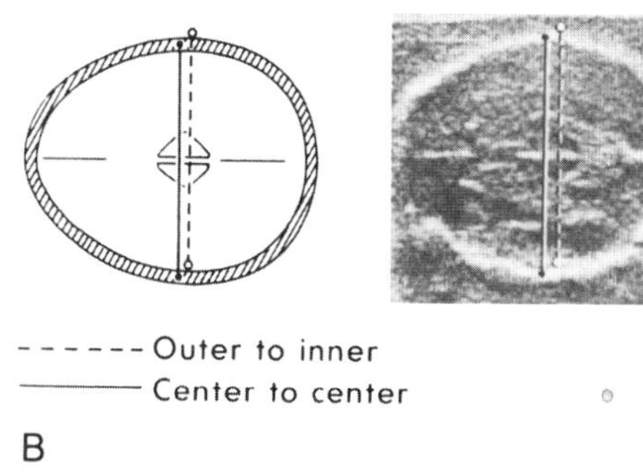

FIGURE 17–6 Measurement of the fetal biparietal diameter. ***A,*** Ultrasound transaxial image of the fetal head, taken with the thalami (t) imaged in the midline, equidistant from the temporoparietal tables of the calvarium. ***B,*** Diagram and image showing the leading edge (outer) to leading edge (inner) measurements of the fetal head, taken at the level of the thalami. SOURCE: Callen PW: *Ultrasonography in Obstetrics and Gynecology,* 2nd ed. Philadelphia: Saunders, 1988, p 51.

Several tables that correlate the BPD with fetal gestational age are available. Serial ultrasounds enable the practitioner to assess fetal growth according to the normal growth curve. If the curve begins to flatten, the physician must assess the fetus for intrauterine growth restriction (IUGR). In this case, additional antenatal surveillance, including Doppler flow studies and biophysical profile with nonstress tests, may be used to assess fetal well-being.

The BPD measurements can be obtained beginning at 11 weeks' gestation, but the BPD is too small for nomograms to be reliable until about 17 weeks. Detection of IUGR and an accurate prediction of fetal age can be most reliably achieved between 20 and 30 weeks' gestation, when the most rapid growth in the BPD occurs. After 40 weeks' gestation, the BPD shows a growth of less than 1mm/week; thus sonograms obtained at this point are of no value. The BPD measurement generally correlates closely with gestational age, especially if serial determinations were obtained beginning early in the pregnancy. However, if only one determination is made late in pregnancy, the gestational age is less accurate and may vary by ± 4 weeks.

Head Circumference The BPD is accurate only if the head is the appropriate ovoid shape. Compression of the fetal skull occurs commonly in fetal malpresentation, such as breech, or in cases of oligohydramnios or multiple gestation. The head circumference is less affected by head compression and is therefore a valuable tool to assess gestational age (Figure 17–7).

Cephalic Index After 28 weeks, the BPD alone should not be relied on to determine gestational age. After this time the *cephalic index* (the ratio of BPD to occipitofrontal [OF] diameter) should be evaluated to assess head shape. The fetal head is normally oval, but there are variations. If the OF diameter is shortened and the BPD is elongated

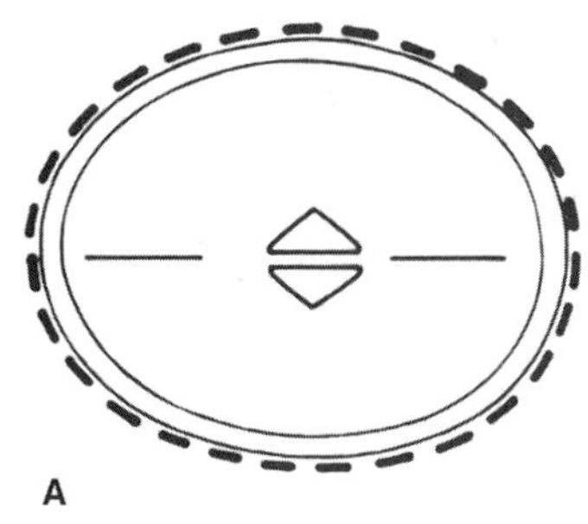

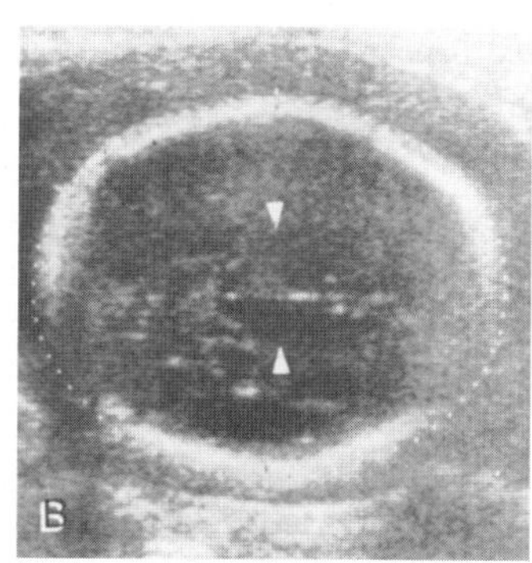

FIGURE 17–7 Measurement of head circumference. ***A,*** Diagram showing a dotted line outlining the head, which indicates the correct place to make a circumference measurement. ***B,*** Ultrasound transaxial scan showing the thalami (arrowheads), positioned in the midline. A dotted line created by a digitizer outlines the correct perimeter, just outside the hyperechoic calvarium, to obtain a circumference measurement. SOURCE: Callen PW: *Ultrasonography in Obstetrics and Gynecology,* 2nd ed. Philadelphia: Saunders, 1988, p 55.

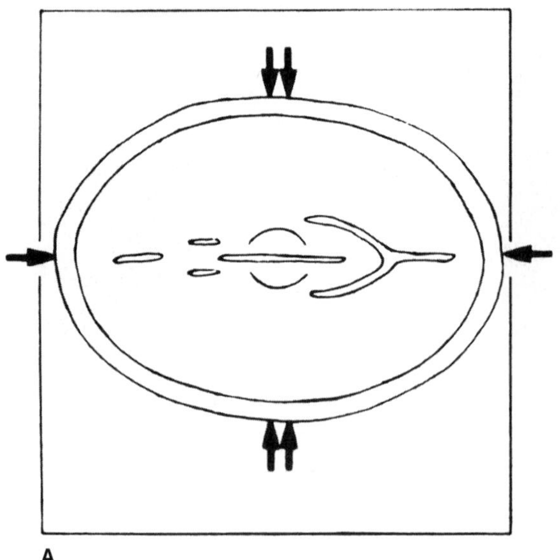

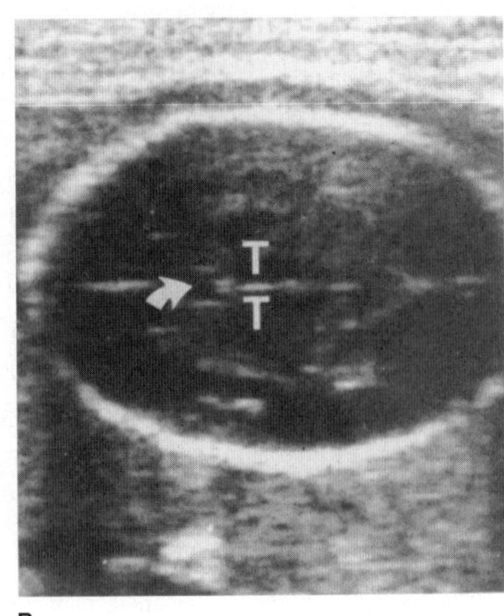

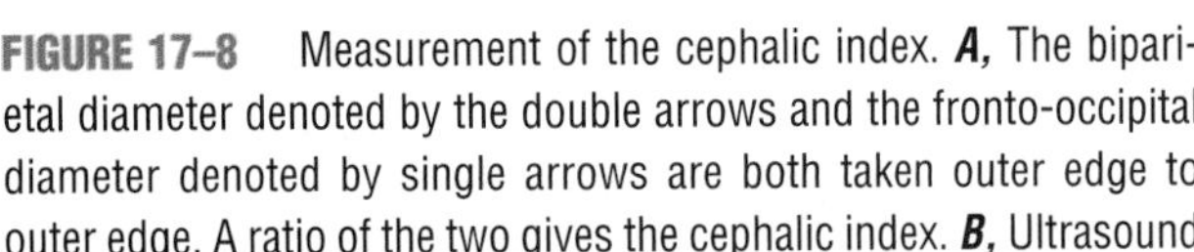

FIGURE 17–8 Measurement of the cephalic index. ***A,*** The biparietal diameter denoted by the double arrows and the fronto-occipital diameter denoted by single arrows are both taken outer edge to outer edge. A ratio of the two gives the cephalic index. ***B,*** Ultrasound transaxial scan of the fetal head at the level of the thalami (T) and cavum septi pellucidi (curved arrow). SOURCE: Callen PW: *Ultrasonography in Obstetrics and Gynecology,* 2nd ed. Philadelphia: Saunders, 1988, p 53.

so that the head is unusually round, the alteration is known as brachycephaly. If the OF diameter is elongated and the BPD is shortened so that the head is unusually elongated, the condition is known as dolichocephaly. If the cephalic index is abnormal, gestational age should be determined by other parameters, and head abnormalities should be considered and further assessed (Figure 17–8).

Femur Length Although any long bone may be used to determine gestational age, the femur is the easiest to image. Femur length is as accurate as BPD in determining gestational age (Callen, 1994). Femur length measurement is made from the major trochanter to the external condyle. Femur length is shortened in the presence of osteogenesis imperfecta or dwarfism (Figure 17–9).

Abdominal Measurements Measurement of the fetal abdominal circumference is useful for monitoring fetal growth and detecting IUGR, macrosomia, and isoimmunization (due to ascites). Fetal abdominal girth ceases to increase in IUGR due to the depletion of glycogen in the fetal liver and diminished accumulation of subcutaneous tissue overlying the fetal abdomen. If the estimated date of birth has been established with early ultrasound measurements, the abdominal circumference measurement may be sufficient to monitor fetal growth. If abdominal circumference is the only measurement that has been taken during the pregnancy, it is meaningless (Figure 17–10).

Head/Abdomen Ratio The head circumference (H) to abdomen circumference (A) ratio is used to assess disproportion between the fetal head and body. Disproportion may be observed in asymmetric IUGR (caused by uteroplacental insufficiency) and congenital anomalies such as microcephaly. The H/A ratio may also be used to estimate fetal weight (Hadlock, 1990).

Third Trimester Pregnancy

The ability to establish gestational age by ultrasound is lost in the third trimester because fetal growth rate is not uniform as it was in the first two trimesters. Without earlier ultrasound measurements, measurements obtained in the third trimester would vary by ± 3 weeks.

Uses of Fetal Ultrasound

Fetal Growth Determination

Serial ultrasound offers a valuable means of assessing intrauterine growth. IUGR is classified as symmetric (primary) or asymmetric (secondary). In symmetric IUGR all organs are reduced in size with equal reduction in body weight and head size; therefore, the fetus has normal head circumference/abdominal circumference (HC/AC) and femur length/abdominal circumference (FL/AC) ratios. At birth all measurements fall below the tenth percentile. Such fetuses comprise approximately 20% to 25% of cases of IUGR. These cases usually are detected by ultrasonography when all growth parameters lag significantly behind those expected based on gestational age confirmed by accurate menstrual history or early ultrasound dating (ACOG, 1994).

It has been estimated that 75% of symmetric IUGR or small for gestational age (SGA) fetuses are constitutionally small, 15% to 20% have uteroplacental insufficiency due to various causes, and 5% to 10% have impaired growth due to perinatal infections or congenital

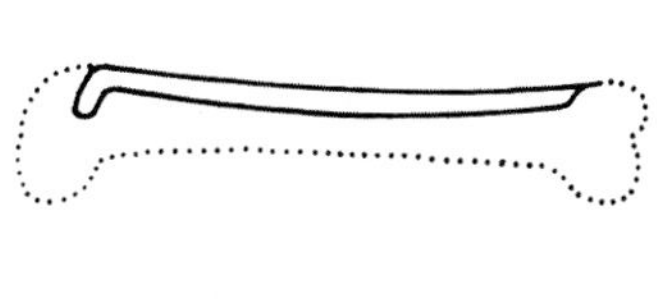

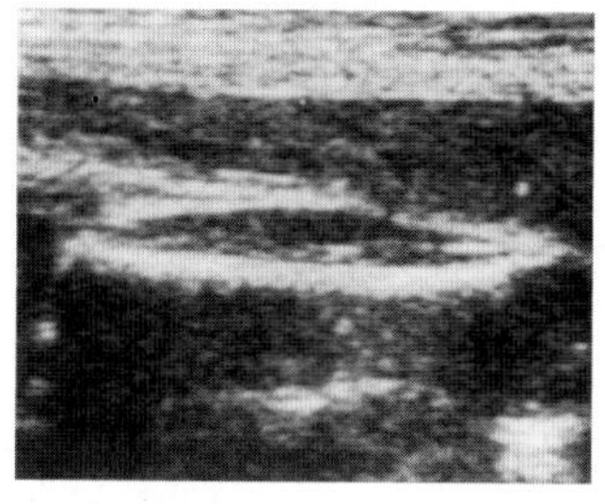

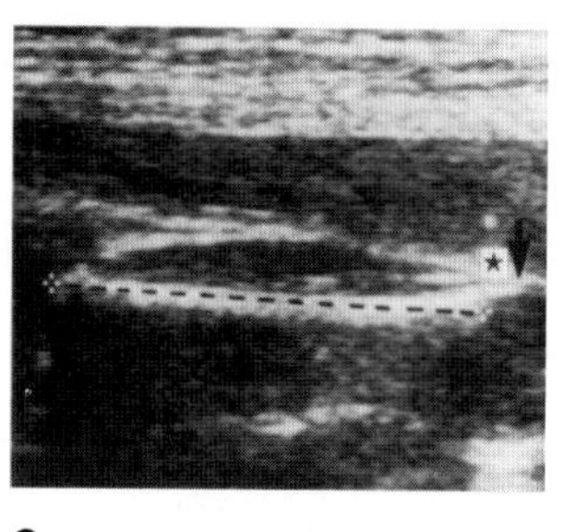

A B C

FIGURE 17–9 Measurement of the femur length. ***A,*** Schematic diagram. ***B,*** Ultrasound image. The hyperechoic line in the ossified lateral margin of the femoral diaphysis. The ends of the bone are the epiphyseal cartilages that have not yet calcified and are therefore hypoechoic. ***C,*** The hyperechoic diaphysis is measured from one end to the other, denoted by the cursors and a dotted line. The "distal femoral point" (* and arrow) is a nonossified extension of the distal epiphyseal cartilage. It should not be included in the measurement. SOURCE: Callen PW: *Ultrasonography in Obstetrics and Gynecology,* 2nd ed. Philadelphia: Saunders, 1988, p 58.

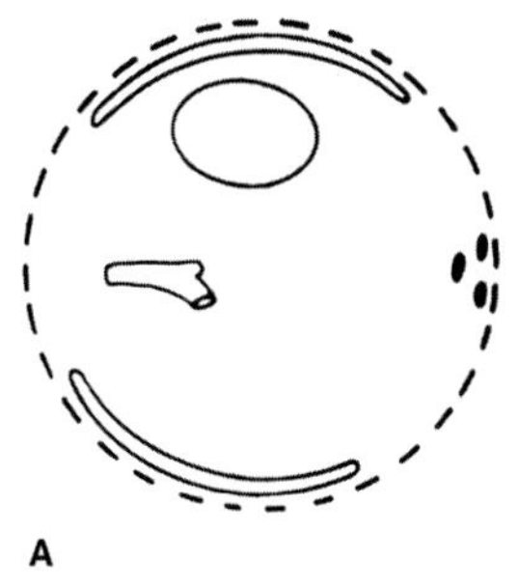

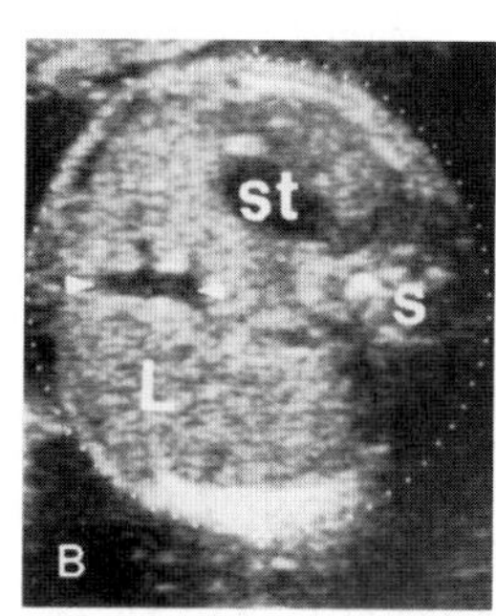

FIGURE 17–10 Measurement of the abdominal circumference. ***A,*** Diagram showing the abdominal circumference as a dotted line traced at the outer margin of the abdomen. ***B,*** Ultrasound transaxial image showing the umbilical portion of the left portal vein (arrowheads) correctly positioned within the liver and equidistant from the lateral walls. (S, spine; L, liver; ST, stomach). A dotted line, created by a digitizer, outlines the outer margins of the abdomen, the correct place to obtain an abdominal circumference measurement. SOURCE: Callen PW: *Ultrasonography in Obstetrics and Gynecology,* 2nd ed. Philadelphia: Saunders, 1988, p 57.

malformations (Manning & Hohler, 1991). This growth retardation is noted in the first half of the second trimester. It may also be associated with chromosomal disorders, chronic hypoxia, teratogens, vascular and renal disease, multiple gestation, maternal malnutrition, and dwarf syndromes.

In asymmetric IUGR, the head and brain sizes are normal, but there is a reduction in abdominal size, apparently caused by a compromise in the uteroplacental blood flow. This is felt to be due to "brain sparing" (the physiologic mechanism present when a restricted amount of oxygen is available to the fetus). The fetus shunts blood to the vital organs (brain, lungs, adrenals, and heart) to spare them the low oxygen concentration of the blood. The lower portion of the body is smaller, due to reduced blood flow, and the kidneys may be affected leading to oligohydramnios (AWHONN, 1997).

The decreased blood flow is associated with PIH, chronic hypertension, diabetes mellitus, and chronic renal disease. This is the more common type of IUGR and is usually not evident prior to the third trimester. Fetuses with asymmetric IUGR are particularly at risk for perinatal asphyxia, hypocalcemia, polycythemia, and hypoglycemia in the neonatal period. Birth weight will be reduced to the tenth percentile, whereas cephalic size is spared and is in the normal range. Perinatal mortality is ten times that of average for gestational age babies (Faranoff & Martin, 1992).

The earlier the gestational age is accurately assessed, the more accurate the prediction of IUGR. If a growth-retarded fetus is suspected, serial ultrasounds should be done every 2 to 3 weeks.

On first examination, the estimated fetal weight (EFW) is figured as a percentile for that fetus. If the percentile is low, serial sonograms are warranted. If on repeat scan the fetus is at the same percentile, no abnormal growth has occurred. If the percentile increases, growth of the fetus has improved. If the fetus is at a lower percentile, fetal growth is slowing, and this fetus should be further assessed with intense antenatal surveillance, including biophysical profiles and Doppler flow studies (Trudinger, 1999).

Management of the growth-retarded fetus depends on fetal well-being and gestational age. After a comprehensive ultrasound survey for structural abnormalities and amniotic fluid index, amniocentesis may be used to evaluate chromosomes and lung maturity. Bed rest and maternal oxygen therapy may be considered to increase fetal oxygenation; increased oral fluids may also be ordered (Battaglia, Artini, D'Ambrogio et al, 1992). The fetus will be assessed with at least weekly biophysical profiles with amniotic fluid index and some type of fetal activity assessment technique.

Serial ultrasounds for EFW growth curve, Doppler flow studies, and antenatal surveillance will help determine the optimal timing for birth (Trudinger, 1999). The

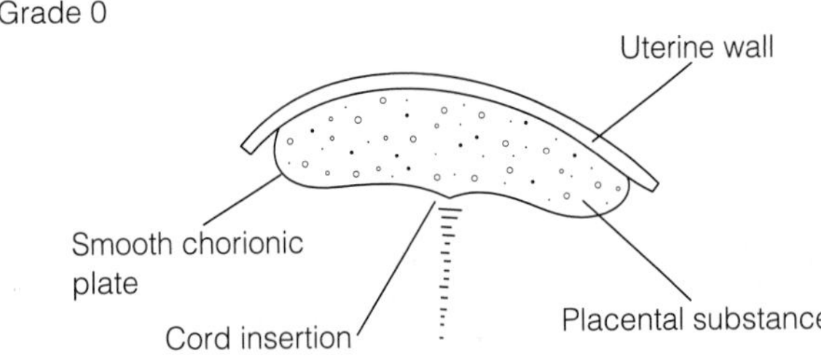

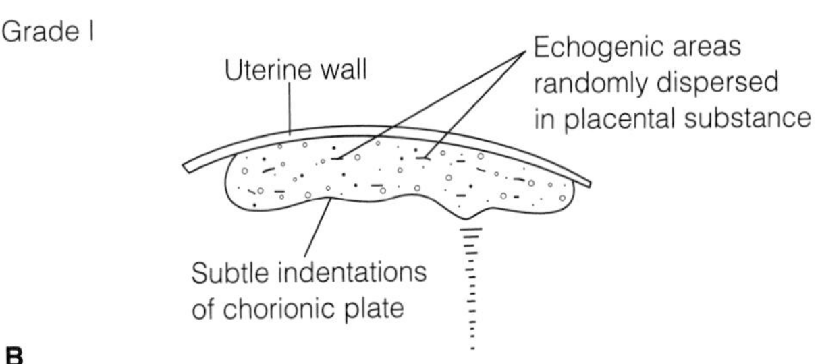

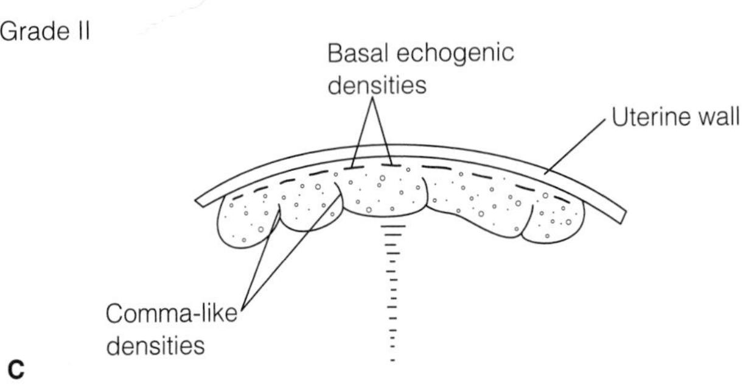

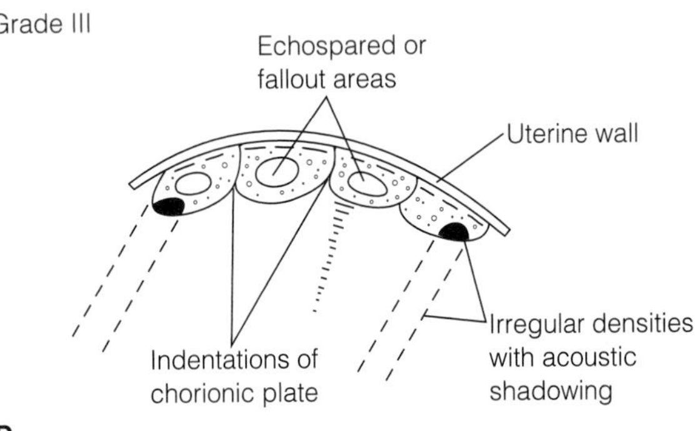

FIGURE 17–11 Placental grading. ***A,*** Diagram showing the ultrasonic appearance of a grade 0 placenta. ***B,*** Diagram showing the ultrasonic appearance of a grade I placenta. ***C,*** Diagram showing the ultrasonic appearance of a grade II placenta. ***D,*** Diagram showing the ultrasonic appearance of a grade III placenta.

timing of birth may depend on gestational age and fetal well-being. If the gestational age of the fetus is greater than 37 weeks, the woman's cervical status will be assessed using Bishop's scoring system (Chapter 20). An amniocentesis to confirm fetal lung maturity may be done before labor is induced.

Detection of Congenital Anomalies

Ultrasound evaluation of fetal anatomy can detect many major and minor structural anomalies, though not with 100% accuracy. A basic ultrasound of fetal anatomy should include evaluation of the following:

- Head shape; size of ventricles to detect hydrocephalus, microcephalus, anencephalus, encephalocele; face for clefts; neck for presence of cystic hygroma
- Spine to detect meningomyelocele or spina bifida
- Chest and heart to detect diaphragmatic hernia, hypoplasia, pericardial teratoma, pleural effusion, congenital heart disease
- Abdomen to detect omphalocele, gastroschisis, tracheoesophageal fistula, hydronephrosis, dilated renal pelves, polycystic kidneys
- Extremities for skeletal dysplasia

Evaluation of the Placenta and Cervix

Placental Maturity The placenta should be evaluated to assess maturity. Grannum, Berkowitz, and Hobbins (1979) noted that throughout gestation the placenta undergoes maturational changes that may be visualized by ultrasound. These morphologic changes in the basal layer, chorionic plate, and intervening placental substance have been classified in terms of grades (0 to III), with increasing changes occurring from 12 weeks' gestation until term. The grade is described according to the presence of echogenic areas in the placental substance, basal layer, and chorionic plate: Grade 0 has a smooth chorionic plate. Grade I has some calcification, which is reflected as some irregularity of the chorionic plate. Grade II has larger indentations that extend down toward the uterine wall. Grade III has extensive calcifications and indentations of the chorionic wall that reach down to the uterine wall (Reed 1994) (Figure 17–11).

The placental grade is a piece of information that adds to the clinical picture. Most decisions to intervene are not based simply on a high grade placenta in a preterm fetus. It is a warning sign that requires further investigation to identify the cause.

Placental Location The placental site should be evaluated in relationship to the cervix. The appearance of the placenta completely covering the internal os of the cervix is called *placenta previa.*

Cervical Length The cervical length can be measured by endovaginal or translabial ultrasound. This assessment has proved to be a more precise means of measuring the length of the cervical canal than a digital cervical exam. It has been used to follow women with cervical cerclage or preterm labor.

Deciding Whom to Screen

Controversy continues regarding whether ultrasound screening of all obstetric clients improves pregnancy outcome. Most recently, a study titled Routine Antenatal Diagnostic Imaging with Ultrasound (RADIUS) involved more than 15,000 women who were at low risk for perinatal problems. Study participants were randomly assigned into a universal screening group and a control group. The universal screen group received ultrasound screening at 15 to 22 weeks and again at 31 to 35 weeks. Women in the control group had ultrasound only when the need was indicated. Overall the study concluded that routine ultrasound screening did not improve perinatal outcome for low-risk women. However, when detection of congenital anomalies was considered, universal screening proved more effective, especially when the screening was completed in a tertiary center. When all data were analyzed, the outcome was still not clear.

At this time, many certified nurse-midwives and physicians tend to use ultrasound early in the pregnancy to establish the presence of a gestational sac and to determine that the gestational sac is in the uterus rather than in the fallopian tube (ectopic pregnancy). Another ultrasound may be scheduled at approximately 20 weeks to assess fetal growth. If all measurements are appropriate no further exams may be done, unless a problem arises.

Who Should Do Ultrasounds?

The American Institute of Ultrasound (AIUM) recommends that only certified ultrasonographers should perform diagnostic ultrasound. In a study by Huffman & Sandelowski (1997), however, nurses revealed that performing cursory ultrasound "enhanced" their practice, expanding their knowledge and skill. The nurses interviewed felt that having the nurse perform ultrasound is helpful to expectant women because it utilizes resources more efficiently in an era of declining numbers of health care providers, enhances opportunities for teaching, and provides opportunities for the expectant parents to bond with their fetus.

Antenatal Fetal Surveillance

The major goal of antepartum fetal surveillance is to reduce fetal demise in those populations at highest risk. Various techniques appear to be effective in reducing perinatal mortality in selected populations. Although antepartum fetal surveillance protocols may in the future also prove effective in reducing perinatal morbidity and improving long-term neurologic outcome, convincing data to support these effects presently do not exist (ACOG, 1994).

Amniotic Fluid Assessment

The volume of amniotic fluid in the uterus serves as an important indicator of fetal well-being. Abnormalities in amniotic fluid volume are associated with adverse perinatal outcomes. Polyhydramnios may indicate a fetal malformation. Oligohydramnios may be encountered with premature rupture of membranes, fetal urinary tract abnormalities, and placental insufficiency, often associated with IUGR or postdate pregnancy. Oligohydramnios has also often been associated with umbilical cord compression and thickened meconium-stained fluid (Moore, 1995).

The amount of amniotic fluid can be evaluated by a technique called *amniotic fluid volume (AFV)* or *amniotic fluid index (AFI)*. AFV is determined by using ultrasound and looking throughout the uterus for pockets of amniotic fluid. (Because the fetus is completely surrounded by amniotic fluid, a pocket of fluid can be visualized in the bend of the fetal arm or between the fetal arm and the face, for example.) When a pocket is visualized, it is measured from top to bottom in centimeters. A pocket of amniotic fluid that measures at least 2 cm across is associated with a normal amount of fluid; a pocket of less than 2 cm is associated with oligohydramnios.

AFI is obtained by measuring pockets of amniotic fluid in four quadrants of the uterus. The landmarks for the quadrants are the maternal umbilicus and the linea nigra (a pigmented vertical line that extends upward from the center of the symphysis pubis to the umbilicus and sometimes beyond the uterus). Within each quadrant the largest pocket of amniotic fluid is identified and measured; then these measurements are added to obtain the AFI. An AFI greater than 20 cm indicates hydramnios; an AFI less than 5 cm indicates oligohydramnios. These cutoff values, which were derived from pregnancies ranging from 36 to 42 weeks, have also been applied, perhaps appropriately, throughout gestation. Because AFV fluctuations have been observed, gestational-age-dependent norms for the AFI were developed. The 5th and 95th percentiles are used to define abnormal AFVs (Cunningham et al, 1997a).

The AFI is a useful measurement in high-risk pregnancies, especially when combined with a nonstress test. AFI identifies the changing amounts of amniotic fluid and especially helps determine the presence of oligohydramnios (low amounts of amniotic fluid). The presence of oligohydramnios indicates possible fetal compromise and the need for further assessment. It also indicates the need for the expectant woman to increase periods of rest (or be on bed rest) and to increase her hydration.

TABLE 17–3 Biophysical Profile Scoring: Technique and Interpretation

Biophysical Variable	Normal (Score = 2)	Abnormal (Score = 0)
Fetal breathing movements	≥1 episode of ≥30 seconds in 30 minutes	Absent or no episode of ≥30 seconds in 30 minutes
Gross body movements	≥3 discrete body/limb movements in 30 minutes (Episodes of active continuous movement considered as single movement.)	≤2 episodes of body/limb movements in 30 minutes
Fetal tone	≥1 episode of active extension with return to flexion of fetal limb(s) or trunk (Opening and closing of hand considered normal tone.)	Either slow extension with return to partial flexion or movement of limb in full extension or absent fetal movement
Reactive fetal heart rate	≥2 episodes of acceleration of ≥15 bpm and of ≥15 seconds associated with fetal movement in 20 minutes	<2 episodes of acceleration of fetal heart rate or acceleration of <15 bpm in 20 minutes
Qualitative amniotic fluid volume	≥1 pocket of fluid measuring ≥1 cm in two perpendicular planes	Either no pockets or a pocket <1 cm in two perpendicular planes

Management Based on Biophysical Profile Score

Attained Score	Intervention
10 of 10 or 8 of 10, with normal amniotic fluid volume	No intervention is needed, normal finding.
8 of 10 with abnormal amniotic fluid volume	If fetal renal function is normal and membranes are intact, delivery is indicated.
6 of 10 with normal amniotic fluid volume	Equivocal (Manning, Snijdeis, Harman, Nicholas, Menticoglov, & Morrison, 1993).
4 of 10, 2 of 10, or 0 of 10	Deliver fetus.

SOURCES: Manning FA et al: Fetal assessment based on fetal biophysical profile scoring: Experience in 12,620 referred high-risk pregnancies. *Am J Obstet Gynecol* 1985; 151(3):344; Manning FA: The biophysical profile: Contemporary use. *Tenth International Symposium on Perinatal Medicine and Obstetrical Ultrasound,* April 9–12, 1990, Las Vegas, NV.

NURSING CARE MANAGEMENT

It is important for the nurse to ascertain whether the woman understands the reason the ultrasound has been ordered. The nurse can provide an opportunity for the woman to ask questions and can act as an advocate if there are questions or concerns that need to be addressed prior to the ultrasound examination. The nurse explains the preparation needed and ensures that adequate preparation is done. If certified to perform a basic or limited ultrasound exam, the nurse provides information regarding the purpose of this particular exam and performs it. After the exam, the nurse can assist with clarifying or interpreting test results for the woman and her partner or other support person.

Biophysical Profile (BPP)

The **biophysical profile (BPP)** represents an assessment of five fetal biophysical variables: breathing movement, body movement, tone, amniotic fluid volume, and FHR reactivity. The BPP is used to assess the fetus at risk for intrauterine compromise. The first four variables are assessed by ultrasound scanning; FHR reactivity is assessed with the nonstress test. By combining these five assessments, the BPP helps to identify the compromised fetus and confirm the healthy fetus.

Specific criteria for normal and abnormal assessments are delineated in Table 17–3. A score of 2 is assigned to each normal finding and 0 to each abnormal one for a maximum score of 10. The absence of a specific activity is difficult to interpret because it may be indicative of central nervous system (CNS) depression or simply the resting state of a healthy fetus. Scores of 8 (with normal amount of amniotic fluid) or 10 are considered normal (Druzin & Gabbe, 1996). A score of 6 is considered equivocal (questionable). If the 4 points that are taken off the score relate to a nonreactive nonstress test and absence of fetal breathing movements, then delivery is not indicated. If the 4 deducted points relate to a nonreactive nonstress test and the amniotic fluid pocket is less than 1 cm or no amniotic fluid is visualized, then the woman is placed on bed rest and is hydrated. The management of a score of 6 (6/10) is not clear and depends on specific conditions present in that situation. A score of 4 or less is abnormal and indicates that the fetus should be born immediately.

The presence of oligohydramnios warrants further evaluation. The correlation of BPP score and perinatal mortality has been studied extensively by Manning (1990, 1995), and the implications of each BPP score are described in Table 17–4. If the BPP test score is 10/10, the perinatal mortality rate in the next 7 days is less than 1/1000 for the fetus. If the BPP score is 2/10, the perinatal mortality rate is 125/1000, which means that if intervention does not occur, the fetus is 125 times as likely to die in the next 7 days than if the score were 10/10.

Clinicians suggest that management not be based solely on BPP scores. Queenan (1996) notes that the biophysical activities of the fetus that develop first are the last to disappear when all activities are arrested due to asphyxia; those that are the last to develop are the most sen-

TABLE 17–4 Interpretation of Fetal Biophysical Profile Score Results and Recommended Clinical Management

Test Score	Interpretation	Perinatal Mortality Within 1 Week Without Intervention	Management
10/10 8/10 (normal fluid) 8/8 (NST not done)	Risk of fetal asphyxia extremely rare	< 1/1000	Intervene only for obstetric and maternal factors. No indication for intervention for fetal disease.
8/10 (abnormal fluid)	Probable chronic fetal compromise	89/1000	Determine that there are functioning renal tissue and intact membranes. If so, birth is indicated for fetal indications.
6/10 (normal fluid)	Equivocal test, possible fetal asphyxia	Variable	If the fetus is mature, birth is indicated. In the immature fetus repeat test within 24 hours. If < 6/10, then birth is indicated.
6/10 (abnormal fluid)	Probable fetal asphyxia	89/1000	Birth is indicated for fetal indications.
4/10	High probability of fetal asphyxia	91/1000	Birth is indicated for fetal indications.
2/10	Fetal asphyxia almost certain	125/1000	Birth is indicated for fetal indications.
0/10	Fetal asphyxia certain	600/1000	Birth is indicated for fetal indications.

SOURCE: Manning FA: The biophysical profile: Contemporary use. *Tenth International Symposium on Perinatal Medicine and Obstetrical Ultrasound.* April 9–12, 1990, Las Vegas, NV.

sitive to hypoxia, and their disappearance can be noted first. For example, fetal tone (exhibited by flexion of the extremities) is the first to develop and the last activity to cease during asphyxia. Other activities in the normal developmental sequence are fetal movement, followed by fetal breathing, and then reactivity of the FHR. Therefore, FHR reactivity is the most sensitive to hypoxia. One of the first indications of fetal compromise is a nonreactive nonstress test.

Indications for BPP include those situations in which the NST and contraction stress test (CST) would be done. Assessment of these fetal biophysical activities is most useful in the evaluation of women who experience decreased fetal movement (who might subsequently have a nonreactive NST) and in the management of IUGR; preterm, diabetic, and postterm pregnancies; and premature rupture of the membranes (PROM) (Manning, 1995).

The two most important components of the BPP are the NST and the AFI. The NST reflects the intactness of the nervous system, and the AFI reflects kidney perfusion. Normal AFI indicates that shunting has not occurred. Reactive NST and normal fluid reflect fetal well-being. The importance of these two tests has led to their use as a modified BPP, especially in the labor and delivery area.

Fetal Echocardiography

Among its many uses, ultrasound may be employed to examine fetal cardiac structures. Echocardiography has made treatment of fetal arrhythmias prior to birth possible, and cases of congenital heart disease have been diagnosed prenatally and managed accordingly.

Fetal echocardiography is recommended for women who have a family history of congenital heart disease, maternal disease that may affect the fetus, history of maternal drug use, evidence of other fetal anomalies, or fetal hydrops. The best timing for fetal echocardiography is 18 to 22 weeks' gestation. There is a 15% occurrence of fetal cardiac arrythmias in this selected population. Premature atrial or ventricular contractions are commonly seen and usually require no treatment. Supraventricular tachycardia can result in hydrops and require in utero treatment to prevent fetal death. Complete heart block, particularly in association with structural heart disease, has poor prognosis for fetal survival (Copel & Kleinman, 1996).

Doppler Velocimetry

Recent advances in ultrasound technology have made it possible to study noninvasively blood flow changes that occur in maternal and fetal circulations to assess placental function. An ultrasound beam, like that provided by the pocket Doppler (a hand-held ultrasound device), is directed at the umbilical artery. The signal is reflected off the red blood cells (RBCs) moving within the vessels, and the subsequent "picture" (waveform) that is received looks like a series of waves. The highest velocity peak of the waves is the systolic measurement, and the lowest point is the diastolic velocity. The umbilical artery waveform can then be analyzed to provide information regarding velocity of blood flow in the vessel.

The most common evaluation of blood flow velocity is the systolic to diastolic (S/D) ratio. The S/D ratio normally decreases as the fetus nears term. This phenomenon reflects the decreasing resistance of placental and umbilical vasculature to allow for greater umbilical blood flow to meet the needs of a growing fetus. The normal range for the S/D ratio is < 3 after 28 weeks' gestation.

The most commonly used index is the umbilical artery S/D ratio. It is considered abnormal in two instances: if it is elevated above the 95th percentile for gestational

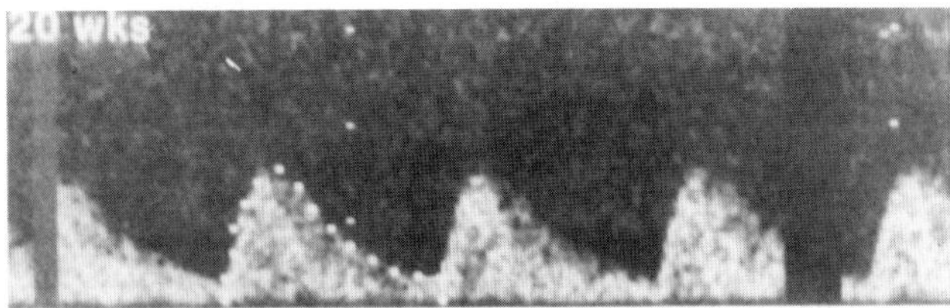

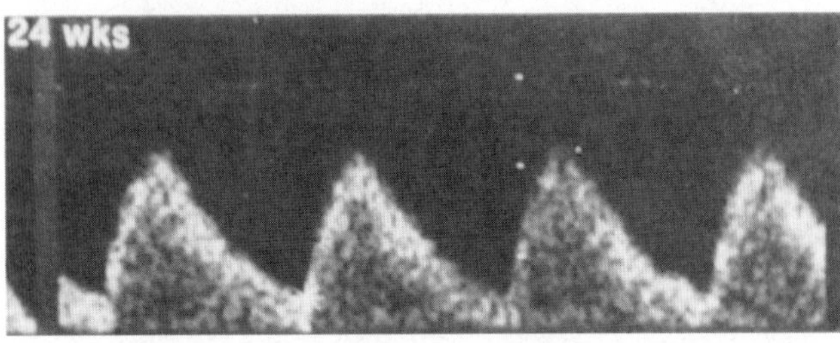

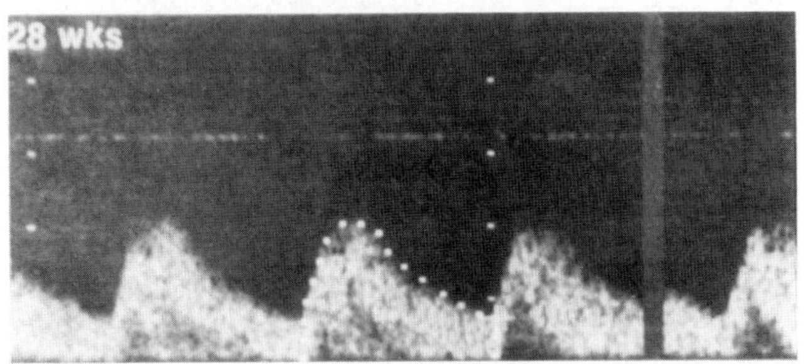

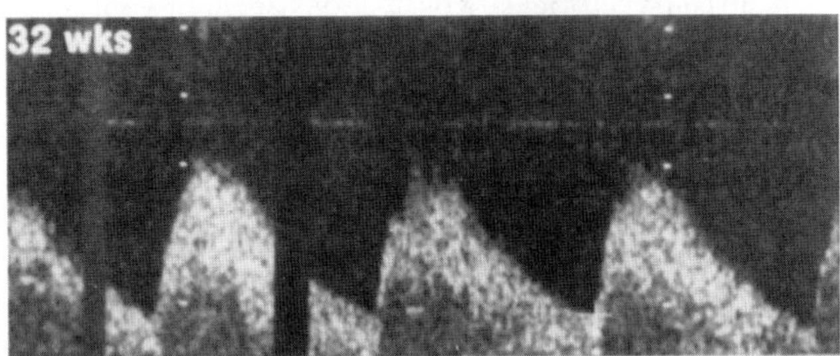

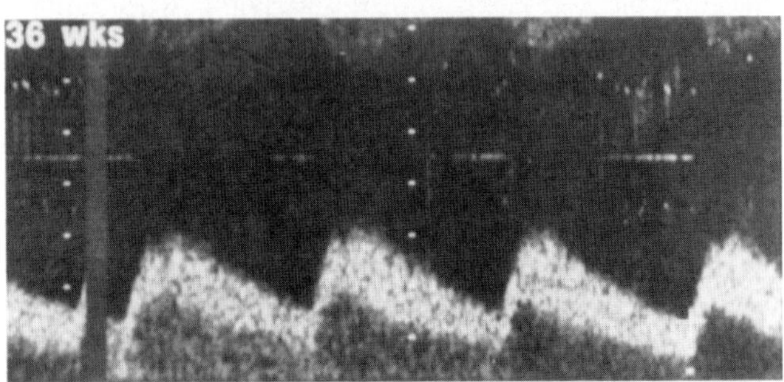

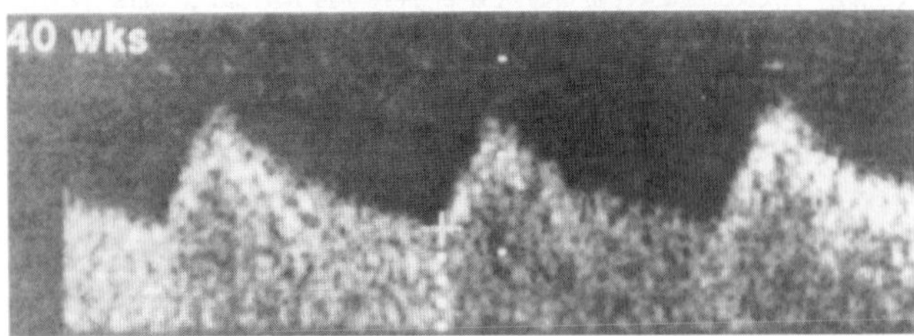

FIGURE 17–12 Serial studies of the umbilical artery velocity waveforms in a normal pregnancy from one client. SOURCE: Cundiff JL, Haybrich KL, Hinzman NG: Umbilical artery Doppler flow studies during pregnancy. SOURCE: *JOGNN* November/December 1990; 19(6): 475, Figure 3.

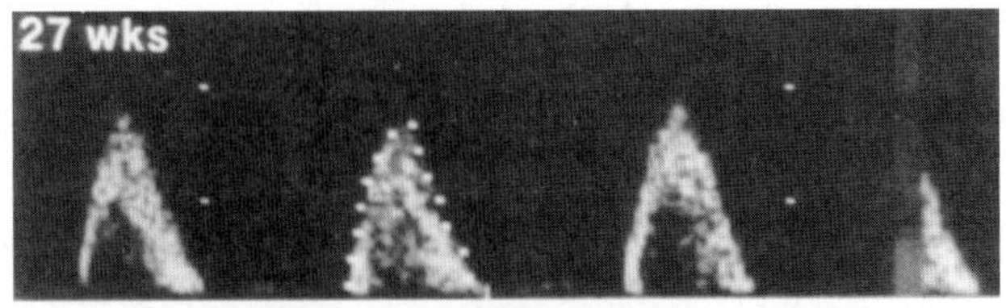

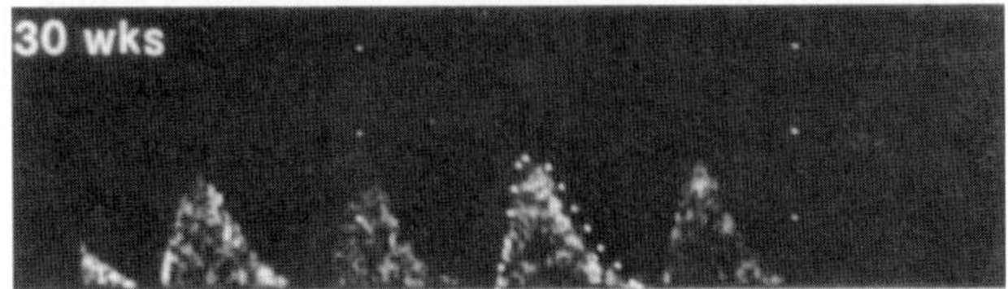

FIGURE 17–13 Two examples of abnormal umbilical artery velocity waveforms taken from a client with intrauterine growth restriction. SOURCE: Cundiff JL, Haybrich KL, Hinzman NG: Umbilical artery Doppler flow studies during pregnancy. SOURCE: *JOGNN* November/December 1990; 19(6): 475, Figure 4.

age, or if it is reversed after 18 to 20 weeks of gestation (ACOG, 1997). An elevated S/D ratio may be associated with fetal growth restriction (Reed, 1996) (Figures 17–12 and 17–13).

The absence of diastolic flow is abnormal, indicating impaired uteroplacental or umbilical circulation. The worst scenario is reverse end diastolic flow, in which the blood flow regurgitates back toward the placenta at each heartbeat. Absence or reversal is not common. It is seen in only the most extreme circumstances and has a very high perinatal mortality rate (ACOG, 1997).

A decrease in fetal cardiac output or an increase in resistance of placental vessels will reduce umbilical artery blood flow. Doppler velocimetry is best used when IUGR is suspected or diagnosed, whether it occurs as an idiopathic process or in the presence of hypertension or preeclampsia (ACOG, 1997).

Nonstress Test (NST)

The **nonstress test (NST)** has become a widely accepted method of evaluating fetal status. The test involves using an electronic fetal monitor to obtain a tracing of the fetal heart rate and observation of acceleration of the FHR with fetal movement. The test is based on the knowledge that the fetus is normally active throughout pregnancy and that good fetal activity will result in acceleration of the fetal heart rate when the normal fetus moves. Accelerations of the FHR imply an intact central and autonomic nervous system that is not being affected by intrauterine hypoxia.

The advantages of the NST are that it is relatively quick, inexpensive, and easy to interpret; it can be done in an outpatient setting; and there are no known side effects. The disadvantages are that it is sometimes difficult to obtain a suitable tracing, the woman has to recline and be relatively still for 20 to 30 minutes, and the fetus may be in a sleep cycle at the time the test is performed.

Fetal age must be considered in the use and evaluation of NSTs. The central nervous system (parasympathetic and sympathetic nervous systems) of the fetus usually matures sufficiently by the 30th week of gestation to allow frequent accelerations of the heart rate when fetal movement occurs (Soffici & Eden, 1994). The NST can be used as an assessment tool in any pregnancy but is especially useful in the presence of diabetes, pregnancy-induced hypertension, intrauterine growth restriction, spontaneous rupture of membranes, multiple gestation, and other high-risk pregnancy problems. Testing intervals may vary, depending on the condition of the mother and baby and recommendations of various experts. Paul and Miller (1995) report most clinicians test twice weekly for high-risk clients and once a week testing for other conditions.

Currently, a *modified NST* may also be used. In this test, a device that sends sound into the fetus (called fetal acoustical stimulation [FAST]) is used after 5 minutes of testing. If there is no acceleration of the fetal heart rate, the sound stimulus is used again (see Fetal Acoustic Stimulation Test [FAST] and Vibroacoustic Stimulation Test [VST] for further discussion).

The NST is a good indicator of fetal well-being but is not an accurate predictor of poor outcomes. The false-negative rate (a reactive NST followed by an unexpected fetal death within 1 week) is 2.5 deaths per 1000. A nonreactive NST is fairly consistent in identifying at-risk fetuses.

NST Procedure

The NST is usually scheduled during the daytime hours, and the woman is asked to eat approximately 2 hours prior to the test. The woman is positioned in a semi-Fowler's position with a small pillow or blanket under the right hip to displace the uterus to the left. Many facilities use a recliner chair, which permits a semi-Fowler's position while providing a leg and foot rest. An electronic fetal monitor is applied (see discussion in Chapter 19). The examiner applies two belts around the woman's abdomen. One belt holds a tocodynamometer that detects uterine or fetal movement. The other belt holds an external transducer that detects the FHR.

Recordings of the FHR are obtained for approximately 20 to 40 minutes. The woman or nurse notes each fetal movement as it is recorded by pushing a button that will record on the monitor strip. If no fetal movements occur after 20 minutes of observation, the test can be extended another 20 minutes (Cunningham et al, 1997).

Interpretation of NST

The results of the NST are interpreted as follows:

- A *reactive* NST shows two or more accelerations of 15 bpm or more within 20 minutes of beginning the test (ACOG, 1994) (Figure 17–14).
- A *nonreactive* test contains a tracing that does not meet the above criteria. For example, the accelerations are less than two in number, the accelerations are less than 15 bpm, or there are no accelerations (Figure 17–15).

It is particularly important that anyone who performs the NST also understands the significance of any spontaneous decelerations of the FHR during testing. If spontaneous decelerations are noted, the physician/certified nurse-midwife should be notified for further evaluation of fetal status (Cunningham et al, 1997).

The NST may also show more subtle signs of fetal deterioration before the interpretation is nonreactive. With increasing levels of anoxia sleep cycles lengthen, accelerations become more uniform, the interval between accelerations increases, variability decreases, and the FHR baseline may increase. This type of subtle change can be noted when serial NSTs are compared. It is important that in this case the fetus be evaluated further with biophysical profile (BPP), amniotic fluid index (AFI), and perhaps Doppler velocimetry studies to assess fetal well-being.

Medical Management

The clinical management may vary somewhat among different clinicians. Paul and Miller (1995) report that most clinicians carry out the following protocol: If the NST is reactive in 20 minutes, the test is concluded and rescheduled as indicated by the condition that is present. If nonreactive, the test time is extended another 20 minutes; if the tracing becomes reactive, the NST is concluded. If the NST is still nonreactive after the additional 20 minutes (40 minutes total), additional testing, such as AFI, is considered. If the gestation is near term and other parameters of the tracing are questionable, a contraction stress test (CST) may be done.

NURSING CARE MANAGEMENT

The nurse ascertains the woman's understanding of the NST, including fetal acoustic stimulation test (FAST) and VST when appropriate and the possible results. The nurse reviews reasons for the NST, the equipment being used, and the procedure prior to beginning the test. The nurse positions the woman and applies the electronic fetal monitor. Maternal blood pressure is monitored during the NST to determine whether hypotension is present. The nurse administers the NST, interprets the results, and reports the findings to the physician or certified nurse-midwife and the expectant woman. The nurse uses this opportunity to assess learning needs concerning the importance of fetal movement and provides information and teaching.

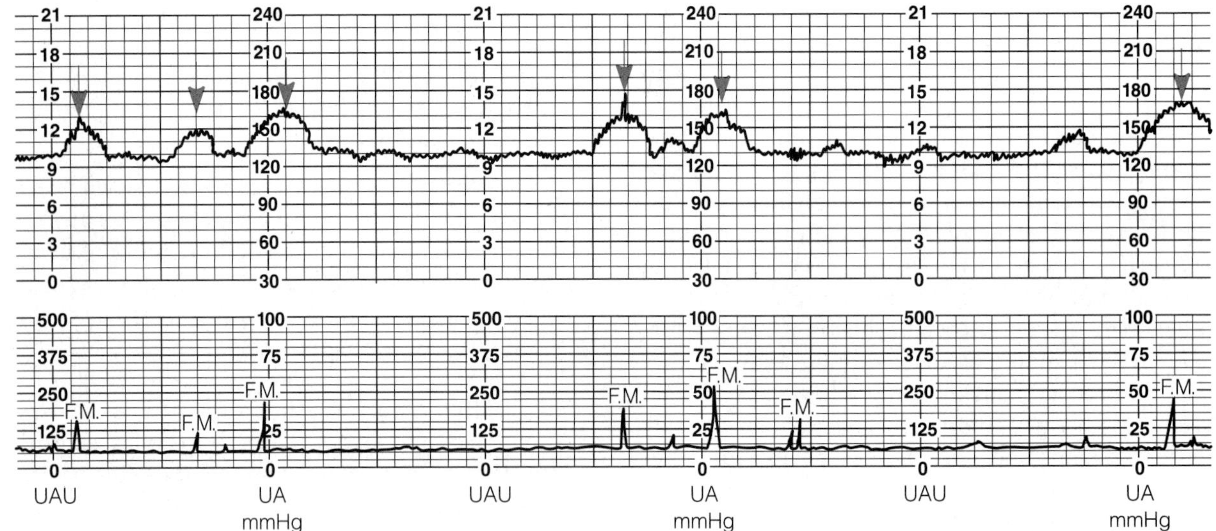

FIGURE 17–14 Example of a reactive nonstress test (NST). Accelerations of 15 bpm lasting 15 seconds with each fetal movement (FM). Top of strip shows fetal heart rate (FHR); bottom of strip shows uterine activity tracing. Note that FHR increases (above the baseline) at least 15 beats and remains at that rate for at least 15 seconds before returning to the former baseline.

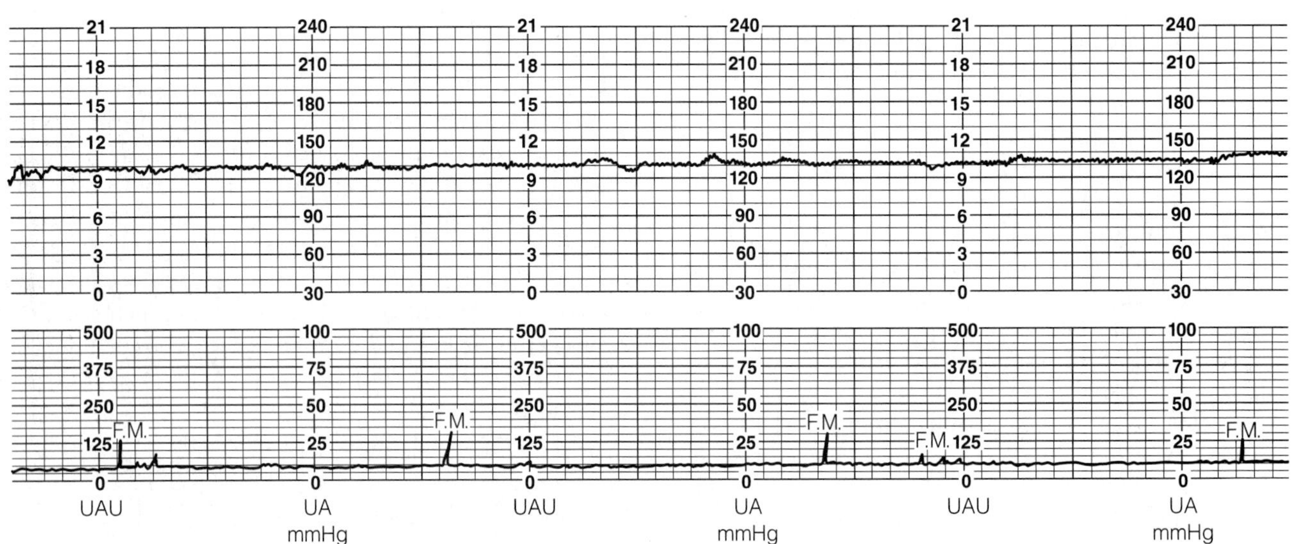

FIGURE 17–15 Example of a nonreactive NST. There are no accelerations of FHR with fetal movement (FM). Baseline FHR is 130 bpm. The tracing of uterine activity is on the bottom of the strip.

Fetal Acoustic Stimulation Test (FAST) and Vibroacoustic Stimulation Test (VST)

Use of acoustic (sound) and vibroacoustic (vibration and sound) stimulation of the fetus is becoming more common as an adjunct to the NST. Several methods have been used (for example, loudspeakers, bells, artificial larynx). Figure 17–16 shows one example. A handheld, self-contained, battery-operated device is applied to the maternal abdomen away from the fetal head, and the sound is delivered for 1 second. This device generates a low-frequency vibration and a buzzing sound, which are intended to induce accelerations of FHR in response to movement in those fetuses who demonstrate nonreactivity during the NST. The **fetal acoustic stimulation test (FAST)** and vibroacoustic stimulation test (VST) offer several advantages. They are noninvasive techniques, results are rapidly available, they allow the NST to be performed in a shorter time, and the tests are easy to perform. A common FHR response to FAST or VST is tachycardia (FHR over 160 beats per minute). It is important to document the return of FHR to baseline. Caution must be exercised when using FAST or VST on a fetus that is already compromised. The response to the stimulation may include bradycardia and fetal distress. The FHR baseline and fetal well-being must be assessed before using FAST or VST.

Contraction Stress Test (CST)

The **contraction stress test (CST)** is a means of evaluating the respiratory function (oxygen and carbon dioxide exchange) of the placenta (ie, uteroplacental function). It enables the health care team to identify the fetus at risk for intrauterine asphyxia by observing the response of the FHR to the stress of uterine contractions (spontaneous or induced). During contractions intrauterine pressure increases. Blood flow to the intervillous space of the placenta is reduced momentarily, thereby decreasing oxygen transport to the fetus. A healthy fetus usually tolerates this reduction well. If the placental reserve is insufficient, fetal hypoxia, depression of the myocardium, and a decrease in FHR occur.

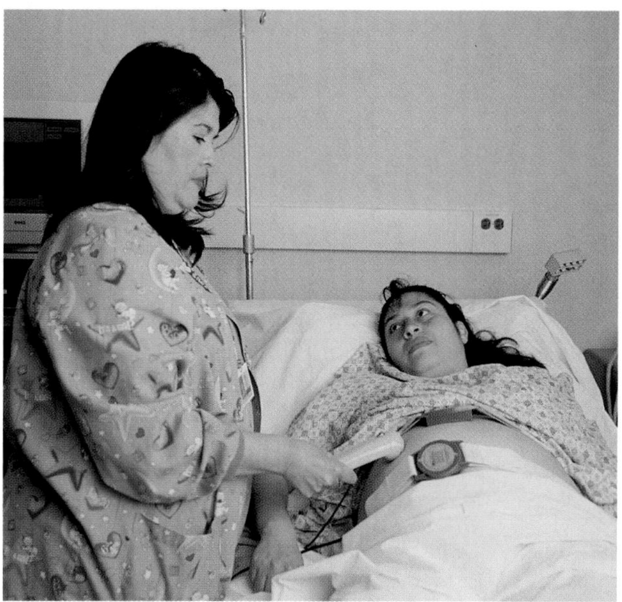

FIGURE 17–16 Fetal acoustic stimulation testing.

Indications and Contraindications

The CST is indicated for pregnancies at risk for placental insufficiency or fetal compromise because of any of the following:

- IUGR
- Diabetes mellitus
- Postdates (42 or more weeks' gestation)
- Nonreactive NST
- Abnormal or suspicious BPP

Contraindications for the CST are the following:

- Third trimester bleeding (placenta previa, marginal abruptio placentae, or unexplained vaginal bleeding)
- Previous cesarean birth with classical uterine incision
- Instances in which the risk of possible preterm labor outweighs the advantage of the CST, including
  - **a.** Premature rupture of the membranes
  - **b.** Incompetent cervix or Shirodkar-Barter operation (cerclage—surgical procedure in which an incompetent cervix is encircled with suture to prevent it from dilating before term)
  - **c.** Multiple gestation

CST Procedure

A necessary component of the CST is the presence of three uterine contractions of at least 40 seconds' duration in 10 minutes. The contractions may occur spontaneously, or they may be induced by oxytocin or nipple stimulation. The most common method of stimulating uterine contractions for a CST has been intravenous administration of oxytocin (Pitocin). Many facilities now use *breast self-stimulation* to obtain a CST. This method is based on the fact that endogenous oxytocin is produced in response to stimulation of the breasts or nipples.

The CST is performed on an outpatient basis by qualified obstetric nurses well acquainted with fetal monitoring and the interpretation of various FHR patterns. Most facilities require the tests be administered in or near the labor and birth unit so that treatment is available in the event that adverse reactions to oxytocin stimulation occur. The procedure, reasons for administering the test, equipment, and normal variations in monitoring that occur during the test should be clearly explained prior to the test to alleviate the woman's apprehension. A consent form may be signed.

During the test, the woman assumes a semi-Fowler's or side-lying position to avoid supine hypotension. The ultrasonic transducer (from the electronic fetal monitor) is placed on the woman's abdomen over the area of the fetal back or chest so that the FHR may be accurately recorded on the monitoring strip. (See Chapter 19 for further discussion of fetal monitoring.) To record uterine contractions, the tocodynamometer (pressure transducer) is placed over the area of the uterine fundus. For the first 15 to 20 minutes, the nurse records baseline measurements, including blood pressure, fetal activity, variations of the FHR during fetal movement, and spontaneous contractions. In addition, pertinent medical and obstetric information may be obtained from the woman to aid in her further management.

After the baseline recording is done, an intravenous oxytocin contraction stress test or breast self-stimulation test (BSST) is done.

Intravenous Oxytocin Contraction Stress Test A CST can also be done by using intravenous oxytocin. In this test an electrolyte solution such as lactated Ringer's

TABLE 17–5 Interpretation of the Contraction Stress Test

Result	Interpretation
Negative	No late decelerations occur after any contractions.
Positive	Late decelerations occur with at least 2 of the 3 contractions.
Equivocal	
Suspicious	Late decelerations occur with a single late deceleration.
Hyperstimulation	Late decelerations occur with hyperstimulation pattern (contractions every 2 minutes, or 5 in a 10 minute window) and there are late decelerations with 5 contractions.

SOURCE: Cunningham, T.G., MacDonald, P.C., Gant, N.F., Leveno, K.J., Gilstrap, L.C., Hankins, G.D.V., & Clark, S.L., (1997). Antepartum Assessment, *Williams Obstetrics*, 20th ed, Chapter 43, pp 1009–1022. Stamford, CT: Appleton & Lange.

solution is started as a primary infusion. A piggyback infusion of oxytocin in a similar solution is attached. An infusion pump is used so that the amount of oxytocin being infused can be measured accurately. The administration procedure is the same as that for inducing labor through oxytocin administration (see Chapter 23). Oxytocin is administered until three uterine contractions lasting 40 to 60 seconds occur in a 10-minute period (called the 10-minute window). If late decelerations occur with all three contractions, the oxytocin infusion is discontinued. The woman's blood pressure and pulse are assessed every 15 minutes and recorded on the tracing.

CST with Breast Self-Stimulation Test (BSST) In BSST, the woman brushes one nipple with the palmar surface of her fingers or rolls the nipple between her finger over her clothing for two minutes. Nipple stimulation is stopped for two minutes and then repeated on the opposite breast. The complete cycle is repeated four times. If contractions do not occur, bilateral stimulation may be used for 10 minutes. Each nipple stimulation is recorded on the monitor strip as well as maternal blood pressure and pulse every 15 minutes. When three uterine contractions occur in 10 minutes, breast stimulation is stopped (Lagrew, 1995). Over time, clinicians have been concerned about nipple stimulation causing a hyperstimulation pattern. Should a hyperstimulation pattern occur (uterine contractions occurring every 2 minutes, which would show on the tracing as three contractions in 6 minutes), the nipple stimulation is immediately stopped. The results are reviewed, recorded, and explained to the woman.

Interpretation and Management

A CST is usually not done prior to 28 weeks' gestation, primarily for two reasons. First, in light of a positive test, birth and extrauterine survival would be questionable at such an early gestational age. Second, sufficient research has not been done to determine whether the same test results apply to a fetus of this gestation. CST is usually done at 32 to 34 weeks' gestation.

Interpretation of CST Results The first step in interpreting results is to analyze the uterine contractions. Three contractions of 40 to 60 seconds' duration should occur in a 10-minute time frame (called the 10-minute window). The FHR is then analyzed for the presence of decelerations (which is the basis of the CST).

- A *negative* CST shows no late decelerations after any contraction (Table 17–5 and Figure 17–17).

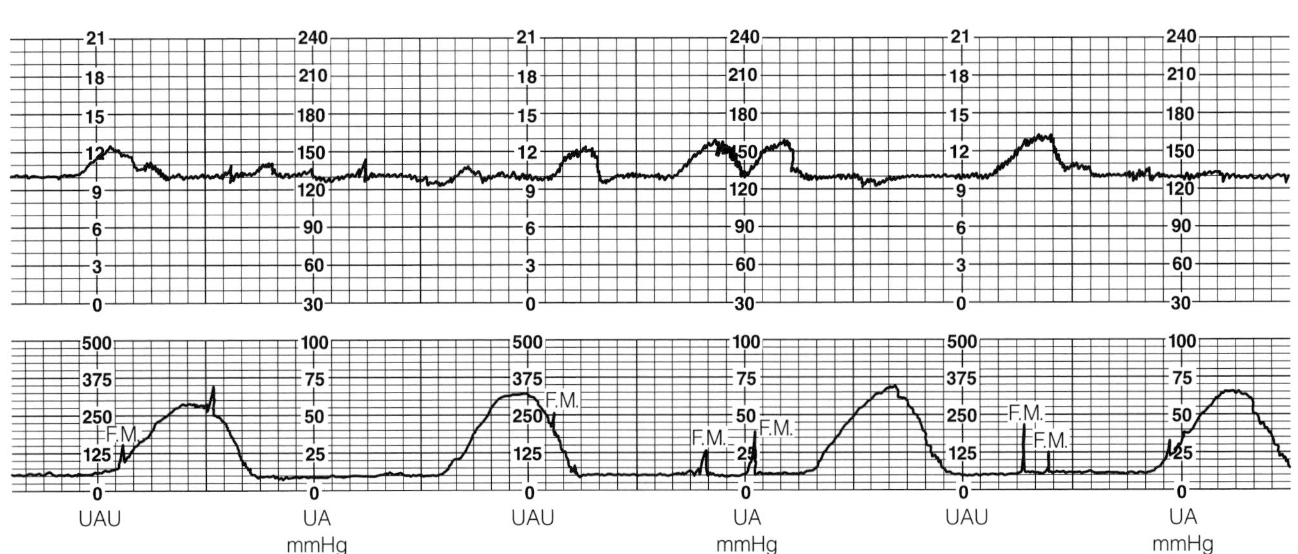

FIGURE 17–17 Example of a negative CST (and reactive NST). The baseline FHR is 130 bpm with acceleration of FHR of at least 15 bpm lasting 15 seconds with each fetal movement (FM). Uterine contractions recorded on bottom half of strip indicate three contractions in 8 minutes.

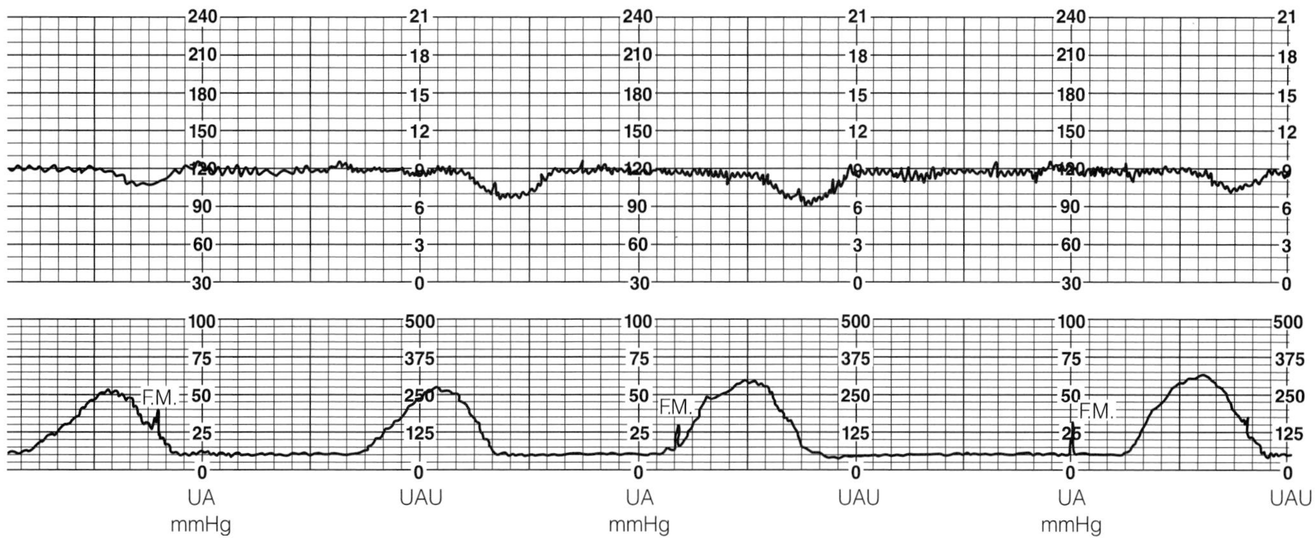

FIGURE 17–18 Example of a positive contraction stress test (CST). Repetitive late decelerations occur with each contraction. Note that there are no accelerations of FHR with three fetal movements (FM). The baseline FHR is 120 bpm. Uterine contractions (bottom half of strip) occurred four times in 12 minutes.

- A *positive* CST shows late decelerations with at least two of the three contractions (Figure 17–18). A positive CST may indicate the possibility of insufficient placental respiratory reserve (Cunningham et al, 1997).
- An *equivocal* (suspicious or difficult to interpret) test may be divided into two subcategories: equivocal suspicious and equivocal hyperstimulation. An equivocal suspicious result is present if there is a single late deceleration. An equivocal hyperstimulation result is present if there has been a hyperstimulation pattern (contractions every 2 minutes, or 5 in a 10-minute window) and there are late decelerations with five contractions.

Contraction stress test results are also evaluated for the presence of accelerations that would meet the criteria of the NST. Combining the CST assessment with NST results and also characteristics of the fetal heart rate, such as variability of the FHR baseline, and the presence of other types of decelerations helps the clinician decide what the best management plan for this fetus would be.

Management Based on CST Results In most cases, a negative CST with a reactive NST would be a desired result. The uteroplacental perfusion is sufficient at this time to allow the fetus to withstand the stress of uterine contractions. Retesting would most likely be rescheduled in 7 days. If the expectant woman is diabetic, the CST schedule would remain the same, except an NST would be done in 3 to 4 days (Lagrew, 1995). A negative CST with a nonreactive NST is more difficult. It should be looked at very carefully for subtle late decelerations. If there are none, then a CST is repeated in 7 days.

Lagrew (1995) suggests that all equivocal tests should be repeated in 24 hours, especially in the presence of a postterm pregnancy. If the gestation is less than 37 weeks, then other surveillance methods should be added.

A positive CST with a nonreactive NST presents evidence that the fetus will probably not withstand the stress of labor. If the gestation is 32 weeks or over, a cesarean delivery should be scheduled (Lagrew, 1995).

NURSING CARE MANAGEMENT

The nurse ascertains the woman's or couple's understanding of the CST and the possible results. The nurse reviews the reasons for the CST and the procedure before beginning the test.

Amniocentesis

Amniocentesis involves inserting a needle through the maternal abdomen into the uterine cavity to withdraw a sample of amniotic fluid. Amniocentesis is a fairly simple procedure, although complications do occur rarely (fewer than 1% of cases).

Early in the pregnancy (usually 16 to 18 weeks' gestation), amniocentesis can make chromosomal and biochemical determinations (enzyme analysis, α-fetoprotein measurement for neural tube defects, blood typing, or cytogenetic, metabolic, or other DNA testing) and can delineate abnormalities detected by ultrasound. Later in pregnancy (from about 30 to 35 weeks' gestation), amniocentesis may be done for lung maturity studies, such as L/S ratio and the presence of phosphatidylglycerol and

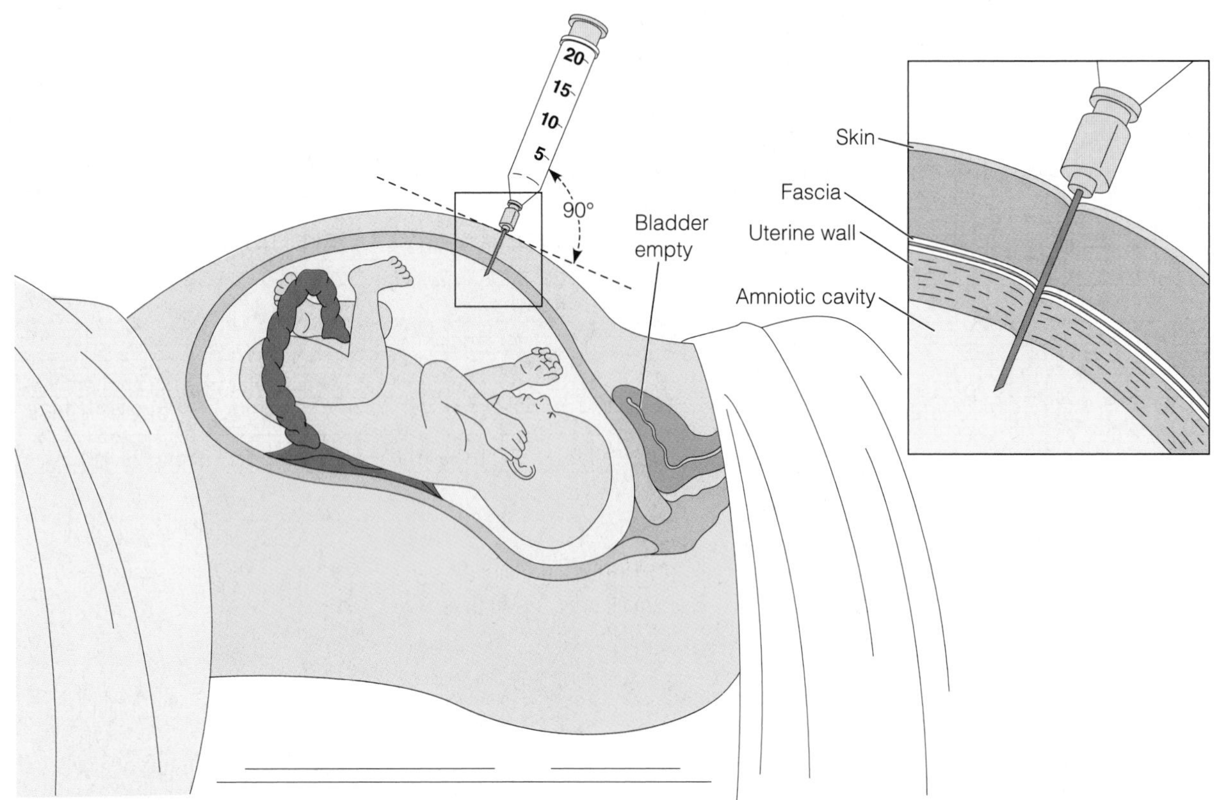

FIGURE 17–19 Amniocentesis. The woman is usually scanned by ultrasound to determine the placental site and to locate a pocket of fluid. As the needle is inserted, three levels of resistance are felt when the needle penetrates the skin, fascia, and uterine wall. When the needle is placed within the uterine cavity, amniotic fluid is withdrawn.

phosphatidylcholine. This procedure is also used to determine the presence or absence of intrauterine infection with premature rupture of the membranes in preterm labor before tocolytic therapy is considered.

Amniotic fluid is obtained by transabdominal amniocentesis. The fetus, umbilical cord, or placenta may be punctured inadvertently, causing injuries ranging from minor scratches of fetal parts to intrauterine hemorrhage, leading to fetal distress and intrauterine fetal death. Placental perforation could result in hemorrhage from the fetal circulation, which could lead to fetal anemia or to increased sensitization of an Rh negative mother. Intra-amniotic infection and induction of preterm labor are also hazards. The above complications are rare (0.5% to 1%), but the woman does need to be informed of them. A consent form is usually signed for this procedure.

CRITICAL THINKING QUESTION

A woman has just come in for her amniocentesis. She appears worried and makes many nervous gestures. When you talk with her, she says she is afraid to have the amniotic fluid removed because then the baby won't have enough for the rest of the pregnancy. How will you answer her?

Procedure

Amniocentesis is done on an outpatient basis but needs to be performed near a birthing area in case acute fetal distress is encountered. The pregnant woman should have a left lateral tilt to prevent hypotension during the procedure.

The abdomen is scanned by ultrasound to locate the placenta, fetus, and an adequate pocket of fluid. The amniocentesis, or "tap," is then done before the fetus has the opportunity to move. The needle insertion site is of the utmost importance because the fetus, placenta, umbilical cord, bladder, and uterine arteries must all be avoided (Figure 17–19). The importance of locating the placenta cannot be stressed enough, especially in cases of Rh isoimmunization, in which trauma to the placenta increases fetal–maternal transfusion and worsens the immunization. In the last few weeks of pregnancy the fetus may occupy what appears to be all the available space in the uterus, and there is a normal decrease in the amount of amniotic fluid. However, with the aid of ultrasound, fluid can be located.

After the abdomen is scanned, the abdominal skin is cleansed with povidone-iodine (Betadine). The woman is given the option of a local anesthetic for the insertion site. A 22-gauge spinal needle is inserted into the uterine cavity. Generally, fluid immediately flows into the needle.

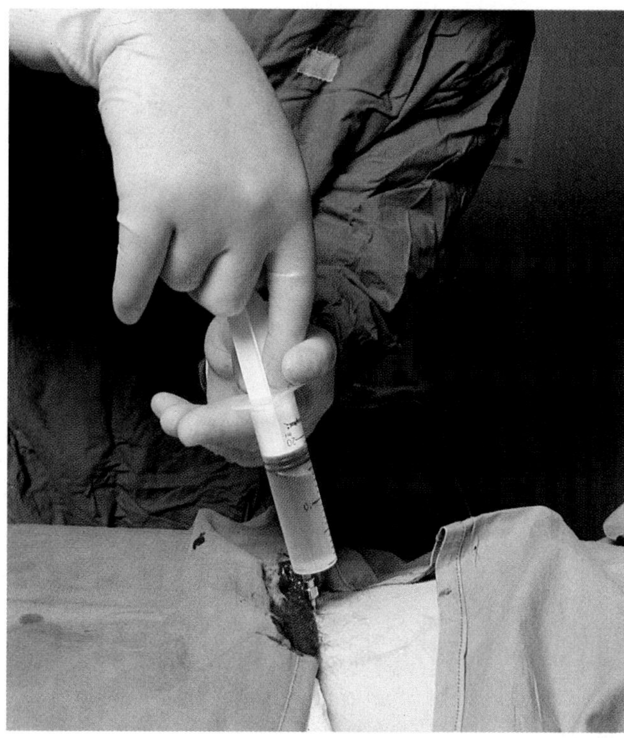

Figure 17–20 During amniocentesis, amniotic fluid is aspirated into a syringe.

The first few drops are discarded; a syringe is then attached to the needle, and the fluid is aspirated (Figure 17–20). From 15 to 20 mL of amniotic fluid are withdrawn, placed in brown-tinted test tubes (to shield the fluid from light to prevent breakdown of bilirubin and other pigments), and sent to the laboratory for analysis. The needle is withdrawn using ultrasound, and the insertion site is evaluated for streaming (movement of fluid), which would indicate bleeding into the amniotic fluid. The FHR is monitored to assess fetal well-being. If the woman's vital signs and the FHR are normal, she is allowed to leave (see Procedure 17–1).

If the collected amniotic fluid is contaminated with blood, the fluid should be centrifuged immediately. The woman is observed for alterations in the FHR. The blood should be tested to determine whether it is maternal or fetal.

Rh negative women are given Rh immune globulin after amniocentesis, provided that they are not already sensitized. If the amniotic fluid from these women is contaminated with blood, the sample should be tested to identify fetal cells. In this situation a larger dose of immune globulin is required.

NURSING CARE MANAGEMENT

The nurse assists the physician during the amniocentesis (Procedure 17–1: Assisting During Amniocentesis on page 460. See also Essential Precautions in Practice: During Amniocentesis on page 462). In addition, the nurse supports the woman undergoing amniocentesis. Women are usually apprehensive about what is about to happen as well as about the information that will be obtained by amniocentesis. The physician explains the procedure before the woman signs the consent form. As it is being performed, the woman may need additional emotional support. She may become anxious during the procedure. She may also become lightheaded, nauseated, and diaphoretic from lying on her back with a heavy uterus compressing the abdominal vessels, so it is important to have her in a lateral tilt. The nurse can provide support to the woman by further clarifying the physician's instructions or explanations, by relieving the woman's physical discomfort when possible, and by responding verbally and physically to the woman's need for reassurance.

Amniotic Fluid Tests

α-Fetoprotein (AFP) Screening

Alpha-fetoprotein (AFP) is a fetal serum protein produced in the yolk sac for the first 6 weeks of gestation and then by the fetal liver. AFP concentration in fetal plasma peaks at about 15 weeks and then declines until term as it is excreted in fetal urine and subsequently into the amniotic fluid (Kochenour, 1994). AFP is found in the amniotic fluid and maternal serum. The concentration of amniotic fluid AFP (AFAFP) parallels the rise and gradual decline of AFP in the fetal serum, but is at a lower level. Maternal serum AFP (MSAFP) rises slowly throughout pregnancy until it peaks at about the 30th week of gestation. Elevated MSAFP levels have been found in women whose fetus has an open neural tube defect (spina bifida or anencephaly), abdominal wall defect (gastroschisis or omphalocele), congenital nephrosis, cystic hygroma, incorrect gestational age (is more advanced in gestation than previously thought), fetal death, and multiple gestation (Kochenour, 1994).

The incidence of neural tube defect (NTD) is approximately 1 in 1000 to 1 in 2000 in the United States. It occurs more frequently in the east than the west and is highest in the Appalachian area (Kochenour, 1994). The incidence in other countries varies, reaching 10 in 1000 (1%) in Ireland, Wales, and the Punjab. In the United States, the recurrence risk for a family with a child with NTD is 2% to 3%; if there have been two affected children, the risk is 6.4%; and if there are three or more affected children the risk is 25% (Kochenour, 1994).

Many researchers suggest that the incidence of neural tube defects can be reduced in low-risk women with the use of folic acid prior to the beginning of pregnancy and during the first trimester. During the preconception period, the woman is advised to take folic acid, 0.4 mg orally every day while attempting pregnancy. Once pregnancy is achieved, the same dose should be continued through the first trimester (13 weeks). Women who have a previous conception with an NTD should take folic acid 4 mg orally each day for one month prior to next

PROCEDURE 17–1 ASSISTING DURING AMNIOCENTESIS

Nursing Action	*Rationale*
Objective: Prepare the woman.	
• Explain the procedure and reassure the woman.	*Explanation of the procedure decreases anxiety.*
• Ask the woman to sign a consent form.	*It is the physician's responsibility to obtain informed consent. The woman's signature indicates her awareness of risks and gives her consent to the procedure.*
Objective: Assemble the equipment.	
Prepare and arrange the following items so they are easily accessible:	
• 22-gauge spinal needle with stylet	
• 10-mL and 20-mL syringes	
• 1% xylocaine	
• Povidone-iodine (Betadine)	
• Three 10-mL test tubes with tops (amber colored or covered with tape)	*Amniotic fluid must be shielded from light to prevent breakdown of bilirubin.*
Objective: Monitor the woman's vital signs.	
Obtain baseline data on maternal BP, temperature, pulse, respirations, and FHR; then monitor every 15 minutes.	
Objective: Locate the fetus and the placenta.	
Assist with real-time ultrasound to assess needle insertion during the procedure.	*Amniocentesis is usually performed laterally in the area of fetal small parts, where pockets of amniotic fluid are often seen. Realtime ultrasound will identify fetal parts and locate pockets of amniotic fluid.*
Objective: Cleanse the woman's abdomen.	*Cleansing the woman's abdomen will decrease the incidence of infection.*
Objective: Collect the amniotic fluid specimen.	
See Essential Precautions in Practice: During Amniocentesis.	
• Obtain the test tubes from the physician.	
• Label the tubes with the correct identification and send to the lab with the appropriate lab slips.	

conception, then during the first trimester (American Academy of Pediatrics [AAP] & American College of Obstetricians [ACOG], 1997 p 67).

Amniotic fluid alpha fetoprotein (AFAFP) peak concentration occurs at about 15 weeks' gestation, and the widest margin between normal and abnormal levels occurs between 16 and 18 weeks. Because concentrations vary at different weeks of gestation, a particular level (called a cutoff level) has been established at each week of gestation. As long as the gestational age assessment is accurate, the identified cutoff level at each week in pregnancy results in an NTD detection rate of 98% and a 0.8% false-positive rate (an abnormality is thought to exist and it does not) (Kochenour, 1994). The number of false-positive results depends on the cutoff level; the higher the cutoff level, the greater the proportion of women who will be suspected of having an abnormal fetus requiring additional testing. Routine screening should be offered to all pregnant women, and the standard cutoff level is recommended as 2.5 multiples of the median (MOM) (AAP & ACOG, 1997). There is contro-

Nursing Action	*Rationale*
Objective: Monitor the woman and reassess her vital signs.	*It is important to determine if the fetus was inadvertently punctured.*
• Determine the woman's BP, pulse, respirations, and FHR.	
• Palpate the woman's fundus to assess for uterine contractions.	
• Monitor the woman with an external fetal monitor for 20–30 minutes after the amniocentesis.	
• Determine a treatment course to counteract any supine hypotension and to increase venous return and cardiac output.	
• Assess the woman's blood type and determine any need for RhoGAM.	
• Have woman lie on her left side.	
Objective: Reassure the woman, and provide self-care education.	
• Instruct the woman to report any of the following side effects to her primary caretaker: **a.** Unusual fetal hyperactivity or lack of movement **b.** Vaginal discharge—clear drainage or bleeding **c.** Uterine contractions or abdominal pain **d.** Fever or chills	*The woman will know how to recognize side effects or conditions that warrant further treatment.*
• Encourage the woman to engage in only light activity for 24 hours.	*A decrease in maternal activity will decrease uterine irritability and increase uteroplacental circulation.*
• Encourage the woman to increase her fluid intake.	*Increased hydration will replace the amniotic fluid through the uteroplacental circulation.*
Objective: Complete the client record.	*Provides a permanent record.*
• Record the type of procedure, the date and time, and the name of the physician who performed the procedure.	
• Record the maternal-fetus response, disposition of the specimen, and discharge teaching.	

versy regarding the necessity for mass screening due to expense of testing, problems related to assay and interpretation of results, the number of false-positive results, and the need for counseling. Women who may choose to be tested include those with a child with an NTD, with a strong family history of NTD, pregnant women with diabetes, and those residing in areas where NTD is prevalent.

MSAFP screening is most accurate when done between weeks 16 and 18. Using the appropriate cutoff number, 90% (AAP & ACOG, 1997) of anencephalic fetuses, 80% of open spina bifida fetuses, and approximately 5% of closed spina bifida (hydrocephalus) fetuses are detected. The levels of MSAFP vary, depending on specific maternal characteristics. Therefore, corrected levels must be established for maternal weight, race, multiple gestation, and diabetes.

Decreased levels of MSAFP have been associated with Down syndrome (Kochenour, 1994). Women at increased risk for having a baby with Down syndrome may

ESSENTIAL PRECAUTIONS IN PRACTICE

During Amniocentesis

Wear goggles or eye covering with side panels, a splash apron, and disposable gloves while assisting with an amniocentesis and handling amniotic fluid specimens. Clearly label the amniotic fluid specimen so that laboratory personnel can take appropriate precautions while handling the specimen.

REMEMBER to wash your hands before putting on the disposable gloves and AGAIN immediately after you remove the gloves.

For further information, consult OSHA and CDC guidelines.

benefit from MSAFP screening to help detect a fetus with Down syndrome.

In the search for an improved screening test for Down syndrome (trisomy 21), trisomy 18, and NTD, the *triple screen* was developed. The triple screen assesses AFP, human chorionic gonadotrophin (hCG), and unconjugated estriol (UE3), in relation to maternal age. The hCG is a glycoprotein produced by the placenta, peaking at 10 weeks' gestation. Elevated levels of hCG have been associated with Down syndrome, hydrops fetalis, and Turner syndrome. Low levels of hCG have been associated with trisomy 18 and fetal demise. UE3 is a short-acting estrogen secreted by the placenta that increases linearly with gestation. Low levels of UE3 have been associated with anencephaly, Down syndrome, trisomy 18, hydrops fetalis, Turner syndrome, and fetal demise. It is important to note that women who will be 35 or older at the time of birth should not have multiple marker testing (triple screen) "recommended as an equivalent alternative to cytogenetic diagnosis for detection of Down syndrome" (AAP & ACOG, 1997 p 79).

Evaluation of Rh-Sensitized Pregnancies

The first studies of amniotic fluid were done in the early 1950s for the evaluation of bilirubin pigment in the amniotic fluid of Rh-sensitized mothers. The analyst could determine the degree to which the fetus was affected by looking at the optical density of the fluid. Liley (1961) produced a graph that is now universally used in determining the severity of hemolytic disease in the fetus.

If a sensitized Rh negative woman produces an incompatible Rh positive fetus, antibodies cross the placenta and cause hemolytic anemia in the fetus. Concentrations of bilirubin and other breakdown products from destroyed red blood cells can be detected in amniotic fluid by spectrophotometry. By plotting their concentration or optical density at ΔOD 450 nm on a Liley curve, the physician can ascertain the degree to which the fetus is affected and the need for intervention or intrauterine transfusion (see Chapter 15).

Liley categorized the degree of hemolytic disease in three zones on the curve. If the optical density falls in zone I (low zone) at 28 to 31 weeks' gestation, the fetus will either be unaffected or have only mild hemolytic disease. Amniocentesis should be repeated in 3 or 4 weeks, although there are no reliable data to determine the optimal frequency for repeating the testing (ACOG, 1996b). When the optical density falls in zone II (midzone), amniocentesis is repeated frequently so that the trend can be determined. The age of the fetus and the trend in optical

RESEARCH IN PRACTICE

What is this study about? Nurses commonly obtain consent to perform procedures after a client has been informed about a procedure and possible consequences. Although no national standard exists in the United States regarding informed consent, accepted elements include disclosure of information, understanding, voluntary consent, and competent decision making. Health care providers may provide pregnant women with the option of screening for birth defects. After information is given and informed consent obtained, the screening tests are completed. One of the commonly offered tests is maternal serum alpha-fetoprotein (MSAFP), a serum marker used to screen for neural tube defects. Either a positive outcome (indicating possibility of spina bifida) or a positive low outcome (possibility of Down syndrome) indicates the need for further testing. Margaret Freda, Nancy DeVore, Nancy Valentine-Adams, Allan Bombard, and Irwin Merkatz designed a study to determine whether pregnant women who received information from their provider and saw a videotape about MSAFP understood enough about the test to meet the criteria for informed consent.

How was the study done? The researchers used a prospective, descriptive, exploratory design. They interviewed 53 women after showing them a videotape about MSAFP. Twelve open-ended interview questions based on the content and vocabulary of the videotape were devised by the authors. All interviews were audiotaped. Data analysis included development of frequency distributions and content analysis of the interviews.

What were the results of the study? Only two of the women answered all of the interview questions correctly, although no one answered all questions incorrectly. Seventy-four percent of the women correctly answered that birth defects or spinal problems could be revealed by the MSAFP test. The women were told in the videotape that a negative result did not mean that the baby was without problems. When asked about a negative finding, 72% gave incorrect replies ranging from stating that the baby was normal to declaring that the baby had a lot of problems. Investigators found no correlation between educational level of the patient, choice of health care provider, and number of incorrect answers.

What additional questions might I have? How did the authors determine the lack of correlation between demographic variables and answers to interview questions? No correlation table was provided in the article.

How can I use this study? As stated by the authors of this study, nurses who request informed consent need to evaluate what their clients really understand about the procedure, both for the client's benefit and for charting purposes.

SOURCE: Freda, M. C., DeVore, N., Valentine-Adams, N., Bombard, A., & Merkatz, I. R. (1998). Informed consent for maternal serum alpha-fetoprotein screening in an inner city population: How informed is it? *JOGNN, 27*(1), 99–106.

density indicate the necessity for fetal transfusion via percutaneous umbilical blood sampling (PUBS) or preterm birth. Optical densities falling in zone III (high zone) indicate that the fetus is severely affected and death is a possibility. Today fetal anemia may be directly assessed through PUBS, and red cells and platelets may be transfused directly into the fetal circulation rather than into the fetal peritoneal space as was done with intrauterine transfusion. Exact degrees of hemolysis can be determined by this method, earlier transfusion is possible, and complete reversal of hydrops fetalis has been reported after direct transfusion (Moise, 1993).

The decision about whether to initiate birth or fetal transfusion depends on the gestational age of the fetus. If the fetal lungs are not mature, packed red blood cells compatible with the mother's serum are transfused into the fetus through the umbilical artery. Fetal transfusions are repeated whenever the fetal hematocrit falls below 30%. After about 32 or 33 weeks of gestation, early birth and extrauterine treatment are probably preferred to performing fetal transfusion.

Evaluation of Fetal Maturity

In managing the woman and fetus at risk, the physician is constantly faced with the possibility of having to induce the birth of an infant prior to term and before the onset of labor. There are many indications for early termination of pregnancy, including repeat cesarean birth, premature rupture of the membranes, diabetes, hypertensive conditions in the pregnant woman, and placental insufficiency. Unfortunately, the most common cause of perinatal mortality is prematurity, especially in infants weighing 1500 g or less and with particular complications arising from pulmonary immaturity (Cunningham et al, 1997). Birth of an infant with immature pulmonary function frequently results in respiratory distress syndrome (RDS), also known as hyaline membrane disease (Chapter 28).

Because gestational age, birth weight, and the rate of development of organ systems do not necessarily correspond, it may be necessary to determine the lung maturation of the fetus by amniotic fluid analysis before elective delivery. Concentrations of certain substances in the amniotic fluid reflect the pulmonary condition of the fetus (see below). In many cases birth of the infant can be delayed until the lungs show maturity.

L/S Ratio The alveoli of the lungs are lined by a substance called **surfactant,** which is composed of phospholipids. Surfactant lowers the surface tension of the alveoli during extrauterine respiratory exhalation. By lowering the alveolar surface tension, surfactant stabilizes the alveoli, and a certain amount of air always remains in the alveoli during expiration. When a newborn with mature pulmonary function takes its first breath, a tremendously high pressure is needed to open the lungs. Upon breathing out, the lungs do not collapse, and about half the air in the alveoli is retained. An infant born too early in his or her development, when synthesis of surfactant is incomplete, is unable to maintain lung stability, resulting in underinflation of the lungs and development of RDS.

Fetal lung maturity can be assessed by determining the ratio of two components of surfactant—lecithin and sphingomyelin. Early in pregnancy the lecithin concentration in amniotic fluid is less than that of sphingomyelin (0.5:1 at 20 weeks), resulting in a low **lecithin/sphingomyelin (L/S) ratio.** At about 30 to 32 weeks' gestation, the amounts of the two substances become equal (1:1). The concentration of lecithin begins to exceed that of sphingomyelin, and at 35 weeks the L/S ratio is 2:1. When at least two times as much lecithin as sphingomyelin is found in the amniotic fluid, respiratory distress syndrome is very unlikely. Clinical outcomes in individual institutions should be correlated before this threshold for pulmonary maturity is accepted (ACOG, 1996b). Infants of diabetic mothers (IDMs) are an exception to this finding and have a high incidence of false-positive results (ie, the L/S ratio is thought to indicate lung maturity, but the baby once born develops RDS). An IDM may also have delayed lung maturation because the high blood sugars interfere with biochemical development. A delay in lung maturation has also been found in babies whose mothers have nonhypertensive renal disease and isoimmunization (ACOG, 1996b).

Some types of chronic intrauterine fetal stress cause an acceleration of lung maturation in the fetus. Prolonged rupture of membranes (over 24 hours) results in acceleration of lung maturation by approximately 1 week and therefore has a protective effect. Although the L/S ratio is the most universally used assay in evaluating pulmonary maturity, the results are not accurate when blood or meconium contaminates the amniotic fluid.

Improper handling can affect results (see discussion of amniocentesis). The L/S ratio remains a cumbersome and labor-intensive test despite numerous changes to the original technique. For this reason, many institutions are looking to other fetal lung maturity (FLM) tests that are being developed.

Phosphatidylglycerol **Phosphatidylglycerol (PG)** is the second most abundant phospholipid in surfactant. Phosphatidylglycerol appears at about 36 weeks' gestation and increases in amount until term. In instances of diabetes complicated by premature rupture of the membranes, vascular disease, or severe PIH, phosphatidylglycerol may be present before 35 weeks' gestation. PG is not measured in specific concentrations; rather, the mere presence of this substance is associated with very low risk of RDS, and the absence of PG is associated with the development of RDS.

Phosphatidylglycerol determination is also useful in blood-contaminated specimens. Because PG is not present in blood or vaginal fluids, its presence in a vaginal specimen is reliable for indicating lung maturity.

In recent years lung maturity has been most frequently assessed by a combination of L/S ratio and PG. Lung maturity apparently can be confirmed in most pregnancies if PG is present in conjunction with an L/S ratio of 2:1.

Identification of Meconium Staining

Any episode of hypoxia in utero may result in an increased fetal peristalsis, relaxation of the anal sphincter, and passage of meconium into the amniotic fluid. The amniotic fluid is normally clear, but the presence of meconium makes the fluid greenish.

Meconium staining may also be observed when amniocentesis is done. After the membranes have ruptured, meconium staining may be observed in the drainage from the vagina.

Once meconium staining is identified, more assessments must be made to determine if the fetus is suffering ongoing episodes of hypoxia.

Other Diagnostic Techniques

Chorionic Villus Sampling

Chorionic villus sampling (CVS) involves obtaining a small sample (5 to 40 mg) of chorionic villi from the edge of the developing placenta. CVS is performed in some medical centers for first trimester diagnosis of genetic, metabolic, and DNA studies. Villi in the chorion frondosum, present from 8 to 12 weeks' gestation, are believed to reflect fetal chromosome, enzyme, and DNA content, thereby permitting earlier diagnosis than can be obtained by amniocentesis. CVS cannot detect neural tube defects, however.

There is an increased risk of pregnancy loss (spontaneous abortion or miscarriage) associated with CVS. There is a higher loss rate reported with CVS than with amniocentesis. There is also an incidence of 1 in 3000 births of fetal limb reduction defects (a portion of a finger or a toe is missing), especially when the CVS is performed before 9.5 weeks' gestation. It is not recommended that CVS be performed before 10 weeks' gestation (AAP & ACOG, 1997). The woman should be aware of the risks and benefits of CVS. Because CVS makes possible an earlier diagnosis of congenital defects, first trimester (prior to 14 weeks' gestation) therapeutic abortion is an option if indicated and desired by the expectant woman or couple.

Before CVS an ultrasound is done to evaluate placental location, uterine position (retroverted or anteverted), and presence of intervening structures (ie, bowel, blood vessels). Various equipment has been used to aspirate chorionic villi from the placenta.

After counseling regarding diagnosis and procedure technique, preliminary blood work may be obtained. The morning of the procedure, the woman is asked to fill her bladder because displacement of an anteverted uterus may aid in positioning the uterus for catheter insertion. Ultrasound is used to determine uterine position, cervical position, gestational sac size, and CRL measurement and to identify the area of placental formation and cord insertion. For the transcervical CVS, the woman is then placed in lithotomy position; the vulva is cleansed with povidone-iodine solution (Betadine); and a sterile speculum is inserted into the vagina. The vaginal vault and cervix are cleansed with the same solution to decrease contamination from the vagina into the uterus. The anterior lip of the cervix is sometimes grasped with a tenaculum to aid in straightening anteflexion of the uterus. The catheter (or cannula) is slowly inserted under ultrasound guidance through the endocervix to the sampling site at the extra-amniotic placental edge (outside the gestational sac). The obturator is withdrawn from the catheter. A 30-mL syringe, containing 3 to 4 mL of tissue culture medium with heparin, is attached, and a sample of villi is aspirated by using a pressure of 20 to 30 mL (Goldberg & Golbus, 1996). The contents of the syringe are flushed into a petri dish containing nutrient medium, and the villi are inspected microscopically and prepared for cell culture.

For the transabdominal sampling, the woman is placed in the supine position. After the skin is cleansed with Betadine and local anesthesia given, an 18- or 20-gauge needle is inserted percutaneously through the maternal abdominal wall and uterine myometrium. The tip of the needle is advanced into the long axis of the chorion frondosum under ultrasound guidance. Chorionic villi are obtained by repeated, rapid aspirations of the syringe containing tissue culture medium and heparin.

Additional risks of CVS include failure to obtain tissue, rupture of membranes, leakage of amniotic fluid, bleeding, intrauterine infection, spontaneous abortion, maternal tissue contamination of the specimen, and Rh isoimmunization. Rh negative women are given $Rh_o(D)$ immune globulin to cover the risk of immunization from the procedure (Goldberg & Golbus, 1996).

Fetal karyotype, diagnosis of hemoglobinopathies (eg, sickle cell anemia and α- and some β-thalassemias), phenylketonuria, α-antitrypsin deficiency, Down syndrome, Duchenne muscular dystrophy, and factor IX deficiency can be detected by this technique. Rapid sex determination can be made so that pregnancies with a male fetus who would be affected in X-linked conditions can be identified early. Because NTDs are not diagnosed by this test, all mothers undergoing this test should be offered MSAFP screening at 15 to 20 weeks' gestation.

One of the greatest advantages to a woman undergoing this procedure is earlier diagnosis and decreased waiting time for results. Whereas amniocentesis is not done until at least 16 weeks' gestation, CVS is performed between 8 and 12 weeks. The CVS results are obtained in 24 hours if the direct preparation method is used and in 7 to 10 days when tissue culture is used. Earlier diagnosis may relieve many of the personal, social, and psychologic concerns of families, particularly if therapeutic abortion is being considered. There may be less emotional stress involved with having an abortion at an earlier stage of gestation. First trimester abortions are also easier to perform, require less time, and are less costly.

Follow-up ultrasound and lab evaluation of each pregnancy must be done after performance of this procedure to evaluate fetal status. Further neonatal follow-up studies are necessary to evaluate the long-term effects of this technique.

NURSING CARE MANAGEMENT

Before the test, the nurse ascertains the woman's understanding of the CVS, its uses, the procedure, and the possible results. The nurse provides opportunities for questions and acts as an advocate when additional questions or concerns are raised. The nurse completes assessments following the procedure.

The nurse plays an important supportive role in helping the woman or couple express any feelings and fears regarding the procedure and also regarding the decision-making process if abortion is being considered. That supportive role continues if abortion is chosen, even though the nurse may not be present for the procedure. It is important that support be provided following the procedure by the nurse who established a relationship with the couple previously.

Fetoscopy

Fetoscopy is a procedure for directly observing the fetus and obtaining a sample of blood or skin. It enables the physician to diagnose such conditions as fetal hemoglobinopathies, immunodeficient diseases, coagulation and metabolic disorders, chromosome abnormalities, Rh isoimmunization, and serious skin defects (Quintero et al, 1994b).

Prior to fetoscopy, women at risk for abnormalities are counseled by the genetic team. Indications, risks, and limitations of the procedure are thoroughly explained, and a consent form is signed for the procedure, which may be done from 11 to 36 weeks' gestation.

Ultrasound is performed prior to and during fetoscopy to determine the gestational age, fetal position, placental location and thickness, location of umbilical cord insertion into the placenta, location of pockets of amniotic fluid, position of the part of the fetus or tissue to be viewed or sampled, and placement of the cannula (Quintero et al, 1994b). Following rapid intravenous sedation of the woman to decrease fetal activity, the abdomen is cleansed with povidone-iodine solution (Betadine), a local anesthetic solution may be injected into the maternal abdomen, and a 0.5 cm incision is made through the abdomen to the peritoneum.

A cannula containing a trochar is inserted through the incision into the uterus and the amniotic cavity to the site previously determined by ultrasound. The trochar is removed, and amniotic fluid is withdrawn for genetic cell analysis and AFP level. A light source is connected to a 15 cm fiber-optic endoscope, which is about the diameter of a 16-gauge needle, and introduced through the cannula to visualize the fetus on a video monitor. Custom-designed miniature (2 mm diameter) surgical instruments have been developed and are used in this procedure. A technique for rapid amniotic fluid exchange with lactated ringers keeps the amniotic fluid pressure change at a minimum through constant monitoring. Simultaneous display of ultrasound and fetoscopic images on a single monitor through a video mixer is helpful (Quintero, Reich, Parder et al, 1994b).

If fetal blood sampling is to be performed, a 26- to 27-gauge needle is inserted through the side channel of the cannula and advanced until the vessel in the umbilical cord is pierced and a sample of blood is obtained.

The numerous indications for fetal blood sampling include suspicion of problems with hemoglobin or coagulation factors and need to assess for rubella, toxoplasmosis, and cytomegalovirus. In those facilities where percutaneous umbilical blood sampling is performed, fetoscopy is rarely performed for these purposes. During fetoscopy blood samples can be taken from vessels in that portion of the cord that is a few centimeters from the placental insertion site. This is usually difficult, however, so a sample (approximately 0.5 mL) is collected from blood that leaks into the amniotic cavity after the needle is withdrawn from the vessel. Because blood aspirated by this method is mixed with amniotic fluid and diagnosis of various inherited diseases requires a pure fetal blood sample, in questionable situations blood is aspirated from a cord vessel at the placental insertion site.

Mother and fetus are monitored for several hours following the procedure for alterations in blood pressure and pulse, FHR abnormalities, uterine activity, vaginal bleeding, and loss of amniotic fluid. The woman is hospitalized until caregivers are sure that no immediate complications have arisen. Rh negative mothers are given Rh_o(D) immune globulin unless the fetal blood is found to be Rh negative; antibiotics and tocolytics may or may not be given prophylactically. The following day, prior to discharge, a repeat ultrasound is performed to confirm the adequacy of amniotic fluid and fetal viability. Women are advised to avoid strenuous activity for 1 to 2 weeks following fetoscopy and to report any pain, bleeding, leakage of amniotic fluid, or fever.

Although amniocentesis permits the prenatal diagnosis of many sex-linked diseases, chromosome defects, and metabolic disturbances, the majority of fetal cells obtained by this procedure are not found to be viable, and culture is difficult and lengthy. Furthermore, many severe congenital abnormalities may be diagnosed only by direct visualization of the fetus or by analyzing fetal blood or skin tissue. Fetoscopy has been used to view the extremities, spine, genitals, and face in situations where the fetus is at risk for development of external abnormalities—such as limb and digital deformities, cleft lip and palate, and hereditary skin disorders—or genetic diseases affecting these structures.

As amniocentesis, ultrasound, and percutaneous umbilical blood sampling techniques become more sophisticated and conclusive for diagnosis of fetal conditions and more widely used, the need for fetoscopy is decreasing except in unusual situations, such as tissue biopsy for diagnosis of genetic skin disorders not detectable by biochemical means, or as a backup measure when other procedures are inadequate.

NURSING CARE MANAGEMENT

The nurse clarifies the woman's understanding of fetoscopy, providing time for questions and acting as an advocate when additional areas of concern arise. Following the test, the nurse completes assessments and continues to provide support.

Percutaneous Umbilical Blood Sampling

Percutaneous umbilical blood sampling (PUBS) (also called cordocentesis) is a technique used to obtain pure fetal blood from the umbilical cord while the fetus is in utero. This procedure has been used for diagnosis of hemophilias, hemoglobinopathies, fetal infections, chromosome abnormalities, nonimmune hydrops, isoimmune hemolytic disorders, and assessment of fetal hemoglobin and hematocrit for calculation of transfusion requirements in the second and third trimesters (Hobbins, 1996).

The indications for fetal blood sampling include the following:

- Rapid fetal karyotyping
- Diagnosis of fetal infection (CMV, toxoplasmosis, parvovirus, rubella)
- Platelet disorders
- Fetal blood grouping
- Diagnosis and treatment of isoimmunization
- Assessment of fetal well-being (pH, PO_2)
- Fetal metabolic disorders

The woman is scanned with a linear-array ultrasound transducer with sterile probe cover, and a 25-gauge spinal needle is inserted into her abdomen through the skin alongside the transducer and into the fetal umbilical vein approximately 1 to 2 cm from the insertion of the cord into the placenta. The stylet is removed from the needle, and fetal blood is aspirated into a syringe containing an anticoagulant. Red blood cell size is determined to distinguish fetal from maternal cells. A paralytic agent, such as pancuronium bromide (Pavulon), may be given to prevent fetal movement during the procedure. If the mother is given a medication to help her relax, care must be given to not oversedate the mother and cause deep breathing. This deep chest/diaphragm movement can interfere with accurate puncture of the umbilical vein.

Within the last 10 years, the improvements in ultrasonographic technique have made PUBS a relatively safe procedure with overall fetal loss rate less than 2%. The complication rate after PUBS is less than 0.5%. Complications include failure to obtain a sample, bleeding from the sampling site, premature rupture of membranes, chorioamnionitis, and fetal bradycardia (Hobbins, 1996).

Caution should, however, be exercised in the decision to use PUBS. Queenan's (1996) development of a chart of spectrophotometric measurements from sensitized pregnancies in middle trimester may reduce the need for PUBS. Advent of the polymerase chain reaction test to ascertain fetal blood type reduces the need for a direct fetal sample (ACOG, 1996).

NURSING CARE MANAGEMENT

The nurse plays an important role in helping women for which PUBS is recommended. Although a genetic counselor explains the risks for genetic defects and chromosome disorders, women and their partners need to be helped to understand the procedure and its risks. They may need anticipatory guidance to help lessen their anxiety, as well as emotional support during the procedure and follow-up evaluation and testing. The nurse may need to assist with coordination of financial and social service resources. The nurse can help promote relaxation during the procedure by instructing the woman in breathing techniques. The nurse completes assessments during and immediately following the procedure and in some cases performs the NST following the procedure.

Magnetic Resonance Imaging (MRI)

Magnetic resonance imaging (MRI) may occasionally be used in the maternal-child area. MRI offers several advantages. It reveals previously inaccessible areas of the body without invasive techniques or risk of ionizing radiation. In addition, MRI can accurately distinguish between normal and impaired or diseased tissue and between fetal and maternal anatomy. Also, MRI could be useful in diagnosing and evaluating the fetal central nervous system and fetal growth restriction. It is also useful in evaluating maternal pelvic masses during pregnancy. Although there are no known adverse effects of MRI during pregnancy, the National Radiological Protection Board advises MRI use only in the second and third trimesters (ACOG, 1995).

Psychologic Reactions to Diagnostic Testing

Little is written regarding the impact of antepartum diagnostic testing on women's anxiety levels; however, the need for testing usually provokes fear.

Ultrasound use during pregnancy has become almost routine, and many women view this antepartum test as an expected part of the prenatal care. They approach the ultrasound with anticipation because it may provide confirmation of the pregnancy through visualization of the fetus with heartbeat, may even identify the sex of the fetus, and promotes psychological preparation for attachment after birth (Colucciello, 1998). However, when more invasive testing is recommended, it may evoke fear and anxiety in the woman and her partner as they consider the reason for the test, the risk to the fetus and woman during the test, and the implications of the test results.

One study (Campbell et al, 1982) noted that being able to see the fetus early in the pregnancy through the use of ultrasound led to more positive attitudes toward the ultrasound procedure and decreased feelings of stress related to the ultrasound. The women who were able to view their fetus on the monitor screen displayed more positive health behavior changes after the ultrasound than those women who were not allowed to view the fetus when the ultrasound was performed. Reading and Platt (1985) studied the reactions of women who had ultrasound examinations for decreased fetal movement. All women approached the ultrasound with anxiety; however, the women who were allowed to view their fetus on the ultrasound screen had a reduction in their anxiety level over other women in the study who were given only verbal communication that their fetus was "okay." This study confirmed that prenatal testing does influence anxiety level (Reading & Platt, 1985) and provides information for caregivers regarding the importance of the test for the woman. The findings also emphasize the importance of providing visual feedback during ultrasound examinations.

FOCUS YOUR STUDY

- Ultrasound offers a valuable means of assessing intrauterine fetal growth because the growth can be followed over a period of time. It is noninvasive and painless, allows the physician to study the gestation serially, is nonradiating to both the woman and her fetus, and to date has no known harmful effects.
- Using ultrasound, the gestational sac may be detected as early as 5 or 6 weeks after the LMP. Measurement of the CRL in early pregnancy is most useful for accurate dating of a pregnancy. The most important and frequently used ultrasound measurements are BPD, HC, AC, and femur length.
- A fetal biophysical profile (BPP) includes five fetal variables (breathing movement, body movement, tone, amniotic fluid volume, and FHR reactivity). It assesses the fetus at risk for intrauterine compromise.
- Maternal assessment of fetal activity is very useful as a screening procedure in evaluation of fetal status.
- A nonstress test (NST) measures fetal heart rate during fetal activity; FHR normally increases in response to fetal activity. The desired result is a reactive test.
- A contraction stress test (CST) provides a method for observing the response of the fetal heart rate to the stress of uterine contractions. The desired result is a negative test.
- Amniocentesis can be used to obtain amniotic fluid for testing. A variety of tests is available to evaluate the presence of disease, genetic conditions, and fetal maturity.
- The L/S ratio of the amniotic fluid can be used to assess fetal lung maturity. The presence of PG may also provide information about fetal lung maturity.
- Chorionic villus sampling is a procedure that obtains fetal karyotyping in the first trimester.
- Fetoscopy is a procedure for observing the fetus directly and obtaining a sample of blood or skin.
- Percutaneous umbilical blood sampling (PUBS) is a technique used in the second and third trimesters for fetal diagnosis, assessment, and therapy.
- Triple screening of AFP, hCG, and estriol in maternal serum provides information about the possibility of open neural tube defects and chromosome abnormalities (trisomy 13, 18, or 21) in the fetus.
- Magnetic resonance imaging (MRI) can be used to assess previously inaccessible areas of the body via a noninvasive process without the risk of ionizing radiation. This procedure can accurately distinguish between normal and impaired or diseased tissues and between fetal and maternal anatomy and pathology.

REFERENCES

American Academy of Pediatrics (AAP) & American College of Obstetricians and Gynecologists (ACOG). (1997). *Guidelines for perinatal care* (4th ed.). Elk Grove Village, IL: Author.

American College of Obstetricians and Gynecologists (ACOG). (1994, Jan.). *Antepartum fetal surveillance.* (Technical Bulletin No. 142). Washington, DC: Author.

American College of Obstetricians and Gynecologists (ACOG). (1995, Sept.). *Guidelines for diagnostic imaging during pregnancy.* (Committee Opinion No. 158). Washington, DC: Author.

American College of Obstetricians and Gynecologists (ACOG). (1996a, Aug.). *Management of isoimmunization in pregnancy.* (ACOG Educational Bulletin No. 227). Washington, DC: Author.

American College of Obstetricians and Gynecologists (ACOG). (1996b, Nov.). *Assessment of fetal lung maturity.* (ACOG Educational Bulletin No. 230). Washington, DC: Author.

American College of Obstetricians and Gynecologists, (ACOG) Committee on Obstetric Practice. (1997, October). *Utility of antepartum umbilical artery Doppler velocimetry in intrauterine growth restriction.* (Committee Opinion No. 188.). Washington, DC: Author.

Arduini, D., Rizzo, G., & Romanini, C. (1992). Changes of pulsatility index from fetal vessels preceding the onset of late decelerations in growth-retarded fetuses. *Obstetrics and Gynecology, 79*, 605.

Association of Women's Health, Obstetrical and Neonatal Nurses (AWHONN). (1993). *Nursing practice competencies and educational guidelines for limited ultrasound examinations in obstetric and gynecologic/infertility settings.*

Association of Women's Health, Obstetrical and Neonatal Nurses (AWHONN). (1997). *Fetal heart monitoring principles and practices* (2nd ed.). Davenport, IA: Kindall/Hunt.

Battaglia, C., Artini, P. G., D'Ambrogio, G. et al. (1992). Maternal hyperoxygenation in the treatment of intrauterine growth retardation. *American Journal of Obstetrics and Gynecology 167*, 430.

Bonnin, P. H. et al. (1992). Relationship between umbilical and fetal cerebral blood flow velocity waveforms and umbilical venous blood gases. *Ultrasound in Obstetrics and Gynecology, 18*(2), 18.

Callen, P. W. (1994). *Ultrasonography in obstetrics and gynecology* (3rd ed.). Philadelphia: Saunders.

Campbell, S. et al. (1982). Ultrasound scanning in pregnancy: The short term psychological effects of early realtime scans. *Journal of Psychosomatic Obstetrics and Gynaecology, 1*, 57.

Chang, T. C., Robson, J. C., Spencer, J. A., et al. (1993). Identification of fetal growth retardation: Comparison of Doppler waveform indices and serial ultrasound measurements of abdominal circumference and fetal weight. *Obstetrics and Gynecology, 82*(2), 230.

Chervenak, F. A., & Gabbe, S. G. (1996). Obstetric ultrasound: Assessment of fetal growth and anatomy. In S. G. Gabbe, J. R. Niebyl, & J. L. Simpson (Eds.), *Obstetrics: Normal and problem pregnancies* (3rd ed.) (pp 279–326). New York: Churchill Livingstone.

Colucciello, M. L. (1998). Pregnant adolescents' perceptions of their babies: Before and after realtime ultrasound. *Journal of Psychosocial Nursing, 36*, 12–19.

Copel, J. A., & Kleinman, C. S. (1996). Fetal echocardiography. In J. T. Queenan & J. C. Hobbins (Eds.), *Protocols for high-risk pregnancies* (4th ed.) (pp 100–106). Cambridge, MA: Blackwell.

Cunningham, T. G., MacDonald, P. C., Gant, N. F., Leveno, K. J., Gilstrap, L. C., Hankins, G. D. V., & Clark, S. L. (1997a). Antepartum assessment. In *Williams obstetrics* (20th ed.). (Chapter 43, pp 1009–1022). Stamford, CT: Appleton & Lange.

Cunningham, T. G., MacDonald, P. C., Gant, N. F., Leveno, K. J., Gilstrap, L. C., Hankins, G. D. V., & Clark, S. L. (1997b). Diseases and abnormalities of the fetal membranes. In *Williams obstetrics* (20th ed.). (Chapter 29, pp 657–667). Stamford, CT: Appleton & Lange.

Druzin, M. L., & Gabbe S. G. (1996). Antepartum fetal evaluation. In S. G. Gabbe, J. R. Neibyl, & J. L. Simpson (Eds.), *Obstetrics: Normal and problem pregnancies* (3rd ed.) (pp 327–367). New York: Churchill Livingstone.

Faranoff, A. A., & Martin, R. J. (1992). *Neonatal-perinatal medicine.* St Louis, MO: Mosby-Year Book.

Goldberg, J. D., & Golbus, M. S. (1996). Chorionic villus sampling. In J. T. Queenan & J. C. Hobbins (Eds.), *Protocols for high-risk pregnancies* (4th ed.) (pp 115–119). Cambridge, MA: Blackwell.

Grannum, P. A.T., Berkowitz, R. I., & Hobbins, J. C. (1979). The ultrasonic changes in the maturing placenta and their relation to fetal pulmonic maturity. *American Journal of Obstetrics and Gynecology, 133*, 915.

Hadlock, F. P. (1990, April 9–12). Ultrasound: Content of the basic U/S examination. *Tenth International Symposium on Perinatal Medicine and Obstetrical Ultrasound.* Las Vegas, NV.

Hobbins, J. C. (1996). Fetal blood sampling. In J. T. Queenan & J. C. Hobbins (Eds.). *Protocols for high-risk pregnancies* (4th ed.) (pp 128–132). Cambridge, MA: Blackwell.

Huffman, C., & Sandelowski, M. (1997). The nurse-technology relationship: The case of ultrasonography. *Journal of Obstetric Gynecologic, Neonatal Nurses, 26*, 673–682.

Kendig, S., & Barron, M. L. (1996). Antenatal care and risk assessment. In K. R. Simpson & P. A. Creehan (Eds.), *AWHONN: Perinatal nursing* (pp 73–107). Philadelphia: Lippincott.

Kochenour, N. K. (1994). Normal pregnancy and prenatal care. In J. R. Scott, P. J. DiSaia, C. B. Hammond, & W. N. Spellacy (Eds.), *Danforth's obstetrics and gynecology* (7th ed.). Philadelphia: Lippincott.

Lagrew, D. C. (1995). The contraction stress test. *Clinical Obstetrics and Gynecology, 38*(1), 11–25.

Liley, A. W. (1961). Liquor amnii analysis in the management of the pregnancy complicated by rhesus sensitization. *American Journal of Obstetrics and Gynecology, 32*, 1359.

Manning, F. A. (1990, April 9–12). The biophysical profile: Contemporary use. *Tenth International Symposium on Perinatal Medicine and Obstetrical Ultrasound.* Las Vegas, NV.

Manning, F. A. (1995). Dynamic ultrasound-based fetal assessment: The fetal biophysical profile score. *Clinical Obstetrics and Gynecology, 38*(1), 26.

Manning, F. A., & Hohler, C. (1991). Intrauterine growth retardation: Diagnosis, prognostication, and management based on ultrasound methods. In A. C. Fleisher et al (Eds.), *The Principles and Practices of Ultrasonography in Obstetrics and Gynecology* (4th ed.). Norwalk, CT: Appleton & Lange.

Manning, F. A., Snijdeis, R., Harman, C. R., Nicholas, K., Menticoglov, S., Morrison, I. (1993). Fetal biophysical profile score 6: Correlation with antepartum umbilical venous pH. *American Journal of Obstetrics and Gynecology, 169*, 775.

Moise, K. (1993). Intrauterine transfusion with red cells and platelets. *Fetal Medicine, 159*, 318.

Moore, T. R. (1995). Assessment of amniotic fluid volume in at-risk pregnancies. *Clinical Obstetrics and Gynecology, 38*(1), 78.

Pardi, G., Ceten, I., Marconi, A. M. et al. (1993). Diagnostic value of blood sampling in fetuses with growth retardation. *New England Journal of Medicine, 328*(10), 692.

Paul, R. H., & Miller, D. A. (1995). Non-stress test. *Clinical Obstetrics and Gynecology, 38*(1), 3–10.

Platt, L. D., & Walla, C. A. (1996). Fetal biophysical profile. In J. T. Queenan & J. C. Hobbins (Eds.), *Protocols for high-risk pregnancies* (4th ed.) (pp 107–112). Cambridge, MA: Blackwell.

Queenan, J. T. (1996). Rh and other blood group immunizations. In J. T. Queenan & J. C. Hobbins (Eds.), *Protocols for high-risk pregnancies* (4th ed.) (pp 523–534). Cambridge, MA: Blackwell.

Queenan, J. T., Tomai, T. P., Ural, S. H., & King, J. C. (1993). Deviation in amniotic fluid optical density at a wavelength of 450 mm in Rh-immunized pregnancies from 14–40 weeks gestation: A proposal for clinical management. *American Journal of Obstetrics and Gynecology, 168*, 1370–1376.

Quintero, R. A., Reich, H., & Miller, D. A. (1994a). Transabdominal thin-gauge embryofetoscopy in continuing pregnancies. *American Journal of Obstetrics and Gynecology, 170*(1), part 2. (SPO Abstract No. 73).

Quintero, R. A., Reich, H., Parder, et al. (1994b). Operative fetoscopy: A new frontier in fetal medicine. *American Journal of Obstetrics and Gynecology, 170*(1), part 2. (SPO Abstract No. 76).

Reading, A. E., & Platt, L. D. (1985). Impact of fetal testing on maternal anxiety. *Journal of Reproductive Medicine, 30*, 907.

Reed, K. L. (1990, April 9–12). Ultrasound: Doppler flow—where does it fit in? *Tenth International Symposium on Perinatal Medicine and Obstetrical Ultrasound.* Las Vegas, NV.

Reed, K. L. (1994). Ultrasound during pregnancy. In J. R. Scott, P. J. DiSaia, C. B. Hammond, & W. N. Spellacy (Eds.), *Danforth's obstetrics and gynecology* (7th ed.). Philadelphia: Lippincott.

Reed, K. L. (1996). Clinical use of Doppler. In J. T. Queenan & J. C. Hobbins (Eds.), *Protocols for high-risk pregnancies* (4th ed.) (pp 92–99). Cambridge, MA: Blackwell.

Richardson, B. S., & Gagnon, R. (1999). Fetal breathing and body movements. In R. K. Creasy, & R. Resnik (Eds.), *Maternal-fetal medicine.* (4th ed.) (pp 231–247). Philadelphia: Saunders.

Simpson, K. R., & Creehan, P. A. (Eds.) (1996). *AWHONN: Perinatal nursing.* Philadelphia: Lippincott.

Soffici, A. R., & Eden, R. D. (1994). Assessment of fetal well-being. In J. R. Scott, P. J. DiSaia, C. B. Hammond, & W. N. Spellacy (Eds.), *Danforth's obstetrics and gynecology* (7th ed.). Philadelphia: Lippincott.

Trudinger, B., (1999) Doppler ultrasound assessment of blood flow. In R. K. Creasy & R. Resnik (Eds.), *Maternal-fetal medicine.* (4th ed.) (pp 216–229). Philadelphia: Saunders.

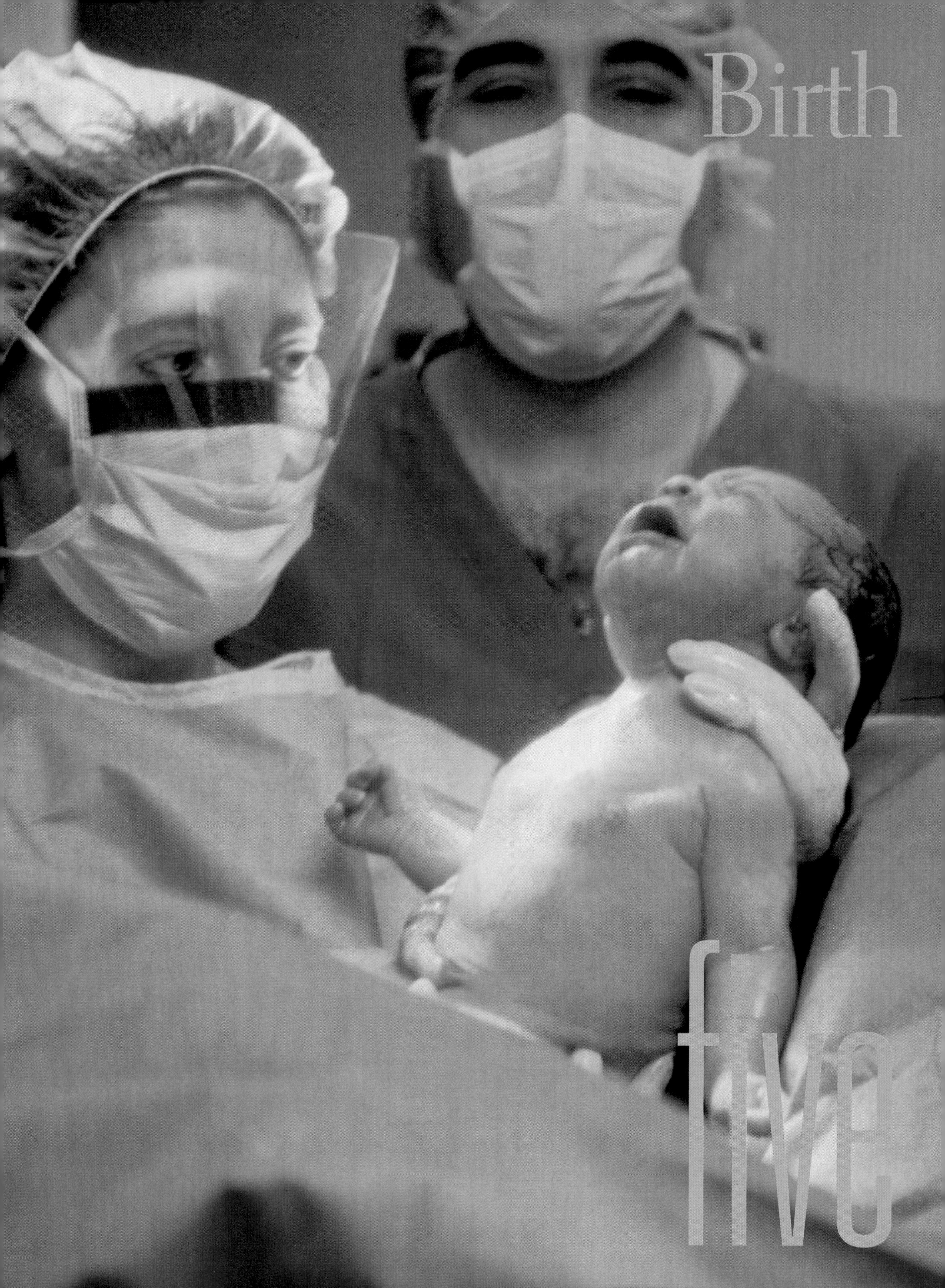
Birth
five

18

Processes and Stages of Labor and Birth

Key Terms

Artificial rupture of membranes (AROM)
Bloody show
Cardinal movements
Cervical dilatation
Crowning
Duration
Effacement
Engagement
Fetal attitude
Fetal lie
Fetal position
Fetal presentation
Fontanelles
Frequency
Intensity
Lightening
Malpositions
Malpresentations
Molding
Presenting part
Spontaneous rupture of membranes (SROM)
Station
Sutures

BIRTH USUALLY FEELS LIKE A STEAMY KITCHEN— similar to holiday preparations, except that the smells are different. The smell of sweat is more acrid, there are some fetid odors, there is the smell and steam rising from blood. The air is thick, pungent, fertile. It is hard not to be reminded of fresh straw and night stars. There is near and heady promise.

~ *A Midwife's Story* ~

Objectives

- Examine four critical factors that influence labor.
- Describe the physiology of labor.
- Discuss premonitory signs of labor.
- Differentiate between false and true labor.
- Describe the physiologic and psychologic changes occurring in each of the phases and stages of labor.
- Summarize maternal systemic responses to labor.
- Discuss fetal responses to labor.

DURING THE WEEKS OF GESTATION the fetus and the expectant woman prepare themselves for birth. The fetus progresses through various stages of growth and development in readiness for the independence of extrauterine life. The expectant woman undergoes various physiologic and psychologic adaptations during pregnancy that gradually prepare her for childbirth and the role of mother. The onset of labor marks a significant change in the relationship between the woman and the fetus.

Critical Factors in Labor

Four factors are important in the process of labor and birth: the birth passage, the fetus, the primary forces of labor, and the woman's psychosocial considerations. Within these areas the following aspects are significant:

1. Birth passage
   a. Size of the maternal pelvis (diameters of the pelvic inlet, midpelvis, and outlet)
   b. Type of maternal pelvis (gynecoid, android, anthropoid, platypelloid, or a combination)
   c. Ability of the cervix to dilate and efface and ability of the vaginal canal and the external opening of the vagina (the *introitus*) to distend
2. Fetus
   a. Fetal head (size and presence of molding)
   b. Fetal attitude (flexion or extension of the fetal body and extremities)
   c. Fetal lie
   d. Fetal presentation (the body part of the fetus entering the pelvis in a single or multiple pregnancy)
   e. Fetal position (relationship of the presenting part to one of the four quadrants of the maternal pelvis)
   f. Placenta (implantation site)
3. Primary forces of labor
   a. Frequency, duration, and intensity of uterine contractions as the fetus moves through the passage
   b. Effectiveness of the maternal pushing effort
   c. Duration of labor
4. Psychosocial considerations
   a. Physical preparation for childbirth
   b. Sociocultural heritage
   c. Previous childbirth experience
   d. Support from significant others
   e. Emotional status

The progress of labor is critically dependent on the complementary relationship of these four factors. Abnormalities in the birth passage, the fetus, the forces of labor, or the psychosocial status of the woman can alter the outcome of labor and jeopardize both the pregnant woman and her fetus. Complications during labor and birth are discussed in Chapter 22.

The Birth Passage

The true pelvis, which forms the bony canal through which the fetus must pass, is divided into three sections: the inlet, the pelvic cavity (midpelvis), and the outlet. (See Chapter 6 for a discussion of each part of the pelvis and Chapter 11 for techniques to assess the pelvis.)

The four classic types of pelvis are gynecoid, android, anthropoid, and platypelloid. Implications of each type for childbirth are described in Table 18–1.

TABLE 18–1 Implications of Pelvic Type for Labor and Birth

Pelvic Type	Pertinent Characteristics	Implications for Birth
Gynecoid	Inlet rounded with all inlet diameters adequate Midpelvis diameters adequate with parallel side walls Outlet adequate	Favorable for vaginal birth
Android	Inlet heart-shaped with short posterior sagittal diameter Midpelvis diameters reduced Outlet capacity reduced	Not favorable for vaginal birth Descent into pelvis is slow Fetal head enters pelvis in transverse or posterior position with arrest of labor frequent
Anthropoid	Inlet oval in shape, with long anteroposterior diameter Midpelvis diameters adequate Outlet adequate	Favorable for vaginal birth
Platypelloid	Inlet oval in shape, with long transverse diameters Midpelvis diameters reduced Outlet capacity inadequate	Not favorable for vaginal birth Fetal head engages in transverse position Difficult descent through midpelvis Frequent delay of progress at outlet of pelvis

NOTE: Description of pelvic shape is exaggerated for easier comprehension.

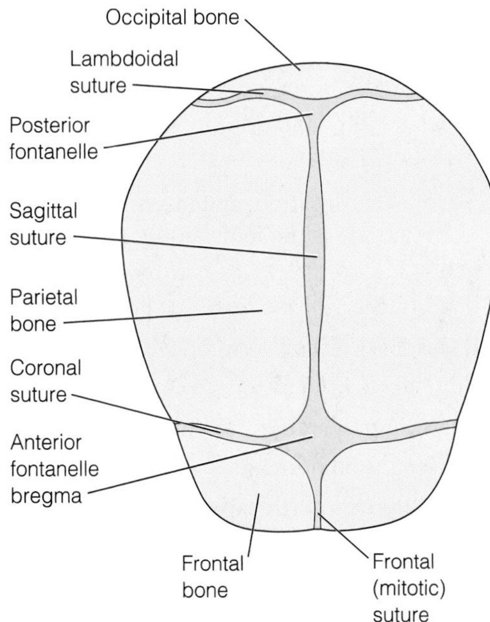

FIGURE 18–1 Superior view of the fetal skull.

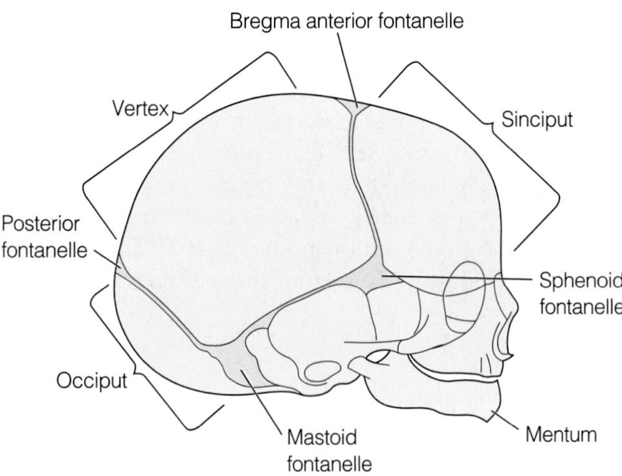

FIGURE 18–2 Lateral view of the fetal skull identifying the landmarks that have significance during birth.

The Fetus

Fetal Head

The fetal head is composed of bony parts, which can either hinder childbirth or make it easier. Once the head (the least compressible and largest part of the fetus) has been born, the birth of the rest of the body is rarely delayed.

The fetal skull has three major parts: the face, the base of the skull (cranium), and the vault of the cranium (roof). The bones of the face and cranial base are well fused and essentially fixed. The base of the cranium is composed of the two temporal bones, each with a sphenoid and ethmoid bone. The bones composing the vault are the two frontal bones, the two parietal bones, and the occipital bone (Figure 18–1). These bones are not fused, allowing this portion of the head to adjust in shape as the presenting part passes through the narrow portions of the pelvis. The cranial bones overlap under pressure of the powers of labor and the demands of the unyielding pelvis. This overlapping is called **molding.**

The **sutures** of the fetal skull are membranous spaces between the cranial bones. The intersections of the cranial sutures are called **fontanelles.** These sutures allow for molding of the fetal head and help the clinician identify the position of the fetal head during vaginal examination. The important sutures of the cranial vault are as follows (Figure 18–1).

- *Frontal (mitotic) suture:* Located between the two frontal bones; becomes the anterior continuation of the sagittal suture
- *Sagittal suture:* Located between the parietal bones; divides the skull into left and right halves; runs anteroposteriorly, connecting the two fontanelles
- *Coronal sutures:* Located between the frontal and parietal bones; extend transversely left and right from the anterior fontanelle
- *Lambdoidal suture:* Located between the two parietal bones and the occipital bone; extends transversely left and right from the posterior fontanelle

The anterior and posterior fontanelles are clinically useful in identifying the position of the fetal head in the pelvis and in assessing the status of the newborn after birth. The anterior fontanelle is diamond-shaped and measures 2 × 3 cm. It permits growth of the brain by remaining unossified for as long as 18 months. The posterior fontanelle is much smaller and closes within 8 to 12 weeks after birth. It is shaped like a small triangle and marks the meeting point of the sagittal suture and the lambdoidal suture.

Following are several important landmarks of the fetal skull (Figure 18–2):

- *Mentum:* The fetal chin
- *Sinciput:* The anterior area known as the brow
- *Bregma:* The large diamond-shaped anterior fontanelle
- *Vertex:* The area between the anterior and posterior fontanelles
- *Posterior fontanelle:* The intersection between posterior cranial sutures
- *Occiput:* The area of the fetal skull occupied by the occipital bone, beneath the posterior fontanelle

The diameters of the fetal skull vary considerably within normal limits. Some diameters shorten and others lengthen as the head is molded during labor. Fetal head diameters are measured between the various landmarks on the skull (Figure 18–3). For example, the suboccipitobregmatic diameter is the distance from the undersurface

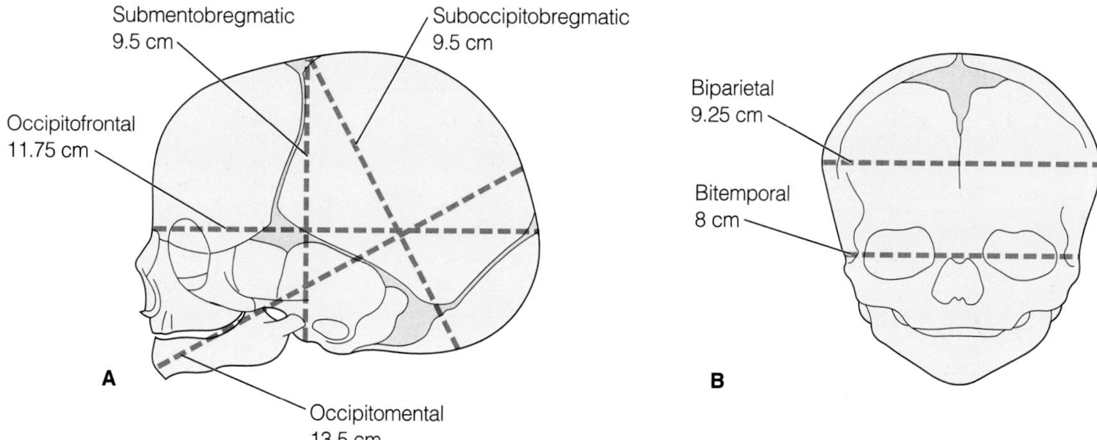

FIGURE 18–3 ***A,*** Anteroposterior diameters of the fetal skull. When the vertex of the fetus presents and the fetal head is flexed with the chin on the chest, the smallest anteroposterior diameter (suboccipitobregmatic) enters the birth canal. ***B,*** Transverse diameters of the fetal skull.

of the occiput to the center of the bregma, or anterior fontanelle. Fetal skull measurements are given in Figure 18–3.

Fetal Attitude

Fetal attitude refers to the relation of the fetal parts to one another. The normal attitude of the fetus is one of moderate flexion of the head, flexion of the arms onto the chest, and flexion of the legs onto the abdomen.

Changes in fetal attitude, particularly in the position of the head, cause the fetus to present larger diameters of the fetal head to the maternal pelvis. These deviations from a normal fetal attitude often contribute to difficult labor (Figure 18–4).

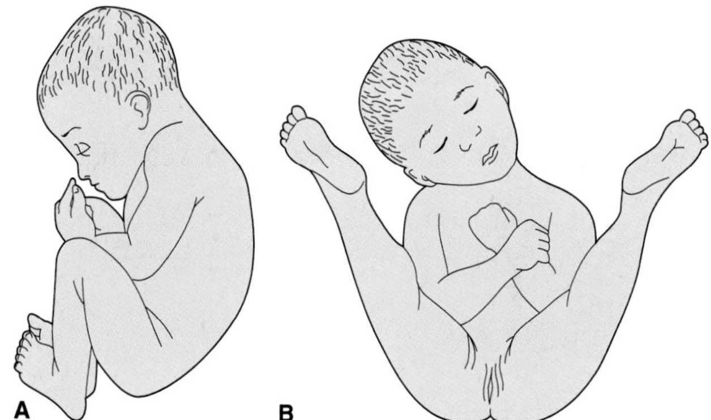

FIGURE 18–4 Fetal attitude. ***A,*** The attitude (or relationship of body parts) of this fetus is normal. The head is flexed forward with the chin almost resting on the chest. The arms and legs are flexed. ***B,*** In this view, the head is tilted to the right. Although the arms are flexed, the legs are extended.

Fetal Lie

Fetal lie refers to the relationship of the cephalocaudal axis (spinal column) of the fetus to the cephalocaudal axis of the woman. The fetus may assume either a longitudinal or a transverse lie. A *longitudinal lie* occurs when the cephalocaudal axis of the fetus is parallel to the woman's spine. A *transverse lie* occurs when the cephalocaudal axis of the fetal spine is at right angles to the woman's spine.

Fetal Presentation

Fetal presentation is determined by fetal lie and by the body part of the fetus that enters the maternal pelvis first. This portion of the fetus is referred to as the **presenting part.** Fetal presentation may be cephalic, breech, or shoulder (Table 18–2).

The most common presentation is cephalic. When this presentation occurs, labor and birth are more likely to proceed normally. Breech and shoulder presentations are associated with difficulties during labor and do not proceed as normal; therefore they are called **malpresentations.** (See Chapter 22 for discussion of malpresentations.)

Cephalic Presentation The fetal head presents to the birth passage in approximately 97% of term births. The cephalic presentation can be further classified according to the degree of flexion or extension of the fetal head (attitude).

Vertex Presentation

- Vertex is the most common type of presentation.
- The fetal head is completely flexed onto the chest.
- The smallest diameter of the fetal head (suboccipitobregmatic) presents to the maternal pelvis (Figure 18–5, *A*).
- The occiput is the presenting part.

TABLE 18–2 Relationship of Fetus to Maternal Pelvis

Presentation	Attitude	Presenting Part	Landmark
Longitudinal lie (99.5%)			
Cephalic (96% to 97%)	Flexion of fetal head onto chest	Vertex (posterior part—occiput)	Occiput (O)
	Military (no flexion, no extension)	Vertex (median part)	Occiput (O)
	Partial extension	Brow	Forehead (frontum) (Fr)
	Complete extension of the head	Face	Chin (mentum) (M)
Breech (3% to 4%)			
Complete	Flexed hips and knees	Buttocks	Sacrum (S)
Frank	Flexed hips, extended knees with legs against abdomen and chest	Buttocks	Sacrum (S)
Footling: single, double	Extended hips and at least one knee extended with foot in cervical canal	Feet (one or two)	Sacrum (S)
Kneeling: single, double	Extended hips, flexed knees	Knees	Sacrum (S)
Transverse or oblique lie (0.5%)			
Shoulder	Variable	Shoulder, arm, trunk	Scapula (Sc or A)

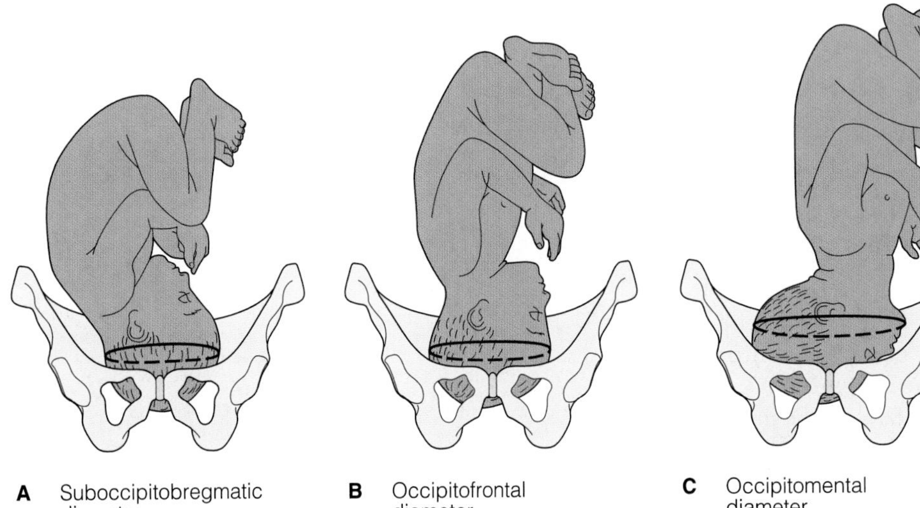

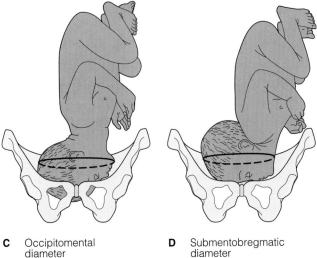

FIGURE 18–5 Cephalic presentation. ***A,*** Vertex presentation. Complete flexion of the head allows the suboccipitobregmatic diameter to present to the pelvis. ***B,*** Military (median vertex) presentation with no flexion or extension. The occipitofrontal diameter presents to the pelvis. ***C,*** Brow presentation. The fetal head is in partial (halfway) extension. The occipitomental diameter, which is the largest diameter of the fetal head, presents to the pelvis. ***D,*** Face presentation. The fetal head is in complete extension, and the submentobregmatic diameter presents to the pelvis.

Military Presentation

- The fetal head is neither flexed nor extended.
- The occipitofrontal diameter presents to the maternal pelvis (Figure 18–5, *B*).
- The top of the head is the presenting part.

Brow Presentation

- The fetal head is partially extended.
- The occipitomental diameter, the largest anteroposterior diameter, is presented to the maternal pelvis (Figure 18–5, *C*).
- The sinciput (see Figure 18–2) is the presenting part.

Face Presentation

- The fetal head is hyperextended (complete extension).
- The submentobregmatic diameter presents to the maternal pelvis (Figure 18–5, *D*).
- The face is the presenting part.

Breech Presentation Breech presentations occur in 3% of term births. These presentations are classified according to the attitude of the fetus's hips and knees. In all variations of the breech presentation the sacrum is the landmark to be noted.

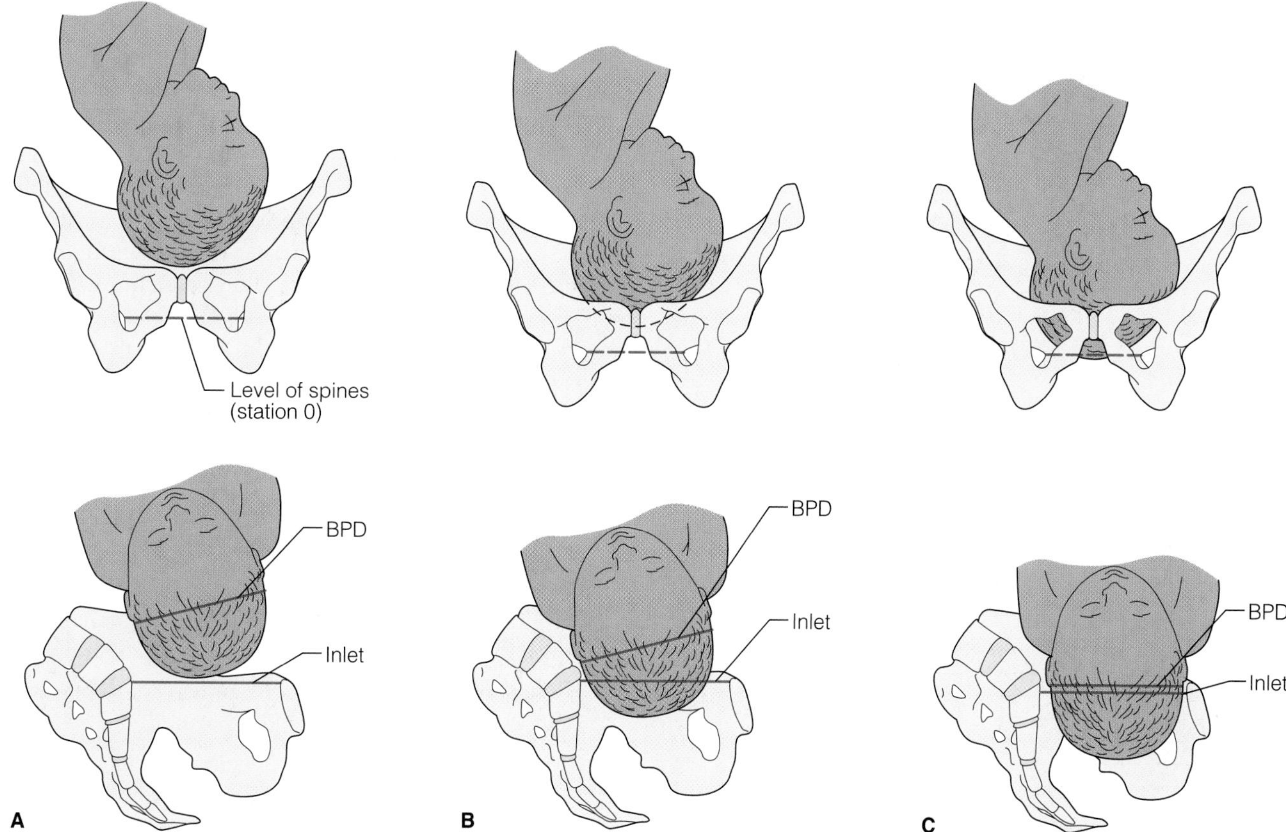

FIGURE 18–6 Process of engagement in cephalic presentation. ***A,*** Floating. The fetal head is directed down toward the pelvis but can still easily move away from the inlet. ***B,*** Dipping. The fetal head dips into the inlet but can be moved away by exerting pressure on the fetus. ***C,*** Engaged. The biparietal diameter (BPD) of the fetal head is in the inlet of the pelvis. In most instances, the presenting part (occiput) will be at the level of the ischial spines (0 station).

Complete Breech

- The fetal knees and hips are both flexed, the thighs are on the abdomen, and the calves are on the posterior aspect of the thighs.
- The buttocks and feet of the fetus present to the maternal pelvis.

Frank Breech

- The fetal hips are flexed, and the knees are extended.
- The buttocks of the fetus present to the maternal pelvis.

Footling Breech

- The fetal hips and legs are extended.
- The feet of the fetus present to the maternal pelvis.
- In a single footling one foot presents; in a double footling both feet present.

Shoulder Presentation A shoulder presentation is also called a *transverse lie.* Most frequently, the shoulder is the presenting part, and the acromion process of the scapula is the landmark to be noted. However, the fetal arm, back, abdomen, or side may present in a transverse lie. See Chapter 22 for further discussion of transverse lie.

Functional Relationships of Presenting Part and Maternal Pelvis

Engagement

Engagement of the presenting part occurs when the largest diameter of the presenting part reaches or passes through the pelvic inlet (Figure 18–6). When the fetal head is flexed, the biparietal diameter is the largest dimension of the fetal skull to pass through the pelvic inlet in a cephalic presentation. The intertrochanteric diameter (transverse diameter between the right and left trochanter) is the largest to pass through the inlet in a breech presentation.

Engagement can be determined by vaginal examination. In primigravidas engagement usually occurs 2 weeks

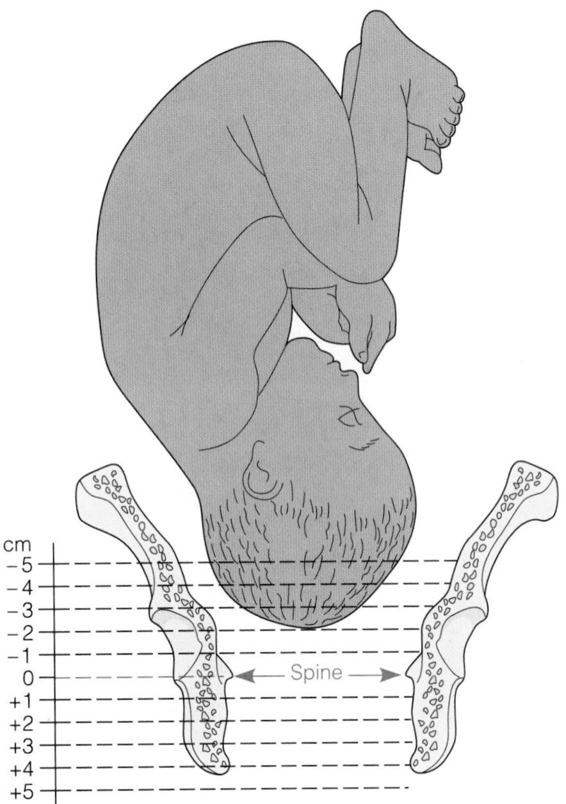

FIGURE 18–7 Measuring the station of the fetal head while it is descending. In this view the station is −2 / −3.

before term. Multiparas, however, may experience engagement several weeks before the onset of labor or during the process of labor.

The presenting part is said to be *floating* (or ballottable) when it is freely movable above the inlet. When the presenting part begins to descend into the inlet, before engagement has truly occurred, it is said to be *dipping* into the pelvis (Figure 18–6).

Station

Station refers to the relationship of the presenting part to an imaginary line drawn between the ischial spines of the maternal pelvis. In a normal pelvis the ischial spines mark the narrowest diameter through which the fetus must pass. These spines are not sharp protrusions but rather blunted prominences at the midpelvis. The ischial spines as a landmark have been designated as zero station (Figure 18–7). If the presenting part is higher than the ischial spines, a negative number is assigned, noting centimeters above zero station. Station −5 is at the inlet, and station +4 is at the outlet. If the presenting part can be seen at the woman's perineum, birth will occur momentarily. During labor the presenting part should move progressively from the negative stations to the midpelvis at zero station and into the positive stations. Failure of the presenting part to descend in the presence of strong contractions may be due to disproportion between the maternal pelvis and fetal presenting part.

Fetal Position

Fetal position refers to the relationship of the landmark on the presenting fetal part to the front (anterior), back (posterior), or sides (right or left) of the maternal pelvis. The landmark on the fetal presenting part is related to four imaginary quadrants of the maternal pelvis: left anterior, right anterior, left posterior, and right posterior. These quadrants designate whether the presenting part is directed toward the front, back, left, or right of the maternal pelvis. The landmark chosen for vertex presentations is the occiput, and the landmark for face presentations is the mentum. In breech presentations the sacrum is the designated landmark, and the acromion process on the scapula is the landmark in shoulder presentations. If the landmark is directed toward the center of the side of the pelvis, fetal position is designated as *transverse*, rather than anterior or posterior. Three notations are used to describe the fetal position:

1. Right (R) or left (L) side of the maternal pelvis
2. The landmark of the fetal presenting part: occiput (O), mentum (M), sacrum (S), or acromion process (A)
3. Anterior (A), posterior (P), or transverse (T), depending on whether the landmark is in the front, back, or side of the pelvis

The abbreviations of these notations help the health care team communicate the fetal position. Thus when the fetal occiput is directed toward the back and to the left of the passage, the abbreviation used is LOP (left-occiput-posterior). The term *dorsal* (D) is used when denoting the fetal position in a transverse lie; it refers to the fetal back. Thus the abbreviation RADA indicates that the acromion process of the scapula is directed toward the woman's right, and the fetus's back is anterior.

Following is a list of positions for various fetal presentations, some of which are illustrated in Figure 18–8.

Positions in vertex presentation:

ROA Right-occiput-anterior
ROT Right-occiput-transverse
ROP Right-occiput-posterior
LOA Left-occiput-anterior
LOT Left-occiput-transverse
LOP Left-occiput-posterior

Positions in face presentation:

RMA Right-mentum-anterior
RMT Right-mentum-transverse
RMP Right-mentum-posterior
LMA Left-mentum-anterior
LMT Left-mentum-transverse
LMP Left-mentum-posterior

Positions in breech presentation:

RSA Right-sacrum-anterior
RST Right-sacrum-transverse
RSP Right-sacrum-posterior
LSA Left-sacrum-anterior

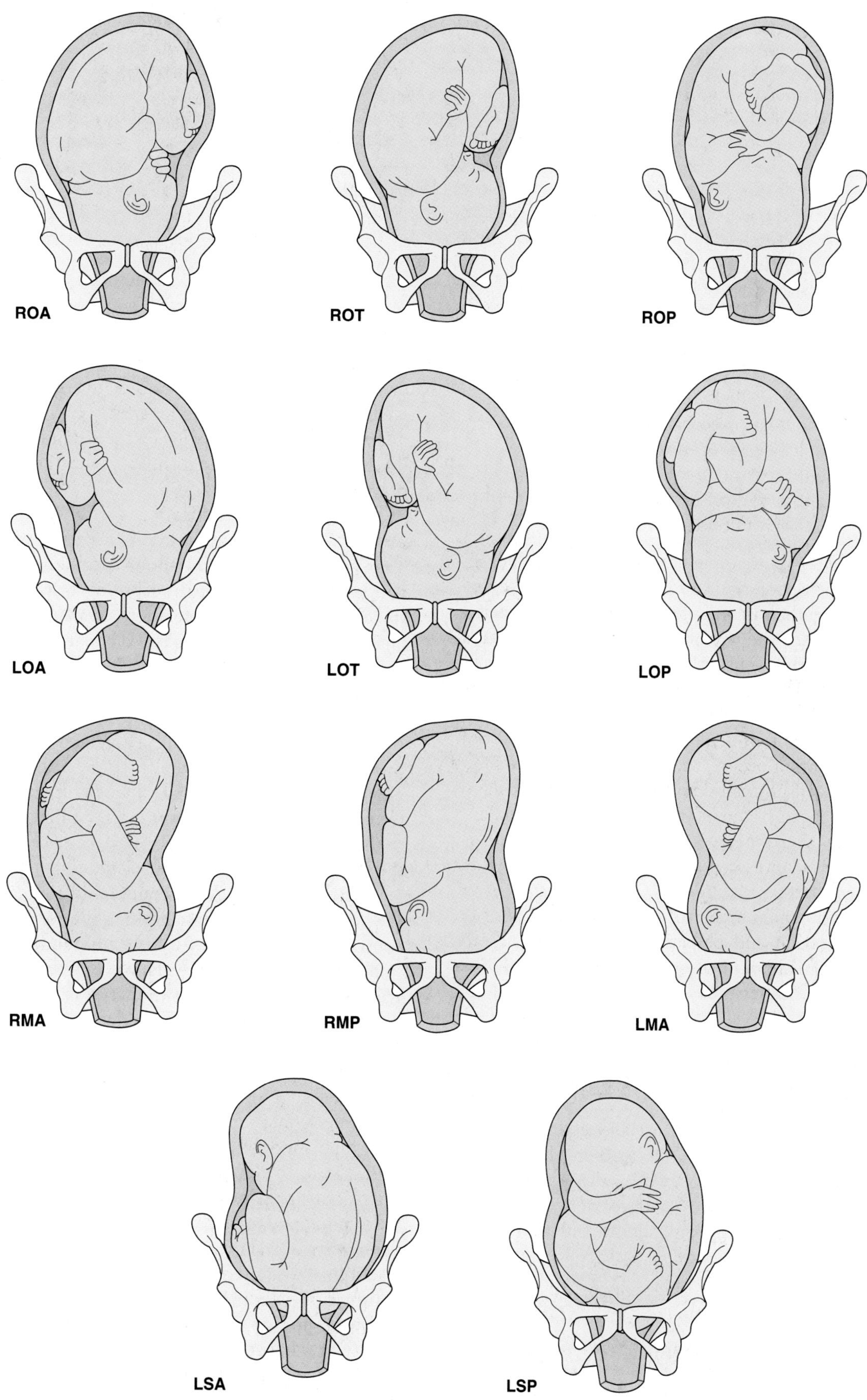

FIGURE 18–8 Categories of presentation. SOURCE: Courtesy Ross Laboratories, Columbus, OH.

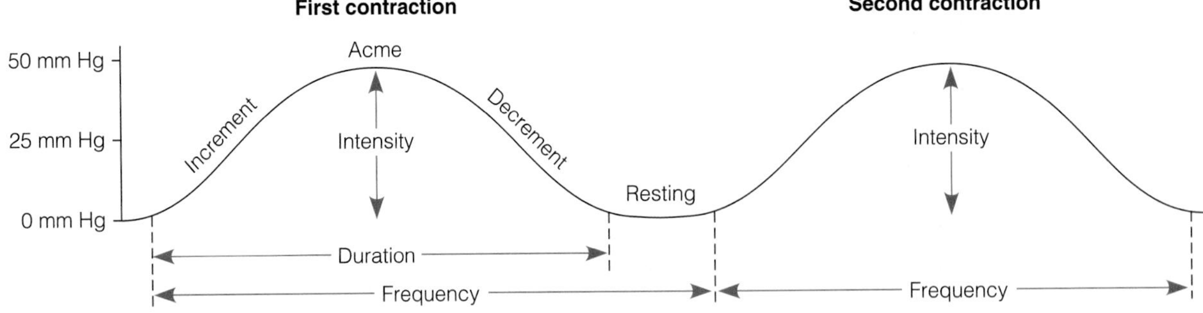

FIGURE 18–9 Characteristics of uterine contractions.

LST Left-sacrum-transverse
LSP Left-sacrum-posterior

Positions in shoulder presentation:

RADA Right-acromion-dorsal-anterior
RADP Right-acromion-dorsal-posterior
LADA Left-acromion-dorsal-anterior
LADP Left-acromion-dorsal-posterior

The fetal position influences labor and birth. For example, in a posterior position the fetal head presents a larger diameter than in an anterior position. A posterior position increases the pressure on the maternal sacral nerves, causing the laboring woman to experience backache and pelvic pressure. As a result, the woman may bear down or feel the urge to push earlier than needed.

The most common fetal position is occiput anterior. When this position occurs, the labor and birth are more likely to proceed normally. Positions other than occiput anterior are more frequently associated with problems during labor; therefore, they are called **malpositions.** (See Chapter 22 for discussion of malpositions and their management.)

Assessment techniques to determine fetal position include inspection and palpation of the maternal abdomen and vaginal examination. (See Chapter 19 for further discussion of assessment of fetal position.)

CRITICAL THINKING QUESTION

You hear the fetal heart rate just above the expectant woman's navel (umbilicus). You read in the prenatal record that 2 weeks ago, at 35 weeks, the fetal presentation was cephalic. What do you think of your findings? Are they consistent with a cephalic presentation? What might you do to gather additional data?

The Forces of Labor

Primary and secondary forces work together to deliver the fetus, the fetal membranes, and the placenta from the uterus into the external environment. The *primary force* is uterine muscular contractions, which cause the changes of the first stage of labor—complete effacement and dilatation of the cervix. The *secondary force* is the use of abdominal muscles to push during the second stage of labor. The pushing adds to the primary power after full dilatation has occurred.

In labor, uterine contractions are rhythmic but intermittent. Between contractions is a period of relaxation. This period of relaxation allows uterine muscles to rest and provides respite for the laboring woman. It also restores uteroplacental circulation, which is important to fetal oxygenation and adequate circulation in the uterine blood vessels.

Each contraction has three phases: (1) *increment*, the "building up" of the contraction (the longest phase); (2) *acme*, or the peak of the contraction; and (3) *decrement*, or the "letting up" of the contraction. When describing uterine contractions during labor, caregivers use the terms *frequency*, *duration*, and *intensity*. **Frequency** refers to the time between the beginning of one contraction and the beginning of the next contraction.

The **duration** of each contraction is measured from the beginning of the contraction to the completion of the contraction (Figure 18–9). In beginning labor the duration is 30 to 40 seconds. As labor continues, duration increases to 60 to 90 seconds (Simpson & Creehan, 1996).

Intensity refers to the strength of the uterine contraction during acme. In most instances the intensity is estimated by palpating the contraction, but it may be measured directly with an intrauterine catheter attached to an electronic fetal monitor. Intensity of uterine contractions cannot be accurately measured by external monitoring with an electronic fetal monitor. When estimating intensity by palpation, the nurse determines whether it is mild, moderate, or strong by judging the amount of indentability of the uterine wall during the acme of a contraction. If the uterine wall can be indented easily, the contraction is considered mild. Strong intensity exists when the uterine wall cannot be indented. Moderate intensity falls between these two ranges. When intensity is measured with an intrauterine catheter, the normal resting tonus (between contractions) is about 10 to 12 mm Hg of pressure. During acme the intensity ranges from 25 to 40 mm Hg in early labor, 50 to 70 mm Hg in active labor, 70 to 90 mm Hg during transition, and 70 to 100 mm Hg while the woman is pushing in the second stage (Creehan, 1996). (See Chapter 19 for further discussion of assessment techniques.)

At the beginning of labor the contractions are usually mild, of short duration, and relatively infrequent. As labor progresses, duration and intensity increase, and the frequency is every 2 to 3 minutes. Because the contractions are involuntary, the laboring woman cannot control their duration, frequency, or intensity.

Psychosocial Considerations

Similar psychosocial factors affect both the mother and the father. Both are making a transition into a new role, and both have expectations of themselves during the labor and birth experience, as caregivers for their child and their new family. Although many prospective mothers and fathers attend childbirth preparation classes, they still tend to be concerned about what labor will be like, whether they will each be able to perform the way they expect, whether the discomfort and pain will be more than the mother expects or can cope with, and whether the father can provide helpful support (McKay & Smith, 1993; Nichols, 1993; Tomlinson & Bryan, 1996).

Every woman is uncertain about what her labor will be like: A woman anticipating her first labor faces a totally new experience, and multiparas cannot be certain what each new labor will bring. The woman does not know whether she will live up to her expectations for herself in relation to her friends and relatives, whether she will be physically injured through laceration, episiotomy, or cesarean incision, or whether significant others will be as supportive as she hopes (Mercer, 1995). The woman faces an irrevocable event—the birth of a new family member—and, consequently, disruption of lifestyle, relationships, and self-image. Finally, the woman must deal with concerns about her loss of control of bodily functions, emotional responses to an unfamiliar situation, and reactions to the pain associated with labor.

Various factors influence a woman's reaction to the physical and emotional crisis of labor (Table 18–3). Her accomplishment of the tasks of pregnancy, usual coping mechanisms in response to stressful life events, support system, preparation for childbirth, and cultural influences are all significant factors.

In her study of the psychosocial adaptations of pregnancy, Lederman (1996) found that expectant women prepared for labor through actions and imaginary rehearsal. The actions frequently consisted of "nesting behavior" (housecleaning, decorating the nursery) and a "psyching up" for the labor, which seemed to vary depending on the woman's self-confidence, self-esteem, and previous experiences with stress. Specific actions to prepare for labor are usually focused on becoming better informed and prepared. Nichols and Humenick (1988) suggest that mastery, or control, of the childbearing experience is the key factor in decreased pain and perceived satisfaction (Lowe, 1996). Childbirth education helps increase positive reactions to the birth experience by giving the laboring woman and her support persons greater opportunities to control the experience of labor. DiMatteo, Kahn, and Berry (1993) suggest that women need to be prepared to face not only areas that are under their personal control, such as patterned breathing and certain comfort measures, but also experiences involving situational control, which include some procedures requested by the certified nurse-midwife/physician or birth-setting institutional protocols.

TABLE 18–3 Factors Associated with a Positive Birth Experience

Motivation for the pregnancy
Attendance at childbirth education classes
A sense of competence or mastery
Self-confidence and self-esteem
Positive relationship with mate
Maintaining control during labor
Support from mate or other person during labor
Not being left alone in labor
Trust in the medical/nursing staff
Having personal control of breathing patterns, comfort measures
Choosing a physician/certified nurse-midwife who has a similar philosophy of care
Receiving clear information regarding procedures

An important developmental step for expectant women is to anticipate the labor in fantasy. Just as a woman "tries on" the maternal role during pregnancy, fantasizing about labor seems to help her understand and become better prepared for it. Fantasies about the excitement of the baby's birth and the sharing of the experience involve the woman in constructive preparation. A woman who has a great deal of apprehension about becoming a mother or great fear of pain during labor is unable to fantasize the labor in positive ways and may have many disturbing thoughts (Lederman, 1996).

Many women fear the pain of contractions. They not only see the pain as threatening but also associate it with a loss of control over their bodies and emotions. When a woman is facing labor, especially for the first time, she may worry about her ability to withstand the pain of labor and maintain self-control.

The laboring woman's support system may also influence the course of labor and birth. For some women, the presence of the father and other significant persons, including the nurse, tends to have a positive effect. In a study by Khazoyan and Anderson (1994), Latina women identified the need for the partner's presence at the bedside for communication and showing love. Communication needs included talking and "affectionate and understanding words" from their partners. Showing love was described as holding hands, hugging, or touching. The partner's presence at the bedside was interpreted as a "loving" gesture.

RESEARCH IN PRACTICE

What is this study about? Guatemalan women view pregnancy as a normal physiologic event rather than as an illness. Only 50% of these women seek medical care and the remainder are attended by traditional midwives or comadronas. In order to explore the meaning of the childbirth experience, Lynn Callister and Rosemarie Vega conducted an ethnographic study using the birth stories and perceptions of Guatemalan women.

How was the study done? The principal investigator and a bilingual Latina nursing student interviewed 30 Guatemalan women who had recently given birth to healthy, full-term infants. Interviews took place in a hospital, clinics, homes, and central plazas. Many of the informants lived in small villages, worked in the fields, and wove fabrics to sell. Data analysis included identifying and classifying core concepts from the translated audiotapes.

What were the results of the study? Participants were evenly divided between 15 multiparae and 15 primiparae. Fourteen women gave birth at home with traditional midwives in attendance and 16 gave birth in the hospital, where primarily physicians in training delivered the child. Using midwives allowed the women to give birth in their own homes with more privacy and family support. Midwives would administer herbs to relieve pain and sometimes a small amount of cooking oil to "soften the pain." Some women gave birth in a kneeling or squatting position. Professional care was viewed as safer and less costly than using the services of the traditional midwives. The midwife's fees might consume the family income for an entire month. Because the women viewed birth as a natural, but painful experience, they vocalized their pain. They also used breathing, rhythmic moaning, or rubbing of thighs and abdomen to relieve or cope with pain. Vaginal births in the professional setting were unmedicated. Many women reported being unhappy when they initially learned of their pregnancy due to their concerns about their ability to provide for the child. Paradoxically, children enhance economic security because children can sometimes earn more than their parents and are obligated to care for elderly parents. Predominant themes found by the researchers included a sense of sacredness related to childbearing, a need to rely on God to provide a positive outcome, and the bittersweet paradox of giving birth.

What additional questions might I have? How did the researchers gain access to the participants? Obtaining access is not described. Did the authors conduct any fieldwork or participant observation? Many ethnographic studies include these methods of data collection.

How can I use this study? As the authors state, the study may assist nurses in the provision of culturally competent care if caring for a Central American immigrant from a similar background as the participants of this study. New immigrants may still be tied to the traditions and customs of their country of origin.

SOURCE: Callister, L. C., & Vega, R. (1998). Giving birth: Guatemalan women's voices. *JOGNN, 27,* 289–295.

How the woman views the childbirth experience in hindsight may have implications for mothering behaviors. Mercer (1995) and Walker and Montgomery (1994) found a significant relationship between the birth experience and mothering behaviors. It appears that any activities by the expectant woman or by health care providers that enhance the birth experience will be beneficial.

The Physiology of Labor

Possible Causes of Labor Onset

Labor usually begins between the 38th and the 42nd week of gestation, when the fetus is mature and ready for birth. Despite medical advances, there is still no full understanding of biochemical substances and interactions that stimulate labor and birth. Some important aspects have been identified: progesterone relaxes uterine smooth muscle; estrogen stimulates uterine muscle contractions; connective tissue loosens to permit softening, stretching, and eventual thinning of the cervix, leading to the formation of the lower uterine segment. At this time, researchers are focusing on fetal membranes (chorion and amnion), the decidua, and the effect of various substances. Hypotheses have been formed about the roles of progesterone withdrawal, of prostaglandin, and of corticotrophin-releasing hormone (Smith, 1999).

Progesterone Withdrawal Hypothesis Progesterone produced by the placenta relaxes uterine smooth muscle by interfering with conduction of impulses from one cell to the next. For this reason, the uterus is usually without coordinated contractions during pregnancy. Biochemical changes toward the end of gestation result in decreased availability of progesterone to myometrial cells. The decrease in availability may be associated with a yet unknown antiprogestin that inhibits the relaxant effect on the uterus but allows other progesterone actions such as lactogenesis (Liggins, 1997).

Prostaglandin Hypothesis Although the exact relationship between prostaglandin and the onset of labor is not yet established, the effect is clinically demonstrated by the successful induction of labor after vaginal application of prostaglandin E. In addition, preterm labor may be stopped by using an inhibitor of prostaglandin synthesis such as indomethacin (Liggins, 1997).

The amnion and decidua are the focus of research on the source of prostaglandins. Once prostaglandin is produced, stimuli for its synthesis may include rising levels of estrogen, decreased availability of progesterone, increased levels of oxytocin or response to oxytocin, platelet-activating factor, and endothelin-1 (Liggins, 1997).

Corticotrophin-Releasing Hormone Hypothesis Corticotrophin-releasing hormone (CRH) is also a focus for researchers. Its possible role in onset of labor is suggested by CRH concentration increases throughout pregnancy, with a sharp increase at term. Also, there is an increase in plasma CRH prior to preterm labor, and CRH levels are elevated in multiple gestation. Finally, CRH is known to stimulate the synthesis of prostaglandin F and prostaglandin E by amnion cells (Smith, 1999).

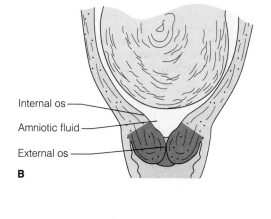

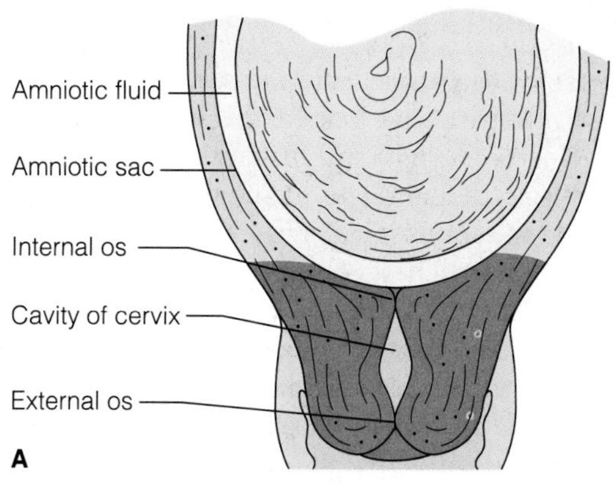

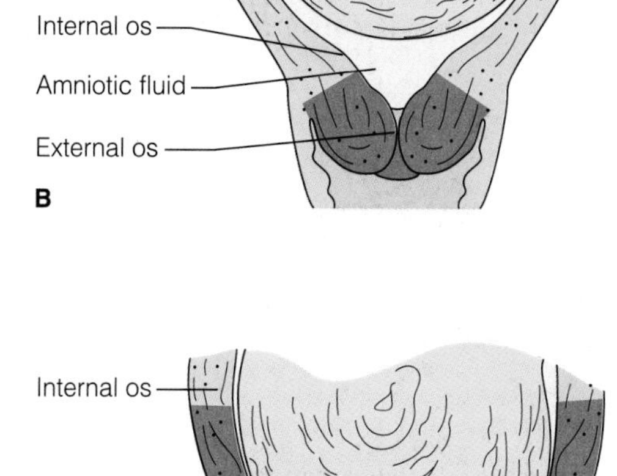

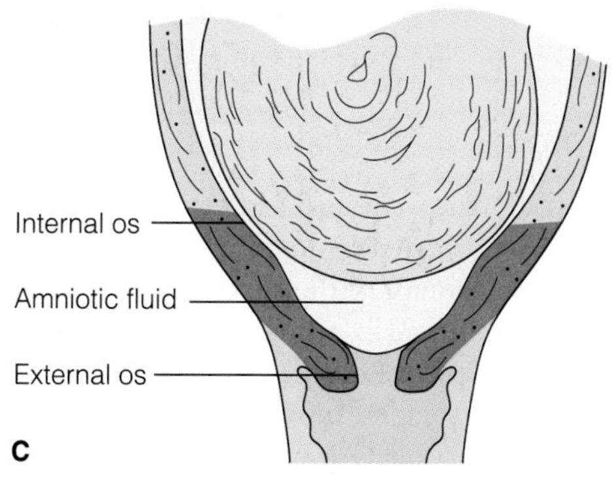

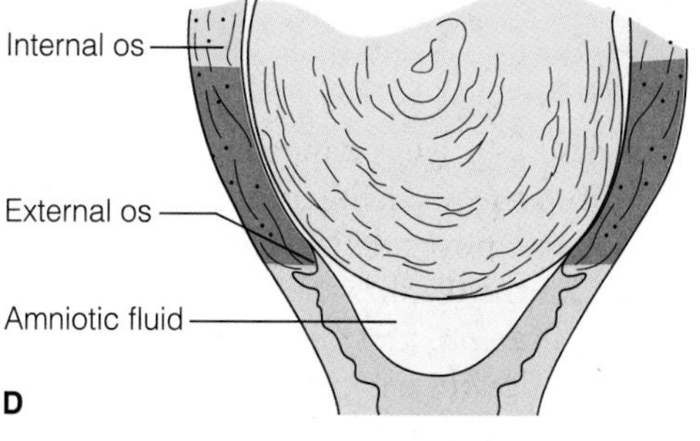

FIGURE 18–10 Effacement of the cervix in the primigravida. ***A,*** At the beginning of labor, there is no cervical effacement or dilatation. The fetal head is cushioned by amniotic fluid. ***B,*** Beginning cervical effacement. As the cervix begins to efface, more amniotic fluid collects below the fetal head. ***C,*** Cervix is about one-half (50%) effaced and slightly dilated. The increasing amount of amniotic fluid below the fetal head exerts hydrostatic pressure on the cervix. ***D,*** Complete effacement and dilatation.

Myometrial Activity

In true labor the uterus divides into two portions. This division is known as the *physiologic retraction ring.* The upper portion, which is the contractile segment, becomes progressively thicker as labor advances. The lower portion, which includes the lower uterine segment and cervix, is passive. As labor continues the lower uterine segment expands and thins out.

With each contraction the muscles of the upper uterine segment shorten and exert a longitudinal traction on the cervix, causing effacement. **Effacement** is the taking up (or drawing up) of the internal os and the cervical canal into the uterine side walls. The cervix changes progressively from a long, thick structure to a structure that is tissue-paper thin (Figure 18–10). In primigravidas effacement usually precedes dilatation. The uterine muscle remains shorter and thicker and does not return to its original length. This phenomenon is known as brachystasis. The space in the uterine cavity decreases as a result of brachystasis, and this places downward pressure on the fetus (Cunningham et al, 1997).

The uterus elongates with each contraction, decreasing the horizontal diameter. This elongation causes a straightening of the fetal body, pressing the part of the fetus in the upper portion of the uterus against the fundus and thrusting the presenting part down toward the lower uterine segment and the cervix. The pressure exerted by the fetus is called *fetal axis pressure.* As the uterus elongates, the longitudinal muscle fibers are pulled upward over the presenting part. This action and the hydrostatic pressure of the fetal membranes cause **cervical dilatation.** The cervical os and cervical canal widen from less than a centimeter to approximately 10 cm, allowing birth of the fetus. When the cervix is completely dilated and retracted up into the lower uterine segment, it can no longer be palpated.

The round ligament pulls the fundus forward, aligning the fetus with the bony pelvis.

Intra-abdominal Pressure

After the cervix is completely dilated, the maternal abdominal musculature contracts as the woman pushes. This pushing is called *bearing down.* The pushing aids in the expulsion of the fetus and the placenta. If the cervix is not completely dilated, bearing down can cause cervical edema (which retards dilatation), possible tearing and bruising of the cervix, and maternal exhaustion.

Musculature Changes in the Pelvic Floor

The levator ani muscle and fascia of the pelvic floor draw the rectum and vagina upward and forward with each contraction, along the curve of the pelvic floor. As the fetal head descends to the pelvic floor, the pressure of the presenting part causes the perineal structure, which was once 5 cm in thickness, to change to a structure less than a centimeter thick. A normal physiologic anesthesia is produced as a result of the decreased blood supply to the area. The anus everts, exposing the interior rectal wall as the fetal head descends forward (Cunningham et al, 1997).

Premonitory Signs of Labor

Most primigravidas and many multiparas experience the following signs and symptoms of impending labor.

Lightening

Lightening describes what happens when the fetus begins to settle into the pelvic inlet (engagement). With its descent the uterus moves downward, and the fundus no longer presses on the diaphragm.

The woman can breathe more easily after lightening. With increased downward pressure of the presenting part, however, she may notice the following:

- Leg cramps or pains due to pressure on the nerves that course through the obturator foramen in the pelvis
- Increased pelvic pressure
- Increased venous stasis leading to edema in the lower extremities
- Increased urinary frequency
- Increased vaginal secretions resulting from congestion of the vaginal mucous membranes

Braxton Hicks Contractions

Prior to the onset of labor, Braxton Hicks contractions—the irregular, intermittent contractions that have been occurring throughout the pregnancy—may become uncomfortable. The pain seems to be in the abdomen and groin but may feel like the "drawing" sensations experienced by some women with dysmenorrhea. When these contractions are strong enough for the woman to believe she is in labor, she is said to be in *false labor.* False labor is uncomfortable and may be exhausting. Because the contractions can be fairly regular, she has no way of knowing whether they are the beginning of true labor. She may come to the hospital/birthing center for a vaginal examination to determine whether cervical dilatation is occurring. Frequent episodes of false labor and trips back and forth to the certified nurse-midwife/physician's office or hospital may frustrate or embarrass the woman, who feels that she should know when she is really in labor. Reassurance by nursing staff can ease embarrassment.

Cervical Changes

Considerable change occurs in the cervix during the prenatal and intrapartal period. At the beginning of pregnancy the cervix is rigid and firm, and it must soften so that it can stretch and dilate to allow fetal passage. This softening of the cervix is called *ripening.*

As term approaches, collagen fibers in the cervix are broken down by the action of enzymes such as collagenase and elastase. As the collagen fibers change, their ability to bind is decreased because of increasing amounts of hyaluronic acid (which loosely binds collagen fibrils) and decreasing amounts of dermatan sulfate (which tightly binds collagen fibrils). There is also an increase in the water content of the cervix, and all these changes result in a weakening and softening of the cervix.

Bloody Show

During the pregnancy cervical secretions have accumulated in the cervical canal to form a mucous plug. With softening and effacement of the cervix the mucous plug is often expelled, resulting in a small amount of blood loss from the exposed cervical capillaries. The resulting pink-tinged secretions are called **bloody show.**

Bloody show is considered a sign of impending labor, usually within 24 to 48 hours. Vaginal examination that includes manipulation of the cervix may also result in a blood-tinged discharge (may be more brownish in color), which is sometimes confused with bloody show.

Rupture of Membranes

In approximately 12% of women the amniotic membranes rupture before the onset of labor. This is called **rupture of membranes (ROM).** After membranes rupture, 80% of women will experience spontaneous labor within 24 hours. If membranes rupture and labor does not begin spontaneously within 12 to 24 hours, labor may be induced to avoid infection (once the membranes have ruptured there is an open pathway into the uterine cavity). An induction of labor is done only if the pregnancy is near term.

When the membranes rupture, the amniotic fluid may be expelled in large amounts. If engagement has not occurred, the danger exists that the umbilical cord may be expelled with the fluid *(prolapsed cord).* Because of these potential problems, the woman is advised to notify her certified nurse-midwife/physician and proceed to the hospital/birthing center. In some instances the fluid is expelled in small amounts and may be confused with episodes of urinary incontinence associated with urinary urgency, coughing, or sneezing. The discharge should be checked to ascertain its source and to determine further action. (See Chapter 19 for assessment techniques used to establish whether membranes are ruptured, for precautions the nurse uses to avoid exposure to amniotic fluid, and for guidelines regarding whether the woman should remain ambulatory.)

Sudden Burst of Energy

Some women report a sudden burst of energy approximately 24 to 48 hours before labor. The cause of the energy spurt is unknown. In prenatal teaching the nurse should warn prospective mothers not to overexert themselves during this energy burst so that they will not be excessively tired when labor begins.

Other Signs

Other premonitory signs include the following:

- Weight loss of 2.2 to 6.6 kg (1 to 3 lb) resulting from fluid loss and electrolyte shifts produced by changes in estrogen and progesterone levels
- Increased backache and sacroiliac pressure from the influence of relaxin hormone on the pelvic joints
- Diarrhea, indigestion, or nausea and vomiting just prior to the onset of labor

The causes of these signs are unknown.

Differences Between True and False Labor

The contractions of true labor produce progressive dilatation and effacement of the cervix. They occur regularly and increase in frequency, duration, and intensity. The discomfort of true labor contractions usually starts in the back and radiates around to the abdomen. The pain is not relieved by ambulation (in fact walking may intensify the pain).

The contractions of false labor do not produce progressive cervical effacement and dilatation. Classically, they are irregular and do not increase in frequency, duration, and intensity. The contractions may be perceived as a hardening or "balling up" without discomfort, or discomfort may occur mainly in the lower abdomen and groin. The discomfort may be relieved by ambulation.

The woman will find it helpful to know the characteristics of true labor contractions as well as the premonitory signs of labor. However, many times the only way to differentiate accurately between true and false labor is to assess dilatation. The woman must feel free to come in for accurate assessment of labor and should never be allowed to feel foolish if the labor is false. The nurse must reassure the woman that false labor is common and that it often cannot be distinguished from true labor except by vaginal examination (Table 18–4).

TABLE 18–4 Comparison of True and False Labor

True Labor	False Labor
Contractions are at regular intervals.	Contractions are irregular.
Intervals between contractions gradually shorten.	Usually no change.
Contractions increase in duration and intensity.	Usually no change.
Discomfort begins in back and radiates around to abdomen.	Discomfort is usually in abdomen.
Intensity usually increases with walking.	Walking has no effect on or lessens contractions.
Cervical dilatation and effacement are progressive.	No change.

Stages of Labor and Birth

There are three stages of labor. The *first stage* begins with the beginning of true labor and ends when the cervix is completely dilated at 10 cm. The *second stage* begins with complete dilatation and ends with the birth of the infant. The *third stage* begins with the expulsion of the infant and ends with the expulsion of the placenta.

Some clinicians identify a *fourth stage* of labor. During this stage, which lasts 1 to 4 hours after expulsion of the placenta, the uterus effectively contracts to control bleeding at the placental site (Cunningham et al, 1997).

The care of the laboring woman is discussed in Chapter 20.

First Stage

The first stage of labor is divided into the *latent*, *active*, and *transition* phases (Table 18–5). Each phase of labor is characterized by physical and psychologic changes.

Latent Phase

The *latent phase* begins with the onset of regular contractions. As the cervix begins to dilate it also effaces, although little or no fetal descent is evident. For a woman in her first labor (nullipara) the latent phase averages 8.6 hours but should not exceed 20 hours. The latent phase in multiparas averages 5.3 hours but should not exceed 14 hours.

Uterine contractions become established during the latent phase and increase in frequency, duration, and intensity. They may start as mild contractions lasting 20 to 40 seconds with a frequency of 3 to 30 minutes. They average 25 to 40 mm Hg by intrauterine pressure catheter (IUPC) at acme (Creehan, 1996).

In the early or latent phase of the first stage of labor, contractions are usually mild. The woman feels able to cope with the discomfort. She may be relieved that labor has finally started. Although she may be anxious, she is able to recognize and express those feelings of anxiety. The woman is often talkative and smiling and is eager to talk about herself and answer questions. Excitement is high, and her partner or other support person is often as elated as she is.

At the beginning of labor the amniotic membranes bulge through the cervix in the shape of a cone. **Spontaneous rupture of membranes (SROM)** generally occurs

TABLE 18–5 Characteristics of Labor

	First Stage			Second Stage
	Latent Phase	**Active Phase**	**Transition Phase**	
Nullipara	8.6 hr	4.6 hr	3.6 hr	Up to 3 hr
Multipara	5.3 hr	2.4 hr	Variable	0–30 min
Cervical dilatation	0–3 cm	4–7 cm	8–10 cm	
Contractions				
Frequency	Every 3–30 min	Every 2–3 min	Every 1 1/2–2 min	Every 1 1/2–2 min
Duration	20–40 sec	40–60 sec	60–90 sec	60–90 sec
Intensity	Begin as mild and progress to moderate; 25–40 mm Hg by intrauterine pressure catheter (IUPC)	Begin as moderate and progress to strong; 50–70 mm Hg by IUPC	Strong by palpation; 70–90 mm Hg by IUPC	Strong by palpation; 70–100 mm Hg by IUPC

at the height of an intense contraction with a gush of the fluid out of the vagina. In many instances the membranes are ruptured by the certified nurse-midwife/physician. This is called *amniotomy*, or **artificial rupture of membranes (AROM).**

Active Phase

During the *active phase* the cervix dilates from about 4 cm to 7 cm. Fetal descent is progressive. The cervical dilatation should be at least 1.2 cm/hour in nulliparas and 1.5 cm/hour in multiparas (Cunningham et al, 1997).

Transition Phase

The *transition phase* is the last part of the first stage. Cervical dilatation slows as it progresses from 8 to 10 cm and the rate of fetal descent increases. The average rate of descent is at least 1 cm/hour in nulliparas and 2 cm/hour in multiparas. The transition phase should not be longer than 3 hours for nulliparas and 1 hour for multiparas (Cunningham et al, 1997). The total duration of the first stage may be increased by approximately 1 hour if epidural anesthesia is used.

During the active and transition phases, contractions become more frequent, are longer in duration, and increase in intensity. At the beginning of the active phase the contractions have a frequency of 2 to 5 minutes, a duration of 40 to 60 seconds, and are strong in intensity. During transition, contractions have a frequency of 1½ to 2 minutes, a duration of 60 to 90 seconds, and are strong in intensity.

When the woman enters the early active phase, her anxiety tends to increase as she senses the fairly constant intensification of contractions and pain. She begins to fear a loss of control and may use coping mechanisms to maintain control. Some women exhibit decreased ability to cope and a sense of helplessness. Women who have support persons available, particularly the baby's father, experience greater satisfaction and less anxiety throughout the birth process than those without these supports.

When the woman enters the transition phase, she may demonstrate significant anxiety. She becomes acutely aware of the increasing force and intensity of the contractions. She may become restless, frequently changing position. She may fear being left alone, and it is crucial that the nurse be available as backup and relief for the support person. By the time the woman enters the transition phase she is inner directed and often tired. At the same time the support person may be feeling the need for a break. The woman should be reassured that she will not be left alone and should always be told where her support people are and how to reach the nurse.

The woman may also fear that she will be "torn open" or "split apart" by the force of the contractions. Many women experience a sensation of pressure so great with the peak of a contraction that it seems to them that their abdomens will burst open. The woman should be informed that this is a normal sensation and reassured that such bursting will not happen.

During transition the woman will most likely withdraw into herself. Increasingly she may doubt her ability to cope with labor. The woman may become apprehensive and irritable. She may be terrified of being left alone, though she does not want anyone to talk to her or touch her. However, with the next contraction she may ask for verbal and physical support. She may need help regaining focus and her breathing pattern. Other characteristics that may accompany this phase include the following:

- Hyperventilation, as the woman increases her breathing rate
- Restlessness
- Difficulty understanding directions
- A sense of bewilderment and anger at the contractions
- Statements that she "can't take it anymore"
- Requests for medication
- Hiccupping, belching, nausea, or vomiting
- Beads of perspiration on the upper lip
- Increasing rectal pressure

The woman in this phase is anxious to "get it over with." She may be amnesic and sleep between her now frequent contractions. Her support persons may start to feel helpless and may turn to the nurse for increased participation as their efforts to alleviate her discomfort seem less effective.

As dilatation approaches 10 cm there may be increased rectal pressure, an uncontrollable desire to bear down, increased amount of bloody show, and rupture of membranes.

Second Stage

The second stage of labor begins when the cervix is completely dilated (10 cm) and ends with birth of the infant. The second stage should be completed within 2 hours after the cervix becomes fully dilated for primigravidas (multiparas average 15 minutes). The use of epidural anesthesia may extend the duration of the second stage an additional 1 hour. Contractions continue with a frequency of 1½ to 2 minutes, a duration of 60 to 90 seconds, and strong intensity. Descent of the fetal presenting part continues until it reaches the perineal floor.

As the fetal head descends the woman has the urge to push because of pressure of the fetal head on the sacral and obturator nerves. As she pushes intra-abdominal pressure is exerted from contraction of the maternal abdominal muscles. As the fetal head continues its descent, the perineum begins to bulge, flatten, and move anteriorly. The amount of bloody show may increase. The labia begin to part with each contraction. Between contractions the fetal head appears to recede. With succeeding contractions and maternal pushing effort, the fetal head descends farther. **Crowning** occurs when the fetal head is encircled by the external opening of the vagina (introitus) and means birth is imminent.

Usually, a childbirth-prepared woman feels relieved that the acute pain she felt during the transition phase is over (see Table 18–5). She also may be relieved that the birth is near and she can now push. Some women feel a sense of control now that they can be actively involved. Others, particularly those without childbirth preparation, may become frightened. They tend to fight each contraction and any attempt of others to persuade them to push with contractions. Such behavior may be frightening and disconcerting to her support persons. The woman may feel she has lost control and become embarrassed and apologetic, or she may demonstrate extreme irritability toward the staff or her supporters in an attempt to regain control over external forces against which she feels helpless. Some women feel acute, increasingly severe pain and a burning sensation as the perineum distends. The woman may continue to fear that she will tear apart.

Spontaneous Birth (Vertex Presentation)

As the head distends the vulva with each contraction, the perineum becomes extremely thin, and the anus stretches and protrudes.

As extension occurs under the symphysis pubis, the head is born. When the anterior shoulder meets the underside of the symphysis pubis, a gentle push by the mother aids in birth of the shoulders. The body then follows (Figure 18–11). Birth of infants in breech presentation is discussed in Chapter 22.

Positional Changes

For the fetus to pass through the birth canal, the fetal head and body must adjust to the maternal pelvis by certain positional changes. These changes, called **cardinal movements** or *mechanisms of labor*, are described in the order in which they occur (Figure 18–12).

Descent Descent is thought to occur because of four forces: (1) pressure of the amniotic fluid, (2) direct pressure of the fundus of the uterus on the breech of the fetus, (3) contraction of the abdominal muscles, and (4) extension and straightening of the fetal body. The head enters the inlet in the occiput transverse or oblique position because the pelvic inlet is widest from side to side. The sagittal suture is an equal distance from the maternal symphysis pubis and sacral promontory.

Flexion Flexion occurs as the fetal head descends and meets resistance from the soft tissues of the pelvis, the musculature of the pelvic floor, and the cervix.

Internal Rotation The fetal head must rotate to fit the diameter of the pelvic cavity, which is widest in the anteroposterior diameter. As the occiput of the fetal head meets resistance from the levator ani muscles and their fascia, the occiput rotates from left to right, and the sagittal suture aligns in the anteroposterior pelvic diameter.

Extension The resistance of the pelvic floor and the mechanical movement of the vulva opening anteriorly and forward assist with extension of the fetal head as it passes under the symphysis pubis. With this positional change the occiput, then brow and face, emerge from the vagina.

Restitution The shoulders of the infant enter the pelvis obliquely and remain oblique when the head rotates to the anteroposterior diameter through internal rotation. Because of this rotation the neck becomes twisted. Once the head emerges and is free of pelvic resistance the neck untwists, turning the head to one side (restitution), and aligns with the position of the back in the birth canal.

External Rotation As the shoulders rotate to the anteroposterior position in the pelvis, the head is turned farther to one side (external rotation).

Expulsion After the external rotation and through expulsive efforts of the laboring woman, the anterior

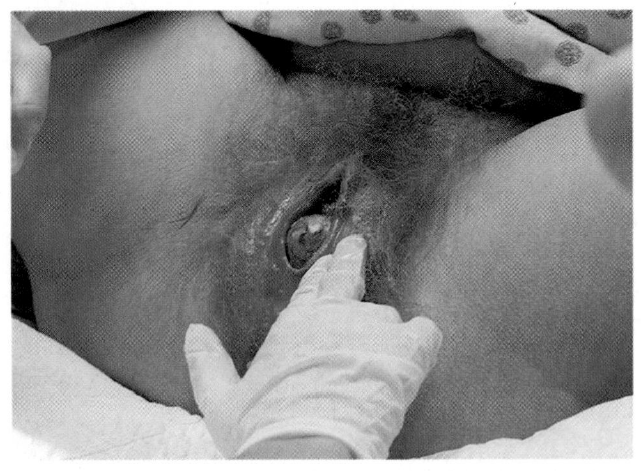
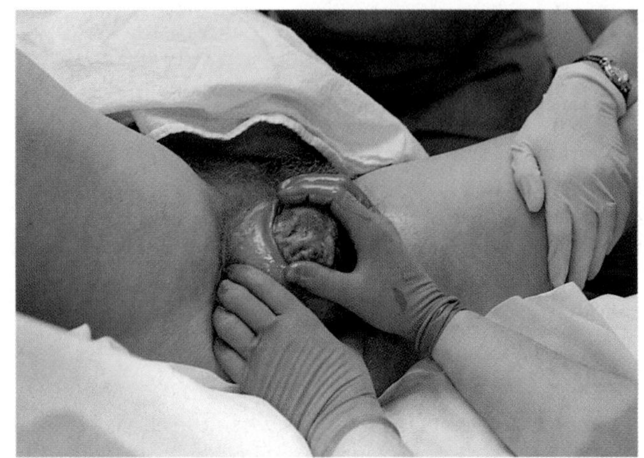
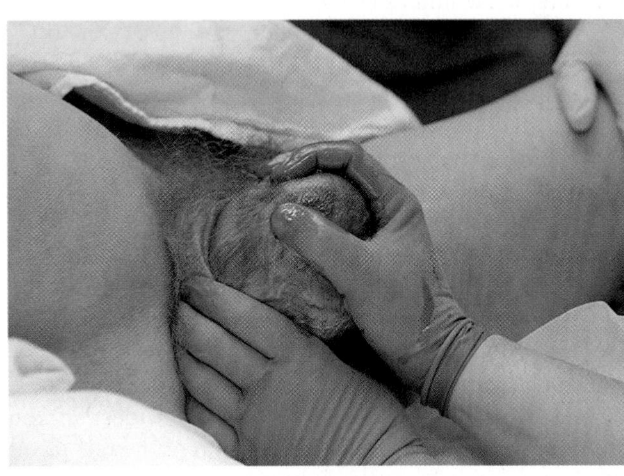
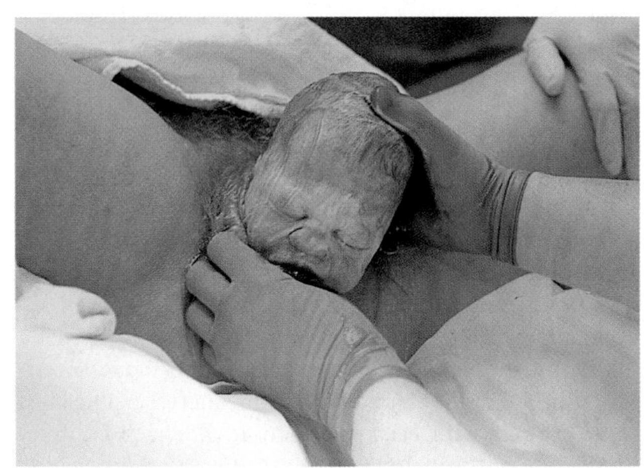
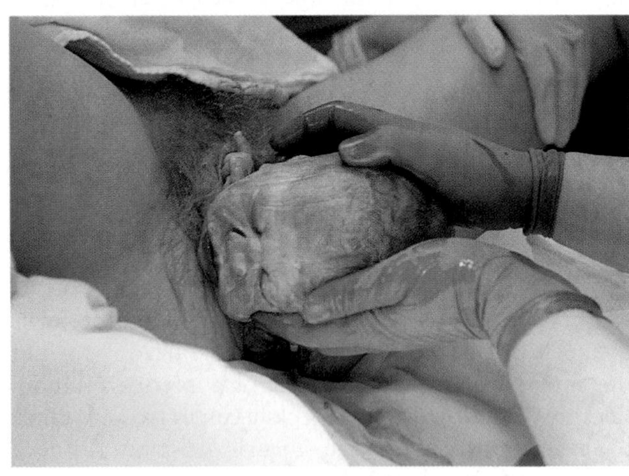
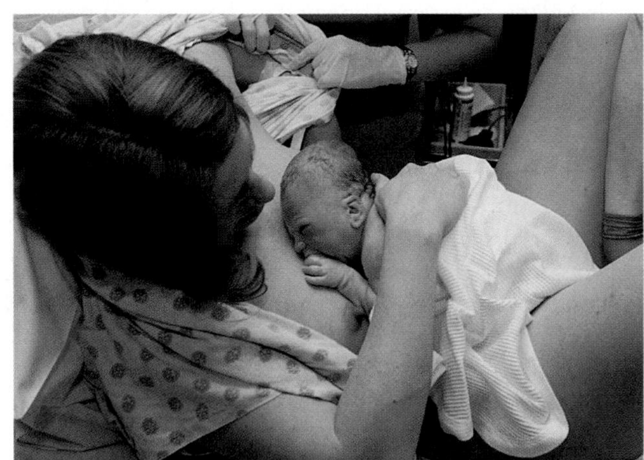

FIGURE 18–11 The birth sequence.

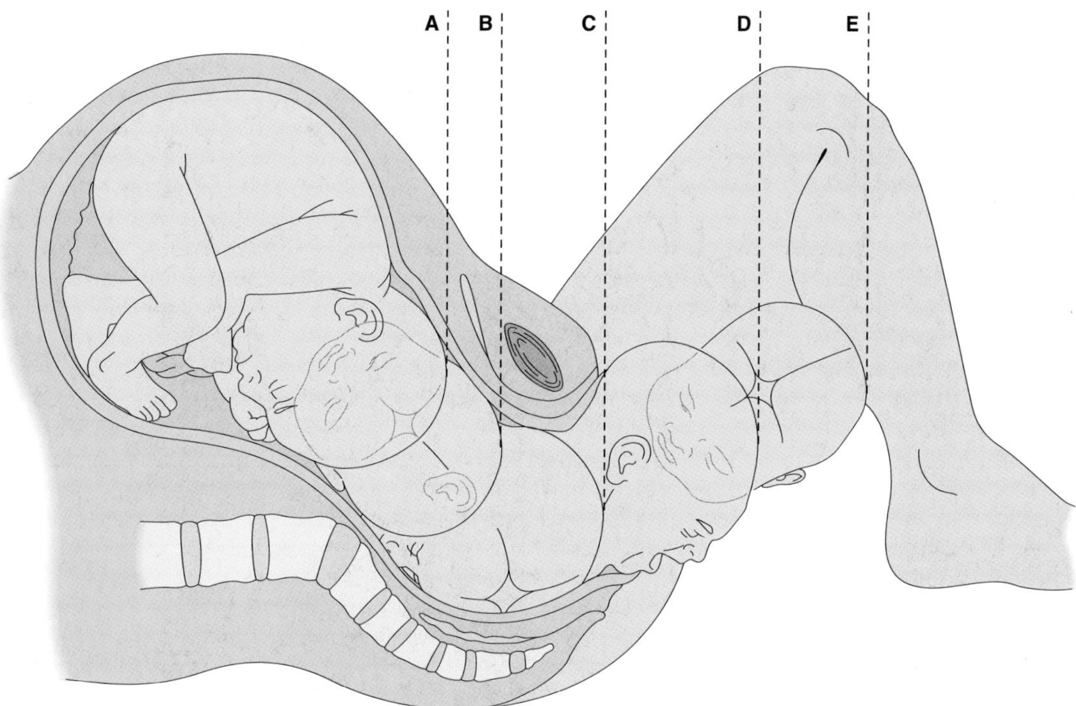

FIGURE 18–12 Mechanisms of labor. ***A, B,*** Descent. ***C,*** Internal rotation. ***D,*** Extension. ***E,*** External rotation.

shoulder meets the under surface of the symphysis pubis and slips under it. As lateral flexion of the shoulder and head occurs, the anterior shoulder is born before the posterior shoulder. The body follows quickly. The adaptations of the newborn to extrauterine life are discussed in Chapter 24.

Third Stage

Placental Separation

After the infant is born the uterus contracts firmly, diminishing its capacity and the surface area of placental attachment. The placenta begins to separate because of this decrease in surface area. As this separation occurs, bleeding occurs, leading to the formation of a hematoma between the placental tissue and the remaining decidua. This hematoma accelerates the separation process. The membranes are the last to separate. They are peeled off the uterine wall as the placenta descends into the vagina.

Signs of placental separation usually appear around 5 minutes after birth of the infant. These signs are (1) a globular-shaped uterus, (2) a rise of the fundus in the abdomen, (3) a sudden gush or trickle of blood, and (4) further protrusion of the umbilical cord out of the vagina.

Placental Delivery

When the signs of placental separation appear, the woman may bear down to aid in placental expulsion. If this fails and the certified nurse-midwife/physician has ascertained that the fundus is firm, gentle traction may be applied to the cord while pressure is exerted on the fundus. The weight of the placenta as it is guided into the placental pan (a basin that holds the placenta once it is expelled) aids in the removal of the membranes from the uterine wall. A placenta is considered to be *retained* if 30 minutes have elapsed from completion of the second stage of labor.

If the placenta separates from the inside to the outer margins, it is expelled with the fetal (shiny) side presenting (Figure 18–13). This is known as the *Schultze mechanism* of placental delivery or more commonly *shiny Schultze.* If the placenta separates from the outer margins inward, it will roll up and present sideways with the maternal surface delivering first. This is known as the *Duncan mechanism* of placental delivery and is commonly called *dirty Duncan* because the placental surface is rough.

Nursing and medical interventions during the third stage of labor are discussed in Chapter 20.

Fourth Stage

The fourth stage of labor is the time from 1 to 4 hours after birth in which physiologic readjustment of the mother's body begins. With the birth hemodynamic changes occur. Blood loss at birth ranges from 250 to 500 mL. With this blood loss and the easing of pressure exerted by the pregnant uterus on the surrounding vessels, blood is redistributed into venous beds. This results in a moderate drop in both systolic and diastolic blood pressure, increased pulse pressure, and moderate tachycardia (Cunningham et al, 1997).

The uterus remains contracted and is in the midline of the abdomen. The fundus is usually midway between

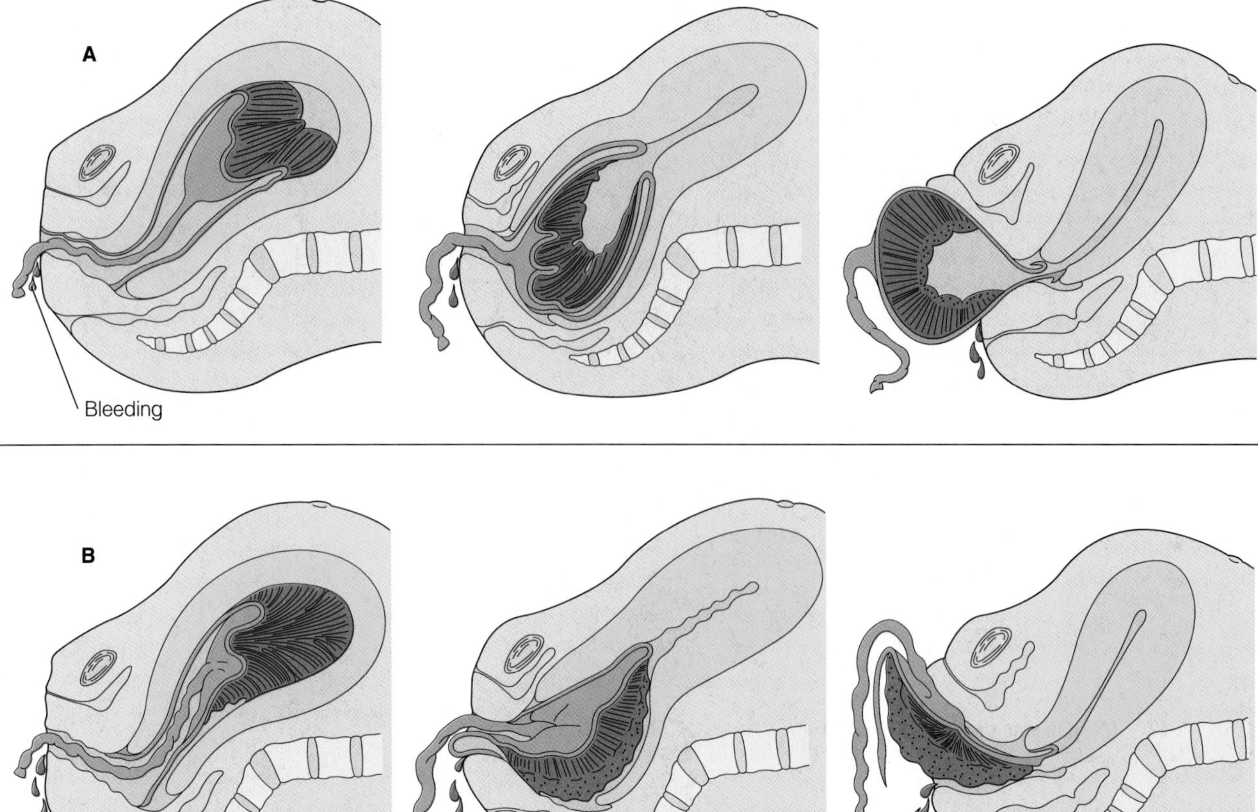

FIGURE 18–13 Placental separation and expulsion. ***A,*** Schultze mechanism. ***B,*** Duncan mechanism.

the symphysis pubis and umbilicus. Its contracted state constricts the vessels at the site of placental implantation. Immediately after birth of the placenta, the cervix is widely spread and thick.

Nausea and vomiting experienced during transition usually cease. The woman may be thirsty and hungry. She may experience a shaking chill, which is thought to be associated with the ending of the physical exertion of labor. The bladder is often hypotonic due to trauma during the second stage and/or the administration of anesthetics that may decrease sensations. Hypotonic bladder leads to urinary retention. Nursing care of this stage is discussed in Chapter 20.

I have had the privilege of practicing nursing in the birthing area for many years. In my head I know all the factors that must work together to bring this new life into the world. But it is in my heart and in working with and watching the laboring woman (and her partner if she has one), that I truly believe each labor and birth is a miracle. I, along with these parents, get to participate in a moment of time that will never occur again for any of us. I will never tire of this, will never get enough.

Maternal Systemic Response to Labor

Cardiovascular System

The woman's cardiovascular system is stressed both by the uterine contractions and by the pain, anxiety, and apprehension the woman experiences. During labor there is a significant increase in cardiac output. Each strong contraction greatly decreases or completely stops the blood flow in the branches of the uterine artery that supply the intervillous space (in the placenta). This leads to a redistribution of about 300 to 500 mL of blood into the peripheral circulation and an increase in peripheral resistance, resulting in increased systolic and diastolic blood pressure, a slowing of the pulse rate, and an increase of about 31% in cardiac output (Blackburn & Loper, 1992).

Maternal position also affects cardiac output, blood pressure, and pulse. When the laboring woman turns to a side-lying position, cardiac output increases by about 22%, the pulse rate decreases by about 6 beats per minute, and stroke volume increases by 27%. When the woman is supine, cardiac output increases 25%, stroke volume increases 33%, pulse pressure increases more than 26%, blood pressure rises significantly, and pulse rate decreases by 15%.

There is an additional effect on hemodynamics during the bearing down efforts in the second stage. When the laboring woman holds her breath and pushes against a closed glottis (Valsalva maneuver), intrathoracic pressure rises. As intrathoracic pressure increases, the venous return is interrupted, increasing venous pressure. In addition the blood in the lungs is forced into the left atrium, which leads to a transient increase in cardiac output, blood pressure, and pulse pressure, and causes bradycardia. As venous return to the lungs continues to be diminished while the breath is held, a decrease in blood pressure, pulse pressure, and cardiac output occurs.

When the next breath is taken (Valsalva maneuver is interrupted), the intrathoracic pressure is decreased. Venous return increases, refilling the pulmonary bed and resulting in recovery of the cardiac output and stroke volume. This process is repeated with each pushing effort.

Immediately after birth cardiac output peaks with an 80% increase over prelabor values. Then in the first 10 minutes it decreases 20% to 25%. Cardiac output further decreases in the first hour after the birth. However, these decreases still leave the woman with an elevated cardiac output for at least 24 hours after the birth.

Blood Pressure

As a result of increased cardiac output, systolic blood pressure rises during uterine contractions. In the first stage, systolic pressure may increase by 35 mm Hg, and there may be further increases in the second stage during pushing efforts. Diastolic pressure also increases by about 25 mm Hg in the first stage and 65 mm Hg in the second stage. These increases begin just before the uterine contraction, with a return to baseline as soon as the contraction ends (Blackburn & Loper, 1992).

Blood pressure may drop precipitously when the woman lies in a supine position and experiences aortocaval compression. In addition to hypotension there is an increase in the pulse rate, diaphoresis, nausea, weakness, and air hunger. These changes are attributed to the decreased cardiac output and a subsequent drop in stroke volume.

Women with the highest risk of developing aortocaval compression are women with hydramnios, multiple gestation, and obese women. Other predisposing factors include hypovolemia, dehydration, hemorrhage, metabolic acidosis, administration of narcotics (which results in vasodilation and inhibits compensatory mechanisms), and administration of epidural anesthesia, which results in *sympathetic blockade* (blocking of the sympathetic nervous system, leading to vasodilation and hypotension).

Fluid and Electrolyte Balance

Profuse perspiration (diaphoresis) occurs during labor. Hyperventilation also occurs, altering electrolyte and fluid balance from insensible water loss. The muscle activity elevates the body temperature, which increases sweating and evaporation from the skin. As the woman responds to the work of labor, the rise in the respiratory rate increases the evaporative water volume because each breath of air must be warmed to the body temperature and humidified. With the increased evaporative water volume, maintaining adequate oral fluids/hydration is important. In some instances parenteral (IV) fluids are administered.

Respiratory System

Oxygen demand and consumption increase at the onset of labor because of the presence of uterine contractions. As anxiety and pain from uterine contractions increase, hyperventilation frequently occurs. With hyperventilation there is a fall in $PaCO_2$, and respiratory alkalosis results (Blackburn & Loper, 1992).

As labor progresses and contractions become more frequent, stronger, and prolonged, the work load, tension, and anxiety of the woman continue to change (Blackburn & Loper, 1992).

By the end of the first stage most women have developed a mild metabolic acidosis compensated by respiratory alkalosis. As she pushes in the second stage of labor, the woman's $PaCO_2$ levels may rise along with blood lactate levels (due to muscular activity), and mild respiratory acidosis occurs. By the time the baby is born (end of second stage) there is metabolic acidosis uncompensated by respiratory alkalosis (Blackburn & Loper, 1992).

The changes in acid-base status that occur in labor are quickly reversed in the fourth stage because of changes in the woman's respiratory rate. Acid-base levels return to pregnancy levels by 24 hours after birth, and nonpregnant values are attained a few weeks after birth (Blackburn & Loper, 1992).

Renal System

During labor there is an increase in maternal renin, plasma renin activity, and angiotensinogen. This elevation is thought to be important in the control of uteroplacental blood flow during birth and the early postpartal period (Blackburn & Loper, 1992).

Structurally, the base of the bladder is pushed forward and upward when engagement occurs. The pressure from the presenting part may impair blood and lymph drainage from the base of the bladder, leading to edema of the tissues (Cunningham et al, 1997).

Gastrointestinal System

During labor gastric motility and absorption of solid food are reduced. Gastric emptying time is prolonged, and gastric volume (amount of contents that remain in the stomach) remains over 25 mL, regardless of the time the last meal was taken. The acidity of the gastric contents increases, and more than half of laboring women have a gastric pH less than 2.5 (Blackburn & Loper, 1992).

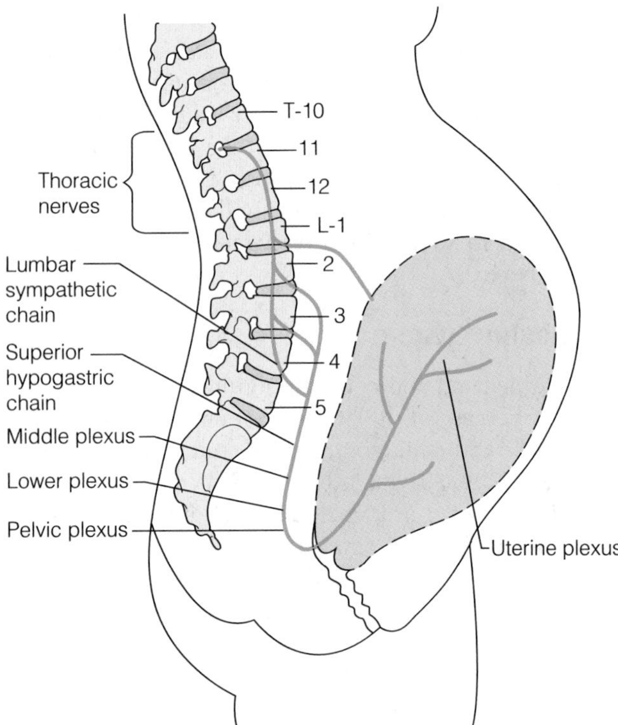

FIGURE 18–14 Pain pathway from uterus to spinal cord. Nerve impulses travel through the uterine plexus, pelvic plexus, inferior hypogastric plexus, middle and superior hypogastric plexus, and lumbar sympathetic chain, and they enter the neuroaxis through the 10th, 11th, and 12th thoracic and 1st lumbar spinal segments. SOURCE: Modified from Bonica, J. J.: *Principles and Practice of Obstetric Analgesia and Anesthesia.* Philadelphia: Davis, 1972, p 492.

Some narcotics also delay gastric emptying time and add to the risk of aspiration should general anesthesia need to be used (Blackburn & Loper, 1992).

The fluid requirements of women in labor have not been clearly established. In some instances oral hydration is the primary goal. In other situations a heparin lock may be inserted so that intravenous access is available if needed. If intravenous fluids are used, it is important to remember that when hypertonic glucose infusions are used, there is an increase in maternal blood glucose; this can lead to fetal hyperglycemia and hyperinsulinemia and to hypoglycemia in the newborn (Blackburn & Loper, 1992).

Immune System and Other Blood Values

The white blood cell (WBC) count increases to 25,000/mm^3 to 30,000/mm^3 during labor and early postpartum (Kuhlmann & Cruikshank, 1994). The change in WBC count is due mostly to increased neutrophils resulting from a physiologic response to stress. The increased WBC count makes it difficult to identify the presence of an infectious process.

Maternal blood glucose levels decrease because glucose is used as an energy source during uterine contractions. The decreased blood glucose levels lead to a decrease in insulin requirements (Blackburn & Loper, 1992).

Pain

Theories of Pain

According to the *gate-control theory*, pain results from activity in several interacting specialized neural systems. The gate-control theory proposes that a mechanism in the dorsal horn of the spinal column serves as a valve or gate that increases or decreases the flow of nerve impulses from the periphery to the central nervous system. The gate mechanism is influenced by the size of the transmitting fibers and by the nerve impulses that descend from the brain. Psychologic processes such as past experiences, attention, and emotion may influence pain perception and response by activating the gate mechanism. The gates may be opened or closed by central nervous system activities, such as anxiety or excitement, or through selective localized activity.

The gate-control theory has two important implications for childbirth: Pain may be controlled by tactile stimulation and can be modified by activities controlled by the central nervous system. These include back rub, sacral pressure, effleurage, suggestion, distraction, and conditioning.

Pain During Labor

The pain associated with the first stage of labor is unique in that it accompanies a normal physiologic process. Even though perception of the pain of childbirth is greatly determined by cultural patterning, there is a physiologic basis for discomfort during labor. Pain during the first stage of labor arises from (1) dilatation of the cervix, (2) hypoxia of the uterine muscle cells during contraction, (3) stretching of the lower uterine segment, and (4) pressure on adjacent structures. The primary source of pain is dilatation or stretching of the cervix. Nerve impulses travel through the uterine plexus, inferior hypogastric (pelvic) plexus, middle hypogastric plexus, superior hypogastric plexus, and lumbar sympathetic and lower thoracic chain and enter the spinal cord through the posterior roots of the 12th, 11th, and 10th thoracic and 1st lumbar nerves (Figure 18–14). As with other visceral pain, pain from the uterus is referred to the dermatomes supplied by the 12th, 11th, and 10th thoracic nerves. The areas of referred pain include the lower abdominal wall and the areas over the lower lumbar region and the upper sacrum (Figure 18–15).

During the second stage of labor discomfort is due to (1) hypoxia of the contracting uterine muscle cells, (2) distention of the vagina and perineum, and (3) pressure on adjacent structures. The nerve impulses from the vagina and perineum are transmitted by way of the pudendal nerve plexus and enter the spinal cord through the

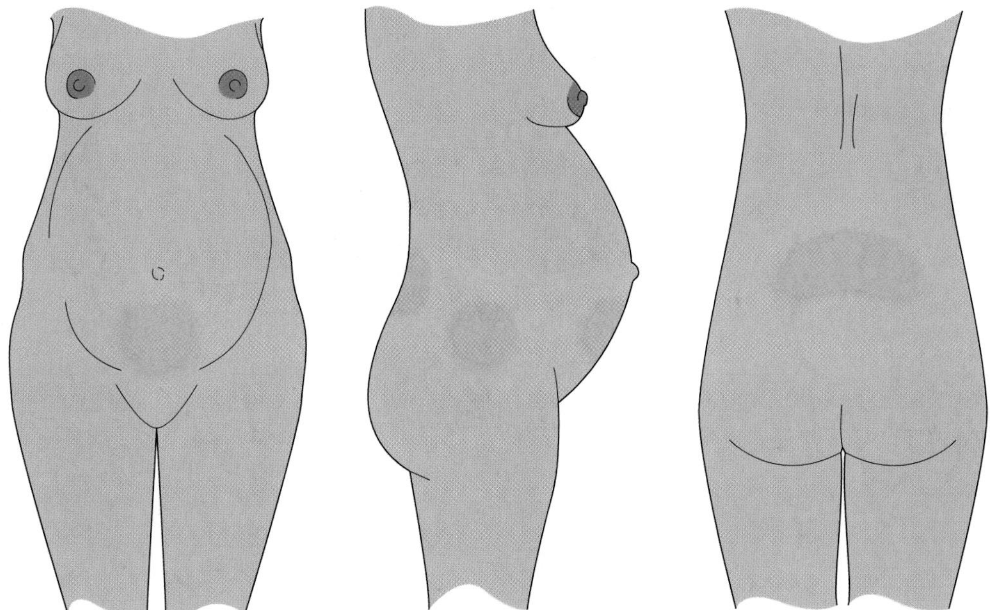

FIGURE 18–15 Area of reference of labor pain during the first stage. Pain is most intense in the darker colored areas. SOURCE: Bonica, J. J.: *Principles and Practice of Obstetric Analgesia and Anesthesia.* Philadelphia: Davis, 1972, p 108.

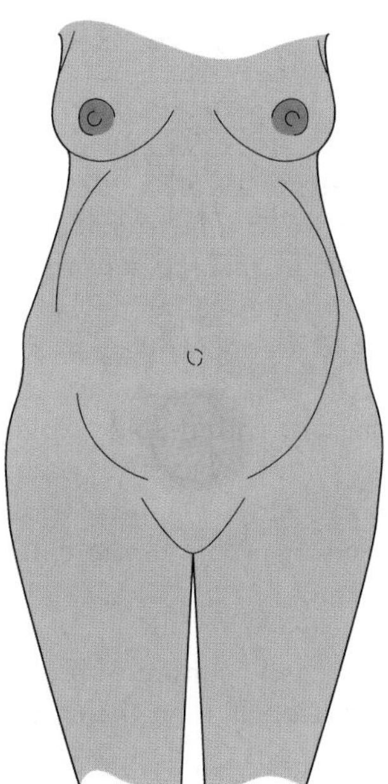

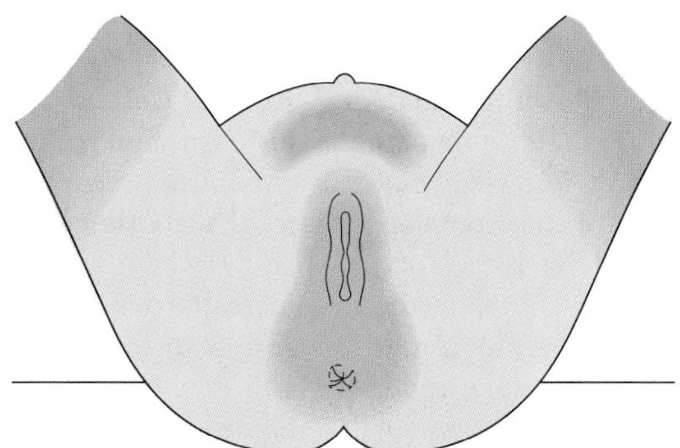

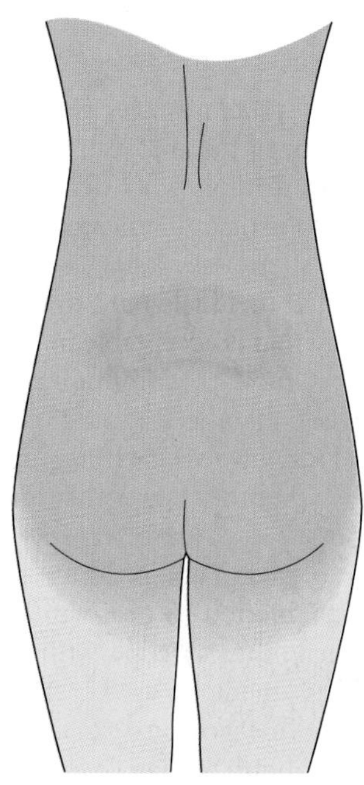

FIGURE 18–16 Distribution of labor pain during the later phase of the first stage and early phase of the second stage. The darkest colored areas indicate the location of the most intense pain; moderate color, moderate pain; and light color, mild pain. The uterine contractions, which at this stage are very strong, produce intense pain. SOURCE: Bonica, J. J.: *Principles and Practice of Obstetric Analgesia and Anesthesia.* Philadelphia: Davis, 1972, p 109.

posterior roots of the 2nd, 3rd, and 4th sacral nerves. The area of pain increases as shown in Figure 18–16.

Pain during the third stage results from uterine contractions and cervical dilatation as the placenta is expelled (Figure 18–17). The mechanism for the transmission of nerve impulses is the same as for the first stage of labor. The third stage of labor is short, and after this phase anesthesia is needed primarily for episiotomy repair.

Factors Affecting Response to Pain

Many factors affect the individual's perception of pain impulses. Some psychologic and environmental influences particularly appropriate to labor are discussed here.

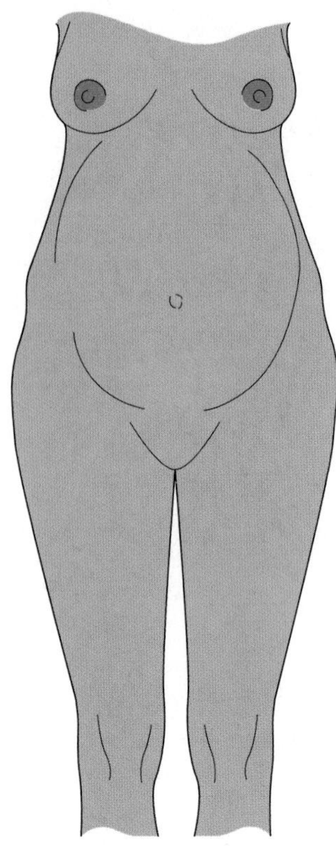
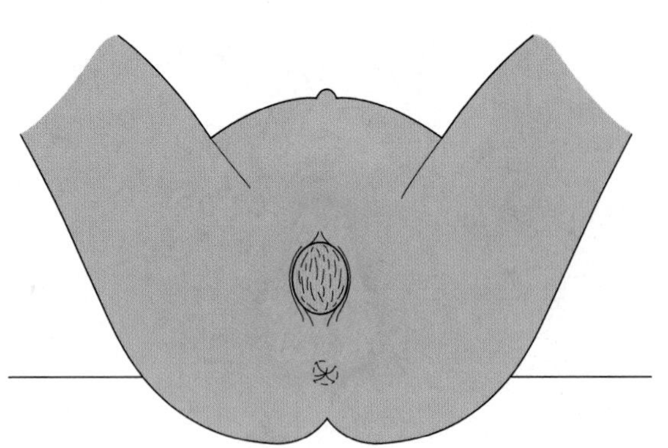
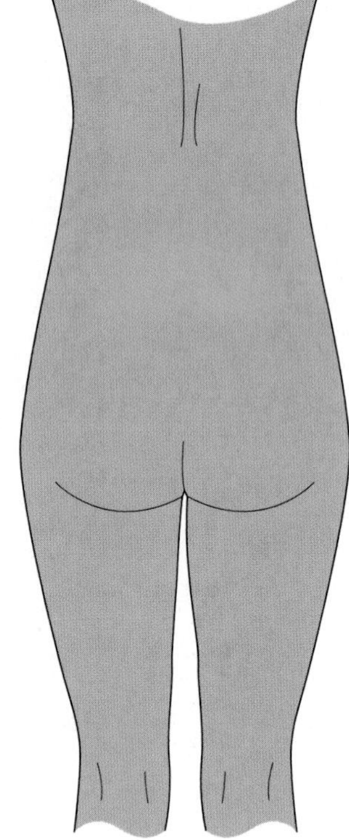

FIGURE 18–17 Distribution of labor pain during the later phase of the second stage and actual birth. The perineal component is the primary cause of discomfort. Uterine contractions contribute much less. SOURCE: Bonica, J. J.: *Principles and Practice of Obstetric Analgesia and Anesthesia.* Philadelphia: Davis, 1972, p 109.

Preparation for childbirth has been shown to reduce the need for analgesia during labor. Lowe (1996) reports that women who demonstrated greater knowledge of childbirth and indicated higher confidence after completing the classes reported a less painful childbirth.

Individuals tend to respond to painful stimuli in the way that is acceptable in their culture. In some cultures, it is natural to communicate pain, no matter how mild, while members of other cultures stoically accept pain out of fear or because it is expected (Weber, 1996).

Another factor that may influence response to pain is *fatigue and sleep deprivation.* The fatigued woman has less energy and ability to use such strategies as distraction or imagination to deal with pain. As a result, she may lose her ability to cope with labor and choose analgesics or other medications to relieve the discomfort.

The woman's *previous experience* with pain also affects her ability to manage current and future pain. Those who have had experience with pain seem more sensitive to painful stimuli than those who have not.

Anxiety can affect a woman's response to pain. Unfamiliar surroundings and events can increase anxiety, as does separation from family and loved ones. Anticipation of discomfort and questions about whether she can cope with the contractions may also increase anxiety.

Both attention and distraction have an influence on the perception of pain. When pain sensation is the focus of attention, the perceived intensity is greater. A sensory stimulus such as a back rub can be a distraction that focuses the woman's attention on the stimulus rather than the pain.

Effect of Childbirth Education Preparing for labor and birth through reading, talking with others, or attending a childbirth preparation class frequently has positive effects for the laboring woman and her partner. The woman who knows what to expect and what techniques she may use to increase comfort tends to be less anxious during the labor. A tour of the birthing center and an opportunity to see and feel the environment also help reduce anxiety because during admission (especially with the first child) many new things are happening and they seem to occur all at once. The more the woman and her partner learn during classes and through their own efforts, the more likely they will reduce some anxiety.

Cultural Background As part of the culture of health care, nursing and medical professionals have their own (collective and individual) expectations of the woman in labor and those who support her. In some settings, the woman is expected to use a breathing technique and relaxation methods, while in other areas most women receive an epidural block, which removes the need for breathing techniques. Value is placed on maintaining self-control and knowing what to expect during labor and birth. Some nurses may believe that the woman and her support persons should take care of themselves and ask for assistance only if really necessary; other nurses may believe that frequent interaction and support are essential as long as the woman and her support persons are comfortable with the interaction.

It is important to know that the health care professional is most likely to interpret pain according to the norms of the health care culture, although various other cultures have different ways of responding to pain. The absence of crying and moaning does not necessarily mean that pain is absent, nor does the presence of crying and moaning necessarily mean that pain relief is desired at that moment. It is very important for the nurse to accept and respect the fact that the pain is whatever the woman says it is and to assist her in decreasing it.

Fetal Response to Labor

When the fetus is normal, the mechanical and hemodynamic changes of normal labor have no adverse effects.

Heart Rate Changes

Fetal heart rate decelerations can occur with intracranial pressures of 40 to 55 mm Hg. The currently accepted explanation of this early deceleration is hypoxic depression of the central nervous system, which is under vagal control. The absence of these head compression decelerations (early decelerations) in some fetuses during labor is explained by the existence of a threshold that is reached more gradually in the presence of intact membranes and lack of maternal resistance. Early decelerations are harmless in the normal fetus.

Acid-Base Status in Labor

The blood flow to the fetus is slowed during the acme of the contraction, which leads to a slow decrease in the fetal pH. During the second stage, as uterine contractions become stronger and last longer and the woman pushes with each contraction, there is a more rapid decrease in fetal pH. There is also an increase in fetal base deficit and in Pco_2, and a drop in fetal oxygen saturation of about 10% (Creasy & Resnik, 1997).

Fetal Movements

When the fetus is between 35 and 40 weeks, episodes of fetal breathing movements increase in the second and third hour following the mother's meals. There is also a marked increase during the night while the mother is asleep, which is thought to be part of a circadian rhythm in fetal breathing activity. In the healthy term fetus there are periods of no breathing movements that last up to 2 hours. It has been noted that the incidence of fetal breathing movements slows markedly and may cease about 3 days before the onset of spontaneous labor (Creasy & Resnik, 1997).

Behavior States

The human fetus develops behavioral states between 36 and 38 weeks of gestation. The behavioral states seem to continue during labor even in the presence of uterine contractions. Two sleep states (quiet and active) are most prevalent, although quiet and active awake states are occasionally observed. A decrease in fetal heart rate variability accompanies the quiet sleep state, and there is also a decrease in fetal breathing movements and other general body activity. The quiet sleep state generally lasts less than 40 minutes.

Hemodynamic Changes

The adequate exchange of nutrients and gases in the fetal capillaries and intervillous spaces depends in part on the fetal blood pressure. Fetal blood pressure is a protective mechanism for the normal fetus during the anoxic periods caused by the contracting uterus during labor. The fetal and placental reserve is enough to see the fetus through these anoxic periods unharmed (Creasy & Resnik, 1997).

FOCUS YOUR STUDY

- Four factors that continually interact during labor and birth are the birth passage, the fetus, the forces of labor (contractions and pushing effort), and factors associated with the woman's psychosocial status.
- Four types of pelves have been identified, and each has a different effect on labor. The diameters of gynecoid and anthropoid pelves are usually large enough for labor and birth to progress normally. In the android and platypelloid types the pelvic diameters are diminished (smaller than in gynecoid and anthropoid), and labor is more likely to be difficult (longer) and a cesarean birth is more likely.
- Important dimensions of the maternal pelvis include the diameters of the pelvic inlet, pelvic cavity, and pelvic outlet.
- The fetal head contains bones in the top portion (cranial vault) that are not fused. This allows them to overlap somewhat in response to the pressures on the fetal head during labor. The pressure and overlapping of the sutures, which are membranous spaces between the cranial bones, result in a change in the shape of the head called molding.
- Fetal attitude refers to the relation of the fetal parts to one another. The head is usually held in midline and not to one side or the other, and the extremities are usually flexed and held close to the body because there is little extra room within the uterine cavity.
- Fetal lie refers to the relationship of the cephalocaudal (head to sacral area) axis of the fetus to the maternal spine. The fetal lie is either longitudinal (both the maternal and fetal spines are vertical) or transverse (the fetal spine is at a right angle to the maternal spine).
- Fetal presentation is determined by the body part lying closest to the inlet of the maternal pelvis. In a longitudinal lie the fetal presentation is usually cephalic (head first) but may also be breech (buttocks or one or both feet first). In a transverse lie the presentation is called transverse, and the fetal shoulder is usually closest to the pelvic inlet.
- Fetal position is the relationship of a specified landmark on the presenting fetal part to the sides, front, or back of the maternal pelvis. Once the position is known, the positions of the fetal head and back can be determined.
- Engagement of the presenting part occurs when the largest diameter of the fetal presenting part reaches or passes through the pelvic inlet.

- Station refers to the relationship of the presenting part to an imaginary line drawn between the maternal ischial spines, which are in the midpoint of the pelvic cavity. The fetal presenting part enters the pelvic inlet at what is termed about a −5 and descends toward the ischial spines, where it is called a 0 (zero) station. Further descent from 0 to +4 occurs as the presenting part descends below the ischial spines toward the vaginal opening.
- Each uterine contraction has an increment, acme, and decrement. Contraction frequency is the time from the beginning of one contraction to the beginning of the next contraction.
- Duration of contractions refers to the period of time from the beginning to the end of one contraction.
- Intensity of contractions refers to the strength of the contraction during acme. Intensity of contractions is termed mild, moderate, or strong.
- Labor stresses the coping skills of women. Women with prenatal education about childbirth usually report more positive responses to labor.
- Possible causes of labor onset include the progesterone withdrawal hypothesis, the prostaglandin hypothesis, and the corticortropin-releasing hormone hypothesis.
- Factors that affect the response to labor pain include education, cultural beliefs, fatigue and sleep deprivation, personal significance of pain, previous experience, anxiety, and the availability of coping techniques.
- Premonitory signs of labor include lightening, Braxton Hicks contractions, cervical softening and effacement, bloody show, sudden burst of energy, weight loss, and sometimes rupture of membranes.
- True labor contractions occur regularly with an increase in frequency, duration, and intensity. The contractions usually start in the back and radiate around the abdomen. The discomfort is not relieved by ambulation. False labor contractions do not produce progressive cervical effacement and dilatation. They are irregular and do not increase in intensity. The discomfort may be relieved by ambulation.
- There are four stages of labor and birth. The first stage is from beginning of true labor to complete dilatation of the cervix. The second stage is from complete dilatation of the cervix to birth. The third stage is from birth to expulsion of the placenta. The fourth stage is from expulsion of the placenta to a period of 1 to 4 hours after.
- Placental separation is indicated by lengthening of the umbilical cord, a small spurt of blood, change in uterine shape, and a rise of the fundus in the abdomen.
- The placenta is expelled by Schultze or Duncan mechanism. This is determined by the way it separates from the uterine wall.
- The fetus accommodates to the maternal pelvis in a series of movements called the cardinal movements of labor, which include descent, flexion, internal rotation, extension, restitution, external rotation, and expulsion.
- Maternal systemic responses to labor involve the cardiovascular, respiratory, renal, gastrointestinal, and immune systems.
- The fetus is usually able to tolerate the labor process with no untoward changes.

REFERENCES

Blackburn, S. T., & Loper, D. L. (1992). *Maternal, fetal and neonatal physiology.* Philadelphia: Saunders.

Challis, J. R. G. (1994). Characteristics of parturition. In R. K. Creasy & R. R. Resnik (Eds.), *Maternal-fetal medicine* (3rd ed.). Philadelphia: Saunders.

Creasy, R. K., & Resnik, R. R. (1997). *Maternal-fetal medicine* (4th ed.). Philadelphia: Saunders.

Creehan, P. A. (1996). Pain relief and comfort measures during labor. In K. R. Simpson & P. A. Creehan (Eds.), *AWHONN perinatal nursing* (pp 227–246). Philadelphia: Lippincott.

Crowe, K., & Baeyer, C. (1989, June). Predictors of a positive childbirth experience. *Birth, 16,* 2.

Cunningham, F. G., MacDonald, P. C., Gant, N. F., Leveno, K. J., Gilstrap, L. C., Hankins, D. V., & Clark, S. L. (1997). *Williams obstetrics* (20th ed.). Stamford, CT: Appleton & Lange.

DiMatteo, M. R., Kahn, K. L., & Berry, S. H. (1993, Dec.). Narratives of birth and the postpartum: Analysis of the focus group responses of new mothers. *Birth, 20*(4), 204.

Khazoyan, C. M., & Anderson, N. L. R. (1994). Latinas' expectations for their partners during childbirth. *Maternal-Child Nursing Journal, 19*(4), 226.

Kuhlmann, R. S., & Cruikshank, D. P. (1994). Maternal trauma during pregnancy. *Clinical Obstetrics and Gynecology, 37*(2), 274.

Lederman, R. P. (1996). *Psychosocial adaptation in pregnancy: Assessment of seven dimensions of maternal development* (2nd ed.). New York: Springer.

Liggins, G. C. (1997). Biology of parturition. In R. K. Creasy (Ed.), *Management of labor and delivery.* Malden, MA: Blackwell.

Lowe, N. K. (1996). The pain and discomfort of labor and birth. *Journal of Obstetric, Gynecologic, and Neonatal Nursing, 25*(1), 82–92.

McKay, S., & Smith, S. Y. (1993). "What are they talking about? Is something wrong?" Information sharing during the second stage of labor. *Birth, 20*(3), 142.

Mercer, R. T. (1995). *Becoming a mother.* New York: Springer.

Nathanielsz, P. W. (1994). A time to be born: Implications of animal studies in maternal-fetal medicine. *Birth, 21*(3), 163.

Nichols, F. H., & Humenick, S. S. (1988). *Childbirth education: Practice, research, and theory.* Philadelphia: Saunders.

Nichols, M. R. (1993). Paternal perspectives of the childbirth experience. *MCN: American Journal of Maternal Child Nursing, 21*(3), 99.

Rubin, R. (1984). *Maternal identity and the maternal experience.* New York: Springer.

Smith, R. (1999). Corticotrophin-releasing hormone and the fetoplacental clock: An Australian perspective. *American Journal of Obstetrics and Gynecology, 180,* s269–s271.

Tomlinson, P. S., & Bryan, A. A. (1996). Family centered intrapartum care: Revisiting an old concept. *Journal of Obstetric, Gynecologic, and Neonatal Nursing, 25*(4), 331–337.

Ueland, K., & Ferguson, J. E. (1990). Cardiorespiratory physiology of pregnancy. In R. Depp, D. A. Eschenbach, & J. J. Sciarra (Eds.), *Gynecology and Obstetrics* (Vol. 3). Philadelphia: Lippincott.

Walker, L. O., & Montgomery, E. (1994). Maternal identity and role attainment: Long-term relations to children's development. *Nursing Research, 43*(2), 105.

Weber, S. E. (1996). Cultural aspects of pain in childbearing women. *Journal of Obstetric, Gynecologic, and Neonatal Nursing, 25*(1), 67–72.

Zlatnik, F. J. (1994). Normal labor and delivery and its conduct. In J. R. Scott, P. J. DiSaia, C. B. Hammond, & W. N. Spellacy, *Danforth's obstetrics and gynecology* (7th ed.). Philadelphia: Lippincott.

Intrapartal Nursing Assessment

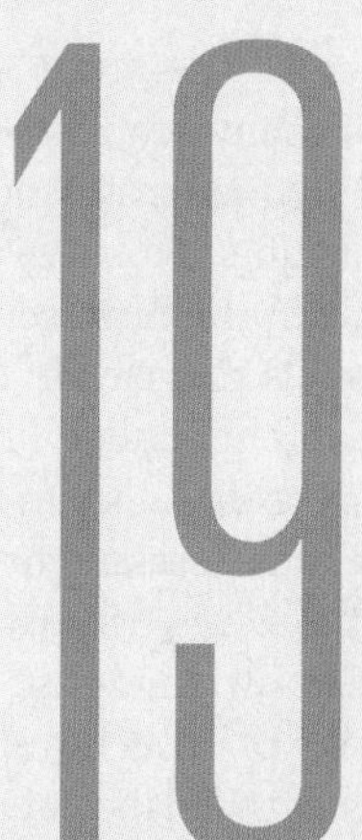

WE KNEW THAT EVERYTHING WAS GOING OK AND that I was making progress, but it was so good to have our nurse come check me to see if I was dilating. It was not very comfortable, but he was as gentle as he could be, and when he told me that I had dilated another two centimeters, I felt that I could keep going on. It was nice for us to know that the birth was getting closer with every contraction.

Objectives

- Summarize intrapartal physical, psychosocial, and cultural assessments necessary for optimum maternal-fetal outcome.
- Define and identify the outer limits of normal progress of each of the phases and stages of labor.
- Compare the various methods of monitoring fetal heart rate and contractions, giving advantages and disadvantages of each.
- Differentiate between baseline and periodic changes in the FHR, and describe the criteria and significance of each.
- Outline the steps to be performed in the systematic evaluation of fetal heart rate tracings, and list factors to consider in evaluation of abnormal findings.
- Identify nonreassuring fetal heart rate patterns and the interventions that should be carried out in the management of each.
- Delineate the indications for fetal blood sampling and guidelines for managing labor for related pH values.
- Discuss information to be taught to the woman and family when electronic fetal monitoring is used, and provide rationale for teaching.
- Discuss the woman's and family's reactions to electronic fetal monitoring and the role of the nurse.

Key Terms

Accelerations
Baseline rate
Baseline variability
Decelerations
Fetal scalp blood sample
Intrauterine catheter
Leopold's maneuvers
Long-term variability (LTV)
Scalp stimulation test
Short-term variability (STV)

THE PHYSIOLOGIC EVENTS THAT OCCUR during labor call for many adaptations by the mother and fetus. Accurate and frequent assessment is crucial because the changes are rapid and involve two individuals, mother and child. The nurse in the birth setting uses a wide variety of assessment skills to provide care for two primary clients, the mother and her child. The expectant mother's partner or support person is also an important part of the birthing experience, and assessments of the couple's coping, interactions, and teamwork are also integral parts of the birthing nurse's knowledge base regarding the family. Nurses use their skills of observation, palpation, and auscultation to ascertain that labor remains within normal parameters. The nurse's physical presence with the laboring woman provides the best opportunity for ongoing assessment, even as the nurse quietly provides comfort measures and gently assists the "coach" in offering support.

In current practice, "hands-on" techniques can be augmented by the use of technology. For example, the nurse or clinician can use Doppler ultrasound to listen to the fetal heart rate (FHR) or an electronic fetal monitor to assist in recording contractions and the FHR. No matter what additional technology is used, however, it is important that the nurse remember that the technology ("the machine" or "the test") only provides information; it is the nurse who monitors the mother and her child. In the birth setting that provides "high touch" nursing care, the "high tech" assessments are easily integrated to provide comprehensive, high-quality care.

This chapter presents the assessments that are an important part of the nursing care in the birth setting.

Maternal Assessment

History

The woman's physiologic history may be obtained in an abbreviated format when the woman is admitted to the labor and birth area. Each agency has its own admission form, but similar information is usually obtained. Relevant data include the following:

- Name and age
- Attending physician or certified nurse-midwife (CNM)
- Personal data: blood type; Rh factor; results of serology testing; HIV testing, Rubella titer; group B streptococci testing; maternal serum alphafetoprotein (MSAFP) testing; prepregnant and present weight; allergies to medications, foods, or substances; and drug and alcohol consumption during pregnancy
- History of previous illness, such as tuberculosis, heart disease, diabetes, convulsive disorders, thyroid disorders
- Problems in the prenatal course, for example, elevated blood pressure, bleeding problems, recurrent urinary tract infection
- Pregnancy data: gravida, para, abortions, term and preterm infants, number of living children, neonatal deaths
- The method chosen for infant feeding
- Type of prenatal education (childbirth preparation classes)
- Requests regarding labor and birth (no enema, no analgesics or anesthetic, father or other support persons in attendance, and so on)
- History of special tests such as nonstress test (NST) or ultrasound and reasons for test administration
- History of any preterm labor requiring tocolytic therapy and corticosteriod
- Pediatrician/family practice physician
- Onset of labor
- Status of amniotic fluid membranes (intact or spontaneously ruptured); time of rupture is critical to group B streptococci (GBS) protocol
- Brief description of previous labor and birth and history of previous infant treated for neonatal infection (see GBS protocol)

Assessment of psychosocial history is a critical component of intrapartal nursing assessment. Because of the prevalence of sexual violence against women in our society (reported incidence is one in three women, regardless of age), the nurse needs to consider the possibility that the woman may have experienced sexual violence at some point in her life. If such is the case, she may be anxious about the labor process, or anxiety may arise during labor. The nurse begins the assessment by reviewing the woman's prenatal record and any previous chart that is available for information that may indicate abuse. In reviewing the records, the nurse keeps in mind questions such as the following:

- Has the woman experienced rape or sexual abuse?
- Does the prenatal record or other admission notes contain any information regarding bruises, teeth marks, or burns to the breasts, abdomen, or genitals? (Note: These areas of the body are frequent targets of abuse during pregnancy.)
- Are there notes of bruising, burns, cuts, teeth marks on upper arms, mutilation of the genitalia, clumps of hair missing, dental trauma, or history of broken bones? Does the woman have a history of increased anxiety, insomnia, frequent headaches, choking sensations, depression, or suicide attempts? Does the prenatal record indicate low weight gain, late entry into prenatal care, or frequent missed appointments?

The presence of any of these factors provides a clue for the nurse that the woman may still be in an abusive relationship. The nurse needs to conduct the psychosocial history interview in private with only the nurse and the woman present. The partner (male or female) should not be present, nor should any child age 2 or older; the child may be verbal enough to report what transpired in the private interview to the partner and thereby further endanger the woman.

The nurse also needs to obtain additional information, such as the following:

- Does the woman have a partner? Who are her support people?
- Is she safe in her relationship with the baby's father? Has there been any physical or emotional abuse prior to or during the pregnancy? If so, what interventions were made? In questioning the woman about safety and abuse issues, the nurse needs to be aware that abuse affects one in six adult women and one in five teenagers during pregnancy (McFarland & Parker, 1994). It is important to ensure that the woman is alone when the questions are asked so that she can answer freely. If she indicates there has been a problem, the nurse must conduct the interview face to face, making sure that the woman can see the written interview questions the nurse is asking. One study found that 29% of women disclosed abuse in a direct face-to-face interview; in contrast, only 8% of women disclosed abuse when asked to complete a written medical form (McFarland & Gondolf, 1998). To encourage the woman to disclose abuse, the nurse can ask the following questions from the Abuse Assessment Screen by McFarland and Parker (1994):
    1. Have you ever been emotionally or physically abused by your partner or someone important to you?
    2. Within the last year, have you been hit, slapped, kicked, or otherwise physically hurt by someone? If yes, by whom? Total number of times?
    3. Since you've been pregnant, have you been hit, slapped, kicked, or otherwise physically hurt by someone? If yes, by whom? Total number of times?
    4. Within the last year, has anyone forced you to engage in sexual activities? If yes, who? Total number of times?
    5. Are you afraid of your partner or anyone you listed above?
- Has she had difficulty or problems with previous pregnancies, labors, or births that would increase her anxiety now?
- Have emotional problems been present during the past few months? What interventions have occurred? (Austin, Gallop, McCay, Peternelj-Taylor, & Bayer, 1999)

As the woman looks at the questions and the nurse reads them aloud, the nurse asks the woman to mark areas of her body that have been involved in any abusive incident. It is important that the nurse document the interview and the woman's responses to the questions, carefully describing in nursing notes any current trauma. The interview provides an opportunity to discus a safety plan (see Chapter 5) and to identify resources within the community. Each nurse will need to identify any state-mandated regulations regarding compulsory reporting. Family services, social services, and/or law enforcement may also need to be contacted. Because psychosocial factors are complex, problems of abuse may not be apparent until later in the labor and birth process. The nurse must be aware of the following aspects of psychosocial history:

- Is there evidence of support between the woman and her partner?
- Is the partner controlling? Does the partner make decisions unilaterally?

I will never forget the 16-year-old single mom who came into the birthing unit. She came in because it was her due date and she thought her labor had started. As I began to work with her, it was difficult to establish rapport. With each question and each action on my part, she seemed to become more uncomfortable. Even my suggestion of placing my hand on her abdomen to palpate contractions became frightening to her. We seemed to be dealing with something far beyond the anxiety that some young women have. She recoiled from me at the mention of any physical assessments.

It took every skill that I had to quietly stay with her, to establish a relationship, and to begin to gain her trust. She was finally able to tell me that the pregnancy was the result of a rape and that there had been continued sexual violence against her throughout the pregnancy. The labor and birth were so very difficult for both of us, each in our own way. She held onto my hand and pleaded with me not to leave her, and together we got through it.

As nurses, if we think of sexual abuse at all, it seems that it is about someone else—a person we read about in the newspaper or in another neighborhood. But we also need to realize that it is us. I teach maternal-child nursing, and each fall as I prepare myself to go back into the birthing area with students, I seem to have to deal again with memories of my own past. There are so many aspects of labor and birthing that are triggers for memories, and I continue to work on dealing with the impact of the memories. In many ways I am lucky because my experience helps keep me in touch with the difficulty that some of the students may have in this area of nursing. It is something that we all work on, one day at a time.

Intrapartal High-Risk Screening

Screening for intrapartal high-risk factors is an integral part of assessing the normal laboring woman. (Note that the preceding discussion of abuse is certainly a high-risk situation.) While obtaining the history, the nurse notes the presence of any factors that may be associated with a high-risk condition. For example, the woman who reports a physical symptom such as intermittent bleeding needs further assessment to rule out abruptio placentae or placenta previa before the admission process continues. In addition to identifying the presence of a high-risk condition, the nurse must recognize the implications of the condition for the laboring woman and her fetus. For example, in the case of an abnormal fetal presentation, the nurse understands that the labor may be prolonged, prolapse of the umbilical cord may be more likely, and there is a greater possibility of a cesarean birth

Some women are at high risk during labor because they have undergone female circumcision (FC), also called female genital mutilation (FGM). FC and FGM are culturally prescribed procedures performed in more than 30 countries; in Africa alone, an estimated 80 to 100 million women are circumcised (Kassindja & Bashir, 1998).

The extent of the mutilation varies significantly. *Sunna*, the mildest form, involves the removal of the prepuce (hood) of the clitoris. Most often, the clitoris and labia minora are excised. The most extreme form of FGM involves the removal of the clitoris, labia minora, and labia majora. The remaining raw tissue edges are then held together using suture, thread, or even thorns. A small pinhole opening is left in the posterior perineum for urine and menses to pass through. Often FGM is performed by untrained people (Miller, 1997). In all cases of FGM except sunna, penile penetration may be impossible, and the scar tissue may have to be cut for intercourse to occur (deinfibulation). This procedure is sometimes performed at home by the husband, and may result in further injury or infection. Women who have undergone FGM also tend to have frequent urinary tract infections.

During labor, use of a speculum may be impossible because the vaginal opening may only admit an index finger. Birth by cesarean may be necessary or the physician may have to further cut the scar tissue to permit vaginal birth.

It is important for the nurse to remember that although FGM has been deemed illegal in many countries, it is still being carried out because it is a cultural expectation for many groups of people. Nonjudgmental acceptance of the woman and her family is critical during this time in their lives.

> *The people of my tribe are good people. But good people can do bad things. They need to think carefully about what they are doing and why, not just keep on doing it because that's how things have always been done in the past. Tradition doesn't make something right. . . . If the people of my tribe stood together and said, "No, this is wrong, it has to stop." Oh, that would make me so proud.*
>
> ~ FAUZIYA KASSINDJA ~ (Kassindja & Bashir, 1998, p 503)

Although physical conditions are frequently listed as the major factors that increase risk in the intrapartal period, sociocultural variables such as poverty, nutrition, the amount of prenatal care, cultural beliefs regarding pregnancy, and communication patterns may also precipitate a high-risk situation in the intrapartal period. The nurse can begin gathering data about sociocultural factors as the woman enters the birthing area. The nurse observes the communication pattern between the woman and her support person(s) and their responses to admission questions and initial teaching. Communication problems can affect the course of labor and the nurse's ability to provide support and education. If the woman and her support persons are not fluent in English or are hearing impaired, the nurse must find some way to provide information in their primary language so that they can make informed decisions. If the nurse or other birthing room staff do not speak the woman's primary language, an appropriate interpreter should be obtained. (See further discussion in Chapter 20, page 544, and Appendices C, D, and E.) Communication may also be affected by cultural standards regarding when it is acceptable to speak, who should ask questions, or whether it is acceptable for the woman to let others know if she is experiencing discomfort (Austin et al, 1999).

The nurse should quickly review the prenatal record for number of prenatal visits, weight gain during pregnancy, progression of fundal height, assistance such as Medicaid and Women, Infants, and Children (WIC), and exposure to environmental agents.

A partial list of intrapartal risk factors appears in Table 19–1. The factors precede the Intrapartal Assessment Guide because they must be kept in mind during the assessment.

Intrapartal Physical and Psychosociocultural Assessment

A physical examination is part of the admission procedure and part of the ongoing care of the client. Although the intrapartal physical assessment is not as complete and thorough as the initial prenatal physical examination (Chapter 11), it does involve assessment of some body systems and the actual labor process. The Intrapartal Assessment Guide on pages 502 to 507 provides a framework the maternity nurse can use when examining the laboring woman.

The physical assessment includes assessments performed immediately on admission as well as ongoing assessments. When labor is progressing very quickly, the nurse may not have time for a complete assessment. In this case, the critical physical assessments would include maternal vital signs, labor status, fetal status, and laboratory findings.

The cultural assessment provides a starting point for this increasingly important aspect of assessment. Recognizing and honoring the laboring woman's values and beliefs can help the nurse plan and implement quality, individualized nursing care. Frequently, however, the nurse

Text continues on page 510.

TABLE 19–1 Intrapartal High-Risk Factors

Factor	Maternal Implication	Fetal-Neonatal Implication
Abnomal presentation	↑ Incidence of cesarean birth ↑ Incidence of prolonged labor	↑ Incidence of placenta previa Prematurity ↑ Risk of congenital abnormality Neonatal physical trauma ↑ Risk of intrauterine growth retardation
Multiple gestation	↑ Uterine distension → ↑ risk of postpartum hemorrhage ↑ Risk of cesarean birth ↑ Risk of preterm labor	Low birth weight Prematurity ↑ Risk of congenital anomalies Feto-fetal transfusion
Hydramnios	↑ Discomfort ↑ Dyspnea ↑ Risk of preterm labor Edema of lower extremities	↑ Risk of esophageal or other high alimentary tract atresias ↑ Risk of CNS anomalies (myelocele)
Oligohydramnios	Maternal fear of "dry birth"	↑ Incidence of congenital anomalies ↑ Incidence of renal lesions ↑ Risk of IUGR ↑ Risk of fetal acidosis ↑ Risk of cord compression Postmaturity
Meconium staining of amniotic fluid	↑ Psychologic stress due to fear for baby	↑ Risk of fetal asphyxia ↑ Risk of meconium aspiration ↑ Risk of pneumonia due to aspiration of meconium
Premature rupture of membranes	↑ Risk of infection (chorioamnionitis) ↑ Risk of preterm labor ↑ Anxiety Fear for the baby Prolonged hospitalization ↑ Incidence of tocolytic therapy	↑ Perinatal morbidity Prematurity ↓ Birth weight ↑ Risk of respiratory distress syndrome Prolonged hospitalization
Induction of labor	↑ Risk of hypercontractility of uterus ↑ Risk of uterine rupture ↑ Length of labor if cervix not ready ↑ Anxiety	Prematurity if gestational age not assessed correctly Hypoxia if hyperstimulation occurs
Abruptio placentae/placenta previa	Hemorrhage Uterine atony ↑ Incidence of cesarean birth	Fetal hypoxia/acidosis Fetal exsanguination ↑ Perinatal mortality
Failure to progress in labor	Maternal exhaustion ↑ Incidence of augmentation of labor ↑ Incidence of cesarean birth	Fetal hypoxia/acidosis Intracranial birth injury
Precipitous labor (< 3 hours)	Perineal, vaginal, cervical lacerations ↑ Risk of PP hemorrhage	Tentorial tears
Prolapse of umbilical cord	↑ Fear for baby Cesarean birth	Acute fetal hypoxia/acidosis
Fetal heart aberrations	↑ Fear for baby ↑ Risk of cesarean birth, forceps, vacuum Continuous electronic monitoring and intervention in labor	Tachycardia, chronic asphyxic insult, bradycardia, acute asphyxic insult Chronic hypoxia Congenital heart block
Uterine rupture	Hemorrhage Cesarean birth for hysterectomy ↑ Risk of death	Fetal anoxia Fetal hemorrhage ↑ Neonatal morbidity and mortality
Postdates (> 42 weeks)	↑ Anxiety ↑ Incidence of induction of labor ↑ Incidence of cesarean birth ↑ Use of technology to monitor fetus ↑ Risk of shoulder dystocia	Postmaturity syndrome ↑ Risk of fetal-neonatal mortality and morbidity ↑ Risk of antepartum fetal death ↑ Incidence/risk of large baby
Diabetes	↑ Risk of hydramnios ↑ Risk of hypoglycemia or hyperglycemia ↑ Risk of pregnancy-induced hypertension	↑ Risk of malpresentation ↑ Risk of macrosomia ↑ Risk of intrauterine growth retardation ↑ Risk of respiratory distress syndrome ↑ Risk of congenital anomalies
Pregnancy-induced hypertension	↑ Risk of seizures ↑ Risk of stroke ↑ Risk of HELLP	↑ Risk of small-for-gestational-age baby ↑ Risk of preterm birth ↑ Risk of mortality
AIDS/STD	↑ Risk of additional infections	↑ Risk of transplacental transmission

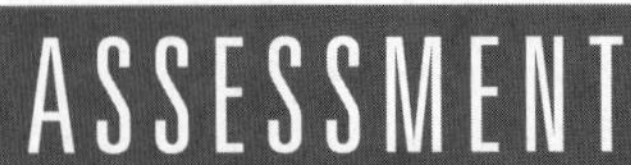 GUIDE: INTRAPARTAL—FIRST STAGE OF LABOR

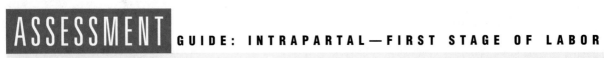

Physical Assessment/ Normal Findings	Alterations and Possible Causes*	Nursing Responses to Data†
Vital Signs		
Blood pressure (BP): < 130 systolic and < 85 diastolic in adult 18 years of age or older or no more than 15–20 mm Hg rise in systolic pressure over baseline BP during early pregnancy (Johannsen, 1993)	High blood pressure (essential hypertension, preeclampsia, renal disease, apprehension or anxiety) Low blood pressure (supine hypotension)	Evaluate history of preexisting disorders and check for presence of other signs of preeclampsia. Do not assess during contractions; implement measures to decrease anxiety and reassess. Turn woman on her side and recheck BP. Provide quiet environment Have 0_2 available.
Pulse: 60–90 bpm	Increased pulse rate (excitement or anxiety, cardiac disorders, early shock)	Evaluate cause, reassess to see if rate continues; report to physician.
Respirations: 14–22/min (or pulse rate divided by 4)	Marked tachypnea (respiratory disease), hyperventilation in transition phase	Assess between contractions; if marked tachypnea continues, assess for signs of respiratory disease.
	Hyperventilation (anxiety)	Encourage slow breaths if woman is hyperventilating.
Pulse ox 95% or greater	>90%: hypoxia, hypotension, hemorrhage	Apply 0_2; notify physician
Temperature: 36.2–37.6C (98–99.6F)	Elevated temperature (infection, dehydration, prolonged rupture of membranes, epidural regional block)	Assess for other signs of infection or dehydration.
Weight		
25–30 lb greater than prepregnant weight	Weight gain > 30 lb (fluid retention, obesity, large infant, diabetes mellitus, PIH), weight gain < 15 lb (SGA)	Assess for signs of edema. Evaluate pattern from prenatal record.
Lungs		
Normal breath sounds, clear and equal	Rales, rhonchi, friction rub (infection), pulmonary edema, asthma	Reassess; refer to physician.
Fundus		
At 40 weeks' gestation located just below xiphoid process	Uterine size not compatible with estimated date of birth (SGA, large for gestational age [LGA], hydramnios, multiple pregnancy)	Reevaluate history regarding pregnancy dating. Refer to physician for additional assessment.
Edema		
Slight amount of dependent edema	Pitting edema of face, hands, legs, abdomen, sacral area (preeclampsia)	Check deep tendon reflexes for hyperactivity; check for clonus; refer to physician.
Hydration		
Normal skin turgor, elastic	Poor skin turgor (dehydration)	Assess skin turgor; refer to physician for deviations.

*Possible causes of alterations are placed in parentheses.

†This column provides guidelines for further assessment and initial nursing intervention.

Physical Assessment/ Normal Findings	Alterations and Possible Causes*	Nursing Responses to Data†
Perineum		
Tissues smooth, pink color (see Prenatal Initial Physical Assessment Guide, Chapter 25)	Varicose veins of vulva, herpes lesions	Exercise care while doing a perineal prep; note on client record need for follow-up in postpartal period; reassess after birth; refer to physician.
Clear mucus; may be blood tinged with earthy or human odor	Profuse, purulent, foul-smelling drainage	Suspected gonorrhea or chorioamnionitis; report to physician; initiate care to newborn's eyes; notify neonatal nursing staff and pediatrician.
Presence of small amount of bloody show that gradually increases with further cervical dilatation	Hemorrhage	Assess BP and pulse, pallor, diaphoresis; report any marked changes. (Note: Gaping of vagina or anus and bulging of perineum are suggestive signs of second stage of labor.) Universal precautions.
Labor Status		
Uterine contractions: regular pattern	Failure to establish a regular pattern, prolonged latent phase Hypertonicity Hypotonicity	Evaluate whether woman is in true labor; ambulate if in early labor. Evaluate client status and contractile pattern. Obtain a 20-minute EFM monitor strip. Notify physician or CNM.
Cervical dilatation: progressive cervical dilatation from size of fingertip to 10 cm (Procedure 19–1)	Rigidity of cervix (frequent cervical infections, scar tissue, failure of presenting part to descend)	Evaluate contractions, fetal engagement, position, and cervical dilatation. Inform client of progress.
Cervical effacement: progressive thinning of cervix (Procedure 19–1)	Failure to efface (rigidity of cervix, failure of presenting part to engage); cervical edema (pushing effort by woman before cervix is fully dilated and effaced, trapped cervix)	Evaluate contractions, fetal engagement, and position. Notify physician/CNM if cervix is becoming edematous; work with woman to prevent pushing until cervix is completely dilated. Keep vaginal exams to a minimum.
Fetal descent: progressive descent of fetal presenting part from station −5 to +4 (Figure 19–4 in Procedure 19–1)	Failure of descent (abnormal fetal position or presentation, macrosomic fetus, inadequate pelvic measurement)	Evaluate fetal position, presentation, and size. Evaluate maternal pelvic measurements.
Membranes: may rupture before or during labor	Rupture of membranes more than 12–24 hours before initiation of labor	Assess for ruptured membranes using Nitrazine test tape before doing vaginal exam. Follow BSI precautions. Instruct woman with ruptured membranes to remain on bed rest if presenting part is not engaged and firmly down against the cervix. Keep vaginal exams to a minimum to prevent infection. When membranes rupture in the birth setting, **immediately assess FHR** to detect changes associated with prolapse of umbilical cord (FHR slows).

*Possible causes of alterations are placed in parentheses

†This column provides guidelines for further assessment and initial nursing intervention.

Physical Assessment/ Normal Findings	Alterations and Possible Causes*	Nursing Responses to Data†
Labor Status *continued*		
Findings on Nitrazine test tape: Membranes probably intact yellow pH 5.0 olive pH 5.5 olive green pH 6.0	False-positive results may be obtained if large amount of bloody show is present, previous vaginal examination has been done using lubricant, or tape is touched by nurse's fingers.	Assess fluid for consistency, amount, odor; assess FHR frequently. Assess fluid at regular intervals for presence of meconium staining. Follow BSI precautions while assessing amniotic fluid.
Membranes probably ruptured blue-green pH 6.5 blue-gray pH 7.0 deep blue pH 7.5		Teach woman that amniotic fluid is continually produced (to allay fear of "dry birth"). Teach woman that she may feel amniotic fluid trickle or gush with contractions. Change Chux pads often.
Amniotic fluid clear, with earthy or human odor, no foul-smelling odor	Greenish amniotic fluid (fetal stress)	Assess FHR; do vaginal exam to evaluate for prolapsed cord; apply fetal monitor for continuous data; report to physician.
	Strong or foul odor (amnionitis)	Take woman's temperature and report to physician.
Fetal Status		
FHR: 120–160 bpm	<120 or >160 bpm (fetal stress); abnormal patterns on fetal monitor: decreased variability, late decelerations, variable decelerations, absence of accelerations with fetal movement	Initiate interventions based on particular FHR pattern.
Presentation: Cephalic, 97% Breech, 3%	Face, brow, breech, or shoulder presentation	Report to physician; after presentation is confirmed as face, brow, breech, or shoulder, woman may be prepared for cesarean birth.
Position: left-occiput-anterior (LOA) most common	Persistent occipital-posterior (OP) position; transverse arrest	Carefully monitor maternal and fetal status.
Activity: fetal movement	Hyperactivity (may precede fetal hypoxia)	Carefully evaluate FHR; apply fetal monitor.
	Complete lack of movement (fetal distress or fetal demise)	Carefully evaluate FHR; apply fetal monitor. Report to physician/CNM.
Laboratory Evaluation		
Hematologic tests Hemoglobin: 12–16 g/dL	<12 g/dL (anemia, hemorrhage)	Evaluate woman for problems due to decreased oxygen-carrying capacity caused by lowered hemoglobin.
CBC Hematocrit: 38%–47% RBC: 4.2–5.4 million/mm^3 WBC: 4500–11,000/mm^3, although leukocytosis to 20,000/mm^3 is not unusual Platelets 150,000–400,000/mm^3	Presence of infection or blood dyscrasias, loss of blood (hemorrhage, disseminated intravascular coagulation [DIC])	Evaluate for other signs of infection or for petechiae, bruising, or unusual bleeding.
Serologic testing STS or VDRL test: nonreactive	Positive reaction (Chapter 25, Initial Prenatal Physical Assessment Guide)	For reactive test notify newborn nursery and pediatrician.

*Possible causes of alterations are placed in parentheses.

†This column provides guidelines for further assessment and initial nursing intervention.

Physical Assessment/ Normal Findings	Alterations and Possible Causes*	Nursing Responses to Data†
Laboratory Evaluation *continued*		
Rh	Rh-positive fetus in Rh-negative woman	Assess prenatal record for titer levels during pregnancy. Obtain cord blood for direct Coombs' at birth.
Urinalysis		
Glucose: negative	Glycosuria (low renal threshold for glucose, diabetes mellitus)	Assess blood glucose; test urine for ketones; ketonuria and glycosuria require further assessment of blood sugars.‡
Ketones: negative	Ketonuria (starvation ketosis)	
Proteins: negative	Proteinuria (urine specimen contaminated with vaginal secretions, fever, kidney disease); proteinuria of 2+ or greater found in uncontaminated urine may be a sign of ensuing preeclampsia	Instruct woman in collection technique; incidence of contamination from vaginal discharge is common.
Red blood cells: negative	Blood in urine (calculi, cystitis, glomerulonephritis, neoplasm)	Assess collection technique (may be bloody show).
White blood cells: negative	Presence of white blood cells (infection in genitourinary tract)	Assess for signs of urinary tract infection.
Casts: none	Presence of casts (nephrotic syndrome)	

Cultural Assessment§	Variations to Consider	Nursing Responses to Data†
Cultural influences determine customs and practices regarding intrapartal care.	Individual preferences may vary.	
Ask the following questions: Who would you like to remain with you during your labor and birth?	She may prefer only her coach to remain or may also want family and/or friends.	Provide support for her wishes by encouraging desired people to stay. Provide information to others (with the woman's permission) who are not in the room.
What would you like to wear during labor?	She may be more comfortable in her own clothes.	Offer supportive materials such as Chux if needed to protect her own clothing. Avoid subtle signals to the woman that she should not have chosen to remain in her own clothes. Have other clothing available if the woman desires. If her clothing becomes contaminated, it will be simple to place it in a plastic bag. The nurse can soak soiled clothing in cool water. The nurse needs to remember to wear disposable gloves and a plastic apron if splashing is anticipated.

§These are only a few suggestions. We do not mean to imply that this is a comprehensive cultural assessment; rather, it is a tool to encourage cultural sensitivity.

*Possible causes of alterations are placed in parentheses.

†This column provides guidelines for further assessment and initial nursing intervention.

‡Glycosuria should not be discounted. The presence of glycosuria necessitates follow-up.

Cultural Assessment[§]	Variations to Consider	Nursing Responses to Data[†]
What activity would you like during labor?	She may want to ambulate most of the time, stand in the shower, sit in the jacuzzi, sit in a chair or on a stool, remain on the bed, and so forth.	Support the woman's wishes; provide encouragement and complete assessments in a manner so her activity and positional wishes are disturbed as little as possible.
What position would you like for the birth?	She may feel more comfortable in lithotomy with stirrups and her upper body elevated, or side-lying or sitting in birthing bed, or standing, or squatting, or on hands and knees.	Collect any supplies and equipment needed to support her in her chosen birthing position. Provide information to the coach regarding any changes that may be needed based on the chosen position.
Is there anything special you would like?	She may want the room darkened or to have curtains and windows open, music playing, a Leboyer birth, her coach to cut the umbilical cord, to save a portion of the umbilical cord, to save the placenta, to videotape the birth, and so forth.	Support requests, and communicate requests to any other nursing or medical personnel (so requests can continue to be supported and not questioned). If another nurse or physician does not honor the request, act as advocate for the woman by continuing to support her unless her desire is truly unsafe.
Ask the woman if she would like fluids, and ask what temperature she prefers.	She may prefer clear fluids other than water (tea, clear juice). She may prefer iced, room-temperature, or warmed fluids.	Provide fluids as desired.
Observe the woman's response when privacy is difficult to maintain and her body is exposed.	Some women do not seem to mind being exposed during an exam or procedure; others feel acute discomfort.	Maintain privacy and respect the woman's sense of privacy. If the woman is unable to provide specific information, the nurse may draw from general information regarding cultural variation: Southeast Asian women may not want any family member in the room during exam or procedures. Her partner may not be involved with coaching activities during labor or birth. Saudi women may need to remain covered during the labor and birth and avoid exposure of any body part. The husband may need to be in the room but remain behind a curtain or screen so he does not view his wife at this time.
If the woman is to breastfeed, ask if she would like to feed her baby immediately after birth.	She may want to feed her baby right away or may want to wait a little while.	

Psychosocial Assessment	Variations to Consider	Nursing Responses to Data[†]
Preparation for Childbirth		
Woman has some information regarding process of normal labor and birth.	Some women do not have any information regarding childbirth.	Add to present information base.
Woman has breathing and/or relaxation techniques to use during labor.	Some women do not have any method of relaxation or breathing to use, and some do not desire them.	Support breathing and relaxation techniques that client is using; provide information if needed.

§These are only a few suggestions. We do not mean to imply that this is a comprehensive cultural assessment; rather, it is a tool to encourage cultural sensitivity.

†This column provides guidelines for further assessment and initial nursing intervention.

Psychosocial Assessment[§]	Variations to Consider	Nursing Responses to Data[†]
Response to Labor		
Latent phase: relaxed, excited, anxious for labor to be well established	May feel unable to cope with contractions because of fear, anxiety, or lack of information	Provide support and encouragement; establish trusting relationship.
Active phase: becomes more intense, begins to tire Transitional phase: feels tired, may feel unable to cope, needs frequent coaching to maintain breathing patterns	May remain quiet and without any sign of discomfort or anxiety, may insist that she is unable to continue with the birthing process	Provide support and coaching if needed.
Coping mechanisms: Ability to cope with labor through utilization of support system, breathing, relaxation techniques	May feel marked anxiety and apprehension, may not have coping mechanisms that can be brought into this experience, or may be unable to use them at this time	Support coping mechanisms if they are working for the woman; provide information and support if she exhibits anxiety or needs alternative to present coping methods.
	Survivors of sexual abuse may demonstrate fear of IVs or needles, may recoil when touched, may insist on a female caregiver, may be very sensitive to bodily fluids and cleanliness, and may be unable to labor lying down (Burrian, 1995)	Encourage participation of coach/significant other if a supportive relationship seems apparent. Establish rapport and a trusting relationship. Provide information that is true and offer your presence.
Anxiety		
Some anxiety and apprehension is within normal limits	May show anxiety through rapid breathing, nervous tremors, frowning, grimacing, clenching of teeth, thrashing movements, crying, increased pulse and blood pressure	Provide support, encouragement, and information. Teach relaxation techniques; support controlled breathing efforts. May need to provide a paper bag to breathe into if woman says her lips are tingling. Note FHR.
Sounds during Labor		
	Some women are very quiet; others moan or make a variety of noises.	Provide a supportive environment. Encourage woman to do what is right for her.
Support System		
Physical intimacy between mother and father (or mother and support person): caretaking activities such as soothing conversation, touching	Some women would prefer no contact, others may show clinging behaviors.	Encourage caretaking activities that appear to comfort the woman; encourage support to the woman; if support is limited, the nurse may take a more active role.
Support person stays in close proximity	Limited interaction may come from a desire for quiet.	Encourage support person to stay close (if this seems appropriate).
Relationship between mother and father (or support person): involved interaction	The support person may seem to be detached and maintain little support, attention, or conversation.	Support interactions; if interaction is limited, the nurse may provide more information and support.
		Assure that coach/significant other has short breaks, especially prior to transition.

[§]These are only a few suggestions. We do not mean to imply that this is a comprehensive cultural assessment; rather, it is a tool to encourage cultural sensitivity.

[†]This column provides guidelines for further assessment and initial nursing intervention.

PROCEDURE 19–1 PERFORMING AN INTRAPARTAL VAGINAL EXAMINATION

Nursing Action	*Rationale*
Objective: Assemble the equipment.	
Prepare and arrange the following items so they are easily accessible:	*Organizing the equipment facilitates the examination.*
• Clean disposable gloves • Slide • Lubricant • Sterile cotton-tipped swab (Q-tip) • Nitrazine test tape	*If membranes are ruptured, sterile disposable gloves are used to decrease the chance of introducing bacteria during the examination. When membranes are intact, clean disposable gloves may be used.*
Objective: Prepare the woman.	
• Explain the procedure, the indications for the exam, what the exam may feel like, and that it may cause discomfort.	*By explaining the procedure, the nurse decreases anxiety and increases relaxation.*
• Assess for latex allergies.	*Select nonlatex gloves if woman is allergic.*
• Position the woman with her thighs flexed and abducted. Instruct her to put the heels of her feet together. Drape the woman with a sheet, leaving a flap to access the perineum.	*Position provides access to the vulvar area.* *The drape provides privacy.*
• Encourage the woman to relax her muscles and legs.	*Relaxation decreases muscle tension and increases comfort.*
• Inform the woman prior to touching her. Use gentleness.	*This action communicates regard for the woman and her privacy.*
Objective: Test for amniotic fluid leakage if indicated.	
If fluid leakage has been reported or noted, use Nitrazine test tape and Q-tip with slide for fern test before performing the exam.	*As long as lubricant has not been used, Nitrazine tape registers a change in pH if amniotic fluid is present.*
• Fern test is done by inserting the swab in the pooling of fluid in the posterior vagina and applying the fluid to a slide.	*Digital exam may be deferred if the woman has ruptured membranes and is not actively laboring (AAP & ACOG, 1997).*
Objective: Use aseptic technique during the exam.	
• Pull glove onto dominant hand.	*If sterile exam is needed, both hands will be gloved with sterile gloves.*
• Using your gloved hand, position the hand with the wrist straight and the elbow tilted downward. Insert your well-lubricated second and index fingers of the gloved hand into the vagina until they touch the cervix. Use care when positioning your hand.	*This positioning allows the fingertips to point toward the umbilicus and find the cervix.*
• If the woman verbalizes discomfort, acknowledge it and apologize.	*This validates the woman's feelings and helps her feel more in control.*
Objective: Determine the status of labor progress.	
• Perform the vaginal examination during and between contractions.	*Cervical dilatation, effacement, and fetal station are affected by the presence of a contraction.*
Objective: Identify the amount of cervical dilatation and effacement (Figure 19–1).	
• Palpate for the opening, or a depression, in the cervix. Estimate the diameter of the depression to identify the amount of dilatation.	*Allows determination of effacement and dilatation.*
Objective: Determine the status of the fetal membranes.	
• Observe for expression of amniotic fluid.	*If fluid is expressed, test for amiotic fluid.*
Objective: Palpate the presenting part (Figure 19–2).	*Provides information regarding fetal descent and cardinal movements.*
Objective: Assess the fetal descent (Figure 19–3).	
• Assess the station, identify the position of the posterior fontanelle.	

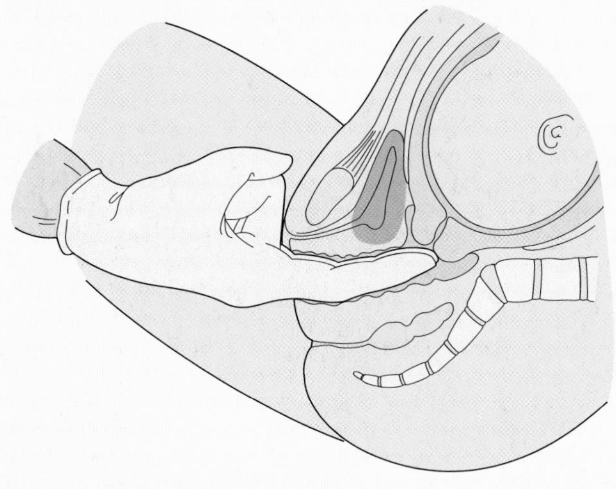

FIGURE 19–1 To gauge cervical dilatation, the nurse places the index and middle fingers against the cervix and determines the size of the opening. Before labor begins, the cervix is long (approximately 2.5 cm), the sides feel thick, and the cervical canal is closed, so an examining finger cannot be inserted. During labor, the cervix begins to dilate, and the size of the opening progresses from 1 cm to 10 cm in diameter.

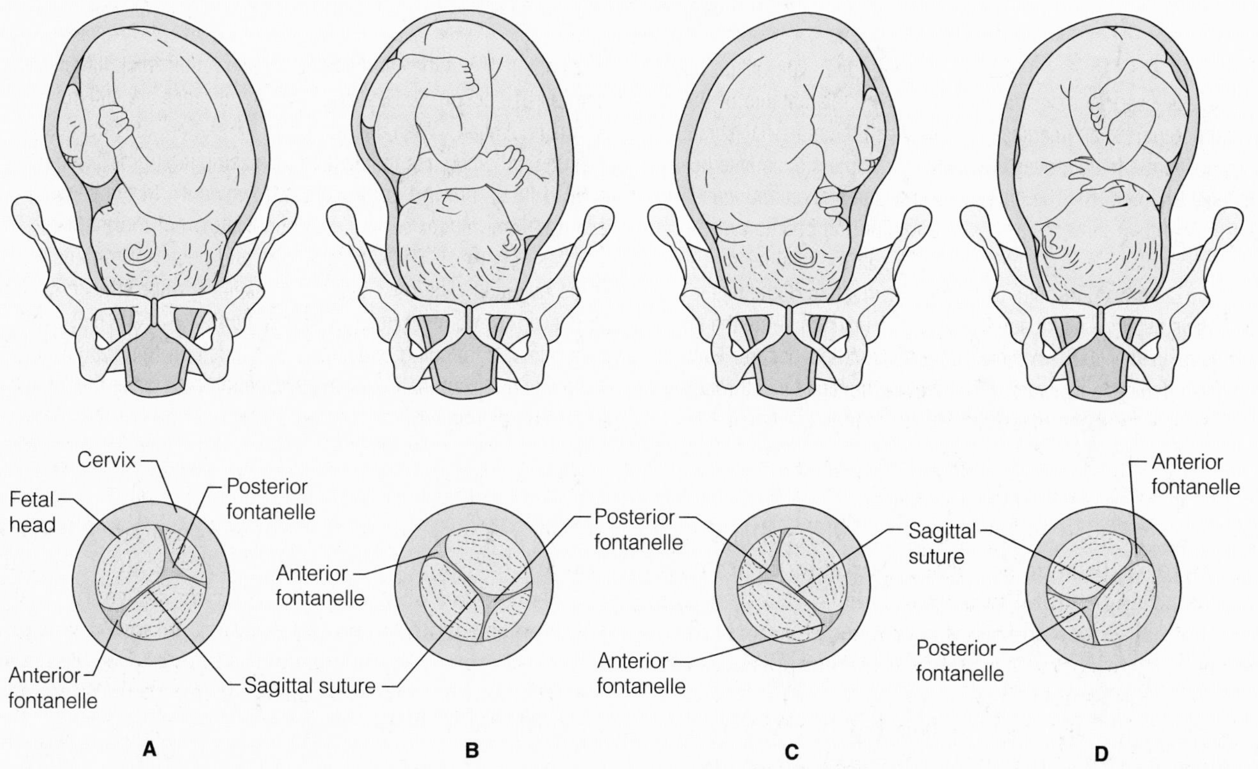

FIGURE 19–2 Palpation of the presenting part (the portion of the fetus that enters the pelvis first). ***A,*** Left occiput anterior (LOA). The occiput (area over the occipital bone on the posterior part of the fetal head) is in the left anterior quadrant of the woman's pelvis. When the fetus is in LOA, the posterior fontanelle (located just above the occipital bone and triangular in shape) is in the upper left quadrant of the maternal pelvis. ***B,*** Left occiput posterior (LOP). The posterior fontanelle is in the lower left quadrant of the maternal pelvis. ***C,*** Right occiput anterior (ROA). The posterior fontanelle is in the upper right quadrant of the maternal pelvis. ***D,*** Right occiput posterior (ROP). The posterior fontanelle is in the lower right quadrant of the maternal pelvis. Note: The anterior fontanelle is diamond shaped. Because of the roundness of the fetal head, only a portion of the anterior fontanelle can be seen in each of the views, so it appears to be triangular in shape.

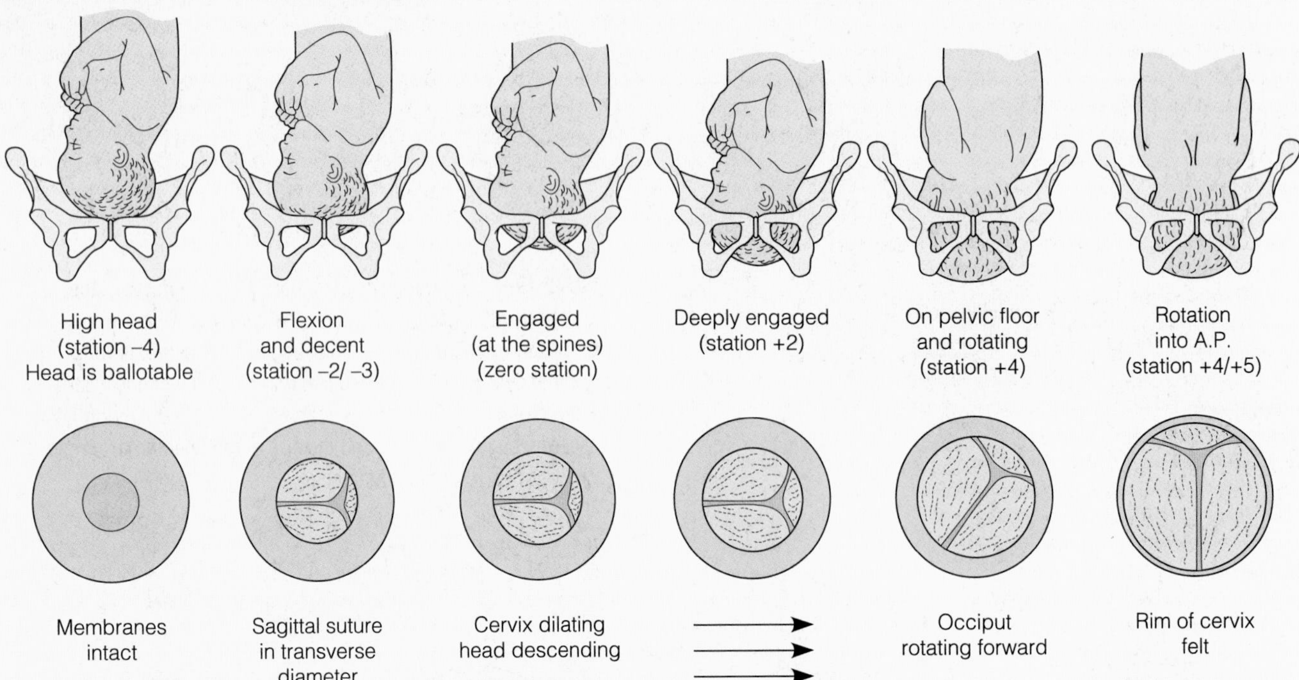

FIGURE 19–3 Descent of the fetus through the maternal pelvis can be assessed by determining station (the relationship of the presenting part to an imaginary line between the maternal ischial spines). As the fetus moves downward, cardinal movements occur (see Chapter 18). The nurse assesses the station and identifies the cardinal movements by determining the position of the posterior fontanelle. The upper panels depict the fetal head progressing downward through the pelvis. From left to right, the first four views depict descent and flexion of the fetal chin onto the fetal chest. In the last two views, internal rotation occurs. Each view also depicts downward movement of the fetal head through the maternal pelvis as measured by the change in station. The lower panels depict the cervix, which is still rather thick (little effacement has occurred). The amniotic membranes are still intact over the fetal head. When the fetus is at −4 station, the fetal head is ballottable (when it is touched by the examining nurse's finger, the head floats upward and resettles downward). In the second view, note the thinner cervix (which indicates that more effacement has occurred). The sagittal suture and posterior fontanelle can be palpated. The next two views depict further effacement and descent of the fetal head from 0 station to +2. The last two views depict continuing effacement and position that would be felt on vaginal examination of the presenting part while the fetal head is completing internal rotation.

feels uncertain about what to ask or consider, perhaps because there has been no personal opportunity to become aware of varying cultural values and beliefs.

The final section addresses psychosocial factors. The laboring woman's psychosocial status is an important part of the total assessment. The woman has previous ideas, knowledge, and fears about childbearing. By assessing her psychosocial status, the nurse can meet the woman's needs for information and support. The nurse can then support the woman and her partner; in the absence of a partner, the nurse may become the support person.

While performing the intrapartal assessment, it is imperative that the nurse follow CDC guidelines to prevent exposure to body substances. The nurse can provide information in a factual manner regarding the precautions. A statement such as the following is helpful: "I will be wearing gloves when I change the Chux on which you are lying. This is to protect my hands from the discharge you are having and to protect you from any organisms that I may have on my hands." Sharing information with the laboring woman and her support person(s) will promote a supportive, caring environment. (See Essential Precautions in Practice: During Intrapartal Assessment for further information.)

CRITICAL THINKING QUESTION

1. You have reason to suspect that the laboring woman who has just been admitted may be in an abusive relationship. If you were the nurse providing care, how could you set up an interview so that the partner would be able to leave the room (and take any

ESSENTIAL PRECAUTIONS IN PRACTICE

During Intrapartal Assessment

Wear disposable gloves when performing the following actions:

- Assisting the woman as she removes any garments moist with bloody show and/or amniotic fluid
- Handling Chux and bedding that are moist with bloody show or amniotic fluid
- Checking amniotic fluid–soaked materials with Nitrazine test tape
- Placing the elastic straps for the electronic monitor around a woman who has been lying in bedding moist with bloody show and/or amniotic fluid
- Assisting with fetal blood sampling and handling the lab tubes

Wear gloves when performing a vaginal examination and when placing fetal scalp electrodes. The gloves protect you from exposure to vaginal secretions, bloody show, and amniotic fluid.

REMEMBER to wash your hands prior to pulling the disposable gloves on and AGAIN immediately after you remove the gloves.

For further information consult, OSHA and CDC guidelines.

accompanying children) and not feel that you are possibly increasing the risk to the woman?

2. What are the laws in your state regarding the obligation of professional health care providers to report possible abuse? What resources would you refer a woman to if she needed them?
3. What is your background? What previous or current experiences do you bring to the childbirth setting? If you are dealing with negative experiences, what support will be important for you? Can you discuss these experiences with your clinical instructor or some other trusted faculty member in your nursing program? It is very important for you to have support now, because maternal-newborn nursing tends to bring to the surface many life experiences that are difficult to re-experience while you are in this area of study. If you can "let another person in," you will increase your chances of receiving support, you won't be as likely to carry your own negative experiences into the clinical area, and you will be able to continue your journey to healing.

Methods of Evaluating Labor Progress

Contraction Assessment

Uterine contractions may be assessed by palpation or continuous electronic monitoring.

Palpation The nurse assesses contractions for frequency, duration, and intensity by placing one hand on the uterine fundus. The hand is kept relatively still because excessive movement may stimulate contractions or cause discomfort. The nurse determines the frequency of the contractions by noting the time from the beginning of one contraction to the beginning of the next. If contractions begin at 7:00, 7:04, and 7:08, for example, their frequency is every 4 minutes. To determine contraction duration, the nurse notes the time when tensing of the fundus is first felt (beginning of contraction) and again as relaxation occurs (end of contraction). During the acme of the contraction, intensity can be evaluated by estimating the indentability of the fundus. The nurse should assess at least three successive contractions to provide enough data to determine the contraction pattern. See Table 19–2 for review of characteristics in different phases of labor.

This is also a good time to assess the laboring woman's perception of pain. What is her affect? Is this contraction more uncomfortable than the last one? Is the nurse's palpation of intensity congruent with the woman's perception? (For instance, the nurse might evaluate a contraction as mild in intensity while the laboring woman evaluates it as very strong.) A nurse's assessment is not complete without the laboring woman's affect and response to the contractions being charted.

Electronic Monitoring of Contractions with External Tocodynamometer Electronic monitoring of uterine contractions provides continuous data. How much an electronic fetal monitor is used depends on many factors: the type of birth setting and associated protocols; the couple's wishes; whether the pregnancy is low risk or high risk; whether other procedures are being done, for example, amnioinfusion (see Chapter 23); and whether other methods, such as frequent use of hand-held Doppler ultrasound, can be used as a substitute. Electronic monitoring may be done externally, with a device that is placed against the maternal abdomen, or internally, with an intrauterine pressure catheter. When monitoring by external means, the clinician places the portion of the

TABLE 19–2 Contraction and Labor Progress Characteristics

Contraction Characteristics	
Latent phase:	Every 10–30 min × 20–40 sec; mild, progressing to Every 5–7 min × 30–40 sec; moderate
Active phase:	Every 2–3 min × 40–60 sec; moderate to strong
Transition phase:	Every 1½–2min × 60–90 sec; strong
Labor Progress Characteristics	
Primipara:	1.2 cm/hr dilatation 1 cm/hr descent <2 hr in second stage
Multipara:	1.5 cm/hr dilatation 2 cm/hr descent <1 hr in second stage

CLINICAL TIP

Learning to assess the intensity of uterine contractions may be difficult when you begin your labor and birth clinical experience. Gently rest your fingers on the fundus of the uterus and occasionally press one fingertip against the abdominal skin to get a sense of how far the skin indents. Resist the temptation to keep your fingers in constant motion. You may ask the woman to let you know when she feels the contraction begin and end; this will help you sense the changes in muscle tension that are occurring in the uterus. During the contraction, push gently against the underlying tissues. During a mild contraction the maternal abdomen indents like a slightly flexed bicep muscle; a moderate contraction feels like a tightly contracted bicep; and a strong or intense contraction feels like the back of your hand.

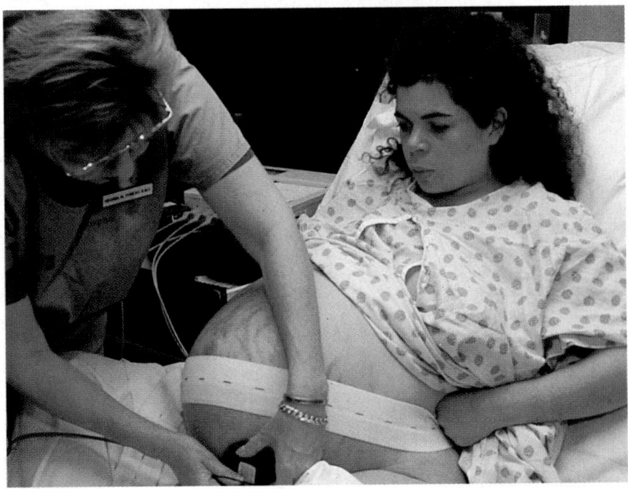

FIGURE 19–4 Woman in labor with external monitor applied. The tocodynamometer placed on the uterine fundus is recording uterine contractions. The lower belt holds the ultrasonic device that monitors the fetal heart rate. The belts can be adjusted for comfort.

monitoring equipment called the *tocodynamometer*, or "toco," against the fundus of the uterus (the area of greatest contractility) and holds it in place with an elastic belt or other adhesive material. The toco contains a flexible disk or a diaphragm (depending on the manufacturer). As the uterus contracts, pressure exerted against the toco is amplified and transmitted to the electronic fetal monitor and recorded on graph paper (Figure 19–4 and Figure 19–11, on page 521). Uterine contractions can be assessed for frequency and duration, but not for intensity. The intensity (as displayed on the graph paper) is a reflection of how tightly the belt is applied around the maternal abdomen. When the belt is tight enough, the nurse should be able to note the beginning of contractions on the monitor just before or at the same time the woman begins to feel them.

The advantages to this method are that it may be used prior to rupture of membranes antepartally and intrapartally and it provides a continuous recording of the duration and frequency of contractions. The major disadvantage is that it cannot assess the intensity of contractions (because the obtained tracing is influenced by how snugly the elastic belt is applied). Intensity of contractions must be assessed by the nurse, who uses the hand to palpate for intensity of the contraction as well as the resting tone of the uterus between contractions. Another disadvantage is that sometimes the belt bothers the woman because it must be snug to monitor uterine contractions accurately—the belt may require frequent readjustment as she changes position, or the woman may feel she needs to remain in one position so as not to disturb the belt.

A beltless tocodynamometer is available. This system consists of an adhesive transducer that is applied to the most prominent part of the woman's abdomen with a double-sided adhesive film. The nonbelted tocodynamometer tends to be preferred by the laboring woman because it allows more freedom of movement and eliminates the need to wear a belt around the abdomen, is easily applied, needs readjustment only infrequently, and generally is more convenient (Figure 19–5).

Electronic Monitoring by Internal Means The **intrauterine catheter** not only provides information regarding frequency and duration of uterine contractions, but also assesses intensity of uterine contractions. (Note: Internal monitoring can be used only if the amniotic membranes are ruptured.) One type of intrauterine catheter, called the INTRAN Plus, has a micropressure transducer (electronic sensor) at the tip. The catheter is slowly inserted through the cervical os into the uterine cavity, usually in the area where fetal small parts (arms or legs) are located. The catheter is advanced only as far as the black marking indicated on the catheter, which should be visualized at the opening to the vagina (Figure 19–6). The catheter is then connected by a cable to the electronic fetal monitor. This catheter incorporates a second lumen and a port for amnioinfusion (an infusion of fluid into the amniotic cavity to provide additional fluid or to dilute amniotic fluid that contains thick meconium). The second port permits amnnioinfusion while simultaneously providing accurate monitoring of intrauterine pressure (Figure 19–7).

In many institutions, the intrauterine catheter is used only during oxytocin augmentation, induction of labor, or vaginal birth after cesarean. It is particularly important to quantitate the intensity and frequency of contractions to avoid hyperstimulation and possible uterine rupture due to overadministration of oxytocin. If the woman's labor is prolonged, internal monitoring can be used to accurately assess the frequency and strength of contractions and resultant FHR pattern response. When an intrauterine catheter is used, there is a 1% risk of infection, but this seems to depend on the duration of ruptured membranes and length of labor.

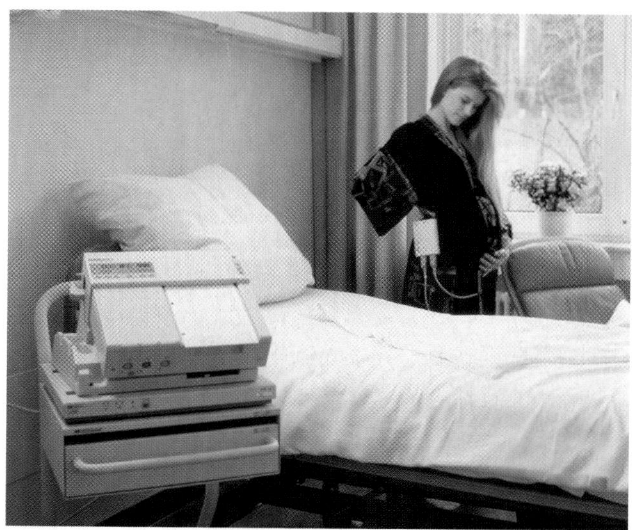

FIGURE 19–5 The beltless tocodynamometer system features remote telemetry. SOURCE: Courtesy of Hewlett-Packard Company.

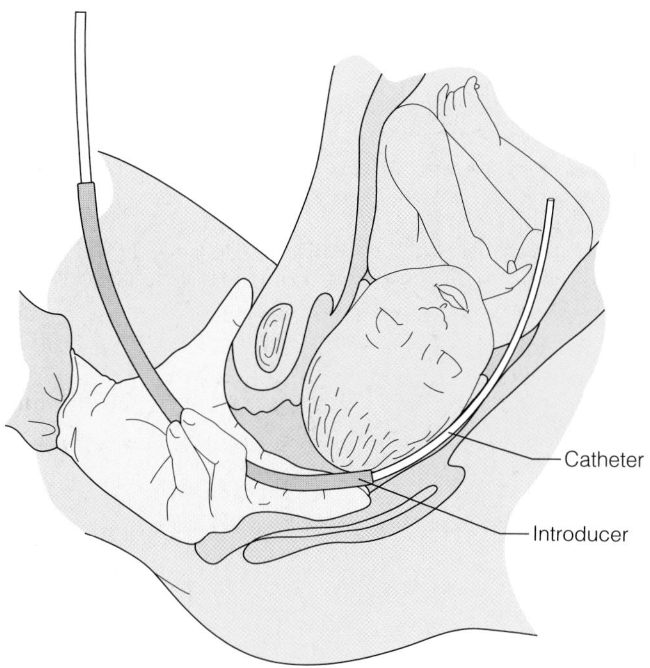

FIGURE 19–6 Technique of inserting a uterine catheter. Note that the introducer (catheter guide) is inserted no farther than beyond the fingertips.

It is of particular importance that the nurse evaluate the woman's labor status by means other than the fetal monitor. As with any type of technology, no machine is flawless, and the monitor cannot fill the role of the nurse. One should never rely solely on data recorded by a machine. Technology is useful only as an adjunct to good nursing assessment. All too often, women are in active labor with adequate contractions that are regarded as being of "poor quality" because the monitor is not functioning properly. The nurse should routinely palpate the intensity of the contractions and the relaxation of the uterus between contractions and compare the assessment with data recorded by the monitor.

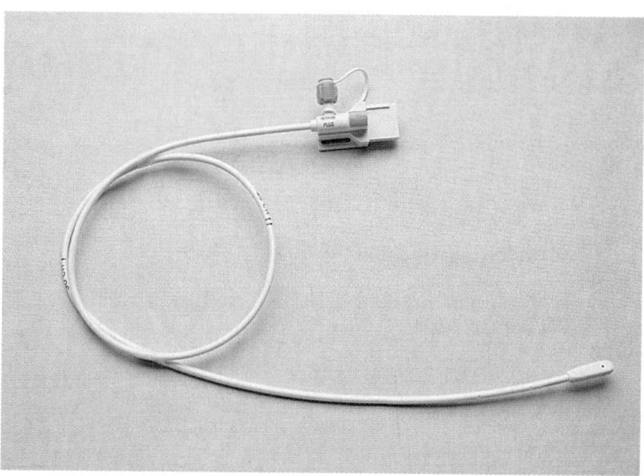

FIGURE 19–7 INTRAN plus intrauterine pressure catheter. There is a micropressure transducer (electronic sensor) located at the tip of the catheter and a port for amnioinfusion at the distal end of the catheter.

Trying to figure out if I was in labor was quite a task. Here I was, a birthing room nurse, and I couldn't decide if my contractions were the real thing. I timed them, and about the time I decided this was It, they would slow down. How exasperating not to be able to really know! It was hard on me because I felt surely a birthing room nurse should know for herself. But now I see that all women are in this spot. They want so much to be right, and we often treat them as if they should be able to know absolutely when it's the real thing. I'd like birthing room nurses to remember this.

Cervical Assessment

Cervical dilatation and effacement are evaluated directly by vaginal examination (see Procedure 19–1: Intrapartal Vaginal Examination). The vaginal examination can also provide information regarding membrane status, fetal position, and station of the presenting part (Procedure 19–2: Assessing for Amniotic Fluid).

CRITICAL THINKING QUESTION

You walk into the birthing center at the beginning of your shift and look at the listing of clients who are in the birthing area. The listing looks like this:

Name	G/P	Contrac	Dil	Efface	Gestation
Brooks	2/1	q10 × 40	4 cm	25%	39
Cole	1/0	q2 × 60	10 cm	100%	40
Johnson	6/5	q5 × 60	4 cm	100%	41
Smith	1/0	q3 × 40	3 cm	30%	27, twins

PROCEDURE 19–2 ASSESSING FOR AMNIOTIC FLUID

Nursing Action	Rationale
Objective: Assemble equipment.	
• Gather Nitrazine test tape and a pair of disposable gloves.	*Nitrazine test tape reacts to alkaline fluids and confirms presence of amniotic fluid.*
• Have microscope and glass slide available if determining ferning of obtained fluid.	*Microscope is used to detect ferning pattern.*
• Obtain a sterile speculum.	
Objective: Set the stage for the assessment.	
Explain the procedure, indications for the procedure, what the woman will feel, and information that may be obtained. Determine whether she has noted the escape of any clear fluid from the vagina.	*Explanation of the procedure decreases anxiety and increases relaxation.*
Objective: Test fluid.	
• Prior to performing a vaginal examination that uses lubricant, put on gloves. With one gloved hand, spread the labia, and with the other hand place a small section of Nitrazine tape (approx. 2 in long) against the vaginal opening. Take care not to touch tape with bare fingers prior to the test.	*Contamination of the Nitrazine test tape with lubricant can make the test unreliable.* *Enough fluid needs to be placed on the test tape to make it wet. Amniotic fluid is alkaline, and an alkaline fluid turns the Nitrazine test tape a dark blue. If the test tape remains a beige color, the test is negative for amniotic fluid.*
• Compare the color on the test tape to the guide on the back of the Nitrazine test tape container to determine the test results.	
• Amniotic fluid may also be obtained by speculum exam. This is indicated in preterm premature rupture of membranes. If fluid is present in sufficient amount to draw some into a syringe, a small amount of fluid can be placed on a glass slide, allowed to dry, and then examined under a microscope. A ferning pattern confirms the presence of amniotic fluid. See Figure 8–4 for an example of ferning.	*Obtaining a specimen by speculum examination reduces the contamination of the fluid with other substances such as blood and reduces chance of infection for the woman who is not actively laboring.*
Objective: Record information on client's record.	
Record on labor record (eg, SROM, Nitrazine positive).	*Nurse documents status of membranes, intact or ruptured.*

After looking at all the data and using the norms that have been provided in Chapters 18 and 19, think through the following questions.

1. Which expectant woman will probably give birth first? Why?
2. Which expectant woman do you not want to continue in labor? Why not?
3. Which of the clients is having her first baby?
4. What stage of labor is each of the women in?
5. Consider the contraction frequency and duration and the cervical dilatation and effacement for each woman. Do the assessments match what you would expect for the stage of labor?
6. Which of the women are at term?

Fetal Assessment

Determination of Fetal Position and Presentation

Fetal position is determined in several ways. The woman's abdomen is inspected and palpated to determine fetal position; auscultation of fetal heart tones also helps determine fetal position. A vaginal examination may be done to determine the presenting part, and ultrasound examination may be used.

Inspection

The nurse should observe the woman's abdomen for size and shape. The lie of the fetus should be assessed by noting whether the uterus projects up and down (longitudinal lie) or left to right (transverse lie).

Palpation: Leopold's Maneuvers

Leopold's maneuvers are a systematic way to evaluate the maternal abdomen (Figure 19–8). Frequent practice increases the examiner's skill in determining fetal position by palpation. Leopold's maneuvers may be difficult to perform on an obese woman or on a woman who has excessive amniotic fluid (hydramnios).

Care should be taken to ensure the woman's comfort during Leopold's maneuvers. The woman should have recently emptied her bladder and should lie on her back with her abdomen uncovered. To aid in relaxation of the abdominal wall, the shoulders should be raised slightly on a pillow and the knees drawn up a little. The procedure should be completed between contractions. The examiner's hands should be warm.

While inspecting and palpating the maternal abdomen, the nurse should consider the following questions:

- Is the fetal lie longitudinal or transverse?
- What is in the fundus? Am I feeling buttocks or head?
- Where is the fetal back?
- Where are the small parts or extremities?
- What is in the inlet? Does it confirm what I found in the fundus?
- Is the presenting part engaged, floating, or dipping into the inlet?
- Is there fetal movement?
- How large is the fetus (appropriate, large, or small for gestational age)?
- Is there one fetus or more than one?
- Is fundal height proportionate to the estimated gestational age?

First Maneuver While facing the woman, the nurse palpates the upper abdomen with both hands (Figure 19–8). The nurse determines the shape, size, consistency, and mobility of the form that is found. The fetal head is firm, hard, and round and moves independently of the trunk. The breech feels softer and symmetric and has small bony prominences; it moves with the trunk.

Second Maneuver After ascertaining whether the head or the buttocks occupies the fundus, the nurse tries to determine the location of the fetal back and notes whether it is on the right or left side of the maternal abdomen. Still facing the woman, the nurse palpates the abdomen with deep but gentle pressure, using the palms (Figure 19–8). The right hand should be steady while the left hand explores the right side of the uterus. The nurse then repeats the maneuver, probing with the right hand and steadying the uterus with the left hand. The fetal back should feel firm and smooth and should connect what was found in the fundus with a mass in the inlet. Once the back is located, the nurse validates the finding by palpating the fetal extremities (small irregularities and protrusions) on the opposite side of the abdomen.

Third Maneuver Next the nurse should determine what fetal part is lying above the inlet by gently grasping the lower portion of the abdomen just above the symphysis pubis with the thumb and fingers of the right hand (Figure 19–8). This maneuver yields the opposite information from what was found in the fundus and validates the presenting part. If the head is presenting and is not engaged, it may be gently pushed back and forth.

Fourth Maneuver For this portion of the examination, the nurse faces the woman's feet and attempts to locate the cephalic prominence or brow. Location of this landmark assists in assessing the descent of the presenting part into the pelvis. The fingers of both hands are moved gently down the sides of the uterus toward the pubis (Figure 19–8). The cephalic prominence (brow) is located on the side where there is greatest resistance to the descent of the fingers toward the pubis. It is located on the opposite side from the fetal back if the head is well flexed. However, when the fetal head is extended, the occiput is the first cephalic prominence felt, and it is located on the same side as the back. Therefore when completing the fourth maneuver, if the first cephalic prominence palpated is on the same side as the back, the head is not flexed. If the first prominence found is opposite the back, the head is well flexed.

CRITICAL THINKING QUESTION

The fetus in Figure 19–8 is in ROA position. Describe what you would feel during Leopold's maneuvers if the fetus were LOA.

Vaginal Examination

The vaginal examination reveals information regarding the fetus such as presentation, position, station, degree of flexion of the fetal head, and any swelling that might be present on the fetal scalp (caput succedaneum).

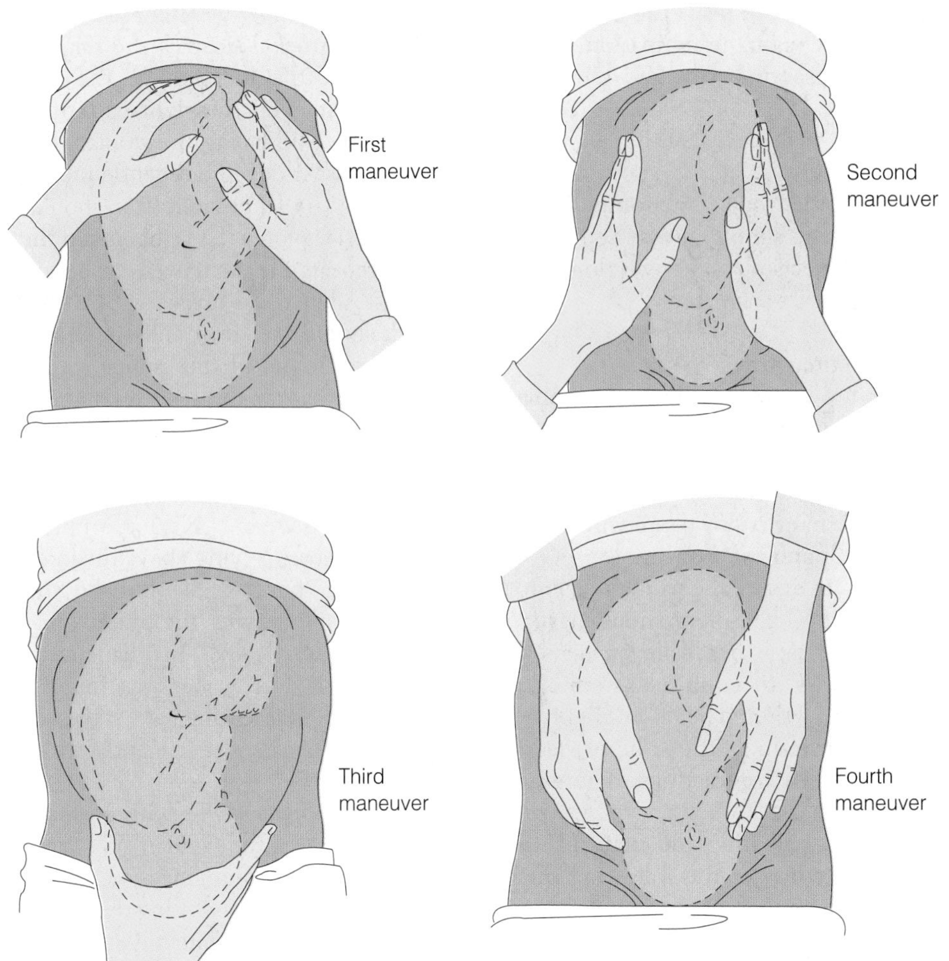

FIGURE 19–8 Leopold's maneuvers for determining fetal position, presentation, and lie. Note: Many nurses do the fourth maneuver first in order to identify the part of the fetus in the pelvic inlet.

Ultrasound

Real-time ultrasound is frequently available in the birth setting and may be used to obtain specific information regarding the fetus. A real-time ultrasound may be done at this time to assess fetal lie, presentation, and position; obtain measurements of biparietal diameter to estimate gestational age; assess for anomalies when a vaginal examination reveals suspicious findings; assess placement of the placenta; and sometimes confirm the presence of more than one fetus. (See Chapter 17 for further discussion of the use of ultrasound for fetal assessment.)

Evaluation of Fetal Status During Labor

Auscultation of Fetal Heart Rate

The fetoscope or a hand-held ultrasound device is used to auscultate the fetal heart rate (FHR) between, during, and immediately after uterine contractions (see Figure 19–9).

Before listening to the FHR the first time, the nurse may choose to perform Leopold's maneuvers and check the maternal heart rate. Leopold's maneuvers not only indicate the probable location of the FHR, but also help determine the presence of multiple fetuses, fetal lie, and fetal presentation. FHR is heard most clearly at the fetal back (Figure 19–10). Thus, in a cephalic presentation, FHR is best heard in the lower quadrant of the maternal abdomen. In a breech presentation it is heard at or above the level of the maternal umbilicus. In a transverse lie FHR may be heard best just above or just below the umbilicus. As the presenting part descends and rotates through the maternal pelvis during labor, FHR tends to descend and move toward the midline.

In some instances, the monitor may track the maternal heart rate instead of the fetal heart rate. However, the nurse can avoid the error by comparing the maternal pulse to the FHR.

After FHR is located, it is usually counted for 30 seconds and multiplied by two to obtain the number of beats per minute. The nurse should occasionally listen for 1 full minute, through and just after a contraction, to detect any abnormal heart rate, especially if the FHR is over 160 (tachycardia), under 120 (bradycardia), or irregular beats are heard. Listening through a contraction may be difficult because of maternal movement or a muffling of the

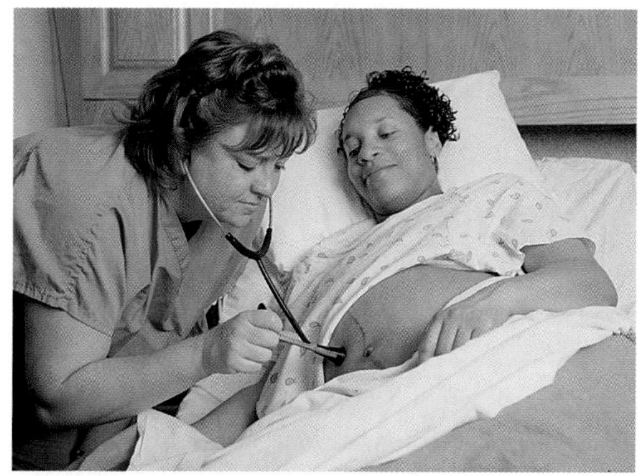
A

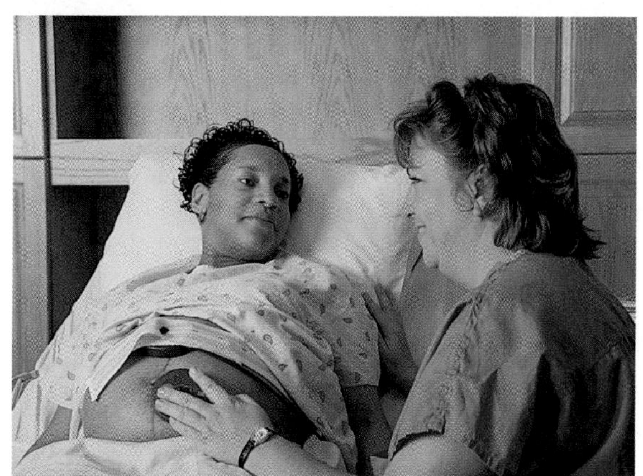
B

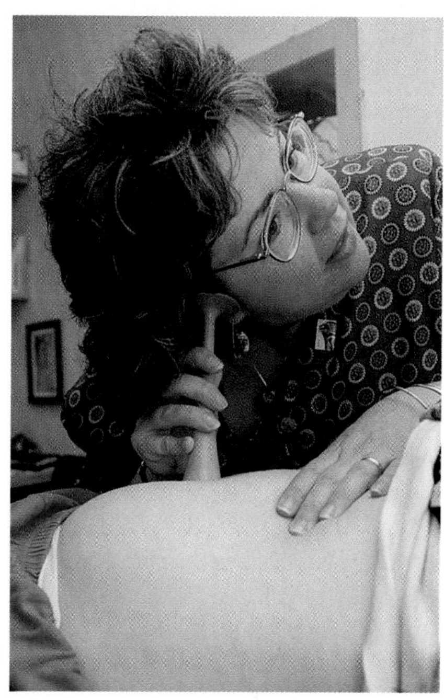
C

FIGURE 19–9 ***A,*** The nurse holds the fetoscope as she places it against the maternal abdomen. ***B,*** When the fetal heart rate is picked up by the electronic monitor, the sound of the heartbeat can be heard by all persons in the room. ***C,*** The Penar fetoscope can be easily used in an outpatient or community setting.

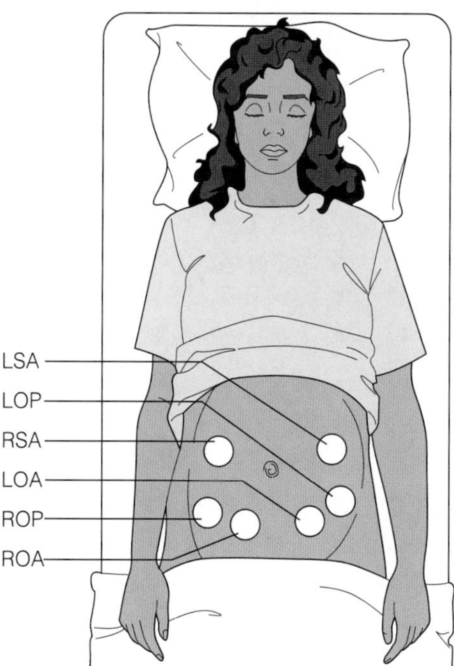

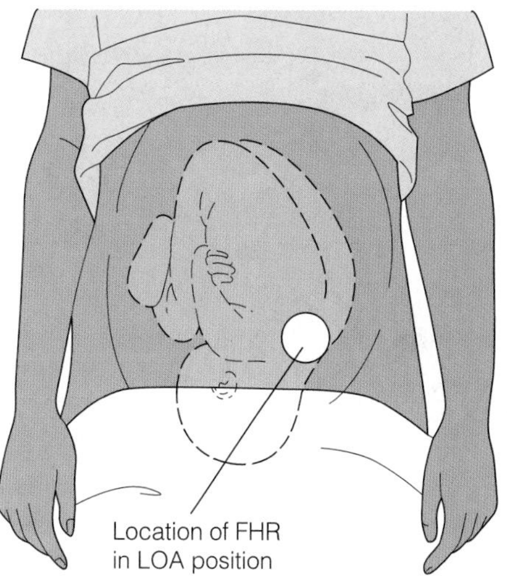

FIGURE 19–10 Location of FHR in relation to the more commonly seen fetal positions. The fetal heart rate is heard more clearly over the fetal back.

FHR sounds. If the FHR is irregular or has changed markedly from the last assessment, the nurse should listen for 1 full minute through and immediately after a contraction. It is especially important to listen during and after the contraction to detect any deceleration that might occur. It is also important to listen immediately after each contraction when the woman is pushing during second stage because fetal bradycardia frequently occurs as pressure is exerted on the fetal head during descent. See Procedure 19–3: Auscultation of Fetal Heart Rate and Table 19–3 for guidelines regarding how often to auscultate FHR.

Text continues on page 520.

PROCEDURE 19–3 AUSCULTATION OF FETAL HEART RATE

Nursing Action	*Rationale*
Objective: Assemble the equipment.	
Obtain a fetoscope or a Doppler.	*These devices amplify the fetal heart rate sounds.*
Objective: Prepare the woman.	
• Explain the procedure, the indications for the procedure, and the information that will be obtained.	*Explaining the procedure decreases anxiety and increases relaxation.*
• Uncover the woman's abdomen.	
Objective: Use the fetoscope or Doppler as indicated and listen carefully for the FHR.	
Objective: Check the woman's pulse, then count the FHR.	
• Check the woman's pulse against the fetal sounds you hear. If the rates are the same, you have probably located maternal pulses and you need to readjust the fetoscope or ultrasound device.	
• If the rates are not similar, count the FHR for 1 full minute. Note that the fetal heart has a double rhythm and just one sound is counted.	
• If you do not find the FHR, move the fetoscope or ultrasound device laterally.	
• Explain to the parents what the FHR is and offer to help them listen if they would like to.	
Objective: Systematically evaluate the FHR.	
Auscultate between, during, and for 30 seconds following a uterine contraction (UC).	*This evaluation provides the opportunity to assess the fetal status and response to the labor process.*
NAACOG (1990) Frequency Recommendations	
• Low-risk women: every 1 hour in the latent phase, every 30 minutes in the active phase, and every 15 minutes in the second stage.	
• High-risk women: every 30 minutes in the latent phase, every 15 minutes in the active phase, and every 5 minutes in the second stage.	
Objective: Record the information on the woman's chart.	
Document FHR data (rate and rhythm), characteristics of uterine activity, and any actions taken as a result of the FHR. Complete documentation is mandatory.	
Sample recordings are shown below.	

Sample Documentation

Entry documenting FHR, rhythm, and response to the labor process:

1-1-02 0730 FHR 140 by auscultation, regular rhythm. Maternal pulse 78. UC q3min × 60 sec strong. No increase or decrease in FHR noted during or following UC. J Smith RN

Nursing Action	Rationale

Sample Documentation *continued*

Entry documenting FHR, response to UC, nursing intervention, and fetal response:

1-1-02 0730 FHR 136 by auscultation with slowing to 130 bpm noted during the acme of UC and for 10 sec following the UC, STV present, LTV average. Client turned to left side. Maternal pulse 80, FHR 140, regular rhythm with no decrease during or following the next two UC. UC q3min 3 60 sec strong. J Smith RN

Using a Fetoscope or a Doppler Ultrasound Device

The Fetoscope

The fetoscope is an older assessment tool; however, some clinicians prefer it because it is "natural" and does not rely on ultrasound.

To use the fetoscope:

- Place the fetoscope earpieces in your ears; use the handpiece to position the bell of the fetoscope on the mother's abdomen.
- Place the diaphragm halfway between the umbilicus and symphysis and in the midline. *You are most likely to hear the FHR in this area.*
- Without touching the fetoscope, listen carefully for the FHR (Figure 19–9A).

The Doppler

To use the Doppler:

- Place "ultrasonic gel" on the diaphragm of the Doppler. Gel is used to maintain contact with the maternal abdomen and enhances conduction of ultrasound.
- Place the diaphragm on the woman's abdomen halfway between the umbilicus and symphysis and in the midline. You are most likely to hear the FHR in this area.
- Listen carefully for the FHR (Figure 19–9B).

TABLE 19–3 Frequency of Auscultation: Assessment and Documentation

Low-Risk Patients	High-Risk Patients
First stage of labor: q1 hr in latent phase q30 min in active phase Second stage of labor: q15 min	First stage of labor: q30 min in latent phase q15 min in active phase Second stage of labor: q5 min

Labor Events

Assess FHR prior to:
- Initiation of labor-enhancing procedures (eg, artificial rupture of membranes)
- Periods of ambulation
- Administration of medications
- Administration or initiation of analgesia/anesthesia

Labor Events *continued*

Assess FHR following:
- Rupture of membranes
- Recognition of abnormal uterine activity patterns, such as increased basal tone or tachysystole
- Evaluation of oxytocin (maintenance, increase, or decrease of dosage)
- Administration of medications (at time of peak action)
- Expulsion of enema
- Urinary catheterization
- Vaginal examination
- Periods of ambulation
- Evaluation of analgesia and/or anesthesia (maintenance, increase, or decrease of dosage)

SOURCE: Nurses' Association of the American College of Obstetricians and Gynecologists (NAACOG): *OGN Nursing Practice Resource, Fetal Heart Rate Auscultation.* Washington, DC: NAACOG, 1990, p 5; American Academy of Pediatrics (AAP), American College of Obstetricians and Gynecologists (ACOG): *Guidelines for Perinatal Care,* 4th ed. Washington, DC :AAP, ACOG, 1997.

The American Academy of Pediatrics (AAP) and the American College of Obstetricians and Gynecologists (ACOG) *Guidelines for Perinatal Care* (1997) indicates that auscultation performed as described earlier is equivalent to electronic fetal monitoring.

If decelerations (discussed later in this chapter) are noted, the woman should be electronically monitored to rule out abnormalities in the FHR.

Electronic Fetal Monitoring

Electronic fetal monitoring (EFM) provides a visual assessment of fetal heart rate. A continuous tracing of the FHR can be obtained, allowing many characteristics of the fetal heart rate to be observed and evaluated. (See Procedure 19–4: Electronic Fetal Monitoring.)

When the FHR is monitored electronically, the interval between two successive fetal heartbeats is measured, and the rate is displayed as if the beats occurred at the same interval for 60 seconds. For example, if the interval between two beats is 0.5 second, the rate for 1 full minute would be 120 beats per minute.

EFM has major advantages over auscultation with the fetoscope. Electronic monitoring is an objective means of evaluating fetal well-being. Fetal distress can be detected by observing the continuous FHR and the periodic responses that occur during and after uterine contractions. Therefore, interventions can be timely and thus more effective.

Indications for Electronic Fetal Monitoring Any woman with previous history of medical or obstetric problems that might affect labor or the health of the fetus should be monitored by continuous electronic fetal monitoring. Some physicians advocate monitoring only those women considered to be at risk or at high risk, but many feel the procedure is mandatory for all women in labor. Table 19–4 lists specific indications for electronic monitoring.

TABLE 19–4 Indications for Electronic Monitoring

Fetal Factors
- Decreased fetal movement
- Abnormal auscultory FHR
- Meconium passage
- Abnormal presentations/positions
- Intrauterine growth restriction (IUGR) or small-for-gestational age (SGA) fetus
- Postdates (>41 weeks)
- Multiple gestation

Maternal Factors
- Fever
- Infections
- PIH
- Disease conditions (eg, hypertension, diabetes)
- Anemia
- Rh isoimmunization
- Previous perinatal death
- Grand multiparity
- Previous cesarean birth
- Borderline/contracted pelvis

Uterine Factors
- Dysfunctional labor
- Failure to progress in labor
- Oxytocin induction/augmentation
- Uterine anomalies

Complications of Pregnancy
- Prolonged rupture of membranes
- Premature rupture of membranes
- Preterm labor
- Marginal abruptio placentae
- Partial placenta previa
- ccult/frank prolapse of cord
- Amnionitis

Regional Anesthesia

Elective Monitoring

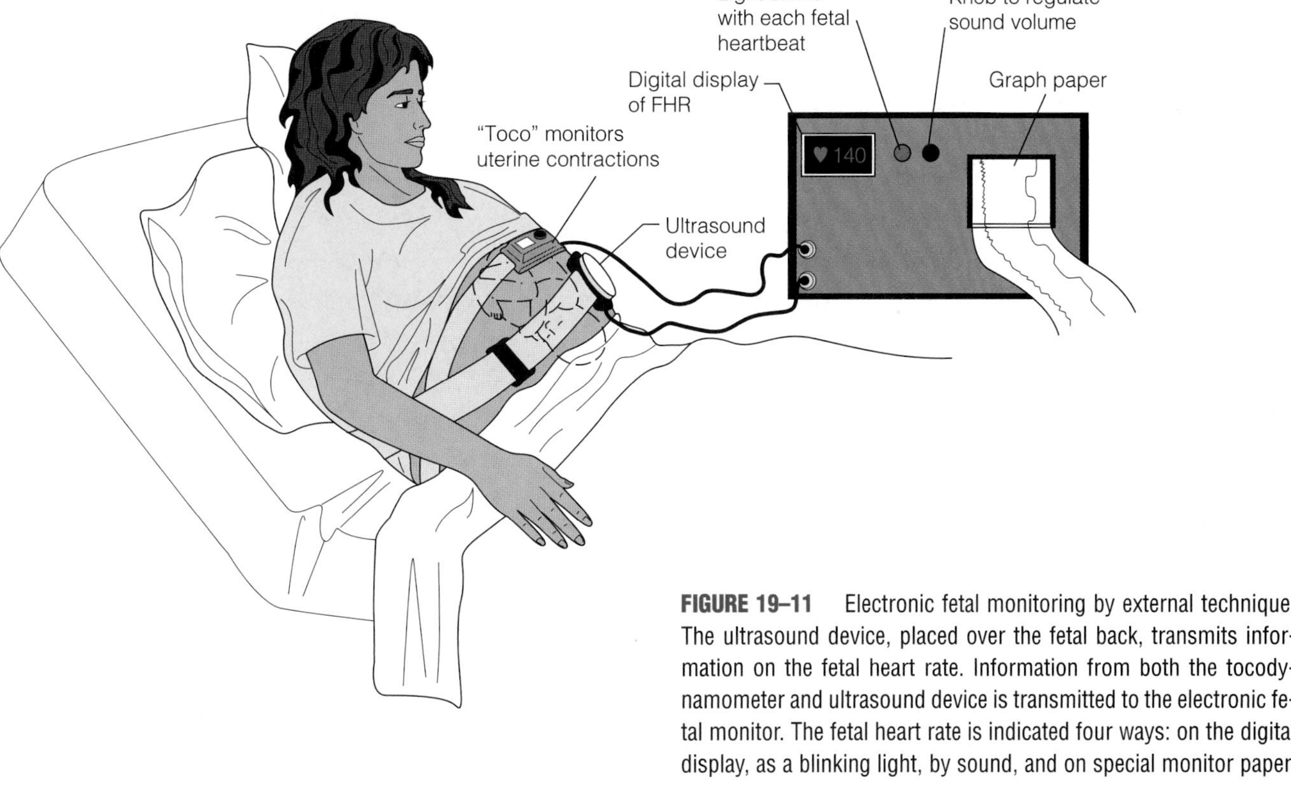

FIGURE 19–11 Electronic fetal monitoring by external technique. The ultrasound device, placed over the fetal back, transmits information on the fetal heart rate. Information from both the tocodynamometer and ultrasound device is transmitted to the electronic fetal monitor. The fetal heart rate is indicated four ways: on the digital display, as a blinking light, by sound, and on special monitor paper. The uterine contractions are displayed on the graph paper.

External Monitoring *External monitoring* of the fetus is usually accomplished by ultrasound. A transducer, which emits continuous sound waves, is placed on the maternal abdomen. A water-soluble gel is applied to the underside of the transducer to aid in conduction of fetal heart sounds. When the transducer is placed correctly, the sound waves bounce off the fetal heart and are picked up by the electronic monitor. The actual moment-by-moment FHR is displayed simultaneously on a screen and on graph paper (Figure 19–11).

The transducer may inadvertently be directed toward a pulsating maternal vessel. In this case there will be a soft swooshing sound (uterine souffle), and the rate will be the same as the maternal pulse.

Disadvantages of monitoring fetal heart rate by external means are similar to those of external uterine contraction monitoring. In addition, the tracing may be poor if the fetus is quite active, if more than a normal amount of amniotic fluid is present (hydramnios), or if the woman is moving about frequently.

Internal Monitoring Internal monitoring is accomplished through use of an internal spiral electrode, which is attached to the skin of the fetal head or buttocks (Figure 19–12). In order for the spiral electrode to be inserted, the cervix must be dilated at least 2 cm, the presenting fetal part must be accessible by vaginal examination, and the membranes must be ruptured. Even though it is not possible to apply the electrode and catheter under strict sterile conditions, the procedure should be performed as aseptically as possible. After determining fetal position by vaginal examination, the examiner (physician or nurse) inserts the electrode, which is encased in a plastic guide, to the level of the internal cervical os and attaches it to the presenting part, being careful not to apply it to the face, suture lines, fontanelles, or perineum if the fetus is in a breech presentation. The electrode is rotated clockwise until it is attached to the presenting part and is then disengaged from the guide tube. The guide tube is removed, and the end wires are connected to a leg plate that is attached to the woman's thigh. The cable from the leg plate is connected to the monitor.

The FHR tracing at the top of Figure 19–13 was obtained by internal monitoring, and the uterine contraction tracing at the bottom by external monitoring. The spiral electrode provides an instantaneous and continuous recording of FHR that is clearer than data provided by external monitoring. Note that the FHR is variable (the tracing moves up and down instead of in a straight line), and the tracing stays close to the line numbered 150. If the graph paper moves through the monitor at 3 cm per minute, each vertical dark lines represents 1 minute. On Figure 19–13 note that the frequency of the uterine contractions is every 2½ to 3 minutes. The duration of the contractions is 50 to 60 seconds.

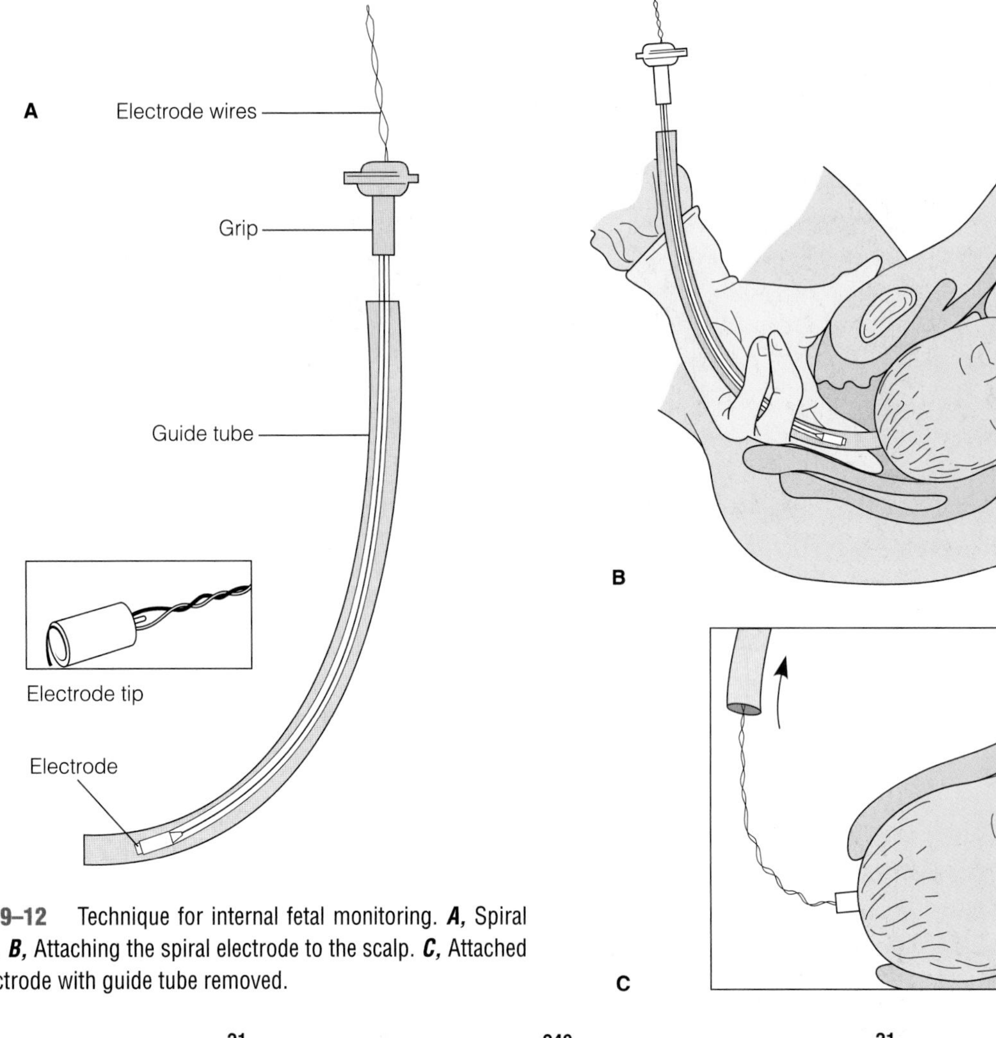

FIGURE 19–12 Technique for internal fetal monitoring. ***A,*** Spiral electrode. ***B,*** Attaching the spiral electrode to the scalp. ***C,*** Attached spiral electrode with guide tube removed.

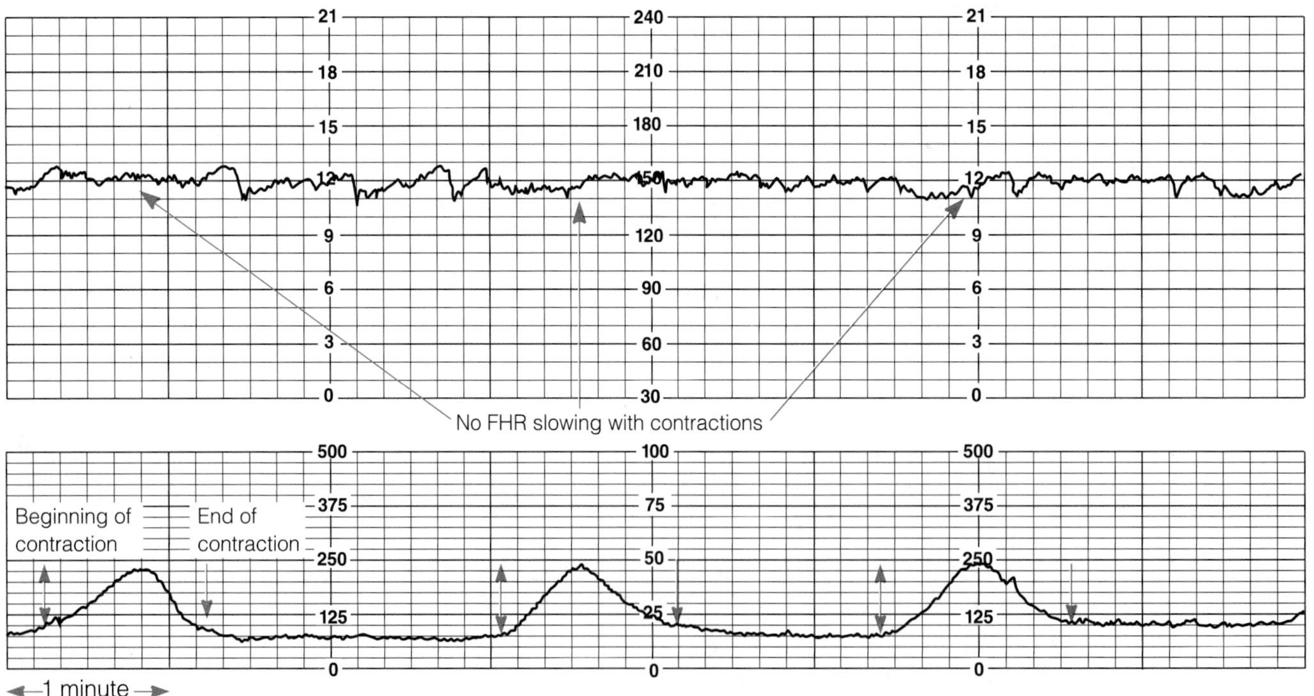

FIGURE 19–13 Normal FHR range is from 120 to 160 beats per minute. The FHR tracing in the upper portion of the graph indicates an FHR range of 140–155 bpm. The bottom portion depicts uterine contractions. Each dark vertical line marks 1 minute, and each small rectangle represents 10 seconds. The contraction frequency is about every 3 minutes, and the duration of the contractions is 50–60 seconds.

PROCEDURE 19–4 ELECTRONIC FETAL MONITORING

Nursing Action	*Rationale*
Objective: Prepare the woman.	
Explain the procedure, the indications for the procedure, and the information that will be obtained.	*Explaining the procedure decreases anxiety and increases relaxation.*
Objective: Place the external fetal monitor.	
• Turn on the monitor.	
• Place two elastic belts around the woman's abdomen.	
• Place the "toco" over the uterine fundus off the midline on the area palpated to be most firm, and secure it with a belt so it fits snugly.	*The uterine fundus is the area of greatest contractility.*
• Note the UC tracing. The resting tone tracing (without uterine contraction) should be recording on the 10 or 15 mm Hg pressure line. Adjust the line to reflect that reading.	*If the tracing is on the zero line, there may be a constant grinding noise.*
• Apply ultrasonic gel to the diaphragm of the ultrasound transducer.	*Ultrasound gel is used to maintain contact with the maternal abdomen. The ultrasonic beam is directed toward the fetal heart.*
• Place the diaphragm on the maternal abdomen in the midline between the umbilicus and the symphysis pubis.	
• Listen for the FHR, which will have a whiplike sound. When the FHR is located, attach the elastic belt snugly. Firm contact is necessary to maintain a continuous tracing.	
Objective: Identify the tracing.	
Place the following information on the beginning of the fetal monitor paper: date, time, client name, gravida, para, membrane status, physician/CNM name. Note: Each birthing area may have specific guidelines regarding additional information to include.	*This ensures accurate identification.*
Objective: Evaluate the EFM tracing.	
See the material below for evaluation guidelines.	
Objective: Report and record your findings.	*Reporting provides a permanent record.*

Sample Documentation

Entry documenting reassuring FHR characteristics and response to UCs:

1-1-02 0700	FHR BL 135–140. STV and LTV present. Two accelerations of 20 bpm × 20 sec with fetal movement in 10 min. UC q3min × 50–60 sec of moderate intensity by palpation, resting tone soft. No decelerations noted. B Burch, RNC

Entry documenting FHR, variability, response of FHR to UC, the intervention used, and subsequent positive fetal response to the intervention.

1-1-02 0730	FHR BL 135–140. STV and LTV present. Late decelerations noted with decrease of FHR to 130 bpm for 20 sec. UC q3min × 50–60 sec of moderate intensity by palpation. Client turned to left side. No further deceleration with three subsequent UC. Two accelerations of 20 bpm × 20 sec noted with fetal movement. Client instructed to remain on left side. B Burch, RNC

PROCEDURE 19–4 ELECTRONIC FETAL MONITORING CONTINUED

Nursing Action	*Rationale*
Guidelines for Evaluating the EFM	
Evaluating the EFM tracing provides an opportunity to assess the fetal status and response to the labor process. The presence of reassuring characteristics is associated with good fetal outcome. Rapid identification of nonreassuring characteristics allows prompt interventions and the opportunity to determine the fetal response to the interventions.	*For high-risk women, NAACOG (1988) recommends evaluating the EFM tracing every 15 minutes in the first stage and every 5 minutes in the second stage; for low-risk women, every 15–30 minutes in the first stage and every 5–15 minutes in the second stage (as long as the FHR has reassuring characteristics) is frequently done. The time interval for evaluation needs to be shortened if any nonreassuring characteristics occur.*

Telemetry Fetal heart rate and uterine activity may also be monitored by a telemetry system. Ultrasound, or fetal ECG, and external uterine pressure transducers are connected to a small battery-operated transducer. Signals are transmitted to a receiver connected to the monitor. The monitor displays FHR and uterine activity data on the oscilloscope and prints it out on graph paper to provide documentation. This system, which can be worn by means of a shoulder strap, allows the woman to ambulate, helping her to feel more comfortable and less confined during labor, yet provides for continuous monitoring. Telemetry provides for direct as well as indirect monitoring of FHR, indirect monitoring of uterine pressure, and dual FHR monitoring of twins. (See a comparison of different methods in Table 19–5.)

Fetal Heart Rate Patterns

Fetal heart rate is evaluated by assessing both baseline and periodic changes. Normal FHR ranges from 120 to 160 beats per minute. More important than FHR are the periodic changes that occur in response to the intermittent stress of uterine contractions and the baseline beat-to-beat variability of the fetal heart rate. A compromised fetus may have a normal heart rate but demonstrate slight periodic changes and decreased variability (the change in FHR over a few seconds to a few minutes) indicative of intrauterine hypoxia.

Baseline Rate The **baseline rate** refers to the range of FHR observed between contractions during a continuous 10-minute period of monitoring. The range does not include the rate during decelerations. There are two abnormal variations of the baseline rate—those above 160 bpm (tachycardia) and those below 120 bpm (bradycardia). Variability also affects the baseline.

Tachycardia *Tachycardia* is defined as FHR above 150 to 160 bpm continuing for 10 minutes or more (Menihan, 1996). Although tachycardia may occur without apparent reason, possible causes include the following (Menihan, 1996):

- Early fetal hypoxia (This leads to stimulation of the sympathetic system as the fetus compensates for reduced blood flow.)
- Maternal fever (Metabolism of the fetus accelerates because of increased maternal temperature.)
- Betasympathomimetic drugs, such as ritodrine, terbutaline, atropine, and isoxsuprine (These drugs have a cardiac stimulant effect.)
- Maternal hyperthyroidism (Thyroid-stimulating hormones may cross the placenta and stimulate the fetal heart rate.)
- Fetal anemia (The heart rate increases as a compensatory mechanism to improve tissue perfusion.)
- Dehydration

Tachycardia is considered an ominous sign if it is accompanied by other FHR patterns such as late deceleration, severe variable decelerations, or decreased variability. If tachycardia is associated with maternal fever, treatment may consist of antipyretics, cooling measures, and antibiotics. Fetal arrhythmia needs to be ruled out. The pediatrician should be notified because tachycardia may cause heart failure in the newborn.

Bradycardia Fetal *bradycardia* is defined as FHR of less than 110 to 120 beats per minute continuing for 10 minutes or more (Menihan, 1996). Causes of fetal bradycardia include the following:

- Late (profound) fetal asphyxia (There is depression of myocardial activity.)
- Maternal hypotension (Maternal hypotension results in decreased blood flow to fetus.)

TABLE 19–5 Advantages and Disadvantages of Various Monitoring Methods

Method	Advantages	Disadvantages
Fetoscope	Inexpensive. Noninvasive. Easy to use. Easily transported.	Intermittent information. Gives no information regarding contractions. Cannot assess variability or periodic changes in FHR unless moderate to severe. Cannot hear FHT until 17–20 weeks' gestation. More difficult to hear during a contraction.
Doppler (pocket-sized ultrasound)	Inexpensive. Noninvasive. Easily transported. Can hear FHT as early as 10–12 weeks.	Gives no information regarding contractions. Cannot assess variability. Cannot assess periodic changes in FHR unless moderate to severe. Intermittent information.
External monitoring (by EFM)	Continuous information. Noninvasive. Uses: antepartal testing and during labor. Gives permanent record. Can assess relative frequency of contractions. Can assess decreased variability and periodic changes. Useful for client teaching.	Equipment is expensive. Subject to artifact. Cannot assess variability unless decreased and then must confirm with internal monitoring. Cannot quantitate contractions. Belts uncomfortable to some women. Subject to double- and half-counting. Needs qualified and knowledgeable personnel to interpret.
Internal monitoring (by EFM)	Accurate, continuous information. Monitors fetal ECG. Not subject to artifact. Client more mobile in bed, chair. Can quantitate contractions. Can assess short-term and long-term variability. Accurate assessment of periodic changes. Useful for client teaching.	Equipment is expensive. Needs qualified and knowledgeable personnel to interpret. Presenting part must be accessible, membranes must be ruptured, and cervix must be dilated enough for application of scalp electrode. Requires knowledgeable personnel to apply equipment. Client confined to bed or chair. Slight increased risk of maternal or fetal infection. Invasive.
Telemetry	Accurate, continuous information. Client can be mobile (out of bed or in hall). Same advantages as internal monitoring.	Equipment is expensive. Not widely used at the present time. Same disadvantages as internal monitoring.

- Prolonged umbilical cord compression (Fetal baroceptors are activated by cord compression, which produces vagal stimulation, and in turn decreases FHR.)
- Fetal arrhythmia (This is associated with complete heart block in fetus.)

Bradycardia may be a benign or ominous (preterminal) sign. If there is average variability present, the bradycardia is considered benign. When bradycardia is accompanied by decreased variability or late decelerations or both, it is considered ominous and a sign of advanced fetal distress (Menihan, 1996).

Baseline Variability One of the most important parameters of fetal well-being is noted in FHR variability. **Baseline variability** is a measure of the interplay (the "push-pull" effect) between the sympathetic nervous system (which acts to increase heart rate) and the parasympathetic nervous system (which acts to decrease heart rate). There are two major types of fetal heart variability—short term and long term (Figure 19–14).

Long-term variability (LTV) refers to the larger rhythmic fluctuations of the FHR that occur from two to six times per minute with a normal range of 6 to 10 beats per minute. The range refers to the difference between the lowest FHR and the highest FHR in each cycle within 1 minute. Long-term variability is increased by fetal movement and decreased or absent when the fetus is in a sleep cycle. Long-term variability has been classified as follows (Hon, 1976 and AWHONN, 1997):

Decreased/minimal variability	0–5 bpm
Moderate/average variability	6–25 bpm
Marked variability (*saltatory*)	>25 bpm

The *saltatory pattern* of marked or excessive variability is characterized by rapid variations in FHR that have a

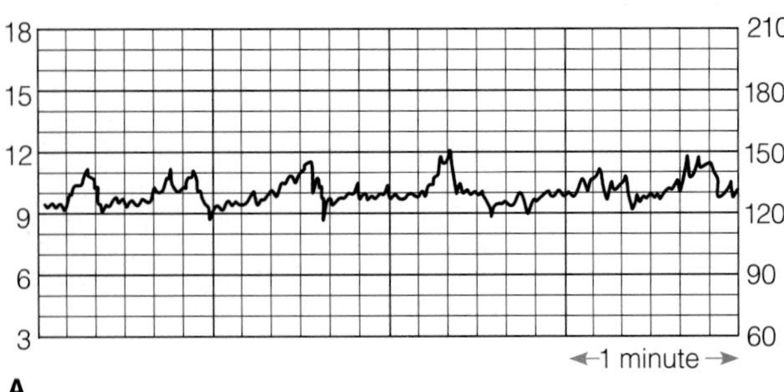

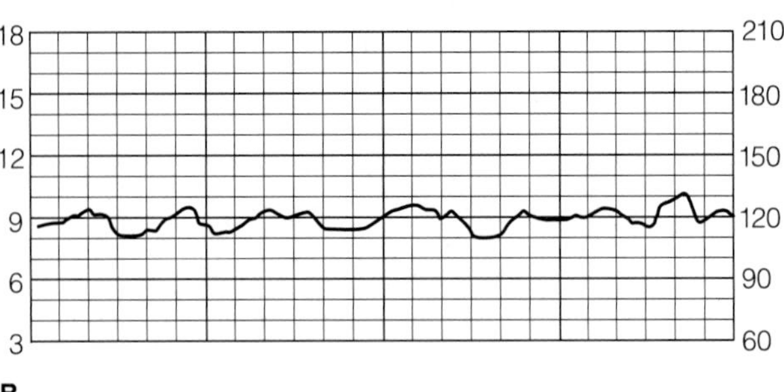

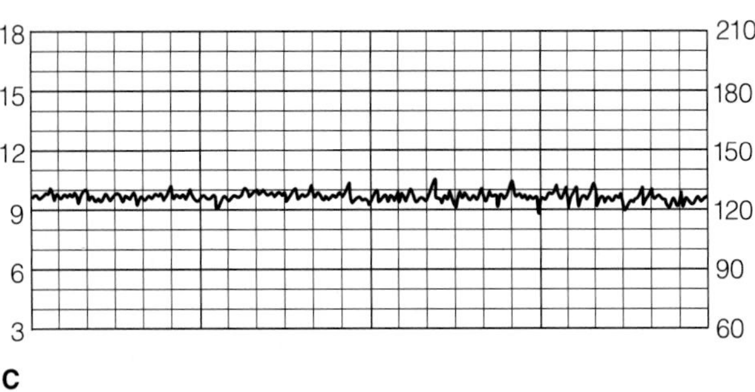

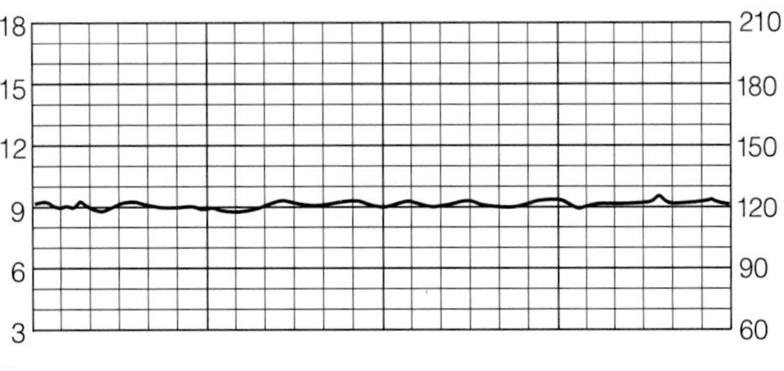

FIGURE 19–14 Short- and long-term variability. ***A,*** Increased LTV; STV present. ***B,*** Average LTV; STV absent. ***C,*** Absent LTV; STV present. ***D,*** Absent LTV; STV absent.

bizarre appearance. LTV occurs with a cycle frequency of three to six per minute, and the amplitude is greater than 25 beats per minute (Figure 19–15). The etiologic origin of this pattern is uncertain. However, it frequently follows moderate to severe variable decelerations (Shifrin, 1990). Attempts to resolve a marked saltatory pattern are appropriate.

An unusual pattern referred to as *sinusoidal* is occasionally seen. It is characterized by an undulant sine wave that is equally distributed above and below the baseline. In a sinusoidal pattern, the FHR usually ranges between 120 and 160 beats per minute. This wavelike baseline FHR usually has an amplitude of 5 to 15 beats per minute and appears to oscillate in a regular, uniform pattern of 2 to 5 cycles per minute (Kang & Boehm, 1999). Fetal activity may be minimal or absent, and there are no FHR accelerations. There is no beat-to-beat short-term variability (Figure 19–16). The pattern does not come and go with periods of normal variability. No fetal accelerations are present, even in response to fetal movement (AWHONN, 1997).

The sinusoidal pattern is associated with Rh isoimmunization, severe anemia, abruptio placentae, fetal-maternal hemorrhage, severe fetal acidosis (AWHONN, 1997) (Kang & Boehm, 1999).

True sinusoidal FHR patterns noted intrapartally suggest fetal anemia or severe asphyxia. If a sinusoidal pattern is noted by external monitoring, internal fetal monitoring should be instituted, and cesarean birth should be considered if the pattern is confirmed. Fetal blood sampling for determination of pH and hematocrit, ultrasound scan for signs of congestive heart failure and hydrops, and biophysical profile may aid in assessment, evaluation, and management of the fetus with this FHR pattern.

Short-term variability (STV) refers to the differences between successive heartbeats as measured by the R-R wave interval of the QRS cardiac cycle and therefore represents actual fluctuation from one heartbeat to the next. STV refers to the tiny fluctuations (tiny ups and downs) in FHR. These fluctuations average 2 to 3 beats per minute. Short-term variability is classified as either present or absent.

Short-term variability indicates fetal central nervous system (CNS) function (previously described), so the presence of STV variability is reassuring. If there is an oxygen deficit in the CNS, the interplay is lost, and STV variability disappears. Thus, short-term variability is a useful indicator of fetal oxygen reserve (Menihan, 1996).

Rather than counting specific beats, the nurse can, with practice, usually become skillful at "eyeballing" the FHR variability and deciding whether it is smooth (absent) or rough (present). When decreased LTV is noted, the nurse must bring careful thought and evaluation to the assessment. Although increased variability is not well understood, there are many associated conditions (pathologic and nonpathologic) that accompany decreased variability. Short-term variability may be decreased in the

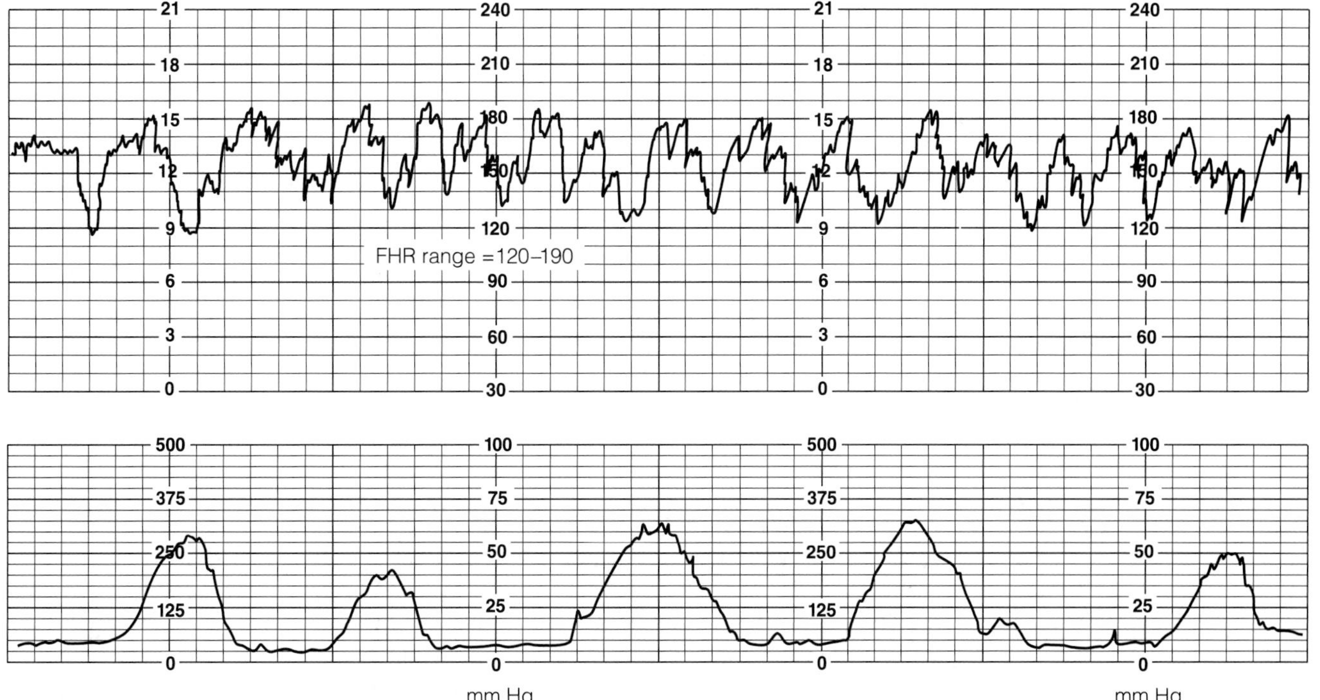

FIGURE 19–15 Saltatory pattern. Note the pattern of marked LTV. FHR varies markedly between 120 and 190 beats per minute. With this type of pattern, it is not possible to determine an average baseline FHR because of the wide, marked variations. STV is present.

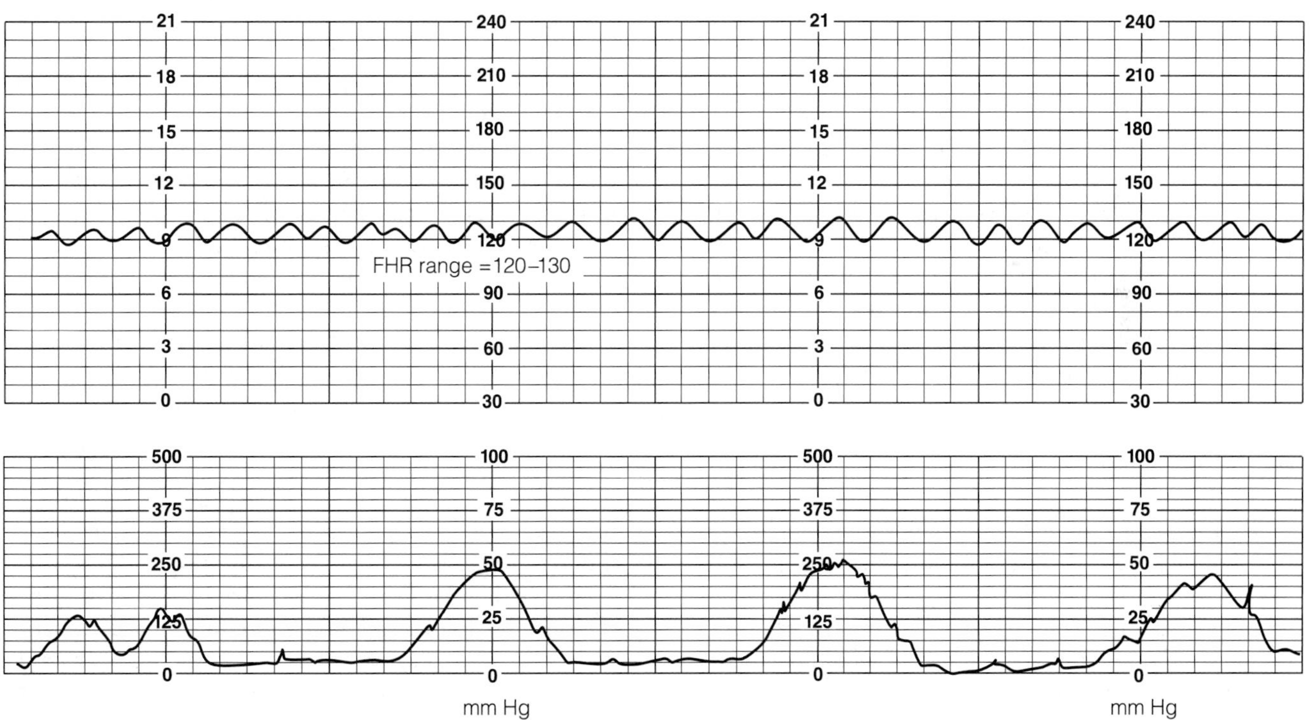

FIGURE 19–16 Sinusoidal pattern. Note the undulating waveform evenly distributed between the 120 and 130 bpm baseline. There is no STV; accelerations or decelerations are not present.

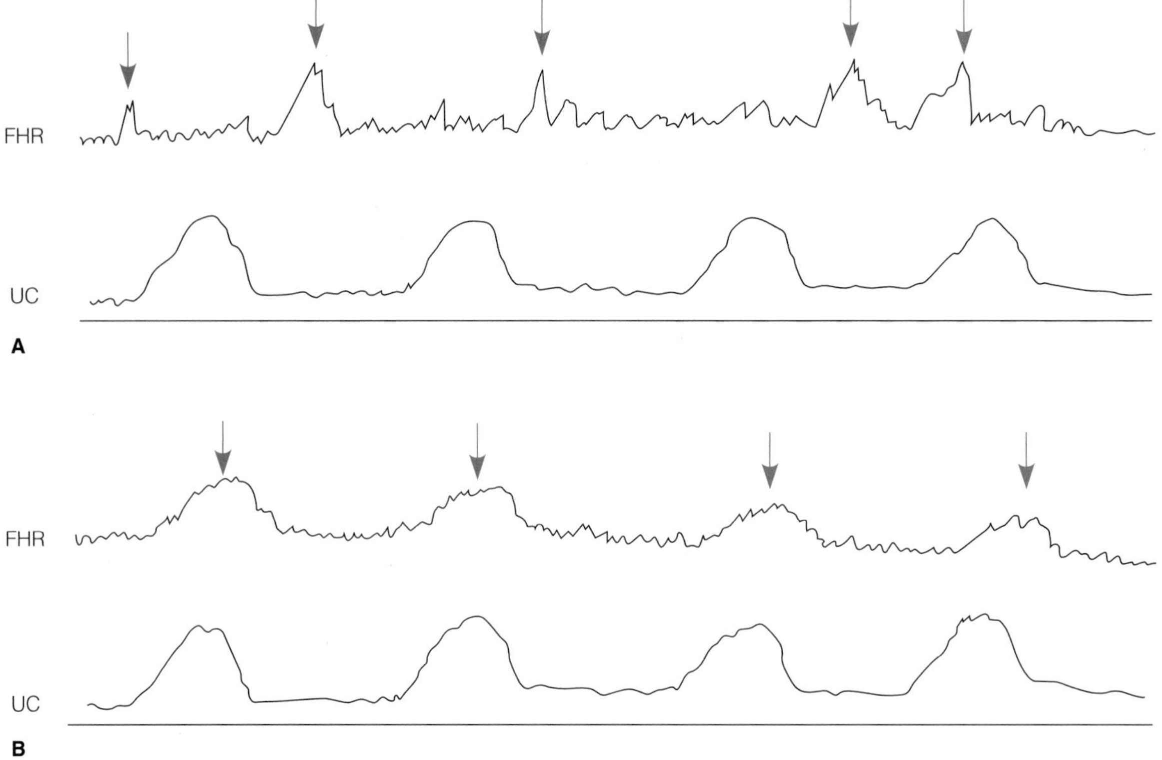

FIGURE 19–17 Types of accelerations. ***A,*** Nonperiodic accelerations. ***B,*** Periodic accelerations.

presence of fetal tachycardia, prematurity, anomalies of the fetal heart and central nervous system, and fetal sleep. Factors that may decrease both LTV and STV include narcotics, tranquilizers, and epidural or spinal anesthetic agents administered to the laboring woman (Menihan, 1996).

The nurse needs to keep in mind that STV can be evaluated only by internal monitoring. The external monitoring may demonstrate "normal" variability due to the presence of artifact when in fact it is decreased. An appearance of decreased variability warrants application of an internal electrode.

Accelerations **Accelerations** are transient increases in the FHR (Figure 19–17). Nonperiodic accelerations are normally caused by fetal movement. As the fetus moves in utero, the heart rate increases, as it does in adults when they exercise. When the fetus quiets down, the heart rate returns to normal. Periodic accelerations are ones that accompany contractions. One theory is that accelerations occur with contractions as a result of fetal movement in response to pressure of the contracting uterine musculature. Accelerations of this type are thought to be a sign of fetal well-being and adequate oxygen reserve. Another explanation that is becoming more important in the intrapartum area is that a mild compression of the umbilical cord with the contraction may occlude the umbilical vein. The resulting decrease in blood flow to the fetus causes a systemic decrease in blood pressure, which triggers a compensatory accelerative response in the fetal heart rate (AWHONN, 1997). This has implications for fetal assessment. It may be an early warning sign of low amniotic fluid or cord compression.

Spontaneous accelerations are symmetric, uniform, nonperiodic increases in FHR. They are benign, represent an intact CNS response to fetal movements or stimulation, and are not associated with contractions or decelerations. This type of acceleration serves as the criterion for a reactive nonstress test (NST).

Deceleration **Decelerations** are periodic decreases in FHR from the normal baseline. Hon and Quilligan (1967) categorized them as early, late, and variable, according to when they occur in the contraction cycle and to their waveform (Figure 19–18).

Early decelerations are due to pressure on the fetal head as it progresses down the birth canal. They have a uniform appearance that inversely mirrors that of the corresponding contraction. Early decelerations begin at the onset of the contraction and end as the contraction ends; the nadir (lowest point) occurs at the peak of the contraction. The nadir is usually within the normal FHR range (120 to 160 bpm) (Figure 19–19).

Early decelerations are generally benign and are seen in early, active labor, when dilatation is 4 to 7 cm. Increased intracranial pressure stimulates the vagus nerve, which in turn slows heart rate (Figure 19–20). If this pattern occurs early in labor, it may be due to head compression from an unengaged presenting part, occiput posterior presentation, or cephalopelvic disproportion. A

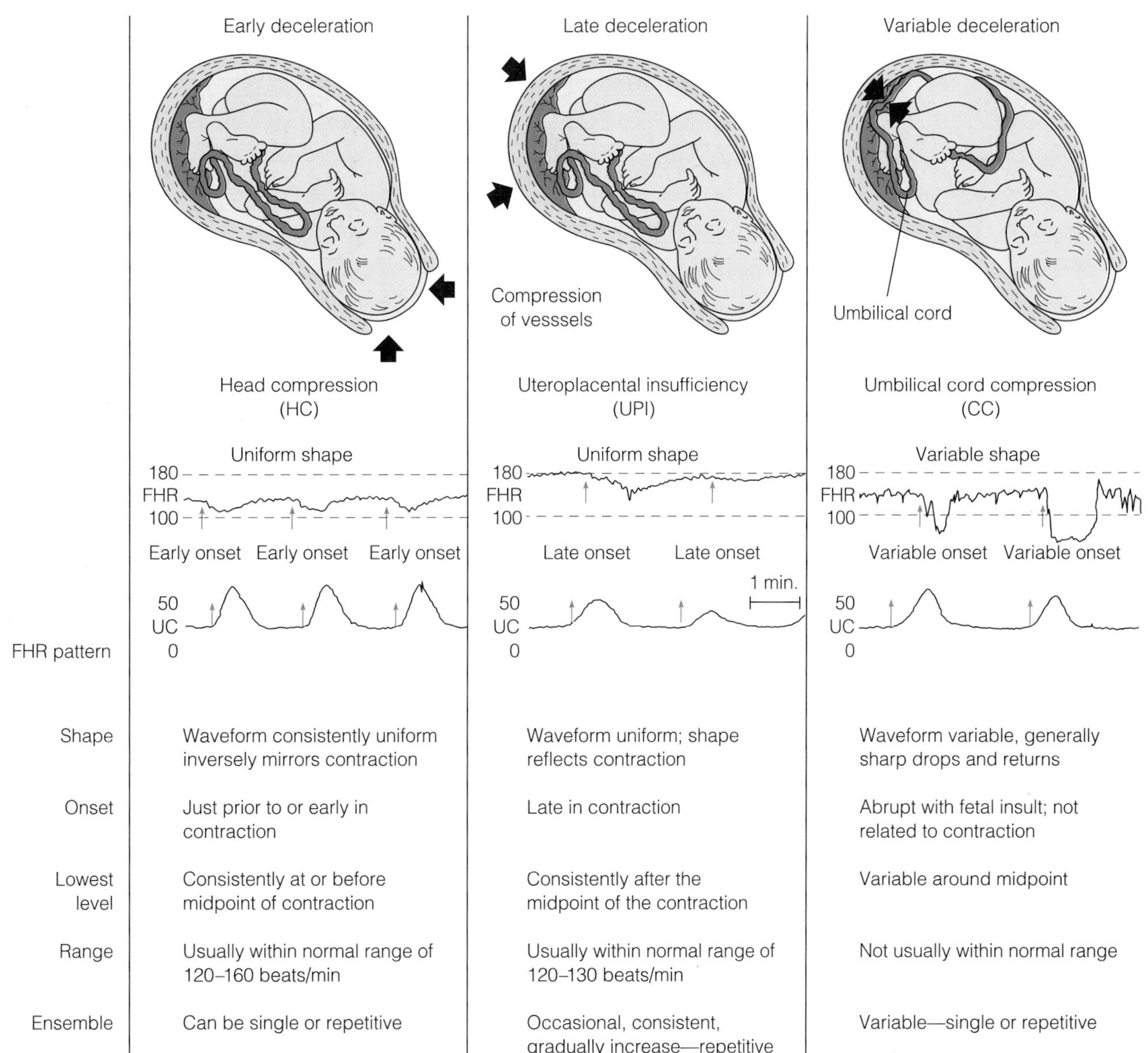

Early deceleration
Late deceleration
Variable deceleration
Compression of vesssels
Umbilical cord
Head compression (HC)
Uteroplacental insufficiency (UPI)
Umbilical cord compression (CC)
Uniform shape
Uniform shape
Variable shape
180
FHR
100
Early onset
Early onset
Early onset
Late onset
Late onset
Variable onset
Variable onset
1 min.
50
UC
0
FHR pattern
Shape
Waveform consistently uniform inversely mirrors contraction
Waveform uniform; shape reflects contraction
Waveform variable, generally sharp drops and returns
Onset
Just prior to or early in contraction
Late in contraction
Abrupt with fetal insult; not related to contraction
Lowest level
Consistently at or before midpoint of contraction
Consistently after the midpoint of the contraction
Variable around midpoint
Range
Usually within normal range of 120–160 beats/min
Usually within normal range of 120–130 beats/min
Not usually within normal range
Ensemble
Can be single or repetitive
Occasional, consistent, gradually increase—repetitive
Variable—single or repetitive

FIGURE 19–18 Types and characteristics of early, late, and variable decelerations. SOURCE: Hon E: *An Introduction to Fetal Heart Rate Monitoring,* 2nd ed. Los Angeles: University of Southern California School of Medicine, 1976, p 29.

nurse must take great care in differentiating this type of deceleration from later decelerations: They look identical yet differ in time of onset.

Early decelerations are not associated with loss of variability, tachycardia, or other FHR changes or with fetal hypoxia, acidosis, or low Apgar scores. Early decelerations are viewed as a reassuring FHR pattern unless seen with lack of descent of the fetal head.

Late decelerations are due to uteroplacental insufficiency. They are the result of decreases in blood flow that impede oxygen transfer to the fetus through the intervillous space during uterine contractions, causing hypoxemia (Figure 19–21). Late decelerations have a smooth, uniform shape that inversely mirrors the contractions (as do early decelerations) and often reflect the strength of the contraction (indicated by the height of the recorded uterine contraction on the graph paper), but they are late in their onset and recovery. Late decelerations begin at or within a few seconds after the peak of the contraction; the nadir is noted near the end of the contraction. When uteroplacental reserve is adequate, the fetus normally tolerates the transient stress of repetitive contractions. If a decrease in uteroplacental blood flow (for example, from maternal hypotension or excessive uterine activity) leads to fetal hypoxia, late decelerations generally occur (Figure 19–22).

This pattern is always considered an ominous sign and requires prompt attention and intervention. Variability in the baseline is of utmost importance. The objective of intervention is to maintain oxygenation (variability)

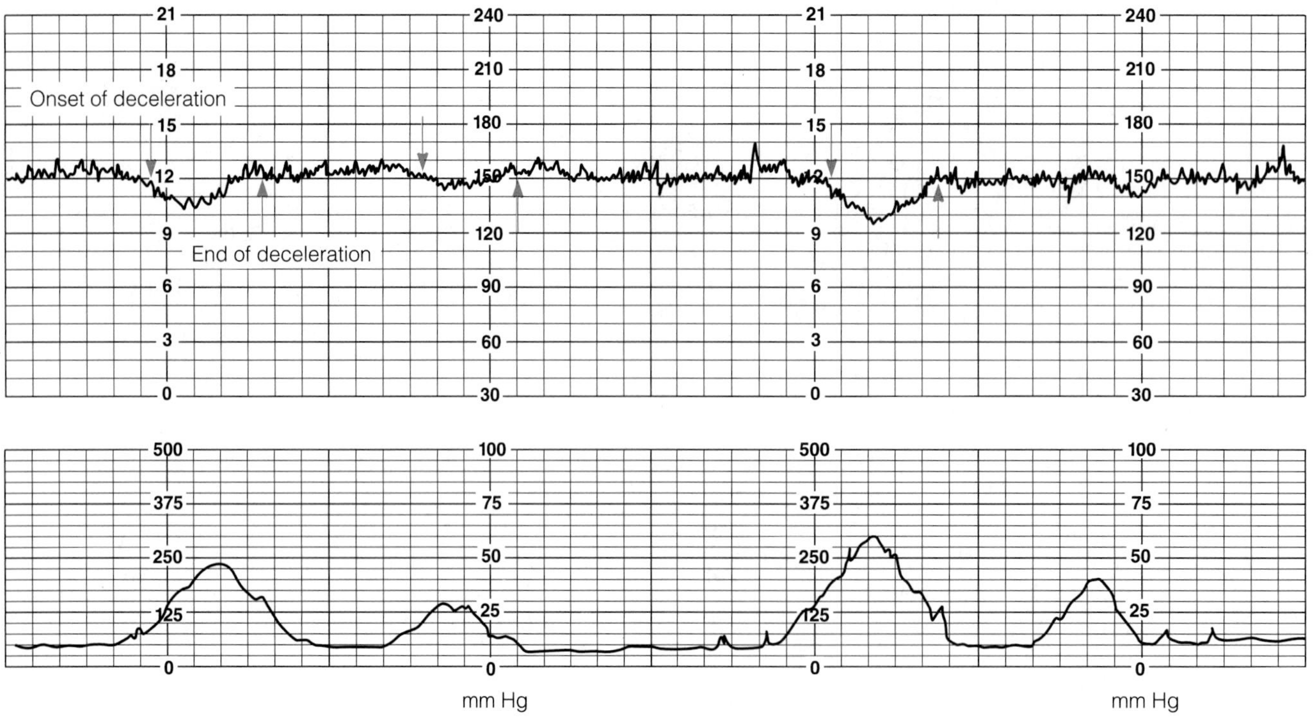

FIGURE 19–19 Early decelerations. Baseline FHR is 150–155 bpm. Nadir (lowest point) of decelerations is 130–145 bpm. LTV is absent; STV is present.

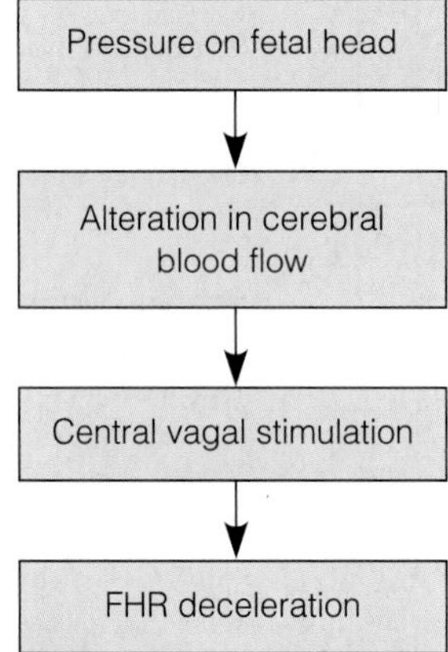

FIGURE 19–20 Mechanism of early deceleration (head compression). SOURCE: Adapted from Freeman RK, Garite TJ: The physiologic basis of fetal monitoring. In *Fetal Heart Rate Monitoring.* Baltimore: Williams & Wilkins, 1981, p 13.

while assessing and eliminating the stressor as reflected by the deceleration. If this is not possible, immediate birth may be indicated.

Sometimes late decelerations are due to the supine position of the laboring woman. In this case, the decrease in uterine blood flow to the fetus may be alleviated by raising the woman's upper trunk or turning her to the side to displace pressure of the gravid uterus on the inferior vena cava. If the woman remains flat on her back, the fetus will continue to have decelerations due to oxygen compromise.

Late decelerations normally occur within the normal heart range (120 to 160 bpm) and may be quite obvious or very subtle and almost indistinguishable. Some fetuses at highest risk demonstrate a flat FHR baseline with late decelerations that are barely noticeable. It must be kept in mind that the depth of the deceleration does not indicate the severity of the insult.

Variable decelerations, as the name suggests, vary in their onset, occurrence, and waveform. They are thought to be due to umbilical cord occlusion, which decreases the amount of blood flow (and therefore oxygen supply) to the fetus (Figure 19–23). Either the fetus squeezes the cord or rolls over onto it, transient pressure is exerted on the cord from compression, or the cord is around the neck of the fetus. An occasional or isolated variable deceleration is usually benign. Variable decelerations that are repetitive and begin to worsen during the course of labor are a cause for concern. Variable decelerations usually fall outside the normal FHR range and are classified as mild, moderate, and severe. They are acute in onset, vary in duration and intensity, and abruptly disappear when the insult of cord compression is relieved (Figure 19–24).

Repetitive decelerations may indicate nuchal cord (umbilical cord around the neck), short cord, or occult

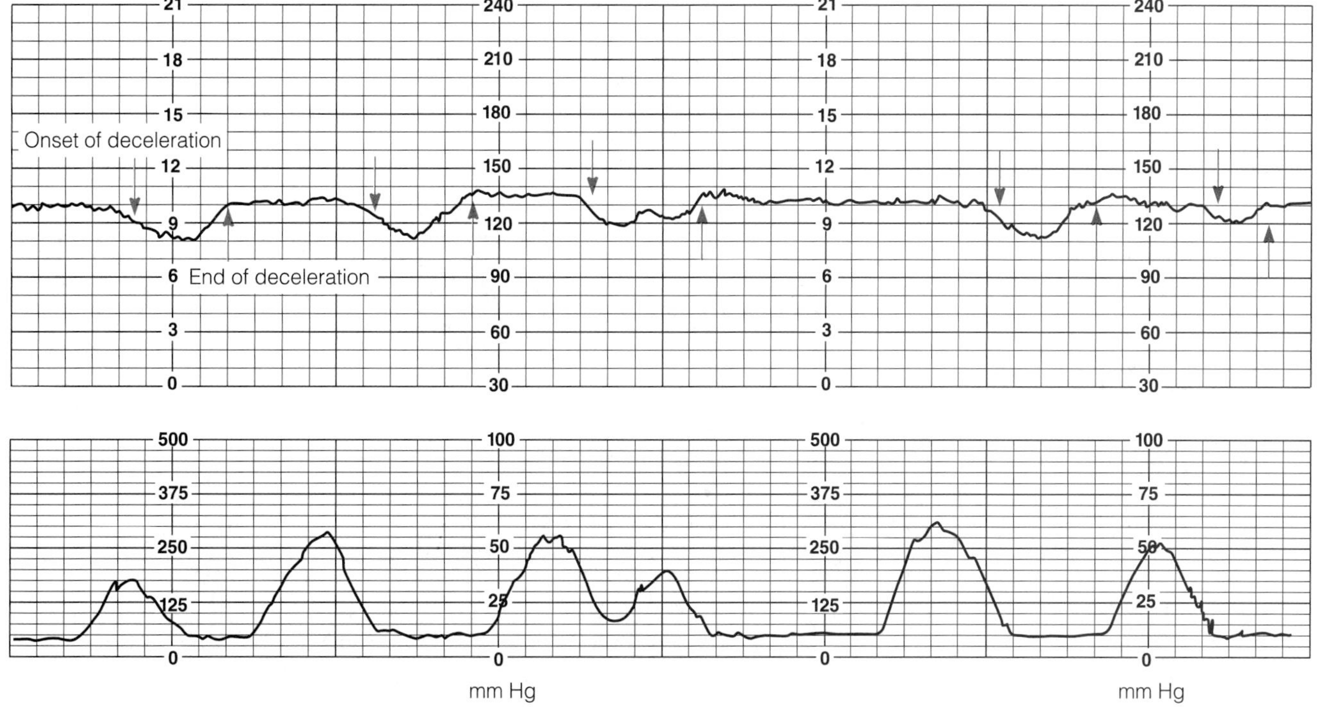

FIGURE 19–21 Late decelerations. Baseline FHR is 130–148 bpm. Nadir (lowest point) of decelerations is 110–120 bpm. LTV and STV are absent.

prolapse of the cord. If this pattern becomes evident early in labor, variable decelerations may subsequently demonstrate a slow return to baseline due to repetitive stress. Acid-base status of the fetus should be assessed because cesarean birth, forceps birth, or vacuum extraction might be indicated.

Decelerations that seem to deviate more from the baseline and widen are ominous and warrant further investigation. When they are prolonged and severe, a significant oxygen deficit develops from myocardial depression (Shifrin, 1990).

With progressively worsening variable decelerations, an overshoot may occur. This is a blunt, smooth acceleration with an increase in rate generally greater than 20 bpm and lasting more than 20 seconds, following the contraction. Overshoot suggests imbalance of the autonomic nervous system of the fetus. It may be seen in neurologically impaired or severely asphyxiated fetuses (Shifrin, 1990) when they are repetitive and STV is absent.

Criteria for evaluating variable decelerations vary from one author to another, and the very nature of these periodic changes can pose considerable anxiety regarding management. Dr Robert Goodlin's "rule of the 60s" (Parer, 1994) describes severe variable deceleration as having the following characteristics: variable decelerations below 60 beats per minute, 60 beats per minute below baseline FHR, or variable decelerations lasting more

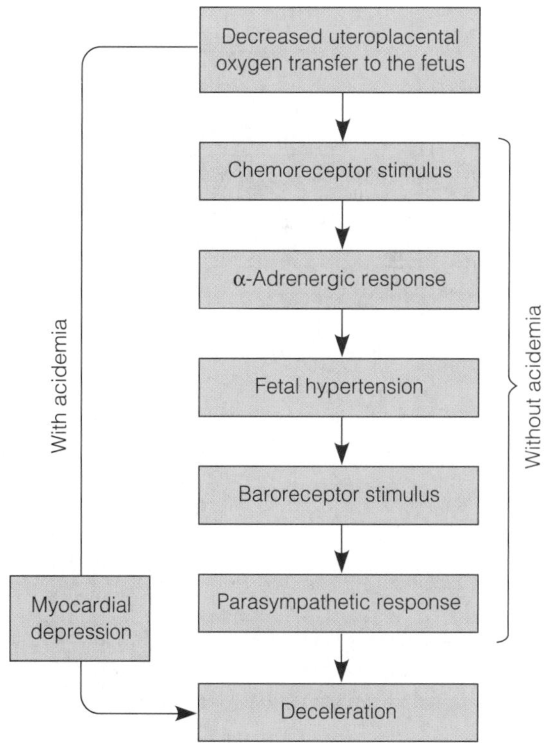

FIGURE 19–22 Mechanism of late deceleration. SOURCE: Freeman RK, Garite TJ: The physiologic basis of fetal monitoring. In *Fetal Heart Rate Monitoring.* Baltimore: Williams & Wilkins, 1981, p 15.

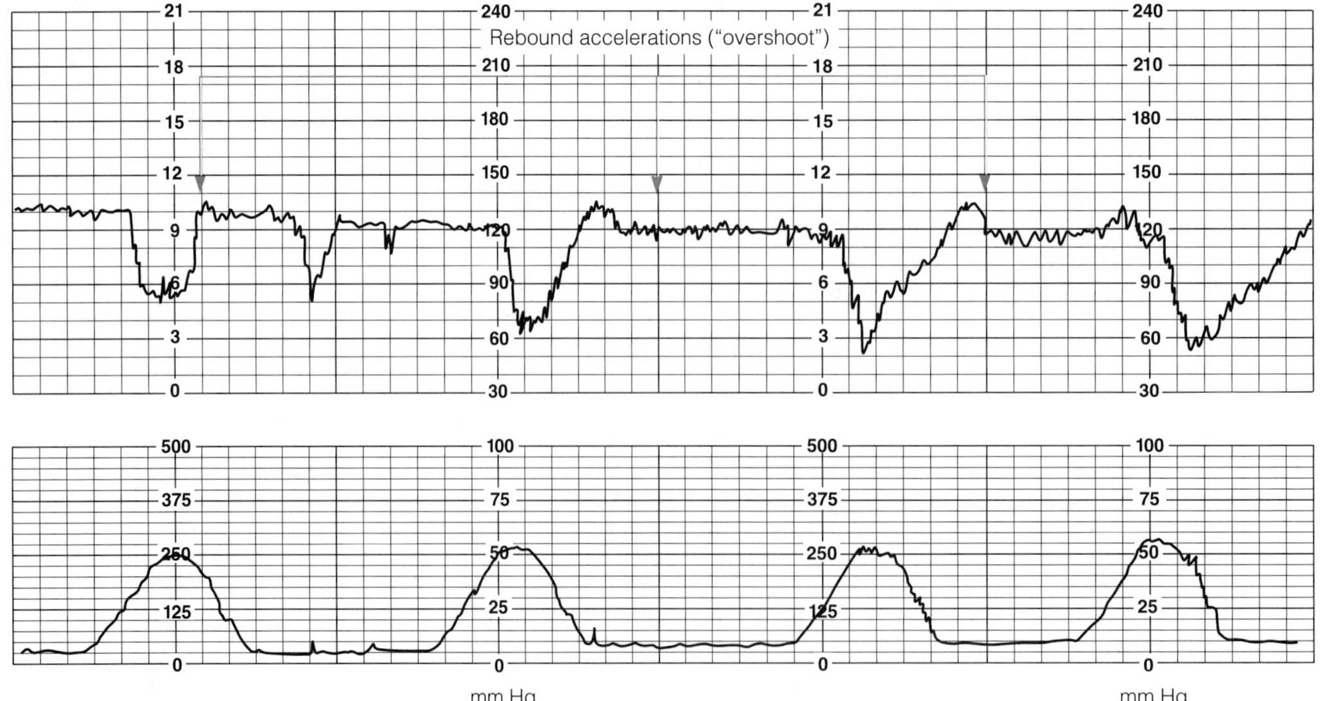

FIGURE 19–23 Variable decelerations with overshoot. The timing of the decelerations is variable, and most have a sharp decline. A rebound acceleration (overshoot) occurs after most of the decelerations. Baseline FHR is 115–130 bpm. Nadir of decelerations is 55–80 bpm. LTV is absent; STV is present.

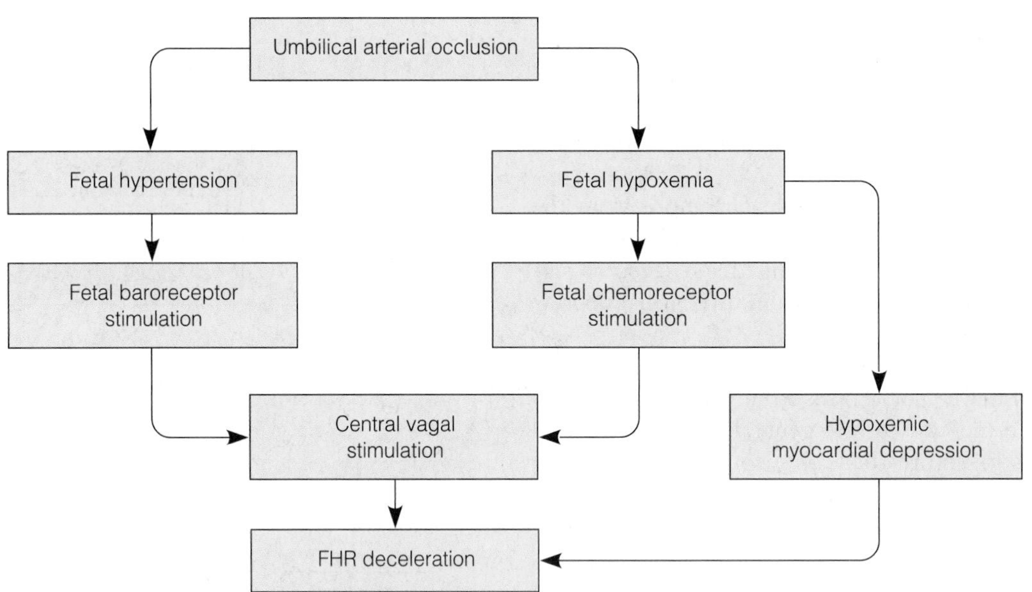

FIGURE 19–24 Mechanism of variable deceleration. SOURCE: Adapted from Freeman RK, Garite TJ: The physiologic basis of fetal monitoring. In *Fetal Heart Rate Monitoring*. Baltimore: Williams & Wilkins, 1981, p 15.

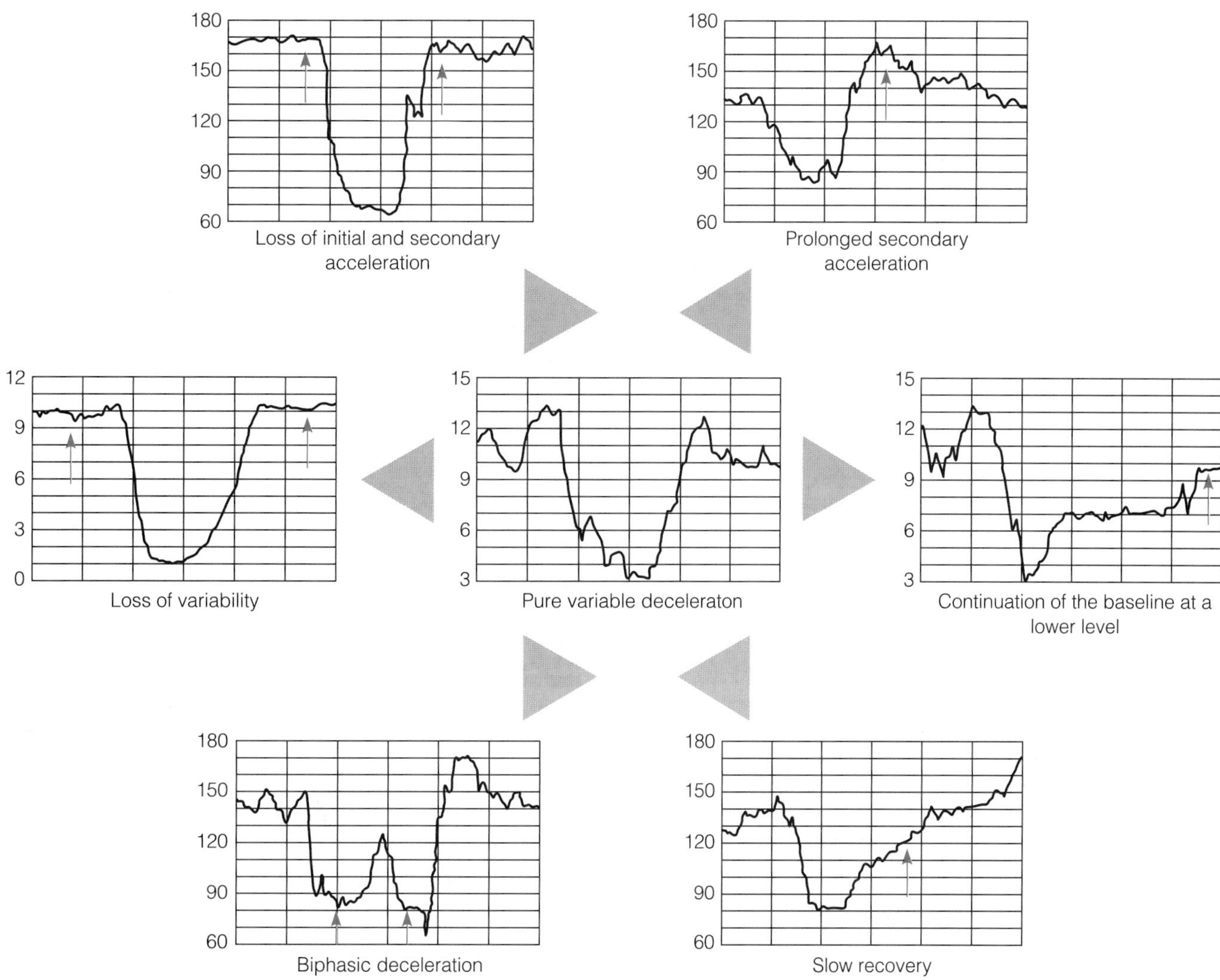

FIGURE 19–25 Atypical variable decelerations. The presence of any of these types of variable decelerations strongly suggests fetal hypoxia, especially when variability is decreased. SOURCE: Krebs HB, Petrie RE, Dunn LJ: Atypical variable decelerations. *Am J Obstet Gynecol,* 1983; 145(3): 298.

than 60 seconds in duration. These criteria seem to be the easiest to remember and perhaps the most practical.

Variable decelerations are frequently seen in labor when the membranes are ruptured. This decreases protection to the cord especially as the fetus descends down the birth canal. Variable decelerations usually do not warrant immediate birth unless a rising baseline, loss of variability, and other ominous signs accompany them. Repositioning the woman often corrects this type of pattern. If it does not, the clinician may attempt to alleviate this pattern by inserting sterile saline via intrauterine catheter (amnioinfusion) to help take pressure off the umbilical cord.

Krebs, Petrie, and Dunn (1983) describe various "atypical variable decelerations," noting that variable decelerations are probably innocuous unless these features are present (Figure 19–25). They note that the presence of these atypical decelerations should be regarded as signs of fetal hypoxia. The nurse should be cognizant of pattern interpretation and be able to recognize severe and "atypical" variables. A point to remember, however, is that in the presence of normal variability of the FHR these variables have not been found to be associated with fetal acidosis and poor outcome.

Prolonged decelerations are those in which the FHR decreases from the baseline for 2 to 10 minutes (Figure 19–26). They may occur suddenly, and if the pattern is promptly corrected, FHR variability will remain good. Rebound tachycardia is an ominous sign implying that a state of hypoxia has occurred. Prolonged decelerations are seen following epidural block due to maternal hypotension. Prolonged decelerations may often be seen with sudden occult or frank prolapse of the umbilical cord. When decelerations occur following administration

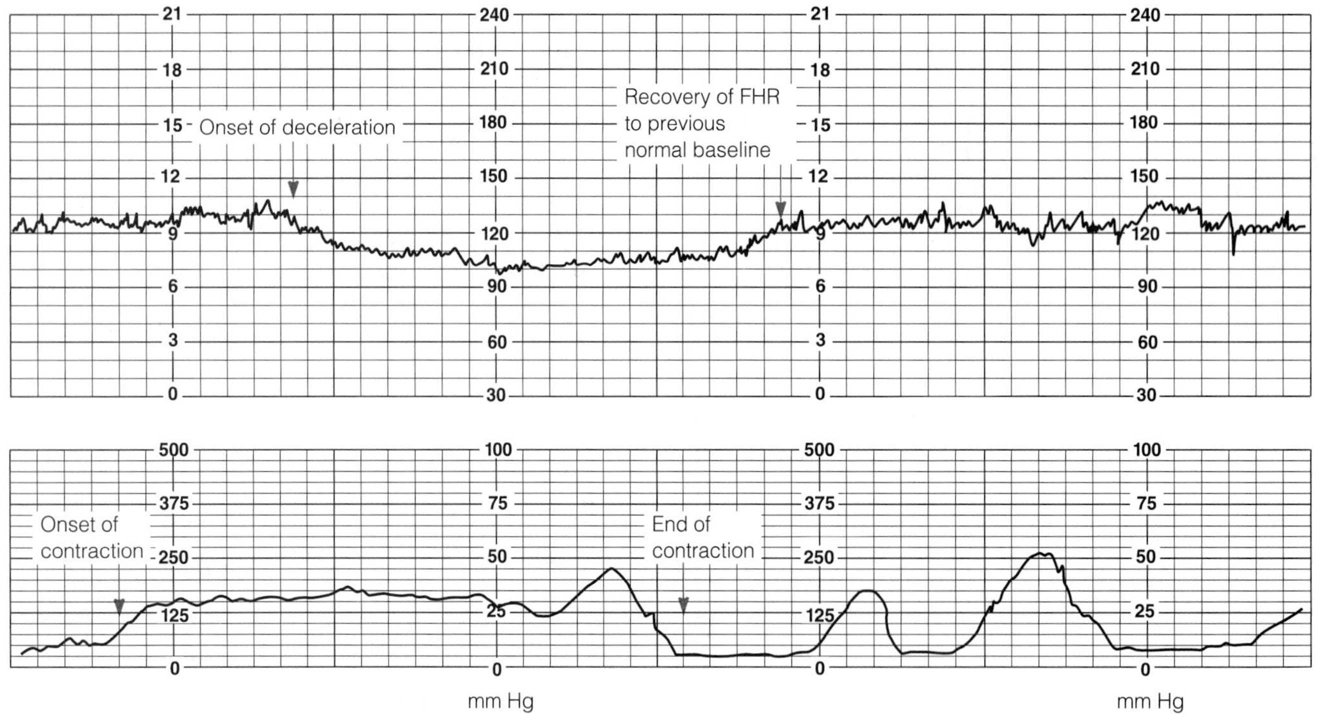

FIGURE 19–26 The prolonged deceleration depicted lasts approximately 160 seconds. Note the prolonged contraction of 120 seconds. The deceleration begins after 80 seconds of uterine contraction. Note the beginning return of FHR 30 seconds after uterine tone returns to normal resting tone (contraction ends). An important aspect of this tracing is that STV is present despite the prolonged deceleration.

of regional anesthesia, the woman should be turned on her side, evaluated for hypotension, and given a bolus of intravenous fluid (500 to 600 mL) to fill the dilated vascular space. This situation can usually be avoided by administering an IV bolus (800 to 900 mL) of lactated Ringer's or normal saline solution to the woman prior to administering regional anesthesia. Solutions containing dextrose should not be given because they may cause fetal hyperglycemia. Other conditions that may result in a prolonged deceleration are extensive abruptio placentae, uterine hypertonus or hyperstimulus, drug reactions, terminal fetal conditions, maternal seizures, maternal death, or something as simple as a vagal response from a vaginal exam. The most important role of the nurse is to look for the cause or the stressor and correct the problem. Intervention may be as simple as a position change.

Combined decelerations may be seen occasionally when two different deceleration patterns occur together (for example, early/late, early/variable, or variable/late). The specific types of patterns must then be ascertained. For instance, variable decelerations with a slow return to baseline should be differentiated from a combined pattern of variable and late decelerations. The former is a sign that the compression of the umbilical cord is worsening; the latter is an indication of cord compression *plus* uteroplacental insufficiency. Initial management should be aimed at treatment of the most ominous pattern first (Shifrin, 1990).

The Family's Responses to Electronic Monitoring

Responses to electronic fetal monitoring can be as complex and varied among women and families as among practitioners in the nursing and medical community. Some women and families view the electronic fetal monitor (EFM) as unneeded technology that interferes with a natural process; they feel that the EFM should not be used unless there are clear indications. Such women who want minimal intervention during labor and birth may carefully develop a birth plan and hire a doula as an advocate (see Chapter 9) to help ensure that their wishes will be met once they arrive in the hospital birthing setting. Other women and families consider the monitor a part of the care surrounding birth and do not realize they may have some personal choice; therefore, they do not object. Such women may not understand how the electronic monitor works or what information it may provide but are willing to allow the nurse or doctor to use it. They are passive receivers of EFM. Still other women and families believe that technology such as EFM represents state-of-the-art practice and may demand it. They may perceive absence of an EFM as withholding of care, perhaps due to financial or other considerations (McConnell, 1998). Lastly, some women and families have a simple response to the EFM; they like it because hearing the fetal heartbeat provides a feeling of reassurance.

At times, laboring women feel that the monitor has become the most important aspect of the labor because so much attention is placed on it. These feelings may be intensified when, for example, the nurse walks into the room and asks, "How are you doing?" while looking at the monitor instead of making eye contact with the woman. Such actions convey an attitude that the only important information emanates from the technologic device. The woman may be left feeling that she is not important and is not even a part of the process—that the machine is all that exists. The machine defines her, how her contractions are doing, whether they appear strong enough for the discomfort or pain she is feeling, and how her baby is reacting to labor. The event seems to feel like a spectacle; her caregivers assess, interpret, intervene, and evaluate what they see on the EFM without looking at her, a live person whose responses are not indicated on the EFM (Sandelowski, 1998).

NURSING CARE MANAGEMENT

As in all interactions with clients, nurses must always be aware of the healing presence that is theirs to bring to the process. The healing presence is more than just the presence of the nurse's physical body; rather, it is the result of the special focus and awareness of the nurse on the client's whole being and the unspoken willingness of both parties to enter into a special healing moment in which both will be changed.

Technology has been advancing at a rapid rate in the labor and birthing area, and each new development further challenges nurses to understand, incorporate, and balance the role of technology into holistic nursing practice. "The practice of nursing in a technological practice setting presents a contrast of strength and vulnerability" (Bernardo, 1998, p 42). A key strength of technology is its ability to explain and predict health patterns or problems with great precision. For instance, the EFM can reveal an ominous FHR pattern in detail. It would be difficult, if not impossible, for the nurse to obtain all of the same data with an auditory device such as a fetoscope. Another strength of some technologies is that they save time (eg, an ear thermometer can obtain a temperature in 1 to 3 seconds, in contrast to an oral mercury thermometer, which must remain in place for 3 minutes). Still other technologic advances have led to more comfortable and less invasive procedures (eg, maternal blood gas levels may now be measured by pulse oximetry instead of requiring blood to be drawn).

Nursing's vulnerability in a technologic environment arises from technology's potential to dehumanize the nurse-client relationship (Bernardo, 1998). First, there is a tendency to allow technology to become the driving force in client care and therefore detach the nurse from meaningful interactions with the client. Second, technology may shift the nurse's focus away from the client's behavior as an indication of health status. Third, technology has the potential to focus attention on a problem or disease process rather than on the individual. Fourth, technology focuses on the tangible and visible rather than on the intuitive, personal nature of each nurse's practice. Lastly, the language used with technology can become contrived and removed from the client's understanding. This "special language" may act as a barrier, isolate the client, and deemphasize the client's experience.

The use of technology will continue to be an integral part of client care and gives rise to many questions about how it changes nursing practice. Experienced nurses recognize that technology can be a tremendously useful tool. However, they never lose sight of the client's perspective about her experiences. How does the nurse learn of the client's actual experience? Although several theories have been proposed, nursing presence seems to best describe the interaction between the nurse and the woman and family in the childbirth setting.

True presence in nursing comes from the "human becoming" theory, which emphasizes that the focus of care must clearly be from the person's perspective, not the nurse's. "The intent of the nurse in true presence is not to change, alter, or intervene but to bear witness to the person's experience in a nonjudgmental manner" (Bernardo, 1998, p 41).

The nurse's awareness and active use of the healing presence help the woman and family develop trust. By sharing their perspectives and expectations, the nurse becomes better able to provide care that meets the needs of the woman and family and to advocate for them.

Additional activities are also required. Prior to applying the monitor, the nurse should fully explain to the woman the reason for using the EFM and the information that can be derived from its use. The nurse explains how the monitor can help identify the beginning of contractions and thus aid in breathing during the various phases of labor. Explaining the information regarding the fetal heart rate is also important. An explanation alleviates apprehensions about equipment that may be totally unfamiliar to the woman. During labor it is advantageous to provide education regarding the use of the internal equipment because the caregiver may quickly decide to convert to this method as a result of examination findings. Women who are informed about the possibility of internal monitoring are better prepared if a quick decision must be made to apply an electrode or catheter.

After the monitor is applied, basic information should be recorded on the monitor strip. The data included are the date, time, woman's name, physician, hospital or agency number, age, gravida, para, estimated date of birth, membrane status, maternal vital signs, and current medical problems. As the monitor strip continues to run and care is provided, it is important that documentation of occurrences during labor should be recorded not only in the nurse's notes on the woman's hospital record, but also on the fetal monitor tracing. The following information should be included on the tracing (AAP & ACOG, 1997):

1. Vaginal examinations (dilatation, effacement, station, and position)
2. Amniotomy or spontaneous rupture of membranes, color of amniotic fluid, presence and consistency of meconium
3. Maternal vital signs
4. Maternal position in bed and changes of position
5. Application of spiral electrode or intrauterine pressure catheter
6. Medications
7. Oxygen administration
8. Maternal behaviors (coughing, hiccuping)
9. Fetal scalp stimulation or fetal scalp blood sampling
10. Vomiting
11. Pushing
12. Administration of anesthesia blocks

In addition, if the monitor does not automatically add the time on the strip at specific intervals, it is important to note the time when recording any information on the strip. If more than one nurse is adding information to the monitor strip, it is wise to initial each note. The tracing is considered a legal part of the woman's medical record and is submissible as evidence in court.

It is important for the laboring woman to feel that what is happening to her is the central focus. The nurse can acknowledge this by always speaking to and looking at the woman when entering the room, before looking at the monitor.

Evaluation of FHR Tracings

The nurse tends to use a systematic approach in evaluating FHR tracings to avoid interpreting findings on the basis of inadequate or erroneous data. With a systematic approach, the nurse can make a more accurate and rapid assessment; easily communicate data to the woman, physician/certified nurse-midwife, and staff; and have a universal language for documenting the woman's record.

Evaluation of the electronic monitor tracing begins with a look at the uterine contraction pattern. To evaluate the contraction pattern, the nurse should:

1. Determine the uterine resting tone.
2. Assess the contractions:
   a. What is the frequency?
   b. What is the duration?
   c. What is the intensity (if internal monitoring)?

The next step is to evaluate the fetal heart rate tracing.

1. Determine the baseline:
   a. Is the baseline within normal range?
   b. Is there evidence of tachycardia?
   c. Is there evidence of bradycardia?
2. Determine FHR variability:
   a. Is short-term variability present or absent?
   b. Is long-term variability average, minimal, or marked?
3. Determine whether a sinusoidal pattern is present.
4. Determine whether there are periodic changes.
   a. Are accelerations present?
   b. Do they meet the criteria for a reactive NST?
   c. Are decelerations present?
   d. Are they uniform in shape? If so, determine if they are early or late decelerations.
   e. Are they nonuniform in shape? If so, determine if they are variable decelerations.

After evaluating the FHR tracing for the factors just listed, the nurse may further classify the tracing as reassuring (normal) or nonreassuring (worrisome). Reassuring patterns contain normal parameters and do not require additional treatment or intervention.

Characteristics of reassuring FHR patterns include the following:

- Baseline rate is 120 to 160 bpm.
- Short-term variability is present.
- Long-term variability ranges from three to five cycles per minute.
- Periodic patterns consist of accelerations with fetal movement, and early decelerations may be present.

Nonreassuring patterns indicate that the fetus is becoming stressed and intervention is needed. Characteristics of nonreassuring patterns include the following:

- Severe variable decelerations (FHR drops below 70 bpm for longer than 30 to 45 seconds and is accompanied by rising baseline or decreasing variability or slow return to baseline.)
- Late decelerations of any magnitude
- Absence of variability (No short-term or long-term variability is present.)
- Prolonged deceleration (Deceleration lasts 60 to 90 seconds or more.)
- Severe (marked) bradycardia (FHR baseline is 70 bpm or less.)

Nonreassuring patterns may require continuous monitoring and more involved treatment and intervention.

It is important to provide information to the laboring woman regarding the FHR pattern and the interventions that will help her fetus. Most women are aware that something is happening, and sharing information with the laboring woman reassures her that a potential or actual problem has been identified and that she is an active participant in the interventions. Occasionally, a problem

TABLE 19–6 Guidelines for Management of Variable, Late, and Prolonged Deceleration Patterns

Pattern	Nursing Interventions
Variable decelerations Isolated or occasional Moderate	Report findings to physician/CNM and document in chart. Provide explanation to woman and partner. Change maternal position to one in which FHR pattern is most improved. Discontinue oxytocin if it is being administered and other interventions are unsuccessful. Perform vaginal examination to assess for prolapsed cord or change in labor progress. Monitor FHR continuously to assess current status and for further changes in FHR pattern.
Variable decelerations Severe and uncorrectable	Give oxygen if indicated. Report findings to physician/CNM and document in chart. Provide explanation to woman and partner. Prepare for probable cesarean birth. Follow interventions listed above. Prepare for vaginal birth unless baseline variability is decreasing or FHR is progressively rising—then cesarean, forceps, or vacuum birth is indicated. Assist physician with fetal scalp sampling if ordered. Prepare for cesarean birth if scalp pH shows acidosis or downward trend.
Late decelerations	Give oxygen if indicated. Report findings to physician/CNM and document in chart. Provide explanation to woman and partner. Monitor for further FHR changes. Maintain maternal position on left side. Maintain good hydration with IV fluids (normal saline or lactated Ringer's). Discontinue oxytocin if it is being administered and late decelerations persist despite other interventions. Administer oxygen by face mask at 7–10 L/min. Monitor maternal blood pressure and pulse for signs of hypotension; possibly increase flow rate of IV fluids to treat hypotension. Follow physician's orders for treatment for hypotension if present. Increase IV fluids to maintain volume and hydration (normal saline or lactated Ringer's). Assess labor progress (dilatation and station). Assist physician with fetal blood sampling: If pH stays above 7.25, physician will continue monitoring and resample; if pH shows downward trend (between 7.25 and 7.20) or is below 7.20, prepare for birth by most expeditious means.
Late decelerations with tachycardia or decreasing variability	Report findings to physician/CNM and document in chart. Maintain maternal position on left side. Administer oxygen by face mask at 7–10 L/min. Discontinue oxytocin if it is being administered. Assess maternal blood pressure and pulse. Increase IV fluids (normal saline or lactated Ringer's). Assess labor progress (dilatation and station). Prepare for immediate cesarean birth. Explain plan of treatment to woman and partner. Assist physician with fetal blood sampling (if ordered).
Prolonged decelerations	Perform vaginal examination to rule out prolapsed cord or to determine progress in labor status. Change maternal position as needed to try to alleviate decelerations. Discontinue oxytocin if it is being administered. Notify physician/CNM of findings/initial interventions and document in chart. Provide explanation to woman and partner. Increase IV fluids (normal saline or lactated Ringer's). Administer tocolytic if hypertonus noted and ordered by physician/CNM. Anticipate normal FHR recovery following deceleration if FHR previously normal. Anticipate intervention if FHR previously abnormal or deceleration lasts > 3 minutes.

arises that requires immediate intervention. In that case, the nurse can say something like, "It is important for you to turn on your left side right now because the baby is having a little difficulty. I'll explain what is happening in just a few moments." This type of response lets the woman know that although an action needs to be accomplished rapidly, information will soon be provided. In the haste to act quickly, the nurse must not forget that it is the woman's body and her baby.

Labor and birth nurses must be skilled and competent in evaluating electronic fetal heart rate patterns and responding appropriately (Table 19–6). Competence can be maintained through frequent inservices, formal courses, and continuing education programs.

Additional Assessment Techniques

Indirect Methods

When there is a question regarding fetal status, indirect methods such as **scalp stimulation** (pressing on the fetal scalp with the examining fingers during a vaginal exam to elicit an acceleration of FHR), acoustic stimulation (using a sound device placed against the maternal abdomen to elicit an acceleration in FHR), or stimulation by maternal abdominal palpation (patting or shaking the abdomen) can be used before more invasive fetal blood sampling. When one of the indirect methods is used, the fetus who

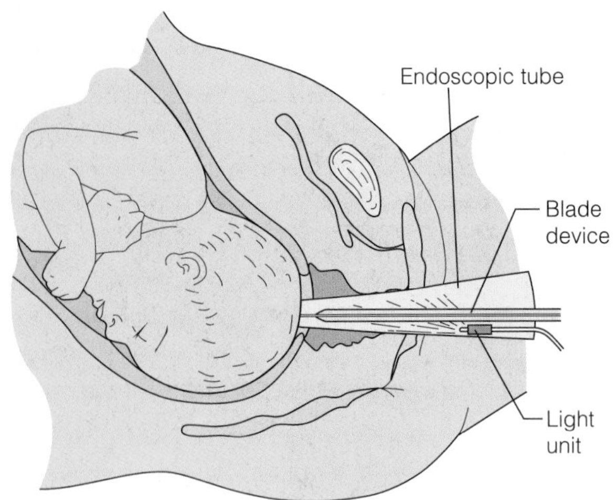

FIGURE 19–27 Technique of obtaining fetal blood from the scalp during labor. SOURCE: Creasy RK, Parer JT: Prenatal care and diagnosis. In *Pediatrics,* 16th ed. Rudolph AM [editor]. Englewood Cliffs, NJ: Appleton-Century-Crofts, 1977.

is not in any stress or distress responds with an acceleration of the FHR, described as a reactive response (acceleration of 15 bpm amplitude with a duration of 15 seconds). Whereas reactivity is associated with fetal well-being, the absence of an acceleration does not diagnose acidemia ore predict fetal compromise. Further observation and assessment measures are indicated.

Fetal Scalp Blood Sampling

When nonreassuring or confusing FHR patterns are noted, additional information about the acid-base status of the fetus must be sought. This may be accomplished by the physician obtaining a **fetal scalp blood sample.** The blood sample is drawn from the fetal scalp. Fetal pH is lower at the end of a contraction, so the sample is best collected before the beginning of the uterine contraction (Swaim & Creasy, 1997).

Swaim and Creasy (1997) recommend the physician consider FBS in two instances. The first instance is in the presence of equivocal FHR patterns. When these patterns are present, knowledge of fetal acid-base status can help care providers determine appropriate choices for managing labor. Examples of such situations may include the following (Swaim & Creasy, 1997):

- Fetal tachycardia with no known complications that does not respond to measures to reduce maternal temperature
- Decreased variability accompanied by a normal baseline for more than 60 minutes, or without periodic changes on admission
- Presence of a high-risk fetus with a normal baseline and no accelerations with scalp or vibroacoustic stimulation
- A premature fetus with an FHR abnormality
- Decreased variability after drug administration and the presence of other concerns regarding the fetus
- An unusual FHR pattern
- Repetitive late decelerations that are unresponsive to fetal stimulation techniques
- Presence of severe variable decelerations

The second instance is the presence of FHR pattern that is known to be compatible with the development of fetal acidosis if the FHR pattern continues over time and the actual birth is close. In this case, knowledge of the fetal acid-base status provides information regarding fetal reserve.

Fetal Blood Sampling Procedure

Equipment needed for fetal blood sampling is available in sterile disposable kits. Items included are heparinized capillary tubes, a short capillary tube holder, a 2 mm micro scalpel on a long handle, a conical vaginal speculum that has an area fitted for placement of a light, clay sealant, silicone gel, and long sponge swabs. An extra overhead light source is needed. The woman's vulva and perineum are cleansed and sterile drapes arranged. The conical speculum is inserted into the vagina and through the cervix to visualize the fetal scalp and the site to be sampled (Figure 19–27). Working through the speculum, the physician cleanses the fetal site to remove vernix, blood, and amniotic fluid. Silicone gel is then applied to the site to enhance beading of the blood once the site is punctured. The site is punctured with the 2 mm micro scalpel in a stab rather than slash motion. A small amount (0.25 mL) of blood is then collected in a long heparinized capillary tube. Two samples should be collected during each procedure to confirm reliability of values. Determinations of pH and base deficit should be readily available in minutes for this procedure to be of value.

The clotting mechanism is compromised when pH is lowered; therefore, blood may ooze at the site for some time. Because loss of even minimal amounts of blood may be harmful to the fetus, pressure is applied to the puncture site throughout the next contraction. Pressure is continued if oozing is prolonged.

Interpretation of FBS Results

An FBS pH of 7.25 or above is considered normal, and the physician will recommend that labor continue as long as the FHR pattern does not become worse. A scalp pH result of 7.20 or lower is an indication for birth without delay. (For instance, if the fetal head is now visible and forceps criteria are met, a forceps-assisted birth is completed; if forceps criteria are not met, a cesarean is performed.) If the scalp pH is between 7.21 and 7.24, it is recommended that serial FBS be done about every 20 minutes until the FHR pattern shows marked improvement or worsening (Swaim & Creasy, 1997).

Although not universally used at present, a pH electrode attached to the fetal scalp tissue can be used to

RESEARCH IN PRACTICE

What is this study about? Dystocia, or labor that does not progress, may result in a cesarean section. According to Patricia McNiven and her colleagues, a diagnosis of dystocia should only be applied in the active, not the latent, phase of labor. A program applying early labor assessment criteria might result in the admission of only women in active labor to the labor unit. Because there may be a correlation between cervical dilatation at the time of hospital admission and the ensuing progression of labor, the authors devised a research study to determine if the relationship was causal. The aim of the study was to ascertain if an early labor assessment would result in a lowered rate of cesarean sections for low-risk nulliparous women.

How was the study done? Investigators recruited 209 low-risk nulliparous women from a hospital in Ontario, Canada and randomly allocated them to either the experimental or the control group. Once the assessment nurse assigned a woman to the control group, the woman was sent to labor and delivery where she received standard care. When a woman was allocated to the experimental group, she received the usual assessments to assure maternal and fetal well-being. If she was not in active labor, the woman received support, advice, and clear instructions about when to return to the hospital, and was sent home or to walk outside until her labor became more active. When labor status was unclear, the woman (and her partner) remained in the assessment area until labor progressed.

What were the results of the study? Investigators obtained feedback about the womens' labor experiences through a questionnaire developed for the study as well as a Labor Agency Scale. The experimental group had a more positive evaluation of labor and delivery based on the questionnaire and the LAS scores (53% exceeded expectations compared to 35% for control). Results for the control group showed a more common diagnosis of slow labor and treatment with oxytocin ($p = 0.001$). The experimental group had a lower use of anesthesia or analgesia ($p = 0.018$), shorter duration of labor in the hospital ($p = 0.001$), and a lower rate of cesarean section (7.6% to 10.6%), although not statistically significant. The investigators found no difference in newborn outcomes as measured by Apgar scores and requirement for active resuscitation.

What additional questions might I have? What were the questions on the Labor Agency Scale? Without more information, it is difficult to understand exactly what was evaluated using this scale.

How can I use this study? When a woman is admitted to the birthing area and not in an active phase of labor (less than 4 cm dilatation, contractions irregular and probably mild in intensity), the nurse can help the woman by strongly encouraging her to be up and walking in the birthing unit. This action may help her advance to active labor and possibly avoid surgery.

SOURCE: McNiven, P. S.; Williams, J. I.; Hodnett, E.; Kaufman, K. & Hannah, M. E. (1998). An early labor assessment program: A randomized, controlled trial. *Birth, 25*(1), 5–10.

monitor fetal pH continuously. This electrode does not measure fetal blood pH level per se, but rather the pH level of subcutaneous tissue. In hypoxia, alpha-adrenergic activity increases initially with accompanying fetal hypertension, causing acidosis to occur in peripheral tissue more rapidly than in the central circulation. Conversely, as hypoxia is corrected, there may be a recovery lag of about 5 minutes in the pH value in the peripheral tissue (Boylan & Parisi, 1994). A great deal of investigation is focused on obtaining continuous fetal O_2 saturation levels. Fetal oximetry monitoring is being tested and refined, and long-term newborn and perinatal outcomes are being studied.

Cord Blood Analysis at Birth

In cases where significant abnormal FHR patterns have been noted prior to birth, amniotic fluid is meconium stained, or the infant is depressed at birth, umbilical cord blood may be analyzed immediately after birth to assess the infant's respiratory status. The cord is usually clamped before the infant takes its first breath to provide an evaluation of blood gas status before the infant interacts with the extrauterine environment because values can change after only a few seconds of neonatal breathing.

An 8- to 10-inch segment of the umbilical cord is double-clamped and cut, and a small amount of blood is aspirated from one of the umbilical arteries (arterial blood seems to provide the most reliable indication of blood gas status and fetal tissue pH). Blood is collected in a heparinized syringe unless it is to be analyzed immediately; it should not be allowed to remain in the segment of cord longer than 30 minutes. Other clinicians may collect a segment of cord and send samples only if the Apgar score is below 7 at 5 minutes, as recommended by the AAP & ACOG (1997). In this instance, values might be used to clarify the cause of a low Apgar score while minimizing any medicolegal exposure and expense. Determination of pH and base deficit values can differentiate whether fetal acidemia is due to hypoperfusion of the placenta or cord compression.

FOCUS YOUR STUDY

- Intrapartal assessment includes attention to both physical and psychosociocultural parameters of the laboring woman, assessment of the fetus, and ongoing assessment for conditions that place the woman and her fetus at increased risk.
- A vaginal examination determines the status of cervical dilatation and effacement, and fetal presentation, position, and station.
- Uterine contractions may be assessed by palpation or by an electronic monitor. The electronic monitor may be used for external or internal monitoring.
- Leopold's maneuvers provide a systematic evaluation of fetal presentation and position.
- Fetal presentation and position may also be assessed by vaginal examination or ultrasound.
- The fetal heart rate may be assessed by auscultation (with a fetoscope) or electronic monitoring.
- Electronic fetal monitoring is accomplished by indirect ultrasound or by direct methods that require the placement of a spiral electrode on the fetal presenting part.

- Indications for electronic monitoring include fetal, maternal, and uterine factors; presence of pregnancy complications; regional anesthesia; and elective monitoring.
- Short-term variability of the FHR can be assessed only by direct electronic monitoring.
- Baseline FHR refers to the range of FHR observed between contractions during a 10-minute period of monitoring.
- The normal range of FHR is 110 to 160 beats per minute.
- Baseline changes of the FHR include tachycardia, bradycardia, and variability.
- Tachycardia is defined as a rate of 160 beats per minute or more for a 10-minute segment of time.
- Bradycardia is defined as a rate of less than 120 beats per minute for a 10-minute segment of time.
- Baseline variability is an important parameter of fetal well-being. It includes both long- and short-term variability.
- Periodic changes are decelerations or accelerations of the FHR from the baseline in response to contractions. Accelerations are normally caused by fetal movement or early cord compression. Decelerations may be termed early, late, variable, or sinusoidal.
- Early decelerations are due to compression of the fetal head during contractions and are considered reassuring.
- Late decelerations are associated with uteroplacental insufficiency.
- Variable decelerations are associated with compression of the umbilical cord.
- Sinusoidal patterns are characterized by an undulant sine wave.
- Psychologic reactions to monitoring vary considerably but tend to reflect one of three responses: 1) the belief that monitoring is invasive and only indicated if a medical reason exists; 2) the belief that monitoring is a necessary part of care; 3) the belief that monitoring is state-of-the-art care and absolutely necessary.
- Birthing room nurses have responsibilities in recognizing and interpreting fetal monitoring patterns, notifying the physician/CNM of problems, and initiating corrective and supportive measures when needed.
- Fetal scalp stimulation can be used when there is a question regarding fetal status.
- Fetal acid-base status may be assessed by fetal blood sampling.

REFERENCES

American Academy of Pediatrics (AAP) and the American College of Obstetricians and Gynecologists (ACOG). (1997). *Guidelines for perinatal care* (4th ed.). Washington, DC: Author.

Austin, W., Gallop, R., McCay, E., Peternelj-Taylor, C., & Bayer, M. (1999). Culturally competent care for psychiatric clients who have a history of sexual abuse. *Clinical Nursing Research 8*, 5–25.

Bernardo, A. (1998). Technology and true presence in nursing. *Holistic Nursing Practice, 12*, 40–49.

Boylan, P. C., & Parisi, V. M. (1994). Acid-base physiology in the fetus. In R. K. Creasy & R. Resnik (Eds.), *Maternal-fetal medicine: Principles and practice* (3rd ed.). Philadelphia: Saunders.

Burrian, J. (1995). Helping survivors of sexual abuse through labor. *Maternal-Child Nursing Journal, 20*(5), 252–255.

Hon, E. H. (1976). An introduction to fetal heart rate monitoring (2nd ed.). Los Angeles: University of Southern California School of Medicine.

Hon, E. H., & Quilligan, E. J. (1967). The classification of fetal heart rate: II. A revised working classification. *Connecticut Medicine, 31*, 779.

Johannsen, J. M. (1993). Update: Guidelines for treating hypertension. *American Journal of Nursing, 93*(3), 42.

Kang, A. H. & Boehm, F. H. (1999). The clinical significance of intermittant sinusoidal fetal heart rate. *American Journal of Obstetrics and Gynecology, 180*, 151–152.

Kassindja, F., & Bashir, L. M. (1998). *Do they hear you when you cry?* New York: Delacorte Press.

Krebs, H. B., Petrie, R. E., & Dunn, L. J. (1983). Atypical variable deceleration. *American Journal of Obstetric and Gynecology, 142*, 297.

McConnell, E. A. (1998). The coalescence of technology and humanism in nursing practice: It doesn't just happen and it doesn't come easily. *Holistic Nursing Practice, 12*, 23–30.

McFarland, J., & Gondolf, E. (1998). Preventing abuse during pregnancy: A clinical protocol. *Maternal-Child Nursing Journal, 23*, 22–26.

McFarland, J., & Parker, B. (1994). Preventing abuse during pregnancy: An assessment and intervention protocol. *MCN; American Journal Maternal/Child Nursing, 19*, 321.

McNiven, P. S., Williams, J. I., Hodnett, E., Kaufman, K., & Hannah, M. E. (1998). An early labor assessment program: A randomized, controlled trial. *Birth, 25*, 5–10.

Menihan, C. A. (1996). Intrapartum fetal monitoring. In K. R. Simpson & P. A. Creehan (Eds.), *AWHONN Perinatal Nursing* (pp 187–225). Philadelphia: Lippincott-Raven.

Nurse's Association of the American College of Obstetricians and Gynecologists (NAACOG). (1990, Mar.). *Fetal heart rate auscultation.* OGN Nursing Practice Resource. Washington, DC.

Parer, J. T. (1994). Fetal heart rate. In R. K. Creasy & R. Resnik (Eds.), *Maternal-fetal medicine.* Philadelphia: Saunders.

Parker, J., & Wiltshire, J. (1995). The handover: Three modes of nursing practice knowledge. In G. Gray & R. Pratt (Eds.), *Scholarship in the discipline of nursing.* Melbourne, Australia: Churchill Livingstone.

Sandelowski, M. (1998). Looking to care or caring to look? Technology and the rise of spectacular nursing. *Holistic Nursing Practice, 12*, 1–11.

Shifrin, B. S. (1990). *Exercises in fetal monitoring.* St Louis: Mosby-Year Book.

Swaim, L. S., & Creasy, R. K. (1997). Fetal assessment and treatment during labor. In R. K. Creasy (Ed.), *Management of labor and delivery* (pp 143–182). Malden, MA: Blackwell.

The Family in Childbirth: Needs and Care

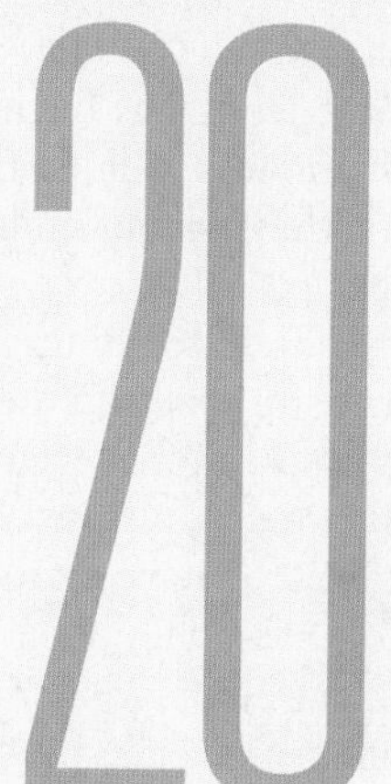

EACH BIRTH IS SO SPECIAL. WHEN THE NEW PARENTS see their baby, it seems that time is suspended. I watch as they gaze at their infant and reach out with their fingers to touch the baby's hands and fingers. I have been so fortunate to be a birthing room nurse and to share this experience with so many new families, but each time is like no other. Every family is unique, and if I can in some way assist them in having a positive caring experience, I believe that it affects their whole life as a family and each of their generations beyond. It's my way of touching the future.

Key Terms

Apgar score
Hyperventilation
Precipitous birth

Objectives

- Compare the advantages and disadvantages of alternative settings for labor and birth.
- Identify options that the childbearing family has during the intrapartal period.
- Identify the database to be created from information obtained upon the woman's admission to the birthing area.
- Review the nursing care that is given during admission.
- Plan strategies to meet the needs of the childbearing family.
- Discuss nursing interventions to meet the needs of the laboring woman and the father during each stage of labor.
- Integrate knowledge of nursing care of the family in the intrapartal period through the use of the nursing process.
- Summarize immediate nursing care of the newborn following birth.
- Discuss initial measures to help the woman and family integrate the newborn into family life.
- Delineate management of a nurse-managed precipitous birth.

IT IS TIME FOR A CHILD TO BE BORN. The waiting is over; labor has begun. The dreams and wishes of the past months fade as the expectant family faces the reality of the tasks of childbearing and child-rearing that are ahead.

The family is about to undergo one of the most meaningful and stressful events in their life together. The adequacy of their preparation for childbirth will now be tested. The coping mechanisms, communication, and support systems that they have established will be put to the test. The childbearing family may feel that their psychologic and physical limits are about to be challenged. The laboring woman may question her ability to cope with the challenges of labor and to meet her expectations for herself. The father may wonder whether he is really ready and able to provide the kind of support and assistance that will be needed. They may worry about the baby's health. Although they look forward to the birth of their baby, the realities of parenthood and incorporating a new family member also present challenges. They both enter a relatively unknown environment where, even with prenatal preparation, many challenges and unknown possibilities await them.

Maternal-newborn nursing has kept pace with the changing philosophy of childbirth. Nurses who choose positions in a birthing area are presented with many opportunities to interact with a wide variety of childbearing families, from those who want maximum decision making and participation in their care, to those who want more interaction with the nurse, to the single woman who enters the birthing experience alone, without support. It is frequently a challenge to provide high-level care in a relaxed atmosphere as well as supportive, culturally sensitive care to such a wide variety of clients.

The previous two chapters present information that lays the foundation for this chapter. Chapter 18 presents a database of information regarding physiologic and psychologic changes during labor and birth, and Chapter 19 discusses intrapartal assessment. This chapter discusses nursing care during labor and birth.

Nursing Diagnosis during Labor and Birth

In devising a plan of care for the intrapartal period, the nurse can develop a general plan that encompasses the whole process, from the beginning of labor through the fourth stage, or the nurse can develop a plan for each stage of labor and birth. An overall plan presents an overview of the whole process, but it is usually general in nature. A plan of care that identifies nursing diagnoses for (at least) each stage provides an opportunity to identify more specific nursing interventions.

In the first stage of labor, nursing diagnoses that may apply include the following:

- ***Fear*** related to discomfort of labor and unknown labor outcome
- ***Ineffective Family Coping*** related to labor process
- ***Pain*** related to uterine contractions, cervical dilatation, and fetal descent
- ***Knowledge*** *Deficit* related to lack of information about normal labor process and comfort measures
- ***Anxiety*** related to unknown birth outcome and anticipated discomfort

Nursing diagnoses for the second and third stages may include the following:

- ***Pain*** related to uterine contractions, birth process, and/or perineal trauma from birth
- ***Knowledge Deficit*** related to lack of information about pushing methods prior to birth
- ***Ineffective Individual Coping*** related to birth process
- ***Fear*** related to outcome of birth process

In the fourth stage, possible nursing diagnoses include the following:

- ***Pain*** related to perineal trauma
- ***Knowledge Deficit*** related to lack of information about involutional process and self-care needs
- ***Altered Family Processes*** related to incorporation of the newborn into the family

Nursing Care Management during Admission

The woman and her support person(s) tend to be concerned about getting to the birthing center or hospital in time for the birth. Sometimes labor occurs so rapidly that birth is imminent upon admission. Usually, the family is advised to arrive at the birth setting at the beginning of the active phase of labor or when the following occur:

- Rupture of membranes (ROM)
- Regular, frequent uterine contractions (nulliparas, about 5 minutes apart for 1 hour; multiparas, 10–15 minutes apart for 1 hour)
- Any vaginal bleeding

If time permits and the family is not familiar with what will occur during labor, the nurse can provide information on admission. (See the Teaching Guide: What To Expect during Labor on the next page.)

The families may be facing a number of unfamiliar procedures that are routine for health care providers. It is important to remember that all women have the right to determine what happens to their bodies. Informed consent should be obtained prior to any procedure that involves touching the body.

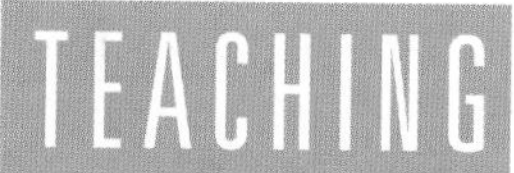

GUIDE: WHAT TO EXPECT DURING LABOR

Assessment As the woman is admitted into the birthing area, assess the woman's knowledge regarding the childbirth experience. Her knowledge base will be affected by previous births, attendance at childbirth education classes, and the amount of information she has been able to gather during her pregnancy by asking questions or reading. You may also assess the factors that affect communication and anxiety level. Assess labor progress to determine what to teach and the time available for teaching. If the woman is in early labor and she needs additional information, proceed with teaching.

Nursing Diagnosis The key nursing diagnosis will probably be ***Knowledge Deficit*** related to lack of information about nursing care during labor.

Nursing Plan and Implementation The teaching plan will focus on the assessments and support the woman will receive during labor.

Client Goals At the completion of teaching, the woman will be able to:

- Verbalize the assessments the nurse will complete during labor.
- Discuss the support and comfort measures that are available.

Teaching Plan

Content	*Teaching Method*
• Describe aspects of the admission process, including: • Taking an abbreviated history • Physical assessment (maternal vital signs [VS], fetal heart rate [FHR], contraction status, status of membranes) • Assessment of uterine contractions (frequency, duration, intensity) • Orientation to surroundings • Introductions to other support staff • Determination of woman's and family support person's expectations of the nurse	*Provide information on the basic assessment and care activities. Allow time for questions and discussion as labor progress permits.*
• Present aspects of ongoing physical care, such as when to expect assessment of maternal VS, FHR, and contractions.	
• If the electronic fetal monitor is used, describe how it works and the information it provides. Orient the woman to the sights and sounds of monitor. Explain what "normal" data will look like and what characteristics are being watched for.	*Demonstrate the fetal monitor.*
• Be sure to note that assessments will increase as the labor progresses, especially during the transition phase (usually the time the woman would like to be left alone) to help keep the mother and baby safe by noting deviations from normal course.	
• Describe the vaginal examination and the information it elicits.	*Use a cervical dilatation chart to illustrate the amount of dilatation.*
• Review comfort techniques that may be used in labor and ascertain what the woman thinks will promote comfort.	*Focus on open discussion.*
• Review the breathing techniques the woman has learned so that you will be able to support her technique.	*Ask the woman to demonstrate the techniques she has learned.*
• Review comfort and support measures, such as positioning, back rub, effleurage, touch, distraction techniques, and ambulation.	*Focus on open discussion.*
• If the woman is in early labor, offer her a tour of the birthing area.	*Provide a tour of birthing area, explaining equipment and routines. Include the woman's partner.*

Evaluation At the end of this teaching session, the woman will be able to describe the assessments that will occur during her labor and to discuss comfort and support measures that may be used.

TABLE 20–1 Improving Communication with a Deaf Woman or Support Person

- Determine how the deaf individual prefers to communicate: speech reading (lip reading), sign language, pantomime, writing, or a combination of methods.
- If speech reading is used, face the person directly, speak with a natural tone and rhythm (exaggerated pronunciation may distort lip movements), and keep your hands away from your face. Do not chew gum.
- Use gestures and pantomime if necessary to enhance your speech.
- Do not assume written communication is the most effective approach. Writing carries a great potential for miscommunication and should not be forced unless the deaf person requests it.
- Most deaf individuals in the United States use American Sign Language (ASL). If the woman signs, call a professional ASL interpreter.
- Only use a family member as an interpreter until the professional interpreter arrives. Family members may not interpret all that is said or may add additional information. Professional ASL interpreters are bound by a code of ethics to maintain strict confidentiality, to transmit accurate messages, and to refrain from editing or adding information.
- Keep the woman's dominant hand and arm free for signing.
- Explain any procedures before they are needed.
- Look at the deaf individual, not the interpreter, when speaking.
- Be alert for signs of "smiling and nodding." Often, when a deaf person does not understand something, the person will simply smile and nod. If that occurs, assess the person's understanding by asking the person to repeat the information to you.

SOURCE: Adapted from Shelp, S. G. (1997). Your patient is deaf, now what? *RN, 60*(2), 37–38, 40.

How the maternity nurse greets the woman and her partner influences the course of her hospital stay. The sudden environmental change and the sometimes impersonal and technical aspects of admission can produce emotional stress. If the family is greeted in a brusque, harried manner, they are less likely to look to the nurse for support. A calm, pleasant manner, in contrast, indicates to the family that they are important. It helps instill in the couple a sense of confidence in the staff's ability to provide quality care and ensure safety during this critical time.

Another important aspect of the initial contact is communicating in the woman and family's primary language. In addition to having interpreters available for Hispanic, Korean, Vietnamese, and other clients who do not speak English fluently, the nurse must consider the special needs of the deaf woman or family. There are more than 400,000 Americans who are deaf in both ears, so there is a good chance that the nurse will work with a deaf expectant mother, father, grandparents, or siblings at some point. Table 20–1 provides suggestions for communicating more effectively with a woman or support person who is deaf.

Following the initial greeting, the woman may be taken into a labor assessment area for evaluation or admitted directly into a birthing room. Some couples prefer to remain together during the admission process, and others prefer to have the partner or support person wait outside. As the nurse helps the woman undress and get into a hospital gown, the nurse can begin to develop rapport and establish the nursing database. The experienced labor and birth nurse can obtain essential information regarding the woman and her pregnancy. By doing an admission assessment, the nurse can initiate any immediate interventions needed and establish individualized priorities. The nurse is then able to make effective nursing decisions regarding intrapartal care:

- Is the woman in labor or should she be sent home with a clear understanding of when to return? The timing of admission of nulliparas may have numerous consequences for the labor and birth, such as the duration of labor and the effect of the hospital environment on the progress of the latent phase of labor (McNiven, Williams, Hodnett, Kaufman, & Hannah, 1998, p 6).
- Are there factors that put the laboring woman or the fetus at risk?
- Should ambulation or bed rest be encouraged?
- Is more frequent monitoring needed?
- What does the woman want during her labor and birth?
- Who will be with her for social support?

The woman is made comfortable. If she wants to rest in bed, a side-lying or semi-Fowler's position rather than a supine position is most comfortable and avoids supine hypotensive syndrome (vena caval syndrome).

After obtaining the essential information from the woman and her prenatal records from her certified nurse-midwife (CNM) or physician, the nurse begins the intrapartal assessment. (Chapter 19 considers intrapartal assessment in depth.) See Essential Precautions in Practice: During Admission and Labor.

Before assessments begin, it is important to establish rapport and to create an environment in which the family feels free to ask questions. The support and encouragement of the nurse in maintaining a caring environment begins with the initial admission but needs to be attended to with all subsequent actions. Before completing assessments, the nurse may provide the opportunity for questions and may explain the environment and the procedures that will be a part of the labor and birthing care. As the assessments begin, the nurse auscultates the fetal heart rate (FHR). (Detailed information on monitoring FHR is presented in Chapter 19.) The woman's blood pressure, pulse, respirations, and oral temperature are assessed. Contraction status (frequency, duration, and intensity), cervical dilatation and effacement, and fetal presentation and station are determined. (See Chapter 19 for discussion of intrapartal vaginal examinations.) If the woman is a nullipara in the early latent phase (for example, contractions are 10 to 30 minutes apart, with mild intensity and very little discomfort; cervix is long and thick, with dilatation of 1 to 2 cm; membranes are intact) she may well be sent home to ambulate and rest in her own surroundings or directed to remain in a birthing center area and ambulate. When further progress is docu-

ESSENTIAL PRECAUTIONS IN PRACTICE

During Admission and Labor

Wear disposable gloves when performing the following actions:

- Assisting the woman as she removes any garments moist with bloody show or amniotic fluid
- Checking amniotic fluid–soaked materials with Nitrazine test tape
- Obtaining and/or handling urine specimens
- Giving an enema or a prep or handling a bedpan
- Handling Chux and bedding that are moist with bloody show and/or amniotic fluid
- Placing elastic belts for the electronic monitor around a woman who has been lying in bedding moist with bloody show and/or amniotic fluid
- Assisting with fetal blood sampling and handling lab tubes

A splash apron and eye covering (such as goggles) must be worn when splashing of body fluids is possible.

REMEMBER to wash your hands prior to putting the disposable gloves on and AGAIN immediately after removing the gloves.

For further information, consult OSHA and CDC guidelines.

TABLE 20–2 Indicators of Normal Labor Process on Admission

Indicator	Normal Characteristics
Uterine contractions	Frequency of not less than 2 minutes Duration of less than 75 seconds Uterine relaxation between contractions Most intense discomfort only with contractions (Some women, especially those with occiput posterior position, complain of less intense lower abdominal and/or back pain between contractions.)
Fetal heart rate	Rate 120–160 with average variability Absence of variability or late decelerations
Maternal vital signs	B/P below 140/90 or less than +30/+15 above prepregnancy readings Pulse 60–100 Temperature between 97.8 and 99.6F (36.5 and 37.5C)
If membranes ruptured	Fluid clear without odor

mented, she is admitted. McNiven et al (1998) found that women who are admitted in the latent phase are much more likely to have longer duration of labor, increased use of epidural analgesia for pain, and increased use of oxytocin to augment labor than women who are clearly in the active phase at admission.

After the vaginal examination, the nurse shares the findings with the couple. If there are signs of advanced labor (frequent contractions, an urge to bear down, and so on), the physician/CNM is notified, and immediate actions are taken to prepare for the birth. If there are signs of excessive bleeding upon admission or if the woman reports episodes of painless bleeding in the last trimester, placenta previa may be present; in such cases, vaginal examination is not performed because it may stimulate copious bleeding.

Results of FHR assessment, uterine contraction evaluation, and the vaginal examination help determine whether the rest of the admission process can proceed at a more leisurely pace or whether additional interventions have higher priority. For example, an FHR of 120 beats per minute (bpm) on auscultation indicates that an electronic fetal monitor (EFM) should be applied immediately to obtain additional data. The woman's vital signs will then be assessed immediately (Table 20–2).

After admission data are obtained, a clean-voided midstream urine specimen is collected. The woman with intact membranes may collect her specimen in the bathroom. If the membranes are ruptured and the presenting part is not engaged, the woman is generally asked to remain in bed to avoid the risk of umbilical cord prolapse. If ambulation is desired to increase the labor contractions, it is generally safe for the woman to walk if the fetal head is well engaged and the monitor strip shows reassuring signs of fetal well-being (Figure 20–1).

The nurse can test the woman's urine for the presence of protein, ketones, and glucose by using a dipstick before sending the sample to the laboratory. This procedure is especially important if nondependent edema or elevated blood pressure is noted on admission. Proteinuria of +1 or more may be a sign of preeclampsia. Glycosuria is found frequently in pregnant women because of the increased glomerular filtration rate in the proximal tubules and the inability of these tubules to increase glucose reabsorption. However, it may also be associated with gestational diabetes and should not be discounted.

If the vaginal examination has established that the fetal head is well engaged, and if the EFM has shown a reassuring FHR pattern, the woman is then encouraged to ambulate to increase her comfort and stimulate labor contractions. In a few areas, the physician/CNM orders a prep and/or enema. Kaczorowski, Levitt, Hanvey, Avard, and Chance (1998) conducted a study of Canadian hospitals and found that in certain regions of the country almost 75% of the hospitals practiced very restricted use of preps, and 61% had very limited use of enemas. In the United States, most regions no longer consider preps or enemas necessary. In the event that a prep is ordered, the perineal hair below the vaginal opening is removed by using a prep set (containing soapy sponges, a receptacle for warm water, disposable razor, and dry sponges); alternatively, the hair can be clipped with sterile scissors. If an enema is prescribed by the physician or CNM, or requested by the client, a small-volume enema such as a Fleets is usually used.

Laboratory tests are often performed in the outpatient setting prior to admission. Hemoglobin and hematocrit values help determine the oxygen-carrying capacity of the circulatory system and the ability of the woman to

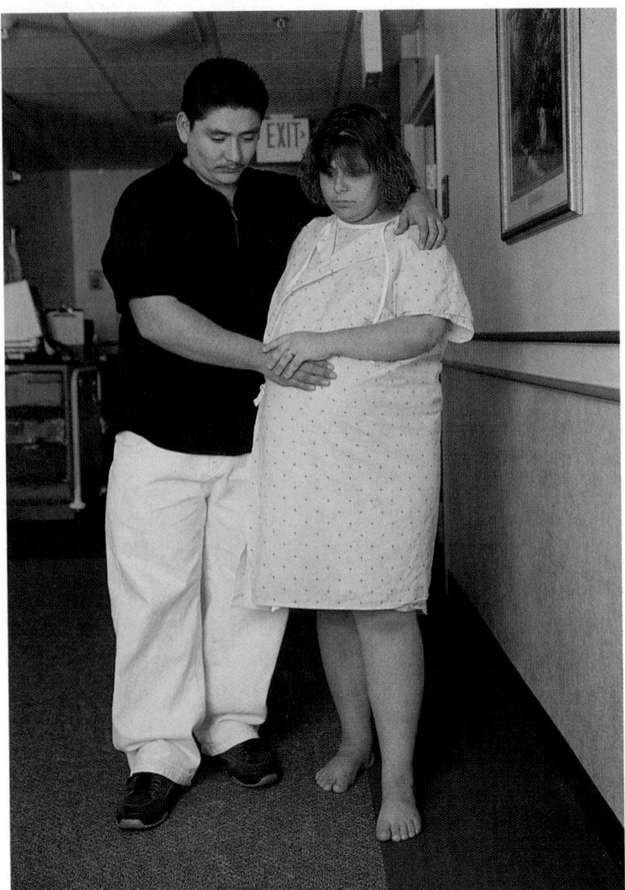

FIGURE 20–1 Woman and her partner walking in the hospital during labor.

withstand blood loss at birth. Elevation of the hematocrit indicates hemoconcentration of blood, which occurs with edema or dehydration. A low hemoglobin, in the absence of other evidence of bleeding, suggests anemia. Blood may be typed and cross-matched if the woman is in a high-risk category. A serology test for syphilis is obtained if one has not been done in the last 3 months or if an antepartal serology result was positive.

In many hospitals, the admission process also includes signing an informed consent for treatment, and the client is given information on arranging advanced directives or instructions about her wishes if she were to become critically ill. In all cases, an identification bracelet is attached to her wrist.

Depending on how rapidly labor is progressing, the nurse notifies the CNM or physician before or after completing the admission procedures. The report should include the following information: cervical dilatation and effacement, station, presenting part, status of the membranes, contraction pattern, FHR, vital signs that are not in the normal range, the woman's wishes, and her response to labor.

A nursing admission note is entered into the computer or the charting system. The admission note should include the reason for admission, the date and time and method of the woman's arrival, notification of the CNM/physician, the condition of the woman and her baby, and labor and membrane status (American Academy of Pediatrics [AAP] & American College of Obstetricians and Gynecologists [ACOG], 1997). Her comfort level and support system should also be addressed.

Screening for psychosocial risk factors is also an integral part of the admission process. Risk factors include family violence, sexual abuse, drugs, alcohol, and sexually transmitted infections. Chapter 19 suggests ways to obtain a psychosocial history regarding family and sexual violence. The nurse should always ask questions regarding family and sexual violence when the woman is alone. The nurse should ask about alcohol and drug use in a straightforward, matter-of-fact manner. For example, a question such as "How many times per week do you drink alcohol?" prompts the woman to be specific in her answer. If the woman reports that she does drink alcohol on a daily basis, the nurse then asks about the amount. Drug use can be assessed in a similar manner. The nurse must maintain a nonjudgmental approach and collect only information relating to the labor and birthing process. This dialogue provides an opportunity for the nurse to continue to build support, to provide information when requested, and to be direct yet supportive.

Nursing Care Management during the First Stage of Labor

Women who have had a chance to look back at their labor have important information to share with birthing nurses regarding the activities and qualities of nursing care that helped them cope with labor and increased their satisfaction with the process.

Research provides information regarding nursing interventions and qualities of the nurse that laboring women have found helpful. Proctor (1998) found that nurse-midwives and laboring women had different views of what determines quality of care. The laboring women in the study revealed that they wanted a clean, homelike environment that conveyed the idea that labor and birth is a normal process, not an "illness." The laboring women also revealed that they wanted information offered to them without their asking for it directly; in some cases, they could not remember to ask questions or were even sure what questions to ask. The women wanted clear, plain, honest explanations about procedures and examinations and information about the choices available for pain relief during labor. Women who had a cesarean wanted to know why the procedure was needed and what factors were involved. The nurse-midwives, in contrast, did not place the same importance on these aspects of the birth experience. Less important to them were such fac-

COMMUNITY IN FOCUS

The Birth Doula

Traditionally, women in labor have been supported by other women who were knowledgeable about childbirth. When childbirth moved from the home to the hospital or birthing center this labor support role became the responsibility of the nurse, partner, or family member. Generally, nurses have the knowledge and skills necessary to be excellent providers of support; however, continuity can be lost when shifts change and a new nurse is assigned to a laboring family. Moreover, should a problem arise, the nurse has many responsibilities in addition to providing comfort and support. Family members are loving supporters, but their knowledge is limited and they may be less effective at promoting comfort than someone who is specially trained for the role. Consequently, many hospitals and birthing centers now offer laboring women the services of a birth doula.

Doula is a Greek term that means "woman's servant." Today's birth doula is a professionally trained labor companion whose role is to provide information and physical and emotional support to a laboring woman and her partner. The doula also acts as a bridge to promote effective communication between the childbearing woman and her caregivers. A doula is an advocate for the couple but is not the decision maker. The doula is not a substitute for a professional nurse, rather the doula's role is nonclinical; her purpose is to enhance the birth experience by working in partnership with the couple and other care providers.

Doulas can provide postpartum services. A postpartum doula may care for the new mother and baby, provide advice and encouragement about breastfeeding, prepare meals, run errands, and even do some cleaning.

In 1992, Doulas of North America (DONA) was established. This nonprofit, international organization seeks to promote the availability and use of well-trained, experienced doulas from all backgrounds, cultures, and socioeconomic levels. To help achieve this goal, DONA has established a certification program for doulas. Certified doulas respect a woman's right to privacy and ascribe to a code of ethics.

Some doulas practice independently and charge a fee for their services. Typically they meet the couple employing them during the prenatal period and are available on call for the labor and birth. They remain with the woman throughout the entire labor and birth process. They can make postpartum visits to give the woman an opportunity to discuss the experience and ask questions.

Other doulas are volunteers or paid employees of a hospital or community agency. Hospital-based doula programs vary widely in organization and approach. In some cases, a couple meets their doula during the prenatal period; in other cases, doulas are part of an on-call rotation and the couple meets the doula when the woman goes into labor. These doulas, too, remain with the couple from the time the doula arrives at the hospital until after the birth. Currently, most doula services are paid for by the couple although there is some third party reimbursement available.

Overall, doulas are received enthusiastically by childbearing women and their families. Many nurses and physicians are also enthusiastic about the role a doula can play in providing comfort measures and support. When each care provider respects the role the others play, a true sense of camaraderie and shared purpose can develop. Moreover, a bilingual doula can help ensure an optimal birth experience for women from different cultures.

Further information about labor doulas is available through DONA at 1-800-206-5440 or through their web site at http://www.dona.com.

SOURCE: Literature and printed materials available through DONA.

tors as continuity of care during labor, providing ongoing information rather than just answering questions as they arose, and introducing the woman to the on-call physician who would come in if difficulties developed (Proctor, 1998).

In a study by Bryanton, Fraser-Davey, and Sullivan (1994), birthing nurses rated making the woman physically comfortable and providing pain medication as important nursing interventions. Laboring women, however, rated these activities much lower in importance. The laboring women identified the most helpful nursing behaviors as "making the woman feel cared about as an individual, giving praise, appearing calm and confident, assisting with breathing and relaxing, treating the woman with respect, explaining hospital routines, answering questions truthfully in an understandable language, providing a sense of security, and accepting what the woman said and did without judging her" (p 641).

Other researchers have validated many similar nursing behaviors that have been identified as helpful. Mackey and Stepans (1993) noted that laboring women wanted the nurse to participate in labor and be there for them, to accept them as individuals, to give information and encouragement, and to be present when the woman desired. Brown and Lumley (1994) in a study of 790 Australian women found that the most important factors regarding satisfaction with nursing care were ready access to information, participation in decision making, and relationships formed with the nurses.

Nurses are recognizing the importance of these aspects of care and therefore are incorporating information gained from research to plan, develop, and deliver more holistic care for each family.

Integration of Family Expectations

Most families come to the birth setting with great anxiety about their capabilities to endure labor and about the safety of their baby. What do they expect of the nurse who will be with them during this important event in their life? Mackey and Lock (1989) conducted a study to identify couples' expectations of the labor and birth nurse. They wanted the nurse to be calm, considerate,

Text continues on page 550.

CRITICAL PATHWAY FOR INTRAPARTAL STAGES

Category	First Stage	Second and Third Stage	Fourth Stage Birth to 1 Hour Past Birth
Referral	**Review prenatal record** **Advise CNM/physician of admission**	**Labor record for first stage**	**Report to recovery room nurse**
Assessments	Admission assessments: Ask about problems since last prenatal visit; labor status (contraction frequency and duration), membrane status (intact or ruptured); coping level; support; woman's desires during labor and birth; ability to verbalize needs; laboratory testing (blood and UA) Intrapartal assessments:Cervical assessment: from 1 to 10 cm dilatation; nullipara (1.2 cm/h), multipara (1.5 cm/h) Cervical effacement: from 0% to 100% Fetal descent: progressive descent from −4 to +4 Membrane assessment: intact or ruptured; when ruptured, Nitrazine positive, fluid clear, no foul odor Comfort level: woman states is able to cope with contractions Behavioral characteristics: facial expressions, tone of voice and verbal expressions are consistent with comfort level and ability to cope Latent Phase: • B/P, P, R q1h if in normal range (B/P 90–140/60–90 or not >30 mm Hg systolic or 15 mm Hg diastolic over baseline; pulse 60–90; respirations 12–20/min, quiet, easy) • Temp q4h unless >37.6C (99.6F) or membranes ruptured then q2h • Uterine contractions q30min (contractions q5–10min, 15–40sec, mild intensity) • FHR q60min (for low-risk women) and q30min (for high-risk women) if reassuring (reassuring FHR has: baseline 120–160, STV present, LTV average, accelerations with fetal movement, no late nor variable decelerations); if nonreassuring, position on side, start O_2, assess for hypotension, monitor continuously, notify CNM/physician Active Phase: • B/P, P, R, q1h if WNL • Temp as above • Uterine contractions q30min: contractions q2–3min, 60 sec, moderate to strong • FHR q30min (for low-risk women) and q15min (for high-risk women) if reassuring; if nonreassuring institute interventions Transition: • B/P, P, R, q30min • Uterine contractions q15–30min: contractions q2min, 60–75 sec, strong • FHR q30min (for low-risk women) and q15min (for high-risk women) if reassuring; if nonreassuring, see above	Second stage assessments: • B/P, P, R q5–15min • Uterine contractions palpated continuously • FHR q15min (for low-risk women) and q5min (for high-risk women) if reassuring; if nonreassuring, monitor continuously Fetal descent: descent continues to birth Comfort level: woman states is able to cope with contractions and pushing Behavioral characteristics: response to pushing, facial expressions, verbalization Third stage assessments: • B/P, P, R q5min • Uterine contractions, palpate occasionally until placenta is delivered, fundus maintains tone and contraction pattern continues to birth of placenta Newborn assessments: • Assess Apgar score of newborn • Respirations: 30–60, irregular • Apical pulse: 120–160 and somewhat irregular • Temperature: Skin temp above 36.5C (97.8F) • Umbilical cord: two arteries, one vein (if one artery, assess for anomalies and urine output) • Gestational age: 38–42 weeks	**Expected Outcomes** Appropriate resources identified and utilized Immediate postbirth assessments of mother q15min for 1h: • B/P: 90–140/60–90; should return to prelabor level • Pulse: slightly lower than in labor; range is 60–90 • Respirations: 12–20/min; easy; quiet • Temperature: 36.2–37.6C (98–99.6F) • Fundus firm, in midline, at the umbilicus • Lochia rubra; moderate amount; <1 pad/h; no free flow or passage of clots with massage • Perineum: sutures intact; no bulging or marked swelling; minimal bruising may be present; no c/o severe pain nor rectal pain • Bladder nondistended; spontaneous void of >100mL clear, straw-colored urine; bladder nondistended following voiding • If hemorrhoids present, no tenseness or marked engorgement; <2 cm diameter Comfort level: <3 on scale of 1 to 10 Energy level: awake and able to hold newborn Newborn assessments if newborn remains with parents: • Respirations: 30–60; irregular • Apical pulse: 120–160 and somewhat irregular • Temperature: skin temp above 36.5C (97.8F); skin feels warm to touch • Skin color noncyanotic • Mucus: small amount, clear, easily suctioned with bulb syringe without skin color change • Behavioral: newborn opens eyes widely if room is slightly darkened • Movements rhythmic; no hand tremors present **Expected Outcomes** Findings indicate normal progression with absence of complications

Category	First Stage	Second and Third Stage	Fourth Stage Birth to 1 Hour Past Birth
Teaching/ psychosocial	Establish rapport Orient to environment, expected assessments and procedures Answer questions and provide information Orient to EFM if used Teach relaxation, visualization & breathing pattern if needed Explain comfort measures available Assume advocacy role for woman/family during labor and birth	Orient to expected assessments and procedures Answer questions and provide information Explain comfort measures available Continue advocacy role	Explain immediate assessments and care after this first hour Teach self-massage of fundus and expected findings Instruct to call for assistance if mother desires to get OOB Begin newborn teaching; bulb syringe, positioning; maintaining warmth Assist parents in exploring their newborn Assist with first breastfeeding experience **Expected Outcomes** Client and partner verbalize/demonstrate understanding of teaching
Nursing care management and report	Straight cath prn if bladder distended If regional block administered monitor B/P, FHR, sensation per protocol Provide continuing status reports to CNM/physician Perineal clip per woman's request Small enema per woman's request Perform sterile vaginal examination as indicated	Straight cath prn if bladder distended Continue monitoring VS, FHR and sensation if regional block has been given	Straight cath if bladder distended Monitor return of motor ability and sensation if regional block has been given Weigh perineal pads if lochia flow >1 saturated pad in 15 min, presence of boggy uterus and clots; ↓B/P, ↑P **Expected Outcomes** • Maternal/fetal well-being maintained and supported • Mother and newborn experience safe labor and birth • Family participates in process as desired
Activity	Encourage ambulation unless contraindicated Maintain bed rest immediately after administration of IV pain medication, or following regional block Woman rests comfortably between contractions	Position comfortably for birth Woman rests comfortably between pushing efforts & while awaiting birth of placenta	Position of comfort **Expected Outcomes** • Activity maintained as desired unless contraindicated • Comfort enhanced by positioning/movement
Comfort	Institute comfort measures: ambulation, frequent position change, effleurage, focal point, patterned paced breathing, visualization, therapeutic touch, back rub, moist cloths to face, holding hand, words of encouragement, changing underpad, shower, whirlpool, staying with the woman/family, warmed blanket at back, sacral pressure Offer pain medication or administer if requested Assist with administration of regional block	Institute comfort measures: • Second stage: cool cloth to forehead, encouragement, coaching, help support legs while pushing, position of comfort for pushing and birth • Third stage: cool cloth to forehead, assist parents to see newborn, position mother to hold newborn, provide encouragement	Institute comfort measures: • Perineal discomfort: gently cleanse and apply ice pack; position to decrease pressure on perineum • Uterine discomfort: palpate fundus gently • Hemorrhoids: ice pack • General fatigue: position of comfort, encourage rest • Administer pain medication ________ **Expected Outcomes** • Optimal comfort level maintained • Active reductionof pain/discomfort achieved
Nutrition	Ice chips and clear fluids Evaluate for signs of dehydration	Ice chips and clear fluids	Regular diet if assessments are WNL Encourage fluids **Expected Outcomes** Nutritional needs met
Elimination	Voids at least q2h; urine clear, straw-colored, negative for protein Bladder nondistended May have bowel movement Monitor I & O with IVs	May void spontaneously with pushing May pass stool with pushing	Voids spontaneously **Expected Outcomes** Urinary bladder and bowel function unimpaired
Medications	Administer pain medication per woman's request	Local infiltration of anesthetic agent for birth by CNM/physician Pitocin 10 units IM, IVP per IV tubing, or added to IV fluids	Continue Pitocin infusion Administer pain medication ____________ **Expected Outcomes** Comfort enhanced by pain relieving techniques, administration of analgesia agent or an analgesic or anesthetic block

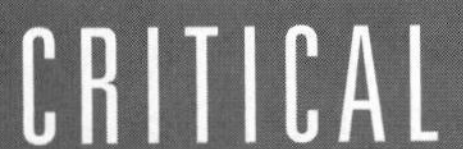

PATHWAY FOR INTRAPARTAL STAGES ***CONTINUED***

Category	First Stage	Second and Third Stage	Fourth Stage Birth to 1 Hour Past Birth
Discharge planning	Evaluate knowledge of labor and birth process Evaluate support system and need for referral after birth		Provide information if mother to be moved from LDR room Provide opportunity for parents to ask questions regarding newborn Evaluate knowledge of normal postpartum, newborn care **Expected Outcomes** Mother and newborn transferred to low-risk postpartal and newborn care
Family involvement	Identify available support person(s) Recognize possible impact of culture on responses Observe interaction between woman and partner Create moment alone with woman to identify possible abuse Assess current parenting skills	Provide opportunities for woman and support person(s) to watch newborn assessments Perform newborn assessment on mother's abdomen/chest if possible	Provide opportunity for parents to be with baby Encourage skin-to-skin contact Darken room to encourage eye-to-eye contact Provide quiet time for new family Parenting: demonstrates early culturally expected parenting behaviors **Expected Outcomes** • Incorporation of newborn into family • Family verbalizes comfort with newborn care
Date			

compassionate, concerned, and friendly—a person who accepts feelings and is interested in the woman as a person. The study revealed seven aspects of the nurse's role that couples considered most important: (1) presence of the nurse in the room during labor, (2) the nurse's accommodation to their desired level of decision making (whether they wanted to make all decisions regarding their care, wanted a collaborative role with the nurse, or expected the nurse to make most of the decisions), (3) assistance with aspects of care, (4) physical assessment by the nurse, (5) information regarding progress and procedures, (6) comfort measures, and (7) support. The study participants also revealed that they had different expectations regarding the amount or level of nursing involvement, and they were divided into three groups: those who wanted limited, moderate, or extensive nurse involvement.

The group who wanted limited nurse involvement expected nurses to complete the necessary assessments and needed procedures, but other than that they wanted to let nurses know when their presence was desired in the room. They wanted to have their decisions respected.

The couples who preferred moderate nurse involvement wanted the nurses' presence intermittently and wanted to collaborate with nurses regarding decisions. They wanted direction, assistance, encouragement, and frequent support.

The couples who favored extensive nurse involvement wanted nurses to be present almost all the time. They wanted the nurses to take responsibility and do what was best. The women wanted a lot of physical contact and wanted the nurses to somehow instill confidence in them that they could handle the labor.

With the variety of expectations clients have of nurses, it becomes a challenge for nurses to provide individualized care. The expert nurse needs to assess the couple's needs and desires and respond in just that manner. There are cues the nurse can look for. When the woman and her coach are admitted, do they seem to take control and know what is going to happen? Do they have a birth plan that they have already worked out, or do they seem hesitant and unsure of the process?

Although these two ends of the spectrum are obvious, they are a starting point. It would be fairly safe to assume that the "situation-is-in-control" couple would want a little less involvement, and the couple who is hesitant and asking questions will want more extensive involvement. The nurse can also gain more information by asking questions such as, "Other than the assessments that I will be making, what kind of involvement would you like from me? Would you like to call me when you need something or have me come in now and then, or would you be more comfortable if I stay in the room most of the time?" This gives the couple an opportunity to make their wishes known. It is also important that the couple knows that the nurse understands that their wishes may change during labor and that the nurse will be available for them throughout the process.

Other family expectations may be communicated by way of a birth plan. The family may have a written plan or may discuss their wishes with the nurse. One aspect of couples' requests is coming under more scrutiny. Photos

RESEARCH IN PRACTICE

What is this study about? Because no Finnish research studies existed about fathers' immediate experiences after childbirth, Katri Vehviläinen-Julkunen and Anja Liukkonen developed a study to describe how fathers present at the birth of their child experienced the event. The researchers wanted to know the fathers' feelings during birth, what being present during birth meant to them, and how they believed midwifery care at birth ought to be developed.

How was the study done? Within 2 hours of birth, midwives approached a convenience sample of 137 fathers to participate in this study. One hundred seven fathers returned the questionnaire that asked about their feelings during delivery and about midwifery procedures. The tool contained both structured, Likert-type questions with preset options as well as open-ended questions.

What were the results of the study? Through factor analysis, investigators identified 11 factors with eigenvalues over 1.0 that described the fathers' feelings during delivery. They then forced the factors to 4: discomfort, pleasure and pride, feelings related to staff members, and feelings related to the maternity environment. Examples of feelings of discomfort included excitement, worries about partner coping, and worry about the baby's welfare. Pleasure and pride incorporated pride related to fatherhood and gratefulness toward partner. Feelings related to staff members encompassed competent staff and a restless environment. Feelings related to maternity environment included "somewhat bleak and dreary" for 36% but "very pleasant" for 73% of the fathers. When the authors analyzed the open-ended questions they found that 80 of the 107 fathers said that being present for the birth was very important for their fatherhood and stressed feelings of responsibility for their partner and baby. The second open-ended question about the best and worst things experienced during birth elicited responses about difficulty watching one's partner in pain. Responses about the best things involved the baby. Regarding improvement of care for the laboring women, the fathers felt that more attention should be paid to the relief of the woman's pain and that the fathers should be better informed about the progress of labor.

What additional questions might I have? What was the number of variables at the beginning of factor analysis? Traditionally, with factor analysis there are at least 5 cases or subjects per variable and that would predicate no more than 21 variables for 107 cases.

How can I use this study? This study illustrates the myriad feelings experienced by the father who participates in the birth of his child. Nurses need to remember to incorporate the father as an equal partner in this important process rather than treat him as an accessory.

SOURCE: Vehviläinen-Julkunen, K., & Liukkonen, A. (1998). Fathers' experiences of childbirth. *Midwifery, 14,* 10–17.

and videocameras in the birthing area are a concern for some health care providers and hospitals because photos and videotapes have been used in malpractice litigation (Cesario, 1998). The result of this use of photos and videotapes has precipitated various reactions; some hospitals have banned the use of cameras and videotapes, and some physicians have become less willing to participate in births that are recorded. This leaves the family disappointed and frustrated that they do not have recorded memories of their birth experience. Some hospitals and birthing centers are establishing programs in which a photographer from their facility is contracted to record the birth. The family can obtain a copy of the video, but the ownership rests with the facility.

The nurse can facilitate discussion regarding recording the birth experience during the admission process. The nurse can ask the mother whether she wishes to be photographed or have a videocamera used. Other questions should include what and whom may be photographed. The nurse needs to assure the woman that she is in control and she can stop filming at any time. Some hospitals are developing a consent form for photography or videotaping, which provides a useful tool not only for purposes of documented consent, but also for providing a mechanism for discussion (Cesario, 1998). After the birth, it is suggested that a brief narrative nursing note be added to document the method of recording, whom and what were recorded, and who maintains ownership of the videotape (Cesario, 1998).

Integration of Cultural Beliefs

Values, customs, and practices of different cultures are as important during labor as they are in the prenatal period. Without this knowledge, a nurse is less likely to understand a family's behavior and may impose personal values and beliefs upon them. As cultural sensitivity increases, so does the likelihood of providing high-quality care.

The following sections briefly present a few possible cultural responses to labor. It is difficult to present even such a limited discussion in a clear, nonjudgmental way because once a statement is made, it may appear stereotypical, and of course no statement of a specific behavior can accurately reflect the preference of all people in a group. The nurse must always remain aware that an individual example of birthing practice will never be pertinent to all women in that group. Within every culture, each person develops his or her own beliefs and value system. Nurses must regard general information about any culture or belief system as background information to help them determine the person's own needs and desires.

Modesty

Modesty is an important consideration for women, regardless of the culture to which they belong. However, some women may be more uncomfortable than others with the degree of exposure needed for some procedures during labor and the birth process. Some women may be particularly uncomfortable when men are present and feel more comfortable with women; others may be uncomfortable with exposure of personal body parts regardless of the gender of the examiner or person who assists them. The nurse needs to be observant of the woman's responses to examinations and procedures and to provide the draping and privacy that the woman needs. It is more prudent to assume that embarrassment will occur with exposure and take measures to provide privacy than to assume that it will not matter to the woman. For example, many Hispanic women may fear loss of privacy, so they labor at home as long as possible (Lipson, Dibble, & Minarik, 1996). Some Asian women are not accustomed to male physicians and attendants, and some Muslims forbid any male (other than the husband) to see a woman who is uncovered. Modesty is of great concern, and exposure of as little of the woman's body as possible is strongly recommended.

Pain Expression

How women deal with the discomfort of labor varies widely. Some turn inward and remain very quiet during the whole process. They speak only to ask others to leave the room or cease conversation. Others may be very vocal, with behaviors such as counting out loud, moaning quietly or loudly, crying, or cursing. They may also turn from side to side or change positions frequently. In the Korean culture it used to be important for the laboring women to be silent during labor so it would not bring shame on the family. However, today women are encouraged to be less passive. Vocalization is more common, although older in-laws or other family members may discourage shouting or outcries as aggressive behavior (Lipson et al, 1996). Hmong women are frequently quiet during labor, although behavior varies from one individual to the next (Lipson et al, 1996). The nurse supports a woman's individual expression of pain, whatever it may be, in order to enhance the birthing experience for mother, baby, and family. European Americans demonstrate a wide variety of behaviors in response to pain. Some stay very quiet and seem to turn inside to "keep control"; others move about in bed, change positions frequently, moan, and cry. Especially in the transitional phase, some women want to squeeze their partner's (or the nurse's) hand, and some may be tempted to bite during the most intense part of the contraction. It is important to inform the woman strongly that biting either the nurse or the partner or support person is not allowed.

Cultural Beliefs: Some Examples

In regard to specific practices related to position and food and drink during labor, some differences between cultures are apparent. In most non-European societies uninfluenced by Westernization, women assume an upright position in childbirth. For example, Hmong women from Laos report that squatting during childbirth is common in their culture (LaDu, 1985). During birth, some Native American women use meditation, self-control, or indigenous plants, and the father may be expected to avoid certain rituals such as eating meat (Lipson et al, 1996).

Hmong women have special customs regarding childbirth. The beginning of labor signifies the beginning of a transition and entails certain dietary restrictions. The woman may want to be active and should be able to move about during labor. The husband is frequently present and actively involved in providing comfort. During labor, the woman usually prefers only "hot" foods, tea made with loose tea leaves, and warm water to drink (Johnson, 1996). Traditionally, the woman prefers that the amniotic membranes not be ruptured until just before birth. It is thought that the escape of fluid at this time makes the birth easier. She may choose to kneel or squat for the birth of her baby. As soon as the baby is born, a soft-boiled egg must be given to the mother to restore her energy. During the postpartum period, the mother prefers "warm" foods, such as chicken prepared with warm water and warm rice (Morrow, 1986).

Vietnamese women also may follow prescribed customs during pregnancy and birth (Calhoun, 1986). While in labor, the woman usually maintains self-control and may smile throughout the labor. She may prefer to walk about during labor and to give birth in a squatting position. She may avoid drinking cold water and prefer fluids at room temperature. The newborn is protected from praise to prevent jealousy.

Latina women often want their partner to stay with them during labor and birth and to reassure them that everything will be all right. The women want the partner to show caring and love as they labor and to speak to them using affectionate words (Khazoyan & Anderson, 1994).

Muslim women may have their husband, a female friend or relative, or a male relative with them during childbirth. Family support may be particularly important but does not preclude the importance of the nurse's presence. The woman may want to retain her head covering (khimar), and two long-sleeved gowns can be offered. It is important to have examinations done by a female nurse, physician, or CNM whenever possible. Some Muslim women are not comfortable in the presence of a male physician or nurse. If a male physician is involved with their care, they may wish for their husband to remain in the room during all care by the physician. It is important to recognize that modesty needs vary, and each individual will need to be assessed. After the birth, Muslim fathers traditionally call praise to Allah (adhan) in the newborn's right ear and clean the newborn. It is helpful if the birthing room personnel are aware of these practices so that this family's expectations and wishes can be incorporated into care (Hutchinson & Baqi-Aziz, 1994).

I am in an area with a very small Muslim population, and one of the clinical nursing students with me had the opportunity to work with a couple during labor, birth, and then in the postpartum area the following day. During labor, the woman's sister remained at her side, and her husband sat on the other side of a drawn curtain inside the labor room and close to the door. He requested that a sign be placed on the door indicating that no males were to enter the room. We took care to ensure that we asked for a female lab tech for blood drawing and informed the neonatal nurse practitioners (NNP) who attend each birth that a female NNP would be needed. A female physician attended the birth. The labor and birth went smoothly, and the woman did not utter any sound, even during pushing. After the birth, the father was shown the child before his wife held the newborn boy. The father was very pleased and talked quietly to his son, with his head down beside the newborn's ear. The next day, the student nurse was once again assigned to this family. The sign remained on the door, and at all times that day, the sister and father remained in the room, the father always sitting away from the bed, close to the door. This was the woman's fifth child, so at first the student thought that the mother would not want much self-care, newborn, or breastfeeding information. But she began to talk to the woman, with her husband interpreting all questions and giving answers, and as each topic was brought up, the mother indicated that she wanted more information. Building on the trust that they had established the previous day in labor, the father told the student to "give the instruction," and he left the room. The mother and sister were full of questions, and it seemed that although this was her fifth baby, the mother had many, many questions, as if she were a first-time mother. The student was so proud that she did not make assumptions and was able to share so much information with them. The student did not emerge from the room for what seemed like hours. Both the mother and sister had an opportunity to learn aspects of their bodies, and to have questions answered that they had had for years. It was an experience that the student and I will always remember with great joy.

In working with women from another culture, the nurse needs an awareness of their beliefs, values, and practices in order to understand their needs. The maternity nurse would do well to make it a priority to become acquainted with the beliefs and practices of the various cultures in the community. In the birthing situation, the nurse supports the family's cultural practices as long as it is safe to do so (eg, meets the standards to which the professional nurse is held).

CRITICAL THINKING QUESTION

What cultural beliefs do you bring to the birthing area? How have your beliefs been influenced by your family and friends? How might you establish the cultural expectations of the birth couple? To what extent should the birth couple request birth options?

Support of the Adolescent during Birth

Each adolescent in labor is different. The nurse must assess what each client brings to the experience by asking the following questions:

- Has the young woman received prenatal care?
- What are her attitudes and feelings about the pregnancy?
- How does her developmental stage influence her behavior, and how are her specific needs different?

CLINICAL TIP

It is best not to assume that women of any culture have the information that they desire regarding labor, birth, self-care, and newborn care, regardless of the number of children they have had. An important aspect of nursing is to teach, so always offer culturally sensitive information. Most nurses are not knowledgeable regarding all cultural practices. So be sensitive, and ask what is important to the mother. For example, ask if there is important clothing for the newborn to wear, or if she has some special ways that she wants the umbilical stump to be cared for. Always be aware that the information that you learned in class and from your text comes primarily from the nursing culture and the Western, chiefly European, culture. To believe that these two cultures have all the answers is an example of ethnocentrism. But remember, you have to start somewhere and then continue to build your information as your clinical practice base grows.

- Who will attend the birth, and what is the person's relationship to her?
- What preparation has she had for the experience?
- What are her expectations and fears regarding labor and birth?
- How has her culture influenced her?
- What are her usual coping mechanisms?
- Does she have adequate social support?
- Does she plan to keep the newborn? If so, does she need to learn parenting skills?

Any adolescent who has not had prenatal care requires close observation during labor. Adolescents are at highest risk for pregnancy and labor complications and must be assessed carefully. The status of the fetus is monitored to promote its well-being. The young woman's prenatal record is carefully reviewed for risks. The adolescent is more likely to have pregnancy-induced hypertension (PIH), cephalopelvic disproportion (CPD), anemia, drugs ingested during pregnancy, sexually transmitted infections, and size-date discrepancies (gestation appears to be less than dates indicate because of minimal weight gain).

The nurse's support role depends on the young woman's support system during labor. When the client is not accompanied by someone who will stay with her during childbirth, it is even more important for the nurse to establish a trusting relationship with her. In this way, the nurse can help her cope with labor and understand what is happening to her. Establishing rapport without recrimination will provide emotional support and encouragement. The adolescent who is given positive reinforcement for "work well done" will leave the experience with increased self-esteem, despite the emotional stress and difficulty of giving birth at so young an age.

The nurse can explain changes in the young woman's behavior that occur during labor and substantiate her wishes. By gentle caring, the nursing staff should reinforce the adolescent's feelings that she is important.

The adolescent who has taken childbirth education classes is generally better prepared than the adolescent who has had no preparation. The nurse must keep in mind, however, that the younger the adolescent, the less she may be able to participate actively in the process.

The very young adolescent (under age 14) has fewer coping mechanisms and less experience to draw on than her older counterparts have. Because her cognitive development is incomplete, the younger adolescent may have fewer problem-solving capabilities. Her ego integrity may be more threatened by the experience, and she may be more vulnerable to stress and discomfort.

The very young woman needs someone to rely on at all times during labor. She may be more childlike and dependent than older teens. The nurse must be sure that instructions and explanations are simple and concrete. During the transition phase, the young teenager may become withdrawn and unable to express her need to be nurtured. Touch, soothing encouragement, and measures to maintain her comfort help her maintain control and meet her needs for dependence. During the second stage of labor, the young adolescent may feel as if she is losing control and may reach out to those around her. By remaining calm and giving directions, the nurse helps her control feelings of helplessness.

One of the most memorable expectant mothers I cared for during my nursing course was a 13-year-old. I met her each week as she came into the OB clinic at our hospital and stayed with her as she waited for her appointment and was then seen by the med student. I noticed that with each passing visit, she became more and more anxious. I did my best to determine the source of her anxiety, provided general teaching and information for all of her questions. I consulted with my professor, and she sat in with me during some visits. But the teenager became more and more anxious. Near term, she began asking if she could just have the baby cut out. Whatever was she afraid of? Finally, in the 38th week, after $2^1/_2$ months of building trust, she told me she was afraid because her baby had gotten too big, and it would never be able to come out through her belly button. I was speechless for a moment. For $2^1/_2$ months, I had answered questions and felt so proud of my support and teaching, and for all this time, she had not been able to ask the most important question of all—the question that paralyzed her with fear. I was finally able to provide specific information, made drawings on a paper towel, had the medical student talk with her, and best of all, was able to be on call and be with her in labor and during birth. The beautiful smile on her face as her baby was born was unbelievable. She wasn't afraid! It's been 39 years since then, and I still remember her name. I think about her and wish her and her beautiful baby girl loving thoughts.

The middle adolescent (age 14 to 16 years) often attempts to remain calm and unflinching during labor. If unable to break through the teenager's stoic barrier, the nurse needs to rise above frustration and realize that a caring attitude will still positively affect the young woman.

Many older adolescents feel that they "know it all," but they may be no more prepared for childbirth than their younger counterparts. The nurse's reinforcement and nonjudgmental manner will help them save face. If the adolescent has not taken classes, she may require preparation and explanations. The older teenager's response to the stresses of labor, however, is similar to that of the adult woman.

Consideration of the adolescent father and mother as parents is a very important aspect of labor and birthing care. As one student nurse wrote of her labor experience with teen parents, "The father probably never expected to wind up on a maternity ward at a time in his life when he should have been picking out a prom tuxedo" (Mills, 1997, p 72). Nurses need to be aware that this is a stressful time for the couple. There are some specific interventions that increase comfort, enhance education, and perhaps decrease stress. The teen father may need encouragement to provide supportive care and to know what actions are acceptable in the birthing area. He may be encouraged to hold the mother's hand, to sit or lie on the bed beside her, to give a back massage, or to stroke her forehead. He may need assistance in how to give a shoulder rub or back rub; he can watch the nurse first and then perform the action himself with the encouragement of the nurse. He may need more encouragement than the older father to share a Jacuzzi or shower or to support the mother in changing positions and ambulating. It is important for the nurse to speak in lay terms and to anticipate questions, to answer all vocalized questions honestly, and to provide opportunities for the parents to ask for further information. In the early part of labor, the nurse can talk with the parents about their expectations for parenting their newborn and what resources are available in the community. It is particularly helpful if the nurse has visited the various community facilities or groups and can tell them the name of a specific person to contact and perhaps to give the parents brochures at this time (Mills, 1997). The attitude of the nurse is important in establishing rapport and gaining trust of this couple with very special needs.

Even if the adolescent is planning to relinquish her newborn, she should be given the option of seeing and holding the infant. She may be reluctant to do this at first, but seeing the infant can facilitate the grieving process. However, seeing or holding the newborn should be the young woman's choice. (See Chapter 30 for further discussion of the relinquishing mother and the adolescent parent.)

Promotion of Comfort in the First Stage

During the first stage of labor, the nurse plans ways to help the woman cope with the intensity and discomfort or pain of labor contractions. Women suffer discomfort from uncomfortable position, lack of position change, diaphoresis, continual leaking of amniotic fluid, a full bladder, a dry mouth, anxiety, and fear. Nursing interventions can minimize the effects of these factors. These interventions are described later in this section.

There are many types of responses to pain, including tension and mental anguish. The most frequent physiologic manifestations are increased pulse and respiratory rates, dilated pupils, increased blood pressure, and muscle tension. In labor, these reactions are transitory because the pain is intermittent. Increased muscle tension is most significant because it may impede the progress of labor. Women in labor frequently tighten skeletal muscles voluntarily during a contraction, remain motionless, and tend to hold their breath. As the intensity of the contraction increases with the progress of labor, the woman is less aware of the environment and may have difficulty hearing verbal instructions. The pattern of coping with labor contractions varies from the use of structured breathing techniques to grimacing, moaning, and loud vocalizations. Sounds are an important part of the labor and birthing process. Some women naturally make sounds and feel that it helps them cope and do the work of labor; they are responding to what their body tells them to do. Others begin to make loud sounds (screams) only as they lose their ability to cope and feel they do not have any other options. The labor is more than they feel they can take.

CRITICAL THINKING QUESTION

When you are in the birthing area, watch how the nurses, physicians, and CNMs respond to laboring women's sounds. Do they appear to take it in stride as a part of labor? Do some appear distressed and feel the need to do something? How many of the labor room doors get shut once the woman becomes vocal? How do you feel when you hear the sounds? What does it make you want to do? How would you explain the sounds to a newly admitted primigravida laboring in an adjacent room?

Some women may want physical contact during contractions (Figure 20–2). They may provide verbal and nonverbal signs, such as crying, moaning, and beseeching the coach or nurse to hold their hand or rub their back. They may look at the support person or reach out for help to indicate their anxiety. A woman generally wants touching and physical contact at times during the first part of labor, but when she moves into the transition phase, she rebuffs all efforts and pulls away. However, some women do not want to be touched at all, regardless of the phase of labor.

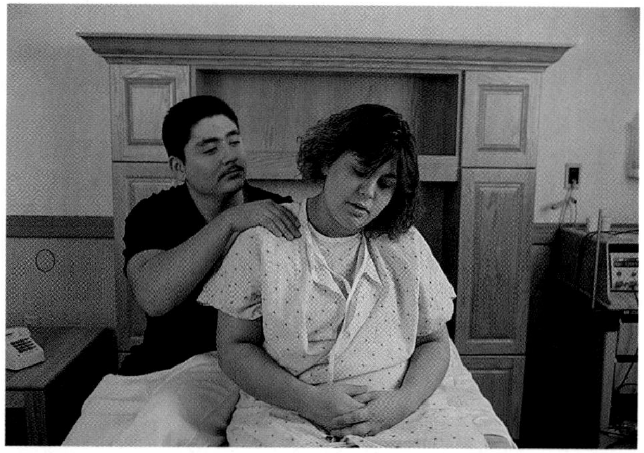

FIGURE 20–2 The woman's partner provides support and encouragement during labor.

Many nurses like to incorporate touch into their nursing care, and they readily respond to the women's cues. Others may be more hesitant, perhaps because of previous experience with being rebuffed or their own personal values regarding touch. Weaver (1990) notes that some labor and birthing nurses avoid the use of touch when caring for another nurse's client or when the woman has a communicable disease or poor hygiene.

A decrease in the intensity of discomfort is one of the goals of nursing support during labor. Nursing measures to decrease pain include the following:

- Using comfort measures
- Decreasing anxiety
- Providing information
- Using specific supportive relaxation techniques
- Encouraging paced breathing
- Administering pharmacologic agents as desired by the woman

Comfort Measures

The woman is encouraged to ambulate if it is not contraindicated. If she stays in bed, she is encouraged to assume any position that she finds comfortable. A side-lying position is generally the most advantageous for the laboring woman, although frequent position changes (at least every hour) seem to achieve more efficient contractions. Care should be taken that all body parts are supported, with the joints slightly flexed. For instance, when the woman is in a side-lying position, pillows may be placed against her chest and under the uppermost arm. A pillow or folded bath blanket is placed between her knees to support the uppermost leg and relieve tension or muscle strain. A pillow (or warmed rolled blanket) placed at the woman's midback also helps provide support. If the woman is more comfortable on her back, the head of the bed should be elevated to relieve the pressure of the uterus on the vena cava. Pillows may be placed under each arm and under the knees to provide support. Because a pregnant woman is at increased risk for thrombophlebitis, excessive pressure behind the knee and calf should be avoided, and frequent assessment of pressure points needs to be made. Back rubs and frequent changes of position contribute to comfort and relaxation. It is also helpful for the woman to ambulate, sit up in a rocking chair, or other comfortable chair or in the shower.

Diaphoresis and the constant leaking of amniotic fluid can dampen the woman's gown and bed linen. Fresh, smooth, dry bed linen promotes comfort. To avoid having to change the bottom sheet following rupture of the membranes, the nurse may replace the underpads at frequent intervals (body substance isolation [BSI] precautions need to be followed). The perineal area should be kept as clean and dry as possible to promote comfort. A full bladder adds to the discomfort during a contraction and may prolong labor by interfering with the descent of the fetus. The bladder should be kept as empty as possible. Even though the woman is voiding, urine may be retained because of the pressure of the fetal presenting part. A full bladder can be detected by palpation directly over the symphysis pubis. Some of the procedures for regional analgesia during labor contribute to the inability to void, and catheterization may be necessary. The woman should be encouraged to empty her bladder about every 1 to 2 hours.

The woman may experience dryness of her mouth. Clear fluids and ice chips are usually offered unless a complication exists that makes cesarean birth a possibility. Popsicles, ice chips, and clear fluids will relieve the discomfort. Some prepared childbirth programs advise the woman to bring lollipops to help combat the dryness that occurs with some of the breathing patterns.

Some women feel discomfort from cold feet. Wearing socks or slippers may increase their comfort. Some women may wish to wear their own nightgown, although they need to know that the gown will most likely be soiled and may be more difficult to move around in than a hospital gown.

Some family members or support persons can assist the woman with comfort measures. They may help with position changes, provide ice chips, walk with the laboring woman, and give effleurage or back rubs. If the family is not already involved in providing comfort measures and seems to want to be, the nurse can act as a role model while providing comfort measures and then invite the support person(s) to join in if they like.

Touch may be used to convey support and enhance comfort for the woman. She may be soothed by a neck or back rub, by holding her partner's or the nurse's hand, by the use of Therapeutic Touch or Healing Touch techniques to enhance relaxation and decrease discomfort from muscle tension. The use of acupressure to maintain balance and harmony of the woman's body may also be employed by nurses who have completed additional study of this therapy (Cook & Wilcox, 1997).

Birth balls are large, heavy plastic balls that accommodate an adult's weight; they are being used by some laboring women to increase comfort. The woman sits on the ball and can roll it back and forth gently. The slow rock is thought to widen the pelvis and enhance fetal descent, while leaning forward on the knees with the head, arms, and chest over the ball simulates a hands-and-knees position and may facilitate rotation of an occiput-posterior. When a birth ball is used, the nurse should remain close by the woman to help provide balance (McCartney, 1998).

Family members also need to be encouraged to maintain their own comfort. As their attention is directed toward the laboring woman, they may forget their own needs. The nurse may have to encourage them to take breaks, maintain food and fluid intake, and rest.

Handling Anxiety

The anxiety experienced by women entering labor is related to a combination of factors inherent to the process. A moderate amount of anxiety about the pain enhances the ability to deal with the pain. But an excessive degree of anxiety decreases the woman's ability to cope with the pain.

To decrease anxiety that is not related to pain, the nurse can give information (which eases fear of the unknown), establish rapport with the couple (which helps them preserve their personal integrity), express confidence in the couple's ability to work with the labor process, and assist with breathing and relaxation techniques. In addition to being a good listener, the nurse must have and demonstrate genuine concern for the laboring woman. Remaining with the woman as much as possible conveys a caring attitude and dispels fear of abandonment. Praise for correct breathing, relaxation efforts, and pushing efforts not only encourages repetition of the behavior but also decreases anxiety about the ability to cope with labor.

Teaching for Self-Care: Providing Information

Providing information about the nature of the discomfort that will occur during labor is important and is best achieved in the early portion of labor. Stressing the intermittent nature and maximum duration of the contractions can be most helpful. The woman can cope with pain better when she knows how far she has progressed and that a period of relief will follow. Describing the type of discomfort and specific sensations that will occur as labor progresses helps the woman recognize these sensations as normal and expected when she does experience them.

During the second stage the woman may interpret rectal pressure as a need to move her bowels. The instinctive response is to tighten muscles rather than bear down (push). The woman may be frightened by a "splitting apart" sensation or an intense "ring of fire" feeling that prevents bearing down with contractions. The woman who expects these sensations and understands that bearing down contributes to progress at this stage is more likely to do so.

> *When I tried to push with the contractions, I felt as if I would tear apart. It hurt so bad that I was shaking. I knew it was time to push and my body was telling me, too, but it hurt so bad. The nurse kept saying, "Just push and you will feel better." I wanted to scream at her. She had no idea what was happening to me.*

The nurse should accompany descriptions of sensations with information on specific comfort measures. Some women experience the urge to push during transition, when the cervix is not fully dilated and effaced. Usually, this sensation can be managed with patterned-paced breathing. The woman will need ongoing support and encouragement from her partner and nurse.

A thorough explanation of surroundings, procedures, and equipment being used also decreases anxiety, thereby reducing pain. Attachment to an electronic monitor can produce fear because equipment of this type is associated with critically ill people. For others, hearing their infant's heartbeat is reassuring. The nurse should explain the monitor and the monitor strip. The nurse can emphasize that the monitor provides information to assess the well-being of the fetus during the course of labor. In addition, the nurse can show the woman and her coach how the monitor can help them use controlled breathing techniques to relieve pain. The monitor may indicate the beginning of a contraction just seconds before the woman feels it. The woman and coach can learn how to read the tracing to identify the beginning of the contraction.

Labor and childbirth may be a critical time for triggering memories of childhood sexual abuse. The literature does not agree on the prevalence of sexual abuse; however, feminist studies note that the incidence is one in three adolescents and women. Although sexual abuse and its incidence remains a topic that the public continues to struggle with, nurses, especially those in the childbirthing area, must become knowledgeable and comfortable in developing assessment and intervention strategies. During the admission process, the nurse can make such statements as, "I am aware that sexual abuse is very common in our society. In working with laboring women, I've learned that some of the experiences of childbirth may trigger uncomfortable feelings. So I ask each woman if there is anything that she recalls about abuse or if there is anything that she would like to ask about. Is there anything you would like to talk about?" (Waymire, 1997). Women may or may not be able to address known abuse with the nurse, because revealing this personal information to a stranger is difficult. The nurse may note that the woman becomes more anxious; unrelenting pain and exposure during vaginal examinations or any other activity may suddenly trigger a memory. She can feel, smell, and sense touch and pain that occurred with that event. She may be totally unaware of the fact that she was sexually abused, so the memory is terrifying in itself. The remembered event is as real as if it were happening at that very moment.

Key interventions that may be helpful include the following (Waymire, 1997):

- *Set the stage.* Ask each adolescent and woman about sexual abuse. Assure them that it is more common in our society than they may be aware of and that events during childbirth may trigger memories.
- *Give the woman control.* As with all women, explain each procedure before it is done and explain why it is needed. In particular, ask for her permission, and wait for permission to be given before proceeding.
- *Give permission to stop.* Tell the woman that it is OK for her to say "Stop!" at any time. She may ask questions about what is happening, even if she does not understand what is happening to her, or may have difficulty describing her feelings or sensations.
- *Affirm her body's abilities.* Assure her that during the labor and birth process, her body is working for her and her baby and that the pain and sensations she feels are "good" in that they are necessary and will bring her baby to her.

Supportive Relaxation Techniques

Tense muscles increase resistance to the descent of the fetus and contribute to maternal fatigue. This fatigue increases pain perception and decreases the woman's ability to cope with the pain. Comfort measures, massage, techniques for decreasing anxiety, and client teaching can conserve energy. The laboring woman needs to be encouraged to use the periods between contractions for rest and to relax her muscles.

Distraction is another method of increasing relaxation and coping with discomfort. During early labor, conversation or activities such as light reading, cards, or other games serve as distractions. One technique that is effective for relieving moderate pain is to have the woman concentrate on a pleasant experience she has had in the past.

Touch is another type of distraction. Although some women regard touching as an invasion of privacy or threat to their independence, others want to touch and be touched during a painful experience. Nurses can make themselves available to the woman who desires touch. The nurse can place a hand on the side of the bed within the woman's reach. The person who needs touch will reach out for contact, and the nurse can pick up and follow through with this behavioral cue.

Visualization techniques enhance relaxation. For example, the nurse might encourage the woman to imagine herself floating in a warm pool of water, fully supported; to imagine the birth canal slowly opening up as the baby descends; or to visualize a rose opening its petals. Table 20–3 describes a simple visualization method.

TABLE 20–3 Simple Visualization Method

Direct a visualization by saying something like the following: "Think about a place you have been that has pleasant memories and feelings around it. A place that was relaxing, where all your stress disappeared. As you think about this place, take in a breath and remember the smells around it. If it was outside, feel the warmth of the sun or the way the breeze felt on your face. Sit in the place again in your mind. Let all your tension and tiredness leave your body as you feel the warmth and breezes."
Give the woman a few moments to think about her special place. Ask if she would like to share information about the setting. If the woman chooses to do this, add the information to help her with the visualization (for example, "Think about the mountain cabin and the warmth of the sun on your face as you sit in the rocking chair on the front porch.").
After the woman has a visualization set up, suggest thinking about it during contractions as a means of increasing relaxation and focusing concentration. You could say, "As each contraction begins, think about this special place for a moment, and let your body relax. Keep a picture of your place in your mind as you breathe with the contraction. When the contraction is over, let your body stay relaxed. Feel the comfort of this room and support of those around you."

Mild to moderate abdominal discomfort during contractions may be relieved or lessened by effleurage. Back pain associated with labor may be relieved more effectively by firm pressure on the lower back or sacral area. To apply firm pressure, the nurse places her hand or a rolled, warmed towel or blanket in the small of the woman's back.

In addition to these measures, the nurse can enhance the woman's relaxation by providing encouragement and support for her controlled breathing techniques.

Patterned-Paced Breathing

Patterned-paced breathing may help the laboring woman. Used correctly, patterned-paced breathing increases the woman's pain threshold, encourages relaxation, enhances the ability to cope with uterine contractions, and allows the uterus to function more efficiently.

Many women learn Lamaze breathing during prenatal education classes. This type of patterned-paced breathing has three levels. The woman tends to begin with the first level and then proceed to the next when she feels the need. Regardless of the level of breathing used, a cleansing breath begins and ends each pattern. A cleansing breath involves only the chest. It consists of inhaling through the nose and exhaling through pursed lips (as if blowing on a spoonful of hot food). See Table 20–4 for information regarding patterned-paced breathing.

Women usually practice the breathing for a number of weeks before birth. If the woman has not learned a patterned-paced breathing method, teaching her may be difficult when she is admitted in active labor. In this instance, the nurse can teach abdominal and pant-pant-blow breathing. In abdominal breathing, the woman moves the abdominal wall upward as she inhales and downward as she exhales (Table 20–4). This method tends to lift the abdominal wall off the contracting uterus and thus may provide some pain relief. The breathing is deep and rhythmic. As transition approaches, the woman may feel the need to breathe more rapidly. To avoid breathing too rapidly, which may occur with deep abdominal breathing, the woman can use the pant-pant-blow breathing pattern.

As the woman uses her breathing technique, the nurse can assess and support the interaction between the woman and her coach or support person. In the absence of a coach, the nurse supports the laboring woman by helping to identify the beginning of each contraction and encouraging her as she breathes through it. Continued encouragement and support with each contraction through labor yield immeasurable benefits.

Hyperventilation may occur when a woman breathes very rapidly over a prolonged period of time. Hyperventilation is the result of an imbalance of oxygen and carbon dioxide (that is, too much carbon dioxide is exhaled, and too much oxygen remains in the body). The signs and symptoms of hyperventilation are tingling or numbness in the tip of nose, lips, fingers, or toes; dizziness; spots before the eyes; or spasms of the hands or feet (carpal-pedal spasms). If hyperventilation occurs, the woman should be encouraged to slow her breathing rate and to take shallow breaths. With instruction and encouragement, many women are able to change their breathing to correct the problem. Encouraging the woman to relax and counting out loud for her so she can pace her breathing during contractions are also helpful. If the signs and symptoms continue or become more severe (that is, if they progress from numbness to spasms), the woman can breathe into a paper surgical mask or into her hands until symptoms abate. Breathing into a mask or her hands causes rebreathing of carbon dioxide. The nurse should remain with the woman to reassure her.

In some instances, analgesic agents or regional anesthetic blocks may be used to enhance comfort and relaxation during labor. See Chapter 21 for a discussion of analgesia and anesthesia. Table 20–5 summarizes labor progress, possible responses of the laboring woman, and support measures.

Provision of Care in the First Stage of Labor

After the admission process is completed, the nurse helps the laboring woman and her partner become comfortable with the surroundings. The nurse assesses the couple's individual needs and plans for this experience. As long as there are no contraindications (such as vaginal bleeding or rupture of membranes [ROM] with the fetus unengaged), the woman may be encouraged to ambulate, because upright positions shorten labor. Many women feel much more at ease and comfortable if they can move around and do not have to remain in bed.

The nurse needs to evaluate physical parameters of the woman and her fetus. Maternal temperature is monitored every 4 hours unless the temperature is over 37.5C (99.6F); in such cases, it must be taken every hour. Blood pressure, pulse, and respirations are monitored every hour. If the woman's blood pressure is over 140/90 mm Hg or her pulse is more than 100, the CNM/physician must be notified. The blood pressure and pulse are then

TABLE 20–4 Nursing Support of Patterned-Paced Breathing

Determine which breathing method the woman (couple) has learned. Provide encouragement as needed in maintaining breathing pattern. Provide support to the labor coach and assist as needed.

Lamaze Breathing Pattern Levels

First level (slow paced)

Pattern begins and ends with a cleansing breath (in through the nose and out through pursed lips as if cooling a spoonful of hot food). While inhaling through the nose and exhaling through pursed lips, slow breaths are taken, moving only the chest. The rate should be approximately 6–9/minute or 2 breaths/15 seconds. The coach or nurse may assist by reminding the woman to take a cleansing breath, and then the breaths could be counted out if needed to maintain pacing. The woman inhales as someone counts "one one thousand, two one thousand, three one thousand, four one thousand." Exhalation begins and continues through the same count.

First level for use during uterine contractions (The level begins and ends with a cleansing breath [CB].)

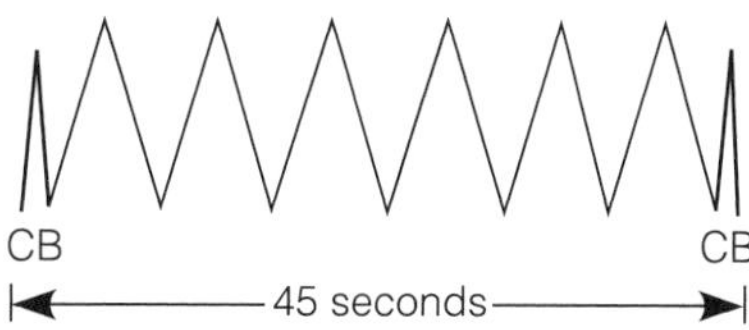

Second level (modified paced)

Pattern begins and ends with a cleansing breath. Breaths are then taken in and out silently through the mouth at approximately 4 breaths/5 seconds. The jaw and entire body need to be relaxed. The rate can be accelerated to 2–2 $\frac{1}{2}$ breaths/second. The rhythm for the breaths can be counted out as "one and two and one and two and..." with the woman exhaling on the numbers and inhaling on "and."

Second level

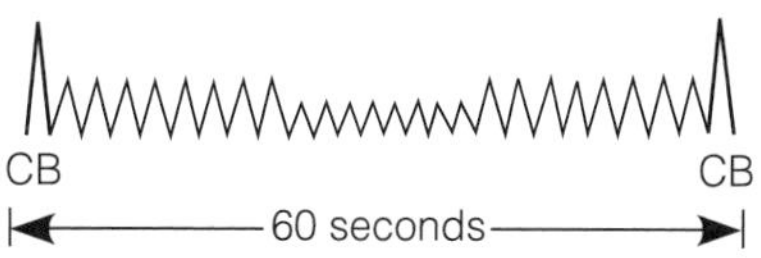

Third level (pattern paced)

Pattern begins and ends with a cleansing breath. All breaths are rhythmical, in and out through the mouth. Exhalations are accompanied by a "hee" or "hoo" sound in a varying pattern, 2:1, which begins as 3:1 (hee hee hee hoo) and can change to 2:1 (hee hee hoo) or 1:1 (hee hoo) as the intensity of the contraction changes. The rate should not be more rapid than 2–2 $\frac{1}{2}$ breaths/second. The rhythm of the breaths would match a "one and two and ..." count.

Third level (Darkened spike represents "hoo.")

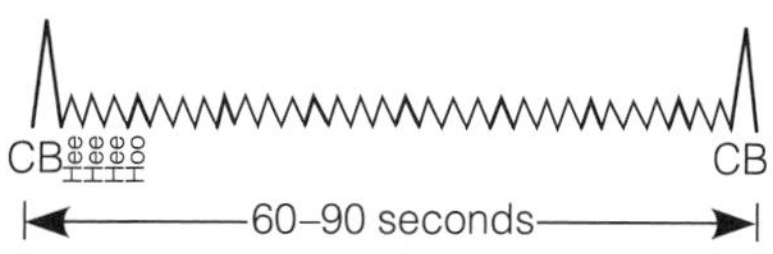

Abdominal Breathing Pattern Cues

The abdomen moves outward during inhalation and downward during exhalation. The rate remains slow with approximately 6–9 breaths/minute.

Breathing sequence for abdominal breathing

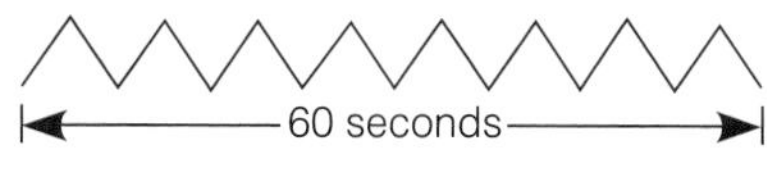

Quick Method

When the woman has not learned a particular method and is in active phase of labor, the nurse may teach her a combination of two patterns. Abdominal breathing may be used until labor is more advanced. Then a more rapid pattern consisting of two short blows from the mouth followed by a longer blow can be used. (This pattern is called "pant-pant-blow" even though all exhalations are a blowing motion.)

Pant-pant-blow breathing pattern

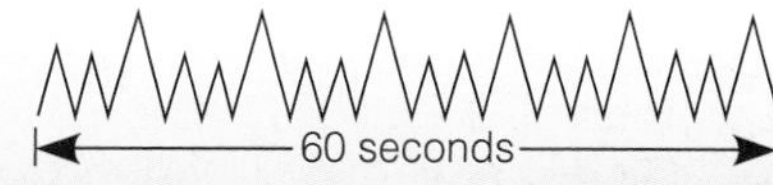

reevaluated more frequently. Uterine contractions are palpated for frequency, intensity, and duration. The FHR is auscultated every 60 minutes for low-risk women and every 30 minutes for high-risk women as long as it remains between 120 and 160 bpm and is reassuring. The FHR should be auscultated throughout one contraction and for about 15 seconds after the contraction to ensure that there are no decelerations. If the FHR is not in the 120 to 160 range and/or decelerations are heard, continuous electronic monitoring is recommended. Table 20–6 summarizes nursing assessments in the first stage of labor.

The laboring woman may feel some discomfort during contractions. The nurse can assist by providing diversions or by repositioning her. The woman may begin to use her breathing method during contractions (see the preceding discussion of pain management).

If the laboring woman has not had childbirth education classes, the latent phase is a time when the nurse can give anticipatory guidance. Most women are not too uncomfortable with contractions at this time and are responsive to teaching about breathing and other techniques for coping with labor contractions. In fact, many women in the latent phase seek information about what to expect. The unprepared woman may hesitate to ask questions and thus can benefit even more from anticipatory guidance by the nurse. If the woman's membranes are intact, a tour of the birthing facility can help decrease anxiety and distract her from her discomfort.

TABLE 20–5 Normal Progress, Psychologic Characteristics, and Nursing Support during First and Second Stages of Labor

Phase	Cervical Dilatation	Uterine Contractions	Woman's Response	Support Measures
Stage 1				
Latent phase	1–4 cm	Every 10–20 minutes, 15–20 seconds' duration Mild intensity *progressing to* Every 5–7 minutes, 30–40 seconds' duration Moderate intensity	Usually happy, talkative, and eager to be in labor Exhibits need for independence by taking care of own bodily needs and seeking information	Establish rapport on admission and continue to build during care. Assess information base and learning needs. Be available to consult regarding breathing technique if needed; teach breathing technique if needed and in early labor. Orient family to room, equipment, monitors, and procedures. Encourage woman and partner to participate in care as desired. Provide needed information. Assist woman into position of comfort; encourage frequent change of position; encourage ambulation during early labor. Offer fluids/ice chips. Keep couple informed of progress. Encourage woman to void every 1 to 2 hours. Assess need for an interest in using visualization to enhance relaxation and teach if appropriate.
Active phase	4–7 cm	Every 2–3 minutes, 40–60 seconds' duration Moderate to strong intensity	May experience feelings of helplessness Exhibits increased fatigue and may begin to feel restless and anxious as contractions become stronger Expresses fear of abandonment Becomes more dependent as she is less able to meet her needs	Encourage woman to maintain breathing patterns. Provide quiet environment to reduce external stimuli. Provide reassurance, encouragement, support; keep couple informed of progress. Promote comfort by giving back rubs, sacral pressure, cool cloth on forehead, assistance with position changes, support with pillows, effleurage. Provide ice chips, ointment for dry mouth and lips. Encourage to void every 1 to 2 hours. Offer shower/whirlpool/warm bath if available.
Transition phase	8–10 cm	Every 2 minutes, 60–75 seconds' duration Strong intensity	Tires and may exhibit increased restlessness and irritability May feel she cannot keep up with labor process and is out of control Physical discomforts Fear of being left alone May fear tearing open or splitting apart with contractions	Encourage woman to rest between contractions. If she sleeps between contractions, wake her at beginning of contraction so she can begin breathing pattern (increases feeling of control). Provide support, encouragement, and praise for efforts. Keep couple informed of progress; encourage continued participation of support persons. Promote comfort as listed above but recognize many women do not want to be touched when in transition. Provide privacy. Provide ice chips, ointment for lips. Encourage to void every 1 to 2 hours.
Stage 2	Complete	Every 2 minutes	May feel out of control, helpless, panicky	Assist woman in pushing efforts. Encourage woman to assume position of comfort. Provide encouragement and praise for efforts. Keep couple informed of progress. Provide ice chips. Maintain privacy as woman desires.

TABLE 20–6 Nursing Assessments in the First Stage

Phase	Mother	Fetus
Latent	Blood pressure, respirations each hour if in normal range Temperature every 4 hours unless over 37.5C (99.6F) or membranes ruptured, then every hour Uterine contractions every 30 minutes	FHR every 60 minutes for low-risk women and every 30 minutes for high-risk women if normal characteristics present (average variability, baseline in the 120–160 bpm range, without late or variable decelerations) (NAACOG, 1990). Note fetal activity. If electronic fetal monitor in place, assess for reactive NST.
Active	Blood pressure, pulse, respirations every hour if in normal range Uterine contractions every 30 minutes	FHR every 30 minutes for low-risk women and every 15 minutes for high-risk women if normal characteristics are present (NAACOG, 1990).
Transition	Blood pressure, pulse, respirations every 30 minutes	FHR every 30 minutes for low-risk women and every 15 minutes for high-risk women if normal characteristics are present (NAACOG, 1990).

CLINICAL TIP

Catheterizing a woman during a contraction is uncomfortable for her and difficult to do because of the increased downward pressure. To avoid these problems, pass the catheter between contractions. If the baby's head is low in the pelvis, you will have to change the direction of the catheter. Visualize passing it up and over the baby's head rather than straight into the urethra.

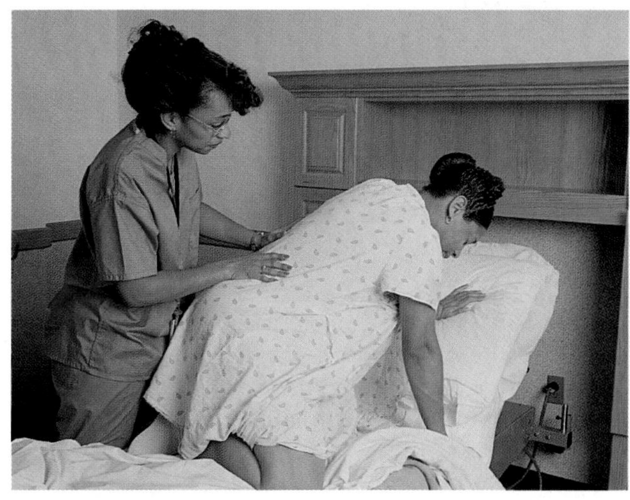

The nurse should offer fluids in the form of clear liquids or ice chips at frequent intervals. Because gastric emptying time is prolonged during labor, solid foods are usually avoided. However, fasting during labor is becoming a controversial practice. Some providers believe that eating and drinking in labor should be an option to women. Many nurse-midwifery practices are now encouraging mothers to eat and drink to toleration (Ludka & Roberts, 1993).

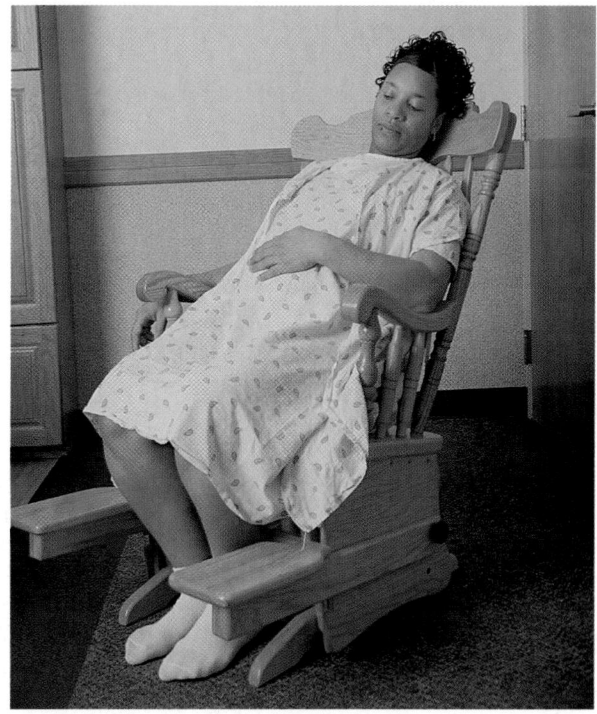

Active Phase

During the active phase, the contractions have a frequency of 2 to 3 minutes, a duration of 50 to 60 seconds, and moderate intensity. Contractions need to be palpated every 15 to 30 minutes. As the contractions become more frequent and intense, vaginal examinations are performed to assess cervical dilatation and effacement and fetal station and position. During the active phase, the cervix dilates from 4 to 7 cm, and vaginal discharge and bloody show increase. Maternal blood pressure, pulse, and respirations should be monitored every hour for low-risk women (unless elevated, as previously noted) and every 30 minutes for high-risk women. The FHR is auscultated and evaluated every 30 minutes for low-risk women and every 15 minutes for high-risk women (Nurses' Association of the American College of Obstetricians and Gynecologists [NAACOG], 1990).

A woman who has been ambulatory up to this point may now wish to sit in a chair or on a bed (Figure 20–3). If the woman wants to lie on the bed, she is encouraged to assume a side-lying position. The nurse can assist her to a position of comfort and may place pillows to support her body. To increase comfort, the nurse can give back rubs or effleurage or place a cool cloth on the woman's forehead or across her neck. The use of hydrotherapy during labor promotes maternal relaxation and pain management and decreases the length of labor. Thus women can be encouraged to use a warm bath or whirlpool (Jacuzzi) to increase comfort during labor.

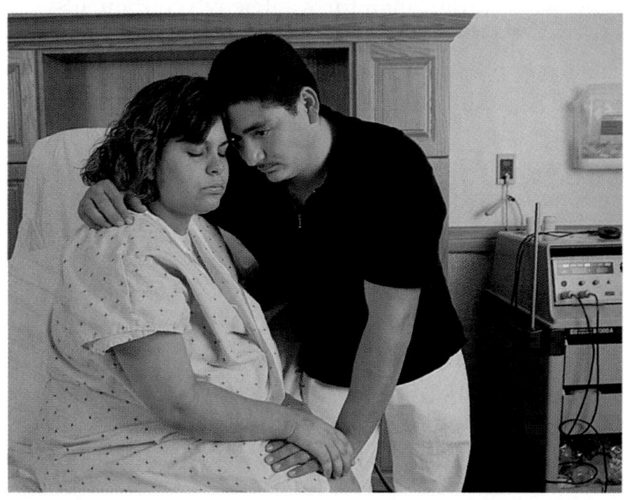

FIGURE 20–3 The laboring woman is encouraged to choose a position of comfort. The nurse modifies assessments and interventions as necessary.

CLINICAL TIP

If the monitor is no longer recording the fetal heart rate tracing, check that there is adequate gel under the transducer and reposition it before you assume that there is a problem with the baby.

Because vaginal discharge increases, the nurse needs to change the underpads frequently. Washing the perineum with warm soap and water removes secretions and increases comfort. The nurse needs to use body substance isolation measures to avoid exposure to vaginal secretions.

Pharmacologic support may be administered at this time if the woman has a well-established contraction pattern and she is not expected to give birth within the next 1 or 2 hours. If an analgesic is given, the woman must remain in bed to promote her safety. If no one can be at the bedside with her, the side rails should be up.

For the woman experiencing slow progress of labor or the inability to tolerate fluids, an intravenous electrolyte solution may be started to provide energy and prevent dehydration. If an IV is started, it becomes even more important to encourage voiding every 1 to 2 hours to prevent bladder distention.

If the amniotic membranes have not ruptured previously, they may do so during this phase. When the membranes rupture, the nurse notes the color and odor of the amniotic fluid and the time of rupture and immediately auscultates the FHR. The fluid should be clear with no odor. Meconium-stained amniotic fluid may be present when the fetus is in a breech presentation. In this case, meconium staining may not indicate any fetal stress. In a cephalic presentation, however, meconium staining may indicate fetal stress. Fetal stress relaxes the intestines and anal sphincter, leading to the release of meconium into the amniotic fluid. Meconium turns the fluid greenish-brown. Whenever the nurse notes meconium-stained fluid, an electronic monitor is applied to continuously assess the FHR. The time of rupture is noted because the incidence of amnionitis increases with rupture over 24 hours. An additional concern is prolapse of the umbilical cord, which occurs when membranes rupture and the fetus is not engaged. The concern is that the amniotic fluid coming through the cervix will propel the umbilical cord through the cervix (prolapsed cord). Prolapsed cord is assessed by monitoring for signs of fetal distress or performing a vaginal examination with a sterile glove. The FHR is auscultated because a drop in the rate might indicate an undetected prolapsed cord. Immediate intervention is necessary to remove pressure on a prolapsed umbilical cord until a cesarean birth can be performed (Chapter 22). See Table 20–7 for additional deviations from normal.

TABLE 20–7 Deviations from Normal Labor Process Requiring Immediate Intervention

Problem	Immediate Action
Woman admitted with vaginal bleeding or history of painless vaginal bleeding	Do not perform vaginal examination. Assess FHR. Evaluate amount of blood loss. Evaluate labor pattern. Notify physician/CNM immediately.
Presence of greenish or brownish amniotic fluid	Continuously monitor FHR. Evaluate dilatation of cervix and determine if umbilical cord is prolapsed. Evaluate presentation (vertex or breech). Maintain woman on complete bed rest on left side. Notify physician/CNM immediately.
Absence of FHR and fetal movement	Notify physician/CNM. Provide truthful information and emotional support to laboring couple. Remain with the couple.
Prolapse of umbilical cord	Relieve pressure on cord manually. Continuously monitor FHR; watch for changes in FHR pattern. Notify physician/CNM. Assist woman into knee-chest position. Administer oxygen.
Woman admitted in advanced labor; birth imminent	Prepare for immediate birth. Obtain critical information: Estimated date of birth (EDB) History of bleeding problems History of medical or obstetric problems Past and/or present use/abuse of prescription/OTC/illicit drugs Problems with this pregnancy FHR and maternal vital signs Whether membranes are ruptured and how long since rupture Blood type and Rh Direct another person to contact physician/CNM. Do not leave woman alone. Provide support to couple. Put on gloves.

Transition

During transition, the contraction frequency is every 2 to 3 minutes, duration is 60 to 90 seconds, and intensity is strong. Cervical dilatation increases from 8 to 10 cm, effacement is complete (100%), and a heavy amount of bloody show is usually present. Contractions are palpated at least every 15 minutes. Sterile vaginal examinations are done more frequently because this stage of labor usually is accompanied by rapid change. Maternal blood pressure, pulse, and respirations are taken at least every 30 minutes, and FHR is auscultated every 15 minutes.

Comfort measures become very important in this phase of labor, but continual assessment is required to intervene appropriately. The woman may rapidly change from wanting a back rub and other "hands-on" care to wanting to be left completely alone. The support person and the nurse need to follow her cues and change interventions as needed. Because the woman is breathing more rapidly, the nurse can offer small spoons of ice chips to moisten her mouth or apply A and D ointment to dry lips. The nurse can encourage the woman to rest between

TABLE 20–8 Nursing Assessments in the Second Stage

Mother	Fetus
Blood pressure, pulse, respirations every 5–15 minutes. Uterine contraction palpated continuously.	FHR every 15 minutes for low-risk women and every 5 minutes for high-risk women (NAACOG, 1990).

contractions. If analgesics have been administered, a quiet environment enhances the quality of rest between contractions. The nurse can awaken the woman just before another contraction starts so that she can begin patterned-paced breathing.

Some women have difficulty coping with the intensity of labor during this time and need help with their breathing. Either the support person or the nurse can breathe along with the woman during each contraction to help her maintain her pattern. It is helpful to encourage her and assure her that she is doing a good job. The woman will begin to feel increased rectal pressure as the fetal presenting part moves down the birth canal and sometimes a burning sensation as the tissues become stretched. The nurse encourages the woman to refrain from pushing until the cervix is completely dilated. This measure helps prevent cervical edema.

The end of transition and beginning of the second stage may be indicated by involuntary passage of flatus and the movement of the fetus from the side of the maternal abdomen to the midline. Other indications include a change in the woman's voice or the sounds she is making. As the fetus moves down and she feels increased pressure and a bearing-down sensation, her voice tends to deepen. A moan during a contraction takes on a more guttural quality. Expert nurses recognize this sound as a sign of changes in the woman.

Nursing Care Management during the Second Stage of Labor

Provision of Care in the Second Stage

The second stage begins when the cervix is completely dilated (10 cm). The uterine contractions continue as in the transition phase. Sterile vaginal examinations are done frequently to assess progress. Maternal pulse, blood pressure, and FHR are assessed every 5 to 15 minutes; some protocols recommend assessment after each contraction. Table 20–8 summarizes nursing assessments in the second stage of labor. As the woman pushes during the second stage she may make a variety of sounds. A low-pitched, grunting sound ("uhhh") usually indicates the woman is working with the pushing (McKay & Roberts, 1990). If she begins to feel she is going to lose control,

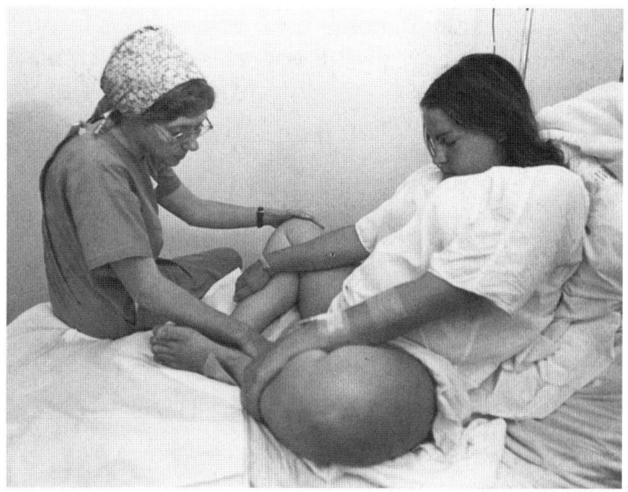

FIGURE 20–4 The nurse provides encouragement and support during pushing efforts.

her sound may change to a high-pitched cry or whimper, or she may even cry out in pain.

Nursing responses to the woman may vary. At times, the sounds are disturbing for nurses and physicians, and they feel the need to help or encourage her to be more quiet. Other nurses feel more comfortable with maternal sounds and use them as cues. The nurse provides support during the woman's pushing effort and stays sensitive to changes in the sounds for clues that the woman needs help coping with her pain. The nurse may encourage her to push harder and not let any breath out or to put all her effort into the push and not into making noise. Nurses and physicians seem to value staying in control, and for some, a childbearing woman's loss of control is a source of embarrassment (McKay & Roberts, 1990).

When the woman feels an uncontrollable urge to push (bear down), the nurse can help by encouraging her and by assisting with positioning (Figure 20–4). The woman can be propped up with pillows to a semireclining position. Other positions might include side-lying, squatting, or hands-and-knees.

When the contraction begins, the nurse tells the woman to take two short breaths, then to take a third breath and hold it while pulling back on her knees and pushing down with her abdominal muscles. Some women prefer to exhale slightly (exhale breathing) while pushing to avoid the physiologic effects of the Valsalva maneuver. With this method the woman takes several deep breaths and then holds her breath for 5 to 6 seconds. Then, through slightly pursed lips, she exhales slowly every 5 to 6 seconds while continuing to hold her breath. The woman takes another breath and continues exhale breathing and pushing during the contraction.

I knew when I was completely dilated. I knew when to push and I did it without tearing. My body told me to listen. I knew what to do.
~ HARRIETTE HARTIGAN, *WOMEN IN BIRTH* ~

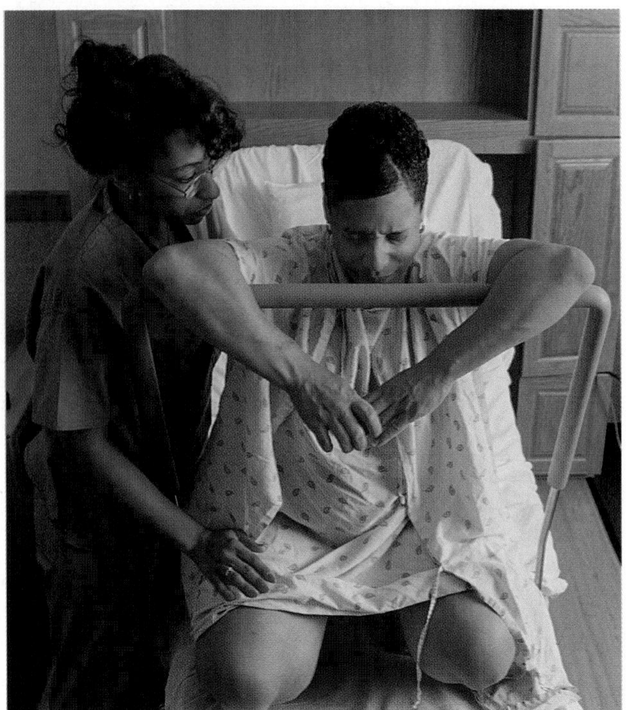

FIGURE 20–5 Using a birthing bar.

The woman is encouraged to rest between contractions. Although the laboring woman may appear exhausted at this time, most experience relief at being able to push with contractions. Perspiration increases with the pushing efforts, and a cold washcloth for forehead and face is most soothing. The birthing woman may also appreciate sips of fluid or ice chips at this time.

When I began pushing, I felt in control because I could do something . . . . I could push the baby out. I knew he was ready to be born.
~ HARRIETTE HARTIGAN, *WOMEN IN BIRTH* ~

Maternal positions, such as standing, squatting while leaning back on a partner or on a birthing bar (Figure 20–5), lying in a lateral or Sims' position, or crouching on hands and knees, may increase comfort and effectiveness of pushing. Some women feel that sitting on a toilet seat is a comfortable position that assists their pushing efforts. This position may cause anxiety in the caregivers, however, for fear that the birth may occur quickly in this most inopportune place.

CRITICAL THINKING QUESTION

What factors might influence a woman's choice of birthing position? What strategies might you use to help the woman try other positions?

Additional comfort measures may be used during this stage. Warm perineal, abdominal, and back compresses may be used to increase muscle relaxation. Perineal massage and stretching with a lubricant (Lubafax) may relieve the tearing and burning sensation as the perineal tissue distends. (At this time, perineal stretching is only done by a CNM and not by other nursing staff.)

Visualization techniques may be helpful. The woman can be encouraged to envision the infant descending the birth canal and the vagina opening up. Phrases such as "Open to your baby" and "Let the baby come; don't try to hold back" can be useful and calming.

If anticipated progress is not made or the laboring woman wants to try other positions for pushing, it is important for the nurse to support her. Some nurses have their own preferences and may be more comfortable with directing the laboring woman to the nurse's preferences. However, it is important to remember who the nurse is there for and that frequent changes in position may assist in the descent of the baby.

Throughout the second stage, it remains important to continue to provide information regarding progress and what is happening in the labor. It is also imperative to address the woman's questions honestly, to acknowledge her concerns, and to continue to provide support.

A nullipara is usually prepared for birth when the perineum begins to bulge. A multipara usually progresses much more quickly, so she may be prepared for the birth when the cervix is dilated 7 to 8 cm.

The woman's blood pressure and the FHR are monitored between contractions, and the contractions are palpated until the birth. The nurse continues to assist the woman in her pushing efforts. Both the woman and the coach are kept informed of procedures and of progress, and both are supported throughout the birth.

In addition to assisting the woman and her partner, the nurse assists the physician or certified nurse-midwife in preparing for the birth. The physician/CNM usually dons a sterile gown and gloves and places sterile drapes over the woman's abdomen and legs. An episiotomy may be done just before birth if there is a need for one. See the discussion of episiotomy in Chapter 23.

Promotion of Comfort in the Second Stage

Most of the comfort measures that have been used during the first stage remain appropriate at this time. Cool cloths to the face and forehead may help provide cooling as the woman is involved in the intense physical exertion of pushing. If she has been diaphoretic, a dry gown may be comforting. The woman may feel hot and want to remove some of the covering. Care still needs to be taken to provide privacy even though covers are removed. The woman can be encouraged to rest and "let all muscles go" during the period between contractions. The nurse and support person(s) can assist the woman into a pushing position with each contraction to further conserve energy. Sips of fluid or ice chips may be used to provide moisture and relieve dryness of the mouth.

ESSENTIAL PRECAUTIONS IN PRACTICE

During Birth

- The labor nurse who continues to provide support for the woman dons disposable gloves and adds further protection by wearing goggles or her own glasses.
- The physician/CNM wears sterile gloves, a protective gown with a splash apron, or a protective plastic apron, glasses or goggles. The nurse also wears a splash apron and eye covering if splashing of fluids is possible.
- The nurse who provides care for the newborn wears disposable gloves when handling the newborn or any objects or bedding that have been used for the newborn.
- All nurses and physicians/CNMs need to avoid exposure to blood, amniotic fluid, urine, feces, and tracheal, esophageal, or gastric aspirate from the baby.
- Immediately after the birth disposable gloves need to be worn when assessing the perineum and lochial flow, changing perineal pads and Chux, placing cold packs, and cleansing the perineum.
- Disposable gloves should be worn when changing any garments, Chux, bedding, pads, or cold packs that have bloody discharge on them.

A splash apron and eye covering (such as goggles) must be worn when splashing of body fluids is possible.

REMEMBER to wash your hands prior to putting the disposable gloves on and AGAIN immediately after removing the gloves.

For further information, consult OSHA and CDC guidelines.

Assisting the Couple and Physician/CNM during Birth

Shortly before the birth, the birthing room or delivery room is prepared with equipment and materials that may be needed. Family members do not need to change into other clothing if the birth occurs in a birthing room; they don a disposable scrub suit if the birth is to occur in a delivery room or surgery suite. Good handwashing is required of the nurses and CNM/physician. Nurses who will be in direct contact with the mother at the time of birth need to wear protective clothing, such as an apron or gown with a splash apron, disposable gloves, and eye covering (see Essential Precautions in Practice: During Birth). The CNM/physician will also need to wear a gown with a splash apron, or plastic apron, eye covering, and sterile gloves.

If the laboring woman is to give birth in a delivery room, she will be moved shortly before birth on her bed or a cart. It is important to preserve her privacy during the transfer, and safety must be provided by raising the side rails into a locked position. In the delivery room, the labor bed or transfer cart must be carefully supported against the delivery table; this ensures the woman's safety during the transfer.

It is important that the woman move from one bed to another between contractions. During the contraction, the woman feels increased discomfort and may be involved in pushing efforts. Perineal bulging may be occurring, which adds to the discomfort and difficulty in moving. All of these factors make moving the woman very uncomfortable. If birth seems imminent (within the next minute), it is safer for the woman to give birth in her labor bed or on the cart. Transfer to the delivery table is then delayed until after the baby is born and the cord has been clamped and cut.

Even though there are differences in the delivery room setting, the family can still be together during the birth. It is important to provide encouragement for family members to participate because the delivery room environment may be unfamiliar and seem less relaxed. The family member may be hesitant to continue to provide support for fear of interfering or being in the way.

Maternal Birthing Positions

The woman is usually positioned for birth on a bed, birthing chair, or delivery table. In some instances, she may give birth standing at the side of the bed or on her hands and knees on the floor. The position the woman assumes is determined not only by her individual wishes but also by the CNM/physician.

Stirrups are not often used, but if they are, they are padded to alleviate pressure, and both legs should be lifted simultaneously to avoid strain on abdominal, back, and perineal muscles. The stirrups should be adjusted to fit the woman's legs. The feet are supported in the stirrup holders. The height and angle of the stirrups are adjusted so there is no pressure on the back of the knees or the calf, which might cause discomfort and postpartal vascular problems. This is particularly true of women with epidural anesthesia. The birthing bed is elevated 30 to 60 degrees to help the woman bear down, and handles are provided so she may pull back on them.

The upright posture for birth was considered normal in most societies until modern times. Squatting, kneeling, standing, and sitting were variously selected by women for birth. Only within the last 200 years has the recumbent position become more usual in the Western world. Its use in this century has been reinforced because of the convenience it offers in applying new technology. The lithotomy position has thus become the conventional manner in which North American women give birth in hospitals. In searching for alternative positions, consumers and professionals alike continue to refocus on the comfort of the laboring woman and the advantages of alternative positions rather than on the convenience of the CNM/physician (Figure 20–6 and Table 20–9).

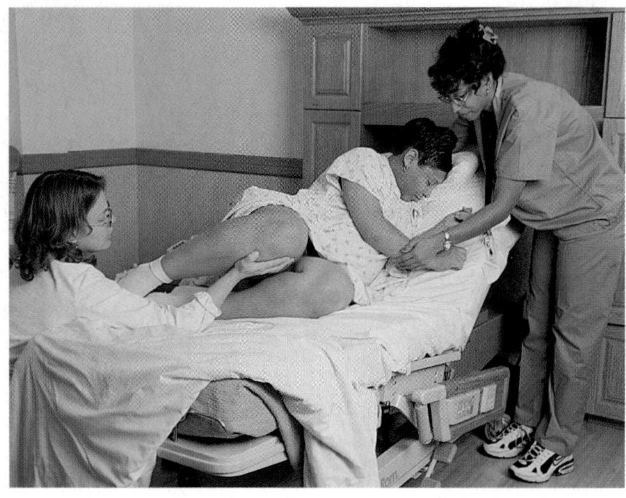

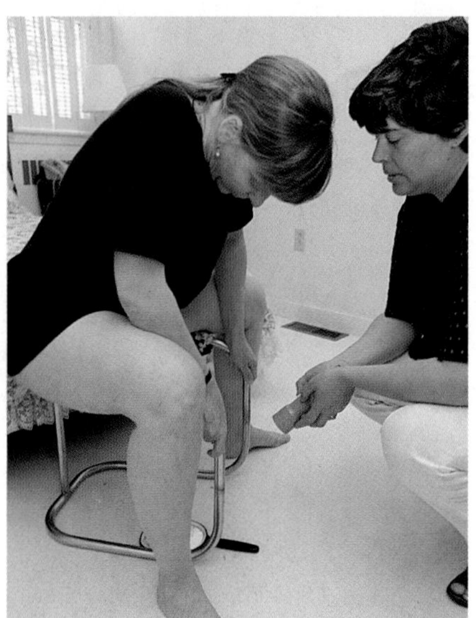

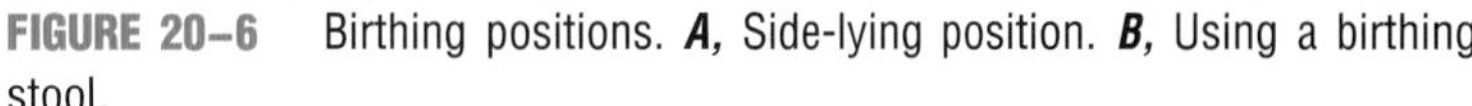

FIGURE 20–6 Birthing positions. ***A,*** Side-lying position. ***B,*** Using a birthing stool.

Recumbent Position The lithotomy position for birth is used sometimes to enhance the maintenance of asepsis, assessment of FHR, and performance of episiotomy and repair. In contrast, when the comfort and well-being of the woman and fetus are considered, the following disadvantages have been noted:

- There is a decrease of as much as 30% in the blood pressure of 10% of women.
- Many women experience difficulty breathing because of pressure of the uterus on the diaphragm.
- The uterine axis is directed toward the symphysis pubis instead of the pelvic inlet.
- Aspiration of vomitus is more likely.
- The woman may feel resentment at being forced to assume an "embarrassing" position.
- Tightening of the vagina and perineum as the thighs are flexed may increase the need for an episiotomy.
- The position may interfere with the frequency and intensity of contractions.
- Stirrups cause excessive pressure on the legs.
- The woman works against gravity.

These disadvantages may be lessened slightly if the woman is in a lithotomy position with her back elevated 30 to 40 degrees.

Left Lateral Sims' Position A common position favored by some women and birth attendants is the left lateral Sims' position (Figure 20–6 *A*). In assuming this position for birth, the woman lies on her left side with her left leg extended and her right knee drawn against her abdomen or flexed by her side or with both legs bent at the knees. Those who favor this position find it increases overall comfort, does not compromise venous return from the lower extremities, and diminishes the chances of aspiration should vomiting occur. Women also perceive the lateral Sims' as a more natural and comfortable position and less intrusive with no stirrups or overhead lights required. Birth attendants have found the position has a positive effect on the management of fetal shoulder dystocias. Fewer episiotomies are required in this position because the perineum tends to be more relaxed. The disadvantages cited relate to the difficulty of cutting and repairing large episiotomies and problems with difficult forceps births.

Squatting Position Squatting is favored by some women primarily for the positive use it makes of gravity. Squatting is thought to facilitate the entrance of the presenting part into the pelvic inlet, thus hastening engagement. A squatting bar (birthing bar) may be used across a bed or on the floor to increase the woman's balance and provide some support (Figure 20–5 *B*). During the second stage of labor, squatting increases the size of the pelvic outlet and helps in the woman's pushing efforts. Some birth attendants object to this position because the perineum is relatively inaccessible, and it is difficult for them to control the birth process. Squatting also increases the difficulty of administering analgesia, using instruments, and monitoring fetal status.

Semi-Fowler's Position Some care providers advocate a semi-Fowler's position as an appropriate middle ground between the recumbent and upright positions. This position enhances the effectiveness of the abdominal muscle efforts while the woman is pushing and thereby shortens the second stage of labor. Raising and supporting the torso helps the woman view the birth process. At the same time the birth attendant has access to the perineum. Supporting a woman in this position is not difficult with most birthing beds.

Sitting Position The sitting position is becoming an option for more women with the increased availability of birthing chairs. The use of birthing chairs or stools can be

TABLE 20–9 Comparison of Birthing Positions

Position	Advantages	Disadvantages	Nursing Actions
Sitting on birthing stool	Gravity aids descent and expulsion of infant. Does not compromise venous return from lower extremities. Woman can view birth process.	It is difficult to provide support for the woman's back.	Encourage woman to sit in a position that increases her comfort.
Semi-Fowler's	Does not compromise venous return from lower extremities. Woman can view birth process.	If legs are positioned wide apart, relaxation of perineal tissues is decreased.	Assess that upper torso is evenly supported. Increase support of body by changing position of bed or using pillows as props.
Left lateral Sims'	Does not compromise venous return from lower extremities. Increases perineal relaxation and decreases need for episiotomy. Appears to prevent rapid descent.	It is difficult for the woman to see the birth.	Adjust position so that the upper leg lies on the bed (scissor fashion) or is supported by the partner or on pillows.
Squatting	Size of pelvic outlet is increased. Gravity aids descent and expulsion of newborn. Second stage may be shortened (Sleep, Roberts, & Chalmers, 1989).	It may be difficult to maintain balance while squatting.	Help woman maintain balance. Use a birthing bar if available.
Sitting in birthing bed	Gravity aids descent and expulsion of the fetus. Does not compromise venous return from lower extremities. Woman can view the birth process. Leg position may be changed at will.		Ensure that legs and feet have adequate support.
Hands and knees	Increases perineal relaxation and decreases need for episiotomy. Increases placental and umbilical blood flow and decreases fetal distress. Improves fetal rotation. Nurse is better able to assess perineum. Nurse has better access to fetal nose and mouth for suctioning at birth. Facilitates birth of infant with shoulder dystocia.	Woman cannot view birth. There is decreased contact with birth attendant. Caregivers cannot use instruments. There may be increased maternal fatigue.	Adjust birthing bed by dropping the foot down. Supply extra pillows for increased support.

traced back to ancient Egypt and was broadly used in ancient Greek, Roman, and Incan civilizations. In the wake of the 19th-century battle against puerperal fever, birthing chairs began to vanish on hygienic grounds. Birthing chairs are being used again during the second stage of labor and are perceived by some women who use them as a positive way to participate in the birth process. A supported sitting position may also be achieved in a birthing bed.

The upright sitting position offers advantages similar to squatting. It has been postulated that the weight of a term fetus is sufficient force in itself to supply much of what is needed to bring the newborn into the world. Proponents of the birthing chair state that it makes possible spontaneous births that would have required operative assistance in the recumbent position. Women experiencing severe back pain have found use of the chair can diminish or eliminate the pain. The woman can curl forward and grasp her knees and ankles during pushing efforts. She can usually see the birth without aid of mirrors, and following birth she can lift the baby up toward her face.

Duration of second stage and fetal outcome is not significantly affected by use of the birthing chair. However, it may carry a potential for increased blood loss.

Hands and Knees Position The hands and knees position is more comfortable for a woman experiencing back labor because there is less pressure on the maternal back from the fetus, and the fetus may be able to rotate more easily from the posterior position. The mother can be well supported by dropping the foot of the birthing bed and supplying extra pillows upon which she can rest her forearms. Because there is less pressure on the perineum, there is less need for an episiotomy. The birth attendant is better able to assess the perineum for stretching and has good access to the fetal nose and mouth for suctioning at the time of birth. This position may also increase placental and umbilical blood flow during episodes of fetal distress. Lastly, the hands and knees position may increase the pelvic diameter and facilitate birth of the infant with shoulder dystocia. Disadvantages of this position include decreased eye-to-eye contact between the mother and birth attendant, the inability to use instruments, and the potential necessity of repositioning the mother for perineal repair. Women may also become easily fatigued in this position.

Cleansing the Perineum

After being positioned for the birth, the woman's vulvar and perineal area is cleansed to increase her comfort and

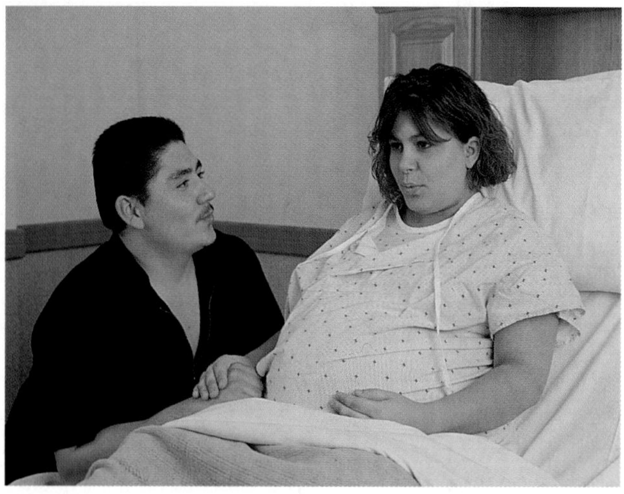

FIGURE 20–7 The partner can provide comfort and assistance during contractions.

to remove the bloody discharge that is present prior to the actual birth. An aseptic technique such as the one that follows is recommended.

After thorough handwashing, the nurse opens the sterile prep tray, dons sterile gloves, and cleans the vulva and perineum with the cleansing solution. Beginning with the mons pubis, the area is cleansed up to the lower abdomen. A second sponge is used to clean the inner groin and thigh of one leg, and a third is used to clean the other leg, moving upward to avoid carrying material from surrounding areas to the vaginal outlet. The last three sponges are used to clean the labia and vestibule with one downward sweep each. The used sponges are discarded. Once the cleansing is completed, the woman returns to the desired birthing position.

Supporting the Couple

The labor coach or support person is made comfortable. Both the woman and the coach are kept informed of procedures and progress and are supported throughout the birth. Some birth settings provide a mirror that can be adjusted so that the couple can watch the birth.

The woman's blood pressure is monitored between contractions, and the contractions are palpated until the birth. FHR is auscultated every 15 minutes for low-risk women and every 5 minutes for high-risk women (NAACOG, 1990). The nurse and support person continue to assist the woman (Figure 20–7).

In addition to assisting the woman and her partner, the nurse assists the physician or certified nurse-midwife in preparing for the birth.

Physician/CNM Interventions

When the fetal head has distended the perineum, the clinician may perform certain hand maneuvers that are believed to prevent undue trauma to the fetal head and maternal soft tissues. The woman may be asked to breathe rapidly to avoid too rapid a birth of the fetal head.

After the infant's head is born, the clinician palpates the neck for the presence of a cord, which can be slipped over the fetal head if it is loose. If the cord is tight, it is double-clamped and cut.

Restitution and external rotation occur after the head is born. The only assistance needed during this time is support of the maternal perineum. While awaiting completion of external rotation, the clinician suctions the newborn's nose and mouth to remove mucus. When the newborn's shoulder appears at the symphysis pubis, the clinician may use both hands to grasp the newborn's head gently and pull downward for release of the anterior shoulder. Gentle upward traction facilitates release of the posterior shoulder.

Birth of the newborn's body may be controlled by grasping the posterior shoulder with one hand, palm turned toward the perineum. The left hand may be used for this if the newborn is left occiput anterior (LOA). The right hand then follows along the infant's back, and the feet are grasped as they are expelled. The newborn's head is kept down and to the side as the feet, legs, and body are tucked under the clinician's left arm in a football hold. The clinician's right hand is then free for further care of the newborn, and the newborn is securely held. Certified nurse-midwives often deliver the newborn directly to the mother's abdomen. The nose and mouth are suctioned with a bulb syringe, and respiratory passages are cleared. Figure 20–8 depicts an entire birthing experience.

There is controversy about when to clamp and cut the cord. If the newborn is held at or below the vagina as cord clamping is delayed, as much as 50 to 100 mL of blood may be shifted from the placenta to the newborn. If the newborn is held 50 to 60 cm above the vagina, blood may be transferred from the neonate to the placenta. The extra amount of blood added to the newborn's circulation by holding the child below the vagina may reduce the frequency of iron deficiency anemia, which can occur later in infancy. However, in some cases the circulatory overload may produce polycythemia and favor hyperbilirubinemia. Cunningham et al (1997) advocate clamping the cord after clearing the newborn's airway, which takes about 30 seconds. The newborn is not elevated above the vagina.

The cord is usually clamped with two Kelly clamps and cut between them, although some birth attendants may ask that the cord be double-clamped so that a section can be made available for the collection of cord blood gases. The clamp on the placental side is placed on the mother's abdomen. A plastic cord clamp or umbilical tape may be applied on the newborn's cord about 2 cm from the newborn's abdomen, and then the Kelly clamp on the newborn's side may be removed. The father or other support person may wish to cut the cord after it has been clamped by the birth attendant.

The sheer pleasure of the feeling of a born baby on one's thighs is like nothing on earth.
~ MARGARET DRABBLE, *EVER SINCE EVE* ~

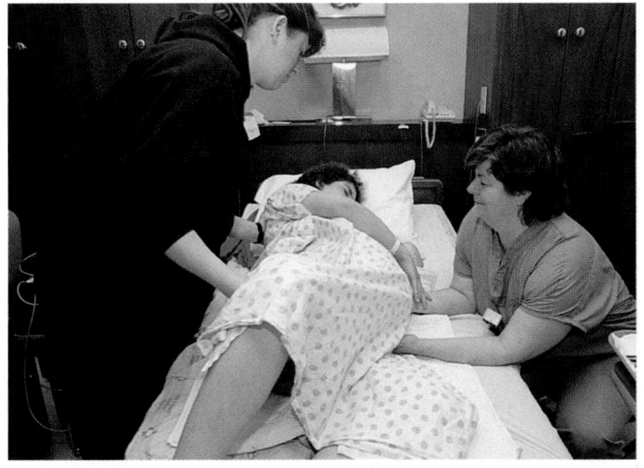
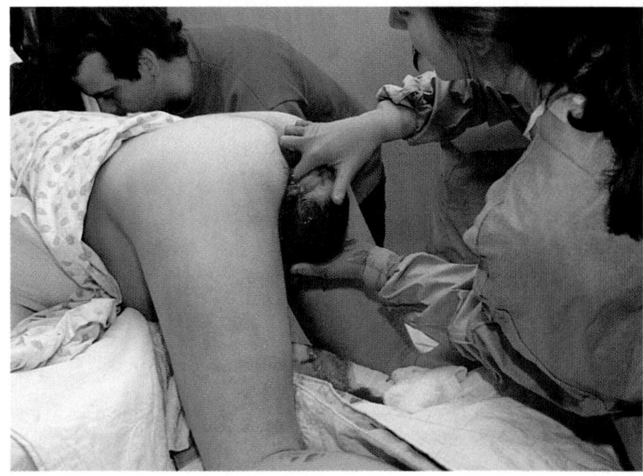
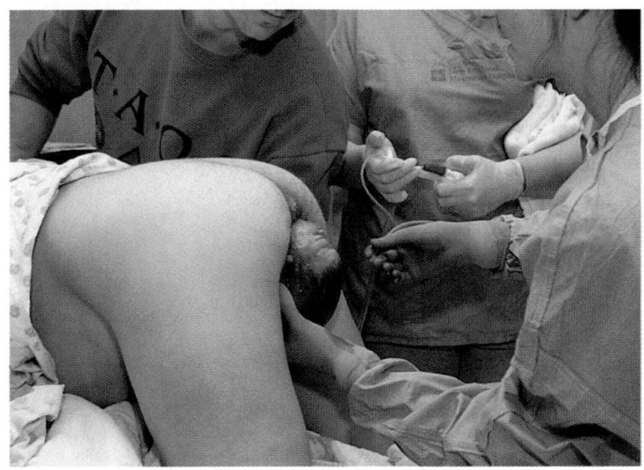
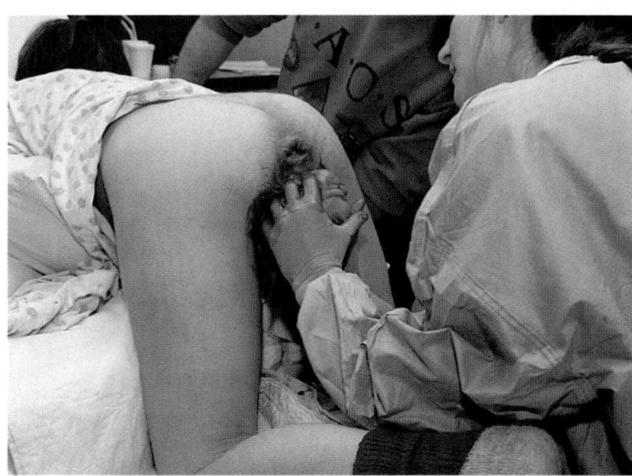
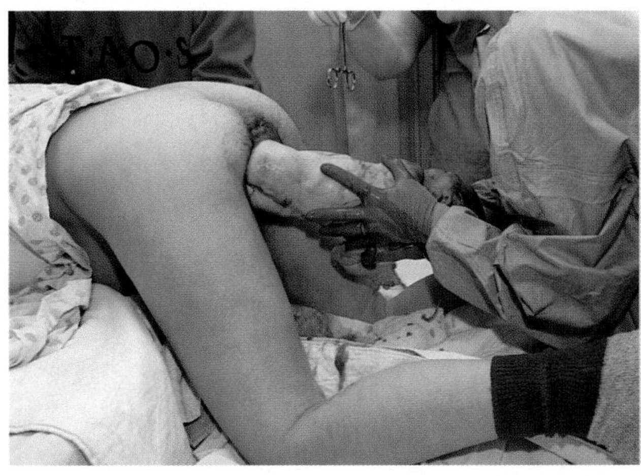
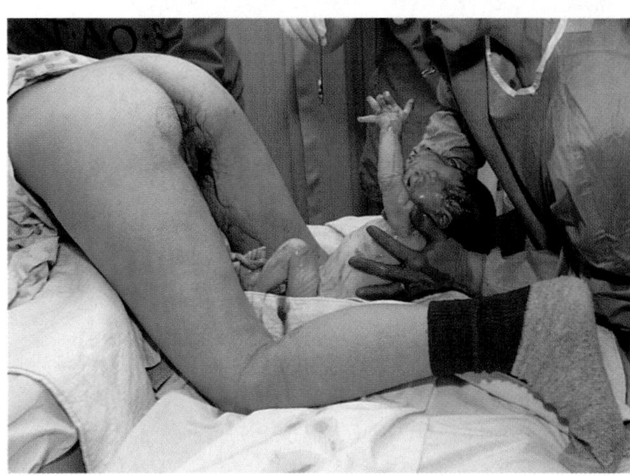

FIGURE 20–8 A birthing sequence.

Nursing Care Management during the Third Stage of Labor

Initial Care of the Newborn

The physician/CNM places the newborn on the mother's abdomen or in the radiant-heated unit to begin the initial care. If the newborn is not placed on the mother's abdomen, the radiant-heated unit is positioned so the parents can see the baby.

Because the first priority is to maintain respirations, the newborn is placed in a modified Trendelenburg position to aid drainage of mucus from the nasopharynx and trachea. The newborn is also suctioned with a bulb syringe or DeLee mucus trap as needed (Procedure 20–1: Performing Nasal Pharyngeal Suctioning).

PROCEDURE 20–1 PERFORMING NASAL PHARYNGEAL SUCTIONING

Nursing Action	*Rationale*
Objective: Clear secretions from the newborn's nose or oropharynx if respirations are depressed or if amniotic fluid was meconium stained.	
• Tighten the lid on the DeLee mucus trap or other suction device collection bottle.	*This avoids spillage of secretions and prevents air from leaking out of the lid.*
• Connect one end of the DeLee tubing to low suction.	
• Insert the other end of the tubing 3 to 5 inches into the newborn's nose or mouth (Figure 20–9).	

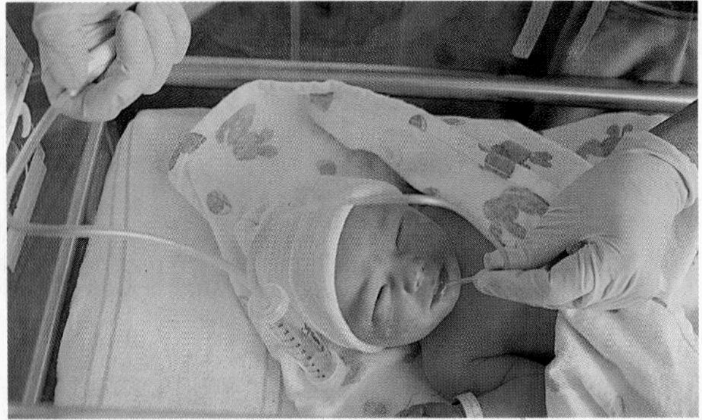

FIGURE 20–9 DeLee mucus trap.

Nursing Action	*Rationale*
• Continue suction as you remove the tube.	*This avoids redepositing secretions in the newborn's nasopharynx.*
• Continue to reinsert the tube and provide suction for as long as fluid is aspirated. Note: *Excessive suctioning can cause vagal stimulation, which decreases heart rate.*	
• If it is necessary to pass the tube into the newborn's stomach to remove meconium secretions that the newborn swallowed before birth, insert the tube into the newborn's mouth and then into the stomach. Provide suction and continue suction as you remove the tube.	
Objective: Record relevant information on the newborn's chart.	
Document completion of the procedure and the amount and type of secretions.	*This provides documentation of intervention and status at birth.*

TABLE 20–10 The Apgar Scoring System

Sign	Score 0	1	2
Heart rate	Absent	Slow—below 100	Above 100
Respiratory effort	Absent	Slow—irregular	Good crying
Muscle tone	Flaccid	Some flexion of extremities	Active motion
Reflex irritability	None	Grimace	Vigorous cry
Color	Pale blue	Body pink, blue extremities	Completely pink

SOURCE: Apgar V: The newborn (Apgar) scoring system, reflections and advice. *Pediatr Clin North Am* August 1966; 13:645.

The second priority is to provide and maintain warmth, so the newborn is dried immediately with warmed soft infant blankets. It is important to begin drying the newborn's head first to minimize heat loss. Warmth can be maintained by putting the newborn in skin-to-skin contact with the mother and placing warmed blankets over both of them. If the newborn is placed in a radiant-heated unit, he or she is dried, laid on a dry blanket, and left uncovered under the radiant heat. Because radiant heat warms the outer surface of objects, a newborn wrapped in blankets will receive no benefit. In many settings a stocking cap is placed on the newborn's head to conserve heat.

Apgar Scoring System

The Apgar scoring system (Table 20–10) was designed in 1952 by Dr Virginia Apgar, an anesthesiologist. The purpose of the **Apgar score** is to evaluate the physical condition of the newborn at birth and the immediate need for resuscitation. The newborn is rated 1 minute after birth and again at 5 minutes and receives a total score ranging from 0 to 10 based on the following criteria:

1. The heart rate is auscultated or palpated at the junction of the umbilical cord and skin. This is the most important assessment. A newborn heart rate of less than 100 beats per minute indicates the need for immediate resuscitation.
2. The respiratory effort is the second most important Apgar assessment. Complete absence of respirations is termed *apnea.* A vigorous cry indicates good respirations.
3. The muscle tone is determined by evaluating the degree of flexion and resistance to straightening of the extremities. A normal term newborn's elbows and hips are flexed, with the knees positioned up toward the abdomen.
4. The reflex irritability is evaluated as the newborn is dried or by lightly rubbing the soles of the feet. A cry is a score of 2. A grimace is 1 point, and no response is 0.
5. The skin color is inspected for cyanosis and pallor. Newborns generally have blue extremities, and the rest of the body is pink, which merits a score of 1. This condition, termed *acrocyanosis,* is present in 85% of normal newborns at 1 minute after birth. A completely pink newborn scores a 2, and a totally cyanotic, pale infant is scored 0. Newborns with darker skin pigmentation will not be pink. Their skin color is assessed for pallor and acrocyanosis, and a score is selected based on the assessment.

A score of 8 to 10 indicates a newborn in good condition who requires only nasopharyngeal suctioning and perhaps some oxygen near the face. An Apgar score between 4 and 7 indicates the need for stimulation; a score under 4 indicates the need for resuscitation. See the discussion in Chapter 28.

Care of the Umbilical Cord

If the physician/CNM has not placed a cord clamp on the newborn's umbilical cord, it is the responsibility of the nurse to do so. Before applying the cord clamp, the nurse examines the cut end for the presence of two arteries and one vein. The umbilical vein is the largest vessel, and the arteries are smaller vessels. The presence of only one artery in the umbilical cord is associated with genitourinary abnormalities. The number of vessels is recorded on the birth and newborn records. The cord is clamped approximately ½ to 1 inch from the abdomen to allow room between the abdomen and clamp as the cord dries (Figure 20–10). Abdominal skin must not be clamped because this will cause necrosis of the tissue. The clamp is removed in the newborn nursery approximately 24 hours after birth if the cord has dried.

Cord Blood Collection for Banking

Growing numbers of parents are arranging for cord blood banking (see discussion in Chapter 1). Immediately after the newborn's umbilical cord is clamped and cut and the placenta is expelled, the CNM/physician withdraws blood from the remaining umbilical cord and the placenta. The blood is placed in a special container that parents receive from the Cord Blood Registry and bring with them for the birth. The parents will have any special directions that are required for storage and care of the container.

Newborn Physical Assessment by the Nurse

An abbreviated systematic physical assessment is performed by the nurse in the birthing area to detect any abnormalities (Table 20–11). First, the nurse notes the size of the newborn and the contour and size of the head in relationship to the rest of the body. The newborn's posture and movements indicate tone and neurologic functioning.

The skin is inspected for discoloration, presence of vernix caseosa and lanugo, and evidence of trauma and

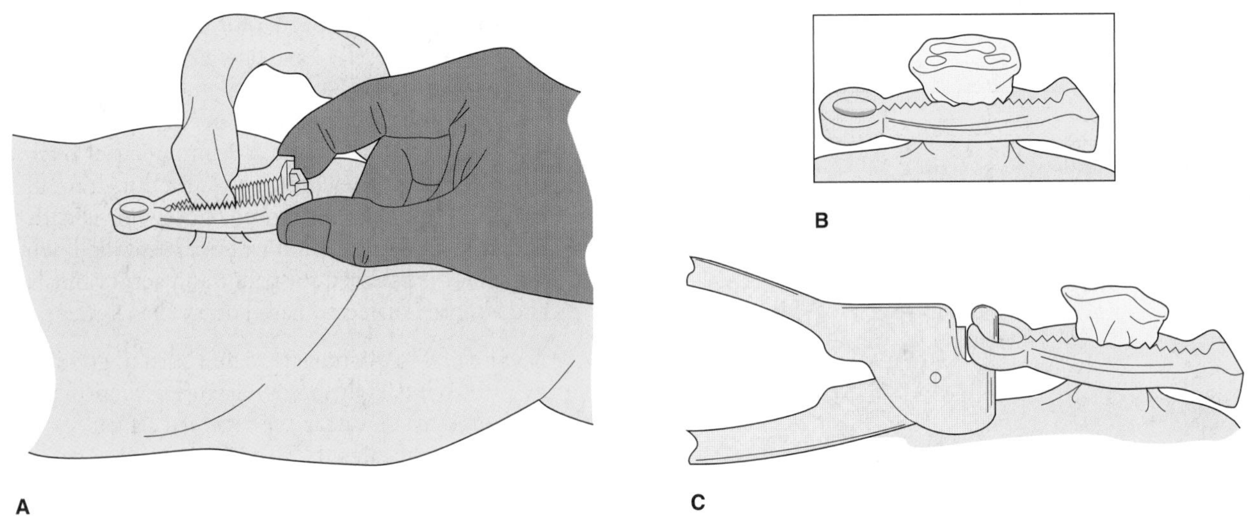

FIGURE 20–10 Hollister cord clamp. ***A,*** Clamp is positioned ½ to 1 inch from the abdomen and then secured. ***B,*** Cut cord. The one vein and two arteries can be seen. ***C,*** Plastic device for removing clamp after cord has dried. After the cord is cut, the nurse grasps the Hollister clamp on either side of the cut area and gently separates it.

desquamation (peeling of skin). Vernix caseosa is a white, cheesy substance normally found on newborns. It is absorbed within 24 hours after birth. Vernix is abundant on preterm infants and absent on postterm newborns. A large quantity of fine hair (lanugo) is often seen on preterm newborns, especially on their shoulders, foreheads, backs, and cheeks. Desquamation of the skin is seen in postterm newborns.

The nares are observed for flaring. As the newborn cries, the palate can be inspected for cleft palate. Mucus in the nose and mouth can be assessed and removed with the bulb syringe as needed. The chest is inspected for respiratory rate and the presence of retractions. If retractions are present, the newborn is assessed for grunting or stridor. A normal respiratory rate is 30 to 40 per minute. The lungs may be auscultated bilaterally for breath sounds. Absence of breath sounds on one side may indicate pneumothorax. Rales may be heard immediately after birth because a small amount of fluid may remain in the lungs; this fluid will be absorbed. Rhonchi indicate aspiration of oral secretions.

The elimination of urine or meconium is noted and recorded on the newborn record.

Newborn Identification

To ensure correct identification, the nurse gives the mother and the newborn matching identification bands in the birthing or delivery room. One bracelet is placed on the mother's wrist and sometimes on the wrist of her partner or a support person whom the mother designates. Two bracelets are placed on the newborn—one on the wrist and one on the ankle. The newborn bands must be applied snugly to prevent their loss.

Most hospitals footprint the newborn and fingerprint the mother for further identification purposes. To prepare the newborn for footprinting, the nurse wipes the soles of both the newborn's feet to remove any vernix caseosa.

Initiation of Attachment

The birth of the baby is usually an emotionally charged time for all members of the family. The sight of the new baby and the sounds of the first cry create an exhilarating and emotional moment for the new parents. They may be filled with utter amazement, and as the baby is placed on the mother's abdomen or chest, she frequently reaches out to touch and stroke her baby. When the newborn is placed in this position, the father also has a very clear, close view and can also reach out to touch his baby. When the parents feel comfortable in the environment, they may talk to the newborn, and some mothers talk to their babies in a high-pitched voice, which seems to soothe newborns. Some couples verbally express amazement and pride when they see they have produced a beautiful, healthy baby. Their verbalization enhances feelings of accomplishment and ecstasy. If lights in the birthing area can be dimmed, the newborn will probably open his or her eyes wide and gaze at the surroundings. In this first hour after birth, the newborn is usually quiet and continues to gaze. This is a wonderful opportunity for eye-to-eye contact with the parents, and many parents are content to gaze quietly at their newborn.

Even though the baby is on the mother's abdomen or chest, the nurse can complete any needed assessments or interventions such as footprinting and applying an identification bracelet to the child. As soon as possible the nurse can assist the mother to a more comfortable position for holding the newborn. Newborns have highly developed sensory skills that allow them to be active participants in interactions from birth (Righard & Alade,

TABLE 20–11 Initial Newborn Evaluation

Assess	Normal Findings
Respirations	Rate 36–60, irregular No retractions, no grunting
Apical pulse	Rate 120–160 and somewhat irregular
Temperature	Skin temp above 36.5C (97.8F)
Skin color	Body pink with bluish extremities
Umbilical cord	Two arteries and one vein
Gestational age	Should be 38–42 weeks to remain with parents for extended time
Sole creases	Sole creases that involve the heel

In general, expect scant amount of vernix on upper back, axilla, groin; lanugo only on upper back; ears with incurving of upper $\frac{2}{3}$ of pinnae and thin cartilage that springs back from folding; male genitals—testes palpated in upper or lower scrotum; female genitals—labia majora larger; clitoris nearly covered

In the following situations, newborns should generally be stabilized rather than remaining with parents in the birth area for an extended period of time:

- Apgar less than 8 at 1 minute and less than 9 at 5 minutes or baby requires resuscitation measures (other than whiffs of oxygen)
- Respirations below 30 or above 60, with retractions and/or grunting
- Apical pulse below 120 or above 160 with marked irregularities
- Skin temperature below 36.5C (97.8F)
- Skin color pale blue or circumoral pallor
- Baby less than 38 or more than 42 weeks' gestation
- Baby very small or very large for gestational age
- Congenital anomalies involving open areas in the skin (meningomyelocele)

1990). Breastfeeding can be encouraged if the mother and baby desire. When the baby is held close to the breast, the baby will seek out the nipple. Even if the newborn does not actively nurse, she or he can lick, taste, and smell the mother's skin. This activity stimulates the maternal release of prolactin, which promotes the onset of lactation.

The initial parental-newborn attachment period can be enhanced if the care providers keep routine investigations to a minimum, delay instillation of ophthalmic antibiotic for 1 hour, keep the room slightly darkened, avoid loud noises, talk in quiet tones, and provide privacy. Both parents need to be encouraged to do whatever they feel most comfortable doing. Parents may have differing wishes concerning contact with their newborn. Some want immediate and unlimited time; some prefer to wait until all birth-related activities are completed (the placenta is expelled and episiotomy repair is completed); others prefer limited contact immediately after birth and quiet time later. Although immediate contact may be important for attachment and initiation of breastfeeding, the parents' wishes need to be supported.

> *I was hungry for the baby as he was born. I wanted to see, hold him. It was hours before I realized or even thought love in relation to him.*
>
> ~ Harriette Hartigan, *Women in Birth* ~

CNM/Physician Interventions

After the cord has been clamped and cut, the physician/CNM observes for the following signs of placental separation:

1. The uterus rises upward in the abdomen because the placenta settles downward into the lower uterine segment.
2. As the placenta proceeds downward, the umbilical cord lengthens.
3. A sudden trickle or spurt of blood appears.
4. The uterus changes from a discoid to a globular shape.

While waiting for these signs, the nurse gently palpates the uterus to check for ballooning caused by uterine relaxation and subsequent bleeding into the uterine cavity.

After the placenta has separated, it may be expelled by various techniques such as maternal bearing-down effort, controlled cord traction, and fundal pressure. Maternal effort allows the placenta to be expelled spontaneously and is best accomplished in an upright position. When the mother is in a dorsal recumbent or lithotomy position, she or the nurse can help the process by splinting or supporting her abdominal muscles. The mother or nurse can place her palms over the lower abdomen, or the mother can flex her thighs over her abdomen. The mother then bears down to expel the placenta.

To help the woman expel her placenta, the physician/CNM first ensures that separation has occurred and then places one hand above the symphysis pubis with the palm against the anterior surface of the uterus. The uterus is displaced upward and backward as the mother is asked to relax her abdominal muscles and breathe through an open mouth. The elevation of the uterus straightens out the birth canal and facilitates expulsion of the placenta, as well as protecting the uterus from invasion. Gentle traction is exerted on the umbilical cord. Excessive pulling may increase the risk of uterine involution. During this procedure, the nurse encourages the mother to continue breathing through an open mouth and to relax her abdominal muscles.

Fundal pressure is not a method of choice because it is very uncomfortable for the mother, may damage uterine supports, and may invert the uterus. If this method is needed, the mother is asked to relax her abdominal muscles, and then the hand of the physician/CNM is placed behind the uterus with the fingers directed downward toward the maternal spine. With a quick "scooping" motion, the contracted uterus is pressed downward in an arc. This motion is different from direct downward pressure, which folds the uterus over the lower segment and does not enhance movement of the placenta. During the procedure, the nurse provides continued encouragement to maintain abdominal relaxation. This is very difficult due to the discomfort of the procedure.

After expulsion of the placenta, the physician/CNM inspects the placental membranes to make sure they are intact and that all cotyledons are present. This inspection is especially important with placentas expelled via the Duncan mechanism (the chance of tearing off a portion of a cotyledon is greatest with this mechanism of placental separation). If there is a defect or a part missing from the placenta, a digital uterine examination is done. The vagina and cervix are inspected for lacerations, and any necessary repairs are made. An episiotomy may be repaired now if it has not been done previously. (See further discussion of episiotomy in Chapter 23.) The fundus of the uterus is palpated; normal position is at the midline and below the umbilicus. If the fundus is displaced, it may be because of a full bladder or a collection of blood in the uterus.

The time and mechanism (Schultze or Duncan) of expulsion of the placenta are noted on the birth record.

The medical-nursing culture tends to refer to the placenta as the "afterbirth" and considers that its value is fulfilled once it is expelled and examined. Disposal of the placenta is prescribed by the hospital or birth center, and no more thought is given to it. However, many cultures have other beliefs regarding the placenta. For instance, in Yucatan, Mexico, the placenta is called "el compañero," the child's companion (Vincent, 1995), and in Korea, the placenta is given different names depending on the month of the birth (Uyoo, 1990). Some clients will have specific beliefs about disposal of the placenta and will ask to take it home with them. Although such requests may not be common, there is usually no reason that their request cannot be honored. Some additional examples of cultural beliefs include the following (Schneiderman, 1998):

- Mexico and southern Texas: The placenta is buried to decrease the mother's pain and to prevent animals from eating it. The burial place differs according to the gender of the newborn: placentas from males are buried far from the house, whereas placentas from females are buried close (Spector, 1996).
- Korea: Future children are affected by the treatment and disposal of the placenta. If the disposal place is far away, the next child will be a long time in coming (Uyoo, 1990).
- Hmong: The gender of the child determines the burial place. The male newborn placenta is buried close to the center of the house, whereas the female newborn's placenta is buried under the parents' bed. The burial place of the placenta is thought to be the "true home," and misfortune can result from burial in the wrong place (Clark, 1996).

Use of Oxytocics

Some CNM and physicians advocate the use of an oxytocic drug (Pitocin) to stimulate uterine contractions after birth and to reduce the incidence of third-stage hemorrhage.

The physician/certified nurse-midwife may request that 10 units of oxytocin be given intramuscularly to the woman when the anterior shoulder of the infant appears at the vaginal opening. Others question whether this method increases the incidence of neonatal hyperviscosity because an additional bolus of blood may be infused into the fetus when the uterus contracts in response to the oxytocin. At other times 10 units of oxytocin may be administered IM at the time of placental expulsion. Both techniques are thought to facilitate expulsion of the placenta. Some prefer to add 10 units of oxytocin to IV fluids administered over a period of hours. Additional information and associated nursing implications are presented in the Drug Guide: Oxytocin (Pitocin) in Chapter 23.

Nursing Care Management during the Fourth Stage of Labor

The period immediately following expulsion of the placenta is referred to as the fourth stage of labor and birth. Actually, the label is misleading because labor and birth are completed with delivery of the placenta, and the next few hours are actually the immediate recovery phase. The fourth stage is usually defined as lasting 1 to 4 hours after the birth or until vital signs are stable. Nursing care in this phase involves the basics of postpartum nursing care. (See Essential Precautions in Practice: During the Fourth Stage.)

Immediately after the placenta is expelled, the episiotomy or vaginal lacerations are repaired. The uterus is palpated at frequent intervals to ensure that it remains firmly contracted. Although labor is completed, the uterus is sensitive to touch. Palpation of the uterine fundus will be uncomfortable for the woman. If the mother has not held her baby yet, immediate newborn care should be completed at her side and within her reach so that she can touch her baby during this time. As soon as immediate care is completed, the new mother is usually eager to cuddle and explore her baby. If she plans to breastfeed and the baby is interested, she should be encouraged and helped to do so right after birth while the baby is awake and alert. Care should be taken not to try to force an uninterested baby to breastfeed because it will just lead to frustration for both mother and baby.

Behavioral characteristics of the mother vary, according to such factors as the length of labor and the extent of interruption in normal sleep patterns. After the initial excitement of becoming acquainted with their new baby and notifying others of the birth, many new mothers are very tired and want to rest. Others are wide awake, eager to talk about their labor and satisfy basic body needs, such as hunger and thirst.

Provisions of Care in the Fourth Stage

As soon as the CNM/physician completes the repair of any perineal lacerations or an episiotomy, drapes (if used) are removed. If the mother is to remain in the birthing bed, the nurse places clean absorbent pads beneath her and applies maternity pads. A cold pack may be placed directly on the perineum if perineal edema is present or an episiotomy has been done. If a mother prefers to shower immediately after birth, the nurse can assist her as needed and change the bed linens while the mother is up.

If stirrups were used, her perineum is cleansed and maternity pads applied before her legs are removed from the stirrups. In order to avoid muscle strain, both legs are removed from the stirrups at the same time. The legs may be held together and gently pushed toward the woman's abdomen, back to a neutral position and then gently lowered toward her right side and then the left side to promote circulation return. If the woman has given birth on a delivery table she is transferred to a recovery room bed. If the mother has not had a chance to hold her infant, she may do so before she is transferred from the birthing room. The nurse ensures that the mother and father or support person and newborn are given time to begin the attachment process.

In addition to encouraging family celebration of the birth, the immediate recovery period involves assessing both maternal bleeding and newborn stabilization. The most significant source of bleeding is from the site where the placenta was implanted and where uterine vessels previously provided pooling of maternal blood to nourish the fetus. It is therefore critical that the fundus stay well contracted in order to clamp off these uterine vessels and prevent hemorrhage. It is the nurse's responsibility to assess the mother's blood pressure, pulse, firmness and position of fundus, and amount and character of vaginal blood flow every 15 minutes for the first 1 or 2 hours. Deviations from the normal ranges require more frequent checking. Table 20–12 summarizes maternal changes following birth. Blood pressure should return to the prelabor level, and pulse rate should be slightly lower than it was in labor. The return of the blood pressure is due to an increased volume of blood returning to the maternal circulation from the uteroplacental shunt. Baroreceptors cause a vagal response, which slows the pulse. The physiologic slowing may be offset by excitement, increased temperature, or dehydration. A rise in the blood pressure may be a response to oxytocic drugs or may be caused by pregnancy-induced hypertension (PIH). Blood loss may be reflected by a lowered blood pressure and a rising pulse rate.

The fundus should be firm at the umbilicus or lower and in the midline. The uterus should be palpated (Figure 20–11) but not massaged unless boggy (atonic). When a uterus becomes boggy, pooling of blood occurs within it, resulting in the formation of clots. Anything left in the uterus prevents it from contracting effectively. Thus if it becomes boggy or appears to rise in the abdomen, the fundus should be massaged until firm; then with one hand supporting the uterus at the symphysis pubis, the nurse should attempt to express retained clots. The uterus at this time is very tender, and palpation and massage cause discomfort. All palpation and massage should be done as gently as possible.

A boggy uterus feels very soft instead of firm and hard. In some cases, the uterus has relaxed so much that it cannot be found when the nurse attempts to palpate it. In this case the nurse places her hand in the midline of the abdomen about at the level of the umbilicus and begins to make kneading motions. This motion stimulates the uterine fundus to contract, and the nurse will feel the fundus tighten to a firm, hard object.

The nurse inspects the bloody vaginal discharge, called lochia, for amount and charts it as minimal, moderate, or heavy. It should be bright red. Because different brands of maternity pads absorb varying amounts of

ESSENTIAL PRECAUTIONS IN PRACTICE

During the Fourth Stage

Wear disposable gloves when performing the following actions:

- Changing any garments, Chux, bedding, pads, or cold packs that have bloody discharge on them
- Assessing the perineum and amount of lochia
- Assisting the woman with urination, emptying bedpans, and so forth
- Cleansing the perineal area
- Handling the newborn (Disposable gloves are required until the newborn has received the first bath.)

REMEMBER to wash your hands prior to putting the disposable gloves on and AGAIN immediately after removing the gloves.

For further information, consult OSHA and CDC guidelines.

TABLE 20–12 Maternal Adaptations Following Birth

Characteristic	Normal Finding
Blood pressure	Returns to prelabor level
Pulse	Slightly lower than in labor
Uterine fundus	In the midline at the umbilicus or 1–2 fingerbreadths below the umbilicus
Lochia	Red (rubra), small to moderate amount (from spotting on pads to $\frac{1}{4}-\frac{1}{2}$ of pad covered in 15 minutes) Doesn't exceed saturation of one pad in first hour
Bladder	Nonpalpable
Perineum	Smooth, pink, without bruising or edema
Emotional state	Wide variation, including excited, exhilarated, smiling, crying, fatigued, verbal, quiet, pensive, and sleepy

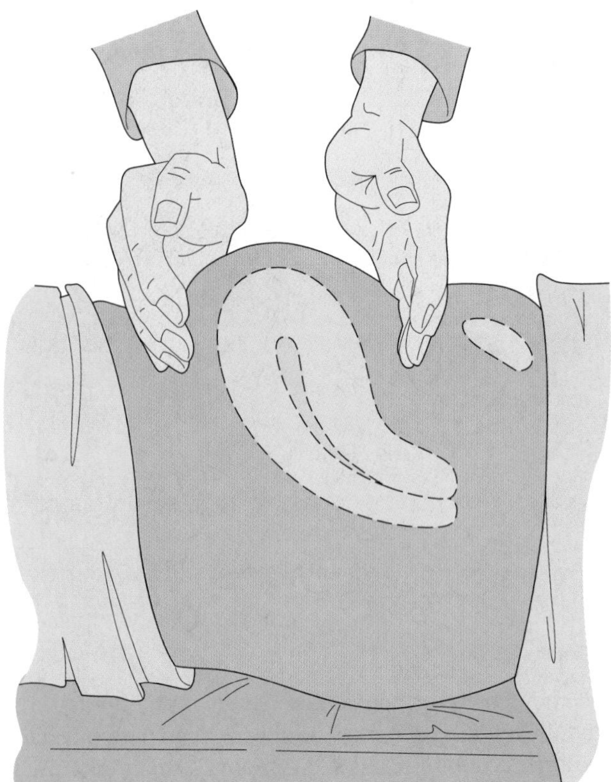

FIGURE 20–11 Suggested method of palpating the fundus of the uterus during the fourth stage. The left hand is placed just above the symphysis pubis, and gentle downward pressure is exerted. The right hand is cupped around the uterine fundus.

blood, it may be necessary to weigh the maternity pad to determine actual blood loss. A gram scale is used, and 1 g is equivalent to approximately 1 mL of blood. If the perineal pad becomes soaked in a 15-minute period or if blood pools under the buttocks, continuous observation is necessary. As long as the woman remains in bed during the first hour, bleeding should not exceed saturation of one pad. Laceration of the vagina, cervix, or an unligated vessel in the episiotomy may be indicated by a continuous trickle of blood even though the fundus remains firm. (See Procedure 20–2: Evaluating Lochia After Birth.)

If the fundus rises and displaces to the right, the nurse palpates the bladder to determine whether it is distended. All measures should be taken to enable the mother to void. If she is unable to void, catheterization is necessary. Postpartal women have decreased sensations to void as a result of the decreased tone of the bladder due to the trauma imposed on the bladder and urethra during childbirth. The bladder fills rapidly as the body attempts to rid itself of the extra fluid volume returned from the uteroplacental circulation and of intravenous fluid that may have been received during labor and birth. If the mother is unable to void, a warm towel placed across the lower abdomen or warm water poured over the perineum or spirits of peppermint poured into a bedpan may help the urinary sphincter relax and thus facilitate voiding. A distended bladder can cause uterine atony, thus increasing postpartal bleeding.

The perineum is inspected for edema and hematoma formation. With an episiotomy or laceration, an ice pack often reduces swelling and alleviates discomfort.

The following conditions should be reported to the CNM/physician: hypotension, tachycardia, uterine atony, excessive bleeding, or a temperature over 38C (100F). The nurse should be aware that the blood pressure may not fall rapidly in the presence of dangerous bleeding in postpartal mothers because of the extra systemic volume. However, an increasing pulse rate may be noted before a decrease in blood pressure is detected. A normal blood pressure with the mother in the Fowler's position is a good confirmation of a normotensive woman.

Women frequently have tremors in the immediate postpartal period. It has been proposed that this shivering response is caused by a difference in internal and external body temperatures (higher temperature inside the body than on the outside). Another theory is that the woman is reacting to the fetal cells that have entered the maternal circulation at the placental site. A heated bath blanket placed next to the woman and perhaps a warm drink tend to alleviate the problem.

The couple may be tired, hungry, and thirsty. Some hospitals serve the couple a meal. The tired mother will probably drift off into a welcome sleep. The father should also be encouraged to rest because his supporting role is physically and mentally tiring. The mother is usually transferred from the birthing unit to the postpartal unit after 2 hours or more, depending on agency policy and whether the following criteria are met: stable vital signs, no bleeding, nondistended bladder, firm fundus, sensations fully recovered from any anesthetic agent received during childbirth.

For some women, the childbirth experience has been extremely painful and filled with hours of being out of control. In this circumstance, the woman is at higher risk of developing posttraumatic stress disorder due to traumatic birth (Reynolds, 1997). See Chapter 22 for further discussion.

Nursing Care Management during Nurse-Attended Birth

Occasionally, labor progresses so rapidly that the maternity nurse is faced with the task of managing the birth of the baby. This is called a **precipitous birth.** The attending maternity nurse has the primary responsibility for providing a physically and psychologically safe experience for the woman and her baby.

A woman whose physician or CNM is not present may feel disappointed, frightened, and abandoned, espe-

PROCEDURE 20–2 EVALUATING LOCHIA AFTER BIRTH

Nursing Action	*Rationale*
Objective: Prepare the woman.	
Explain the procedure, the reason for performing the procedure, and the information that will be obtained.	*Explaining the procedure decreases anxiety and increases relaxation.*
Objective: Obtain and evaluate maternal vital signs.	
Assess maternal temperature, blood pressure, and pulse.	*This provides information regarding the woman's physiologic status.*
Objective: Accurately evaluate the amount of lochia after birth.	
• Don disposable gloves.	*Universal precautions and body substance isolation require use of gloves when exposed to body secretions.*
• Lower the perineal pad so that you can visualize the amount of lochia.	
• Palpate the uterine fundus, located in the midline at the umbilicus or one to two fingerbreadths below the umbilicus, by placing one hand on the fundus and the other hand just over the symphysis pubis and pressing downward. Use your other hand to palpate the fundus.	*Downward pressure exerted just above the symphysis pubis will prevent excessive downward movement of the uterus during assessment.*
• Determine the firmness of the fundus.	*The uterus must remain firmly contracted to prevent excessive blood loss.*
• If the fundus is boggy, massage by rubbing in a circular motion.	*Manual pressure stimulates uterine contractions.*
• Evaluate the color and amount of lochia, and observe for clots.	
Lochia Evaluation Guidelines	
Small: Smaller than a 4-inch stain on the pad; 10 to 25 mL	
Moderate: Smaller than a 6-inch stain; 25 to 50 mL	
Large: Larger than a 6-inch stain; 50 to 80 mL (Leugenbiehl et al, 1990)	
If blood loss exceeds the above guidelines, weigh the perineal pads and the Chux to estimate the blood loss more accurately (1 g = 1 mL).	*Weighing the pads and Chux can provide important information. Because some blood loss is normal, care providers may not otherwise detect excessive blood loss.*

cially if she is not prepared through childbirth education. The nurse can support the woman by keeping her informed about the labor progress and assuring her that the nurse will stay with her. If birth is imminent, the nurse must not leave the mother alone. Auxiliary personnel can be directed to contact the attending physician or CNM, or other physicians/CNMs who are in the facility. The auxiliary personnel should also retrieve the emergency pack ("precip pack"), which should be readily accessible to the birthing/labor rooms. A typical pack contains the following items: a small drape that can be placed under the woman's buttocks to provide a sterile field; a bulb syringe to clear mucus from the newborn's mouth; two sterile clamps (Kelly or Rochester) to clamp the umbilical cord before applying a cord clamp; sterile scissors to cut the umbilical cord; a sterile umbilical cord clamp; a baby blanket to wrap the newborn in after birth; a package of sterile gloves.

As the materials are being gathered, the nurse must remain calm. The woman is reassured by the nurse's composure and feels that the nurse is competent. The primary goal of nursing care is the safe birth of the fetus.

Birth of Infant in Vertex Presentation

The nurse manages precipitous birth in the hospital by encouraging the woman to assume a comfortable position. If time permits, the nurse scrubs her hands with soap and water and puts on sterile gloves. Sterile drapes are placed under the woman's buttocks.

At all times during the birth, the nurse gives clear instructions to the woman, supports her efforts, and provides reassurance. The nurse needs to remain calm and proceed in a slow, confident manner.

When the infant's head crowns, the nurse instructs the woman to breathe rapidly, which decreases her urge to push. The nurse checks whether the amniotic sac is intact. If it is, the nurse tears the sac with a clamp so that the newborn will not breathe in amniotic fluid with the first breath.

The nurse may place an index finger inside the lower portion of the vagina and the thumb on the outer portion of the perineum and gently massage the area to aid in stretching of perineal tissues and to help prevent perineal lacerations. This is called "ironing the perineum."

With one hand, the nurse applies gentle pressure against the fetal head to maintain flexion and prevent it from popping out rapidly. The nurse does not hold the head back forcibly. Rapid birth of the head may tear the woman's perineal tissues. The rapid change in pressure within the fetal head may cause subdural or dural tears. The nurse supports the perineum with the other hand and allows the head to be delivered between contractions.

As the woman continues to breathe rapidly, the nurse inserts one or two fingers along the back of the fetal head to check for the umbilical cord. If the cord is around the neck, the nurse bends her fingers like a fish hook, grasps the cord, and pulls it over the baby's head, loosens it, or slips it down over the shoulders. It is important to check that the cord is not wrapped around more than one time. If the cord is tightly looped and cannot be slipped over the baby's head, the nurse places two clamps on the cord, cuts it between the clamps, and unwinds the cord.

Immediately after birth of the head, first the mouth, throat, and then the nasal passages are suctioned. The nurse places the hand on each side of the head and instructs the woman to push gently so that the rest of the body can be expelled quickly. The newborn must be supported as it emerges.

The newborn is held at the level of the uterus to facilitate blood flow through the umbilical cord. The combination of amniotic fluid and vernix makes the newborn very slippery, so the nurse must be careful to avoid dropping the newborn. The nurse suctions the nose and mouth of the newborn again, using a bulb syringe. The nurse then dries the newborn quickly to prevent heat loss.

As soon as the nurse determines that the newborn's respirations are adequate, the infant can be placed on the mother's abdomen. The newborn's head should be slightly lower than the body to aid drainage of fluid and mucus. The weight of the newborn on the mother's abdomen stimulates uterine contractions, which aid in placental separation. The umbilical cord should not be pulled. The Apgar is assessed at 1 and 5 minutes.

The nurse is alert for signs of placental separation. When these signs are present, the nurse places one hand just above the symphysis pubis to guard the uterus and uses the other hand to maintain gentle downward traction on the cord while instructing the mother to push so that the placenta can be expelled. In some instances the mother can squat, and this usually helps expel the placenta. The nurse inspects the placenta to determine whether it is intact.

The nurse checks the firmness of the uterus. The fundus may be gently massaged to stimulate contractions and decrease bleeding. Putting the newborn to breast also stimulates uterine contractions through release of oxytocin from the pituitary gland.

The umbilical cord may now be cut. Two sterile clamps are placed approximately 2 to 4 inches from the newborn's abdomen. The cord is cut between them with sterile scissors. A sterile cord clamp (Hollister or Hesseltine) can be placed adjacent to the clamp on the newborn's cord, between the clamp and the newborn's abdomen. The clamp must not be placed snugly against the abdomen because the cord will dry and shrink.

The area under the mother's buttocks is cleaned, and her perineum is inspected for lacerations. Bleeding from lacerations may be controlled by pressing a clean perineal pad against the perineum and instructing the woman to keep her thighs together.

If the arrival of the physician or CNM is delayed or if the newborn is having respiratory distress, the newborn should be transported immediately to the nursery. The newborn must be properly identified before he or she leaves the birthing area.

Record Keeping

The following information is noted and placed on a birth record:

1. Position of fetus at birth
2. Presence of cord around neck or shoulder (nuchal cord)
3. Time of birth
4. Apgar scores at 1 and 5 minutes after birth
5. Gender of newborn
6. Time of expulsion of placenta
7. Method of placental expulsion
8. Appearance and intactness of placenta
9. Mother's condition
10. Any medications that were given to mother or newborn (per agency protocol)

Postbirth Interventions

Postbirth interventions are the same as those listed under Nursing Care Management during the Third Stage.

Birth of Infant in Breech Presentation

A significant factor in a breech birth is that the smallest part of the fetus presents first; succeeding parts are progressively larger. The cervix is not as effectively dilated when the fetus is in breech presentation as it is when the fetus is in the vertex position. Therefore, descent is usually slow and may not occur until the cervix is fully dilated and the membranes rupture.

The primary concern in a breech birth is to prevent the entrapment of the head in the cervix. The nurse is advised to avoid intervening until the buttocks are born. Then the nurse pulls down a loop of cord (to avoid stress on its point of insertion) and supports the breech in both hands. The infant's body is lifted slightly upward for birth of the posterior shoulder and arm. The newborn may then be lowered, and the anterior shoulder and arm will pass under the symphysis pubis.

Suprapubic pressure should be applied to maintain the normal flexion of the baby's head and should be continued until the baby is born. The nape of the neck pivots under the symphysis, and the rest of the head is born over the perineum by a movement of flexion.

The remaining birth and postbirth interventions for breech birth are described in the preceding section on precipitous birth of an infant in vertex presentation.

Evaluation

Evaluation provides an opportunity to determine the effectiveness of nursing care. As a result of comprehensive nursing care during the intrapartal period, the following outcomes may be anticipated:

- The mother's physical needs and the psychologic well-being of the family have been maintained and supported.
- The baby's physical and psychologic well-being has been protected and supported.
- The family has had input into the birth process, and members have participated as much as they desired.
- The birth was safe and promoted family cohesiveness.

FOCUS YOUR STUDY

- Admission to the birth setting involves assessment of many physiologic and psychologic factors. The information gained helps the nurse establish priorities of care.
- Before initiating care, the nurse explains what will be done, the reasons, potential benefits and risks, and possible alternatives if appropriate. This helps the woman determine what happens to her body and is a critical element in the process of obtaining informed consent.
- Behavioral responses to labor vary with the phase of labor, the woman's preparation and previous experience, cultural beliefs, and developmental level.
- The adolescent has special needs in the birth setting. Her developmental needs require specialized nursing care.
- Each woman's cultural beliefs affect her need for privacy, expression of discomfort, expectations for the birth, and the role she wishes the father to play in the birth event.
- The laboring woman's comfort may be increased by general comfort measures, supportive relaxation techniques, methods of handling anxiety, controlled breathing, and support by a caring person.
- The laboring woman fears being alone during labor. Even though there is a support person available, the woman's anxiety may be decreased when the nurse remains with her.
- Maternal birthing positions include a wide variety of possibilities, from recumbent to side-lying to sitting, to squatting, to crouching on hands and knees.
- Immediate assessments of the newborn include evaluation of the Apgar score and an abbreviated physical assessment. These early assessments help determine whether there is a need for resuscitation and whether the newborn's adaptation to extrauterine life is progressing normally. The newborn who is not experiencing problems may remain with the parents for an extended period of time following birth.
- Immediate care of the newborn following birth also includes maintaining respirations, promoting warmth, preventing infection, and accurate identification.
- The new parents and their baby are given time together as soon as possible after birth.
- Nursing assessments continue after the birth and are important to ensure that normal physiologic adaptations are taking place.

REFERENCES

American Academy of Pediatrics (AAP) and the American College of Obstetricians and Gynecologists (ACOG) (1997). *Guidelines for perinatal care* (2nd ed.). Washington, DC: Author.

Brown, S., & Lumley, J. (1994). Satisfaction with care in labor and birth: A survey of 790 Australian women. *Birth, 21,* 4.

Bryanton, J., Fraser-Davey, H., & Sullivan, P. (1994). Women's perceptions of nursing support during labor. *Journal of Obstetric, Gynecologic, and Neonatal Nursing, 23,* 638–642.

Calhoun, M. A. (1986). The Vietnamese woman: Health/illness attitudes and behaviors. In P. N. Stern (Ed.), *Women, health and culture.* Washington, DC: Hemisphere.

Cesario, S. K. (1998). Should cameras be allowed in the delivery room? *Maternal-Child Nursing Journal, 23,* 87–91.

Clark, M. J. (1996). *Nursing in the community.* Stamford, CT: Appleton & Lange.

Cook, A., & Wilcox, G. (1997, April). Pressuring pain. *AWHONN Lifelines, 1,* 36–41.

Cunningham, F. G., MacDonald, P. C., Gant, N. F., Leveno, K. J., Gilstrap, L. C., Hankins, G. D. V., & Clark, S. L. (1997). *Williams obstetrics* (20th ed.) (pp 261–378). Stamford, CT: Appleton & Lange.

dePaula, T., Lagana, K., & Gonzalez-Ramirez, L. (1996). Mexican Americans. In L. G. Lipson, L. L. Dibble, & R. A. Minarik (Eds.), *Culture and nursing care: A pocket guide* (chapter 20, pp 203–221). San Francisco: UCSF Nursing Press.

Gannon, J. M. (1992). Delivery on the hands and knees. *Journal of Nurse-Midwifery, 37,* 48.

Hutchinson, M. K., & Baqi-Aziz, M. (1994). Nursing care of the childbearing Muslim family. *Journal of Obstetric, Gynecologic, and Neonatal Nursing, 23,* 67.

Johnson, S. (1996). Hmong. In L. G. Lipson, S. L. Dibble, & R. A. Minarik (Eds.), *Culture and nursing care: A pocket guide* (chapter 16, pp 161–168). San Francisco: UCSF Nursing Press.

Kaczorowski, J., Levitt, C., Hanvey, L., Avard, D., & Chance, K. (1998). A national survey of use of obstetric procedures and technologies in Canadian hospitals: Routine or based on existing evidence? *Birth, 25,* 11–18.

Kennell, J. H. (1994). The time has come to reassess delivery room routines. *Birth, 21,* 49.

Khazoyan, C. M., & Anderson, N. L. R. (1994). Latinas' expectations for their partners during childbirth. *Maternal-Child Nursing Journal, 19,* 226.

Kramer, J. (1996). American Indians. In J. G. Lipson, S. L. Dibble, & R. A. Minarik (Eds.), *Culture and nursing care: A pocket guide* (chapter 3, pp 11–22). San Francisco: UCSF Nursing Press.

LaDu, E. B. (1985). Childbirth care for Hmong families. *Maternal-Child Nursing Journal, 10,* 382.

Lipson, J. G., Dibble, S. L., & Minarik, P. A. (1996). *Culture and nursing care: A pocket guide.* San Francisco: UCSF Nursing Press.

Ludka, L. M., & Roberts, C. C. (1993). Eating and drinking in labor: A literature review. *Journal of Nurse-Midwifery, 38,* 199.

Leugenbiehl, D. L., Brophy, G. H., Artigue, G. S., Phillips, K. E., & Flak, R. J. (1990). Standardized assessment of blood loss. *Maternal-Child Nursing Journal 15*(4), 241–244.

Mackey, M. C., & Lock, S. E. (1989). Women's expectations of the labor and delivery nurse. *Journal of Obstetric, Gynecologic, and Neonatal Nursing, 18,* 505.

Mackey, M. C., & Stepans, M. E. (1993). Women's evaluation of their labor and delivery nurses. *Journal of Obstetric, Gynecologic, and Neonatal Nursing, 23,* 413.

McCartney, P. R. (1998). The birth ball—are you using it in your practice setting? *Maternal-Child Nursing Journal, 23,* 218.

McKay, S., & Roberts, J. (1990). Obstetrics by ear: Maternal and caregiver perceptions of the meaning of maternal sounds during second stage of labor. *Journal of Nurse-Midwifery, 35,* 266.

McKay, S., & Smith S. (1993). "What are they talking about? Is something wrong?" Information sharing during the second stage of labor. *Birth 20,* 142.

McNiven, P. S., Williams, J. I., Hodnett, E., Kaufman, K., & Hannah, M. E. (1998). An early labor assessment program: A randomized, controlled trial. *Birth, 25,* 5–10.

Mills, C. B. (1997). Taking time to care: Making ways to help teen parents. *AWHONN Lifelines, 1,* 70–71.

Morrow, K. (1986). Transcultural midwifery: Adapting to Hmong birthing customs in California. *Journal of Nurse-Midwifery, 31,* 285.

Nurses' Association of the American College of Obstetricians and Gynecologists (NAACOG OGN) Nursing Practice Resource. (1990). *Fetal heart rate auscultation.* Washington, DC: NAACOG.

Proctor, S. (1998). What determines quality in maternity care? Comparing the perceptions of childbearing women and midwives. *Birth, 25,* 85–93.

Reynolds, J. L. (1997). Post-traumatic stress disorder after childbirth: The phenomenon of traumatic birth. *Canadian Medical Association Journal, 156,* 831–835.

Righard, L., & Alade, M. O. (1990, November 3). Effect of delivery room routines on success of first breast-feed. *Lancet, 336*(8723), 1105–1107.

Schneiderman, J. U. (1997). Rituals of placenta disposal. *AWHONN Lifelines, 23,* 142–143.

Shelp, S. G. (1997). Your patient is deaf, now what? *RN, 60*(2), 37–38, 40.

Sleep, J., Roberts, J., & Chalmers, I. (1989). Care during the second stage of labor. In I. Chalmers, M. Enkin, & M. J. N. C. Keirse (Eds.), *Effective care in pregnancy and childbirth: Vol. 2. Childbirth.* New York: Oxford University Press.

Spector, R. E. (1996). *Cultural diversity in health and illness.* Stamford, CT: Appleton & Lange.

Strong, T. H. (1997). The effect of amnioinfusion on the duration of labor. *Obstetrics and Gynocology, 89,* 1044–1046.

Uyoo, A. (1990). *Korean traditional childbearing.* Seoul, S. Korea: Seoul University Publishing.

Vincent, P. (1995). Traditional and modern thought about the placenta. *Midwives, 108,* 325–327.

Waymire, V. (1997). A triggering time: Childbirth may recall sexual abuse memories. *AWHONN Lifelines, 23,* 47–50.

Weaver, D. F. (1990). Nurses' views on the meaning of touch in obstetrical nursing practice. *Journal of Obstetric, Gynecologic, and Neonatal Nursing, 19,* 157.

Weigers, T. A., van der Zee, J., & Keirse, J. N. J. (1998). Transfer from home to hospital: What is its effect on the experience of childbirth? *Birth, 25,* 14–19.

Wuitchik, M., Bakal, D., & Lipshitz, J. (1989). The clinical significance of pain and cognitive activity in latent labor. *Obstetrics and Gynecology, 73*(1), 35.

Pain Management during Birth

21

WE HAD ATTENDED ALL OF OUR CLASSES AND PRACTICED through the last few weeks, but I was not ready for the amount of discomfort that I felt during my labor. I had hoped to go through the whole labor and birth without any medications, but we had talked about it and knew that if I felt I needed something, that it would be all right. My nurse was also helpful and supportive of my decision. She helped me feel that I was making a good decision and that I wasn't failing somehow.

Key Terms

Epidural block
Local anesthesia
Pudendal block
Regional analgesia
Regional anesthesia
Spinal block

Objectives

- Describe the use of systemic drugs to promote pain relief during labor.
- Compare the major types of regional analgesia and anesthesia, including area affected, advantages, disadvantages, techniques, and nursing implications.
- Discuss possible complications of regional anesthesia.
- Describe the major inhalation and intravenous anesthetics used to provide general anesthesia.
- Delineate the major complications of general anesthesia.

THE CHILDBEARING WOMAN EXPERIENCES many demanding sensations and discomforts during labor and birth. The nurse can assist her to have a positive childbirth experience by providing effective comfort measures. Nursing interventions directed toward pain relief begin with nonpharmacologic measures, such as providing information, support, and physical comfort. Measures to promote comfort include back rubs, the application of cool cloths to her forehead, showers, whirlpool (Jacuzzi), and encouragement in practicing breathing techniques. Some laboring women need no further interventions. For other women, the progression of labor brings increasing discomfort that interferes with their ability to perform breathing techniques and maintain any sense of comfort. Pharmacologic analgesics may be used to decrease discomfort, increase relaxation, and reestablish the woman's ability to participate in her labor.

Methods of Pain Relief

Pain and discomfort during labor may be relieved by several different methods. In addition to the nursing measures and patterned-paced breathing discussed in Chapter 20, systemic drugs, regional nerve blocks (epidural, spinal, and combined epidural-spinal), and local anesthesic blocks (pudendal and local anesthesia of the perineum) are available.

The methods are not mutually exclusive, and any one may be used in combination with other comfort measures. Systemic drugs such as butorphanol tartrate (Stadol) promote the woman's comfort during contractions and increase her ability to rest between the contractions. Regional nerve blocks, such as an epidural, may be used to relieve the discomfort of labor contractions, and because the epidural does not cause drowsiness, the laboring woman can remain awake and be involved in the labor and birth process.

Although systemic analgesics and local anesthetic agents affect the fetus, so do the pain and stress experienced by the laboring woman. The pain and stress of labor increase the woman's ventilation and oxygen consumption, which decreases the amount of oxygen available to the fetus. In addition, the pain and stress can lead to metabolic acidosis and the release of catecholamine, which cause the maternal vessels to constrict, which in turn decreases oxygen and nutrient supply to the fetus (Russell & Reynolds, 1997).

Plasma epinephrine and norepinephrine levels are higher during labor than in the last trimester of pregnancy. The body's response to the pain and stress of labor causes a release of high levels of catecholamines. When discussing medication alternatives with any couple, the nurse should take a positive approach to help them understand that if the woman's pain and anxiety are more than she can cope with, the adverse physiologic effects on the fetus may be as great as would occur with the administration of a small amount of an analgesic agent.

Many couples who have had childbirth education approach childbirth confident that the psychoprophylactic techniques they have learned will enable them to cope with the discomforts of labor. Many expectant parents experience a great deal of "peer pressure" from many sources to have the "ideal" birth experience. The parents may plan a natural childbirth with no medications, except perhaps local infiltration anesthesia for episiotomy repair. If the labor is more intensive and painful than expected, the desire for analgesia may elicit a sense of inadequacy and a feeling of guilt. The nurse plays a very special role in assisting a woman and her partner to explore alterations in their original plan. Reassuring the woman that accepting analgesia for discomfort is not a failure is important in maintaining the woman's self-esteem. The emphasis should be placed on the goal of a healthy, satisfying outcome for the family.

Pharmacologic Methods

The goal of pharmacologic analgesia during labor is to provide maximal pain relief with minimal risk for the woman and fetus. Three factors must be considered in the use of analgesic agents: (1) the effects on the woman, (2) the effects on the fetus, and (3) the effects on the labor contractions.

The effects on the mother are of primary importance because the well-being of the fetus depends on adequate functioning of the maternal cardiopulmonary system. Any alteration of function that disturbs the woman's homeostatic mechanism affects the fetal environment. Maintaining the maternal respiratory rate and blood pressure within normal range is thus of prime importance. The use of electronic fetal monitoring (EFM) provides a means of accurately assessing the effects of pharmacologic agents on uterine contractions.

All systemic drugs used for pain relief during labor cross the placental barrier by simple diffusion, with some agents crossing more readily than others. Drug action in the body depends on the rate at which the substance is metabolized by liver enzymes and excreted by the kidneys. The fetal liver enzymes and renal systems are inadequate to metabolize analgesic agents, so high doses remain active in fetal circulation for a prolonged period of time. The fetal brain receives a greater amount of the cardiac output than the neonatal brain. The percentage of blood volume flowing to the brain increases even further during intrauterine stress, so the hypoxic fetus receives an even larger amount of a depressant drug. The blood–brain barrier is more permeable at the time of birth, a factor that also increases the amount of drug carried to the central nervous system.

Administration of Pharmacologic Analgesic Agents

The optimal time for administering analgesia is determined after a complete assessment of many factors. In general, an analgesic agent is administered to nulliparas when the active phase of labor is well established (cervix has dilated to 5 or 6 cm) and to multiparas when the cervix has reached 3 or 4 cm dilatation. This is only a generalization, however; the character of each labor must be taken into account. Analgesia given too early may prolong labor and depress the fetus. Analgesia given too late is of no value to the woman and may cause neonatal respiratory depression. In many institutions, the nurse decides when to give the analgesic agent prescribed by the physician or certified nurse-midwife (CNM) or certified registered nurse-anesthetist. This decision is based on a complete assessment of the woman and the progress of labor.

Maternal Assessment

- The woman is willing to receive medication after being advised about it.
- Vital signs are stable.

Fetal Assessment

- The fetal heart rate (FHR) is between 120 and 160 beats/minute, reactive nonstress test (NST) (accelerations of FHR are present with fetal movement), short-term variability is present, long-term variability is average, and periodic late decelerations or nonperiodic (variable) decelerations are absent.
- The fetus is at term.
- Meconium staining is not present.

Assessment of Labor

- The contraction pattern is well established.
- The cervix is dilated at least 4 to 5 cm in nulliparas and 3 to 4 cm in multiparas.
- The fetal presenting part is engaged.
- There is progressive descent of the fetal presenting part. No complications that would preclude administering an analgesic agent are present.

If normal parameters are absent, the nurse may need to complete further assessments with the physician/CNM.

Prior to administering the medication, the nurse once again ascertains whether the woman has a history of any drug reactions or allergies and provides information regarding the medication (Table 21–1). After giving the medication, the nurse records the drug name, dose, route, site, and the woman's blood pressure and pulse (before and after) on the electronic fetal monitor strip and on the woman's record. If the woman is alone, side rails should be raised to provide safety. The FHR is assessed for possible effects of the medication. See Essential Precautions in Practice: During Administration of Analgesia and Anesthesia.

TABLE 21–1 What Women Need to Know About Pain Relief Medications

Before receiving medications, the woman should understand the following:

- Type of medication administered
- Route of administration
- Expected effects of medication
- Implications for fetus/neonate
- Safety measures needed (for example, remain in bed with side rails up)

Oral analgesics are not used because they are poorly absorbed and gastric emptying time is prolonged during labor. The intramuscular and intravenous routes are used instead. For intramuscular administration, the needle must be of sufficient length to penetrate the muscle rather than only the subcutaneous fat. The intravenous route is preferred because it results in prompt, smooth, and more predictable action with a smaller total dose than the intramuscular route. When an agent is given intravenously, it is suggested that the intravenous injection be given with the onset of a contraction, when the blood flow to the uterus and the fetus is normally decreased.

When an analgesic medication is administered by intramuscular or subcutaneous route, it will take a few minutes for the effect to be felt. The nurse can continue with other supportive measures to enhance comfort, such as ensuring a quiet environment in the room, providing a back rub or cool cloth, assisting with relaxation exercises and visualizations, or providing therapeutic touch until the effect of the medication is felt. When the medication begins to take effect, the woman may sleep between contractions. This short period of rest helps her relax and can

ESSENTIAL PRECAUTIONS IN PRACTICE

During Administration of Analgesia and Anesthesia

Wear disposable gloves when performaing the following actions:

- Administering intravenous medications for analgesia to prevent exposure to blood.
- Starting intravenous fluids prior to regional blocks.
- Assisting the woman into position for an epidural or spinal. While the nurse assists the woman into position, the nurse may inadvertently be exposed to vaginal fluids or amniotic fluid.

REMEMBER to wash your hands prior to putting on the disposable gloves and AGAIN immediately after you remove the gloves.

For further information, consult OSHA and CDC guidelines.

restore her energy. When an intravenous route is prescribed by the CNM/physician, the woman will feel the effect of the drug within a couple of minutes, so if any change of position is necessary or if the woman needs to void, the nurse may suggest that these activities be completed before the drug is administered. Some women may be so uncomfortable that they do not want anything except the medication. In this case, administering the medication first would be more helpful for the woman.

Narcotic Analgesics

Narcotic analgesic agents that are injected into the circulation have their primary action at sites in the brain. Specifically, a narcotic that diffuses out of cerebral capillaries and reaches the periventricular/periaqueductal gray area of the brain will activate the neurons that descend to the spinal cord and inhibit the transmission of pain impulses in the substantia gelatinosa (Paradise, 1994). Nausea and vomiting are produced by stimulation of the medullary chemoreceptor trigger zone.

A brief discussion of some selected narcotic analgesic agents appears in the next section.

Butorphanol Tartrate (Stadol)

Butorphanol tartrate (Stadol) is a mixed agonist-antagonist agent. The analgesic potency is 30 to 40 times that of meperidine and 7 times that of morphine (*PDR Nurse's Handbook*, 1999). Administration of butorphanol will reverse the analgesic effect of other opioids or narcotics in the woman's body and precipitate withdrawal in drug-dependent individuals. For this reason, it is important to assess each woman's history of drug use during the admission assessment; if she has been using drugs, she should not receive butorphanol.

For the woman in labor, butorphanol is most frequently given by the intravenous route; however, it can also be given by intramuscular injection. When administered intravenously, the recommended dose is 1 to 2 mg (the smallest dose is most frequently used); the onset of action is rapid; peak analgesia occurs in 30 to 60 minutes (*PDR Nurse's Handbook*, 1999), and duration is 3 to 4 hours (Karch, 1999). If given by intramuscular route, the recommended dose is 1 to 2 mg, although 2 mg is the most usual dose; onset of action occurs in 10 to 15 minutes; peak analgesia occurs in 30 to 60 minutes (*PDR Nurse's Handbook*, 1999); and duration is 3 to 4 hours (Karch, 1999).

Respiratory depression of both the mother and fetus/newborn can occur. The effects of butorphanol (Stadol) can be reversed with naloxone (Narcan).

NURSING CARE MANAGEMENT

Administering butorphanol with other central nervous system depressants, such as sedatives, phenothiazides, and other tranquilizers, hypnotic agents, and general anesthetics, exacerbates respiratory depression and other effects. For this reason, the nurse should evaluate the woman's respiratory and cardiac status by careful observation of vital signs and pulse oximetry. The woman's level of consciousness should also be checked frequently. Continuous electronic monitoring of the fetal heart rate pattern is recommended. Respiratory depression in the mother or fetus/newborn can be reversed by naloxone (Narcan), which is a specific antagonist for this agent. A slightly depressed newborn is not likely to have prolonged drowsiness or sluggishness, however, because the metabolites of butorphanol are inactive.

Although urinary retention is rare, the nurse should be alert for bladder distention when a woman has received this drug for analgesia during labor, has intravenous fluids infusing, and receives regional anesthesia (epidural or subarachnoid block) for the birth.

Nalbuphine Hydrochloride (Nubain)

Like butorphanol, nalbuphine hydrochloride (Nubain) is a synthetic agonist-antagonist narcotic analgesic and may precipitate drug withdrawal if the woman is physically dependent on narcotics (*PDR Nurse's Handbook*, 1999). Nalbuphine crosses the placenta to the fetus and can cause fetal distress and neonatal respiratory depression (Karch, 1999). Nalbuphine may be given by the intramuscular (IM), subcutaneous (SC), or intravenous (IV) route. It is most frequently given by the intravenous route in the birth setting. The usual dose for adults is 10 mg/70 kg (Karch, 1999). If given intravenously, onset of action occurs in 2 to 3 minutes, peak of action occurs in 15 to 20 minutes, and duration is 3 to 6 hours (Karch, 1999). When given by the IM or SC route, the onset of action occurs in less than 15 minutes, peak of action occurs in 30 to 60 minutes, and duration is 3 to 6 hours (Karch, 1999). When given by the IV route, nalbuphine may be given directly into the tubing of a running IV infusion; 10 mg should be administered over 3 to 5 minutes (Karch, 1999). Adverse effects in the woman include respiratory depression, drowsiness, dizziness, crying, blurred vision, nausea, diaphoresis, and urinary urgency (Karch, 1999).

CRITICAL THINKING IN PRACTICE

Luisa Silva, a 33-year-old G1 P0, is 32 weeks pregnant. She is trying to decide whether she should accept any analgesia during her labor. She has finished childbirth education classes and wants an unmedicated labor and birth. She says, "I want to do this on my own, but I'm afraid it may be too much. Will it be OK if I need to take something?" What will you tell her?

Answers can be found in Appendix I.

NURSING CARE MANAGEMENT

The nurse assesses the woman's history to identify contraindications to use of nalbuphine, such as the possibility of current narcotic drug dependence, sensitivity to sulfites, and history of asthma (*PDR Nurse's Handbook*, 1999). If no contraindications exist, the intravenous route is frequently used during labor. The woman's respiratory rate and quality of respirations and characteristics of the FHR must be carefully assessed. Anticipation of urinary urgency is important. Because the woman may experience dizziness and sedation, use of a bedpan may be necessary.

Opiate Antagonist: Naloxone (Narcan)

Because naloxone (Narcan) is an antagonist with little or no agonistic effect, it exhibits little pharmacologic activity in the absence of narcotic agents. Naloxone can be used to reverse the mild respiratory depression, sedation, and hypotension following small doses of opiates (Karch, 1999). Naloxone (Narcan) exerts its effect by competing for opiate receptors and taking the place of the opiate on the receptor. In this manner, naloxone blocks or reverses the action of the narcotic analgesic (*PDR Nurse's Handbook*, 1999). The drug is useful for respiratory depression caused by butorphanol (Stadol) and nalbuphine (Nubain) (Karch, 1999). Naloxone is the drug of choice when the depressant is unknown because it will cause no further depression. Naloxone's duration of action is less than that of most narcotic analgesics, however, respiratory depression may return as the antagonistic effect of naloxone wears off.

The expected action is reversal of narcotic-induced respiratory depression. Adverse actions include nausea and vomiting, sweating, and hypertension due to reversal of the narcotic depression. When used postoperatively, excessive dosages of naloxone may cause ventricular tachycardia and fibrillation, hypotension or hypertension, and pulmonary edema (Karch, 1999; *PDR Nurse's Handbook*, 1999).

For the laboring adult woman, initial recommended dosage is 0.4 mg to 2 mg intravenously; if necessary, the dose may be repeated at 2- to 3-minute intervals (Karch, 1999; *PDR Nurse's Handbook*, 1999). If no response is obtained after a total of 10 mg has been administered, diagnosis should be questioned. When naloxone is administered intravenously, onset of action occurs in 2 minutes, peak effect occurs in 5 to 15 minutes, and the duration of action varies depending on the dose but may be as short as 45 minutes (*PDR Nurse's Handbook*, 1999) or as long as 4 to 6 hours (Karch, 1999). If the expectant mother is very young, or of low weight, the appropriate dosage may need to be calculated on the basis of milligrams per kilogram of weight. Initial dose for a child is 0.005 to 0.01 mg IV at 2- to 3-minute intervals until the respiratory depression is relieved (*PDR Nurse's Handbook*, 1999). When the age or size of the laboring mother brings up questions, the nurse should calculate the expected dosage and compare it to the physician-prescribed dosage. If the prescribed dosage exceeds the mg per kg dose, the nurse must consult with the physician prior to administering the medication.

Naloxone may also be administered to the newborn immediately after birth if needed (see Drug Guide: Naloxone [Narcan] in Chapter 28 for discussion of neonatal dosages). After naloxone administration, the newborn should be observed for at least 4 hours in a special care area (such as an admission nursery) before transfer to regular care.

NURSING CARE MANAGEMENT

When naloxone is administered to the laboring mother or to the newborn just after birth, resuscitative measures and trained personnel should be readily available in the event that additional respiratory support is needed. When administered to the laboring mother, naloxone may be injected undiluted at a rate of 0.4 mg over 15 seconds into the tubing of a running IV infusion. Naloxone may also be diluted in an IV infusion of 5% dextrose or normal saline for a titrated dose. Titrated doses of naloxone are more likely to be used in a postoperative setting, when epidural analgesia has been given with a cesarean birth. After the direct IV administration, maternal vital signs should be obtained at 5-minute intervals until the respiratory rate has been stabilized and then every 30 minutes (Karch, 1999). The duration of the drug is shorter (minutes to hours) than the analgesic drug it is acting as an antagonist for, so the nurse must be alert to the return of respiratory depression and the need for repeated doses. Naloxone should be given with caution in women with known or suspected opiate dependence because it may precipitate severe withdrawal symptoms in the mother and the newborn.

Sedatives

In current labor and birth practice, barbiturates are used primarily in the very early latent phase of labor, when the cervix is long, closed, and thick and rest is prescribed for the expectant woman. An oral dose of secobarbital (Seconal) or pentobarbital (Nembutal) promotes relaxation and allows the woman to sleep for a few hours. Upon the woman's awakening, contractions have either ceased (ie, the woman was in false labor) or contractions return and take on a regular pattern that effects changes in cervical dilatation and effacement.

Regional Analgesia and Anesthesia

Regional anesthesia is the temporary and reversible loss of sensation produced by injecting an anesthetic agent (called a local anesthetic) into an area that will bring the agent into direct contact with nervous tissue. Loss of sensation occurs because the local agents stabilize the cell membrane, which prevents initiation and transmission of nerve impulses. The regional anesthetic blocks most commonly used in childbearing include epidural, spinal, or combined epidural-spinal. Epidural blocks may be used for analgesia during labor and vaginal birth and for anesthesia during cesarean birth. A combined epidural-spinal block may also be used. With this approach, the epidural is used to provide analgesia for labor, and the spinal provides anesthesia for birth or analgesia following birth.

An epidural relieves pain associated with the first stage of labor by blocking the sensory nerves supplying the uterus. Pain associated with the second stage of labor and with birth can be alleviated with epidural, combined epidural-spinal, and pudendal blocks (see Figure 21–1 and Table 21–2).

Until fairly recently, the same anesthetic agents used for regional epidural anesthesia were also used to produce **regional analgesia** (pain relief) during labor. This approach was somewhat problematic because anesthetic agents alter the transmission of impulses to the bladder, making voiding difficult. The agents also interfere with the woman's ability to maintain her blood pressure and move her lower extremities. In addition, the descent of the fetus may be slowed because the agents also decrease the woman's ability to push effectively during the second stage of labor (Thorpe & Breedlove, 1996; Youngstrom, Baker, & Miller, 1996). To address these problems, regional analgesia is now obtained by injecting a narcotic agent such as fentanyl along with only a small amount of a local anesthetic agent. This approach yields effective pain relief without the troubling side effects of epidural anesthesia. The woman's pain is relieved, her blood pressure remains stable, and, because there is no motor blockage, she is able to move about freely and ambulate. At times she may have difficulty urinating, but this can be relieved by bladder catheterization (Youngstrom et al, 1996).

The intrathecal injection of narcotics results in another type of regional analgesia. In this case, the narcotic is injected into the subarachnoid space. Fentanyl citrate and preservative-free morphine are the most frequently used narcotic agents. The woman's pain is usually relieved; however, she may experience urinary retention. Delayed respiratory depression may also occur and seems to be more frequent with the use of morphine (Karch, 1999).

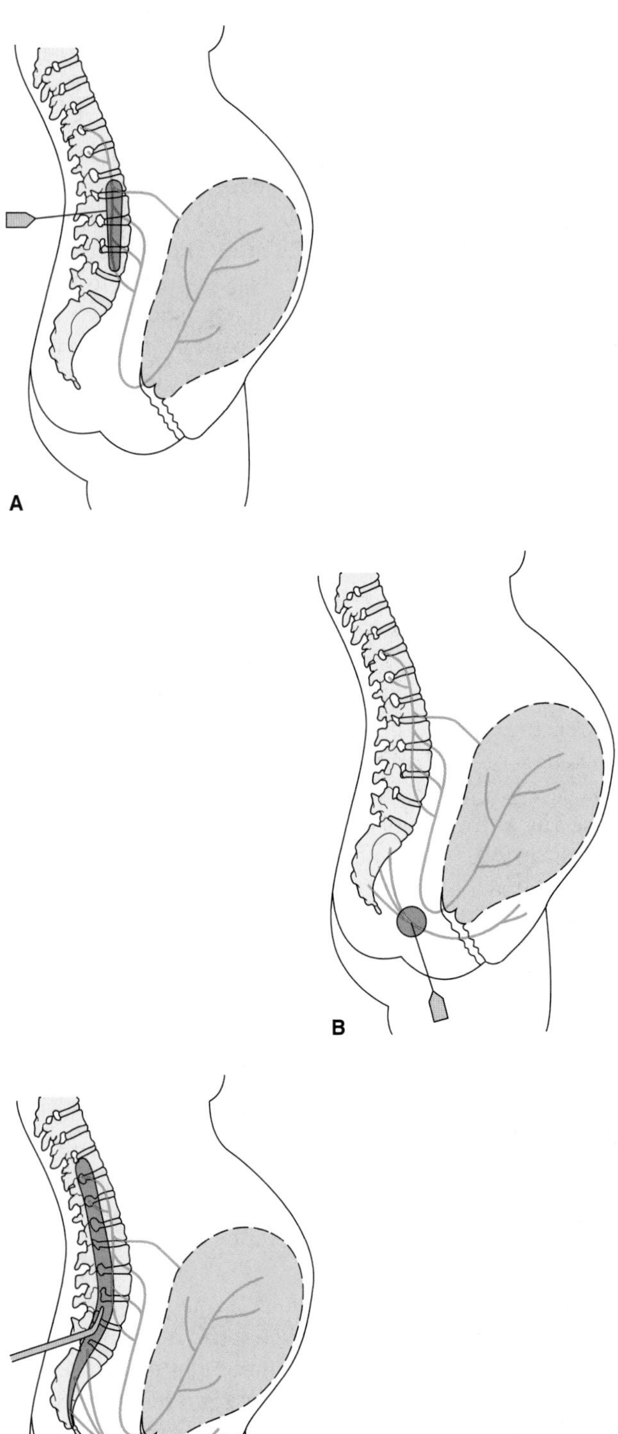

FIGURE 21–1 Schematic diagram showing pain pathways and sites of interruption. ***A,*** Lumbar sympathetic (spinal) block: relief of uterine pain only. ***B,*** Pudendal block: relief of perineal pain. ***C,*** Lumbar epidural block: Dark area demonstrates peridural (epidural) space and nerves affected, and the gray tube represents a continuous plastic catheter. SOURCE: Bonica JJ: *Principles and Practice of Obstetric Analgesia and Anesthesia.* Philadelphia: Davis, 1972, pp 492, 512, 521, 614.

TABLE 21–2 Summary of Commonly Used Regional Blocks

Type of Block	Areas Affected	Use during Labor and Birth	Nursing Actions
Lumbar epidural	Uterus, cervix, vagina, and perineum	Given in first stage and second stage of labor.	Assess woman's knowledge regarding the block. Act as advocate to help her obtain further information if needed. Monitor maternal blood pressure to detect the major side effect, which is hypotension. Provide support and comfort. See Lumbar Epidural Critical Pathway for further nursing actions.
Combined spinal epidural	Uterus, cervix, vagina, and perineum	Spinal analgesia may be given in latent phase for pain relief. Epidural is given when active labor begins.	Assess woman's knowledge regarding the block. Monitor maternal vital signs and FHR staus. Provide comfort measures.
Pudendal	Perineum and lower vagina	Given in the second stage just prior to birth to provide anesthesia for episiotomy or for low forceps birth.	Assess woman's knowledge regarding the block. Act as advocate to help her obtain further information if needed.
Local infiltration	Perineum	Administered just before birth to provide anesthesia for episiotomy.	Assess woman's knowledge regarding the block. Provide information as needed. Provide comfort and support. Observe perineum for bruising or other discoloration in the recovery period.

It is important for the laboring woman to have information regarding the regional analgesia or anesthesia that is to be administered. As with other procedures, the woman needs to know how the block is given, the expected effect on her and the fetus, advantages and disadvantages, and possible risks. Many women discuss possible analgesic and anesthetic blocks with their physician/CNM during the pregnancy. If they have not, it will be important for them to have an opportunity to ask questions and obtain information prior to receiving any regional analgesia or anesthesia while in labor.

Anesthetic Agents for Regional Blocks

Local anesthetic agents block nerve conduction by impairing propagation of the action potential in axons. The agents interact directly with specific receptors on the sodium channel, inhibiting sodium ion influx (Russell & Reynolds, 1997). The types of nerve fibers are differentially sensitive to the various anesthetic agents. In general, the smaller the fiber, the more sensitive it is to local agents. For example, it is possible to block the small C and A delta fibers, which transmit pain, touch, and temperature, without blocking the larger A alpha, A beta, and A gamma fibers, which continue to maintain a sense of pressure, muscle tone, position sense, and motor function (Russell & Reynolds, 1997).

Absorption of local anesthetic agents depends primarily on the vascularity of the area of injection. The agents also increase blood flow by causing vasodilation. High concentrations cause greater vasodilation. Good maternal physical condition or a high metabolic rate aids absorption. Malnutrition, dehydration, electrolyte imbalance, and cardiovascular and pulmonary problems increase the potential for toxic effects. The pH of tissues affects the rate of absorption, which has implications for fetal complications, such as acidosis. The addition of vasoconstrictors, such as epinephrine, delays absorption and prolongs the anesthetic effect. Recent studies have demonstrated that epinephrine decreases uteroplacental blood flow, making it an undesirable additive in many situations. The breakdown of local anesthetics in the body is accomplished by the liver and plasma esterase, and the resulting substance is eliminated by the kidneys. It is important to use the weakest concentration and the smallest amount necessary to produce the desired results.

Types of Local Anesthetic Agents

Three types of local anesthetic agents are currently available—esters, amides, and opiates. The ester type includes procaine hydrochloride (Novocain), chloroprocaine hydrochloride (Nesacaine), and tetracaine hydrochloride (Pontocaine). Esters are rapidly metabolized; therefore, toxic maternal levels are not as likely to be reached, and placental transfer to the fetus is prevented. Amide types include bupivacaine hydrochloride (Marcaine), mepivacaine hydrochloride (Carbocaine) and lidocaine hydrochloride (Xylocaine). Amide types are more powerful and longer-acting agents. They readily cross the placenta, can be measured in the fetal circulation, and affect the fetus for a prolonged period.

Opioids are used with epidural blocks to produce anagelsia for labor. Some of the agents being used include morphine, fentanyl, butorphanol, and meperidine (Russell & Reynolds, 1997). When only opioids are used epidurally, the amount of pain relief is not as effective, especially toward the end of labor; therefore, a combination of opioids and a low dose of a local anesthetic agent are given (Russell & Reynolds, 1997). The mechanism of action seems to involve specific opiate receptors in the spinal cord (Russell & Reynolds, 1997).

A variety of anesthetic agents and a wide range of doses have been used for epidural anesthesia with varying results. The most commonly used agents are lidocaine 2% with epinephrine 1:200,000, bupivacaine 0.5%, and 2-chloroprocaine 3%. Each agent provides adequate anesthesia with 15 to 20 mL of the solution, but each has been identified with side effects. The pharmacology of each drug must be understood before it is used.

Adverse Maternal Reactions to Anesthetic Agents

Reactions to local anesthetic agents range from mild symptoms to cardiovascular collapse. Mild reactions include palpitations, vertigo, tinnitus, apprehension, confusion, headache, and a metallic taste in the mouth. Moderate reactions include more severe degrees of mild symptoms plus nausea and vomiting, hypotension, and muscle twitching, which may progress to convulsions and loss of consciousness. The severe reactions are sudden loss of consciousness, coma, severe hypotension, bradycardia, respiratory depression, and cardiac arrest. High concentrations of the agents may also cause local toxic effects on tissues. It is important to remember that when the mother experiences an adverse reaction, the fetus is also affected.

Systemic toxic reactions most commonly occur with an excessive dose through too great a concentration or too large a volume. Accidental intravenous injection that suddenly increases the amount of the drug in maternal circulation results in depression of vasomotor, respiratory, and other medullary centers of the brain. It also depresses the heart and peripheral vascular bed. A massive intravascular dose can result in sudden circulatory collapse within 1 minute. Reactions to subcutaneous and extradural injection occur in 5 to 40 minutes. The short-acting agent (procaine) can produce toxic reactions in 10 to 15 minutes, and the long-acting agents (mepivacaine) in 20 to 40 minutes. It is imperative that the woman is under close supervision by knowledgeable personnel throughout the time that the agent is being used and that an intravenous line is in place.

If epinephrine has been added to the anesthetic agent to prolong the anesthesia, it is necessary to differentiate between reaction to the anesthetic agent and to the epinephrine. Reaction to epinephrine is characterized by pallor, perspiration, a greater increase in blood pressure and pulse than occurs with reactions to anesthetic agents, and dyspnea.

Psychogenic reactions such as severe anxiety, hallucinations, inability to move or speak, or catatonic appearance can also occur, with symptoms similar to those occurring with systemic toxic reactions. This phenomenon may occur as the procedure is begun and prior to the injection of the anesthetic agent. Regardless of the cause, the symptoms must be treated.

Allergic reactions to anesthetic agents may also occur. The manifestations of the antigen-antibody reaction include urticaria, laryngeal edema, joint pain, swelling of the tongue, and bronchospasm.

Interventions

Treatment of Systemic Toxicity Preferred treatment of mild toxicity involves the administration of oxygen by mask and intravenous injection of a short-acting barbiturate to decrease anxiety. The clinician should anticipate the possibility of convulsions or cardiovascular collapse and make appropriate preparations to treat them. Specific nursing interventions in the treatment of systemic toxicity are included in the Critical Pathway for Epidural Anesthesia on pages 595 to 597.

Treatment of Convulsions The best treatment for convulsions is to establish the airway and administer 100% oxygen. Thiopental or diazepam may be administered to stop convulsions. Small doses are adequate and help avoid cardiorespiratory depression.

Treatment of Sudden Cardiovascular Collapse In sudden cardiovascular collapse, an airway must be established as cardiopulmonary resuscitation begins. Intravenous fluids are increased, and emergency cesarean birth may be started immediately.

Adverse Maternal Reactions to Epidural or Intrathecal Opioids

The most common side effects include pruritus, nausea and vomiting, vertigo, drowsiness, respiratory depression, and urinary retention. During administration, the woman may also experience respiratory depression and urinary retention.

Lumbar Epidural Block

A lumbar **epidural block** involves injection of a local anesthetic agent into the epidural space. The epidural space is a potential space between the dura mater and the ligamentum flavum extending from the base of the skull to the end of the sacral canal (Figure 21–2). It contains areolar tissue, fat, lymphatics, and the internal vertebral venous plexus. Access to the space is through the lumbar area. The technique is most often used as a continuous block to provide analgesia and anesthesia from active labor through the birth and episiotomy repair.

Lumbar epidural block has become fairly common during labor and birth. In the United States, more than 50% of cesarean births are performed under epidural block (Downing, Johnson, Gonzalez, Arney, Herman, & Johnson, 1997). Use of epidural blocks in Great Britain averages around 25%. However, the rate varies greatly

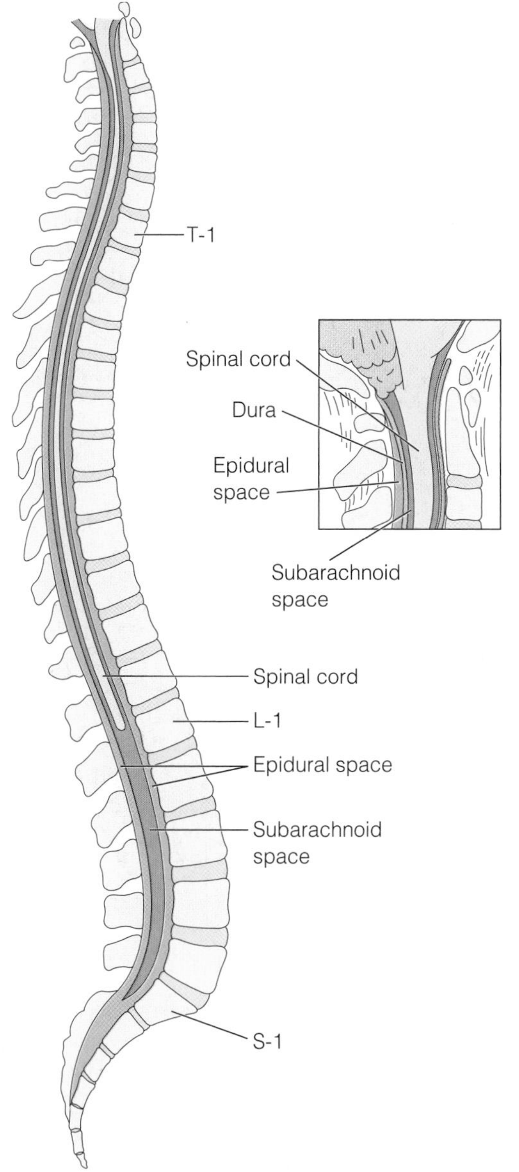

FIGURE 21–2 The epidural space lies between the dura mater and the ligamentum flavum, extending from the base of the skull to the end of the sacral canal.

from one area to another; the rate is greater than 80% in the southeast of England but only 10% in Northern Ireland (Seymour, 1997). The varying use of epidural block raises questions regarding how and to whom the procedure is offered. In the United States, there have been some cases in which a third party payor or managed care company deemed a woman ineligible for an epidural block (Chestnut, 1997). The American College of Obstetricians and Gynecologists (ACOG) has stated, "There is no other circumstance where it is considered acceptable for a person to experience severe pain, amenable to safe intervention, while under a physician's care" (ACOG, 1993, p 1). ACOG supports the woman's request as sufficient justification for providing an epidural (ACOG, 1993).

Epidural blocks can be administered in a number of ways. To provide analgesia and anesthesia during labor, the block can be administered as a single dose with an epidural needle, a single dose through an epidural catheter with additional doses (called "top-ups") given as needed, or as a continuous epidural. Some procedures require that the woman remain in bed, whereas others—called "walking," "ambulatory," or "mobile" epidurals (Seymour, 1997)—are given with analgesic agents, anesthetic agents (or both) that leave the woman with sufficient motor control to be out of bed. When an epidural block is used for cesarean birth, an epidural catheter is inserted and a single dose is usually given. The catheter provides access to the epidural space, so that additional anesthetic agents and opioids may be administered if needed and so that opioids may be given to provide pain relief for the 24 hours following birth.

When used during labor, the block may be administered as soon as active labor is established (nullipara is 5 to 6 cm, multipara is 3 to 4 cm) and the fetal vertex is engaged (zero station) (Holt, Diehl, & Wright, 1999).

Advantages

The lumbar epidural block produces good analgesia that alters maternal physiologic responses to pain. The woman is fully awake during labor and birth. The continuous technique allows different blocking for each stage of labor so that internal rotation of the fetus can be accomplished. In many cases, the dose of anesthetic agent can be adjusted to preserve the woman's reflex urge to bear down.

Disadvantages

The most common complication of an epidural block is maternal hypotension. This is generally prevented by preloading with a rapid infusion of intravenous fluids, then providing intravenous fluids continuously. Another disadvantage is that the onset of analgesia may not occur for up to 30 minutes. Epidural block requires skilled personnel for administration and close observation of the woman and her fetus. The anesthesiologist must be careful while administering the block to avoid perforating the dura mater, which would place the needle in the subarachnoid space; if the error is not recognized, the anesthetic agent would be injected into the spinal canal. Skilled nurses are also required to maintain close observation of the laboring woman and her fetus. Variability of the FHR may decrease, and late decelerations may occur if maternal hypotension develops. Some clinicians believe that epidural blocks lengthen the first and second stage of labor and increase the incidence of cesarean birth; however, this belief is controversial (Chestnut, 1997). Most health care providers assert that epidural analgesia does not prolong the first stage of labor and may even shorten the active and transition phases because of the pain relief.

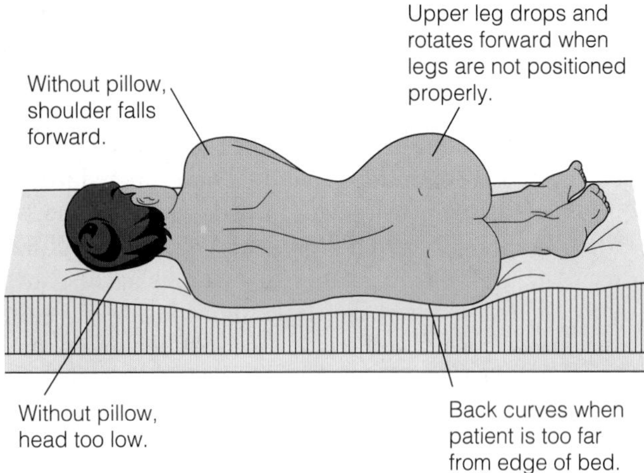
Without pillow, shoulder falls forward.
Upper leg drops and rotates forward when legs are not positioned properly.
Without pillow, head too low.
Back curves when patient is too far from edge of bed.

A

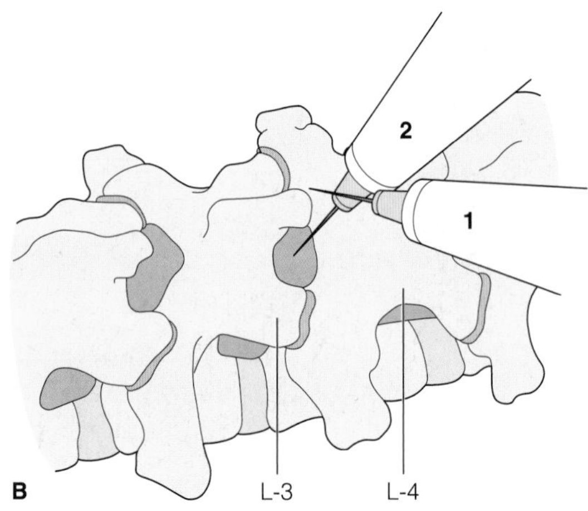
2
1
B
L-3
L-4

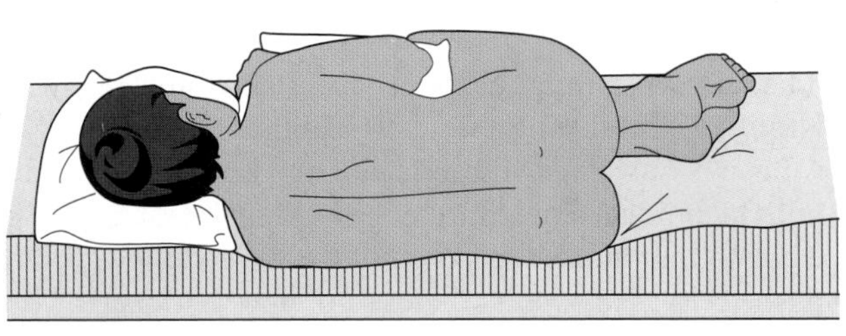
C

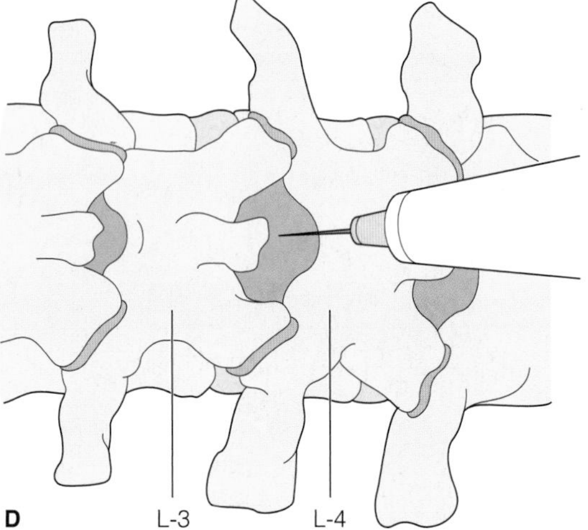
D
L-3
L-4

FIGURE 21–3 Positioning woman for epidural anesthesia block. ***A,*** Incorrect maternal positioning for placing subarachnoid or epidural block. The upper shoulder has fallen forward, upper leg has rotated forward, and the client is positioned on the center of the bed so that there is no support from the edge and the back can curve. ***B,*** Vertebral position with client in incorrect position. The vertebrae rotate forward and, if the needle is inserted in the usual way, (1) the apophyseal joints are encountered. The direction that the needle must follow is shown in D. ***C,*** Correct maternal positioning. The back is straight and vertical, the shoulders are square, and the upper leg is prevented from rolling forward. ***D,*** Vertebral position with the woman correctly positioned. SOURCE: Shnider SM, Levinson G: *Anesthesia for Obstetrics,* 3rd ed. Baltimore: Williams & Wilkins, 1993, figs 9.0, 9.10, 9.11, 9.12.

Contraindications

The absolute contraindications for epidural block are maternal refusal, local or systemic infection, coagulation disorders, hypovolemia, allergy to a specific class of local anesthetic agents, and lack of trained staff (Russell & Reynolds, 1997).

Technique for Continuous Lumbar Epidural Block

The following steps must be taken by the anesthesiologist in administering a continuous lumbar epidural block:

1. Maternal and fetal status and labor progress. Because maternal blood pressure and pulse will be taken frequently, an automatic blood pressure device may be useful. FHR is continuously monitored by an electronic fetal monitor.
2. Oxygen and resuscitative equipment is readied.
3. An intravenous infusion is begun, and a preload of 500 to 1000 mL of balanced salt solution (eg, 0.45% normal saline) is given over approximately 15 to 30 minutes.
4. The woman is placed on her left or right side, at the edge of the bed (the mattress is firmer and provides more support), with her legs slightly flexed. The spinal column is not kept convex, as it is for a spinal block, because the convex position reduces the peridural space to a greater degree and stretches the dura mater, making it more susceptible to puncture. (The epidural space is decreased during pregnancy because of venous engorgement. It is also smaller in obese and short individuals.) A small pillow may be placed under her head and in front of her chest to provide support for her arms (Figure 21–3). A sitting position may be used for obese women (Shnider & Levinson, 1993).

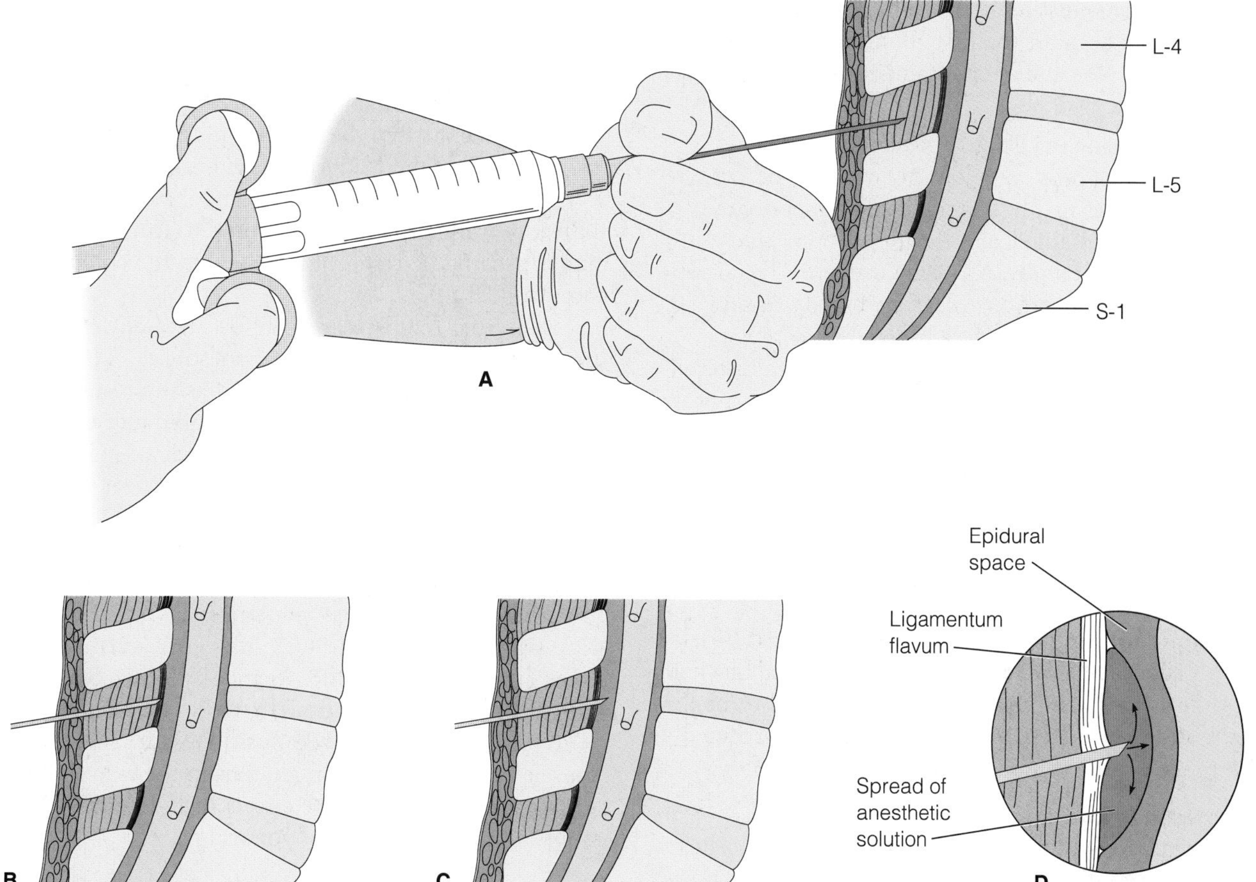

FIGURE 21–4 Technique for lumbar epidural block. ***A,*** Proper position of insertion. ***B,*** Needle in the ligamentum flavum. ***C,*** Tip of needle in epidural space. ***D,*** Force of injection pushing dura away from tip of needle. SOURCE: Bonica JJ: *Principles and Practice of Obstetric Analgesia and Anesthesia.* Philadelphia: Davis, 1972, p 631.

5. The skin is prepared with an antiseptic agent.
6. A skin wheal is made to anesthetize the supraspinous and interspinous ligaments.
7. A short, beveled 16- to 18-gauge needle with stylet is passed to the ligamentum flavum in the widest interspace below the second lumbar vertebrae (usually in the third or fourth lumbar interspace) (Figure 21–4). The ligamentum flavum is identified by its resistance to injection of saline or air (called loss of resistance technique). Resistance disappears as the peridural space is entered.
8. Aspiration for blood (indicating that a vessel has been inadvertently entered) and cerebrospinal fluid (indicating the dura mater has been punctured) is performed.
9. Five mL of preservative-free saline is injected in order to pass the catheter into the epidural space more easily.
10. The catheter is inserted approximately 1 to 2 cm into the epidural space. The needle is removed. Aspiration for blood or cerebrospinal fluid is attempted, and, if negative, a test dose of local anesthetic agent containing epinephrine 1:200,000 concentration is injected. If the catheter has penetrated a blood vessel, the maternal pulse rate will increase by 20% to 30%. (Taylor, 1993). If the subarachnoid space has been entered, sensory and motor changes in the woman's extremities will occur within 3 to 5 minutes (Taylor, 1993). If there are no untoward effects, additional anesthetic agent is injected. The catheter is securely taped so that its placement will not be disturbed.
11. The woman is placed in a semireclining position with left lateral tilt of uterus for 10 minutes to allow for distribution of the block. She is then maintained in a side-lying position to maximize uteroplacental perfusion. If she needs to be turned to a supine position for fetal blood sampling or other procedures, the nurse turns the woman as quickly as possible and repositions her on her side.
12. The nurse monitors the maternal blood pressure every 1 to 2 minutes for the first 10 minutes past the injection and then every 5 to 15 minutes until the block wears off. Maternal vital signs are evaluated against baseline readings obtained just prior to the beginning of the procedure.

13. The woman must be attended by a nurse, anesthesiologist, or both for the first 20 minutes following the initial dose and after administration of any additional dose.
14. If hypotension (a 20% to 30% fall in systolic pressure or a drop to below 100 mm Hg) occurs, the nurse ensures that left lateral displacement of the uterus is maintained, and the intravenous fluids are infused more rapidly. A 10- to 20-degree Trendelenburg position may be used. If the blood pressure is not restored within 1 to 2 minutes, a vasopressor such as ephedrine, 5 to 15 mg, may be administered intravenously.
15. The maternal blood pressure and pulse and the FHR continue to be monitored.
16. If the epidural is not being administered by continuous pump, the anesthesiologist aspirates the catheter prior to administering subsequent doses.

Technique for Single-Dose Lumbar Epidural Block

The procedure of a single-dose lumbar epidural block is the same as for the lumbar block just described through step 8, after which steps 9 and 10 should be substituted with the following (Shnider & Levinson, 1993):

9. A test dose of 2 to 3 mL of anesthetic agent is injected to make sure the dura mater has not been penetrated.
10. After checking again to confirm the dura mater has not been perforated, the clinician injects a single dose of 10 to 12 mL to provide anesthesia for birth. (Note: Subsequent care is described in steps 11 through 15 of the Technique for Continuous Lumbar Epidural Block, pages 591 and 592.)

Problems and Adverse Effects

The major adverse effect of epidural anesthesia is maternal hypotension caused by a spinal blockade, which lowers peripheral resistance, decreases venous return to the heart, and subsequently lessens cardiac output and lowers blood pressure. The risk of hypotension can be minimized by hydrating the vascular system with 500 to 1000 mL of crystalloid IV solution (Ezekiel, 1997) prior to the procedure and changing the woman's position and/or increasing the IV rate afterward.

A potentially distressing maternal problem is an inadequate block, unilateral block, or block failure. Epidural anesthesia has a higher failure rate than spinal anesthesia because the catheter must be properly placed to produce adequate anesthesia. A one-sided block is fairly common and can be overcome by having the woman lie on the unanesthetized side and injecting more of the local anesthetic agent. If the woman has a continuous epidural block, she should turn from side to side every hour to avoid a one-sided block. A block may be effective except for a "spot" or "window" of pain in the inguinal or suprapubic area. Breakthrough pain may occur at any time during the epidural infusion. It usually occurs when the continuous infusion rate of the anesthetic agent is below the recommended rate for a therapeutic dose. It may also occur when the infusion pump rate is altered or the integrity of the epidural line is broken.

Pruritus may occur at any time during the epidural infusion. It usually appears first on the face, neck, or torso and is usually the result of the agent in the epidural infusion.

Maternal temperature may be elevated to 37.8C or higher with the use of epidural anesthesia. The increase in temperature has been suggested as the result of a decrease in heat loss due to the woman's failure to hyperventilate. In addition, sympathetic blockade may decrease sweat production and, in turn, diminish heat loss. It has also been suggested that heat loss may result from a failure of the central nervous system to regulate temperature (Mayer, Chescheir, & Spielman, 1997).

Short-term localized tenderness at the needle puncture site occurs in about 40% of women during the first week after birth (Russell & Reynolds, 1997). Backache is fairly common and is thought to result from inadvertently maintaining stressed positions during periods of muscle relaxation and pain relief from the epidural block. Other problems or adverse effects include urinary retention, shivering, nausea, and vomiting.

Complications

One of the most serious complications of regional anesthesia, systemic toxic reaction, has been discussed in Adverse Maternal Reactions to Anesthetic Agents. Toxic reactions following a lumbar epidural block may be caused by unintentional placement of the drug in the arachnoid or subarachnoid space, excessive amount of the drug in the epidural space (massive epidural), or accidental intravascular injection. Because large quantities of anesthetic agent are used for epidural block, the likelihood of toxic reactions is higher than with some of the other regional procedures. The incidence of drug reactions is relatively low, but the possibility is always present.

Pain during cesarean birth with epidural anesthesia has been reported by a growing number of women. In light of this, some anesthesiologists use both temperature and pinprick to assess sensory loss. Bourne, de Melo, Bastianpillai, and May (1997) recommend that all dermatomes from T_4 to S_3 be tested for sensory loss before beginning a cesarean. The method of assessment and results should be documented in the anesthesia record.

NURSING CARE MANAGEMENT

The nurse assesses the maternal vital signs and FHR for baseline information and to ensure that both maternal and fetal vital signs are within normal limits. (Note: All information regarding assessments, procedures, and other activities are to be recorded on the fetal electronic monitor strip as well as in the nursing notes.) Labor progress is also assessed. The procedure and expected results are explained, and the woman's questions are answered. If questions arise that indicate the need for the woman, father, or other support person to talk with the anesthesiologist, then the nurse will act as an advocate and arrange that conversation. The laboring woman will need to give informed consent for the epidural, so she must clearly understand all aspects of the procedure.

The nurse starts an IV infusion, if one is not already in place. If directed by the anesthesiologist or agency protocol, the nurse preloads at a rapid infusion rate to increase both blood volume and cardiac output. The greater circulating blood volume will counteract the loss of peripheral resistance that occurs with sympathetic blockade. It is recommended that dextrose-free solutions be used because dextrose can cause fetal hyperglycemia with rebound hypoglycemia the first few hours after birth. It is helpful to provide an opportunity for the woman to void just before administering the block because her urge to urinate will be decreased. The nurse assists the woman with positioning on either lateral side. After the epidural block is given, the woman may be positioned in a semireclining position (head at 25 degrees) with lateral uterine tilt to provide equal distribution of the block; then she is turned to a side-lying position. If she is supine for procedures such as sterile vaginal examinations or fetal scalp blood sampling, the nurse places a wedge under her right hip to help eliminate aortocaval compression. The nurse takes maternal blood pressure and pulse every 5 minutes for at least 30 minutes and then at least every 30 minutes thereafter while the block is present (Russell & Reynolds, 1997). An automatic blood pressure measurement device is helpful. The FHR is monitored and assessed by continuous electronic fetal monitor.

If hypotension (systolic blood pressure below 100 mm Hg) occurs, the nurse assists with corrective measures such as positioning the woman in a left-side-lying position, increasing the flow rate of the intravenous infusion, and placing the bed in a 10- to 20-degree Trendelenburg position. If maternal blood pressure does not increase within 1 to 2 minutes, 5 to 15 mg of ephedrine may be administered intravenously per physician or protocol order. These measures are usually sufficient; however, if hypotension persists, oxygen by mask at 7 to 10 L/minute and additional vasopressors may be needed (Shnider & Levinson, 1993). Administration of oxygen helps decrease the nausea associated with a drop in blood pressure, increases fetal oxygenation, and reassures the mother. With severe or prolonged hypotension added treatment includes elevating the woman's legs for 2 or 3 minutes to increase blood return from the extremities.

If additional local anesthetic agents are injected, the regimen of assessing maternal blood pressure and initial surveillance should be repeated each time the epidural catheter is reinjected. If the woman's legs have been in stirrups during a vaginal birth, her blood pressure should be assessed as soon as her legs are taken out of the stirrups. While the legs were elevated, circulating blood volume in the trunk increased. Restoring circulation to the legs decreases the overall blood volume and may precipitate hypotension.

Throughout the administration of the block, the nurse provides continued support by offering information and reassurance and remaining with the woman. Additional nursing care following the block includes frequent assessment of the bladder to avoid bladder distention. Catheterization may be necessary because most women are unable to void. Shivering may be caused by heat loss from increased peripheral blood flow or alteration of thermal input to the central nervous system when warm but not cold sensations have been suppressed. Applying warmed blankets and reassuring her may make the woman feel more comfortable.

The nurse assesses the woman's comfort and whether she has adequate pain relief. The nurse can promote equal distribution by assessing the temperature of the woman's feet. If one foot warms more quickly than the other, the woman should be positioned with the cooler side dependent (Russell & Reynolds, 1997). If a "spot" or "window" of pain exists or a unilateral block, the woman may be turned to the unanesthetized side. It is important for the woman to turn from side to side every hour to promote equal distribution of the anesthetic agent. If positioning changes do not help and the woman has inadequate pain relief, the anesthetist needs to be notified. During a continuous epidural block, the anesthesiologist should titrate the infusion to maintain a sensory level of T_{10}, and the presence of motor block and height of sensory block should be documented at least hourly (Russell & Reynolds, 1997).

Nausea and vomiting may be associated with hypotension, so the nurse needs to ensure that maternal blood pressure is within normal limits. Also, an antiemetic may be ordered to increase the woman's comfort.

Respiratory rate and quality of the respirations should be assessed at least every 15 to 30 minutes. The nurse should notify the anesthetist of any significant decreases in respiratory rate or respiratory pattern changes. If the respiratory rate falls below 14 respirations per minute, naloxone (Narcan) may be given to remove the effect of the anesthetic agent; respirations will then return to a normal rate.

The nurse asks the woman if she is experiencing pruritus (itching) and is alert for signs of scratching, especially on the face, neck, and torso. If present, it is usually treated with diphenhydramine (Benadryl), 25 mg administered intravenously or 50 mg intramuscularly. Should no standing order exist, the nurse should notify the anesthetist. Epidural infusion may need to be discontinued.

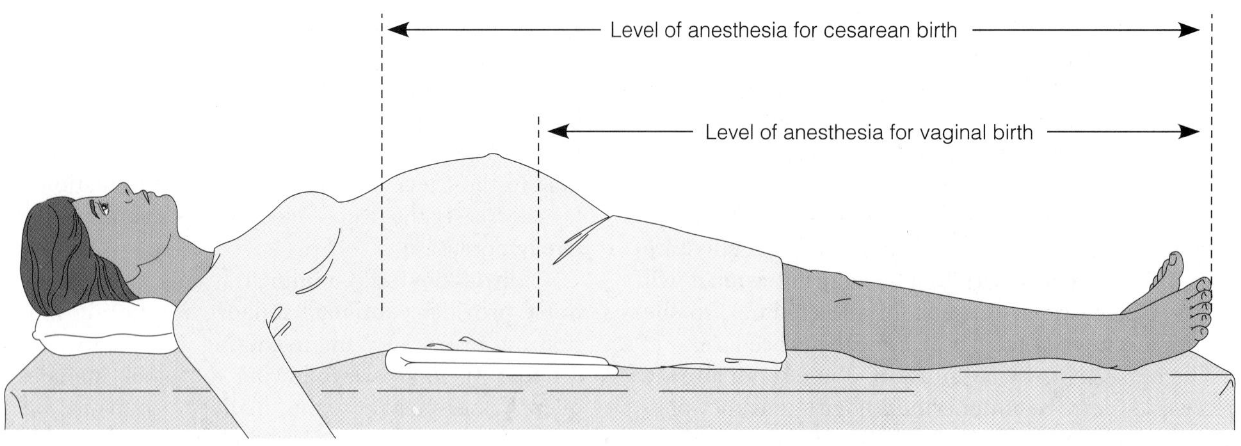

FIGURE 21–5 Levels of anesthesia for vaginal and cesarean births. SOURCE: Reprinted with permission of Ross Laboratories, Columbus, OH. From Clinical Education Aid No. 17.

During the second stage of labor, the woman may require assistance with pushing because she may not feel her contractions or experience the urge to push. She may also need assistance holding or controlling her legs in order to push. (Women with epidurals may have decreased sensation and decreased ability to move their legs or may have essentially no control over movement.)

Ambulation should be delayed until the anesthesia has worn off. This may take several hours, depending on the agent and the total dose. Motor control of the legs is weak but not totally absent after birth. Return of complete sensation and the ability to control the legs are essential before ambulation is attempted. The woman must also be able to maintain blood pressure in a sitting and then standing position. For further discussion of nursing care, see Critical Pathway: Epidural Anesthesia on pages 595 to 597.

Epidural Analgesia after Birth

To provide analgesia for approximately 24 hours after the birth, the anesthesiologist may inject an opioid, such as Duramorph 5.0 mg or 7.5 mg, into the epidural space immediately following the birth. The analgesic effect of Duramorph begins approximately 30 to 60 minutes after the injection (*PDR Nurse's Handbook*, 1999). The side effects include pruritus, nausea and vomiting, and urinary retention (*PDR Nurse's Handbook*, 1999). (See Drug Guide: Postbirth Epidural Morphine.)

Meperidine may be injected during an epidural block for birth, and then continued through use of patient-controlled epidural analgesia (PCEA). Ngan Kee, Khaw, and Ma (1997) found that epidural meperidine was rated as more effective than PCEA using fentanyl or than patient-controlled intravenous analgesia and had fewer side effects than epidural morphine. Grass, Sakima, Schmidt, Michitsch, Zuckerman, and Harris (1997) conducted a study comparing epidural fentanyl and sufentanil following birth managed by epidural using 2% lidocaine with epinephrine (1:200,000). Findings indicated no significant difference in perceived pain relief, duration of pain relief, effectiveness, level of sedation, or side effects.

Spinal Block

In a **spinal block,** a local anesthetic agent is injected directly into the spinal fluid in the spinal canal to provide anesthesia for cesarean birth. Cesarean birth requires anesthetic blockade to the T_8 dermatome (Figure 21–5).

The subarachnoid space is the fluid-filled area between the dura and the spinal cord. During pregnancy the space decreases because of the distention of the epidural veins. Thus a specific dose of anesthetic produces a much higher level of anesthesia in the pregnant woman than in the nonpregnant woman. When a low spinal block is properly administered, failure rate is low.

Advantages

The advantages of spinal block are immediate onset of anesthesia, relative ease of administration, a smaller drug volume, and maternal compartmentalization of the drug.

Disadvantages

The primary disadvantage is intense blockade of sympathetic fibers, resulting in a high incidence of hypotension. This leads to a greater potential for fetal hypoxia. In addition, uterine tone is maintained, which makes intrauterine manipulation difficult. The level of spinal blockage is less predictable in laboring women.

Contraindications

Spinal anesthesia is contraindicated for women with severe hypovolemia, regardless of cause; central nervous system disease; infection over the site of puncture; maternal coagulation problems; and allergy to local anesthetic agents. Sepsis and active genital herpes may be considered relative rather than absolute contraindications. Spinal block is also contraindicated for women who do

Text continues on page 598.

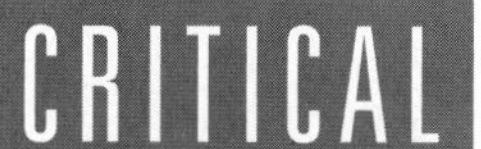

CRITICAL PATHWAY FOR EPIDURAL ANESTHESIA

Category	First Stage	Second and Third Stage	Fourth Stage Birth to 1 Hour Past Birth
Referral	**Review prenatal record** **Advise CNM/physician of admission**	**Labor record for first stage**	**Report to recovery room nurse**
Assessments	Admission assessments: Ask about problems since last prenatal visit; labor status (contraction frequency and duration cervical dilatation, and effacement), membrane status; coping level; support; woman's desires during labor and birth; ability to verbalize needs; laboratory testing (blood and UA) Woman's request for epidural Intrapartal assessment: timing *Latent Phase:* • B/P, P, R, q1h if in normal range (B/P 90–140/60–90 or no increase >30 mm Hg systolic or 15 mm Hg diastolic over baseline; pulse 60–90; respirations 12–20/min, quiet, easy) • Temp q4h unless >37.6C (99.6F) or membranes ruptured; then q2h. Uterine contractions q30min: contractions q5–10min, 15–40sec, mild intensity) • FHR q60min (for low-risk women) and q30min for high-risk women if reassuring (FHR baseline 120–160, STV present, LTV average, accelerations with fetal movement, no late nor variable decelerations); if nonreassuring, position on side, start O_2, assess for hypotension, monitor continuously, notify CNM/physician *Active Phase:* • B/P, P, R, q1h if WNL • Temp as above • Uterine contractions assessed continuously • FHR assessed continuously per EFM • Pulse ox >95% *Transition Phase:* • B/P, P, R, q30min if in normal range • Uterine contractions q15–30min • FHR q30min (for low-risk women) and q15min (for high-risk women) if reassuring: if nonreassuring, see above • Pulse ox >95% Cervical assessment: from 1–10 cm dilatation; nullipara (1.2 cm/h), multipara (1.5 cm/h) Cervical effacement: from 0% to 100% Fetal descent: progressive descent from −4 to +4 Membrane assessment: when ruptured, Nitrazine positive, fluid clear, no foul odor Behavioral characteristics: response to labor process, facial expressions, verbalizations, tone of voice, changes in behavior during contractions, body movement	Second stage assessments: • B/P, P, R q5–15min • Uterine contractions palpated continuously • FHR q15min (for low-risk women) and q5min (for high-risk women) if reassuring; if nonreassuring, monitor continuously Fetal descent: descent continues to birth Behavioral characteristics: response to pushing, facial expressions, verbalization Third stage assessments: • B/P, P, R q5min • Uterine contractions, palpate occasionally until placenta is delivered, fundus maintains tone and contraction pattern continues to birth of placenta Newborn assessments: • Assess Apgar score of newborn • Respirations: 30–60, irregular • Apical pulse: 120–160 and somewhat irregular • Temperature: skin temp above 36.5C (97.8F) • Umbilical cord: 2 arteries, 1 vein (if 1 artery, assess for anomalies and urine output) • Gestational age: 38 to 42 weeks	**Expected Outcomes** Appropriate resources identified and utilized Immediate post-birth assessments q15 min for one hour • B/P: 90–140/60–90; should return to prelabor level • Pulse: slightly lower than in labor; range is 60–90 • Respirations: 12–20/min; easy; quiet • Temperature: 36.2–37.6C (98-99.6F) • Fundus firm, in midline, at the umbilicus or 1–2 fingerbreadths below the umbilicus • Lochia rubra; moderate amount; <1 pad/h; no free flow or passage of clots with massage • Perineum: sutures intact; no bulging or marked swelling; minimal bruising may be present; no c/o severe pain nor rectal pain • Bladder nondistended; spontaneous void of >100 mL clear, straw-colored urine; bladder nondistended following voiding (catheterize if necessary) • If hemorrhoids present, no tenseness or marked engorgement; <2 cm diameter Comfort level: <3 on scale of 1 to 10 Energy level: awake and able to hold newborn Newborn assessments if newborn remains with parents: • Respirations: 30–60; irregular • Apical pulse: 120–160 and somewhat irregular • Temperature: skin temp above 36.5C (97.8F); skin feels warm to touch • Skin color noncyanotic • Mucus: small amount, clear, easily suctioned with bulb syringe without skin color change • Behavioral: newborn opens eyes widely if room is slightly darkened • Movements rhythmic; no hand tremors present **Expected Outcomes** • Assessment findings indicate labor is progressing WNL, maternal vital signs stable and within established parameters, and reassuring fetal heart rate • Maternal/fetal well-being unimpaired

Category	First Stage	Second and Third Stage	Fourth Stage Birth to 1 Hour Past Birth
Teaching/ psychosocial	Establish rapport Orient to environment, expected assessments and procedures Answer questions and provide information/give emotional support Orient to EFM Teach relaxation, visualization and breathing pattern if needed Explain comfort measures available. Provide information regarding the reason for the block, possible side effects and nursing care that may be expected Assume advocacy role for woman/family during labor and birth Explain possible delayed effects of anesthetic agents on fetus	Orient to expected assessments and procedures Answer questions and provide information Continue advocacy role Instruct woman to maintain bed rest until full function of lower extremities returns	Explain immediate assessments and care after this first hour Teach self-massage of fundus and expected findings Instruct to call for assistance if mother desires to get OOB Begin newborn teaching; bulb syringe, positioning, maintaining warmth Assist with first breastfeeding experience **Expected Outcomes** Woman verbalizes/demonstrates understanding of teaching
Nursing care management and reports	Straight cath PRN if bladder distended If regional block administered monitor B/P, FHR, sensation per protocol and obtain consent for procedure Provide continuing status reports Perineal clip per woman's request Small enema per woman's request Perform sterile vaginal examination as indicated Position woman correctly for regional block Assess maternal status: • Obtain baseline vital signs before any anesthetic agent is given • Monitor blood pressure q1–2min for 10 min and then q5–15min following administration of anesthetic agent • Monitor pulse and respiration • Monitor FHR continuously Observe, record, and report complications of anesthesia, including hypotension, fetal stress, respiratory paralysis, changes in uterine contractility, decrease in voluntary muscle effort, trauma to extremities, nausea and vomiting, and loss of bladder tone Observe, record, and report symptoms of hypotension, including systolic pressure $<$ 100 mm Hg or a 20–30% fall in systolic pressure, apprehension, restlessness, dizziness, tinnitus, headache Initiate treatment measures: • Place woman in left lateral position or position as directed with the foot of the bed elevated • Increase IV fluid rate • Administer oxygen by face mask at 7–10 L/min as needed • Administer vasopressors as ordered (usually ephedrine 5–15 mg IV) • Manually displace uterus laterally to left • Keep woman supine (semireclining) for 5–10 min following administration of block to allow drug to diffuse bilaterally. After 5–10 min position woman on side Observe, record, and report fetal bradycardia (FHR $<$120 bpm) and loss of beat-to-beat variability	Straight cath PRN if bladder distended Continue monitoring VS, FHR, and sensation Assess for potential problems of epidural infusion: sedation, nausea, vomiting, pruritus, hypotension, and "breakthrough pain"	Straight cath if bladder distended Monitor return of motor ability and sensation if regional block has been given Weigh perineal pads if lochia flow $>$1 saturated pad in 1 h; presence of boggy uterus and clots; decreased B/P, increased P **Expected Outcomes** Mother and fetus experience safe labor and birth Actual/potential complication identified and minimized Woman and family actively participate in decision making and plan of care

Category	First Stage	Second and Third Stage	Fourth Stage Birth to 1 Hour Past Birth
Activity	Encourage ambulation unless contraindicated Maintain bed rest immediately after administration of IV pain medication, or following regional block Woman rests comfortably between contractions	Position comfortably for birth Woman rests comfortably between pushing efforts, and while awaiting birth of placenta	Position of comfort **Expected Outcomes** Activity maintained per protocol. Comfort and uterine perfusion enhanced by position/movement
Comfort	Woman states that she desires regional anesthesia Assist with administration of epidural block	Second stage: assess and inform woman of progress of labor. Provide reassurance throughout labor. Assist with "sitting dose" reinjection for birth. Encouragement, coaching, help support legs while pushing, position of comfort for pushing and birth. Third stage: cool cloth to forehead, assist parents to see newborn, position mother to hold newborn, provide encouragement	Institute comfort measures: Perineal discomfort: gently cleanse and apply ice pack; position to decrease pressure on perineum Uterine discomfort: palpate fundus gently Hemorrhoids: ice pack General fatigue: position of comfort, encourage rest Administer pain medication **Expected Outcomes** Optimal comfort maintained
Nutrition	Ice chips and clear fluids Evaluate for signs of dehydration	Ice chips and clear fluids	Regular diet if assessments are WNL Encourage fluids **Expected Outcomes** Nutrition and hydration needs met
Elimination	Voids at least q2h; urine clear, straw-colored, negative for protein Bladder nondistended; empty before regional block administered May have bowel movement Monitor I & O with IVs	Monitor bladder at frequent intervals	Monitor bladder status with each assessment **Expected Outcomes** Intake and output WNL
Medications	Hydrate the woman receiving an epidural block with 500–1000 mL fluid prior to procedure (dextrose-free solution is recommended)	Local infiltration of anesthetic agent for birth by CNM/physician Pitocin 10 units IM, IVP per IV tubing, or added to IV fluids	Continue Pitocin infusion Administer pain medication **Expected Outcomes** Perfusion and hydration supported Uterine hemorrhage prevented or successfully treated
Discharge planning/ home care	Evaluate knowledge of labor and birth process Evaluate support system and need for referral after birth		Provide information if mother to be moved from LDR room Provide opportunity for parents to ask questions regarding newborn Evaluate knowledge of normal postpartum, newborn care **Expected Outcomes** Individualized discharge teaching completed
Family involvement	Identify available support person(s) Recognize possible impact of culture on responses Observe interaction between woman and partner Create moment alone with woman to identify possible abuse Assess current parenting skills	Provide opportunities for woman and support person(s) to watch newborn assessments Perform newborn assessment on mother's abdomen/chest if possible	Provide opportunity for parents to be with baby Encourage skin-to-skin contact Darken room to encourage eye-to-eye contact Provide quiet time for new family Parenting: demonstrates early culturally expected parenting behaviors **Expected Outcomes** Family demonstrates support of family members Family able to identify supportive resources in the community
Date			

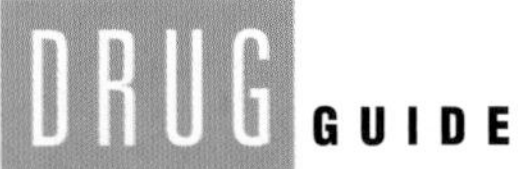

Postbirth Epidural Morphine

Overview of Action

Epidural morphine is used to provide relief of pain associated with cesarean birth, extensive episiotomies (mediolaterals), or third- and fourth-degree lacerations. Epidural morphine pain relief results directly from its effect on the opiate receptors in the spinal cord (it depresses pain impulse transmission). Morphine binds opiate receptors, thereby altering both the perception of and the emotional response to pain. Women experience little or no discomfort or pain during recovery and for up to 24 hours afterward. There is no motor or sympathetic block or associated hypotension. Onset of analgesia is slower, but duration is longer.

Dosage, Route

5–10 mg of morphine is injected through a catheter into the epidural space, providing relief for about 24 hours (Wilson, Shannon, & Strang, 1997).

Maternal Contraindications

Hypersensitivity to opiates
Narcotic addiction
Chronic debilitating respiratory disease
Reduced blood volume

Maternal Side Effects

Late onset respiratory depression (rare but may occur 8–12 hours after administration)
Nausea and vomiting (occurring between 4 and 7 hours after injection)
Itching (begins within 3 hours and lasts up to 10 hours)
Urinary retention
Somnolence (rarely)
Side effects can be managed with naloxone (Cunningham et al, 1997)

Effect on Fetus/Neonate

No adverse effects since medication is injected after birth of baby

Nursing Considerations

Assess client's sensitivity to narcotics on admission.
Monitor and evaluate analgesic effect. Ask client about comfort level and notify anesthesiologist of inadequate pain relief.
If present, check epidural catheter for obvious knots, breaks, and leakage at insertion site and catheter hub.
Assess for pruritus (scratching and rubbing, especially around the face and neck).
Administer comfort measures for narcotic-induced pruritus, such as lotion, back rubs, cool/warm packs, or diversional activities. If the itching can be tolerated, naloxone should be avoided, especially because it counteracts the pain relief.
If allergic reaction (urticaria, edema, or respiratory difficulties) occurs, administer naloxone or diphenhydramine per physician order.
Provide comfort measures for nausea or vomiting, such as frequent oral hygiene or gradual increase in activity; administration of naloxone, trimethobenzamide, or metoclopramide HCl per physician order.
Assess postural blood pressure and heart rate before ambulation.
Assist client with her first ambulation and then as needed.
Assess respiratory function frequently for the first 24 hours, then every 2–8 hours as needed. Also assess level of consciousness and mucous membrane color. May need to monitor client via apnea monitor for 24 hours and use continuous pulse oximetry.
Monitor urinary output and assess bladder for distention. Assist client to void.

not wish to have spinal procedures (Cunningham et al, 1997).

Technique

The following steps are followed in administering a subarachnoid block:

1. Place the woman in a sitting or left lateral position. Because the procedure is not done until the presenting part is on the perineum, sitting on the edge of the operating room bed may be very difficult for the laboring woman.
2. Intravenous infusion should be checked for patency.
3. The woman places her arms between her knees, bows her head, and arches her back to widen the intervertebral space.
4. Prepare skin carefully, maintaining sterility.
5. A skin wheal is made over L3 or L4.
6. An 18- or 19-gauge needle is introduced through the skin and into the intraspinous ligament. Then, a 24- to 27-gauge pencil-point needle is introduced inside the larger needle and inserted into interspinous ligament, ligamentum flavum, and epidural space into the subarachnoid space (Figure 21–6).
7. Upon removal of the introducer, a drop of fluid can be seen in the hub of the needle if the spinal canal has been entered.
8. The appropriate amount of anesthetic agent is injected slowly, and both needles are removed.
9. With hyperbaric solutions, the woman remains sitting up for 45 seconds.
10. Place the woman on her back with a pillow under her head. Position changes can alter the dermatome

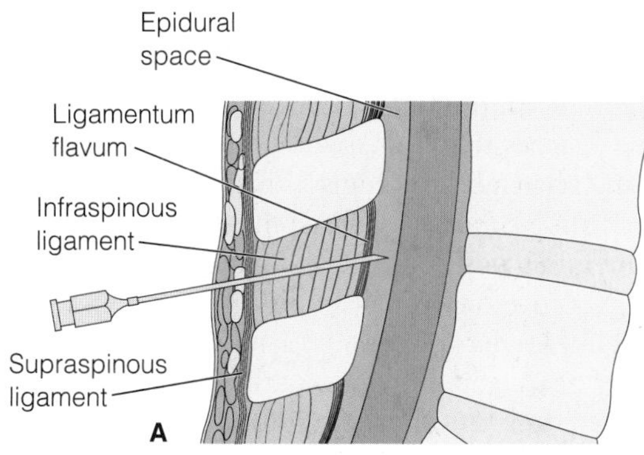

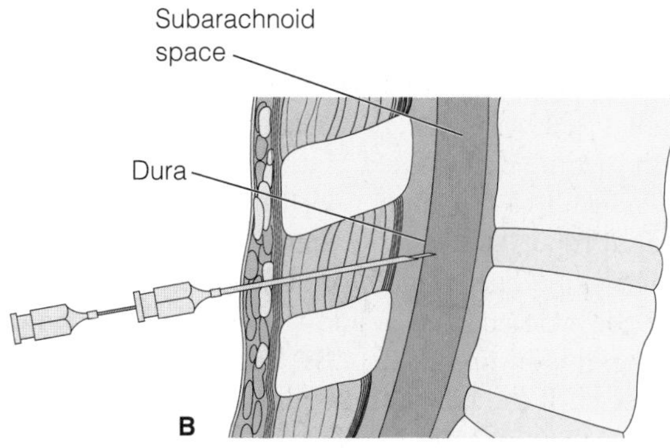

FIGURE 21–6 Double-needle technique for spinal injection. ***A,*** Large needle in epidural space. ***B,*** 25-gauge needle in larger needle entering the spinal canal. SOURCE: Bonica JJ: *Principles and Practice of Obstetric Analgesia and Anesthesia.* Philadelphia: Davis, 1972, p 563.

level if done within 3 to 5 minutes. After 10 minutes, a position change will not affect the level of anesthesia.

11. Blood pressure, pulse, and respiration must be monitored every 1 to 2 minutes for the first 10 minutes, then every 5 to 10 minutes.

The nurse helps the woman into position and provides encouragement and support during the procedure. The nurse informs the physician when a contraction is beginning so the anesthetic agent will not be injected at that time.

In the absence of maternal hypotension or toxic reaction, a spinal blocks exerts no direct effect on the fetus. The amount of anesthetic used is too small to reach fetal circulation in a quantity that might cause fetal depression. Spinal anesthesia has been shown to be well tolerated by a healthy fetus when a maternal IV fluid preload in excess of 500 to 1000 mL precedes the administration of the spinal.

Complications

The complications of spinal anesthesia include hypotension, drug reaction, total spinal neurologic sequelae, and spinal headache. The side effects include nausea, shivering, and urinary retention.

RESEARCH IN PRACTICE

What is this study about? In order to provide pain control for laboring women, anesthesiologists or nurse anesthetists sometimes use regional anesthesia. Regional anesthesia includes intrathecal analgesia, epidural analgesia, or a combined spinal-epidural technique. Intrathecal analgesia involves the injection of opioid and local anesthetic into the spinal fluid, and epidural analgesia entails the injection of medication into the epidural space just outside the spinal column. Combined analgesia incorporates an initial intrathecal injection followed by a continuous epidural infusion of a low-dose local anesthetic. Controversy exists about whether or not regional anesthesia impacts the length and progression of labor. Caroline Cutbush and her colleagues conducted a retrospective study of 213 women to determine how regional anesthesia influenced the length of labor.

How was the study done? The researchers reviewed anesthetic records in a military hospital and selected low-risk women (50 per group) who had received epidural, intrathecal, combined, or no regional anesthesia. All members of the anesthesia department followed standardized procedures during the provision of each type of regional anesthesia. The investigators used multiple analysis of variance to compare age, height, weight, gestational age, parity, infant weight, use of oxytocin, delivery type, and anesthetic type to the length of the first and second stage of labor.

What were the results of the study? The rates of spontaneous vaginal birth ranged from 95% for the no-anesthesia group to 53% for the women who received an epidural. Researchers reported the following mean lengths of labor in minutes for stage one and two for each group: Combined, 195 and 74; epidural, 204 and 62; intrathecal, 83 and 44; none, 320 and 25. The shortened length of stage one was statistically significant when comparing the first three groups to the no-anesthetic group ($p < .05$). When compared to the combined and the epidural groups, the no-anesthesia group had a statistically shorter second stage ($p < .05$). The comparison of rates of cervical dilatation after initial injection of regional anesthesia showed a statistically significant greater rate for the intrathecal group when compared to the combined group ($p < .05$). No significant differences were found between other groupings.

What additional questions might I have? Was the difference in spontaneous vaginal birth rates statistically significant? The authors might have provided a results table for the multiple analysis of variance to enhance reader interpretation; however, journals restrict space.

How can I use this study? Nurses caring for women who receive regional anesthesia should be prepared for a possible effect on both the first and second stages of labor.

SOURCE: Cutbush, C.M., McDonough, J.P., Clark, K., & McCarthy, E.J. (1998). The effect of intrathecal and epidural narcotic analgesia on the length of labor. *CRNA: The Clinical Forum for Nurse Anesthetists, 9*(3), 106–112.

Hypotension can be minimized by prehydrating with 500 to 1000 mL of non-dextrose-containing fluids and displacing the uterus to the left. The practice of placing an already hypotensive woman in a sitting position following injection to prevent upward spread of hyperbaric solution is dangerous because it will cause venous pooling in the lower extremities, further decreasing the maternal blood pressure. The normal curve of the thoracic spine prevents cranial spread of an intrathecal agent. A pillow is placed under the woman's head to exaggerate the curve.

Treatment of hypotension is the same as with an epidural block: positioning the woman in a left lateral, head-down position and rapidly infusing intravenous fluids. Preventing cardiovascular collapse requires early detection, supplemental oxygen, assisted ventilation, and measures to maintain the blood pressure. The extent to which the fetus is affected relates to the degree of maternal hypotension. When maternal hypotension has been reversed, it is best to delay the birth for 4 to 5 minutes to allow the fetus to recover. Resuscitative equipment and trained personnel must be available to treat the mother and baby.

A total spinal occurs when there is paralysis of the respiratory muscles. It is a relatively rare but critical event. The symptoms are apnea, dilation of pupils, loss of consciousness, and absence of blood pressure. The onset of symptoms usually occurs within minutes of the injection but can occur in a span of time ranging from 30 seconds to 45 minutes. Resuscitative treatment, airway control, and support of blood pressure must begin immediately. If this complication occurs, it is important to remember that this woman is not asleep; although she may be paralyzed, she is aware of everything going on around her. She requires assurance that her respiration is being maintained and will continue to be maintained until she can breathe on her own.

Neurologic complications may occur coincidentally with spinal anesthesia, for example, with preexisting disease or faulty positioning of the woman. Genuine neurologic sequelae, such as paralysis, is extremely rare.

Although much less serious than other complications, headache may be an unpleasant aftermath of spinal anesthesia. It is the most frequent complication. Leakage of spinal fluid at the site of dural puncture is thought to be the cause. Several techniques have been suggested to decrease the possibility of headache. The use of a narrow-gauge pencil-point anesthesia needle (24- to 27-gauge) reduces the incidence of spinal headache (Wildman, Mohl, Cassel, Houston, & Allerheiligen, 1997). The incidence of spinal headache is only about 2% (Russell & Reynolds, 1997). Hyperhydration and keeping the woman flat in bed for 6 to 12 hours after birth have been recommended as preventive measures, but there is no evidence that these procedures are effective.

NURSING CARE MANAGEMENT

The nurse should assist in positioning the woman, provide oxygen via nasal cannula or mask, assess and record baseline vital signs of the mother and fetus, and start an intravenous infusion prior to administration of the block. After the block is instilled, the nurse should continue to monitor maternal blood pressure, pulse and respiration, and FHR at least every 5 minutes until the anesthesiologist takes over monitoring of the mother and the FHR is no longer accessible because an abdominal surgical prep is begun. The anesthesiologist is responsible for assessing and recording the level of the spinal block.

The nurse positions the woman correctly on the operating room table, usually upright with her legs on a stool. The woman places her arms between her knees, bows her head (shoulders should be even with hips), and arches her back to widen the intervertebral spaces. The nurse supports the woman in this position and palpates the uterus to detect the beginning of a contraction. Intrathecal agents are not administered during a contraction because the increased pressure could cause a higher level of anesthesia than desired. After the agent has been administered, the woman is asked to sit upright for the length of time determined by the anesthesiologist and is then assisted to the supine position with a wedge under her right hip to displace the uterus; a pillow is placed under her head. The spinal block may also be administered when the woman is in a side-lying position. The nurse monitors blood pressure, pulse, and respirations every 5 minutes until the birth. Some physicians administer oxygen as a prophylactic measure. The woman should be kept informed of everything that is going on in the birthing area, particularly if she is receiving mask oxygen. Placing her legs in stirrups will facilitate venous return from the extremities. Both legs should be raised at the same time to avoid undue tension and possible injury to back muscles.

If hypotension should occur, the intravenous fluids should be increased and the uterus displaced manually to the left. If the woman reports that she is having difficulty breathing, she needs to be assessed very carefully. Total spinal rarely occurs, but the possibility must always be kept in mind. The woman should be observed for apnea, unconsciousness, pupil dilation, and unobtainable blood pressure. Prompt treatment, which may include the use of a vasopressor (such as ephedrine), may avert a catastrophe for the woman or baby. It is essential to establish an airway and give oxygen with positive pressure until the woman can be intubated and other emergency measures instituted.

Following the birth, the woman is kept flat. Although the effectiveness of the supine position to avoid headache following a spinal is controversial, the physician's orders may include lying flat for 6 to 12 hours.

Combined Spinal-Epidural Block

Spinal anesthesia may be combined with an epidural block. The combined spinal-epidural (CSE) can be used for labor analgesia and for cesarean birth. The anesthetic and analgesic agents used differ according to the purpose of the CSE. A CSE is accomplished by inserting an epidural needle into the epidural space. A narrow-gauge atraumatic (24- to 27-gauge pencil point) is inserted through the epidural needle, through the dura, and into the cerebral spinal fluid. A small amount of local anesthetic agent, opioid, or both, is injected, and the needle is withdrawn. An epidural catheter is then threaded through the epidural needle into the epidural space. The epidural needle is removed and the epidural catheter is securely placed against the woman.

An advantage of CSE is that the spinal (intrathecal) anesthetic and/or analgesic agent will have a faster onset than medications that are injected into the epidural. Most drugs are used in low dose, so spinal analgesia may be given in early labor to assist with labor pain. The epidural is activated when active labor begins (Ezekiel, 1997). Motor function is preserved, and most women are able to ambulate (Russell & Reynolds, 1997).

Pudendal Block

The **pudendal block** technique provides perineal anesthesia for the second stage of labor, birth, and episiotomy repair. An anesthetic agent is injected below the pudendal plexus, which arises from the anterior division of the second and third sacral nerves and the entire fourth sacral nerve. The pudendal nerve crosses the sacrosciatic notch and passes the tip of the ischial spine, where it divides into the perineal, dorsal, and inferior hemorrhoidal nerves. The perineal nerve, which is the largest branch of the pudendal plexus, supplies the skin of the vulvar area, the perineal muscles, and the urethral sphincter. The dorsal nerve supplies the clitoris, and the inferior hemorrhoidal nerve supplies the skin and muscles of the perineal region as well as the internal anal sphincter. Pudendal block provides relief of pain from perineal distention but does not relieve pain of uterine contractions (Figure 21–7).

Advantages and Disadvantages

The advantages of pudendal block are ease of administration and absence of maternal hypotension. It also allows the use of low forceps or vacuum extraction for birth.

A moderate dose of anesthetic agent (10 mL per side) has minimal ill effects on the woman and the course of labor. The urge to bear down during the second stage of labor may be decreased, but the woman is able to do so with appropriate coaching. There is usually little effect on the uncompromised fetus unless overly rapid or intravascular injection occurs. The block may be done by a transvaginal or transperineal approach. Transvaginal injection is simpler, safer, and more direct, making it the procedure of choice.

Complications

Systemic toxic reaction can occur from accidental vascular injection. Other possible maternal complications specific to pudendal block include broad ligament hematoma, perforation of the rectum, and trauma to the sciatic nerve.

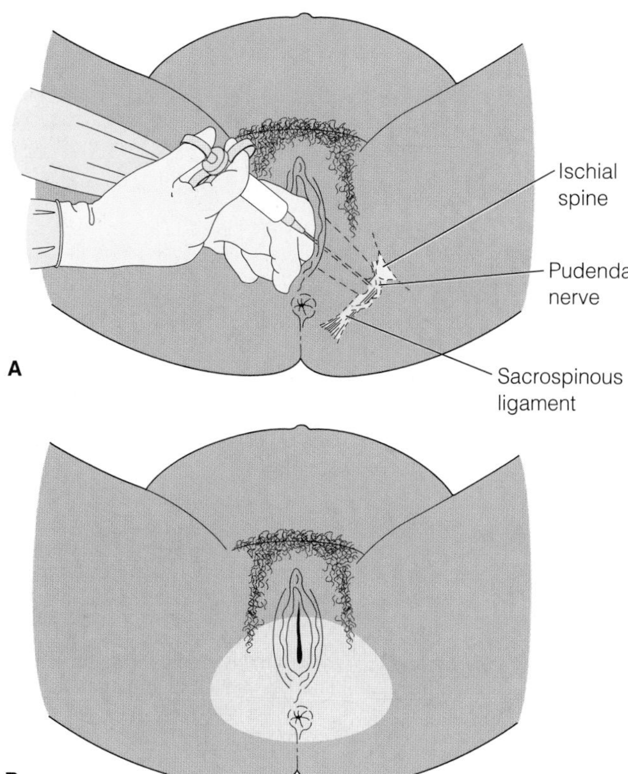

FIGURE 21–7 *A,* Pudendal block by the transvaginal approach. *B,* Area of perineum affected by pudendal block.

NURSING CARE MANAGEMENT

The nurse explains the procedure and the expected effect and answers any questions. Pudendal block does not alter maternal vital signs or FHR, so assessments in addition to the expected ones are not necessary.

Local Infiltration Anesthesia

Local anesthesia is accomplished by injecting an anesthetic agent into the intracutaneous, subcutaneous, and intramuscular areas of the perineum (Figure 21–8). It is generally used at the time of birth for episiotomy repair and is especially useful for women giving birth by psychoprophylactic methods of childbirth. The procedure is essentially free from complications.

Advantages

The major advantage of the local block is that it involves the use of the least amount of anesthetic agent. It can be done only if an episiotomy is needed just prior to the birth.

Disadvantages

The major disadvantage is that large amounts of solution must be used. Although any local anesthetic may be used, chloroprocaine (Nesacaine), lidocaine (Xylocaine), and

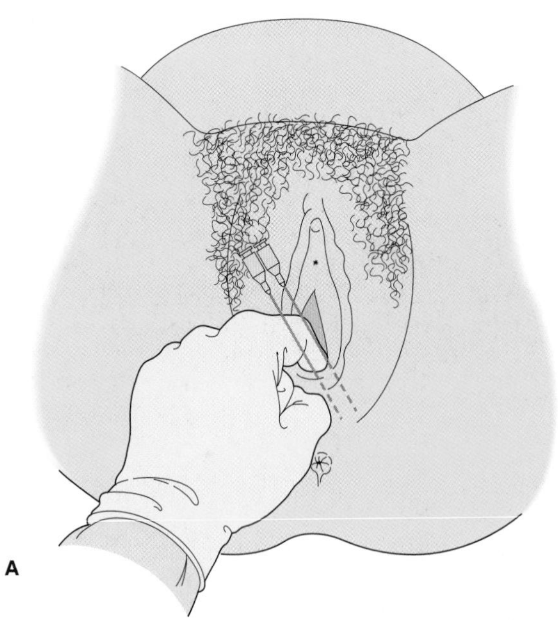

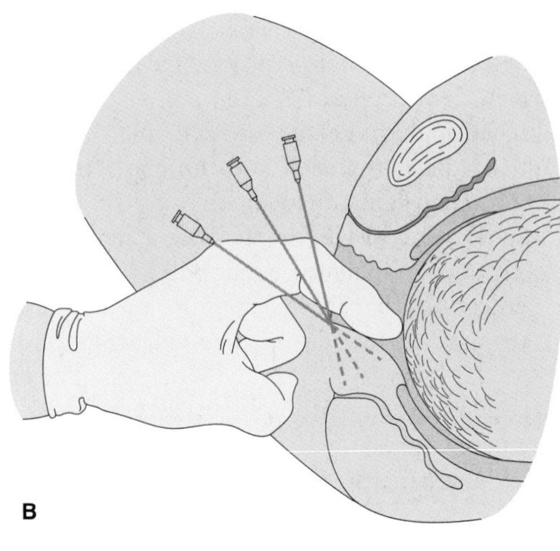

FIGURE 21–8 Local infiltration anesthesia. ***A,*** Technique of local infiltration for episiotomy and repair. ***B,*** Technique of local infiltration showing fan pattern for the fascial planes. SOURCE: Bonica JJ: *Principles and Practice of Obstetric Analgesia and Anesthesia.* Philadelphia: Davis, 1972, p 505.

mepivacaine (Carbocaine) are the agents of choice in local infiltration because of their capacity for diffusion.

NURSING CARE MANAGEMENT

The nurse explains the procedure and the expected effect and answers any questions. Local anesthetic agents have no effect on maternal vital signs or FHR, so additional assessments are unnecessary.

General Anesthesia

General anesthesia may be needed for cesarean birth and surgical intervention with some obstetric complications. The method used to achieve general anesthesia may be intravenous injection, inhalation of anesthetic agents, or a combination of both methods.

Intravenous Anesthetics

Sodium thiopental (Pentothal) is an ultra–short-acting barbiturate, which means that it exerts its effect rapidly and has a brief duration of action. Sodium thiopental produces narcosis within 30 seconds after intravenous administration. Induction and emergence from its effects are smooth and pleasant, with little incidence of nausea and vomiting. Sodium thiopental is most frequently used for induction and as an adjunct to other more potent anesthetics.

Complications of General Anesthesia

A primary danger of general anesthesia is fetal depression. Most general anesthetic agents reach the fetus in about 2 minutes. The depression is the fetus is directly proportional to the depth and duration of the anesthesia. The long-term significance of fetal depression in a normal birth has not been determined. The poor fetal metabolism of general anesthesic agents is similar to that of analgesic agents administered during labor. General anesthesia is not advocated when the fetus is considered to be at high risk, particularly in premature delivery.

Most general anesthetic agents cause some degree of uterine relaxation. They may also cause vomiting and aspiration.

Pregnancy results in decreased gastric motility, and the onset of labor halts the process almost entirely. Food eaten hours earlier may remain undigested in the stomach. Even when food and fluids have been withheld, the gastric juice produced during fasting is highly acidic and can produce chemical pneumonitis if aspirated. This pneumonitis is known as Mendelson's syndrome. The signs and symptoms are chest pain, respiratory distress, cyanosis, fever, and tachycardia.

Care during General Anesthesia

Prophylactic antacid therapy to reduce the acidic content of the stomach before general anesthesia is given. Administration of a nonparticulate antacid (such as Bicitra) may be used. Cimetidine (Tagamet) may also be used (Cunningham et al, 1997).

Before the induction to anesthesia, the woman should have a wedge placed under her right hip to displace the uterus and avoid vena caval compression in the supine position. She should also be preoxygenated with 3 to 5 minutes of 100% oxygen. Intravenous fluids should be started so that access to the intravascular space is immediately available.

During the process of rapid induction of anesthesia, the nurse applies cricoid pressure. This is accomplished by depressing the cricoid cartilage 2 to 3 cm posteriorly so that the esophagus is occluded. Cricoid pressure is continued until the anesthesiologist has placed the cuffed endotracheal tube and indicates that the pressure can be released. Figure 21–9 shows the appropriate technique. The woman's neck should be supported by the nurse's other hand.

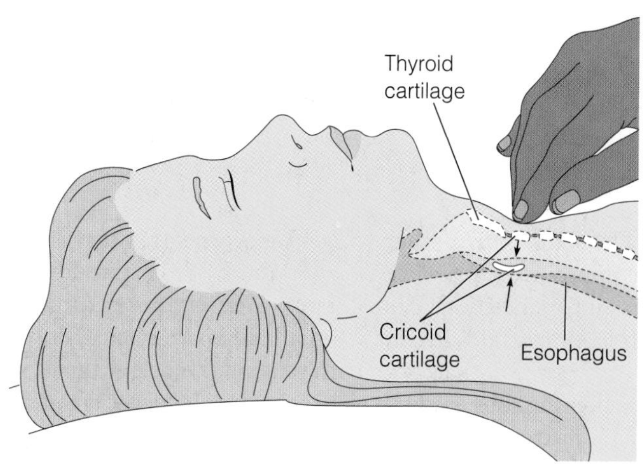

FIGURE 21–9 Proper position for fingers in applying cricoid pressure until a cuffed endotracheal tube is placed by the anesthesiologist or certified nurse-anesthetist. The cricoid cartilage is depressed 2–3 cm posteriorly so that the esophagus is occluded.

Neonatal Neurobehavioral Effects of Anesthesia and Analgesia

Studies have focused on the neurobehavioral effects on the newborn of pharmacologic agents used during labor and birth. Although analgesic and anesthetic agents may alter the behavioral and adaptive function of the newborn, physiologic factors such as hunger, degree of hydration, and time within the sleep-wake cycle may also exert an influence (Ezekiel, 1997). The long-range importance of these findings has not been well established.

Analgesic and Anesthetic Considerations for the High-Risk Mother and Fetus

Up to this point the discussion of obstetric analgesia and anesthesia has dealt with the healthy woman and healthy fetus. Pain relief for high-risk women during labor and birth requires skill in decision making, close observation, and awareness of potential threats to the woman and fetus. Safety for all involved requires the close cooperation of obstetrician, anesthesiologist, pediatrician, and labor nurse. The pathophysiologic changes that accompany maternal disorders have a direct influence on the choice of agent or technique. It is difficult to separate maternal and fetal complications because whatever alters the woman's response will also affect the fetus. The effects on the woman cannot be considered without the potential effects on the fetus.

Preterm Labor

The preterm fetus has special risks and requirements. An immature fetus is more susceptible to depressant drugs because it has less protein available for binding; has a poorly developed blood-brain barrier, which increases the likelihood that pharmacologic agents will attain a higher concentration in the central nervous system; and has a decreased ability to metabolize and excrete drugs after birth. Analgesia during labor should be avoided whenever possible. If it becomes necessary, the smallest dose that will provide relief should be administered. Emotional support will be very valuable to the woman in this situation.

Pregnancy-Induced Hypertension

Pregnancies complicated by pregnancy-induced hypertension (PIH) are high-risk situations, as indicated in Chapter 16. The potential for chronic placental insufficiency or preterm birth is also present. The woman with mild PIH usually may have the analgesia or anesthesia of choice, although the incidence of hypotension with epidural anesthesia is increased. If hypotension occurs with the epidural block, it provides further stress on an already compromised cardiovascular system. Hypotension can usually be managed with judicial fluid increase and positioning (Ezekiel, 1997).

The woman with severe PIH poses a real challenge. Regional anesthesia seems to be the preferred method as long as hypotension can be avoided. Raising the central venous pressure by 3 to 4 cm H_2O with intravenous fluids helps avoid hypotension, but it must be remembered that this woman is already threatened with heart failure. The effect of fluid intake can be monitored with a central venous pressure (CVP) line or pulmonary catheter. It is important to monitor and record the fluid intake and output. Some physicians use vasopressors; others avoid them because of the possible decrease in uterine blood flow to an already compromised fetus and the threat of a maternal cerebral vascular accident. Spinal anesthesia is rarely used because of the greater potential for hypotension.

The use of general anesthesia poses a risk of aggravating maternal hypertension. The safest method for general anesthesia includes intubation, which may cause a hypertensive episode.

Diabetes Mellitus

The fetus of a mother with diabetes mellitus may have compromised placental reserve, and hypotension during regional anesthesia can deplete this reserve even further. If labor can be managed without fetal distress, small doses of intravenous narcotics with pudendal block at birth or the continuous epidural technique may be undertaken. If fetal distress occurs, cesarean birth may be necessary.

Anesthesia for cesarean birth requires special consideration in this case. The diabetic woman is more likely to experience cardiovascular depression during a regional block because of higher sympathetic blockade (Datta, 1995). If a regional block is selected, it is recommended that acute hydration (preload) be provided by administering dextrose-free solution. In addition, left uterine displacement is initiated prior to the administration of the block and maintained throughout the surgery. Hypotension is treated promptly.

Cardiac Disease

Pregnancy imposes significant risk for the woman with cardiac disease. With mild mitral stenosis, the preferred anesthetic is continual epidural anesthesia with low forceps birth. This method avoids the cardiovascular changes associated with contractions and the Valsalva maneuver during bearing down in the second stage of labor. Hypotension can be avoided with carefully controlled intravenous fluids and measuring CVP to avoid overload. Epidural block or general anesthesia may be used in cesarean birth. Ketamine should be avoided because it produces tachycardia.

Bleeding Complications

The current trend in treating bleeding complications during labor is to schedule cesarean birth when possible. When the maternal cardiovascular system is stable and there is no evidence of fetal distress, an epidural may be given for birth. However, when either of these conditions results in active bleeding, the threat of hypovolemia must be treated immediately. Maternal hypovolemia and shock produce fetal hypoxia, acidosis, and possible fetal death.

Regional blocks are contraindicated during active bleeding because the sympathetic block causes vasodilattion and further reduction of the vascular volume. General anesthesia is recommended for these cases. Sodium thiopental may be used, but it is a cardiac depressant and vasodilator, and ketamine may be a more appropriate choice for induction. Following birth of the infant and placenta, oxytocin should not be given as an intravenous bolus to contract the uterus because it causes vasodilation, which in turn causes a decrease in blood pressure and in total peripheral resistance. Oxytocin should be given as a dilute infusion to gain an oxytocic effect to treat uterine atony (relaxation) and to control postpartum bleeding.

FOCUS YOUR STUDY

- Pain relief during labor may be enhanced by psychoprophylactic methods and administration of analgesic agents and regional anesthesia blocks.
- The goal of pharmacologic analgesia during labor is to provide maximal pain relief with minimal risk for the woman and fetus.
- The optimal time for administering analgesia is determined after a complete assessment of many factors. An analgesic agent is generally administered to nulliparas when the cervix has dilated 5 to 6 cm and to multiparas when the cervix has reached 3 to 4 cm dilatation.
- Two common analgesic agents are butorphanol (Stadol) and nalbuphine (Nubain).
- Opiate antagonists, such as naloxone (Narcan), counteract the respiratory depressant effect of the opiate narcotics by acting at specific receptor sites in the CNS.
- Regional anesthesia is achieved by injecting local anesthetic agents into an area that will bring the agent into direct contact with nerve tissue. Methods most commonly used in childbearing include lumbar epidural, spinal block, pudendal block, and local infiltration.
- Three types of local anesthetic agents used in regional blocks are amides, esters, and opiates. The amides are absorbed quickly and can be found in maternal blood within minutes after administration. The esters are metabolized more rapidly and have only limited placental transfer. Opiates act on specific opiate receptors in the spinal cord and have a greater analgesic effect when combined with a low dose of local anesthetic.
- New agents in use for intrathecal and epidural routes include the opiods morphine and fentanyl. Adverse reactions of the woman to local anesthetic agents range from mild symptoms, such as palpitations, to cardiovascular collapse.
- The goal of general anesthesia is to provide maximal pain relief with minimal side effects to the woman and her fetus.
- Complications of general anesthesia include fetal depression, uterine relaxation, vomiting, and aspiration.
- The choice of analgesia and anesthesia for the high-risk woman and fetus requires careful evaluation.

REFERENCES

American College of Obstetricians and Gynecologists (ACOG). ACOG Committee Opinion No. 118. (1993). Pain relief during labor. Washington, DC: Author.

Bourne, T. M., deMelo, A. E., Bastianpillai, B. A., & May, A. E. (1997). A survey of how British obstetric anesthetists test regional anaesthesia before Caesarean section. *Anaesthesia, 52,* 896–913.

Briggs, G., Freeman, R. K., & Yaffe, S. J. (1999). *Drugs in pregnancy and lactation* (5th ed.). Baltimore: Williams & Wilkins.

Chestnut, D. H. (1997). Epidural analgesia and the incidence of cesarean section. *Anesthesiology, 87,* 472–476.

Cunningham, F. G., MacDonald, P. C., Gant, N. F., Leveno, K. J., Gilstrap, L. C., Hankins, G. V. D., & Clark, S. L. (1997). Analgesia and anesthesia. In *Williams obstetrics* (20th ed.) (pp 379–398). Stamford, CT: Appleton & Lange.

Datta, S. (1995). *The obstetric anesthesia handbook.* St Louis: Mosby.

Downing, J. W., Johnson, H. V., Gonzalez, H. F., Arney, T. L., Herman, N. L., & Johnson, R. F. (1997). The pharmacokinetics of epidural lidocaine and bupivacaine during cesarean section. *Anesthesia and Analgesia, 84,* 527–532.

Ezekiel, M. R. (1997). *Handbook of anesthesiology.* Laguna Hills, CA: Current Clinical Strategies Publishing.

Grass, J. A., Sakima, N. T., Schmidt, R., Michitsch, R., Zuckerman, R. L., & Harris, A. P. (1997). A randomized, double-blind, dose-response comparison of epidural fentanyl versus sufentanil analgesia after cesarean section. *Anesthesia and Analgesia, 85,* 365–371.

Gutsche, B. R., & Cheek, T. G. (1993). Anesthetic considerations in preeclampsia-eclampsia. In S. M. Shnider & G. Levinson (Eds.), *Anesthesia for obstetrics* (3rd ed.). Baltimore: Williams & Wilkins.

Holt, R. O., Diehl, S. J., & Wright, J. W. (1999). Station and cervical dilation at epidural placement in predicting cesarean risk. *Obstetrics Gynecology, 93,* 281–284.

Karch, A. M. (1999). *Lippincott's nursing drug guide.* Philadelphia: Lippincott.

Levinson, G., & Shnider, S. M. (1993). Systemic medication for labor and delivery. In S. M. Shnider & G. Levinson (Eds.), *Anesthesia for obstetrics* (3rd ed.). Baltimore: Williams & Wilkins.

Mayer, D. C., Chescheir, N. C., & Spielman, F. J. (1997). Increased intrapartum antibiotic administration associated with epidural analgesia in labor. *American Journal of Perinatology, 14,* 83–86.

Ngan Kee, W. D., Khaw, K. S., & Ma, M. L. (1997). Patient-controlled epidural analgesia after cesarean section using meperidine. *Canadian Journal of Anaesthesia, 44,* 702–706.

Paradise, N. F. (1994). Personal communication.

PDR nurse's handbook. (1999). Montvale, NJ: Demar Publishers and Medical Economics Co., Inc.

Russell, R., & Reynolds, F. (1997). Pain relief and anesthesia during labor. In R. K. Creasy (Ed.), *Management of labor and delivery* (pp 183–222). Malden, MA: Blackwell.

Seymour, J. (1997). Pain relief in childbirth. *Nursing Times, 93,* 55–56.

Sharma, S. K., Sidawi, J. E., Ramin, S. M., Lucas, M. J., Leveno, K. J., & Cunningham, F. G. (1997). Cesarean delivery: A randomized trial of epidural versus patient-controlled meperidine analgesia during labor. *Anesthesiology, 87,* 487–494.

Shnider, S. M., & Levinson, G. (1993). *Anesthesia for obstetrics* (3rd ed.). Baltimore: Williams & Wilkins.

Shnider, S. M., Levinson, G., & Ralston, D. H. (1993). Regional anesthesia for labor and delivery. In S. M. Shnider & G. Levinson (Eds.), *Anesthesia for obstetrics* (3rd ed.). Baltimore: Williams & Wilkins.

Taylor, T. (1993). Epidural anesthesia in the maternity patient. *Maternal-Child Nursing Journal, 18,* 86.

Thorpe, J., & Breedlove, G. (1996). Epidural analgesia in labor: An evaluation of risks and benefits. *Birth, 23,* 63.

Wildman, K. M., Mohl, V. K., Cassel, J. H., Houston, R. E., & Allerheiligen, D. A. (1997). Intrathecal analgesia for labor. *Journal of Family Practice, 44,* 535–540.

Wilson, B. A., Shannon, M. J., & Strang, C. L. (1997). *Nurse's drug guide.* Stamford, CT: Appleton & Lange.

Youngstrom, P., Baker, S. W., & Miller, J. L. (1996). Epidurals redefined in analgesia and anesthesia: A distinction with a difference. *Journal of Obstetrics, Gynecology, and Neonatal Nursing, 25,* 350.

22 Childbirth at Risk

Key Terms

Abruptio placentae
Active management of labor (AMOL)
Amniotic fluid embolism
Cephalopelvic disproportion (CPD)
Dystocia
Hydramnios
Macrosomia
Oligohydramnios
Persistent occiput-posterior (OP) position
Placenta previa
Postterm pregnancy
Precipitate labor and birth
Prolapsed cord

SINCE THE DAY I BEGAN MY NURSING PROGRAM, I had been waiting for this rotation in the birthing center. At last I would be able to be with a couple during their labor and birth. My first family had such wonderful plans for the labor and birth. I was able to be with them and could even assist with helping her breathe when she got to transition. Then suddenly the fetal heart rate dropped, and I recognized a variable deceleration. It lasted 20 seconds, but it felt like it was forever. The nurse and I helped the mother onto her other side, and we waited expectantly. I felt like time had stopped, but I realized at that moment that if I was feeling like this, so were the parents. I looked at them, and their faces were so tense. I reached out and took her hand. I didn't know what to say, but I knew that at least I could stay with her. There were no further problems, but I will never forget that moment.

Objectives

- Describe psychologic factors that may contribute to complications during labor and birth.
- Discuss dysfunctional labor patterns.
- Describe the impact of postterm pregnancy on the childbearing family.
- Explore the causes and management of uterine rupture.
- Summarize various types of fetal metabolism and malpresentation and possible associated problems.
- Discuss the identification, management, and care of fetal developmental abnormalities such as macrosomia and hydrocephalus.
- Discuss the nursing care that is indicated in the event of fetal distress.
- Discuss intrauterine fetal death, including etiology, diagnosis, management, and the nurse's role in assisting the family.
- Compare abruptio placentae and placenta previa.
- Identify variations that may occur in the umbilical cord and insertion into the placenta.
- Discuss the identification, management, and nursing care of women with amniotic fluid embolus, hydramnios, and oligohydramnios.
- Delineate the effects of pelvic contractures on labor and birth.
- Discuss complications of the third and fourth stages of labor.

THE SUCCESSFUL COMPLETION OF THE 40-week gestational period requires the harmonious functioning of four components: psychosocial factors, contractile forces, fetus, and maternal pelvis or birth passage (these components are described in depth in Chapter 18). The psychosocial factors are the intellectual and emotional processes of the pregnant woman as influenced by heredity, environment, and her life experiences and include her feelings about pregnancy and motherhood. The contractile forces of labor are the myometrial forces of the contracting uterus. The fetus, in this case, includes all the products of conception: the fetus, placenta, umbilical cord, membranes, and amniotic fluid. The birth passage comprises the vagina and bony pelvis. Disruptions in any of the four components may affect the others and cause **dystocia** (at-risk or difficult labor). Some of the most common at-risk conditions are discussed in this chapter.

Care of the Woman at Risk Due to Anxiety and Fear

Stress, anxiety, and fear have a profound effect on labor, particularly when complications that imply maternal or fetal jeopardy occur. A labor process that was initially viewed with confidence and happiness may provoke anxiety and a variety of physiologic and psychologic responses once labor has begun.

In the laboring woman, anxiety and fear may exacerbate pain; continued pain may then increase her anxiety and fear, producing a vicious cycle. The resulting increase in catecholamine release in turn increases physical distress and may result in myometrial dysfunction and ineffectual labor (Figure 22–1).

Anxiety may affect the woman and family in a variety of ways. Some families are in denial; they prefer to focus on the positive and act as though everything were normal, even though they have been informed that there may be a problem with the labor, the birth, or the baby. They may ask no questions, seek no assistance, seem happy, and act almost as though they do not understand that there could be a problem.

Other families may have dealt with so much stress during the pregnancy that they are emotionally exhausted by the time they come in for the birth. Their ability to cope has long since been expended. They may be demanding, argumentative, strongly assertive, angry, passive, or a mixture of all these emotions. If a particular aspect of the labor and birth has been fearfully anticipated, the parents' anxiety may rise as that event nears.

I am a nurse-midwife, and many of my clients are special, but Ann and Dave really stand out. They worked hard together, attending classes and practicing all the breathing and relaxation techniques. When Ann was in labor, Dave was there helping her breathe and encouraging her at every step. When Ann was pushing, Dave said he wished so much that he could see their baby be born—you see, Dave was blind. I quickly had a nurse help him into gloves, and he stood beside me. The baby was crowning, and I placed his hands on his baby's head. My hands held his, and his hands touched the baby. He kept his hands there for the whole birth and was able to cut the umbilical cord with the help of Ann and myself. Tears streamed down all our cheeks. Dave said, "Thank you for letting me 'see' my baby be born."

RESEARCH IN PRACTICE

What is this study about? Each pregnancy, labor, and birth constitute an important event in a woman's life. An obstetrically complicated delivery may cause the woman to feel less positive about her childbirth encounter. Marie Berg and Karin Dahlberg undertook a phenomenologic study to describe the experience of complicated childbirth.

How was the study done? The sample comprised ten women who had given birth at a Swedish hospital. Two women were multiparous and eight were primiparous (one with twins). Complications among the women included the following: two diabetics, one renal transplant patient, five emergency cesarian sections, two vacuum extractions, two perineal suturing under general anesthesia, two deliveries ending in manual removal of the placenta, three premature babies, and seven women observed in the intensive care unit postdelivery. The researchers conducted and audiotaped interviews 1 to 2 days postpartum. The investigators analyzed transcribed interviews, identified meaning units, and organized the units into themes. Through reflection, they explicated five themes and formulated an essential structure or essential meaning of the experience.

What were the results of the study? The five themes that Marie Berg and Karin Dahlberg identified were (1) to be seen; (2) trust; (3) dialogue; (4) control; and (5) mothering. The theme *to be seen* incorporated a strong need to be seen and respected, with caregivers listening to the woman's thoughts and desires. Giving of *trust* involved confidence in the caregivers' professional knowledge as well as their pliancy, calmness, consideration, and conveyance of feelings of safety. The theme of *dialogue* included feelings of affirmation developed as a result of receiving sincere verbal communication from the caregivers. *Control* consisted of increased self-esteem and self-confidence resulting from having control of the situation, including pain. *Mothering* encompassed development of the mother character throughout pregnancy until the ultimate affirmation of the baby's birth. The essential structure of the experience of complicated childbirth incorporated the woman's desire to be recognized and affirmed as a genuine subject. When confirmation or affirmation occurred, the woman felt capable as a childbearing woman and mother-to-be.

What additional questions might I have? Did the researchers return to their informants for affirmation that the findings accurately reflected the actual experience?

How can I use this study? If caregivers provide affirmation and control, even during difficult situations, they may profoundly affect the woman's experience of childbirth.

SOURCE: Berg, M., & Dahlberg, K. (1998). A phenomenological study of women's experiences of complicated childbirth. *Midwifery, 14,* 23–29. Lincoln, Y. S., & Guba, E. G. (1985). *Naturalistic inquiry.* Beverly Hills: Sage Publications.

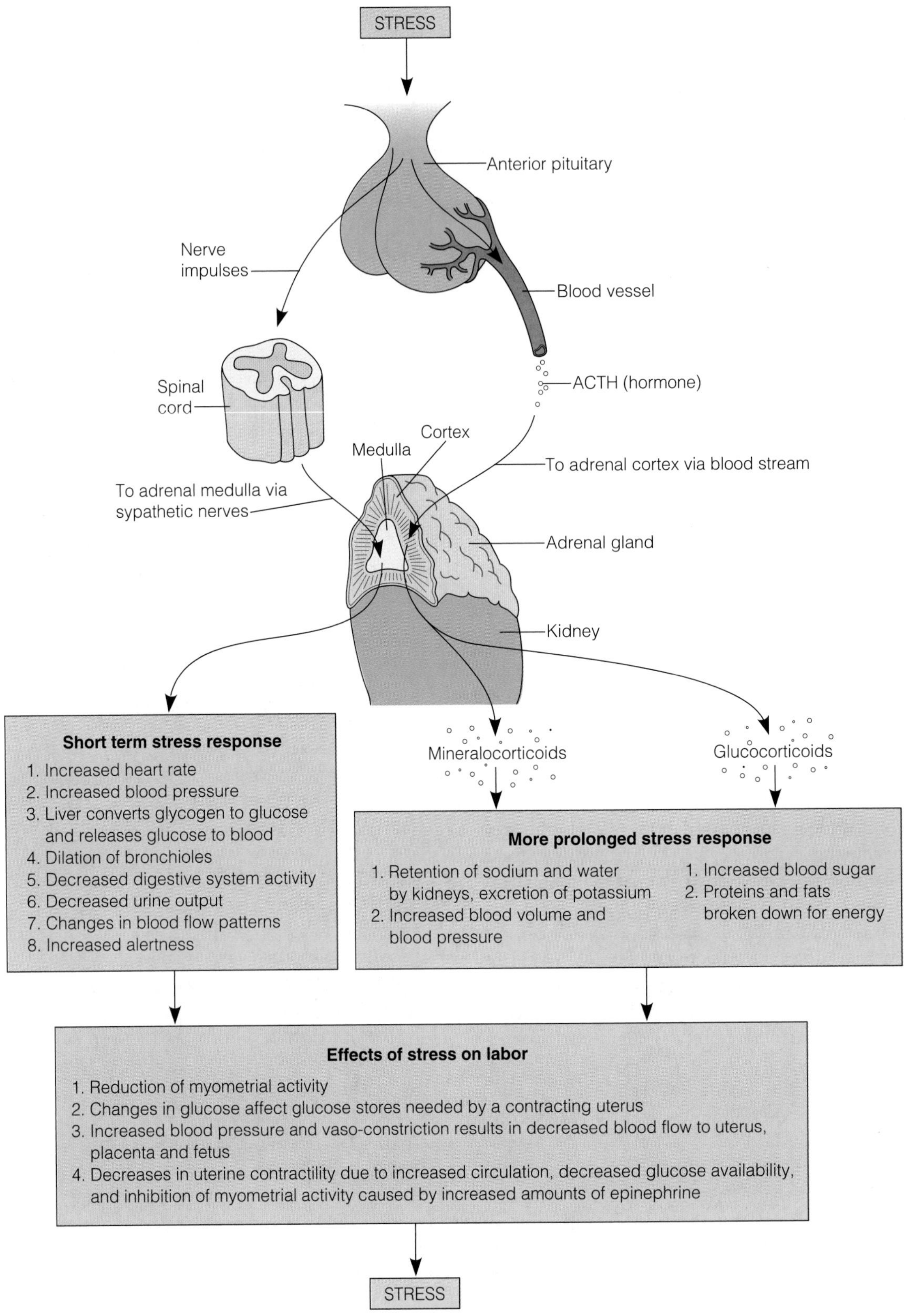

STRESS
Anterior pituitary
Nerve impulses
Blood vessel
Spinal cord
ACTH (hormone)
Cortex
Medulla
To adrenal cortex via blood stream
To adrenal medulla via sypathetic nerves
Adrenal gland
Kidney
Mineralocorticoids
Glucocorticoids
Short term stress response
1. Increased heart rate
2. Increased blood pressure
3. Liver converts glycogen to glucose and releases glucose to blood
4. Dilation of bronchioles
5. Decreased digestive system activity
6. Decreased urine output
7. Changes in blood flow patterns
8. Increased alertness
More prolonged stress response
1. Retention of sodium and water by kidneys, excretion of potassium
2. Increased blood volume and blood pressure
1. Increased blood sugar
2. Proteins and fats broken down for energy
Effects of stress on labor
1. Reduction of myometrial activity
2. Changes in glucose affect glucose stores needed by a contracting uterus
3. Increased blood pressure and vaso-constriction results in decreased blood flow to uterus, placenta and fetus
4. Decreases in uterine contractility due to increased circulation, decreased glucose availability, and inhibition of myometrial activity caused by increased amounts of epinephrine
STRESS

FIGURE 22–1 Effects of stress on labor. SOURCE: Adapted from Campbell N: *Biology,* 2nd ed. Redwood City, CA: Benjamin/Cummings, 1990.

Women who are in an abusive relationship may be especially passive during labor and birth, looking to their partner for all direction and letting the partner answer all questions. The woman follows the partner's directions and exhibits a need to please. She may exhibit anxiety or be more passive.

At times, a woman will exhibit rather exaggerated behaviors during labor. She may need absolute control of everything that happens and will not participate until she feels sure that she knows what will happen. She may be very anxious and not able to articulate her fears or needs and may not respond to supportive nursing measures. She may be unaware of what will happen in labor and birth, may be unable to understand, or may be dealing with memories of sexual abuse from earlier in her life that suddenly are brought back by the labor process and some of the procedures that are performed (Waymire, 1997).

One young woman I worked with was in preterm labor. I was evaluating her, and she was cooperative but anxious. The on-call physician came to examine her, and when he began the vaginal exam, her face changed, and she began screaming and yelling over and over: "Don't hurt me, I'll do anything you want. No, keep the fire away, please please, please." She was not with us in the room, she was in another event in her life, and she was terrified! I didn't know what to do. I stayed right beside her and kept talking softly. "It's all right Cheryl, you are here in the birth center. I'm Sally, your nurse. I will stay with you, and I won't let anyone hurt you. There is no fire here with me. Can you look at me? Hold my hand. You are safe here." She held my hand and finally was able to look at me. She finally became less anxious and was present in the room with us. She would not accept an exam and immediately left the birthing center. I still wonder what happened to her. I still have Cheryl with me in my heart.

Clinical Therapy

The goal of clinical therapy is to provide adjunctive therapies that will help decrease the woman's anxiety. The physician or certified nurse-midwife (CNM) may prescribe a sedative as needed to help allay anxiety and may seek to talk with the woman to answer questions. The physician/CNM may also provide written orders for analgesic medications that address pain and discomfort. Relieving the pain may decrease the woman's anxiety.

NURSING CARE MANAGEMENT

Nursing Assessment and Diagnosis

Unless birth is imminent or severe complications exist, the nurse begins the assessment by reviewing the woman's background. Factors such as age, parity, family support, culture, past and present experiences, and knowledge of the labor process contribute to the woman's psychologic response to labor.

As labor progresses, the nurse remains alert for the woman's verbal and nonverbal behavioral responses to the pain and anxiety of labor. The woman who is agitated and seems uncooperative or too quiet and compliant may require further appraisal for anxiety. Verbal statements such as, "Is everything okay?" "I'm really nervous," or "What's going on?" usually indicate some degree of anxiety and concern. Other women may be irritable, require frequent explanations, or repeat the same questions. The nurse further observes for nonverbal cues, including a tense posture, clenched hands, or pain out of context to the stage of labor (Roberts, Reardon, & Rosenfeld, 1999). Recognizing the impact of fatigue on pain and anxiety is another important nursing observation.

Nursing diagnoses may include the following:

- ***Ineffective Individual Coping*** related to increased anxiety and stress associated with labor and birth process
- ***Ineffective Family Coping*** related to anxiety associated with labor and birth
- ***Fear*** related to unknown outcome of the birth process
- ***Pain*** related to increased anxiety and stress
- ***Sensory/Perceptual Alteration*** related to reactivation of traumatic memories

Nursing Plan and Implementation

Hospital-Based Nursing Care

Primary nursing interventions center on supporting the laboring woman and her family and support persons. Families/couples who have attended childbirth preparation classes can be offered support and encouragement as they employ the techniques they have learned. If the woman begins to lose her ability to cope, the nurse can often assist the partner in helping the woman regain control. If anxiety is evident, the nurse should acknowledge the anxiety and offer methods to promote relaxation and comfort (see Chapter 20).

The woman or family who has not been able to attend prenatal classes can be taught breathing techniques and comfort measures at the time of admission, especially if active labor has not begun. The nurse can provide clear but succinct information about the labor process, medical procedures, the environment, simple breathing exercises, and relaxation techniques, thereby preventing or relieving some apprehension and fear. Even a woman in active labor who has had no prior childbirth preparation can achieve a great deal of relaxation from physical comfort measures, touch, frequent attention, therapeutic interaction, and possibly analgesic agents.

The nurse's ability to support the woman and her partner as they deal with the stress of labor is directly related to the rapport established among them. By employing a calm, caring, confident, nonjudgmental approach, the nurse can not only acknowledge the anxiety, but also identify the source of the distress. Once the causative

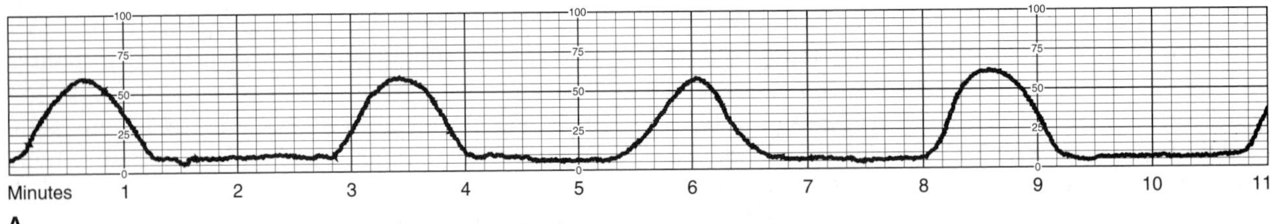

A

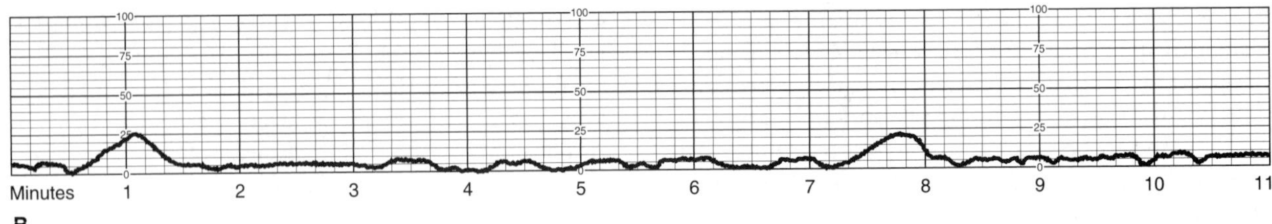

B

FIGURE 22–2 Comparison of labor patterns. ***A,*** Normal uterine contraction pattern. Note that the contraction frequency is every 3 minutes; duration is 60 seconds. The baseline resting tone is below 10 mm Hg. ***B,*** Hypotonic uterine contraction pattern. Note in this example that the contraction frequency is every 7 minutes with some uterine activity between contractions, duration is 50 seconds, and intensity increases approximately 25 mm Hg during contractions.

factors are known, the nurse can implement appropriate interventions, such as information, comfort measures, touch, therapeutic communication, and therapeutic use of self.

Providing emotional support and comfort measures has been demonstrated to make a difference in outcomes. Randomized controlled trials of nulliparous women in labor who receive this support during labor have demonstrated lower rates of analgesia/anesthesia, lower operative birth rates, lower episiotomy rates, shorter labors, and fewer newborns with a 5-minute Apgar score of less than 7 (Hodnett et al, 1997).

CRITICAL THINKING QUESTION

What constitutes emotional support and comfort measures? How can you implement these strategies in today's high-technology-oriented facilities? Is there scientific support for the use of technology, such as electronic fetal monitoring (EFM), with women in labor? How does the use of technology affect the obstetric outcome? Can you support your answer by citing relevant data?

Evaluation

Expected outcomes of nursing care include the following:

- The woman experiences a decrease in physiologic and psychologic stress and an increase in physiologic and psychologic comfort.
- The woman uses effective coping mechanisms to manage her stress and anxiety in labor.
- The woman's and the family's fear is decreased.
- The woman verbalizes feelings about her labor. ●

Care of the Woman Experiencing Dystocia Related to Dysfunctional Uterine Contractions

Dystocia, or difficult labor, encompasses many problems in labor, the most common of which is dysfunctional (or uncoordinated) uterine contractions that result in a prolongation of labor (Bowes, 1997). Contractions associated with normal progress in labor tend to occur regularly, at 2 to 4 contractions per 10 minutes with a mean amplitude of 35 mm Hg in early labor. Later in a normal labor, the contractions progress to 4 to 5 in 10 minutes with a mean amplitude of 40 to 50 mm Hg (Bowes, 1997). Dysfunctional uterine contractions typically are irregular, of low amplitude, and slow progress (less than 1 cm dilatation per hour). Alternatively, cervical dilatation may be arrested; that is, contractions continue but cervical dilatation progresses to a certain point and then remains the same. Figure 22–2 depicts normal and hypotonic uterine contraction patterns.

The specific cause of dysfunctional contractions is unknown; however, Dizon-Townson and Ward (1997) have suggested that genetic factors may control the normal physiologic processes of labor. Cesarean birth and operative vaginal birth (use of forceps or vacuum extractor), for example, tend to run in families. If the laboring woman's parents were born by cesarean, there is a high probability that the woman herself was born by cesarean and that she will also give birth by cesarean because of dysfunctional labor.

The familial tendencies for difficult labor give rise to the theory that genetic processes control normal labor. It is hypothesized that there may be an inheritable tendency toward poor uterine contractions and/or soft-tissue relaxation (Dizon-Townson & Ward, 1997). In one study, nulliparas who underwent cesarean birth because of prolonged labor had a "significantly higher concentration of collagen, with a decrease in solubility, in the uterine isthmus and cervix" (Dizon-Townson & Ward, 1997, p 480). Further research may establish additional evidence of a familial alteration in collagen composition.

Clinical Therapy

When uterine contractions are irregular and of low amplitude and there is less than 1 cm cervical dilatation per hour (called *protracted labor*) or there has been no change of cervical dilatation for 2 hours *(arrest of progress)*, the physician evaluates the woman for the presence of any factor that would preclude the use of oxytocin (Pitocin) augmentation. The physician evaluates the size of the maternal pelvis, the position and presentation of the fetus, and fetal weight. The physician carefully considers the possibility of **cephalopelvic disproportion (CPD),** which is a disparity between the size of the maternal pelvis and the size of the presenting fetal head due to position, presentation, or increased fetal weight that precludes a vaginal birth. If CPD exists, oxytocin (Pitocin) augmentation should not be used.

When CPD is ruled out, an amniotomy (AROM) is performed if membranes are intact. Studies of the effectiveness of amniotomy have not demonstrated conclusive results. However, it is an accepted procedure with the diagnosis of dystocia secondary to uterine hypocontractility (American College of Obstetricians and Gynecologist [ACOG], 1995). Oxytocin (Pitocin) augmentation is then begun (see Drug Guide: Oxytocin in Chapter 23). Lopez-Zeno (1997) recommends that the oxytocin infusion be initiated at 1 mU/minute. If needed, the dose may then be increased by 1 to 2 mU/min every 15 minutes with the goal of obtaining 8 contractions per 20 minutes. Continuous electronic fetal monitoring (EFM) is used to provide ongoing information regarding fetal response to the augmentation. If second stage labor is present, fetal scalp pH may be measured to assess fetal acid-base balance. With augmentation of labor, the contraction pattern and progressive cervical contraction pattern should improve, and fetal descent (measured by station) should occur. If there is no improvement in these areas, cesarean birth may be necessary.

Some physicians support the use of **active management of labor (AMOL),** a process whereby labor is managed from the beginning with amniotomy, timed cervical examinations, and augmentation of labor with intravenous oxytocin if adequate progress is not made. Supporters of AMOL contend that it is preventive treatment that reduces the potential for protracted labor or arrest of progress. AMOL has been studied around the world since the mid 1960s and has been found to be effective in decreasing the length of labor (less than 12 hours for nulliparas), decreasing the incidence of febrile complications that may be associated with prolonged labor, and decreasing the cesarean birth rate (Lopez-Zeno, 1997). AMOL begins with careful assessment of the laboring woman, artificial rupture of membranes (if the membranes are still intact) within 1 hour of diagnosis of the presence of actual labor, and hourly cervical examinations for the first 3 hours. Thereafter cervical examinations are performed every 2 hours, and at least 1 additional cm of dilatation is expected at each examination. If cervical dilatation is less than expected, augmentation with an intravenous oxytocin infusion is begun (Lopez-Zeno, 1997). AMOL also incorporates a strong one-to-one nursing care program, in which the nurse remains with the woman. This permits ongoing assessment and provides the beneficial aspect of constant nursing support (Lopez-Zeno, 1997). Proponents of AMOL believe that its use can avoid dysfunctional labor patterns, instrumental delivery, and cesarean birth. Those who oppose AMOL, in contrast, contend that labor needs to be considered as a normal process and allowed to progress without automatic intervention. Only if problems occur should the labor be augmented.

CRITICAL THINKING IN PRACTICE

A fetal heart tracing demonstrates the following: baseline heart rate of 140 with variability of 6–10 bpm. When you compare the FHR with the uterine contractions, you note that there is a slowing of the FHR at the time of the contraction and that the FHR tracing looks like the contraction curve, but it is upside down. *Based on this tracing, what would you do?*

Answers can be found in Appendix I.

NURSING CARE MANAGEMENT

Nursing Assessment and Diagnosis

Assessing maternal vital signs, contractions, cervical dilatation, fetal descent, and fetal heart rate characteristics provides the nurse with data to evaluate maternal-fetal status. During the vaginal examination, the fetal presenting part (usually vertex) is assessed for the development of a caput. If the fetal vertex presses down on the cervix during contractions without further descent, a caput succedaneum may occur. In this case, the caput continues to increase in size; it seems that the head is descending, but it is not (Figure 23–3).

Because labor progress may be slow, the nurse assesses the woman's stress and coping, noting whether anxiety is having a deleterious effect on labor progress. Evidence of increasing frustration and discouragement on the part of the mother and her partner may become apparent as labor continues.

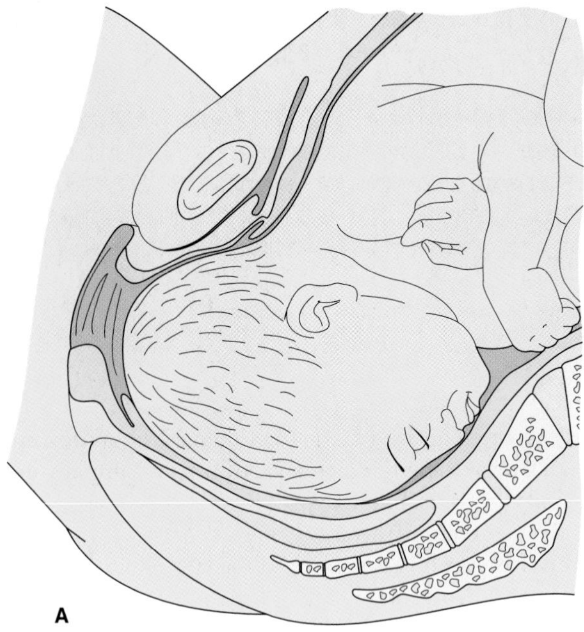

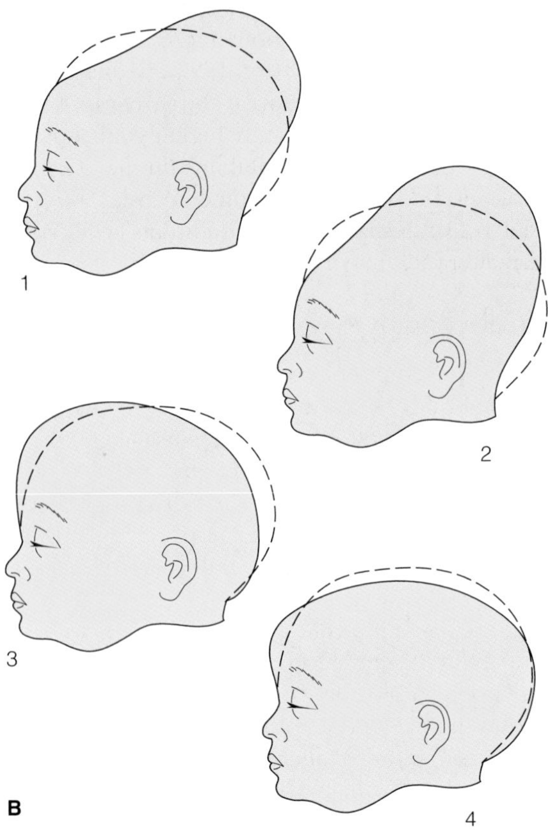

FIGURE 22–3 Effects of labor on the fetal head. ***A,*** Caput succedaneum formation. The presenting portion of the scalp area is encircled by the cervix during labor, causing swelling of the soft tissue. ***B,*** Molding of the fetal head in cephalic presentations: (1) occiput anterior, (2) occiput posterior, (3) brow, (4) face.

Nursing diagnoses that may apply to the woman experiencing dysfunctional labor include the following:

- ***Pain*** related to woman's difficulty in relaxing secondary to uterine contractions
- ***Risk for Ineffective Individual Coping*** related to ineffectiveness of breathing techniques to relieve discomfort
- ***Anxiety*** related to slow labor progress
- ***Knowledge Deficit*** related to lack of information about dysfunctional labor patterns

Nursing Plan and Implementation

Hospital-Based Nursing Care

The woman experiencing a dysfunctional labor pattern will probably be very uncomfortable because of protracted labor and the disappointment associated with the lack of progress. Her anxiety level and that of her partner may be high. The nurse attempts to reduce the woman's discomfort and promote a more effective labor pattern.

The nurse may suggest supportive measures such as a change of position: left lateral side-lying, high-Fowler's, on her knees in the bed with her arms up around the top of the bed while it is in high-Fowler's, rocking in a rocking chair, sitting up, and walking. Soothing measures such as a warm shower, whirlpool, quiet environment, music the woman finds soothing, back rub, therapeutic touch, and visualization may also be helpful. Comfort measures may also be utilized: mouth care, change of linens, effleurage, and relaxation exercises. The woman should be encouraged to void every 2 hours, and her bladder should be checked for distention. If the bladder is distended and the woman cannot void, catheterization will be necessary. (See Essential Precautions: During Care of the Woman at Risk for Intrapartal Complications.) The labor coach may also need assistance in helping the woman cope.

The nurse helps the woman and her partner cope with this difficult labor. Additional nursing measures include taking a warm, calm, caring approach coupled with techniques to reduce anxiety, such as using comfort measures (position changes, ambulation, sitting in a shower or whirlpool, back rub, use of touch), encouraging stress-reducing activities (breathing patterns, relaxation techniques, visualizations), and staying with the couple. It is important to note that in active management of labor, an integral part of the process is one-to-one nursing and the nurse remains with the woman. The positive value of the nurse's presence with the laboring woman has been well documented by numerous studies.

The laboring woman needs information about the dysfunctional labor pattern and the possible implications for her and her baby. It is particularly important to address the couple's concerns and questions with clear, ac-

ESSENTIAL PRECAUTIONS IN PRACTICE

During Care of the Woman at Risk for Intrapartal Complications

Wear disposable gloves when performing the following actions:

- Handling Chux and bedding that are moist with bloody show or amniotic fluid
- Cleansing the perineum
- Assessing the perineum

REMEMBER to wash your hands prior to putting the disposable gloves on and AGAIN immediately after you remove the gloves.

For further information, consult OSHA and CDC guidelines.

curate information. They need to be informed of progress and possible treatment measures. Disadvantages and treatment alternatives also need to be discussed and understood by the woman and her support person.

Evaluation

Expected outcomes of nursing care include the following:

- The woman and her partner understand the labor pattern and its possible implications.
- The woman and her partner are able to cope with the labor.
- The woman's comfort increases and her anxiety decreases.
- The woman experiences a more effective labor pattern.
- The father's supportive role is respected and maintained, and he is included in all planning if he chooses to be involved. ●

Precipitate Labor and Birth

Precipitate labor and birth is extremely rapid labor and birth within 3 hours. The most common causes are abnormally low resistance in maternal soft tissues, which allows for rapid cervical dilatation and fetal descent, and abnormally strong uterine contractions (Cunningham et al, 1997). In precipitate labor, cervical dilatation is 5 cm or more per hour in the primigravida and up to 10 cm in an hour for the multipara. The labor and birth may also be associated with cocaine abuse, abruptio placentae, meconium-stained fluid, low Apgar scores in the newborn, and postpartal hemorrhage.

Precipitate labor and birth and precipitous birth are not the same. A precipitous birth is a sudden, and often unattended, birth. See page 576 in Chapter 20 for discussion of precipitous birth.

CLINICAL TIP

As you know, normal cervical dilatation in a first-time mother—commonly known as a "primip"—is just over 1.0 cm/hour, and dilatation in a "multip" is about 1.5 cm/hour. If your assessments reveal that this expected pattern is not occurring, consider that a problem may be developing. The most likely causes of the problem are related to either the contractions or to fetal position or size.

Maternal risks may include abuptio placentae due to the abnormally strong contractions. If maternal tissues are not soft, extensive lacerations of the cervix, vagina, and perineum may occur. Fetal risks include meconium-stained fluid that may be aspirated at birth, low Apgar scores, and intracranial trauma resulting from the rapid birth and resistance of the birth canal to the fetal head (Cunningham et al, 1997).

Clinical Therapy

Any woman with a history of precipitate labor requires close medical monitoring and preparation for precipitate birth to facilitate a safe outcome for the mother and fetus. Drugs such as magnesium sulfate or a tocolytic agent such as terbutaline may be used to slow the uterine contractions (Cunningham et al, 1997). (See Drug Guide: Magnesium Sulfate in Chapter 16.)

NURSING CARE MANAGEMENT

Nursing Assessment and Diagnosis

During the intrapartal nursing assessment, the nurse can identify a woman at increased risk of precipitate labor. (For example, a previous history of precipitate or short labor places a woman at risk.) During the labor, accelerated cervical dilatation and fetal descent and intense contractions with little uterine relaxation between contractions are indicative of precipitate labor.

Nursing diagnoses that may apply to the woman with precipitate labor include the following:

- ***Risk for Injury*** related to rapid labor and birth
- ***Pain*** related to rapid labor process

Nursing Plan and Implementation

Hospital-Based Nursing Care

If the woman has a history of precipitate labor, it is imperative that the nurse establish rapport quickly because the nurse and woman may be involved in another precipitate labor and birth and the situation has the potential to be tense. Rapport and support from the nurse will enhance all other interventions. The nurse closely monitors the woman's contractions and cervical dilatation, and an emergency birth pack is kept near the bed. The nurse stays in constant attendance if at all possible and promotes comfort by assisting the woman to a comfortable position and providing a quiet environment. The nurse provides information and support before and after the birth. See page 576, Chapter 20, for discussion of nurse-managed birth.

The fetus is monitored for signs of hypoxia and other indications of fetal stress or distress. If meconium staining of the amniotic fluid is present, the fetal nares and mouth will be suctioned just after the head is born to prevent the baby from drawing more meconium-stained fluid into the lungs with the first breath. After the birth of the baby, the cords will be visualized and additional suctioning carried out as needed.

Evaluation
Expected outcomes of nursing care include the following:

- The woman and her baby are closely monitored during labor, and a safe birth occurs.
- The couple feels support and enhanced comfort during labor and birth. ●

Care of the Woman with Postterm Pregnancy

Postterm pregnancy is one that extends more than 294 days or 42 completed weeks past the first day of the last menstrual period. It is important to understand the phrase "42 completed weeks." "Pregnancies between 41 weeks 1 day and 41 weeks 6 days, although in the 42nd week, do not complete 42 weeks until the 7th day has elapsed" (Cunningham et al, 1997, p 827). The incidence of postterm pregnancy is approximately 3% to 7% of all pregnancies in the United States (Quilligan, 1996) and 4% to 14% in England (Hilder, Costeloe, & Thilaganathan, 1997). Postterm pregnancy occurs more frequently in primigravidas and women over 35 (Quilligan, 1996).

The cause of true postterm pregnancy is unknown. The most frequent cause is error in determining the time of ovulation and conception according to the first day of the last menstrual period (ACOG, 1997). This error can be corrected by performing ultrasound scans between 14 and 22 weeks. The scan reveals the biparietal diameter of the fetal head, which is then compared to conventional dating tables (Gardosi, Banner, & Francis, 1997).

Maternal Risks

Although postterm pregnancy does not pose any significant risk to the woman during the pregnancy, the labor and birth process may be affected. In many instances, labor is induced. Postterm pregnancy is associated with an increased incidence of large-for-gestational age (LGA) or macrosomic (weight in excess of 4000 g) fetuses, and vaginal birth is frequently associated with the use of forceps or vacuum extractor. Maternal hemorrhage may occur (Campbell, Ostbye, & Irgens, 1997). Cesarean birth may also be necessary.

Fetal-Neonatal Risks

True postterm pregnancies are frequently associated with placental changes that cause a decrease in the uterine-placental-fetal circulation. This decrease reduces the blood supply, oxygen, and nutrition for the fetus. Oligohydramnios (decreased amount of amniotic fluid) is frequently present and may increase the risk of umbilical cord compression (because the cord does not have as much fluid to float in). The fetus is more likely to be small-for-gestational-age (SGA) due to decreased nutrition associated with decreased utero-placental-fetal circulation. If utero-placental-fetal circulation is not compromised, the fetus continues to gain weight until the 42nd week; therefore, the fetus is often large-for-gestational-age (LGA) and macrosomic (weight in excess of 4000 g). The LGA or macrosomic fetus has a higher incidence of birth trauma or shoulder dystocia (difficulty or inability to deliver the baby's shoulders) (Cunningham et al, 1997). During labor, the postterm fetus may have meconium staining of the amniotic fluid which can lead to fetal stress or distress and meconium aspiration at birth (Cunningham et al, 1997). Perinatal mortality is slightly increased (Campbell, Ostbye, & Irgens, 1997).

Clinical Therapy

When the 40th week of gestation is completed and birth has not occurred, most obstetricians begin using the nonstress test (NST), biophysical profile (BPP) (especially the amniotic fluid volume portion of the BPP), and Doppler flow studies as assessment tools. The tests may be done two to three times a week. Any time that tests indicate fetal problems or there is decreased amniotic fluid volume, induction of labor is recommended (Cunningham et al, 1997).

NURSING CARE MANAGEMENT

Nursing Assessment and Diagnosis
When the woman is admitted into the birthing area, it is important to establish the estimated date of birth (EDB) and ascertain the type of antenatal testing that has been

completed. During labor, ongoing assessments of the FHR by continuous electronic fetal monitoring (EFM) are important to identify reassuring characteristics (presence of short-term and long-term variability, accelerations with fetal movement) and to determine the presence of nonperiodic variable decelerations so that corrective actions may be taken. When amniotic membranes rupture, the nurse assesses the fluid for the presence of meconium. Ongoing assessments of labor progress (contractions, progressive cervical dilatation and effacement, and fetal descent) may provide clues to the presence of a macrosomic fetus because labor may be lengthened.

Possible nursing diagnoses for the woman with postterm pregnancy include the following:

- *Knowledge Deficit* related to lack of information about postterm pregnancy
- *Fear* related to the unknown outcome for the baby
- *Risk for Ineffective Individual Coping* or *Ineffective Family Coping* related to concern regarding the status of the baby

Nursing Plan and Implementation

Community-Based Nursing Care

If the woman has not been assessing fetal activity every day, the nurse teaches her how to do it so that she can identify inadequate fetal movement and contact her health provider (see Chapter 17 for further discussion of techniques to detect fetal movement). The nurse encourages the woman to keep all appointments for biophysical profiles and other testing and provides information regarding the postterm pregnancy and the antenatal testing that will be indicated. In addition, the nurse addresses the implications and associated risks for the baby, as well as possible treatment plans, and provides the woman and her partner opportunities to ask questions and clarify information.

Hospital-Based Nursing Care

In the birth setting, the response of the fetus during labor is assessed carefully. Continuous electronic fetal monitoring of FHR is important to determine whether reassuring characteristics are present and to detect variable decelerations, especially if oligohydramnios is present. If variable decelerations are present, the laboring woman's position is changed to attempt to take pressure off the umbilical cord, and FHR is reevaluated. When an amnioinfusion is performed to increase the volume of fluid or to dilute meconium-stained fluid, the nurse assists with the procedure and monitors the infusion and the response of the FHR. (See Chapter 23 for further discussion.)

Evaluation

Expected outcomes of nursing care include the following:

- The woman has knowledge regarding the postterm pregnancy.
- The woman and her partner and family feel supported and able to cope with the labor and birth.
- Fetal problems are identified quickly. ●

Care of the Woman and Fetus at Risk Due to Fetal Malposition

Occiput-Posterior Position

Persistent occiput-posterior (OP) position of the fetus occurs in approximately 25% of pregnancies at term. This position may be normal in some races, particularly those whose women tend to have a small pelvis. For a fetus in an occiput-posterior position to rotate to an occiput-anterior position, it must rotate 135 degrees (ROP to ROT to ROA to OA), and in most cases this rotation is accomplished. In others, however, it is not. Labor progress may cease or the fetus may be born in a posterior position.

Maternal-Fetal-Neonatal Risks

The woman usually experiences intense pain in the small of her back throughout the labor, unless the baby rotates. At birth, if the fetus remains in a posterior position, the woman may suffer a third- or fourth-degree perineal laceration or extension of a midline episiotomy. There is no increased risk of fetal mortality due to the occiput-posterior position unless labor is protracted or an operative birth is performed.

Clinical Therapy

Medical treatment focuses on close monitoring of both maternal and fetal status and labor progress to determine whether vaginal or cesarean birth is the safer method. According to Cunningham et al (1997), vaginal birth is possible as follows:

1. Await spontaneous birth
2. Forceps-assisted birth with the occiput directly posterior
3. Forceps rotation of the occiput to the anterior position and birth (Scanzoni maneuver; Figure 22–4)
4. Manual rotation to the anterior position followed by forceps-assisted birth (Figure 22–5)

If the pelvis has larger diameters and the perineal muscles are relaxed, as found in grandmultiparity, the fetus may have no particular problem emerging spontaneously in the occiput-posterior position. If, however, the perineum is rigid, the second stage of labor may be prolonged. A prolonged second stage is one that lasts over an hour in multiparas and 2 hours or more in nulliparas.

In the event of a prolonged second stage with arrest of descent due to occiput-posterior position, a midforceps or manual rotation may be done if no CPD is present. In cases of CPD, cesarean birth is the preferred treatment.

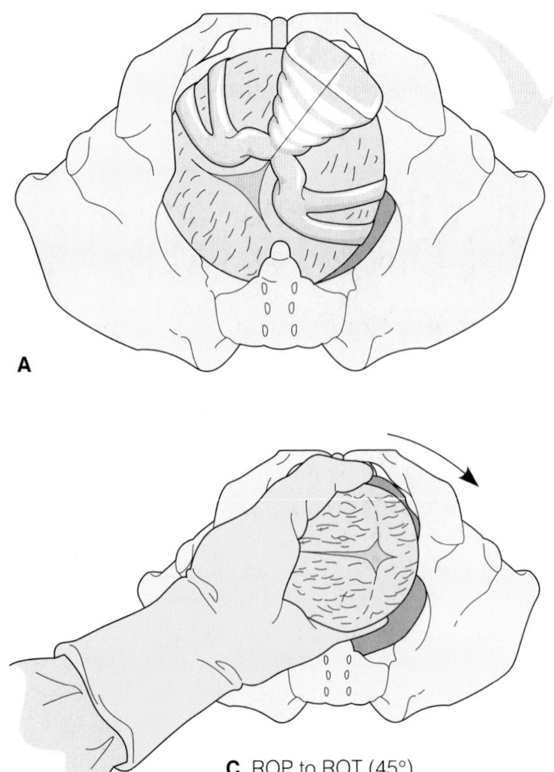

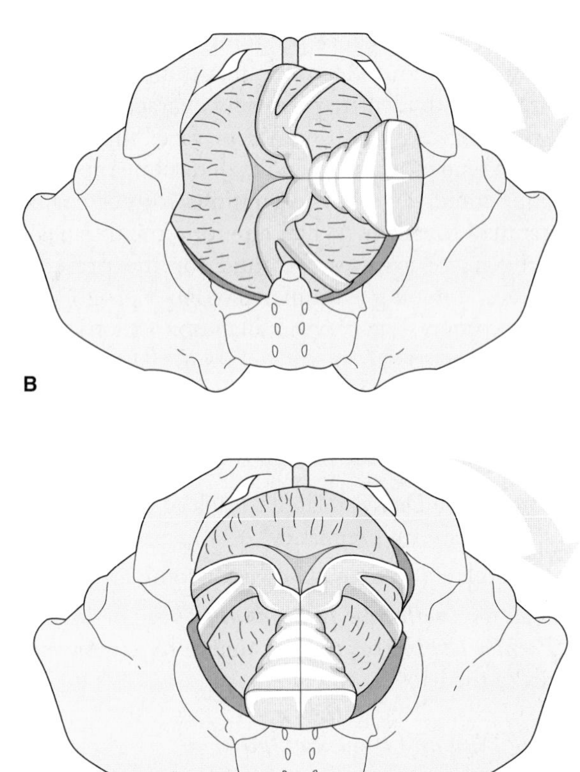

FIGURE 22–4 Scanzoni maneuver, anterior rotation. In clockwise order: ***A,*** Forceps are applied to the fetal head, which is in ROP position. ***B,*** Fetal head is rotated 45 degrees to ROT. ***C,*** Fetal head is rotated another 45 degrees to ROA. ***D,*** Fetal head is rotated another 45 degrees to OA. The fetal position has changed from ROP to ROT to ROA to OA for a rotation of 135 degrees. The forceps are now upside down, so they are removed and reapplied to provide the traction necessary for a forceps-assisted birth. SOURCE: Oxorn J: *Human Labor and Birth,* 5th ed. Norwalk, CT: Appleton & Lange, 1986, p 401.

NURSING CARE MANAGEMENT

Nursing Assessment and Diagnosis

The first sign of occiput-posterior position is intense back pain in the first stage of labor. The back pain is caused by the fetal occiput compressing the sacral nerves. Other signs and symptoms may include a dysfunctional labor pattern, a prolonged active phase, secondary arrest of dilatation, or arrest of descent. Further assessment may reveal a depression in the maternal abdomen above the symphysis pubis (because the fetal face, rather than the back of its head, is turned up against the symphysis). Fetal heart rate may be heard far laterally on the maternal abdomen, and on vaginal examination the nurse will find the wide diamond-shaped anterior fontanelle in the anterior portion of the pelvis. This fontanelle may be difficult to feel because of molding of the fetal head.

Nursing diagnoses that may apply to women with persistent OP position include the following:

- ***Pain*** related to back discomfort secondary to occiput-posterior position
- ***Ineffective Individual Coping*** related to persistent back pain

Nursing Plan and Implementation

Hospital-Based Nursing Care

Changing maternal posture has been used for many years to enhance rotation of OP or OT to OA. The woman may be placed on one side and then asked to move to the other side as the fetus begins to rotate. This side-lying position may promote rotation; it also enables the support persons to apply counterpressure on the sacral area to decrease discomfort. A knee-chest position provides a downward slant to the vaginal canal, directing the fetal head downward on descent. Andrews and Andrews (1983) suggest that a hands-and-knees position is often effective in rotating the fetus. In addition to maintaining a hands-and-knees position on the bed, the woman may do pelvic rocking, and the support person may perform firm stroking motions on the abdomen. The stroking begins over the fetal back and swings around to the other side of the abdomen. After the fetus has rotated, the woman lies in Sims' position on the side opposite the fetal back. In

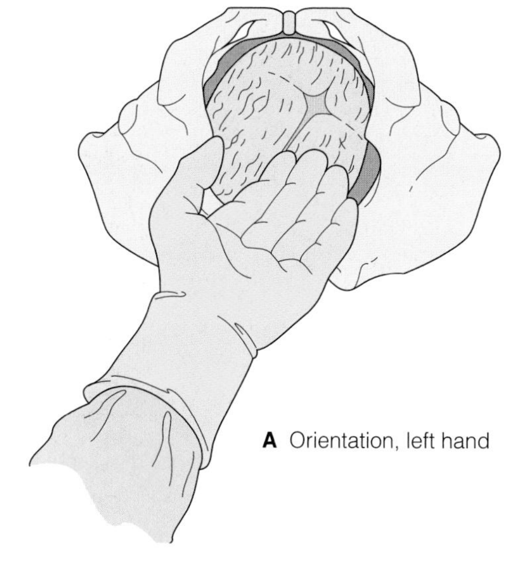

A Orientation, left hand

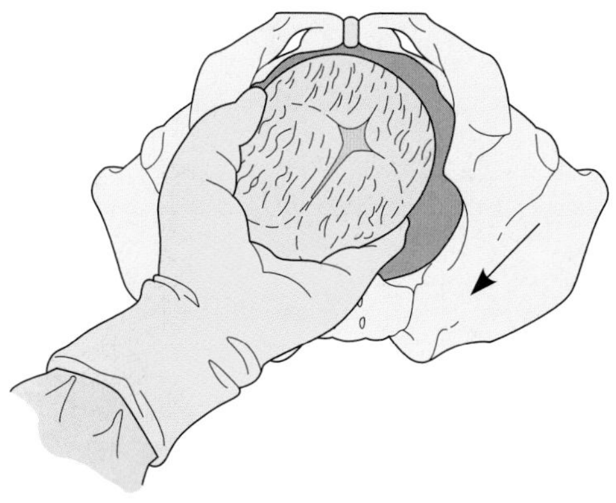

B Grasping the head

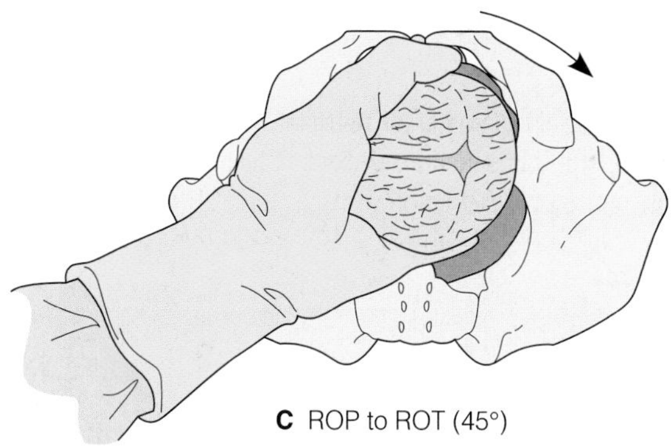

C ROP to ROT (45°)

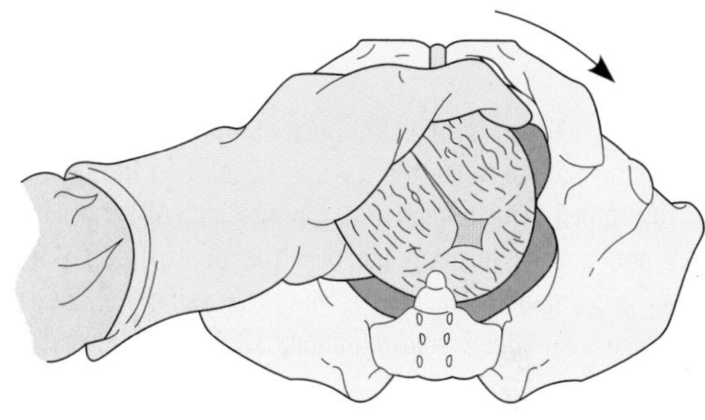

D Manual rotation using left hand: ROT to ROA (45°)

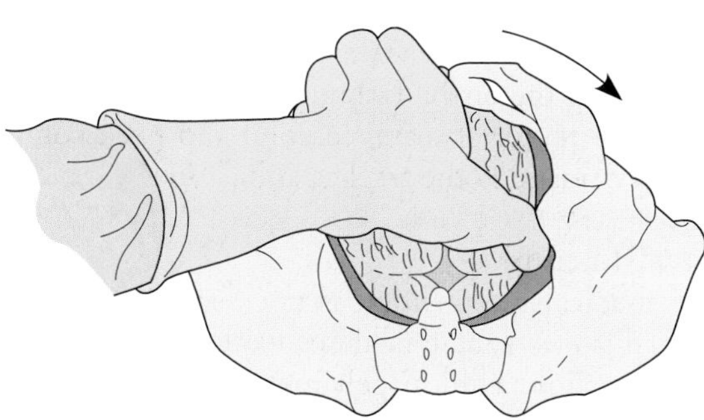

E The manual rotation is completed as the head is rotated another 45° from ROA to OA

FIGURE 22–5 Manual rotation of ROP to OA. ***A,*** The physician's left hand is inserted into the vagina. ***B,*** The back of the fetal head is grasped. ***C,*** The head is flexed and then rotated 45 degrees to ROT. ***D,*** The head is rotated another 45 degrees to ROA. ***E,*** The manual rotation is completed as the head is rotated another 45 degrees from ROA to OA. During the manual rotation, the physician's other hand is placed on the maternal abdomen, and the body is turned in the same direction by applying pressure to the fetal breech or shoulders.

addition to assuming these positions, the woman may want to sit on the toilet, walk around the room, stand beside the bed and lean forward with her hands on the bed and do the pelvic rock, rest in a whirlpool, or lie on her side in the bed.

Evaluation

Expected outcomes of nursing care include the following:

- The woman's discomfort is decreased.
- The woman and her partner understand comfort measures and position changes that may assist her.
- The woman's coping abilities are strengthened.
- The woman and her partner feel supported and encouraged. ●

Care of the Woman and Fetus at Risk Due to Fetal Malpresentation

Three vertex attitudes of the fetus are classified as abnormal presentations: the sinciput (military), brow, and face

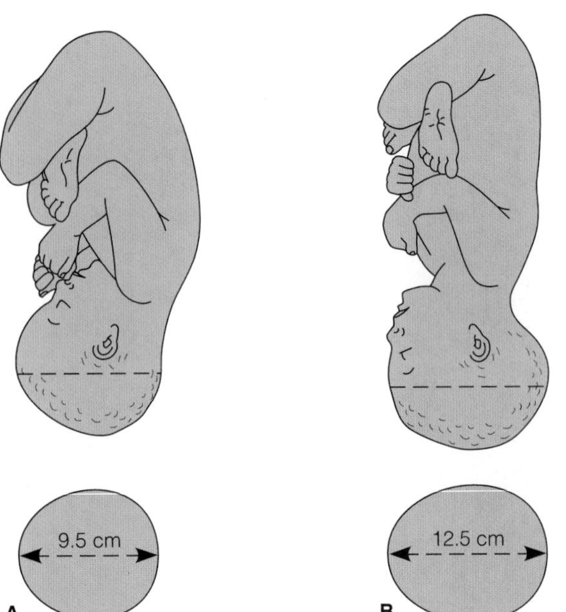

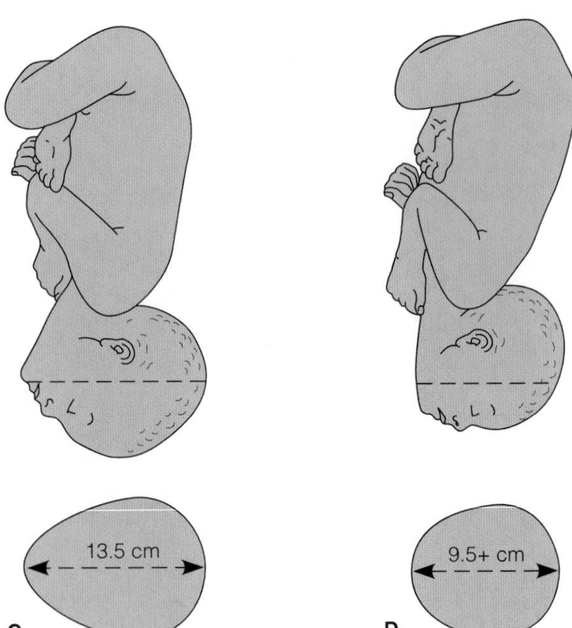

FIGURE 22–6 Types of cephalic presentations. ***A,*** The occiput is the presenting part because the head is flexed and the fetal chin is against the chest. The largest anteroposterior (AP) diameter that presents and passes through the pelvis is approximately 9.5 cm. ***B,*** Military presentation. The head is neither flexed nor extended. The presenting AP diameter is approximately 12.5 cm. ***C,*** Brow presentation. The largest diameter of the fetal head (approximately 13.5 cm) presents in this situation. ***D,*** Face presentation. The AP diameter is 9.5 cm. SOURCE: Danforth DN, Scott JR (editors): *Obstetrics and Gynecology,* 5th ed. New York: Lippincott: 1990, Fig 8–9, p 170.

(Figure 22–6). The fetal body straightens out in these presentations from the classic fetal position to an S-shaped position. The sinciput presentation is probably the least difficult for the woman and fetus. In most cases, as soon as the head reaches the pelvic floor, flexion occurs and a vaginal birth results.

In addition to the vertex malpresentation, the breech, shoulder (transverse lie), and compound presentations can cause significant difficulty during labor. These and the vertex presentations are discussed here.

Brow Presentation

In a brow presentation, the forehead of the fetus becomes the presenting part. The fetal head is slightly extended instead of flexed, with the result that the fetal head enters the birth canal with the widest diameter of the head (occipitomental) foremost (Figure 22–6). Although no specific cause can be identified, proposed causes include high parity, placenta previa, uterine anomaly, hydramnios, fetal anomaly, low birth weight or large fetus, and nuchal cord (Thorp, 1997, p 379). The incidence varies in different studies. Cunningham et al (1997) report that brow presentation occurs at a rate of 1 in 360 births at Parkland Hospital. Approximately 50% of brow presentations spontaneously convert to face or normal vertex presentation (Thorp, 1997).

Cesarean birth is preferred in the presence of CPD or failure of a brow presentation to convert to a normal vertex or face presentation. If a vaginal birth is attempted, the woman will probably have an episiotomy and may require extension of the episiotomy at the moment of birth.

Fetal mortality is increased because of injuries received during the birth. Trauma during the birth process can include tentorial tears, cerebral and neck compression, and damage to the trachea and larynx.

Clinical Therapy

Active medical intervention is not necessary as long as cervical dilatation and fetal descent are occurring. If labor progress is slow, clinical pelvimetry findings and ultrasound to determine the presence of fetal anomalies are important. Oxytocin is used with caution in multiparas because if CPD is present, the continued contractions may cause an obstructed labor that can lead to uterine rupture. Epidural analgesia and instrumental delivery may be used (Thorp, 1997). If problems occur, cesarean birth is selected.

NURSING CARE MANAGEMENT

Nursing Assessment and Diagnosis

Leopold's maneuvers suggest a brow presentation when both the chin and occiput are palpable. A brow presentation may be detected on vaginal examination by palpation of the diamond-shaped anterior fontanelle and orbital ridges (Figure 22–7).

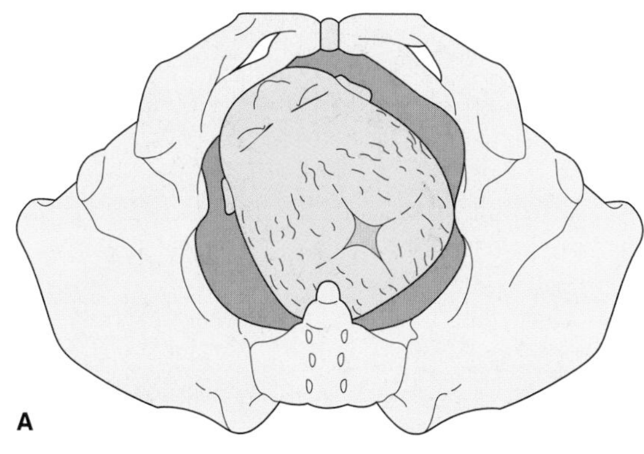

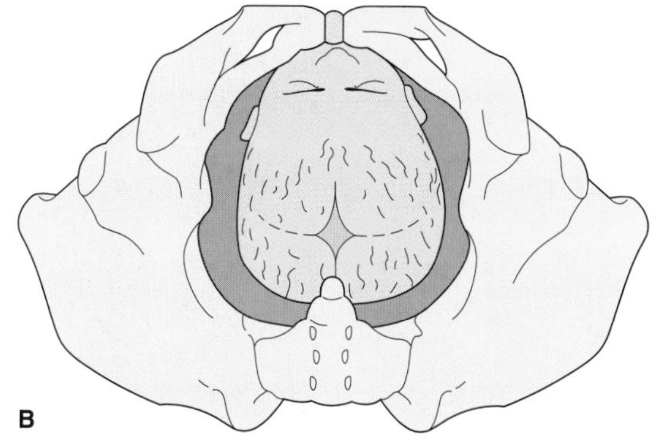

FIGURE 22–7 Brow presentation. ***A,*** Descent. ***B,*** Internal rotation in the pelvic cavity.
SOURCE: Oxorn H: *Human Labor and Birth,* 5th ed. Norwalk, CT: Appleton & Lange 1986, p 211.

Nursing diagnoses that may apply to brow presentation include the following:

- ***Anxiety or Fear*** related to outcome for fetus
- ***Knowledge Deficit*** related to lack of information about possible maternal-fetal effects of brow presentation
- ***Risk for Injury*** to the fetus related to pressure on fetal structures secondary to brow presentation

Nursing Plan and Implementation

Hospital-Based Nursing Care

Nursing management of abnormal cephalic presentations includes close observation of the woman for labor aberrations and of the fetus for signs of stress. The fetus should be observed closely during labor for signs of hypoxia as evidenced by periodic (late) decelerations.

The nurse may need to explain the position of the fetus to the laboring couple or to interpret what the physician/CNM has told them. The nurse should stay close at hand to reassure the couple, inform them of any changes, and assist them with labor-coping techniques.

In brow and face presentation, the appearance of the newborn may be affected. The couple may need help in beginning the attachment process because of the newborn's facial appearance. After the infant is inspected for gross abnormalities, the pediatrician and nurse can assure the couple that the facial edema and excessive molding are only temporary and will subside in a few days.

Evaluation

Expected outcomes of nursing care include the following:

- The woman and her partner understand the implications and associated problems of brow presentation.
- The mother and her baby have a safe labor and birth. ●

Face Presentation

In a face presentation, the face of the fetus is the presenting part. The fetal head is hyperextended even more than in the brow presentation. Face presentation occurs most frequently in multiparas, in preterm birth, and in the presence of anencephaly. The incidence of face presentation is about 1 in 500 births (Thorp, 1997).

The risks of CPD and prolonged labor are increased with face presentation. As with any prolonged labor, the chance of infection is increased.

The fetus may develop caput succedaneum of the face during labor, and after birth the edema gives the newborn an unusual appearance. As with the brow presentation, the neck and internal structures may swell as a result of trauma received during descent. Petechiae and ecchymoses are often seen in the superficial layers of the facial skin because of the birth trauma.

Clinical Therapy

If no CPD is present, the chin (mentum) is anterior, and the labor pattern is effective, the objective of medical treatment is a vaginal birth (Figure 22–8). Mentum posteriors can become wedged on the anterior surface of the sacrum (Figure 22–9). In this case as well as in the presence of CPD, cesarean birth is the preferred method of management.

NURSING CARE MANAGEMENT

Nursing Assessment and Diagnosis

When performing Leopold's maneuvers, the nurse finds that the back of the fetus is difficult to outline, and a deep furrow can be palpated between the hard occiput and the fetal back (Figure 22–10). Fetal heart tones can be heard on the side where the fetal feet are palpated. It may be difficult to determine by vaginal examination whether a breech or face is presenting, especially if facial edema is

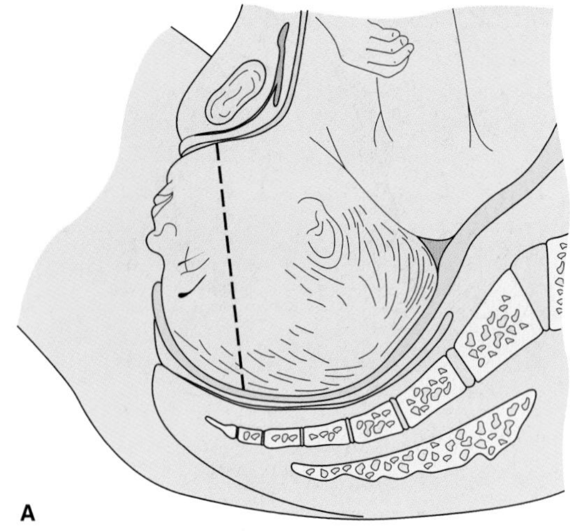

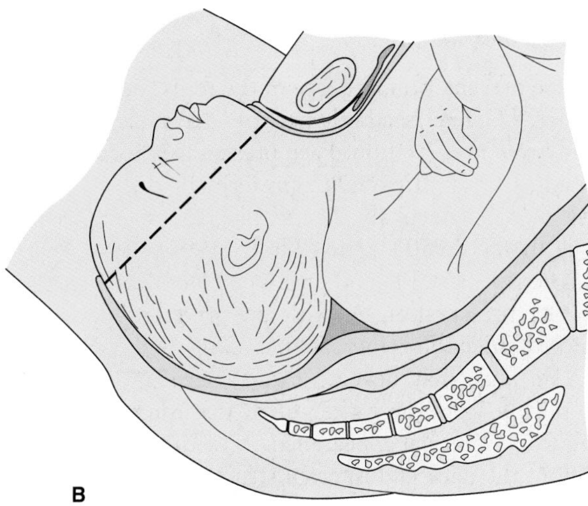

FIGURE 22–8 Mechanism of birth in face (mentoanterior) position. ***A,*** The submentobregmatic diameter at the outlet. ***B,*** The fetal head is born by movement of flexion.

already present. During the vaginal examination, palpation of the saddle of the nose and the gums should be attempted. When assessing engagement, the nurse needs to remember that the face has to be deep within the pelvis before the biparietal diameter has entered the inlet.

Nursing diagnoses that may apply to the woman with a fetus in face presentation include the following:

- ***Fear*** related to unknown outcome of the labor and appearance of the baby
- ***Risk for Injury*** to the newborn's face related to edema secondary to the birth process

Nursing Plan and Implementation

Hospital-Based Nursing Care

Nursing interventions are the same as for the brow presentation.

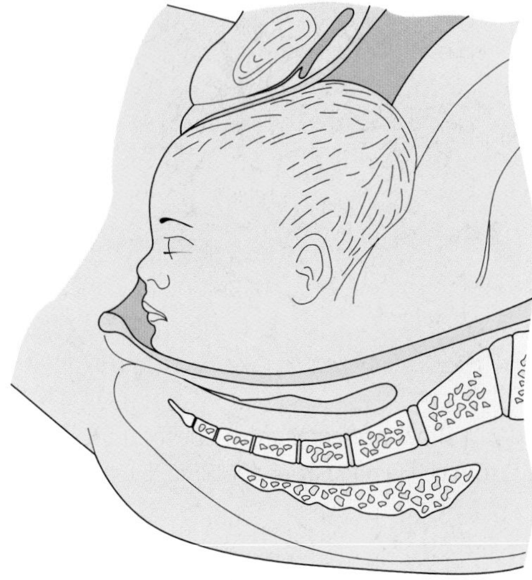

FIGURE 22–9 Face presentation. Mechanism of birth in mentoposterior position. Fetal head is unable to extend farther. The face becomes impacted.

Evaluation

Expected outcomes of nursing care include the following:

- The woman and her partner understand the implications and problems of face presentation.
- The mother and her baby have a safe labor and birth. ●

Breech Presentation

Breech presentation is the most common malpresentation, with an overall incidence of approximately 4% of births. The incidence of breech presentation is directly related to gestational age. At 25 to 26 weeks' gestation, the incidence of breech presentation is about 21%, and after 28 weeks, the incidence decreases to 1.8% at 40 weeks' gestation (Thorp, 1997).

Frank breech is the most common type of breech (especially at term) and occurs in about 60% of breech births. Single or double footling (incomplete breech) accounts for about 35% of breech births and occurs more frequently in preterm fetuses. The remaining 5% of breech presentations are complete breech presentations (Figure 22–11). Breech presentation is most frequently associated with placenta previa, implantation of the placenta in either cornual area, hydramnios, multiple gestation, and fetal anomalies (Thorp, 1997). Because the presenting part does not completely fill the space in the lower uterine segment, once membranes rupture, cord prolapse is more likely. The incidence of cord prolapse is approximately 4% as compared to an incidence of 0.5% with cephalic presentations at term (Thorp, 1997).

Fetal anomalies are three times more likely to be present in a breech versus a cephalic presentation. Major congenital malformations have been reported in 17% of

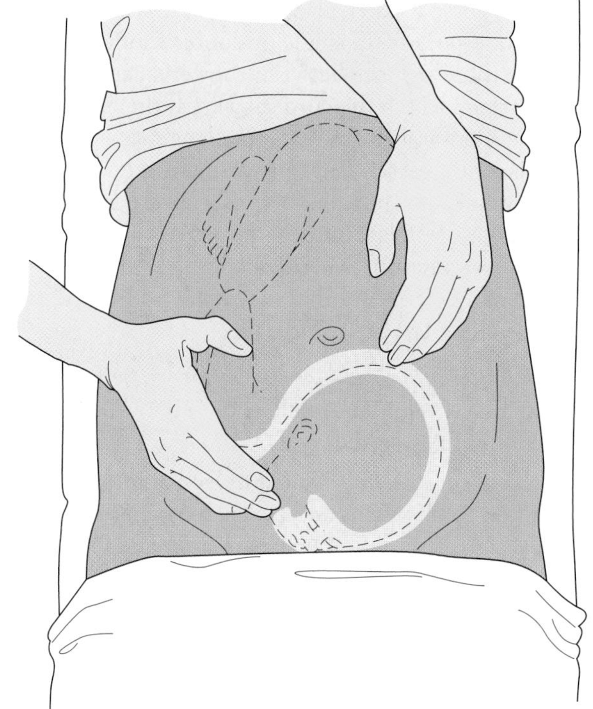

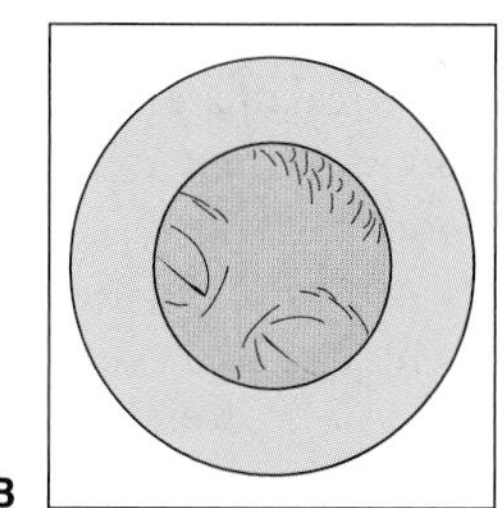

FIGURE 22–10 Face presentation. ***A,*** Palpation of the maternal abdomen with the fetus in right mentum posterior (RMP). ***B,*** Vaginal examination may permit palpation of facial features of the fetus.

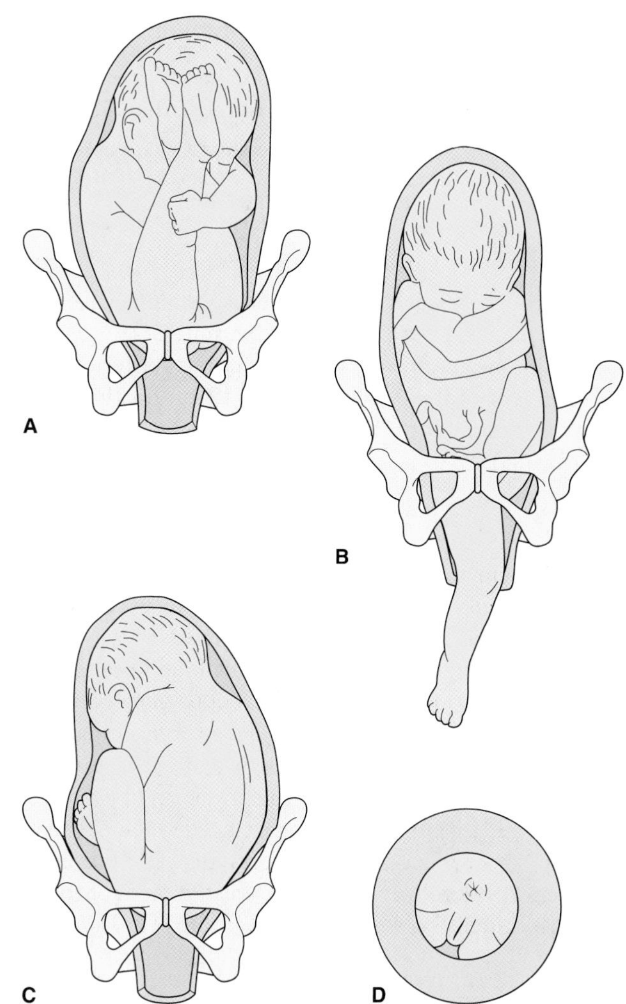

FIGURE 22–11 Breech presentation. ***A,*** Frank breech. ***B,*** Incomplete (footling) breech. ***C,*** Complete breech in left sacral anterior (LSA) position. ***D,*** On vaginal examination, the nurse may feel the anal sphincter. The tissue of the fetal buttocks feels soft.

preterm breech fetuses, in 9% of term breech fetuses, and in 50% of term breech babies who die just before birth, at birth, or within 28 days after birth (Thorp, 1997).

Head trauma during vaginal birth is more likely in breech presentation because it does not allow for the slow molding that occurs in a cephalic presentation as the fetal head moves through the birth canal. The head is the largest and least resilient part of the fetal body. It is the last to come through the maternal pelvis, and molding does not occur. In the case of a preterm breech, a single or double footling and the body may deliver through a cervix that is not completely dilated, and the larger head can be trapped by the cervix (called entrapment). Entrapment may also occur with cesarean birth if the incision is inadequate or uterine relaxation is less than optimum (Cruikshank, 1994).

A difference of opinion exists regarding the implication of breech presentation on length of labor. Some believe that labor progresses at the same rate as cephalic presentation; others believe labor may be slowed because the softer buttocks do not exert as much pressure on the cervix as the firm fetal head.

Clinical Therapy

An external version is usually attempted at 37 to 38 weeks' gestation. If the version is unsuccessful or the fetus spontaneously turns back into a breech presentation, the physician will evaluate the possibility of a vaginal birth or plan a cesarean birth. A woman with little prenatal care who arrives in labor with a breech presentation needs to be carefully evaluated to determine whether labor should continue and vaginal birth should occur. If the woman has not had a previous cesarean birth, the physician will first estimate fetal weight. If fetal weight is between 1500 g and 3600 to 3800 g, the physician will use computed tomography (CT), ultrasound, or x-ray pelvimetry to evaluate the fetal head for hyperextension, extension of the fetal arms over the head, fetal measurements, presence of fetal anomalies, and maternal pelvic measurements. Contraindications for labor and vaginal birth include the following:

- Fetal weight less than 1500 g or more than 3800 g
- Hyperextension of the fetal neck of more than 90 degrees
- Extension of the fetal arms over the head
- Anomalies, such as hydrocephalus
- Diminished maternal pelvic measurements (Average measurements are 10 cm for the transverse [bispinous] diameter, 11 cm for anteroposterior diameter of the pelvic inlet, and 12 cm for the transverse diameter of the inlet—this is called the 10, 11, 12 rule.)

Once active labor is reached, the nullipara should have 1.2 cm cervical dilatation per hour, and the multipara 1.5 cm per hour, with progressive fetal descent. Narcotic agents or an epidural block may be used for pain relief. Epidural anesthesia may be advantageous during the later portion of labor because it will help prevent the pushing sensation the woman may feel prior to complete dilatation. If the woman pushes before cervical dilatation is complete, the fetal body may be expelled and the head entrapped. At the time of birth the physician may have an assistant available in case forceps are needed. Once the fetal body is born, an assistant supports the fetal body as the physician applies Piper forceps to assist in birth of the fetal head (called aftercoming head) (Thorp, 1997).

NURSING CARE MANAGEMENT

Nursing Assessment and Diagnosis

At times, the nurse is the first person to recognize a breech presentation. On palpation using Leopold's manuevers, the nurse feels the hard vertex in the fundus and can perform ballottement of the head independently of the fetal body. The wider sacrum is palpated in the lower part of the abdomen. If the sacrum has not descended, on ballottement the entire fetal body will move. Furthermore, fetal heart tones (FHTs) are usually auscultated above the umbilicus. Passage of meconium from compression of the infant's intestinal tract during descent may occur.

CRITICAL THINKING QUESTION

Try to visualize what your hands would feel if you did Leopold's maneuvers when the fetus is in a breech presentation. If there was hyperextension of the fetal head, how would it feel? How would you explain ballottement to someone who does not know what it means? Compare the findings to those of a transverse lie.

The nurse is particularly alert for a prolapsed umbilical cord, especially in single or double footling breeches, because there is space between the cervix and presenting part through which the cord can slip. If the infant is small and the membranes rupture, the danger is even greater. This is one reason why any woman admitted to the birthing area with a history of ruptured membranes should not ambulate until a full assessment, including vaginal examination, is performed.

Nursing diagnoses that may apply to breech presentation include the following:

- ***Risk for Impaired Gas Exchange*** in the fetus related to interruption in umbilical blood flow secondary to compression of the cord
- ***Knowledge Deficit*** related to lack of information about implications and associated complications of breech presentation on the mother and fetus

Nursing Plan and Implementation

Hospital-Based Nursing Care

During labor, the fetus is at increased risk for prolapse of the cord. Some agency protocols may therefore call for continuous fetal monitoring even though there are no current research studies to support the use of EFM. Ongoing assessments of contractions, cervical dilatation, and effacement and fetal descent are also important to monitor labor progress. Emotional support and sharing of information are critical to the childbearing woman and her support person. They need to be kept apprised of the labor's current status as well as the possible treatment plans so they can continue to make informed choices.

During a vaginal birth, the nurse continues to assess the FHR and to provide encouragement and support for the couple. Piper forceps need to be readily available to the physician; the nurse may assist the physician if the forceps are needed for the birth.

Evaluation

Expected outcomes of nursing care include the following:

- The woman and her partner understand the implications and associated problems with breech presentation.
- The mother and baby have a safe labor and birth.
- Major complications are recognized early, and corrective measures are instituted. ●

Shoulder Presentation (Transverse Lie)

A transverse lie occurs in approximately 1 in 360 term births (Cunningham et al, 1997). The infant's long axis lies across the woman's abdomen, and on inspection the contour of the maternal abdomen appears widest from side to side (Figure 22–12).

Maternal conditions associated with a transverse lie are grandmultiparity with lax uterine musculature (the most common cause); obstructions such as bony dystocia, placenta previa, neoplasms, and fetal anomalies; hydramnios; and preterm fetus. It is not uncommon in multiple gestations for one or more of the fetuses to be in a transverse lie. Vaginal birth is impossible with a transverse lie. Labor should not be allowed to continue, and a cesarean birth is done quickly. Frequently a vertical incision is made in the uterus because the fetal head and fetal feet lie in the upper portion of the uterus; a low transverse incision may lead to difficulties in extracting the fetus (Cunningham et al, 1997).

If labor is allowed to continue, the fetal shoulder is forced down into the pelvis. As labor continues, the fetus becomes impacted. With no relief, uterine rupture may occur (Cunningham et al, 1997).

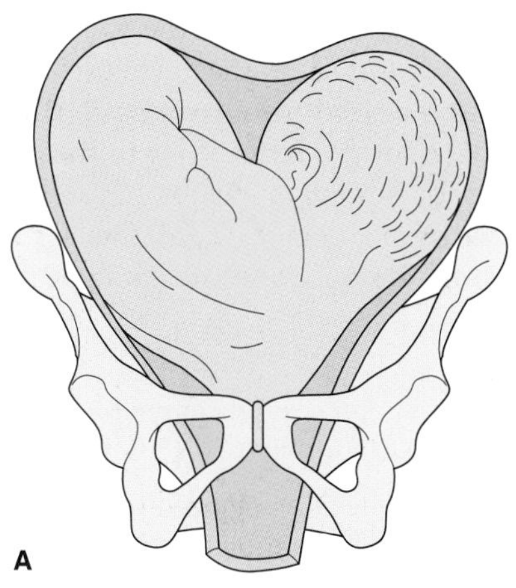

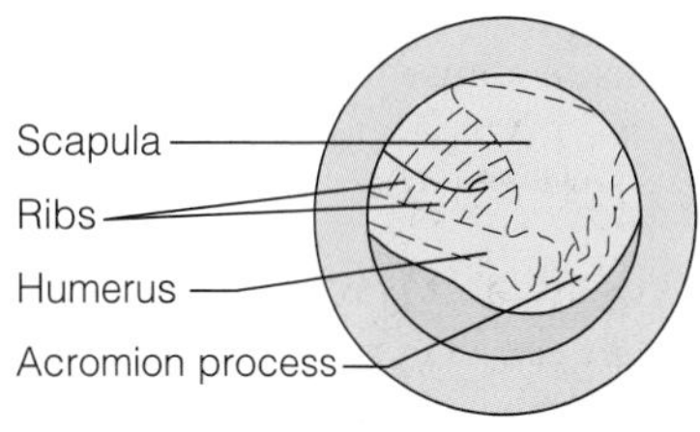

FIGURE 22–12 Transverse lie. ***A,*** Shoulder presentation. ***B,*** On vaginal examination, the nurse may feel the acromion process as the fetal presenting part.

Clinical Therapy

Transverse lie may be diagnosed using Leopold's maneuvers and can then be confirmed by ultrasound. At the time of the ultrasound examination, it is important to confirm fetal position, fetal biparietal diameters (to confirm gestational age), and location of the placenta and to carry out an examination for the presence of fetal anomalies and structural abnormalities of the uterus such as leimyomata (fibroid tumor) or adnexal tumors (King, 1994).

Management varies, depending on the length of gestation, because many transverse lies convert to either cephalic or breech presentation by term (38 weeks). If the fetus is still in a transverse lie at term, an external cephalic version (ECV) may be done if (1) there is no contraindication to vaginal birth (for example, a fetal anomaly, complete placenta previa, or a structural problem in the uterus); and (2) fetal pulmonary lung maturity is confirmed either by ultrasound measurements or by amniocentesis for assessment of phospholipids (2:1 lecithin/sphingomyelin [L/S] ratio and the presence of phosphatidylglycerol). An external cephalic version is most likely to be successful close to term. Spontaneous version will likely occur by 37 weeks. The use of tocolytics for the procedure may be helpful for nulliparas. The fetus is assessed with a nonstress test or biophysical profile prior to the procedure. If the version is successful, the woman may be induced if she is at term and her cervix is favorable. However, scientific studies do not support immediate induction as a routine to minimize the chance the fetus will return to the original position (ACOG, 1997).

NURSING CARE MANAGEMENT

Nursing Assessment and Diagnosis

The nurse can identify a transverse lie by inspection and palpation of the abdomen, by auscultation of FHTs in the midline of the abdomen (not conclusive), and by vaginal examination.

On palpation, no fetal part is felt in the fundal portion of the uterus or above the symphysis pubis. The head may be palpated on one side and the breech on the other. Fetal heart tones are usually auscultated just below the midline of the umbilicus. On vaginal examination, if a presenting part is palpated, it is the ridged thorax or possibly an arm that is compressed against the chest.

Nursing diagnoses that may apply when transverse lie is present include the following:

- ***Knowledge Deficit*** related to lack of information about implications and problems associated with transverse lie
- ***Risk for Impaired Gas Exchange*** in the fetus related to decrease in blood flow secondary to cord compression associated with prolapsed cord
- ***Risk for Ineffective Individual Coping*** or ***Ineffective Family Coping*** related to unknown outcome
- ***Fear*** related to unknown outcome of birth

Nursing Plan and Implementation

Hospital-Based Nursing Care

The primary nursing actions are to help evaluate the fetal presentation and to provide information and support to the couple. If an ECV has been accomplished and an induction is done, the nurse completes all interventions related to the induction. (See discussion in Chapter 23.) If transverse lie is discovered when the woman is admitted to the birthing unit in labor, the nurse provides information regarding the need for a cesarean birth and assists with preparation for the birth. Prior to the cesarean, the nurse watches for rupture of membranes and the possibility of prolapse of the umbilical cord. (See Chapter 23 for further information regarding teaching with cesarean birth.)

Evaluation

Expected outcomes of nursing care include the following:

- The transverse lie is recognized promptly, and crucial assessments are completed.
- The mother and baby have a safe birth.
- The couple understands the implications and associated problems of transverse lie. ●

Compound Presentation

A compound presentation is one in which there are two presenting parts. It can occur when the pelvic inlet is not totally occluded by the primary presenting part. If the prolapsed part is a hand, the birth is generally not difficult. Sometimes the hand slips back, and occasionally it is born alongside the head. This may increase the chance of laceration. If the prolapsed part is left alone, the birth is generally not difficult. Cesarean birth is indicated in the presence of uterine dysfunction or fetal distress (Cunningham et al, 1997).

Care of the Woman and Fetus at Risk Due to Developmental Abnormalities

Macrosomia

Fetal **macrosomia** is defined as weight of more than 4000 g (8 lb, 14 oz) at birth. Some sources, however, suggest that the fetus not be considered macrosomic unless it weighs 4500 g or more (Cunningham et al, 1997). In a study of more than 104,000 births, the incidence of newborns who weighed more than 4000 g was 5.3%, but only 0.4% weighed more than 4500 g (Cunningham et al, 1997). It is important to remember that the mean birth weight varies among various peoples of the world. For instance, mean birth weight of the Lumi of New Guinea is 2400 g; for the Cheyenne Indians of North America it is 3830 g (Cunningham et al, 1997). The definition of macrosomia will thus differ according to the ethnic grouping being discussed.

A woman who is obese is 3 to 4 times more likely to have a macrosomic fetus (>4000 g) (Zlatnik, 1997). Obesity has been defined a number of ways; however, recent guidelines suggest basing the definition on body mass index (BMI). To obtain BMI, the woman's weight in kilograms is divided by the square of her height in meters. The advantage of using BMI is that it takes height into account in determining whether a person is obese. Obesity is diagnosed if the BMI exceeds 29.0 (Zlatnik, 1997). A woman with undiagnosed or uncontrolled gestational diabetes is also at risk for having a macrosomic baby (Coustan, 1997).

A woman's pelvis that is adequate for an average-sized fetus may be disproportionately small for an oversized fetus. Distention of the uterus causes overstretching of the myometrial fibers, which may lead to dysfunctional labor and an increased incidence of postpartal hemorrhage. If the oversized fetus is not able to descend, the chance of uterine rupture during labor increases. Vaginal birth poses an increased risk of perineal lacerations and extensions of an episiotomy.

Fetal prognosis is guarded. If a macrosomic fetus is unsuspected and labor is allowed to continue in the presence of disproportion, the fetus can receive cerebral trauma from intermittent forceful contact with the maternal bony pelvis. During difficult operative procedures performed at the time of vaginal birth, the fetus may become asphyxiated or experience neurologic damage from pressure exerted on its head.

Shoulder dystocia is an obstetric emergency. However, shoulder dystocia may occur with fetuses weighing less than 4000 g, and risk factors are not reliable predictors (ACOG, 1997). Following delivery of the head, the anterior shoulder does not deliver either spontaneously or with gentle traction (Bowes, 1994). If shoulder dystocia is not managed correctly, permanent injury to the baby may result. Brachial plexus injury (due to improper or excessive traction applied to the fetal head) and fractured clavicles may occur.

Clinical Therapy

The occurrence of the maternal and fetal problems associated with macrosomic infants may be somewhat lessened by identifying macrosomia prior to the onset of labor. If a large fetus is suspected, the maternal pelvis should be evaluated carefully. An estimation of fetal size can be made by palpating the crown–rump length of the fetus in utero, but the greatest errors in estimation occur on both ends of the spectrum—the macrosomic fetus and the very small fetus. Fundal height can give some clue. Ultrasound measurements have limited accuracy (ACOG, 1997). Whenever the uterus appears excessively large, hydramnios, an oversized fetus, or a multiple pregnancy must be considered.

Labor may proceed within normal limits, or there may be a slowing of fetal descent (change of station) and a prolonged second stage (Cunningham et al, 1997). Even though these problems are present, it is still not possible to anticipate shoulder dystocia that results in trauma to the newborn. If difficulty extracting the shoulders occurs during the birth, the obstetrician/CNM may direct the woman to sharply flex her thighs up against her abdomen (McRoberts maneuver). This position is thought to change the maternal pelvic angle and therefore reduce the force needed to extract the shoulders and decrease the incidence of brachial plexus stretching and clavicular fracture (Figure 22–13) (Cunningham et al, 1997). McRoberts maneuver has a high success rate (ACOG, 1997). In addition, the obstetrician/CNM may incorporate other interventions, such as checking the placement of the shoulder, enlarging the episiotomy, asking the labor and birth nurse to apply suprapubic pressure, and using the Woods Screw maneuver (which consists of rotating the anterior shoulder 180 degrees to the posterior position).

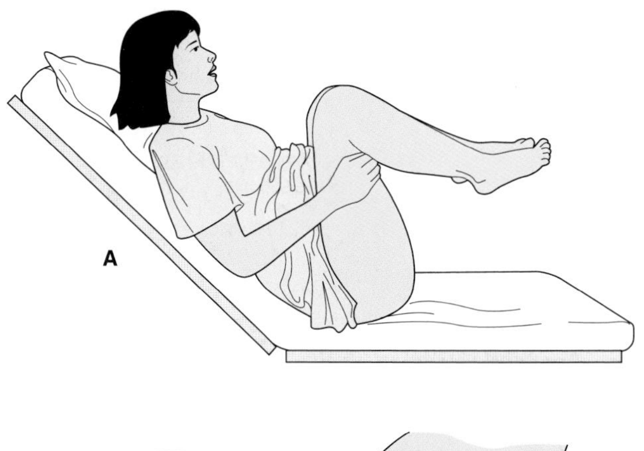

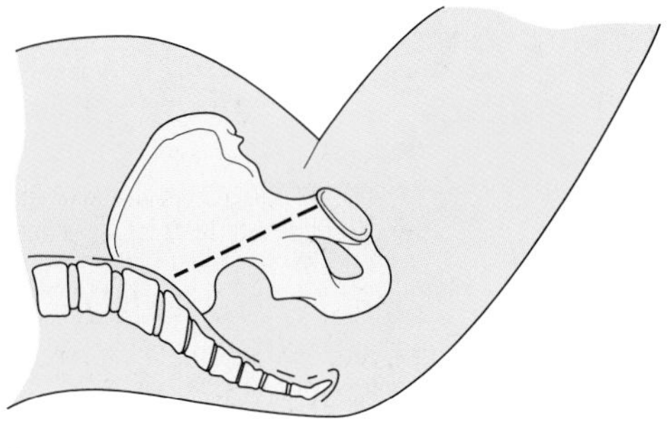

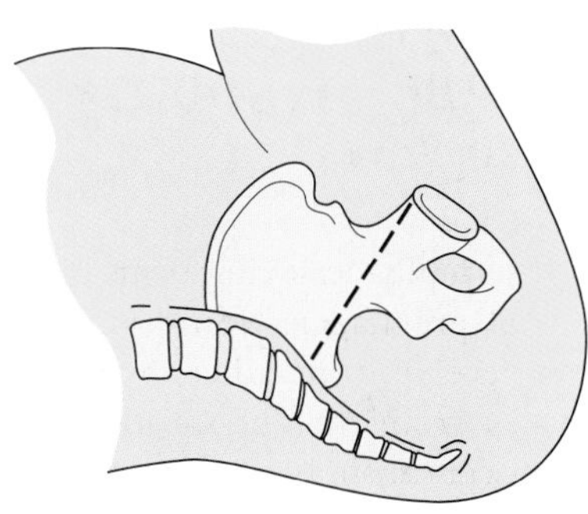

FIGURE 22–13 McRoberts maneuver. ***A,*** The woman flexes her thighs up onto her abdomen. ***B,*** The angle of the maternal pelvis prior to McRoberts maneuver. ***C,*** The angle of the pelvis with McRoberts maneuver.

NURSING CARE MANAGEMENT

Nursing Assessment and Diagnosis

The nurse assists in identifying factors associated with macrosomic infants, which include multiparity, maternal obesity, excessive weight gain during this pregnancy, maternal diabetes, history of a large infant or previous shoulder dystocia, and pregnancy that extends to 42 weeks or beyond. During the intrapartum period, the risk factors include slow descent of the fetus and prolonged second stage. Because women with these risk factors are prime candidates for dystocia and its complications, the nurse frequently assesses the FHR for indications of fetal stress and evaluates the rate of cervical dilatation and fetal descent.

Nursing diagnoses that may apply to the woman with a macrosomic fetus include the following:

- ***Risk for Injury*** to the fetus related to trauma during the birth process
- ***Risk for Infection*** related to traumatized tissue secondary to maternal tissue damage during birth
- ***Knowledge Deficit*** related to lack of information about the implications and possible problems associated with birth of a macrosomic baby

Nursing Plan and Implementation

Hospital-Based Nursing Care

The nurse monitors labor closely for a dysfunctional pattern, assessing fetal heart rate and reporting any sign of labor dysfunction or fetal stress to the physician/CNM.

The nurse provides support for the laboring woman and her partner and information regarding the implications and possible associated problems. During the birth, the nurse continues to provide support and encouragement to the couple.

After the birth, the nurse inspects the newborn for cephalhematoma, Erb palsy (caused by overstretching of the brachial plexus and damage to C5, C6, C7), and fractured clavicles (exhibited by nonmovement of one arm) and informs the admission nursery of any problems. The newborn will need to be observed closely for cerebral and neurologic damage.

Postpartally, the nurse checks the uterus for potential atony and the maternal vital signs for deviations suggesting hypovolemic shock.

Evaluation

Expected outcomes of nursing care include the following:

- The woman and her partner understand the implications and possible associated problems.
- The mother and baby have a safe labor and birth. ●

TABLE 22–1 Characteristics of Twin Pregnancy

Type	Time of Division	Characteristics	Frequency	Mortality Rate
Dizygotic				
(Two separate ova) Fraternal twins dichorionic-diamniotic	Develop from two ova released at the same time.	Each twin has own placenta, chorion, amnion. Dizygotic twins are called fraternal twins. They may be the same or different sex.	99% of all twins	11.5%
Monozygotic				
(Single ovum) Identical twins			1% of all twins	
Dichorionic-diamniotic twins	Division occurs within 72 hours past fertilization.* Inner cell mass not yet developed.	Each twin has own chorion, amnion, placenta.	30% of monozygotic twins	9%
Monochorionic-diamniotic twins	Division occurs at blastocyst stage, 4 to 8 days after fertilization.* Inner cell mass divides in two.	Placenta has one chorion and two amnions. Each twin lies in own sac.	68% of monozygotic twins	25%
Monochorionic-monoamniotic twins	Division occurs in primitive germ disk, 9 to 13 days past fertilization.*	Twins lie in the same amniotic sac. Increased risk of umbilical cords becoming tangled or knotted.	2% of monozygotic twins	>50%

*Chasen, S.T., & Chervenak, F.A. (1998). What is the relationship between the universal use of ultrasound, the rate of detection of twins, and outcome differences? *Clinical Obstetrics and Gynecology,* 41, pp 67–77.

Care of the Woman with a Multiple Pregnancy

Twin Pregnancy

The incidence of naturally occurring twins in the United States is 2% of all pregnancies (Simpson & D'Alton, 1996). Twins can develop from either the fertilization of two separate ova or from the division of one fertilized ovum. Twins that occur from two separate ova are called dizygotic, and they may be the same sex or different sexes. In this type of twinning, there are two amnions (diamniotic) and two chorions (dichorionic).

Twins from one fertilized ovum are called monozygotic and are always of the same sex (Table 22–1). One percent of twins are monozygotic twins (Keith, Papiernik, & Oleszczuk, 1998). If the fertilized ovum (zygote) divides within the first 72 hours past fertilization, the twins will be diamniotic and dichorionic. If the division occurs from the fourth to the eighth day past fertilization, the embryos will develop with two separate amnions and one chorion (monochorionic). If the division happens after the eighth day, the two fetuses will share both a common amniotic sac and chorion (monoamniotic, monochorionic). The terminology is important because the perinatal morbidity and mortality rates differ greatly among different types of twins (Keith et al, 1998; Chasen & Chervenak, 1998).

The development of sensitive human chorionic gonadotrophin (hCG) assays has made it possible to determine more accurately the early pregnancy loss rate of twins. The calculation of pregnancy loss must include both complete pregnancy loss and spontaneous resorption of one twin. The resorption of one twin has been called the "vanishing twin" phenomenon and can now be documented with ultrasound examination. In a study of a Japanese government database, it was found that the fetal loss rate in twins was 11.5%, which is triple the rate found in singleton gestations (Grobman & Peaceman, 1998). In further analysis of their data, it was found that the twinning rate was 1 in 30 conceptions, which is a much higher rate than previously thought. Evidence suggests that approximately 30% of pregnancies are lost before the woman is even aware that she is pregnant. Sixty-five percent of single gestations do not survive to 4 weeks of gestational age, and 74.6% of twin pregnancies are lost before the end of the first trimester (Grobman & Peaceman, 1998). Causative factors in twin gestation loss in the first trimester include environmental factors, infectious organisms, trophoblast dysfunction, poor embryo quality, or a lower concentration of placentally produced substances. Marginal and velamentous insertions are more likely to be present when there is a vanishing twin, and the presence of a monochorionic placenta is more likely to result in either a singleton gestation (because of a vanishing twin) or complete pregnancy loss (Grobman & Peaceman, 1998).

Pregnancy loss of twins in the second trimester is associated with congenital anomalies, growth restriction, and chromosomal abnormalities. Marginal and velamentous cord insertions occur with increased frequency in twin gestations and are more likely associated with the death of one twin. In a monochorionic placenta, there may be a vascular anastamosis that leads to twin-to-twin transfusion syndrome. When this syndrome is present, blood is chronically drained from one fetus to the other. The donor fetus becomes growth restricted, and oligohydramnios develops. The recipient fetus becomes polycythemic and hydropic, and hydramnios develops. If the fetuses become severely affected during the second trimester, untreated mortality may be 100% (Grobman & Peaceman, 1998). Cervical incompetence is more likely to occur in twin gestations and consists of silent cervical effacement and dilatation during the second trimester. Treatment with cervical cerclage is controversial with a multiple gestation (Grobman & Peaceman, 1998). The incidence of preterm birth is higher in multiple gestations. The percentage of preterm births is 5.9 times more likely in twins than in singletons, and 10.7 times more likely in triplets (Keith & Papiernik, 1998). Recent reports from Japan have suggested that optimal perinatal survival occurs at earlier gestational ages in multiple births than in singletons (Keith & Papiernik, 1998). In singletons, the perinatal mortality is at the lowest point at 40 weeks' gestation; for twins, in contrast, the perinatal mortality rate decreases until 38 weeks and then increases steadily from 39 to 42 weeks (Keith & Papiernik, 1998).

During the prenatal period, a fundal height greater than expected for the weeks of gestation and auscultation of two heartbeats that differ by at least 10 bpm are the most likely clues of twin pregnancy. Some women experience severe nausea and vomiting and develop severe anemia despite the intake of multiple-vitamin therapy. The α-fetoprotein level may be elevated (Kochenour, 1992).

Women with a multiple gestation are more likely to develop complications, which include the following (Senat, Ancel, Bouvier-Colle, & Breart, 1998; Keith et al, 1998):

- Spontaneous abortions are more common, as previously discussed.
- Hypertension is the major maternal complication. The risk of developing severe hypertension or preeclampsia is two to three times greater in a twin pregnancy than in a singleton.
- Maternal anemia occurs because of demands of the twin gestation. The hemoglobin averages 10 g/dL from the 20th week on. Anemia is indicated by hemoglobin levels below 11 g/dL in the first or third trimester or below 10.5 g/dL in the second trimester. When decreased hemoglobin is accompanied by serum ferritin concentration of less than 12 μg/dL, iron deficiency anemia is diagnosed.
- Hydramnios may be due to increased renal perfusion from cross-vessel anastomosis of monozygotic twins.
- Complications during labor include preterm labor, uterine dysfunction due to an overstretched myometrium, abnormal fetal presentations, instrumental or cesarean birth, and postpartum hemorrhage.

The woman pregnant with twins may experience more physical discomfort during her pregnancy, such as shortness of breath, dyspnea on exertion, backaches, and pedal edema, because of the oversized uterus.

Clinical Therapy

The goals of medical care are to promote normal fetal development for both fetuses, to prevent preterm birth, and to diminish fetal trauma during labor.

Ultrasound examinations play a crucial role in the care and treatment of multiple gestations. Ultrasound assists with identifying the presence of more than one fetus early in the pregnancy, providing accurate dating of the pregnancy, and detecting fetal anomalies. Because the incidence of perinatal mortality and morbidity is increased in twins, use of ultrasound in the first and second trimester can be particularly helpful. Ultrasound allows the assessment of additional aspects, such as chorionicity in the first trimester. Knowledge of chorionicity is essential in differentiating twin-to-twin transfusion from fetal growth restriction secondary to abnormal placental blood flow. Knowledge of chorionicity is also important in determining the management of a twin pregnancy in which one twin is sonographically abnormal. If the twins are dichorionic/diamniotic (DC/DA), then selective termination could be considered. Determination of amnionicity is based on ultrasound visualization or the lack of visualization of an intertwin membrane. Visualization of this membrane becomes more difficult as the gestation advances because of progressive thinning of the intertwin membrane, fetal crowding, and an increasing incidence of oligohydramnios. Knowledge regarding the presence of one amnion is crucial, because management of monochorionic/monoamniotic (MC/MA) twins requires more intensive surveillance and earlier birth, usually by cesarean (Chasen & Chervenak, 1998).

Preventing preterm labor is a major goal. Prenatal care should begin early, and more frequent visits are usually scheduled. Roberts & Morrison (1998) support vaginal examinations at each visit to identify cervical changes, such as cervical lengthening, effacement, or dilatation, or the beginning of bulging membranes. An ultrasound vaginal probe may be used to measure the dimensions of the cervix and changes in the lower uterine segment. Roberts & Morrison (1998) demonstrated that the dimensions of the cervix were different when the woman was reclining as opposed to standing. In the standing position, the cervix was shorter and wider. These changes may be associated with the suggestion that prolonged standing is a high-risk factor for preterm labor (Manning, 1999).

Evidence-based practice has precipitated questions regarding the effectiveness of prior management strategies, including bed rest, betamimetics, cerclage, and

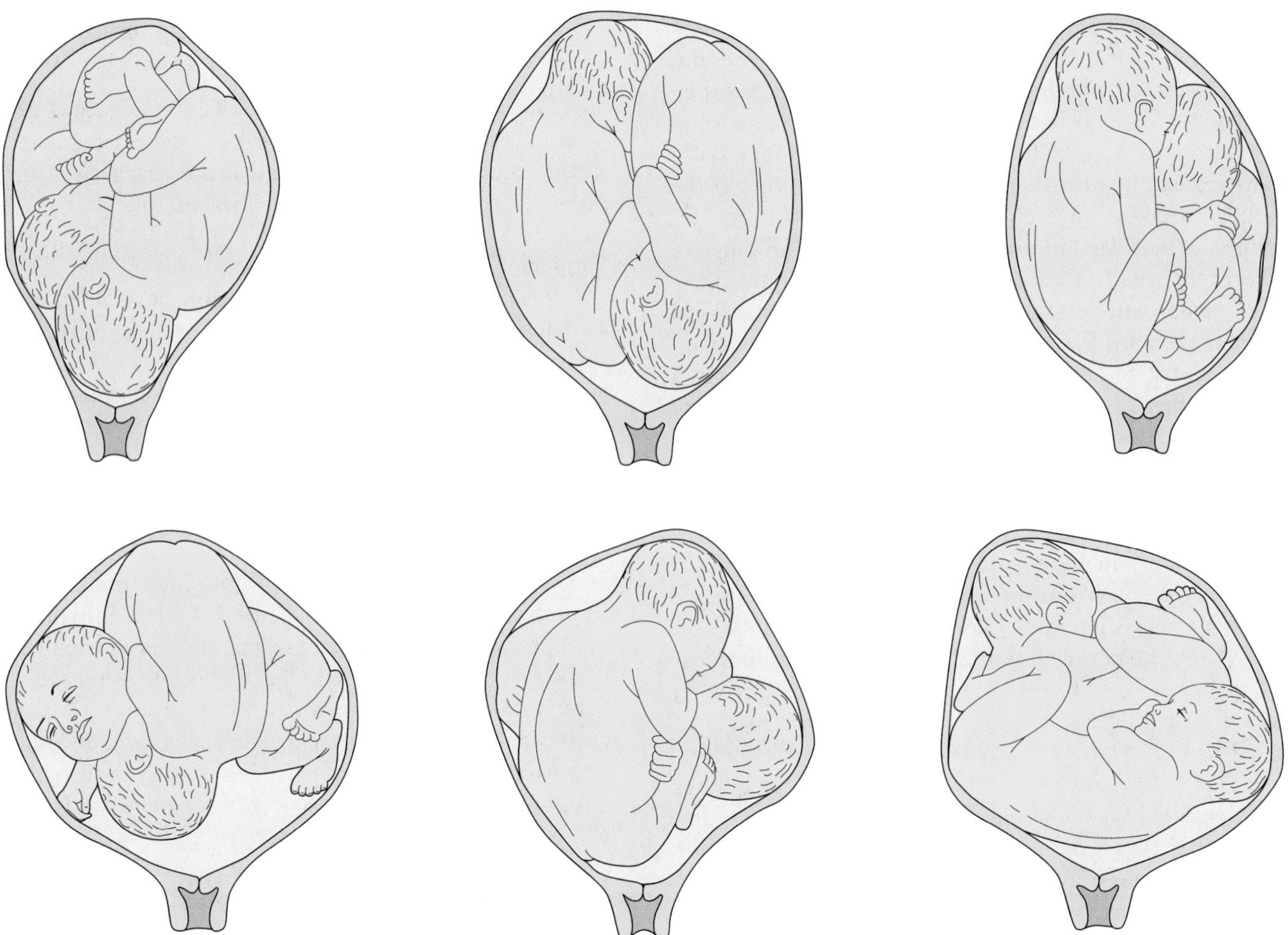

FIGURE 22–14 Twins may be in any of these presentations while in utero.

progestins (Papiernik, Keith, Oleszczuk, & Cervantes, 1998). More recent strategies include work leave, lifestyle modifications, and achieving optimal weight gain. Work leave and lifestyle modifications include avoiding standing for prolonged periods of time and avoiding working 40 hours or more a week. It is recommended that the physician prescribe reduction of work effort and medically indicated work leave earlier in the pregnancy; in France, for example, work leave begins at 22 weeks for twin gestations (Papiernik et al, 1998). Maternal weight gain of 40 to 50 pounds is associated with good outcomes of both twins (Papiernik et al, 1998).

Home monitors have been helpful in identifying uterine hyperactivity and the presence of contractions. Early detection of contractions can provide an opportunity for the woman to seek assistance more quickly (Roberts & Morrison, 1998).

Some areas offer twin clinics, which provide many advantages for the woman with multiple gestation. These advantages include consistent evaluation, intensive prenatal education, counseling and support from the same health care providers.

Intrapartal management and assessment require careful attention to maternal and fetal status. The mother should have an intravenous infusion in place with a large-bore needle. Anesthesia and cross-matched blood should be readily available. The twins are monitored by dual electronic fetal monitoring. The labor may progress very slowly or very quickly.

The decision about method of birth may not be made until labor occurs, and the method depends on a variety of factors. The presence of maternal complications such as placenta previa, abruptio placentae, or severe pregnancy-induced hypertension (PIH) usually indicates the need for cesarean birth. Fetal factors such as severe intrauterine growth restriction (IUGR), preterm birth, fetal anomalies, fetal stress, or unfavorable fetal position or presentation also require cesarean birth.

Any combination of presentations and positions can occur with twins (Figure 22–14). Approximately 50% of twins are born by cesarean, which is chosen in the hope of reducing complications for the twins, especially birth asphyxia (Cunningham et al, 1997).

The placentas are examined after the birth. If the twins are of the same sex, the placentas are sent to the pathology laboratory for examination to determine whether they are monozygotic or dizygotic twins.

NURSING CARE MANAGEMENT

Nursing Assessment and Diagnosis

When obtaining a maternal history at the beginning of antenatal care, the nurse should identify any family history of twinning. Equally important is a history of medication taken to enhance fertility. These facts should be noted on the antepartal record.

At each antepartal clinic visit, the nurse should measure the fundal height. Any growth, fetal movement, or heart tone auscultation out of proportion to gestational age by dates is indicative of twins. During palpation, the nurse may feel many small parts on all sides of the abdomen (Figure 22–15). If twins are suspected, the nurse should attempt to auscultate two separate heartbeats in different quadrants of the maternal abdomen. Use of the Doppler device may be helpful. Conclusive evidence of twins is found on sonography.

During the prenatal visits the nurse should determine the family's level of preparation for integrating more than one new member. Although the thought of having twins can be very exciting, the reality of the stress of attaching to two infants and the parental role may be a difficult adjustment.

During labor it is important to monitor both twins. An external electronic monitor can be applied to both twins, or if conditions permit, the internal monitor can be applied to twin A and the external monitor to twin B. The heart rates may be auscultated on different quadrants of the maternal abdomen, but continuous monitoring is more beneficial. Signs of distress should be reported to the obstetrician.

After a multiple birth, the mother is closely monitored for postpartal hemorrhage. Nursing diagnoses that may apply to a woman with a twin pregnancy include the following:

- ***Fear*** related to unknown outcome of the birth process
- ***Ineffective Individual Coping*** or ***Ineffective Family Coping*** related to uncertainty about the labor and birth plan
- ***Knowledge Deficit*** related to implications and problems associated with twin pregnancy
- ***Risk for Impaired Gas Exchange*** in the twins related to decreased oxygenation secondary to cord compression

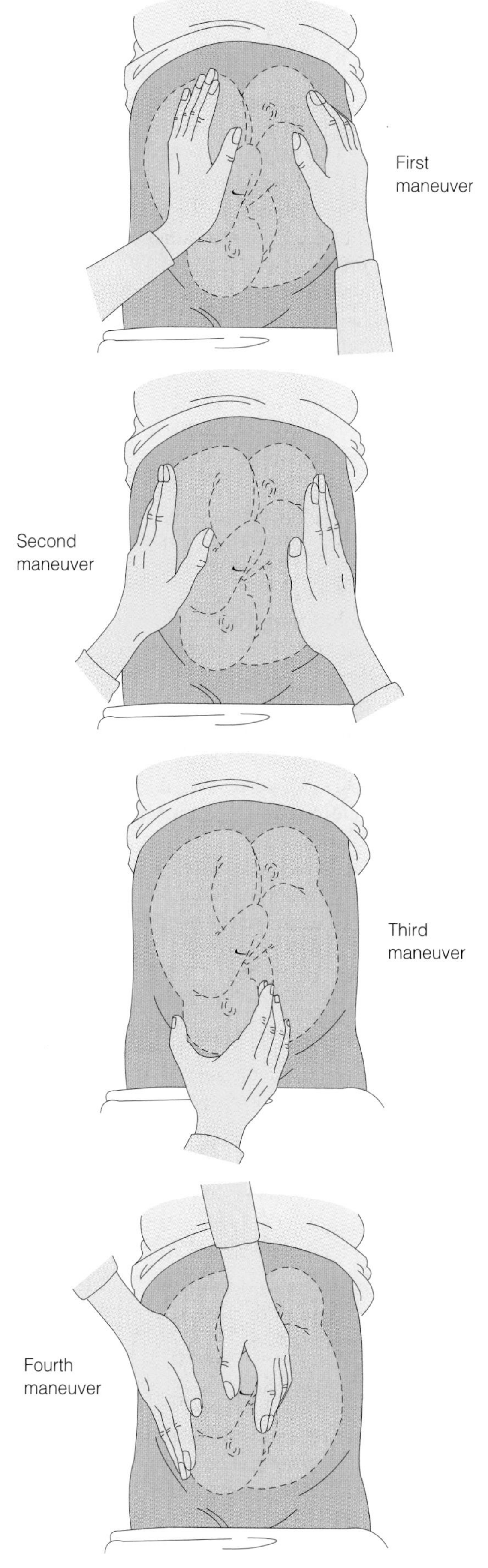

FIGURE 22–15 Leopold's maneuvers in twin pregnancy. The fetus on the mother's right side is in cephalic presentation, and the fetus on the left is in breech presentation.

Nursing Plan and Implementation

Community-Based Nursing Care

Antepartally, the woman may need counseling about diet and daily activities. The nurse can help her plan meals to meet her increased needs. A daily intake of 4000 kcal (minimum) and 135 g of protein is recommended for optimal weight gain and fetal growth. A prenatal vitamin and 1 mg of folic acid should also be taken daily. A weight gain of 40 to 50 lbs has been recommended, with a 15- to 20-lb weight gain by 20 weeks.

Maternal hypertension is treated with bed rest in the lateral position to increase uterine and kidney perfusion. The nurse can help the woman schedule frequent periods of rest during the day. Family members or friends may be willing to care for the woman's other children periodically to allow her time to get rest. Back discomfort can be alleviated by pelvic rocking, good posture, and good body mechanics.

Teaching regarding prevention and recognition of preterm labor is very important. For further discussion see Chapter 16.

Hospital-Based Nursing Care

The nurse needs to prepare to receive two neonates. This means a duplication of resuscitation equipment and newborn identification papers and bracelets. The newborns may be placed in individual radiant warmers or in the same one once identification bands have been applied. Two staff members should be available for newborn resuscitation. While one nurse is monitoring the second twin in utero, the other nurse is caring for the first newborn and preparing to ensure correct identification of the neonates. Special precautions should be observed to ensure correct identification of the neonates. The first born is usually tagged Baby A; the second, Baby B.

Evaluation

Expected outcomes of nursing care include the following:

- The woman is knowledgeable regarding the implications and problems associated with twin pregnancy.
- The woman feels she is able to cope with the pregnancy and birth.
- The woman understands the treatment plan and how to gain further information.
- The mother, father, and babies have a safe prenatal course, labor, and birth and a safe postpartal and newborn course. ●

Three or More Fetuses

When three or more fetuses are present, maternal and fetal problems are increased. The more fetuses conceived, the smaller they tend to be at the time of birth. Birth of three or more fetuses is best accomplished by cesarean because of the risk of fetal insult due to decreased placental perfusion and hemorrhage from the separating placenta during the intrapartal period (Cunningham et al, 1997). Complicated obstetric maneuvers, such as breech extraction and podalic version, the risk of prolapse of the cord, and an increase in fetal collision provide additional reasons for cesarean birth.

Care of the Woman and Fetus in the Presence of Fetal Distress

When the oxygen supply is insufficient to meet the physiologic demands of the fetus, fetal distress may result. The condition may be acute, chronic, or a combination of both. A variety of factors may contribute to fetal distress. The most common are related to cord compression and uteroplacental insufficiency associated with placental abnormalities and preexisting maternal or fetal disease. If the resultant hypoxia persists and metabolic acidosis follows, the situation can be life threatening to the fetus.

The most common initial signs of fetal stress are meconium-stained amniotic fluid (in a vertex presentation) and changes in the FHR. The presence of ominous FHR patterns, such as late or severe variable decelerations, decrease in or lack of variability, and progressive acceleration in the FHR baseline, are indicative of hypoxia. Fetal scalp blood samples demonstrating a pH value of 7.20 or less provide a more sophisticated indication of fetal problems and are generally obtained when questions about fetal status arise. (See also Chapter 19.)

Clinical Therapy

When there is evidence of possible fetal stress, treatment centers on relieving the hypoxia and minimizing the effects of anoxia on the fetus. Initial interventions include changing the mother's position and administering oxygen by mask at 6 to 10 L per minute. If electronic fetal monitoring has not yet been used, it is usually instituted at this time. If oxytocin is in use, it should be discontinued. Fetal scalp blood samples are taken. Figure 22–16 depicts intrapartal management of fetal distress.

NURSING CARE MANAGEMENT

Nursing Assessment and Diagnosis

The nurse reviews the woman's prenatal history to anticipate the possibility of fetal distress. When the membranes rupture, it is important to assess FHR and to observe for meconium staining. As labor progresses, the nurse is particularly alert for even subtle changes in the

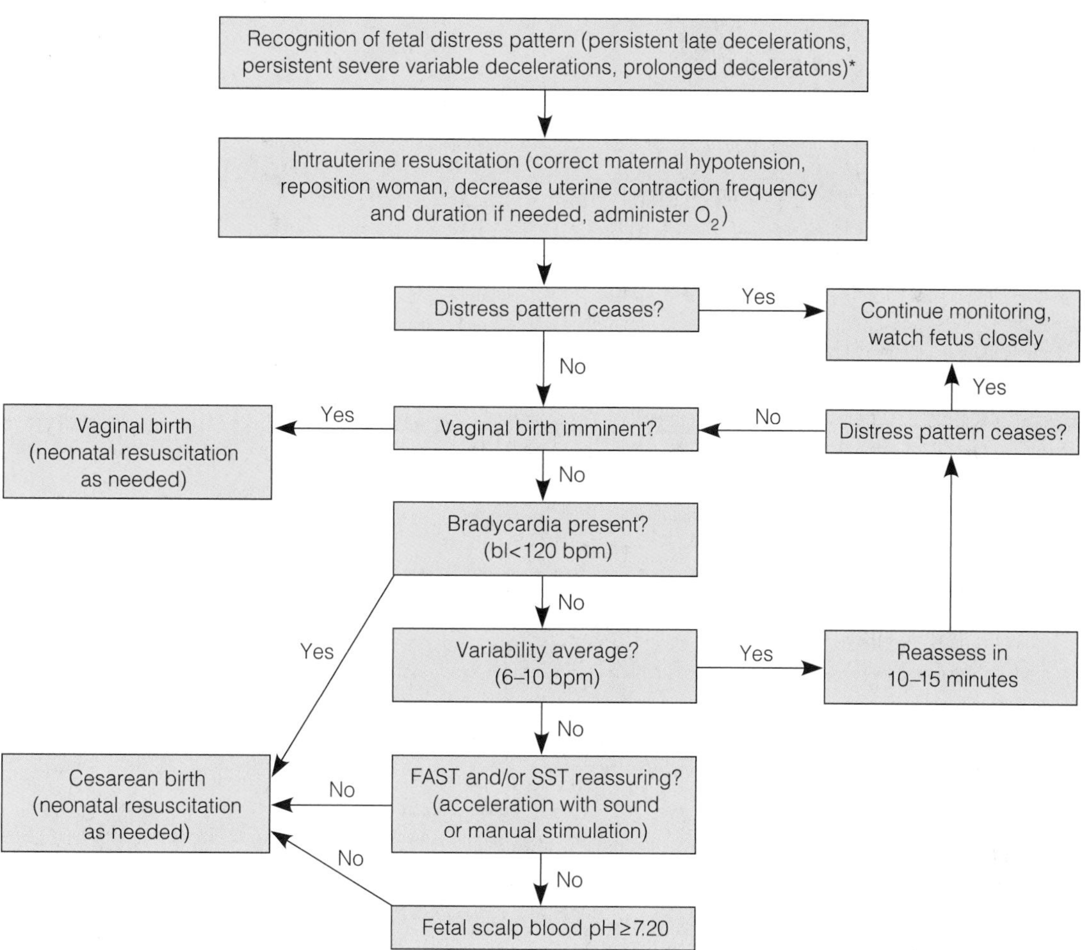

FIGURE 22–16 Intrapartal management of fetal distress. Note: bl = baseline; FAST = fetal acoustic stimulation test; SST = scalp stimulation test. SOURCES: Based on information from Strong TH: Fetal distress in the intrapartum period. In: *Current Therapy in Obstetrics and Gynecology,* 3rd ed. Quilligan EJ, Zuspan FP (editors). Philadelphia: WB Saunders, 1990; *Huddleston JF, Freeman RK: Estimation of fetal well-being. In: *Neonatal–Perinatal Medicine: Diseases of the Fetus and Newborn,* 5th ed. Fanaroff AA, Martin RS (editors). St Louis: Mosby-Year Book, 1992.

FHR pattern and the fetal scalp pH, if available. Reports by the mother of increased or greatly decreased fetal activity may also be associated with fetal distress. For further discussion of FHR patterns and characteristics, see Evaluation of Fetal Status during Labor in Chapter 19.

Nursing diagnoses may include the following:

- ***Decreased Cardiac Output*** in fetus related to decreased uteroplacental perfusion secondary to maternal hypotension, decreased blood volume, vasoconstriction with PIH
- ***Anxiety*** related to knowledge of fetal stress

Nursing Plan and Implementation

Hospital-Based Nursing Care

The professional staff may become so involved in assessing fetal status and initiating corrective measures that they fail to give explanations and emotional support to the woman, her partner, and other family members. It is imperative to provide both full explanations of the problem and comfort to the couple. In many instances, if birth is not imminent, the woman must undergo cesarean birth. This operation may cause fear and frustration for the couple, especially if they were committed to a shared, prepared birth experience.

Evaluation

Expected outcomes of nursing care include the following:

- The woman and her family become less anxious and more able to cope with their situation.
- The fetal heart rate remains in normal range, or, alternatively, supportive measures maintain the FHR as normal as possible. ●

COMMUNITY IN FOCUS

RTS Parent Support Group

The death of an infant during the perinatal period is a devastating experience for families, and dealing with the loss is a lengthy, painful process. Eight years ago, as a nurse at a hospital in central Georgia worked to assist parents to cope during the initial days following a stillbirth or newborn death, she recognized the tremendous need for ongoing support. To help meet this need in her community, the nurse, Cheryl Pope Kish, attended the intensive national training program offered by RTS (Resolve Through Sharing) Bereavement Services of LaCrosse, Wisconsin, and became certified as a perinatal grief counselor and coordinator of a perinatal loss support program. She then returned to her community, enlisted the assistance of a colleague, Leta (Frankie) Holder, RN, a psychiatric/mental health clinical specialist, and created the RTS Parent Support Group of Central Georgia. The group now serves a six-county area.

The support group meets once a month in the evening. A local hospital helped with start-up of the group by providing stationery and helping to print and distribute pamphlets. Currently the hospital provides space for the group to meet. Additional funding has come from contributions made by family and friends. For example, following their baby's death, one family requested that, in lieu of flowers, donations be made to the group. The money has been used to augment library holdings on grief and loss and to send remembrance cards to families on the anniversary of a death.

Nationwide, on average, about 10% of people who have suffered a perinatal loss choose to participate in a support group. The Parent Support Group of Central Florida reflects the national trend for participation. The number of participants varies each month but typically includes about 10 to 12 people. People generally attend for a minimum of 6 months. Often both parents participate at first; however, the fathers tend to drop out of the group before their partners. The mothers seem to be more interested in telling and retelling their stories as new members join and seem to find healing in the process. Fathers often prefer to tell their stories once and then move on. These differences may reflect differences in the socialization of men and women.

Originally the program was designed to begin with an educational session followed by a time for sharing. Over the years the approach has become more flexible based on group needs and the educational component tends to be more integrated. A variety of topics are covered, such as the stages of grief; rituals and activities to remember the lost child; dealing with holidays, and so forth.

The initial meeting and the day following the meeting are often the most painful for the grieving couple because they have had to revisit their tragedy. The group facilitators, recognizing this, encourage the couple to return rather than let the pain of the first session deter them. Over time, established members become a source of support for newer members, often giving their home phone numbers so that a new member has someone to call between meetings. Because the common bond of the group is loss, group diversity does not become an issue and participants from different ethnic backgrounds and socioeconomic status work well together.

For many couples who have experienced a loss, another pregnancy becomes a primary goal. Because there is fear associated with the pregnancy, women who become pregnant often remain in the group until they begin to show. Subsequently, if they give birth to a healthy child, they may return to the group with their infant. These meetings tend to give hope to other members and are well received.

The RTS Parent Support Group of Central Georgia is a direct result of the work of two nurses who recognized an important community need and who have given generously of their time to meet that need. Their community is richer because of their efforts.

SOURCE: Personal communication with Cheryl Pope Kish, RNC, EdD, WHNP and Professor of Nursing, Georgia College and State University.

Care of the Family at Risk Due to Intrauterine Fetal Death

Fetal death, often referred to as fetal demise, accounts for one-half of perinatal mortality after 20 weeks' gestation. Intrauterine fetal death (IUFD) results from unknown causes or a number of physiologic maladaptations, including PIH, abruptio placentae, placenta previa, diabetes, infection, congenital anomalies, and isoimmune disease.

Prolonged retention of the fetus may lead to the development of disseminated intravascular coagulation (DIC), also referred to as consumption coagulopathy. After the release of thromboplastin from the degenerating fetal tissues into the maternal bloodstream, the extrinsic clotting system is activated, triggering the formation of multiple tiny blood clots. Fibrinogen and factors V and VII are subsequently depleted, and the woman begins to display symptoms of DIC. Fibrinogen levels begin a linear descent 3 to 4 weeks after the death of the fetus and continue to decrease without appropriate medical intervention.

Clinical Therapy

Abdominal ultrasound may reveal Spalding's sign (an overriding of the fetal cranial bones). Diagnosis of IUFD is confirmed by absence of heart action on ultrasonography. In addition, maternal estriol levels fall.

Most women have spontaneous labor within 2 weeks of fetal death. If other complications are not present, some physicians wait for labor to begin spontaneously (Cunningham et al, 1997).

NURSING CARE MANAGEMENT

Nursing Assessment and Diagnosis

Cessation of fetal movement reported by the mother to the nurse is frequently the first indication of fetal death. It is followed by a gradual decrease in the signs and symptoms of pregnancy. Fetal heart tones are absent, and fetal movement is no longer palpable. Once fetal demise is established by the physician, ongoing support and communication become even more important. Open communication among the mother, her partner, and the health care team members contributes to a more realistic understanding of the medical condition and its associated treatments. The nurse may discuss prior experiences the family has had with stress and what they feel were their coping abilities at that time. Determining the family's social supports and resources is also important.

> *Birth and death together. It's confusing and frightening enough for adults, but how are young children to understand it? For them the baby never really existed, or lived only briefly. What does this mean for them? Why are the parents so distraught? Too often, children's feelings about these issues are ignored or misunderstood. When parents are struggling to deal with their own feelings, they find it even harder to respond to the emotional needs of their other children.*
> ~ *WHEN PREGNANCY FAILS* ~

Nursing diagnoses that may apply to the woman experiencing intrauterine fetal death include the following:

- ***Grieving*** related to an actual loss
- ***Altered Family Processes*** related to loss of a family member
- ***Ineffective Individual Coping*** related to depression in response to loss of child
- ***Ineffective Family Coping*** related to death of a child

> *A friend asked if we had named our stillborn baby. After telling her the name, we both began referring to the baby by her name, Sarah. It felt good to call her a name.*
> ~ *WHEN PREGNANCY FAILS* ~

Nursing Plan and Implementation

Hospital-Based Nursing Care

The parents of a stillborn infant suffer a devastating experience, precipitating an intense emotional trauma. During the pregnancy, the couple has already begun the attachment process, which now must be terminated through the grieving process. The behaviors that couples exhibit while mourning may be associated with the five stages of grieving described by Elizabeth Kübler-Ross (1969). Often, the first stage is denial of the death of the fetus. Even when the initial health care provider suspects fetal demise, the couple is hoping that a second opinion will be different. Some couples may not be convinced of the death until they view and hold the stillborn infant. The second stage is anger, resulting from the feelings of loss, loneliness, and perhaps guilt. The anger may be projected at significant others and health care team members, or it may be absent when the death of the fetus is sudden and unexpected. Bargaining, the third stage, may or may not be present, depending on the couple's preparation for the death of the fetus. If the death is unanticipated, the couple may have no time for bargaining. In the fourth stage, depression is evidenced by preoccupation, weeping, and withdrawal. Physiologic postpartal depression appearing 24 to 48 hours after the stillbirth may compound the depression associated with grief. The final stage is acceptance, which involves the process of resolution. This is a highly individualized process that may take months to complete.

In some facilities, a checklist is used to make sure important aspects of working with the parents are addressed. The checklist becomes a communication tool between staff members to share information particular to this couple (Brown, 1992). Such a checklist might include the following items:

- When the fetal death is known before admission, inform the admission department and nursing staff so that inappropriate remarks are not made.
- Allow the woman and her partner to remain together as much as they wish. Provide privacy by assigning them to a private room.
- Stay with the couple, and do not leave them alone and isolated.
- As much as possible, have the same nurse provide care to increase the support for the couple. Develop a care plan to provide for continuity of care. Encourage family members to visit support persons.
- Have the most experienced labor and birth nurse auscultate for fetal heart tones. This avoids the searching that a more inexperienced nurse might feel compelled to do. Avoid the temptation to listen again "to make sure."
- Listen to the couple; do not offer explanations. They require solace without minimizing the situation.
- Facilitate the woman and her partner's participation in the labor and birth process. When possible, allow them to make decisions about who will be present and what ritual will occur during the birth process. Allow the woman to make the decision regarding whether to have sedation during labor and birth. Provide a quiet supportive environment; ideally, the labor and birth should occur in a labor room or possibly a birthing room rather than the delivery room.
- Give parents accurate information regarding plans for labor and birth.

- Provide ongoing opportunities for the couple to ask questions.
- Arrange for the woman to be assigned to a room that is away from new mothers and babies if she requests it. It is important to let the woman decide whether she wants to be on another unit. If early discharge is an option, allow the family to make that selection.
- Encourage the couple to experience the grief that they feel. Accept the weeping and depression. A couple may have intense feelings that they are unable to share with each other. Encourage them to talk together, and allow emotions to show freely. Help them understand that they may each experience different feelings (Cordell & Thomas, 1989).
- Give the couple and family an opportunity to see and hold the stillborn infant in a private quiet location. (Advocates of seeing the stillborn believe that viewing assists in dispelling denial and enables the couple to progress to the next step in the grieving process.) If they choose to see their stillborn infant, prepare the couple for what they will see by saying, "The baby is cold," "The baby is blue," "The baby is bruised," or other appropriate statements (Furrh & Copley, 1989).
- Some families may elect to bathe or dress their stillborn; support them in their choice.
- Take a photograph of the infant, and let the family know it is available if they want it now or some time in the future.
- Offer a card with footprints, crib card, ID band, and possibly a lock of hair to the parents. These items may be kept with the photo if the parents do not want them at this time.
- Prepare the couple for returning home. If there are siblings, each will usually progress through age-appropriate grieving. Provide the parents with information about normal mourning reactions, both psychologic and physiologic.
- Furnish the mother with educational materials that discuss the changes she will experience in returning to the nonpregnant state.
- Provide information about community support groups, including group name, contact person if possible, and phone number. Use materials such as the book *When Hello Means Goodbye* by Schwiebert and Kirk (1985).
- Remember it is not so important to "say the right words." The caring support and human contact that a couple receives is important and can be conveyed through silence and your presence.
- Contact religious support systems if parents desire.
- Discuss further care of the stillborn baby (dress, rituals).

The nurse experiences many of the same grief reactions as the parents of a stillborn infant. It is important to have support persons and colleagues available for counseling and support.

Evaluation

Expected outcomes of nursing care include the following:

- The family members express their feelings about the death of their baby.
- The family participates in decisions regarding whether to see their baby and in other decisions regarding the baby.
- The family knows what community resources are available and has names and phone numbers to use if they choose.
- The family moves into and through the grieving process. ●

I knew something was wrong just by the way everyone was scurrying around in the delivery room and by that terrible silence. Then we knew the baby was dead. The doctor's only comment was, "It must be congenital," as if to say it certainly must be my fault, not his. Then a nurse said: "It would be worse if you had a five-year-old that died." I suppose she was right, but it certainly didn't make me feel any better. Later, the doctor said, "You're young, you'll have lots more kids." I was appalled—I was thirty-three already. Where do they learn all these stupid comments?
~ *When Pregnancy Fails* ~

Care of the Woman and Fetus at Risk Due to Placental Problems

Maintaining placental function is paramount to ensure fetal well-being and continuation of the pregnancy. Because the placenta is highly vascular, problems that develop are usually associated with maternal and possible fetal hemorrhage. Causes and sources of hemorrhage are reviewed in Table 22–2.

Abruptio Placentae

Abruptio placentae is the premature separation of a normally implanted placenta from the uterine wall. The incidence of abruptio placentae is 1 in 120 births but accounts for 15% of perinatal mortality (Gabbe, Niebyl, & Simpson, 1996). It is more frequent in pregnancies complicated by cocaine abuse (Cunningham et al, 1997). The risk of recurrence is much higher than for the general population. The recurrence rate varies between 5% and 17%. In the woman with a history of 2 previous abruptions, the chance of recurrence is 25% (Gabbe, 1996).

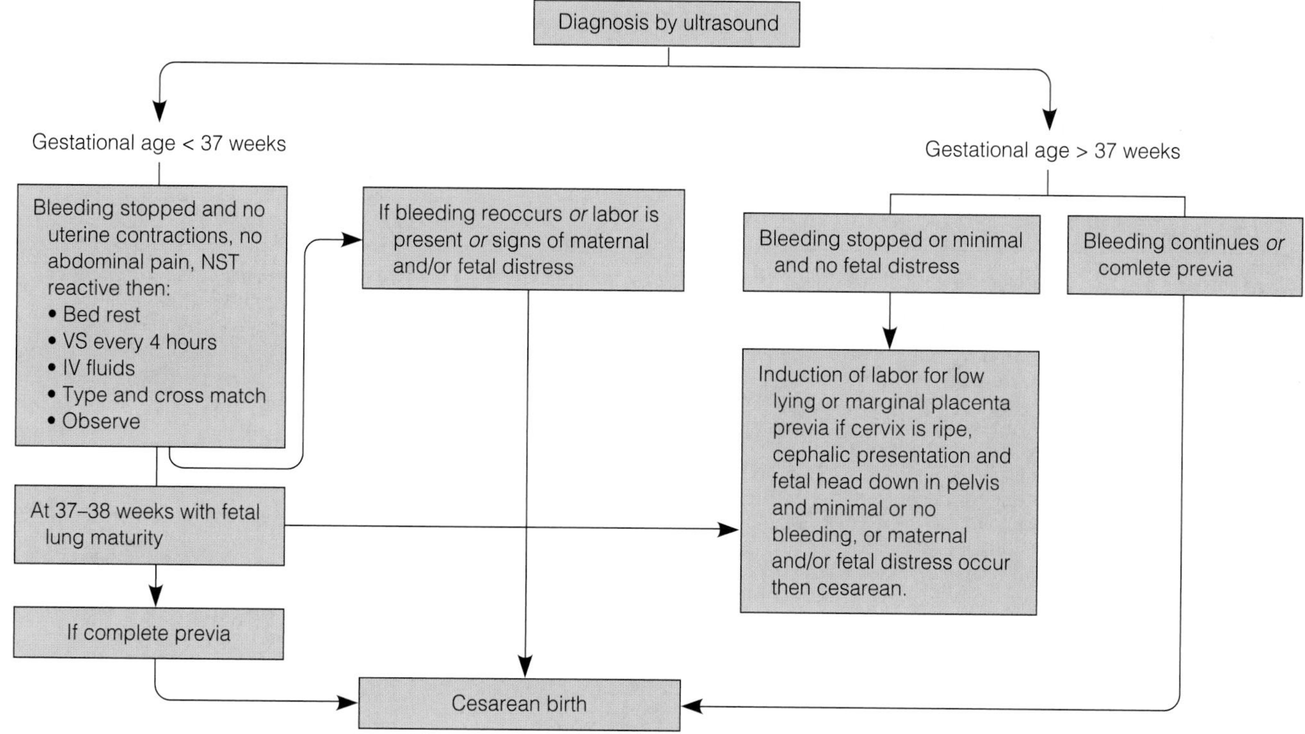

FIGURE 22–20 Management of placenta previa. SOURCE: Based on information from Barker RK, Fields DH, Kaufman SA: *Quick Reference to OB-GYN Procedures,* 3rd ed. New York: Lippincott/Harper & Row, 1990.

6. Complete laboratory evaluation: hemoglobin, hematocrit, Rh factor, and urinalysis
7. Intravenous fluid (lactated Ringer's solution) with drip rate monitored
8. Two units of cross-matched blood available for transfusion

If frequent, recurrent, or profuse bleeding persists or if fetal well-being appears threatened, a cesarean birth will need to be performed.

NURSING CARE MANAGEMENT

Nursing Assessment and Diagnosis

Assessment of the woman with placenta previa must be ongoing to prevent or treat complications that are potentially lethal to the mother and fetus. Painless, bright red vaginal bleeding is the best diagnostic sign of placenta previa. If this sign should develop during the last 3 months of a pregnancy, placenta previa should always be considered until ruled out by examination. The first bleeding episode is generally scanty. If no vaginal examinations are performed, it often subsides spontaneously. However, each subsequent hemorrhage is more profuse.

The uterus remains soft, and if labor begins, it relaxes fully between contractions. The FHR usually remains stable unless profuse hemorrhage and maternal shock occur. As a result of the placement of the placenta, the fetal presenting part is often unengaged, and transverse lie is common.

Blood loss, pain, and uterine contractility are appraised by the nurse from both subjective and objective perspectives. Maternal vital signs and the results of blood and urine tests provide the nurse with additional data about the woman's condition. FHR is evaluated with an external fetal monitor. Another nursing responsibility is observing and verifying the family's ability to cope with the anxiety associated with an unknown outcome.

Nursing diagnoses that may apply to the woman experiencing placenta previa are as follows:

- ***Fluid Volume Deficit*** related to hypovolemia secondary to excessive blood loss
- ***Risk for Altered Tissue Perfusion*** related to blood loss secondary to uterine atony following birth
- ***Anxiety*** related to concern for own personal status and the baby's safety
- ***Risk for Impaired Gas Exchange*** related to decreased blood volume and hypotension

Nursing Plan and Implementation

Hospital-Based Nursing Care

The nurse continues to monitor the woman and her fetus to determine the status of the bleeding and to determine

CRITICAL PATHWAY FOR HEMORRHAGE IN THIRD TRIMESTER AND AT BIRTH

Category	Immediate Care	Outcomes
Referral	Perinatologist Neonatologist Psychiatric Clinical Nurse Practitioner	**Expected Outcomes** Appropriate resources identified and utilized
Assessments	Obtain history to identify if any factors are present predisposing to hemorrhage: • Presence of preeclampsia-eclampsia (PIH) • Overdistension of the uterus; multiple pregnancy; hydramnios • Grandmultiparity • Advanced age • Uterine contractile problems: hypotonicity; hypertonicity • Painless vaginal bleeding after seventh month • Presence of hypertension • Presence of diabetes • History of previous hemorrhage or bleeding problems, blood coagulation defects, abortion • Retention of placental fragments • Cervical and/or vaginal lacerations Determine religious preference to establish whether client will permit a blood transfusion	**Expected Outcomes** • Potential/actual hemorrhage identified • Related complications minimized
Teaching/ psychosocial	Keep woman informed of present status Provide accurate information Provide opportunities for questions Establish a trusting relationship with client Encourage the woman to participate in decision making if at all possible Instruct client to keep bladder empty Notify RN if vag bleeding or leaking noted, decreased fetal movement, abdominal pain/discomfort or uterine contractions Report saturation $>$ 1 pad within 1 h or less	**Expected Outcomes** Woman verbalizes/demonstrates understanding of teaching
Nursing care management and reports	Observe, record, and report blood loss Evaluate using the following parameters: • Monitor rate and quality of respirations frequently • Measure pulse rate • Assess pulse quality by direct palpation • Determine pulse deficit by comparing apical-radial rates • Compare present BP with woman's baseline BP; note pulse pressure • Inspect skin for presence of pallor and cyanosis, coldness, and clamminess • Evaluate state of consciousness frequently • Measure CVP: normal CVP is 5–10 cm H_2O • Assess amount of blood loss: • Count pads • Weigh pads and Chux (1 g = approximately 1 mL blood) • Record amount in a specific amount of time (eg, 50 mL bright red blood on pad in 20 min) Relieve decreased blood pressure by administering whole blood per physician order While waiting for whole blood to be available, infuse isotonic fluids, plasma, plasma expanders, or serum albumin, per physician order If marginal abruptio placentae is present: • Evaluate blood loss • Assess uterine contractile pattern, tenderness, and height • Start continuous monitoring of uterine contractions by EFM • Monitor maternal vital signs • Assess fetal status per continuous EFM • Assess cervical dilatation and effacement to determine labor progress if uterine contractions are present • Rule out placenta previa • Assist with amniotomy, and begin oxytocin infusion per physician order if labor does not start immediately or is ineffective • Review and evaluate diagnostic lab tests (hemoglobin, hematocrit, PT, APPT, fibrin split products, fibrinogen, platelets)	**Expected Outcomes** • Blood loss reduced and controlled or halted • Perfusion and oxygenation supported

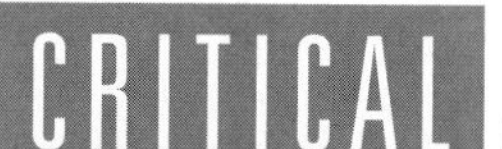 PATHWAY *CONTINUED*

Category	Immediate Care	Outcomes
Nursing care management and reports *continued*	If central abruptio placentae with severe blood loss is present: • Perform same assessments as for marginal abruptio placentae • Monitor CVP • Replace blood loss • Effect immediate birth • Observe for signs and symptoms of disseminated intravascular coagulation (DIC) Woman is at risk for uterine atony following birth: • Assess contractility of uterus and amount of vaginal bleeding • Assess uterus q15min × 4, q30min × 2, q60min × 2–4. Evaluate more frequently if uterus is boggy or not in the midline. Administer oxytocin per protocol or physician order.	
Activity	Complete bed rest Diversional activity	**Expected Outcomes** No exacerbation of hemorrhage occurs
Comfort	Assess comfort of woman	**Expected Outcomes** Woman's comfort maintained
Nutrition	IV fluids infusing NPO	**Expected Outcomes** Optimal hydration and blood volume maintained
Elimination	Monitor urine output (decrease to less than 30 mL/h is sign of shock): • Insert Foley catheter • Measure output hourly • Measure specific gravity to determine concentration of urine	**Expected Outcomes** Urinary output maintained
Medications	IV—lactated Ringer's at 150 mL/h If premature—Betamethasone O_2 as indicated	**Expected Outcomes** Circulation and perfusion maintained
Discharge planning/ home care	Determine need for assistance in the home Provide information regarding community resources	**Expected Outcomes** Woman is discharged with plan for follow-up care related to fatigue and blood loss
Family involvement	Establish a trusting relationship with family	**Expected Outcomes** Family development and newborn attachment unimpaired
Date		

the mother's and baby's responses. Vital signs, intake and output, and other pertinent assessments must be made frequently. The nurse evaluates the electronic monitor tracing to evaluate the fetal status.

Emotional support for the family is an important nursing care goal. When active bleeding is occurring, the assessments and management must be directed toward physical support. However, emotional aspects need to be addressed simultaneously. The nurse can explain the assessments being completed and the treatment measures that need to be done. Time can be provided for questions, and the nurse can act as an advocate in obtaining information for the family. Emotional support can also be offered by staying with the family and by the use of touch.

The newborn's hemoglobin, cell volume, and erythrocyte count should be checked immediately and then monitored closely. The newborn may require oxygen and administration of blood and admission into a neonatal intensive care unit.

Additional information regarding nursing care is addressed in the Critical Pathway for Hemorrhage in Third Trimester and at Birth.

Evaluation

Expected outcomes of nursing care include the following:

- The cause of hemorrhage is recognized promptly, and corrective measures are taken.

TABLE 22–4 Placental and Umbilical Cord Variations

Placental Variation	Maternal Implications	Fetal-Neonatal Implications	
Succenturiate placenta One or more accessory lobes of fetal villi will develop on the placenta.	Postpartal hemorrhage from retained lobe	None, as long as all parts of the placenta remain attached until after birth of the fetus	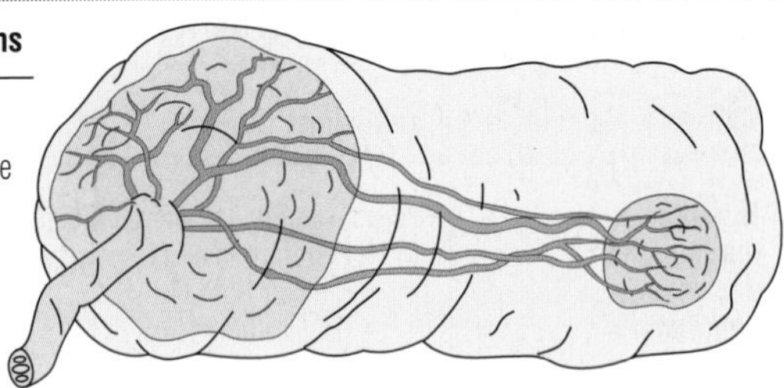
Circumvallate placenta A double fold of chorion and amnion form a ring around the umbilical cord, on the fetal side of the placenta.	Increased incidence of late abortion, antepartal hemorrhage, and preterm labor	Intrauterine growth restriction, prematurity, fetal death	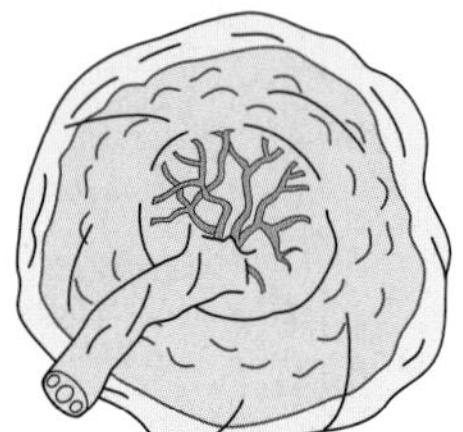
Battledore placenta The umbilical cord is inserted at or near the placental margin.	Increased incidence of preterm labor and bleeding	Prematurity, fetal distress	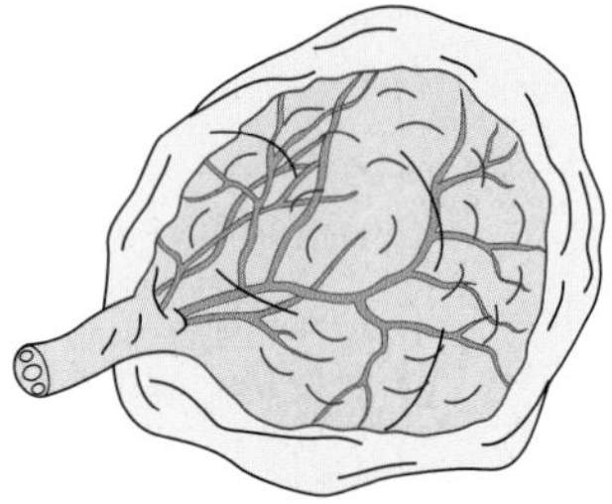
Velamentous insertion of the umbilical cord The vessels of the umbilical cord divide some distance from the placenta in the placental membranes.	Hemorrhage if one of the vessels is torn	Fetal distress, hemorrhage	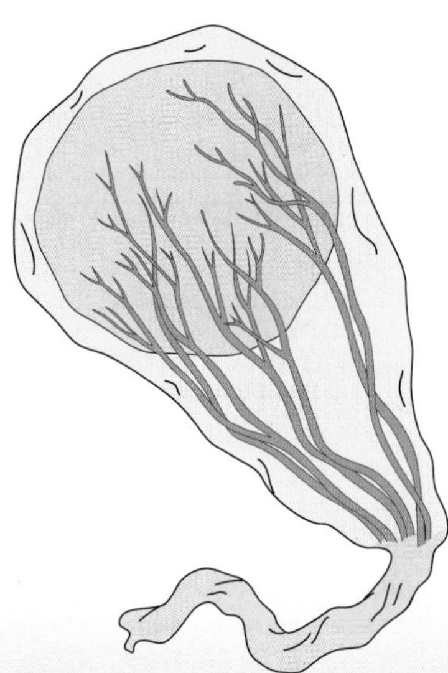

- The woman's vital signs remain in the normal range.
- The woman and her baby have a safe labor and birth.
- The family understands what has happened and the implications and associated problems of placenta previa. ●

Other Placental Problems

Other problems of the placenta can be divided into those that are developmental and those that are degenerative. Developmental problems of the placenta include placental lesions, succenturiate placenta, circumvallate placenta, and battledore placenta (Table 22–4). Degenerative changes include infarcts and placental calcification.

Succenturiate Placenta

In succenturiate placenta, one or more accessory lobes of fetal villi have developed on the placenta, with vascular connections of fetal origin (Table 22–4). Vessels from the major to the minor lobe(s) are supported only by the membranes, thus increasing the risk of the minor lobe's being retained during the third stage of labor.

The gravest maternal danger is postpartal hemorrhage if this minor lobe is severed from the placenta and remains in the uterus. All placentas should be examined closely for intactness. If vessels appear to be severed at the margin of the placenta, the uterus should be explored for retained placental tissue. This condition is not usually diagnosed until after the birth of the placenta. If the vascular connections rupture between the lobes, life-threatening fetal hemorrhage can result. Examination of the fetal membrane following birth may reveal a small hole with vessels running toward it. This is another indication of a retained lobe (Cunningham et al, 1997). At birth, the infant should be inspected for pallor, cyanosis, retractions, tachypnea, tachycardia, and feeble pulse. The infant's cry will be weak and the muscle tone flaccid.

Circumvallate Placenta

In circumvallate placenta, the fetal surface of the placenta is exposed through a ring opening around the umbilical cord (Table 22–4). The vessels descend from the cord and end at the margin of the ring instead of coursing through the entire surface area of the placenta. The ring is composed of a double fold of amnion and chorion with some degenerative decidua and fibrin between. The cause of this condition is unknown. Maternal-fetal problems include an increased incidence of late abortion or fetal death, antepartal hemorrhage, prematurity, and abnormal maternal bleeding during or following the third stage of labor, resulting from improper placental separation or shearing of membranes from the placenta.

Battledore Placenta

In battledore placenta, the umbilical cord is inserted at or near the placental margin (Table 22–4). As a result, all fetal vessels transverse the placental surface in the same direction. The chances of preterm labor are high because of interference with fetal circulation and nutrition. Fetal distress or bleeding during labor is also likely because of cord compression or vessel rupture.

Placental Infarcts and Calcifications

In the aging process, the placenta may develop infarcts and calcifications. They become significant if they cover a large enough area to interfere with the uterine-placental-fetal exchange. Altered exchange can also occur with certain maternal disease processes, such as hypertension. Infarcts are most often seen in cases of severe pregnancy-induced hypertension and in women who smoke.

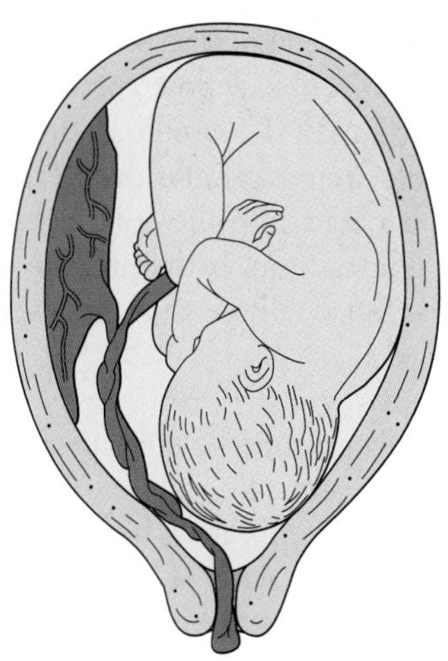

FIGURE 22–21 Prolapse of the umbilical cord.

Care of the Woman and Fetus at Risk Due to Problems Associated with the Umbilical Cord

Prolapsed Umbilical Cord

When the umbilical cord precedes the fetal presenting part, it is known as a **prolapsed cord.** In this situation, pressure is placed on the umbilical cord as it is trapped between the presenting part and the maternal pelvis. Consequently, the vessels carrying blood to and from the fetus are compressed. The cord falls or is washed down through the cervix into the vagina and in rare circumstances may be visible at the lower edge of the vagina. In other cases the umbilical cord lies beside or just ahead of the fetal head; this is called occult cord prolapse.

Any time that the pelvic inlet is not completely filled by the fetus or the presenting part is not firmly against the cervix, and the membranes rupture, the umbilical cord can be washed down into the birth canal in front of the presenting part (Figure 22–21). The incidence of prolapse of the cord is 20 times greater with abnormal axis lie (Gabbe, 1996)—especially footling breech and shoulder presentations—low birth weight, a multipara with more than five previous births, multiple gestation, obstetric manipulation (amniotomy), and the presence of a long cord (longer than 80 cm). Approximately 50% of cord prolapses occur in the second stage. The incidence of cord prolapse is 0.2% to 0.6% of births (Cruikshank, 1994).

Maternal-Fetal-Neonatal Risks

Although a prolapsed cord does not directly precipitate physical alterations in the woman, her immediate concern for the baby creates enormous stress. The woman may need to deal with some unusual interventions, a cesarean birth, and in some circumstances death of the baby.

The fetus is affected because compression of the umbilical cord occludes blood flow through the umbilical vessels. Bradycardia (FHR baseline below 120 beats per minute) and persistent variable decelerations may develop. If labor is occurring, the cord is compressed further with each contraction. If the pressure on the cord is not relieved, the fetus will die.

Clinical Therapy

Preventing the occurrence of cord prolapse is the preferred medical approach. For all laboring women with a history of ruptured membranes, bed rest is usually indicated until engagement with no cord prolapse has been documented. If the prolapse does occur, it is most usually discovered by the nurse, and relieving the compression of the cord is critical for the fetus. The method of birth will most likely be cesarean.

NURSING CARE MANAGEMENT

Nursing Assessment and Diagnosis

In the intrapartal area, the nurse reviews the nursing history and ascertains whether the woman is likely to be at risk for prolapse of the cord. Particularly when the presenting part is not engaged and spontaneous or artificial rupture of the membranes occurs, the nurse observes the perineum and assesses the FHR for bradycardia and severe, recurrent, variable decelerations.

Nursing diagnoses that may apply to the woman with a prolapsed cord include the following:

- ***Risk for Impaired Gas Exchange*** in the fetus related to decreased blood flow secondary to compression of the umbilical cord
- ***Fear*** related to unknown outcome

Nursing Plan and Implementation

Hospital-Based Nursing Care

Because there are few outward signs of cord prolapse, each pregnant woman is advised to call her physician or certified nurse-midwife when the membranes rupture and to go to the office, clinic, or birthing facility. A sterile vaginal examination determines whether there is danger of cord prolapse. If the presenting part is well engaged, the risk is minimal, and ambulation may be encouraged. If the presenting part is not well engaged, bed rest is recommended to prevent cord prolapse. Maintaining bed rest after rupture of membranes can lead to conflict if the laboring woman and her partner do not hold the same opinions. The nurse can ease this situation by helping communication between the physician/CNM and the couple.

If membranes have not yet ruptured when the woman arrives at the facility, at the time of spontaneous rupture or amniotomy (artificial rupture of the membranes) the FHR should be monitored by electronic fetal monitoring or auscultated for at least a full minute and again at the end of a contraction and after a few contractions. In the presence of cord prolapse, EFM tracings show baseline bradycardia or severe, moderate, or prolonged nonperiodic decelerations. If these patterns are found, the nurse completes a vaginal examination.

If a loop of cord is discovered, the nurse's gloved fingers are left in the vagina, and the presenting part is gently pushed upward to lift the fetal part off the cord and relieve cord compression until the physician/CNM arrives. This is a life-saving measure. Oxygen is administered, and FHR is monitored by EFM to see if the cord compression is adequately relieved (baseline will rise above 120 beats per minute, and variable decelerations are lessened or relieved). The nurse may also feel pulsation in the cord; however, in some instances a pulsation cannot be felt, and FHR can be detected only by EFM.

In some cases, another nurse may insert an indwelling bladder catheter and, using a sterile asepto syringe or infusion device, fill the bladder with approximately 350 to 500 mL of warmed, sterile normal saline. The filled bladder lifts the fetal head upward and relieves pressure on the umbilical cord (Griese & Prickett, 1993). Filling her bladder and maintaining the woman in a side-lying position may be all that is needed to relieve the pressure on the cord. If the bladder is not filled, the force of gravity can be incorporated. In this instance, the nurse maintains pressure on the presenting part while performing a vaginal examination and instructs the woman to move into a knee-chest position or adjusts the bed to the Trendelenburg position. The nurse maintains pressure on the presenting part, and the woman is transported to the birthing or operating room in this position.

Evaluation

Expected outcomes of nursing care include the following:

- The FHR remains in normal range with supportive measures.
- The fetus is born safely.
- The woman and her partner feel supported.
- The woman and her partner understand the problem and the corrective measures that are undertaken. ●

Umbilical Cord Abnormalities

Umbilical cord abnormalities include congenital absence of an umbilical artery, insertion variations, cord length variations, and knots and loops of the cord. Insertion variations include velamentous insertion and vasa previa, and cord length problems include long and short cords.

Congenital Absence of Umbilical Artery

Absence of an umbilical artery may have serious fetal implications. The incidence of all types of fetal anomalies is 25% in infants born with two-vessel cords.

Immediately after the umbilical cord is cut, it should be inspected to determine whether the correct number of vessels is present. If an artery is absent, the nurse should examine the newborn more closely for anomalies and gestational age problems.

Insertion Variations

In a velamentous insertion, the vessels of the umbilical cord divide some distance from the placenta in the placental membranes (Table 22–4). Velamentous insertions occur more frequently in multiple gestations than in singletons. Other placental anomalies, such as succenturiate placenta, often accompany this condition. The velamentous insertion is more easily compressed or kinked during pregnancy or labor because of the lack of Wharton's jelly to protect it. If the vessels become torn during labor, fetal hemorrhage can occur, and the blood can escape from the vagina. When fetal hemorrhage occurs, it results in FHR abnormalities.

When the vessels of a velamentous insertion transverse the internal os and appear in front of the fetus, a vasa previa has occurred. Fetal hemorrhage with asphyxia is likely to result because as the fetal blood escapes out of the vagina the hemorrhage will probably be diagnosed as maternal.

Cord Length Variations

The average length of the umbilical cord is 55 cm. Although short cords rarely cause complications directly, they have been associated with umbilical hernias in the fetus, abruptio placentae, and cord rupture. Long cords tend to twist and tangle around the fetus, causing transient variable decelerations. A long cord rarely causes fetal death, however, because it is generally not pulled tight until descent at the time of birth. With a long cord and an active fetus, one or more true knots can result. Again, these knots usually are not pulled tight enough to cause fetal stress until the infant has been born, and the cord can then be clamped and cut.

Clinical Therapy

The goals of medical treatment are to prevent serious fetal complications and to examine the newborn for anomalies that coexist with umbilical cord abnormalities.

Any vaginal bleeding during labor warrants continuous monitoring of the fetus, preferably with an external electronic monitor. Any signs of fetal stress should be reported immediately. In the presence of bleeding, laboratory tests may be used to differentiate fetal from maternal red blood cells. Fetal hemorrhage is resolved by terminating the pregnancy vaginally or through cesarean birth and by correcting neonatal anemia. Expediting the birth, whether vaginally or surgically, is paramount when severe fetal stress is apparent. Following the birth, the pediatric team identifies and treats any neonatal complications or anomalies.

NURSING CARE MANAGEMENT

Nursing Assessment and Diagnosis

Umbilical abnormalities may not become evident until the birth of the fetus. During labor the nurse should observe for signs of fetal distress and excessive bleeding (with velamentous insertion and vasa previa).

Nursing diagnoses that may apply include the following:

- *Risk for Impaired Gas Exchange* in the fetus related to decreased blood flow secondary to placental abnormalities
- *Knowledge Deficit* related to lack of information about implications and associated problems of placental abnormalities

Nursing Plan and Implementation

Hospital-Based Nursing Care

The nurse is alert for an unusual amount of bleeding during the labor and birth. Following the birth, the placenta is inspected for abnormalities.

Often any mild or moderate variable deceleration can be successfully managed by the nurse. Repositioning of the woman often alleviates pressure on the cord if this is the reason for the deceleration.

Evaluation

Expected outcomes of nursing care include the following:

- The mother and baby have a safe labor and birth.
- The woman's bleeding is assessed quickly, and corrective measures are taken.
- The family is able to cope successfully with fetal or neonatal anomalies, if they exist. ●

Care of the Woman and Fetus at Risk Due to Amniotic Fluid–Related Complications

Amniotic Fluid Embolism/Anaphalactoid Syndrome of Pregnancy

Amniotic fluid embolism occurs when a bolus of amniotic fluid enters the maternal circulation and then the maternal lungs. The cause of this obstetric emergency is unknown. Earlier suggestions that uterine hyperstimulation was a causative factor cannot be supported with evidence; fewer than 10% of cases with this diagnosis experienced hyperstimulation (Gabbe, 1996). Current investigation suggests this is an immune response that is similar to anaphylactic shock (Foley & Strong, 1997). Because amniotic fluid embolism is a rare complication a National Registry was initiated in 1988 in order to collect retrospective data for analysis.

Hydramnios

Hydramnios (also called *polyhydramnios*) occurs when there is over 2000 mL of amniotic fluid. The exact cause of hydramnios is unknown; however, it often occurs in cases of major congenital anomalies. It is postulated that a major source of amniotic fluid is found in special amnion cells that lie over the placenta (Cunningham et al, 1997). During the second half of the pregnancy, the fetus begins to swallow and inspire amniotic fluid and to urinate, which contributes to the amount present. In cases of hydramnios, no pathology has been found in the amniotic epithelium. However, hydramnios is associated with fetal malformations that affect the fetal swallowing mechanism and neurologic disorders in which the fetal meninges are exposed in the amniotic cavity.

This condition is also found in cases of anencephaly, in which the fetus is thought to urinate excessively due to overstimulation of the cerebrospinal centers. When a monozygotic twin manifests hydramnios, it is possible that the twin with the increased blood volume urinates excessively. The weight of the placenta has been found to be increased in some cases of hydramnios, indicating that increased functioning of the placental tissue may contribute to the problem.

There are two types of hydramnios: chronic and acute. In the chronic type, the fluid volume gradually increases and is a problem of the third trimester. Most cases are of this variety. In acute cases, the volume increases rapidly over a period of a few days. The acute type is usually diagnosed between 20 and 24 weeks' gestation.

When the amount of amniotic fluid is over 3000 mL, the woman experiences shortness of breath and edema in the lower extremities from compression of the vena cava. If hydramnios is severe enough, she can experience intense pain. The acute form of hydramnios tends to be more severe. Milder forms of hydramnios occur more frequently and are associated with minimal symptoms. Hydramnios is associated with such maternal disorders as diabetes and Rh sensitization.

Fetal malformations and preterm birth are common with hydramnios; thus there is a fairly high rate of perinatal mortality. Prolapsed umbilical cord can occur when the membranes rupture, which adds a further complication for the fetus. The incidence of malpresentations is also increased.

Clinical Therapy

Hydramnios is managed with supportive treatment unless the intensity of the woman's distress and symptoms dictate otherwise.

If the accumulation of amniotic fluid is severe enough to cause maternal dyspnea and pain, hospitalization and removal of the excessive fluid are required. This can be done vaginally by AROM or by amniocentesis. The dangers of performing the technique vaginally are prolapsed cord and the inability to remove the fluid slowly. If amniocentesis is performed, it should be done with the aid of sonography to prevent inadvertent damage to the fetus and placenta.

Prostaglandin synthesis inhibitor (indomethacin) is often utilized to treat hydramnios. Indomethacin has been shown to decrease amniotic fluid volume by decreasing fetal urine output (Cunningham et al, 1997).

NURSING CARE MANAGEMENT

Nursing Assessment and Diagnosis

Hydramnios should be suspected when the fundal height increases out of proportion to the gestational age.

With increased fluid, the nurse may have difficulty palpating the fetus and auscultating the FHR. In more severe cases the maternal abdomen appears extremely tense and tight on inspection. On sonography large spaces can be identified between the fetus and the uterine wall.

Nursing diagnoses that may apply include the following:

- ***Risk for Impaired Gas Exchange*** related to pressure on the diaphragm secondary to hydramnios
- ***Fear*** related to unknown outcome of the pregnancy

Nursing Plan and Implementation

Hospital-Based Nursing Care

When amniocentesis is performed, sterile technique is used to prevent infection. The nurse can offer support to the couple by explaining the procedure to them.

If the fetus has been diagnosed with a congenital defect in utero or is born with the defect, psychologic support is needed to assist the family. Often the nurse collaborates with social services to offer the family this additional help.

Evaluation

Expected outcomes of nursing care include the following:

- The woman and her partner understand the procedure, implications, risks, and characteristics that need to be reported to the caregiver. ●

Oligohydramnios

Oligohydramnios is defined as a less than normal amount of amniotic fluid (approximately 500 mL is considered normal). Although no exact amount of fluid has been definitively identified as diagnostic of oligohydramnios, oligohydramnios is diagnosed when the largest vertical pocket of amniotic fluid visible on ultrasound examination is 5 cm or less (Cunningham et al, 1997). The exact cause of this condition is unknown. It is found in cases of postmaturity, with IUGR secondary to placental insufficiency, and in fetal conditions associated with major renal malformations, including renal aplasia with dysplastic kidneys and obstructive lesions of the lower urinary tract. If oligohydramnios occurs in the first part of pregnancy, there is a danger of fetal adhesions (one part of the fetus may adhere to another part).

During the gestational period, fetal skin and skeletal abnormalities may occur because fetal movement is impaired as a result of inadequate amniotic fluid volume. Because there is less fluid available for the fetus to use during fetal breathing movements, pulmonary hypoplasia may develop. During the labor and birth, the lessened amounts of fluid reduce the cushioning effect for the umbilical cord, and cord compression is more likely to occur.

Clinical Therapy

During the antepartum period, oligohydramnios may be suspected when the uterus does not increase in size in accordance with established gestational dating, the fetus is easily palpated and outlined by the examiner, and the fetus is not ballottable. The fetus can be assessed by biophysical profiles, nonstress tests, and serial ultrasound. During labor the fetus will be monitored by continuous electronic fetal monitoring to detect cord compression, which will be indicated by nonperiodic decelerations. Amnioinfusion can replace some fluid volume and remove pressure on the umbilical cord (see Chapter 23).

NURSING CARE MANAGEMENT

Continuous electronic fetal monitoring is an important part of assessment during the labor and birth. The nurse evaluates the EFM tracing for the presence of nonperiodic decelerations or other nonreassuring signs (such as increasing or decreasing baseline, decreased variability, or presence of periodic decelerations). If nonperiodic decelerations are noted, the nurse can change the woman's position (to relieve pressure on the umbilical cord) and must then notify the physician/CNM. If position changes are insufficient to relieve the pattern, an amnioinfusion may be performed. After the birth, the newborn is evaluated for signs of congenital anomalies, pulmonary hypoplasia, or postmaturity.

Care of the Woman with Cephalopelvic Disproportion

The birth passage includes the maternal bony pelvis, beginning at the pelvic inlet and ending at the pelvic outlet, and the maternal soft tissues within these anatomic areas.

TABLE 22–5 Clues to Contractures of Maternal Pelvis

Diagonal conjugate <11.5 cm (contracture of inlet), outlet <8 cm (contracture of outlet)
Unengaged fetal head in early labor in primigravidas (consider contracture of inlet, malpresentation, or malposition)
Hypotonic uterine contraction pattern (consider contracted pelvis)
Deflexion of fetal head (fetal head not flexed on fetal chest; may be associated with occiput posterior)
Uncontrollable pushing prior to complete dilatation of cervix (may be associated with occiput posterior)
Failure of fetal descent (consider contracture of inlet, midpelvis, or outlet)
Edema of anterior portion (lip) of cervix (consider obstructed labor at the inlet)

A contracture in any of the described areas can result in cephalopelvic disproportion (CPD). Abnormal fetal presentations and positions occur in CPD as the fetus moves to accommodate passage through the maternal pelvis.

The gynecoid and anthropoid pelvic types are usually adequate for vertex birth, but the android and platypelloid types predispose to CPD. Certain combinations of types also can result in pelvic diameters inadequate for vertex birth. (See Chapter 11 for a description of the types of pelves and their implications for childbirth.) Clues that may lead to suspicion of contractures of the maternal pelvis are presented in Table 22–5.

Types of Contractures

Contractures of the Inlet

The pelvic inlet is contracted if the shortest anterior-posterior diameter is less than 10 cm or the greatest transverse diameter is less than 12 cm. The anterior-posterior diameter may be approximated by measuring the diagonal conjugate, which in the contracted inlet is less than 11.5 cm. Clinical and x-ray pelvimetry are used to determine the smallest anterior-posterior diameter through which the fetal head must pass.

The treatment goal is to allow the natural forces of labor to push the biparietal diameter of the fetal head beyond the potential interspinous obstruction. Although forceps may be used, they cause difficulty because pulling on the head destroys flexion and because they further diminish the available space. A bulging perineum and crowning indicate that the obstruction has been passed.

Contractures of the Outlet

An interischial tuberous diameter of less than 8 cm constitutes an outlet contracture. Outlet and midpelvic contractures frequently occur simultaneously. Whether vaginal birth can occur depends on the woman's interischial tuberous diameters and the fetal posterosagittal diameter.

Implications of Pelvic Contractures

Labor is prolonged and protracted in the presence of CPD, and premature rupture of the membranes (PROM) can result from the force of the unequally distributed contractions being exerted on the fetal membranes. In obstructed labor (the fetus is not able to pass through the birth canal) uterine rupture can also occur. With delayed descent, necrosis of maternal soft tissues can result from pressure exerted by the fetal head. Eventually, necrosis can cause fistulas from the vagina to other nearby structures. Difficult forceps-assisted births can also result in damage to maternal soft tissue.

If the membranes rupture and the fetal head has not entered the inlet, there is a danger of cord prolapse. Extreme molding of the fetal head can result. Traumatic forceps-assisted births can damage the fetal skull and central nervous system.

Clinical Therapy

Fetopelvic relationships can be assessed by comparing the estimated weight of the fetus as obtained by ultrasound measurements to pelvic measurements obtained by a manual examination prior to labor and by computed tomography (CT). Although it is only used occasionally, x-ray pelvimetry may be obtained. The x-ray pelvimetry provides measurements for the maternal pelvic inlet, midpelvis, outlet, degree of fetal descent, and selected diameters of the fetal head. Occasionally, in high-risk centers magnetic resonance imaging (MRI) is used to identify adequacy of pelvic diameters.

When the pelvic diameters are borderline or questionable, a trial of labor (TOL) may be advised. In this process the woman continues to labor, and careful assessments of uterine contractions, cervical dilatation, and fetal descent are made by the physician and nurse. As long as there is continued progress, the TOL continues. If progress ceases, the decision for a cesarean birth is made.

NURSING CARE MANAGEMENT

Nursing Assessment and Diagnosis

The adequacy of the maternal pelvis for a vaginal birth should be assessed intrapartally as well as antepartally. During the intrapartal assessment, the size of the fetus and its presentation, position, and lie must also be considered. (See Chapter 19 for intrapartal assessment techniques.)

The nurse should suspect CPD when labor is prolonged, cervical dilatation and effacement are slow, and engagement of the presenting part is delayed.

Nursing diagnoses that may apply include the following:

- ***Knowledge Deficit*** related to lack of information about implications and associated complications of CPD
- ***Fear*** related to unknown outcome of labor

Nursing Plan and Implementation

Hospital-Based Nursing Care

Nursing actions during the TOL are similar to care during any labor, with the exception that the assessments of cervical dilatation and fetal descent are done more frequently. Contractions should be monitored and the labor progress charted. The fetus should also be monitored frequently. Any signs of fetal distress are reported to the physician/CNM immediately.

The woman may be positioned in a variety of ways to increase the pelvic diameters. Sitting or squatting increases the outer diameters and may be effective in instances where there is failure of or slow fetal descent. Changing from one side to the other or maintaining a hands-and-knees position may assist the fetus in occiput-posterior position to change to an occiput-anterior position. The woman may instinctively want to assume one of these positions. If not, the nurse may encourage a change of position.

A couple may need help in coping with the stresses of complicated labor. The nurse should keep the couple informed of what is happening and explain the procedures that are being used. This should reassure the couple that measures are being taken to resolve the problem.

Evaluation

Expected outcomes of nursing care include the following:

- The woman's fear is lessened.
- The woman has additional knowledge regarding the problems, implications, and treatment plans. ●

Care of the Woman at Risk Due to Complications of Third and Fourth Stages of Labor

Lacerations

Lacerations of the cervix or vagina may be indicated when bright red vaginal bleeding persists in the presence of a well-contracted uterus. The incidence of lacerations is higher among childbearing women who are young, are nulliparous, have an epidural block, undergo forceps-assisted birth, or undergo an episiotomy. Vaginal and perineal lacerations are often categorized in terms of degree:

- First-degree laceration is limited to the fourchet, perineal skin, and vaginal mucous membrane.
- Second-degree laceration involves the perineal skin, vaginal mucous membrane, underlying fascia, and muscles of the perineal body; it may extend upward on one or both sides of the vagina.
- Third-degree laceration extends through the perineal skin, vaginal mucous membranes, and perineal

body and involves the anal sphincter; it may extend up the anterior wall of the rectum.

- Fourth-degree laceration is the same as the third degree but extends through the rectal mucosa to the lumen of the rectum; it may be called a third-degree laceration with a rectal wall extension.

Placenta Accreta

In placenta accreta, the chorionic villi attach directly to the myometrium of the uterus. Two other types of placental adherence are placenta increta, in which the myometrium is invaded, and placenta percreta, in which the myometrium is penetrated. The adherence itself may be total, partial, or focal, depending on the amount of placental involvement. The incidence of placenta accreta is 1 in 2500 births (Cunningham et al, 1997). Placenta accreta is the most common type of adherent placenta.

The primary complication of placenta accreta is maternal hemorrhage and failure of the placenta to separate following birth of the infant. An abdominal hysterectomy may be the necessary treatment, depending on the amount and depth of involvement. Chapter 33 discusses hemorrhage following birth.

FOCUS YOUR STUDY

- Anxiety during labor may be associated with a variety of factors such as worry about the fetal condition or the presence of a maternal complication. Women with a history of sexual abuse may be very anxious during labor because of their association of past experiences with activities of labor such as vaginal examinations, procedures that are done without explanation, being uncovered with other people in the room, or being watched by unknown people such as students, nurses from the nursery who appear just before birth to care for the newborn, and so on.
- Hypotonic labor patterns begin normally and then progress to infrequent, less intense contractions. If there are no contraindications, oxytocin is administered intravenously as treatment.
- Precipitate labor is extremely rapid labor that lasts less than 3 hours. It is associated with an increased risk to the mother and newborn infant.
- Postterm pregnancy is one that extends more than 294 days, or 42 weeks, past the first day of the last menstrual period.
- The occiput posterior position of the fetus during labor prolongs the labor process, causes severe back discomfort in the laboring woman, and predisposes her to vaginal and perineal trauma and lacerations during birth.
- The types of fetal malpresentations include face, brow, breech, and shoulder.
- A fetus or newborn weighing more than 4000 g (8 lb, 13 oz) is termed macrosomic. Macrosomia may lead to problems during labor, birth, and in the early neonatal period.
- If the presence of twins has been detected, preventing and treating problems that infringe on the development and birth of normal fetuses are significant medical-nursing activities.
- Fetal distress is indicated by persistent late decelerations, persistent severe variable decelerations, and prolonged decelerations. If fetal distress is recognized and treated appropriately, the fetus may be spared any permanent damage.
- Intrauterine fetal death poses a major nursing challenge to provide support and caring for the parents.
- Major bleeding problems in the intrapartal period are abruptio placentae and placenta previa.
- Abruptio placentae is the separation of the placenta from the side of the uterus prior to birth of the infant. Abruptio placentae may be central, marginal, or complete.
- Placenta previa occurs when the placenta implants low in the uterus near or over the cervix. A low-lying or marginal placenta is one that lies near the cervix. In partial placenta previa, part of the placenta lies over the cervix. In complete placenta previa, the cervix is completely covered.
- Prolapsed umbilical cord results when the umbilical cord precedes the fetal presenting part. When this occurs, pressure is placed on the umbilical cord, and blood flow to the fetus is diminished.
- Amniotic fluid embolism occurs when a bolus of amniotic fluid enters the maternal circulation and then enters the maternal lungs. Maternal mortality is very high with this complication.
- Hydramnios (also called polyhydramnios) is the presence of over 2000 mL of amniotic fluid contained within the amniotic membranes. Hydramnios is associated with fetal malformations that affect fetal swallowing and with maternal diabetes mellitus, Rh sensitization, and multiple gestations.
- Oligohydramnios is a severely reduced volume of amniotic fluid. Oligohydramnios is associated with IUGR, postterm pregnancy, and fetal renal or urinary malfunctions. The fetus is more likely to experience variable decelerations because the amniotic fluid is insufficient to keep pressure off the umbilical cord.
- Cephalopelvic disproportion (CPD) occurs when there is a narrowed diameter in the maternal pelvis. The narrowed diameter is called a contracture, and it may occur in the pelvic inlet, midpelvis, or outlet. If pelvic measurements are borderline, a trial of labor (TOL) may be attempted. Failure of cervical dilatation or fetal descent would then necessitate a cesarean birth.
- Third- and fourth-stage complications usually involve a hemorrhage. Causes of hemorrhage include lacerations of the birth canal or cervix and placenta accreta.

REFERENCES

American Association of Pediatrics (AAP) & American Association of Obstetricians and Gynecologists (ACOG). (1997). *Guidelines for perinatal care* (4th ed.). Washington, DC: Author.

American College of Obstetricians and Gynecologists (ACOG). (1995). (Technical Bulletin No. 218) Washington, DC: Author.

American College of Obstetricians and Gynecologists (ACOG). (1997). (Practice Patterns, No. 7). Washington, DC: Author.

Andrews, C. M., & Andrews, E. C. (1983). Nursing, maternal postures, and fetal positions. *Nursing Research*, *32*, 6.

Blackburn, C., & Copley, R. (1989). Precious moment: What you can offer when a newborn infant dies. *Nursing*, *19*, 52.

Bowes, W. A. (1994). Clinical aspects of normal and abnormal labor. In R. K. Creasy & R. Resnik (Eds.), *Maternal-fetal medicine: Principles and practice* (3rd ed.). Philadelphia: Saunders.

Bowes, W. A. (1997). Dystocia. In R. K. Creasy (Ed.), *Management of labor and delivery* (pp 328–357). Malden, MA: Blackwell.

Boyle, J. G., & O'Shaughnessy, R. (1996). Twins, triplets, and beyond. In J. T. Queenan & J. C. Hobbins (Eds.), *Protocols for high-risk pregnancies* (3rd ed.) (pp 624–632). Cambridge, MA: Blackwell.

Brown, Y. (1992, June). The crisis of pregnancy loss: A team approach to support. *Birth*, 82.

Campbell, M. K., Ostbye, T., & Irgens, L. M. (1997). Post-term birth: Risk factors and outcomes in a 10-year cohort of Norwegian births. *Obstetrics and Gynecology, 89*, 543–548.

Chasen, S. T., & Chervenak, F. A. (1998). What is the relationship between the universal use of ultrasound, the rate of detection of twins, and outcome differences? *Clinical Obstetrics and Gynecology, 41*, 67–77.

Clark, S. L. (1994). Care of the critically ill obstetric patient. In J. R. Scott, P. J. DiSaia, C. B. Hammond, & W. N. Spellacy, *Danforth's obstetrics and gynecology* (7th ed.). Philadelphia: Lippincott.

Cordell, A. S., & Thomas, N. (1989). Fathers and grieving: Coping with infant death. *Journal of Perinatology, 10*, 75.

Coustan, D. R. (1997). Gestational diabetes. In J. T. Queenan & J. T. Hobbins (Eds.), *Protocols for high-risk pregnancies* (pp 249–252). Cambridge, MA: Blackwell.

Cruikshank, D. P. (1994). Malpresentations and umbilical cord complications. In J. R. Scott, P. J. DiSaia, C. B. Hammond, & W. N. Spellacy, *Danforth's obstetrics and gynecology* (7th ed.). Philadelphia: Lippincott.

Cunningham, F. G., MacDonald, P. C., Gant, N. F., Leveno, K. J., Gilstrap, L. C., Hankins, G. D. V., & Clark, S. L. (1997). *Williams obstetrics* (20th ed.). Stamford, CT: Appleton & Lange.

Dizon-Townson, D., & Ward, K. (1997). The genetics of labor. *Clinical Obstetrics and Gynecology, 40*, 479–484.

Evans, M. I., & Johnson, M. P. (1996). Fetal reduction. In J. T. Queenan & J. C. Hobbins (Eds.), *Protocols for high-risk pregnancies* (3rd ed.) (pp 133–137). Cambridge, MA: Blackwell.

Furrh, C. B., & Copley, R. (1989). One precious moment. *Nursing 9*, 52.

Gardosi, J., Banner, R., & Francis, A. (1997). Gestational age and induction of labour for prolonged pregnancy. *British Journal of Obstetrics and Gynaecology, 104*, 792–797.

Gabbe, S. G. (1996). Diabetes mellitus. In J. T. Queenan & J. C. Hobbins (Eds.), *Protocols for high-risk pregnancies* (3rd ed.) (pp 253–263). Cambridge, MA: Blackwell.

Gabbe, S., Niebyl, J., & Simpson, J. (1996). *Obstetrics: Normal and problem pregnancies* (3rd ed.). New York: Churchill Livingstone.

Gillogley, K. (1991). Abnormal labor and delivery. In K. R. Niswander (Ed.), *Manual of obstetrics*. Boston: Little, Brown.

Griese, M. E., & Prickett, S. A. (1993). Nursing management of umbilical cord prolapse. *Journal of Obstetric, Gynecologic, and Neonatal Nursing, 22*, 311.

Grobman, W. A., & Peaceman, A. M. (1998). What are the rates and mechanisms of first and second trimester pregnancy loss in twins? *Clinical Obstetrics and Gynecology, 41*, 37–45.

Hilder, L., Costeloe, K., & Thilaganathan, B. (1997). Prolonged pregnancy: Evaluating gestation-specific risks of fetal and infant mortality. *British Journal of Obstetrics and Gynaecology, 105*, 169–173.

Hodnett, E. D., Hannah, M. E., Weston, J. A., Ohlsson, A., Myhr, T. L., Wang, E. E. I., Hewson, S. A., Willan, A. R., & Farine, D. (1997). Women's evaluations of induction of labor versus expectant management for prelabor rupture of the membranes at term. *Birth, 24*, 214–220.

Iam, J. D., Goldenberg, R. L., Meis, P. J., et al (1996). The length of the cervix and the risk of spontaneous premature delivery. *New England Journal of Medicine, 334*, 567.

Keith, L., & Papiernik, E. (1998). Multiple gestation. *Clinical Obstetrics and Gynecology, 41*, 1.

Keith, L., Papiernik, E., & Oleszczuk, J. J. (1998). How should the efficacy of prenatal care be tested in twin gestations? *Clinical Obstetrics and Gynecology, 41*, 85–93.

Kiely, J. L. (1998). What is the population-based risk of preterm birth among twins and other multiples? *Clinical Obstetrics and Gynecology, 41*, 3–11.

King, J. C. (1994). Transverse and oblique lie. In P. V. Dilts & J. J. Sciarri (Eds.). *Gynecology and obstetrics*, Vol 2. Philadelphia: Lippincott.

Kochenour, N. K. (1992). Postterm pregnancy. In A. A. Fanaroff & R. J. Martin (Eds.). *High risk pregnancy: A team approach*. (2nd ed.). St. Louis: Mosby.

Kübler-Ross, E. (1969). *On death and dying*. New York: Macmillan.

Lopez-Zeno, J. A. (1997). Active management of labor: The American experience. *Clinical Obstetrics and Gynecology, 40*, 510–515.

Manning, F. A. (1999). General principles and applications of ultrasonography. In R. K. Creasy & R. Resnik (Eds), *Maternal-fetal medicine* (4th ed.) (pp 169–206). Philadelphia: Saunders .

Papiernik, E., Keith, L., Oleszczuk, & Cervantes, A. (1998). What interventions are useful in reducing the rate of preterm delivery in twins? *Clinical Obstetrics and Gynecology, 41*, 13–23.

Quilligan, E. J. (1996). Postdate pregnancies. In J. T. Queenan & J. C. Hobbins (Eds.), *Protocols for high-risk pregnancies* (3rd ed.) (pp 633–635). Cambridge, MA: Blackwell.

Resnik, R. (1997). Amniotic fluid embolus. In J. T. Queenan & J. C. Hobbins (Eds.), *Protocols for high-risk pregnancies* (3rd ed.) (pp 574–576). Cambridge, MA: Blackwell.

Resnik, R. (1994). Post-term pregnancy. In R. K. Creasy & R. Resnik (Eds.), *Maternal-fetal medicine: Principles and practice* (3rd ed.). Philadelphia: Saunders.

Roberts, S. J., Reardon, K. M., & Rosenfeld, S. (1999). Childhood sexual abuse: Surveying its impact on primary care. *AWHONN Lifelines, 3*, 39–45.

Roberts, W. E., & Morrison, J. C. (1998). How has the use of home monitors, fetal fibronectin, and measurement of cervical length helped predict labor and/or prevent preterm delivery in twins? *Clinical Obstetrics and Gynecology, 41*, 95–102.

Schwiebert, P., & Kirk, P. (1985). *When hello means goodbye*. Eugene, OR: Oregon Health Sciences University.

Senat, M. V., Ancel, P. Y., Bouvier-Colle, M. H., & Breart, G. (1998). How does multiple pregnancy affect maternal mortality and morbidity? *Clinical Obstetrics and Gynecology, 41*, 79–83.

Simpson, L., & D'Alton, M. E. (1996). Multiple pregnancy. In R. K. Creasy (Ed.), *Management of labor and delivery* (pp 395–413). Cambridge, MA: Blackwell.

Thorp, J. A. (1997). Malpresentations and special situations. In R. K. Creasy (Ed), *Management of labor and delivery*. Cambridge, MA: Blackwell.

Waymire, V. (1997). A triggering time: Childbirth may recall sexual abuse memories. *AWHONN Lifelines*, 47–50.

Zlatnik, F. J. (1997). Obesity. In J. T. Queenan & J. C. Hobbins (Eds), *Protocols for high-risk pregnancy* (3rd ed.) (pp 245–248). Cambridge, MA: Blackwell.

Birth-Related Procedures

23

WITH OUR FIRST BABY ALL OF A SUDDEN I HAD TO have a cesarean. Everything happened so fast, but our son was OK, and that's all that mattered. With our second baby I wanted to try a vaginal birth. Even though I wanted to, I was afraid. I don't know what I would have done without my nurse. She stayed with me the whole time and kept giving me support. She explained what was happening and gave me encouragement. I felt safe. I had a beautiful baby girl after 8 hours of labor. Everything went fine, and I am so glad that I was able to avoid another cesarean. We don't plan to have another baby, but if we did, I wouldn't be so afraid.

Key Terms

Amnioinfusion
Amniotomy
Cervical ripening
Episiotomy
External cephalic version
Forceps-assisted birth
Internal version
Labor induction
Vacuum extraction
Vaginal birth after cesarean (VBAC)

Objectives

- Incorporate an understanding of the impact of selected procedures on the childbearing woman and her family or support system.
- Examine the methods of external cephalic version and internal version and the related nursing management.
- Discuss the use of amniotomy in current maternal-newborn care.
- Compare methods for inducing labor, explaining their advantages and disadvantages.
- Discuss the use of transcervical intrapartum amnioinfusion.
- Describe the types of episiotomies performed, the rationale for each, and the associated nursing interventions.
- Summarize the indications for forceps-assisted birth, types of forceps that may be used, complications, and related interventions.
- Discuss the use of vacuum extraction, including indications, procedure, complications, and related nursing management.
- Explain the indications for cesarean birth, impact on the family unit, preparation and teaching needs, and associated nursing management.
- Discuss vaginal birth following cesarean birth.

MOST BIRTHS OCCUR WITHOUT THE need for operative obstetric intervention. In some instances, however, obstetric procedures are necessary to maintain safety for the woman and the fetus. The most common obstetric procedures are amniotomy, induction of labor, episiotomy, cesarean birth, and vaginal birth following a previous cesarean birth.

Generally, women are aware of the possible need for an obstetric procedure during their labor and birth, and many women accept whatever procedure is recommended based on the belief that the caregiver knows what is needed and that it is in the baby's best interest. However, some women expect to have a "natural" labor and birth and do not anticipate the need for any medical intervention. This conflict between expectation and the need for intervention presents a challenge to maternity nurses. The nurse can provide information regarding any procedure to enhance the woman and her partner's understanding of what is proposed, the anticipated benefits and possible risks, and any possible alternative treatments.

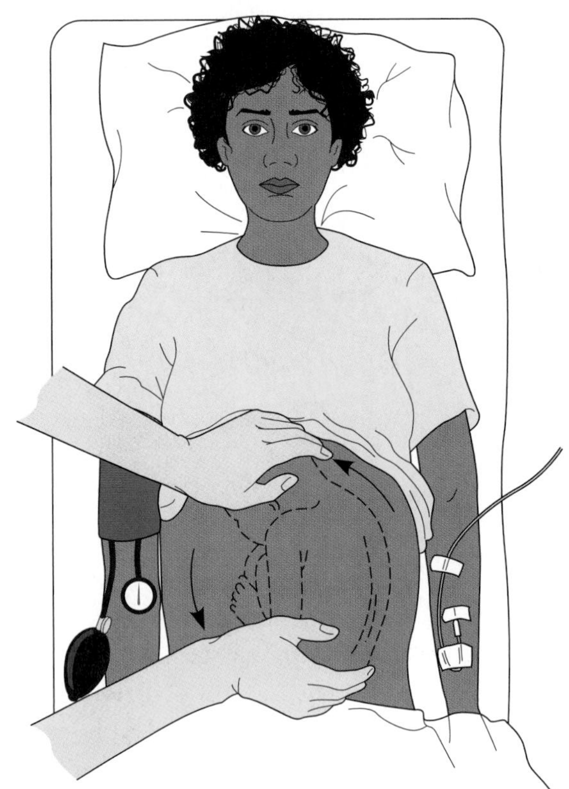

FIGURE 23–1 External (or cephalic) version of the fetus. A new technique involves applying pressure to the fetal head and buttocks so that the fetus completes a "backward flip" or "forward roll."

Care of the Woman during Version

Version, or turning the fetus, is a procedure used to change the fetal presentation by abdominal or intrauterine manipulation. The most common type of version is external (or cephalic) version. In an **external cephalic version** (ECV) the presentation of the fetus is changed from a breech to a cephalic presentation by external manipulation of the maternal abdomen (Figure 23–1). The other type of version, called **internal version,** or *podalic version*, is used only with the second twin during a vaginal birth. In an internal version the obstetrician places a hand inside the uterus, grabs the fetus's feet, and then turns the fetus from a transverse or cephalic presentation to a breech presentation (Figure 23–2).

External Version

If breech or shoulder presentation (transverse lie) is detected in the later weeks of pregnancy, an external version may be attempted. The version is usually done after 37 weeks' gestation because most fetuses still in breech presentation at this time will not spontaneously change back to a vertex presentation. Successful external version rates have ranged from 41% to 77% over the past few years (Lau, Lo, & Rogers, 1997) and average 63% in Western countries (Thorp, 1997). The success rate for external cephalic versions varies, depending upon factors such as the experience of the clinical practitioner, components of the procedure (eg, whether a tocolytic agent such as ritodrine is used), and factors associated with the woman, fetus, and pregnancy. As a result of a prospective study, Lau, Lo, and Rogers (1997) reported there were eight factors that could serve as predictors of a successful external version: parity, maternal obesity, placental site, type of breech, position of fetal spine, amniotic fluid volume, engagement, station, and estimated fetal weight. In addition, Lau, Lo, Wan, and Rogers (1997) found three independent variables that significantly affected the success rate. First was the ease with which the fetal head could be found prior to the ECV. This factor had not been identified before; however, the researchers felt that it was logical as pressure exerted on both fetal poles (head and buttocks) during the version would be more equal. Second, the presence of an engaged presenting part was the most significant indicator of failure of ECV. The third and last variable was a tense uterus on palpation that persisted after a tocolytic agent had been administered. This was also significantly associated with failure of ECV. The researchers suggest that if predictive criteria could be discovered, planning and resources for breech presentations could be used more effectively.

The following criteria should be met prior to performing external version (Lau, Lo, & Rogers, 1997):

- A single fetus (also called a singleton) must be present. If a multiple gestation exists, a variety of concerns preclude an external version. For example, a cesarean rather than vaginal birth may need to be considered, and the fetuses might become entangled during a version.

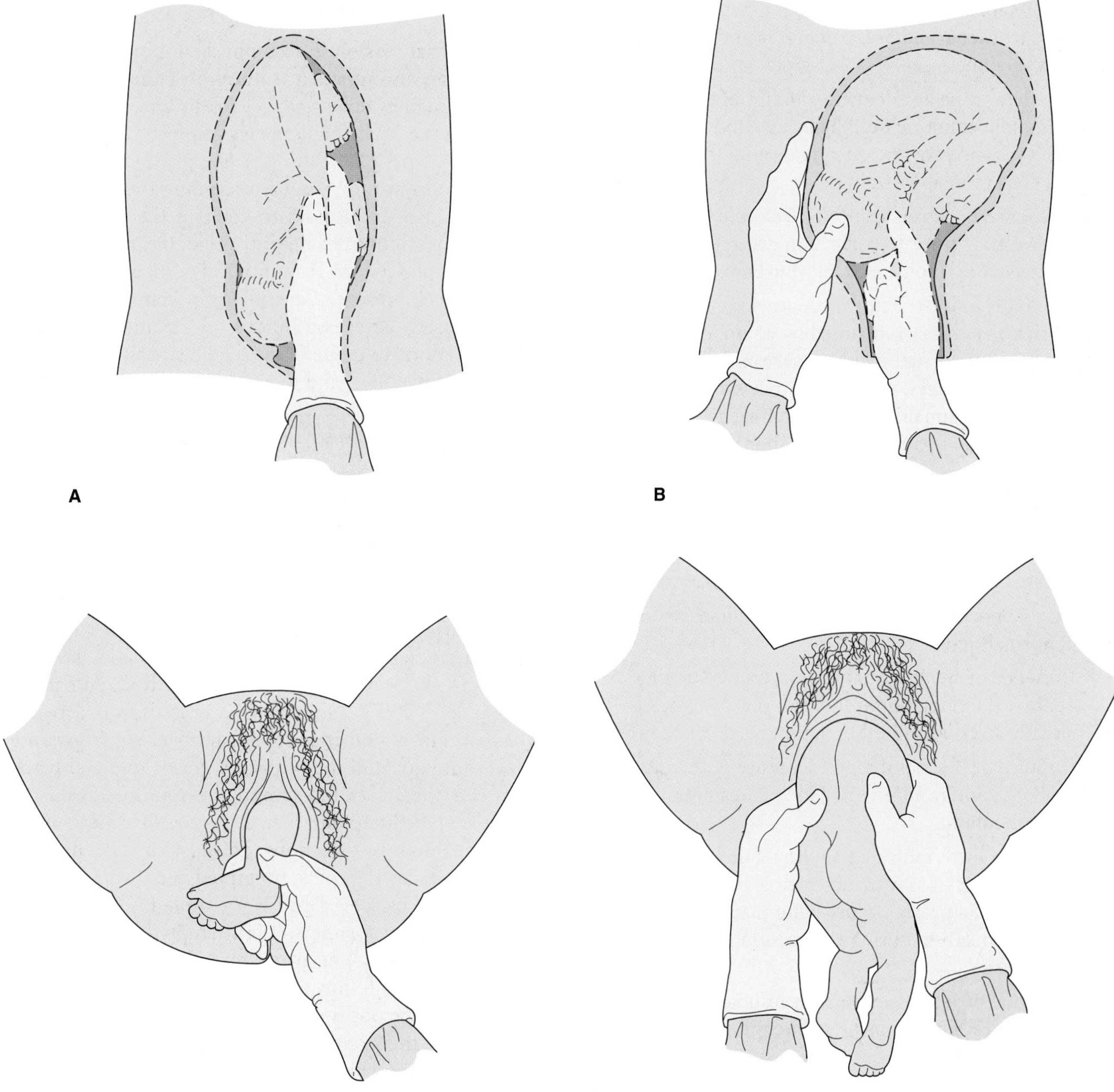

FIGURE 23–2 Use of podalic version and extraction of the fetus to assist in the vaginal birth of the second twin. ***A,*** The physician reaches into the uterus and grasps a foot. Although a vertex birth is always preferred in a singleton birth, in this instance of assisting in the birth of a second twin it is not possible to grasp any other fetal part. The fetal head would be too large to grasp and pull downward, and grasping the fetal arm would result in a transverse lie and make vaginal birth impossible. ***B,*** While applying pressure on the outside of the abdomen to push the baby's head up toward the top of the uterus with one hand, the physician pulls the baby's foot down toward the cervix. ***C,*** Both feet have been pulled through the cervix and vagina. ***D,*** The physician now grasps the baby's trunk and continues to pull downward on the baby to assist the birth.

- The fetal breech is not engaged. Once the presenting part is engaged, it is difficult if not impossible to do a version.
- There must be an adequate amount of amniotic fluid. The amniotic fluid helps ease movement of the fetus and provides adequate room for the umbilical cord to float without being compressed.
- A reactive nonstress test (NST) should be obtained immediately prior to performing the version. A reactive NST indicates fetal well-being.
- The fetus must be 38 or more weeks' gestation. A version may be accompanied by complications that require immediate birth by cesarean. If gestation is less than 38 weeks, a preterm birth would result. (Note: Occasionally, a physician may do an external version while the woman is in labor.)

Absolute contraindications include the following (Lau, Lo, & Rogers, 1997):

- Intrauterine growth restriction. The fetus has been stressed and amniotic fluid may be decreased.
- Fetal abnormality. This category includes major abnormalities.
- Presence of an abnormal fetal heart rate tracing. An abnormal tracing might indicate that the fetus is already stressed and other action needs to be taken.
- Rupture of the membranes. Rupture of the membranes would result in an inadequate amount of amniotic fluid.
- Cesarean birth indicated anyway. For example, if a complete previa is present, birth will be by cesarean. If a marginal previa or low-lying placenta is present, the manipulation during the version may precipitate bleeding.
- Maternal problems such as gestational diabetes that has required insulin or pregnancy-induced hypertension (PIH).

Relative contraindications include the following:

- Oligohydramnios (amniotic fluid index < 5 cm). Decreased fluid makes the fetus difficult to maneuver and increases risk of umbilical cord compression.
- Hydramnios (amniotic fluid index > 25 cm). Increased amount of amniotic fluid stretches the uterine walls increasing pressure and decreasing the chance the fetus will remain in a cephalic presentation.
- Previous lower uterine segment cesarean birth. Prior scarring of the uterus may increase the risk of uterine tearing.
- Nuchal cord. A nuchal cord may tighten around the fetal neck and decrease circulation to the fetus.

External Version Procedure

The external version is accomplished in a birthing unit, rather than an outpatient setting, in case further intervention (such as emergency cesarean birth) is necessary. Although the "risk of emergency intervention is probably less than 1% to 2%" (Thorp, 1997, p 371), the woman is instructed to fast for 8 hours preceding the version. The physician uses ultrasound to confirm the presence of a single fetus, amount of amniotic fluid, location of the placenta, the position of the umbilical cord, and to confirm that a breech presentation still exists. Maternal vital signs are assessed, and continuous electronic monitoring (EFM) is done to evaluate the fetal heart rate (FHR), obtain a reactive NST, and to evaluate the presence of uterine contractions or uterine wall tenseness. An intravenous line is established to be ready to administer medications in case of difficulty. A β-mimetic agent (intravenous infusion of ritodrine or a subcutaneous dose of terbutaline) or intravenous infusion of magnesium sulfate (if a β-mimetic agent is contraindicated because of a medical condition) is administered to achieve uterine relaxation. Occasionally, some physicians do not use a β-mimetic agent during the version, although the use of a tocolytic agent increases chances of a successful version and much enhances the comfort of the woman (Healey, Porter, & Galimberti, 1997). Once uterine relaxation is achieved, the maternal abdomen is copiously covered with warmed ultrasound gel, and the physician grasps the fetal breech between the index finger and the thumb. If the fetal breech can be lifted out, then the breech and head are rotated in opposite directions. In most cases, a direction similar to a forward roll is attempted initially. If that is not successful, a backward roll is attempted. Occasionally a lateral direction for the roll is attempted if the other efforts have failed. The procedure should be concluded when any of the following occur: the fetal head is moved to a head-down position, no more than two attempts have been made, the woman had indicated that the procedure has become too painful or stressful, or signs of maternal or fetal problems occur (Thorp, 1997). The intravenous tocolytic agent is discontinued, and frequently the fetus is held in the new presentation until the uterus regains tone. The version is discontinued immediately in the presence of severe maternal discomfort or significant FHR bradycardia or decelerations (Lau, Lo, & Rogers, 1997). If the woman is Rh negative, an adequate amount of anti-D immunoglobulin must always be administered after the version (Thorp, 1997). A vaginal examination is done to evaluate cervical dilatation and fetal descent.

NURSING CARE MANAGEMENT

The nurse begins by ensuring that the expectant woman understands the procedure, knows that the procedure may be uncomfortable or very painful, and realizes that she can tell the physician to stop the procedure if the pain is too great. The possibility of failure of the ECV and the slight risk of a cesarean birth if the fetus becomes stressed or exhibits distress should also be discussed. Explaining what will occur in either of these circumstances will better prepare the woman and partner if intervention becomes necessary. The nurse also answers any further questions. Prior to the version, the nurse completes initial maternal and fetal assessments, provides ongoing evaluation of FHR, and performs the NST. The nurse continues to monitor maternal blood pressure and pulse about every 2 minutes throughout the period of time the β-mimetic agent is used and for about 30 minutes after. The FHR is monitored for approximately 1 to 2 hours following the ECV. Assessment of the maternal-fetal response to the tocolytic agent is also performed. The nurse continues to provide information by reiterating aftercare instructions, such as monitoring for uterine contractions and being aware of fetal movement (fetal kick counts).

ESSENTIAL PRECAUTIONS IN PRACTICE

During Procedures

Wear disposable gloves when performing the following actions:

- Handling amniotic fluid–soaked Chux pads and bedding at the time of an amniotomy and the cleansing of the perineum afterward
- Inserting the intravenous catheter to induce labor with oxytocin
- During the abdominal-perineal preparation of the woman for cesarean birth (Note: Sterile gloves also are worn during insertion of an indwelling bladder catheter. This provides asepsis for the woman and also protects the nurse from exposure to the perineal area and to urine.)

REMEMBER to wash your hands prior to putting the disposable gloves on and AGAIN immediately after you remove the gloves.

For further information, consult OSHA and CDC guidelines.

Care of the Woman during an Amniotomy

Amniotomy is the artificial rupture of the amniotic membranes (AROM). It is probably the most common operative procedure in obstetrics. Because the amniotomy requires that an instrument be inserted through the cervix, at least 2 cm of cervical dilatation must be present. The amniotomy may be performed as a method of induction of labor (to stimulate the beginning of labor), or it may be done at any time during the first stage of labor with the goal of accelerating the labor. If an amniotomy is done after 3 cm of cervical dilatation, the labor will probably be shortened by 1 to 2 hours (Ferguson, 1997). Amniotomy may also be performed during labor to allow access to the fetus in order to apply an internal fetal heart monitoring electrode to the scalp, to insert an intrauterine pressure catheter, or to obtain a fetal scalp blood sample for acid-base determination.

Amniotomy as a method of labor induction has the following advantages:

1. The contractions elicited are similar to those of spontaneous labor.
2. There is usually no risk of hypertonus or rupture of the uterus, as with intravenous oxytocin induction.
3. The woman does not require the same intensive monitoring as with intravenous oxytocin induction.
4. EFM is facilitated because once the membranes are ruptured, a fetal scalp electrode may be applied, an intrauterine catheter may be inserted, and scalp blood sampling for pH determinations may be done to assist in evaluating a fetal heart rate pattern.
5. The color and composition of amniotic fluid can be evaluated.

The disadvantages of amniotomy are as follows:

1. Once an amniotomy is done, birth must occur because microorganisms can now invade the intrauterine cavity and cause amnionitis.
2. The danger of a prolapsed cord is increased once the membranes have ruptured, especially if the fetal presenting part is not firmly pressed down against the cervix.
3. Compression and molding of the fetal head are increased due to loss of the cushioning effect of the amniotic fluid for the fetal head during uterine contractions.

AROM Procedure

Before an amniotomy is performed, the fetus is assessed for presentation, position, and station. Unless the fetal head is well engaged in the pelvis, some obstetricians do not advocate an amniotomy because of the danger of prolapsed cord. Other risks are abruptio placentae (due to rapid decompression of the uterus with the rapid loss of amniotic fluid), infection (due to the introduction of organisms into the cervix and intrauterine cavity), and amniotic fluid embolus (due to rapid decompression of the uterus and small amounts of fluid entering the maternal vascular system from under the edge of the placenta). These complications may also be associated with spontaneous rupture of membranes.

While performing a sterile vaginal examination, the physician/CNM introduces an amnihook (or other rupturing device) into the vagina, through the cervix, and against the amniotic membrane which is in front of the fetal presenting part. A small tear is made in the amniotic membrane. Following rupture of the membranes, amniotic fluid is allowed to escape slowly.

NURSING CARE MANAGEMENT

The nurse explains the AROM procedure to the woman. The fetal presentation, position, and station are assessed because amniotomy is usually delayed until engagement has occurred (to decrease the risk of a prolapsed cord when the fluid is expelled). The woman is positioned in a semireclining position and draped to provide privacy. The FHR is assessed just prior to and immediately after the amniotomy, and the two FHR assessments are compared. If there are marked changes, the nurse should check for prolapse of the cord. The amniotic fluid is inspected for amount, color, odor, and the presence of meconium or blood. While wearing disposable gloves, the nurse cleanses and dries the perineal area and changes the disposable underpads. (See Essential Precautions in Practice: During Procedures.) Because there is now an open pathway for organisms to ascend into the uterus, strict sterile technique must be observed during vaginal examinations. In addition, the number of vaginal examinations must be kept to a minimum in order to reduce the chance of introducing an infection, and the woman's temperature should be monitored every 2 hours. Bed rest is maintained unless the presenting part is engaged and is firmly against the cervix (to decrease the risk of prolapsed cord). The nurse needs to provide information regarding the amniotomy and the expected effects. Some couples may worry that all the amniotic fluid will be gone and that they will experience a "dry birth." It is important for them to know that amniotic fluid is constantly produced.

Care of the Woman during Prostaglandin Administration at Term

Prostaglandin (PGE_2) gel for **cervical ripening** (softening and effacing the cervix) may be used for the pregnant woman at or near term when there is a medical or obstetric indication for induction of labor. Two types of gel are Prepidil and Cervidil. Prepidil gel contains 0.5 mg dinoprostone (a form of prostaglandin E_2 for intracervical application). Cervidil is packaged in a pessary form and provides a slow release of 10 mg dinoprostone at a rate of 0.3 mg/hr over 12 hours (Chyu & Strassner, 1997). These preparations have been demonstrated to cause cervical ripening, shorter labor, and lower requirements for oxytocin during labor induction, and vaginal birth is achieved within 24 hours for most women (Chyu & Strassner, 1997; Stemple, Prins, & Dean, 1997). Most research had not found an improvement in the failed induction rate or a decrease in the overall cesarean birth rate when the gel is used (American College of Obstetricians and Gynecologists [ACOG], 1993).

Contraindications to the use of PGE gel include evidence of cephalopelvic disproportion (CPD), placenta previa, vasa previa, unexplained vaginal bleeding, and obstetric emergencies that may require surgical intervention (ACOG, 1993). Prostaglandin should be used with caution in women with compromised cardiovascular, hepatic, or renal function and in women with asthma or glaucoma (Chyu & Strassner, 1997).

Possible maternal side effects of prostaglandin administration for cervical ripening prior to induction of labor include hyperstimulation of uterine contractions (more than five contractions in 10 minutes or two or more contractions lasting more than 2 minutes [Arias, 1993]), nausea, and vomiting (Chyu & Strassner, 1997).

Prostaglandin Gel Insertion Procedure

At this time it is recommended that prostaglandin gel be used only in a hospital birthing unit and that an obstetrician be readily available in case an emergency cesarean birth is needed. The use of PGE in outpatient settings and birth centers is currently under study. When Prepidil is used, it is introduced by means of a prefilled syringe with a catheter attached to the hub. The catheter is inserted through the vagina and into the endocervix, where the gel is injected. The catheter has a small shield at the top so that the gel cannot be deposited above the internal os. Dinoprostone is also available as a gel that may be placed in a diaphragm and applied to the cervix and as a suppository that is placed in the posterior fornix.

NURSING CARE MANAGEMENT

Physicians, certified nurse-midwives (CNMs), and birthing room nurses who have had special education and training may administer PGE products. Maternal vital signs are assessed for a baseline, and an electronic fetal monitor is applied for at least 30 minutes to obtain an external tracing of uterine activity, FHR pattern, and a reactive nonstress test (NST). If a nonreactive test is obtained, consultation with the physician/CNM is required. After insertion, the woman is instructed to remain supine with a rolled blanket or hip wedge under her right hip to tip the uterus slightly to the left for 1 hour to minimize leakage of the gel from the endocervix (Association of Women's Health, Obstetric, and Neonatal Nurses [AWHONN], 1993) . The nurse monitors the woman for uterine hyperstimulation and FHR abnormalities (changes in baseline rate, variability, and presence of decelerations) for 30 minutes to 2 hours (AWHONN, 1993). If tachysystole (hyperstimulation) of the uterus greater than five contractions in 10 minutes occurs, the woman is positioned on her left side and oxygen is administered if fetal stress is noted. The administration of a tocolytic agent (such as a subcutaneous injection of 0.25 mg terbutaline) should be considered if the uterine hy-

DRUG GUIDE

Dinoprostone (Cervidil) Vaginal Insert

Pregnancy Risk Category: C

Overview of Maternal-Fetal Action

Dinoprostone is a naturally occurring form of prostaglandin E_2. Dinoprostone can be used at term to ripen the cervix and can stimulate the smooth muscle of the uterus to enhance uterine contractions. A single vaginal insert may be used to ripen the cervix and then oxytocin can be administered 30 minutes later (Zatuchi & Slupik, 1996; Forrest Pharmaceuticals, Inc. Drug Insert, 1995).

Route, Dosage, Frequency

The vaginal insert contains 10 mg of dinoprostone. The insert is placed transversely in the posterior fornix of the vagina, and the client is kept supine for 2 hours but then may ambulate. The dinoprostone is released at approximately 0.3 mg/hour over a 12-hour period. The vaginal insert should be removed by pulling on the retrieval string upon onset of uterine contractions or after 12 hours (Forrest Pharmaceuticals, Inc. Drug Insert, 1995).

Contraindications

- Client with known sensitivity to prostaglandins
- Presence of fetal distress
- Unexplained bleeding during pregnancy
- Strong suspicion of cephalopelvic disproportion
- Client already receiving oxytocin
- Client with 6 or more previous term pregnancies
- Client who is not anticipated to be able to give birth vaginally

Dinoprostone vaginal insert should be used with CAUTION in clients with ruptured membranes, a fetus in breech presentation, presence of glaucoma, or history of asthma (Forrest Pharmaceuticals, Inc., 1995).

Maternal Side Effects

Uterine hyperstimulation with or without fetal distress has occurred in a very small number (2.8–4.7%) of clients. Fewer than 1% of clients have experienced fever, nausea, vomiting, diarrhea, or abdominal pain (Forest Pharmaceuticals, Inc., 1995).

Effects on Fetus/Neonate

Fetal distress (Zatuchi & Slupik, 1996).

Nursing Considerations

- Assess for presence of contraindications.
- Monitor maternal vital signs, cervical dilatation, and effacement carefully.
- Monitor fetal status for presence of reassuring fetal heart rate pattern (baseline 120–160 bpm, presence of short-term variability, average variability, presence of accelerations with fetal movement, absence of late or variable decelerations).
- Remove vaginal insert if uterine hyperstimulation, sustained uterine contractions, fetal distress, or any other maternal adverse actions occur.

perstimulation pattern continues (ACOG, 1993). The gel may be removed if severe nausea, vomiting, or tachysystole develops (Arias, 1993).

Care of the Woman during Misoprostol (Cytotec) Administration

Misoprostol (Cytotec) is a synthetic PGE_1 analogue that has the ability to ripen the cervix when there is a Bishop score of 5 or less (2 cm dilatation, 50% effacement, and −1 station) and to induce labor for medical indications. (See Table 23–1 on page 658.) Misoprostol is contraindicated under the following conditions (*Memorial Hospital Guidelines*, 1998):

- Uterine contractions three times in 10 minutes
- Significant asthma
- History of previous uterine scar or bleeding during the pregnancy
- Placenta previa
- Nonreassuring fetal heart rate tracing

NURSING CARE MANAGEMENT

The nurse provides the woman and her support persons information regarding the procedure and answers any questions. Maternal vital signs are obtained and a continuous EFM tracing is obtained for a minimum of 30 minutes. The EFM tracing should indicate a reassuring FHR pattern and reactive NST. If uterine contractions are not occurring regularly, a 25-μg misoprostol tablet is inserted into the posterior vaginal fornix. The woman is requested

TABLE 23–1 Prelabor Status Evaluation Scoring System

Factor	Assigned Value 0	1	2	3
Cervical dilatation	Closed	1–2 cm	3–4 cm	5 cm or more
Cervical effacement	0% to 30%	40% to 50%	60% to 70%	80% or more
Fetal station	−3	−2	−1, 0	+1, or lower
Cervical consistency	Firm	Moderate	Soft	
Cervical position	Posterior	Midposition	Anterior	

SOURCE: Bishop EH: Pelvic scoring for elective inductions. *Obstet Gynecol* 1964; 24:266.

to lie supine with a hip wedge under her right hip for at least 1 hour. The dose of misoprostol may be repeated every 3 hours unless the Bishop score is greater than 5, cervical dilatation increases more than 3 cm, or uterine contractions are three or more in 10 minutes (*Memorial Hospital Guidelines*, 1998). The nurse should note that there are additional methods of cervical ripening. A 14 gauge Foley catheter is inserted into the cervical canal (intracervical) and the balloon is inflated. The pressure of the balloon stimulates the release of prostaglandins. The physcian/CNM may instill extra-amniotic saline through the Foley catheter. Goldman and Wigton (1999) report the use of extra-amniotic saline infusion was more effective than intracervical Dinoprostone gel for cervical ripening and was as safe.

Care of the Woman during Induction of Labor

The American College of Obstetricians and Gynecologists defines **labor induction** as the stimulation of uterine contractions before the spontaneous onset of labor, with or without ruptured fetal membranes, for the purpose of accomplishing birth (ACOG, 1995). Induction may be indicated in the presence of the following:

- Diabetes mellitus
- Renal disease
- Pregnancy-induced hypertension (PIH)
- Premature rupture of membranes (PROM)
- Chorioamnionitis
- Fetal demise
- Postterm gestation
- Intrauterine growth restriction (IUGR)
- Isoimmunization
- History of rapid labor (precipitous labor and birth)
- Mild abruptio placentae, no fetal stress or distress

The most frequently used methods of induction selected by physicians are stripping (also called sweeping) the amniotic membranes, amniotomy, intravenous oxytocin (Pitocin) infusion, nipple self-stimulation, and administration of misoprostol. (See prior discussion of amniotomy in this chapter). Oxytocin infusion is discussed later in this section.

Contraindications

All contraindications to spontaneous labor and vaginal birth are contraindications to the induction of labor. Relative maternal contraindications include the following (ACOG, 1995):

- Client refusal
- Placenta previa or vasa previa
- Transverse fetal lie
- Prolapsed umbilical cord
- Prior classic uterine incision (vertical incision in the upper portion of the uterus)
- Active genital herpes infection

Before induction is attempted, appropriate assessment must indicate that both the woman and fetus are ready for the onset of labor. This includes evaluation of fetal maturity and cervical readiness.

Fetal Maturity

The gestational age of the fetus is best evaluated by accurate menstrual dating, visualization of the gestational sac between 5 and 6 weeks, quickening at 18 to 20 weeks. Serial ultrasounds are helpful in validating gestational age. When needed, amniotic fluid studies looking for lecithin/sphingomyelin (L/S) ratio and phoshatidylglycerol are also beneficial in assessing fetal maturity.

Cervical Readiness

The findings on vaginal examination will help determine whether cervical changes favorable for induction have occurred. Bishop (1964) developed a prelabor scoring system that is still helpful in predicting the inductibility of women (Table 23–1). Components evaluated are cervical dilatation, effacement, consistency, and position, as well as the station of the fetal presenting part. A score of 0, 1, 2, or 3 is given to each assessed characteristic. The higher the total score for all the criteria, the more likely that labor will occur. The lower the total score, the higher the failure rate. A favorable cervix is the most important criterion for a successful induction (Cunningham et al, 1997b). The presence of a cervix that is anterior, soft, 50% effaced, and dilated at least 2 cm, with the fetal head at +1 station or lower (Bishop score of 9) is favorable for successful induction (ACOG, 1995).

If the cervix is unfavorable, a method to enhance cervical ripening may be tried. In addition to the use of PGE_2 gel and misoprostol, another method is *stripping (or sweeping) the amniotic membranes.* This is usually done in the office of the physician or CNM during a prenatal visit at term (38 through 41 weeks' gestation). The CNM or physician inserts a gloved finger as far as possible into the internal cervical os and rotates the finger 360 degrees, twice. This motion separates the amniotic membranes that are lying against the lower uterine segment and internal os from the distal part of the lower uterine segment. The stripping or sweeping is thought to release PGF_{2a} from the amniotic membranes or PGE_2 from the cervix (Summers, 1997, p 78).

Methods of Inducing Labor

In traditional medical (allopathic) practice, labor is usually accomplished by ripening the cervix (if the Bishop score is unfavorable), performing an amniotomy (if the cervix is ripe and the presenting part is down against the cervix), and then administering an oxytocin infusion or misoprostol insertion.

Oxytocin Infusion

Intravenous administration of oxytocin is an effective method of initiating uterine contractions to induce labor. The goal is to achieve three uterine contractions with a duration of 40 to 60 seconds in 10 minutes with good uterine relaxation and return to the baseline tone between contractions.

Clinical Therapy Ten units of oxytocin (Pitocin) are added to 1 L of intravenous fluid (usually 5% dextrose in balanced saline solution—for example, 5% dextrose in lactated Ringer's solution). The resulting mixture will contain 10 mU of oxytocin per milliliter (1 mU/minute, or 6 mL/hour), and the prescribed dose can be calculated easily. Other dosage concentrations are presented in the Drug Guide: Oxytocin (Pitocin) on page 660.

A second bottle of intravenous fluid is prepared and used to start and maintain the infusion. This avoids infusing a large dose of oxytocin as the line is begun and provides additional fluids while the oxytocin solution is being kept at a low infusion rate. After the infusion is started, the oxytocin solution is piggybacked into the primary tubing port closest to the catheter insertion. This allows only a small amount of oxytocin to backflow into the tubing and ensures greater dosage accuracy. The oxytocin should be administered with a device that permits precise control of the flow rate. Over the past few years, differences in opinion regarding oxytocin dosage have surfaced. ACOG (1995) recommends two protocols for oxytocin infusion. The first utilizes an initial dose of 1 to 2 mU/minute with increases of 1 mU/minute every 15 minutes until the desired contraction pattern is obtained. The second protocol starts the initial dose at 0.5 to 1 mU/minute with increases every 40 to 60 minutes in increments of 1 to 2 mU/minute. The physician can choose either protocol.

A maximum oxytocin infusion rate of 2 to 8 mU/minute has been reported to be sufficient to achieve cervical dilatation of at least 1 cm/hour (ACOG, 1991). Studies suggest that smaller dose regimens are as effective as previous larger dose regimens and that adverse effects of oxytocin are dose related (Solomon & D'Alton, 1997). Once labor is established and cervical dilatation reaches 5 to 6 cm, oxytocin may be reduced by similar increments (ACOG, 1988).

Oxytocin induction is not without some associated risks: hyperstimulation of the uterus, resulting in uterine contractions that are too frequent (more often than every 2 minutes), uterine contractions that are too intense, or an increased uterine resting tone. Other risks include uterine rupture and water intoxication (*PDR Nurse's Handbook*, 1999).

Researchers continue to investigate a new method of labor induction with pulsatile oxytocin administration by a computer-controlled pump.

CRITICAL THINKING IN PRACTICE

You are a birthing center nurse caring for Wendy Johnson, gravida 2, para 1, during an oxytocin infusion to induce her labor. Wendy has been receiving the medication via infusion pump for 4 hours and currently is receiving 6 mU/minute (36 mL/hour). You have just completed your assessments and found the following: BP 120/80, pulse 80, respirations 16; contractions every 3 minutes lasting 60 seconds and of strong intensity; the FHR baseline is 144–150 with average long-term variability; and cervical dilatation is 6 cm. Will you continue the same infusion rate, increase the rate, or decrease the rate?

Answers can be found in Appendix I.

NURSING CARE MANAGEMENT

Close observation and accurate assessments are mandatory to provide safe, optimal care for both woman and fetus. Baseline data (maternal temperature, pulse, respiration, blood pressure, FHR, and NST) should be obtained before beginning the infusion. A fetal monitor is used to provide continuous data. Induction protocols recommend obtaining a 20- to 30-minute EFM recording

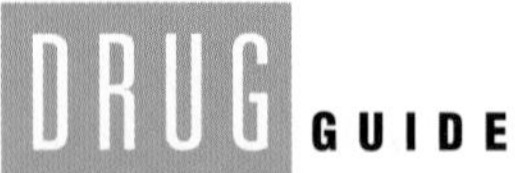

Oxytocin (Pitocin)

Overview of Obstetric Action

Oxytocin (Pitocin) exerts a selective stimulatory effect on the smooth muscle of the uterus and blood vessels. Oxytocin affects the myometrial cells of the uterus by increasing the excitability of the muscle cell, increasing the strength of the muscle contraction, and supporting propagation of the contraction (movement of the contraction from one myometrial cell to the next). Its effect on the uterine contraction depends on the dosage used and on the excitability of the myometrial cells. During the first half of gestation, there is little excitability of the myometrium, and the uterus is fairly resistant to the effects of oxytocin. However, from midgestation on, the uterus responds increasingly to exogenous intravenous oxytocin. Cautious use of diluted oxytocin administered intravenously at term results in a slow rise of uterine activity.

The circulatory half-life of oxytocin is 3 to 5 minutes. It takes approximately 40 minutes for a particular dose of oxytocin to reach a steady-state plasma concentration (Arias, 1993).

The effects of oxytocin on the cardiovascular system can be pronounced. Blood pressure initially may decrease but after prolonged administration increase by 30% above the baseline. Cardiac output and stroke volume increase. With doses of 20 mU/minute or above, oxytocin exerts an antidiuretic effect, decreasing free water exchange in the kidney and markedly decreasing urine output.

Oxytocin is used to induce labor at term and to augment uterine contractions in the first and second stages of labor. Oxytocin may also be used immediately after birth to stimulate uterine contraction and thereby control uterine atony.

Route, Dosage, Frequency

For induction of labor: Add 10 units of Pitocin (1 mL) to 1000 mL of intravenous solution. (The resulting concentration is 10 mU oxytocin per 1 mL of intravenous fluid.) Using an infusion pump, administer IV, starting at 0.5–1 mU/minute and increase by 1–2 mU/minute every 40–60 minutes. Alternatively, start at 1–2 mU/minute and increase by 1 mU/minute every 15 minutes until a good contraction pattern (every 2–3 minutes and lasting 40–60 seconds) is achieved.

Maternal Contraindications

- Severe preeclampsia-eclampsia (pregnancy-induced hypertension [PIH])
- Predisposition to uterine rupture (in nullipara over 35 years of age, multigravida 4 or more, overdistention of the uterus, previous major surgery of the cervix or uterus)
- Cephalopelvic disproportion
- Malpresentation or malposition of the fetus, cord prolapse
- Preterm infant
- Rigid, unripe cervix; total placenta previa
- Presence of fetal distress

Maternal Side Effects

Hyperstimulation of the uterus results in hypercontractility, which in turn may cause the following:

- Abruptio placentae
- Impaired uterine blood flow, leading to fetal hypoxia
- Rapid labor, leading to cervical lacerations
- Rapid labor and birth, leading to lacerations of cervix, vagina, or perineum; uterine atony; fetal trauma
- Uterine rupture
- Water intoxication (nausea, vomiting, hypotension, tachycardia, cardiac arrhythmia) if oxytocin is given in electrolyte-free solution or at a rate exceeding 20 mU/minute; hypotension with rapid IV bolus administration postpartum

Effect on Fetus-Neonate

- Fetal effects are primarily associated with the presence of hypercontractility of the maternal uterus. Hypercontractility decreases the oxygen supply to the fetus, which is reflected by irregularities or decrease in fetal heart rate (FHR).
- Hyperbilirubinemia (Arias, 1993)
- Trauma from rapid birth

Nursing Considerations

- Explain induction or augmentation procedure to client.
- Apply fetal monitor, and obtain 15- to 20-minute tracing and nonstress test (NST) to assess FHR before starting IV oxytocin.
- For induction or augmentation of labor, start with primary IV, and piggyback secondary IV with oxytocin and infusion pump.
- Ensure continuous monitoring of the fetus and uterine contractions.
- The maximum rate is 40 mU/minute (ACOG, 1988). Not all protocols recommend a maximum dose. When indicated, the maximum dose is generally between 16 and 40 mU/minute. Decrease oxytocin by similar increments once labor has progressed to 5–6 cm dilatation (Arias, 1993). Protocols may vary from one agency to another.

  0.5 mU/min = 3 mL/hr
  1.0 mU/min = 6 mL/hr
  1.5 mU/min = 9 mL/hr
  2 mU/min = 12 mL/hr
  4 mU/min = 24 mL/hr
  6 mU/min = 36 mL/hr
  8 mU/min = 48 mL/hr
  10 mU/min = 60 mL/hr
  12 mU/min = 72 mL/hr
  15 mU/min = 90 mL/hr
  18 mU/min = 108 mL/hr
  20 mU/min = 120 mL/hr

- Assess FHR, maternal blood pressure, pulse, frequency and duration of uterine contractions, and uterine resting tone before each increase in the oxytocin infusion rate.
- Record all assessments and IV rate on monitor strip and on client's chart.
- Record oxytocin infusion rate in mU/minute and mL/hour (eg, 0.5 mU/minute [3 mL/hour]).
- Record on monitor strip all client activities (such as change of position, vomiting), procedures done (amniotomy, sterile vaginal examination), and administration of analgesic agents to allow for interpretation and evaluation of tracing.
- Assess cervical dilatation as needed.
- Apply nursing comfort measures.
- Discontinue IV oxytocin infusion and infuse primary solution when (1) fetal distress is noted (bradycardia, late or variable decelerations); (2) uterine contractions are more frequent than every 2 minutes; (3) duration of contractions exceeds more than 60 seconds; or (4) insufficient relaxation of the uterus between contractions or a steady increase in resting tone are noted (ACOG, 1991). In addition to discontinuing IV oxytocin infusion, turn client to side, and if fetal distress is present, administer oxygen by tight face mask at 7–10 L/minute; notify physician.
- Maintain intake and output record.

For augmentation of labor:

Prepare and administer IV Pitocin as for labor induction. Increase rate until labor contractions are of good quality. The flow rate is gradually increased at no less than every 30 minutes to a maximum of 10 mU/minute (Cunningham et al, 1997b). In some settings or in a situation when limited fluids may be administered, a more concentrated solution may be used. When 10 U Pitocin are added to 500 mL IV solution, the resulting concentration is 1 mU/minute = 3 mL/hour. If 10 U Pitocin are added to 250 mL IV solution, the concentration is 1 mU/minute = 1.5 mL/hour.

For administration after delivery of placenta:

- One dose of 10 units of Pitocin (1 mL) is given intramuscularly or added to IV fluids for continuous infusion.
- Assess FHR, maternal blood pressure, pulse, frequency and duration of uterine contractions, and uterine resting tone before each increase in oxytocin infusion rate.
- Record all assessments and IV rate on monitor strip and on client's chart. Record oxytocin infusion rate in mU/minute and mL/hour (eg, 0.5 mU/minute [3 mL/hour]).
- Record on monitor strip all client activities (such as change of position, vomiting), procedures done (amniotomy, sterile vaginal examination), and administration of analgesic agents to allow for interpretation and evaluation of tracing.
- Assess cervical dilatation as needed.
- Apply nursing comfort measures.
- Discontinue IV oxytocin infusion and infuse primary solution when (1) fetal stress or distress is noted (tachycardia or bradycardia, late or variable decelerations), (2) uterine contractions are more frequent than every 2 minutes, (3) duration of contractions exceeds 60 seconds, or (4) insufficient relaxation of the uterus between contractions or a steady increase in resting tone are noted (ACOG, 1988). In addition to discontinuing IV oxytocin infusion, turn client to side, and if fetal distress is present, administer oxygen by tight face mask at 7–10 L/minute; notify physician.
- Maintain intake and output record. Assess intake and output every hour.

demonstrating a reassuring FHR and reactive NST and contraction status before the infusion is started.

Before each advancement of the infusion rate, assessments of the following should be made:

- Maternal blood pressure and pulse
- Uterine contraction status, including frequency, duration, intensity, resting tone between contractions, and maternal response to the contractions
- FHR baseline, variability (short term and long term), presence of accelerations with fetal movement, and periodic or nonperiodic decelerations

As contractions are established, vaginal examinations are performed to evaluate cervical dilatation, effacement, and station. The frequency of vaginal examinations depends primarily on the woman's parity and on characteristics of contractions. For example, a nullipara with contractions every 5 to 7 minutes, each lasting 30 seconds, who does not perceive her contractions does not usually require a vaginal examination. But when her contractions occur every 2 to 3 minutes, lasting 50 to 60 seconds with good intensity, a vaginal examination will be needed to evaluate her progress.

When evaluating the need for analgesia, a vaginal examination should be performed to avoid giving the medication too early and increasing the risk of prolonging labor and to identify advanced dilatation and imminent birth.

Labor Induction by Misoprostol

Uterine contraction and FHR status are continuously monitored by EFM to determine the presence of contractions and a reassuring FHR pattern and reactive NST. The nurse documents the Bishop score and assesses the fetal presentation and position. If no contraindications are present, an intravenous infusion is started to provide access if needed later, and a 25-μg misoprostol tablet is inserted in the posterior vaginal fornix. The dose may be repeated every 3 to 4 hours until uterine contractions are at least three in 10 minutes or the Bishop score is equal to or greater than 5. An oxytocin infusion may be started if there is no adequate contraction pattern, the Bishop score is greater then 5, and it has been at least 3 hours since the last dose of misoprostol.

NURSING CARE MANAGEMENT

During the oxytocin infusion, the woman needs skilled care. A qualified obstetrician should be readily accessible to manage any complication that may occur (ACOG, 1995).

Aspects to address during client teaching include the purpose and procedure for the induction, nursing care that will be provided, assessments during the induction procedure, comfort measures, and a review of breathing techniques that may be used during labor.

For additional information regarding nursing interventions during the use of oxytocin, see Drug Guide: Oxytocin (Pitocin) on page 660 and Critical Pathway for Induction of Labor on the facing page.

Intravenous oxytocin may also be given for augmentation of labor; see Drug Guide: Oxytocin (Pitocin) on page 660 for further discussion.

Additional Methods for Cervical Ripening, Inducing Labor, and Augmenting Labor

In addition to the allopathic medical cervical ripening and induction methods previously discussed, there are a variety of more "natural" and noninvasive methods that certified nurse-midwives tend to use either in the home setting or in tertiary care centers. These methods include the following (Summers, 1997): sexual intercourse/lovemaking; self or partner nipple and breast stimulation; the use of herbs, such as blue/black cohosh, evening primrose oil, and red raspberry leaves; the use of homeopathic solutions, such as caulophyllum or pulsatilla; castor oil; enemas; and acupuncture. Mechanical dilation of the cervix with balloon catheters is another technique used. Pharmacologic hormonal preparations may also be used; these include oxytocin and misoprostol (Cytotec) (already discussed), mifeprestone (RU486), and relaxin.

Prior to recommending any of these methods, the clinician assesses the woman for the presence of contraindications (Summers, 1997):

- Prior classic uterine incision for cesarean birth
- Active genital herpes infection in the mother
- Placenta previa, vasa previa, or transverse fetal lie

Conditions that require caution include the following (Summers, 1997):

- Fetal factors such as presenting part above the pelvic outlet, breech presentation, multiple gestation, and abnormal FHR pattern not requiring emergency delivery
- Maternal factors such as cardiac disease, grandmultiparity, or hydramnios

Summers (1997) points out that although they are not frequently presented in medical (allopathic) or nursing texts, the natural methods are very effective and are often the preferred choice of many certified nurse-midwives and their clients. It is important for basic nursing students, nurses, and consumers to be aware of all aspects of pregnancy care.

Sexual intercourse is a logical method of stimulating cervical ripening and uterine contractions; female orgasm stimulates uterine contractions, and the male ejaculate contains a rich source of natural prostaglandins. Breast and nipple stimulation is also a frequent part of lovemaking, and this stimulates endogenous oxytocin, which in turn stimulates the uterus to contract. Until recently, most literature regarding sexual intercourse and lovemaking during pregnancy has focused on the possible harmful effects that may arise; however, more current research is dispelling the older beliefs (Summers, 1997).

Nipple stimulation for cervical ripening may be done at term. The woman gently massages her breasts with a warm wash cloth for 30 to 60 minutes, three times a day. In one study, nipple stimulation increased most women's Bishop score, and some women went into labor (Summers, 1997).

Herbal preparations have not been scientifically studied to the same extent as other natural methods. For further information, see S. S. Weed, *Wise Woman Herbal for the Childbearing Year*, Woodstock, New York: AshTree Publishing, 1985.

Homeopathic solutions, such as caulophyllum, cimicifuga, pulsatilla, and others, are used for cervical ripening and induction of labor. The caregiver needs thorough personal knowledge of homeopathic remedies or ongoing consultation with a homeopathic physician. The solutions are prepared in dilutions according to two scales, the decimal scale (abbreviated X, such as 1 X, 3 X) or by the centesimal scale (abbreviated C, such as 5C or 6C).

Castor oil has been used for many years but has not frequently been studied as a method of labor induction. The method by which castor oil stimulates uterine contractions is not understood. Some practitioners consider castor oil an old-fashioned and nonuseful substance, whereas others have noted that it is especially useful for primigravidas at term (Summers, 1997).

Acupuncture is not as accepted in the United States as it is in other countries. However, the rising interest in and use of holistic practices and alternative medicine is

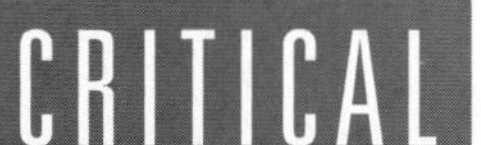

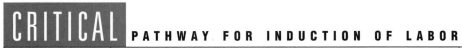

CRITICAL PATHWAY FOR INDUCTION OF LABOR

Category	Immediate Care	Outcomes
Referral	Review prenatal record Advise CNM/physician of admission Anesthesia	**Expected Outcomes** Appropriate resources identified and utilized
Assessments	Previous pregnancies, present pregnancy, and childbirth preparation Estimated gestational age of the fetus Assess woman's feelings regarding induction as well as knowledge base regarding the induction process Assess knowledge of breathing techniques. If woman does not have a method to use, teach breathing techniques before starting oxytocin infusion.	**Expected Outcomes** Potential/actual complications identified
Teaching/ psychosocial	Provide emotional support through teaching and answering all questions	**Expected Outcomes** Woman verbalizes/demonstrates understanding of information given
Nursing care management and reports	Examination of pregnant uterus (Leopold's maneuvers to determine fetal size and position) Vaginal examination to evaluate cervical readiness: • Ripe cervix feels soft to the examining finger, is located in a medial to anterior position, is more than 50% effaced, and is 2–3 cm dilated • Unripe cervix feels firm to the examining finger, is long and thick, is perhaps in a posterior position, and is dilated little or not at all Presence of contractions Membranes intact or ruptured Maternal vital signs and a 20 min baseline fetal monitoring strip prior to induction to determine fetal well-being Diagnostic studies: • Fetal maturity tests (L/S ratio, creatinine concentrations, ultrasonography), NST, CST, BPP • Maternal blood studies (CBC, hemoglobin, hematocrit, blood type, Rh factor) • Urinalysis Monitor for nausea, vomiting, hypotension, tachycardia, cardiac arrhythmias, headache, mental confusion, decreased urinary output Monitor FHR by continuous electronic fetal monitoring. Do not start infusion or advance rate (if induction has already begun) if FHR is not in range of 120–160 bpm, if decelerations are present, or if variability decreases. Evaluate and document maternal BP and pulse before beginning induction and then before each increase in infusion rate. Do not advance infusion rate in presence of maternal hypertension or hypotension or radical changes in pulse rate. If the woman becomes hypotensive: • Keep her on her side. May change to other side. • Discontinue oxytocin infusion • Increase rate of primary IV • Monitor FHR • Notify physician • Assess for cause of hypotension Evaluate and document contraction frequency, duration, and intensity prior to each increase in infusion rate Discontinue oxytocin infusion if: • Contractions are more frequent than q2min • Contraction duration exceeds 90 sec • Uterus does not relax between contractions Increase oxytocin IV infusion rate q20min until adequate contractions are achieved. Do not exceed an infusion rate of 20–40 mL/min. (Note: Protocols directing how often oxytocin is increased may vary from 15–60 min. See ACOG 1991 guidelines and institutional protocol.) Check infusion pump to assure oxytocin is infusing. Check whether pump is on, chamber refills and empties, level of fluid in IV bottle becomes lower. If problem is found, correct and restart infusion at beginning dose. Check main IV site frequently. Check piggyback connection to primary tubing to assure solution is not leaking. Evaluate cervical dilatation by vaginal examination as indicated.	**Expected Outcomes** • Progression of labor and birth without difficulty • Potential/actual complications minimized

➤

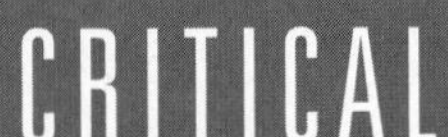 PATHWAY FOR INDUCTION OF LABOR *CONTINUED*

Category	Immediate Care	Outcomes
Nursing care management and reports *continued*	Monitor FHR continuously (normal range is 120–160 bpm). In episodes of bradycardia (<120 bpm) lasting for more than 30 sec, administer oxygen by face mask at 7–10 L/min. Stop oxytocin infusion. Position woman on left side if quick recovery of FHR does not occur. Carefully evaluate fetal tachycardia (>160 bpm). Sustained tachycardia may necessitate discontinuation of oxytocin infusion. Assess for presence of meconium staining. Notify physician.	
Activity	Ambulate until 5–10 cm then bed Position woman in left lateral or semi-Fowler's position Encourage her to avoid supine position	**Expected Outcomes** Activity individualized for woman
Comfort	Provide support to woman as she uses breathing techniques Encourage use of effluerage, back rub, and other supportive measures Assess need for analgesia or anesthesia	**Expected Outcomes** Optimal comfort level maintained
Nutrition	IV/lactated Ringer's Ice chips, clear fluids	**Expected Outcomes** Nutritional and hydration needs met
Elimination	Encourage voiding q2h. Monitor and record I/O.	**Expected Outcomes** Intake and output WNL
Medications	Start primary IV as ordered Administer oxytocin in electrolyte solution (Piggyback oxytocin onto primary IV at closest site to IV needle insertion.) Pain meds prn	**Expected Outcomes** Induction/augmentation of labor occurs within expected parameters
Disharge planning/home care	Photo packet Birth certificate worksheet Sibling visitation Car seat	**Expected Outcomes** Individualized discharge teaching completed
Family involvement	Family visitation policy per institutional protocol Encourage significant other to stay close and assist with breathing of woman	**Expected Outcomes** Family/support person involvement maximized
Date		

prompting a closer look at acupuncture as a method of inducing labor and relieving labor pain (Summers, 1997). Although acupuncture requires extensive education and training, some certified nurse-midwives can work with an acupuncturist to learn manual massage of acupuncture and acupressure points, shiatsu, and other touch techniques (Summers, 1997).

Balloon catheters have been used for cervical ripening for many years. Currently, a Foley catheter with a 25 to 50 mL balloon is passed through the undilated cervix and then inflated. The pressure of the weighted balloon applies pressure on the internal os of the cervix and acts to ripen the cervix (soften and efface). Summers (1997) reports studies that have found that this method is effective, is less costly, and does not require continuous EFM. Balloon catheter use is primarily an option in developing countries.

Evaluation

Expected outcomes of nursing care include the following:

- The woman and family understand the induction process and are able to relate the advantages, disadvantages, and possible outcomes.
- The woman's labor is successfully induced.
- The labor and birth process are within normal limits, and the woman and her baby do not experience any complications.

Care of the Woman during Amnioinfusion

Amnioinfusion (AI) is a technique by which a volume of warmed, sterile, normal saline or Ringer's lactate solution is introduced into the uterus through the use of an intrauterine pressure catheter (IUPC). Amnioinfusion can be used intrapartally to increase the volume of fluid when oligohydramnios is present and the physician either wants to prevent the possibility of nonperiodic (variable) decelerations by increasing the volume of amniotic fluid or to treat nonperiodic decelerations that are already occurring. The AI increases the volume of fluid, relieving pressure on the umbilical cord and promoting increased perfusion to the fetus. When AI is used for this indication or for prolonged decelerations in FHR patterns, the abnormal FHR pattern is usually relieved in 20 to 30 minutes (Schmidt, 1997). Amnioinfusion used for meconium dilution in the presence of medium to heavy meconium staining has resulted in a significant decrease of meconium below the cords (vocal cords when viewed with a laryngoscope) after birth and a decrease in meconium aspiration. It is not known whether the decreased incidence is due to dilution of the meconium in the amniotic fluid or to the decreased incidence of nonperiodic decelerations (Swaim & Creasy, 1997). Amnioinfusion is also indicated for preterm labor with premature rupture of membranes (Miyazaki, 1996). Contraindications include ominous fetal heart rate patterns, such as flat baseline or tachycardia of 180 bpm or more in the absence of maternal fever; umbilical cord prolapse; significant maternal vaginal bleeding with suspected abruptio placentae or placenta previa; and uterine hypertonia (Miyazaki, 1996).

There is no one accepted protocol for amnioinfusion. However, most procedures involve infusing from 250 to 500 mL of warmed normal saline through an intrauterine catheter using an infusion pump.

NURSING CARE MANAGEMENT

The nurse is frequently the first person to detect changes in FHR associated with cord compression or to observe thick, meconium-stained amniotic fluid. When cord compression is suspected, the immediate intervention is to assist the laboring woman to another position in an effort to relieve the compression (see Chapter 22 for further discussion). If this intervention is not successful, an amnioinfusion will be considered. The nurse helps with the amnioinfusion and monitors the woman's vital signs (blood pressure, pulse, and respiration) and contraction status (frequency, duration, intensity, resting tone, and associated maternal discomfort). FHR is monitored by continuous EFM. It is very important to provide ongoing information to the laboring woman and her partner and to answer questions as they arise. Comfort measures and positioning will be very important because AI requires the woman to be on bed rest.

The amnioinfusion should not cause pain or discomfort for the laboring woman other than the need for bed rest. The amnioinfusion should decrease the incidence and severity of nonperiodic (variable) decelerations. The meconium-stained fluid should appear less thick and lighter in color.

Care of the Woman during an Episiotomy

An **episiotomy** is a surgical incision of the perineal body that is perceived by some physicians and CNMs to prevent damage to the periurethra, perineum, anal sphincter, and rectum from lacerations during the birth (Keane, 1997), to prevent damage to the posterior wall of the vagina, to prevent jagged tears from lacerations, to reduce mechanical and metabolic risk to the fetus/neonate, to protect the maternal bladder, and to prevent future perineal relaxation (Helewa, 1997).

Episiotomy is the second most common procedure in maternal-child care (Maier & Maloni, 1997). It is estimated that in the United States the incidence of episiotomies is 50% to 90% in primigravidas (Keane, 1997). In Canada, the incidence is approximately 37.8%, which reflects a decline of 29.1% since the early 1980s, with most of the decline occurring in the early 1990s (Graham & Graham, 1997). In the same period of time, the incidence in the United States decreased only 13.6%. Even though the procedure is very common, its routine use has been questioned. Research suggests that rather than protecting the perineum from lacerations, the presence of an episiotomy makes it more likely that the woman will have deep perineal tears. It has also been suggested that perineal lacerations heal more quickly in the absence of episiotomy (Keane, 1997). In clinical practice, research has shown that the incidence of major perineal trauma (extension to or through the anal sphincter) is four times more likely to occur if a midline episiotomy is performed (Maier & Maloni, 1997). Ecker, Tan, Bansal, Bishop, and Kilpatrick (1997) found that the decreased use of episiotomy resulted in more lacerations and fewer fourth-degree extensions, but the rate of third-degree lacerations stayed the same. The researchers note that the third-degree laceration rate probably was not affected because a midline incision was used for operative deliveries. Additional complications associated with an episiotomy are blood loss, infection, pain, and perineal discomfort that may continue for days or weeks past birth, including dyspareunia (painful intercourse), psychologic trauma, feelings of loss of control, and increased health care costs (Maier & Maloni, 1997). In light of the debate over the value of episiotomy, it is now suggested that an episiotomy be used selectively to facilitate birth in the

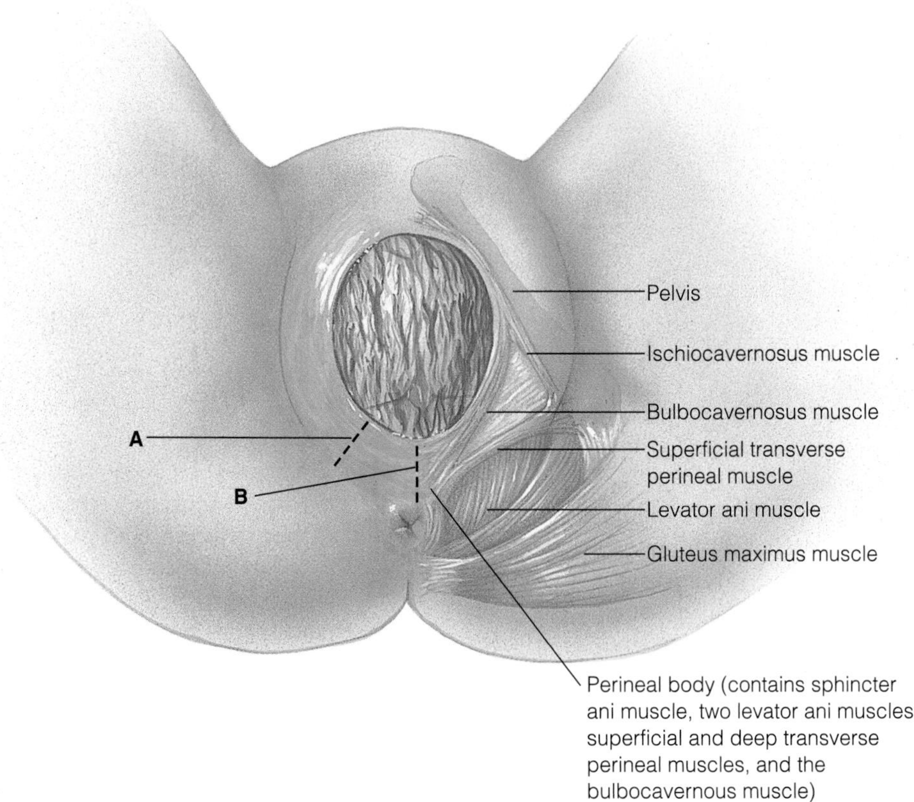

FIGURE 23–3 The two most common types of episiotomies are midline and mediolateral. ***A,*** Right mediolateral. ***B,*** Midline.

presence of maternal or fetal distress, to create more room in the presence of a breech presentation or multiple gestation, or for the use of an instrument (forceps or vacuum extractor) to assist birth (Keane, 1997).

Risk Factors that Predispose Women to Episiotomy

Overall factors that place a woman at increased risk are primigravid status, large or macrosomic fetus, occiput posterior position, use of forceps or vacuum extractor, and shoulder dystocia. Other factors that predispose a woman to episiotomy may be mitigated by nurses and physician/CNMs. These include the following (Maier & Maloni, 1997):

- Use of lithotomy position or other recumbent position (causes excessive perineal stretching)
- Encouraging or requiring sustained breath holding during second-stage pushing (causes excessive perineal stretching, can adversely affect blood flow in mother and fetus, and encourages women to be responsive to caregiver directions rather than to her own urges to push spontaneously)
- Arbitrary time limit placed by the physician/CNM on the length of the second stage

Episiotomy Procedure

The episiotomy is performed with sharp scissors that have rounded points, just before birth, when approximately 3 to 4 cm of the fetal head is visible during a contraction (Cunningham et al, 1997b). There are two types in current practice: midline and mediolateral (Figure 23–3). A midline episiotomy is performed along the median raphe of the perineum. It extends down from the vaginal orifice to the fibers of the rectal sphincter. This type of episiotomy avoids muscle fibers and major blood vessels because it divides the insertions of the superficial perineal muscles. A midline episiotomy is preferred if the perineum is of adequate length and no difficulty is anticipated during the birth because it entails less blood loss, is easy to repair, and heals with less discomfort for the mother. The major disadvantage is that a tear of the midline incision may extend through the anal sphincter and rectum.

In the presence of a short perineum, macrosomia, and instrumental delivery (use of forceps or vacuum extractor), a mediolateral episiotomy provides more room and decreases the possibility of a traumatic extension into the rectum. The mediolateral episiotomy begins in the midline of the posterior fourchette (in order to avoid incision into the Bartholin's gland) and extends at a 45-

degree angle downward to the right or left (the direction depending on the handedness of the clinician). The mediolateral episiotomy may be complicated by greater blood loss, a longer healing period, and more postpartal discomfort.

The episiotomy is usually performed with regional or local anesthesia but may be performed without anesthesia in emergency situations. It is generally proposed that as crowning occurs, the distention of the tissues causes numbing. Adequate anesthesia must be given for the repair.

Repair of the episiotomy (episiorrhaphy) and any lacerations is performed either during the period between birth of the neonate and before expulsion of the placenta or after expulsion of the placenta.

NURSING CARE MANAGEMENT

The woman needs to be supported during the episiotomy and the repair because she may feel some pressure sensations. In the absence of adequate anesthesia she may feel pain. Placing a hand on her shoulder and talking with her can provide comfort and distraction from the repair process. If the woman is having more discomfort than she can comfortably handle, the nurse needs to act as an advocate in communicating the woman's needs to the physician/CNM. At all times, the woman needs to be the one who decides whether the amount of discomfort is tolerable, and she should never be told, "This doesn't hurt." She is the person experiencing the discomfort, and her evaluation needs to be respected. If there are just a few (three to five) stitches left, she may choose to forego more local anesthesia, but she should be given the choice.

The nurse notes the type of episiotomy on the birth record. This information should also be included in a report to the recovery room so that adequate assessments can be made and relief measures can be instituted if necessary.

Pain relief measures may begin immediately after birth with application of an ice pack to the perineum. For optimal effect, the ice pack should be applied for 20 to 30 minutes and removed for at least 20 minutes before being reapplied because the ice causes vasoconstriction. If the ice pack is left in place more than 30 minutes, vasodilation and subsequent edema may occur. The perineal tissues should be assessed frequently to prevent injury from the ice pack. The episiotomy site should be inspected every 15 minutes during the first hour after the birth for redness, swelling, tenderness, and hematomas. As a part of postpartal care, the mother will need instruction in perineal hygiene care and comfort measures. (See Chapter 31 for additional discussion of relief measures for the immediate postpartum period.)

It is important for nurses to recognize that perineal pain continues for a period of time. Glazener (1997) reported that 42% of women still experienced significant pain for a week after the birth, 22% continued to have pain at 8 weeks postpartum, and 10% of women had pain for a much longer period. Women who experienced prolonged pain tended to have other problems, such as breastfeeding difficulties and depression, and were reluctant to reestablish sexual activity. Nursing advocacy is needed to promote selective rather than routine episiotomies. The nurse can begin by educating pregnant women to read about prenatal perineal preparation and to talk with the physician or CNM regarding their personal beliefs and incidence of episiotomy in their practice. Nurses can share current research with nursing colleagues through staff meetings and explore and strongly encourage nursing care interventions that avoid lithotomy. Support of the woman during the second stage to respond to her body's urges to push will promote spontaneous pushing. Just as clients ask physicians and CNMs about their episiotomy philosophy and incidence, clients may at some time in the future ask labor and birthing nurses to provide information regarding their actions to help decrease episiotomy rates. It is imperative that each nurse continue to stay current regarding new information and research in order to maintain current practice standards.

CRITICAL THINKING QUESTION

1. A pregnant woman tells you she does not want an episiotomy and asks whether there is anything she can do during pregnancy to help avoid one. What will you tell her?
2. As a new mother's episiotomy is repaired, she says that she can feel the procedure and that it hurts. What will you do?

Care of the Woman during Forceps-Assisted Birth

Forceps are designed to assist the birth of a fetus by providing traction or by providing the means to rotate the fetal head to an occiput-anterior position. In medical literature and practice, **forceps-assisted birth** is also known as *instrumental delivery*, *operative delivery*, or *operative vaginal delivery*. To better understand the use of forceps, it is important to recognize that there are many different types, each with special functions. For example, Piper forceps are designed to be used with a breech presentation (buttocks as presenting part); they are applied after the birth of the body, when the fetal head is still in the birth canal and assistance is needed. In conversational language, Piper forceps are said to be applied to the aftercoming head. All other forceps are used in situations when the fetus is in a cephalic (head down) presentation. In such situations, the forceps are applied to the sides of the head.

RESEARCH IN PRACTICE

What is this study about? Laboring in water increases feelings of relaxation for some women and may increase their feelings of being in control of the birthing process. Water births have been introduced in many hospital maternity units in the United Kingdom. Susan Hall conducted a study to examine womens' experience of labor in water and collaborated with Immy Holloway to publish the study.

How was the study done? The study sample consisted of nine women who had experienced a normal pregnancy, delivered a healthy baby, and used water as part of their childbirth process. The investigator conducted in-depth, unstructured interviews 48 hours postpartum. She analyzed the interviews using a constant comparative technique to generate constructs and formulate theoretical ideas. The process of open coding, axial coding, and theoretical sampling guided subsequent interviews and development of categories.

What were the results of the study? The researcher identified the core category as personal control with dimensions of gaining mastery of the situation, making decisions, and negotiating support. Gaining mastery included retaining or regaining control. Making decisions involved an interplay between feelings of being in control and the opportunity to make decisions regarding care. Negotiating support incorporated a balance between having support from the midwife and being in personal control. The four other major categories extracted from the data but not explained in the article are as follows: exercising choice, releasing inhibitions, coping with pain, and experiencing fulfillment.

What additional questions might I have? What was contained in the other categories discovered in the study and how were these categories related to the core category of staying in control? Although the other categories were mentioned in the article, it is very difficult to understand a qualitative study without examining and comprehending the whole study. What was the theory generated from this study? Grounded theory should result in the generation of a theory that is inextricably related to the core variable and based on the discovery and conceptualization of complex interactional processes (Hutchinson, 1986).

How can I use this study? Students and others who care for a laboring woman can try to devise strategies to help the woman remain in control. The philosophical stance of the patient remaining in control differs greatly from the idea of "giving" the woman control.

SOURCE: Hall, S. M., & Holloway, I. M. (1998). Staying in control: Women's experiences of labor in water. *Midwifery, 14,* 30–36. Hutchinson, S. A. (1986). Grounded theory: The method. In P. L. Munhall, & C. J. Oiler, *Nursing research: A qualitative perspective.* Norwalk: Appleton-Century-Crofts.

Nearly a decade ago, the American College of Obstetricians and Gynecologists (ACOG, 1991) revised the definitions of forceps applications into three categories: outlet, low, and midforceps. Criteria for *outlet forceps* application are as follows:

1. Forceps are applied when the fetal skull has reached the perineum. (There is bulging of the perineum.)
2. The scalp is visible between contractions. (Earlier in labor, as the woman pushes during the contraction, the fetal scalp may be visible, but when the pushing effort ceases, the scalp recedes and is no longer visible. This criterion indicates that the scalp remains visible even when the woman is not pushing.)
3. The sagittal suture is not more than 45 degrees from the midline. The sagittal suture is the anterior-posterior suture on the top of the fetal head. At this point in a spontaneous birth, extension has almost been completed, external rotation is beginning, and the sagittal suture is between the midline and 45 degrees from the midline. (For example, think of a clock face. If 12:00 is the maternal symphysis pubis and the fetus is in LOA, the sagittal suture and the occiput are between 12:00 and 1:30.) The important aspect of this criterion is that with outlet forceps, the fetal head is moving naturally from extension to external rotation, and the forceps are being used to guide or lift the head out.

The criterion for *low forceps* application is that the leading edge (presenting part) of the fetal skull must be at a station of +2 or below (for example, +3) but not on the pelvic floor. The rotation (internal rotation, which is part of the cardinal movements) of the fetal head is less than 45 degrees (right or left occiput anterior to occiput anterior, or right or left occiput posterior to occiput posterior) (ACOG, 1991). The criterion for *midforceps* application is that the fetal head must be engaged (largest diameter of the head reaches or passes through the pelvic inlet), but the leading edge (presenting part) of the fetal skull is above a +2 station (for example +1, 0, −1, −2). When midforceps are used, the goal is to apply traction, and, frequently, to rotate the head and facilitate the vaginal birth. Types of forceps are depicted in Figure 23–4.

Indications

Indications for the use of forceps include the presence of any condition that threatens the mother or fetus and that can be relieved by birth. Conditions that put the woman at risk include heart disease, acute pulmonary edema, intrapartal infection, or exhaustion. Fetal conditions include premature placental separation and fetal distress. Forceps may be used electively to shorten the second stage of labor and spare the woman's pushing effort (when exhaustion or heart disease is present) or when regional anesthesia has affected the woman's motor innervation and she cannot push effectively. In the past, outlet forceps have been used to protect the head of a preterm infant during birth; however, the advantages of this practice are now being questioned (ACOG, 1991; Cunningham et al, 1997b).

In a study by Turcot, Marcoux, Fraser, and the Canadian Early Amniotomy Study Group (1997) involving low-risk nulliparous women, independent variables were found at admission and then later during active labor that were predictive of the need for forceps- or vacuum-assisted birth (instrumental delivery) or for cesarean birth

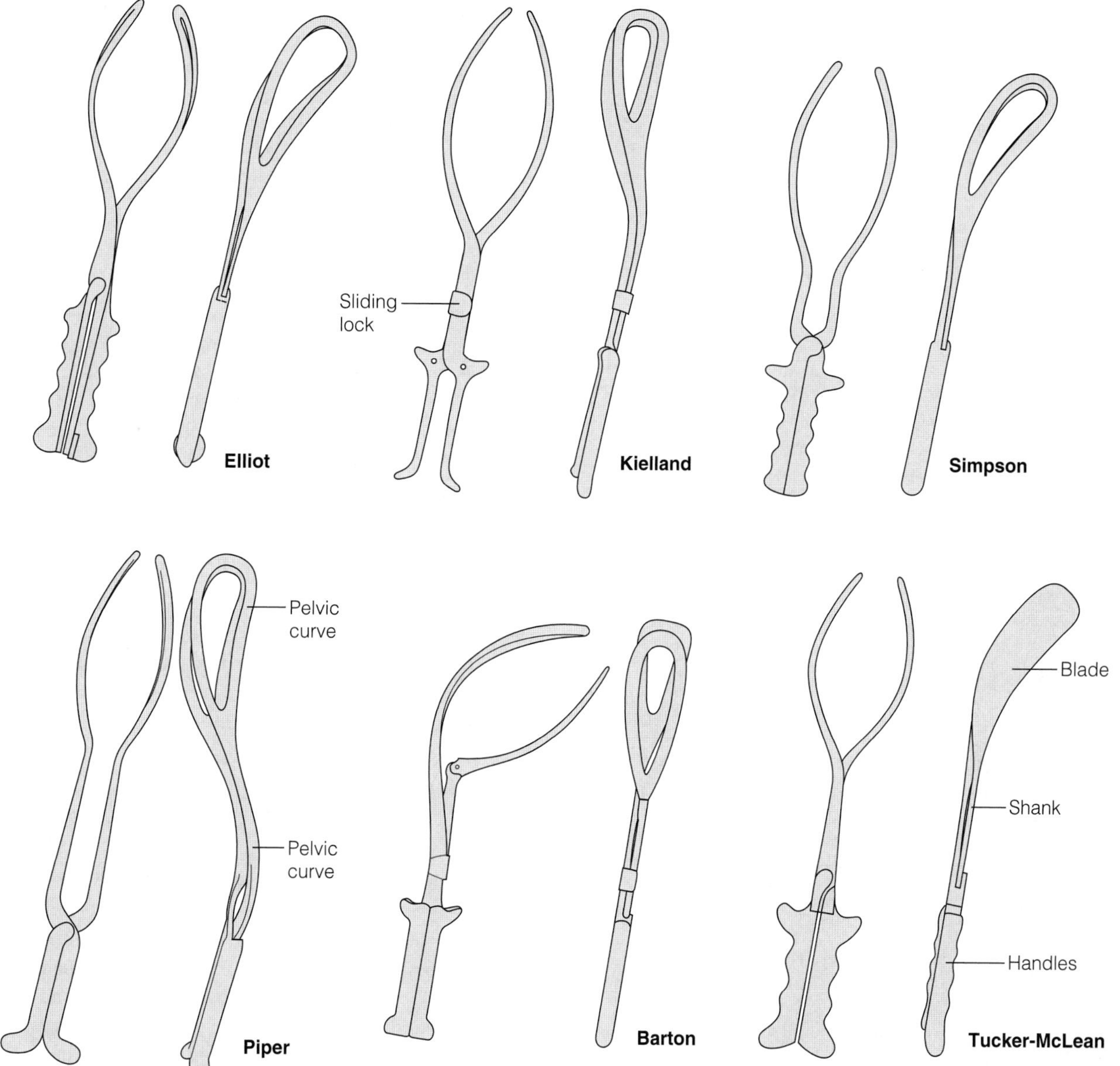

FIGURE 23–4 Forceps are composed of a blade, shank, and handle and may have a cephalic and pelvic curve. (Note labels on Piper and Tucker-McLean forceps.) The blades may be fenestrated (open) or solid. The front and lateral views of these forceps illustrate differences in blades, open and closed shanks, and cephalic and pelvic curves. Elliot, Simpson, and Tucker-McLean forceps are used as outlet forceps. Kielland and Barton forceps are used for midforceps rotations. Piper forceps are used to provide traction and flexion of the aftercoming head (the head comes after the body) of a fetus in breech presentation.

(operative delivery) if the forceps or vacuum extractor failed. The most accurate predictors were found to be a combination of variables present at admission and some that developed during active labor. The predictive variables were as follows (Turcot et al, 1997):

- Maternal age (A woman 35 or over was six times more likely to have an operative delivery than a woman under 20.)
- Maternal height (A woman whose height was less than 150 cm [4 ft 11 in.] was 2.5 times more likely to have an operative delivery.)
- Pregnancy weight gain of more than 15 kg [33 lb]
- Smoking status (Women who smoked were at less risk.)
- Gestational age (Women with a gestation age of 41 weeks or more had an 85% increase in the risk of operative delivery.)
- Epidural anesthesia (Women who received an epidural block more than 1 hour before birth had an incidence of operative delivery four times greater than that of women who had other types of analgesia or no analgesia.)

- Presence of dystocia (The incidence of operative delivery among women who received an oxytocin infusion was twice that of women who did not.)
- Abnormal fetal heart rate tracing (Abnormal tracing was associated with a 65% higher incidence of operative delivery.)
- Racial origin (The incidence of operative delivery among black women was 40% less than that of white women; the incidence among Asian women was 63% greater than that of white women.)

Neonatal and Maternal Risks

Some neonates may develop a small area of ecchymosis or edema or both along the sides of the face as a result of forceps application. Caput succedaneum or cephalhematoma (and subsequent hyperbilirubinemia) may occur as well as transient facial paralysis.

Maternal risks may include lacerations of the birth canal, periurethal lacerations, and extensions of a median episiotomy into the anus, resulting in increased bleeding, bruising, and perineal edema.

Prerequisites for Forceps Application and Delivery

It is very important that all of the prerequisites be met before the forceps procedure is attempted. The prerequisites are as follows (Charles, 1997):

- The physician must be knowledgeable about the advantages and disadvantages of different types of forceps and their use.
- The cervix must be completely dilated.
- The fetal head must be engaged, and the station, presentation, and exact position of the head should be known.
- Amniotic membranes must be ruptured to allow a firm grasp on the fetal head.
- The type of pelvis should be identified, because certain pelvic types do not permit rotation. In addition, there must be no disproportion between the fetal head and the maternal pelvis (Cunningham et al, 1997b).
- Maternal bladder should be empty.
- There must be no obstructions to the delivery below the fetal head, such as an incurving coccyx that will not allow the fetus to pass (Keane, 1997).
- Adequate anesthesia must be given (Revah, Ezra, Farine, & Ritchie, 1997) for the type of forceps procedure that is anticipated. For instance, low forceps may be done with a pudendal block; however, midforceps or a rotation of more than 45 degrees requires an epidural, spinal-epidural, or general anesthesia.

The use of forceps is an operative procedure, and it requires the same degree of respect and care as any other operative procedure (Charles, 1997).

Keane (1997) notes that the average biparietal diameter of the full-term fetal head is 9.5 cm and some forceps are not able to accommodate this diameter. The physician needs to carefully adjust the force applied to the handles to avoid excessive fetal head compression.

Trial or Failed Forceps Procedure

In a trial forceps procedure, the physician attempts to use forceps with the knowledge that there is a degree of CPD. A complete setup for immediate cesarean birth needs to be available before the forceps are applied. If a good application cannot be obtained or if no descent occurs with the application, cesarean birth is the method of choice. Revah et al (1997) suggest that all forceps applications be considered a trial and that the health care team are prepared to perform a cesarean birth within 10 minutes if the forceps-assisted birth is not accomplished in three pulls. In their study, Revah et al (1997) found there was no increase in maternal or neonatal morbidity or mortality when Keilland's or Simpson's forceps were applied at station 0 or lower, provided that cesarean birth was possible within 10 minutes.

NURSING CARE MANAGEMENT

Using information from the study by Turcot et al (1997), the nurse may note those variables that are associated with increased risk of operative delivery. The nurse could then direct nursing care measures toward the variable(s) that may be positively affected by nursing care measures. For instance, dystocia may be corrected by changing maternal position, ambulation, rocking, frequent bladder emptying, and so on. Fetal heart rate abnormalities may be affected by utero-placental-fetal circulation, so the nurse could support ambulation (if not contraindicated), frequent position changes, intake of adequate fluids, and monitoring to detect early FHR changes.

If a forceps-assisted birth is required, the nurse explains the procedure briefly to the woman. With adequate regional anesthesia, the woman should feel some pressure but no pain. The nurse encourages her to maintain breathing techniques to prevent her from pushing during application of the forceps. (Figure 23–5 depicts the application of forceps.) The nurse monitors contractions and advises the physician when one is present because traction is applied only with a contraction. During the contraction, as the forceps are applied, the nurse encourages the woman to use her breathing technique to avoid pushing. With each contraction, after the forceps are in place, the physician provides traction on the forceps as the woman pushes. It is not uncommon to observe mild bradycardia as traction is applied to the forceps. This bradycardia results from head compression and is transient.

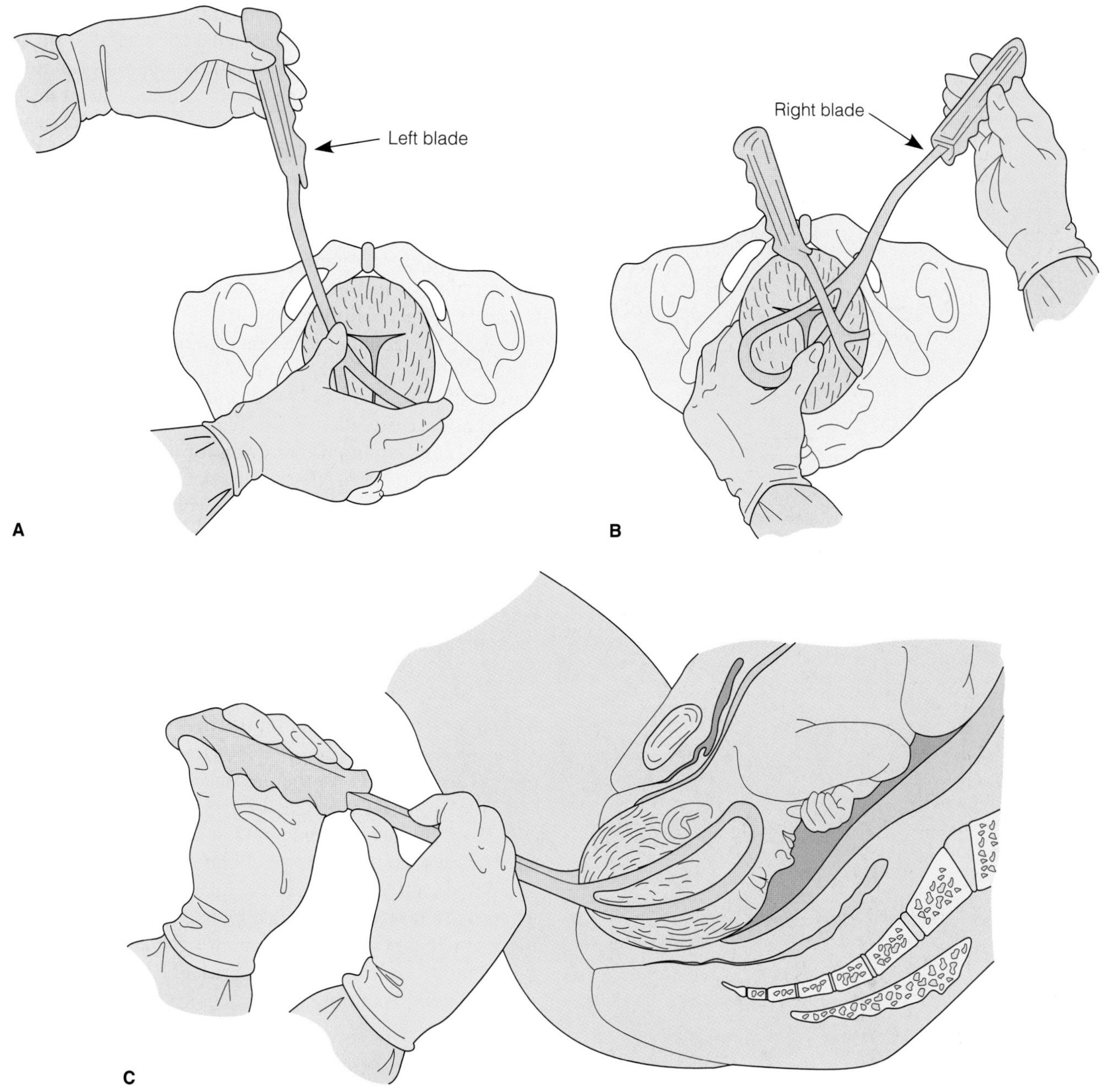

FIGURE 23–5 Application of forceps in occiput anterior (OA) position. ***A,*** The left blade is inserted along the left side wall of the pelvis over the parietal bone. ***B,*** The right blade is inserted along the right side wall of the pelvis over the parietal bone. ***C,*** With correct placement of the blades, the handles lock easily. During uterine contractions, traction is applied to the forceps in a downward and outward direction to follow the birth canal.

The newborn is assessed for facial edema, bruising, caput succedaneum, cephalhematoma, and any sign of cerebral edema. In the fourth stage, the nurse assesses the woman for perineal swelling, bruising, hematoma, excessive bleeding, and hemorrhage. In the postpartum period it is important to assess for signs of infection if lacerations occurred during the procedure.

The nurse answers questions and reiterates explanations provided, reviews nursing assessments of the woman and her newborn, and provides opportunities for the woman and family to ask further questions.

Care of the Woman during Vacuum Extraction

Vacuum extraction is an obstetric procedure used to assist the birth of a fetus by applying suction to the fetal head. The vacuum extractor is composed of a soft suction cup attached to a suction bottle (pump) by tubing. The suction cup, which comes in various sizes, is placed against the occiput of the fetal head. Care must be taken to ensure that no cervical or vaginal tissue is trapped under the cup. The pump is used to create negative pressure

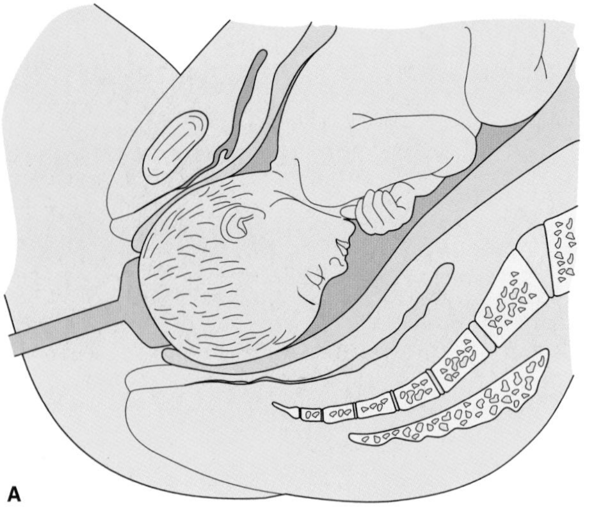

A

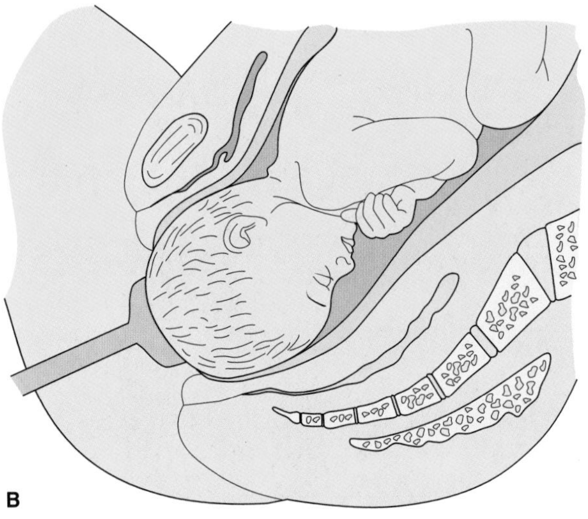

B

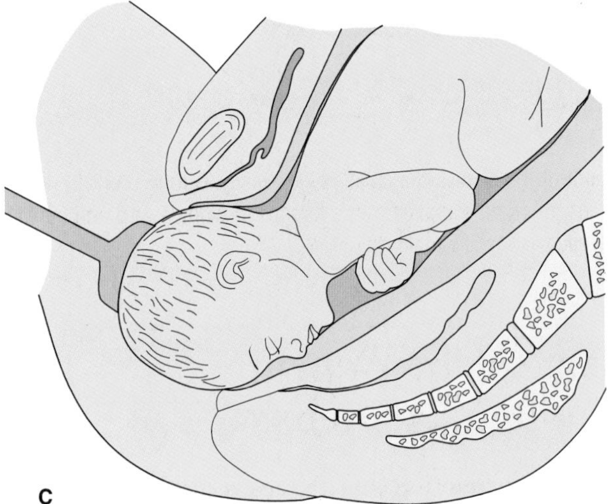

C

FIGURE 23–6 Vacuum extractor traction. ***A,*** The cup is placed on the fetal occiput creating suction. Traction is applied in a downward and outward direction. ***B,*** Traction continues in a downward direction as the fetal head begins to emerge from the vagina. ***C,*** Traction is maintained to lift the fetal head out of the vagina.

(suction) of approximately 50 to 60 mm Hg, and an artificial caput ("chignon") is formed as the fetal scalp is pulled into the cup. The physician then applies traction in coordination with uterine contractions, the fetal head should descend with each contraction, and the fetal head is born (Figure 23–6). Teng and Sayre (1997) report the duration of time the negative suction is applied varies from 0.5 to 26 minutes, with a median of 3 minutes. Negative suction applied for more than 10 minutes was associated with a greater incidence of scalp injury. The longer the duration of suction, the more likely the neonate will have scalp injury. Although the ACOG does not specify a time limit for vacuum extraction procedures, general recommendations are that there should be progressive descent with the first two pulls and that the procedure should not exceed 30 minutes (Teng & Sayre, 1997).

The most common indication for use of the vacuum extractor is a prolonged second stage of labor. Vacuum extraction is also used to relieve the woman of pushing effort or when analgesia or fatigue interfere with her ability to push effectively. The vacuum extractor is preferred to forceps in cases of borderline CPD, when successful passage of the fetal head requires all potential space inside the vaginal canal. CPD is an absolute contraindication to vacuum extraction. Relative contraindications include suspected fetal macrosomia, high fetal station, face or breech presentation, gestation less than 35 weeks, incompletely dilated cervix, and previous fetal scalp blood sampling (Keane, 1997). In the presence of a preterm gestation, risk of periventricular-intraventricular hemorrhage (PV-IVH) has been a concern, and some studies provide conflicting recommendations. Thomas, Morgan, Asrat, and Weeks (1997) in a retrospective study found that when there is an indicated use for vacuum extraction using a silicone cup and the fetus weighs 2000 g or less, there appears to be no associated risk of PV-IVH or other neonatal complications.

NURSING CARE MANAGEMENT

There are different types of vacuum extractors. The nurse should be familiar with the types used within the birthing setting and learn the pressure limits of each type.

The nurse should inform the woman about what is happening during the procedure. If adequate regional anesthesia has been administered, the woman feels only pressure during the procedure. The FHR should be auscultated at least every 5 minutes or assessed by continuous electronic fetal monitoring. The parents need to be informed that the caput (chignon) on the baby's head will disappear within 2 to 3 days.

The nurse should continue to assess the newborn for cephalhematomas, intracranial hemorrhage, and retinal hemorrhages (Sachs, Kobelin, Castro, & Frigoletto, 1999).

Care of the Family during Cesarean Birth

Cesarean birth is the birth of the infant through an abdominal and uterine incision. Cesarean birth is one of the oldest surgical procedures known. Until the 20th century, cesareans were primarily equated with an attempt to save the fetus of a dying woman. As the maternal and perinatal morbidity and mortality rates associated with cesarean birth steadily decreased throughout the 20th century, the rate of cesarean births increased. In 1970, cesarean births comprised 5.5% of all births and progressed to a high of 24.7% in 1988 (Sachs et al, 1999). Then, as a result of concern about the high rates and about the associated increase in health care costs, the rates decreased to 21% in 1995 (Curtin & Kozak, 1997). Internationally, the incidence has been much lower throughout the 20th century; England, Scotland, and Sweden have rates of approximately 10% to 12% and the rate in Japan is 7% (Depp, 1996).

Many factors affect the cesarean birth rate, and they need to be considered in discussions about decreasing the current rate in the United States. These factors include changing philosophies regarding the best method of delivering breech presentation, interpretations of EFM tracings, changing practice related to vaginal birth after cesarean birth, increased use of epidural anesthesia, and physician convenience (Sachs et al, 1999).

Indications

Cesarean births are performed in the presence of a variety of maternal and fetal conditions. Commonly accepted indications include complete placenta previa, cephalic pelvic disproportion, placental abruption, active genital herpes, umbilical cord prolapse, failure to progress in labor, proven fetal distress, benign and malignant tumors that obstruct the birth canal, and cervical cerclage (Keane, 1997). Indications that are more controversial include breech presentation, previous cesarean birth, major congenital anomalies, and severe Rh isoimmunization.

Maternal Mortality and Morbidity

Cesarean births have a higher maternal mortality rate than vaginal births. Approximately 5.8 women per 100,000 live births die, and about half of the deaths are attributed to the operation and a coexisting medical condition (Bowes, 1999). Perinatal morbidity is primarily associated with infection, reactions to anesthesia agents, blood clots, and bleeding.

Surgical Techniques

Skin Incisions

The skin incision for a cesarean birth is either transverse (Pfannenstiel) or vertical and is not indicative of the type of incision made into the uterus. The transverse incision

COMMUNITY IN FOCUS

ICAN (International Cesarean Awareness Network)

The International Cesarean Awareness Network (ICAN) is a volunteer organization committed to three broad goals: (1) to lower the high cesarean birth rate through education; (2) to provide a forum through which individuals can express their thoughts and concerns about the birth experience; and (3) to provide a support network for women who are healing from past birth experiences and those who are preparing for future births. With headquarters in Redondo Beach, California, the organization currently has approximately 32 chapters throughout the United States including ICAN of Southeast Minnesota, New York City, Los Angeles, Northeast Ohio, Houston, Washington DC, and Denver, to name a few.

ICAN was founded in 1982 by Esther Zorn, a woman who had a traumatic cesarean birth experience and wanted to have a vaginal birth in a subsequent pregnancy. At the time, VBAC (vaginal birth after cesarean) was extremely rare, but Ms Zorn persevered and was able to find a like-minded caregiver to enable her to give birth vaginally.

Members of ICAN typically are women who have had a cesarean birth experience and are pregnant or planning another pregnancy, which they hope to complete by VBAC. They join ICAN for information, support, and referral to caregivers who agree with a generally non-interventionist approach to childbirth. Other participants include childbirth educators, nurses, other health care providers, and community members who are opposed to unnecessary cesarean births and supportive of organizations that empower women.

ICAN chapters hold monthly meetings that feature a variety of educational topics. The meetings also provide a forum for the exchange of ideas and a safe place in which to explore feelings and attitudes. Phone counseling is also available for women who are in need of information or emotional support. In addition, all members receive a quarterly newsletter, the *Clarion*.

It is difficult to evaluate the overall effect of an organization like ICAN. Historically, the impact of concerned citizens on the birth experience has been significant. Consumers have actively sought the opportunity for the family to participate more fully in the birth experience and changes such as the presence of a partner or other loved ones at birth, rooming-in, and early discharge have resulted. Moreover, the incidence of VBAC has risen markedly over the past 10 years as women actively challenged the old axiom, "Once a cesarean, always a cesarean." It is exciting, however, to see how a grassroots effort such as ICAN can take hold and flourish because it provides a valuable service to childbearing women and their families.

SOURCE: Personal communication with April Kubachka, President of ICAN, and ICAN literature.

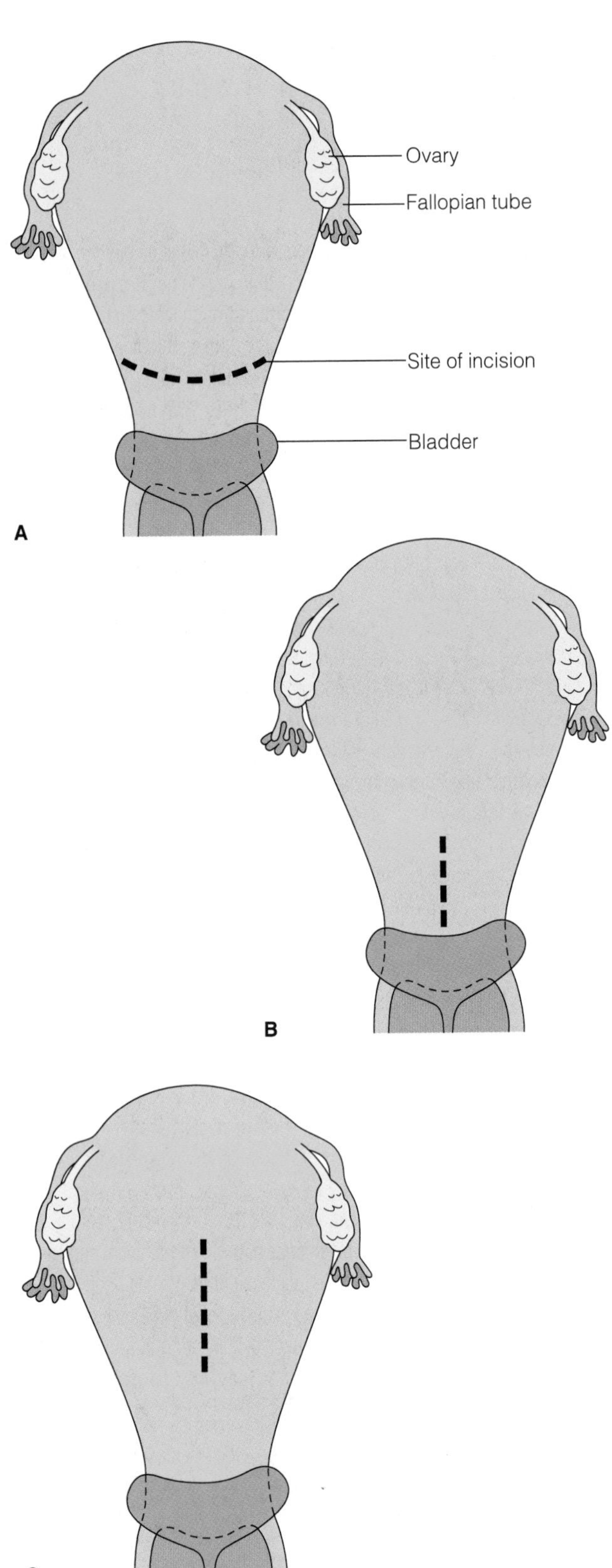

FIGURE 23–7 Uterine incisions for a cesarean birth. ***A,*** This transverse incision in the lower uterine segment is called a Kerr incision. ***B,*** The Sellheim incision is a vertical incision in the lower uterine segment. ***C,*** This view illustrates the classic uterine incision that is done in the body (corpus) of the uterus. The classic incision was commonly done in the past and is associated with increased risk of uterine rupture in subsequent pregnancies and labor.

is made across the lowest and narrowest part of the abdomen. Because the incision is made just below the pubic hair line, it is almost invisible after healing. The limitations of this type of skin incision are that it does not allow for extension of the incision if needed. Because it usually requires more time, this incision is used when time is not of the essence (eg, with failure to progress and no fetal or maternal distress).

The vertical (infraumbilical midline) incision is made between the navel and the symphysis pubis. This incision is quicker and is therefore preferred in cases of fetal distress when rapid birth is indicated, preterm or macrosomic infants, or when the woman is obese (Cunningham et al, 1997a). The type of skin incision is determined by time factor, client preference, or physician preference.

Uterine Incisions

The type of uterine incision depends on the need for the cesarean. The choice of incision affects the woman's opportunity for a subsequent vaginal birth and her risks of a ruptured uterine scar with a subsequent pregnancy.

The two major locations of uterine incisions are the lower uterine segment and the upper segment of the uterine corpus.

The most common lower uterine segment incision is a transverse incision, although a vertical incision may also be used (Figure 23–7). The transverse incision is preferred for the following reasons (Cunningham et al, 1997a):

1. The lower segment is the thinnest portion of the uterus and involves less blood loss.
2. It requires only moderate dissection of bladder from underlying myometrium.
3. It is easier to repair, although repair takes longer.
4. The site is less likely to rupture during subsequent pregnancies.
5. There is a decreased chance of adherence of bowel or omentum to the incision line.

The disadvantages include the following:

1. It takes longer to make a transverse incision.
2. It is limited in size because of the presence of major blood vessels on either side of the uterus.
3. It has a greater tendency to extend laterally into the uterine vessels.
4. The incision may stretch and become a thin window, but it usually does not create problems clinically until subsequent labor ensues.

The lower uterine segment vertical incision is preferred for multiple gestation, abnormal presentation, placenta previa, fetal distress, and preterm and macrosomic fetuses. Disadvantages of this incision are as follows:

1. The incision may extend downward into the cervix.
2. More extensive dissection of the bladder is needed to keep the incision in the lower uterine segment.

3. If the incision extends upward into the upper segment, hemostasis and closure are more difficult.
4. The vertical incision carries a higher risk of rupture with subsequent labor.

One other incision, the classic incision, was the method of choice for many years but is used infrequently now. This vertical incision was made into the upper uterine segment. More blood loss resulted, and it was more difficult to repair. Most important, it carried an increased risk of uterine rupture with subsequent pregnancy, labor, and birth because the upper uterine segment is the most contractile portion of the uterus.

Nursing Care

Preparation for Cesarean Birth

Because one out of every five births is a cesarean, preparing the woman and family for this possibility should be an integral part of prenatal education. Nurses should encourage all pregnant women and their partners to discuss with their obstetrician/CNM what approach would be taken in the event of a cesarean. They can also discuss their needs and desires as a couple under those circumstances. Their preferences may include the following:

- Participating in the choice of anesthetic
- Presence of the father (or significant other) during the procedures and/or birth
- Presence of the father (or significant other) in the recovery or postpartum room
- Audio recording and/or taking pictures of the birth
- Delayed instillation of eye drops to promote eye contact between parent and infant in the first hours after birth
- Physical contact or holding the newborn while on the operating room table or in the recovery room (If the mother cannot hold the newborn, the father can hold the baby for her.)
- Breastfeeding immediately after birth

Information that couples need about cesarean birth includes the following:

- Preparation that may be done, such as abdominal prep, insertion of an indwelling bladder catheter, and starting an intravenous infusion
- Description or viewing of the delivery room
- Types of anesthesia for birth and analgesia available postpartum
- Sensations that may be experienced
- Roles of significant others
- Interaction with newborn
- Immediate recovery phase
- Postpartal phase

The context in which this information is given should be "birth oriented" rather than surgery oriented.

Preparation for Repeat Cesarean Birth

When a couple is anticipating a cesarean birth, they have time to analyze and synthesize the information they are given and to prepare for the experience. Many hospitals or local groups provide preparation classes for cesarean birth. The instructor should impart factual information and a feeling of normality, which will allow a couple to make choices and participate in their birth experience. Couples who have had previous negative experiences need an opportunity to describe what they felt contributed to these events. They should be encouraged to identify what they would like to have altered and to list interventions that would make the experience more positive. Those who have had positive experiences need reassurance that their needs and desires will be met in the same manner. In addition, the nurse should provide an opportunity for the couple to discuss any fears or anxieties.

Preparation for Emergency Cesarean Birth

The period preceding surgery must be used to its greatest advantage. The couple needs some time for privacy to assimilate the information given to them and to ask for additional information. It is imperative that caregivers use their most effective communication skills. The nurse must address what the couple may anticipate during the next few hours. Asking the couple, "What questions do you have about the decision?" gives the couple an opportunity for further clarification. The nurse can prepare the woman in stages, giving her information and the rationale for each procedure before commencing. Before carrying out a procedure, it is essential to tell the woman (1) what is going to happen, (2) why it is being done, and (3) what sensations she may experience. This allows the woman to be informed and to consent to the procedure. The woman experiences a sense of control and therefore less helplessness and powerlessness.

Preparing the woman for surgery involves more than the procedures of establishing intravenous lines and urinary indwelling catheter or doing an abdominal prep. As discussed previously, good communication skills are essential in assisting the couple. Therapeutic use of touch and eye contact (if culturally acceptable and possible) do much to maintain reality orientation and control. These measures reduce anxiety for the woman during the stressful preparatory period.

If the cesarean birth is scheduled and not an emergency, the nurse has ample time for preoperative teaching. The woman needs to practice her turning, coughing, and deep breathing. It is helpful if she is taught to splint her abdominal muscles when she coughs. An informed consent for surgery will need to be signed.

To prepare the woman for the surgery, she is given nothing by mouth. To reduce the likelihood of serious pulmonary damage should aspiration of gastric contents occur, antacids may be administered within 30 minutes of surgery. If epidural anesthesia is used, the nurse may assist with the procedure, monitor the woman's blood pressure and response, and continue EFM. An abdominal and perineal prep is done, and an indwelling catheter is inserted to prevent bladder distention. An intravenous line is started with a needle of adequate size to permit blood administration, and preoperative medication may be ordered. The pediatrician should be notified and adequate preparation made to receive the infant. The nurse should make sure that the infant warmer is functional and that appropriate resuscitation equipment is available.

The nurse assists in positioning the woman on the operating table. Fetal heart rate should be ascertained before surgery and during preparation because fetal hypoxia can result from aortocaval compression. The operating table may be adjusted so it slants slightly to one side, or a wedge (folded blanket or towels) may be placed under the right hip. The uterus should be displaced about 15 degrees from the midline. This helps relieve the pressure of the heavy uterus on the vena cava and lessens the incidence of vena caval compression and supine maternal hypotension. The suction should be in working order, and the urine collection bag should be positioned under the operating table to ensure proper urinary drainage. Auscultation or electronic monitoring of the fetal heart rate needs to continue until immediately prior to the surgery. A last-minute check is done to ensure that the fetal scalp electrode has been removed if the fetus was internally monitored.

Birth

Every effort should be made to include the father/partner in the birth experience. When the father attends the cesarean birth, he must scrub and wear a surgical gown and mask as do others in the operating suite. The father can sit on a stool placed beside the woman's head to provide physical touch, visual contact, and verbal reassurance to his partner.

Other measures, such as the following, can be taken to promote the participation of the father who chooses not to be in the delivery room:

1. Allowing the father to be near the delivery/operating room, where he can hear the newborn's first cry
2. Encouraging the father to carry or accompany the infant to the nursery for the initial assessment
3. Involving the father in postpartal care in the recovery room

After birth, the nurse assesses the Apgar score and completes the initial assessment and identification procedures as after a vaginal birth. Every effort must be made to assist the parents in bonding with the infant. If the mother is awake, one of her arms should be freed to enable her to touch and stroke the infant. The baby can be given to the father to hold until she or he must be taken to the nursery.

Analgesia and Anesthesia

There is no perfect anesthesia for cesarean birth. Each has its advantages, disadvantages, possible risks, and side effects. Goals for analgesia and anesthesia administration include safety, comfort, and emotional satisfaction for the client. See Chapter 21.

Immediate Postpartal Recovery Period

The nurse caring for the postpartal woman should check the mother's vital signs every 5 minutes until they are stable, then every 15 minutes for an hour, then every 30 minutes until she is discharged to the postpartal unit. The nurse should remain with the woman until she is stable.

The dressing and perineal pad must be checked every 15 minutes for at least an hour, and the fundus should be gently palpated to determine whether it is remaining firm. The fundus may be palpated by placing a hand to support the incision. Intravenous oxytocin is usually administered to promote the contractility of the uterine musculature. If the woman has been under general anesthesia, she should be positioned on her side to facilitate drainage of secretions, turned, and assisted with coughing and deep breathing every 2 hours for at least 24 hours. If she has received a spinal or epidural anesthetic, the level of anesthesia should be checked every 15 minutes. It is important to monitor intake and output and to observe the urine for bloody tinge, which could mean surgical trauma to the bladder. The physician prescribes medication to relieve the mother's pain and nausea, and this should be administered as needed. Some physicians use a single dose of epidural morphine (5 to 7.5 mg) for postsurgical pain relief. Facilitation of parent-infant interaction following birth and postpartal care is discussed in Chapter 31. Pertinent areas of nursing care are addressed in the Cesarean Birth Critical Pathway in Chapter 32.

Care of the Woman Undergoing Vaginal Birth after Cesarean (VBAC)

There is an increasing trend to have a trial of labor and **vaginal birth after cesarean (VBAC)** birth in cases of nonrecurring indications (for example, umbilical cord accident, placenta previa, fetal distress). This trend has been influenced by consumer demand and studies that support VBAC as a viable alternative (Keane, 1997).

The 1988 ACOG guidelines state that the following aspects need to be considered for VBAC:

- A woman with one previous cesarean birth and a low transverse uterine incision should be counseled and encouraged to attempt VBAC.
- A woman with two or more previous cesareans may attempt VBAC.
- A classic uterine incision is a contraindication.
- It must be possible to do a cesarean within 30 minutes.
- A physician who is able to do a cesarean needs to be available.

The most common risks associated with VBAC are hemorrhage and uterine scar separation (uterine rupture). The risk of uterine rupture is approximately 1% (Sachs et al, 1999).

Success rates for VBAC have been encouraging. Women whose previous cesarean was performed because of fetal distress, twins, or breech presentation have been reported to have approximately a 70% chance of success with VBAC (Depp, 1996).

NURSING CARE MANAGEMENT

The nursing care of a woman undergoing VBAC varies according to institutional protocols. Generally, if the woman is at very low risk (has had one previous cesarean with a lower uterine segment incision), her blood count, type, and screen are obtained on admission; a heparin lock is inserted for intravenous access if needed; continuous EFM is used; and clear fluids may be taken. If the woman is at higher risk, NPO status should be maintained and, in addition to the care listed above, an intrauterine catheter may be inserted to monitor intrauterine pressures during labor.

Supportive and comfort measures are very important. The woman may be excited about this opportunity to experience labor and vaginal birth, or she may be hesitant and frightened about the possibility of complications. The presence of the nurse is important in providing information and encouragement for the laboring woman and her partner.

FOCUS YOUR STUDY

- An external (or cephalic) version may be done after 37 weeks' gestation to change a breech presentation to a cephalic presentation, thereby making a lower-risk vaginal birth more possible.The version is accomplished with the use of tocolytic agents to relax the uterus. An internal (podalic) version is used only when needed during the vaginal birth of a second twin.
- Amniotomy (AROM) is performed to hasten labor. The risks are prolapse of the umbilical cord and infection.
- Prostaglandin E_2 may be used before an induction of labor to soften the cervix (called cervical ripening). The gel is inserted into the vagina and held in place with a diaphragm.
- Labor is induced for many reasons. The methods include amniotomy and intravenous oxytocin infusion. Nursing responsibilities are heightened during an induced labor.
- An episiotomy may be performed just before birth of the fetus. Although it is very prevalent in the United States, it is becoming somewhat controversial.
- Forceps-assisted birth can be accomplished using outlet forceps, low forceps, or midforceps. Outlet forceps are the most common and are associated with few maternal-fetal complications. Midforceps are associated with more complications but, when needed, are an important aid to birth.
- A vacuum extractor is a soft, pliable cup attached to suction that can be applied to the fetal head and used in much the same way as forceps.
- At least one in five births is now accomplished by cesarean. The nurse has a vital role in providing information, support, and encouragement to the couple participating in a cesarean birth.
- Vaginal birth after cesarean (VBAC) is becoming more popular. Overcoming the old fears of uterine rupture is a high priority for both the parents and the medical and nursing community.

REFERENCES

American College of Obstetricians and Gynecologists (ACOG). (1988). *Guidelines for vaginal birth after previous cesarean birth.* (ACOG Committee Opinion, No. 64). Washington, DC: Author.

American College of Obstetricians and Gynecologists (ACOG). (1991). *Operative vaginal delivery.* (ACOG Technical Bulletin, No. 152). Washington, DC: American College of Obstetricians and Gynecologists.

American College of Obstetricians and Gynecologists (ACOG). (1993). *Prostaglandin E gel for cervical ripening.* (ACOG Committee Opinion, No. 123). Washington, DC: Author.

American College of Obstetricians and Gynecologists (ACOG). (1995). *Induction of labor.* (ACOG Technical Bulletin, No. 217). Washington, DC: Author.

Arias, F. (1993). *Practical guide to high-risk pregnancy and delivery.* St. Louis: Mosby-Year Book.

Association of Women's Health, Obstetric, and Neonatal Nurses (AWHONN). (1993). *Cervical ripening and induction and augmentation of labor.* Washington, DC: Author.

Bishop, E. H. (1964). Pelvic scoring for elective induction. *Obstetrics Gynecology, 24,* 266.

Bowes, W. A. (1999). Clinical aspects of normal and abnormal labor. In R. K. Creasy & R. Resnik (Eds.), *Maternal-fetal medicine* (4th ed.) (pp 541–568) Philadelphia: Saunders .

Charles, A. G. (1997). Forceps delivery and vacuum extraction. In P. V. Dilts & J. J. Sciarri (Eds.), *Gynecology and obstetrics* (Vol. 2). Philadelphia: Lippincott.

Chyu, J. K., & Strassner, H. T. (1997). Prostaglandin E_2 for cervical ripening: A randomized comparison of Cervidil versus Prepidil. *American Journal of Obstetrics and Gynecology, 177,* 606–611.

Cunningham, F. G., MacDonald, P. C., Gant, N. F., Leveno, L. J., Gilstrap, L. C., Hankins, G. V., & Clark, S. L. (1997a). Cesarean delivery and cesarean hysterectomy. In *Williams obstetrics* (20th ed.) (pp 509–533). Norwalk, CT: Appleton & Lange.

Cunningham, F. G., MacDonald, P. C., Gant, N. F., Leveno, K. J., Gilstrap, L. C., Hankins, G. V., & Clark, S. L. (1997b). Operative vaginal delivery. In *Williams obstetrics* (20th ed.) (pp 473–494). Norwalk, CT: Appleton & Lange.

Curtin, S. C., & Kozak, L. J. (1997). Cesarean delivery rates in 1995 continue to decline in the United States. *Birth, 24,* 194–196.

Ecker, J. L., Tan, W. M., Bansal, R. K., Bishop, J. T., & Kilpatrick, S. J. (1997). Is there a benefit to episiotomy at operative vaginal delivery? Observations over ten years in a stable population. *American Journal of Obstetrics and Gynecology, 176,* 411–414.

Farah, L. A., Sanchez-Ramos, L., Rosa, D., Del Valle, G. O., Gaudier, F., Delke, E., & Kaunitz, A. M. (1997). Randomized trial of two doses of the prostaglandin E_1 analog misoprostol for labor induction. *American Journal of Obstetrics and Gynecology, 177,* 364–371.

Ferguson, W. G. L. (1997). Management of labor and delivery in low-risk patients. In R. K. Creasy (Ed.), *Management of labor and delivery* (pp 92–142). Malden, MA: Blackwell.

Flamm, B. L., Berwick, D. M., & Kabacenell, A. (1998). Reducing cesarean section rates safely: Lessons from a "breakthrough series" collaborative. *Birth, 25,* 117–125.

Forrest Pharmaceuticals, Inc. (1995). *Cervidil Dinoprostone 10 mg. vaginal insert.* Forrest Pharmaceuticals. St. Louis, MO. UAB Laboratories.

Glazener, C. M. A. (1997). Sexual function after childbirth: Women's experiences, persistent morbidity and lack of professional recognition. *British Journal of Obstetrics and Gynaecology, 104,* 330–335.

Goldman, J. B., & Wigton, T. R. (1999). A randomized comaprison of extra-amniotic saline infusion and intracervical Dinoprostone gel for cervical ripening. *Obstetrics Gynecology, 93,* 271–274.

Graham, I. D., & Graham, D. F. (1997). Episiotomy counts: Trends and prevalence in Canada, 1981/1982 to 1992/1994. *Birth, 24,* 141–147.

Healey, M., Porter, M., & Galimberti, A. (1997). Introducing external cephalic version at 36 weeks or more in a district general hospital: A review and an audit. *British Journal of Obstetrics and Gynaecology, 104,* 1073–1079.

Helewa, M. E. (1997). Episiotomy and severe trauma: Of science and fiction. *Canadian Medical Association, 156,* 811–813.

Kaczorowski, J., Levitt, C., Hanvey, L., Avard, D., & Chance, G. A. (1998). National survey of use of obstetric procedures and technologies in Canadian hospitals: Routine or based on existing evidence? *Birth, 25,* 11–18.

Keane, D. P. (1997). Operative procedures. In R. K. Creasy (Ed.), *Management of labor and delivery* (pp 414–457). Malden, MA: Blackwell.

Lau, T. K., Lo, L. W. K., & Rogers, M. S. (1997). Pregnancy outcome after successful external cephalic version for breech presentation at term. *American Journal of Obstetrics and Gynecology, 176,* 218–223.

Lau, T. K., Lo, L. W. K., Wan, D., & Rogers, M. S. (1997). Predictors of successful external cephalic version at term: A prospective study. *British Journal of Obstetrics and Gynaecology, 104,* 798–802.

Maier, J. S., & Maloni, J. A. (1997). Nurse advocacy for selective versus routine episiotomy. *Journal of Obstetrics, Gynecology, and Neonatal Nursing, 26,* 155–161.

Memorial Hospital guidelines for the use of misoprostol (Cytotec) for induction of labor. (1998). Memorial Hospital Family Birthing Center, Colorado Springs, CO.

Miyazaki, F. S. (1996). Saline amnioinfusion indications and technique. In J. T. Queenan & J. C. Hobbins (Eds.), *Protocols for high-risk pregnancies* (3rd ed.) (pp 161–164). Cambridge, MA: Blackwell.

PDR nurse's handbook. (1999). Montvale, NJ: Demar Publishers and Medical Economics Co., Inc.

Reva, A., Ezra, Y., Farine, D., & Ritchie, K. (1997). Failed trial of vacuum or forceps—maternal and fetal outcome. *American Journal of Obstetrics and Gynecology, 176,* 200–204.

Sachs, B. P., Kobelin, C., Castro, M. A., & Frigoletto, F. (1999). Sounding board: The risks of lowering the cesarean-delivery rate. *The New England Journal of Medicine, 340,* 54–57.

Schmidt, J. (1997). Fluid check: Making the case for intrapartum amnioinfusion. *AWHONN Lifelines (1),* 47–51.

Solomon, J. E., & D'Alton, M. E. (1997). Induction of labor. In R. K. Creasy (Ed.), *Management of labor and delivery* (pp 293–315). Malden, MA: Blackwell.

Stemple, J. E., Prins, R. P., & Dean, S. (1997). Preinduction cervical ripening: A randomized prospective comparison of the efficacy and safety of intravaginal and intracervical prostaglandin E_2 gel. *American Journal of Obstetrics and Gynecology, 176,* 1305–1312.

Summers, L. (1997). Methods of cervical ripening and labor induction. *Journal of Nurse-Midwifery, 42,* 71–82.

Swaim, L. S., & Creasy, R. K. (1997). Fetal assessment and treatment during labor. In R. K. Creasy (Ed.), *Management of labor and delivery* (pp 143–182). Malden, MA: Blackwell.

Teng, F. Y., & Sayre, J. W. (1997). Vacuum extraction: Does duration predict scalp injury? *Obstetrics and Gynecology, 89,* 281–285.

Thomas, S. J., Morgan, M. A., Asrat, T., & Weeks, J. W. (1997). The risk of periventricular-intraventricular hemorrhage with vacuum extraction of neonates weighing 2000 grams or less. *Journal of Perinatology, 17,* 37–41.

Thorp, J. A. (1997). Malpresentations and special situation. In R. K. Creasy (Ed.), *Management of labor and delivery* (pp 358–394). Malden, MA: Blackwell.

Turcot, L., Marcoux, S., Fraser, W. D., & the Canadian Early Amniotomy Study Group. (1997). Multivariate analysis of risk factors for operative delivery in nulliparous women. *American Journal of Obstetrics and Gynecology, 176,* 395–402.

Weed, S. S. (1985). *Wise woman herbal for the childbearing year.* Woodstock, NY: AshTree Publishing.

Wing, D. A. (1997). A comparison of intermittent vaginal administration of misoprostol with continuous dinoprostone for cervical ripening and labor induction. *American Journal of Obstetrics and Gynecology, 177,* 612–618.

Zatuchi, G. L., & Slupik, R. I. (1996). *Obstetrics and gynecology drug handbook* (2nd ed.) St. Louis: Mosby.

The Newborn

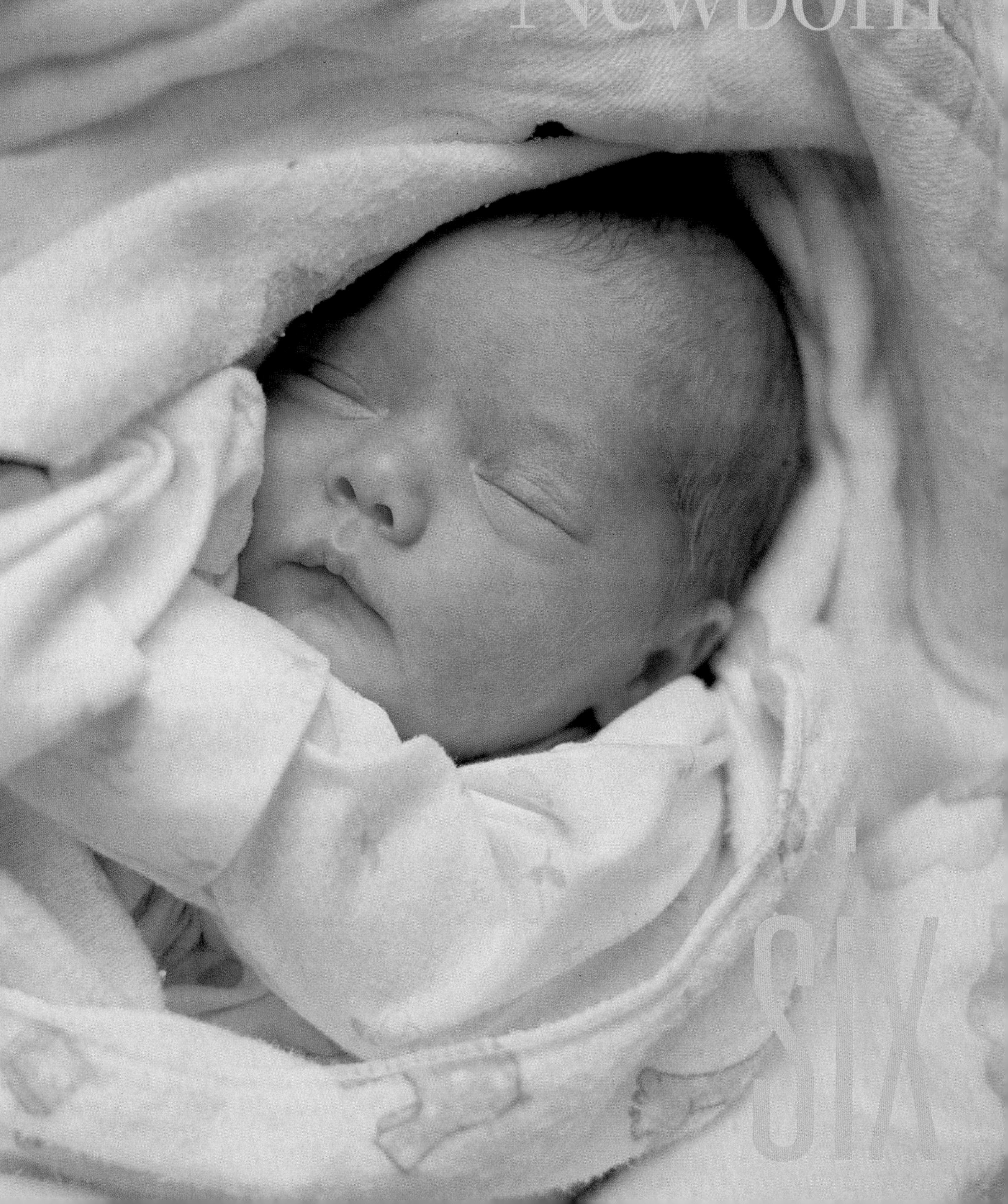

SIX

24 Physiologic Responses of the Newborn to Birth

Key Terms

Active acquired immunity
Brown adipose tissue (BAT)
Cardiopulmonary adaptation
Conduction
Convection
Evaporation
Habituation
Meconium
Neonatal transition
Orientation
Passive acquired immunity
Periodic breathing
Periods of reactivity
Physiologic anemia of infancy
Physiologic jaundice
Radiation
Self-quieting ability
Surfactant
Thermal neutral zone (TNZ)
Total serum bilirubin

THE INCREDIBLE ATTRIBUTES OF THE NEWBORN HAVE a major purpose. They prepare the baby for interaction with the family and for life in the world.
~ *The Amazing Newborn* ~

Objectives

- Summarize the respiratory and cardiovascular changes that occur during the transition to extrauterine life.
- Describe how various factors affect the newborn's blood values.
- Correlate the major mechanisms of heat loss in the newborn to the process of thermogenesis in the newborn.
- Explain the steps involved in conjugation and excretion of bilirubin in the newborn.
- Discuss the reasons why the newborn may develop jaundice.
- Delineate the functional abilities of the newborn's gastrointestinal tract and liver.
- Identify the reasons the newborn's kidneys have difficulty maintaining fluid and electrolyte balance.
- List the immunologic responses available to the newborn.
- Explain the physiologic and behavioral responses of newborns during the periods of reactivity, and identify possible interventions.
- Describe the normal sensory/perceptual abilities and behavioral states present in the newborn period.

THE NEWBORN PERIOD IS THE TIME from birth through the first 28 days of life. During this period, the newborn adjusts from intrauterine to extrauterine life. The nurse needs to be knowledgeable about a newborn's normal physiologic and behavioral adaptations and be able to recognize alterations from normal.

To begin life as a separate being, the baby must immediately establish respiratory gas exchange, which occurs in conjunction with marked circulatory changes. These radical and rapid changes are crucial to the maintenance of extrauterine life. The first few hours of life, in which the newborn stabilizes respiratory and circulatory functions, are called **neonatal transition.** All other newborn body systems change their level of functioning or become established over a longer period of time during the neonatal period.

Respiratory Adaptations

Although the significant respiratory events occur at birth, certain intrauterine factors also enhance the newborn's ability to breathe.

Intrauterine Factors Supporting Respiratory Function

Fetal Lung Development

The respiratory system is in a continuous state of development during fetal life, and lung development continues into early childhood. During the first 20 weeks of gestation, lung development is limited to the differentiation of pulmonary, vascular, and lymphatic structures. At 20 to 24 weeks, alveolar ducts begin to appear, followed by primitive alveoli at 24 to 28 weeks. During this time, the alveolar epithelial cells begin to differentiate into type I cells (structures necessary for respiratory gas exchange) and type II cells (structures that provide for the synthesis and storage of surfactant). **Surfactant** is composed of a group of surface-active phospholipids (lecithin and sphingomyelin), which are critical for alveolar stability.

At 28 to 32 weeks of gestation, the number of type II cells increases further, and surfactant is produced by choline pathway within type II cells. Surfactant production by this pathway peaks at about 35 weeks of gestation and remains high until term, paralleling late fetal lung development. At this time, the lungs are structurally developed enough to maintain good lung expansion and adequate exchange of gases.

Clinically, the peak production of lecithin corresponds closely to the marked decrease in incidence of idiopathic respiratory distress syndrome for babies born after 35 weeks' gestation. Production of sphingomyelin (one component of surfactant) remains constant during gestation. The newborn born before the lecithin/sphingomyelin (L/S) ratio is 2:1 will have varying degrees of respiratory distress. (See discussion of L/S ratio in Chapters 17 and 29.)

Fetal Breathing Movements

The newborn's ability to breathe immediately on exposure to air in the extrauterine environment appears to be the consequence of weeks of intrauterine practice. In this respect, breathing can be regarded as a continuation of an intrauterine process in which the lungs convert from fluid-filled to gas-filled organs. Fetal breathing movements (FBM) occur as early as 11 weeks' gestation (see Chapter 17 for discussion). These breathing movements are essential for developing the chest wall muscles and the diaphragm and, to a lesser extent, for regulating lung fluid volume and resultant lung growth.

Initiation of Breathing

To maintain life, the lungs must function immediately after birth. Two radical changes must take place for the lungs to function:

1. Pulmonary ventilation must be established through lung expansion following birth.
2. A marked increase in the pulmonary circulation must occur.

The first breath of life—the gasp in response to mechanical, chemical, thermal, and sensory changes associated with birth—initiates the serial opening of the alveoli. So begins the transition from a fluid-filled environment to an air-breathing, independent, extrauterine life. Figure 24–1 summarizes the initiation of respiration.

Mechanical Events

During the latter half of gestation, the fetal lungs continuously produce fluid. This fluid production expands the lungs almost completely, filling the air spaces. Some of the lung fluid moves up into the trachea and into the amniotic fluid. The amniotic fluid is then swallowed by the fetus.

Production of lung fluid diminishes 2 to 4 days before onset of labor. However, approximately 80 to 110 mL of fluid remains in the respiratory passages of a normal term fetus at the time of birth. This fluid must be removed from the lungs to permit adequate movement of air.

The primary mechanical events that initiate respiration involve removal of fluid from the lungs as the fetus passes through the birth canal. During the birth process the fetal chest is compressed, increasing intrathoracic pressure, and approximately one-third of the fluid is squeezed out of the lungs. After the birth of the newborn's trunk, the chest wall recoils. This chest recoil creates negative intrathoracic pressure, which is thought to

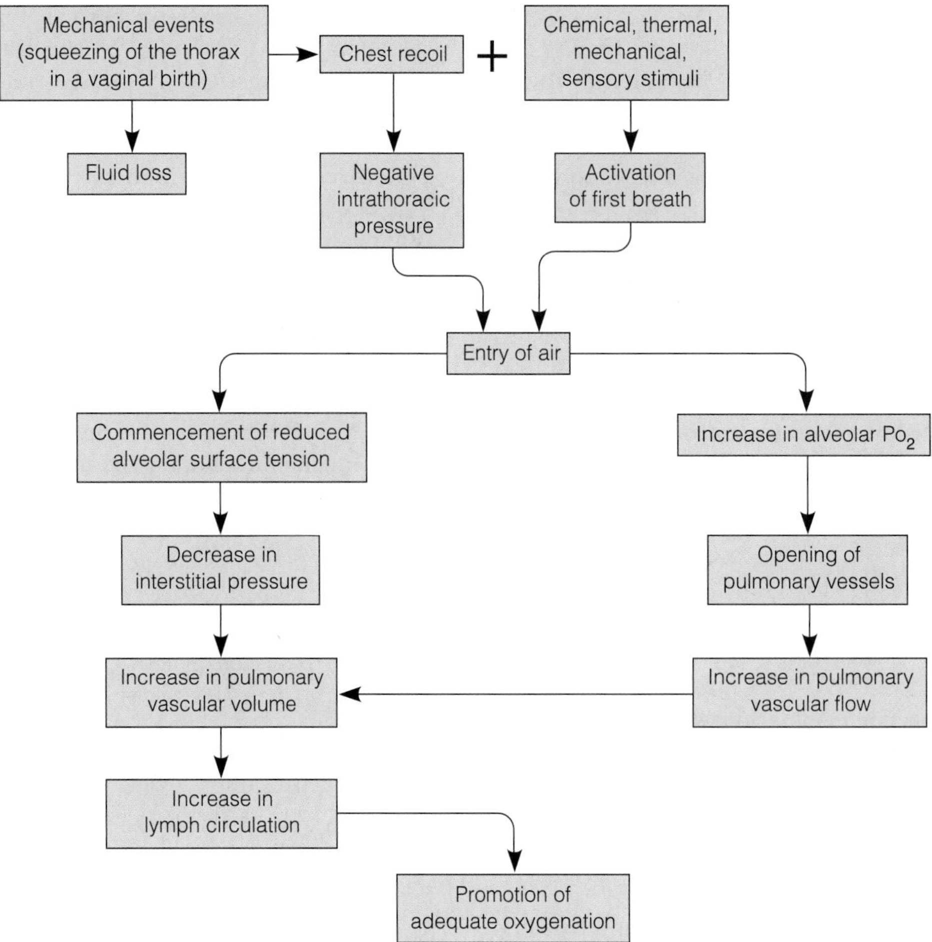

FIGURE 24–1 Initiation of respiration in the neonate.

produce a small, passive inspiration of air that replaces the fluid that was squeezed out.

After this first inspiration, the newborn exhales, with crying, against a partially closed glottis, creating a positive intrathoracic pressure. The high positive intrathoracic pressure distributes the inspired air throughout the alveoli and begins the establishment of *functional residual capacity (FRC)*, the air left in the lungs at the end of a normal expiration. The higher intrathoracic pressure also increases absorption of lung fluid via the capillaries and lymphatic system. The negative intrathoracic pressure resulting from downward movement of the diaphragm with inspiration causes lung fluid to flow from the alveoli across the alveolar membranes into the pulmonary interstitial tissue.

With each succeeding breath, the lungs expand, stretching the alveolar walls and increasing the alveolar volume. Because the protein concentration is higher in the pulmonary capillaries, oncotic pressure draws the interstitial fluid into the capillaries and lymphatic tissue. The expansion of the lung facilitates movement of the remaining lung fluid into the interstitial tissue. As pulmonary vascular resistance decreases, pulmonary blood flow increases, and more interstitial fluid is absorbed into the bloodstream. In the normal term newborn, lung fluid moves rapidly into the interstitial tissue but may take several hours to move into the lymph and blood vessels. Figure 24–2 depicts the changes in fetal lung fluid with the first and subsequent breaths. About 80% of the fluid is reabsorbed within 2 hours after birth, and it is completely absorbed within 12 to 24 hours after birth.

Although the initial chest compression and recoil should clear the airways of accumulated fluid and permit further inspiration, most clinicians feel it is wise to suction mucus and fluid from the newborn's mouth and oropharynx. They use a mucus trap attached to suction as soon as the newborn's head and shoulders are born and again as the newborn adapts to extrauterine life and stabilizes (see Procedure 20–1, and Chapter 20).

Problems associated with lung fluid clearance or initiation of respiratory activity may be caused by a variety of factors. The lymphatic system may be underdeveloped, thus decreasing the rate at which the fluid is absorbed from the lungs. Complications that occur antenatally or during labor and birth can interfere with adequate lung expansion, causing failure to decrease pulmonary vascular resistance, resulting in decreased pulmonary blood flow. These complications include inadequate compression of

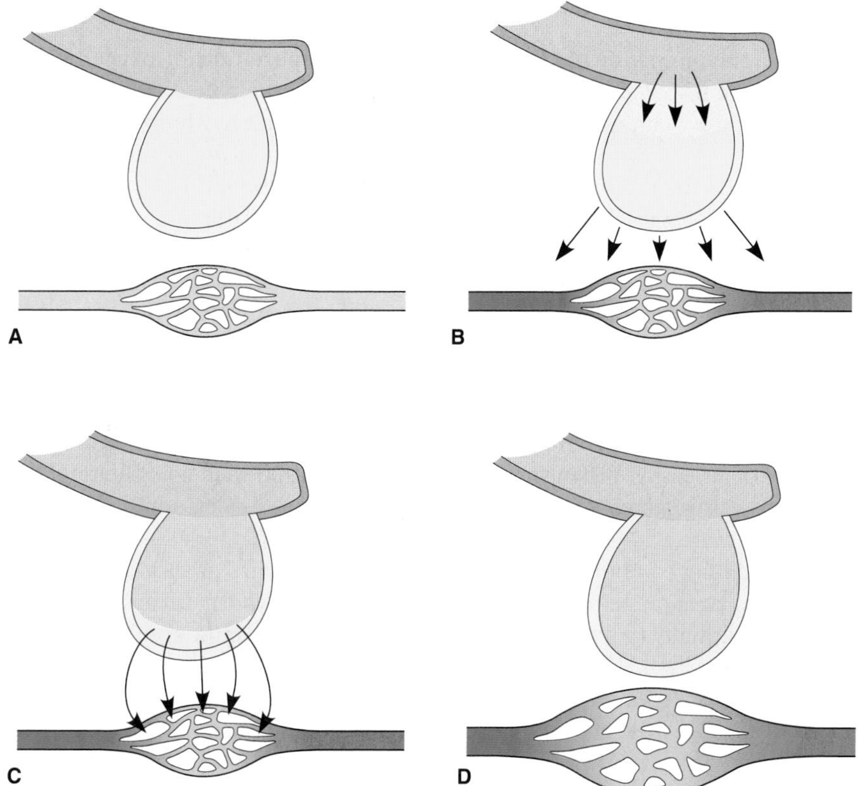

FIGURE 24–2 Process of absorption of fetal lung fluid during breathing after birth. ***A,*** Fetal alveoli filled to functional residual capacity with fetal lung fluid. Fetal lung fluid is produced by the alveoli, fills the airways, and eventually enters the amniotic fluid. ***B,*** After fetal chest compression, one-third of the fetal lung fluid is squeezed out, allowing air to enter passively as the chest recoils. ***C,*** With each subsequent breath, the lungs expand, facilitating the movement of the remaining fetal lung fluid into the capillaries and lymphatic system. Pulmonary blood flow is increasing. ***D,*** Normal alveoli after removal of fetal lung fluid and dilatation of pulmonary arteries. Surfactant has lined the inside of the alveoli to prevent collapse.

the chest wall in a very small newborn, the absence of the chest wall compression in the newborn born by cesarean birth, respiratory depression secondary to maternal anesthesia, or aspiration of amniotic fluid or meconium.

Chemical Stimuli

An important chemical stimulator that contributes to the onset of breathing is transitory asphyxia of the fetus and newborn. The first breath is really an inspiratory gasp triggered by the elevation in PCO_2 and decrease in pH and PO_2, which are the natural result of normal vaginal birth with cessation of placental gas exchange when the cord is clamped. These changes, present in all newborns to some degree, stimulate the aortic and carotid chemoreceptors, initiating impulses that trigger the medulla's respiratory center. Although this brief period of asphyxia is a significant stimulator, prolonged asphyxia is abnormal and acts as a CNS respiratory depressant.

Thermal Stimuli

A significant decrease in ambient temperature after birth—from 37C to 21 to 23.9C (98.6F to 70 to 75F)—also stimulates the initiation of breathing. The cold stimulates nerve endings of the skin, and the newborn responds with rhythmic respirations. Normal temperature changes that occur at birth are apparently within acceptable physiologic limits. Excessive cooling, however, may result in profound respiratory depression and evidence of cold stress (see Chapter 29 for discussion of cold stress).

Sensory Stimuli

As the fetus moves from a familiar, comfortable environment, a number of sensory and physical influences help initiate respiration. They include the numerous tactile, auditory, and visual stimuli of birth. During intrauterine life, the fetus is in a dark, sound-dampened, fluid-filled environment and is nearly weightless. After birth the newborn experiences light, sounds, and the effects of gravity for the first time. Joint movement results in enhanced proprioreceptive stimulation to the respiratory center to sustain respirations. Historically, vigorous stimulation was provided by slapping the buttocks or heels of the newborn, but today greater emphasis is placed on gentle physical contact. Thoroughly drying the newborn and placing it in skin-to-skin contact with the mother's chest and abdomen provides stimulation in a far more comforting way and also decreases heat loss.

Factors Opposing the First Breath

Three major factors may oppose the initiation of respiratory activity: (1) alveolar surface tension, (2) viscosity of lung fluid within the respiratory tract, and (3) degree of lung compliance.

The contracting force between the moist surfaces of the alveoli is called *alveolar surface tension.* This tension, which is necessary for healthy respiratory function, would nevertheless cause the small airways and alveoli to collapse after each inspiration were it not for the presence of surfactant. By reducing the attracting force between alveoli, surfactant prevents the alveoli from completely collapsing with each expiration and thus promotes lung expansion. Similarly, surfactant promotes lung compliance, the ability of the lung to fill with air easily. When surfactant is decreased, compliance is also decreased, and the pressure needed to expand the alveoli with air increases. Resistive forces of the fluid-filled lung combined with the small radii of the airways necessitates pressures of 30 to 40 cm of water to open the lung initially (Thureen, Deacon, O'Neill, & Hernandez, 1999).

The first breath usually establishes functional residual capacity (FRC) that is 30% to 40% of the fully expanded lung volume. This FRC allows alveolar sacs to remain partially expanded on expiration. Thus the air that remains in the lung after expiration (FRC) decreases the need for continuous high pressures for each of the following breaths. Subsequent breaths require only 6 to 8 cm H_2O pressure to open alveoli during inspiration. Thus, the first breath of life is usually the most difficult.

Cardiopulmonary Physiology

The onset of respiration stimulates in the cardiovascular system changes that are necessary for the successful transition to extrauterine life, hence the term **cardiopulmonary adaptation.** As air enters the lungs, Po_2 rises in the alveoli, which stimulates the relaxation of the pulmonary arteries and triggers a decrease in the pulmonary vascular resistance. As pulmonary vascular resistance decreases, the vascular flow in the lung increases very rapidly and achieves 100% normal flow volume at 24 hours of life. This delivery of greater blood volume to the lungs contributes to the conversion from fetal circulation to newborn circulation.

After pulmonary circulation is established, blood is distributed throughout the lung, although the alveoli may or may not be fully open. For adequate oxygenation to occur, sufficient blood must be delivered by the heart to the functioning open alveoli. Shunting of blood is common in the early newborn period. Bidirectional blood flow, or right-to-left shunting through the ductus arteriosus, may divert a significant amount of blood away from the lungs, depending on the pressure changes of respiration, crying, and the cardiac cycle. This shunting in the newborn period is also responsible for the unstable transitional period in cardiopulmonary function.

Oxygen Transport

The transportation of oxygen to the peripheral tissues depends on the type of hemoglobin in the red blood cell. In the fetus and newborn, a variety of hemoglobins exists, the most significant being fetal hemoglobin (HbF) and adult hemoglobin (HbA). Approximately 70% to 90% of hemoglobin in the fetus and newborn is fetal hemoglobin. The greatest difference between HbF and HbA is related to the transport of oxygen.

The oxygen-carrying capacity of fetal hemoglobin is lower than that of adult hemoglobin. Although each gram of fetal hemoglobin carries less oxygen, it has a greater affinity for the oxygen molecules it carries. At any given arterial oxygen level, fetal hemoglobin has a greater oxygen saturation than adult hemoglobin. Thus the oxygen-hemoglobin dissociation curve for fetal hemoglobin lies to the left of that for adult hemoglobin (Figure 24–3). Fetal hemoglobin's greater affinity for oxygen benefits the fetus and newborn because it facilitates oxygen transfer across the placenta and into the newborn's tissues. In utero, the fetus has an arterial oxygen tension (Pao_2) between 30 and 40 mm Hg. Due to the nature of the fetal hemoglobin as depicted in the curve, small changes in fetal Pao_2 result in a great amount of oxygen loading in the placenta or unloading to the tissues as compared to the adult. Fetal hemoglobin's greater affinity for oxygen also requires that a lower tissue oxygen level exist prior to oxygen unloading than required by adult hemoglobin. Due to this phenomenon, the newborn will have both a lower arterial oxygen level and lower oxygen saturation than the adult before cyanosis becomes clinically apparent.

In addition to the specific characteristics of fetal hemoglobin, other conditions affect the transport of oxygen. Alkalosis and hypothermia result in increased oxygen affinity and thus less oxygen availability to the tissues; acidosis, hypercarbia, and hyperthermia result in decreased oxygen affinity, resulting in greater oxygen release to the tissues. Therefore, as blood is perfusing active tissues that are producing acids and carbon dioxide, hemoglobin's affinity for oxygen decreases, allowing oxygen unloading and carbon dioxide and acid uptake. This blood is then transferred to the placenta or the lungs, where its lower carbon dioxide and acid content results in uploading of these waste products from hemoglobin and the uptake of oxygen to be transferred to the tissues.

Other factors that regulate oxygen delivery to the tissues are oxygen-carrying capacity and cardiac output. The oxygen-carrying capacity of blood is defined as the product of the hemoglobin concentration and the maximum amount of oxygen that 1 g of hemoglobin can hold when it is fully saturated. The amount of oxygen bound to hemoglobin divided by the oxygen-carrying capacity yields a percentage that signifies oxygen saturation. Oxygen saturation usually reaches a value between 96% and 98% after several hours of life. Although fetal hemoglobin can hold only 1.26 mL of oxygen per gram of hemo-

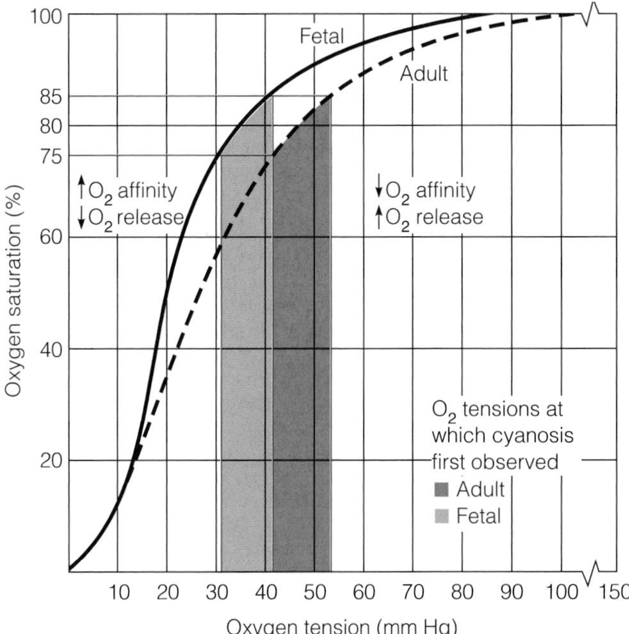

FIGURE 24–3 Fetal oxygen-hemoglobin dissociation curve. SOURCE: Modified from Klaus M, Fanaroff AA: *Care of the High Risk Infant,* 3rd ed. Philadelphia: Saunders, 1986, p 234.

globin, compared to 1.34 mL of oxygen per gram of adult hemoglobin, the newborn's hemoglobin level at birth (17 g/dL) is substantially greater than in adults (13 g/dL). Therefore, the absolute oxygen-carrying capacity of fetal blood (21.42 vol%) is greater than in adult blood (17.42 vol%) and allows the fetus to tolerate the relatively hypoxic intrauterine environment.

A significant reduction in the oxygen-carrying capacity results in an increased cardiac output to compensate for hemoglobin's decreased oxygen concentration. Lastly, cardiac output of the fetus and newborn is relatively greater per body weight than in the adult, which contributes to the rapid delivery of oxygenated blood to tissues with high metabolic demands.

Maintaining Respiratory Function

The lungs' ability to maintain oxygen and carbon dioxide exchange (ventilation) is influenced by such factors as lung compliance and airway resistance. Lung compliance is influenced by the elastic recoil of the lung tissue and by anatomic differences in the newborn. The newborn has a relatively large heart as well as mediastinal structures that reduce available lung space. Also, the newborn chest is equipped with weak intercostal muscles, a rib cage with horizontal ribs, and a high diaphragm that restricts the space available for lung expansion. The large abdomen further encroaches on the high diaphragm to decrease lung space. Another factor that limits ventilation is airway resistance, which depends on the radii, length, and number of airways.

CRITICAL THINKING IN PRACTICE

Thomas and David Smith are monoamniotic, monochorionic twins born by cesarean birth to a 29-year-old, gravida 1, para 0 woman at 36 weeks' gestation. Shortly after birth, Thomas, whose birth weight was 2750 g, is noted to have acrocyanosis and has a respiratory rate of 62. His hemoglobin is 20 g/dL; his hematocrit is 59%; the oxygen saturation monitor is reading 93%. David, whose birth weight was 2670 g, is pale and has a respiratory rate of 88. David's hemoglobin is 11 g/dL; his hematocrit is 32%; his oxygen saturation monitor is reading 100%. Which of these two infants is at greater risk for developing tissue hypoxia?

Answers can be found in Appendix I.

Characteristics of Newborn Respiration

The normal newborn respiratory rate is 30 to 60 breaths per minute. Initial respirations may be largely diaphragmatic, shallow, and irregular in depth and rhythm. The abdomen's movements are synchronous with chest movements. When the breathing pattern is characterized by pauses lasting 5 to 15 seconds, **periodic breathing** is occurring. Periodic breathing is rarely associated with differences in skin color or heart rate changes, and it has no prognostic significance. Tactile or other sensory stimulation stimulates the respiratory center and converts periodic breathing patterns to normal breathing patterns during neonatal transition. With deep sleep, the pattern is reasonably regular. Periodic breathing occurs with rapid eye movement (REM) sleep, and grossly irregular breathing is evident with motor activity, sucking, and crying. Cessation of breathing lasting more than 20 seconds is defined as apnea and is abnormal in term newborns. Apnea may or may not be associated with changes in skin color or heart rate (drop below 100 beats per minute). Apnea always needs to be further evaluated.

The newborn is an obligatory nose breather, and any obstruction will cause respiratory distress, so it is important to keep the throat and nose clear. Immediately after birth and for about 2 hours after birth respiratory rates of 60 to 70 breaths per minute are normal. Some cyanosis and acrocyanosis are normal for several hours; thereafter, a steady improvement in color occurs. If respirations drop below 30 or exceed 60 per minute when the baby is at rest, or if dyspnea, cyanosis, or nasal flaring and expiratory grunting occur, the clinician should be notified. Any increased use of the intercostal muscle (retracting) may indicate respiratory distress. (See Chapter 29 and Table 29–2 for signs of respiratory distress.)

Cardiovascular Adaptations

As described earlier, the onset of respiration triggers increased pulmonary blood flow after birth, which contributes to the transition from fetal to neonatal circulation.

Fetal-Newborn Transitional Physiology

During fetal life, blood with the highest oxygen content is directed to the heart and brain. Blood in the descending aorta is less oxygenated and supplies the kidneys and intestinal tract before it is returned to the placenta. Limited amounts of blood, pumped from the right ventricle toward the lungs, enters the pulmonary vessels. In the fetus, increased pulmonary resistance forces most of the blood through the ductus arteriosus into the descending aorta (Table 24–1).

Marked changes occur in the cardiovascular system at birth. Expansion of the lungs with the first breath decreases the pulmonary vascular resistance and increases pulmonary blood flow. Pressure in the left atrium increases as blood returns from the pulmonary veins. Pressure in the right atrium drops, and systemic vascular resistance increases as umbilical venous flow is halted when the cord is clamped.

These physiologic mechanisms mark the beginning of transition from fetal to neonatal circulation and show the interplay of the cardiovascular and respiratory systems (Figure 24–4) (Sansoucie & Cavaliere, 1997). There are five major areas of change in cardiopulmonary adaptation (Figure 24–5):

TABLE 24–1 Fetal and Neonatal Circulation

System	Fetal	Neonatal
Pulmonary blood vessels	Constricted with very little blood flow; lungs not expanded	Vasodilation and increased blood flow; lungs expanded; increased oxygen stimulates vasodilation.
Systemic blood vessels	Dilated with low resistance; blood mostly in placenta	Arterial pressure rises due to loss of placenta; increased systemic blood volume and resistance.
Ductus arteriosus	Large with no tone; blood flow from pulmonary artery to aorta	Reversal of blood flow. Now from aorta to pulmonary artery because of increased left atrial pressure. Ductus is sensitive to increased oxygen and body chemicals and begins to constrict.
Foramen ovale	Patent with large blood flow from right atrium to left atrium	Increased pressure in left atrium attempts to reverse blood flow and shuts one-way valve.

1. *Increased aortic pressure and decreased venous pressure.* Clamping of the umbilical cord eliminates the placental vascular bed and reduces the intravascular space. Consequently, aortic (systemic) blood pressure increases. At the same time, blood return via the inferior vena cava decreases, resulting in decreased right atrial pressure and a small decrease in pressure within the venous circulation.
2. *Increased systemic pressure and decreased pulmonary artery pressure.* With the loss of the low-resistance placenta, systemic resistance increases, resulting in greater systemic pressure. At the same time, lung

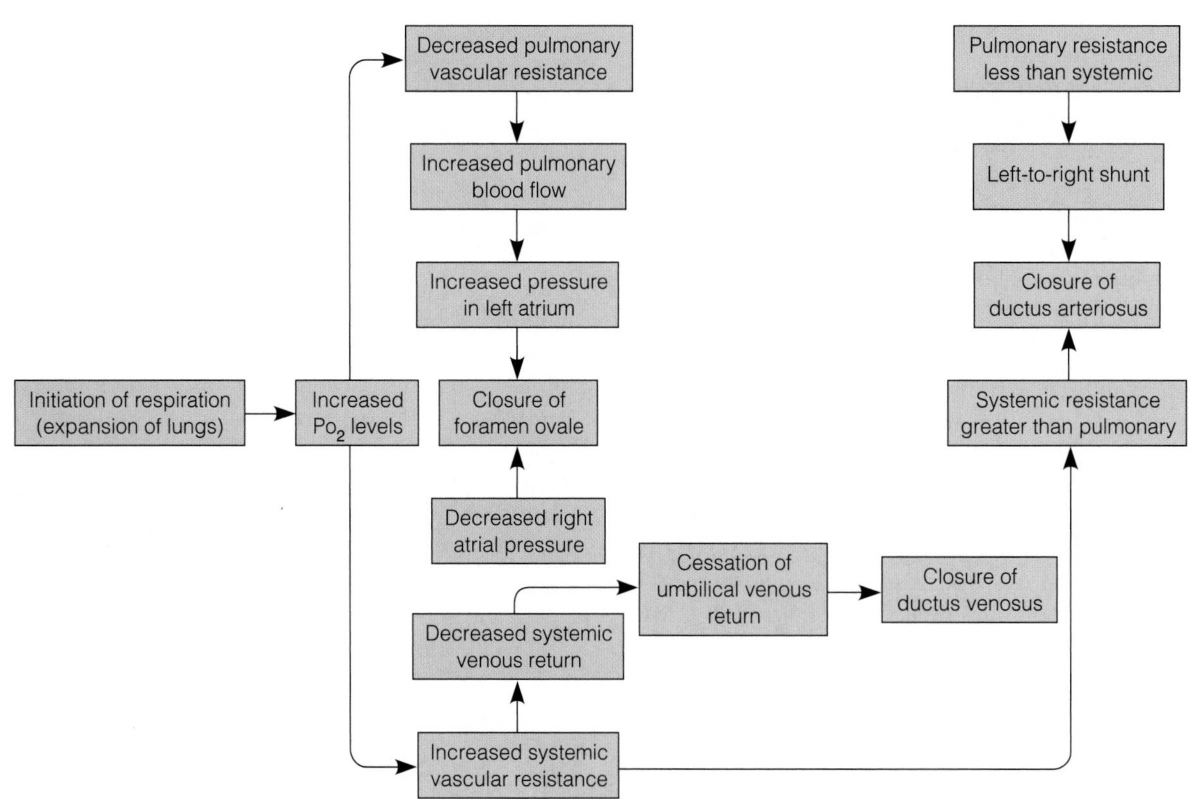

FIGURE 24–4 Transitional circulation: conversion from fetal to neonatal circulation.

expansion increases pulmonary blood flow, and the increased blood Po_2 associated with initiation of respirations dilates pulmonary blood vessels. The combination of vasodilation and increased pulmonary blood flow decreases pulmonary artery resistance. As the pulmonary vascular beds open, the systemic vascular pressure increases, enhancing perfusion of the other body systems.

3. *Closure of the foramen ovale.* Closure of the foramen ovale is a function of changing atrial pressures. In utero, pressure is greater in the right atrium, and the foramen ovale is open after birth. Decreased pulmonary resistance and increased pulmonary blood flow increase pulmonary venous return into the left atrium, thereby increasing left atrial pressure slightly. The decreased pulmonary vascular resistance and the decreased umbilical venous return to the right atrium also cause a decrease in right atrial pressure. The pressure gradients across the atria are now reversed, with left atrial pressure greater, and the foramen ovale is functionally closed 1 to 2 hours after birth. However, a slight right-to-left shunting may occur in the early neonatal period. Any increase in pulmonary resistance or right atrial pressure, such as occurs in crying, acidosis, cold stress, or induced hypoxia, may cause the foramen ovale to reopen, causing a right-to-left shunt. Permanent closure of the foramen ovale occurs within 6 months.
4. *Closure of the ductus arteriosus.* Initial elevation of the systemic vascular pressure above the pulmonary vascular pressure increases pulmonary blood flow by reversing the flow through the ductus arteriosus. Blood now flows from the aorta into the pulmonary artery. Furthermore, although the presence of oxygen causes the pulmonary arterioles to dilate, an increase in blood Po_2 triggers the opposite response in the ductus arteriosus—it constricts.

   In utero the placenta produces prostaglandin E_2 (PGE_2), which causes ductus vasodilation. With the loss of the placenta and increased pulmonary blood flow, PGE_2 levels drop, leaving the active constriction by Po_2 unopposed. If the lungs fail to expand or if Po_2 levels drop, the ductus remains patent. Functional closure is accomplished within 15 hours of birth, and fibrosis of the ductus occurs within 3 weeks after birth (Nelson, 1994).
5. *Closure of the ductus venosus.* Although the mechanism of initiating closure of the ductus venosus is not known, it appears to be related to mechanical pressure changes that result from severing of the cord, redistribution of blood, and cardiac output. Closure of the bypass forces perfusion of the liver. Fibrotic closure occurs within 2 months (Long, 1990). Figure 24–6 depicts the changes in blood flow and oxygenation as the fetal cardiopulmonary circulation adapts to extrauterine life.

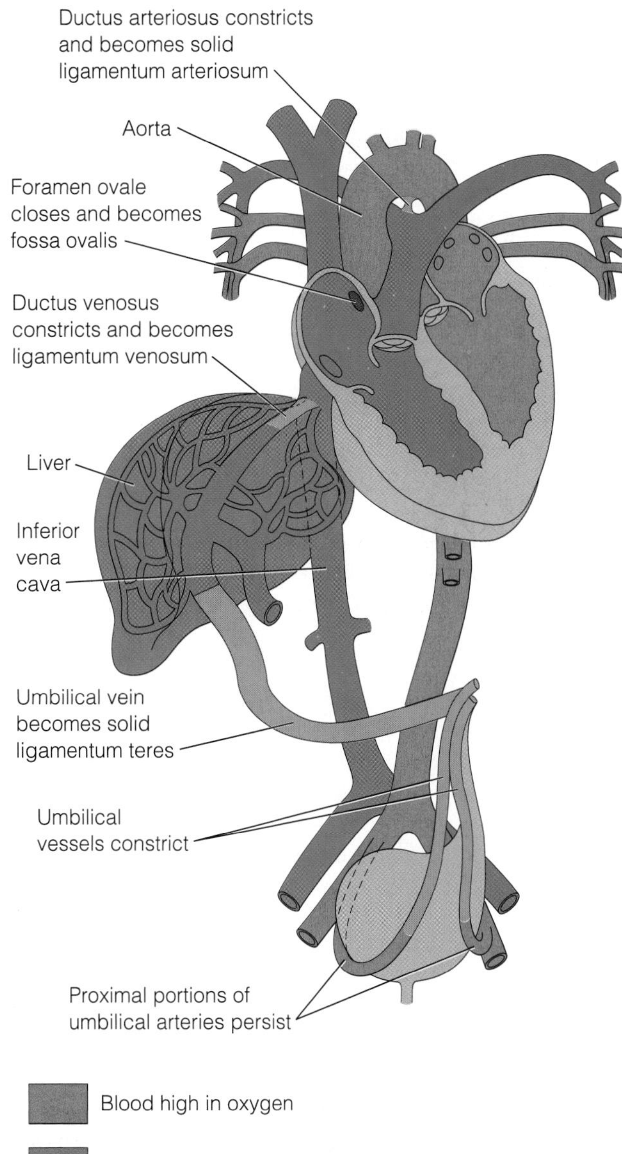

FIGURE 24–5 Major changes that occur in the newborn's circulatory system. SOURCE: Hole JW: *Human Anatomy and Physiology,* 5th ed. Dubuque, IA: William C Brown, 1990. All Rights Reserved.

Characteristics of Cardiac Function

Heart Rate

Shortly after the first cry and the start of changes in cardiopulmonary circulation, the newborn heart rate accelerates to 175 to 180 beats per minute (bpm). The average resting heart rate in the first week of life is 125 to 130 bpm in a quiet, full-term newborn (Fanaroff & Martin, 1997). In full-term newborns, heart rates range from 100 bpm while asleep to 120 to 160 bpm while awake. Resting heart rates may be as low as 85 to 90 bpm; when the newborn cries, the heart rate may exceed 180 bpm.

Apical pulse rates should be obtained by auscultation for a full minute, preferably when the newborn is asleep.

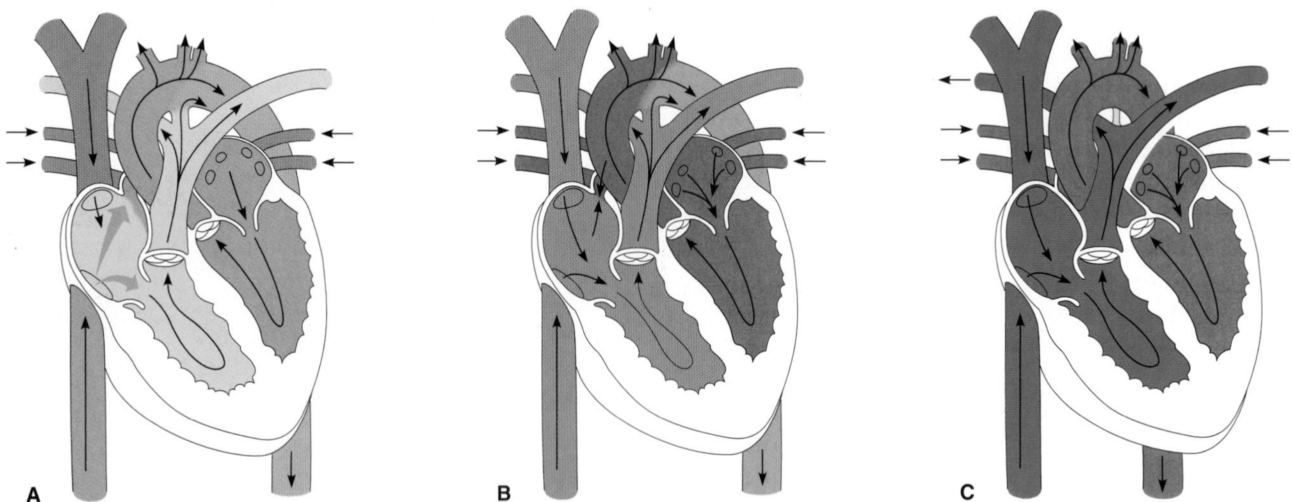

FIGURE 24–6 Fetal-neonatal circulation. *A,* Pattern of blood flow and oxygenation in fetal circulation. *B,* Pattern of blood flow and oxygenation in transitional circulation of the newborn. *C,* Pattern of blood flow and oxygenation in neonatal circulation.

The heart rate should be evaluated for abnormal rhythms or beats. Peripheral pulses of all extremities should also be evaluated to detect any lags or unusual characteristics. Peripheral radial pulses are difficult to palpate in the newborn. They can be assessed when blood pressure is measured if blood pressure readings are taken on all four extremities.

Blood Pressure

The blood pressure tends to be highest immediately after birth, and then it descends to its lowest level at about 3 hours of age. By 4 to 6 days of life, the blood pressure rises and plateaus at a level approximately the same as the initial level. Blood pressure is sensitive to the changes in blood volume that occur in the transition to newborn circulation. Figure 24–7 diagrams this response. Peripheral perfusion pressure is a particularly sensitive indicator of the newborn's ability to compensate for alterations in blood volume prior to changes in blood pressure. Capillary refill should be less than 2 to 3 seconds when the skin is blanched.

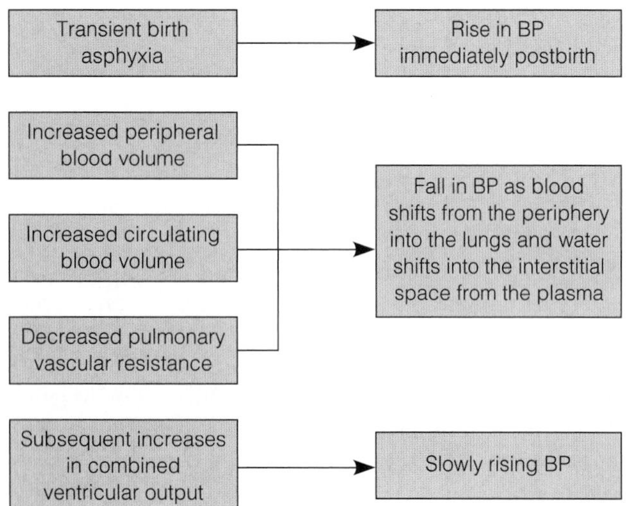

FIGURE 24–7 Response of blood pressure (BP) to changes in neonatal blood volume.

Blood pressure values during the first 12 hours of life vary with the birth weight. In the full-term resting newborn, the average blood pressure is 72/47 mm Hg and 64/39 mm Hg for the preterm newborn (Fanaroff & Martin, 1997). Crying may cause an elevation of 20 mm Hg in both the systolic and diastolic blood pressure; thus accuracy is more likely in the quiet newborn. The measurement of blood pressure is best accomplished by using the Doppler technique or a 1- to 2-inch cuff and a stethoscope over the brachial artery.

Heart Murmurs

Murmurs are usually produced by turbulent blood flow. Murmurs may be heard when blood flows across an abnormal valve or across a stenosed valve, when there is an atrial septal or ventricular septal defect, or when there is increased flow across a normal valve.

In newborns, 90% of all murmurs are transient and not associated with anomalies. They usually involve incomplete closure of the ductus arteriosus or foramen ovale. Soft murmurs may be heard as the pulmonary branch arteries increase their blood flow from 7% to 50% of the combined ventricular output during transition, causing a physiologic peripheral pulmonary stenosis. Because of the current practice of early discharge, murmurs associated with ventricular septal defect and patent ductus arteriosus are often not detected until the first well-baby checkup at 4 to 6 weeks of age. Murmurs are sometimes absent in seriously malformed hearts (Johnston, 1998). Clicks may normally be heard at the lower left sternal border as the great vessels dilate to accommodate systolic blood flow in the first few hours of life (Verklan, 1997).

Cardiac Work Load

In the first 2 hours after birth, when the ductus arteriosus remains mostly patent, about one-third of the left ventricular output is returned to the pulmonary circulation. As a result, the left ventricle has a significantly greater volume load than the right ventricle after birth. In the adult, right and left ventricular outputs are equal; in the newborn, right ventricular output reflects systemic venous return, and left ventricular output reflects pulmonary venous return. Systemic blood volume and pulmonary blood volume are not equal in the neonate. The newborn's combined cardiac output (left and right ventricular) is greater per unit of body weight than it will be in later childhood.

Before birth, the right ventricle does approximately two-thirds of the cardiac work, resulting in increased size and thickness of the right ventricle at birth. After birth, the left ventricle must assume a larger share of the cardiac workload, and it progressively increases in size and thickness. This may explain why right-sided heart defects are better tolerated than left-sided lesions and why left-sided heart defects rapidly become symptomatic after birth.

Hematologic Adaptations

Fetal blood (umbilical vein) in utero is 50% oxygen saturated; this relative hypoxia causes increased amounts of erythropoietin to be secreted, resulting in active erythropoiesis (an increase in nucleated red blood cells and reticulocytes). After birth, the increases in oxygen saturation and arterial oxygen levels shut off the production of erythropoietin. In the first days of life, hemoglobin concentration may rise 1 to 2 g/dL above fetal levels as a result of placental transfusion, low oral fluid intake, and diminished extracellular fluid volume. By 1 week postnatally, peripheral hemoglobin is comparable to fetal blood counts. The hemoglobin level declines progressively thereafter during the first 2 to 3 months after birth (Polin & Fox, 1998). This initial decline in hemoglobin creates a phenomenon known as **physiologic anemia of infancy.** A factor that influences the degree of physiologic anemia is the nutritional status of the neonate. Supplies of vitamin E, folic acid, and iron may be inadequate given the amount of growth in the later part of the first year of life. Hemoglobin values fall, mainly from a decrease in red cell mass rather than from the dilutional effect of increasing plasma volume. The fact that red cell survival is lower in newborns than in adults, and that red cell production is less, also contributes to this anemia. Neonatal red blood cells have a life span of 80 to 100 days, approximately two-thirds of an adult's red blood cell life span. About 5% of neonatal RBCs retain their nucleus.

Leukocytosis is a normal finding because the stress of birth stimulates increased production of neutrophils during the first few days of life. Neutrophils then decrease to 35% of the total leukocyte count by 2 weeks of age. Lymphocytes play a role in antibody formation and eventually become the predominant type of leukocyte, and the total white blood count falls. Also, megakaryocytes appear in the liver and spleen as platelets at about 11 weeks' gestation and approach adult values by 30 weeks.

Blood volume of the term infant is estimated to be 80 to 85 mL/kg of body weight. For example, a 3.6 kg (8 lb) newborn has a blood volume of 290 to 309 mL. Blood volume varies according to the amount of placental transfusion received during the delivery of the placenta as well as other factors, including the following:

1. *Delayed cord clamping and the normal shift of plasma to the extravascular spaces.* Newborn hemoglobin and hematocrit values are higher when a placental transfusion occurs at birth. Placental vessels contain about 100 mL of blood at term, most of which can be transfused into the newborn by holding the newborn below the level of the placenta and by delaying clamping of the cord (Figure 24–8). Blood volume increases by 50% with delayed cord clamping (Polin & Fox, 1998). The increase is reflected by a rise in hemoglobin level and an increase in the hematocrit to about 65% after birth (compared with 48% when the cord is clamped immediately). For greatest accuracy, the initial hemoglobin and hematocrit levels should be measured in the cord blood, although this is not a routine practice.
2. *Gestational age.* There appears to be a positive association between gestational age, red blood cell numbers, and hemoglobin concentration.
3. *Prenatal or perinatal hemorrhage.* Significant prenatal or perinatal bleeding decreases the hematocrit level and causes hypovolemia.
4. *The site of the blood sample.* Hemoglobin and hematocrit levels taken simultaneously are significantly higher in capillary blood than in venous blood. Sluggish peripheral blood flow creates stasis of red blood cells, thereby increasing their concentration in the capillaries. Because of this, blood samples taken from venous blood sites are more accurate.

The concentration of serum electrolytes in the blood indicates the fluid and electrolyte status of the newborn. See Table 24–2 for normal electrolyte and blood values of the full-term newborn.

Temperature Regulation

Temperature regulation is the maintenance of balance between the loss of heat to the environment and the production of heat. Newborns are homeothermic; they attempt to stabilize their internal (core) body temperatures within a narrow range in spite of significant temperature

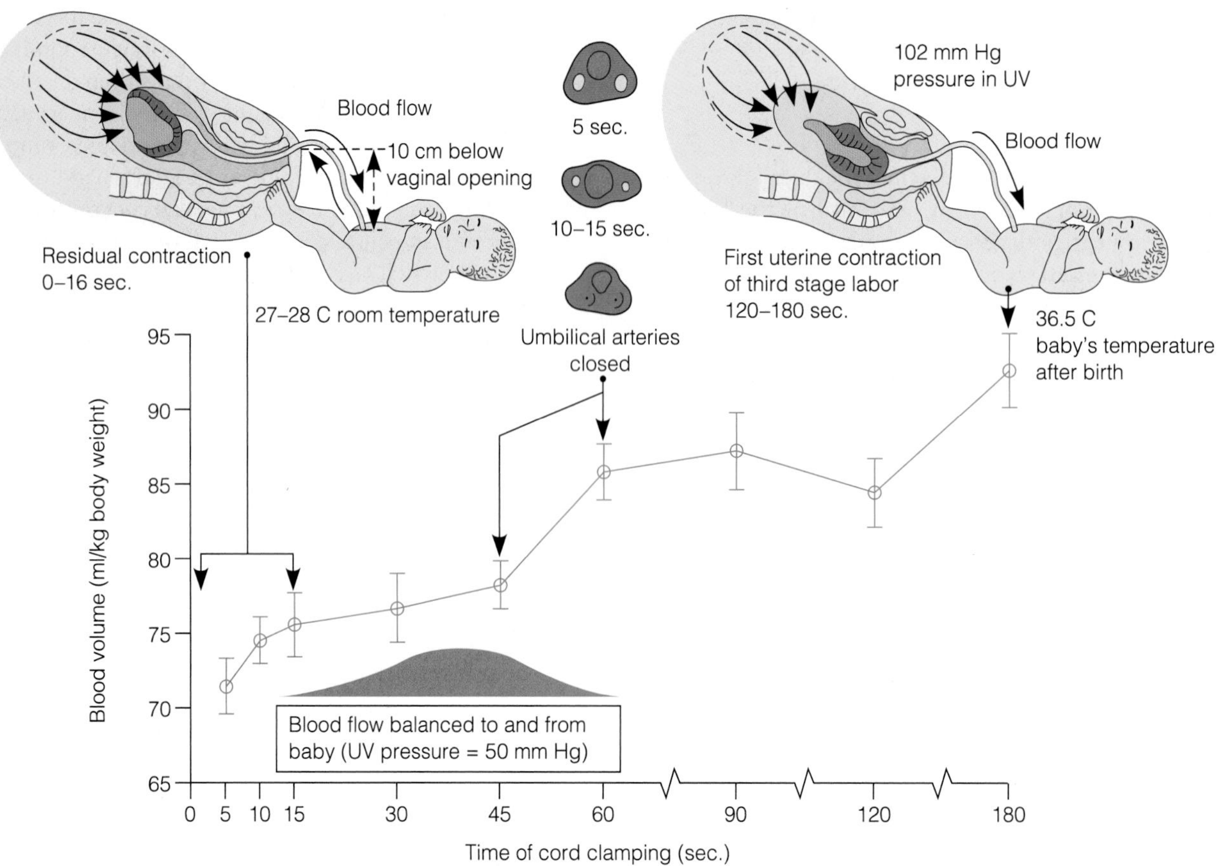

FIGURE 24–8 Schematic illustration of the mechanisms in placental transfusion (normal term births). The mean neonatal blood volume at 30 minutes is plotted against the time of cord clamping after birth (mean +1 SE, data from 114 full-term infants). Note episodic, stepwise increments in blood volume at 10, 60, and 180 seconds. SOURCE: Yao AC, Lind J: *Placental Transfusion: A Clinical and Physiological Study.* Springfield, IL: Charles C Thomas, 1982.

TABLE 24–2 Normal Term Newborn Blood Values

Laboratory Data	Normal Range
Hemoglobin	15–20 g/dL
Hematocrit	43%–61%
WBC	10,000–30,000/mm^3
Neutrophils	40%–80%
Immature WBC	3%–10%
Platelets	100,000–280,000/mm^3
Reticulocytes	3%–6%
Blood volume	82.3 mL/kg (third day after early cord clamping)
	92.6 mL/kg (third day after delayed cord clamping)
Sodium	124–156 mmol/L
Potassium	5.3–7.3 mmol/L
Chloride	90–111 mmol/L
Calcium	7.3–9.2 mg/dL
Glucose	40–97 mg/dL

variations in their environment. At birth, the fetus moves from a warm intrauterine environment to the relatively colder extrauterine environment. The newborn's temperature may fall 2C to 3C after birth mainly because of evaporative losses; this triggers cold-induced metabolic responses and heat production. Term newborns can increase their metabolic rate by 100% by 15 to 30 minutes after birth (Blackburn & Loper, 1992).

Thermoregulation in the newborn is closely related to the rate of metabolism and oxygen consumption. Within a specific environmental range called the **thermal neutral zone (TNZ),** the rates of oxygen consumption and metabolism are minimal, and internal body temperature is maintained because of thermal balance (Table 24–3). For an unclothed full-term newborn, the TNZ range is an ambient environmental temperature of 32 to 34C (89.6 to 93.2F). The limits for an adult are 26 to 28C (78.8 to 82.4F) (Polin & Fox, 1998). Thus the normal newborn requires higher environmental temperatures to maintain a thermoneutral environment.

Several newborn characteristics affect the establishment of a TNZ. The newborn has less subcutaneous fat than an adult and a thin epidermis. Blood vessels of the newborn are closer to the skin than those of an adult. Therefore, the circulating blood is influenced by changes in environmental temperature and in turn influences the hypothalamic temperature-regulating center.

The flexed posture of the term infant decreases the surface area exposed to the environment, thereby reducing heat loss. Other newborn characteristics such as size, ratio of surface area to body weight, and age may also affect the establishment of a TNZ. The preterm small-for-gestational-age (SGA) newborn has less adipose tissue and is hypoflexed and therefore require higher environmental temperatures to achieve a thermal neutral environment. A larger, well-insulated newborn may be able to cope with lower environmental temperatures. If the environmental temperature falls below the lower limits of the TNZ, the newborn responds with increased oxygen consumption and raised metabolism, which results in greater heat production. Prolonged exposure to the cold may result in depleted glycogen stores and acidosis. Oxygen consumption also increases if the environmental temperature is above the TNZ.

Heat Loss

A newborn is at a distinct disadvantage in maintaining a normal temperature. With a large body surface in relation to mass and a limited amount of insulating subcutaneous fat, the full-term newborn loses about four times as much heat as an adult (Cunningham et al, 1997). The newborn's poor thermal stability is due primarily to excessive heat loss rather than to impaired heat production. Because of the risk of hypothermia and possible cold stress, minimizing heat loss in the newborn after birth is essential. (See Chapters 20 and 26 for nursing measures.)

Two major routes of heat loss are from the internal core of the body to the body surface and from the external body surface to the environment. Usually the core temperature is higher than the skin temperature, resulting in continuous transfer or conduction of heat to the surface (Fanaroff & Martin, 1997). The greater the difference in temperatures between core and skin, the more rapid the transfer. The transfer is accomplished through an increase in oxygen consumption, depletion of glycogen stores, and metabolizing of brown fat.

TABLE 24–3 Neutral Thermal Environmental Temperatures

Age and Weight	Range of Temperature (C)
0–6 Hours	
Under 1200 g	34.0–35.4
1200–1500 g	33.9–34.4
1501–2500 g	32.8–33.8
Over 2500 (and >36 weeks)	32.0–33.8
6–12 Hours	
Under 1200 g	34.0–35.4
1200–1500 g	33.5–34.4
1501–2500 g	32.2–33.8
Over 2500 (and >36 weeks)	31.4–33.8
12–24 Hours	
Under 1200 g	34.0–35.4
1200–1500 g	33.3–34.3
1501–2500 g	31.8–33.8
Over 2500 (and >36 weeks)	31.0–33.7
24–36 Hours	
Under 1200 g	34.0–35.0
1200–1500 g	33.1–34.2
1501–2500 g	31.6–33.6
Over 2500 (and >36 weeks)	30.7–33.5
36–48 Hours	
Under 1200 g	34.0–35.0
1200–1500 g	33.0–34.1
1501–2500 g	31.4–33.5
Over 2500 (and >36 weeks)	30.5–33.3
48–72 Hours	
Under 1200 g	34.0–35.0
1200–1500 g	33.0–34.0
1501–2500 g	31.2–33.4
Over 2500 (and >36 weeks)	30.1–33.2
72–96 Hours	
Under 1200 g	34.0–35.0
1200–1500 g	33.0–34.0
1501–2500 g	31.1–33.2
Over 2500 (and >36 weeks)	29.8–32.8
4–12 Days	
Under 1500 g	33.0–34.0
1501–2500 g	31.0–33.2
Over 2500 (and >36 weeks)	
4–5 days	29.5–32.6
5–6 days	29.4–32.3
6–8 days	29.0–32.2
8–10 days	29.0–31.8
10–12 days	29.0–31.4
12–14 Days	
Under 1500 g	32.6–34.0
1500–2500 g	31.0–33.2
Over 2500 (and >36 weeks)	29.0–30.8
2–3 Weeks	
Under 1500 g	32.2–34.0
1500–2500 g	30.5–33.0
3–4 Weeks	
Under 1500 g	31.6–33.6
1500–2500 g	30.0–32.7
4–5 Weeks	
Under 1500 g	31.2–33.0
1500–2500 g	29.5–32.2
5–6 Weeks	
Under 1500 g	30.6–32.3
1500–2500 g	29.0–31.8

*Generally speaking, the smaller infants in each weight group will require a temperature in the higher portion of the temperature range. Within each time range, the younger the infant, the higher the temperature required.

SOURCE: Adapted from Scopes and Ahmed (1966) (For his table Scopes had the walls of the incubator 1 to 2 degrees warmer than the ambient air temperatures.) Reproduced, with permission, from Klaus MH, Fanaroff, AA: *Care of the High-Risk Neonate*, 3rd ed. Philadelphia: Saunders, 1986, p 103.

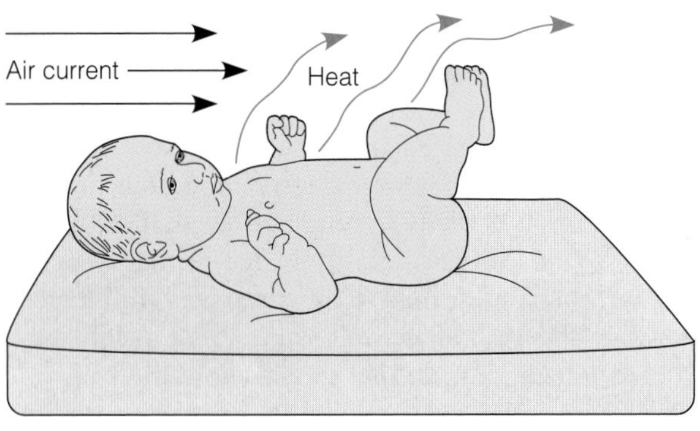

A

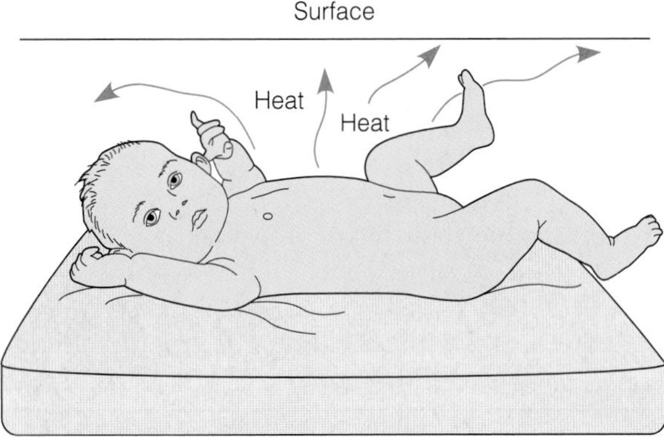

B

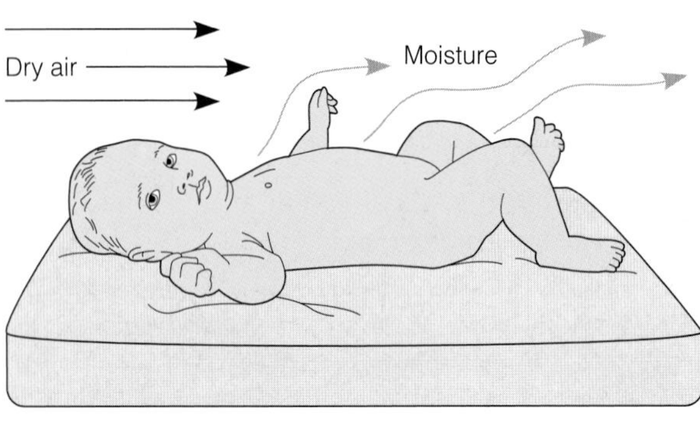

C

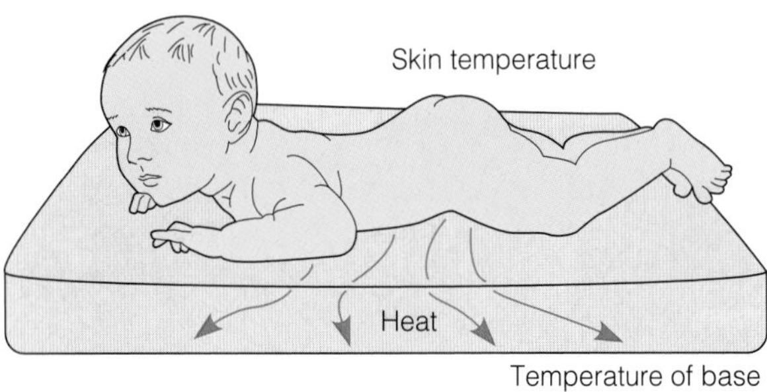

D

FIGURE 24–9 Methods of heat loss. ***A,*** Convection. ***B,*** Radiation. ***C,*** Evaporation. ***D,*** Conduction.

Heat loss from the body surface to the environment takes place by four avenues—convection, radiation, evaporation, and conduction (Figure 24–9).

- **Convection** is the loss of heat from the warm body surface to the cooler air currents. Air-conditioned rooms, air currents with a temperature below the infant's skin temperature, oxygen by mask, and removal of the infant from an incubator for procedures increases convective heat loss of the newborn.
- **Radiation** losses occur when heat transfers from the heated body rise to cooler surfaces and objects not in direct contact with the body. The walls of a room or of an incubator are potential causes of heat loss by radiation, even if the ambient temperature of the incubator is within the thermal neutral range for the infant. Placing cold objects (such as ice for blood gases) onto the incubator or near the infant in the radiant warmer will increase radiant heat losses.
- **Evaporation** is the loss of heat incurred when water is converted to a vapor. The newborn is particularly prone to heat loss by evaporation immediately after birth, when the baby is wet with amniotic fluid, and during baths; thus drying the newborn is critical.
- **Conduction** is the loss of heat to a cooler surface by direct skin contact. Chilled hands, cool scales, cold examination tables, and cold stethoscopes can cause heat loss by conduction. Even if objects are warmed to the incubator temperature, there still may be a significant temperature difference between the infant's core temperature and the ambient temperature. This results in heat transfer.

Once the infant has been dried after birth, the highest losses of heat generally result from radiation and convection because of the newborn's large ratio of body surface to weight, and from thermal conduction because of the marked difference between core temperature and skin temperature. The newborn can respond to the cooler environmental temperature with adequate peripheral vasoconstriction, but this mechanism is less effective because of the minimal amount of fat insulation present, the large body surface, and ongoing thermal conduction. Because of these factors, minimizing the baby's heat loss and preventing hypothermia are imperative. Nursing measures for preventing hypothermia are described in Chapter 26.

Heat Production (Thermogenesis)

When exposed to a cool environment, the newborn requires additional heat. The newborn has several physiologic mechanisms that increase heat production, or *thermogenesis.* These include increased basal metabolic rate, muscular activity, and chemical thermogenesis (also called *nonshivering thermogenesis [NST]*) (Hey, 1994).

Nonshivering thermogenesis, an important mechanism of heat production, is unique to the newborn. NST occurs when skin receptors perceive a drop in environmental temperature and transmit sensations to the CNS, which in turn stimulates the sympathetic nervous system, which in turn uses the newborn's stores of **brown adipose tissue (BAT)** (also called *brown fat*) as the primary source of heat in the cold-stressed newborn. It first appears in the fetus at 26 to 30 weeks' gestation and continues to increase until 2 to 5 weeks after the birth of a term infant, unless it is depleted by cold stress. Brown fat is deposited in the midscapular area, around the neck, and in the axillas, with deeper placement around the trachea, esophagus, abdominal aorta, kidneys, and adrenal glands (Figure 24–10). BAT constitutes 2% to 6% of the newborn's total body weight. Brown fat receives its name from its dark color, which is due to its enriched blood supply, dense cellular content, and abundant nerve endings. The large numbers of fat cells facilitate the speed with which triglycerides can be metabolized to produce heat. These characteristics promote rapid metabolism, heat generation, and heat transfer to the peripheral circulation.

In addition, brown fat possesses a rich blood supply to enhance distribution of heat throughout the body and a nerve supply for initiation of metabolic activity. Release of norepinephrine by the adrenal gland and at local nerve endings in the brown fat causes triglycerides to be metabolized into glycerol and fatty acids. The oxidation of fatty acids is highly exothermic (heat producing); thus heat is distributed to the body. Brown fat is a major producer of heat for the cold-stressed newborn.

Shivering, a form of muscular activity common in the cold adult, is rarely seen in the newborn, although it has been observed at ambient temperatures of 15C (59F) or less (Polin & Fox, 1998). If the newborn does shiver, it means the newborn's metabolic rate has already doubled. The extra muscular activity does little to produce needed heat.

Thermographic studies of newborns exposed to cold show an increase in the skin heat over the brown fat deposits in the neonate between 1 and 14 days of age. If the brown fat supply has been depleted, the metabolic response to cold will be limited or lacking. An increase in basal metabolism as a result of hypothermia results in an increase in oxygen consumption. A decrease in the environmental temperature of 2C, from 33C to 31C, is a drop sufficient to double the oxygen consumption of a term newborn. Keeping the normal newborn warm promotes normal oxygen requirements, whereas chilling can cause the newborn to show signs of respiratory distress.

When exposed to cold, the normal term neonate is usually able to cope with the increase in oxygen requirements, but the preterm neonate may be unable to increase ventilation to the necessary level of oxygen consumption. (See Chapter 29 for discussion of cold stress.) Because oxidation of fatty acids depends on the availability of oxygen, glucose, and adenosine triphosphate (ATP), the newborn's ability to generate heat can be altered by pathologic events such as hypoxia, acidosis, and hypoglycemia or by medications that block the release of norepinephrine. The effect of certain drugs such as meperidine (Demerol) may also prevent metabolism of brown fat. Meperidine given to the laboring woman leads to a greater fall in the newborn's body temperature during the neonatal period. Neonatal hypothermia prolongs as well as potentiates the effects of many analgesic and anesthetic drugs in the newborn.

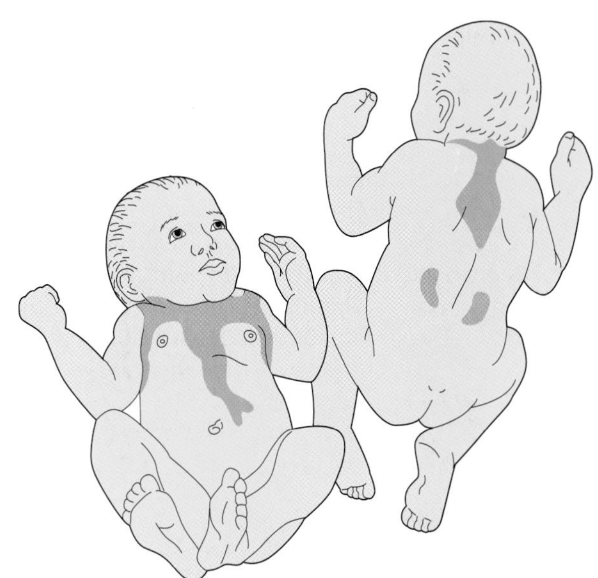

FIGURE 24–10 The distribution of brown adipose tissue (brown fat) in the neonate. SOURCE: Adapted from Davis V: Structure and function of brown adipose tissue in the neonate. *JOGNN* November/December 1980; 9:364.

Response to Heat

Sweating is the usual initial response of the term newborn to hyperthermia. The newborn has six times as many sweat glands as the adult, but the capacity of the sweat gland is one-third that of the adult. The glands have limited function until after the fourth week of extrauterine life. Heat is dissipated by peripheral vasodilation and evaporation of insensible water loss. In term small-for-gestational-age infants, the onset of sweating is delayed; it is virtually nonexistent in preterm infants of less than 30 weeks' gestation because of the underdevelopment of the sweat glands (Hey, 1994). Oxygen consumption and metabolic rate also increase in response to hyperthermia. Severe hyperthermia can lead to death or to gross brain damage if the baby survives.

Hepatic Adaptations

In the newborn, the liver is frequently palpable 2 to 3 cm below the right costal margin. It is relatively large and occupies about 40% of the abdominal cavity. The neonatal liver plays a significant role in iron storage, carbohydrate metabolism, conjugation of bilirubin, and coagulation.

Iron Storage and Red Blood Cell Production

As red blood cells (RBCs) are destroyed after birth, the iron is stored in the liver until needed for new red blood cell production. Newborn iron stores are determined by total body hemoglobin content and length of gestation. The term newborn has about 270 mg of iron at birth, and about 140 to 170 mg of this amount is in the hemoglobin. If the mother's iron intake has been adequate, enough iron will be stored to last until 5 months of age. After about 6 months of age, foods containing iron or iron supplements must be given to prevent anemia.

Carbohydrate Metabolism

At term, the newborn's cord blood glucose is 70% to 80% of the maternal blood glucose level. Neonatal carbohydrate reserves are relatively low. One-third of this reserve is in the form of liver glycogen. Neonatal glycogen stores are twice that of the adult.

The newborn enters an energy crunch at the time of birth with the removal of the maternal glucose supply and the increased energy expenditure associated with the birth process and extrauterine life. Fuel sources are consumed at a faster rate because of the work of breathing, loss of heat when exposed to cold, activity, and activation of muscle tone. Glucose is the main source of energy in the first 4 to 6 hours after birth. The blood glucose level falls rapidly and then stabilizes at values of 50 to 60 mg/dL; by the third day postnatally, the mean values increase to 60 to 70 mg/dL (Karp, Scardino, & Butler, 1995).

Glucose level is assessed by using a Chemstrip method on the infant's admission to the neonatal nursery and at 4 hours of age. As stores of liver and muscle glycogen and blood glucose decrease, the newborn compensates by changing from a predominantly carbohydrate metabolism to fat metabolism. Energy is derived from fat and protein as well as from carbohydrates. The amount and availability of each of these "fuel substrates" depends on the ability of immature metabolic pathways (ie, lacking specific enzymes or hormones) to function in the first few days of life.

Conjugation of Bilirubin

Conjugation of bilirubin is the conversion of yellow lipid-soluble pigment into water-soluble pigment. Unconjugated (indirect) bilirubin is a breakdown product derived from hemoglobin that is released primarily from destroyed red blood cells. Unconjugated bilirubin is not in an excretable form and is a potential toxin. **Total serum bilirubin** is the sum of conjugated (direct) and unconjugated (indirect) bilirubin.

Fetal unconjugated bilirubin crosses the placenta to be excreted, so the fetus doesn't need to conjugate bilirubin. Total bilirubin at birth is less than 3 mg/dL unless an abnormal hemolytic process has been present. After birth, the newborn's liver must begin to conjugate bilirubin. This produces a rise in serum bilirubin in the first few days of life. The newborn liver has relatively less glucuronyl transferase activity at birth and in the first few weeks of life than an adult liver. This reduction in hepatic activity, along with a relatively large bilirubin load, decreases the liver's ability to conjugate bilirubin and increases susceptibility to jaundice.

The bilirubin formed after red blood cells are destroyed is transported in the blood bound to albumin. The bilirubin is transferred into the hepatocytes and bound to two intracellular proteins. These two proteins determine the amount of bilirubin that is held in the liver cells for processing and consequently determine the amount of bilirubin uptake into the liver. The activity of glucuronyl transferase enzyme results in the attachment of unconjugated bilirubin to glucuronic acid (product of liver glycogen), producing conjugated, direct bilirubin. Direct bilirubin is excreted into the tiny bile ducts, then into the common duct and duodenum. The (direct) conjugated bilirubin then progresses down the intestines, where bacteria transform it into urobilinogen. This product is not reabsorbed but is excreted as a yellow-brown pigment in the stools.

Even after the bilirubin has been conjugated and bound, it can be changed back to unconjugated bilirubin via the enterohepatic circulation. In the intestines, β-glucuronidase enzyme acts to split off (deconjugate) the bilirubin from glucuronic acid if it has not first been acted upon by gut bacteria to produce urobilinogen; the free bilirubin is reabsorbed through the intestinal wall and brought back to the liver via portal vein circulation. This recycling of the bilirubin and decreased ability to clear bilirubin from the system are prevalent in babies who have very high β-glucuronidase activity levels as well as delayed bacterial colonization of the gut (such as with the use of antibiotics) and further increases the newborn's susceptibility to jaundice. Conjugation of bilirubin in newborns is depicted in Figure 24–11.

Physiologic Jaundice

Physiologic jaundice is caused by accelerated destruction of fetal RBCs, impaired conjugation of bilirubin, and increased bilirubin reabsorption from the intestinal tract. This condition does not have a pathologic basis, but rather is a normal biologic response of the newborn.

Maisels (1994) describes six factors whose interactions may give rise to physiologic jaundice:

1. *Increased amounts of bilirubin delivered to the liver.* The increased blood volume due to delayed cord clamping combined with faster RBC destruction in the newborn leads to an increased bilirubin level in the blood. A proportionately larger amount of non-erythrocyte bilirubin is formed in the newborn.

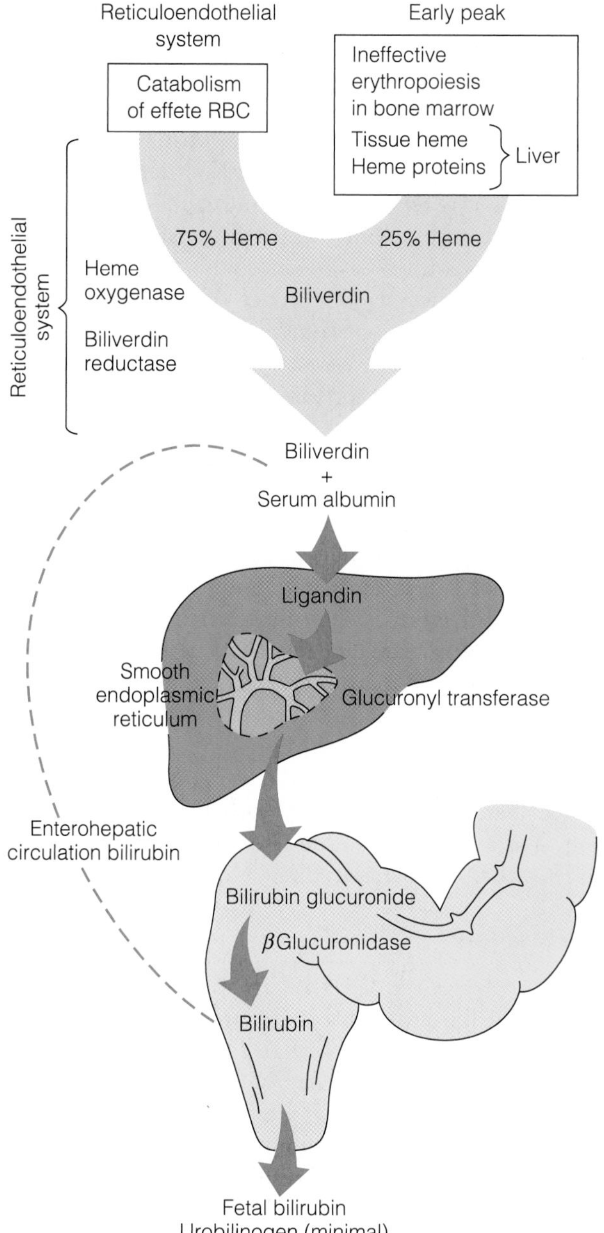

FIGURE 24–11 Conjugation of bilirubin in newborns. SOURCE: Avery GB, Fletcher MA, MacDonald MG: *Neonatology: Pathophysiology and Management of the Newborn,* 4th ed. Philadelphia: Lippincott, 1994, p 635.

Therefore, newborns have two to three times greater production or breakdown of bilirubin. The use of forceps, which sometimes causes facial bruising or cephalhematoma (entrapped hemorrhage), can increase the amount of bilirubin to be handled by the liver.

2. *Defective uptake of bilirubin from the plasma.* If the newborn does not ingest adequate calories, the formation of hepatic intracellular binding proteins diminishes, resulting in higher bilirubin levels.
3. *Defective conjugation of the bilirubin.* Decreased glucuronyl transferase activity, as in hypothryoidism, and inadequate caloric intake causes the intracellular binding proteins to remain saturated and results in greater unconjugated bilirubin levels in the blood. The fatty acids in maternal breast milk compete with bilirubin for albumin binding sites; this process is thought to impede bilirubin processing.
4. *Defect in bilirubin excretion.* A congenital infection may cause impaired excretion of conjugated bilirubin. Delay in introduction of bacterial flora and decreased intestinal motility can also delay excretion and increase enterohepatic circulation of bilirubin.
5. *Inadequate hepatic circulation.* Decreased oxygen supplies to the liver associated with neonatal hypoxia or congenital heart disease lead to a rise in the bilirubin level.
6. *Increased reabsorption of bilirubin from the intestine.* Reduced bowel motility, intestinal obstruction, or delayed passage of meconium increases the circulation of bilirubin in the enterohepatic pathway, thereby resulting in higher bilirubin values.

About 50% of full-term and 80% of preterm newborns exhibit physiologic jaundice on about the second or third day after birth. The characteristic yellow color results from increased levels of unconjugated bilirubin, which are a normal product of RBC breakdown and reflect a temporary inability of the body to eliminate bilirubin. Serum levels of bilirubin are about 4 to 6 mg/dL before yellow coloration of the skin and sclera appears. The signs of physiologic jaundice appear *after* the first 24 hours postnatally. This differentiates physiologic jaundice from pathologic jaundice (Chapter 29), which is clinically seen at birth or within the first 24 hours of postnatal life.

In the past, it was thought that during the first week, unconjugated bilirubin levels in physiologic jaundice should not exceed 13 mg/dL in the full-term or preterm newborn. Peak bilirubin levels are reached between days 3 and 5 in the full-term infant and between days 5 and 7 in the preterm infant. These values are established for European and American Caucasian newborns. Chinese, Japanese, Korean, and Native American newborns have considerably higher bilirubin levels that are not as apparent and that persist for longer periods with no apparent ill effects (MacMahon, Stevenson, & Oski, 1998). Some studies propose levels up to 22 mg/dL (300 to 375 μmol/L) in well babies (Newman & Maisels, 1992).

The nursery or postpartum room environment, including lighting, can hinder the early detection of the degree and type of jaundice. Pink walls and artificial lights mask the beginning of jaundice in newborns. Daylight assists the observer in early recognition by eliminating distortions caused by artificial light.

If jaundice is suspected, the nurse can quickly assess the newborn's coloring by pressing the skin, generally on the forehead or nose, with a finger. As blanching occurs, the nurse can observe the icterus (yellow coloring).

There are several newborn care procedures designed to decrease the probability of high bilirubin levels:

- Maintain the newborn's skin temperature at 36.5C (97.8F) or above, because cold stress results in acidosis. Acidosis in turn decreases available serum albumin-binding sites, weakens albumin-binding powers, and causes elevated unconjugated bilirubin levels.
- Monitor stool for amount and characteristics. Bilirubin is eliminated in the feces; inadequate stooling may result in reabsorption and recycling of bilirubin. Encourage early breastfeeding because the laxative effect of colostrum increases excretion of stool.
- Encourage early feedings to promote intestinal elimination and bacterial colonization and to provide caloric and protein intake necessary for the formation of hepatic binding proteins.

If jaundice becomes apparent, nursing care is directed toward keeping the newborn well hydrated and promoting intestinal elimination. For specific nursing management and therapies, see the Critical Pathway for the Newborn with Hyperbilirubinemia in Chapter 29.

Physiologic jaundice may be very upsetting to parents; they require emotional support and thorough explanation of the condition. If the baby is placed under phototherapy, a few additional days of hospitalization may be required. This may also be disturbing to parents. They should be encouraged to provide for the emotional needs of their newborn by continuing to feed, hold, and caress the infant. If the mother is discharged, the parents should be encouraged to return for feedings and feel free to telephone or visit whenever possible. In many instances the mother, especially if she is breastfeeding, may elect to remain hospitalized with her newborn; this decision should be supported. As an alternative to continued hospitalization, some newborns are treated in home phototherapy programs.

Breast Milk Jaundice

Breastfeeding is implicated in prolonged jaundice in some newborns. From 1% to 5% of breastfed newborns will develop breastfeeding jaundice. The breastfed jaundiced newborn's bilirubin level begins to rise after the first week of life, when physiologic jaundice is waning and the mother's mature milk has come in. The level peaks at 2 to 3 weeks of age and may reach 20 to 25 mg/dL without intervention.

Some women's breast milk may contain several times the normal concentration of certain free fatty acids. These free fatty acids may compete with bilirubin for binding sites on albumin and inhibit the conjugation of bilirubin or increase lipase activity, which disrupts the red blood cell membrane. Increased lipase activity enhances absorption of bile across the GI tract membrane, thereby increasing the enterohepatic circulation of bilirubin. In the past it was thought that the breast milk of women whose newborns have breastfeeding jaundice contained an enzyme that inhibited glucuronyl transferase.

Newborns with breastfeeding jaundice appear well, and at present there is an absence of documented kernicterus with this type of jaundice. Temporary cessation of breastfeeding may be advised if bilirubin reaches presumed toxic levels of approximately 20 mg/dL or if the interruption is necessary to establish the cause of the hyperbilirubinemia. Within 24 to 36 hours after breastfeeding is discontinued, the newborn's serum bilirubin levels begin to fall dramatically (Rebar, 1999).

Many physicians believe that breastfeeding may be resumed once other causes of jaundice have been ruled out and breastfeeding is determined to be the cause. The bilirubin concentration may rise 2 to 3 mg/dL with a subsequent decline. Nursing mothers need encouragement and support in their desire to breastfeed their infants, assistance and instruction regarding pumping and expressing milk during the interrupted nursing period, and reassurance that nothing is wrong with their milk or their mothering abilities. Table 24–4 summarizes key factors in physiologic and breastfeeding jaundice.

Coagulation

The liver plays an important part in blood coagulation during fetal life and continues this function following birth. Coagulation factors II, VII, IX, and X (synthesized in the liver) are activated under the influence of vitamin K and therefore are considered vitamin K dependent. The absence of normal intestinal flora needed to synthesize vitamin K in the newborn gut results in low levels of vitamin K and creates a transient blood coagulation alteration between the second and fifth day of life. From a low point at about 2 to 3 days after birth, these coagulation factors rise slowly but do not approach adult levels until 9 months of age or later. Other coagulation factors with low cord blood levels are XI, XII, and XIII. Fibrinogen and factors V and VII are near adult ranges.

Although newborn bleeding problems are rare, an injection of vitamin K (AquaMEPHYTON) is given prophylactically on the day of birth to combat potential clinical bleeding problems. (Hemorrhagic disease of the newborn is discussed in more depth in Chapter 29.)

Platelet counts at birth are in the same range as for older children, but newborns may manifest mild transient difficulty in platelet aggregation functioning. This platelet problem is accentuated by phototherapy. Prenatal maternal therapy with phenytoin sodium (Dilantin) or phenobarbital also causes abnormal clotting studies and newborn bleeding in the first 24 hours after birth. Infants

TABLE 24–4 Jaundice

Physiologic Jaundice
Physiologic jaundice occurs *after* the first 24 hours of life.
During the first week of life, bilirubin should not exceed 13 mg/dL. Some pediatricians allow levels up to 15 mg/dL.
Bilirubin levels peak at 3 to 5 days in term infants.
Breast Milk Jaundice
Bilirubin levels begin to rise about the fourth day after mature breast milk comes in.
Peak of 20–25 mg/dL is reached at 2 to 3 weeks of age.
It may be necessary to interrupt nursing for a short period when bilirubin reaches 20 mg/dL.

born to mothers receiving Coumadin (warfarin) compounds may bleed because these agents cross the placenta and accentuate existing vitamin K–dependent factor deficiencies. Transient neonatal thrombocytopenia may occur in infants born to mothers with severe hypertension or HELLP syndrome (hemolysis, elevated liver enzymes, and low platelet count) and in mothers who have idiopathic isoimmune thrombocytopenic purpura.

Gastrointestinal Adaptations

By 36 to 38 weeks of fetal life, the gastrointestinal tract is adequately mature, with the presence of enzymatic activity and the ability to transport nutrients. The term newborn has adequate intestinal and pancreatic enzymes to digest most simple carbohydrates, fat, and proteins.

The carbohydrates requiring digestion in the newborn are usually disaccharides (lactose, maltose, sucrose), which are split into monosaccharides (galactose, fructose, and glucose) by the enzymes of the intestinal mucosa. Lactose is the primary carbohydrate in the breastfeeding newborn and is generally easily digested and well absorbed. The only enzyme lacking at birth is pancreatic amylase, which remains relatively deficient during the first few months of life. Newborns have trouble digesting starches (changing more complex carbohydrates into maltose). Therefore, starches should not be introduced into the diet until after the first few months of life.

Although proteins require more digestion than carbohydrates, they are well digested and absorbed from the newborn intestine. The newborn digests and absorbs fats less efficiently because of the minimal activity of pancreatic lipase. The neonate excretes 10% to 20% of the dietary fat intake, compared with 10% for the adult. The fat in breast milk is absorbed more completely by the newborn than is the fat in cow's milk because it consists of more medium-chain triglycerides and contains lipase. (See Chapter 27 for a more detailed discussion of infant nutrition.)

By birth, the newborn has experienced swallowing, gastric emptying, and intestinal propulsion. In utero, swallowing is accompanied by gastric emptying and peristalsis of the fetal intestinal tract. By the end of gestation, peristalsis becomes much more active in preparation for extrauterine life. Fetal peristalsis is also stimulated by anoxia, causing the expulsion of meconium into the amniotic fluid in more mature fetuses.

Air enters the stomach immediately after birth. The small intestine is air filled within 2 to 12 hours, and the large bowel within 24 hours. The salivary glands are immature at birth, and little saliva is manufactured until the infant is about 3 months old. The newborn's stomach has a capacity of 50 to 60 mL. It empties intermittently, starting within a few minutes of the beginning of a feeding and ending between 2 and 4 hours after feeding. The newborn's gastric pH becomes less acidic about a week after birth and remains less acidic than that of adults for the next 2 to 3 months.

The cardiac sphincter is immature, as is neural control of the stomach, so some regurgitation may be noted in the neonatal period. Regurgitation of the first few feedings during the first day or two of life can usually be lessened by avoiding overfeeding and by burping the newborn well during and after the feeding.

When no other signs and symptoms are evident, vomiting is limited and ceases within the first few days of life. Continuous vomiting or regurgitation should be monitored closely. If the newborn has swallowed bloody or purulent amniotic fluid, lavage of the stomach may be indicated in the term newborn to relieve the problem. Bilious vomiting is abnormal and must be evaluated thoroughly because it might represent a condition that warrants prompt surgical intervention.

Adequate digestion and absorption are essential for newborn growth and development. If optimal nutritional support is available, postnatal growth ideally should parallel intrauterine growth; that is, after 30 weeks of gestation the fetus gains 30 g per day and adds 1.2 cm to body length daily. To gain weight at the intrauterine rate, the term newborn requires 120 kcal/kg/day. Following birth, caloric intake is often insufficient for weight gain until the newborn is 5 to 10 days old. During this time there may be a weight loss of 5% to 10% in term newborns. Shift of intracellular water to extracellular space and insensible water loss account for the 5% to 10% weight loss. Thus failure to lose weight when caloric intake is limited may indicate fluid retention.

Term newborns normally pass **meconium** within 8 to 24 hours of life—and almost always within 48 hours. Meconium is formed in utero from the amniotic fluid and its constituents, with intestinal secretions and shed mucosal cells. It is recognized by its thick, tarry, black (or dark green) appearance. Transitional (thinner brown to green) stools consisting of part meconium and part fecal material are passed for the next day or two, after which the stools become entirely fecal. Generally, the stools of a breastfed newborn are pale yellow (but may be pasty green); they are more liquid and more frequent than those of formula-fed newborns, whose stools are paler (Figure 24–12). Frequency of bowel movement varies but

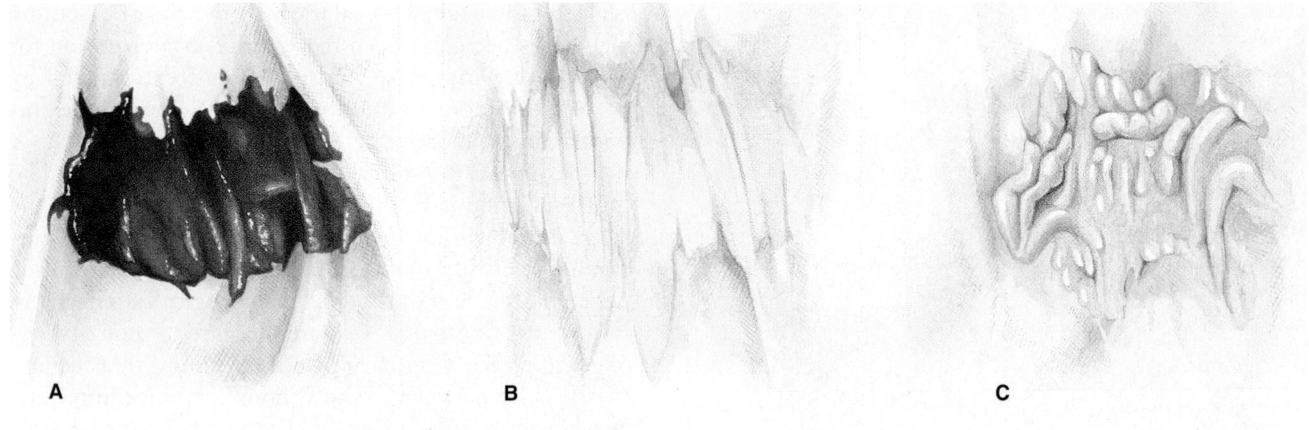

FIGURE 24–12 Newborn stool samples. *A,* Meconium stool. *B,* Breast milk stool. *C,* Cow's milk stool.

initially ranges from one every 2 to 3 days to as many as ten daily. Totally breastfed infants often progress to stools that occur every 5 to 7 days. Mothers should be counseled that this is not constipation as long as the bowel movement remains soft. Table 24–5 describes the progression of stools and other physiologic adaptations to extrauterine life.

When the nurse took my first child and put him to my breast his tiny mouth opened and reached for me as if he had known forever what to do.
~ LESLIE KENTON, *ALL I EVER WANTED WAS A BABY* ~

Urinary Adaptations

Kidney Development and Function

Certain physiologic features of the newborn's kidneys may affect the newborn's ability to handle body fluids and excrete urine:

1. The term newborn's kidneys have a full complement of functioning nephrons by 34 to 36 weeks of gestation (Seaman, 1995).
2. The glomerular filtration rate of the newborn's kidneys is low in comparison with the adult rate. Because of this physiologic inefficiency, the newborn's kidneys are unable to dispose of water rapidly when necessary because it favors reabsorption of sodium (Seaman, 1995).
3. The juxtamedullary portion of the nephron has limited capacity to reabsorb HCO_3 and H^+ and concentrate urine. The limitation of tubular reabsorption can lead to inappropriate loss of substances present in the glomerular filtrate, such as amino acids, bicarbonate, glucose, and sodium.

TABLE 24–5 Physiologic Adaptations to Extrauterine Life

Periodic breathing may be present.
Desired skin temperature 36–36.5C (96.8–97.7F), stabilizes 4 to 6 hours after birth.
Desired blood glucose level reaches 60–70 mg/dL by third postnatal day.
Stools (progress from): Meconium (thick, tarry, black) Transitional stools (thin, brown to green) Breastfed infants (yellow gold, soft, or mushy) Bottle-fed infants (pale yellow, formed, and pasty)

Full-term newborns are less able than adults to concentrate urine (reabsorb water back into the blood) because the tubules are short and narrow. The newborn's capacity for glomerular filtration is greater than the capacity for tubular reabsorption-secretion. Although feeding practices may affect the osmolarity of the urine, the newborn can concentrate urine only to a maximum specific gravity of 1.025. The inability to concentrate urine is caused by the limited tubular reabsorption of water and limited excretion of solutes (principally sodium, potassium, chloride, bicarbonate, urea, and phosphate) in the growing newborn. The ability to concentrate urine fully is attained by 3 months of age.

Because the newborn has difficulty concentrating urine, the effect of excessive insensible water loss or restricted fluid intake is unpredictable. The newborn kidney is also limited in its dilutional capabilities; it can dilute only to a maximum specific gravity of 1.001. Concentrating and dilutional limitations of renal function are important considerations in monitoring fluid therapy to avoid dehydration and overhydration (Seaman, 1995).

Characteristics of Newborn Urinary Function

Many newborns void immediately after birth, and the voiding frequently goes unnoticed. Among normal newborns, 93% void by 24 hours after birth, and 98% void by 48 hours (Thureen, Deacon, O'Neill & Hernandez,

TABLE 24–6 Newborn Urinalysis Values

Protein < 5–10 mg/dL
WBC < 2–3
RBC 0
Casts 0
Bacteria 0
Specific gravity 1.001–1.025
Color pale yellow

1999). A newborn who has not voided by 48 hours should be assessed for adequacy of fluid intake, bladder distention, restlessness, and symptoms of pain. The appropriate clinical personnel should be notified if indicated.

The initial bladder volume is 6 to 44 mL of urine. Unless edema is present, normal urinary output is often limited, and the voidings are scanty until fluid intake increases. (The fluid of edema is eliminated by the kidneys, so infants with edema have a much higher urinary output.) The first 2 days postnatally the newborn voids two to six times daily, with a urine output of 15 mL/kg/day. The newborn subsequently voids 5 to 25 times every 24 hours, with a volume of 25 mL/kg/day.

Following the first voiding, the newborn's urine frequently appears cloudy (due to mucus content) and has a high specific gravity, which decreases as fluid intake increases. Occasionally, pink stains ("brick dust spots") appear on the diaper. These are caused by urates and are innocuous. Blood may occasionally be observed on the diapers of female infants. This *pseudomenstruation* is related to the withdrawal of maternal hormones. Males may have bloody spotting from a circumcision. In the absence of apparent causes for bleeding, the clinician should be notified. During early infancy, normal urine is straw colored and almost odorless, although odor occurs when there is a metabolic disorder or when infection is present. Table 24–6 summarizes urinalysis values of the normal newborn.

RESEARCH IN PRACTICE

What is the study about? Although reference values for leukocyte and neutrophil cell counts in normal full-term infants over the first 72 hours of life have been published and referenced, they are being challenged as normal for all infants in the clinical setting. The infant's gestational age and weight have been studied as variables that may alter laboratory tests. This study was designed to test the adequacy of previously established leukocyte indices in very low birthweight (VLBW) infants.

How was the study done? All charts of infants born in a large metropolitan hospital and admitted to the NICU over a six-month period served as a sample for this study. Laboratory results including leukocyte indices were obtained for the first 72 hours of life from the charts of 131 infants who met the study criteria (≤32 weeks gestation, ≤1200 birth weight, no maternal history of infection, no delivery room resuscitation, and no congenital anomalies).

What were the results of the study? None of the variables (sex of the infant, weight, gestational age, use of steroids during labor) obtained from the chart audit significantly affected the total leukocyte and absolute neutrophil counts. Ranges for total leukocyte count, absolute neutrophil count, and immature/total neutrophil (I:T) ratio were found to vary and change over time.

What additional questions might I have? (1) Are the reference values presently used for CBC and differential indices too restrictive for VLBW infants? (2) How different are the differential values in the infected and non-infected infant who is VLBW?

How can I use this study? This study represents the largest number of healthy newborn infant values for CBC and differential to date. A very large range of leukocyte and neutrophil counts were discovered for this study group of VLBW infants. this leads the clinician to question the index of values presently used to interpret CBC and differential values in the VLBW infants. Further study is needed to evaluate the ranges clinicians should use in practice.

SOURCE: Nash, P. & Kwon, I. (1998). CBC and differential in VLBW infants. *Neonatal Network, 17*(7), 17–22.

Immunologic Adaptations

The newborn possesses varying degrees of impairment of the nonspecific and specific immune responses. The inflammatory response and phagocytosis are altered in newborns primarily because functional limitations of their polymorphonuclear neutrophils (PMNs) affect leukocyte metabolic activities, mobilization, chemotaxis, opsonization, phagocytic activity, and intracellular killing. Newborns, particularly preterm infants, have decreased serum opsonization activity (the process of coating invasive bacteria to prepare them for phagocytic ingestion), resulting from low levels of immunoglobins and complement components. These limitations in the newborn's inflammatory response result in failure to recognize, localize, and destroy invasive bacteria. Thus the signs and symptoms of infection are often subtle and nonspecific in the newborn. The newborn also has a poor hypothalamic response to pyrogens; therefore fever is not a reliable indicator of infection. In the neonatal period, hypothermia is a more reliable sign of infection.

Of the three major types of immunoglobulins primarily involved in immunity—IgG, IgA, and IgM—only IgG crosses the placenta. The pregnant woman forms antibodies in response to illness or immunization. This process is called **active acquired immunity.** When IgG antibodies are transferred to the fetus in utero, **passive acquired immunity** results because the fetus does not produce the antibodies itself. IgG is very active against bacterial toxins.

Because the maternal immunoglobin is transferred primarily during the third trimester, preterm newborns (especially those born prior to 34 weeks) may be more susceptible to infection. In general newborns have maternally induced immunity to tetanus, diphtheria, smallpox, measles, mumps, poliomyelitis, and a variety of other bacterial and viral diseases. The period of resistance varies: Immunity against common viral infections such as measles may last 4 to 8 months, whereas immunity to certain bacteria may disappear within 4 to 8 weeks.

The normal newborn does produce antibodies in response to an antigen, but not as effectively as an older child would. It is customary to begin immunization at 2 months of age so the infant can develop active acquired immunity.

IgM immunoglobulins are produced in response to blood group antigens, gram-negative enteric organisms, and some viruses in the expectant mother. Because IgM does not normally cross the placenta, most or all is produced by the fetus beginning at 10 to 15 weeks' gestation. Elevated levels of IgM at birth may indicate placental leaks or, more commonly, fetal antigenic stimulation in utero. Consequently, elevations suggest that the infant was exposed to an intrauterine infection such as syphilis or a TORCH (toxoplasmosis, rubella, cytomegalovirus, herpes virus hominis type 2) infection. (For in-depth discussion, see Table 29–6.) The lack of available maternal IgM in the newborn also accounts for the infant's susceptibility to gram-negative enteric organisms such as *Escherichia coli.*

The functions of IgA immunoglobins are not fully understood. IgA appears to provide protection mainly on secreting surfaces such as the respiratory tract, gastrointestinal tract, and eyes. Serum IgA does not cross the placenta and is not normally produced by the fetus in utero. Unlike the other immunoglobins, IgA is not affected by gastric action. Colostrum, the forerunner of breast milk, is very high in the secretory form of IgA. Consequently, it may be of significance in providing some passive immunity to the infant of a breastfeeding mother. Newborns begin to produce secretory IgA in their intestinal mucosa at about 4 weeks after birth.

Neurologic and Sensory/Perceptual Functioning

The newborn's brain is about one-quarter the size of an adult's, and myelination of nerve fibers is incomplete. Unlike the cardiovascular or respiratory systems, which undergo tremendous changes at birth, the nervous system is minimally influenced by the actual birth process.

Because many biochemical and histologic changes have yet to occur in the newborn's brain, the postnatal period is considered a time of risk in regard to the development of the brain and nervous system. For neurologic development—including development of intellect—to proceed, the brain and other nervous system structures must mature in an orderly, unhampered fashion. For discussion of cranial nerves, see Chapter 25.

Intrauterine Factors Influencing Newborn Behavior

Newborns respond to and interact with the environment in a predictable pattern of behavior that is shaped somewhat by their intrauterine experience. This intrauterine experience is affected by intrinsic factors such as maternal nutrition and external factors such as the mother's physical environment. Depending on the newborn's intrauterine experience and individual temperament, newborn behavioral responses to different stresses vary. Some newborns react quietly to stimulation; others become overreactive and tense; and some may exhibit a combination of the two.

Brazelton and colleagues (1977) found a positive association between newborn behavior and nutritional status of the pregnant woman. Newborns with higher birth weight attended to and responded to visual and auditory cues and exhibited more mature motor activity than newborns with low birth weight.

Factors such as exposure to intense auditory stimuli in utero can eventually be manifested in the behavior of the newborn. For example, the fetal heart rate initially increases when the pregnant woman is exposed to an auditory stimuli, but repetition of the stimuli leads to decreased FHR. Thus the newborn who was exposed to intense noise during fetal life is significantly less reactive to loud sounds postnatally.

Characteristics of Newborn Neurologic Function

Partially flexed extremities with the legs near the abdomen is the usual position of the normal newborn. When awake, the newborn may exhibit purposeless, uncoordinated bilateral movements of the extremities. The organization and intensity of the newborn's motor activity are influenced by a number of factors, including the following (Brazelton, 1984): (1) sleep-wake states; (2) presence of environmental stimuli, such as heat, light, cold, and noise; (3) conditions causing a chemical imbalance, such as hypoglycemia; (4) hydration status; (5) state of health; and (6) recovery from the stress of labor and birth.

Eye movements are observable during the first few days of life. An alert neonate is able to fixate on faces and geometric objects or patterns such as black and white stripes. A bright light shining in the newborn's eyes elicits the blinking reflex.

The cry of the newborn should be lusty and vigorous. High-pitched cries, weak cries, or no cries are all causes for concern.

Growth of the newborn's body progresses in a cephalocaudal (head-to-toe), proximal-distal fashion.

The newborn is somewhat hypertonic; that is, there is resistance to extending the elbow and knee joints. Muscle tone should be symmetric. Diminished muscle tone and flaccidity may indicate neurologic dysfunction.

Specific symmetric deep tendon reflexes can be elicited in the newborn. The knee jerk is brisk; a normal ankle clonus may involve three or four beats. Plantar flexion is present. Other reflexes, including the Moro, grasping, rooting, Babinski, and sucking reflexes, are characteristics of neurologic integrity. (For further discussion, see Chapter 25.)

Performance of complex behavioral patterns reflects the newborn's neurologic maturation and integration. The newborn who can bring a hand to the mouth is demonstrating motor coordination as well as a self-quieting technique, thus increasing the complexity of the behavioral response. Newborns also possess complex organized defensive motor patterns as exhibited by the ability to remove an obstruction, such as a cloth across the face.

Periods of Reactivity

The baby usually shows a predictable pattern of behavior during the first several hours after birth, characterized by two **periods of reactivity** separated by a sleep phase.

First Period of Reactivity

The first period of reactivity lasts approximately 30 minutes after birth. During this period the newborn is awake and active and may appear hungry and have a strong sucking reflex. This is a natural opportunity to initiate breastfeeding if the mother has chosen it (Figure 24–13). Bursts of random, diffuse movements alternating with relative immobility may occur. Respirations are rapid, as high as 80 breaths/minute, and there may be retraction of the chest, transient flaring of the nares, and grunting. The heart rate is rapid, and rhythm may be irregular. Bowel sounds are usually absent.

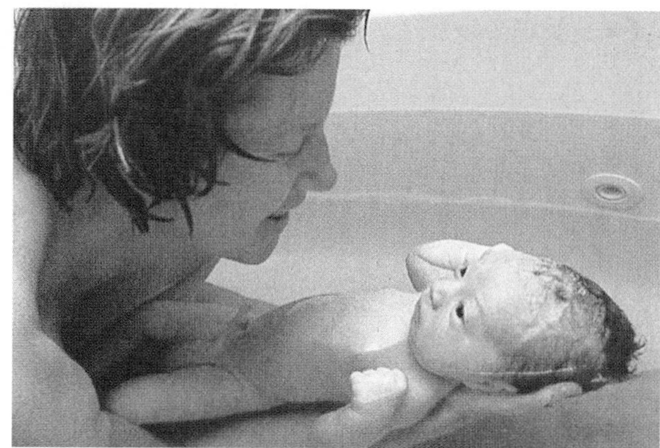

FIGURE 24–13 Mother and baby gaze at each other. This quiet alert state is the optimal state for interaction.

Period of Inactivity to Sleep Phase

After approximately half an hour, the newborn's activity gradually diminishes, and the heart rate and respirations decrease as the newborn enters the sleep phase. The sleep phase may last from a few minutes to 2 to 4 hours. During this period the newborn will be difficult to awaken and will show no interest in sucking. Bowel sounds become audible, and cardiac and respiratory rates return to baseline values.

Second Period of Reactivity

During the second period of reactivity, the newborn is again awake and alert. This period lasts 4 to 6 hours in the normal newborn. Physiologic responses are variable during this stage. The heart and respiratory rates increase; however, the nurse must be alert for apneic periods, which may cause a drop in the heart rate. The newborn is stimulated to continue breathing during such times. The newborn may develop rapid color changes and become mildly cyanotic or mottled during these fluctuations. Production of respiratory and gastric mucus increases, and the newborn responds by gagging, choking, and regurgitating.

Continued close observation and intervention may be required to maintain a clear airway during this period of reactivity. The gastrointestinal tract becomes more active. The first meconium stool is frequently passed during this second active stage, and the initial voiding may also occur at this time. The newborn will indicate readiness for feeding by such behaviors as sucking, rooting, and swallowing. If feeding was not initiated in the first period of reactivity, it is done at this time. See Chapter 27 for further discussion of this first feeding.

Behavioral States of the Newborn

The behavior of the newborn can be divided into two categories: the sleep state and the alert state (Brazelton, 1984). These postnatal behavioral states are similar to those that have been identified during pregnancy. Subcategories are identified under each major category.

Sleep States

The sleep states are as follows:

1. *Deep or quiet sleep.* Deep sleep is characterized by closed eyes with no eye movements, regular even breathing, and jerky motion or startles at regular intervals. Behavioral responses to external stimuli are likely to be delayed. Startles are rapidly suppressed, and changes in state are not likely to occur. Heart rate may range from 100 to 120 beats per minute.
2. *Active REM.* Irregular respirations, eyes closed with REM, irregular sucking motions, minimal activity, and irregular but smooth movement of the extremities can be observed in active REM sleep. Environmental and internal stimuli initiate a startle reaction and a change of state.

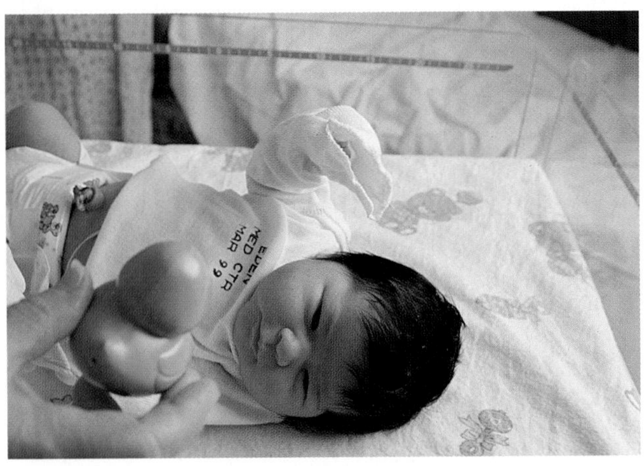

FIGURE 24–14 Head turning to follow an object.

Sleep cycles in the newborn have been recognized and defined according to duration. The length of the cycle depends on the age of the newborn. At term, REM active sleep and quiet sleep occur in intervals of 45 to 50 minutes. About 45% to 50% of the total sleep of the neonate is active sleep, 35% to 45% is quiet (deep) sleep, and 10% of sleep is transitional between these two periods. It is hypothesized that REM sleep stimulates the growth of the neural system. Over a period of time, the newborn's sleep-wake patterns become diurnal; that is, the newborn sleeps at night and stays awake during the day. (See Chapter 25 for in-depth discussion of assessment of neonatal states.)

Alert States

In the first 30 to 60 minutes after birth, many newborns display a quiet alert state, characteristic of the first period of reactivity. Nurses should use these alert states to encourage bonding and breastfeeding. These periods of alertness tend to be short the first 2 days after birth to allow the baby to recover from the birth process. Subsequently, alert states are of choice or of necessity (Brazelton, 1984). Increasing choice of wakefulness by the newborn indicates a maturing capacity to achieve and maintain consciousness. Heat, cold, and hunger are but a few of the stimuli that can cause wakefulness by necessity. Once the disturbing stimuli are removed, sleep tends to recur.

The following are subcategories of the alert state (Brazelton, 1984):

1. *Drowsy or semidozing.* The behaviors common to the drowsy state are open or closed eyes, fluttering eyelids, semidozing appearance, and slow, regular movements of the extremities. Mild startles may be noted from time to time. Although the reaction to a sensory stimulus is delayed, a change of state often results.
2. *Wide awake.* In the wide awake state, the newborn is alert and follows and fixates on attractive objects, faces, or auditory stimuli. Motor activity is minimal, and the response to external stimuli is delayed.
3. *Active awake.* The eyes are open, and motor activity is quite intense, with thrusting movements of the extremities in the active awake state. Environmental stimuli increase startles or motor activity, but discrete reactions are difficult to distinguish because of generalized high activity level.
4. *Crying.* Intense crying is accompanied by jerky motor movements. Crying serves several purposes for the newborn. It may be used as a distraction from disturbing stimuli such as hunger and pain. Fussiness often allows the newborn to discharge energy and reorganize behavior. Most important, crying elicits an appropriate response of help from the parents.

Behavioral and Sensory Capacities of the Newborn

Habituation is the newborn's ability to process and respond to complex visual and auditory stimulation. For example, when a bright light is flashed into the newborn's eyes, the initial response is blinking, constriction of the pupil, and perhaps a slight startle reaction. However, with repeated stimulation the newborn's response repertoire gradually diminishes and disappears. The capacity to ignore repetitious disturbing stimuli is a neonatal defense mechanism readily apparent in the noisy, well-lighted nursery.

Orientation is the newborn's ability to be alert to, to follow, and to fixate on complex visual stimuli that have a particular appeal and attraction. The newborn prefers the human face and eyes and bright shiny objects. As the face or object is brought into the line of vision, the neonate responds with bright, wide eyes, still limbs, and fixed staring. This intense visual involvement may last several minutes, during which time the newborn is able to follow the stimulus from side to side. Figure 24–14 illustrates this response. The newborn uses this sensory capacity to become familiar with family, friends, and surroundings.

Self-quieting ability refers to newborns' ability to use their own resources to quiet and comfort themselves. Their repertoire includes hand-to-mouth movements, sucking on a fist or tongue, and attending to external stimuli. Neurologically impaired newborns are unable to use self-quieting activities and require more frequent comforting from caregivers when stimulated. For example, drug-positive newborns often exhibit abnormal sleep and feeding patterns and irritability.

Auditory Capacity

The newborn responds to auditory stimulation with a definite, organized behavior repertoire. The stimulus used to assess auditory response should be selected to match the state of the newborn. A rattle is appropriate for light sleep, a voice for an awake state, and a clap for deep sleep. As the newborn hears the sound, the cardiac rate rises, and a minimal startle reflex may be seen. If the sound is appealing, the newborn will become alert and search for the site of the auditory stimulus.

Olfactory Capacity

Newborns are apparently able to select people by smell. In one study, newborns were able to distinguish their mothers' breast pads from those of other mothers at just 1 week postnatally (Brazelton, 1984).

Taste and Sucking

The newborn responds differently to varying tastes. Sugar, for example, increases sucking. Sucking pattern variations also exist in newborns fed with a rubber nipple versus the breast. When breastfeeding, the newborn sucks in bursts with frequent regular pauses. The bottle-fed newborn tends to suck at a regular rate with infrequent pauses.

When awake and hungry, the newborn displays rapid searching motions in response to the rooting reflex. Once feeding begins, the newborn establishes a sucking pattern according to the method of feeding. Finger sucking is present not only postnatally, but also in utero. The newborn frequently uses nonnutritive sucking as a self-quieting activity, which assists in the development of self-regulation. Nonnutritive sucking with a pacifier should not be discouraged if the infant is bottle-fed. Pacifiers should be offered to breastfed infants only after breastfeeding is well established. If the pacifier is offered too soon, a phenomenon called "nipple confusion" may occur in which the breastfed infant has difficulty learning to suck from the breast. (See Chapter 27 for a more in-depth discussion.)

Tactile Capacity

The newborn is very sensitive to being touched, cuddled, and held. Often a mother's first response to an upset or crying newborn is touching or holding. Swaddling, placing a hand on the abdomen, or holding the arms to prevent a startle reflex are other methods of soothing the newborn. The settled newborn is then able to attend to and interact with the environment.

FOCUS YOUR STUDY

- Newborn respiration is initiated primarily by chemical and mechanical events in association with thermal and sensory stimulation.
- The production of surfactant is crucial to keeping the lungs expanded during expiration by reducing alveolar surface tension.
- The newborn is an obligatory nose breather. Respirations move from being primarily shallow, irregular, and diaphragmatic to synchronous abdominal and chest breathing.
- Normal respiratory rate is 30 to 60 breaths/minute.
- Periodic breathing is normal, and newborn sleep states affect breathing patterns.
- The status of the cardiopulmonary system may be measured by evaluating the heart rate, blood pressure, and presence or absence of murmurs. The normal heart rate is 120 to 160 bpm.
- Oxygen transport in the newborn is significantly affected by the presence of greater amounts of HbF (fetal hemoglobin) than HbA (adult hemoglobin). HbF holds oxygen more efficiently but releases it to the body tissues only at low Po_2 levels.
- Blood values in the newborn are modified by several factors, such as site of the blood sample, gestational age, prenatal or perinatal hemorrhage, and the timing of the clamping of the umbilical cord.
- Blood glucose levels should reach 60 to 70 mg/dL by the third postnatal day.
- The newborn is considered to have established thermoregulation when oxygen consumption and metabolic activity are minimal.
- Evaporation is the primary heat loss mechanism in newborns who are wet from amniotic fluid or a bath. In addition, excessive heat loss occurs from radiation and convection because of the newborn's larger surface area compared to weight and from thermal conduction because of the marked difference between core temperature and skin temperature.
- The primary source of heat in the cold-stressed newborn is brown adipose tissue.
- The normal newborn possesses the ability to digest and absorb nutrients necessary for newborn growth and development.
- The newborn's liver plays a crucial role in iron storage, carbohydrate metabolism, conjugation of bilirubin, and coagulation.
- The newborn's stools change from meconium (thick, tarry, black) to transitional stools (thinner, brown to green) and then to the distinct forms for either breastfed newborns (yellow-gold, soft, or mushy) or bottle-fed newborns (pale yellow, formed, and pasty).
- Most newborns pass their first stool within 24 hours of birth.
- Controversy continues about the relationship of breastfeeding and the development of prolonged jaundice.
- The newborn's kidneys are characterized by a decreased rate of glomerular flow, limited tubular reabsorption, limited excretion of solutes, and limited ability to concentrate urine.
- Most newborns void within 24 hours of birth.
- The immune system in the newborn is not fully activated until sometime after birth, but the newborn does possess some immunologic abilities.
- Neurologic and sensory perceptual functioning in the newborn is evident from the newborn's interaction with the environment, presence of synchronized motor activity, and well-developed sensory capacities.
- The first period of reactivity lasts for 30 minutes after birth. The newborn is alert and hungry at this time, making this a natural opportunity to promote attachment.
- The second period of reactivity requires close monitoring by the nurse because apnea, decreased heart rate, gagging, choking, and regurgitation are likely to occur and require nursing intervention.
- Behavioral states in the newborn can be divided into sleep states and alert states.

REFERENCES

Blackburn, S. T., & Loper, D. L. (1992). *Maternal, fetal, and neonatal physiology: A clinical perspective.* Philadelphia: Saunders.

Brazelton, T. B. (1984). *Neonatal behavioral assessment scale* (2nd ed.). London: Heineman.

Brazelton, T. B., Tronick, E., Lechtig, A., Lasky, R. E., & Klein, R. E. (1977). The behavior of nutritionally deprived Guatemalan neonates. *Developmental Medicine and Child Neurology, 19,* 364–372.

Cunningham, F. G., MacDonald, P. C., Gant, N. G., Leveno, K. J., Gilstrap, L. C. III, Hankins, G. D. V., & Clark, S. L. (1997). *Williams obstetrics* (20th ed.). Stamford, CT: Appleton & Lange.

Fanaroff, A. A., & Martin, R. J. (1997). *Neonatal-perinatal medicine* (6th ed.). St. Louis: Mosby.

Fletcher, M. E. (1994). Physical assessment and classification. In G. B. Avery, M. A. Fletcher, & M. G. MacDonald (Eds.), *Neonatology: Pathophysiology and management of the newborn* (4th ed.). Philadelphia: Lippincott.

Hey, E. (1994). Thermoregulation. In G. B. Avery, M. A. Fletcher, & M. G. MacDonald (Eds.), *Neonatology: Pathophysiology and management of the newborn* (4th ed.). Philadelphia: Lippincott.

James, L. S., & Adamsons, K. (1994). The neonate and resuscitation. In J. R. Scott, P. J. DiSaia, C. B. Hammond, & W. N. Spellacy (Eds.), *Danforth's obstetrics and gynecology* (7th ed.). Philadelphia: Lippincott.

Johnston, P. G. B. (1998). *The newborn child* (8th ed.). New York: Churchill.

Karp, T. B., Scardino, C., & Butler, L. A. (1995). Glucose metabolism in the neonate: The short and sweet of it. *Neonatal Network, 14*(8), 17–23.

Long, W. A. (1990). *Fetal and neonatal cardiology.* Philadelphia: Saunders.

MacMahon, J. R., Stevenson, D. K., & Oski, F. A. (1998). Physiologic jaundice. In H. W. Taeusch & R. A. Ballard (Eds.), *Avery's diseases of the newborn* (7th ed.). Philadelphia: Saunders.

Maisels, M. J. (1994). Jaundice. In G. B. Avery, M. A. Fletcher, & M. G. MacDonald (Eds.), *Neonatology: Pathophysiology and management of the newborn* (4th ed.). Philadelphia: Lippincott.

Nelson, N. (1994). Physiology of transition. In G. B. Avery, M. A. Fletcher, & M. G. MacDonald (Eds.), *Neonatology: Pathophysiology and management of the newborn* (4th ed.). Philadelphia: Lippincott.

Newman, T. B., & Maisels, M. J. (1992). Evaluation and treatment of jaundice in the term newborn: A kinder, gentler approach. *Pediatrics, 89*(5 Pt. 1), 809–818.

Polin, R. A., & Fox, W. W. (1998). *Fetal and neonatal physiology* (2nd ed.). Philadelphia: Saunders.

Rebar, R. W. (1999). The breast and the physiology of lactation. In R. K. Creasy & R. Resnik (Eds.), *Maternal fetal medicine* (4th ed.). Philadelphia, Saunders.

Sansoucie, D. A., & Cavaliere, T. A. (1997). Transition from fetal to extrauterine circulation. *Neonatal Network, 16*(2), 5–12.

Seaman, S. L. (1995). Renal physiology. II. Fluid and electrolyte regulation. *Neonatal Network, 14*(5), 5–11.

Thureen, P. J., Deacon, J., O'Neill, P., & Hernandez, J. (1999). *Assessment and care of the well newborn.* Philadelphia: Saunders.

Verklan, M. T. (1997). Diagnostic techniques in cardiac disorders: Pt 1. *Neonatal Network, 16*(4), 9–15.

Nursing Assessment of the Newborn

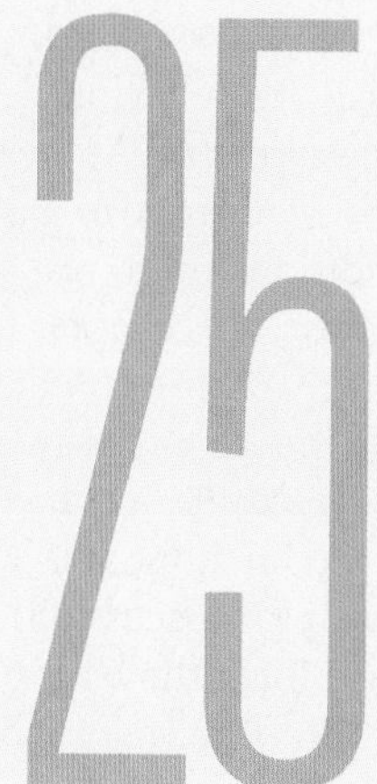

SOMETHING VERY SPECIAL OCCURS WITHIN THE FIRST hour after birth. If the environment is quiet, the birthing without complications, the lights lowered, the handling diminished, newborn infants—aside from all the physiological adaptations they must make—begin in a uniquely human way to adapt to the new experience of being in the world.
~ *The Amazing Newborn* ~

Objectives

- Describe the normal physical and behavioral characteristics of the newborn.
- Summarize the components of a complete newborn assessment and the significance of normal variations and abnormal findings.
- Explain the various components of the gestational age assessment.
- Discuss the neurologic and neuromuscular characteristics of the newborn and the reflexes that may be present at birth.
- Describe the categories of the newborn behavioral assessment.

Key Terms

Acrocyanosis
Babinski reflex
Barlow's maneuver
Brazelton's neonatal behavioral assessment
Caput succedaneum
Cephalhematoma
Chemical conjunctivitis
Epstein's pearls
Erb-Duchenne paralysis (Erb's palsy)
Erythema toxicum
Gestational age assessment tools
Grasping reflex
Harlequin sign
Milia
Molding
Mongolian spots
Moro reflex
Mottling
Nevus flammeus (port wine stain)
Nevus vasculosus (strawberry mark)
Ortolani's maneuver
Pseudomenstruation
Rooting reflex
Skin turgor
Subconjunctival hemorrhage
Sucking reflex
Telangiectatic nevi (stork bites)
Thrush
Tonic neck reflex
Trunk incurvation (Galant reflex)
Vernix caseosa

Unlike adults, newborns communicate their needs primarily by behavior. Because nurses are the most consistent observers of the newborn, they must be able to interpret this behavior to gain information about the newborn's condition and to respond with appropriate nursing interventions. This chapter focuses on the assessment of the newborn and interpretation of findings.

Assessment of the newborn is a continuous process used to evaluate development and adjustments to extrauterine life. In the birthing area, Apgar scoring procedure (see Chapter 20 for discussion) and careful observation of the newborn form the basis of the assessment and are correlated with information such as the following:

- Maternal prenatal care history
- Birthing history
- Maternal analgesia and anesthesia
- Complications of labor or birth
- Treatment instituted in birthing room, in conjunction with determination of clinical gestational age
- Consideration of the newborn's classification by weight and gestational age and by neonatal mortality risk
- Physical examination of the newborn

The nurse incorporates data from these sources with the assessment findings during the first 1 to 4 hours after birth to formulate a plan for nursing intervention.

The various newborn assessments and the data obtained from them are only as effective as the degree to which the findings are shared with the parents. The parents must be included in the assessment process from the moment of their child's birth. The Apgar score and its meaning should be explained immediately to the family. As soon as possible, the parents should be a part of the physical and behavioral assessments, as well.

The nurse encourages the parents to identify the unique behavioral characteristics of their newborn and to learn nurturing activities. Attachment is promoted when parents have the opportunity to explore their newborn in private, identifying individual physical and behavioral characteristics. The nurse's supportive responses to the parents' questions and observations are essential throughout the assessment process. The newborn physical examination therefore is the beginning of newborn health surveillance and health education for the newborn's family that continues into the community (Fowlie & Forsyth, 1995).

Timing of Newborn Assessments

The first 24 hours of life are significant because during this period the newborn makes the critical transition from intrauterine to extrauterine life. The risk of mortality and morbidity is statistically high during this period. Assessment of the newborn is essential to ensure that the transition is proceeding successfully.

TABLE 25–1 Timing and Types of Newborn Assessments

Assess immediately after birth: need for resuscitation or if newborn is stable and can be placed with parents to initiate early attachment/bonding
Assessments within 1 to 4 hours after birth:
Progress of newborn's adaptation to extrauterine life
Determination of gestational age
Ongoing assessment for high-risk problems
Assessment procedures within first 24 hours or prior to discharge:
Complete physical examination (Depending on agency protocol, the nurse may complete some components independently with the certified nurse-midwife/physician/nurse practitioner completing the exam prior to discharge.)
Nutritional status and ability to bottle-feed or breastfeed satisfactorily.
Behavioral state organization abilities

There are three major time frames for assessing newborns while they are in the birth facility. The first assessment is done in the birthing area immediately after birth to determine the need for resuscitation or other interventions. The newborn who is stable can stay with the family after birth to initiate early attachment. The newborn who has complications is usually taken to the nursery for further evaluation and intervention.

A second assessment is done in the first 1 to 4 hours after birth as part of the routine admission procedures. During this assessment, the nurse carries out a brief physical examination to evaluate the newborn's adaptation to extrauterine life and to estimate gestational age. No later than 2 hours after birth, the admitting nursery nurse should evaluate the newborn's status and any problems that place the newborn at risk (American Academy of Pediatrics [AAP] & the American College of Obstetricians and Gynecologists [ACOG], 1997).

Prior to discharge, a certified nurse-midwife, physician, or nurse practitioner carries out a behavioral assessment and a complete physical examination to detect any emerging or potential problems. A general assessment is also done at this time (Table 25–1).

This chapter presents the procedures for estimating gestational age and performing the complete physical examination and behavioral assessment. Chapter 20 discusses the immediate postbirth assessment. Chapter 26 describes the brief assessment performed during the first 4 hours of life.

Estimation of Gestational Age

The nurse must establish the newborn's gestational age in the first 4 hours after birth so that careful attention can be given to age-related problems (Alexander & Allen, 1996). Traditionally, a newborn's gestational age was determined from the date of the pregnant woman's last menstrual period. This method was accurate only 75% to 85% of the time. Because of the problems that develop with the newborn who is preterm or whose weight is inappropriate for gestational age, a more accurate system was developed to evaluate the newborn. Once learned, the procedure can be done in a few minutes. *It is essential that the nurse wear gloves when assessing the newborn in these early hours after birth prior to the first bath.*

Clinical **gestational age assessment tools** have two components: external physical characteristics and neurologic or neuromuscular development evaluations. Physical characteristics generally include sole creases, amount of breast tissue, amount of lanugo, cartilaginous development of the ear, testicular descent, and scrotal rugae or labial development. These objective clinical criteria are not influenced by labor and birth and do not change significantly within the first 24 hours after birth.

During the first 24 hours of life, the newborn's nervous system is unstable; thus neurologic evaluation findings based on reflexes or assessments dependent on the higher brain centers may not be reliable. If the neurologic findings drastically deviate from the gestational age derived by evaluation of the external characteristics, a second assessment is done in 24 hours.

The neurologic assessment components (excluding reflexes) can aid in assessing the gestational age of newborns of less than 34 weeks' gestation. Between 26 and 34 weeks, neurologic changes are significant, whereas significant physical changes are less evident. The important neurologic changes consist of replacement of extensor tone by flexor tone in a *caudocephalad* (tail-to-head) progression. Neurologic examination facilitates assessment of functional or physiologic maturation in addition to physical development.

Ballard and colleagues' (1979) *estimation of gestational age by maturity* rating is a simplified version of the well-researched Dubowitz tool (Dubowitz & Dubowitz, 1977). The Ballard tool omits some of the neuromuscular tone assessments, such as head lag, ventral suspension (which is difficult to assess in very ill newborns or those on respirators), and leg recoil. In Ballard's tool, each physical and neuromuscular finding is given a value, and the total score is matched to a gestational age (Figure 25–1). The maximum score on the Ballard's tool is 50, which corresponds to a gestational age of 44 weeks.

For example, on completing a gestational assessment of a 1-hour-old newborn, the nurse gives a score of 3 to all the physical characteristics, for a total of 18, and gives a score of 3 to all the neuromuscular assessments, for a total neurologic score of 18. The physical characteristics score of 18 is added to the neurologic score of 18 for a total score of 36, which correlates with 38+ weeks' gestation. Because all newborns vary slightly in the development of physical characteristics and maturation of neurologic function, scores will usually vary instead of all being 3, as in the example.

Current postnatal gestational age assessment tools can overestimate preterm gestational age and underestimate postterm gestational age (Gardosi, 1997). The tools have been shown to lose accuracy when newborns of fewer than 28 weeks' or more than 43 weeks' gestation are assessed. Ballard and colleagues (1991) added criteria for more accurate assessment of the gestational age of newborns 20 to 28 weeks old and less than 1500 g. They suggest that the assessment be made within 12 hours of birth to optimize accuracy, especially in infants of less than 26 weeks' gestational age (Ballard, Khoury, Wedig, Wang, Eilers-Walsman, & Lipp, 1991).

In carrying out gestational age assessments, the nurse keeps in mind that some maternal conditions, such as pregnancy-induced hypertension (PIH), diabetes, and maternal analgesia and anesthesia, may affect certain gestational assessment components and warrant further study. Maternal diabetes, although it appears to accelerate fetal physical growth, seems to retard maturation. Maternal hypertensive states, which retard fetal physical growth, seem to speed maturation.

Newborns of women with PIH have a poor correlation with the criteria involving active muscle tone and edema. Maternal analgesia and anesthesia may cause the baby to have respiratory depression. Babies with respiratory distress syndrome (RDS) tend to be flaccid and edematous and to assume a "froglike" posture. These characteristics affect the scoring of the neuromuscular components of the assessment tool used.

Assessment of Physical Characteristics

The nurse first evaluates observable characteristics without disturbing the baby. Selected physical characteristics common to both gestational assessment tools are presented here in the order in which they might be evaluated most effectively:

1. *Resting posture,* although a neuromuscular component, should be assessed as the baby lies undisturbed on a flat surface (Figure 25–2).
2. *Skin* in the preterm newborn appears thin and transparent, with veins prominent over the abdomen early in gestation. As term approaches, the skin appears opaque because of increased subcutaneous tissue. Disappearance of the protective vernix caseosa promotes skin desquamation and is commonly seen in postmature infants (infants of more than 42 weeks' gestational age and showing signs of placental insufficiency; see Chapter 28).
3. *Lanugo,* a fine hair covering, decreases as gestational age increases. The amount of lanugo is greatest at 28 to 30 weeks and then disappears, first from the face, then from the trunk and extremities.
4. *Sole (plantar) creases* are reliable indicators of gestational age in the first 12 hours of life. After this the skin of the foot begins drying, and superficial creases appear. Development of sole creases begins at the top (anterior) portion of the sole and, as gestation progresses, proceeds to the heel (Figure 25–3).

NEWBORN MATURITY RATING & CLASSIFICATION

ESTIMATION OF GESTATIONAL AGE BY MATURITY RATING

Symbols: X - 1st Exam O - 2nd Exam

NEUROMUSCULAR MATURITY

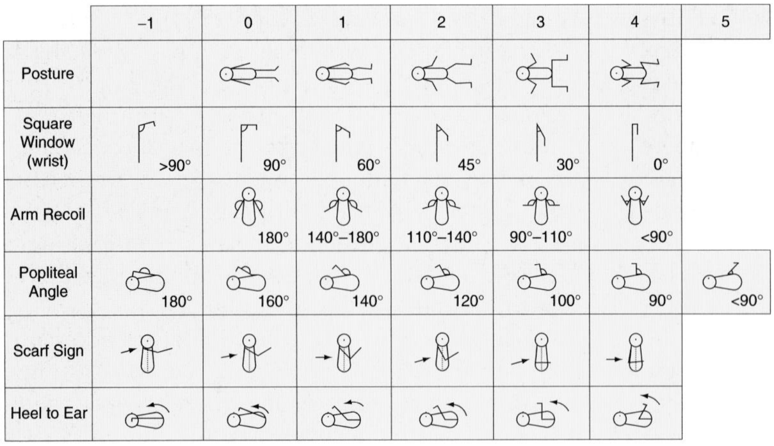

	–1	0	1	2	3	4	5
Posture							
Square Window (wrist)	>90°	90°	60°	45°	30°	0°	
Arm Recoil		180°	140°–180°	110°–140°	90°–110°	<90°	
Popliteal Angle	180°	160°	140°	120°	100°	90°	<90°
Scarf Sign							
Heel to Ear							

Gestation by Dates ________________ wks

____

Birth Date __________ Hour __________ am pm

APGAR __________ 1 min __________ 5 min

MATURITY RATING

score	weeks
–10	20
–5	22
0	24
5	26
10	28
15	30
20	32
25	34
30	36
35	38
40	40
45	42
50	44

PHYSICAL MATURITY

Skin	sticky friable transparent	gelatinous red, translucent	smooth pink, visible veins	superficial peeling &/or rash, few veins	cracking pale areas rare veins	parchment deep cracking no vessels	leathery cracked wrinkled
Lanugo	none	sparse	abundant	thinning	bald areas	mostly bald	
Plantar Surface	heel-toe 40–50mm:–1 <40mm:–2	>50mm no crease	faint red marks	anterior transverse crease only	creases ant. 2/3	creases over entire sole	
Breast	imperceptible	barely perceptible	flat areola no bud	stippled areola 1–2mm bud	raised areola 3–4mm bud	full areola 5–10mm bud	
Eye/Ear	lids fused loosely:–1 tightly:–2	lids open pinna flat stays folded	sl. curved pinna; soft; slow recoil	well curved pinna; soft but ready recoil	formed & firm instant recoil	thick cartilage ear stiff	
Genitals male	scrotum flat, smooth	scrotum empty faint rugae	testes in upper canal rare rugae	testes descending few rugae	testes down good rugae	testes pendulous deep rugae	
Genitals female	clitoris prominent labia flat	prominent clitoris small labia minora	prominent clitoris enlarging minora	majora & minora equally prominent	majora large minora small	majora cover clitoris & minora	

SCORING SECTION

	1st Exam = X	2nd Exam = 0
Estimating Gest Age by Maturity Rating	______Weeks	______Weeks
Time of Exam	Date ________ Hour ______ am pm	Date ________ Hour ______ am pm
Age at Exam	______ Hours	______ Hours
Signature of Examiner	____________ M.D.	____________ M.D.

FIGURE 25–1 Newborn maturity rating and classification. If a 1-hour-old newborn is given a score of 3 for each of the physical characteristics and neuromuscular assessments, the newborn's total score would be 36. A total score of 36 correlates with 38 or more weeks' gestation.
SOURCE: Ballard JL et al: New Ballard score, expanded to include extremely premature infants. *J Pediatr* 1991; 119:417.

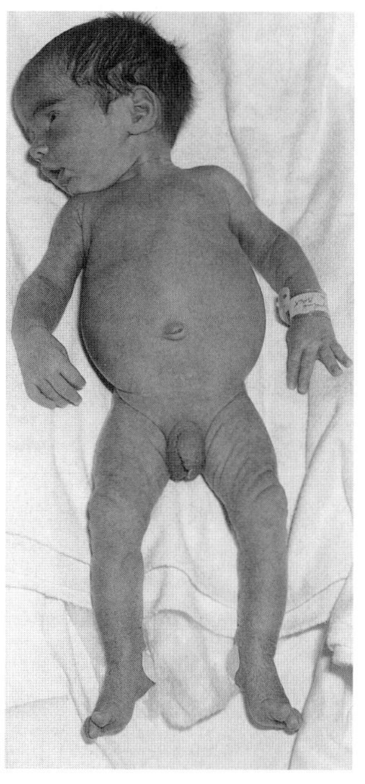

A

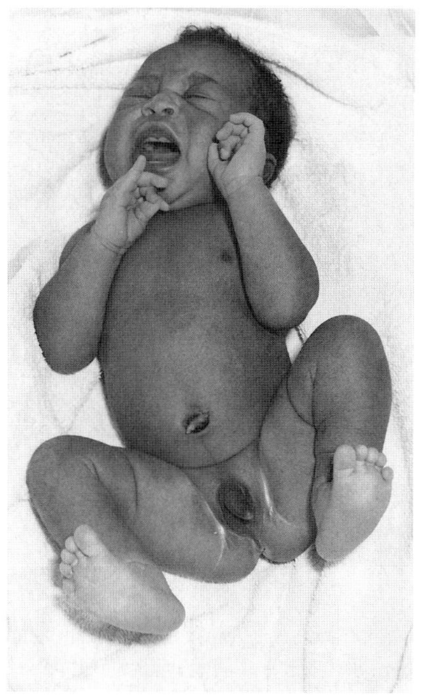

B

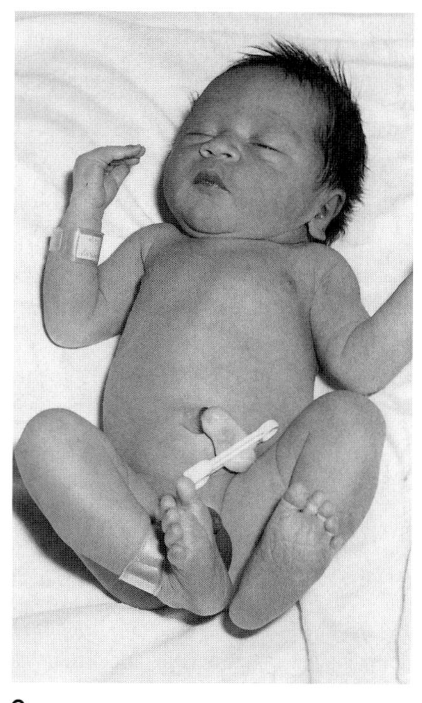

C

FIGURE 25–2 Resting posture. ***A,*** Infant exhibits beginning of flexion of the thigh. The gestational age is approximately 31 weeks. Note the extension of the upper extremities. ***B,*** Infant exhibits stronger flexion of the arms, hips, and thighs. The gestational age is approximately 35 weeks. ***C,*** The full-term infant exhibits hypertonic flexion of all extremities. SOURCE: Dubowitz L, Dubowitz V: *The Gestational Age of the Newborn.* Menlo Park, CA: Addison-Wesley, 1977. Reprinted by permission of V Dubowitz, MD, Hammersmith Hospital, London, England.

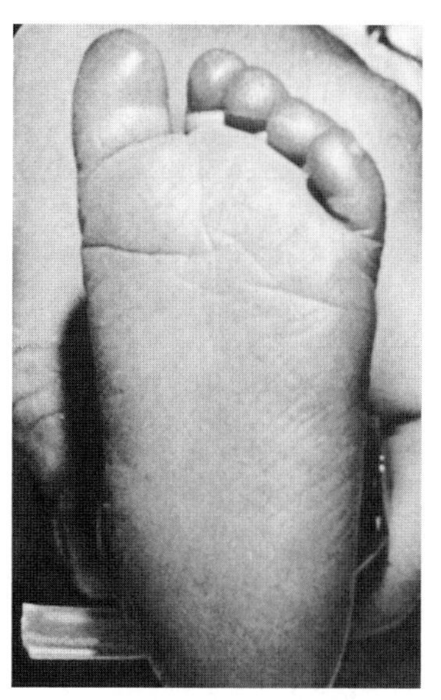

A

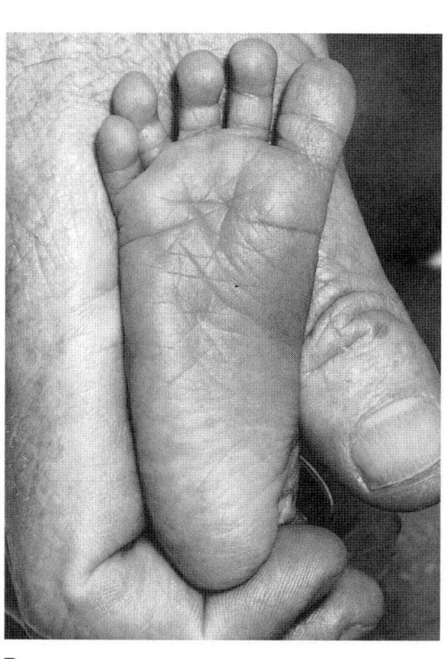

B

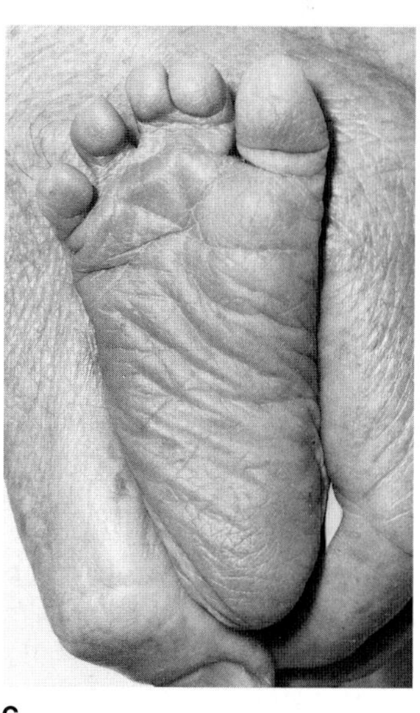

C

FIGURE 25–3 Sole creases. ***A,*** Infant has a few sole creases on the anterior portion of the foot. Note the slick heel. The gestational age is approximately 35 weeks. ***B,*** Infant has a deeper network of sole creases on the anterior two-thirds of the sole. Note the slick heel. The gestational age is approximately 37 weeks. ***C,*** The full-term infant has deep sole creases down to and including the heel as the skin loses fluid and dries after birth. Sole (plantar) creases can be seen even in preterm newborns. SOURCE: Dubowitz L, Dubowitz V: *Gestational Age of the Newborn.* Menlo Park, CA: Addison-Wesley, 1977. Reprinted by permission of V Dubowitz, MD, Hammersmith Hospital, London, England.

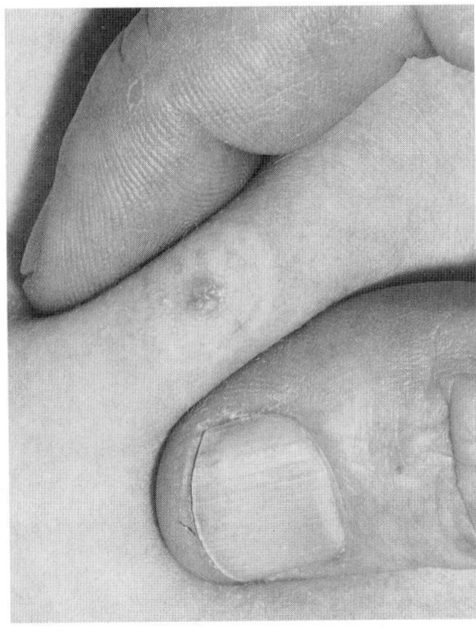

A

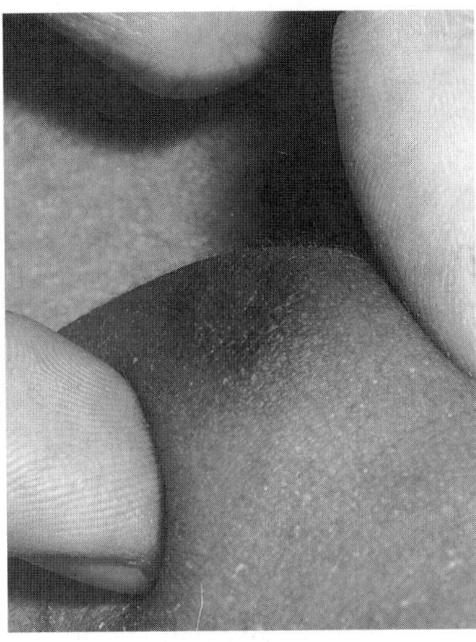

B

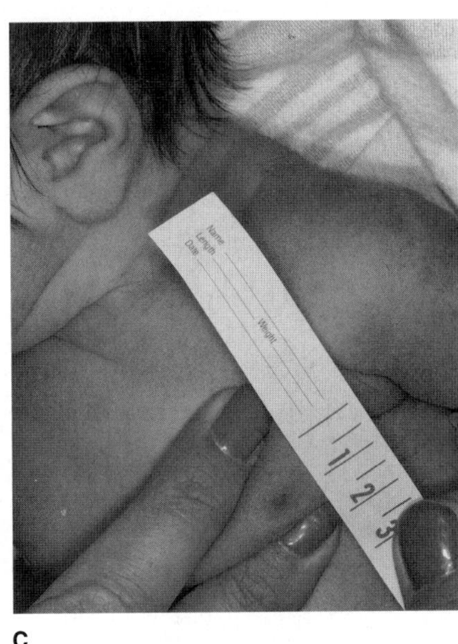

C

FIGURE 25–4 Breast tissue. ***A,*** Newborn has a visible raised area. On palpation the area is 4 mm. The gestational age is 38 weeks ***B,*** Newborn has a breast tissue area of 10 mm. The gestational age is 40 to 44 weeks. ***C,*** To measure breast tissue, gently compress the tissue between the middle and index fingers, and measure the tissue in centimeters or millimeters. Absence of or decreased breast tissue often indicates premature or SGA newborn. SOURCE: Dubowitz L, Dubowitz V: *Gestational Age of the Newborn.* Menlo Park, CA: Addison-Wesley, 1977. Reprinted by permission of V Dubowitz, MD, Hammersmith Hospital, London, England.

Peeling may also occur. Plantar creases vary with race. In newborns of African descent, sole creases may be less developed at term.

5. The nurse inspects the *areola* and gently palpates the *breast bud tissue* by applying the forefinger and middle finger to the breast area and measuring the tissue between them in centimeters or millimeters (Figure 25–4). At term gestation, the tissue will measure between 0.5 and 1 cm (5 to 10 mm). During the assessment, the nipple should not be grasped firmly because skin and subcutaneous tissue will prevent accurate estimation of size. The nurse must do this procedure gently to avoid causing trauma to the breast tissue.

   As gestation progresses, the breast tissue mass and areola enlarge. However, a large breast tissue mass can occur as a result of conditions other than advanced gestational age or the effects of maternal hormones on the baby. The infant of a diabetic mother may be large for gestational age (LGA), and the accelerated development of breast tissue is a reflection of subcutaneous fat deposits. Small-for-gestational-age (SGA) term or postterm newborns may have used subcutaneous fat (which would have been deposited as breast tissue) to survive in utero; as a result their lack of breast tissue may indicate a gestational age of 34 to 35 weeks, even though other factors indicate a term or postterm newborn.

6. *Ear form and cartilage distribution* develop with gestational age. The cartilage gives the ear its shape and substance (Figure 25–5). In a newborn of less than 34 weeks' gestation, the ear is relatively shapeless and flat; it has little cartilage, so the ear folds over on itself and remains folded. By approximately 36 weeks' gestation, some cartilage and slight incurving of the upper pinna are present, and the pinna springs back slowly when folded. (The nurse tests this response by holding the top and bottom of the pinna together with the forefinger and thumb and then releasing it, or by folding the pinna of the ear forward against the side of the head and releasing it, and observing the response.) By term, the newborn's pinna is firm, stands away from the head, and springs back quickly from the folding.

7. *Male genitals* are evaluated for size of the scrotal sac, the presence of rugae, and descent of the testes (Figure 25–6). Prior to 36 weeks, the small scrotum has few rugae, and the testes are palpable in the inguinal canal. By 36 to 38 weeks, the testes are in the upper scrotum, and rugae have developed over the anterior portion of the scrotum. By term, the testes are generally in the lower scrotum, which is pendulous and covered with rugae.

8. The appearance of the *female genitals* depends in part on subcutaneous fat deposition and therefore relates to fetal nutritional status (Figure 25–7). The clitoris varies in size and occasionally is so large that it is difficult to identify the sex of the newborn. This may be caused by adrenogenital syndrome, which causes the adrenals to secrete excessive amounts of androgen and other hormones. At 30 to 32 weeks'

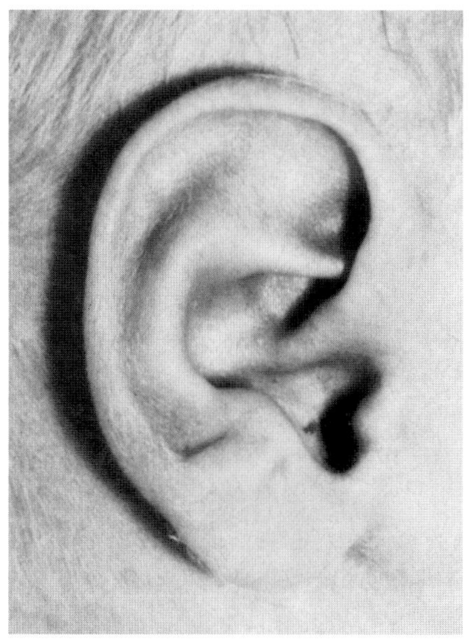

A

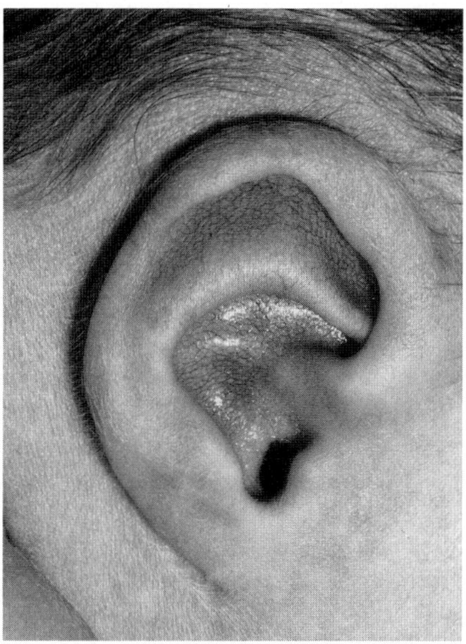

B

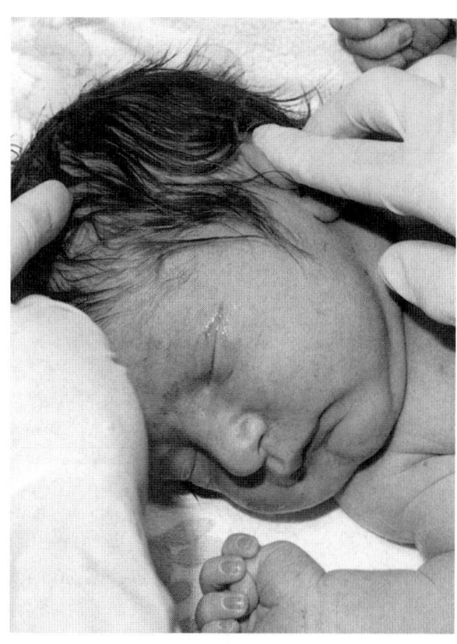

C

FIGURE 25–5 Ear form and cartilage. ***A,*** The ear of the infant at approximately 36 weeks' gestation shows incurving of the upper two-thirds of the pinna. ***B,*** Infant at term shows well-defined incurving of the entire pinna. ***C,*** If the auricle stays in the position in which it is pressed or returns slowly to its original position, it usually means that the gestational age is less than 38 weeks. SOURCE: *A* and *C;* Dubowitz L, Dubowitz V: *Gestational Age of the Newborn.* Menlo Park, CA: Addison-Wesley, 1977. Reprinted by permission of V Dubowitz, MD, Hammersmith Hospital, London, England.

gestation, the clitoris is prominent, and the labia majora are small and widely separated. As gestational age increases, the labia majora increase in size. At 36 to 40 weeks, they nearly cover the clitoris. At 40 weeks and beyond, the labia majora cover the labia minora and clitoris.

Other physical characteristics assessed by some gestational age scoring tools include the following:

1. *Vernix* covers the preterm newborn. The postterm newborn has no vernix. After noting vernix distribution, the birthing area nurse (wearing gloves) dries the newborn to prevent evaporative heat loss, thus disturbing the vernix and potentially altering this gestational age criterion. The birthing area nurse must communicate to the neonatal nurse the amount of vernix and the areas of vernix coverage.
2. *Hair* of the preterm newborn has the consistency of matted wool or fur and lies in bunches rather than in the silky, single strands of the term newborn's hair.
3. *Skull firmness* increases as the fetus matures. In a term newborn, the bones are hard, and the sutures are not easily displaced. The nurse should not attempt to displace the sutures forcibly.

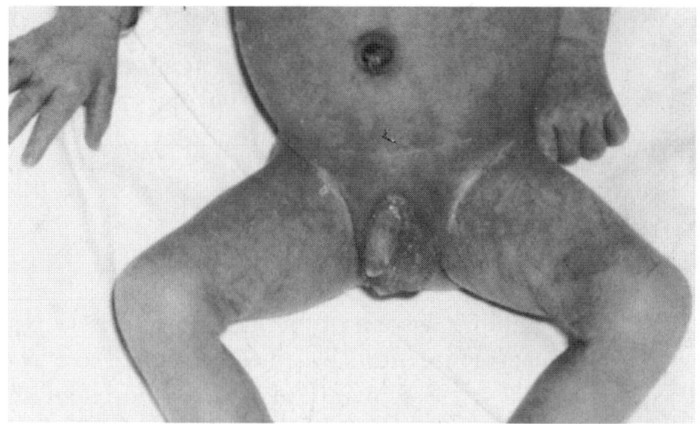

A

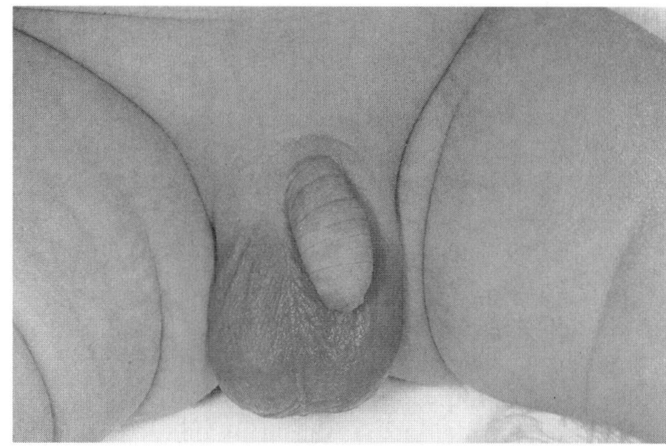

B

FIGURE 25–6 Male genitals. ***A,*** Preterm infant's testes are not within the scrotum. The scrotal surface has few rugae. ***B,*** Term infant's testes are generally fully descended. The entire surface of the scrotum is covered by rugae. SOURCE: Dubowitz L, Dubowitz V: *Gestational Age of the Newborn.* Menlo Park, CA: Addison-Wesley, 1977. Reprinted by permission of V Dubowitz, MD, Hammersmith Hospital, London, England.

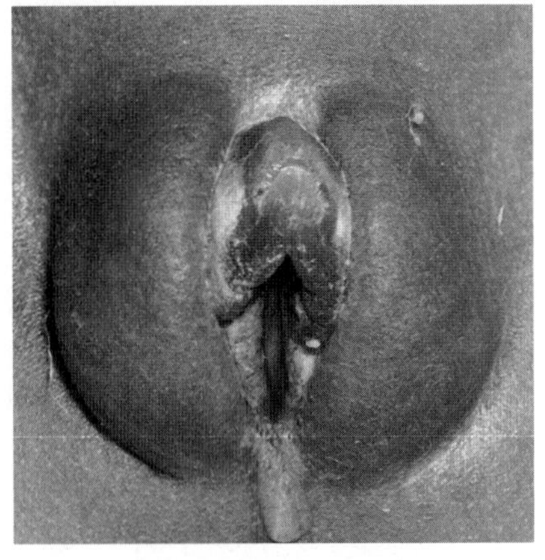

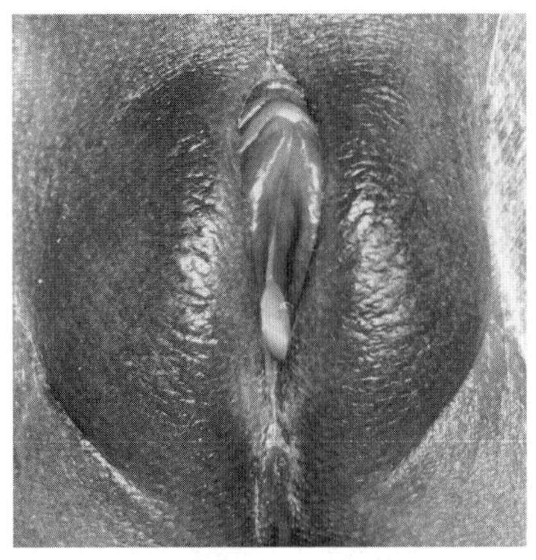

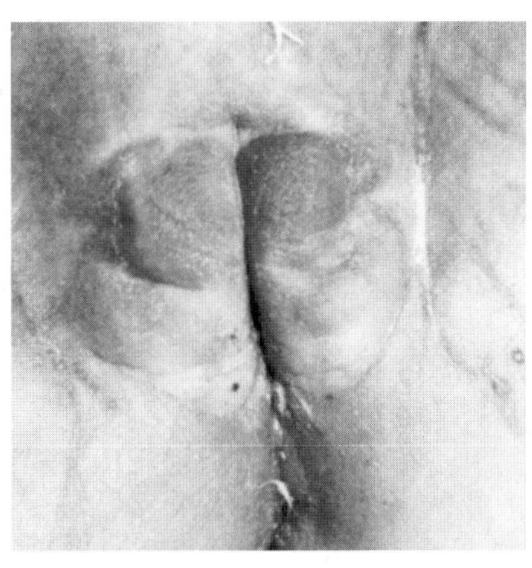

FIGURE 25–7 Female genitals. ***A,*** Infant has a prominent clitoris. The labia majora are widely separated, and the labia minora, viewed laterally, would protrude beyond the labia majora. The gestational age is 30 to 36 weeks. ***B,*** The clitoris is still visible. The labia minora are now covered by the larger labia majora. The gestational age is 36 to 40 weeks. ***C,*** The term infant has well-developed, large labia majora that cover both clitoris and labia minora. SOURCE: Dubowitz L, Dubowitz V: *Gestational Age of the Newborn.* Menlo Park, CA: Addison-Wesley, 1977. Reprinted by permission of V Dubowitz, MD, Hammersmith Hospital, London, England.

4. *Nails* appear and cover the nail bed at about 20 weeks' gestation. Nails extending beyond the fingertips may indicate a postterm newborn.

Assessment of Neuromuscular Maturity Characteristics

The central nervous system of the human fetus matures at a fairly constant rate. Tests have been designed to evaluate neurologic status as manifested by development of neuromuscular tone. In the fetus, neuromuscular tone develops from the lower to the upper extremities. The neurologic evaluation requires more manipulation and disturbances than the physical evaluation of the newborn.

The neuromuscular evaluation (Figure 25–1) is best performed when the infant has stabilized. The following characteristics are evaluated:

1. The *square window sign* is elicited by flexing the baby's hand toward the ventral forearm until resistance is felt. The angle formed at the wrist is measured (Figure 25–8).
2. *Recoil* is a test of flexion development. Because flexion first develops in the lower extremities, recoil is first tested in the legs. The newborn is placed on its back on a flat surface. With a hand on the newborn's knees and while manipulating the hip joint, the nurse places the baby's legs in flexion, then extends them parallel to each other and flat on the surface. The response to this maneuver is recoil of the newborn's legs. According to gestational age, they may not move, or they may return slowly or quickly to the flexed position. Preterm infants have less muscle tone than term infants, so preterm infants have less recoil.

   Arm recoil is tested by flexion at the elbow and extension of the arms at the newborn's side. While the baby is in the supine position, the nurse completely flexes both elbows, holds them in this position for 5 seconds, extends the arms at the baby's side, and releases them. Upon release, the elbows of a full-term newborn form an angle of less than 90 degrees and rapidly recoil back to flexed position. The elbows of preterm newborns have slower recoil time and form a greater than 90-degree angle. Arm recoil is also slower in healthy but fatigued newborns after birth; therefore arm recoil is best elicited after the first hour of birth, when the baby has had time to recover from the stress of birth. The deep sleep state also decreases the arm recoil response. Assessment of arm recoil should be bilateral in order to rule out brachial palsy.
3. The *popliteal angle* (degree of knee flexion) is determined with the newborn flat on its back. The thigh is flexed on the abdomen and chest, and the nurse places the index finger of the other hand behind the newborn's ankle to extend the lower leg until resistance is met. The angle formed is then measured. Results vary from no resistance in the very immature newborn to an 80-degree angle in the term newborn.
4. The *scarf sign* is elicited by placing the newborn supine and drawing an arm across the chest toward the newborn's opposite shoulder until resistance is met. The location of the elbow is then noted in relation to the midline of the chest (Figure 25–9).
5. The *heel-to-ear extension* is performed by placing the newborn in a supine position and then gently draw-

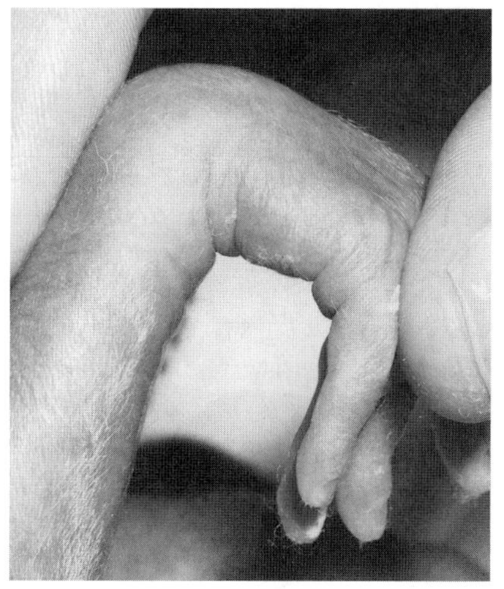
A

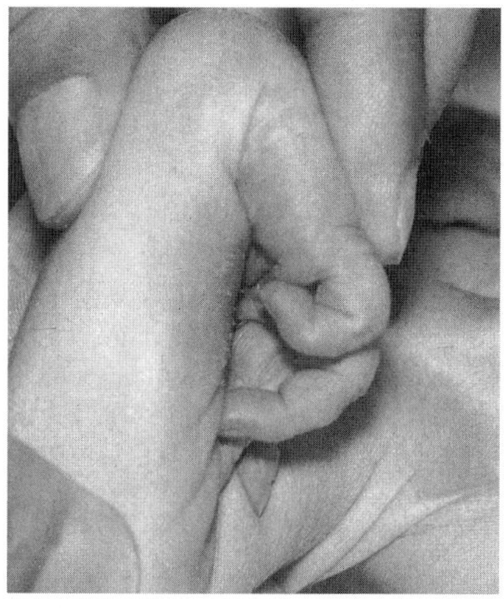
B

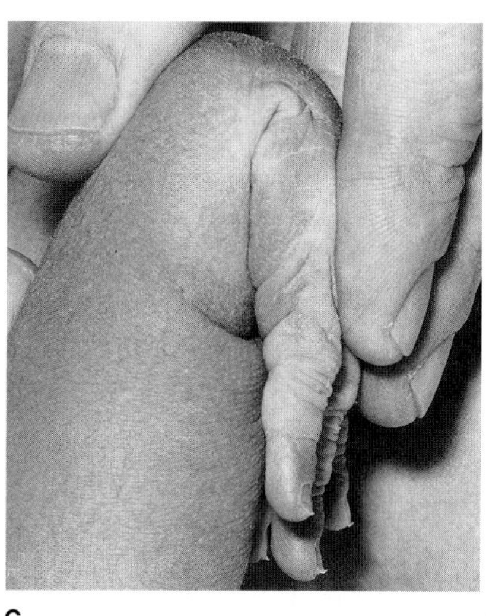
C

FIGURE 25–8 Square window sign. ***A,*** This angle is 90 degrees and suggests an immature newborn of 28 to 32 weeks' gestation. ***B,*** A 30-degree angle is commonly found in newborns from 38 to 40 weeks' gestation. ***C,*** A 0-degree angle occurs in newborns from 40 to 42 weeks' gestation. SOURCE: Dubowitz L, Dubowitz V: *Gestational Age of the Newborn.* Menlo Park, CA: Addison-Wesley, 1977. Reprinted by permission of V Dubowitz, MD, Hammersmith Hospital, London, England.

ing the foot toward the ear on the same side until resistance is felt. The nurse should allow the knee to bend during the test. It is important to hold the buttocks down to keep from rolling the baby. Both the proximity of foot to ear and degree of knee extension are assessed. A preterm, immature newborn's leg will remain straight, and its foot will go to the ear or beyond. With advancing gestational age, the newborn demonstrates increasing resistance to this maneuver. Maneuvers involving the lower extremities of newborns who had frank breech presentation should be delayed to allow for resolution of leg positioning (Ballard, Novak, & Driver, 1979).

6. *Ankle dorsiflexion* is determined by flexing the ankle on the shin. The examiner uses a thumb to push on the sole of the newborn's foot while the fingers support the back of the leg. Then the angle formed by the foot and the interior leg is measured (Figure 25–10). This sign can be influenced by intrauterine position and congenital deformities.

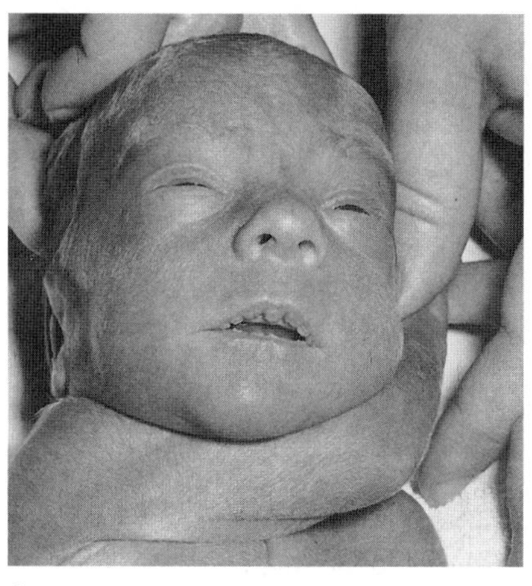
A

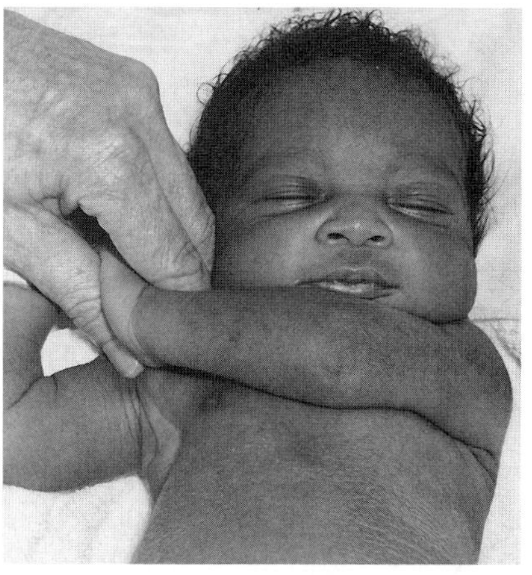
B

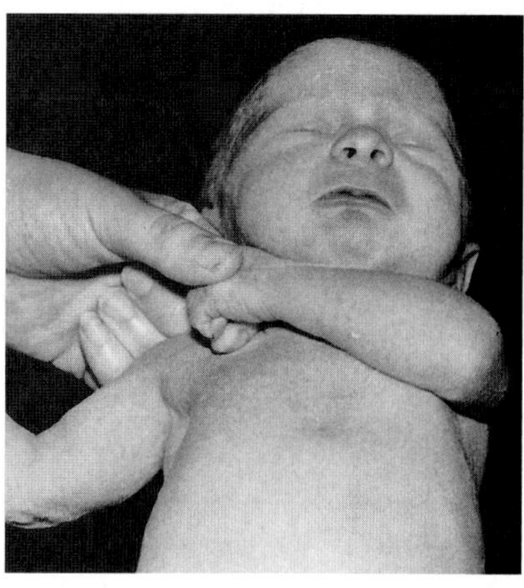
C

FIGURE 25–9 Scarf sign. ***A,*** No resistance is noted until after 30 weeks' gestation. The elbow can be readily moved past the midline. ***B,*** The elbow is at midline at 36 to 40 weeks' gestation. ***C,*** Beyond 40 weeks' gestation, the elbow will not reach the midline. SOURCE: Dubowitz L, Dubowitz V: *Gestational Age of the Newborn.* Menlo Park, CA: Addison-Wesley, 1977. Reprinted by permission of V Dubowitz, MD, Hammersmith Hospital, London, England.

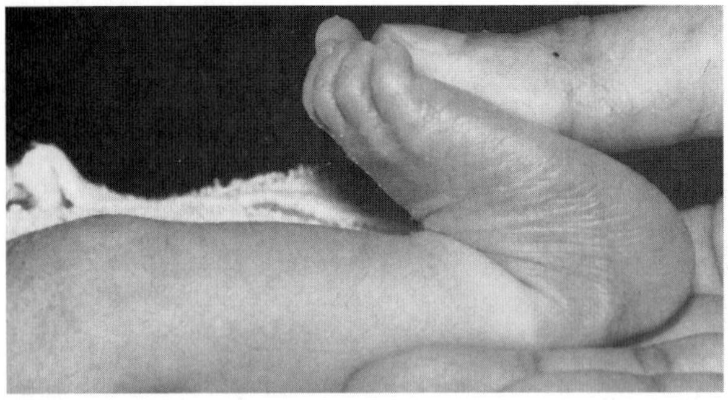

A

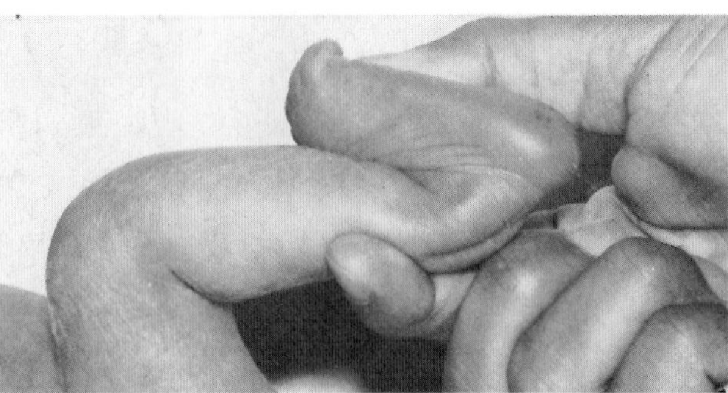

B

FIGURE 25–10 Ankle dorsiflexion. ***A,*** A 45-degree angle indicates 32 to 36 weeks' gestation. A 20-degree angle indicates 36 to 40 weeks' gestation. ***B,*** A 0-degree angle is common at gestational age of 40 weeks or more. SOURCE: Dubowitz L, Dubowitz V: *Gestational Age of the Newborn.* Menlo Park, CA: Addison-Wesley, 1977. Reprinted by permission of V Dubowitz, MD, Hammersmith Hospital, London, England.

7. *Head lag* (neck flexors) is measured by pulling the baby to a sitting position and noting the degree of head lag. Total lag is common in infants up to 34 weeks' gestation, whereas the postmature newborn (42+ weeks) will hold the head in front of the body line. Full-term newborns are able to support their heads momentarily.
8. *Ventral suspension* (horizontal position) is evaluated by holding the newborn prone on the examiner's hand. The position of head and back and degree of flexion in the arms and legs are then noted. Some flexion of arms and legs indicates 36 to 38 weeks' gestation; fully flexed extremities, with head and back even, are characteristic of a term newborn.
9. *Major reflexes* such as sucking, rooting, grasping, Moro, tonic neck, Babinski, and others are also evaluated during the newborn exam.

A supplementary method for estimating gestational age (done by the physician or nurse practitioner) is to view the vascular network of the cornea with an ophthalmoscope. The amount of vascularity present over the surface of the lens has excellent correlation with infants of 27 through 34 weeks' gestational age. In babies of less than 27 weeks' gestation, the cornea is cloudy, and the vascular network is not visible; after 34 weeks' gestation the vascular network has generally disappeared completely.

When the gestational age determination and birth weight are considered together, the newborn can be identified as one whose *growth is below the tenth percentile,* or *small for gestational age (SGA); appropriate for gestational age (AGA);* or *above the 90th percentile,* or *large for gestational age (LGA)* (Figure 25–11). This determination enables the nurse to anticipate possible physiologic problems. This information is used in conjunction with a complete physical examination to establish a plan of care appropriate for the individual newborn (Dodd, 1996). For example, an SGA newborn often requires frequent glucose monitoring and early feedings. See Chapter 28 for discussion of these categories and their potential problems.

The nurse also plots the gestational age against the newborn's length, head circumference, and weight on the appropriate growth chart to determine whether these measurements fall within the average range—the tenth to 90th percentile for the corresponding gestational age (Figure 25–12). These correlations further document the level of maturity and appropriate category for the newborn. The comparison of the newborn's ratio of weight to length further facilitates identification of SGA newborns as being symmetrically or asymmetrically [growth retarded] undergrown. See Chapter 28 for more detail.

Physical Assessment

After the initial determination of gestational age and related potential problems, a more extensive physical assessment is carried out. The nurse should choose a warm, well-lighted area that is free of drafts. Completing the physical assessment in the presence of the parents provides an opportunity to acquaint them with their unique newborn. The examination is performed in a systematic, head-to-toe manner, and all findings are recorded. When assessing the physical and neurologic status of the newborn, the nurse should first consider general appearance and then proceed to specific areas.

The Newborn Physical Assessment Guide on pages 734–748 outlines how to systematically assess the newborn. Normal findings, alterations, and related causes are presented and correlated with suggested nursing responses. The findings are typical for a full-term newborn.

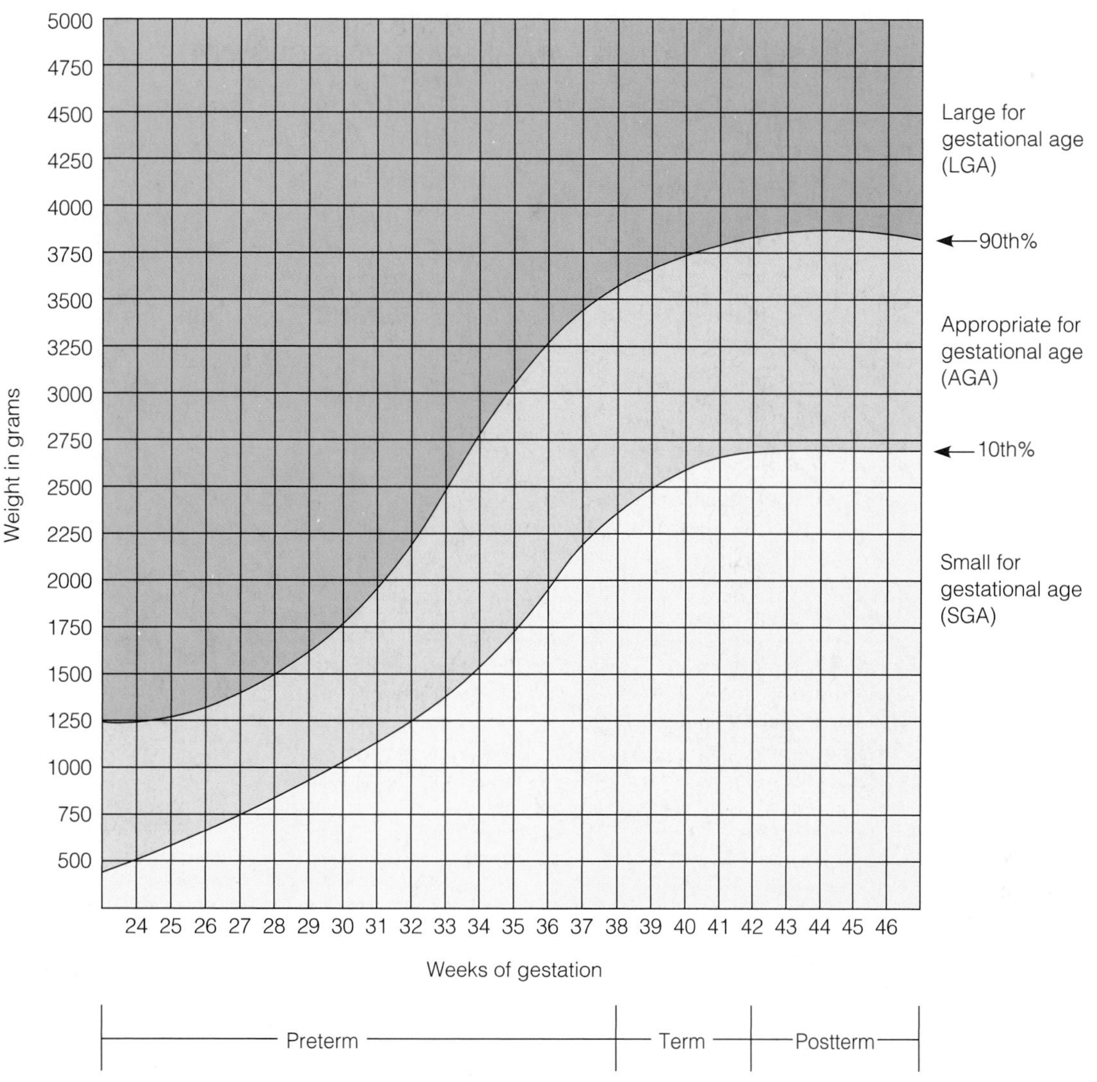

FIGURE 25–11 Classification of newborns by birth weight and gestational age. The newborn's birth weight and gestational age are placed on the graph. The newborn is then classified as large for gestational age (LGA), appropriate for gestational age (AGA), or small for gestational age (SGA). SOURCE: Battaglia FC, Lubchenco LO: A practical classification of newborn infants by weight and gestational age. *J Pediatr* 1967; 71:161.

General Appearance

The newborn's head is disproportionately large for the body. The center of the baby's body is the umbilicus rather than the symphysis pubis, as in the adult. The body appears long and the extremities short. The flexed position that the newborn maintains contributes to the short appearance of the extremities. The hands are tightly clenched. The neck looks short because the chin rests on the chest. Newborns have a prominent abdomen, sloping shoulders, narrow hips, and rounded chests. They tend to stay in a flexed position similar to the one maintained in utero and will offer resistance when the extremities are straightened. After a breech birth, the feet are usually dorsiflexed, and it may take several weeks for the newborn to assume typical newborn posture.

Weight and Measurements

The normal full-term Caucasian newborn has an average birth weight of 3405 g (7 lb, 8 oz). Newborns of African and Asian descent are usually somewhat smaller (Brooks, Johnson, Steer, Pawson, & Abdella, 1995; Wen, Kramer, & Usher, 1995). Other factors that influence weight are age and size of parents, health of mother (smoking and malnutrition decrease birth weight), and interval between pregnancies (pregnancies that occur too close together, such as every year, tend to result in lower birth weight) (Basso, Olsen, Knudsen, & Christensen, 1998; Cogswell & Yip, 1995). After the first week and for the first 6 months, the newborn's weight will increase about 198 g (7 oz) weekly.

Approximately 70% to 75% of the newborn's body weight is water. During the initial newborn period (the

CLASSIFICATION OF NEWBORNS—BASED ON MATURITY AND INTRAUTERINE GROWTH

Symbols: X-1st Exam O-2nd Exam

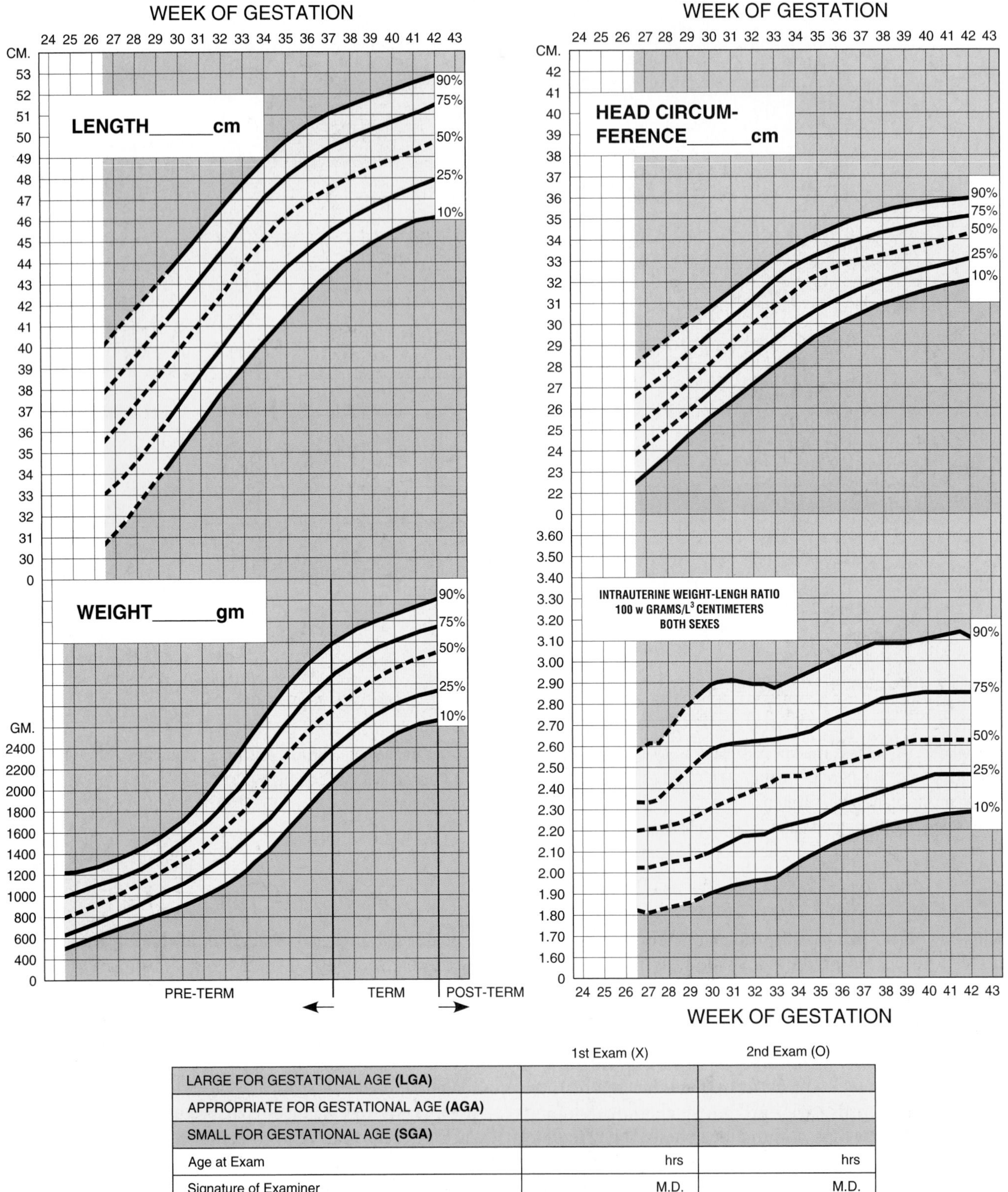

	1st Exam (X)	2nd Exam (O)
LARGE FOR GESTATIONAL AGE **(LGA)**		
APPROPRIATE FOR GESTATIONAL AGE **(AGA)**		
SMALL FOR GESTATIONAL AGE **(SGA)**		
Age at Exam	hrs	hrs
Signature of Examiner	M.D.	M.D.

FIGURE 25–12 Classification of newborns based on maturity and intrauterine growth. SOURCES: Adapted from Lubchenco LO, Hansman C, Boyd E: *Pediatrics* 1966; 37:403; Battaglia FC, Lubchenco LO: A practical classification of newborn infants by weight and gestational age. *J Pediatr* 1967; 71:159.

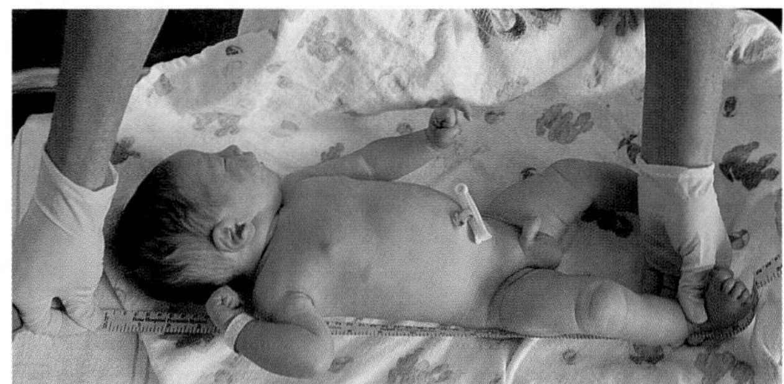

FIGURE 25–13 Measuring the length of the newborn.

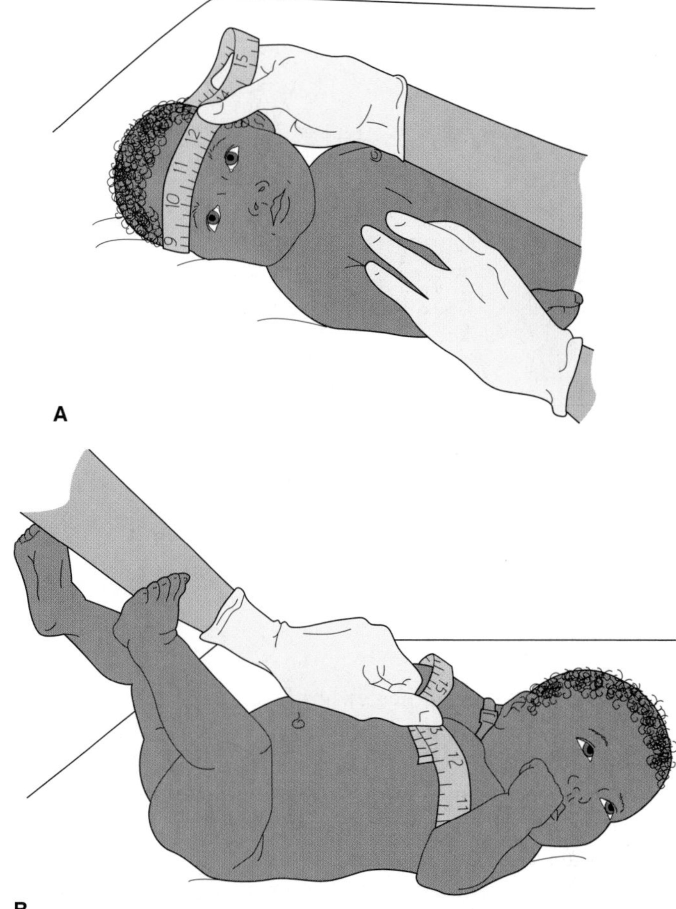

FIGURE 25–14 ***A,*** Measuring the head circumference of the newborn. ***B,*** Measuring the chest circumference of the newborn.

first 3 or 4 days), there is a physiologic weight loss of 5% to 10% for term newborns due to fluid shifts. This weight loss may reach 15% for preterm newborns. Large babies may tend to lose more weight. If weight loss is greater than 10%, clinical reappraisal is necessary. Factors contributing to weight loss include small fluid intake resulting from delayed breastfeeding or a slow adjustment to formula, increased volume of meconium excreted, and urination. Weight loss may be marked in the presence of temperature elevation (because of associated dehydration) or consistent chilling (because of nonshivering thermogenesis).

The length of the normal newborn is difficult to measure because the legs are flexed and tensed. To measure length, the nurse should place newborns flat on their backs with legs extended as much as possible (Figure 25–13). The average length is 50 cm (20 in), with the range being 48 to 52 cm (18 to 22 in). The newborn will grow approximately 1 inch a month for the next 6 months. This is the period of most rapid growth.

At birth, the newborn's head is one-third the size of an adult's head. The circumference of the newborn's head is 32 to 37 cm (12.5 to 14.5 in). For accurate measurement, the tape is placed over the most prominent part of the occiput and brought to just above the eyebrows (Figure 25–14, *A*). The circumference of the newborn's head is approximately 2 cm greater than the circumference of the newborn's chest at birth and will remain in this proportion for the next few months. (Factors that alter this measurement are discussed under Head section.) It is best to take another head circumference on the second day if the newborn experienced significant head molding or caput from the birth process.

The average circumference of the chest at birth is 32 cm (12.5 in) and ranges from 30 to 35 cm. Chest measurements should be taken with the tape measure at the lower edge of the scapulas and brought around anteriorly directly over the nipple line (Figure 25–14, *B* and Table 25–2). The abdominal circumference or girth may also be measured at this time by placing the tape around the newborn's abdomen at the level of the umbilicus, with the bottom edge of the tape at the top edge of the umbilicus.

TABLE 25–2 Newborn Measurements

Weight
Average: 3405 g (7 lb, 8 oz)
Range: 2500–4000 g (5 lb, 8 oz–8 lb, 13 oz)
Weight is influenced by racial origin and maternal age and size.
Physiologic weight loss: 5%–10% for term newborns, up to 15% for preterm newborns
Growth: 198 g (7 oz) per week for first 6 months
Length
Average: 50 cm (20 in)
Range: 48–52 cm (18–22 in)
Growth: 2.5 cm (1 in) per month for first 6 months
Head Circumference
32–37 cm (12.5–14.5 in)
Approximately 2 cm larger than chest circumference
Chest Circumference
Average: 32 cm (12.5 in)
Range: 30–35 cm (12–14 in)

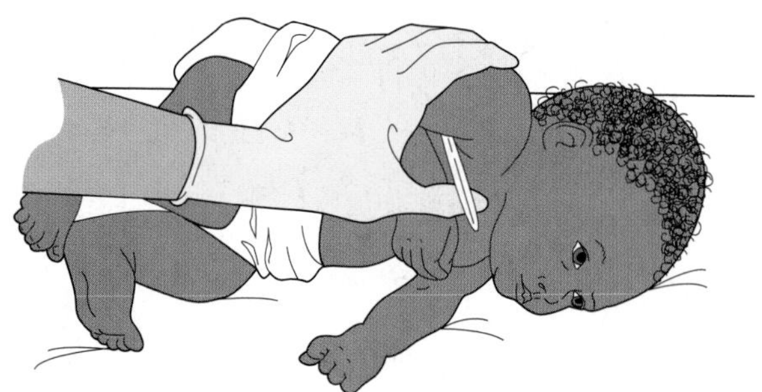

FIGURE 25–15 Axillary temperature measurement. The axillary temperature should be taken for 3 minutes. The newborn's arm should be tightly but gently pressed against the thermometer and the newborn's side, as illustrated.

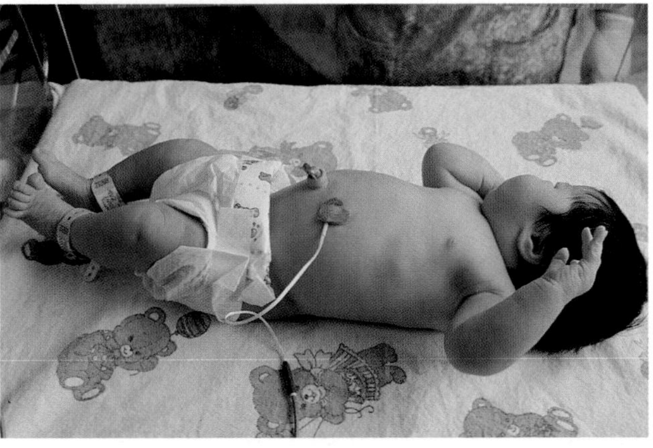

FIGURE 25–16 Temperature monitoring for the newborn. A skin thermal sensor is placed on the newborn's abdomen, upper thigh, or arm and secured with porous tape or a foil-covered foam pad.

Temperature

Initial assessment of the newborn's temperature is critical. In utero, the temperature of the fetus is about the same as or slightly higher than the expectant mother's. When babies enter the outside world, their temperatures can suddenly drop as a result of exposure to cold drafts and the skin's heat loss mechanisms.

If no heat conservation measures are started, the normal term newborn's deep body temperature falls 0.1C (0.2F) per minute; skin temperature lowers 0.3C (0.5F) per minute. Skin temperature markedly decreases within 10 minutes after exposure to room air. The temperature should stabilize within 8 to 12 hours. Temperature should be monitored when the newborn is admitted to the nursery and at least every 30 minutes until the newborn's status has remained stable for 2 hours. Thereafter the nurse should assess temperature at least once every 8 hours or according to institutional policy (AAP & ACOG, 1997). (See Chapter 24 for a discussion of the physiology of temperature regulation.)

Temperature can be assessed by the axillary skin method, a continuous skin probe, the rectal route, or a tympanic thermometer. Axillary temperature reflects body (core) temperature and the body's compensatory response to the thermal environment. Axillary temperatures are the preferred method and are considered to be a close estimation of the rectal temperature. In preterm and term newborns there is less than 0.1C (0.2F) difference between temperatures taken by the axillary and rectal route. If the axillary method is used, the thermometer must remain in place at least 3 minutes, unless an electronic thermometer is used (Figure 25–15). Axillary temperature ranges from 36.5C to 37.0C (97.7F to 98.6F). Keep in mind that axillary temperatures can be misleading because the friction caused by apposition of the inner arm skin and upper chest wall and the nearness of brown fat to the probe may elevate the temperature. Parents need to be aware that current research on forehead strip thermometers indicates that they do not reflect core temperature as accurately as the axillary method does (Shann & Mackenzie, 1996).

Skin temperature is measured most accurately by continuous skin probe, especially for small newborns or newborns maintained in incubators or under radiant warmers. Normal skin temperature is 36C to 36.5C (96.8F to 97.7F). Assessing skin temperature allows time for interventions to be initiated before a more serious fall in core temperature occurs (Figure 25–16).

Rectal temperature is assumed to be the closest approximation to core temperature, but the accuracy of this method depends on the depth to which the thermometer is inserted. Normal rectal temperature is 36.6C to 37.2C (97.8F to 99F). The rectal route is not recommended as a routine method because it may predispose to rectal mucosal irritation and increase chances of perforation. If the temperature must be taken rectally, the nurse inserts the lubricated thermometer to a depth of no greater than 0.5 in (1.27 cm) into the rectum and continuously holds it in place while stabilizing the infant's lower extremities.

Some institutions are now using tympanic thermometers. These are portable sensor probes with disposable covers that are placed in the auditory canal. The probe uses infrared technology to measure the temperature of the internal carotid artery blood flow within several seconds. Early research findings indicate that tympanic temperatures are as accurate an estimation of body temperature in the newborn as axillary temperatures (Hicks, 1996).

Temperature instability, a deviation of more than 1C (2F) from one reading to the next, or a subnormal temperature may indicate an infection. In contrast with an elevated temperature in older children, an increased tem-

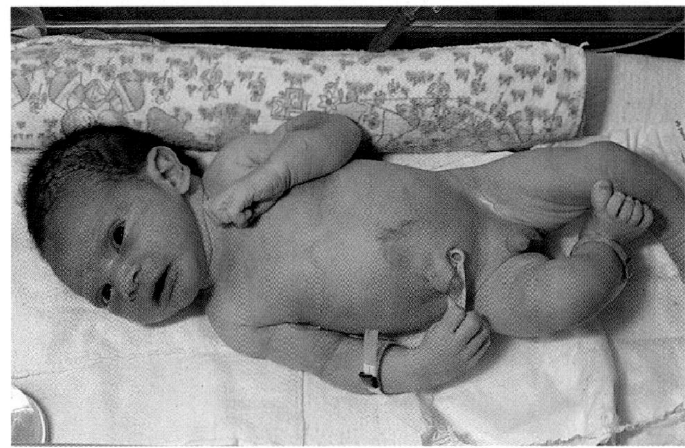

FIGURE 25–17 Acrocyanosis.

perature in a newborn may indicate reactions to too much covering, too hot a room, or dehydration. Dehydration, which tends to increase body temperature, occurs in newborns whose feedings have been delayed for any reason. Newborns respond to overheating (temperature greater than 37.5C or 99.5F) by increased restlessness and eventually by perspiration. The perspiration is initially seen on the head and face, then on the chest. Many newborns initially cannot perspire, so they increase their respiratory and heart rates, which increases oxygen consumption.

Skin Characteristics

Although the newborn's skin color varies with genetic background, all healthy newborns have a pink tinge to their skin. The ruddy hue results from increased red blood cell concentrations in the blood vessels and from limited subcutaneous fat deposits.

Skin pigmentation is slight in the newborn period, so color changes may be seen even in darker skinned babies. A newborn who is cyanotic at rest and pink only with crying may have choanal atresia (congenital blockage of the passageway between the nose and pharynx). If crying increases the cyanosis, heart or lung problems may be suspected. Very pale newborns may be anemic or have hypovolemia (low BP) and are evaluated for these problems.

CRITICAL THINKING QUESTION

How do you differentiate central cyanosis from peripheral cyanosis?

Acrocyanosis

Acrocyanosis (bluish discoloration of the hands and feet) may be present in the first 2 to 6 hours after birth (Figure 25–17). This condition is due to poor peripheral circulation, which results in vasomotor instability and capillary stasis, especially when the baby is exposed to cold. If the central circulation is adequate, the blood supply should return quickly to the extremity after the skin is blanched with a finger. Blue hands and nails are a poor indicator of oxygenation in a newborn. The face and mucous membranes should be assessed for pinkness reflecting adequate oxygenation.

Mottling (lacy pattern of dilated blood vessels under the skin) occurs as a result of general circulation fluctuations. It may last several hours to several weeks or may come and go periodically. Mottling may be related to chilling or prolonged apnea.

Harlequin Sign

Harlequin sign (clown) color change is occasionally noted: A deep color develops over one side of the newborn's body while the other side remains pale, so that the skin resembles a clown's suit. This color change results from a vasomotor disturbance in which blood vessels on one side dilate while the vessels on the other side constrict. It usually lasts from 1 to 20 minutes. Affected neonates may have single or multiple episodes, but they are transient and not of clinical significance.

Jaundice

Jaundice is first detectable on the face (where skin overlies cartilage) and the mucous membranes of the mouth. It is evaluated by blanching the tip of the nose, the forehead, or the gum line. This procedure must be carried out in appropriate lighting. If jaundice is present, the area will appear yellowish immediately after blanching. Another area to assess for jaundice is the sclera. Jaundice must be evaluated and its cause determined immediately to prevent possibly serious sequelae. The jaundice may be related to breastfeeding (in a few cases), hematomas, immature liver function, or bruises from forceps, or it may be caused by blood incompatibility, oxytocin (Pitocin) augmentation or induction, or severe hemolytic process. Any jaundice noted before 24 hours of age should be reported to the physician or nurse practitioner. For a detailed discussion of the causes and assessment of jaundice, see Chapter 29.

Erythema Toxicum

Erythema toxicum is a perifollicular eruption of lesions that are firm, vary in size from 1 to 3 mm, and consist of a white or pale yellow papule or pustule with an erythematous base. It is often called "newborn rash" or "flea bite" dermatitis. The rash may appear suddenly, usually over the trunk and diaper area, and is frequently widespread (Figure 25–18). The lesions do not appear on the palms of the hands or the soles of the feet. The peak incidence is at 24 to 48 hours of life. The condition rarely presents at birth or after 5 days of life. The cause is unknown and no treatment is necessary. Some clinicians feel it may be caused by irritation from clothing. The lesions disappear in a few hours or days. Should a maculopapular rash (eruption consisting of both macules and papules) appear, a smear of the aspirated papule will show numerous eosinophils on staining; no bacteria will be cultured.

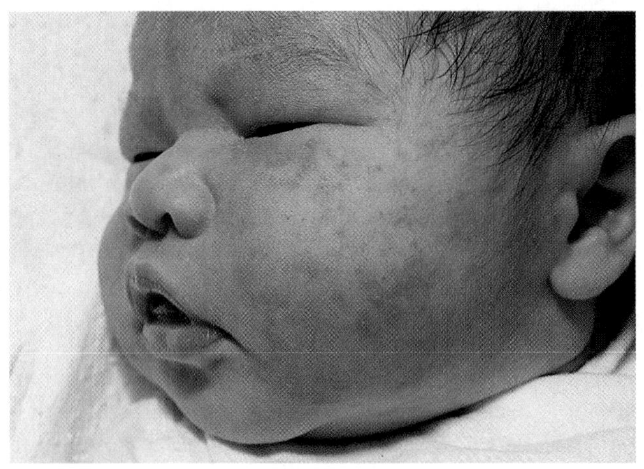

FIGURE 25–18 Erythema toxicum.

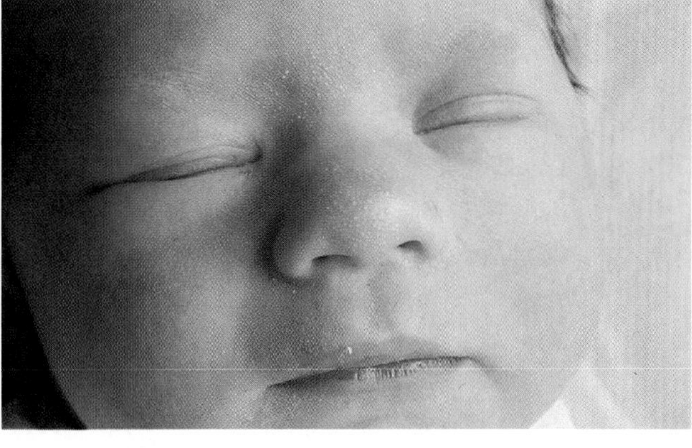

FIGURE 25–19 Facial milia.

Milia

Milia, which are exposed sebaceous glands, appear as raised white spots on the face, especially across the nose (Figure 25–19). No treatment is necessary, because they will clear up spontaneously within the first month. Infants of African heritage have a similar condition called transient neonatal pustular melanosis (Taeusch & Ballard, 1998).

Skin Turgor

Skin turgor is assessed to determine hydration status, the need to initiate early feedings, and the presence of any infectious processes. The usual place to assess skin turgor is over the abdomen or the thigh. Skin should be elastic and should return rapidly to its original shape.

Vernix Caseosa

Vernix caseosa, a whitish cheeselike substance, covers the fetus while in utero and lubricates the skin of the newborn. The skin of the term or postterm newborn has less vernix and is frequently dry; peeling is common, especially on the hands and feet.

Forceps or Vacuum Extractor Marks

Forceps marks may be present after a difficult forceps birth. The newborn may have reddened areas over the cheeks and jaws. It is important to reassure the parents that these will disappear, usually within 1 or 2 days. Transient facial paralysis resulting from the forceps pressure is a rare complication. Suction marks on the vertex of the scalp are often seen when vacuum extractors are used to assist with the birth. These are benign and do not indicate any underlying brain lesions.

Birthmarks

Telangiectatic Nevi

Telangiectatic nevi (stork bites) appear as pale pink or red spots and are frequently found on the eyelids, nose, lower occipital bone, and nape of the neck (Figure

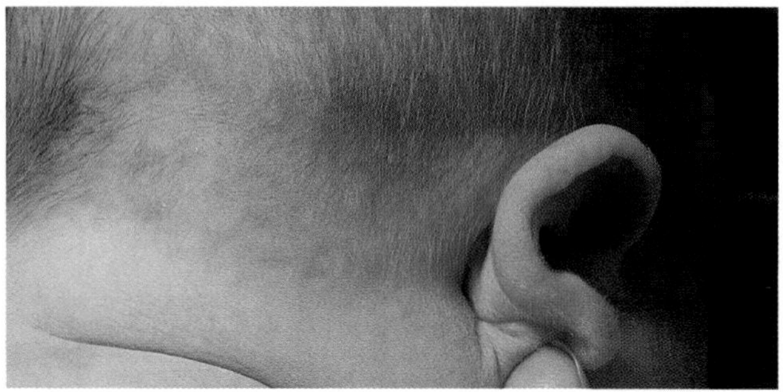

FIGURE 25–20 Stork bites.

25–20). These lesions are common in light-complexioned newborns and are more noticeable during periods of crying. These areas have no clinical significance and usually fade by the second birthday.

Mongolian Spots

Mongolian spots are macular areas of bluish-black or gray-blue pigmentation found on the dorsal area and the buttocks (Figure 25–21). They are common in newborns of Asian and African descent and other dark-skinned races. They gradually fade during the first or second year of life. They may be mistaken for bruises and should be documented in the newborn's chart.

Nevus Flammeus

Nevus flammeus (port wine stain) is a capillary angioma directly below the epidermis. It is a nonelevated, sharply demarcated, red to purple area of dense capillaries (Figure 25–22). In infants of African descent it may appear as a purple-black stain. The size and shape varies, but it commonly appears on the face. It does not grow in size, does not fade with time, and does not blanch as a rule. The birthmark may be concealed by an opaque cosmetic cream. If convulsions and other neurologic prob-

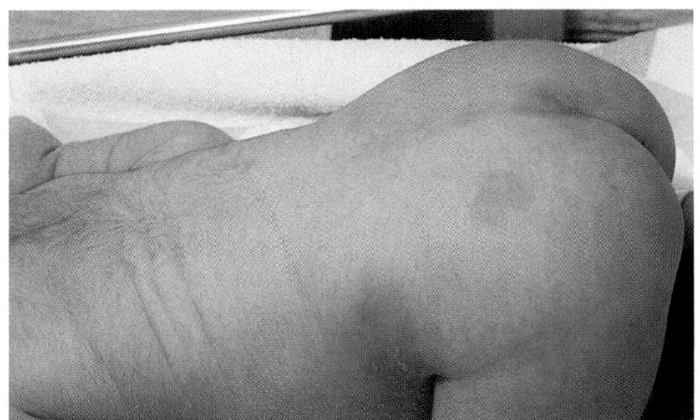

FIGURE 25–21 Mongolian spots.

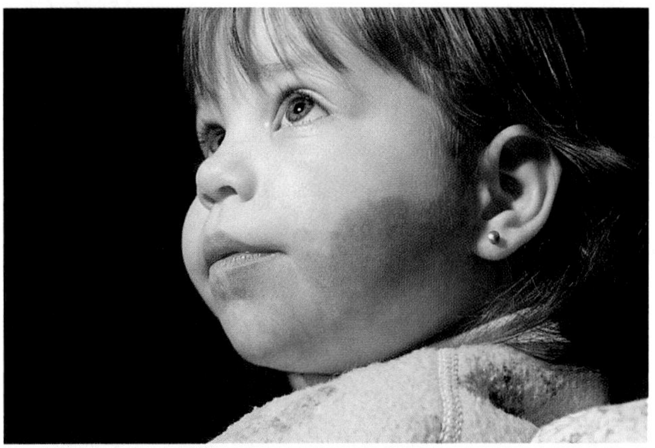

FIGURE 25–22 Port wine stain.

lems accompany the nevus flammeus, the clinical picture is suggestive of Sturge-Weber syndrome with involvement of the fifth cranial nerve (the ophthalmic branch of the trigeminal nerve).

Nevus Vasculosus

Nevus vasculosus (strawberry mark) is a capillary hemangioma. It consists of newly formed and enlarged capillaries in the dermal and subdermal layers. It is a raised, clearly delineated, dark red, rough-surfaced birthmark commonly found in the head region. Such marks usually grow (often rapidly) for several months, and become fixed in size by 8 months. They then begin to shrink and start to resolve spontaneously several weeks to months after peak growth is reached. About 90% of cases resolve by the time the child is 10 years old (Kane, Page-Salyards, & Keith-Perry, 1997). Parents can be told that resolution is heralded by a pale purple or gray spot on the surface of the hemangioma. The best cosmetic effect is achieved when the lesions are allowed to resolve spontaneously.

Birthmarks are frequently a cause of concern for the parents. The mother may be especially anxious, fearing that she is to blame. ("Is my baby marked because of something I did?") Guilt feelings are common in the presence of misconceptions about the cause. Birthmarks should be identified and explained to the parents. By providing appropriate information about the cause and course of birthmarks, the nurse frequently relieves the fears and anxieties of the family. The nurse should note any bruises, abrasions, or birthmarks seen on the newborn's admission to the nursery.

Head

General Appearance

The newborn's head is large (approximately one-fourth of the body size), with soft, pliable skull bones. The head may appear asymmetric in the newborn of a vertex delivery. This asymmetry, called **molding,** is caused by overriding of the cranial bones during labor and birth (Figure 25–23). The degree of molding varies with the amount and length of pressure exerted on the head. Within a few days after birth, the overriding usually diminishes, and the suture lines become palpable. Because head measurements are affected by molding, a second measurement is indicated a few days after birth. The heads of breech-born newborns and those born by elective cesarean birth are characteristically round and well shaped because pressure was not exerted on them during birth. Any extreme differences in head size may indicate microcephaly or hydrocephalus. Variations in the shape, size, or appearance of the head may be due to *craniostenosis* (premature closure of the cranial sutures), which is corrected through surgery to allow brain growth, or *plagiocephaly* (asymmetry caused by pressure on the fetal head during gestation).

Two *fontanelles* ("soft spots") may be palpated on the newborn's head. Fontanelles, which are openings at the juncture of the cranial bones, can be measured with the fingers. Accurate measurement necessitates that the examiner's finger be measured in centimeters. The assessment should be carried out with the newborn in sitting position and not crying. The diamond-shaped *anterior fontanelle* is 3 to 4 cm long by 2 to 3 cm wide. It is located at the juncture of the frontal and parietal bones. The *posterior fontanelle*, smaller and triangular, is formed by the parietal bones and the occipital bone and is 0.5 cm by 1 cm. Because of molding, the fontanelles tend to be

CLINICAL TIP

Vital sign assessments are most accurate if the newborn is at rest, so measure pulse and respirations first if the baby is quiet. To soothe a crying baby, try placing your moistened gloved finger in the baby's mouth, and then complete your assessment while the baby suckles.

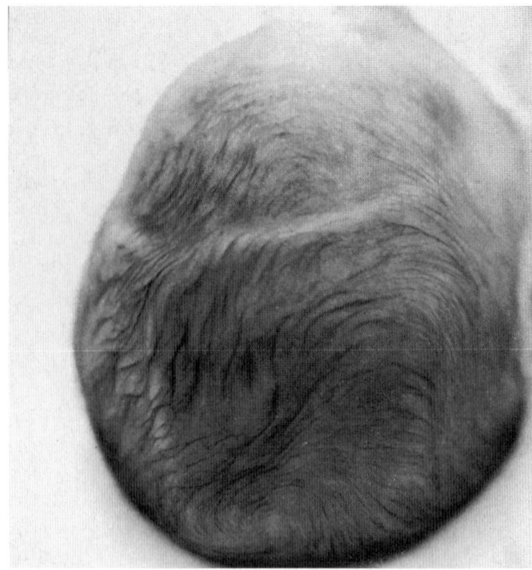

FIGURE 25–23 Overlapped cranial bones produce a visible ridge in a small premature infant. Easily visible overlapping does not occur often in term infants. SOURCE: Korones SB: *High-Risk Newborn Infants,* 4th ed. St Louis: Mosby, 1986.

smaller immediately after birth than several days later. The anterior fontanelle closes within 18 months, whereas the posterior fontanelle closes within 8 to 12 weeks.

The fontanelles are a useful indicator of the newborn's condition. The anterior fontanelle may swell when the newborn cries or passes a stool or may pulsate with the heartbeat, which is normal. A bulging fontanelle usually signifies increased intracranial pressure, and a depressed fontanelle indicates dehydration.

The sutures between the cranial bones should be palpated for amount of overlap. In growth-retarded newborns, the sutures may be wider than normal, and the fontanelles may also be larger because of impaired fetal growth of the cranial bones. In addition to being inspected for degree of molding and size, the head should be evaluated for soft tissue edema and bruising.

Cephalhematoma

Cephalhematoma is a collection of blood resulting from ruptured blood vessels between the surface of a cranial bone (usually parietal) and the periosteal membrane (Figure 25–24). The scalp in these areas feels loose and slightly edematous. These areas emerge as defined hematomas between the first and second day. Although external pressure may cause the mass to fluctuate, it does not increase in size when the newborn cries. Cephalhematomas may be unilateral or bilateral and do not cross suture lines. They are relatively common in vertex births and may disappear within 2 to 3 weeks or slowly over subsequent months. They may be associated with physiologic jaundice, because there are extra red blood cells being destroyed within the cephalhematoma.

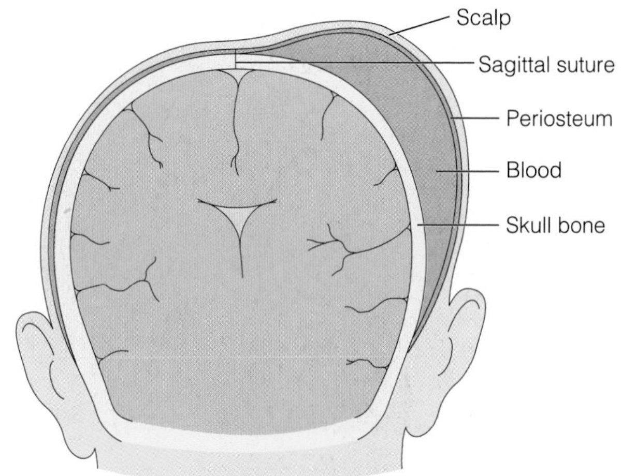

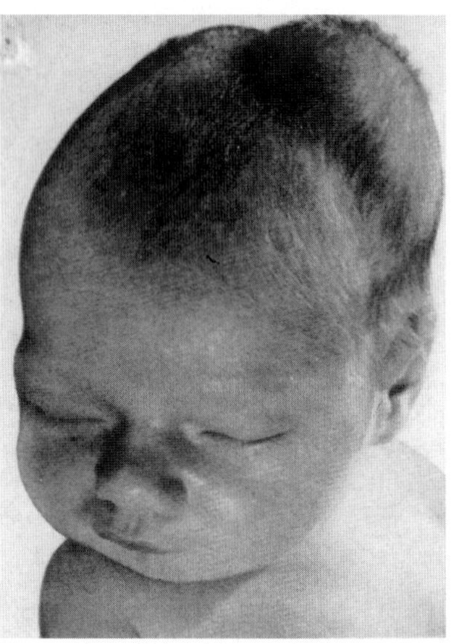

FIGURE 25–24 Cephalhematoma is a collection of blood between the surface of a cranial bone and the periosteal membrane. This is a cephalhematoma over the left parietal bone. SOURCE: Photo reproduced with permission from Porter EL, Craig JM: *Pathology of the Fetus and Infant,* 3rd ed. Chicago: Year Book Medical Publishers, 1975.

Caput Succedaneum

Caput succedaneum is a localized, easily identifiable soft area of the scalp, generally resulting from a long and difficult labor or vacuum extraction. The sustained pressure of the presenting part against the cervix results in compression of local blood vessels, and venous return is slowed. This causes an increase in tissue fluids, an edematous swelling, and occasional bleeding under the periosteum. The caput may vary from a small area to a large area covering a severely elongated head. The fluid in the caput is reabsorbed within 12 hours to a few days after birth. Caputs resulting from vacuum extractors are sharply outlined, circular areas up to 2 cm thick. They disappear more slowly than naturally occurring edema. It is possible to distinguish between a cephalhematoma and a caput because the caput overrides suture lines (Figure

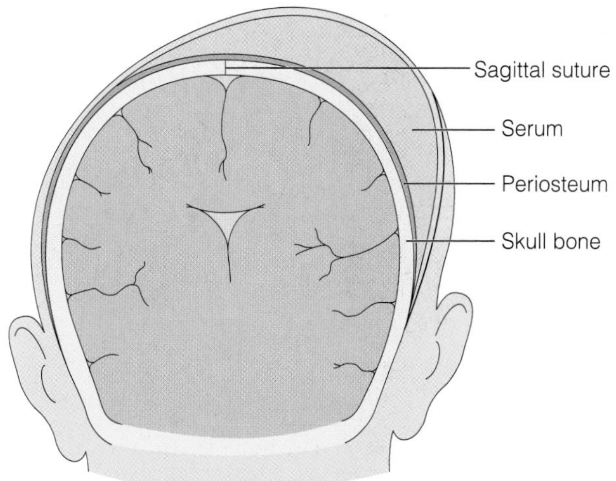

TABLE 25–3 Comparison of Cephalhematoma and Caput Succedaneum
Cephalhematoma
Collection of blood between cranial (usually parietal) bone and periosteal membrane
Does not cross suture lines
Does not increase in size with crying
Appears on first and second day
Disappears after 2 to 3 weeks or may take months
Caput Succedaneum
Collection of fluid, edematous swelling of the scalp
Crosses suture lines
Present at birth or shortly thereafter
Reabsorbed within 12 hours or a few days after birth

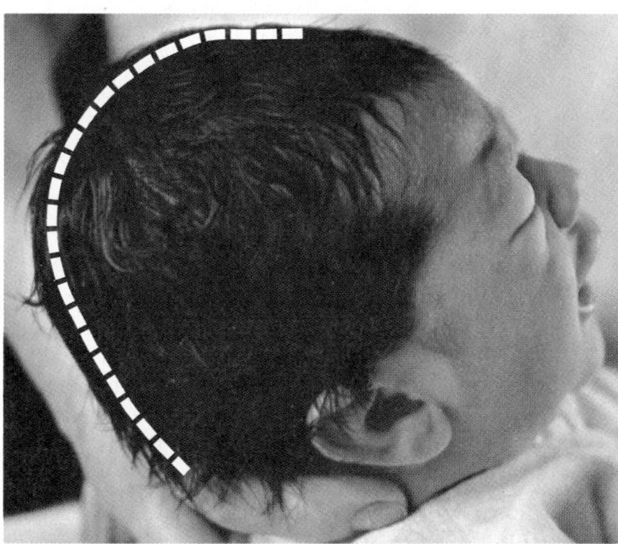

FIGURE 25–25 Caput succedaneum is a collection of fluid (serum) under the scalp. SOURCE: Photo courtesy Mead Johnson Laboratories, Evansville, IN.

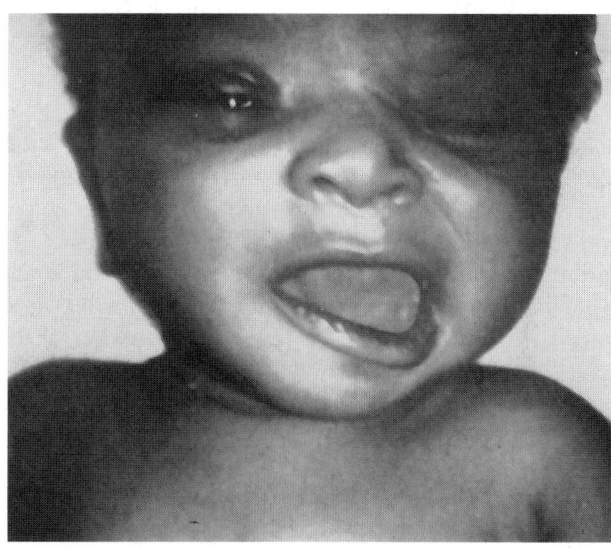

FIGURE 25–26 Paralysis of the right side of the face from an injury to the right facial nerve. SOURCE: Potter EL, Craig JM: *Pathology of the Fetus and Infant,* 3rd ed. Chicago: Year Book Medical Publishers, 1975. Courtesy Dr Ralph Platow.

25–25), whereas the cephalhematoma, because of its location, never crosses a suture line (Table 25–3). Caput succedaneum is present at birth, whereas cephalhematoma generally is not.

Face

The newborn's face is well designed to help the infant suckle. Sucking (fat) pads are located in the cheeks, and a labial tubercle (sucking callus) is frequently found in the center of the upper lip. The chin is recessed, and the nose is flattened. The lips are sensitive to touch, and the sucking reflex is easily initiated.

Symmetry of the eyes, nose, and ears is evaluated. See the Newborn Physical Assessment Guide for deviations in symmetry and variations in size, shape, and spacing of facial features. Facial movement symmetry should be assessed to determine the presence of facial palsy.

Facial paralysis appears when the newborn cries; the affected side is immobile, and the palpebral (eyelid) fissure widens (Figure 25–26). Paralysis may result from forceps-assisted birth or pressure on the facial nerve from the maternal pelvis during birth. Facial paralysis usually disappears within a few days to 3 weeks, although in some cases it may be permanent.

Eyes

The eyes of newborns of northern European descent are a blue or slate blue-gray. Scleral color tends to be white to bluish-white because of its relative thinness. A blue sclera is associated with osteogenesis imperfecta (Tappero & Honeyfield, 1996). The infant's eye color is usually established at approximately 3 months, but it may change any time up to 1 year. Dark-skinned neonates tend to have dark eyes at birth.

The eyes should be checked for size, equality of pupil size, reaction of pupils to light, blink reflex to light, and edema and inflammation of the eyelids. The eyelids can be edematous during the first few days of life because of the pressure associated with birth. Erythromycin and tetracycline are now frequently used prophylactically instead of silver nitrate and usually don't cause chemical irritation of the eye. The instillation of silver nitrate drops in the newborn's eyes may cause edema and **chemical conjunctivitis,** which may appear a few hours after instillation and disappear in 1 to 2 days. If infectious conjunctivitis exists, the newborn has the same purulent (greenish-yellow) discharge as in chemical conjunctivitis, but it is caused by gonococcus, *Chlamydia*, staphylococci, or a variety of gram-negative bacteria and requires treatment with ophthalmic antibiotics. Onset is usually after the second day. Edema of the orbits or eyelids may persist for several days until the newborn's kidneys can evacuate the fluid.

Small **subconjunctival hemorrhages** appear in about 10% of newborns and are commonly found on the sclera. These hemorrhages are caused by the changes in vascular tension or ocular pressure during birth. They will remain for a few weeks and are of no pathologic significance. Parents need reassurance that the infant is not bleeding from within the eye and that vision will not be impaired.

The newborn may demonstrate transient strabismus (pseudostrabismus) or squinting caused by neuromuscular control of eye muscles (Figure 25–27). It gradually regresses in 3 to 4 months. The "doll's eye" phenomenon is also present for about 10 days after birth: As the newborn's head position is changed to the left and then to the right, the eyes move to the opposite direction. "Doll's eye" results from underdeveloped integration of head-eye coordination.

The nurse should observe the newborn's pupils for opacities or whiteness and for the absence of a normal red retinal reflex. Red retinal reflex is a red-orange flash of color observed when an ophthalmoscope light reflects off the retina. In a newborn with dark skin color, the retina may appear paler or more grayish. Absence of red reflex occurs with cataracts. Congenital cataracts should be suspected in infants of mothers with a prenatal history of rubella, cytomegalic inclusion disease, or syphilis.

The cry of the newborn is commonly tearless because the lacrimal structures are immature at birth and are not usually fully functional until the second month of life. However, some babies may produce tears during the newborn period. Poor oculomotor coordination and absence of accommodation limit visual abilities, but newborns do have peripheral vision and can fixate on near objects (10 to 20 in) in front of their faces for short periods, can accommodate to large objects (3 in tall by 3 in wide), and can seek out high-contrast geometric shapes (Ludington-Hoe & Golani, 1988). Newborns can perceive faces, shapes, and colors and begin to show visual preferences early. Visual acuity has been reported to be 20/400 (Reed & Davidhizar, 1997). Newborns generally blink in response to bright lights, to a tap on the bridge of the nose (glabellar reflex), or to a light touch on the eyelids. Pupillary light reflex is also present. The eye is best examined by rocking the newborn from an upright position to the horizontal a few times or by other methods, such as diminishing overhead lights, which will elicit an opened-eye response.

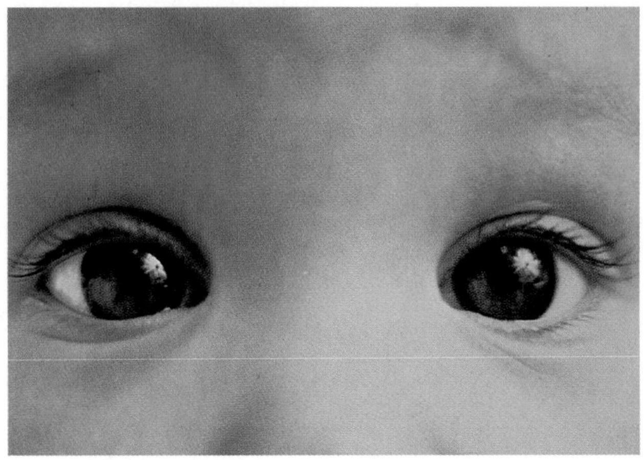

FIGURE 25–27 Transient strabismus in the newborn may be due to poor neuromuscular control. SOURCE: Courtesy Mead Johnson Laboratories, Evansville, IN.

Nose

The newborn's nose is small and narrow. Infants are characteristically nose breathers for the first few months of life. The newborn generally removes obstructions by sneezing. Nasal patency is assured if the baby breathes easily with mouth closed. If respiratory difficulty occurs, the nurse checks for *choanal atresia* (congenital blockage of the passageway between nose and pharynx).

The newborn has the ability to smell after the nasal passages are cleared of amniotic fluid and mucus. This ability is demonstrated by the search for milk. Newborns will turn their heads toward the milk source, whether bottle or breast. Newborns react to strong odors, such as alcohol, by turning their heads away or blinking.

Mouth

The lips of the newborn should be pink, and a touch on the lips should produce sucking motions. Saliva is normally scant. The taste buds are developed prior to birth, and the newborn can easily discriminate between sweet and bitter flavors.

The easiest way to examine the mouth completely is to stimulate infants gently to cry by depressing their tongue, thereby causing them to open the mouth fully. It is extremely important to observe the entire mouth to look for a cleft palate, which can be present even in the

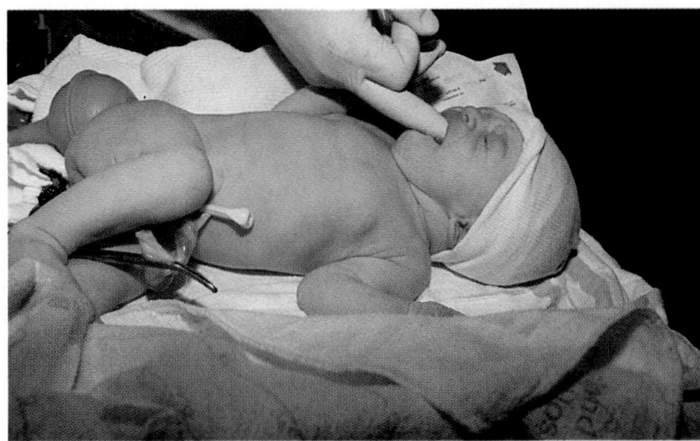

FIGURE 25–28 The nurse inserts the index finger into the newborn's mouth and feels for any openings along the hard and soft palates. Note that gloves are worn to examine the palate.

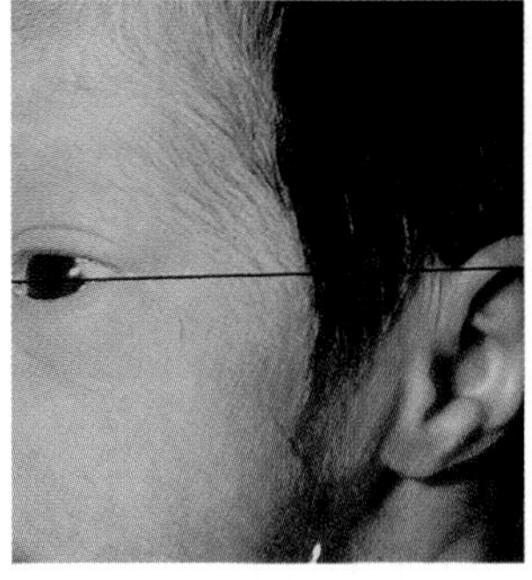

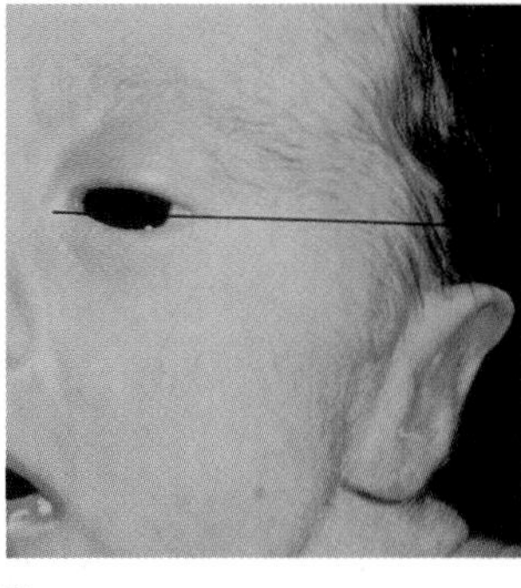

A B

FIGURE 25–29 The position of the external ear may be assessed by drawing a line across the inner and outer canthus of the eye to the insertion of the ear. ***A,*** Normal position. ***B,*** True low-set position. SOURCE: Courtesy Mead Johnson Laboratories, Evansville, IN.

absence of a cleft lip (Thureen, Deacon, O'Neill, & Hernandez, 1999). The examiner moves a gloved index finger along the hard and soft palate to feel for any openings (Figure 25–28). Glove powder should always be removed before examining the newborn's mouth.

Occasionally, an examination of the gums will reveal *precocious teeth* on the lower central incisor. If they appear loose, they should be removed to prevent aspiration. Gray-white lesions (inclusion cysts) on the gums may be confused with teeth. On the hard palate and gum margins, **Epstein's pearls,** small glistening white specks (keratin-containing cysts) that feel hard to the touch are often present. These usually disappear in a few weeks and are of no significance. **Thrush** may appear as white patches that look like milk curds adhering to the mucous membranes and cause bleeding when removed. Thrush is caused by *Candida albicans,* often acquired from an infected vaginal tract during birth or if the mother uses poor hand washing when handling her newborn. Thrush is treated with a preparation of nystatin (Mycostatin).

A newborn who is tongue-tied has a ridge of frenulum tissue attached to the underside of the tongue at varying lengths from its base, causing a heart shape at the tip of the tongue. "Clipping the tongue," or cutting the ridge of tissue, is not recommended. This ridge does not affect speech or eating, but cutting does create an entry for infection.

Transient nerve paralysis resulting from birth trauma may be manifested by asymmetric mouth movements when the newborn cries or by difficulty with sucking and feeding.

Ears

The ears of the newborn should be soft and pliable and should recoil readily when folded and released. In the normal newborn, the top of the ear (pinna) should be parallel to the outer and inner canthus of the eye. The ears should be inspected for shape, size, position, and firmness of ear cartilage. *Low-set ears* are characteristic of many syndromes and may indicate chromosomal abnormalities (especially trisomies 13 and 18), mental retardation, or internal organ abnormalities, especially bilateral renal agenesis as a result of embryologic developmental deviations (Figure 25–29). A *preauricular skin tag* may be present just in front of the ear. Preauricular tags are ligated at the base and allowed to slough off.

Visualization of the tympanic membranes is not usually done soon after birth because blood and vernix block the ear canal.

Following the first cry, the newborn's hearing becomes acute as mucus from the middle ear is absorbed, the eustachian tube is aerated, and the tympanic membrane becomes visible. Risk factors (AAP & ACOG, 1998) associated with potential hearing loss include the following:

- The presence of hearing loss in any family member prior to the age of 50 years
- Serum bilirubin level greater than 20 mg/dL for the full-term newborn or hyperbilirubinemia with a level exceeding indications for exchange transfusion due to toxic drugs
- Suspected maternal rubella infection during pregnancy, resulting in congenital rubella syndrome
- Congenital infection with herpes, cytomegalovirus, toxoplasmosis, or syphilis
- Bacterial meningitis
- Congenital defects of the ear, nose, or throat
- Small neonatal size, particularly less than 1500 g at birth
- Perinatal asphyxia

The newborn's hearing is evaluated by response to loud or moderately loud noises unaccompanied by vibrations. The sleeping newborn should stir or awaken in response to the nearby sounds. (This is not a very accurate test, but it may help to alert the examiner to possible problems.) The newborn can discriminate the individual characteristics of the human voice and is especially sensitive to sound levels within the normal conversation range (Merenstein & Gardner, 1998). The newborn in a noisy nursery may be able to habituate to the sounds and not stir unless the sound is sudden or much louder.

Neck

A short neck, creased with skin folds, is characteristic of the normal newborn. Because muscle tone is not well developed, the neck cannot support the full weight of the head, which rotates freely. The head lags considerably when the newborn is pulled up from a supine to a sitting position, but the prone newborn is able to raise the head slightly. The neck is palpated for masses and presence of lymph nodes and is inspected for webbing. Adequacy of range of motion and neck muscle function is determined by fully extending the head in all directions. Injury to the sternocleidomastoid muscle (congenital torticollis) must be considered in the presence of neck rigidity.

The clavicles are evaluated for evidence of fractures, which occasionally occur during difficult births or in neonates with broad shoulders. The normal clavicle is straight. If fractured, a lump and a grating sensation (crepitus) during movements may be palpated along the course of the side of the break. The Moro reflex (page 732) is also elicited to evaluate bilateral equal movement of the arms. If the clavicle is fractured, this response will be demonstrated only on the unaffected side.

Chest

The thorax is cylindrical and symmetric at birth, and the ribs are flexible. The general appearance of the chest should be assessed. A protrusion at the lower end of the sternum, called the *xiphoid cartilage*, is frequently seen. It is under the skin and will become less apparent after several weeks as the infant accumulates adipose tissue.

Engorged breasts occur frequently in both male and female newborns. This condition, which appears by the third day, is a result of maternal hormonal influences and may last up to 2 weeks (Figure 25–30). A whitish secretion from the nipples may also be noted. The infant's breast should not be massaged or squeezed because this practice may cause a breast abscess. Extra nipples or *supernumerary nipples* are occasionally noted below and medial to the true nipples. These harmless pink or brown (in darker skinned newborns) spots vary in size and do not contain glandular tissue. Accessory nipples can be differentiated from a pigmented nevus (mole) by placing the fingertips alongside the accessory nipple and pulling the adjacent tissue laterally. The accessory nipple will appear dimpled. At puberty the accessory nipple may darken.

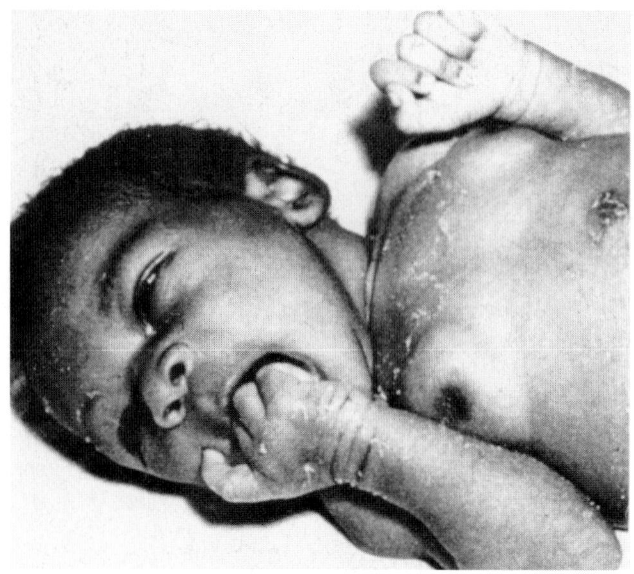

FIGURE 25–30 Breast hypertrophy. SOURCE: Korones SB: *High-Risk Newborn Infants,* 4th ed. St Louis: Mosby, 1986.

Cry

The newborn's cry should be strong, lusty, and of medium pitch. A high-pitched, shrill cry is abnormal and may indicate neurologic disorders or hypoglycemia. Periods of crying vary in length after consoling measures are used. Babies' cries are an important method of communication and alert caregivers to changes in the baby's condition and needs.

Respiration

Normal breathing for a term newborn is 30 to 60 respirations per minute and predominantly diaphragmatic, with associated rising and falling of the abdomen during inspiration and expiration. Any signs of respiratory distress, nasal flaring, intercostal or xiphoid retractions, expiratory grunting or sigh, seesaw respirations, or tachypnea (sustained or greater than 60 respirations per minute) should be noted. Hyperexpansion (chest appears high) or hypoexpansion (chest appears low) of the anteroposterior diameter of the chest should also be noted. Both the anterior and posterior chest are auscultated. Some breath sounds are heard better when the newborn is crying, but localizing and identifying breath sounds are difficult in the newborn. Upper airway noises and bowel sounds may also be heard over the chest wall and make auscultation difficult. Because sounds may be transmitted from the unaffected lung to the affected lung, the absence of breath sounds may not be diagnosed. Air entry may be noisy in the first couple of hours until lung fluid resolves, especially in cesarean births. Brief periods of apnea (episodic breathing) occur, but no color or heart rate changes occur in healthy, term newborns.

Heart

Heart rates can be as rapid as 180 beats per minute in newborns and fluctuate a great deal, especially if the baby moves or is startled. Normal range is 120 to 160 beats per minute. Auscultation provides the nurse with valuable assessment data. The heart is examined for rate and rhythm, position of the apical impulse, and heart sound intensity. Dysrhythmias should be reassessed by the physician.

The pulse rate is variable and is influenced by physical activity, crying, state of wakefulness, and body temperature. Auscultation is performed over the entire heart region (precordium), below the left axilla, and below the scapula. Apical pulse rates are obtained by auscultation for a full minute, preferably when the newborn is asleep.

The placement of the heart in the chest should be determined when the newborn is in a quiet state. The heart is relatively large at birth and is located high in the chest, with its apex somewhere between the fourth and fifth intercostal spaces.

A shift of heart tones in the mediastinal area to either side may indicate pneumothorax, dextrocardia (heart placement on the right side of the chest), or a diaphragmatic hernia. The experienced nurse can diagnose these and many other problems early with a stethoscope. Normally, the heartbeat has a "toc tic" sound. A slur or slushing sound (usually after the first sound) may indicate a murmur. Although 90% of all murmurs are transient and are considered normal, they should be monitored closely by a physician. Many murmurs are related to a patent ductus arteriosus, which closes in about 1 to 2 days.

In newborns, a low-pitched, musical murmur heard just to the right of the apex of the heart is fairly common. Occasionally, significant murmurs will be heard, including the murmur of a patent ductus arteriosus, aortic or pulmonary stenosis, or small ventricular septal defect. See Chapter 28 for a discussion of congenital heart defects.

Peripheral pulses (brachial, femoral, pedal) are also evaluated to detect any lags or unusual characteristics. Brachial pulses are palpated bilaterally for equality and compared with the femoral pulses. Femoral pulses are palpated by applying gentle pressure with the middle finger over the femoral canal (Figure 25–31). Decreased or absent femoral pulses indicate coarctation of the aorta and require additional investigation. A wide difference in blood pressure between the upper and lower extremities also indicates coarctation. The measurement of blood pressure is best accomplished by using the Doppler technique or a 1- to 2-inch cuff and a stethoscope over the brachial artery (Figure 25–32). If a Doppler device is used, the newborn's extremities must be immobilized during the assessment, and the cuff should cover two-thirds of the upper arm or upper leg. Movement, crying, and inappropriate cuff size can give inaccurate measurements of the blood pressure.

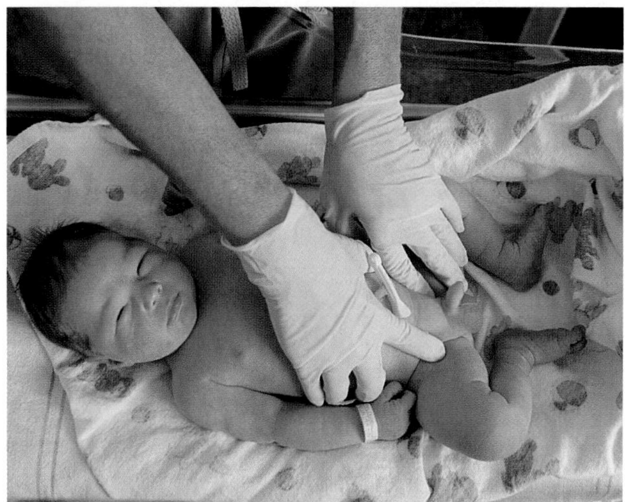

A

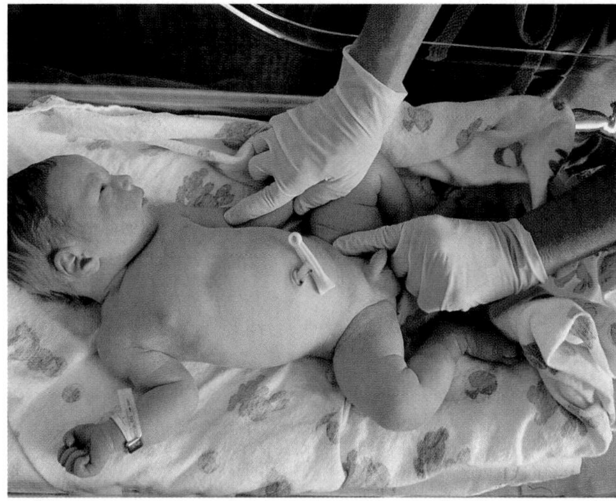

B

FIGURE 25–31 ***A,*** Bilaterally palpate the femoral arteries for rate and intensity of the pulses. Press fingertip gently at the groin as shown. ***B,*** Compare the femoral pulses to the brachial pulses by palpating the pulses simultaneously for comparison of rate and intensity.

Blood pressure may not be measured routinely on healthy newborns but is a routine measurement on newborns who are having distress, are premature, or are suspected of cardiac anomaly (Taeusch & Ballard, 1998). Infants who have birth asphyxia and are on ventilators have significantly lower systolic and diastolic blood pressures

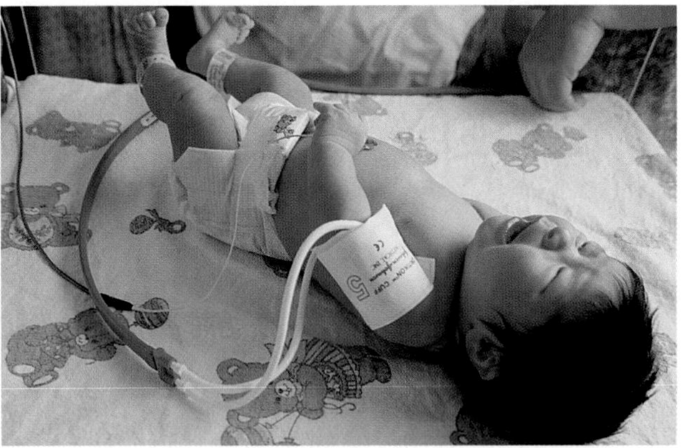

FIGURE 25–32 Blood pressure measurement using the Dinemapp and Doppler devices. The cuff can be applied to either the neonate's upper arm or thigh.

TABLE 25–4 Newborn Vital Signs

Pulse	**Blood Pressure**
120–160 bpm	80–60/45–40 mm Hg at birth
During sleep as low as 100 bpm; if crying, up to 180 bpm	100/50 mm Hg at day 10
Apical pulse counted for 1 full minute	**Temperature**
Respirations	Normal range: 36.5–37.5C (97.7–99.4F)
30–60 respirations/minute	Axillary: 36.4–37.2C (97.5–99F)
Predominantly diaphragmatic but synchronous with abdominal movements	Skin: 36–36.5C (96.8–97.7F)
Respirations are counted for 1 full minute	Rectal: 36.6–37.2C (97.8–99F)

than healthy infants (Hegyi et al, 1996). If cardiac anomaly is suspected, blood pressure is palpated in all four extremities (Table 25–4). At birth, systolic values usually range from 80 to 45 mm Hg and diastolic values from 60 to 40 mm Hg. By the tenth day of life, blood pressure rises to 100/50 mm Hg.

Abdomen

The nurse can learn a great deal about the newborn's abdomen without disturbing the infant. The abdomen should be cylindrical, protrude slightly, and move with respiration. A certain amount of laxness of the abdominal muscles is normal. A scaphoid (hollow-shaped) appearance suggests the absence of abdominal contents. No cyanosis should be present, and few if any blood vessels should be apparent to the eye. There should be no gross distention or bulging. The more distended the abdomen, the tighter the skin becomes, and engorged vessels appear. Distention is the first sign of many of the abnormalities found in the gastrointestinal tract.

Before palpation of the abdomen, the nurse should auscultate the presence or absence of bowel sounds in all four quadrants. Bowel sounds should be present by 1 hour after birth. Palpation can cause a transient decrease in bowel sound intensity.

Abdominal palpation should be carried out systematically. The nurse palpates each of the four abdominal quadrants, moving in a clockwise direction, checking for softness, tenderness, and the presence of masses. When palpating the abdomen, the nurse may feel for the liver. The newborn's liver is large in proportion to the rest of the body and can usually be felt between 1 and 2 cm below the right costal margin. Depending on institutional protocol, palpation of the kidney may be performed by the staff nurse. Kidneys are more difficult to feel but can be more easily examined within 4 to 6 hours after birth, before the intestines become distended with air and feedings are initiated. By placing a finger at the posterior flank and pushing upward while pressing downward with the opposite hand, each kidney may be palpated as a firm oval mass between the examiner's finger and hand. The lower pole of the kidney is usually found 1 to 2 cm above the umbilicus. The spleen tip may be palpated in the lateral aspect of the left upper quadrant in the normal newborn.

Umbilical Cord

Initially, the umbilical cord is white and gelatinous in appearance, with the two umbilical arteries and one umbilical vein readily apparent. Because a single umbilical artery is frequently associated with congenital anomalies, the vessels should be counted as part of the newborn assessment. The cord begins drying within 1 or 2 hours after birth and is shriveled and blackened by the second or third day. Within 7 to 10 days it sloughs off, although a granulated area may remain for a few days longer.

Cord bleeding is abnormal and may result because the cord was inadvertently pulled or because the cord clamp was loosened. Foul-smelling drainage is also abnormal and is generally caused by infection, which requires immediate treatment to prevent septicemia. If the neonate has a patent urachus (abnormal connection between the umbilicus and bladder), moistness or draining urine may be apparent at the base of the cord.

Serous or serosanguineous drainage that continues after the cord falls off may indicate a granuloma. It appears as a small, red button deep in the umbilicus. Treatment involves cauterization by a physician with a silver nitrate stick. Another umbilical cord anomaly that must be assessed before cord clamping is umbilical cord hernia and associated patent omphalomesenteric duct (O'Donnell, Glick, & Coty, 1998).

Genitals

Female Infants

The nurse examines the labia majora, labia minora, and clitoris, noting the size of each as appropriate for gestational age. A vaginal tag or hymenal tag is often evident and will usually disappear in a few weeks. During the first week of life, the newborn may have a vaginal discharge composed of thick whitish mucus. This discharge, which can become tinged with blood, is referred to as **pseudomenstruation** and is caused by the withdrawal of maternal hormones. Smegma, a white cheeselike substance, is often present between the labia. Removing it may traumatize tender tissue.

Male Infants

The penis is inspected to determine whether the urinary orifice is correctly positioned. *Hypospadias* occurs when the urinary meatus is located on the ventral surface of the penis. It occurs most commonly among Western Europeans in the United States. *Phimosis* is a condition occurring in newborn males in which the opening of the foreskin (prepuce) is small, and the foreskin cannot be pulled back over the glans at all. This condition may interfere with urination, so the adequacy of the urinary stream should be evaluated.

The scrotum is inspected for size and symmetry and should be palpated to verify the presence of both testes and to rule out *cryptorchidism* (failure of testes to descend). The testes are palpated separately between the thumb and forefinger, with the thumb and forefinger of the other hand placed together over the inguinal canal. Scrotal edema and discoloration are common in breech births. *Hydrocele* (a collection of fluid surrounding the testes in the scrotum) is common in newborns and should be identified. It usually resolves without intervention. The presence of a hard testis should raise the suspicion of perinatal torsion (Taeusch & Ballard, 1998).

Anus

The anal area is inspected to verify that it is patent and has no fissure. Imperforate anus and rectal atresia may be ruled out by observation. Digital examination, if necessary, is done by a physician. The passage of the first meconium stool is also noted. Atresia of the gastrointestinal tract or meconium ileus with resultant obstruction must be considered if the newborn does not pass meconium in the first 24 hours of life.

Extremities

Extremities are examined for gross deformities, extra digits or webbing, clubfoot, and range of motion. Normal newborn extremities appear short, are generally flexible, and move symmetrically.

Arms and Hands

Nails extend beyond the fingertips in term newborns. Fingers and toes should be counted. *Polydactyly* is the presence of extra digits on either the hands or the feet. *Syndactyly* refers to fusion (webbing) of fingers or toes. Hands should be inspected for normal palmar creases. A single palmar crease, called simian line (see also Figure 8–19), is frequently present in children with Down syndrome.

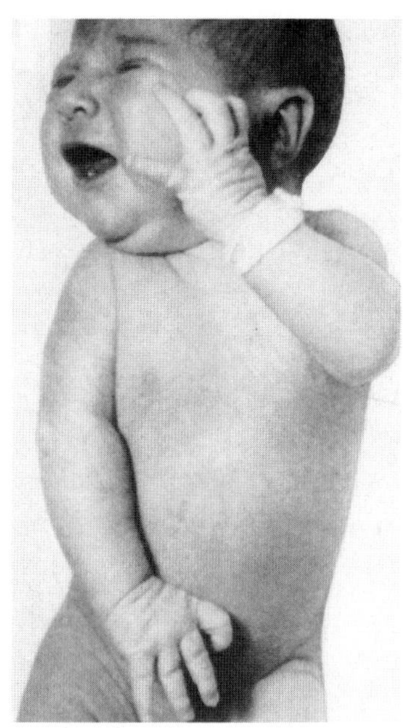

FIGURE 25–33 Right Erb palsy resulting from injury to the fifth and sixth cervical roots of brachial plexus. SOURCE: Potter EL, Craig JM: *Pathology of the Fetus and Infant,* 3rd ed. Chicago: Year Book Medical Publishers, 1975. Reproduced with permission.

Brachial palsy, which is partial or complete paralysis of portions of the arm, results from trauma to the brachial plexus during a difficult birth. It occurs most commonly when strong traction is exerted on the head of the newborn in an attempt to deliver a shoulder lodged behind the symphysis pubis in the presence of shoulder dystocia. Brachial palsy may also occur during a breech birth if an arm becomes trapped over the head and traction is exerted.

The portion of the arm affected is determined by the nerves damaged. **Erb-Duchenne paralysis (Erb's palsy)** involves damage to the upper arm (fifth and sixth cervical nerves) and is the most common type. Injury to the eighth cervical and first thoracic nerve roots and the lower portion of the plexus produces the relatively rare *lower arm injury.* The *whole arm type* results from damage to the entire plexus.

With Erb-Duchenne paralysis, the newborn's arm lies limply at the side (Figure 25–33). The elbow is held in extension, with the forearm pronated. The newborn is unable to elevate the arm, and therefore the Moro reflex cannot be elicited on the affected side. When lower arm injury occurs, paralysis of the hand and wrist results; complete paralysis of the limb occurs with the whole arm type.

The nurse carefully instructs the parents in the correct method of performing passive range-of-motion exercises (to prevent muscle contractures and restore function) and arranges supervised practice sessions. In more

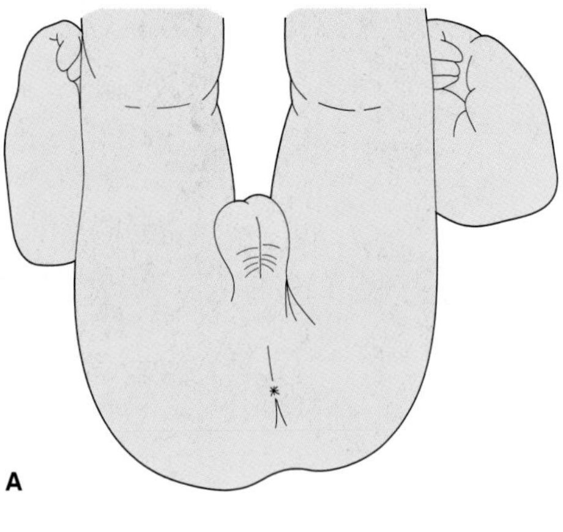

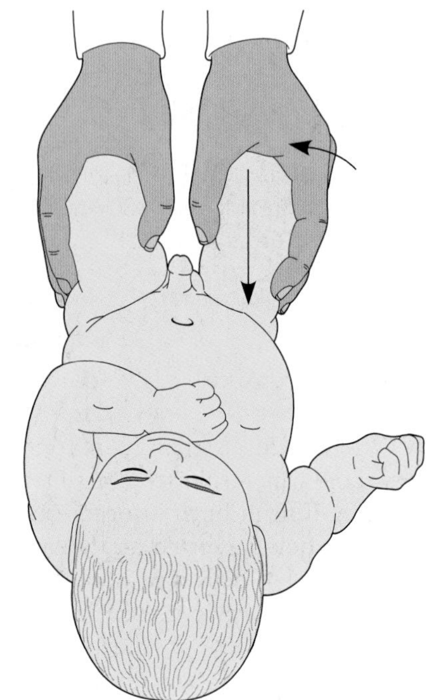

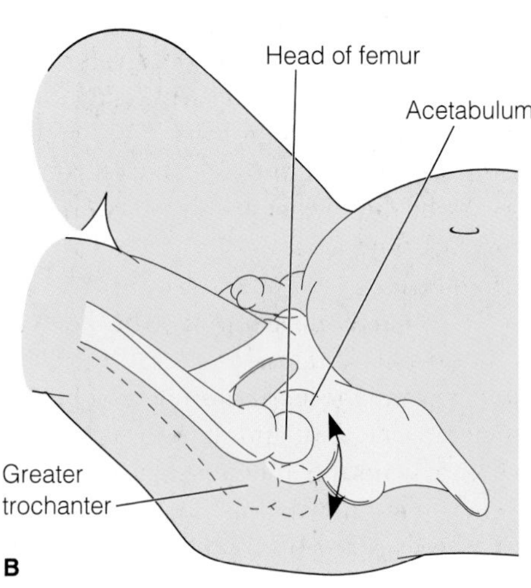

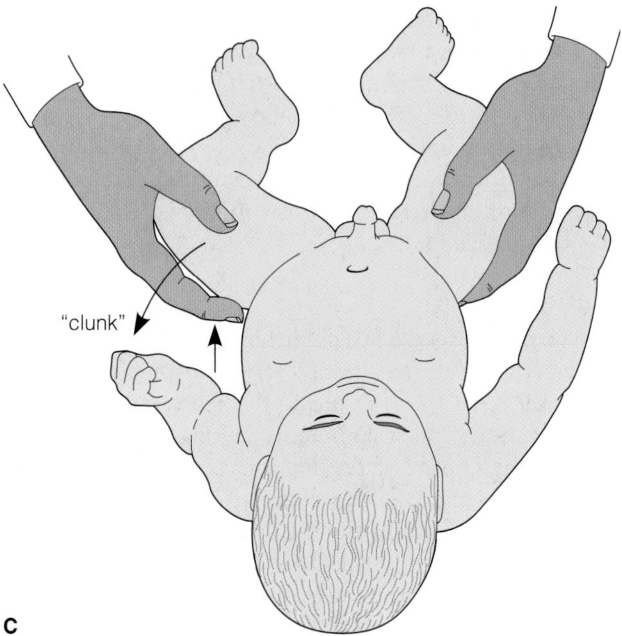

FIGURE 25–34 ***A,*** Congenitally dislocated right hip in a young infant as seen on gross inspection. ***B,*** Barlow's (dislocation) maneuver. Baby's thigh is grasped and adducted with gentle downward pressure. Dislocation is palpable as femoral head slips out of acetabulum. ***C,*** Ortolani's maneuver puts downward pressure on the hip and then inward rotation. If the hip is dislocated, this maneuver will force the femoral head back into the acetabular rim with a noticeable "clunk."

severe cases, splinting of the arm is indicated until the edema decreases. The arm is held in a position of abduction and external rotation with the elbow flexed 90 degrees. The "Statue of Liberty" splint is commonly used, although similar results are obtained by attaching a strip of muslin to the head of the crib and tying the other end around the wrist, thereby holding the arm up.

Prognosis is related to the degree of nerve damage resulting from trauma and hemorrhage within the nerve sheath. Complete recovery occurs within a few months with minimal trauma. Moderate trauma may result in some partial paralysis. Recovery is unlikely with severe trauma, and muscle wasting may develop.

Legs and Feet

The legs of the newborn should be of equal length, with symmetric skin folds. However, they may assume a "fetal posture" secondary to position in utero, and it may take several days for the legs to relax into normal position.

To evaluate for hip dislocation or hip instability, Ortolani's and Barlow's maneuvers are performed (Figure 25–34). The nurse performs **Ortolani's maneuver** to rule out the possibility of congenital hip dysplasia (hip dislocatability). With the newborn relaxed and quiet on a firm surface, the hips and knees flexed at a 90-degree angle, the nurse grasps the infant's thigh with the middle finger over the greater trochanter and lifts the thigh to bring the femoral head from its posterior position toward the acetabulum. With gentle abduction of the thigh, the femoral head is returned to the acetabulum. Simultaneously, the examiner feels a sense of reduction or a "clunk" as the femoral returns. This reduction is palpable and cannot be heard. With **Barlow's maneuver,** the nurse grasps and adducts the infant's thigh and applies gentle downward pressure. Dislocation is felt as the femoral head slips out of the acetabulum. The femoral head is then returned to the acetabulum using Ortolani's maneuver, confirming the diagnosis of an unstable or dislocatable hip.

The feet are then examined for evidence of a talipes deformity (clubfoot). Intrauterine position frequently causes the feet to appear to turn inward (Figure 25–35); this is termed a "positional" clubfoot. If the feet can easily be returned to midline by manipulation, no treatment is indicated. Range-of-motion exercises can be taught to the family. Further investigation is indicated when the foot will not turn to the midline position or align readily. This is considered the most severe type of "true clubfoot," or talipes equinovarus.

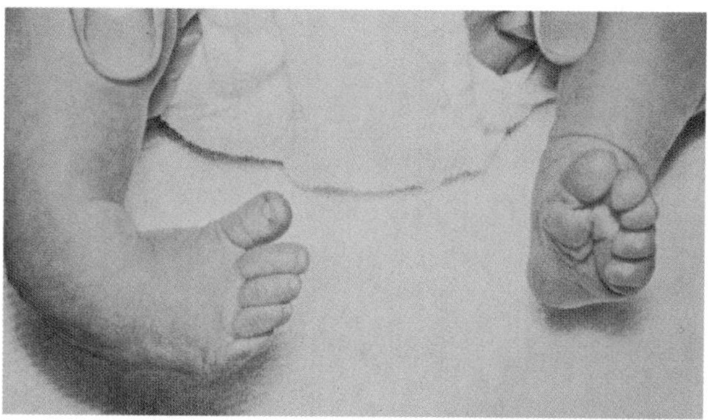

A

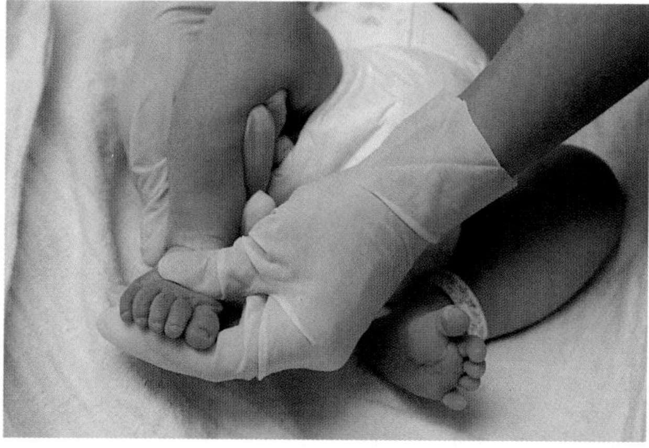

B

FIGURE 25–35 ***A,*** Unilateral talipes equinovarus (clubfoot). ***B,*** To determine the presence of clubfoot, the nurse moves the foot to the midline. Resistance indicates true clubfoot.

Back

With the baby prone, the nurse examines the back. The spine should appear straight and flat because the lumbar and sacral curves do not develop until the infant begins to sit. The base of the spine is then examined for a dermal sinus. The nevus pilosus ("hairy nevus") is only occasionally found at the base of the spine in newborns, but it is significant because it is frequently associated with spina bifida. A pilonidal dimple should be examined to ascertain that there is no connection to the spinal canal.

Assessment of Neurologic Status

The nurse should begin the neurologic examination with a period of observation, noting the general physical characteristics and behavior of the newborn. Important behaviors to assess are the *state of alertness, resting posture, cry,* and *quality of muscle tone and motor activity.*

The usual position of the newborn is with partially flexed extremities with the legs abducted to the abdomen. When awake, the newborn may exhibit purposeless, uncoordinated bilateral movements of the extremities. If these movements are absent, minimal, or obviously asymmetric, neurologic dysfunction should be suspected. Eye movements are observable during the first few days of life. An alert neonate is able to fixate on faces and brightly colored objects. Shining a bright light in the newborn's eyes elicits the blinking response.

The nurse evaluates muscle tone by moving various parts of the body while the head of the newborn remains in a neutral position. The newborn is somewhat hypertonic; that is, the newborn resists the examiner's attempts to extend the elbow and knee joints. Muscle tone should be symmetric. Diminished muscle tone and flaccidity require further evaluation.

Tremors or jitteriness is common in the full-term newborn and must be evaluated to differentiate it from a convulsion. A fine jumping of the muscle is likely to be a central nervous system disorder and requires further evaluation. Jitteriness may be related to hypoglycemia, hypocalcemia, or substance withdrawal. Environmental stimuli may initiate tremors. Holding or flexing the involved extremity will stop the tremor. Neonatal seizures may consist of no more than chewing or swallowing movements, deviations of the eyes, rigidity, or flaccidity because of CNS immaturity. Seizures are not usually initiated by stimuli, and cannot be stopped by holding.

Specific deep tendon reflexes can be elicited in the newborn but have limited value unless they are obviously asymmetric. The knee jerk is brisk; a normal ankle clonus may involve three or four beats. Plantar flexion is present.

The central nervous system of the newborn is immature and characterized by a variety of reflexes. Because the newborn's movements are uncoordinated, methods of communication are limited, and control of bodily functions is drastically limited, the reflexes serve a variety of purposes. Some are protective (blink, gag, sneeze); some

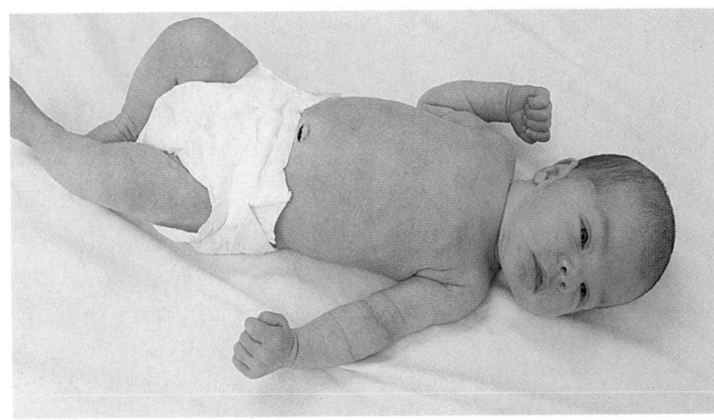

FIGURE 25–36 Tonic neck reflex.

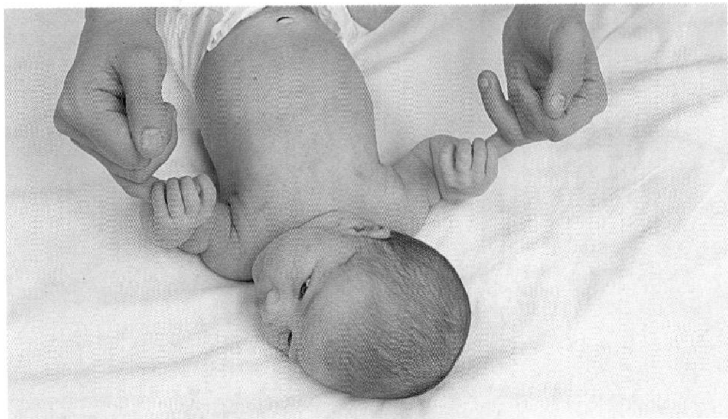

FIGURE 25–37 Grasping reflex.

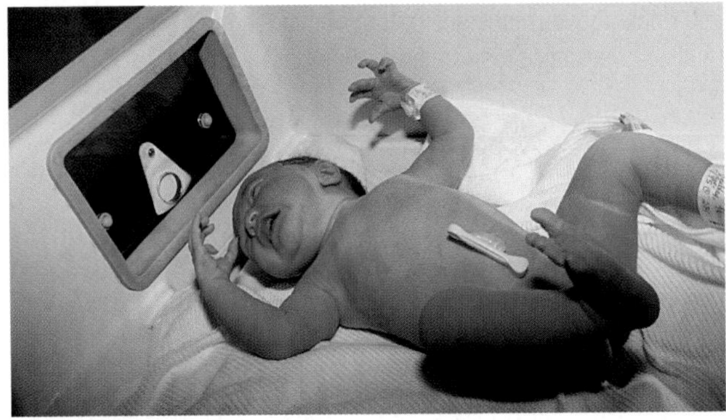

FIGURE 25–38 Moro reflex.

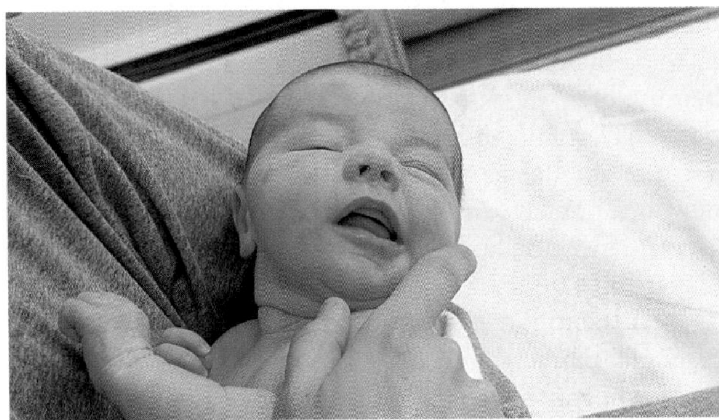

FIGURE 25–39 Rooting reflex.

aid in feeding (rooting, sucking) and may not be very active if the infant has eaten recently; some stimulate human interaction (grasping). Neonatal reflexes and general neurologic activity should be carefully assessed (Pressler & Hepworth, 1997).

The most common reflexes found in the normal newborn are the following:

- The **tonic neck reflex** (fencer position) is elicited when the newborn is supine and the head is turned to one side. In response, the extremities on the same side straighten, whereas on the opposite side they flex (Figure 25–36). This reflex may not be seen during the early newborn period, but once it appears, it persists until about the third month.
- The **grasping reflex** is elicited by stimulating the newborn's palm with a finger or object. The newborn will grasp and hold the object or finger firmly enough to be lifted momentarily from the crib (Figure 25–37).
- The **Moro reflex** is elicited when the newborn is startled by a loud noise or is lifted slightly above the crib and then suddenly lowered. In response the newborn straightens arms and hands outward while the knees flex. Slowly, the arms return to the chest, as in an embrace. The fingers spread, forming a C, and the newborn may cry (Figure 25–38). This reflex may persist until about 6 months of age.
- The **rooting reflex** is elicited when the side of the newborn's mouth or cheek is touched. In response the newborn turns toward that side and opens the lips to suck (if not fed recently) (Figure 25–39).
- The **sucking reflex** is elicited when an object is placed in the newborn's mouth or anything touches the lips. Newborns suck even while sleeping; this is called nonnutritive sucking, and it can have a quieting effect on the baby.
- The **Babinski reflex,** or fanning and hyperextension of all toes, occurs when the lateral aspect of the sole is stroked from the heel upward across the ball of the foot. In adults, by contrast, the toes flex.
- **Trunk incurvation (Galant reflex)** is seen when the newborn is prone. Stroking the spine causes the pelvis to turn to the stimulated side.

In addition to these reflexes, newborns can *blink*, *yawn*, *cough*, *sneeze*, and *draw back from pain* (protective reflexes). They can even move a little on their own. When placed on their stomachs, they push up and try to crawl *(prone crawl)*. When held upright with one foot touching a flat surface, the newborn puts one foot in front of the other and "walks" *(stepping reflex)* (Figure 25–40). This reflex is more pronounced at birth and is lost in 4 to 5 months. Table 25–5 summarizes the stimulus for and response of the common newborn reflexes.

TABLE 25–5 Common Reflexes of the Newborn

Reflex Name	Evoking Stimulus	Response
Blinking reflex	Light flash	Eyelids close.
Pupillary reflex	Light flash	Pupil constricts.
Rooting reflex	Light touch of finger on cheek close to mouth	Head rotates toward stimulation; mouth opens and attempts to suck finger. Disappears by about 4 months of age.
Sucking reflex	Finger (or nipple) inserted into mouth	Rhythmic sucking occurs.
Moro reflex	Infant lying on back: slightly raised head suddenly released; infant held horizontally, lowered quickly about 6 in, and stopped abruptly	Arms are extended, head is thrown back, fingers are spread wide; arms are then brought back to center convulsively with hands clenched; spine and lower extremities are extended. Disappears by about 6 months of age.
Startle reflex	Loud noise	Similar to Moro reflex flexion in arms; fists are clenched.
Grasping reflex	Finger placed in palm of hand	Infant's fingers close around and grasp object.
Tonic neck reflex	Head turned to one side while infant lies on back	Arm and leg are extended on the side the infant faces. Opposite arm and leg are flexed.
Abdominal reflex	Tactile stimulation or tickling	Abdominal muscles contract.
Withdrawal reflex	Slight pinprick to the sole of the infant's foot	Leg flexes.
Walking reflex	Infant supported in an upright position with feet lightly touching a flat surface	Rhythmic stepping movement. Disappears at about 4 months of age.
Babinski reflex	Gentle stroking on the sole of each foot	Fanning and extension of the toes (adults respond to this stimulation with flexion of toes).
Plantar, or toe-grasping, reflex	Pressure applied with the finger against the balls of the infant's feet	A plantar flexion of all toes. Disappears by the end of the first year of life.

SOURCE: Adapted from Mott SR, James SR, Sperhac AM: *Nursing Care of Children and Families: A Holistic Approach,* 2nd ed. Menlo Park, CA: Addison-Wesley Nursing, 1990.

Text continues on page 749.

Brazelton (1984) recommends the following steps as a means of assessing central nervous system integration:

1. Insert a gloved finger into the newborn's mouth to elicit a sucking reflex.
2. As soon as the newborn is sucking vigorously, assess hearing and vision responses by noting sucking changes in the presence of a light, a rattle, and a voice.
3. The newborn should respond with a brief cessation of sucking followed by continuous sucking with repeated stimulation.

This examination demonstrates auditory and visual integrity as well as complex behavioral interactions.

Newborn Physical Assessment Guide

Following is a guide for systematically assessing the newborn. Normal findings, alterations, and related causes are presented in correlation with suggested nursing responses. The findings are typical for a full-term newborn.

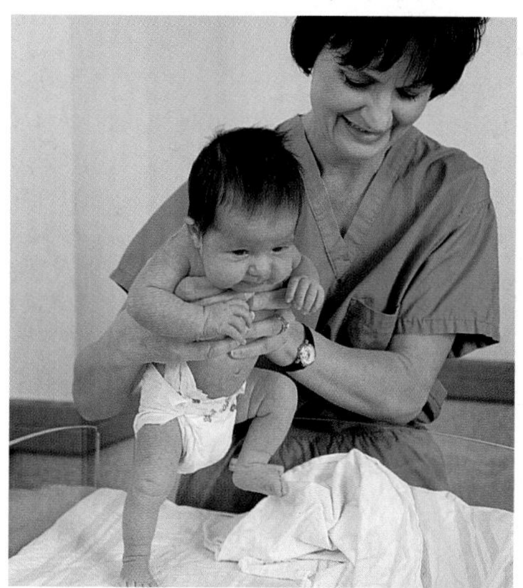

FIGURE 25–40 The stepping reflex disappears after 4 to 5 months.

ASSESSMENT GUIDE: NEWBORN PHYSICAL ASSESSMENT

Physical Assessment/ Normal Findings	Alterations and Possible Causes*	Nursing Responses to Data†
Vital Signs		
Blood pressure (BP) At birth: 80–60/45–40 mm Hg Day 10: 100/50 mm Hg (may be unable to measure diastolic pressure with standard sphygmomanometer)	Low BP (hypovolemia, shock)	Monitor BP in all cases of distress, prematurity, or suspected anomaly. Low BP: Refer to physician immediately so measures to improve circulation are begun.
Pulse 120–160 bpm (if asleep 100 bpm; if crying, up to 180 bpm)	Weak pulse (decreased cardiac output)	Assess skin perfusion by blanching (capillary refill test).
	Bradycardia (severe asphyxia, arrhythmia)	Correlate finding with BP assessments; refer to physician.
	Tachycardia (over 160 bpm at rest) (infection, central nervous system problems, arrhythmia)	Carry out neurologic and thermoregulation assessments.
Respirations 30–60 breaths/minute Synchronization of chest and abdominal movements Diaphragmatic and abdominal breathing	Tachypnea (pneumonia, respiratory distress syndrome [RDS]) Rapid, shallow breathing (hypermagnesemia due to large doses given to mothers with PIH) Respirations below 30 breaths/minute (maternal anesthesia or analgesia)	Identify sleep-wake state; correlate with respiratory pattern. Evaluate for all signs of respiratory distress; report findings to physician.
Transient tachypnea	Expiratory grunting, subcostal and substernal retractions; flaring of nares (respiratory distress); apnea (cold stress, respiratory disorder)	Evaluate for cold stress. Report findings to physician/nurse practitioner.
Crying Strong and lusty Moderate tone and pitch Cries vary in length from 3 to 7 minutes after consoling measures are used	High pitched, shrill (neurologic disorder, hypoglycemia) Weak or absent (CNS disorder, laryngeal problem)	Discuss newborn's use of cry for communication. Assess and record abnormal cries. Reduce environmental noises.
Temperature Axilla 36.4–37.2C (97.5–99F) Rectal 36.6–37.2C (97.8–99F); 36.8C (98.8F) desired Heavier neonates tend to have higher body temperatures	Elevated temperature (room too warm, too much clothing or covers, dehydration, sepsis, brain damage) Subnormal temperature (brain stem involvement, cold, sepsis) Swings of more than 2F from one reading to next or subnormal temperature (infection)	Notify physician of elevation or drop. Counsel parents on possible causes of elevated or low temperatures, appropriate home-care measures, when to call physician. Teach parents how to take rectal and/or axillary temperature; assess parents' information regarding use of thermometer; provide teaching as needed.
Weight 2500–4000 g (5 1b, 8 oz–8 1b, 13 oz)	$<$ 2748 g ($<$ 6 lb) = SGA or preterm infant $>$ 4050 g ($>$ 9 lb) = LGA or infants of diabetic mothers	Plot weight and gestational age on growth chart to identify high-risk infants. Ascertain body build of parents. Counsel parents regarding appropriate caloric intake.

*Possible causes of alterations are placed in parentheses.

†This column provides guidelines for further assessment and initial nursing interventions.

Physical Assessment/ Normal Findings	Alterations and Possible Causes*	Nursing Responses to Data†
Within first 3 to 4 days, normal weight loss of 5%–10% Large babies tend to lose more due to greater fluid loss in proportion to birth weight except infants of diabetic mother	Loss greater than 15% (small fluid intake, loss of meconium and urine, feeding difficulties)	Notify physician of net losses or gains. Calculate fluid intake and losses from all sources (insensible water loss, radiant warmers, and phototherapy lights).
Length		
48–52 cm (18–22 in) Grows 10 cm (3 in) during first 3 months	Less than 45 cm (congenital dwarf) Short/long bones proximally (achondroplasia) Short/long bones distally (Ellis-Van Creveld syndrome)	Assess for other signs of dwarfism. Determine other signs of skeletal system adequacy. Plot progress at subsequent well-baby visits.
Posture		
Body usually flexed, hands may be tightly clenched, neck appears short as chin rests on chest In breech births feet are usually dorsiflexed	Only extension noted, inability to move from midline (trauma, hypoxia, immaturity) Constant motion (maternal caffeine intake)	Record spontaneity of motor activity and symmetry of movements. If parents express concern about newborn's movement patterns, reassure and evaluate further if appropriate.
Skin		
Color		
Color consistent with genetic background Newborns of European descent: pink-tinged or ruddy color over face, trunk, extremities Newborns of African or Native American descent: pale pink with yellow or red tinge Newborns of Asian descent: pink or rosy red to yellow tinge	Pallor of face, conjunctiva (anemia, hypothermia, anoxia) Beefy red (hypoglycemia, immature vasomotor reflexes, polycythemia)	Discuss with parents common skin color variations to allay fears. Document extent and time of occurrence of color change.
Common variations: acrocyanosis, circumoral cyanosis, or harlequin color change	Meconium staining (fetal distress) Jaundice (hemolytic reaction from blood incompatibility within first 24 hours, sepsis)	Obtain Hb and hematocrit values; obtain bilirubin levels. Assess for respiratory difficulty. Differentiate between physiologic and pathologic jaundice.
Mottled when undressed	Cyanosis (choanal atresia, CNS damage or trauma, respiratory or cardiac problem, cold stress)	Assess degree of (central or peripheral) cyanosis and possible causes; refer to physician.
Minor bruising over buttocks in breech presentation and over eyes and forehead in facial presentations		Discuss with parents cause and course of minor bruising related to labor and birth.
Texture		
Smooth, soft, flexible; may have dry, peeling hands and feet	Generalized cracked or peeling skin (SGA or postterm; blood incompatibility; metabolic, kidney dysfunction) Seborrheic-dermatitis (cradle cap) Absence of vernix (postmature) Yellow vernix (bilirubin staining)	Report to physician. Instruct parents to shampoo the scalp and anterior fontanelle areas daily with soap; rinse well; avoid use of oil.

*Possible causes of alterations are placed in parentheses.

†This column provides guidelines for further assessment and initial nursing interventions.

Physical Assessment/ Normal Findings	Alterations and Possible Causes*	Nursing Responses to Data†
Turgor		
Elastic, returns to normal shape after pinching	Maintains tent shape (dehydration)	Assess for other signs and symptoms of dehydration.
Pigmentation		
Clear; milia across bridge of nose, forehead, or chin will disappear within a few weeks		Advise parents not to pinch or prick these pimplelike areas.
Café-au-lait spots (one or two)	Six or more (neurologic disorder such as Von Recklinghausen disease, cutaneous neurofibromatosis)	If there are six or more café-au-lait spots, refer for genetic and neurologic consult.
Mongolian spots common over dorsal area and buttocks in dark-skinned infants		Assure parents of normalcy of this pigmentation; it will fade in first year or two.
Erythema toxicum	Impetigo (group A β-hemolytic streptococcus or *Staphylococcus aureus* infection)	If impetigo occurs, instruct parents about hand washing and linen precautions during home care.
Telangiectatic nevi	Hemangiomas: Nevus flammeus (port wine stain) Nevus vascularis (strawberry hemangioma) Cavernous hemangiomas	Collaborate with physician. Counsel parents about birthmark's progression to allay misconceptions. Record size and shape of hemangiomas. Refer for follow-up at well-baby clinic.
Rashes	Rashes (infection)	Assess location and type of rash (macular, papular, vesicular). Obtain history of onset, prenatal history, and related signs and symptoms.
Petechiae of head or neck (breech presentation, cord around neck)	Generalized petechiae (clotting abnormalities)	Determine cause; advise parents if further health care is needed.
Head		
General appearance, size, movement Round, symmetric, and moves easily from left to right and up and down; soft and pliable	Asymmetric, flattened occiput on either side of the head (plagiocephaly) Head held at angle (torticollis)	Instruct parents to change infant's sleeping positions frequently.
	Unable to move head side to side (neurologic trauma)	Determine adequacy of all neurologic signs.
Circumference: 32–37 cm (12.5–14.5 in); 2 cm greater than chest circumference Head one-fourth of body size	Extreme differences in size may be microencephaly (Cornelia de Lange syndrome, cytomegalic inclusion disease [CID]), rubella, toxoplasmosis, chromosome abnormalities), hydrocephalus (meningomyelocele, achondroplasia), anencephaly (neural tube defect) Head is 3 cm or more larger than chest circumference (preterm, hydrocephalus)	Measure circumference from occiput to frontal area using metal or paper tape. Measure chest circumference using metal or paper tape and compare to head circumference. Record measurements on growth chart. Reevaluate at well-baby visits.

*Possible causes of alterations are placed in parentheses.

†This column provides guidelines for further assessment and initial nursing interventions.

Physical Assessment/ Normal Findings	Alterations and Possible Causes*	Nursing Responses to Data†
Common variations		
Molding Breech and cesarean newborns' heads are round and well shaped	Cephalhematoma (trauma during birth, persists up to 3 weeks) Caput succedaneum (long labor and birth; disappears in 1 week)	Evaluate neurologic response. Observe for hyperbilirubinemia. Reassure parents regarding common manifestations due to birth process and when they should disappear.
Fontanelles		
Palpation of juncture of cranial bones Anterior fontanelle: 3–4 cm long by 2–3 cm wide, diamond shaped Posterior fontanelle: 1–2 cm at birth, triangle shaped	Overlapping of anterior fontanelle (malnourished or preterm newborn) Premature closure of sutures (craniostenosis) Late closure (hydrocephalus)	Discuss normal closure times with parents and care of "soft spots" to allay misconceptions. Refer to physician. Observe for signs and symptoms of hydrocephalus.
Slight pulsation	Moderate to severe pulsation (vascular problems)	Refer to physician.
Moderate bulging noted with crying, stooling, or pulsations with heartbeat	Bulging (increased intracranial pressure, meningitis) Sunken (dehydration)	Evaluate hydration status. Evaluate neurologic status. Report to physician.
Hair		
Texture		
Smooth with fine texture variations (Note: Variations depend on ethnic background.)	Coarse, brittle, dry hair (hypothyroidism) White forelock (Waardenburg syndrome)	Instruct parents regarding routine care of hair and scalp.
Distribution		
Scalp hair high over eyebrows (Spanish-Mexican hairline begins mid-forehead and extends down back of neck.)	Low forehead and posterior hairlines may indicate chromosomal disorders.	Assess for other signs of chromosomal aberrations. Refer to physician.
Face		
Symmetric movement of all facial features, normal hairline, eyebrows and eyelashes present		Assess and record symmetry of all parts, shape, regularity of features, sameness or differences in features.
Spacing of features		
Eyes at same level, nostrils equal size, cheeks full, and sucking pads present	Eyes wide apart—ocular hypertelorism (Apert syndrome, cri-du-chat, Turner syndrome)	Observe for other signs and symptoms indicative of disease states or chromosomal aberrations.
Lips equal on both sides of midline	Abnormal face (Down syndrome, cretinism, gargoylism)	
Chin recedes when compared to other bones of face	Abnormally small jaw—micrognathia (Pierre Robin syndrome, Treacher Collins syndrome)	Maintain airway; do not position supine. Initiate surgical consultation and referral.

*Possible causes of alterations are placed in parentheses.

†This column provides guidelines for further assessment and initial nursing interventions.

Physical Assessment/ Normal Findings	Alterations and Possible Causes*	Nursing Responses to Data†
Movement		
Makes facial grimaces	Inability to suck, grimace, and close eyelids (cranial nerve injury)	Initiate neurologic assessment and consultation.
Symmetric when resting and crying	Asymmetry (paralysis of facial cranial nerve)	Assess and record symmetry of all parts, shape, regularity of features, and sameness or differences in features.
Eyes		
General placement and appearance		
Bright and clear; even placement; slight nystagmus (involuntary cyclical eye movements)	Gross nystagmus (damage to third, fourth, and sixth cranial nerves)	
Concomitant strabismus	Constant and fixed strabismus	Reassure parents that strabismus is considered normal up to 6 months.
Move in all directions		
Blue- or slate-blue gray	Lack of pigmentation (albinism) Brushfield spots may indicate Down syndrome (a light or white speckling of the outer two-thirds of the iris)	Discuss with parents any necessary eye precautions. Assess for other signs of Down syndrome.
Brown color at birth in dark-skinned infants		Discuss with parents that permanent eye color is usually established by 3 months of age.
Eyelids		
Position: above pupils but within iris, no drooping	Elevation or retraction of upper lid (hyperthyroidism)	Assess for signs of hydrocephalus and hyperthyroidism.
	"Sunset sign" lid retraction and downward gaze (hydrocephalus), ptosis (congenital or paralysis of oculomotor muscle)	Evaluate interference with vision in subsequent well-baby visits.
Eyes on parallel plane Epicanthal folds in Asian and 20% of newborns of northern European descent	Upward slant in non-Asians (Down syndrome) Epicanthal folds (Down syndrome, cri-du-chat syndrome)	Assess for other signs of Down syndrome.
Movement		
Blink reflex in response to light stimulus Eyes open wide in dimly lighted room	Blink absent (CNS injury)	Evaluate neurologic status. Refer to physician.
Inspection		
Edematous for first few days of life, resulting from birth and instillation of silver nitrate (chemical conjunctivitis); no lumps or redness	Purulent drainage (infection); infectious conjunctivitis (gonococcus, chlamydia, staphylococcus, or gram-negative organisms) Marginal blepharitis (lid edges red, crusted, scaly)	Initiate good hand washing. Refer to physician. Evaluate infant for seborrheic dermatitis; scales can be removed easily.

*Possible causes of alterations are placed in parentheses.

†This column provides guidelines for further assessment and initial nursing interventions.

Physical Assessment/ Normal Findings	Alterations and Possible Causes*	Nursing Responses to Data†
Cornea		
Clear Corneal reflex present	Ulceration (herpes infection); large cornea or corneas of unequal size (congenital glaucoma) Clouding, opacity of lens (cataract)	Refer to ophthalmologist. Assess for other manifestations of congenital herpes; institute nursing care measures.
Sclera		
May appear bluish in newborn, then white; slightly brownish color frequent in newborns of African descent	True blue sclera (osteogenesis imperfecta)	Refer to physician.
Pupils		
Pupils equal in size, round, and react to light by accommodation	Anisocoria—unequal pupils (CNS damage) Dilation or constriction (intracranial damage, retinoblastoma, glaucoma) Pupils nonreactive to light or accommodation (brain injury)	Refer for neurologic examination.
Slight nystagmus in newborn who has not learned to focus Pupil light reflex demonstrated at birth or by 3 weeks of age	Nystagmus (labyrinthine disturbance, CNS disorder)	
Conjunctiva		
Chemical conjunctivitis Subconjunctival hemorrhage	Pale color (anemia)	Obtain hematocrit and hemoglobin. Reassure parents that chemical conjunctivitis will subside in 1 to 2 days and subconjunctival hemorrhage disappears in a few weeks.
Palpebral conjunctiva (red but not hyperemic)	Inflammation or edema (infection, blocked tear duct)	
Vision		
20/150 Tracks moving object to midline Fixed focus on objects at a distance of about 10–20 in; may be difficult to evaluate in newborn Prefers faces, geometric designs, and black and white to colors	Cataracts (congenital infection)	Record any questions about visual acuity, and initiate follow-up evaluation at first well-baby checkup.
Lashes and lacrimal glands		
Presence of lashes (lashes may be absent in preterm newborns)	No lashes on inner two-thirds of lid (Treacher Collins syndrome); bushy lashes (Hurler syndrome); long lashes (Cornelia de Lange syndrome)	
Cry commonly tearless	Excessive tearing (plugged lacrimal duct, natal narcotic withdrawal), glaucoma	Demonstrate to parents how to milk blocked tear duct. Refer to ophthalmologist if tearing is excessive before third month of life.

*Possible causes of alterations are placed in parentheses.

†This column provides guidelines for further assessment and initial nursing interventions.

Physical Assessment/ Normal Findings	Alterations and Possible Causes*	Nursing Responses to Data†
Nose		
Appearance of external nasal aspects		
May appear flattened as a result of birth process	Continued flat or broad bridge of nose (Down syndrome)	Arrange consultation with specialist.
Small and narrow in midline, even placement in relationship to eyes and mouth	Low bridge of nose, beaklike nose (Apert syndrome, Treacher Collins syndrome) Upturned (Cornelia de Lange syndrome)	Initiate evaluation of chromosomal abnormalities.
Patent nares bilaterally (nose breathers)	Blockage of nares (mucus and/or secretions), choanal atresia	Inspect for obstruction of nares.
Sneezing common to clear nasal passages	Flaring nares (respiratory distress)	Maintain oral airway until surgical correction is made.
Responds to odors, may smell breast milk	No response to stimulating odors	Inspect for obstruction of nares.
Mouth		
Function of facial, hypoglossal, glossopharyngeal, and vagus nerves		
Symmetry of movement and strength	Mouth draws to one side (transient seventh cranial nerve paralysis due to pressure in utero or trauma during birth, congenital paralysis) Fishlike shape (Treacher Collins syndrome)	Initiate neurologic consultation. Administer eye care if eye on affected side of face is unable to close.
Presence of gag, swallowing, coordinated with sucking reflexes Adequate salivation	Suppressed or absent reflexes	Evaluate other neurologic functions of these nerves.
Palate (soft and hard)		
Hard palate dome-shaped Uvula midline with symmetrical movement of soft palate	High-steepled palate (Treacher Collins syndrome), bivid uvula (congenital anomaly)	Assess for other congenital anomalies.
Palate intact, sucks well when stimulated	Clefts in either hard or soft palate (polygenic disorder)	Initiate a surgical consultation referral.
Epithelial (Epstein's) pearls appear on mucosa		Assure parents that these are normal and will disappear at 2 or 3 months of age.
Esophagus patent, some drooling common in newborn	Excessive drooling or bubbling (esophageal atresia)	Test for patency of esophagus.
Tongue		
Free moving in all directions, midline	Lack of movement or asymmetric movement (neurologic damage) Tongue-tied	Further assess neurologic functions. Test reflex elevation of tongue when depressed with tongue blade.
	Deviations from midline (cranial nerve damage)	Check for signs or weakness or deviation.

*Possible causes of alterations are placed in parentheses.

†This column provides guidelines for further assessment and initial nursing interventions.

Physical Assessment/ Normal Findings	Alterations and Possible Causes*	Nursing Responses to Data†
Pink color, smooth to rough texture, non-coated	White cheesy coating (thrush) Tongue has deep ridges	Differentiate between thrush and milk curds. Reassure parents that tongue pattern may change from day to day.
Tongue proportional to mouth	Large tongue with short frenulum (cretinism, Down syndrome, other syndromes)	Evaluate in well-baby clinic to assess development delays. Initiate referrals.
Ears		
External ear		
Without lesions, cysts, or nodules	Nodules, cysts, or sinus tracts in front of ear Adherent earlobes Low set	Evaluate characteristics of lesions. Counsel parents to clean external ear with washcloth only; discourage use of cotton-tip applicators.
	Preauricular skin tags	Refer to physician for ligation.
Hearing		
Eustachian tubes are cleared with first cry Absence of all risk factors	Presence of one or more risk factors	Assess history of risk factors for hearing loss.
Attends to sounds; sudden or loud noise elicits Moro reflex	No response to sound stimuli (deafness)	Test for Moro reflex.
Neck		
Appearance		
Short, straight, creased with skin folds	Abnormally short neck (Turner syndrome) Arching or inability to flex neck (meningitis, congenital anomaly)	Report findings to physician.
Posterior neck lacks loose extra folds of skin	Webbing of neck (Turner syndrome, Down syndrome, trisomy 18)	Assess for other signs of the syndromes.
Clavicles		
Straight and intact	Knot or lump on clavicle (fracture during difficult birth)	Obtain detailed labor and birth history; apply figure-8 bandage.
Moro reflex elicitable	Unilateral Moro reflex response on unaffected side (fracture of clavicle, brachial palsy, Erb-Duchenne paralysis)	Collaborate with physician.
Symmetric shoulders	Hypoplasia	

*Possible causes of alterations are placed in parentheses.

†This column provides guidelines for further assessment and initial nursing interventions.

Physical Assessment/ Normal Findings	Alterations and Possible Causes*	Nursing Responses to Data[†]
Chest		
Appearance and size		
Circumference: 32.5 cm, 1–2 cm less than head		Measure at level of nipples after exhalation.
Wider than it is long Normal shape without depressed or prominent sternum Lower end of sternum (xiphoid cartilage) may be protruding; is less apparent after several weeks Sternum 8 cm long	Funnel chest (congenital or associated with Marfan syndrome) Continued protrusion of xiphoid cartilage (Marfan syndrome, "pigeon chest") Barrel chest	Determine adequacy of other respiratory and circulatory signs. Assess for other signs and symptoms of various syndromes.
Expansion and retraction		
Bilateral expansion	Unequal chest expansion (pneumonia, pneumothorax, respiratory distress)	Assess respiratory effort regularity, flaring of nares, difficulty on both inspiration and expiration.
No intercostal, subcostal, or supracostal retractions	Retractions (respiratory distress) See-saw respirations (respiratory distress)	Record and consult physician.
Auscultation		
Breath sounds are louder in infants	Decreased breath sounds (decreased respiratory activity, atelectasis, pneumothorax)	Perform assessment and report to physician any positive findings.
Chest and axilla clear on crying	Increased breath sounds (resolving pneumonia or in cesarean births)	
Bronchial breath sounds (heard where trachea and bronchi closest to chest wall, above sternum and between scapulae): Bronchial sounds bilaterally Air entry clear Rales may indicate normal newborn atelectasis Cough reflex absent at birth, appears in 2 or more days	Adventitious or abnormal sounds (respiratory disease or distress)	Evaluate color for pallor or cyanosis. Report to physician.
Breasts		
Flat with symmetric nipples Breast tissue diameter 5 cm or more at term Distance between nipples 8 cm Breast engorgement occurs on third day of life; liquid discharge may be expressed in term newborns	Lack of breast tissue (preterm or SGA) Discharge Enlargement Breast abscesses	Evaluate for infection. Reassure parents of normality of breast engorgement.
Nipples	Supernumerary nipples Dark-colored nipples	No intervention is necessary.

*Possible causes of alterations are placed in parentheses.

[†]This column provides guidelines for further assessment and initial nursing interventions.

Physical Assessment/ Normal Findings	Alterations and Possible Causes*	Nursing Responses to Data†
Heart		
Auscultation		
Location: lies horizontally, with left border extending to left of midclavicle		
Regular rhythm and rate	Arrhythmia (anoxia), tachycardia, bradycardia	Refer all arrhythmia and gallop rhythms.
Determination of point of maximal impulse (PMI) Usually lateral to midclavicular line at third or fourth intercostal space	Malpositioning (enlargement, abnormal placement, pneumothorax, dextrocardia, diaphragmatic hernia)	Initiate cardiac evaluation.
Functional murmurs No thrills	Location of murmurs (possible congenital cardiac anomaly)	Evaluate murmur: location, timing, and duration; observe for accompanying cardiac pathology symptoms; ascertain family history.
Horizontal groove at diaphragm shows flaring of rib cage to mild degree	Marked rib flaring (vitamin D deficiency) Inadequacy of respiratory movement	Initiate cardiopulmonary evaluation; assess pulses and blood pressures in all four extremities for equality and quality.
Abdomen		
Appearance		
Cylindrical with some protrusion, appears large in relation to pelvis, some laxness of abdominal muscles No cyanosis, few vessels seen Diastasis recti—common in infants of African descent	Distention, shiny abdomen with engorged vessels (gastrointestinal abnormalities, infection, congenital megacolon) Scaphoid abdominal appearance (diaphragmatic hernia) Increased or decreased peristalsis (duodenal stenosis, small bowel obstruction)	Examine abdomen thoroughly for mass or organomegaly. Measure abdominal girth. Report deviations of abdominal size. Assess other signs and symptoms of obstruction.
	Localized flank bulging (enlarged kidneys, ascites, or absent abdominal muscles)	Refer to physician.
Umbilicus		
No protrusion of umbilicus (protrusion of umbilicus common in infants of African descent) Bluish-white color Cutis navel (umbilical cord projects), granulation tissue present in navel	Umbilical hernia Patent urachus (congenital malformation) Omphalocele Gastroschisis Redness or exudate around cord (infection) Yellow discoloration (hemolytic disease, meconium staining)	Measure umbilical hernia by palpating the opening and record; it should close by 1 year of age; if not, refer to physician. Cover omphalocele with sterile, moist dressing. Instruct parents on cord care and hygiene.
Two arteries and one vein apparent Begins drying 1 to 2 hours after birth No bleeding	Single umbilical artery (congenital anomalies) Discharge or oozing of blood from the cord	Refer anomalies to physician.
Auscultation and percussion Soft bowel sounds heard shortly after birth every 10–30 seconds	Bowel sounds in chest (diaphragmatic hernia) Absence of bowel sounds Hyperperistalsis (intestinal obstruction)	Collaborate with physician. Assess for other signs of dehydration and/or infection.
Femoral pulses		
Palpable, equal, bilateral	Absent or diminished femoral pulses (coarctation of aorta)	Monitor blood pressure in upper and lower extremities.

*Possible causes of alterations are placed in parentheses.

†This column provides guidelines for further assessment and initial nursing interventions.

➤

Physical Assessment/ Normal Findings	Alterations and Possible Causes*	Nursing Responses to Data†
Inguinal area		
No bulges along inguinal area No inguinal lymph nodes felt	Inguinal hernia	Initiate referral. Continue follow-up in well-baby clinic.
Bladder		
Percusses 1–4 cm above symphysis Emptied about 3 hours after birth; if not, at time of birth Urine—inoffensive, mild odor	Failure to void within 24–48 hours after birth Exposure of bladder mucosa (exstrophy of bladder) Foul odor (infection)	Check whether baby voided at birth. Obtain urine specimen if infection is suspected. Consult with clinician.
Genitals		
Gender clearly delineated	Ambiguous genitals	Refer for genetic consultation.
Male		
Penis		
Slender in appearance, about 2.5 cm long, 1 cm wide at birth Normal urinary orifice, urethral meatus at tip of penis	Micropenis (congenital anomaly) Meatal atresia Hypospadias, epispadias	Observe and record first voiding. Collaborate with physician in presence of abnormality. Delay circumcision.
Noninflamed urethral opening	Urethritis (infection)	Palpate for enlarged inguinal lymph nodes and record painful urination.
Foreskin adheres to glans	Ulceration of meatal opening (infection, inflammation)	Evaluate whether ulcer is due to diaper rash; counsel regarding care.
Uncircumcised foreskin tight for 2 to 3 months	Phimosis—if still tight after 3 months	Instruct parents on how to care for uncircumcised penis.
Circumcised Erectile tissue present		Teach parents how to care for circumcision.
Scrotum		
Skin loose and hanging or tight and small; extensive rugae and normal size Normal skin color Scrotal discoloration common in breech	Large scrotum containing fluid (hydrocele) Red, shiny scrotal skin (orchitis) Minimal rugae, small scrotum	Shine a light through scrotum (transilluminate) to verify diagnosis. Assess for prematurity.
Testes		
Descended by birth; not consistently found in scrotum	Undescended testes (cryptorchidism)	If testes cannot be felt in scrotum, gently palpate femoral, inguinal, perineal, and abdominal areas for presence.
Testes size 1.5–2 cm at birth	Enlarged testes (tumor) Small testes (Klinefelter syndrome or adrenal hyperplasia)	Refer and collaborate with physician for further diagnostic studies.

*Possible causes of alterations are placed in parentheses.

†This column provides guidelines for further assessment and initial nursing interventions.

Physical Assessment/ Normal Findings	Alterations and Possible Causes*	Nursing Responses to Data†
Female		
Mons		
Normal skin color, area pigmented in dark-skinned infants		
Labia majora cover labia minora in term and postterm newborns; symmetric size appropriate for gestational age	Hematoma, lesions (trauma) Labia minora prominent	Evaluate for recent trauma. Assess for prematurity.
Clitoris		
Normally large in newborn Edema and bruising in breech birth	Hypertrophy (hermaphroditism)	Refer for genetic workup.
Vagina		
Urinary meatus and vaginal orifice visible (0.5 cm circumference) Vaginal tag or hymenal tag disappears in a few weeks	Inflammation; erythema and discharge (urethritis) Congenital absence of vagina	Collect urine specimen for laboratory examination. Refer to physician.
Discharge; smegma under labia	Foul-smelling discharge (infection)	Collect data and further evaluate reason for discharge.
Bloody or mucoid discharge	Excessive vaginal bleeding (blood coagulation defect)	
Buttocks and Anus		
Buttocks symmetric	Pilonidal dimple	Examine for possible sinus. Instruct parents about cleansing this area.
Anus patent and passage of meconium within 24–48 hours after birth	Imperforate anus, rectal atresia (congenital gastrointestinal defect)	Evaluate extent of problems. Initiate surgical consultation. Perform digital examination to ascertain patency if patency uncertain.
No fissures, tears, or skin tags	Fissures	
Extremities and Trunk		
Short and generally flexed, extremities move symmetrically through range of motion but lack full extension	Unilateral or absence of movement (spinal cord involvement) Fetal position continued or limp (anoxia, CNS problems, hypoglycemia)	Review birth record to assess possible cause.
All joints move spontaneously; good muscle tone, of flexor type, birth to 2 months	Spasticity when infant begins using extensors (cerebral palsy, lack of muscle tone, "floppy baby" syndrome) Hypotonia (Down syndrome)	Collaborate with physician.

*Possible causes of alterations are placed in parentheses.

†This column provides guidelines for further assessment and initial nursing interventions.

Physical Assessment/ Normal Findings	Alterations and Possible Causes*	Nursing Responses to Data†
Arms		
Equal in length Bilateral movement Flexed when quiet	Brachial palsy (difficult birth) Erb-Duchenne paralysis Muscle weakness, fractured clavicle Absence of limb or change of size (phocomelia, amelia)	Report to clinician.
Hands		
Normal number of fingers	Polydactyly (Ellis-Van Creveld syndrome) Syndactyly—one limb (developmental anomaly) Syndactyly—both limbs (genetic component)	Report to clinician.
Normal palmar crease	Simian line on palm (Down syndrome)	Refer for genetic workup.
Normal size hands	Short fingers and broad hand (Hurler syndrome)	
Nails present and extend beyond fingertips in term newborn	Cyanosis and clubbing (cardiac anomalies) Nails long or yellow stained (postterm)	Evaluate for history of distress in utero.
Spine		
C-shaped spine Flat and straight when prone Slight lumbar lordosis Easily flexed and intact when palpated At least half of back devoid of lanugo Full-term infant in ventral suspension should hold head at 45-degree angle, back straight	Spina bifida occulta (nevus pilosus) Dermal sinus Myelomeningocele Head lag, limp, floppy trunk (neurologic problems)	Evaluate extent of neurologic damage; initiate care of spinal opening.
Hips		
No sign of instability	Sensation of abnormal movement, jerk, or snap of hip dislocation	Examine all newborn infants for dislocated hip prior to discharge from birthing center.
Hips abduct to more than 60 degrees		If this is suspected, refer to orthopedist for further evaluation. Reassess at well-baby visits.
Inguinal and buttock skin creases		
Symmetric inguinal and buttock creases	Asymmetry (dislocated hips)	Refer to orthopedist for evaluation. Counsel parents regarding symptoms of concern, and discuss therapy.
Legs		
Legs equal in length Legs shorter than arms at birth	Shortened leg (dislocated hips) Lack of leg movement (fractures, spinal defects)	Refer to orthopedist for evaluation. Counsel parents regarding symptoms of concern, and discuss therapy.

*Possible causes of alterations are placed in parentheses.

†This column provides guidelines for further assessment and initial nursing interventions.

Physical Assessment/ Normal Findings	Alterations and Possible Causes*	Nursing Responses to Data†
Feet		
Foot is in straight line Positional clubfoot—based on position in utero	Talipes equinovarus (true clubfoot)	Discuss differences between positional and true clubfoot with parents. Teach parents passive manipulation of foot.
Fat pads and creases on soles of feet	Incomplete sole creases in first 24 hours of life (premature)	Refer to orthopedist if not corrected by 3 months of age.
Talipes planus (flat feet) normal under 3 years of age		Reassure parents that flat feet are normal in infants.
Neuromuscular		
Motor function		
Symmetric movement and strength in all extremities	Limp, flaccid, or hypertonic (CNS disorders, infection, dehydration, fracture)	Appraise newborn's posture and motor functions by observing activities and motor characteristics.
May be jerky or have brief twitchings	Tremors (hypoglycemia, hypocalcemia, infection, neurologic damage)	Evaluate electrolyte imbalance, hypoglycemia, and neurologic functioning.
Head lag not over 45 degrees	Delayed or abnormal development (preterm, neurologic involvement)	
Neck control adequate to maintain head erect briefly	Asymmetry of tone or strength (neurologic damage)	Refer for genetic evaluation.
Reflexes		
Blink		
Stimulated by flash of light; response is closure of eyelids	Lack of blink response (damage to cranial nerve, CNS injury)	Assess neurologic status.
Pupillary reflex		
Stimulated by flash of light; response is constriction of pupil	Lack of reflex (damage to cranial nerve, CNS injury)	
Moro		
Response to sudden movement or loud noise should be one of symmetric extension and abduction of arms with fingers extended; then return to normal relaxed flexion Infant lying on back: slightly raised head suddenly released; infant held horizontally, lowered quickly about 6 in, and stopped abruptly Fingers form a C Present at birth; disappears by 6 months of age	Asymmetry of body response (fractured clavicle, injury to brachial plexus) Consistent absence (brain damage)	Discuss normality of this reflex in response to loud noises and/or sudden movements. Absence of reflex requires neurologic evaluation.

*Possible causes of alterations are placed in parentheses.

†This column provides guidelines for further assessment and initial nursing interventions.

Physical Assessment/ Normal Findings	Alterations and Possible Causes*	Nursing Responses to Data†
Rooting and sucking		
Turns in direction of stimulus to cheek or mouth; opens mouth and begins to suck rhythmically when finger or nipple is inserted into mouth; difficult to elicit after feeding; disappears by 4 to 7 months of age Sucking is adequate for nutritional intake and meeting oral stimulation needs; disappears by 12 months	Poor sucking or easily fatigable (preterm, breastfed infants of barbiturate-addicted mothers, possible cardiac problem) Absence of response (preterm, neurologic involvement, depressed newborns)	Evaluate strength and coordination of sucking. Observe newborn during feeding, and counsel parents about mutuality of feeding experience and newborn's responses.
Palmar grasp		
Fingers grasp adult finger when palm is stimulated and held momentarily; lessens at 3 to 4 months of age	Asymmetry of response (neurologic problems)	Evaluate other reflexes and general neurologic functioning.
Plantar grasp		
Toes curl downward when sole of foot is stimulated; lessens by 8 months	Absent (defects of lower spinal column)	Assess for other lower extremity neurologic problems.
Stepping		
When held upright and one foot touching a flat surface, will step alternately; disappears at 4 to 5 months of age	Asymmetry of stepping (neurologic abnormality)	Evaluate muscle tone and function on each side of body. Refer to specialist.
Babinski		
Fanning and extension of all toes when one side of sole is stroked from heel upward across ball of foot; disappears at about 12 months	Absence of response (low spinal cord defects)	Refer for further neurologic evaluation.
Tonic neck		
Fencer position—when head is turned to one side, extremities on same side extend and on opposite side flex; this reflex may not be evident during early neonatal period; disappears at 3 to 4 months of age Response often more dominant in leg than in arm	Absent after 1 month of age or persistent asymmetry (cerebral lesion)	Assess neurologic functioning.
Prone crawl		
While on abdomen, neonate pushes up and tries to crawl	Absence or variance of response (preterm, weak, or depressed newborns)	Evaluate motor functioning. Refer to specialist.
Trunk incurvation (Galant)		
In prone position stroking of spine causes pelvis to turn to stimulated side	Failure to rotate to stimulated side (neurologic damage)	

*Possible causes of alterations are placed in parentheses.

†This column provides guidelines for further assessment and initial nursing interventions.

Newborn Behavioral Assessment

Two conflicting forces influence parents' perceptions of their newborn. One is the parents' preconceptions, based on hopes and fears, of what their newborn will be like. The other is their initial reaction to their baby's temperament, behaviors, and physical appearance. Nurses can assist parents in identifying their baby's specific behaviors.

> *One of the newborn's first responses is to move into a quiet but alert state of consciousness. The baby is still; his body molds to yours; his hands touch your skin; his eyes open wide and are bright and shiny. He looks directly at you.*
>
> *This special alert state, this innate ability to communicate, may be the initial preparation for becoming attached to other human beings. One feels awed by the intensity and appealing power of this little bud of humanity meeting the world for the first time.*
>
> ~ *The Amazing Newborn* ~

Brazelton's neonatal behavioral assessment scale provides valuable guidelines for assessing the newborn's state changes, temperament, and individual behavior patterns. It furnishes a means by which the health care provider, in conjunction with the parents (primary caregivers), can identify and understand the individual newborn's states and capabilities. Families learn which responses, interventions, or activities best meet the special needs of their newborn, and this understanding fosters positive attachment experiences.

The assessment tool attempts to identify the newborn's repertoire of behavioral responses to the environment and also documents the newborn's neurologic adequacy and capabilities. The examination usually takes 20 to 30 minutes and involves about 30 tests. Some items are scored according to the newborn's response to specific stimuli. Others, such as consolability and alertness, are scored as a result of continuous behavioral observations throughout the assessment. For a complete discussion of all test items and maneuvers, see Brazelton's *Neonatal Behavioral Assessment Scale* (1973.)

Because the first few days after birth are a period of behavioral disorganization, the complete assessment should be done on the third day after birth. The nurse should make every effort to elicit the best response. This may be accomplished by repeating tests at different times or by testing during situations that facilitate the best possible response, such as when parents are holding, cuddling, rocking, and singing to their baby.

The assessment of the newborn should be carried out initially in a quiet, dimly or softly lighted room, if possible. The nurse should determine the newborn's state of consciousness, because scoring and introduction of the test items correlate with the sleep or awake state. The newborn's state depends on physiologic variables, such as the amount of time from the last feeding, positioning, environmental temperature, and health status; presence of such external stimuli as noises and bright lights; and the sleep-wake cycle of the infant. An important characteristic of the neonatal period is the pattern of states, as well as the transitions from one state to another. The pattern of states is a predictor of the newborn's receptivity and ability to respond to stimuli in a cognitive manner. Babies learn best in a quiet, alert state and in an environment that is supportive and protective and that provides appropriate stimuli.

The nurse should observe the newborn's sleep-wake patterns (as discussed in Chapter 24) and the rapidity with which the newborn moves from one state to another, the newborn's ability to be consoled, and the newborn's ability to diminish the impact of disturbing stimuli. The following questions may provide the nurse with a framework for assessment:

- Does the newborn's response style and ability to adapt to stimuli indicate a need for parental interventions that will alert the newborn to the environment so that the baby can grow socially and cognitively?
- Are parental interventions necessary to lessen the outside stimuli, as in the case of the baby who responds to sensory input with intensity?
- Can the baby control the amount of sensory input to be dealt with?

The behaviors and the sleep-wake states in which they are assessed are categorized as follows:

- *Habituation.* The newborn's ability to diminish or shut down innate responses to specific repeated stimuli, such as a rattle, bell, light, or pinprick to heel.
- *Orientation to inanimate and animate visual and auditory assessment stimuli.* How often and where the newborn attends to auditory and visual stimuli are observed. Orientation to the environment is determined by an ability to respond to cues given by others and by a natural ability to fix on and to follow a

CRITICAL THINKING IN PRACTICE

Maria Reyes, a 19-year-old G2 now P2 mother, delivered a 40-week-old female neonate 24 hours ago. The newborn exam was normal. Mrs Reyes asks about the newborn's exam. She says she has noticed that the baby cries more than her first child and seems to require holding for longer periods of time after feeding before "quieting down." She is concerned that there is something she is doing wrong and wants to know when her newborn will start to act like her first baby. What should you discuss with her about newborn behavior?

Answers can be found in Appendix I.

visual object horizontally and vertically. This capacity and parental appreciation of it are important for positive communication between infant and parents; the parents' visual *(en face)* and auditory (soft, continuous voice) presence stimulates their infant to orient to them. Inability or lack of response may indicate visual or auditory problems. It is important for parents to know that their newborn can turn to voices usually soon after birth or by 3 days of age and can become alert at different times with a varying degree of intensity in response to sounds.

- *Motor activity.* Several components are evaluated. Motor tone of the newborn is assessed in the most characteristic state of responsiveness. This summary assessment includes overall use of tone as the neonate responds to being handled—whether during spontaneous activity, prone placement, or horizontal holding—and overall assessment of body tone as the newborn reacts to all stimuli.
- *Variations.* Frequency of alert states, state changes, color changes (throughout all states as examination progresses), activity, and peaks of excitement are assessed.
- *Self-quieting activity.* Assessment is based on how often, how quickly, and how effectively newborns can use their resources to quiet and console themselves when upset or distressed. Considered in this assessment are such self-consolatory activities as putting hand to mouth, sucking on a fist or the tongue, and attuning to an object or sound. The newborn's need for outside consolation must also be considered—for example, seeing a face; being rocked, held, or dressed; using a pacifier; and being swaddled.
- *Cuddliness or social behaviors.* This area encompasses the infant's need for and response to being held. Also considered is how often the newborn smiles. These behaviors influence the parents' self-esteem and feelings of acceptance or rejection. Cuddling also appears to be an indicator of personality. Cuddlers appear to enjoy, accept, and seek physical contact; are easier to placate; sleep more; and form earlier and more intense attachments. Noncuddlers are active, restless, have accelerated motor development, and are intolerant of physical restraint. Smiling, even as a grimace reflex, greatly influences parent-infant feedback. Parents identify this response as positive.

FOCUS YOUR STUDY

- A perinatal history, determination of gestational age, physical examination, and behavior assessment form the basis for complete newborn assessment.
- The common physical characteristics included in the gestational age assessment are skin, lanugo, sole (plantar) creases, breast tissue and size, ear form and cartilage, and genitals.
- The neuromuscular components of gestational age scoring tools are usually posture, square window sign, popliteal angle, arm recoil, heel-to-ear extension, and scarf sign.
- By assessing the physical and neuromuscular components specified in a gestational age tool, the nurse can determine the gestational age of the newborn.
- After determining the gestational age of the baby, the nurse can assess how the newborn will make the transition to extrauterine life and can anticipate potential physiologic problems.
- The nurse identifies the newborn as small for gestational age (SGA), appropriate for gestational age (AGA), or large for gestational age (LGA), and prioritizes individual needs.
- Normal ranges for vital signs assessed in newborns are heart rate of 120 to 160 beats per minute; respiratory rate of 30 to 60 respirations per minute; axillary temperature of 36.4C to 37.2C (97.5F to 99F); skin temperature of 36C to 36.5C (96.8F to 97.7F); rectal temperature of 36.6C to 37.2C (97.8F to 99F); and blood pressure of 80/45 to 60/40 mm Hg (at birth).
- Normal newborn measurements include weight from 2500 to 4000 g (5 lb, 8 oz to 8 lb, 13 oz), with weight dependent on maternal size and age; length from 48 to 52 cm (18 to 22 in); and head circumference from 32 to 37 cm (12.5 to 14.5 in). Head circumference is approximately 2 cm larger than the chest circumference.
- Commonly elicited newborn reflexes are tonic neck, Moro, grasping, rooting, sucking, and blink.
- Newborn behavioral abilities include habituation, orientation to visual and auditory stimuli, motor activity, cuddliness, and self-quieting activity.
- An important role of the nurse during the physical and behavioral assessments of the newborn is to teach parents about their newborn and involve them in their baby's care. This facilitates the parents' identification of their newborn's uniqueness and allays their concerns.

REFERENCES

American Academy of Pediatrics (AAP) Committee on Fetus and Newborn & American College of Obstetricians and Gynecologists (ACOG) Committee on Obstetrics (1998). *Guidelines for perinatal care* (4th ed.). Evanston, IL: Author.

Alexander, G. R., & Allen, M. C. (1996). Conceptualization, measurement, and use of gestational age: I. Clinical and public health practice. *Journal of Perinatology, 16*(1), 53–59.

Ballard, J. L. , Khoury, J. C., Wedig, K., Wang, L., Eilers-Walsman, B. L., & Lipp, R. (1991). New Ballard score, expanded to include extremely premature infants. *Journal of Pediatrics, 119*(3), 417–423.

Ballard, J. L., Novak, K. K., & Driver, M. (1979). A simplified score for assessment of fetal maturation of newly born infants. *Journal of Pediatrics, 95*(5 Pt 1), 769–774.

Basso, O., Olsen, J., Knudsen, L. B. & Christensen, K. (1998). Low birth weight and preterm birth after short interpregnancy intervals. *American Journal of Obstetrics and Gynecology, 178*(2), 259–263.

Brazelton, T. (1973). *The neonatal behavioral assessment scale.* Philadelphia: Lippincott.

Brazelton,T. (1984). Neonatal behavior and its significance. In M. E. Avery & H. W. Taeusch, Jr. (Eds.). *Schaffer's diseases of the newborn.* Philadelphia: Saunders.

Brooks, A. A., Johnson, M. R., Steer, P. J., Pawson, M. E., & Abdella, H. I. (1995). Birth weight: Nature or nurture? *Early Human Development, 42*(1), 29–35.

Cogswell, M. E., & Yip, R. (1995).The influence of fetal and maternal factors on the distribution of birthweight. *Seminars in Perinatology, 19*(3), 222–240.

Dodd, V. (1996). Gestational age assessment. *Neonatal Network, 15*(1), 27.

Dubowitz, L., & Dubowitz, V. (1977). *Gestational age of the newborn.* Menlo Park, CA: Addison-Wesley.

Fowlie, P., & Forsyth, S. (1995). Examination of the newborn infant. *Modern Midwife, 5*(1), 15–18.

Gardosi, J. (1997). Customized growth curves. *Clinical Obstetrics and Gynecology, 40*(4), 715–722.

Hegyi, T., Anwar, M., Carbone, M. T., Ostfeld, B., Hiatt, M., Koons, A., Pinto-Martin, J., & Paneth, N. (1996). Blood pressure ranges in premature infants: II. The first week of life. *Pediatrics, 97*(3), 336–342.

Hicks, M. A. (1996). A comparison of the tympanic and axillary temperatures of the preterm and term infant. *Journal of Perinatology, 16*(4), 261–267.

Kane, J., Page-Salyards, W., & Keith-Perry, C. R. (1997). Congenital hepatic hemangioma in the neonate. *MCN; American Journal of Maternal Child Nursing, 22*(4), 187–193.

Ludington-Hoe, S. M., & Golani, S. (1988). *How to have a smarter baby.* New York: Bantam.

Merenstein, G. B., & Gardner, S. L. (1998). *Handbook of neonatal intensive care* (4th ed.). St. Louis: Mosby.

O'Donnell, K. A., Glick, P. L., & Coty, M. G. (1998). Pediatric umbilical problems. *Pediatric Clinics of North America, 45*(4), 791–799.

Pressler, J. L., & Hepworth, J. T. (1997). Newborn neurologic screening using NBAS reflexes. *Neonatal Network, 16*(6), 33–46.

Reed, B., & Davidhizar, R. (1997, Feb.). Setting their sights: Visual development in newborns. *Advances for Nurse Practitioner,* 67–68, 70.

Shann, F., & Mackenzie, A., (1996). Comparison of rectal, axillary, and forehead temperatures. *Archives of Pediatric and Adolescent Medicine, 150*(1), 74–78.

Taeusch, H. W., & Ballard, R. A. (1998). *Avery's diseases of the newborn* (7th ed.). Philadelphia: Saunders.

Tappero, E. P., & Honeyfield, M. E. (1996). *Physical assessment of the newborn* (2nd ed.). Petaluma, CA: NICU Ink.

Thureen, P. J., Deacon, J., O'Neill, P. & Hernandez, J. (1999). *Assessment and care of the well newborn.* Philadelphia: Saunders.

Wen, S. W., Kramer, M. S., & Usher, R. H. (1995). Comparison of birth weight distribution between Chinese and Caucasian infants. *American Journal of Epidemiology, 141*(12), 1177–1187.

26

The Normal Newborn: Needs and Care

Key Terms

Circumcision

Normal screening tests

Parent-newborn attachment

THIS MOMENT OF MEETING SEEMED TO BE A BIRTHTIME for both of us; her first and my second life. Nothing, I knew, could ever be the same again.

~ *Laurie Lee*, Two Women ~

Objectives

- Summarize the essential areas of information to be obtained about a newborn's birth experience and immediate postnatal period.
- Explain the physiologic and behavioral responses of newborns and possible interventions needed.
- Discuss the major nursing considerations and activities to be carried out during the first 4 hours after birth (admission and transitional period) and subsequent daily care.
- Identify activities that should be included in a daily care plan for a normal newborn.
- Determine common concerns of families regarding their newborns.
- Describe topics and related content to be included in parent teaching classes on newborn and infant care.
- Identify opportunities to individualize parent teaching and enhance each parent's abilities and confidence while providing infant care in the birthing unit.
- Delineate information to be included in discharge planning with the newborn's family.

AT THE MOMENT OF BIRTH, NUMEROUS physiologic adaptations begin to take place in the newborn's body. Because of these dramatic changes, newborns require close observation to determine how smoothly they are making the transition to extrauterine life. Newborns also require special care that enhances their chances of making the transition successfully.

The two broad goals of nursing care during this period are to promote the physical well-being of the newborn and to enhance the establishment of a well-functioning family unit. The nurse meets the first goal by providing comprehensive care to newborns while in the mother-baby unit. The nurse meets the second goal by teaching family members how to care for their new baby and by supporting their parenting efforts so that they feel confident and competent.

Thus the nurse must be knowledgeable about family adjustments that need to be made, as well as the health care needs of the newborn. It is important that the family return home with the positive feeling that they have the support, information, and skills to care for their newborn. Equally important is the need for each member of the family to begin a unique relationship with the newborn. The cultural and social expectations of individual families and communities affect the way normal newborn care is carried out.

The previous two chapters discussed physiologic and behavioral changes occurring in the newborn and the pertinent nursing assessments that are needed. This chapter discusses nursing care managment while the newborn is in the birthing unit. The Critical Pathway for Newborn Care starts on page 754.

Nursing Care Management During Admission and the First Four Hours of Life

Nursing Assessment and Diagnosis

During the first 4 hours after birth, the nurse carries out a preliminary physical examination, including an assessment of the newborn's physiologic adaptations. In many facilities, the nurse performs and documents the initial head-to-toe physical assessment during the first hour of transition. The nurse is responsible for notifying the physician or nurse practitioner of any deviations from normal. A complete physical examination is also performed later by the physician or nurse practitioner, within the first 24 hours after birth and within 24 hours before discharge. This can be accomplished with one physical examination (American Academy of Pediatrics [AAP], 1997) (see Chapter 25 and Table 25–1).

Nursing diagnoses are based on an analysis of the assessment findings. Physiologic alterations of the newborn form the basis of many nursing diagnoses, as does the family's incorporation of them in caring for their new baby. Nursing diagnoses that may apply to the newborn include the following:

- ***Ineffective Airway Clearance*** related to presence of mucus and retained lung fluid
- ***Risk for Altered Body Temperature*** related to evaporative, radiant, conductive, and convective heat losses
- ***Altered Peripheral Tissue Perfusion*** related to decreased thermoregulation
- ***Pain*** related to vitamin K injection or heel sticks for glucose or hematocrit

Many of these nursing diagnoses and associated interventions must be identified and implemented very quickly during this period. As discussed in Chapter 24, the newborn's physiologic adaptation to extrauterine life occurs rapidly. All body systems are affected. Thus the newborn requires close monitoring during the first few hours of life so that any deviation from normal can be identified immediately and appropriate interventions made.

CRITICAL THINKING QUESTION

Which critical perinatal and neonatal assessments have the most significant impact on the newborn's care during the first 4 hours after birth?

Nursing Plan and Implementation

The nurse initiates newborn admission procedures and evaluates the newborn's need to remain under observation. The nurse monitors the newborn's ability to maintain a clear airway and stable vital signs, maintain body temperature, demonstrate normal neurologic status and no observable complications, and tolerate the first feeding. If these criteria are met, it indicates a successful beginning adaptation to extrauterine life, and the baby is moved back to the mother's room or to a regular nursery. This transfer usually takes place between 2 and 6 hours after birth.

Initiation of Admission Procedures

After birth, the baby is formally admitted to the health care facility. The admission procedures include gestational age assessment and an assessment to ensure that the newborn's adaptation to extrauterine life is proceeding normally. This evaluation of the newborn's status and for risk factors must be done no later than 2 hours after birth (AAP, 1997). See Essential Precautions in Practice: During Newborn Care on page 756.

If the initial assessment indicates that the newborn is not at risk physiologically, the nurse performs many of the routine admission procedures in the presence of the

Text continues on page 756.

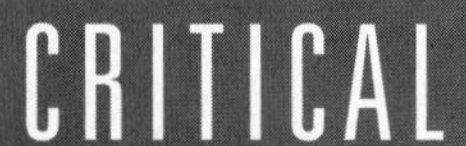

CRITICAL PATHWAY FOR NEWBORN CARE

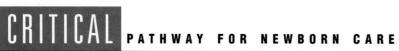

Category	First 4 Hours	4–8 Hours Past Birth	8–24 Hours Past Birth
Referral	Review labor/birth record Review transitional nursing record Check ID bands PRN Consults: Orthopedics, Genetics, Infectious Disease	Check ID bands Transfer to mother/baby care at 4–6 hours of age if stable. As parents desire, obtain circumcision permit after their discussion with physician. Lactation Consult prn	Check ID bands q shift **Expected Outcomes:** Mother/baby ID bands correlate at time of discharge. Consults completed prn.
Assessments	Continue assessments begun first hour after birth. Vital signs: TPR, B/P prn, q1h × 4 (skin temp 97.8-98.6F, resp may be irregular but within 30-60 per min) **Newborn Assessments:** • Respiratory status with resp distress scale × 1 then prn. If resp distress, assess q 5-15 min • Cord-bluish white color, clamp in place • Color: skin, mucous membranes, extremities. Trunk pink with slight acrocyanosis of hands and feet • Wt (5lb 8oz-8lb 13oz), Length (18-22 in), HC (12.5-14.5 in), CC (32.5cm, 1-2 in less than head) • Extremity movement—may be jerky or brief twitches • Gestational age classification—Term AGA • Anomalies (cong. anomalies can interfere with normal extrauterine adaptation)	Assess newborn's progress through periods of reactivity Vital signs: TPR q8h and prn, B/P prn **Newborn Assessments:** • Skin color q4h prn (circulatory system stabilizing, acrocyanosis decreased) • Eyes for drainage, redness, hemorrhage • Ausculate lungs q4h (noisy, wet resp normal) • Increased mucus production (normal in 2nd period of reactivity) • Check apical pulse q4h • Umbilical cord base for redness, drainage, foul odor, drying, clamp in place • Extremity movement q4h • Check for expected reflexes (suck, rooting, Moro, grasp, blink, yawn, sneeze, tonic neck, Babinski) • Note common normal variations • Assess suck and swallow during feeding • Note behavioral characteristics • Temp before and after admission bath	VS q8h. Normal ranges: T, 97.5–99F; P 120-160; R, 30-60; B/P, 60–80/45-40 mm Hg **Continue Newborn Assessments:** • Skin color q4h • Signs of drying or infection in cord area • Check cord clamp in place until removed before discharge • Check circ for bleeding after procedure, then q30min × 2, then q4h and prn **Expected Outcomes** Vital signs medically acceptable, color pink, assessments WNL, circ site without s/s infection, cord site without s/s infection and clamp removed; newborn behavior WNL
Teaching/ psychosocial	Admission activities performed at mother's bedside if possible, orient to nursery prn, handwashng, assess teaching needs Teach parents use of bulb syringe, signs of choking, positioning, and when to call for assistance Teach reasons for use radiant warmer, infant hat and warmed blankets when out of warmer Discuss/teach infant security, identification	Reinforce teaching about choking, bulb syringe use, positioning, temperature maintenance with clothing and blankets Teach infant positioning to facilitate breathing and digestion Teach new parents holding and feeding skills Teach parents soothing and calming techniques	Final Discharge Teaching: diapering, normal void and stool patterns, bathing, nail and cord care, circumcision/uncircumcised penis/genital care and normal characteristics, rashes, jaundice, sleep/wake cycles, soothing activities, taking temperatures, thermometer reading Explain s/s of illness and when to call health care provider Infant safety: car seats, immunizations, metabolic screening **Expected Outcomes** Mother/family verbalize comprehension of teaching; demonstrates care capabilities
Nursing care management and reports	Place unde'r radiant warmer Place hat on newborn (decreases convection heat loss) Suction nares/mouth with bulb syringe prn Keep bulb syringe with infant Attach security sensor Obtain lab tests: blood glucose; as needed obtain blood type, Rh, Coombs on cord blood, HSV culture if parental hx Notify physician's office or exchange of infant's birth and status Maintain Universal Precautions	Wean from radiant warmer (T98F axillary) Chemstrips prn; B/P prn Oxygen saturation prn Bathe infant if temp >97.8R Position on side Suction nares prn (esp during 2nd period of reactivity) Obtain peripheral Hct per protocol Cord care per protocol (alcohol or triple dye prn) Fold diaper below cord (for plastic diapers, turn plastic layer away from skin)	Check for hearing test results Weigh before discharge Cord care q shift DC cord clamp before discharge Perform newborn metabolic screening blood tests before discharge Circumcision if indicated. Circumcision care: change diaper prn noting ability to void, follow policy for Gomco or Plastibell care **Expected Outcomes** Newborn maintains temp, lab test WNL, cord dry without s/s infection and clamp removed, screening tests accomplished, circ site without s/s infection or bleeding

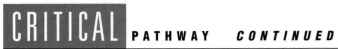

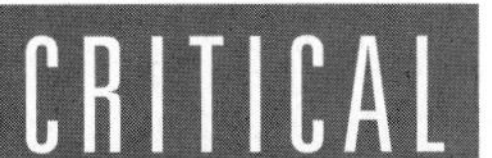
PATHWAY CONTINUED

Category	First 4 Hours	4–8 Hours Past Birth	8–24 Hours Past Birth
Activity and comfort	Place under radiant warmer or wrap in pre-warmed blankets until stable Soothe baby as needed with voice, touch, cuddling, nesting in warmer	Leave in warmer until stable, then swaddle Position on side after each feeding	Place in open crib Swaddle to allow movement of extremities in blanket, including hands to face **Expected Outcomes** Infant maintains temp WNL in open crib; infant attempts self calming
Nutrition	Assist newborn to breastfeed as soon as mother/baby condition allows Supplement breast only when medically indicated or per agency policy Initiate bottle-feeding within first hour Gavage feed if necessary to prevent hypoglycemia	Breastfeed on demand, at least q3–4h. Teach positions, observe/assist with feeding, breast/nipple care, establishing milk supply, breaking suction, feeding cues, latching on techniques, nutritive suck, burping. Bottlefeed on demand, at least q3–6h Determine readiness to feed and feeding tolerance	Continue breast/bottlefeeding pattern Assess feeding tolerance q4h Discuss normal feeding requirements, signs of hunger and satiation, handling feeding problems, and when to seek help **Expected Outcomes** Mother verbalizes knowledge of feeding information; breastfeeds on demand without supplement; bottle - tolerates formula feeding, nipples without problems
Elimination	Note first void and stool if not noted at birth	Note all voids, amount and color of stools q4h	Evaluate all voids and stools color q8h **Expected Outcomes** Voids qs; stools qs without difficulty; stool character WNL; diaper area without s/s skin breakdown or rashes
Medication	Prophylactic ophthalmic ointment OU after baby makes eye contact with parents within 1 h after birth Administer Aquamephyton IM, dosage according to infant weight per MD/NP order	Hepatitis B injection as ordered by physician after consent signed by parents	Hepatitis B vaccine before discharge **Expected Outcomes** Baby has received ophthalmic ointment and vitamin K injection; baby has received first Hep B vaccine if ordered and parental permission received
Discharge planning/ home care	Hepatitis B consent signed Hearing screen consent signed Plan discharge call with parent or guardian in 24 hrs to 2 days Assess parents' discharge plans, needs and support systems	Review/reinforce teaching with mother and significant other Review home preparedness Present birth certificate instructions	Initial newborn screening tests (hearing, blood tests, ie, PKU) before discharge Bath and feeding classes, videos, or written information given Give written copy of discharge instructions Newborn photographs Set up appointment for follow-up PKU test Have car seat available before discharge All discharge referrals made, follow up appt. scheduled **Expected Outcomes** Infant discharged home with family; mother verbalizes follow up appt. time/date
Family involvement	Facilitate early investigation of baby's physical characteristics (maintain temp during unwrapping), hold infant en face Dim lights to help infant keep eyes open	Assess parents' knowledge of newborn behaviors, such as alertness, suck and rooting, attention to human voice, response to calming techniques	Assess mother-baby bonding/interaction Incorporate father and siblings in care Enhance parent-infant interaction by sharing characteristics and behavioral assessment Support positive parenting behaviors Identify community referral needs and refer to community agencies **Expected Outcomes** Demonstrates caring and family incorporation of infant
Date			

ESSENTIAL PRECAUTIONS IN PRACTICE

During Newborn Care

Examples of procedures for which disposable gloves are recommended include the following:

- Handling baby prior to first bath and removal of all blood and amniotic fluid
- Oral or nasal suctioning after birth when blood or amniotic fluid is present in secretions
- Carrying out blood work (ie, glucose, hematocrit, newborn screen)
- Administer vitamin K and eye prophylaxis
- Changing linen soiled with blood or amniotic fluid
- Breast milk
- Urine
- Stool
- Vomitus
- Nasal secretions
- Oral secretions
- Diaper change

REMEMBER to wash your hands prior to putting the disposable gloves on and AGAIN immediately after you remove the gloves.

For further information, consult OSHA and CDC guidelines.

parents in the birthing area. The care measures indicated by the assessment findings may be performed by the nurse or by the parents under the guidance of the nurse in an effort to educate and support the family. Other interventions may be delayed if the newborn is transferred to an observational nursery.

The nurse responsible for the newborn first checks and confirms the newborn's identification with the mother's identification and then obtains and records all significant information. The essential data to be recorded as part of the newborn's chart include the following:

1. *Condition of the newborn.* Pertinent information includes the newborn's Apgar scores at 1 and 5 minutes, resuscitative measures required in the birthing area, physical examination, vital signs, voidings, and passing of meconium. Complications to be noted include excessive mucus, delayed spontaneous respirations or responsiveness, abnormal number of cord vessels, and obvious physical abnormalities.
2. *Labor and birth record.* A copy of the labor and birth record should be placed in the newborn's chart or be accessible on computer. The record contains all the significant data about the birth, for example, duration, course, and status of mother and fetus throughout labor and birth and any analgesia or anesthesia administered to the mother. Particular care is taken to note any variation or difficulties such as prolonged rupture of membranes, abnormal fetal position, meconium-stained amniotic fluid, signs of fetal distress during labor, nuchal cord (cord around the newborn's neck at birth), precipitous birth, use of forceps, vacuum extraction, maternal analgesia and anesthesia received within 1 hour of birth, and administration of antibiotics during labor.
3. *Antepartal history.* Any maternal problems that may have compromised the fetus in utero—such as pregnancy-induced hypotension (PIH), spotting, illness, recent infections, rubella status, serology results, hepatitis B screen results, exposure to group B streptococci, or a history of maternal substance abuse—are of immediate concern in newborn assessment (AAP, 1997). The chart should also include information about maternal age, estimated date of birth (EDB), previous pregnancies, and presence of any congenital anomalies. Human immunodeficiency virus (HIV) test result, if obtained, is also relevant. State statutes vary as to who may have access to this information (AAP, 1997).
4. *Parent-newborn interaction information.* The nurse notes parents' interactions with their newborn and their desires regarding care, such as rooming-in, circumcision, and type of feeding. Information about other children in the home, available support systems, and patterns of interaction within each family unit assists the nurse in providing comprehensive care.

Table 26–1 summarizes normal findings for the newborn during transition.

As part of the admission procedure, the nurse weighs the newborn in both grams and pounds; parents understand weights best when stated in pounds and ounces (Figure 26–1). The nurse cleans and covers the scales each time a newborn is weighed to prevent cross-infection and heat loss from conduction.

The nurse then measures the newborn, recording the measurements in both centimeters and inches. Three routine measurements are length, circumference of the head, and circumference of the chest. In some facilities, abdominal girth may also be measured. The nurse rapidly assesses the baby's color, muscle tone, alertness, and general state. Remember that the first period of reactivity may have concluded, and the baby may be in the sleep-inactive phase, which makes the infant hard to arouse. The nurse does basic assessments for estimating gesta-

TABLE 26–1 Signs of Newborn Transition

Normal findings for the newborn during the first few days of life include the following:
Pulse: 120–160 beats/minute
  During sleep as low as 100 beats/minute
  If crying, up to 180 beats/minute
  Apical pulse is counted for 1 full minute because rate may fluctuate
Respirations: 30–60 respirations/minute
  Predominantly diaphragmatic but synchronous with abdominal movements
  Brief periods of apnea (5–10 seconds) with no color or heart rate changes
Temperature: axillary: 36.5–37C (97.5–98.6F)
Skin: 36–36.5C (96.8–97.7F)
Blood pressure: 80–60/45–40 mm Hg at birth; 100/50 mm Hg at day 10
Chemstrip: greater than 40 mg%
Hematocrit: less than 65%–70% central venous sample

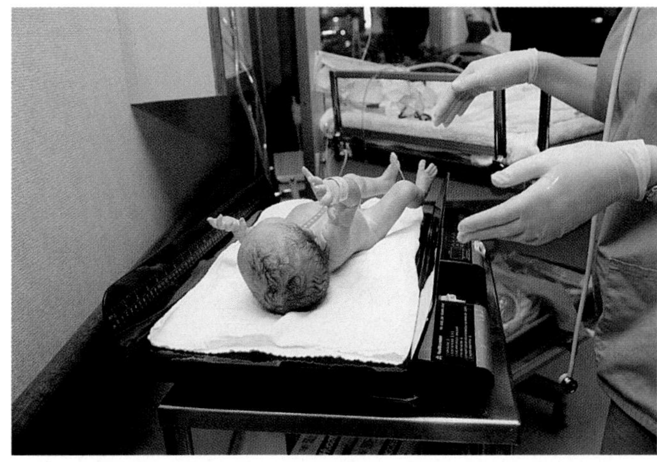

FIGURE 26–1 Weighing a newborn. The scale is balanced before each weighing, with the protective pad in place. The caregiver's hand is poised above the infant as a safety measure.

tional age and completes the physical assessment. (For more discussion of the process of newborn assessment, see Chapter 25.)

In addition to obtaining vital signs, the nurse performs hematocrit and blood glucose evaluations on at-risk newborns or as clinically indicated (such as for small-for-gestational-age [SGA] or large-for-gestational-age [LGA] infants or if the newborn is jittery). These procedures may be done on admission or within the first 4 hours after birth (AAP, 1997). (See Procedure 29–1.)

Maintenance of a Clear Airway and Stable Vital Signs

The nurse positions the newborn on his or her side. If necessary, a bulb syringe or DeLee wall suction (Procedure 20–1) is used to remove mucus from the nasal passages and oral cavity. A DeLee catheter attached to suction may be used to remove mucus from the stomach to help prevent possible aspiration. This procedure also ensures that the esophagus is patent prior to the newborn's first feeding. Gastric suctioning can cause vagal nerve stimulation, which may result in bradycardia and apnea in the unstabilized newborn.

In the absence of any newborn distress, the nurse continues with the admission by taking the newborn's vital signs. The initial temperature is taken by the axillary method. A wider range of normal exists for axillary temperature, specifically 36.5C to 37.0C (97.7F to 98.6F) (Merestein & Gardner, 1998).

Once the initial temperature is taken, the nurse monitors the core temperature either by obtaining axillary temperatures at intervals or by placing a skin sensor on the newborn for continuous reading. The usual skin sensor placement site is on the newborn's abdomen, but placement on the upper thigh or arm can give a reading closely correlated with the mean body temperature. The vital signs for a healthy term newborn should be monitored at least every 30 minutes until the newborn's condition has remained stable for 2 hours (AAP, 1997). The newborn's respirations may be irregular yet still be normal. Brief periods of apnea, lasting only 5 to 10 seconds with no color or heart rate changes, are considered normal. The normal pulse range is 120 to 160 beats per minute (bpm), and the normal respiratory range is 30 to 60 respirations per minute.

Maintenance of a Neutral Thermal Environment

A neutral thermal environment is essential to minimize the newborn's need for increased oxygen consumption and use of calories to maintain body heat in the optimal range of 36.4C to 37.2C (97.5F to 99F). If the newborn becomes hypothermic, the body's response can lead to metabolic acidosis, hypoxia, and shock.

The nurse can best achieve a neutral thermal environment by performing the assessment and interventions with a newborn unclothed and under a radiant warmer. The thermostat of the radiant warmer is controlled by the thermal skin sensor taped to the newborn's abdomen, upper thigh, or arm. The sensor indicates when the newborn's temperature exceeds or falls below the acceptable temperature range. The nurse should be aware that leaning over the newborn may block the radiant heat waves from reaching the newborn. It is common practice in some institutions to cover the neonate's head with a cap made of wool lined with gauze and cotton, Thinsulate, or cotton and polyester fill terry cloth to prevent further heat loss in addition to placing the baby under a radiant warmer ("Neonatal Thermoregulation," 1997).

When the newborn's temperature is normal and vital signs are stable (about 2 to 4 hours after birth), the baby may be given a sponge bath. However, this admission bath may be postponed for some hours if the newborn's condition dictates or the parents wish to give the first bath. Recent research provides some reassurances, in light of early discharge practices (12 to 48 hours), that healthy term infants can be safely bathed immediately after the admission assessment is completed (Penny-MacGillivray, 1996). The baby is bathed while still under

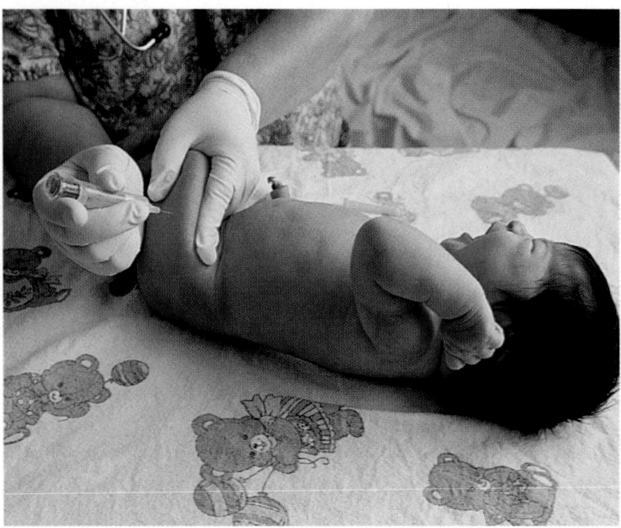

FIGURE 26–2 Procedure for vitamin K injection. Cleanse area thoroughly with alcohol swab, and allow skin to dry. Bunch the tissue of the upper thigh (vastus lateralis muscle) and quickly insert a 25-gauge ⅝-inch needle at a 90-degree angle to the thigh. Aspirate, then slowly inject the solution to distribute the medication evenly and minimize the baby's discomfort. Remove the needle and massage the site with an alcohol swab.

the radiant warmer. This may be done in the parents' room. Bathing the newborn offers an excellent opportunity for teaching and welcoming parent involvement in the care of their baby.

The nurse rechecks the temperature after the bath, and if it is stable, dresses the newborn in a shirt, diaper, and cap; wraps the baby; and places the baby in an open crib at room temperature. If the baby's axillary temperature is below 36.4C (97.5F), the nurse returns the baby to the radiant warmer. The rewarming process should be gradual to prevent the possibility of hyperthermia. Slow rewarming is accomplished by maintaining a difference between the ambient temperature and the infant's skin temperature of less than 1.5C (3F) ("Neonatal Thermoregulation," 1997). When this new skin temperature is reached, the nurse increases the air temperature in hourly increments of 1.0C until the desired skin temperature is reached and the infant's temperature is stable. Once the newborn is rewarmed, the nurse implements measures to prevent further neonatal heat loss, such as keeping the newborn dry, swaddled in one or two blankets with hat on, and away from cool surfaces or instruments. The nurse also protects the newborn from drafts, open windows or doors, or air conditioners. Blankets and clothing are stored in a warm place. See Temperature Regulation in Chapter 25 and Procedure 26–1 on page 760 to 761.

Prevention of Complications of Hemorrhagic Disease of Newborn

A prophylactic injection of vitamin K_1 (AquaMEPHYTON) is given to prevent hemorrhage, which can occur due to low prothrombin levels in the first few days of life (see the Drug Guide: Vitamin K_1, Phytonadione [AquaMEPHYTON] on page 761). The potential for hemorrhage results from the absence of gut bacterial flora, which influences the production of vitamin K in the newborn. (See Chapter 29 for further discussion.) Controversy exists over whether the administration of vitamin K may predispose the newborn to significant hyperbilirubinemia. However, Cunningham and colleagues (1997) indicate there is no evidence to support this concern as long as a standard dose of 1 mg parenterally is given. All newborns should receive a single parenteral dose of 0.5 to 1.0 mg of natural vitamin K_1 oxide (phytonadione) within 1 hour of birth (AAP, 1997). Some people have questioned the need to give vitamin K to newborns who have had a nontraumatic birth.

Currently oral vitamin K preparations are not recommended for use in the United States (AAP, 1997). However, parents may request that vitamin K be given orally. To ensure an adequate dose, 2 mg of an oral preparation of vitamin K is given by mouth. This dosage should be administered orally again at 1 to 2 weeks and at 4 weeks of age. Oral vitamin K has not been shown to be as efficacious as parenteral administration.

Vitamin K injection is given intramuscularly in the middle third of the vastus lateralis muscle located in the lateral aspect of the thigh (Figure 26–2). Before injecting, the nurse must clean the newborn's skin site for the injection thoroughly with a small alcohol swab. The nurse uses a 25-gauge, ⅝-inch needle for the injection. An alternative site is the rectus femoris muscle in the anterior aspect of the thigh. However, this site is near the sciatic nerve and femoral artery and should be used with caution (Figure 26–3). When stored, vitamin K_1 needs to be protected from light.

Prevention of Eye Infection

The nurse is also responsible for giving the legally required prophylactic eye treatment for *Neisseria gonorrhoea*, which may have infected the newborn of an infected mother during the birth process. A variety of topical agents appear to be equally effective. Ophthalmic ointments that are used include 1% silver nitrate, 0.5% erythromycin (Ilotycin Ophthalmic) (see the Drug Guide: Erythromycin [Ilotycin Ophthalmic] on page 762), and 1% tetracycline. All are also effective against chlamydia, which has a higher incidence than gonorrhea. Bell and associates (1993) showed that either one of the possible eye prophylaxis medications or no prophylaxis at all is reasonable for newborns born to women who received prenatal care and had no sexually transmitted infection during pregnancy.

Successful eye prophylaxis requires that the medication be instilled into the lower conjunctival sac of each

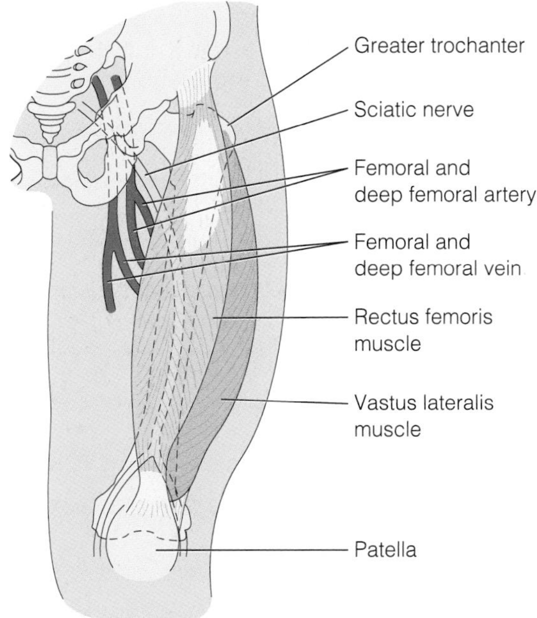

FIGURE 26–3 Injection sites. The middle third of the vastus lateralis muscle is the preferred site for intramuscular injection in the newborn. The middle third of the rectus femoris is an alternative site, but its proximity to major vessels and the sciatic nerve necessitates caution in using this site for injection.

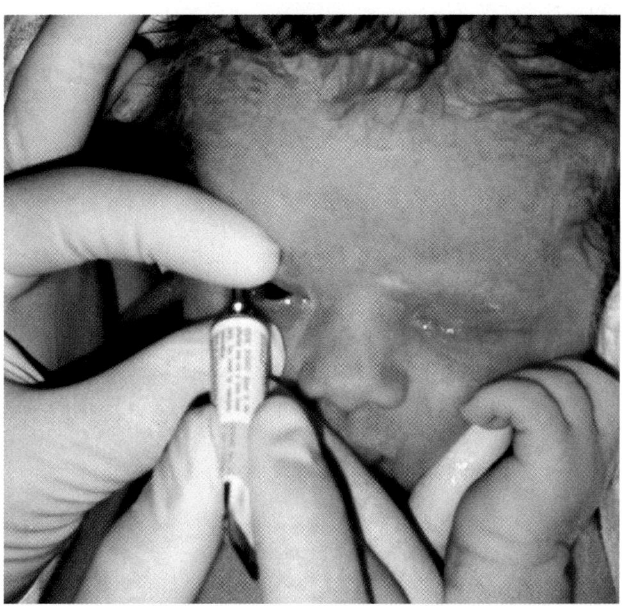

FIGURE 26–4 Ophthalmic ointment. Retract lower eyelid outward to instill a ¼-inch strand of ointment from a single-dose ampule along the lower conjunctival surface.

eye (Figure 26–4). It may be delayed up to 1 hour after birth to allow eye contact during parent-newborn bonding (AAP, 1997) (Procedure 26–2 on page 763.).

Eye prophylaxis medication can cause chemical conjunctivitis, which gives the newborn some discomfort and may interfere with the baby's ability to focus on the parents' faces. The resulting edema, inflammation, and discharge may cause concern if the parents have not been informed that the side effects will clear in 24 to 48 hours and that this prophylactic eye treatment is necessary for the newborn's well-being.

Early Assessment of Neonatal Distress

During the first 24 hours of life, nurses are constantly alert for signs of distress. If the newborn is with the parents during this period, the nurse must take extra care to teach them how to maintain their newborn's temperature, recognize the hallmarks of newborn distress, and respond immediately to signs of respiratory problems. The parents should learn to observe the newborn for changes in color or activity, rapid breathing with chest retractions, or facial grimacing. Their interventions should include nasal and oral suctioning with bulb syringe, positioning, and vigorous fingertip stroking of the newborn's spine to stimulate respiratory activity if necessary. The nurse also must be available immediately should the newborn develop distress (Table 26–2).

A common cause of neonatal distress is early-onset group B streptococcal (GBS) disease. The case–fatality rate for GBS disease is estimated to be 5% to 20% for newborns (Centers for Disease Control and Prevention, 1996). The disease in newborns usually occurs as bacteremia, pneumonia, or meningitis. Infected mothers transmit GBS infection to their infants during labor and birth; thus it is recommended that at-risk mothers receive intrapartum antimicrobial prophylaxis (IAP) for GBS disease. All infants of mothers identified as at risk should be assessed and observed for signs and symptoms of sepsis.

TABLE 26–2 Signs of Neonatal Distress
Increased respiratory rate (more than 60/minute) or difficult respirations
Sternal retractions
Nasal flaring
Grunting
Excessive mucus
Facial grimacing
Cyanosis (central: skin, lips, tongue)
Abdominal distention or mass
Vomiting of bile-stained material
Absence of meconium elimination within 24 hours of birth
Absence of urine elimination within 24 hours of birth
Jaundice of the skin within 24 hours of birth or due to hemolytic process
Temperature instability (hypothermia or hyperthermia)
Jitteriness or glucose less than 40 mg%

SOURCE: Adapted from Tappero EP, Honeyfield ME: *Physical Assessment of the Newborn,* 2nd ed. Petaluma, CA: NICU Ink, 1996.

PROCEDURE 26–1 THERMOREGULATION OF THE NEWBORN

Nursing Action	*Rationale*
Objective: Prepare the warming equipment.	
• Prewarm the incubator or radiant warmer. Make sure warmed towels and/or lightweight blankets are available. • Maintain the birthing room at 22C (71F), with a relative humidity of 60%–65%.	*The change from a warm, moist intrauterine environment to a cool, dry, drafty environment stresses the newborn's immature thermoregulation mechanisms.*
Objective: Establish a stable temperature after birth.	
• Wipe the newborn free of blood and excessive vernix, especially from the head, with prewarmed towels.	*This prevents loss of body heat from a large surface area through evaporation.*
• Place the newborn under the radiant warmer.	*The radiant warmer creates a heat-gaining environment.*
• Wrap the newborn in a prewarmed blanket and transfer the newborn to the mother.	*Use of the prewarmed blanket reduces convective heat loss and facilitates maternal-infant contact without compromising the newborn's thermoregulation.*
• Place the infant skin-to-skin with the mother under a warmed blanket.	*Skin-to-skin contact with the mother or father helps maintain the newborn's temperature.*
Objective: Maintain a stable infant temperature.	
• Diaper the newborn and place a stocking hat on its head. Place the newborn uncovered (except for diaper and hat) under the radiant warmer.	*Radiant heat warms the outer surface skin, so the skin needs to be exposed.*
• Tape a servocontrol probe on the newborn's anterior abdominal wall, with the metal side next to the skin, and cover the probe with an aluminum heat deflector patch.	*The aluminum cover prevents heating of the probe directly and overheating the infant.*
• Turn the heater to servocontrol mode so that the abdominal skin is maintained at 36.5–37C (97.5–98.6F).	
• Monitor the newborn's axillary and skin probe temperature per institution's protocol. • When the newborn's temperature reaches 37C (98.6F), remove the infant from the radiant warmer, and place a T-shirt, diaper, and stocking hat on the newborn. • Double wrap (2 blankets) the newborn and place the newborn in an open crib.	*The temperature indicator on the radiant warmer continually displays the newborn's probe temperature, so the axillary temperature is checked to ensure that the machine accurately reports the newborn's temperature.*
• Recheck the newborn's axillary temperature in 1 h.	*It is important to monitor the infant's ability to maintain its own thermoregulation.*
Objective: Rewarm the newborn gradually if temperature drops below 36.1C (97F).	
• Assess axillary temperature frequently, per agency routine; usually every 2–4h. • If the newborn needs rewarming, place the newborn (unclothed except for diaper) under the radiant warmer with a servocontrol probe on the abdomen.	*Frequent assessment may detect hypothermia, which predisposes the newborn to cold stress.*
• Gradually rewarm back to normal temperature.	*Rapid heating can lead to hyperthermia, which is associated with apnea, increased insensible water loss, and increased metabolic rate.*

PROCEDURE 26–1 *CONTINUED*

Nursing Action	***Rationale***
• Recheck the newborn's temperature in 30 min, then hourly. When the temperature reaches 37C (98.6F), remove the newborn from the radiant heater, dress the newborn, double wrap, and place in the open crib. Recheck the temperature in 1 h.	
Objective: Prevent drops in the newborn's temperature.	
The nurse carries out the following activities:	
• Keep the newborn's clothing and bedding dry.	
• Double wrap the newborn and put a stocking hat on.	
• Use the radiant warmer during procedures.	
• Reduce the newborn's exposure to drafts.	
• Warm objects that will come in contact with the newborn (eg, stethoscopes).	
• Encourage the mother to snuggle with the newborn under blankets or breastfeed the newborn with hat and light cover on.	

DRUG GUIDE

Vitamin K_1 Phytonadione (AquaMEPHYTON)

Overview of Neonatal Action

Phytonadione is used in prophylaxis and treatment of hemorrhagic disease of the newborn. It promotes liver formation of the clotting factors II, VII, IX, and X. At birth, the neonate does not have the bacteria in the colon that are necessary for synthesizing fat-soluble vitamin K_1; therefore, the newborn may have decreased levels of prothrombin during the first 5 to 8 days of life, reflected by a prolongation of prothrombin time.

Route, Dosage, Frequency

Intramuscular injection is given in the vastus lateralis thigh muscle. A one-time-only prophylactic dose of 0.5 to 1 mg is given intramuscularly in the birthing area or on admission to the newborn nursery.

If the mother received anticoagulants during pregnancy, an additional dose may be ordered by the physician and is given at 6 to 8 hours post first injection. A dose of 2 mg is given if the route of administration is by mouth. This dosage should be administered orally again at 1 to 2 weeks and at 4 weeks of age to ensure an adequate dose (American Academy of Pediatrics, Vitamin K Ad Hoc Task Force,1993).

Neonatal Side Effects

Pain and edema may occur at injection site. Allergic reactions, such as rash and urticaria, may also occur.

Nursing Considerations

- Observe for bleeding (usually occurs on second or third day). Bleeding may be seen as generalized ecchymoses or bleeding from umbilical cord, circumcision site, nose, or gastrointestinal tract. Results of serial PT and PTT should be assessed.
- Observe for jaundice and kernicterus, especially in preterm infants.
- Observe for signs of local inflammation.
- Protect drug from light.
- Give vitamin K_1 before circumcision procedure.

DRUG GUIDE

Erythromycin Ophthalmic Ointment (Ilotycin Ophthalmic)

Overview of Neonatal Action

Erythromycin (Ilotycin Ophthalmic) is used as prophylactic treatment of ophthalmia neonatorum, which is caused by the bacteria *Neisseria gonorrhoeae.* Preventive treatment of gonorrhea in the newborn is required by law. Erythromycin is also effective against ophthalmic chlamydial infections. It is either bacteriostatic or bactericidal, depending on the organisms involved and the concentration of drug.

Route, Dosage, Frequency

Ophthalmic ointment (0.5%) is instilled as a narrow ribbon or strand, ¼ inch long, along the lower conjunctival surface of each eye, starting at the inner canthus. It is instilled only once in each eye. The ointment may be administered in the birthing area or, alternatively, later in the nursery so that eye contact between infant and parent is facilitated and the bonding process immediately after birth is not interrupted. After administration, gently close eye and manipulate to ensure spread of ointment.

Neonatal Side Effects

Sensitivity reaction; may interfere with ability to focus and may cause edema and inflammation. Side effects usually disappear in 24 to 48 hours.

Nursing Considerations

- Wash hands immediately prior to instillation to prevent introduction of bacteria.
- Do not irrigate the eyes after instillation. Use new tube or single-use container for ophthalmic ointment administration shortly after birth. May wipe away excess after 1 minute.
- Observe for hypersensitivity.
- Teach parents about need for eye prophylaxis. Educate them regarding side effects and signs that need to be reported to the health care provider.

Initiating First Feeding

The timing of the first feeding varies, depending on whether the newborn is to be breastfed or bottle-fed and whether there were any complications during pregnancy or birth, such as maternal diabetes, intrauterine growth restriction (IUGR), and so forth. Mothers who choose to breastfeed their newborns may seek to put their baby to breast while in the birthing area. This practice should be encouraged because successful, long-term breastfeeding during infancy appears to be related to beginning breastfeedings in the first few hours of life. Bottle-fed newborns usually begin the first feedings by 5 hours of age, during the second period of reactivity, when they awaken and appear hungry.

Signs indicating newborn readiness for the first feeding are active bowel sounds, absence of abdominal distention, and a lusty cry that quiets with rooting and sucking behaviors when a stimulus is placed near the lips.

Facilitating Parent-Newborn Attachment

Eye-to-eye contact between the parents and their newborn is extremely important during the early hours after birth, when the newborn is in the first period of reactivity. The newborn is alert during this time, the eyes are wide open, and often direct eye contact is made with human faces within optimal range for visual acuity (7 to 8 in). It is theorized that this eye contact is an important foundation in establishing attachment in human relationships (Klaus & Klaus, 1985). Consequently, the prophylactic eye medication is often delayed, but no more than 1 hour, to provide an opportunity for this period of eye contact between parents and their newborn, thus facilitating the attachment process (AAP, 1997).

Nursing Care Management of Newborn During Stay in Birthing Unit

Nursing Diagnosis

Examples of nursing diagnoses that may apply during daily care of the newborn include the following:

- ***Risk for Ineffective Breathing Pattern*** related to periodic breathing
- ***Altered Nutrition: Less than Body Requirements*** related to limited nutritional or fluid intake and increased caloric expenditure
- ***Altered Urinary Elimination*** related to meatal edema secondary to circumcision
- ***Risk for Infection*** related to umbilical cord healing, circumcision site, or immature immune system
- ***Knowledge Deficit*** related to lack of information about male circumcision or pros and cons of breastfeeding and bottle-feeding
- ***Altered Family Processes*** related to integration of newborn into family unit or demands of newborn feeding schedule

Nursing Plan and Implementation

Maintenance of Cardiopulmonary Function

The nurse assesses *vital signs* every 6 to 8 hours or more, depending on the newborn's status. The newborn should be placed in a propped, side-lying position when left unattended to prevent aspiration and facilitate drainage of mucus. A bulb syringe is kept within easy reach should the baby need oral-nasal suctioning. If the newborn has

PROCEDURE 26–2 INSTILLING OPHTHALMIC ILOTYCIN OINTMENT

Nursing Action	*Rationale*
Objective: Provide newborn prophylactic eye care.	
• Wash your hands and put on gloves.	*This prevents introduction of bacteria.*
• Clean the infant's eyes to remove any drainage.	*Removal of exudate will facilitate instillation and absorption of the ointment.*
• Retract the lower eyelid outward with your forefinger.	
• Instill ¼-inch strand of ointment along the lower conjunctival surface, beginning at the inner canthus.	*This maximizes the absorption.*
• Repeat the above process on the other eye. Instill only a single dose per eye.	*Prophylaxis requires only a single dose.*
• Wipe excess ointment away after 1 min (American Academy of Pediatrics, 1997). Do not irrigate eyes.	*Irrigation will remove the ointment.*
• Assess for any sensitivity reaction such as edema, inflammation, or drainage.	*Sensitivity reactions may interfere with the infant's ability to focus and with the bonding process.*
Objective: Explain the procedure to the parents.	
Explain the rationale for eye prophylaxis. Explain that it may interfere with the newborn's ability to focus on the parents' faces and that there may be temporary side effects, which usually disappear in 24 to 48 hrs.	*The parents should understand that the instillation of ointment is required by law and is preventive treatment of gonorrhea and chlamydia infection, both of which can cause blindness.*
Objective: Record the completion of the procedure on the newborn's chart.	*This provides a permanent record to meet the legal requirements.*

respiratory difficulty, the airway is cleared. Vigorous fingertip stroking of the baby's spine will frequently stimulate respiratory activity. A cardiorespiratory monitor can be used on newborns who are not being observed at all times and are at risk for decreased respiratory or cardiac function. Indicators of risk are pallor, cyanosis, ruddy color, apnea, or other signs of instability. Changes in skin color may indicate the need for closer assessment of temperature, cardiopulmonary status, hematocrit, glucose, and bilirubin levels.

Maintenance of a Neutral Thermal Environment

The nurse makes every effort to maintain the newborn's temperature within the normal range. The nurse must make certain the newborn is dressed and exposed to the air as little as possible. A head covering should be used for the small newborn, who has less subcutaneous fat to act as insulation in maintaining body heat. The ambient temperature of the room where the newborn is kept should be monitored routinely and kept at approximately 32.5C to 33.9C (90.5F to 93.1F) for large babies and 35.4C +/− 0.5C for smaller babies (Merenstein & Gardner, 1998). Parents may be advised to dress the newborn in one more layer of clothing than is necessary for an adult to maintain thermal comfort.

A newborn whose temperature falls below optimal levels will use calories to maintain body heat rather than for growth. Chilling also decreases the affinity of serum albumin for bilirubin, thereby increasing the likelihood of newborn jaundice. It also increases oxygen use and may cause respiratory distress.

An overheated newborn will increase activity and respiratory rate in an attempt to cool the body. Both measures deplete caloric reserves. In addition, the increased respiratory rate leads to increased insensible fluid loss ("Neonatal Thermoregulation," 1997).

CRITICAL THINKING IN PRACTICE

A mother calls you to her room. She sounds frightened and says her baby can't breathe. You find the mother cradling her infant in her arms. The infant is mildly cyanotic, waving her arms, and has mucus coming from her nose and mouth. What would you do?

Answers can be found in Appendix I.

RESEARCH IN PRACTICE

What is the study about? Neonatal thermoregulation is a vital function that reflects physiologic status and the infant's adaptation to extrauterine life. Obtaining accurate measurement of body temperature and instituting appropriate nursing interventions to maintain a stable temperature in the neonate are important aspects of nursing care. Interventions aimed at achieving infant thermoregulation require that temperature measurements be accurate and reliable. The purposes of this study were: (1) to explore the use of commercially available instruments as well as other standard methods for measuring temperatures in hospitalized infants, and (2) to determine the possible effects of environmental, developmental, and pharmacologic factors on readings obtained from these instruments.

How was this study done? The study design was descriptive. A convenience sample of 220 infants who weighed ≥1500 gm (average weight of 2715 gm ± 743 gm) with an average age of 17 ± 22 days of life and who were being cared for in a nursery provided the sample for this study. The infants were term and preterm. Excluded from the study were infants with skin conditions that would not tolerate application and removal of a skin probe or adhesive patches. The outcomes were comparisons between the "reference" axillary, glass, mercury thermometer readings and axillary, skin, and tympanic membrane measurements obtained from Tempa Dot Single Use Clinical Thermometers, Mon-a-Therm Model 1000 skin temperature monitor, IVAC Core Check tympanic thermometers, and IncuTemp3 radiant warmer skin temperature sensor measurements. Each infant had temperatures checked with each of the thermometers under study. In addition, information was collected about environmental, developmental, and pharmacologic factors that might affect the readings.

What were the results of the study? The B-D Digital Fever thermometer had the highest correlation with the glass, mercury thermometer. Tempa Dot measurements showed the next highest correlation with the glass, mercury thermometer. Skin temperatures were influenced by nesting, clothing, swaddling, and probe site placement. Tympanic readings show effects of bed type and environmental temperature.

What additional questions do I have? (1)Why is the tympanic thermometer less accurate in the neonatal population? (2) What environmental influences and application techniques affect temperature readings on a servo warmer?

How can I use this study? Results of this study appear to support the use of the B-D Digital Fever thermometer and the Tempa Dot Single Use Clinical Thermometer as reliable and useful instruments. As results in this study indicate, nurses need to be aware that skin temperature readings vary with probe site placement, bed type, the associated environmental temperature, and the presence of clothing. Further study is needed to determine the most accurate sites for skin probe placement.

SOURCE: Leick-Rude, M. & Bloom, L. (1998). A comparison of temperature taking methods in neonates. *Neonatal Network, 17*(5), 21–37.

CLINICAL TIP

You may be surprised by the difficulty you encounter when attempting to put a T-shirt on a newborn. This is most easily done by placing your fingers through the sleeve, grasping the infant's hand, and drawing it back through the sleeve. This technique keeps the baby from grasping the fabric.

Promotion of Adequate Hydration and Nutrition

Newborn nutrition is addressed in depth in Chapter 27. The nurse records the newborn's caloric and fluid intake and enhances adequate hydration by maintaining a neutral thermal environment and offering early and frequent feedings. Early feedings promote gastric emptying and increase peristalsis, thereby decreasing the degree of hyperbilirubinemia by limiting the amount of time fecal material is in contact with the enzyme β-glucuronidase in the small intestine. This enzyme acts to free the bilirubin from the stool, allowing bilirubin to be reabsorbed into the vascular system. The nurse records voiding and stooling patterns. The first voiding should occur within 24 hours and passage of stool within 48 hours. When they do not occur, the nurse continues the normal observation routine while assessing for abdominal distention, bowel sounds, hydration, fluid intake, voiding pattern, and temperature stability.

The newborn should be weighed at the same time each day for accurate comparisons and must be kept warm during the weighing. A weight loss of up to 10% for term newborns is considered within normal limits during the first week of life. This is the result of limited intake, loss of excess extracellular fluid, and passage of meconium. Parents should be told about the expected weight loss, the reason for it, and the expectations for regaining the birth weight. Birth weight should be regained by 2 weeks if feedings are adequate.

Excessive handling of the newborn can cause an increase in the newborn's metabolic rate and calorie use and cause fatigue. The nurse should be alert to the baby's subtle cues of fatigue. These include a decrease in muscle tension and activity in the extremities and neck and loss of eye contact, which may be manifested by fluttering or closing the eyelids or turning the head away. The nurse quickly ceases stimulation when signs of fatigue appear. The nurse's care should demonstrate to the parents the need to be aware of newborn cues of fatigue and to wait for periods of alertness in the baby for contact and stimulation. The nurse is also responsible for assessing the woman's comfort and latching-on techniques in breastfeeding or bottle-feeding.

Promotion of Skin Integrity

Newborn skin care, including bathing, is important for the health and appearance of the individual newborn and for infection control within the nursery. Ongoing skin care involves cleansing the buttock and perianal areas with fresh water and cotton, or with a mild soap and water, with diaper changes.

The umbilical cord is assessed for signs of bleeding or infection, such as oozing and foul smell. A triple-dye or antimicrobial agent such as bacitracin is applied to the normal newborn's cord. The skin absorption and toxicity of triple-dye agents in newborns have not been carefully studied (AAP, 1997). Alcohol is probably not effective in preventing microbial colonization of the cord and omphalitis. The nurse is responsible for giving cord care each time the diaper is changed.

Prevention of Complications and Promoting Safety

Newborns are at continued risk for the complications of hemorrhage, late-onset cardiac symptoms, and infection. Pallor may be an early sign of hemorrhage and must be reported to the physician. The newborn is placed on a cardiorespiratory monitor to permit continuous assessment. Several newborn conditions put the newborn at risk for bleeding. Cyanosis that is not relieved by oxygen administration requires emergency intervention, may indicate a congenital cardiac condition or shock, and requires ongoing assessment.

The circumcision is assessed for signs of hemorrhage and infection. The first voiding after a circumcision is also a significant assessment to evaluate for possible urinary obstruction due to trauma and edema. Vaseline™ gauze is applied to the circumcision site to prevent bleeding; the gauze can easily be removed and replaced if it becomes soiled.

Infection in the nursery is best prevented by requiring that all personnel having direct contact with newborns scrub for 2 to 3 minutes from fingertips to and including elbows at the beginning of each shift. The hands must be washed with soap and rubbed vigorously for 15 seconds ("Neonatal Skin Care," 1992) before and after contact with every newborn or after touching any soiled surface, such as the floor or one's hair or face. Parents are often instructed to use an antiseptic hand cleaner before touching the baby. Anyone with an infection should refrain from working with newborns until the infection has cleared. A few agencies ask family members to wear a gown (preferably disposable) over their street clothes. Parents need to be taught that people who handle the baby should wash their hands before doing so, even after the baby is home.

Safety of the newborn is provided through a variety of nursing interventions and institutional security measures. It is essential that the nurse verify the identity of the newborn by checking and comparing the numbers and names on the identification bracelets of mother and newborn before giving a baby to a parent and to follow institutional policies for identification of all nursery personnel. Individual birthing units should practice safety measures to prevent infant abduction and provide teaching and information to parents regarding their role in this area (Nelson, 1999).

Circumcision

Circumcision is a surgical procedure in which the prepuce, an epithelial layer covering the tip of the penis, is separated from the glans penis and excised. This permits exposure of the glans for easier cleaning.

Circumcision was originally a religious rite practiced by Jews and Muslims. The practice gained widespread cultural acceptance in the United States but is done infrequently in many European countries. Many parents choose circumcision because they want the male child to have a physical appearance similar to that of the father or the majority of other children, or they may feel that it is expected by society. Another frequently cited reason for circumcising newborn males is to prevent the need for anesthesia, hospitalization, pain, and trauma should the procedure be needed later in life (American Academy of Pediatrics Task Force on Circumcision, 1999).

Families make the decision about circumcision for their newborn male child. In most cases, the choice is based on cultural, social, and family tradition. To ensure informed consent, parents should be informed about possible long-term medical effects of circumcision and noncircumcision during the prenatal period.

Current Recommendations In the past, recommendations regarding circumcision have varied. In 1999, however, the American Academy of Pediatrics published a policy statement recommending against circumcision. The policy also includes a suggestion that analgesia (e.g., emula cream, DPNB, or subcutaneous ring block) be used during circumcision to decrease procedural pain (American Academy of Pediatrics Task Force on Circumcision, 1999).

Circumcision should not be performed if the newborn is premature or compromised, has a known bleeding problem, or is born with a genitourinary defect, such as hypospadias or epispadias, that may necessitate the use of the foreskin in future surgical repairs (Reynolds, 1996).

Nurse's Role The nurse plays an essential role in providing parents with current information about circumcision. Nurses can facilitate parental informed consent because of their knowledge of the medical, social, and psychologic aspects of newborn circumcision (L'Archevesque & Goldstein-Lohman, 1996). A well-informed nurse can allay parents' anxiety by sharing information and allowing them to express their concerns. Parents must be informed about potential risks and outcomes of circumcision. Hemorrhage, infection, difficulty in voiding, separation of the edges of the circumcision, pain, and restlessness are early potential problems. Later there is the risk that the glans and

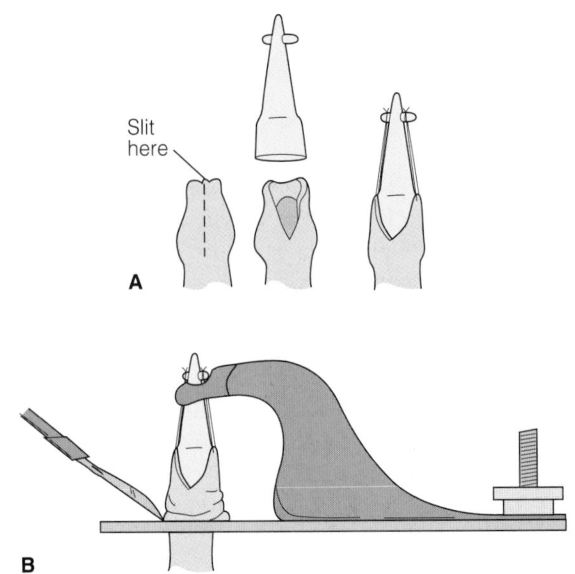

FIGURE 26–5 Circumcision using the Yellen or Gomco clamp. ***A,*** The prepuce is drawn over the cone. ***B,*** The clamp is applied. Pressure is maintained for 3 to 4 minutes, and then excess prepuce is cut away.

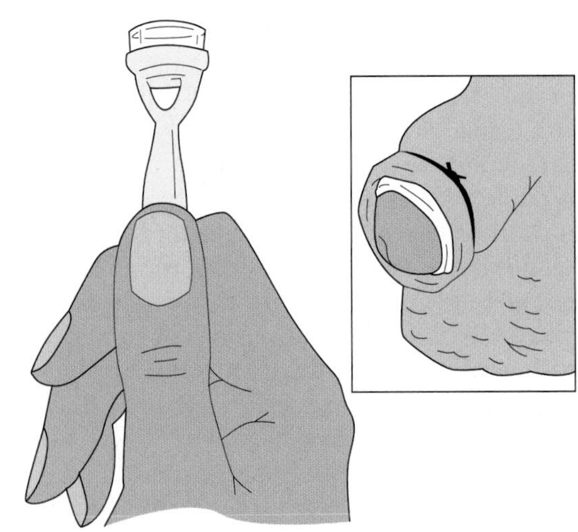

FIGURE 26–6 Circumcision using the Plastibell. The bell is fitted over the glans. A suture is tied around the bell's rim, and the excess prepuce is cut away. The plastic rim remains in place for 3 to 4 days until healing occurs. The bell may be allowed to fall off; it is removed if still in place after 8 days.

urethral meatus can become irritated and inflamed from contact with ammonia from urine. Ulcerations and progressive stenosis may develop. Adhesions, entrapment of the penis, and damage to the urethra are all potential complications that could require surgical correction (American Academy of Pediatrics Task Force on Circumcision, 1999).

The parents of an uncircumcised male infant require information from the nurse about good hygiene practices. They should be told that the foreskin and glans are two similar layers of cells that separate from each other. The separation process begins prenatally and is normally completed at between 3 and 5 years of age. In the process of separation, sterile sloughed cells build up between the layers. This buildup looks similar to the smegma secreted after puberty, and it is harmless. Occasionally during the daily bath, the parents can gently test for retraction. If retraction has occurred, daily gentle washing of the glans with soap and water is sufficient to maintain adequate cleanliness. The parents should teach the child to incorporate this practice into his daily self-care activities. Most uncircumcised males have no difficulty incorporating this into daily practice. If circumcision is desired, the procedure should be performed after the newborn is well stabilized and has received his initial physical examination by a health care provider. The parents may also choose to have the circumcision done after discharge. However, they need to be advised that if the baby is older than 1 month, the current practice is to hospitalize him for the procedure.

Prior to a circumcision, the nurse ascertains that the physician has explained the procedure, determines whether the parents have any further questions about the procedure, and checks that the circumcision permit is signed. The nurse gathers the equipment and prepares the newborn by removing the diaper and placing him on a circumcision board or some other type of restraint, but restraining only the legs (O'Grady, 1996). In Jewish circumcision ceremonies, the infant is held by the father or grandfather and given wine before the procedure (Reynolds, 1996).

There are a variety of techniques for circumcision (Figures 26–5 and 26–6), and all produce minimal bleeding. Therefore the nurse should make special note of infants with family history of bleeding disorders or with mothers who took anticoagulants, including aspirin, prenatally (Williamson, 1997). During the procedure, the nurse assesses the newborn's response. One important consideration is pain experienced by the newborn. Some physicians use local anesthesia for this procedure. The American Academy of Pediatrics Committee on the Fetus and Newborn and Committee on Drugs (1987) has published a policy statement endorsing the administration of local or systemic anesthesia to infants undergoing surgical procedures. A dorsal penile nerve block (DPNB) using 1% lidocaine without epinephrine significantly minimizes the pain and the shifts in behavioral patterns, such as crying, irritability, and erratic sleep cycles associated with circumcision. Other studies are investigating the use of topical anesthetic applied 60 to 90 minutes prior to prepuce removal, acetaminophen, and cryoanalgesia (American Academy of Pediatrics Task Force on Circumcision, 1999).

During the procedure, the nurse can provide comfort measures such as lightly stroking the baby's head, providing a pacifier, and talking to him. Following the circumcision, the infant should be held and comforted by a family member or the nurse. The nurse must be alert to any cues that these measures are overstimulating the newborn instead of comforting him. Such cues include turning away of the head, increased generalized body movement, skin color changes, hyperalertness, and hiccuping.

After the circumcision, the nurse assesses the infant every 30 minutes for at least 2 hours and every 2 hours thereafter, particularly to identify any abnormal bleeding (Williamson, 1997). A and D ointment is placed on the penis to keep the diaper from adhering to the site in all procedures except those using the Plastibell. New ointment is applied with each diaper change or at least four to five times a day for at least 24 to 48 hours. Petroleum jelly or an antibiotic ointment may be used instead of A and D ointment. Parents should assess the newborn's voiding for amount, adequacy of stream, and presence of blood. If bleeding does occur, light pressure is applied intermittently to the site with a sterile gauze pad, and the physician is notified (Narchi & Kulaylat, 1998).

The newborn may cry when he voids after circumcision. He is best positioned on his side with the diaper fastened loosely to prevent undue pressure. He may remain fussy for several hours and be less interested in feedings. The parents should be instructed to squeeze water gently over the penis and pat it dry after each diaper change. The diaper is loosely fastened for 2 to 3 days because the glans remains tender for this length of time. Before discharge, the parents are instructed to observe the penis for bleeding or possible signs of infection. A whitish-yellow exudate that adheres to the glans is granulation tissue. It is normal and not indicative of an infection. The exudate may be noted for about 2 or 3 days and should not be removed.

If the Plastibell is used, parents are informed that it can remain in place for up to 8 days and then falls off. If it is still in place after 8 days, it may require manual removal by the clinician.

Enhancing Parent-Newborn Attachment

Parent-newborn attachment is promoted by encouraging all family members to be involved with the new member of the family. Some specific interventions are examined in Chapters 20 and 31 and the accompanying Teaching Guide: Enhancing Attachment. Infant massage is a common child care practice in many parts of the world, especially Africa and Asia, and has recently gained attention in the United States. Parents can be taught to use infant message as a method to facilitate the bonding process and to reduce the stress and pain associated with teething, inoculations, constipation, and colic. Infant massage induces relaxation not only for the infant, but also provides a calming and "feel good" interaction for the parents that fosters the development of warm, positive relationships (Field, 1992). The nurse plays a vital role in fostering parent-infant attachment (Figure 26–7).

Nursing Plan and Implementation in Preparation for Discharge

Parent Teaching

To meet parent needs for information, the nurse who is responsible for the daily care of the mother and newborn should assume the primary responsibility for parent education. Nearly every contact with the parents presents an opportunity for sharing information that can facilitate their sense of competence in newborn care. The nurse also needs to recognize and respect the fact that there are many good ways to provide safe care. Unless their care methods are harmful to the newborn, the parents' methods of giving care should be reinforced rather than contradicted. The nurse also needs to be sensitive to the cultural beliefs and values of the family (Table 26–3).

The information that follows is provided to increase the nurse's knowledge of newborn care and is used to meet parents' needs for information. Parents may be familiar with handling and caring for infants, or this may be their first time to interact with a newborn. If they are new parents, the sensitive nurse gently teaches them by example and provides instructions geared to their needs and previous knowledge about the various aspects of newborn care.

The length of stay in the birthing unit for mother and baby after birth is often 48 hours or less. The challenge for the nurse is to use every opportunity to teach, guide, and support parents, fostering the parents' capabilities and confidence in caring for their newborn. Including mother-baby care and home care instruction on the night shift can help meet the teaching needs of early discharge parents.

CRITICAL THINKING QUESTION

What factors should you consider when providing parents with information about their baby's care needs?

The nurse observes how parents interact with their infant during feeding and caregiving activities. Even during a short stay, there will be opportunities for the nurse

Text continues on page 770.

A Letter From Your Baby

Dear Parents:

I come to you a small, immature being with my own style and personality. I am yours for only a short time; enjoy me.

1. Please take time to find out who I am, how I differ from you and how much I can bring you joy.
2. Please feed me when I am hungry. I never knew hunger in the womb, and clocks and time mean little to me.
3. Please hold, cuddle, kiss, touch, stroke, and croon to me. I was always held closely in the womb and was never alone before.
4. Please don't be disappointed when I am not the perfect baby that you expected, nor disappointed with yourselves that you are not the perfect parents.
5. Please don't expect too much from me as your newborn baby, or too much from yourself as a parent. Give us both six weeks as a birthday present—six weeks for me to grow, develop, mature and become more stable and predictable, and six weeks for you to rest and relax and allow your body to get back to normal.
6. Please forgive me if I cry a lot. Bear with me and in a short time, as I mature, I will spend less and less time crying and more time socializing.
7. Please watch me carefully and I can tell you the things that soothe, console and please me. I am not a tyrant who was sent to make your life miserable, but the only way I can tell you that I am not happy is with my cry.
8. Please remember that I am resilient and can withstand the many natural mistakes you will make with me. As long as you make them with love, you cannot ruin me.
9. Please take care of yourself and eat a balanced diet, rest and exercise so that when we are together, you have the health and strength to take care of me.
10. Please take care of your relationship with others. Relationships that are good for you, support both you and me.

Although I may have turned your life upside down, please realize that things will be back to normal before long.

Thank you,

Your Loving Child

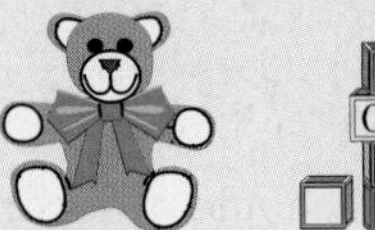

FIGURE 26–7 A letter from your baby.

TABLE 26–3 Examples of Cultural Beliefs and Practices Regarding Baby Care*

Umbilical Cord

People of Latin American or Filipino cultural background may use an abdominal binder or bellyband to protect against dirt, injury, and umbilical hernia. They may also apply oils to the stump of the cord or tape metal to the umbilicus to ward off evil spirits.

People of northern European ancestry may expect a sterile cutting of the cord at birth. They may allow the stump to air dry and discard the cord once it falls off.

Parent-Infant Contact

People of Asian ancestry may pick up the baby as soon as it cries, or they may carry the baby at all times.

Some Native Americans, notably the Navajos, may use cradle boards.

Korean mothers may be reluctant to pick up or touch their infant, deferring infant care to the paternal grandmother (Schneiderman, 1996).

The Muslim father traditionally calls praise to Allah in the newborn's right ear, and cleans the infant after birth (Hutchinson & Baqi-Aziz, 1994).

Feeding

Some people of Asian heritage may breastfeed their babies for the first 1 to 2 years of life.

Many Cambodian refugees practice breastfeeding on demand without restriction, or, if bottle-feeding, provide a "comfort bottle" in between feedings (Rasbridge & Kulig, 1995).

People of Iranian heritage may breastfeed female babies longer than males.

Some people of African ancestry may wean their babies after they begin to walk.

Most Korean mothers resist breastfeeding in the hospital, contending that they do not have "milk," and state that they will begin breastfeeding at home (Schneiderman, 1996).

Circumcision

People of Muslim and Jewish ancestry practice circumcision as a religious ritual (Hutchinson & Baqi-Aziz, 1994).

Many natives of Africa and Australia practice circumcision as a puberty rite.

Most Native Americans and people of Asian and Latin American cultures rarely perform circumcision.

Only 15% of the world's male population is circumcised.

Health/Illness

Some people from Latin American cultural backgrounds may believe that touching the face or head of an infant when admiring it will ward off the "evil eye." They may also neglect to cut the baby's nails to avoid nearsightedness and instead put mittens on the baby's hands to prevent scratching. They also may believe that fat babies are healthy.

Some people of Asian heritage may not allow anyone to touch the baby's head without asking permission.

Some Orthodox Jews believe that saying the baby's name before the formal naming ceremony will harm the baby.

Some people of Vietnamese ancestry believe that cutting a baby's hair or nails will cause illness.

*NOTE: The above are meant only as examples of some of the behaviors that may be found within certain cultures. Not all members of a culture will practice the behaviors described.

SOURCES: Adapted from Andrews MM: Transcultural perspectives in the nursing care of children and adolescents. In: *Transcultural Concepts in Nursing Care,* 2nd ed, Andrews MM, Boyle JS (editors). Philadelphia: Lippincott, 1995; Riordan J, Auerbach KG: *Breastfeeding and Human Lactation.* (2nd ed.) Boston: Jones & Bartlett, 1999.

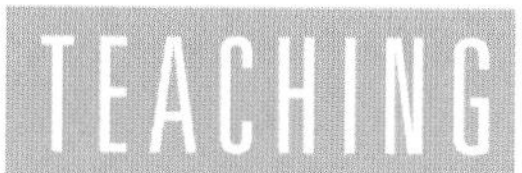

TEACHING GUIDE: ENHANCING ATTACHMENT

Assessment Observe and document the interactions between the parents and their baby immediately after birth to determine the family's needs for teaching, support, or interventions.

Nursing Diagnoses The key nursing diagnoses will probably be ***Altered Family Processes*** related to addition of a new baby to the family or ***Knowledge Deficit*** related to lack of information about emotional needs of newborn.

Nursing Plan and Implementation The teaching plan will include information about the infant's physical status and normal characteristics, comforting techniques, and the baby's emotional needs immediately after birth and during the newborn period. Encourage the parents to maintain continuous contact with the baby through rooming-in, thus providing maximum opportunity for them to interact with their infant.

Client Goals At the completion of teaching, the parents will be able to:

- Demonstrate appropriate nurturing behaviors such as touching, bonding, talking to, kissing, and holding their baby.
- Discuss the normal characteristics and emotional needs of the newborn.
- List at least three comforting techniques.

Teaching Plan

Content	*Teaching Method*
• Present information on periods of reactivity and expected newborn responses.	*Focus on open discussion.*
• Describe normal physical characteristics of newborn.	*Present slides showing newborn characteristics.*
• Explain the bonding process, its gradual development, and the reciprocal interactive nature of the process.	
• Discuss the infant's capabilities for interaction, such as nonverbal communication abilities. The nonverbal communications include movement, gaze, touch, facial expressions, and vocalizations—including crying. Emphasize that eye contact is considered one of the cardinal factors in developing infant-parent attachment and will be integrated with touching and vocal behaviors.	*Show a video on the interactive capabilities of newborns.*
• Explain that touching, including stroking, patting, massaging, and kissing, will progress to interactive touch between the parents and their infant; discuss their need to assimilate these behaviors into their daily routine with the baby.	*Provide handouts, and use a doll to demonstrate behaviors.*
• Describe and demonstrate comforting techniques, including the use of sound, swaddling, rocking, and stroking.	*Demonstrate the techniques and ask for a return demonstration.*
• Describe the progression of the infant's behaviors as the infant matures, and the importance of the parents' consistent response to their infant's cues and needs.	*Allow time for questions and discussion.*
• Provide information about available pamphlets, videos, and support groups in the community.	

Evaluation Evaluate the learning by providing time for discussion, questions, and return demonstrations in the birthing unit, and during the postpartal return visit or home visit. Continue to observe the parents' positive interaction with their baby during the remainder of their stay in birthing unit.

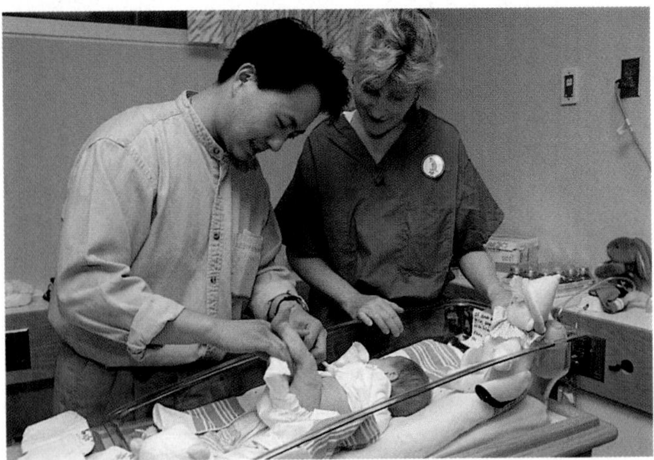

FIGURE 26–8 Individualizing parent education. Father returns demonstration of diapering his son.

to provide information and evaluate whether the parents are comfortable with changing diapers and wrapping, handling, and feeding their newborn. Do both parents get involved in the infant's care? Is the mother depending on someone else to help her at home? Does the mother give excuses ("I am too tired," "My stitches hurt," or "I will learn later") for not wanting to be involved in her baby's care? As the family provides care, the nurse can enhance parental confidence by giving them positive feedback. If the family encounters problems, the nurse can express confidence in the family's abilities to master the new skill or information, suggest alternatives, and serve as a role model. All these considerations need to be taken into account when evaluating the educational needs of the parents.

Several methods may be used to teach parents about newborn care. Daily child care classes are a nonthreatening way to convey general information. Individual instruction is helpful to answer specific questions or to clarify an item that may have been confusing in class (Figure 26–8). See the Self-Care Guide at the back of the book that provides new parents with guidelines on infant care. Both first-time and experienced postpartum mothers rated individual teaching as the most effective method of instruction (Beger & Loveland Cook, 1998). Bordman and Holzman (1996) found that many women pose questions about their baby's care to confirm that they are doing the right thing, not to receive absolute answers. With shorter stays, most teaching unfortunately tends to focus on infant feeding and immediate physical care needs of the mothers, with limited anticipatory guidance provided in other areas (Brown & Johnson, 1998).

> *With the new life come new rhythms. Or perhaps I should say no rhythms. The day is divided into phone calls, meals eaten on the run, visitors who've come to see the baby, trips from hospital to home to walk the dog.*
>
> *The new life brings new thoughts, new perceptions of the world.*
>
> *Why don't men take paternity leave? Why is time off, if any, basically reserved for women? Why don't we take a month off. In those first few chaotic days, filled with ecstasy and fear, the family needs to be together. Being together in times of joy and sadness is what a family is. A month's distance from the office grind, from the bottom line could not help but create a healthier world.*
>
> ~ DENNIS DONZIGER, *DADDY* ~

CLINICAL TIP

You'll find that left-handed people tend to hold the baby over their right shoulder, and right-handed people do the opposite. This keeps the dominant hand free. However, most health personnel wear their name tags on the left side. To avoid scratching the baby's face, wear your name tag on the same side as your dominant hand.

General Instructions for Newborn Care

How to pick up a newborn is one of the first concerns of anyone who has not had experience. The newborn is easily picked up by sliding one hand under the neck and shoulders and the other hand under the buttocks or between the legs, then gently lifting the newborn. This technique provides security and support for the head (which the baby is unable to support until 3 or 4 months of age).

The American Academy of Pediatrics (1997) recommends that healthy term infants be placed on their back or side to decrease the risk of sudden infant death syndrome. The nurse should demonstrate the proper positioning of the newborn and correct use of the bulb syringe. The baby should never be left alone anywhere but in the crib. The mother is reminded that while she and the newborn are together in the birthing unit, she should never leave the baby alone for security reasons and because newborns spit up frequently the first day or two after birth.

Demonstrating a bath, cord care, and temperature assessment is the best way for the nurse to provide information on these topics to parents (see Chapter 32). Parents should be told to call their health care provider if bright red bleeding or pus-like drainage occurs at the cord site or if the area remains unhealed 2 to 3 days after the cord stump has sloughed off. See the Self-Care Guide entitled How to Care for Your Baby's Umbilical Cord at the back of this book.

The nurse demonstrates for the family how to take axillary temperature and discusses the different types of thermometers. It is important that families understand the differences and know how to select the appropriate one. The newborn's temperature needs to be taken only

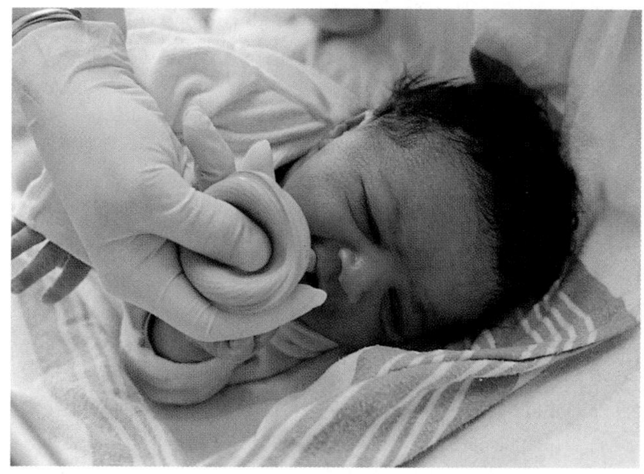

FIGURE 26–9 Nasal and oral suctioning. The bulb is compressed, the tip is placed in either the mouth or the nose, and the bulb is released.

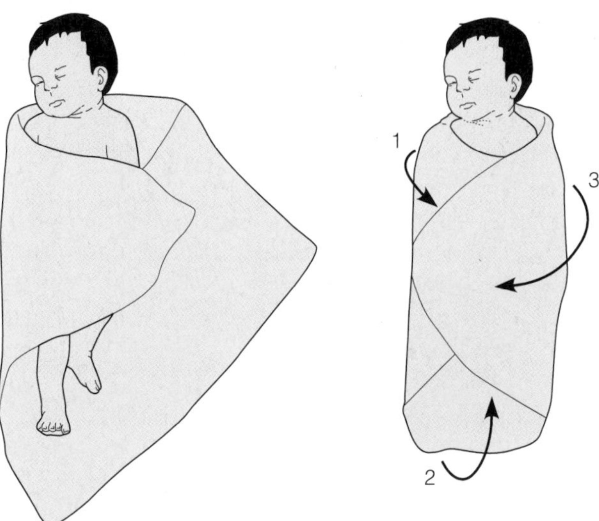

FIGURE 26–10 Steps in wrapping a baby.

when signs of illness are present. Parents are advised to call their physician or pediatric nurse practitioner immediately if any signs of illness become apparent.

Nasal and Oral Suctioning

Most newborns are obligatory nose breathers for the first months of life. They generally maintain air passage patency by coughing or sneezing. During the first few days of life, however, the newborn has increased mucus, and gentle suctioning with a bulb syringe may be indicated. The nurse can demonstrate the use of the bulb syringe in the nose and mouth and have the parents do a return demonstration. The parents should repeat this demonstration before discharge so they will feel more confident and comfortable with the procedure. Care should be taken to apply only gentle suction so nasal bleeding does not occur.

To suction the newborn, the bulb syringe is compressed and the tip is placed in the nostril. The nurse or parent must take care not to occlude the passageway. The bulb is permitted to reexpand slowly by releasing the compression on the bulb (Figure 26–9). The bulb syringe is removed from the nostril, and drainage is then compressed out of the bulb onto a tissue. The bulb syringe may also be used in the mouth if the newborn is spitting up and unable to handle the excess secretions. The bulb is compressed; the tip of the bulb syringe is placed about 1 inch to one side of the newborn's mouth; and compression is released. This draws up the excess secretions. The procedure is repeated on the other side of the mouth. The roof of the mouth and back of the throat are avoided because suction in these areas might stimulate the gag reflex. The bulb syringe should be washed in warm, soapy water and rinsed in warm water daily and as needed after use. A bulb syringe should always be kept near the newborn. New parents and nurses who are inexperienced with babies may fear that the baby will choke and may be relieved if they know how to take action if such an event occurs. They should be advised to turn the newborn's head to the side or down as soon as there is any indication of gagging or vomiting and to use the bulb syringe as needed.

Wrapping the Newborn

Wrapping (swaddling) helps the newborn maintain body temperature, provides a feeling of closeness and security, and may be effective in quieting a crying baby. A blanket is placed on the crib (or secure surface) in the shape of a diamond. The top corner of the blanket is folded down slightly, and the newborn's body is placed with the head at the upper edge of the blanket. The right corner of the blanket is wrapped around the infant and tucked under the left side (not too tightly—newborns need a little room to move). The bottom corner is then pulled up to the chest, and the left corner is wrapped around the baby's right side (Figure 26–10). The nurse can show this wrapping technique to a new mother so she will feel more skilled in handling her baby.

Sleep and Activity

Perhaps nothing is more individual to each baby than the sleep-activity cycle. It is important for the nurse to recognize the individual variations of each newborn and to assist parents as they develop sensitivity to their infant's communication signals and rhythms of activity and sleep. See Chapter 25 for more detailed discussion of sleep-wake activity.

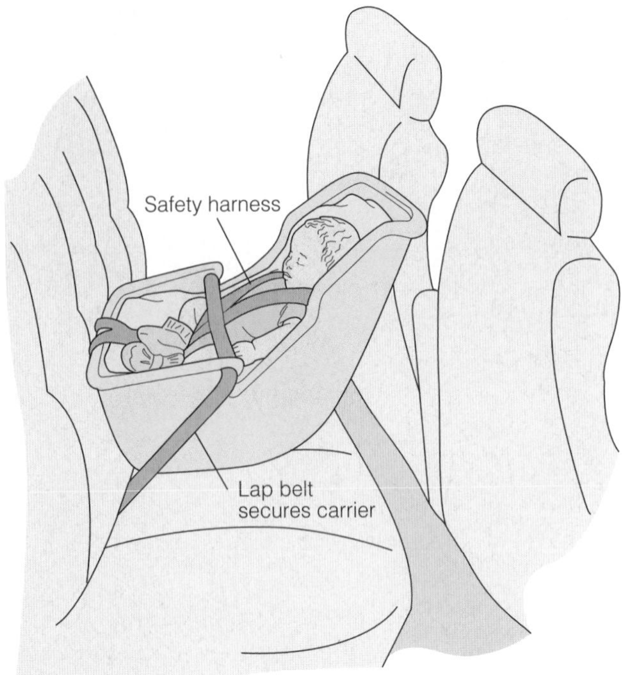

FIGURE 26–11 Infant car restraint for use from birth to about 12 months of age. SOURCE: Mott SR, James SB, Sperhac AM: *Nursing Care of Children and Families,* 2nd ed. Redwood City, CA: Addison-Wesley Nursing, 1990, p 530.

Safety Considerations

Half the children killed or injured in automobile accidents could have been protected by the use of a federally approved car seat. Newborns should go home from the birthing unit in a car seat adapted to fit newborns (Figure 26–11). Babies should never be in the front seat of a car equipped with a passenger-side air bag. The car seat should be placed in the back seat and positioned to face the rear of the car until the baby is a year old or weighs 20 pounds (9.09 kg). In many states, the use of car seats for children up to the age of 4 is mandatory. Nurses need to ensure that all parents are knowledgeable about the benefits of child safety seat use (Block, 1997).

Newborn Screening and Immunization Program

Before the newborn and mother are discharged from the birthing unit, the nurse informs the parents about the **normal screening tests** for newborns and tells them when to return to the birthing center or clinic if further tests are needed. The disorders that can be identified from a drop of blood obtained by a heel stick are cystic fibrosis, galactosemia, homocystinuria, hypothyroidism, maple syrup urine disease, phenylketonuria (PKU), and hemoglobinopathies. Early newborn discharge puts infants at risk for delayed or even missed diagnosis of PKU and congenital hypothyroidism because of decreased sensitivity of screening and should be retested by 2 weeks of

COMMUNITY IN FOCUS

The Stork's Nest

The Stork's Nest is an innovative educational program co-sponsored by the National March of Dimes Birth Defects Foundation and the Zeta Phi Beta, Inc. sorority, an organization of African-American professional women. Designed primarily for low income women of African-American descent, the program provides incentives for women to attend perinatal educational seminars. In addition to the education provided, women earn points for attending a seminar. These points can then be used to shop for baby clothes at a "store" or Stork's Nest located on site. Individual chapters of the March of Dimes can adopt the basic program as designed or modify it based on their community's needs. The two Stork's Nests sponsored by the Northern Ohio Chapter of the March of Dimes are examples of successful program implementation.

The Stork's Nests located in Cleveland and Akron, which began in 1994 and 1997 respectively, truly represent a community partnership. Each Nest is located in a church that serves a predominantly African-American population. The churches provide space for the seminars and for housing the baby clothes, which are actually arranged as though part of a small store. The Zetas, members of the sorority, staff the Stork's Nests, handle logistics on the day of each seminar, keep track of the points each woman earns, and run the store. Clothing is donated by Gymboree, a nationwide chain of children's clothing stores.

The Northern Ohio Chapter of the March of Dimes has developed the seminars using a nationally developed curriculum, and coordinates the volunteer faculty and clothing donations. Seminars, offered monthly on a Saturday, cover a variety of topics such as "Taking care of oneself during pregnancy," "Caring for a newborn," "Exercise during pregnancy," "Nutrition during pregnancy," and so forth. These seminars cover each topic in depth but in a relaxed atmosphere with time for questions and discussion. Seminar leaders, all volunteers, are often nurses from the prenatal clinics and hospitals that serve this population. These classes are not designed to replace preparation for childbirth classes but to supplement them. On average, 25 women participate in a seminar, although some sessions have had as many as 60 participants. Some women come for one or two seminars, others attend the entire series of classes. Many bring their partners for some sessions. Women can continue to participate for up to one year postpartum. Women learn of the Stork's Nest program from a variety of sources including the clinics where they receive prenatal care, through WIC offices, and from friends. Over 1000 women have participated to date.

Partnerships are an important way of addressing community needs. The Stork's Nests are an example of collaboration at its best and meet an important community need.

SOURCE: Personal communication with John G. Ladd, Director of Program Services, March of Dimes Northern Ohio Chapter.

age if the first test was done prior to 24 hours of age (Wallman, 1998).

Immunization programs against the hepatitis B virus during the newborn period and infancy are in place in many states, at least 20 countries, and high-incidence areas such as Alaska and American Samoa. Universal hepatitis B vaccination for all infants, regardless of maternal HB_SAg status, is currently recommended by the Centers for Disease Control and Prevention (CDC) and American Academy of Pediatrics (Woodruff et al, 1996). The current recommendation is that newborns receive the first vaccine dose within 12 hours of birth (0.5 mL of either vaccine preparation) and then a second dose at 1 month of age and the last dose at 6 months of age. See the Drug Guide: Recombinant Hepatitis B Vaccine. Parents need to be advised whether their birthing center provides newborn hepatitis vaccination so that an adequate follow-up program can be set in motion (Zola, Smith, Goldman, & Woodruff, 1997).

Early discharge has affected both the timing of newborn metabolic screening tests and the acquisition of subsequent immunization. For example, the accuracy of the test for PKU is directly related to the newborn's age. The likelihood of detecting PKU increases as the infant grows older; and the infant must be at least 24 hours old for a valid test (Wallman, 1998).

The nurse should teach the family all necessary caregiving methods before discharge. A checklist may be helpful to determine whether the teaching has been completed and to verify the parents' knowledge on leaving the birthing unit (Figure 26–12). The nurse needs to review all areas for understanding or any outstanding questions with the mother and father, without rushing, taking time to answer all queries. Any concerns of the parents or nurse are noted.

CRITICAL THINKING QUESTION

What behaviors would you consider indicative of new parents' readiness for discharge and for the integration of the baby into the family?

Community-Based Nursing Care

By discussing with parents ways to meet their newborns' needs, ensure safety, and appreciate the newborn's unique characteristics and behaviors, and by assisting parents in establishing links with their community-based health care provider, the nurse can get the new family off to a good start. Parents also need to know the signs of illness, how to reach the pediatrician or after-hours clinic, and the importance of follow-up after discharge. See Table 26–4 on page 775. Parents should also check with their clinician for advice about over-the-counter medications to be kept in the medicine cabinet.

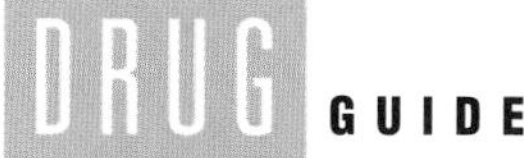

GUIDE

Recombinant Hepatitis B Vaccine

Overview of Neonatal Action

Recombinant Hepatitis B vaccine is used as a prophylactic treatment against all subtypes of hepatitis B virus. It provides passive immunization for newborns of HBsAg negative and HBsAg positive mothers. Hepatitis B can be transmitted across the placenta, but most newborns are infected during birth. It is produced from baker's yeast and plasmid containing the HBsAg gene.

Hepatitis B vaccine contains more than 95% HBsAg protein and is an inactivated (noninfective) product. Universal immunization is recommended.

Infants of HBsAg positive mothers should concurrently receive 0.5 mL of hepatitis B immunoglobulin (HBIG) prophylaxis.

Route, Dosage, Frequency

The first dose of 0.5 mL (10μg) is given intramuscularly into the anterolateral thigh within 12 hours of birth for infants born to HBsAg positive mothers. The second dose of vaccine is given at 1 month of age and followed by a final dose at 6 months of age.

Infants born to HBsAg negative mothers receive their first dose of vaccine at birth, the second dose at 1 to 2 months, and the third dose at 6 to 18 months (American Academy of Pediatrics, 1997).

Infants whose mother's HBsAg status is unknown receive the same doses of vaccine as infants born to HBsAg positive mothers.

Neonatal Side Effects

The only common side effect is soreness at the injection site. Occasionally, there is erythema, swelling, warmth, and induration at the injection site or a low-grade fever.

Nursing Considerations

Delay administration during active infection; the vaccine will not prevent infection during its incubation period.

- The vaccine should be used as supplied. Do not dilute.
- Do not inject intravenously or interdermally.
- Monitor for adverse reactions. Monitor temperature closely.
- Have epinephrine available to treat possible allergic reactions.
- Responsiveness to the vaccine is age dependent. Preterm infants weighing less than 1000 g have lower seroconversion rates. Consider delaying the first dose until the infant is term PCA (postconceptual age) or use a four-dose schedule.

					FOR NURSES ONLY
NURSERY TEACHING CHECKLIST Please read the *Mother/Baby* information booklet given to you after delivery. After reading it, please go through the following list and check whether you understand each topic or need to know more.		I know this already	Doesn't apply to me	I need to know more	Taught/ reviewed/ demonstrated
Baby Care	What to do if baby is choking or gagging				
	Safety				
	How to do skin care/cord care				
	How to take care of the circumcision or genital area				
	How to know if my baby is sick and what to do				
	What is jaundice and how to detect it				
	Use of thermometer				
	Use of bulb syringe				
	How and when to burp baby				
	Newborn behavior: crying/comforting				
	How to position baby after feeding				
	What does demand scheduling mean				
Breastfeeding	I attended breastfeeding class/watched breastfeeding video	YES ☐	NO ☐		
	How to position baby for feeding				
	How to get baby to latch on to my nipple properly				
	When and how long to nurse				
	Removal of baby from my nipple				
	What is the supply and demand concept				
	What is the let down reflex				
	When does breast milk come in				
	Supplementing				
	Proper diet for breastfeeding mothers				
	Prevention and comfort measures for sore nipples				
	Prevention and comfort measures for engorgement				
	When and how to use a breast pump				
	How to express milk by hand				
	How to go back to work and continue to breastfeed				
Bottle Feeding	How to feed my baby a bottle				
	Reasons for NOT propping bottles				
	How to clean nipple/bottle				
	How to mix formula				
	What formula should my baby drink				
	State Law requires use of infant car seat				
	I have a baby/infant car seat and know how to use it	YES ☐	NO ☐		

Other information:

____

____

____

____

____

I have received and understand the instructions given on the above topics.

______________________________ ______________

MOTHER'S SIGNATURE DATE

Videos viewed/ Literature given:

____

____

____

____

Nurse's Signature(s):

____

____

____

FIGURE 26–12 An infant teaching checklist is completed by the time of discharge.
SOURCE: Adapted from Presbyterian/St. Luke's Medical Center, Denver, CO.

TABLE 26–4 When Parents Should Call Their Health Care Provider
Temperature above 38.4C (101F) rectally or 38C (100.4F) axillary or below 36.1C (97F) rectally or 36.6C (97.8F) axillary
Continual rise in temperature
More than one episode of forceful vomiting or frequent vomiting over a 6-hour period
Refusal of two feedings in a row
Lethargy (listlessness), difficulty in awakening baby
Cyanosis with or without a feeding
Absence of breathing longer than 15 seconds
Inconsolable infant (quieting techniques are not effective) or continuous high-pitched cry
Discharge or bleeding from umbilical cord, circumcision, or any opening (except vaginal mucus or pseudomenstruation)
Two consecutive green, watery stools
No wet diapers for 18 to 24 hours or fewer than six to eight wet diapers per day after 4 days of age
Development of eye drainage

The family should have the certified nurse-midwife/nurse practitioner/physician's phone number, address, and any specific instructions. Having the birthing unit or nursery phone number is also reassuring to a newborn's family. They are encouraged to call with questions. Follow-up calls or visits after discharge lend added support by providing another opportunity for parents to have their questions answered. Several programs link the birthing center and the community-based nursing care to better meet the new family's educational and support needs. Programs such as Birth Care Home Advantage, for example, provide a model where experienced birthing/mother-baby nurses are able to meet the family's ongoing education and support needs in the home setting (Mendler, Scallen, Kovtun, Balesky, & Lewis, 1996). Other programs have the birthing unit staff nurses visit new families in their home within a few hours or days of discharge to bridge the gap between early discharge and routine health care checkups (Brown & Johnson, 1998).

To assist parents in caring for their newborn at home, some physicians encourage pediatric prenatal visits so that this contact is established before the birth. Public health nurses have long been involved in newborn care and parent education. Birthing units are now expanding their primary care functions to the new family to include one home visit by the primary nurse who cared for the family in the birthing unit. Some institutions have initiated postpartum visits (PPV) as a solution to early discharge problems for parents where a home visit is not an option. The PPV program offers parents a return visit to the birthing unit within 48 to 72 hours after discharge at no additional charge (Weinberg, 1994). Physical examinations of mother and baby are completed, teaching and emotional support provided, and, if necessary, referrals are made during this visit. Both parents have an opportunity to share how the family is managing at home. A follow-up telephone call is made 2 weeks later.

Routine well-baby visits should be scheduled with the clinic, pediatric nurse practitioner, or physician. One study of a poor and low-income client population identified the following predictors of nonattendance at the first newborn health visit: a multiparous mother, no telephone in the home, and an unmarried teenage mother (Specht & Bourquet, 1994). Although these predictors are easily identified from the baby's record, successful, cost-effective interventions will be more difficult to develop. An assessment of the adequacy of social environment and parenting skills should play an important part in the early discharge decision-making process (Britton et al, 1994).

Education is a wonderful aspect of family-centered maternity care. The nurse who takes the time to get the family off to a good start can feel the satisfaction that optimal care is being provided.

Evaluation

When evaluating the nursing care provided during the newborn period, the nurse may anticipate the following outcomes:

- The newborn baby's adaptation to extrauterine life is supported and complete.
- The baby's physiologic and psychologic integrity is supported.
- The newborn feeding pattern will be satisfactorily established.
- The parents demonstrate safe techniques for caring for their newborn.
- The parents express understanding of the bonding process and display attachment behaviors.
- The parents verbalize developmentally appropriate behavioral expectations of and community-based follow-up care for their newborn.

FOCUS YOUR STUDY

- The overall goal of newborn nursing care is to provide comprehensive care while promoting the establishment of a well-functioning family unit.
- The period immediately following birth, during which adaptation to extrauterine life occurs, requires close monitoring to identify any deviations from normal.
- Nursing goals during the first 4 hours after birth (admission period) are to maintain a clear airway, maintain a neutral thermal environment, prevent hemorrhage and infection, initiate oral feedings, and facilitate attachment.
- The newborn is routinely given prophylactic vitamin K to prevent possible hemorrhagic disease of the newborn.

- Prophylactic eye treatment for *Neisseria gonorrhoeae* is legally required on all newborns.
- Nursing goals in daily newborn care include maintaining cardiopulmonary function, maintaining a neutral thermal environment, promoting adequate hydration and nutrition, preventing complications, promoting safety, and enhancing attachment and family knowledge of child care.
- Essential daily care includes assessing vital signs, weight, overall color, intake, output, umbilical cord and circumcision, newborn nutrition, parent education, and attachment.
- Following a circumcision, the newborn must be observed closely for signs of bleeding, inability to void, and signs of infection.
- Signs of illness in newborns include temperature above 38.4C (101F) or below 36.1C (97F), more than one episode of forceful vomiting, refusal of two feedings in a row, lethargy, cyanosis with or without a feeding, and absence of breathing for longer than 15 seconds.
- Newborn screening for cystic fibrosis, galactosemia, homocystinuria, hypothyroidism, maple syrup urine disease, phenylketonuria, and hemoglobinopathies is done on all newborns in the first 1 to 3 days.

REFERENCES

American Academy of Pediatrics (AAP). (1997). *Guidelines for perinatal care* (4th ed.). Chicago: Author.

American Academy of Pediatrics (AAP). Committee on Fetus and Newborn. (1989). Report of the Ad Hoc Task Force on Circumcision. [Published erratum appears in *Pediatrics, 84*(5), 761 (1989).] *Pediatrics, 84*(2), 388–391.

American Academy of Pediatrics (AAP). Committee on Fetus and Newborn and Committee on Drugs. (1987). Neonatal anesthesia. *Pediatrics, 80*(3), 446.

American Academy of Pediatrics (AAP) Committee on Genetics. (1992). Issues in newborn screening. *Pediatrics, 89*(2), 345–349.

American Academy of Pediatrics Vitamin K Ad Hoc Task Force. (1993). Controversies concerning vitamin K and the newborn. *Pediatrics, 91*(5), 1001–1003.

Andrews, M. M. (1995). Transcultural perspectives in the nursing care of children and adolescents. In M. M. Andrews. & J. S. Boyle (Eds.), *Transcultural concepts in nursing care* (2nd ed. pp 123–179). Philadelphia: Lippincott.

Beger, D., & Loveland Cook, C. A. (1998). Postpartum teaching priorities: The viewpoints of nurses and mothers. *Journal of Obstetric, Gynecologic, and Neonatal Nursing, 27*(2), 161–168.

Bell, T. A., Grayston, J. T., Krohn, M. A., & Kronmal, R. A. (1993). Randomized trial of silver nitrate, erythromycin, and no eye prophylaxis for the prevention of conjunctivitis among newborns not at risk for gonococcal ophthalmitis. *Pediatrics, 92*(6), 755–760.

Block, D. (1997). Child safety seat use in a midwestern Hmong community. *American Journal of Maternal Child Nursing, 22,* 304–307.

Bordman, H. B., & Holzman, U. R. (1996). Infant care knowledge of primiparous urban mothers. *Journal of Perinatology, 16*(2 Pt. 1), 107–110.

Britton, J. R., Britton, H. L., & Beebe, S. A. (1994). Early discharge of the term newborn: A continued dilemma. *Pediatrics, 94*(3), 291–295.

Brown, S. G., & Johnson, B. T. (1998). Enhancing early discharge with home follow-up: A pilot project. *Journal of Obstetric, Gynecologic, and Neonatal Nursing, 27*(1), 33–38.

Centers for Disease Control and Prevention. (1996, May 31). Prevention of perinatal group B streptococcal disease: A public health perspective [published erratum appears in *MMWR (Morbidity & Mortality Weekly Report), 45*(31), 679. (1996, August 9).]. *MMWR (Morbidity & Mortality Weekly Report), 45*(RR-7), 1–24.

Cunningham, F. G., MacDonald, P. C., Gant, N. F., Leveno, K. J., Gilstrap, L. C. III, Hankins, G. D. V., & Clark, S. L. (1997). *Williams obstetrics* (20th ed.). Stamford, CT: Appleton & Lange.

Field, T. (1992, Oct./Nov.). Infant massage. *Zero to Three,* 8.

Hutchinson, M. K., & Baqi-Aziz, M. (1994). Nursing care of the childbearing Muslim family. *Journal of Obstetric, Gynecologic, and Neonatal Nursing, 23*(9), 767–771.

Klaus, M., & Klaus, P. (1985). *The amazing newborn.* Menlo Park, CA: Addison-Wesley.

L'Archevesque, C. I., & Goldstein-Lohman, H. (1996). Ritual circumcision: Educating parents. *Pediatric Nursing, 22*(3), 228, 230–234.

Mendler, V. M., Scallen, D. J., Kovtun, L. A., Balesky, J., & Lewis, C. (1996). The conception, birth, and infancy of an early discharge program. *American Journal of Maternal Child Nursing, 21*(5), 241–246.

Merestein, G. B., & Gardner, S. L. (1998). *Handbook of neonatal intensive care* (4th ed.). St. Louis: Mosby.

Narchi, H., & Kulaylat, N. (1998). Neonatal circumcision: When can infants reliably be expected to void? *Pediatrics, 102*(1) 150–152.

Neonatal Skin Care. (1992, Jan.). *NAACOG-OGN Nursing Practice Resource.*

Neonatal Thermoregulation. (1997). In *NANN guidelines for practice.*

O'Grady, J. P. (1996). Circumcision: Ritual and surgery. In J. J. Sciarra, & T. J. Watkins (Eds.), *Gynecology and obstetrics* (Vol. 2). Philadelphia: Harper & Row.

Penny-MacGillivray, T. (1996). A newborn's first bath: When? *Journal of Obstetric, Gynecologic, and Neonatal Nursing, 25*(6), 481–487.

Perlmutter, D. F., Lawrence, J. M., Krauss, A. N., & Auld, P. A. (1995). Voiding after neonatal circumcision. *Pediatrics, 96*(6), 1111–1112.

Rasbridge, L. A., & Kulig, J. C. (1995). Infant feeding among Cambodian refugees. *MCN; American Journal of Maternal Child Nursing, 20*(4), 213–218.

Reynolds, R. D. (1996). Use of the Mogen clamp for neonatal circumcision. *American Family Physician, 54*(1), 177–182.

Riordan, J., & Auerbach, K. G. (1999). *Breastfeeding and human lactation.* (2nd ed.). Boston: Jones & Bartlett.

Schneiderman, J. U. (1996). Postpartum nursing for Korean mothers. *MCN; American Journal of Maternal Child Nursing, 21*(3), 155–158.

Specht, E. M., & Bourquet, C. C. (1994). Predictors of nonattendance at the first newborn health supervision visit. *Clinical Pediatrics, 33*(5), 273–279.

Tappero, E. P., & Honeyfield, M. E. (1996). *Physical assessment of the newborn* (2nd ed.). Petaluma, CA: NICU Ink.

Wallman, C. M. (1998). Newborn genetic screening. *Neonatal Network, 17*,(3), 55–60.

Weinberg, S. H. (1994). An alternative to meet the needs of early discharge: The tender beginnings postpartum visit. *MCN; American Journal of Maternal Child Nursing, 19*(6), 339–342.

Williamson, M. L. (1997). Circumcision anesthesia: A study of nursing implications for dorsal penile nerve block. *Pediatric Nursing, 23*(1), 59–63.

Woodruff, B. A., Stevenson, J., Yusuf, H., Kwong, S. L., Todoroff, K. P., Hadler, J. L., Hoyt, M. A., & Mahoney, F. J. (1996). Progress toward integrating hepatitis B vaccine into routine infant immunization schedules in the United States, 1991 through 1994. *Pediatrics, 97*(6 Pt. 1), 798–803.

Zola, J., Smith, N., Goldman, S., & Woodruff, B. A. (1997). Attitudes and educational practices of obstetric providers regarding infant hepatitis B vaccination. *Obstetrics and Gynecology, 89*(1), 61–64.

27 Newborn Nutrition

Key Terms

Colostrum
Foremilk
Hindmilk
La Leche League
Let-down reflex
Mature milk
Milk/plasma ratio
Oxytocin
Prolactin
Transitional milk
Weaning

I HAD BEEN TOLD THAT MOST BABIES ATE EVERY three or four hours and slept the rest of the time. Not mine! She wanted to nurse every two hours, and sometimes more often than that. Sometimes she would sleep for an hour, sometimes for fifteen minutes. I loved her, but I also felt consumed by her needs. It was hard to adjust to the fact that I couldn't get anything finished, whether it was an article I was reading or folding the laundry. At the end of the day I would realize I hadn't accomplished anything. Once I accepted the fact that I was not going to function at my old efficient rate (at least for a while) and stopped feeling guilty about what I wasn't getting done, I felt free to enjoy the time I was spending with my baby.

~ *The New Our Bodies, Ourselves* ~

Objectives

- Compare the nutritional value and composition of breast milk and formula preparations.
- Discuss the advantages and disadvantages of breastfeeding and formula-feeding for both mother and newborn.
- Develop guidelines for helping both breastfeeding and bottle-feeding mothers to feed their infants successfully.
- Delineate nursing responsibilities for client teaching about problems the breastfeeding mother may encounter at home.
- Describe an appropriate process for weaning an infant from breastfeeding.
- Incorporate knowledge of newborn nutrition and normal growth patterns into parent education and infant assessment.
- Recognize the influence of cultural values on infant care, especially feeding practices.

FEEDING THEIR NEWBORN IS AN EXCITING, satisfying, and often worrisome task for parents. Meeting this essential need of their new child helps parents strengthen their attachment to their baby and fosters their self-images as nurturers and providers. Whether a woman chooses to breastfeed or bottle-feed, she can be reassured that she can adequately meet her infant's needs. As questions arise about feeding, the nurse works with the woman to help her develop skill in her chosen method. In every interaction it is the nurse's responsibility to support the parents and promote the family's sense of confidence.

Nutritional Needs of the Newborn

The newborn's diet must supply nutrients to meet the rapid rate of physical and mental growth and development. A neonatal diet should provide adequate calories and include protein, carbohydrate, fat, water, vitamins, and minerals. The recommended dietary allowances (RDAs) for birth through the first 6 months have been established.

The calories (105 to 108 kcal/kg/day or 50 to 55 kcal/lb/day) in the newborn's diet are divided among protein, carbohydrate, and fat. Protein is needed for rapid cellular growth and maintenance. Carbohydrates provide energy. The fat portion of the diet provides calories, regulates fluid and electrolyte balance, and is necessary for the normal development of the neonatal brain and neurologic system.

Water requirements are high (140 to 160 mL/kg/day or 64 to 73 mL/lb/day) because of the newborn's inability to concentrate urine. Fluid needs are further increased in illness or hot weather.

The infant's iron needs will be affected by the accumulation of iron stores during the fetal life and by the mother's iron and other food intake if she is breastfeeding. Ascorbic acid (usually in the form of fruit or fruit juices) and meat, poultry, and fish are known to enhance absorption of iron in the mother just as it does later in the infant. Adequate minerals and vitamins are needed by the newborn to prevent deficiency states such as scurvy, cheilosis, and pellagra.

Formula-fed babies do gain weight faster than breastfed babies because of the higher protein content in commercially prepared formula and the larger volumes of formula that are needed to obtain the necessary nutrients. (Because breast milk is digested more easily than formula, the nutrients are more readily available.) Bottle-fed infants tend to regain their birth weight by 10 days after birth and may gain as much as 30 g (1 oz) per day up to 6 months of age. Healthy breastfed babies, however, tend to regain their birth weight about 14 days after birth and gain approximately 15 g (0.5 oz) per day in the first 6 months of life. Formula-fed infants generally double their weight in 3.5 to 4 months, whereas nursing infants double their weight at about 5 months of age.

Breast Milk

The composition of human milk varies with the stage of lactation, the time of day, the time during the feeding, maternal nutrition, and gestational age of the newborn at birth. During the establishment of lactation there are three stages of human milk: colostrum, transitional milk, and mature milk.

Colostrum is a yellowish or creamy-appearing fluid that is thicker than later milk and contains more protein, fat-soluble vitamins, and minerals (Wagner, Anderson, & Pittard, 1996). It also contains high levels of immunoglobulins (antibodies, such as IgA) and can be a source of passive immunity for the newborn. Colostrum production begins early in pregnancy and may last for several days after birth. However, in most cases colostrum is replaced by transitional milk within 2 to 4 days after birth.

Transitional milk is produced from the end of colostrum production until approximately 2 weeks postpartum. This milk contains more fat, lactose, water-soluble vitamins, and calories than colostrum contains.

The final milk produced, **mature milk,** contains about 10% solids (carbohydrates, proteins, fats) for energy and growth; the rest is water, which is vital for maintaining hydration. The composition of mature milk varies according to the time during the feeding. **Foremilk** is the milk obtained at the beginning of the feeding. It is high in water content and contains vitamins and protein. **Hindmilk** is released after the initial let-down, or release of milk, and has higher fat concentration.

Although mature milk appears similar to skim milk (watery and somewhat bluish in color) and may cause mothers to question whether their milk is "rich enough," mature breast milk provides 20 kcal/oz, as do most prepared formulas. However, the percentage of calories derived from protein is lower in breast milk than in formulas, and a greater proportion of calories is derived from fat (P. B. Lawrence, 1994). In breastfed babies, protein metabolism produces less nitrogen waste, which has a positive effect on the infant's immature renal system.

The American Academy of Pediatrics (AAP) and American College of Obstetricians and Gynecologists (AGOG) (1997) recommended breast milk as the optimal food for the first 6 to 12 months of life. It is believed that breastfeeding provides newborns and infants with specific immunologic, nutritional, and psychosocial advantages.

Immunologic Advantages

Immunologic advantages include varying degrees of protection from respiratory and gastrointestinal infections, otitis media, meningitis, sepsis, and allergies (AAP, 1997). This protection provides coverage for the breastfed baby during the neonatal period until the baby's own immunoglobulins become active by 18 months of age.

Secretory IgA, an immunoglobulin present in colostrum and breast milk, has antiviral, antibacterial, and antigenic-inhibiting properties. Secretory IgA plays a role in decreasing the permeability of the small intestine to antigenic macromolecules (Xanthou, 1998). Other properties in colostrum and breast milk that act to inhibit the growth of bacteria or viruses are *Lactobacillus bifidus*, lysozymes, lactoperoxidase, lactoferrin, transferrin, and various immunoglobulins. Immunoglobulins to the poliomyelitis virus are also present in the breast milk of mothers who have immunity to this virus. Because the presence of these immunoglobulins may inhibit the desired intestinal infection and immune response of the infant, some clinics suggest that breastfeedings be withheld for 30 to 60 minutes following the administration of the Sabin oral polio vaccine. In addition to its immunologic properties, breast milk is known to be nonallergenic.

Nutritional Advantages

Breast milk is composed of lactose, lipids, polyunsaturated fatty acids, and amino acids, especially taurine, and has a whey:casein protein ratio that facilitates its digestion, absorption, and full use compared to formulas (Xanthou, 1998). Some researchers contend that the high concentration of cholesterol and the balance of amino acids in breast milk make it the best food for myelination and neurologic development. High cholesterol levels in breast milk may stimulate the production of enzymes that lead to more efficient metabolism of cholesterol, thereby reducing its harmful long-term effects on the cardiovascular system (P. B. Lawrence, 1994).

Human milk is also considered the ideal first food because its composition varies according to gestational age and stage of lactation. For example, the milk of a preterm mother has more long-chain polyunsaturated fatty acids (LC-PUFA) than mothers of full-term babies. LC-PUFA are essential for brain growth (McVeagh & Brand Miller, 1997), and preterm infants are born with very low LC-PUFA reserves.

Breast milk provides newborns with minerals in more appropriate doses than do formulas (R. A. Lawrence, 1994). The iron found in breast milk, even though much lower in concentration than that of prepared formulas, is much more readily and fully absorbed and appears sufficient to meet the infant's iron needs for the first 4 to 6 months. The American Academy of Pediatrics (1997) states that there is generally no need to give supplemental iron to full-term breastfed newborns before the age of 6 months. Furthermore, supplemental iron may decrease the ability of breast milk to protect the newborn by interfering with lactoferrin, an iron-binding protein that enhances the absorption of iron and has anti-infective properties.

Another advantage of breast milk is that all its components are delivered to the infant in an unchanged form, and vitamins are not lost through processing and heating. If the breastfeeding mother is taking daily multivitamins and her diet is adequate, the only supplements the infant will need until after the age of 6 months are vitamin D and fluoride (American Academy of Pediatrics [AAP], 1997). If the mother's diet or vitamin intake is inadequate or questionable, caregivers may choose to prescribe additional vitamins for the infant.

Psychosocial Advantages

Psychophysiologic reactions during nursing have been shown to affect maternal-infant attachment. The mother's level of oxytocin generally increases with breastfeeding, and studies indicate that this hormonal change coincides with more even mood responses and increased feelings of maternal well-being (Rogers, Golding & Emmett, 1997).

Breastfeeding enhances attachment by providing the opportunity for frequent, direct skin contact between the newborn and the mother. The newborn's sense of touch is highly developed at birth and is a primary means of communication. The tactile stimulation associated with breastfeeding can communicate warmth, closeness, and comfort. The increased closeness provides both newborn and mother with the opportunity to learn each other's behavioral cues and needs. The mother's sense of accomplishment in being able to satisfy her baby's needs for nourishment and comfort is enhanced when the newborn suckles vigorously and is satiated and calmed by the breastfeeding. Some mothers prefer breastfeeding as a means of extending the close, unique, nourishing relationship between mother and baby that existed prior to birth.

In the event of a twin birth, breastfeeding not only is possible but also enhances the mother's individualization and attachment to each newborn. The fantasized single baby is replaced more readily with the reality of two individual babies when the mother has close and frequent contact with each. Fathers can also be actively involved with the feeding experience by offering fresh pumped or thawed (frozen) breast milk to the baby at one or more feedings daily.

Contraindications and Disadvantages

There are some medical contraindications to breastfeeding. A mother with a diagnosis of breast cancer should not breastfeed so that she may begin treatment immediately. With regard to AIDS, the recommendation is to counsel the mother against breastfeeding except in a country where the risk of neonatal death from diarrhea and other disease (excluding AIDS) is high (Golding, 1997). Breastfeeding is also contraindicated for the infant suffering from galactosemia (AAP, 1997).

Maternal medications may preclude breastfeeding, as discussed in Chapters 15 and 28. Medications such as metronidazole (Flagyl) used to treat trichomoniasis pass into breast milk and may be harmful to the breastfeeding infant (Banta-Wright, 1997). Management of jaundice in the newborn may include suspension of breastfeeding (see Chapter 29).

In the dominant Western culture, where women actively pursue activities outside the home, being "tied down" to an infant for 9 to 12 feedings every day may be considered inconvenient and stressful. Another often cited disadvantage of breastfeeding is exclusion of the father from the nurturing involved in feeding the infant. But because nurturing encompasses more than just feeding, the father can comfort and attend to the baby in many other ways (Figure 27–1).

Opinion varies as to the advisability of continuing breastfeeding in the event of another pregnancy. Some feel the nutritional demands on the pregnant mother are too great and advocate gradual weaning. Others suggest that with adequate rest, a proper diet, and strong emotional support, continued breastfeeding during pregnancy is a valid choice. The practice of nursing one infant throughout pregnancy and then breastfeeding both infants after birth is called *tandem nursing.* When pregnancy occurs, the decision of how to handle nursing is best made on an individual basis after considering maternal health and motivation and the age of the first child.

Even though many mothers obtain information about breastfeeding from written sources, family and friends, and the **La Leche League** (an international breastfeeding support and information group), the nurse needs to be a ready source of information, encouragement, and support, as well. The nurse can be helpful when parents are deciding whether to breastfeed, after birth when breastfeedings are just being established, and after the family returns home.

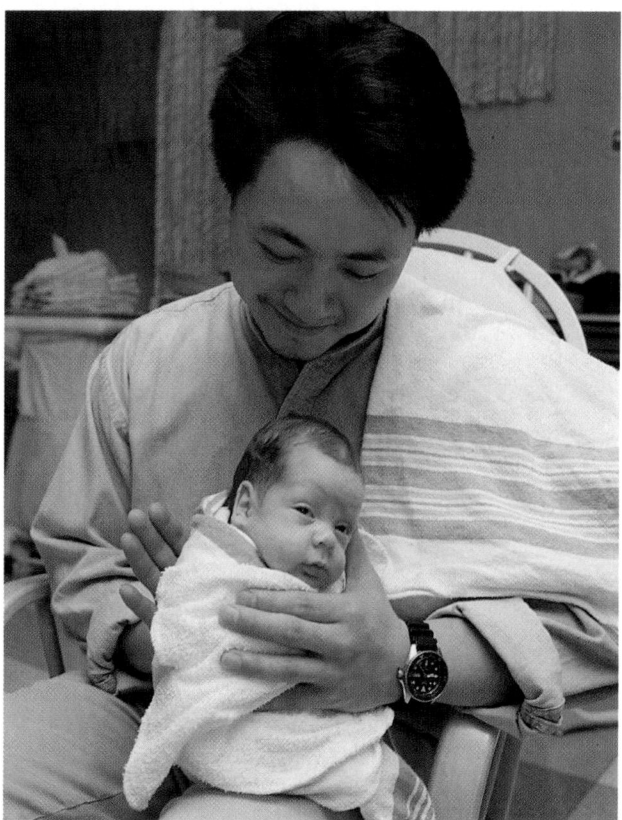

FIGURE 27–1 A father can nurture his baby in many ways.

Formula Feeding

Although breastfeeding is increasing in popularity, formula-feeding continues to be a nurturing choice, particularly in developed countries, and meets the goal of successful growth of the baby. The closeness and warmth that can occur during breastfeeding is also an integral part of bottle-feeding. An advantage of bottle-feeding is that parents can share equally in this nurturing, caring experience with their baby. Numerous types of commercially prepared lactose formulas meet the nutritional needs of the infant. These formulas contain tyrosine and phenylalanine and less taurine than breast milk does.

Because many commercial formulas use a cow's milk base, they tend to have a higher renal solute load, high protein and casein content, high proportion of saturated fats, low amounts of linoleic acid, poorer mineral bioavailablity, and increased risk for allergy to cow's milk proteins (Tigges, 1997). Commercial formulas have been developed to minimize the harmful components of cow's milk. The formulas have been enriched with carnitine and/or taurine; some of them with long-chain polyunsaturated fatty acids; all of them with vitamins and, in particular, with vitamin D (Piacentini, Boner, Richelli, & Gaburro, 1995).

There are three categories of infant formulas: formulas with cow's milk base, soy protein–based formulas, and specialized or therapeutic formulas. The specialized formulas are categorized as casein-hydrolysated or whey-hydrolysated formulas. Some of the common cow's milk–based formulas are Similac, Enfamil, and Gerber. These formulas contain nonfat cow's milk, demineralized whey, vegetable oils to replace butterfat, and carbohydrates in the form of lactose to increase the percentage of carbohydrate calories.

Soy protein–based formulas (eg, Isomil, Prosobee, Gerber Soy) substitute soy protein supplemented with methionine for cow's milk protein. Carbohydrates are in the form of glucose polymers and/or sucrose, and vegetable oils provide calories from fat. Soy formulas are used for primary lactase deficiency or galactosemia conditions. The AAP recommends hydrolysated formulas for infants with allergy or intolerance to cow's milk protein to avoid risk of concomitant allergy to soy protein (Tigges, 1997). Specialized formulas such as casein-hydrolysated formulas (eg, Nutramigen, Pregestimil, Alimentum) are used when an infant has an allergy or intolerance to cow's milk protein. Casein hydrolysate is essentially a "predigested" protein that presents protein fragments too small to be recognized by the infant's immune system as an antigen, thereby decreasing the baby's allergic response. Corn syrup products and corn, soy, and

TABLE 27–1 Comparison of Breastfeeding and Bottle-Feeding

Breast	Bottle (Feeding Iron-Enriched Formula)
Nutrition	
Breast milk is species specific (ie, perfect balance of proteins, carbohydrates, fats, vitamins, and minerals for human infants).	Formula is as close to human milk as possible, but nutrients are not as efficiently utilized.
Breast milk contains higher levels of lactose, cystine, and cholesterol, which are necessary for brain and nerve growth.	Nutritional adequacy depends on proper preparation (overdilution results in decreased nutrients delivered to infant).
Proteins are easily digested and fats are well absorbed.	Some babies cannot tolerate the fats or carbohydrates found in regular formula. Companies offer alternative formulas.
Composition varies according to gestational age and stage of lactation, thereby meeting the changing nutritional requirements of individual infants as they grow.	
Infants determine the volume of milk consumed.	Pediatrician or caregiver determines the volume consumed. Overfeeding may occur if caregiver is determined that baby empty bottle.
Frequency of feeding is determined by infant cues.	Feeding is determined by infant's cues.
Anti-Infective and Antiallergic Properties	
Breast milk contains immunoglobulins, enzymes, and leukocytes that protect against pathogens.	Formula is linked to an increased number of GI and respiratory infections.
Bacteriostatic properties permit storage at room temperature up to 6 hours, in refrigerator for 24 hours, and freezing for 6 months.	Potential for bacterial contamination exists during preparation and storage.
Breast milk decreases the incidence of allergy by eliminating exposure to potential antigens (cow and soy protein).	Some babies are allergic to cow or soy protein. Formula companies are offering alternative formulas suitable for babies who develop allergies.
Psychosocial Aspects	
Skin-to-skin contact enhances closeness.	Bottle-feeding provides an opportunity for positive parent-infant interaction.
Hormones of lactation promote maternal feelings and sense of well-being.	
The value system of an industrial society can create barriers to successful breastfeeding: Mother may feel ashamed or embarrassed. Breastfeeding after return to work may be difficult.	
Father is not able to breastfeed, but he can feed expressed breast milk from a bottle and nurture the infant in ways other than feeding.	Father can feed the baby.
Cost	
Healthy diet for mother.	Formula is an expense.
Optional, but recommended, items include nursing pads, nursing bras.	Bottles or disposable nursers with plastic liners, nipples, and nipple caps must be purchased.
A breast pump may be needed.	
Refrigeration is necessary for storing expressed milk.	A refrigeration system is necessary if mixing formula for more than one feeding at a time or using large containers of ready-to-feed formula.
Convenience	
The milk is always the perfect temperature.	Varying amounts of time are involved in formula preparation.
No preparation time is needed.	Anyone can feed the baby.
The mother must be available to feed or provide expressed milk to be given in her absence.	
If she misses a feeding, the mother must express milk to maintain lactation.	
The mother may experience slight discomfort in the early days of lactation.	
Maternal medication may interrupt breastfeeding.	

coconut oils serve as substitute carbohydrate and fat sources for babies with carbohydrate intolerance or fat malabsorption. Whey-hydrolysated formulas, such as Carnation Good Start, can also be used with cow's milk allergy but not if the child has an IgE-mediated allergy to cow's milk. Whey-hydrolysated formulas are less expensive than casein-hydrolystated formulas (Tigges, 1997).

Potential Contraindications

If formula is prepared improperly (such as by adding excessive powder), the excess salts (ie, sodium) may be detrimental to the newborn's immature kidneys and may lead to thirst in the formula-fed infant, causing overfeeding. If formula is overdiluted, the infant will not receive adequate nutrients.

Another potential problem with cow's milk–based formulas is an allergic reaction in the newborn. The small intestine of the infant is permeable to macromolecules such as those found in some cow's milk–based formulas. The introduction of these foreign proteins in formula may cause an allergic reaction, with signs such as vomiting, colic, diarrhea, colitis, reluctance to feed, and eczema (Table 27–1).

Clinicians recommend that parents who are bottle-feeding use iron-fortified formulas or supplements because iron deficiency anemia still occurs. The RDA for iron is 6 mg per day from birth to 6 months. However, the nurse must be aware that too much iron in the form of iron-fortified cereal may interfere with the infant's natural ability to defend against disease. Many companies make enriched formulas that are similar to breast milk. These formulas have sufficient levels of carbohydrate, protein, fat, vitamins, and minerals to meet the newborn's nutritional needs.

The AAP (1997) has recommended that infants be given breast milk or iron-fortified formula rather than whole milk until 1 year of age. Neither unmodified cow's milk (ie, whole milk) nor skim milk is an acceptable alternative for newborn feeding. The levels of protein in cow's milk is much higher (50% to 75% greater) than in human milk, is poorly digested, and may cause bleeding of the gastrointestinal tract. It also has higher levels of calcium, phosphorus, sodium, and potassium, which increase the renal solute load and result in greater obligatory water loss. Skim milk lacks adequate calories, fat content, and essential fatty acids necessary for proper development of the neonate's neurologic system. Nutritionists advise against use of whole milk, cow's milk with decreased fat content (2% milk), or skim milk for children under 2 years of age.

RESEARCH IN PRACTICE

What is this study about? Although infant irritability is not associated with serious disease, the behavior of these infants is often disturbing to nurses and families. Colic or idiopathic infant irritability is unique in that no cause has been established for this disease that affects one in four infants. The purpose of this study was to identify newborn behaviors that may predict infant irritability commonly referred to as colic.

How was this study done? This prospective, correlational study was conducted in a private hospital of a large metropolitan city. Sixty infants who were low risk and full term and whose weight loss was appropriate for gestational age were recruited as subjects during their postpartum stay in a level I nursery. Infants with congenital anomalies, signs of illness, or high-risk factors were excluded from the study. During the infants' one to four day stay, their crying was assessed and reported by their nurses and a neonatal behavior scale was completed on each infant. At one month of age irritability scores were assessed using the fussiness rating scale.

What were the results of the study? The cluster of variables for the neonatal behavioral scale representing motor activity and supplemental items measuring the persistence necessary on the part of the examiner to get the infant to attend to stimuli were significantly related to the newborns' development of colic or irritability at one month of age. The infants classified as irritable at one month of age by the parents were described as more active and attentive to stimuli in the first few days of life. The infants' cries as rated by the nurses were not related to the infants' later development of colic.

What additional questions might I have? (1) What part does the neonate's environment play in the development of colic as an infant and (2) are certain stimui within the neonates environment more predictive of later development of colic or is it the infant's activity and attentiveness early on that are the true predictors of colic?

How can I use this study? Little is known about the factors that predispose neonates to the development of colic. In this study, newborn infants with high motor activity and attentiveness to stimuli went on to develop colic. These factors may indeed be predictors of colic and should be assessed in all newborns. Further research into behavior and human interaction cues as well as environmental factors that contribute to the development of colic are needed.

SOURCE: Keefe, M., Foese-Frietz, A., & Kotzer, A. (1998). Newborn predictors of infant irritability. *JOGNN, 27*(5), 513–520.

Newborn Feeding

Initial Feeding

The timing of the first feeding is determined by the physiologic and behavioral cues of the newborn. The nurse should assess for active bowel sounds, absence of abdominal distention, and a lusty cry that quiets and is replaced with rooting and sucking behaviors when a stimulus is placed near the lips. These signs are indicators that the newborn is hungry and physically ready to tolerate the feeding.

The first feeding provides an opportunity for the nurse to assess the effectiveness of the newborn's suck, swallow, and gag reflexes. The mother who plans to breastfeed should be encouraged to nurse her newborn immediately following birth, allowing the baby to nurse to satiety. Because colostrum is not irritating if aspirated (which may occur because of the newborn's initially uncoordinated sucking and swallowing abilities) and is readily absorbed by the respiratory system, breastfeeding can usually begin immediately after birth. Contraindications to immediate nursing include heavy sedation of the mother and physical compromise of either mother or baby. Bottle-feeding newborns are offered formula as soon as they show an interest.

Early feedings benefit the breastfeeding pair because oxytocin helps expel the placenta and prevent excessive maternal blood loss, lactation is accelerated, and the infant receives the immunologic protection of colostrum. For both breastfed and formula-fed infants, early feedings stimulate peristalsis, facilitating elimination of the by-products of bilirubin conjugation, which decreases the risk of jaundice, and enhances maternal-infant attachment.

TABLE 27–2 Infant Feeding Behaviors

Age	Hunger Behavior	Feeding Behavior	Satiety Behavior
Birth to 13 weeks (0–3 months)	Cries; hands fisted; body tense	Rooting reflex; medial lip closure; strong suck reflex; suck-swallow pattern; tongue thrust and retraction; palmomental reflex, gags easily, needs burping	Withdraws head from nipple; falls asleep; hands relaxed; relief of body tension
14–24 weeks (4–6 months)	Eagerly anticipates; grasps and draws bottle or breast to mouth; reaches with open mouth	Aware of hands; generalized reaching; intentional hand to mouth; tongue elevation; lips purse at corners—pucker; shifts food in mouth—prechewing; tongue protrudes in anticipation of nipple; tongue holds nipple firm; tongue projection strong; suck strength increases; coughs and chokes easily; preference for tastes	Tosses head back; fusses or cries; covers mouth with hands; ejects food; distracted by surroundings

SOURCE: Mott S et al: *Nursing Care of Children and Families,* 2nd ed. Redwood City, CA: Addison-Wesley Nursing, 1990, p 155.

Throughout the first 2 hours after birth, but especially during the first 20 to 30 minutes, the infant is usually alert and ready to nurse. However, newborn suckling patterns vary, and although many babies are eager to suckle at this time, many will simply lick or nuzzle the nipple. This behavior is beneficial because the licking stimulates the release of oxytocin, which aids uterine involution and lactation (let-down). The mother should be encouraged to interpret this as a positive breastfeeding interaction (Riordan & Auerbach, 1999).

Assessment of the newborn's physiologic status is of primary and ongoing concern to the nurse throughout the first feeding. Extreme fatigue coupled with rapid respiration, circumoral cyanosis, and diaphoresis of the head and face may indicate cardiovascular complications and should be assessed further. The initial feeding also requires assessment of the infant for rare congenital anomalies such as tracheoesophageal fistula and esophageal atresia (Chapter 28). Findings associated with esophageal anomalies include maternal polyhydramnios and increased oral mucus in the infant. In cases of esophageal atresia, the feeding is taken well initially, but as the esophageal pouch fills, the feeding is quickly regurgitated unchanged by stomach contents. If a fistula is present, the infant gags, chokes, regurgitates mucus, and may become cyanotic as fluid passes through the fistula into the lungs.

It is not unusual for the newborn to regurgitate some mucus, water, or colostrum following a feeding, even if it was taken without difficulty. Consequently, the newborn is observed closely and positioned on the right side after a feeding to aid drainage and facilitate gastric emptying.

Establishing a Feeding Pattern

An "on demand" feeding program facilitates each baby's own rhythm and assists a new mother in establishing lactation. The newborn rapidly digests breast milk and may desire to nurse eight to ten times in a 24-hour period. After the initial period of alertness and eagerness to suckle, the infant progresses to light sleep, then deep sleep, followed by increased wakefulness and interest in nursing. As wakefulness and interest in nursing increase, the infant will often cluster five to ten feeding episodes over 2 to 3 hours, followed by a 4- to 5-hour deep sleep. After this cluster of minifeeds and deep sleep, the infant will feed frequently, but at more regular intervals. Maternal medications received during labor may affect newborn feeding behavior by delaying these early cluster feedings. Delays in normal feeding patterns depend on the specific drug and its half-life. Newborns whose mothers received epidural analgesia have been noted to be irritable and demonstrate reduced motor organization, poor self-quieting skills, and decreased visual skills and alertness (Riordan & Auerbach, 1999).

Couplet care permits the mother to learn about and respond to her infant's early feeding cues. Early cues that indicate a newborn is interested in feeding include hand-to-mouth or hand-passing-mouth motion, whimpering, sucking, and rooting (Mulford, 1992). Crying is a late sign of hunger. When couplet care is not available, a supportive nursing staff and flexible nursery policies allow the mother to feed her infant on cue. It is very frustrating to a new mother to attempt to feed a newborn who is sound asleep because he or she is either not hungry or exhausted from crying. Table 27–2 can be used to help parents identify their baby's cues for hunger and satiation.

Although society accepts crying as normal and healthy behavior for newborns, it may actually delay the transition to extrauterine life. Crying involves a Valsalva maneuver that results in increased pulmonary vascular pressure, which may cause unoxygenated blood to be shunted into systemic circulation through the foramen ovale and ductus arteriosus. Therefore, it may be advantageous for the baby to be in the room with the mother because she will respond to the baby's needs more quickly than the nursery staff may be able to, resulting in less infant crying.

Formula-fed newborns may awaken for feedings every 2 to 5 hours but are frequently satisfied with feedings every 3 to 4 hours. Because formula is digested more slowly, the bottle-fed infant may go longer between feedings but should not go longer than 4 hours. Babies may begin skipping the night feeding at about 8 to 12 weeks of age (Riordan & Auerbach, 1999). This is very individualized, depending on the infant's size and development.

Both breastfed and bottle-fed infants experience growth spurts at certain times and required increased feeding. The mother of a breastfed infant will meet these increased demands by nursing more frequently to increase her milk supply. It will take about 24 hours for the milk supply to increase adequately to meet the new demand (R. A. Lawrence, 1994). A slight increase in the amount of formula given at each feeding will meet the needs of the formula-fed infant.

Providing nourishment for her newborn is a major concern for the new mother. Her feelings of success or failure may influence her self-concept as she assumes her maternal role. With proper instruction, support, and encouragement from health care providers, feeding becomes a source of pleasure and satisfaction to both parents and infant.

Community-Based Nursing Care

Promotion of Successful Infant Feeding

Parents may see the task of feeding their baby as the center of their relationship with the new family member. Whether the mother has chosen to bottle-feed or breastfeed, the nurse can help the mother have a successful experience while in the birthing center and during the early days at home. Feeding and caring for newborns may be routine tasks for the nurse, but the success or lack of success that a mother achieves the first few times may determine her feelings about herself as an adequate mother.

The newborn's response to caring is an expression of personality but often has great significance for parents. A parent may interpret the newborn's behavior as rejection, which may alter the parent-child relationship. A parent may also interpret the sleepy infant's refusal to suck or inability to retain formula as evidence of his or her incompetence as a parent. The breastfeeding mother may deduce that the newborn does not like her if the baby fails to take her nipple readily. Conversely, infants pick up messages from the muscular tension of those holding them.

A nurse who is sensitive to the needs of the mother can form a relationship with her that permits sharing of knowledge about techniques and emotions connected with feeding. Breastfeeding women frequently express disappointment in the help given to them by birthing unit or hospital nurses, saying they would like more encouragement, support, and practical information about feeding their newborns, especially in the case of early discharge. This need also applies to nonnursing mothers. Consistency in teaching by nursing personnel is paramount. A new mother becomes very frustrated if she is shown a number of different methods of feeding her newborn. With the technologic advances in formula production and the availability of knowledge about breastfeeding techniques, the mother should be confident that the choice she makes will promote normal growth and development of her newborn.

The decision by the mother about whether to breastfeed or bottle-feed is usually made by the sixth month of pregnancy and often even before conception. The final decision, however, may not be made until the mother's admission to the birth center. The decision is frequently influenced by relatives, especially the baby's father and maternal grandmother (Sharma & Petosa, 1997), and by friends and social customs, rather than being based on knowledge about the nutritional and psychologic needs of herself and her newborn.

The goals of Healthy People 2000 are to have 75% of infants breastfeeding at birth and 50% continuing to consume at least some human milk until 6 months (AAP, 1997). It is the health care provider's responsibility to provide the parents with accurate information regarding the distinct advantages of breastfeeding to the mother and infant. In times of short stays, the Baby Friendly Hospital Initiative program promotes breastfeeding by designing hospitals as centers for breastfeeding education (Pascale, Brittian, Lenfestey, & Jarrett-Pulliam, 1996). Parents have a right to hear about the data so they can make their own informed choice.

Once an *informed choice* has been made, the nurse's primary responsibility is to support the family's decision and to help the family achieve a positive result. No woman should be made to feel inadequate or superior because of her choice in feeding (Gigliotti, 1995). There are advantages and disadvantages to breastfeeding and bottle-feeding, but positive bonds in parent-child relationships may be developed with either method.

CRITICAL THINKING QUESTION

What are the key actions that promote a successful mother-infant feeding experience?

Before feeding, the mother should be made as comfortable as possible. Preparations may include voiding, washing her hands, and assuming a position of comfort. The woman who has had a cesarean birth needs support so that the newborn does not rest on her abdomen for long periods of time. When she is breastfeeding, she may be more comfortable lying on her side with a pillow behind her back and one between her legs. The nurse can position the newborn next to the woman's breast and place a rolled towel or small pillow behind the infant for support. Initially the mother will need assistance turning from side to side and burping the newborn. She may prefer to breastfeed sitting up with a pillow on her lap and the infant resting on the pillow rather than directly on her abdomen. It may be helpful to place a rolled pillow

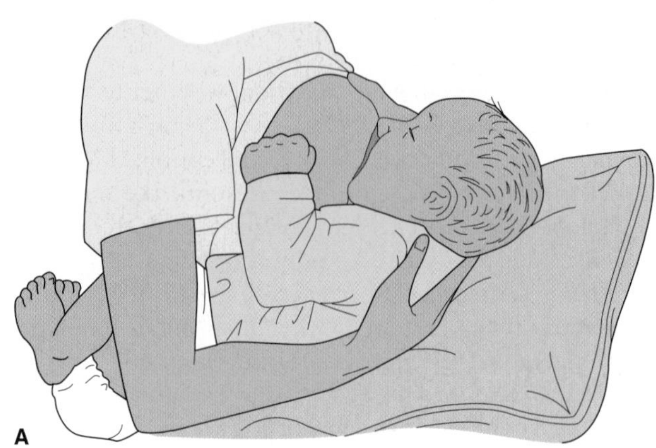

- Hold the baby's back and shoulders in the palm of your hand.
- Tuck the baby up under your arm, lining up the baby's lips with your nipple.
- Support the breast to guide it into the baby's mouth.
- Hold your breast until the baby nurses easily.

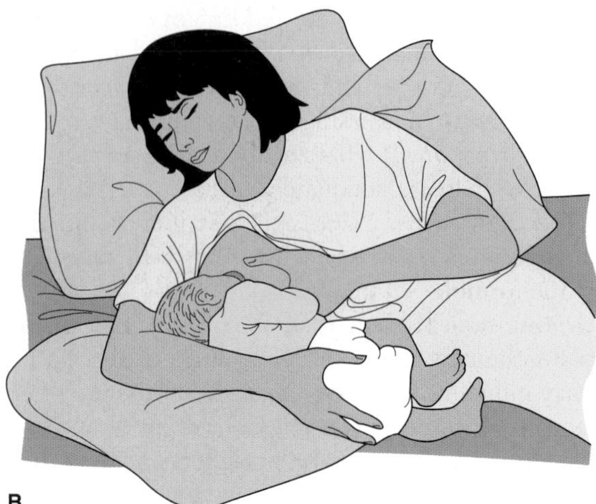

- Lie on your side with a pillow at your back and lay the baby so you are facing each other.
- To start, prop yourself up on your elbow and support your breast with the opposite hand.
- Pull the baby close to you, lining up the baby's mouth with your nipple.
- Lie back down once the baby is nursing well.

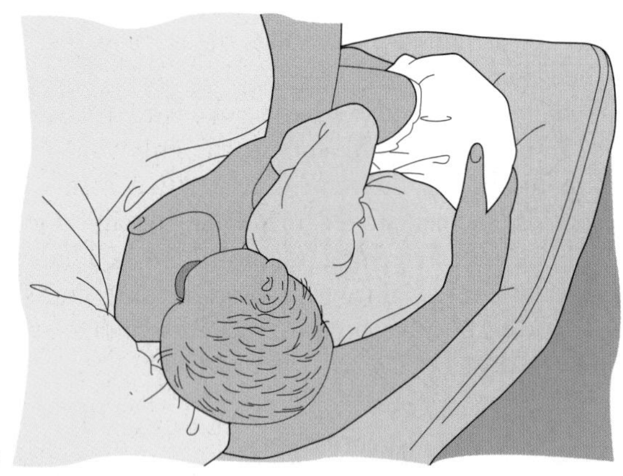

- Cradle the baby in the arm closest to the breast, with the baby's head in the crook of the arm.
- Have the baby's body facing you, tummy-to-tummy.
- Use your opposite hand to support the breast.

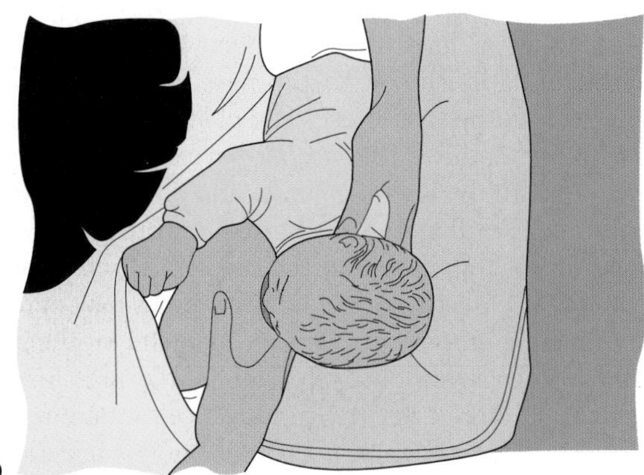

- Lay your baby on pillows across your lap.
- Turn the baby facing you.
- Reach across your lap to support the baby's back and shoulders with the palm of your hand.
- Support your breast from underneath to guide it into the baby's mouth.

FIGURE 27–2 Four common breastfeeding positions. ***A,*** Football hold. ***B,*** Lying down. ***C,*** Cradling. ***D,*** Across the lap. SOURCE: *Breastfeeding: A Special Relationship.* Eagle Video Productions, Raleigh, NC. Copyright Lactation Consultants of NC.

under the arm supporting the infant's head. An alternative position that avoids pressure on the incision while allowing for maximum visualization of the infant's face is the football hold. See Figure 27–2 for a variety of breastfeeding positions. Bottle-feeding mothers who have undergone cesarean birth frequently use the sitting position also. If incisional pain makes this position difficult, the bottle-feeding mother may also find it helpful to assume the side-lying position. The infant can be positioned in a semisitting position against a pillow close to the mother.

Depending on the newborn's level of hunger, the parents may want to use the time before feeding to get acquainted with their infant. The presence of the nurse during part of this time to answer questions and provide reinforcement of parenting skills will be helpful for the family. For the sleepy baby, a period of playful activity—such as gently rubbing the feet and hands or adjusting clothing and loosening coverings to expose the infant to room air—may increase alertness so that, when the feeding is initiated, the infant is ready and sucks eagerly. If an infant is overly hungry and upset, talking quietly and rocking gently may provide the baby with an opportunity to calm down so that he or she can find and grasp the nipple effectively. After the feeding, when the infant is satisfied and asleep, parents may explore the characteristics unique to their newborn. Routines must be flexible enough to allow this time for the family. Couplet care offers spontaneous, frequent encounters for the family and provides opportunities to practice handling skills, thereby increasing confidence in care after discharge. It also encourages feeding in response to cues from the baby, rather than feeding by a fixed schedule. A study by Brandt, Andrews, and Kvale (1998) indicated that women who continue to breastfeed are more aware of and/or responsive to their infant's cues and state (eg, quiet alert) than are mothers who wean earlier than planned.

It is also important to understand and support the mother who chooses to have her newborn cared for in the nursery so that she can rest. This is especially important if she must care for herself, the newborn, and other children without adult help at home.

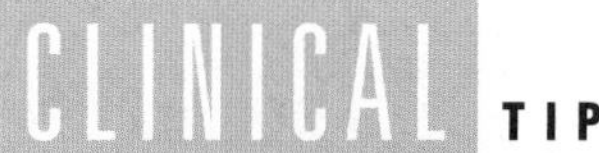

TIP

As you assist new mothers with breastfeeding, it is important to create a relaxed environment and approach to breastfeeding. Encourage mom to get into a comfortable position, well supported with pillows. Remind her to bring the baby to her breast rather than leaning forward to the baby.

Cultural Considerations in Infant Feeding

It is important for the nurse to understand how culture and society influence infant feeding. Motherhood itself changes the woman's lifestyle. Perceptions of the mother's role and of breastfeeding as a biologic act also influence the mother's comfort with breastfeeding. Some mothers identify shame, modesty, and embarrassment as reasons they chose not to breastfeed. The amount of body contact considered acceptable also influences parental behaviors (Figure 27–3). North American and European societies sometimes consider it indecent to expose the breast, believe that too much handling spoils children, and regard weaning as a sign of infant development (R. A. Lawrence, 1994).

The nurse also needs to understand the impact of the culture on the idiosyncrasies of specific feeding practices. For example, in many cultures (Mexican American, Navajo, Filipino, and Vietnamese) and in some countries (Guinea, Pakistan, Bangladesh), colostrum is not offered to the newborn (Riordan & Auerbach, 1999). Breastfeeding begins only after the milk flow is established. In some Asian cultures, the newborn is given boiled water until the mother's milk flows. The newborn is fed on demand, and cries are responded to immediately. If the crying continues, evil spirits may be blamed, and a priest's blessing may be sought. Although many of the Hmong women of Laos combine breastfeeding with some bottle-feeding, they find expressing their milk or pumping their breasts unacceptable. Thus other methods of providing relief should be suggested if breast engorgement develops. Most Muslim mothers breastfeed because the Qur'an encourages it until the child is 2 years old (Hutchinson & Baqi-Aziz, 1994). Japanese women are returning to

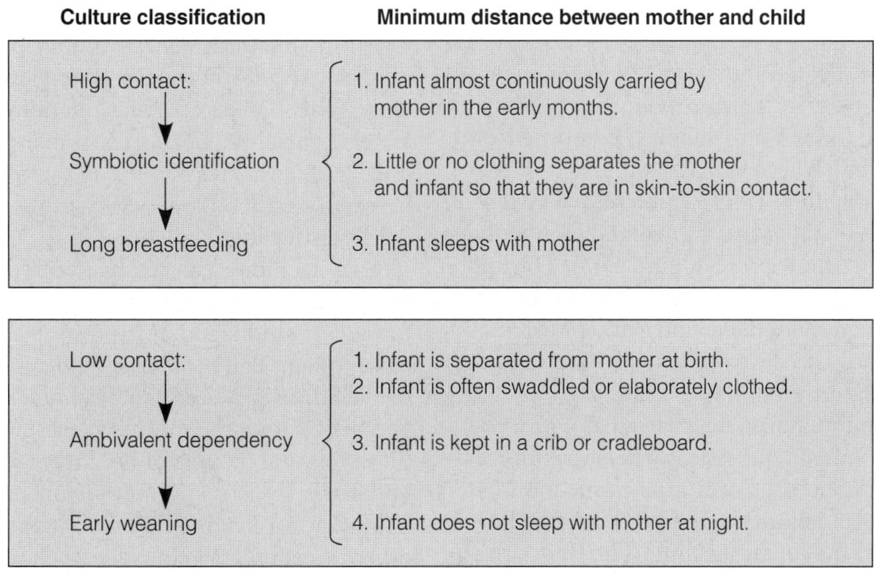

FIGURE 27–3 Culturally determined mother-child body interaction and implications for breastfeeding practices. The amount of contact and degree of closeness between mother and infant is often culturally determined and may influence how long the mother will breastfeed. SOURCE: Lawrence RA: *Breastfeeding: A Guide for the Medical Profession,* 4th ed. St Louis: Mosby, 1994, p 185.

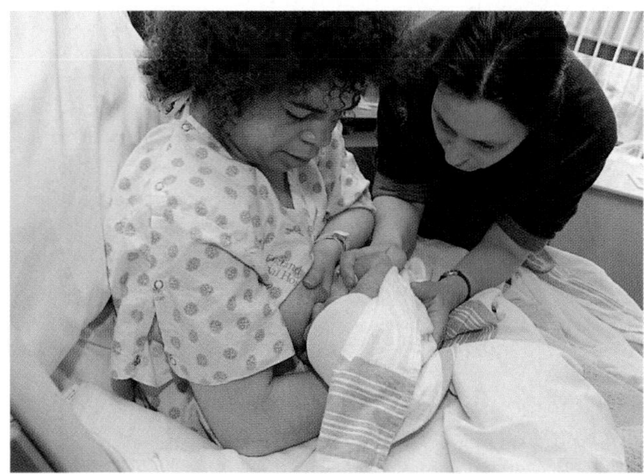

FIGURE 27–4 For many mothers, the nurse's support and knowledge are instrumental in establishing successful breastfeeding.

breastfeeding as the method of feeding for the baby's first year (Riordan & Auerbach, 1999).

The African American culture tends to emphasize plentiful feeding. Solid foods are introduced early and may even be added to the infant's formula. African American mothers view frequent feeding as an expression of hardiness and a positive behavior characteristic for the future (Vezeau, 1991). For the traditional Mexican, a fat baby is considered healthy and infants are fed on demand. "Spoiling" is encouraged.

These are but a few of the cultured practices related to feeding. When faced with an infant care practice different from the ones to which they are accustomed, nurses need to evaluate the effect of the practice. Just because a practice is different does not mean it is inferior. The nurse should intervene only if the practice is actually harmful to the mother or baby.

Physiology of the Breasts and Lactation

The female breast is divided into 15 to 24 lobes, separated from one another by fat and connective tissue. These lobes are subdivided into lobules, composed of small units called alveoli where milk is synthesized by the alveolar secretory epithelium. The lobules have a system of lactiferous ductiles that join larger ducts and eventually open onto the nipple surface (see Figure 6–6). During pregnancy, increased levels of estrogen stimulate breast duct proliferation and development, and elevated progesterone levels promote the development of lobules and alveoli in preparation for lactation.

Birth results in a rapid drop in estrogen and progesterone with a concomitant increase in the secretion of **prolactin.** This hormone promotes milk production by stimulating the alveolar cells of the breasts. Prolactin levels rise in response to the infant suckling. The newborn's suckling also stimulates the release of **oxytocin** from the pituitary gland. This hormone increases the contractility of the myoepithelial cells lining the walls of the mammary ducts, and a flow of milk results. This is called the **let-down reflex,** or milk injection. Mothers have described the let-down reflex as a prickling or tingling sensation during which they feel the milk coming down. Other signs of let-down include increased uterine cramps and increased lochia (during the early postpartum period), milk leaking from the other breast, and a feeling of relaxation. It is not unusual for the breasts to leak some milk prior to feeding.

The let-down reflex can be stimulated by the newborn's suckling, presence, or cry, or even by maternal thoughts about her baby. It may also occur during sexual orgasm because oxytocin is released. Conversely, the mother's lack of self-confidence or fear of, embarrassment about, or pain connected with breastfeeding may prevent the milk from being ejected into the duct system.

Milk production is decreased with repeated inhibition of the milk ejection reflex. Failure to empty the breasts frequently and completely also decreases production because as milk accumulates and is not withdrawn, the buildup of pressure in the alveoli suppresses secretion. Once lactation is well established, prolactin production decreases. Oxytocin and suckling continue to be the facilitators of milk production.

Client Education for Breastfeeding

Breastfeeding Process

The nurse caring for the breastfeeding mother should help the woman achieve independence and success in her feeding efforts (Figure 27–4). Prepared with a knowledge of the anatomy and physiology of the breast and lactation, the components and positive effects of breast milk, and the techniques of breastfeeding, the nurse can help the woman and her family use their own resources to achieve a successful experience. The objectives of breastfeeding are (1) to provide adequate nutrition, (2) to facilitate maternal-infant attachment, and (3) to prevent trauma to the nipples. All information and support are aimed toward these goals. When assisting the mother with breastfeeding, the nurse should use disposable gloves because breast milk and newborn saliva are body substances that call for precautions. (See Essential Precautions in Practice: During Breastfeeding.)

To facilitate successful breastfeeding, the nurse should arrange for privacy, help the mother find a comfortable position, and help position the baby comfortably close to her. The mother should support her breast with her hand, using either the C-hold or the scissors hold. For the C-hold, the mother places her thumb well above the areola and the rest of her fingers below the areola and under the breast. The mother may also use the scissors hold, placing her index finger above the areola and her other three fingers below the areola and under the breast. Either method of presenting the breast to the infant is acceptable as long as the hands are well away from the nipple so the baby can "latch on" to the breast (Figure 27–5).

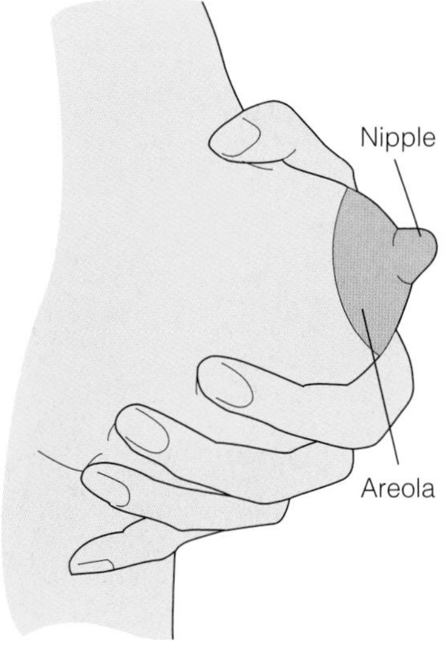

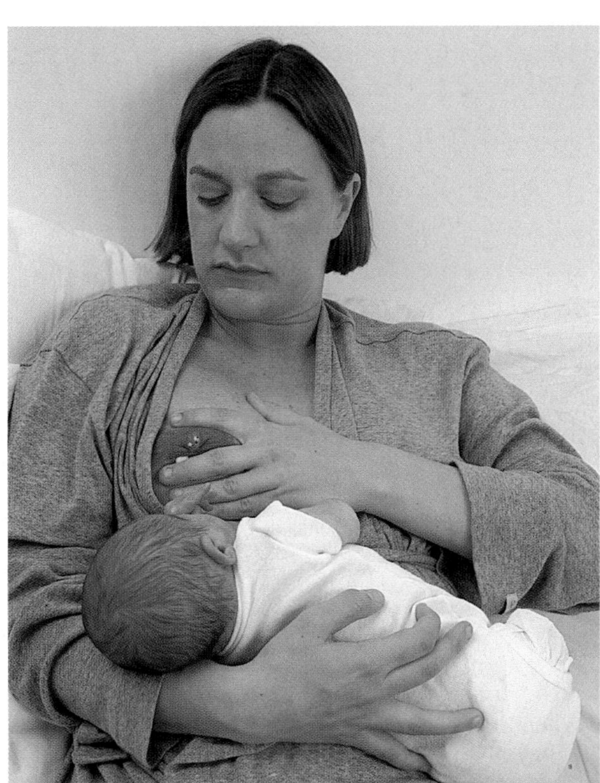

FIGURE 27–5 ***A,*** C-hold. SOURCE: Courtesy Childbirth Graphics Ltd., Rochester, NY. ***B,*** Scissors hold.

The mother should position the baby so that her or his nose is at the level of the nipple. She then lightly tickles the baby's lower lip with her nipple until the baby opens his or her mouth wide, and then brings the baby to the breast. The baby needs to take the whole nipple into the mouth so that the gums are on the areola. This allows the jaws to compress the milk ducts directly beneath the areola when the baby suckles (Figure 27–6). The baby's nose and chin should touch the breast. If the breast occludes the baby's airway, simply lifting up on the breast will usually clear the nares. The baby's lips should be relaxed and flanged outward with the tongue over the lower gum. At this point, the baby should be facing the mother (tummy to tummy or chest to chest), with the ear, shoulder, and hip aligned (Figure 27–7).

During these early feedings, the infant should be offered both breasts at each feeding to stimulate the supply-demand response. In some cases, the neonate will suckle only one breast well before falling asleep. As long as each breast is offered frequently (at least every 2 hours), single-breast feeds of whatever duration the baby wishes are an appropriate option until the baby shows a desire for both breasts (Woolridge, Phil, & Baum, 1993). The mother should feed until she becomes relaxed to the point of sleepiness—a delightful side effect of oxytocin secretion (Mulford, 1990)—or until she notes cues from the infant suggesting satiety (suckling activity ceases or the baby falls asleep). The length of the feedings is up to the mother; she need not watch a clock. Literature suggests that imposing time limits for breastfeeding does not prevent nipple soreness and in fact interferes with successful feeding. For example, the length of nursing time necessary to stimulate the milk ejection reflex varies with the individual. If the mother feeds according to the clock and disengages the baby prior to let-down, the baby will not get the hindmilk. Because the hindmilk is higher in fat

ESSENTIAL PRECAUTIONS IN PRACTICE

During Breastfeeding

Examples of times when disposable gloves should be worn include:

- Assisting the mother to breastfeed the newborn immediately after birth
- Handling breast milk for breast milk banking
- Assisting with manual expression of breast milk
- Handling used breastfeeding pads

Excellent handwashing is essential when assisting a breastfeeding mother.

REMEMBER to wash your hands prior to putting the disposable gloves on and AGAIN immediately after you remove the gloves.

For further information, consult OSHA and CDC guidelines.

CLINICAL TIP

Sleepy baby: Unwrap baby, encourage lots of skin-to-skin contact between mom and baby, have mom rest with baby near breast so baby can feel and smell the breast. Encourage mom to watch for feeding cues, such as hand-to-mouth activity, fluttering eyelids, vocalization but not necessarily crying, and mouthing activities.

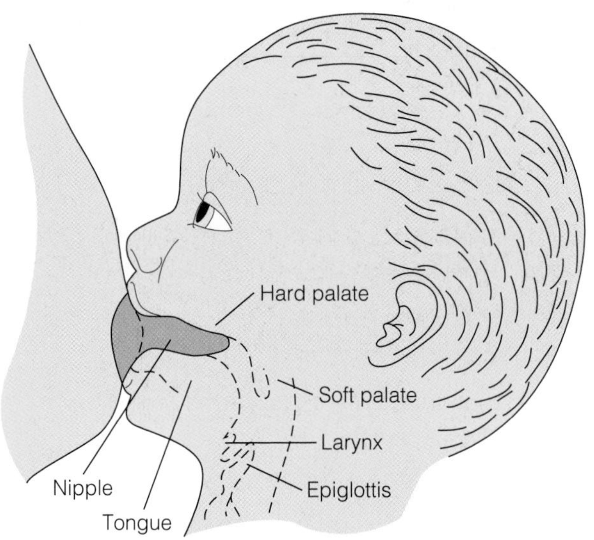

FIGURE 27–6 Baby properly positioned at the breast with good latch-on. Nose is near the breast, gums are on the areola, lips are flanged out, tongue is over the bottom gum. SOURCE: Adapted from Lawrence RA: *Breastfeeding: A Guide for Medical Profession,* 4th ed. St Louis: Mosby, 1994, p 219.

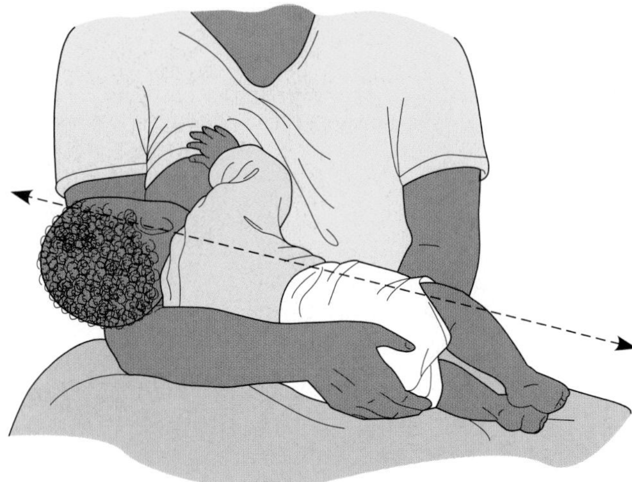

FIGURE 27–7 Infant in good breastfeeding position: tummy-to-tummy; ear, shoulder, and hip aligned. SOURCE: Adapted from Riordan J, Auerbach K: *Breastfeeding and Lactation.* Boston: Jones & Bartlett, 1993, p 248.

and calories than the foremilk, the baby will be less satisfied, will need to nurse again sooner, and will gain less weight. The mother should be encouraged to feed in response to the cues from her baby and her body, not in accordance with an arbitrary time schedule. If the mother wishes to end the feeding before the infant falls asleep or detaches himself or herself, she should break the suction by gently inserting her finger between the baby's gums. Burping between feedings on each breast and at the end of the feeding continues to be necessary. If the infant has been crying, it is also advisable to burp before beginning feeding.

Breastfeeding Assessment

During the birthing unit stay, the nurse must carefully monitor the progress of the breastfeeding pair. A systematic assessment of several breastfeeding episodes provides the opportunity to teach the new mother about lactation and the breastfeeding process, provide anticipatory guidance, and evaluate the need for follow-up care after discharge. Criteria for evaluating a breastfeeding session include maternal and infant cues, latch-on, position, let-down, nipple condition, infant response, and maternal response. The literature provides various tools to guide the assessment and documentation of the breastfeeding efforts (Riordan & Koehn, 1997). The LATCH Scoring Table is one example (Figure 27–8).

Leaking

Initially, more milk is produced than the infant requires. During the first few weeks, infant needs and maternal responses are not yet well attuned, daily variabilities of feeding frequency and duration are greatest, and most women experience breast leaking. Stimuli that result in let-down or leaking breast milk include hearing a baby cry and or even thinking about the baby. The mother should be forewarned of this and use breast pads in her bra to absorb the secretions. She should be cautioned to remove wet pads frequently to avoid irritation of the nipples or infection. (Breast pads with plastic liners interfere with air circulation; the mother should remove the plastic before using them.) Once breastfeeding is well established—usually after the first month—the mother may also be taught to apply direct pressure to the breast with her hand or forearm when leaking occurs.

Supplementary Feedings

Using supplementary bottle-feedings for the breastfeeding infant may weaken or confuse the suckling reflex or decrease the infant's interest in nursing. To grasp the

CLINICAL TIP

Digital suck training: If baby is pulling tongue back, humping tongue, or thrusting tongue, you can use digital suck training to bring the tongue down and forward. Place a finger in baby's mouth, pad side up. When baby starts sucking well, turn finger so the pad is down. If the baby is sucking correctly, the tongue will come forward and cup the finger, and baby will continue to suckle. Performing this technique prior to feedings encourages the baby to use the tongue correctly.

	0	1	2
L Latch	Too sleepy or reluctant No latch achieved	Repeated attempts Hold nipple in mouth Stimulate to suck	Grasps breast Tongue down Lips flanged Rhythmic sucking
A Audible swallowing	None	A few with stimulation	Spontaneous and intermittent <24 hrs old Spontaneous and frequent >24 hrs old
T Type of nipple	Inverted	Flat	Everted (after stimulation)
C Comfort (breast/ nipple)	Engorged Cracked, bleeding, large blisters or bruises Severe discomfort	Filling Reddened/small blisters or bruises Mild/moderate discomfort	Soft Tender
H Hold (positioning)	Full assist (staff holds infant at breast)	Minimal assist (ie, elevate head of bed, place pillows for support) Teach one side; mother does other Staff holds and then mother takes over	No assist from staff Mother able to position/hold infant

FIGURE 27–8 LATCH: a breastfeeding charting and documentation tool. LATCH was created to provide a systematic method for breastfeeding assessment and charting. It can be used to assist the new mother in establishing breastfeeding and define areas of needed intervention. SOURCE: Jensen D et al: LATCH: A breastfeeding charting system and documentation tool *JOGNN* 1994; 23(1):27.

mother's nipple, the newborn has to open her or his mouth wider than needed to grasp a bottle nipple. The shape of the mouth and lips and the sucking mechanism are also different for sucking the breast and the bottle nipple. While suckling at the breast, the infant's tongue moves in a peristaltic manner from front to back, squeezing the milk from the nipple. While sucking on a rubber nipple, the tongue pushes forward against the nipple to control the milk flow. Some breastfeeding babies who are given supplementary bottles cannot adjust to these different techniques and push the mother's nipple out of their mouth in subsequent breastfeeding attempts. This can be frustrating for both mother and baby. Breastfeeding mothers should avoid introducing bottles until breastfeeding is well established.

Parents are often concerned because they have no visual assurance of the amount of breast milk consumed. The mother should be taught the signs of milk transfer to the infant (ie, audible swallowing, milk appearing in the baby's mouth, her breasts feeling soft after feeding, milk leaking from the opposite breast) (Mulford, 1992). In addition, if the infant gains weight and has six or more wet diapers a day without supplemental feedings of water or formula, he or she is receiving adequate amounts of milk. Parents should know that because breast milk is more easily digested than formula, the breastfed infant becomes hungry sooner. Thus the frequency of breastfeeding will be greater. The parents may also expect the infant to demand more frequent nursing during growth spurts, such as 10 days to 2 weeks, 5 to 6 weeks, and 2.5 to 3 months.

Expression of Milk

If the mother who desires to breastfeed is unable to nurse her baby for medical or workplace reasons, she needs to know about other means of stimulating milk production and storing the breast milk. The choice of method may depend on the mother's physiologic capabilities to produce the desired amount of milk and her personal preference. During the early postpartum period, if the baby can't nurse at the breast (as in the case of some premature or sick infants), the mother needs frequent breast stimulation to establish and increase her milk supply to prepare for later breastfeeding. She should use an electric breast pump at least eight times in each 24-hour period (Riordan & Auerbach, 1999). Research has shown that a pulsatile electric pump and double setup (allowing both breasts to be stimulated simultaneously) results in higher prolactin levels and a greater volume of milk than does manual expression (Corbett-Dick & Bezek, 1997) (Figure 27–9). After lactation is established, milk expression may be accomplished by the method that the mother finds most effective and convenient.

To express her milk manually, the woman washes her hands, then massages her breast to stimulate let-down. To massage her breast, the woman grasps the breast with

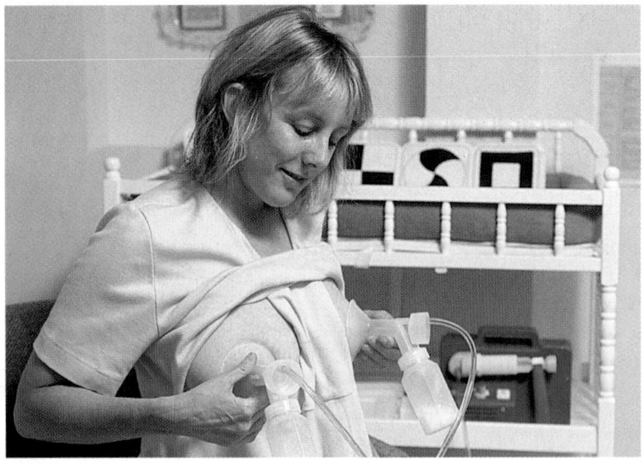

FIGURE 27–9 Mother using electric breast pump and double setup.

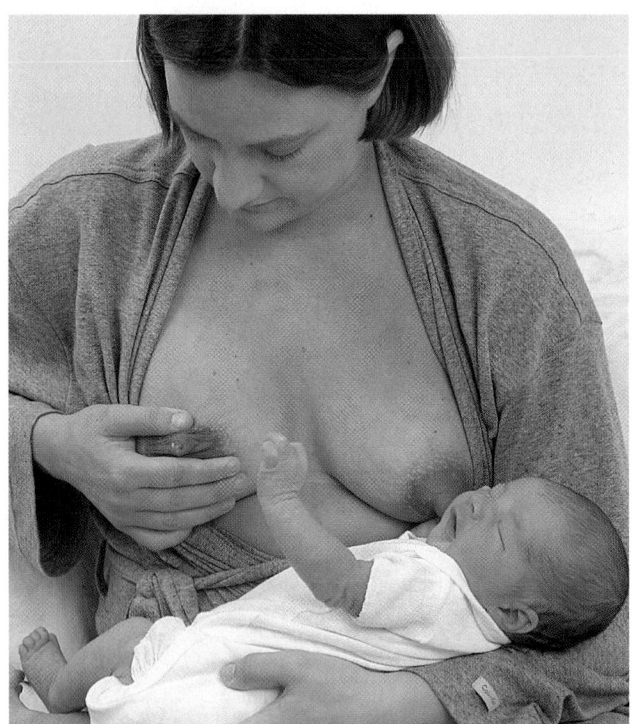

FIGURE 27–10 Hand position for manual expression of milk.

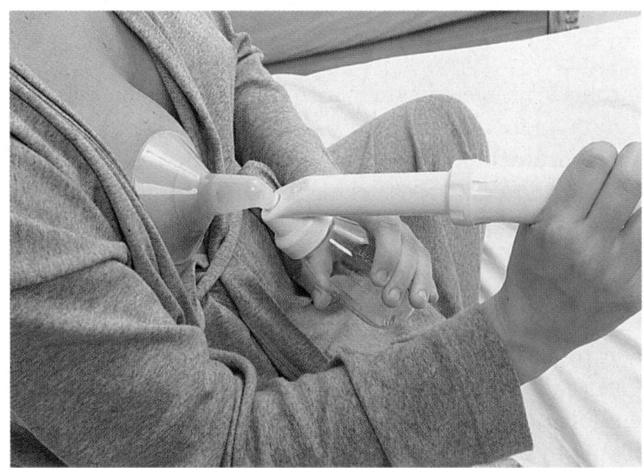

FIGURE 27–11 A mother expresses milk with her Kaneson hand pump.

both hands at the base of the breast near the chest wall. Using the palms of her hands, she firmly slides her hands toward her nipple. She repeats this process several times. Then she is ready to begin hand expression. The woman generally uses her left hand for her right breast and right hand for her left breast. However, some women find it preferable to use the hand on the same side as the breast. The nurse should encourage the woman to use the method she finds most effective. The woman grasps the areola with her thumb on the top and her first two fingers on the lower portion (Figure 27–10). Without allowing her fingers to slide on her skin, she pushes inward toward the chest and then squeezes her fingers together while pulling forward on the areola. She can use a container to catch any fluid that is squeezed out. She then repositions her hand by rotating it slightly so that she can repeat the process. She continues to reposition her hand and repeat the process to empty all the milk sinuses.

Breast pumps use suction to express the milk. Some have collection systems to conveniently store the milk. Hand pumps are portable and inexpensive. Battery-operated pumps are more efficient than hand pumps but are also more expensive. Electric pumps are the most efficient but are bulky and expensive; however, they may be rented in many areas. Many agencies have a variety of pumps available and provide instruction on correct use (Figure 27–11). Videotapes or photographs are also useful in demonstrating the process to new mothers (Table 27–3).

Storing Breast Milk

Breast milk has bacteriostatic qualities because of the presence of IgA and IgG antibodies, which retard bacterial growth. Breast milk can be stored for up to 6 hours at room temperature or up to 8 days in a refrigerator (Bocar, 1997). If breast milk is to be refrigerated and then fed to the infant, it should be stored in clean plastic containers because the white blood cells in the milk will adhere to glass, and their protective effect will be lost. Breast milk may be frozen in either glass or plastic because freezing destroys the white blood cells anyway. Breast milk may be stored in a freezer compartment inside the refrigerator for up to 2 weeks, in a self-contained freezer unit of a refrigerator up to 1 month, and in a separate deep freeze unit at 0 degrees up to 6 months. Frozen breast milk can be thawed by running warm water over the container. The container should be shaken well to return to suspension the fat molecules that separate during freezing.

TABLE 27–3 Recommendations for the Nursing Mother Who Uses a Pump

General Pumping Recommendations	Recommendations for Specific Types of Pumps
1. Read the instructions on the use and cleaning of a pump before expressing milk with any product. **2.** Wash hands before each pumping session. **3.** Frequency: For occasional pumping, pump during, after, or between feedings, whichever gives the best results. Most mothers tend to express more milk in the morning. Working mothers should use the pump on a regular basis for the number of nursings that are missed. For premature or ill babies who are not at breast, the number of pumpings should total eight or more in 24 hours. Initiation of pumping should be delayed no longer than 6 hours following birth unless medically indicated. This ensures appropriate development and sensitivity of prolactin receptors. More frequent pumping will avoid the buildup of excessive back pressure of milk during engorgement. **4.** Duration: With single-sided pumping, optimal duration is 10 to 15 minutes with an electric pump and 10 to 20 minutes with a manual pump. If double pumping with an electric or two battery-operated pumps, 7 to 15 minutes is optimal. Encourage mothers to tailor these times to their own situation. **5.** Technique: • Elicit the milk ejection reflex before using any pump. • Use only as much suction as is needed to maintain milk flow. • Massage the breast in quadrants during pumping to increase intramammary pressure. • Allow enough time for pumping to avoid anxiety. • Use inserts or different flanges if needed to obtain the best fit between pump and breast. • Avoid long periods of uninterrupted vacuum. • Stop pumping when the milk flow is minimal or has ceased.	**1.** Avoid pumps that use rubber bulbs to generate vacuum; they can cause bruising. **2.** Cylinder pumps: • When "O" rings are used, they must be in place for proper suction. • Remove gaskets *after each use* for cleaning to avoid harboring bacteria in the pump. • Roll the gasket on the inner cylinder back and forth to restore it to its original shape. • The pump stroke may need to be shortened as the outer cylinder fills with milk. • The user may need to empty the outer cylinder once or twice during pumping. • Hand position should be palm up with the elbow held close to the body. **3.** Battery-operated pumps: • Use alkaline batteries. • Replace batteries when cycles per minute decrease. • Interrupt vacuum frequently to avoid nipple pain and damage. • Use an AC adapter when possible, especially if the pump generates fewer than six cycles per minute. • Consider renting an electric pump for pumping that will continue for longer than 1 or 2 months. • Use two pumps simultaneously if pumping time is limited or to increase the quantity of milk obtained. • Choose a pump in which the vacuum can be regulated. • Massage the breast by quadrants during pumping. **4.** Semiautomatic pumps: • Vacuum may be easier to control if the mother does not lift her finger completely off the hole but rolls it back and forth rhythmically so that the vacuum is efficient but not painful. **5.** Automatic electric pumps: • Use the lowest pressure setting that is efficient. • Use a double setup (simultaneous pumping) when time is limited to increase the milk supply and for prematurity, maternal or infant illness, or other special situations.

SOURCE: Riordan J, Auerbach K: *Breastfeeding and Human Lactation.* (2nd ed.), Boston: Jones & Bartlett, 1999, page 397.

External Supports

Childbirth and the beginning of motherhood are a critical time in a woman's life, so physical, psychologic, and social supports are of paramount importance. The father or other partner is the most important support person for her, although the baby can also provide some support in the form of positive feedback. However, extensive family support systems may not be available. Mothers, sisters, and other females who could mentor and care for the new mother may live at a distance or work full time. As evidenced by the frequent discontinuation of breastfeeding in the early postpartum weeks, there is a need for assistance and follow-up in this area. Nurses, dietitians, childbirth educators, certified nurse-midwives, lactation consultants, mother-to-mother support groups, and physicians must collaborate to provide consistent, timely information and support and to attend to the new mother's special needs. Breastfeeding mothers who work outside the home and who receive support for their decision tend to breastfeed their infants for longer periods of time (Bocar, 1997).

La Leche League International is an organized group of volunteers who work to provide education about breastfeeding and assistance to women who are breastfeeding. Organized as small, neighborhood-based groups, it sponsors activities, offers printed material, offers electric breast pumps for rental, offers one-to-one counseling to mothers with questions or problems, and provides group support to breastfeeding mothers. Lactation consultants offer a wide range of services through private practice and health care facilities. A variety of lactation education programs are offered with differing prerequisites and objectives. Numerous books, pamphlets, and educational videos are also available to help the breastfeeding mother. The mother needs the support of all family members, her certified nurse-midwife/physician, pediatrician or certified nurse practitioner, and all nursing personnel because it is often the attitudes of these people that lead the woman to success or failure.

Drugs and Breastfeeding

It has long been recognized that certain medications taken by the mother may have an effect on her infant. It should be noted that (1) most drugs pass into breast milk; (2) almost all medications appear in only small amounts in human milk (usually less than 1% of the maternal dosage); and (3) very few drugs are contraindicated for breastfeeding women. Concerns about the consequences of the presence of drugs in breast milk focus on the effect on the infant and on the milk volume.

Characteristics of a drug that influence its passage into breast milk include the following:

1. *Degree of protein binding.* Unbound drugs are most likely to enter the breast milk.
2. *Degree of ionization.* Drugs tend to cross into breast milk in un-ionized form.
3. *Molecular weight.* Drugs with a molecular weight greater than 200 will not cross into breast milk.
4. *Degree of solubility in fat and water.* Alveolar epithelium is a lipid barrier with water-filled pores, but colostrum makes epithelium more permeable to lipid-soluble drugs.
5. *Mechanism of transport.* Drugs enter breast milk by active transport, simple diffusion, or carrier-mediated diffusion.
6. *The pH.* Breast milk, which is acidic, attracts drugs that are weak bases.
7. *Half-life.* Rates of absorption, metabolism, and excretion determine a drug's half-life, or how fast it leaves the body. The longer the half-life, the greater the risk of accumulation in tissues.
8. *Milk/plasma ratio.* The higher the **milk/plasma ratio,** the higher the drug concentration in the breast milk compared to the drug concentration in the plasma. An M/P ratio of 1.0 indicates that the milk and plasma contain equal concentrations of the drug. An M/P ratio of less than 1.0 indicates that the concentration of the drug in the milk is lower than its plasma concentration, whereas an M/P ratio greater than 1.0 indicates that the drug's concentration in milk is greater than in plasma.

Other variables that affect the passage of drugs into breast milk include the amount of the drug taken, the frequency and route of administration, and the timing of the dose in relationship to infant feeding. A drug's effects are influenced by the infant's age, the feeding frequency, the volume of milk taken, and the degree of absorption through the gastrointestinal tract.

Four adjustments should be made when administering drugs to a nursing mother to decrease the effects on the infant (Banta-Wright, 1997):

1. Long-acting forms of drugs should be avoided. The infant may have difficulty metabolizing and excreting them, and accumulation may be a problem.
2. Absorption rates and peak blood levels should be considered in scheduling the administration of the drugs. Less of the drug crosses into the milk if the medication is given immediately after the woman has nursed her baby.
3. The infant should be closely observed for any signs of drug reaction, including rash, fussiness, lethargy, or changes in sleeping habits or feeding pattern.
4. Whenever alternatives are available, the drug that shows the least tendency to pass into breast milk should be selected.

The mother should be given information about the potential of most drugs to cross into breast milk (AAP, 1997). She should also be advised to tell any physician who may prescribe medications for her that she is breastfeeding.

The effect of maternal medication on milk volume is also a concern for the breastfeeding mother. Barbiturates, antihistamines, diuretics, ergot alkaloids, and oral contraceptives high in estrogen generally decrease milk output. Some psychotherapeutic drugs increase the milk supply (Banta-Wright, 1997).

In counseling the nursing mother, the health care provider should weigh the benefits of the medication against the possible risk to the infant and its possible effects on the breastfeeding process. The potential risk to the infant must also be weighed against the effect of interrupting breastfeeding.

Selected Potential Problems in Breastfeeding

Because mothers are discharged from the hospital before breastfeeding is well established, they are frequently alone when they encounter changes in the breastfeeding process. Many women stop nursing if the situations they encounter seem to pose problems. Nurses can offer anticipatory guidance regarding common breastfeeding phenomena and provide resources for the woman's use after discharge. Table 27–4 summarizes self-care measures the nurse can suggest to a woman with a breastfeeding problem.

Nipple Soreness The mother should be made aware that often some discomfort occurs initially with breastfeeding, peaking between the third and sixth days, and then receding (Riordan & Auerbach, 1999). The infant should not be switched to bottle-feeding or have feedings delayed because these measures will only cause engorgement and more soreness. Discomfort that lasts throughout the feeding or past the first week demands attention. Health care providers should educate breastfeeding mothers in ways to minimize engorgement and nipple trauma (Brent, Rudy, Redd, Rudy, & Roth, 1998).

TABLE 27–4 Breastfeeding Problems and Remedies

Nipples Not Graspable

Flat or inverted nipples

- Use Hoffman technique to break adhesions.
- Wear milk cups to encourage nipples to protrude.
- Use nipple tug and roll to increase protractility.
- Form the nipple prior to nursing by hand shaping, ice, wearing milk cups a half-hour before feeding.
- As a last resort, use nipple shield for first few minutes of feeding to draw out nipple; then place baby on breast.

Engorged breasts

Treat engorgement by relieving fullness with hand expression of milk prior to nursing and instituting frequent feeding so nipple is more prominent.

Large breasts

- Support breast with opposite hand, or use rolled towel under breast to bring nipple to the level of baby's mouth.
- Use C-hold to make nipple accessible to baby.

Engorgement

Missed or infrequent feedings

- Nurse frequently (every $1\frac{1}{2}$ hours).
- Massage and hand express or pump to empty breasts completely when feedings are missed or when a full feeling develops in breasts and baby is not available or willing to nurse.

Breasts not emptied at feedings

- Nurse long enough to empty breasts (10–15 minutes on each side at each feeding).
- If baby will not nurse long enough to empty breasts, hand express or pump after feeding.

Inadequate let-down

- Use relaxation techniques, massage, and warm or cool compresses before nursing.
- Relax in warm shower with water running from back over shoulders and breasts, hand expressing to relieve fullness.
- If due to anxiety, try to eliminate the source of tension.

Baby sleepy or not eager to nurse

- Use rousing techniques (eg, hold baby upright, unwrap blanket, change diaper).
- Pre-express milk onto nipple or baby's lips to entice baby.
- Avoid use of bottles of water or formula; these will decrease baby's willingness to suckle.

Inadequate Let-Down

Let-down not well established

- Give the baby ample time at the breast (at least 15 minutes per side) to allow for let-down and complete emptying.
- Nurse in a quiet spot away from distractions.
- Massage breasts before nursing.
- Drink juice, water, tea (no caffeine) before and during nursing.
- Condition let-down by setting up a routine for beginning feedings.
- Use relaxation and breathing techniques.
- Stimulate the nipple manually before nursing.
- Concentrate thought on the baby and milk flow; turn on a faucet so that the sound of running water helps stimulate let-down.
- Use synthetic oxytocin nasal spray several times during a feeding. (This should condition let-down within 24 hours. Then it is no longer needed. Spray must be prescribed by a doctor.)

Mother overtired or overextended

- Nap or rest when the baby rests.
- Lie down to nurse.
- Nurse the baby in bed at night.
- Simplify daily chores; set priorities.

Mother tense, pressured

- Identify the causes of tensions and eliminate or minimize them.
- Decrease fatigue.

Mother caught in cycle of little milk, worry, less milk

- Try all the actions above.
- Develop confidence in mothering skills. (A home visit by a counselor may help.)

Cracked Nipples

All causes of sore nipples carried to extreme

- Refer to all actions for sore nipples.
- Consult doctor about using aspirin, acetaminophen (Tylenol), or other painkiller.
- Improve nutritional status, increasing protein, vitamin C, zinc.

Local infection (baby with staph or other organism may have infected mother's nipples)

Refer to physician.

Plugged Ducts

Poor positioning

Try a variety of positions for complete emptying.

Incomplete emptying of breast

- Nurse at least 10 minutes per side after let-down.
- Alternate nursing positions.
- If baby does not empty breasts, pump or express milk after feedings.

External pressure on breast

- Use larger size bras, insert bra extender, or go braless.
- Use nursing bra instead of pulling up conventional bra to nurse to avoid pressure on ducts.
- Avoid bunching up sweater or nightgown under arm during nursing.

Sore Nipples

Poor positioning

- Alternate nursing positions throughout the day.
- Bring the baby close to nurse so the baby does not pull on the breast.
- Place the nipple and some of the areola in the baby's mouth.
- Check to ensure the baby is put on and off the breast properly.
- Check to ensure the nipple is back far enough in the baby's mouth.
- Hold the baby closely during nursing so the nipple is not constantly being pulled.

Baby chewing or nuzzling onto nipple

- Form the nipple for the baby.
- Set up a pattern of getting the baby onto the breast using the rooting reflex.

Baby nursing on end of nipple

- Ensure the nipple is way back in the baby's mouth by getting the baby properly onto the breast.
- Check for an inverted nipple.
- Check for engorgement.

Baby chewing his or her way off the nipple (nipple being pulled out of baby's mouth at end of feeding)

- Remove the baby from the breast by placing a finger between the baby's gums to ensure suction is broken.
- End feeding when the baby's suckling slows, before he or she has a chance to chew on the nipple.

➤

Sore Nipples ***continued***

Baby overly eager to nurse
- Nurse more often.
- Pre-express milk to hasten let-down, avoiding vigorous suckling.

Dry colostrum or milk causing nipple to stick to bra or breast pads
Moisten bra or pads before taking off so as not to remove keratin.

Nipples not allowed to dry
- Remove plastic liners from milk pads.
- Air dry breast completely after nursing.
- Change milk pads frequently.

Improper use of breast shield
- Use shield only to draw out nipple; then have the baby nurse on the breast.
- Cut tip of shield back bit by bit and eventually discard.

Nipple skin not resistant to stress
- Improve diet, especially adding fresh fruits and vegetables and vitamin supplements.
- Eliminate or decrease use of sugary foods, alcohol, caffeine, cigarettes.
- Check use of cleansing or drying agents.

Natural oils removed or keratin layers broken down by drying agents (soap, alcohol, shampoo, deodorant)
- Eliminate irritants.
- Wash breasts with water only.

SOURCE: Adapted from Lauwers J, Woessner C: *Counseling the Nursing Mother: A Reference Handbook for Health Care Providers and Lay Counselors,* 2nd ed. Garden City Park, NY: Avery, 1990, pp 385–397.

The baby's position at the breast is one of the most critical factors in nipple soreness. The mother's hand should be off the areola, and the baby should be facing the mother's chest with ear, shoulder, and hip aligned (see Figure 27–7).

Because the area of greatest stress to the nipple is in line with the newborn's chin and nose, nipple soreness may be decreased by encouraging the mother to rotate positions when feeding the infant. Changing position alters the focus of greatest stress and promotes more complete breast emptying.

Nipple soreness may also develop if the infant has faulty sucking habits. Nipples may be bruised, scabbed, or blistered from the nipple entering the baby's mouth at an upward angle and rubbing against the roof of the mouth (Riordan & Auerbach, 1999). Soreness may also result from continuous negative pressure if the infant falls asleep with the breast in his or her mouth.

Chewed nipples, which result from improper positioning, lead to cracking or tenderness at or near the base. In these cases, the baby's jaws close only on the nipple instead of the areola, or the baby's mouth is not opened wide enough, or the infant's mouth has slipped down to the nipple from the areola as a result of engorgement. Soreness on the underside of the nipple is caused by the infant's nursing with her or his bottom lip tucked in rather than out, causing a friction burn. Vigorous sucking produces little milk because the milk sinuses under the areola are not compressed. This results in a frustrated infant and marked soreness for the mother. The problem is overcome by positioning the infant with as much areola as possible in his or her mouth and rotating the baby's positions at the breast.

Nipple soreness is especially pronounced during the first few minutes of the feeding. If the mother is not expecting this, she may become discouraged and quickly stop. The let-down reflex may take a few minutes to activate, and it may not occur if the mother stops nursing too quickly. The problem is compounded if the infant is unsatisfied, and the possibility of breast engorgement increases.

Because nipple soreness can also result from an overeager infant, the mother may find it helpful to nurse more frequently or hand express a few drops of milk to alleviate the initial discomfort. This helps ease the vigorous sucking of a ravenous infant. The woman can also apply ice to her nipples and areola for a few minutes prior to feeding. This promotes nipple erectness and numbs the tissue to ease the initial discomfort. To prevent excoriation and skin breakdown, the nipples and areola should be washed with water and then allowed to dry thoroughly. Drying may be accomplished by leaving the bra flaps down for several minutes after feeding or by exposing the nipples to sunlight or ultraviolet light for 30 seconds at first and gradually increasing to 3 minutes. Drying the nipples with a hair dryer on low heat setting also facilitates drying and promotes healing, especially if breast milk is allowed to dry on the nipples (Riordan & Auerbach, 1999).

The use of substances such as lanolin, Masse breast cream, Eucerin cream, or A and D ointment on the nipples between feedings should be discouraged. These preparations may cause allergic reactions or increase irritation if they need to be washed off prior to nursing. The substance may also be contaminated. In very dry environments, however, cream may be appropriate. Lanolin is most hazardous to women with wool allergy (R. A. Lawrence, 1994). Lansinoh is a purified, alcohol-free, and "allergen-free" ointment that is considered safe if an ointment is indicated.

Alternatively, applying breast milk and allowing it to dry on the nipples has been shown to heal sore nipples rapidly. Breast milk is high in fat, fights infection, and will not irritate the nipples (Brent et al, 1998). An obvious advantage is that it is readily available at no cost to the mother.

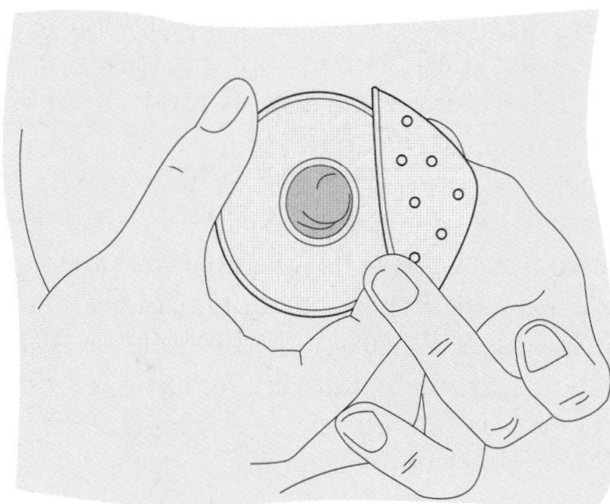

FIGURE 27–12 Breast shells can help correct flat or inverted nipples. SOURCE: Courtesy Medela, Inc: *Breastfeeding Information Guide.* McHenry, IL, p 5.

CRITICAL THINKING IN PRACTICE

Ann calls you from home in tears on her third postpartum day. She states that, although breastfeeding was going well in the hospital, her breasts are now swollen, hard, and very painful, and her baby is refusing to suckle. Ann expresses extreme disappointment that "the breastfeeding didn't work" because she truly believes that breast milk is best for babies and she had enjoyed her breastfeeding experience in the hospital, especially nursing the baby immediately after delivery. But she also states she has not been able to stop crying all day and can no longer tolerate her painful breasts. In addition she says that the baby "seems happier" with the bottle. What would you do?

Answers can be found in Appendix I.

If the woman finds that her bra or clothing rubs against her nipples and adds to her discomfort, she may insert shields into her bra. Both Medela shells and Woolrich shields, for example, relieve friction and promote air circulation. If a woman uses breast pads inside her bra to keep milk from leaking onto her clothes, the pads should be changed frequently so that the nipples remain dry.

Older remedies for nipple soreness are receiving renewed acceptance. For instance, tea bags may be moistened in warm water and applied to the nipples. The tannic acid seems to help toughen the nipples, and the warmth is soothing and promotes healing. However, tannic acid can cause drying and cracking and so is not appropriate in all situations (R. A. Lawrence, 1994).

Nipple dermatitis causes swollen, erythematous, burning nipples. It is most commonly caused by thrush or by allergic response to breast creams. If the nipple soreness has a sudden onset, accompanied by burning or itching, shooting pains through the breast, and a deep pink coloration of the nipple, it may be caused by a thrush infection transmitted from the infant. White patches or streaks in the infant's mouth indicate a need for treatment of the mouth and nipple infection. The disease can be treated with a variety of antifungal preparations and does not preclude breastfeeding.

Flat or Inverted Nipples If the mother does not have a prominent nipple or if she has an inverted nipple, she may try rolling the nipple between her thumb and forefinger or stretching it by pressing inward and outward around the nipple prior to feeding (Hoffman's technique). Breast shells, or milk cups, are made of hard, formed plastic and fit over the nipple, causing it to protrude (Figure 27–12). The mother wears the shells prenatally and between feedings so that the nipple is more prominent at the beginning of the feeding. Use of an electric breast pump will quickly stimulate the nipple to become more prominent, and when a few drops of colostrum are expressed, the infant becomes more eager to latch on.

The use of an all-rubber nipple shield after the baby's birth to correct nipple position may reduce the transfer of milk from the breast to the infant by 58% while increasing the infant's suck effort and rate, thereby increasing the time the baby needs to rest during the feeding. New thin latex shields do not affect sucking patterns, but they reduce milk transfer (Riordan & Auerbach, 1999). A shield should be used as a last resort and preferably after consultation with a lactation expert. Any rubber or artificial nipple is more pliable than the breast and thus allows more milk to pass through it per suck. As a result of the different milking actions required, the infant may experience "nipple confusion" and refuse the breast when it is offered again (Riordan & Auerbach, 1999).

Cracked Nipples Nipple soreness is frequently coupled with cracked nipples. Whenever a breastfeeding mother complains of soreness, the nipples must be carefully examined for fissures or cracks, and the mother should be observed during breastfeeding to see whether the infant is correctly positioned at the breast and latched onto the nipple. If the positioning is correct but cracks exist, further interventions are necessary. The mother's first reaction may be to cease nursing on the sore breast, but this may aggravate the problem if engorgement and plugged ducts result. All the interventions described for sore nipples may be used. It may also help the mother to begin nursing sessions using the breast that is less sore. This allows the let-down reflex to occur in the affected breast, and the infant does more vigorous sucking on the less tender breast, which decreases trauma to the cracked nipple. With severe cases, the temporary use of a nipple shield for nursing may be appropriate. For the mother's comfort, analgesics may be taken after nursing.

Breast Engorgement A distinction should be made between breast fullness and engorgement. All lactating women experience a transient fullness at first. This is caused by venous congestion and later by accumulating milk. However, this generally lasts only 24 hours, the breasts remain soft enough for the newborn to suckle, and there is no pain. Engorged breasts are hard, painful, and appear taut and shiny. In this case, nursing is difficult for the infant and painful for the mother.

The infant should suckle for an average of 15 minutes per feeding and should feed at least eight times in 24 hours (Riordan & Auerbach, 1999). If the baby is unable to nurse more frequently, the mother may express some milk manually or with a pump, being careful not to traumatize the breast tissue. Warm or cool compresses before nursing stimulate let-down and soften the breast so that the infant can more easily grasp the areola. The mother should be encouraged to wear a well-fitting nursing bra 24 hours a day. The bra supports the breasts and prevents further discomfort from tension and pulling on the Cooper's ligament. Analgesics such as acetaminophen or aspirin, alone or in combination with codeine, are appropriate, especially if taken just prior to nursing. The pain will be relieved, but the medication will not reach the milk for at least 30 minutes (R. A. Lawrence, 1994).

Plugged Ducts Some mothers experience plugging of one or more ducts, especially in conjunction with or following engorgement. This is often referred to as "caked breasts." Manifested as an area of tenderness or "lumpiness" in an otherwise well woman, plugging may be relieved by the use of heat and massage. The mother can be encouraged to massage her breasts from her chest wall forward to the nipple while standing in a warm shower or following the application of moist heat to the breast (Riordan & Auerbach, 1999). She should then nurse her infant, starting on the unaffected breast if the plugged breast is tender. Frequent nursing and trying a variety of positions to ensure complete emptying will help prevent the problem. She should also avoid bras with underwires, bras that are too tight or bind, or straps on a baby carrier (Riordan & Auerbach, 1999).

Breastfeeding and the Working Mother

The best preparation for maintaining lactation after return to work is frequent, unlimited breastfeeding and enjoying the baby. Even when planned, the first day back to work may be fraught with emotional and physical distresses (Riordan & Auerbach, 1999). Anticipatory guidance from the nurse may facilitate the transition from maternity leave to work (Bocar, 1997). The earlier the breastfeeding mother returns to work, the more often she will need to pump her breasts to express the breast milk. Because milk production follows the principle of supply and demand, if breasts are not pumped, the milk supply will decrease. An electric breast pump and double collection system are considered the optimal means of milk expression. But this is not the only method; use of mechanical pumps may not suit some women.

Sometimes a mother has a flexible schedule and can return home to nurse at lunchtime or have the baby brought to her. If this is not possible, the infant may be fed expressed milk. For proper storage of breast milk, see Storing Breast Milk earlier in this chapter. While the mother is absent, the infant can be bottle-fed or spoon-fed. If the baby is 3 months or older, cup-feeding is an option. The mother should wait until lactation is well established before introducing the bottle. Most babies will adjust to the bottle within 7 to 10 days.

To maintain an adequate milk supply, the working mother must pay special attention to her fluid intake. She can ensure an adequate intake by drinking extra fluid at each break whenever possible during the day. In addition, it is helpful to nurse more on weekends, to nurse during the night, to eat a nutritionally sound diet, and to continue manual expression or pumping when not nursing (Bocar, 1997).

Night nursing presents a dilemma in that it may help a working mother maintain her milk supply but may also contribute to fatigue. Some women choose to have the infant sleep with her so that breastfeeding is more easily accomplished. If a woman finds it difficult to sleep soundly when the infant is in the same bed, she might put the crib in her room. Another alternative is to limit breastfeeding to the morning and evening, with supplemental feeding at other times. In a study by Pinella and Birch (1993), the use of focal feeds (feeding between 10 PM and midnight) and teaching parents to help their babies develop self-soothing activities was found to promote infant sleeping for longer intervals at night.

Weaning

The decision to wean a baby from the breast may be made for a variety of reasons, including family or cultural pressures, change in the home situation, pressure from the woman's partner, or a personal opinion about when **weaning** should occur. For the woman who is comfortable with breastfeeding and well-informed about the process, the appropriate time to wean her infant will become evident if she is sensitive to the child's cues. Often weaning falls between periods of great developmental activity for the child. Thus weaning commonly occurs at 8 to 9 months, 12 to 14 months, 18 months, 2 years, or 3 years of age. In the United States, however, weaning commonly occurs before the child is 9 months old, although it may occur any time from soon after birth to 4 years of age. The infant may give weaning signals as early as 5 or 6 months of age (Furman, 1995).

If weaning is timed to respond to the child's cues and if the mother is comfortable with the timing, it can be accomplished with less difficulty than if the process is be-

CLINICAL TIP

When you help a mother bottle-feed her baby for the first time, there are many potential frustrations you can help her avoid. The first is often "flying arms" as the baby waves his or her arms in the air. The second is the "chin plunge" as the baby's head falls forward in the mother's tentative hold. To avoid this, assist the mother with positioning. A third frustration may arise when she tries to get the nipple correctly placed in the mouth. To do this, put your index finger on the baby's chin, and gently pull downward while quickly sliding the nipple in over the tongue.

gun before both mother and child are ready emotionally. Nevertheless, weaning is a time of emotional separation for mother and baby; it may be difficult for them to give up the closeness of their nursing sessions. The nurse who is understanding about this possibility can help the mother see that her infant is growing up and plan other comforting, consoling, and play activities to replace breastfeedings. A gradual approach is the easiest and most comforting way to wean the child from breastfeeding. Other activities can enhance the parent-infant attachment process. If a mother needs to terminate breastfeeding earlier than planned, she may experience a sense of failure. To avoid this, nurses need to pay special attention to mother-infant interaction and the mother's perception of the earlier-than-planned breastfeeding termination (Brandt et al, 1998).

During weaning, the mother should substitute one cup-feeding or bottle-feeding for one breastfeeding session over several days to a week so that her breasts gradually produce less milk. Eliminating the breastfeedings associated with meals first facilitates the mother's ability to wean the infant as satiation with food lessens the desire for milk. Over a period of several weeks she should substitute more cup-feedings or bottle-feedings for breastfeedings. Many mothers continue to nurse once a day in the early morning or late evening for several months until the milk supply is gone. The slow method of weaning prevents breast engorgement, allows infants to alter their eating methods at their own rates, and allows time for psychologic adjustment.

Client Teaching for Bottle-Feeding

With the great emphasis placed on successful breastfeeding, the teaching needs of the bottle-feeding new mother may be overlooked. If she has had only limited experience in feeding infants, she may need some guidelines to feed her newborn successfully. The following information is helpful for parents to facilitate adequate nutrition and foster attachment.

The baby is held for all feedings in order to prevent positional otitis media. Positional otitis media may develop when the infant is fed horizontally because milk and nasal mucus may occlude the eustachian tube. Holding the infant provides social and close physical contact for the baby and an opportunity for parent-infant interaction and bonding (Figure 27–13).

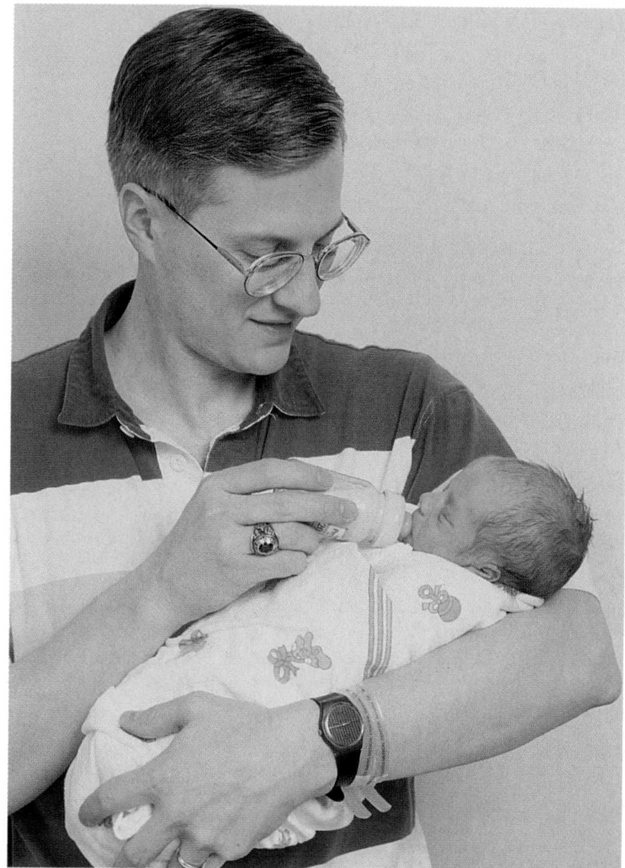

FIGURE 27–13 An infant is supported comfortably during bottle-feeding.

Nipples should have a hole big enough to allow milk to flow in drops when the bottle is inverted. Too large an opening may cause regurgitation because of rapid feeding. If feeding is too fast, the nipple should be changed, and the infant should be helped to eat more slowly by stopping the feeding frequently for burping and cuddling. The nipple is pointed directly into the mouth, not toward the palate or tongue, and is placed on top of the tongue. The nipple needs to be full of liquid at all times to avoid ingestion of air, which decreases the amount of feeding and increases gastric discomfort. Nipples vary in shape, amount of energy needed to obtain the formula. and rate of formula flow through the nipple unit (Fadavi, Punwani, Jain, Vidyasagar, 1997).

The infant is burped at intervals, preferably at the middle and end of the feeding. The infant who seems to swallow a great deal of air while sucking may need more frequent burping. If the infant has cried before being fed, air may have been swallowed; in such cases, the infant is burped before beginning to feed or after taking just

TABLE 27–5 Formula Preparation

Ready to Feed (20 kcal/oz; available in 32 oz cans or 4 oz bottles):

Use within 30 minutes to 1 hour once opened.

Do not dilute. Use directly from can, no mixing required.

Just add clean nipple to bottle.

Most expensive type of formula preparation.

Formula Concentrate (available in 13 oz cans):

Mix equal amounts of concentrate and water from uncontaminated source. This provides a 20 kcal/30 mL (1 oz) dilution. For example, for a 4 oz feeding mix 2 oz of formula concentrate with 2 oz water.

Wash punch-type can opener and top of formula can before opening.

Prepare a single feeding by measuring water and liquid directly into nursing bottle.

Cover opened concentrate formula cans with foil or plastic wrap and refrigerate until next bottle is made up.

Powdered Formula (52 scoops per can):

Mix one unpacked level scoop of powdered formula with each 60 mL (2 oz) of warm water.

Always pour water into bottle first; then add powder and stir well.

Make sure the powder and water are well mixed to ensure the formula composition is 20 kcal/30 mL (1 oz).

After opening, keep can tightly covered and use contents within 1 month to assure freshness.

Will keep in refrigerator for up to 24 hours.

Least expensive type.

enough to calm down. Burping is done by holding the infant upright on the shoulder or by holding the infant in a sitting position on the feeder's lap with chin and chest supported on one hand. The back is then gently patted or stroked with the other hand. Too frequent burping may confuse a newborn who is attempting to coordinate sucking, swallowing, and breathing simultaneously.

Newborns frequently regurgitate small amounts of feedings. This may look like a large amount to the inexperienced parent, however, and she or he may require reassurance that this is normal. Initially, regurgitation may be due to excessive mucus and gastric irritation from foreign substances such as aspirated blood in the stomach from birth. Later, regurgitation may result when the infant feeds too rapidly and swallows air. It may also occur when the infant is overfed; the cardiac sphincter allows the excess to be regurgitated. Because this is such a common occurrence, experienced parents and nurses generally keep a "burp cloth" available. Although regurgitation is normal, vomiting or a forceful expulsion of fluid is not. When forceful expulsion occurs, further evaluation may be indicated, especially if other symptoms are present.

Parents should be encouraged to avoid overfeeding or feeding infants every time they cry. Infants should be encouraged to feed and should be allowed to set their own pace once feedings are established. Parents sometimes set artificial goals—"The baby must take all 5 ounces"—and tend to keep feeding the child until those goals are met, even though the infant may not be hungry. During early feedings, however, the infant may need simple tactile stimulation—such as gently rubbing feet and hands, adjusting clothing, and loosening coverings—to maintain adequate sucking for a sufficient time to complete a full feeding.

The desirable amount and frequency of formula feeding vary with postnatal age of the infant. From birth to 2 months of age, the baby takes six to eight feedings of approximately 2 to 4 ounces of formula at each feeding within a 24-hour period (Tigges, 1997). There are three forms of formula (Table 27–5). They are ready-to-feed, liquid concentrate, and powdered.

Formula preparation is always important to discuss with families. Cleanliness is essential, but sterilization is necessary only if the water source is questionable. Bottles may be effectively prepared in dishwashers or washed thoroughly in warm soapy water and rinsed well. Nipples may be weakened by the temperature of dishwashers and therefore should be washed thoroughly by hand and rinsed well. Tap water, if from an uncontaminated source, may be used for mixing powdered formulas, which are less expensive than the concentrated or ready-to-use prepared formulas. Honey should not be used as a "sugar source" because of the danger of infant botulism.

Bottles may be prepared individually, or up to one day's supply of formula may be prepared at one time. Extra bottles are stored in the refrigerator and should be warmed slightly before feeding. Ready-to-use disposable bottles of formula are very convenient but are also expensive. Formula left in bottles after a feeding should be discarded.

The WIC program provides 8 pounds of powdered formula or 403 ounces of concentrated liquid formula per month. Individual states make provisions about when WIC nutritionists may distribute soy formulas and whether prescriptions are needed for special or therapeutic formulas.

Nutritional Assessment of the Infant

During the early months of life, the food offered to and consumed by infants will be instrumental to their proper growth and development. The infant's nutritional status is assessed at each well-baby visit. Assessment should include four components:

- Nutritional history from the parent
- Weight gain since the last visit
- Growth chart percentiles
- Physical examination

The nutritional history reports the type, amount, and frequency of milk and supplemental foods, vitamins, and minerals being given to the infant on a daily basis. If the baby is taking formula, the history also includes how the formula is mixed (checking for underdilution or overdilution) and stored. The healthy formula-fed infant should generally gain 30 g (1 oz) per day for the first 6 months of life and 15 g (0.5 oz) per day for the second 6 months. Individual charts show the infant's growth with respect to height, weight, and head circumference. The important consideration is that infants continue to grow at their own individual rates.

For a mother who is concerned about whether her infant is getting adequate nutrition, the nurse can recommend looking for an appearance of weight gain and counting the number of wet and soiled diapers in a 24-hour period. Approximately six wet diapers or more and frequent stools in a day indicate adequate nutrition is being attained in the totally breastfed infant. If additional water is ingested, the diaper count should be higher. The presence of urine can most accurately be assessed when the diaper is free of feces. The diaper is most likely to be free of feces prior to feedings because the gastrocolic reflex often stimulates stooling following a feeding. For the anxious parent, another means of reassurance of adequate intake and output is to keep a record of the frequency and duration of feedings, amount of swallowing, and the exact number of wet and/or soiled diapers. Keeping a record tends to give the worried parent a sense of control and a tangible indication on which to rule out or base concern (Table 27–6).

The physical examination will help identify any nutritional disorders. Iron deficiency should be suspected in an infant who is pale, diaphoretic, and irritable.

By calculating the nutritional needs of infants, the nurse can recommend a diet that supplies appropriate nutrition for infant growth and development. The assessment is especially helpful in counseling mothers of infants under 6 months of age, because there is a tendency to add too many supplemental foods or offer too much formula to infants of this age. Clinicians generally advise that an infant not be given more than 32 oz of formula in 1 day. If additional calories are needed, supplemental foods should be added to the diet. Conversely, if the caloric intake is adequate, formula alone gives the infant enough calories, and introduction of solid foods can be delayed.

Appropriate nutritional intake can be identified by comparing the infant's dietary intake with the desired caloric intake for the infant's weight and age. Most commercial formulas prescribed for the normal healthy newborn contain 20 kcal per 30 mL (1 oz). If the infant is eating solids, the caloric value of those foods must be determined and included in the calculations of nutritional intake. With knowledge of the number of calories needed by the infant according to weight (108 kcal/kg/day [55 kcal/lb/day]), the nurse can counsel the parents about how many ounces per day the infant needs to meet caloric requirements. The following example shows the effectiveness of these assessments and interventions.

TABLE 27–6 Successful Breastfeeding Evaluation

Babies are probably getting enough milk if

- They are nursing at least eight times in 24 hours.
- In a quiet room, their mothers can hear them swallow while nursing.
- Their mothers' breasts appear to soften after nursing.
- The number of wet diapers increases by the fourth or fifth day after birth, or there are at least six to eight wet diapers every 24 hours after day 5.
- The baby's stools are yellow or are beginning to lighten in color by the fourth or fifth day after birth.

Offering a supplemental bottle is not a reliable indicator because most babies will take a few ounces even if they are getting enough breast milk (Neifert, 1994).

Jamie Adams, age 1 week, is visited at home by the nurse associated with her family's health maintenance organization. Jamie is Mrs Adams's first child, and Mrs Adams is concerned about whether Jamie is getting adequate nourishment. Jamie weighed 7 lb at birth and has regained her birth weight after an 11 oz (10%) loss. Mrs Adams reports that Jamie takes 3 oz of formula every 3 hours, does not spit up any formula, and has eight to ten wet diapers a day with one to two soft bowel movements per day. Jamie is a contented baby who sleeps between feedings.

Based on requirements of 108 kcal/kg/day, the nurse calculates 1-week-old Jamie's dietary needs as follows:

- Jamie's weight = 7 lb. Converting weight into kg (2.2 lb/kg), Jamie weighs 3.2 kg.
- Jamie's 24-hour caloric need = 3.2 kg (Jamie's weight) × 108 kcal/kg/day = 346 kcal/day.
- Amount of formula (at 20 kcal/oz) needed in 24 hours =17 oz.
- Jamie's 24-hour intake × 24 oz (3 oz every 3 hours) × 20 kcal/oz = 480 kcal.

The nurse makes the following nursing diagnoses:

- ***Knowledge Deficit*** related to lack of information about assessing adequacy of food intake
- ***Altered Nutrition: More than Body Requirements*** related to formula intake that is greater than necessary to meet Jamie's growth needs

The nursing plan outlines the following actions:

- Discuss Jamie's feeding cues with Mrs Adams. How does Mrs Adams decide when to feed Jamie? Is she feeding in response to Jamie or in response to a time schedule? Explain that infants have a need for non-nutritive sucking that can be met with a pacifier.
- Explain normal infant sleep-wake cycles and how babies can self-regulate in phases of light sleep, although they may make stirring noises.
- Explain that Jamie is ingesting more calories than necessary, and point out the need to reduce her intake by approximately 7 oz/day. Mrs Adams can

accomplish this by feeding Jamie a little less frequently and feeding slightly less formula (approximately 0.5 oz or less) each feeding. Giving Jamie 75 mL (2.5 oz) at each of seven feedings provides 350 cal/day. Teach Mrs Adams how to feed Jamie in response to feeding cues, such as rooting and hand-to-mouth activity. When Jamie has taken 75 to 90 mL (2.5 to 3 oz) of formula, substitute a pacifier to provide nonnutritive sucking. Explain that if Jamie takes 2.5 to 3 oz and seems to want to eat again before 3 to 4 hours, Mrs Adams should try other comfort measures, such as changing Jamie's diaper, rocking her, giving her a pacifier, or putting her in a swing, before resorting to feeding.

- Discuss with Mrs Adams the behaviors that indicate satiation. These include minimal sucking with release of the nipple and falling asleep with hands and body relaxed. She should not attempt to force the remaining milk, if any, but should discard it because of the potential for bacterial growth even if refrigerated.
- Formula amounts can be increased gradually to meet Jamie's changing caloric needs and growth without excessive caloric intake. Once Jamie is ingesting 32 oz a day, the addition of solid foods can be considered after discussion with the health provider.
- Explore alternative methods for providing comfort to a newborn.

On a follow-up well-baby visit, Jamie is weighed and is gaining 30 g (1 oz) per day. Jamie continues to have approximately eight to ten wet diapers a day and is alert and responsive.

FOCUS YOUR STUDY

- The RDA for calories for the newborn is 105 to 108 kcal/kg/day (50 to 55 kcal/lb/day).
- The nurse must monitor the first feeding because this is when the newborn may initially manifest signs of cardiac complications or anomalies of the upper GI tract.
- Breast milk has immunologic and nutritional properties that make it the optimal food for the first year of life.
- Signs indicating newborn readiness for the first feeding are active bowel sounds, absence of abdominal distention, and a lusty cry that quiets with rooting and sucking behaviors when a stimulus is placed near the lips.
- Mature breast milk and commercially prepared formulas (unless otherwise noted) provide 20 kcal/oz.
- Breastfed infants need supplements of vitamin D and fluoride. However, there is no need to give supplemental iron to breastfed infants before 6 months of age.
- Nurses must recognize that cultural values influence infant feeding practices, be sensitive to ethnic backgrounds of minority populations, and understand that the dominant culture in any society defines "normal" maternal-infant feeding interaction.
- Breastfed infants are getting adequate nutrition if they are gaining weight and have at least six wet diapers a day when not receiving additional water supplements.
- Most maternal medications are transmitted through breast milk. The effects on the infant and lactation depend on a variety of factors, including route of administration, timing of the dose with respect to feeding time, and multiple properties of the medication.
- Breastfeeding mothers should be encouraged to ensure that the infant is correctly positioned at the breast, with a large portion of areola in the mouth and not under the tongue. The mother is advised to rotate the baby's position periodically to ensure that all ducts are emptied.
- To prevent sore nipples the nurse can encourage the breastfeeding mother to allow her breasts to air dry after feeding.
- Formula-fed infants regain their birth weight by 10 days of age and gain 1 oz/day for the first 6 months and 0.5 oz/day for the second 6 months; birth weight is doubled at 3.5 to 4 months of age. Healthy breastfed babies gain approximately 0.5 oz/day in the first 6 months of life, regain their birth weight by about 14 days of age, and double their birth weight at approximately 5 months of age.
- Formula-fed infants need no vitamins or mineral supplements other than iron, if it is not already in the formula, and fluoride, if it is not in the water system.
- The bottle-feeding mother may need help feeding and burping her infant. She will also benefit from information about feeding schedules and types of formula.
- The use of skim milk, cow's milk with lowered fat content, or unmodified cow's milk is not recommended for children under 2 years old.
- Nutritional assessment of the infant includes nutritional history from the parent, measurement of weight gain, determination of growth chart percentiles, and physical examination.

REFERENCES

American Academy of Pediatrics, Work Group on Breastfeeding. (1997). Breastfeeding and the use of human milk. *Pediatrics, 100*(6), 1035–1039.

American Academy of Pediatrics (AAP) and the American College of Obstericians and Gynecologists (ACOG). (1997). *Guidelines for perinatal care* (4th ed.). Washington, DC: Author.

Banta-Wright, S. A. (1997). Minimizing infant exposure to and risks from medication while breastfeeding. *Journal of Perinatal and Neonatal Nursing, 11*(2), 71–84.

Bear, K., & Tigges, B. B. (1993). Management strategies for promoting successful breastfeeding. *Nurse Practitioner, 18*(6), 50, 53–54, 56–58 passim.

Bocar, D. L. (1997). Combining breastfeeding and employment: Increasing success. *Journal of Perinatal and Neonatal Nursing, 11*(2), 23–43.

Brandt, K. A., Andrews, C. M., & Kvale, J. (1998). Mother-infant interaction and breastfeeding outcome 6 weeks after birth. *Journal of Obstetric, Gynecologic, and Neonatal Nursing, 27*(2), 169–174.

Brent, N., Rudy, S. J., Redd, B., Rudy, T. E., & Roth, L. A. (1998). Sore nipples in breast-feeding women. *Archives of Pediatric Adolescent Medicine 152* (Nov.), 1077–1082.

Corbett-Dick, P., & Bezek, S. K. (1997). Breastfeeding promotion for the employed mother. *Journal of Pediatric Health Care, 11*(1), 12–19.

Fadavi, S., Punwani, I. C., Jain, L., & Vidyasagar, D. (1997). Mechanics and energetics of nutritive sucking: A functional comparison of commercially available nipples. *Journal of Pediatrics, 130*(5), 740–745.

Furman, L. (1995). A developmental approach to weaning. *American Journal of Maternal Child Nursing, 20*(6), 322–325.

Gigliotti, E. (1995). When women decide not to breastfeed. *American Journal of Maternal Child Nursing, 20*(6), 315–321.

Golding, J. (1997). Unnatural constituents of breast milk—medication, lifestyle, pollutants, viruses. *Early Human Development, 49,* S29–S43.

Hutchinson, M. K., & Baqi-Aziz, M. (1994). Nursing care of the childbearing Muslim family. *Journal of Obstetric, Gynecologic, and Neonatal Nursing, 23*(9), 767–771.

Jensen, D., Wallace, S., & Kelsay, P. (1994). LATCH: A breastfeeding charting system and documentation tool. *Journal of Obstetric, Gynecologic, and Neonatal Nursing, 23*(1), 27–32.

Lawrence, P. B. (1994). Breast milk. Best source of nutrition for term and preterm infants. *Pediatric Clinics of North America, 41*(5), 925–941.

Lawrence, R. A. (1994). *Breastfeeding: A guide for the medical profession* (4th ed.). St. Louis: Mosby.

Littler, C. (1997). Beliefs about colostrum among women from Bangladesh and their reasons for not giving it to the newborn. *Midwives 110*(1308), 3–6.

Littman, H., Medendorp, S. V., & Goldfarb, J. (1994). The decision to breastfeed. The importance of father's approval. *Clinical Pediatrics, 33*(4), 214–219.

McVeagh, P., & Brand Miller, J. (1997). Human milk oligosaccharides: Only the breast. *Journal of Paediatrics/Child Health 33,* 281–286.

Mulford, C. (1990). Subtle signs and symptoms of the milk ejection reflex. *Journal of Human Lactation, 6*(4), 177–178.

Mulford, C. (1992). The mother-baby assessment (MBA): An "Apgar score" for breastfeeding. *Journal of Human Lactation, 8*(2), 79–82.

Neifert, M. (1994). *Criteria for assessing early breastfeeding.* Denver, CO: The Lactation Program.

Pascale, J. A., Brittian, L., Lenfestey, C. C., & Jarrett-Pulliam, C. (1996). Breastfeeding, dehydration, and shorter maternity stays. *Neonatal Network, 15*(7), 37–43.

Piacentini, G. L., Boner, A. L., Richelli, C. C., & Gaburro, D. (1995). Artificial feeding: Progresses and problems. *Annali dell Istituto Superiore di Sanita, 31*(4), 411–418.

Pinella, T., & Birch, L. L. (1993). Help me make it through the night: Behavioral entrainment of breast-fed infants' sleep patterns. *Pediatrics, 91*(2), 436–444.

Riordan, J., & Auerbach, K. (1999). *Breastfeeding and human lactation.* (2nd ed.). Boston: Jones & Bartlett.

Riordan, J. M., & Koehn, M. (1997). Reliability and validity testing of three breastfeeding assessment tools. *Journal of Obstetric, Gynecologic, and Neonatal Nursing, 26*(2), 181–187.

Rogers, I. S., Golding, J., & Emmett, P. M. (1997). The effects of lactation on the mother. *Early Human Development, 49* suppl, S191–S203.

Sharma, M., & Petosa, R. 1997. Impact of expectant fathers in breast-feeding decisions. *Journal of the American Diatetic Association, 97*(11), 1311–1313.

Tigges, B. B. (1997). Infant formulas: Practical answers for common questions. *Nurse Practitioner 22*(8), 70, 73, 77–80, 82, 83, 86–87.

Vezeau, T. M. (1991). Investigating "greedy." *American Journal of Maternal Child Nursing, 16*(6), 337–338.

Wagner, C. L., Anderson, D. M., & Pittard, W. B., III. (1996). Special properties of human milk. *Clinical Pediatrics, 35*(6), 283–293.

Woolridge, M. W., Phil, D., & Baum, J. D. (1993). Recent advances in breast feeding. *Acta Paediatrica Japonica, 35*(1), 1–12.

Xanthou, M. (1998). Immune protection of human milk. *Biology of the Neonate 74,* 121–133.

28 The Newborn at Risk: Conditions Present at Birth

Key Terms

Drug-dependent infants
Fetal alcohol effects (FAE)
Fetal alcohol syndrome (FAS)
Grief work
Inborn errors of metabolism
Infant of diabetic mother (IDM)
Intrauterine growth restriction (IUGR)
Large for gestational age (LGA)
Neonatal morbidity
Neonatal mortality risk
Phenylketonuria (PKU)
Postterm newborn
Postmaturity
Preterm infant
Small for gestational age (SGA)

The rhythmic tides of her sleeping and feeding spaciously measured her days and nights. Her frail absorption was a commanding presence, her helplessness strong as a rock.
~ Laurie Lee, Two Women ~

Objectives

- Identify factors present at birth that help identify an at-risk newborn.
- Compare the underlying etiologies of the physiologic complications of small-for-gestational-age (SGA) newborns and preterm appropriate-for-gestational-age (Pr AGA) newborns.
- Describe the impact of maternal diabetes mellitus on the newborn.
- Compare the characteristics and underlying etiologies of potential complications of the postterm newborn and the newborn with postmaturity syndrome.
- Discuss the physiologic characteristics of the preterm newborn that predispose each body system to various complications.
- Identify the data used in developing the nursing diagnoses required to plan interventions for the care of the Pr AGA newborn.
- Explain the special care needed by an alcohol- or drug-exposed newborn.
- Relate the consequences of maternal HIV/AIDS to the management of the infant in the neonatal period.
- Identify physical examination findings during the early newborn period that would make the nurse suspect a congenital cardiac defect.
- Discuss the nursing assessments of and initial interventions for a newborn born with congenital anomalies.
- Explain the special care needed by a newborn with an inborn error of metabolism.
- Describe interventions to facilitate parental attachment with the at-risk newborn.
- Identify the nursing actions that provide support to family members dealing with the birth of an at-risk infant.

WITHIN THE PAST THREE DECADES, THE field of neonatology has expanded greatly. Many levels of nursery care have evolved in response to increasing knowledge about the newborn: special care; convalescent/transitional care; low-risk and high-risk care. The nurse is an important caregiver in all these settings. As a member of the multidisciplinary health care team, the nurse contributes to the high-touch care necessary in today's high-tech perinatal environment.

In addition to the availability of a high level of newborn care, a variety of other factors influences the outcomes of these at-risk infants, including the following:

- Birth weight
- Gestational age
- Type and length of newborn illness
- Environmental factors
- Maternal factors
- Maternal-infant separation

Identification of At-Risk Newborns

An at-risk infant is one who is susceptible to illness (morbidity) or even death because of dysmaturity, immaturity, physical disorders, or complications during or after birth. In most cases, the infant is the product of pregnancy involving one or more predictable risk factors, including the following:

- Low socioeconomic level of the mother and limited access to health care
- Exposure to environmental dangers, such as toxic chemicals and illicit drugs
- Preexisting maternal conditions, such as heart disease, diabetes, hypertension, and renal disease
- Maternal factors, such as age or parity
- Medical conditions related to pregnancy and their associated complications

Various risk factors and their specific effects on the pregnancy outcome are listed in Table 11–2. Because these factors and the perinatal risks associated with them are known, the birth of at-risk newborns can often be anticipated. The pregnancy can be closely monitored, treatment can be instituted as necessary, and arrangements can be made for birth to occur at a facility with appropriate resources to care for both mother and baby.

At-risk infants cannot always be identified before the onset of labor because the course of labor and birth and the infant's ability to withstand the stress of labor are not known beforehand. Thus during labor, electronic fetal heart monitoring or frequent monitoring by fetoscope by the nurse has played a significant role in detecting distress in the fetus. Immediately after birth, the Apgar score is a helpful tool in identifying the at-risk newborn, but it is not the only indicator of possible long-term outcome.

The newborn classification and neonatal mortality risk chart is another useful tool in identifying newborns at risk (Figure 28–1). Before this classification tool was developed, birth weight of less than 2500 g was the sole criterion for determination of immaturity. It was eventually recognized that an infant could weigh more than 2500 g but still be immature. Conversely, an infant weighing less than 2500 g might be functionally mature at term or beyond. Thus birth weight and gestational age together became the criteria used to assess neonatal maturity and mortality risk.

According to the newborn classification and neonatal mortality risk chart, gestation is divided as follows:

- Preterm: less than 37 (completed) weeks
- Term: 38 to 41 (completed) weeks
- Postterm: greater than 42 weeks

As shown in Figure 28–1, large-for-gestational-age (LGA) infants are those that plot above the 90th percentile curve. Appropriate-for-gestational-age (AGA) infants are those that plot between the 10th percentile and 90th percentile curve. Small-for-gestational-age (SGA) infants are those that plot below the 10th percentile curve. A newborn is assigned to a category depending on birth weight and gestational age. For example, a newborn classified as Pr SGA is preterm and small for gestational age. The full-term newborn whose weight is appropriate for gestational age is classified F AGA. It should be noted that intrauterine growth charts are influenced by altitude and the ethnicity of the population the charts were based upon. There is a correlation between an increase in altitude and a decrease in birth weight (Nagey & Viscardi, 1993).

Neonatal mortality risk is the chance of death within the newborn period, that is, within the first 28 days of life. As indicated in Figure 28–1, the neonatal mortality risk decreases as both gestational age and birth weight increase. Infants who are preterm and small for gestational age have the highest neonatal mortality risk. The previously high mortality rates for LGA infants have decreased at most perinatal centers because of improved management of diabetes in pregnancy and increased recognition of potential complications of LGA newborns.

Neonatal morbidity can be anticipated based on birth weight and gestational age. In Figure 28–2, the infant's birth weight is located on the vertical axis, and the gestational age in weeks is found along the horizontal axis. The area where the two meet on the graph identifies common problems. This tool assists in determining the needs of particular infants for special observation and care. For example, an infant of 2000 g at 40 weeks' gestation should be carefully assessed for evidence of fetal distress, hypoglycemia, congenital anomalies, congenital infection, and polycythemia.

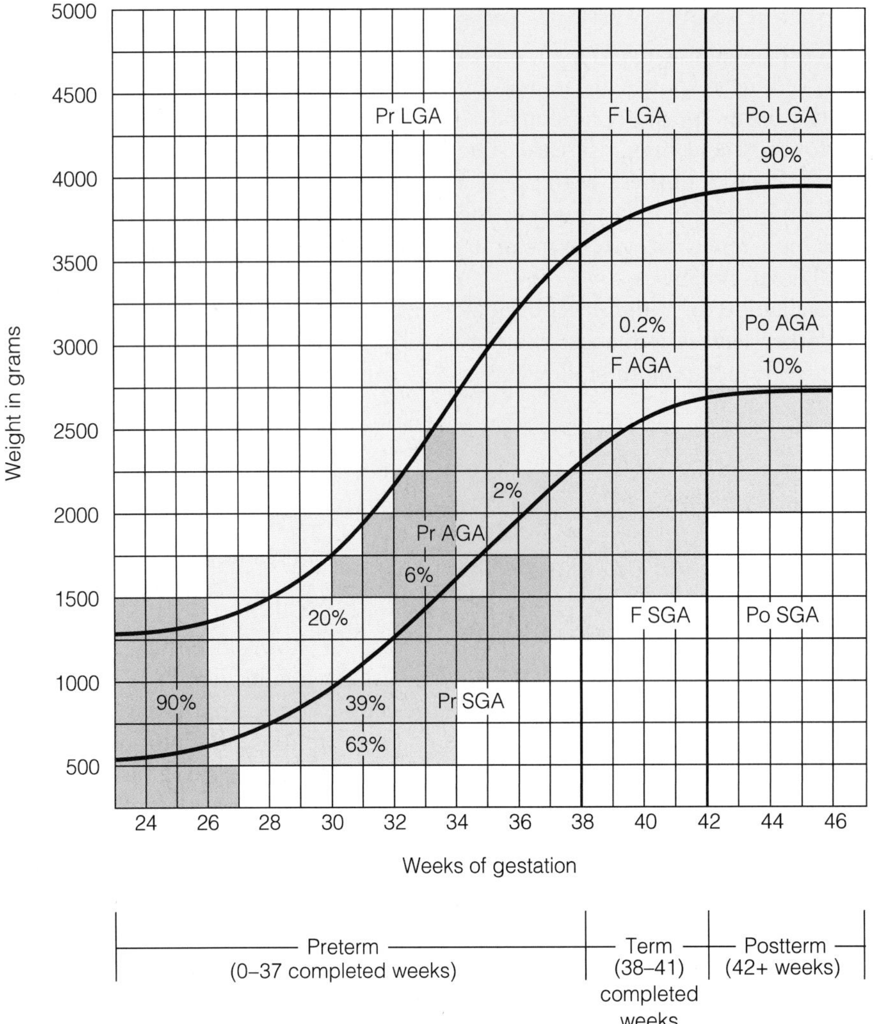

FIGURE 28–1 Newborn classification and neonatal mortality risk chart. Infants are classified according to weight as small for gestational age (SGA), appropriate for gestational age (AGA), or large for gestational age (LGA) and by weeks of newborn as preterm (Pr), term (F), or postterm (Po). Corresponding neonatal mortality risks are indicated by the percentages in the various colored regions. SOURCE: Koops BL, Morgan LP, Battaglia FC: Neonatal mortality risk in relationship to birth weight and gestational age. *J Pediatr* 1982; 101(6):969.

Identifying the nursing care needs of the at-risk newborn depends on minute-to-minute observations of the changes in the newborn's physiologic status. It is essential to a baby's survival that the nurse understand the basic physiologic principles that guide nursing management of the at-risk newborn. The nursing care management must be directed toward the following:

- Decreasing physiologically stressful situations
- Constantly observing for subtle signs of change in clinical condition
- Interpreting laboratory data and coordinating interventions
- Conserving the infant's energy for healing and growth
- Providing for developmental stimulation and maintenance of sleep cycles
- Assisting the family in developing attachment behaviors
- Involving the family in the planning and providing care

Care of the Small-for-Gestational-Age Newborn

Any newborn who at birth is at or below the 10th percentile for weight (intrauterine growth curves) on the newborn classification chart is considered **small for gestational age (SGA)** (Figure 28–1). For purposes of assigning SGA classification to a newborn, birth weight charts should be based on the local population into which the newborn is born (Bakketeig, 1998). A SGA newborn

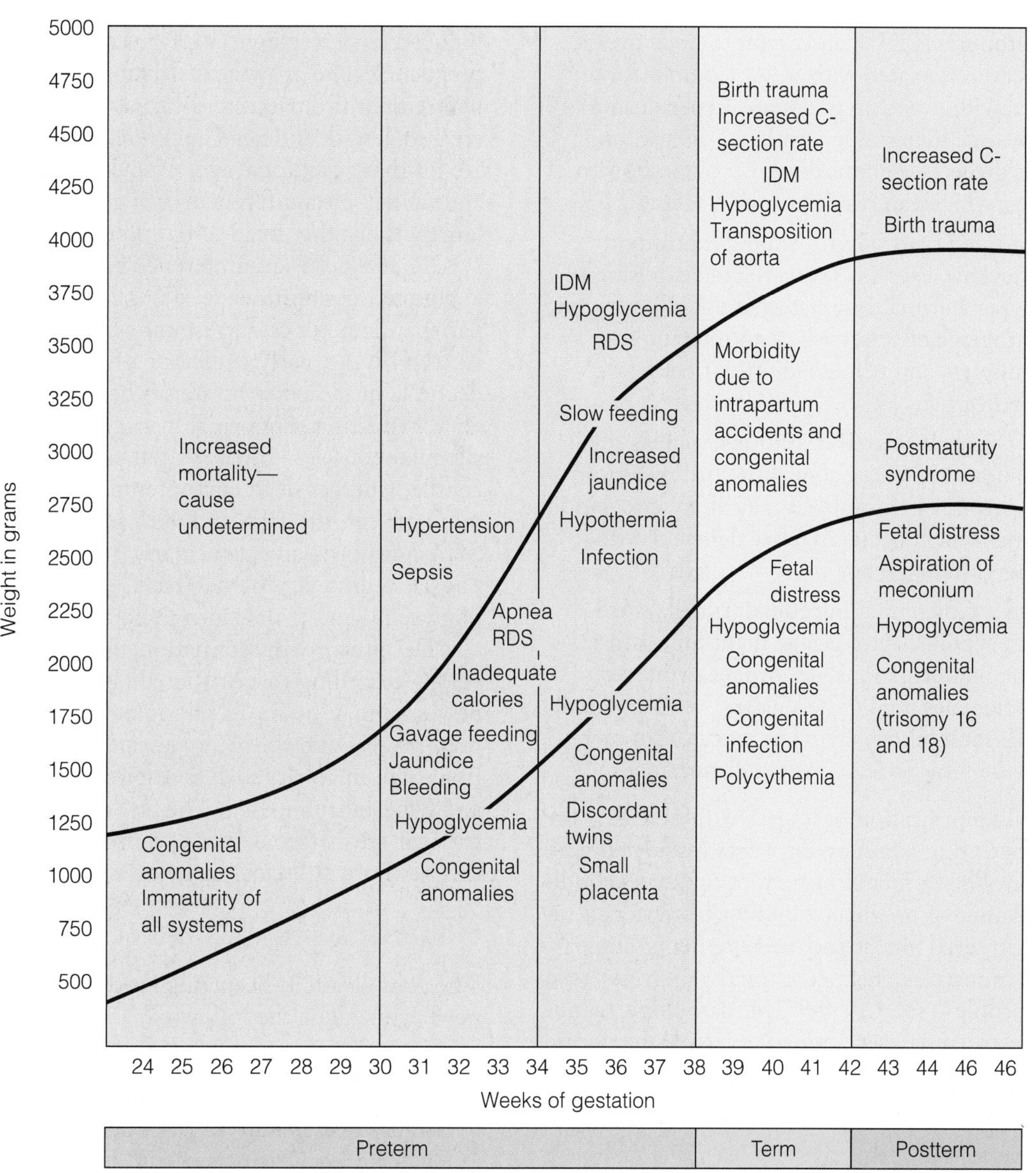

FIGURE 28–2 Neonatal morbidity by birth weight and gestational age. SOURCE: Lubchenco LO: *The High Risk Infant.* Philadelphia: Saunders, 1976, p 122.

may be preterm, term, or postterm. Other terms used to designate an undergrown newborn include **intrauterine growth restriction (IUGR),** which describes the pregnancy circumstance of advanced gestation and limited fetal growth. The terms SGA and IUGR are used interchangeably.

Small-for-gestational-age infants have an incidence of perinatal asphyxia five times that of AGA infants, and a perinatal mortality rate eight times that of AGA infants (Sohl & Moore, 1998). The incidence of polycythemia and hypoglycemia are also higher in this group of infants.

Factors Contributing to Intrauterine Growth Restriction (IUGR)

IUGR may be caused by maternal, placental, or fetal factors and may not be apparent antenatally. Intrauterine growth is linear in the normal pregnancy from approximately 28 to 38 weeks' gestation. After 38 weeks, growth is variable, depending on the genetic growth potential of the fetus and placental function. The most common factors affecting growth restriction are the following:

- *Maternal factors.* Primiparity, grand multiparity, multiple pregnancy (twins, triplets, and so on), smoking, lack of prenatal care, age extremes (under 16 or over 40), and low socioeconomic status (which can result in inadequate health care, inadequate education, and inadequate living conditions) affect IUGR (Spinillo, Capuzzo, Piazzi, Nicola, Colonna, & Iasci, 1994). Before the third trimester, the nutritional supply to the fetus far exceeds its needs. Only in the third trimester is maternal malnutrition a limiting factor in fetal growth.
- *Maternal disease.* Maternal heart disease, substance abuse (drugs, smoking, alcohol), sickle cell anemia,

phenylketonuria (PKU), and asymptomatic pyelonephritis are associated with SGA. Complications associated with pregnancy-induced hypertension (PIH), chronic hypertensive vascular disease, and advanced diabetes mellitus diminish blood flow to the uterus, which can result in a SGA infant.

- *Environmental factors.* High altitude, exposure to x-rays, excessive exercise, work-related exposure to toxins, hyperthermia, and maternal use of drugs that have teratogenic effects, such as antimetabolics, anticonvulsants, and trimethadione, affect fetal growth (Kliegman, 1997).
- *Placental factors.* Placental conditions, such as small placenta, infarcted areas, abnormal cord insertions, placenta previa, or thrombosis may affect circulation to the fetus, which becomes more deficient with increasing gestational age.
- *Fetal factors.* Congenital infections (rubella, toxoplasmosis, syphilis, cytomegalic inclusion disease), congenital malformations, discordant twins, sex of the fetus (females tend to be smaller), chromosomal syndromes, and inborn errors of metabolism can predispose a fetus to fetal growth disturbances.

Antenatal identification of fetuses with IUGR is the first step in detecting common disorders associated with this newborn. The perinatal history of maternal conditions, early dating of pregnancy by first trimester ultrasound and then serial ultrasound measurements, antepartal testing (nonstress test, contraction stress test, biophysical profile—see Chapter 17), pathology examination of the placenta, gestational age assessment, and the physical and neurologic assessment of the newborn are also important (Sohl & Moore, 1998).

Patterns of IUGR

Intrauterine growth occurs by an increase in cell number and by an increase in cell size. If insult occurs early during the critical period of organ development in the fetus, fewer new cells are formed, organs are small, and organ weight is subnormal. In contrast, growth failure that begins later in pregnancy does not affect the total number of cells, only their size. The organs are normal, but their size is diminished. There are two clinical pictures of SGA newborns.

Symmetric (proportional) IUGR is caused by long-term maternal conditions (such as chronic hypertension, severe malnutrition, chronic intrauterine infection, substance abuse, and anemia) or fetal genetic abnormalities (Sohl & Moore, 1998). Symmetric IUGR can be noted by ultrasound in the first half of the second trimester. In symmetric IUGR there is chronic prolonged restriction of growth in size of organs, body weight, body length, and, in severe cases, head circumference.

Asymmetric (disproportional) IUGR is associated with an acute compromise of uteroplacental blood flow. Some associated causes are placental infarcts, pregnancy-induced hypertension (PIH), and poor weight gain in pregnancy. The growth retardation is usually not evident before the third trimester because although weight is decreased, length and head circumference remain appropriate for that gestational age. After 36 weeks' gestation, the abdominal circumference of a normal fetus becomes larger than the head circumference. In asymmetric IUGR, the head circumference remains larger than the abdominal circumference. Thus measuring only the biparietal diameter on ultrasound will not reveal asymmetric IUGR. An early indicator of asymmetric SGA is a decrease in the growth rate of the abdominal circumference, reflecting subnormal liver growth and a paucity of subcutaneous fat. Birth weight is below the 10th percentile, whereas head circumference, and/or length, may plot between the 10th and 90th percentiles. Asymmetric SGA newborns are particularly at risk for perinatal asphyxia, pulmonary hemorrhage, hypocalcemia, and hypoglycemia in the newborn period.

Despite growth retardation, physiologic maturity develops according to gestational age. Therefore the SGA newborn may be more physiologically mature than the preterm AGA newborn and less predisposed to complications of prematurity such as respiratory distress syndrome and hyperbilirubinemia. The SGA newborn's chances for survival are better because of organ maturity, although this newborn still faces many other potential difficulties.

Common Complications of the SGA Newborn

The complications occurring most frequently in the SGA newborn include the following:

- *Perinatal asphyxia.* The SGA infant suffers chronic hypoxia in utero, which leaves little reserve to withstand the demands of labor and birth. Thus intrauterine asphyxia occurs with its potential systemic problems. Cesarean birth may be necessary.
- *Aspiration syndrome.* In utero, hypoxia can cause the fetus to gasp during birth, resulting in aspiration of amniotic fluid into the lower airways. It can also lead to relaxation of the anal sphincter and passage of meconium. This may result in aspiration of the meconium in utero or with the first breaths after birth.
- *Heat loss.* Diminished subcutaneous fat (used for survival in utero), depletion of brown fat in utero, and a large surface area decrease the IUGR newborn's ability to conserve heat. The effect of surface area is diminished somewhat because of the flexed position assumed by the term SGA newborn.
- *Hypoglycemia.* An increase in metabolic rate in response to heat loss and poor hepatic glycogen stores cause hypoglycemia. In addition, the infant is compromised by inadequate supplies of enzymes to activate gluconeogenesis (conversion of nonglucogen sources, such as fatty acids and proteins, to glucose).

- *Polycythemia.* The number of red blood cells is increased in the SGA newborn. This finding is considered a physiologic response to in utero chronic hypoxic stress.

Newborns who have significant IUGR tend to have a poor prognosis, especially when born before 37 weeks' gestation. Factors contributing to poor outcome include:

- *Congenital malformations.* Congenital malformations occur 10 to 20 times more frequently in SGA infants than in AGA infants. The more severe the IUGR, the greater the chance for malformation as a result of impaired mitotic activity and cellular hypoplasia.
- *Intrauterine infection.* When fetuses are exposed to intrauterine infections such as rubella and cytomegalovirus, they are profoundly affected by direct invasion of the brain and other vital organs by the offending virus, resulting in IUGR.
- *Continued growth difficulties.* It is generally agreed that SGA newborns tend to be shorter than newborns of the same gestational age. Asymmetric IUGR infants can be expected to catch up in weight to normal growth infants by 3 to 6 months of age. Symmetric SGA infants reportedly have varied growth potential but tend not to catch up to their peers (Sohl & Moore, 1998).
- *Learning difficulties.* Often SGA newborns exhibit poor brain development and subsequent failure to catch up, and learning disabilities are not uncommon. The disabilities are characterized by hyperactivity, short attention span, and poor fine motor coordination (reading, writing, and drawing). Poor scholastic performance is also a common problem (Kliegman, 1997). Some hearing loss and speech defects also occur.

Studies have determined that the quality of the home environment of a preterm SGA infant predicts developmental outcome better than any single biologic risk factor (Strauss & Dietz, 1997).

Clinical Therapy

The goal of medical therapy for SGA infants is early recognition and implementation of medical management of the potential problems.

NURSING CARE MANAGEMENT

Nursing Assessment and Diagnosis

The nurse is responsible for assessing gestational age and identifying signs of potential complications associated with SGA infants.

All body parts of the symmetric IUGR infant are in proportion, but they are below normal size for the baby's gestational age. Therefore the head does not appear overly large or the length excessive in relation to the other body parts. These newborns are generally vigorous.

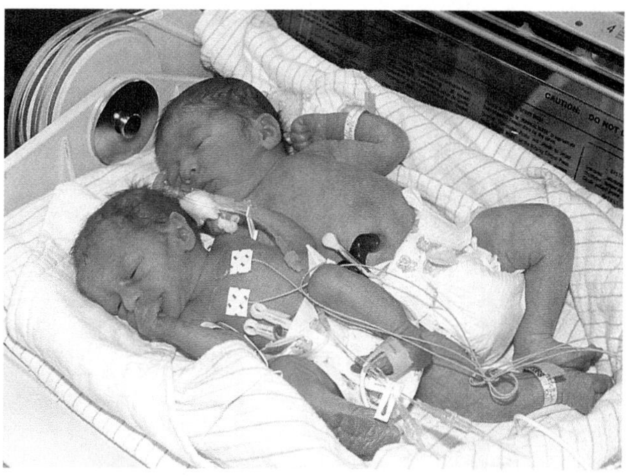

FIGURE 28–3 Thirty-five week gestational age twins. Twin B is SGA and weighs 1260 grams and Twin A is AGA and weighs 2605 grams. SOURCE: Courtesy of Carol Harrigan, RNC, MSN, NNP.

The asymmetric IUGR infant appears long, thin, and emaciated, with loss of subcutaneous fat tissue and muscle mass (Figure 28–3). The baby may have loose skin folds; dry, desquamating skin; and a thin and often meconium-stained cord. The head appears relatively large (although it approaches normal size) because the chest size and abdominal girth are decreased. The baby may have a vigorous cry and appear alert and wide eyed.

Nursing diagnoses that may apply to the small-for-gestational-age newborn include the following:

- ***Impaired Gas Exchange*** related to aspiration of meconium
- ***Hypothermia*** related to decreased subcutaneous fat
- ***Risk for Injury*** to tissues related to decreased glycogen stores and impaired gluconeogenesis
- ***Altered Nutrition: Less than Body Requirements*** related to SGA's increased metabolic rate
- ***Risk for Altered Tissue Perfusion*** related to increased blood viscosity
- ***Risk for Altered Parenting*** related to prolonged separation of newborn from parents secondary to illness

Nursing Plan and Implementation

Hospital-Based Nursing Care

Hypoglycemia, the most common metabolic complication of IUGR, can produce CNS abnormalities and mental retardation. Conditions such as asphyxia, hyperviscosity, and cold stress may also affect the baby's outcome. Meticulous attention to physiologic parameters is essential for immediate nursing management and reduction of long-term disorders (see the Critical Pathway for Small-for-Gestational-Age Newborns on page 810).

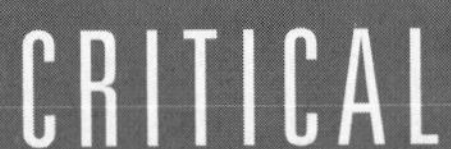

CRITICAL PATHWAY FOR SMALL-FOR-GESTATIONAL-AGE NEWBORNS

Category	Day of Birth—First 4 Hours	Remaining Day of Birth
Referral	Report from L&D, neonatal nurse practitioner Check ID bands Prn consults: high-risk peds, genetics	Check ID bands q shift As parents desire, obtain circumcision permit after their discussion with MD Lactation consult prn
Assessments	(Refer to Newborn Critical Pathway, pp. 754 to 755) • Complete set of VS • Admission wt, length, HC • Assess skin color • Gestational age assessment • Assess for s/s hypoglycemia. Chemstrip ASAP after birth, then follow SGA policy and procedure for blood glucose monitoring • Assess for polycythemia: follow policy for treatment prn	Vital signs: T/P/R q4h and prn, BP prn Newborn assessment q shift (See Newborn Critical Pathway, pp. 754 to 755) Continue hypoglycemia assessments, chemstrips per SGA protocol Assess mother/baby interaction
Teaching/ psychosocial	(See Newborn Critical Pathway, pp. 754 to 755) Admission activities performed at mother's bedside if possible, orient to nursery, handwashing, assess teaching needs Teach parents rationale for SGA protocol	(See Newborn Critical Pathway, pp. 754 to 755) Reinforce previous teaching Teach parent/guardian feeding methods, burping, diapering, calming techniques, s/s of stress, elimination norms
Nursing care management and reports	Diagnostic Tests: blood type, Rh, Coombs' on cord blood when applicable, chemstrip within 1 h of birth and q1–2h until feedings initiated per protocol Check chemstrip before at least two feedings or until condition stabilizes (chemstrip $>$ 40mg/dL x2)	Femoral pulse or BP all 4 extremities if early DC Hct per policy Baer hearing screen Cord care per policy (triple dye x1, then alcohol q diaper change) Bathe per policy
Activity and comfort	Place under radiant warmer, attach skin probe to maintain NTE Soothe baby as needed with voice, touch, nesting in warmer	Leave in radiant warmer until stable, then swaddle in open crib Incubator if temp instability; adjust incubator for infant size and gestation to maintain NTE
Nutrition	Initiate breast- or bottle-feeding as soon as mother and baby condition allows Lavage and gavage prn Supplement breast when medically indicated or ordered by MD per policy Feed SGA infants q3–4h Monitor feeding tolerance, suck	Continue feeding schedule: small frequent feedings, high calorie formula, nutritional fortifiers
Elimination	Note first void and stool if not at birth	Note all voids, amount and color of stools q4h
Medication	Aquamephyton IM, dosage according to infant wt per MD orders Ilotycin ophth ointment OU	Hep B vaccine as ordered by MD after consent signed by parent
Discharge planning/ home care	Hep B consent reviewed with parents Plan DC with parent/guardian in 1–3 days Evaluate for social services/home care/discharge planning needs	Hep B consent signed by parents Birth certificate instructions/worksheet Car seat for DC
Family involvement	Evaluate psychosocial needs Evaluate parent teaching. Access community resources prn, ie, Teen "Healthy Starts"	Assess parents' knowledge of newborn behavior and reflexes Encourage family involvement in infant's care as possible and as infant tolerates
Date		

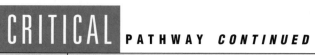

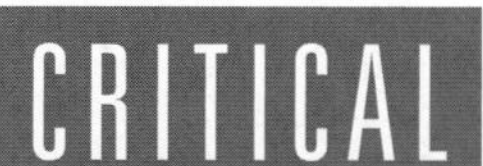

PATHWAY *CONTINUED*

Category	Day 1	Day 2/3 (if applicable)
Referral	Check ID bands q shift	Check ID bands q shift **Expected Outcomes** Mother/baby ID bands correlate at time of discharge. Consults completed prn.
Assessments	Assess thermoregulation Assess for potential complications: perinatal asphyxia, aspiration syndrome, hypoglycemia, hypocalcemia, polycythemia Assess mother/baby interaction	Assess color for jaundice Assess for apnea Assess mother/baby interaction **Expected Outcomes** Physical assessments, VS WNL; no complications of SGA noted
Teaching/ psychosocial	(See Newborn Critical Pathway, pp. 754 to 755) Reinforce previous teaching Parent teaching: bathing, cord care, skin/nail care, use of thermometer, activity, sleep patterns, soothing, reflexes, jaundice, growth/feeding patterns	Final Discharge Teaching (See Newborn Critical Pathway, pp. 754 to 755) Review infant safety, s/s of illness and when to call health care provider with parents **Expected Outcomes** Mother verbalizes comprehension of instructions, demonstrates care capabilities
Nursing care management and reports	Scalp treatment BID Daily wt Newborn assessment q shift Check circumcision site q diaper change Unclamp cord clamp Cord care per policy Total bilirubin level prn	Newborn assessment q shift Daily wt Check circumcision site Cord care per policy Note Baer hearing test results Femoral pulse or BP all 4 extremities **Expected Outcomes** Physical assessments WNL; cord unclamped and dry without s/s of infection; circ site unremarkable; gaining wt or wt stabilized to not >10% loss, labs WNL
Activity and comfort	Swaddled in open crib Incubator if temp instability; adjust incubator for infant size and gestation to maintain NTE	**Expected Outcomes** Maintains temp WNL swaddled in open crib
Nutrition	Continue enhanced feeding schedule, gavage prn per MD orders Supplement breast only when medically indicated/policy or ordered by MD/NP Encourage on demand feeds, minimally q3–4h, breast or bottle	Continue enhanced feeding schedule, gavage prn per MD/NP orders **Expected Outcomes** Infant tolerates feedings, feeds on demand, breastfeeds without supplement, nipples without problems; regaining lost wt or wt stabilized
Elimination	Evaluate all voids and stool color q8h **Expected Outcomes** Voids and stools without difficulty	Note all voids and stool color q shift **Expected Outcomes** Voids qs, stools without difficulty and WNL
Medication	Hep B vaccine before discharge	**Expected Outcomes** Infant has received ophth ointment OU and Aquamephyton injection; received first Hep B vaccine if ordered and parental consent given
Discharge planning/ home care	Newborn photographs Complete birth certificate packet If vag birth, complete DC teaching	If C/S birth complete DC instructions (See Newborn Critical Pathway, pp. 754 to 755) **Expected Outcomes** Infant DC home with mother; mother verbalizes follow-up appointment time/date
Family involvement	Bath, newborn care and feeding classes Newborn channel as available Assess mother/baby bonding and interaction Incorporate significant others and siblings in care Support positive parenting behaviors Evaluate mother/parent teaching	Assess mother/baby bonding and interaction Identify community referral needs and refer to community agencies **Expected Outcomes** Demonstrates caring and family incorporation of infant
Date		

Community-Based Nursing Care

The long-term needs of the SGA newborn include careful follow-up evaluation of patterns of growth and possible disabilities that may later interfere with learning or motor functioning. Long-term follow-up care is especially necessary for those infants with congenital malformations, congenital infections, and obvious sequelae from physiologic problems. In addition, the parents of the IUGR baby need support because a positive atmosphere can enhance the baby's growth potential and the child's ultimate outcome.

Evaluation

Expected outcomes of nursing care include the following:

- The SGA newborn is free from respiratory compromise.
- The SGA newborn maintains a stable temperature and glucose hemostasis.
- The SGA newborn gains weight and takes nipple- or bottle-feedings without physiologic distress or fatigue.
- The parents verbalize their concerns surrounding their baby's health problems and understand the rationale behind management of their newborn.

Care of the Large-for-Gestational-Age Newborn

A neonate whose birth weight is at or above the 90th percentile on the intrauterine growth curve (at any week of gestation) is considered **large for gestational age (LGA).** The classification of LGA may vary according to the intrauterine growth curve chart used; therefore, the chart used should correlate with the characteristics of the client population (Harrington & Campbell, 1993). Some LGA newborns have been incorrectly categorized as LGA because of miscalculation of the date of conception due to postconceptional bleeding. Careful gestational age assessment is therefore essential to identify the potential needs and problems of such infants.

The best known condition associated with excessive fetal growth is maternal diabetes (White's classes A through C; see Table 15–2); however, only a small fraction of LGA newborns are born to diabetic mothers. The cause of the majority of cases of LGA infants is unclear, but certain factors or situations have been found to correlate with their births:

- Genetic predisposition is correlated proportionally to the mother's prepregnancy weight and to weight gain during pregnancy. Large parents tend to have large infants.
- Multiparous women have two to three times the number of LGA infants as primigravidas.
- Male infants are typically larger than female infants.
- Infants with erythroblastosis fetalis, Beckwith-Wiedemann syndrome (a genetic condition associated with macroglossia, omphalocele, and newborn hypoglycemia and hyperinsulinemia), or transposition of the great vessels are usually large.

The increase in the LGA infant's body size is characteristically proportional, although head circumference and body length are in the upper limits of intrauterine growth. The exception to this rule is the infant of the diabetic mother, whose body weight is higher but whose length and head circumference may be in the normal range. Macrosomic infants have poor motor skills and have more difficulty in regulating behavioral states. LGA infants tend to be more difficult to arouse and may have problems maintaining a quiet alert state. They may also have feeding difficulties (Pressler & Hepworth, 1997).

Common Complications of the LGA Newborn

Disorders of the LGA infant can include the following:

- *Birth trauma due to cephalopelvic disproportion (CPD).* Often these newborns have a biparietal diameter greater than 10 cm (4 in) or are associated with a maternal fundal height measurement greater than 42 cm (16 in) without the presence of hydramnios. Because of their excessive size, there are more breech presentations and shoulder dystocias. These complications may result in asphyxia, fractured clavicles, brachial plexus palsy, facial paralysis, phrenic nerve palsy, depressed skull fractures, hematomas, and bleeding of the head due to birth trauma.
- *Increased incidence of cesarean births and oxytocin-induced births due to fetal size.* These births are accompanied by all the risk factors associated with cesarean births.
- *Hypoglycemia, polycythemia, and hyperviscosity.* These disorders are most often seen in infants of diabetic mothers and infants with erythroblastosis fetalis or Beckwith-Wiedemann syndrome.

NURSING CARE MANAGEMENT

The perinatal history, in conjunction with ultrasonic measurement of fetal skull and gestational age testing, is important in identifying an at-risk LGA newborn. Nursing care is directed toward early identification and immediate treatment of the common disorders. Essential components of the nursing assessment are monitoring vital signs, screening for hypoglycemia and polycythemia, and observing for signs and symptoms related to birth trauma. The nurse should address parental concerns about the visual signs of birth trauma and the potential for continuation of the overweight pattern. The nurse should help parents learn to arouse and console their newborn and facilitate nutritional intake and attachment behaviors. Mothers of LGA infants with bruising of the face or head may be reluctant to interact with their infants because they fear increasing the bruising or causing their infants pain (Pressler & Hepworth, 1997). The nursing care involved in the complications associated with LGA newborns is the same as the care needed by the infant with a diabetic mother and will be discussed in the next section.

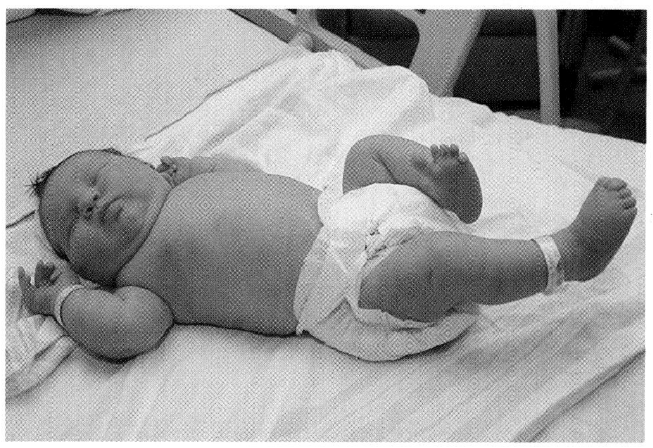

FIGURE 28–4 Macrosomic infant of a diabetic mother. X-ray examination of these infants often reveals caudal regression of the spine.

Care of the Infant of a Diabetic Mother

Infants of diabetic mothers (IDMs) are considered at risk and require close observation the first few hours to the first few days of life. Mothers with severe diabetes or diabetes of long duration (type I or White's classes D through F, associated with vascular complications; see Table 15–2) may give birth to SGA infants. The typical IDM (Type I or White's classes A and C), however, is LGA. The infant is macrosomic, ruddy in color, and has excess adipose fat tissue (Figure 28–4). The umbilical cord and placenta are large. There is a higher incidence of macrosomic infants born to certain ethnic groups (Native Americans, Mexican Americans, African Americans, and Pacific Islanders) (Doshier, 1995; Homko, Sivan, Nyirjesy, & Reece, 1995).

CRITICAL THINKING QUESTION

What information would you provide to a diabetic woman prior to conception that could decrease the possible complications for her baby?

IDMs have decreased total body water, particularly in the extracellular spaces, and are therefore not edematous. Their excessive weight is due to increased weight of the visceral organs, cardiomegaly (hypertrophy), and increased body fat. The only organ not affected is the brain.

The excessive fetal growth of the IDM is caused by exposure to high levels of maternal glucose, which readily crosses the placenta. The fetus responds to these high glucose levels with increased insulin production and hyperplasia of the pancreatic beta cells. The main action of insulin is to facilitate the entry of glucose into muscle and fat cells in a function similar to a cellular growth hormone. Once in the cells, glucose is converted to glycogen and stored. Insulin also inhibits the breakdown of fat to free fatty acids, thereby maintaining lipid synthesis; increases the uptake of amino acids; and promotes protein synthesis. Insulin is an important regulator of fetal metabolism and has a "growth hormone" effect that results in increased linear growth. There has been an association between IDM and childhood obesity (Doshier, 1995).

Common Complications of the IDM

Although IDMs are usually large, they are immature in physiologic functions and exhibit many of the problems of the preterm (premature) infant. The complications most often seen in an IDM are as follows:

- *Hypoglycemia.* After birth, the most common problem of an IDM is hypoglycemia. Even though the high maternal blood sugar supply is lost, this newborn continues to produce high levels of insulin, which deplete the infant's blood glucose within hours after birth. IDMs also have less ability to release glucagon and catecholamines, which normally stimulate glucagon breakdown and glucose release. The incidence of hypoglycemia in IDMs varies from 20% to 40% (Tyrala, 1996). The incidence of hypoglycemia also varies according to the degree of success in controlling the maternal diabetes, the maternal blood sugar level at the time of birth, the length of labor, the class of maternal diabetes, and early versus late feedings of the newborn.
- *Hypocalcemia.* Tremors are the obvious clinical sign of hypocalcemia. This may be due to the IDM's increased incidence of prematurity and to the stresses of difficult pregnancy, labor, and birth. Diabetic women tend to have decreased serum magnesium levels at term secondary to increased urinary calcium excretion, which causes secondary hypoparathyroidism in their infants. Other factors may include vitamin D antagonism, which results from

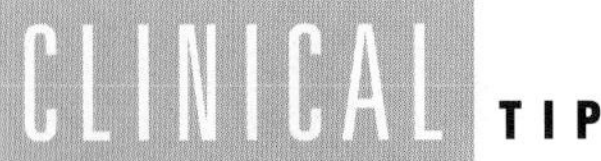 TIP

When beginning fluids on an IDM, it is sometimes best to start at a higher concentration of dextrose to avoid hypoglycemia episodes.

elevated corticol levels, hypophosphatemia from tissue catabolism, and decreased serum magnesium levels.

- *Hyperbilirubinemia.* This condition may be seen at 48 to 72 hours after birth. It may be caused by slightly decreased extracellular fluid volume, which increases the hematocrit level, and the presence of hepatic immaturity (Tyrala, 1996). Enclosed hemorrhages resulting from complicated vaginal birth may also cause hyperbilirubinemia. There may also be an increase in the rate of bilirubin production in the presence of polycythemia.
- *Birth trauma.* Because most IDMs are LGA, trauma may occur during labor and birth.
- *Polycythemia.* This condition may be caused by the decreased extracellular fluid volume in IDMs. Fetal hyperglycemia and hyperinsulinism results in increased oxygen consumption, leading to fetal hypoxia (Tyrala, 1996). Research has focused on the ability of hemoglobin A_{1c} to bind to oxygen, which decreases the oxygen available to the fetal tissues. This tissue hypoxia stimulates increased erythropoietin production, which increases both the hematocrit level and the potential for hyperbilirubinemia.
- *Respiratory distress syndrome (RDS).* This complication occurs especially in newborns of White's classes A through C diabetic mothers. Insulin antagonizes the cortisol-induced stimulation of lecithin synthesis that is necessary for lung maturation. Therefore IDMs may have lungs that are less mature than expected for their gestational age. There is also a decrease in the phospholipid phosphatidylglycerol (PG), which stabilizes surfactant. The insufficiency of PG increases the incidence of respiratory distress syndrome (RDS). Therefore it is important to test for the presence of phosphatidylglycerol in the amniotic fluid. RDS does not appear to be a problem for infants born to diabetic mothers in White's classes D through F; instead, the stresses of poor uterine blood supply may lead to increased production of steroids, which accelerates lung maturation. IDMs may also have a delay in closure of the ductus arteriosus and decreases in postnatal pulmonary artery pressure (Seppänen, Ojanperä, Kääpä, & Kero, 1997).
- *Congenital birth defects.* Congenital anomalies that may occur in IDMs include transposition of the great vessels, ventricular septal defect, patent ductus arteriosus, small left colon syndrome, and sacral agenesis (caudal regression) (Tyrala, 1996). Early and careful control of maternal glucose prior to and during pregnancy decreases the risk of birth defects. See Chapter 16.

Clinical Therapy

The goal of clinical therapy is the early detection of and intervention in the problems associated with infants born to diabetic mothers. Prenatal management is directed toward controlling maternal glucose levels, which minimizes the common complications of IDMs.

Because the onset of hypoglycemia occurs between 1 and 3 hours after birth in IDMs (with a spontaneous rise to normal levels by 4 to 6 hours), blood glucose determinations should be performed on cord blood hourly during the first 4 hours after birth and then at 4-hour intervals until the risk period (about 24 hours) has passed or per agency protocol (Ogata, 1994).

IDMs whose serum glucose falls below 40 mg/dL should have early feedings with formula or breast milk (colostrum). The infant may need to be gavage-fed if lethargic. If normal glucose levels cannot be maintained with oral feeding or if seizures occur, an intravenous infusion of glucose will be necessary. The rate of 4 to 6 mg/kg/minute usually maintains normoglycemia in the IDM (Tyrala, 1996). Once the blood glucose has been stable for 24 hours, the infusion rate can be decreased as oral feedings are increased. The newborn's blood glucose levels must be carefully monitored. Dextrose (25% to 50%) as a rapid infusion is contraindicated because it may lead to severe rebound hypoglycemia following an initial brief increase in glucose level.

NURSING CARE MANAGEMENT

Nursing Assessment and Diagnosis

The nurse should not be lulled into thinking that a big baby is a mature baby. In almost every case, because of the infant's large size, the IDM will appear older than gestational age scoring indicates. The nurse must consider both the gestational age and whether the baby is AGA or LGA in planning and providing safe care. In caring for the IDM, the nurse assesses for signs of respiratory distress, hyperbilirubinemia, birth trauma, and congenital anomalies.

Nursing diagnoses that may apply to IDMs include the following:

- ***Altered Nutrition: Less than Body Requirements*** related to increased glucose metabolism secondary to hyperinsulinemia
- ***Impaired Gas Exchange*** related to respiratory distress secondary to impaired production of surfactant

- ***Alteration in Calcium Homeostasis*** related to inappropriate parathyroid response
- ***Increased Incidence of Congenital Anomalies*** related to poor maternal metabolic control
- ***Alteration in Hematologic Status: Polycythemia*** related to increased synthesis of erythropoietin secondary to hypoxia due to increased metabolic rate
- ***Ineffective Family Coping: Compromised,*** related to the illness of the baby

Nursing Plan and Implementation

Nursing care of the IDM is directed toward early detection and ongoing monitoring of hypoglycemia (by performing glucose tests) and polycythemia (by obtaining central hematocrits), respiratory distress, and hyperbilirubinemia. For specific nursing interventions for respiratory distress syndrome, hypoglycemia, hyperbilirubinemia, and polycythemia, see Chapter 29.

Parent teaching is directed toward preventing macrosomia and the resulting fetal-newborn problems and instituting early and ongoing diabetic control. Parents are advised that with early identification and care, most IDMs' complications have no significant sequelae.

Evaluation

Expected outcomes of nursing care include the following:

- The IDM's respiratory and metabolic alteration problems are minimized.
- The parents understand the etiology of the baby's health problems and preventive steps they can initiate to decrease the impact of maternal diabetes on subsequent fetuses.
- The parents verbalize their concerns surrounding their baby's health problems and understand the rationale behind management of their newborn.

Care of the Postterm Newborn

The **postterm newborn** is any newborn born after 42 weeks' gestation. In the past, the terms *postterm* and *postmature* were used interchangeably. The term **postmaturity** now applies only to the infant who is born after 42 completed weeks of gestation and also demonstrates characteristics of the *postmaturity syndrome.*

Postterm or prolonged pregnancy occurs in approximately 3% to 12% of all pregnancies (McMahon, Kuller, & Yankowitz, 1996). The cause of most postterm pregnancies is not completely understood, but several factors are known to be associated with it, including primiparity, high multiparity (five or more pregnancies), and a history of prolonged pregnancies. Many pregnancies classified as prolonged are thought to be a result of inaccurate determination of the estimated date of birth (EDB) (McMahon et al, 1996). A positive correlation exists between postterm pregnancy and Australian, Greek, and Italian ethnic groups.

Most babies born as a result of prolonged pregnancy are of normal size and health; some keep on growing and are over 4000 g at birth, which supports the contention that the postterm fetus can remain well nourished (Harrington & Campbell, 1993). Intrapartal problems for these healthy but large fetuses include cephalopelvic disproportion (CPD) and shoulder dystocia. At birth about 5% of postterm newborns show signs of postmaturity syndrome. The major portion of the following discussion will address the fetus who is not tolerating the prolonged pregnancy, is suffering from uteroplacental compromise to blood flow and resultant hypoxia, and is therefore considered to have postmaturity syndrome.

Common Complications of the Newborn with Postmaturity Syndrome

The truly postmature newborn is at high risk for morbidity and has a mortality rate two to three times higher than that of term infants. Although today the percentages are extremely low, the majority of postmature fetal deaths occur during labor because by that time the fetus has used up necessary reserves. Decreased placental function impairs oxygenation and nutrition transport, leaving the fetus prone to hypoglycemia and hypoxemia when the stresses of labor begin. These infants often do not tolerate labor and are born by cesarean. The following are other common disorders of the postmature newborn:

- Hypoglycemia from nutritional deprivation and resultant depleted glycogen stores.
- Meconium aspiration in response to in utero hypoxia. The presence of oligohydramnios increases the danger of aspirating thick meconium. Severe meconium aspiration syndrome increases the baby's chance of developing persistent pulmonary hypertension, pneumothorax, and pneumonia.
- Polycythemia due to increased production of red blood cells (RBCs) in response to hypoxia.
- Congenital anomalies of unknown cause.
- Seizures due to hypoxic insult.
- Cold stress due to loss or poor development of subcutaneous fat.

The long-term effects of postmaturity syndrome are unclear. At present, studies do not agree on the effect of postmaturity syndrome on weight gain and IQ scores.

Prolonged pregnancy by itself is not responsible for the postmaturity syndrome. The characteristics of the postmature newborn are caused primarily by a combination of placental aging and subsequent insufficiency and continued exposure to amniotic fluid.

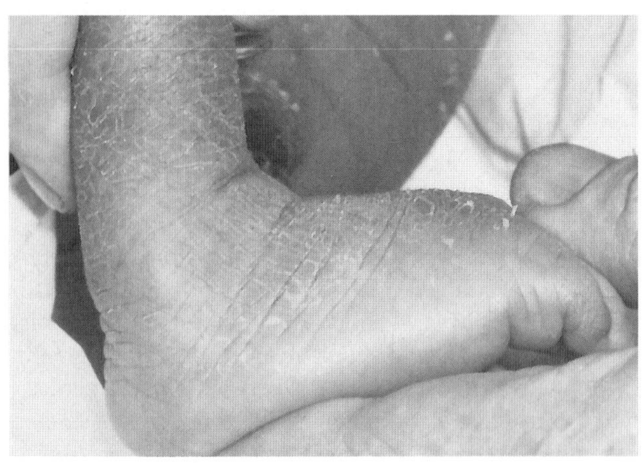

FIGURE 28–5 The skin of the postterm infant exhibits deep cracking and peeling. SOURCE: Dubowitz L, Dubowitz V: *The Gestational Age of the Newborn.* Menlo Park, CA: Addison-Wesley, 1977. Reprinted by permission of V Dubowitz, MD, Hammersmith Hospital, London, England.

Clinical Therapy

The aim of antenatal management is to differentiate the fetus who has postmaturity syndrome from the fetus who is large, well-nourished, and alert and who is tolerating the prolonged (postterm) pregnancy.

Antenatal tests that can be done to evaluate fetal status and determine obstetric management include fetal ultrasound, fetal biophysical profile (refer to Chapter 17), measurement of serum placental hormones, such as human chorionic gonadotropin (hCG) and human placental lactogen (hPL), and the nonstress test (NST) and contraction stress test (CST). These tests and their use in postterm pregnancy are discussed in more depth in Chapter 22.

If the amniotic fluid is meconium stained, an amnioinfusion can be done using 300 to 500 mL of normal saline infused directly into the amniotic sac during labor. This procedure "thins" the meconium and thereby decreases the risk of meconium aspiration syndrome. During birth, to minimize the chance of meconium aspiration syndrome, the physician/CNM should suction the nose and mouth of the baby twice: prior to birth of the chest and trunk; and, most important, before the baby takes its first breath. In some cases, direct suctioning of the trachea is needed. For detailed discussion of medical management and nursing assessments and care of this condition, see Chapter 29.

Hypoglycemia is monitored by serial glucose determinations as per agency protocols. The baby may be placed on glucose infusions or given early feedings if respiratory distress is not present, but these measures must be instituted with caution because of the frequency of asphyxia in the first 24 hours (Kochenour, 1997). Postmature newborns are often voracious eaters.

As with SGA infants, peripheral and central hematocrits are determined to assess the presence of polycythemia. Fluid resuscitation can be initiated, and in extreme cases a partial exchange transfusion may be necessary to prevent polycythemia and adverse sequelae such as hyperviscosity. Oxygen is provided for respiratory distress. Also, temperature instability and excessive loss of body heat can result from decreased liver glycogen stores (Kochenour, 1997). See Chapter 26 for thermoregulation techniques.

NURSING CARE MANAGEMENT

Nursing Assessment and Diagnosis

The newborn with postmaturity syndrome appears alert. This wide-eyed, alert appearance is not necessarily a positive sign because it may indicate chronic intrauterine hypoxia.

The infant has dry, cracking, parchmentlike skin without vernix or lanugo (Figure 28–5). Fingernails are long, and scalp hair is profuse. The infant's body appears long and thin. The wasting involves depletion of previously stored subcutaneous tissue, causing the skin to be loose. Fat layers are almost nonexistent.

Postmature newborns frequently have meconium staining, which colors the nails, skin, and umbilical cord. The varying shades (yellow to green) of meconium staining can give some clue about whether the expulsion of meconium was a recent or a chronic problem. Green coloring indicates a more recent event.

Nursing diagnoses that may apply to the postmature newborn include the following:

- ***Hypothermia*** related to decreased liver glycogen and brown fat stores
- ***Altered Nutrition: Less than Body Requirements*** related to increased use of glucose secondary to stress in utero and decreased placental perfusion
- ***Impaired Gas Exchange*** in the lungs and at the cellular level related to airway obstruction from meconium aspiration
- ***Risk for Altered Tissue Perfusion*** related to increased blood viscosity

Nursing Plan and Implementation

Hospital-Based Nursing Care

Nursing interventions are primarily supportive measures. They include the following:

- Monitor cardiopulmonary status because the stresses of labor are poorly tolerated and can result in hypoxemia in utero and possible asphyxia at birth.
- Provide warmth to counterbalance the infant's poor response to cold stress and decreased liver glycogen and brown fat stores.
- Frequently monitor blood glucose and initiate early feeding (at 1 or 2 hours of age) or intravenous glucose per physician order.

- Obtain a central line hematocrit to determine accurately the presence of polycythemia.

The nurse encourages parents to express their feelings and fears regarding the newborn's condition and potential long-term problems. The nurse also gives careful explanations of procedures, includes the parents in developing care plans for their baby, and encourages follow-up care as needed.

Evaluation

Expected outcomes of nursing care include the following:

- The postterm newborn establishes effective respiratory function.
- The postmature baby is free of metabolic alterations (hypoglycemia) and maintains a stable temperature.

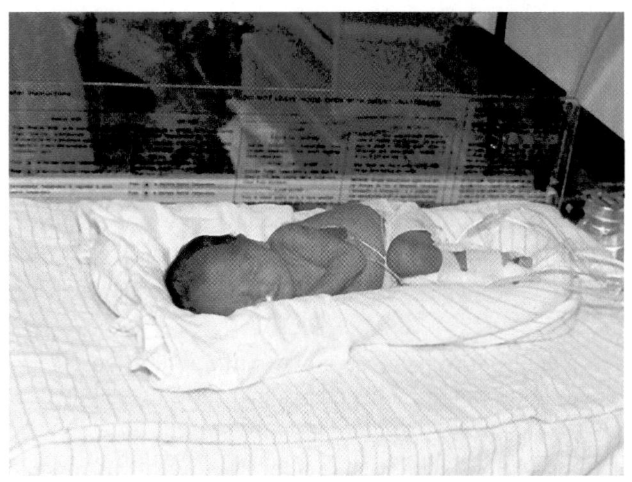

FIGURE 28–6 A six day old, 28 weeks gestational age, 960 gram preterm infant. SOURCE: Courtesy of Carol Harrigan, RNC, MSN, NNP.

Care of the Preterm (Premature) Newborn

A **preterm infant** is an infant born before the completion of 37 weeks' gestation. The length of gestation and thus the level of maturity vary even in the "premature" population. Figure 28–6 shows a preterm newborn.

The incidence of preterm births in the United States is approximately 8%. In socioeconomically deprived populations, it is 15% (American Academy of Pediatrics [AAP] & the American College of Obstetricians and Gynecologists [ACOG], 1997). A higher incidence of prematurity is also seen in single women and adolescents. Prematurity and low birth weight are two common outcomes of pregnancy in young mothers.

The causes of preterm labor are poorly understood, but more of the factors that influence preterm labor and birth are being identified. (See also Chapter 16.) With the help of modern technology, infants are surviving at younger gestational ages.

The major problem of the preterm newborn is variable immaturity of all systems. The degree of immaturity depends on the length of gestation. Maintenance of the preterm newborn falls within narrow physiologic parameters. The preterm newborn must traverse the same complex, interconnected pathways from intrauterine to extrauterine life as the term newborn. Because of immaturity, the premature newborn is ill equipped to make this transition smoothly.

Alteration in Respiratory and Cardiovascular Physiology

The preterm newborn is at risk for respiratory problems because the lungs are not fully mature and not fully ready to take over the process of oxygen and carbon dioxide exchange until 37 to 38 weeks' gestation. The most critical influencing factor in the development of respiratory distress is the preterm infant's inability to produce adequate amounts of surfactant. (See Chapter 24 for discussion of respiratory adaptation and development.) Inadequate surfactant lessens compliance (ability of the lung to fill with air easily), and the inspiratory pressure needed to expand the lungs with air increases. The collapsed (or atelectatic) alveoli will not facilitate an exchange of oxygen and carbon dioxide, resulting in hypoxia, inefficient pulmonary blood flow and decreased tissue perfusion, and depletion of the preterm newborn's available energy.

The muscular coat of the pulmonary blood vessels is incompletely developed. Because of this, the pulmonary arterioles do not constrict as well in response to decreased oxygen levels. This lowered pulmonary vascular resistance leads to increased left-to-right shunting through the ductus arteriosus, which steps up the blood flow back into the lungs.

The ductus arteriosus usually responds to increasing oxygen levels and prostaglandin E levels by vasoconstriction; in the preterm infant, who has higher susceptibility to hypoxia, the ductus may remain open. A patent ductus increases the blood volume to the lungs, causing pulmonary congestion, increased respiratory effort, carbon dioxide retention, and bounding femoral pulses. Congestive heart failure is common.

The common complications of the cardiopulmonary system in preterm infants include respiratory distress syndrome, patent ductus arteriosus, and pulmonary air leaks.

Alteration in Thermoregulation

Heat loss is a major problem that the nurse can do much to prevent. Two limiting factors in heat production, however, are the availability of glycogen in the liver and the amount of brown fat available for metabolism. Both of these limiting factors appear in the third trimester. In the cold-stressed newborn, norepinephrine is released which in turn stimulates the metabolism of brown fat for heat production. As a complicating factor, the hypoxic newborn cannot increase oxygen consumption in response to cold stress because of the already limited reserves and thereby becomes progressively colder. Because the muscle mass is small in preterm infants and voluntary muscular activity is diminished (they are unable to shiver), little heat is produced.

Heat loss occurs as a result of five physiologic and anatomic factors:

1. The preterm baby has a high ratio of body surface to body weight. This means that the baby's ability to produce heat (based on body weight) is much less than the potential for losing heat (based on surface area). The loss of heat in a preterm infant weighing 1500 g is five times greater per unit of body weight than in an adult.
2. The preterm baby has very little subcutaneous fat, which is the human body's insulation. Without adequate insulation, heat is easily conducted from the core of the body (water temperature) to the surface of the body (cooler temperature). Heat is lost from the body as the blood vessels, which lie close to the skin surface in the preterm infant, transport blood from the body core to the subcutaneous tissues.
3. The preterm baby has thinner, more permeable skin than the term infant. This increased permeability contributes to a greater insensible water loss as well as heat loss.
4. The posture of the preterm baby influences heat loss. Flexion of the extremities decreases the amount of surface area exposed to the environment. Extension increases the surface area exposed to the environment and thus increases heat loss. The gestational age of the infant influences the amount of flexion, from completely hypotonic and extended at 28 weeks to strong flexion displayed by 36 weeks.
5. The preterm baby has a decreased ability to vasoconstrict superficial blood vessels and conserve heat in the body core.

In summary, gestational age is directly proportional to the ability to maintain thermoregulation; thus the more preterm the newborn, the less the infant is able to maintain heat balance. Preventing heat loss by providing a neutral thermal environment is one of the most important considerations in nursing management of the preterm infant. Cold stress, with its accompanying severe complications, can be prevented (see Chapter 29).

Alteration in Gastrointestinal Physiology

The basic structure of the gastrointestinal (GI) tract is formed early in gestation. Maturation of the digestive and absorptive processes is more variable, however, and occurs later in gestation.

As a result of GI immaturity, the preterm newborn has the following ingestion, digestion, and absorption problems:

- A marked danger of aspiration and its associated complications due to the infant's poorly developed gag reflex, incompetent esophageal cardiac sphincter, and poor sucking and swallowing reflexes.
- Difficulty in meeting high caloric and fluid needs for growth due to small stomach capacity.
- Limited ability to convert certain essential amino acids to nonessential amino acids. Certain amino acids, such as histidine, taurine, and cysteine, are essential to the preterm infant but not to the term infant.
- Inability to handle the increased osmolarity of formula protein due to kidney immaturity. The preterm infant requires a higher concentration of whey protein than casein.
- Difficulty absorbing saturated fats due to decreased bile salts and pancreatic lipase. Severe illness of the newborn may also prevent intake of adequate nutrients.
- Difficulty with lactose digestion initially because processes may not be fully functional during the first few days of a preterm infant's life. The preterm newborn can digest and absorb most simple sugars.
- Deficiency of calcium and phosphorus may exist because two-thirds of these minerals are deposited in the last trimester. Rickets and significant bone demineralization due to deficiency of calcium and phosphorus, which are deposited primarily in the last trimester.
- Increased basal metabolic rate and increased oxygen requirements due to fatigue associated with sucking.
- Feeding intolerance and necrotizing enterocolitis (NEC) due to diminished blood flow and tissue perfusion to the intestinal tract due to prolonged hypoxia and hypoxemia at birth.

Alteration in Renal Physiology

The kidneys of the preterm infant are immature in comparison with those of the full-term infant, which poses clinical problems in the management of fluid and electrolyte balance. Specific characteristics of the preterm infant include the following:

- The glomerular filtration rate (GFR) is lower because of decreased renal blood flow. The GFR is directly related to lower gestational age, so the more preterm the newborn, the lower the GFR. The GFR is also decreased in the presence of diseases or conditions that decrease the renal blood flow or oxygen content, such as severe respiratory distress and perinatal asphyxia. Anuria or oliguria may be observed in the preterm infant after severe asphyxia with associated hypotension.

- The preterm infant's kidneys are limited in their ability to concentrate urine or to excrete excess amounts of fluid. This means that if excess fluid is administered, the infant is at risk for fluid retention and overhydration. If too little is administered, the infant will become dehydrated because of the inability to retain adequate fluid.
- The kidneys of the preterm infant begin excreting glucose at a lower serum glucose level than those of the term infant. Therefore glycosuria with hyperglycemia is common.
- The buffering capacity of the kidney is reduced, predisposing the infant to metabolic acidosis. Bicarbonate is excreted at a lower serum level, and acid is excreted more slowly. Therefore, after periods of hypoxia or insult, the preterm infant's kidneys require a longer time to excrete the lactic acid that accumulates. Sodium bicarbonate is frequently required to treat the metabolic acidosis.
- The immaturity of the renal system affects the preterm infant's ability to excrete drugs. Because excretion time is longer, many drugs are given over longer intervals (for example, every 12 hours instead of every 8 hours). Urine output must be carefully monitored when the infant is receiving nephrotoxic drugs, such as gentamicin, vancomycin, and others. In the event of oliguria, drugs can become toxic in the infant much more quickly than in the adult.

Alteration in Hepatic and Hematologic Physiology

Immaturity of the preterm newborn's liver predisposes the infant to several problems. After birth, the glycogen stores in the liver are rapidly used for energy. Glycogen deposits are affected by asphyxia in utero and after birth by both asphyxia and cold stress. The baby born preterm has decreased glycogen stores at birth and frequently experiences stress, which rapidly uses up these limited stores. Therefore the preterm newborn is at high risk for hypoglycemia and its complications.

Iron is also stored in the liver, especially during the last trimester of pregnancy. Therefore the preterm newborn is born with low iron stores. If subject to hemorrhage, rapid growth, and excess blood sampling, the preterm infant is likely to become iron depleted more quickly than the term infant. Many preterm babies require transfusions of packed cells to replace the blood withdrawn by frequent blood sampling.

Conjugation of bilirubin in the liver is impaired in the preterm infant. Thus bilirubin levels increase more rapidly and to a higher level than in the full-term infant. Early clinical assessment of jaundice at nontoxic bilirubin levels is more difficult in preterm newborns because they lack subcutaneous fat.

The normal cord hemoglobin in an infant of 34 weeks' gestation is approximately 16.8 g/dL, and total blood volume ranges from 85 mL/kg to 110 mL/kg (Taeusch & Sniderman, 1998). Due to the small total blood volume, any blood loss is highly significant to the preterm infant. For this reason, all blood taken for sampling must be recorded. When the infant has lost 10% of total blood volume, clinical status is assessed, and a decision is made whether or not to replace the lost blood volume.

Alteration in Immunologic Physiology

The preterm infant is at a much greater risk for infection than the term infant. This increased susceptibility is partially attributable to an underdeveloped cellular immune system but may also be the result of an infection acquired in utero, which precipitates preterm labor and birth. The preterm infant has immature specific and nonspecific immaturity.

In utero the fetus receives passive immunity against a variety of infections from maternal IgC immunoglobulins, which cross the placenta (see Chapter 24). Because most of this immunity is acquired in the last trimester of pregnancy, the preterm infant has few antibodies at birth. These provide less protection and become depleted earlier than in a full-term infant. This may be a contributing factor in the higher incidence of recurrent bacterial infection during the first year of life as well as in the immediate neonatal period.

The other immunoglobulin significant for the preterm infant is secretory IgA, which does not cross the placenta but is found in breast milk in significant concentrations. Breast milk's secretory IgA provides immunity to the mucosal surfaces of the gastrointestinal tract, protecting the newborn from enteric infections such as those caused by *Escherichia coli* and *Shigella.* Ill preterm infants may be unable to have breast milk and thus are at risk for enteric infection.

Another altered defense against infection in the preterm infant is the skin surface. In very small infants the skin is easily excoriated, and this factor, coupled with many invasive procedures, places the infant at great risk for nosocomial infections. It is vital to use good handwashing techniques in the care of these infants to prevent unnecessary infection.

Alteration in Neurologic Physiology

The general shape of the brain is formed during the first 6 weeks of gestation. Between the second and fourth months of gestation the brain's total complement of neurons proliferate; these neurons migrate to specific sites throughout the central nervous system, and nerve impulse pathways organize. The final step in neurologic development is the covering of these nerves with myelin, which begins in the second trimester of gestation and continues into adult life (Volpe, 1995).

Because the period of most rapid brain growth and development occurs during the third trimester of pregnancy, the closer to term an infant is born, the better the neurologic prognosis. A common interruption of neurologic development in the preterm infant is caused by intraventricular hemorrhage (IVH) and intracranial hemorrhage (ICH).

Alteration in Reactivity Periods and Behavioral States

The newborn infant's response to extrauterine life is characterized by two periods of reactivity, as discussed in Chapter 27. The preterm infant's periods of reactivity are delayed. In the very ill infant, these periods of reactivity may not be observed at all because the infant may be hypotonic and unreactive for several days after birth.

As the preterm newborn grows and the condition stabilizes, identifying behavioral states and traits unique to each infant becomes increasingly possible. This is a very important part of nursing management of the high-risk infant because it facilitates parental knowledge of their infant's cues for interaction.

In general, stable preterm infants do not demonstrate the same behavioral states as term infants. Preterm infants are more disorganized in their sleep-wake cycles and are unable to attend as well to the human face and objects in the environment. Neurologically, their responses (sucking, muscle tone, states of arousal) are weaker than full-term infants' responses.

By observing each infant's patterns of behavior and responses, especially the sleep-wake states, the nurse can teach parents optimal times for interacting with their infant. The parents and nurse can plan nursing care around the times when the infant is alert and best able to attend. In addition, the more knowledge parents have about the meaning of their infant's responses and behaviors, the better prepared they will be to meet their newborn's needs and to form a positive attachment with their child. See discussion of developmental care for the preterm newborn later in this section.

Management of Nutrition and Fluid Requirements

Providing adequate nutrition and fluids for the preterm infant is a major concern of the health care team. Early feedings are extremely valuable in maintaining normal metabolism and lowering the possibility of such complications as hypoglycemia, hyperbilirubinemia, hyperkalemia, and azotemia. However, the preterm newborn is at risk for complications that may develop because of immaturity of the digestive system.

Nutritional Requirements

Oral (enteral) caloric intake necessary for growth in an uncompromised healthy preterm infant is 110 to 130 kcal/kg/day. In addition to these relatively high caloric needs, the preterm infant requires more protein: 3 to 3.5 g/kg/day, as opposed to 2.0 to 2.5 g/kg/day for the full-term infant (Merenstein & Gardner, 1998). To meet these needs, many institutions use breast milk or special preterm formulas.

Whether breast milk or formula is used, feeding regimens are established based on the infant's weight and estimated stomach capacity (Table 28–1). Initial formula feedings are gradually increased as the infant tolerates them. In many institutions, it is necessary to supplement the oral feedings with parenteral fluids to maintain adequate hydration and caloric intake until the baby is on full oral feedings. Those preterm infants who cannot tolerate any oral (enteral) feedings are given nutrition by total parenteral nutrition (TPN).

In addition to a higher calorie and higher protein formula, preterm infants should receive supplemental multivitamins, including vitamin E and trace minerals. The requirement for vitamin E is increased by a diet high in polyunsaturated fats (which preterm infants tolerate best). Preterm infants fed iron-fortified formulas have higher red cell hemolysis and lower vitamin E concentrations and thus require additional vitamin E. Preterm formulas also need to contain medium-chain triglycerides (MCT) and additional amino acids such as cysteine, as well as calcium, phosphorus, and vitamin D supplements to increase mineralization of bones. Rickets and significant bone demineralization have been documented in very-low-birth-weight infants and otherwise healthy preterm infants.

Nutritional intake is considered adequate when there is consistent weight gain of 20 to 30 g per day. Initially, no weight gain may be noted for several days, but total weight loss should not exceed 15% of the total birth weight or more than 1% to 2% per day. Some institutions add the criteria of head circumference growth and increase in body length of 1 cm/week once the newborn is stable.

Methods of Feeding

The preterm infant is fed by various methods, depending on the infant's gestational age, health and physical condition, and neurologic status. The three most common oral feeding methods are bottle, breast, and gavage.

Bottle-Feeding Preterm infants who have a coordinated suck and swallow reflex are usually at least 34 weeks' gestation, and those showing continued weight gain (20 to 30 g/day) may be fed by bottle. To avoid excessive expenditure of energy, a soft, smaller nipple is usually used. The infant is fed in a semisitting position and burped gently after each half ounce or ounce. The feeding should take no longer than 15 to 20 minutes (nippling requires more energy than other methods).

Preterm infants often progress from parenteral feedings to complete oral or nipple feedings in five or six phases (Pickler, Mauck, & Geldmaker, 1997). Babies who

TABLE 28–1 Oral Feeding Schedule for the Low-Birth-Weight Infant

		≤ 1000 g		1001–1500 g		1501–2000 g		> 2000 g	
Time	Substance*	Amount	Frequency	Amount	Frequency	Amount	Frequency	Amount	Frequency
First feeding	½-strength human milk or ¼-strength formula	1–2 mL/kg	1–2 hours	2–3 mL/kg	2 hours	3–4 mL/kg	2–3 hours	10 mL/kg (full strength)	3 hours
Subsequent feedings, 12–72 hours	Formula or ½ to full-strength human milk	Increase 1 mL† every other feeding to maximum of 5 mL	2 hours	Increase 1 mL† every other feeding to maximum of 10 mL	2 hours	Increase 2 mL every other feeding to maximum of 15 mL	2–3 hours	Increase 5 mL every other feeding to maximum of 20 mL	3 hours
Final feeding schedule	Full-strength formula or human milk	10–15 mL	2 hours	20–28 mL	2–3 hours	28–37 mL	3 hours	37–50 mL, then ad libitum	3–4 hours
Total time to full oral feeds			10–14/day or more for infants <750 g		7–10/day		5–7/day		3–5/day

*Supplemental IV fluids should be given to fulfill requirements of 140–160 mL/kg (urine specific gravities 1.008–1.010) and caloric requirements of 90–130 cal/kg.

†Strength should be increased alternately with volume.

SOURCE: Modified from Avery GB, Fletcher MA, MacDonald MG (editors): *Neonatology: Pathophysiology and Management of the Newborn*, 4th ed. Philadelphia: Lippincott, 1994, p 334.

are progressing from gavage feedings to bottle-feeding should be started with one session of bottle-feeding a day, and the number of times a day a bottle is given should be increased slowly until the baby tolerates all feedings from a bottle.

The nurse also assesses the infant's ability to suck. Sucking may be affected by age, asphyxia, sepsis, intraventricular hemorrhage, or other neurologic insult. Before initiating nipple feeding, the nurse observes the infant for any signs of stress, such as tachypnea (more than 60 respirations/minute), respiratory distress, or hypothermia, which may increase the risk of aspiration. During the feeding, the infant should be observed for signs of difficulty with feeding (tachypnea, cyanosis, bradycardia, lethargy, and uncoordinated suck and swallow). In addition, Pickler, Mauck and Geldmaker (1997) suggest that the longer an infant continues to receive assisted ventilation, the older the infant will be at the initial bottle-feeding and subsequent feedings until discharge.

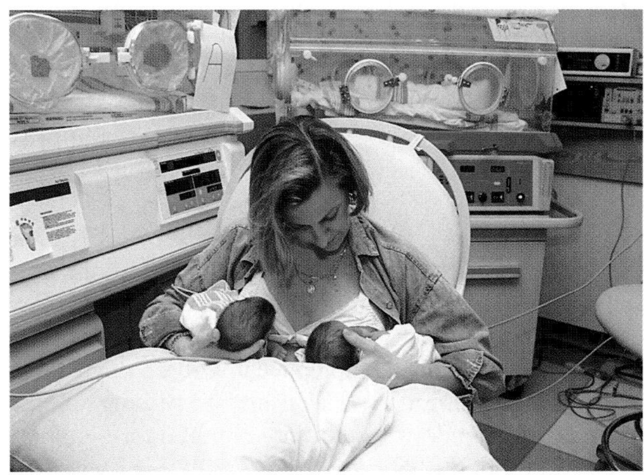

FIGURE 28–7 Mother visits neonatal intensive care unit to breastfeed her infants.

Breastfeeding Mothers who wish to breastfeed their preterm infants should be given the opportunity to put the infant to breast as soon as the infant has demonstrated a coordinated suck and swallow reflex, is showing consistent weight gain, and can control body temperature outside of the incubator. Besides breast milk's many benefits for the infant, it allows the mother to contribute actively to the infant's well-being (Figure 28–7). The nurse should encourage mothers to breastfeed if they choose to do so. It is important for the nurse to be aware of the advantages of breastfeeding as well as the possible disadvantages if breast milk is the sole source of food for the preterm infant. See Chapter 27 for a detailed discussion of the advantages and disadvantages of breastfeeding. Even if the infant can't be put to the breast, mothers can pump their breasts, and the breast milk can be given via gavage. Use of the double-pumping system produces higher levels of prolactin than sequential pumping of the breasts (Figure 27–9). Delaying transition from bottle to breast results in the infant developing a sucking mechanism specific to the artificial nipple that impedes subsequent transfer to the breast (Jaeger, Lawson & Filteau, 1997).

By initiating skin-to-skin holding of low-birth-weight infants in the early intensive care phase, mothers can significantly increase milk volume, thereby overcoming lactation problems (Hurst, Valentine, Renfro, Burns, & Ferlic, 1997). Also preterm infants tolerate breastfeeding with higher transcutaneous oxygen pressure and better maintenance of body temperature than during bottle-feeding.

The infant is placed at the mother's breast. It has been suggested that the football hold is a convenient position for preterm babies. Feeding time may take up to 45 minutes, and babies should be burped as they alternate breasts. Length of feeding time must be monitored so that the preterm does not burn too many calories.

The nurse should coordinate a flexible feeding schedule so babies can nurse during alert times and be allowed to set their own pace. Feedings should be on demand, but a maximum number of hours between feedings should be set. A similar regimen should be used for the baby who is progressing from gavage feeding to breastfeeding. The mother should begin with one feeding at the breast and then gradually increase the number of times during the day that the baby breastfeeds. When breastfeeding is not possible because the infant is too small or too weak to suck at the breast, an option for the mother may be to express her breastmilk into a cup. The milk touches the infant's lips and is lapped by the protruding motions of the tongue.

Gavage Feeding The gavage feeding method is used with preterm infants (less than 34 weeks' gestation) who lack or have a poorly coordinated suck and swallow reflex or are ill and ventilator dependent. Gavage feeding may be used as an adjunct to nipple feeding if the infant tires easily or as an alternative if an infant is losing weight because of the energy expenditure required for nippling. See Procedure 28–1: Performing Gavage Feedings. Gavage feedings are administered by either the nasogastric or orogastric route and by intermittent bolus or continuous drip method.

Transpyloric Feeding An alternative method of feeding is transpyloric feeding (a method in which the stomach is bypassed). This feeding method should be used only in specially equipped and staffed high-risk nurseries because it can perforate the stomach or intestines during passage of the tube.

Total Parenteral Nutrition Total parenteral nutrition (TPN) is used in situations that contraindicate feeding the infant through the gastrointestinal tract. Contraindications include gastrointestinal anomalies requiring surgical intervention, necrotizing enterocolitis, intolerance of feedings, and extreme prematurity.

The TPN method provides complete nutrition to the infant intravenously. TPN includes use of hyperalimentation and intralipids. Hyperalimentation provides calories, vitamins, minerals, protein, and glucose. Intralipids must also be administered to provide essential fatty acids.

The nurse needs to monitor serum glucose levels and serum chemistries carefully during TPN. Urine is checked for protein, sugar, and specific gravity at least every 8 hours. The intravenous rate is monitored hourly to maintain accurate intake. The rate should not be increased to "catch up" if administration lags behind. The intravenous site should be observed hourly for signs of infiltration—hyperalimentation is extremely caustic and causes severe tissue destruction if it infiltrates. Intake and output are carefully monitored (hyperglycemia causing an osmotic diuresis can lead to dehydration). The nurse observes for signs of reaction to intralipids (eg, dyspnea, vomiting, elevated temperature, or cyanosis). Infants can also develop fat emboli.

Fluid Requirements

Calculation of fluid requirements takes into account the infant's weight and postnatal age. Recommendations for fluid therapy in the preterm infant are approximately 80 to 100 mL/kg/day for day 1, 100 to 120 mL/kg/day for day 2, and 120 to 150 mL/kg/day by day 3 of life. These amounts may be increased up to 200 mL/kg/day if the infant is very small, receiving phototherapy, or under a radiant warmer because of increased insensible water losses. Fluid losses can be minimized through the use of heat shields and humidity, or "swamping."

Common Complications of Preterm Newborns and Their Clinical Management

The goals of clinical therapy are to meet the growth and development needs of the preterm newborn and to anticipate and manage the complications associated with prematurity. Complications associated with prematurity that require clinical intervention are respiratory distress syndrome (RDS), patent ductus arteriosus (PDA), apnea, and intraventricular hemorrhage (IVH) and sepsis. Long-term problems include retinopathy of prematurity (ROP), bronchopulmonary dysplasia (BPD), pulmonary interstitial emphysema (PIE), and posthemorrhagic hydrocephalus.

An in-depth discussion of RDS, BPD and sepsis, including pathophysiology, clinical management, and nursing care, is contained in Chapter 29. Patent ductus arteriosus, apnea, intraventricular hemorrhage, retinopathy of prematurity, and other complications are discussed below.

Patent Ductus Arteriosus

The incidence of symptomatic patent ductus arteriosus is related to birth weight in preterm infants and has been

PROCEDURE 28–1 PERFORMING GAVAGE FEEDING

Nursing Action	*Rationale*
Objective: Assemble and prepare the equipment.	
• No. 5 or no. 8 Fr. feeding tube. See the material below for guidelines for choosing tube size.	*Equipment organization facilitates the procedure.*
• 10- to 30-mL syringe, for aspirating stomach contents	
• 1/4-inch paper tape, to mark the tube for insertion depth and to secure the catheter during feeding	
• Stethoscope, for auscultating the rush of air into the stomach when testing the tube placement	
• Appropriate formula	
• Small cup of sterile water to test for tube placement and to act as lubricant	
Objective: Explain the procedure to the parents.	
Objective: Insert the tube accurately into the stomach.	
See the material below for step-by-step instructions.	
Objective: Maximize the feeding pleasure of the infant.	
• Whenever possible, hold the infant during gavage feeding. If it is too awkward to hold the infant during feeding, be sure to take time for holding after the feeding.	*Feeding time is important to the infant's tactile sensory input.*
• Offer a pacifier to the infant during the feeding.	*Sucking during feeding comforts and relaxes the infant, making the formula flow more easily. Infants can lose their sucking reflexes when fed by gavage for long periods.*

Gavage Feeding Guidelines

Choosing a Catheter Size

When choosing the catheter size, consider the size of the infant, the area of insertion (oral or nasal), and the desired rate of flow. The size of the catheter will influence the rate of flow.

The very small infant (less than 1600 g) requires a 5 Fr. feeding tube; an infant greater than 1600 g may tolerate a larger tube.

Orogastric insertion is preferable to nasogastric because most infants are obligatory nose breathers. If nasogastric is used, a 5 Fr. catheter should be used to minimize airway obstruction.

Inserting and Checking the Tube

- Elevate the head of the bed and position the infant on the back or side to allow easy passage of the tube.
- Measure the distance from the tip of the ear to the nose to the xiphoid process, and mark the point with a small piece of paper tape (Figure 28–8) to ensure enough tubing to enter the stomach.

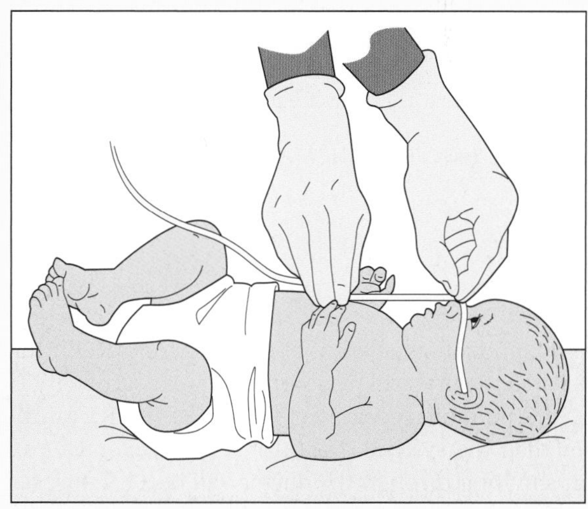

FIGURE 28–8 Measuring gavage tube length.

Inserting and Checking the Tube continued

- If inserting the tube nasally, lubricate the tip in a cup of sterile water. Use water instead of an oil-based lubricant, in case the tube is inadvertently passed into a lung. Shake any excess drops to prevent aspiration.
- If inserting the tube orally, the oral secretions are enough to lubricate the tube adequately.
- Stabilize the infant's head with one hand and pass the tube via the mouth (or nose) into the stomach to the point previously marked. If the infant begins coughing or choking or becomes cyanotic or phonic, remove the tube immediately as the tube has probably entered the trachea.
- If no respiratory distress is apparent, lightly tape the tube in position, draw up 0.5–1.0 mL of air in the syringe, and connect the syringe to the tubing. Place the stethoscope over the epigastrum and briskly inject the air (Figure 28–9). You will hear a sudden rush as the air enters the stomach.

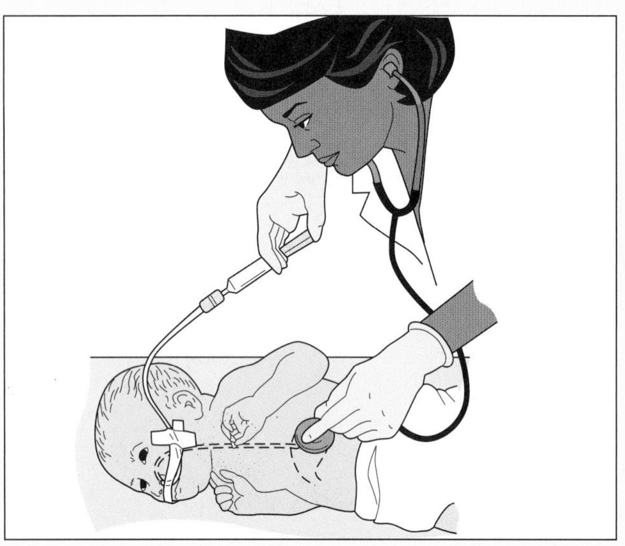

FIGURE 28–9 Auscultation for placement of gavage tube.

- *Aspirate the stomach contents with the syringe, and note the amount, color, and consistency to evaluate the infant's feeding tolerance. Return the residual to the stomach unless you are asked to discard it. It is usually not discarded because of the potential for electrolyte imbalance.*
- *If the aspirated contents contain only a clear fluid or mucus and if it is unclear whether or not the tube is in the stomach, test the aspirate for pH. Stomach aspirate has a pH between 1 and 3.*

Administering the Feeding

- *Hold the infant for feeding, or position the infant on the right side, to decrease the risk of aspiration in case of emesis during feeding.*
- *Separate the syringe from the tube, remove the plunger from the barrel, reconnect the barrel to the tube, and pour the formula into the syringe.*
- *Elevate the syringe 6–8 inches over the infant's head, and allow the formula to flow by gravity at a slow, even rate. You may need to initiate the flow of formula by inserting the plunger of the syringe into the barrel just until you see formula enter the feeding tube. Do not use pressure.*
- *Regulate the rate to prevent sudden stomach distention leading to vomiting and aspiration. Continue adding formula to the syringe until the infant has absorbed the desired volume.*

Clearing and Removing the Tube

- *Clear the tubing with 2–3 mL sterile water or with air. This ensures that the infant has received all of the formula. If the tube is going to be left in place, clearing it will decrease the risk of clogging and bacterial growth in the tube.*
- *To remove the tube, loosen the tape, fold the tube over on itself, and quickly withdraw the tube in one smooth motion to minimize the potential for fluid aspiration as the tube passes the epiglottis. If the tube is to be left in, position it so that the infant is unable to remove it. Replace the tube every 24 hours.*

shown to decrease with increase in birth weight. Symptomatic PDA is often seen around the third day of life, when the premature infant is recovering from RDS. Initially, when the preterm newborn is hypoxic secondary to RDS, the pulmonary vascular resistance (PVR) can be higher than the systemic vascular resistance, and right-to-left shunting through the ductus will occur. However, as the RDS improves and adequate oxygenation is maintained, the lungs open up, and more blood flows into them, leading to ventricular volume overload, pulmonary edema, and congestive failure. Oxygenation is again compromised, and ventilator requirements will increase, leading to the possible difficulty in weaning from the ventilator and long-term pulmonary sequelae.

Early identification of symptomatic infants and prompt clinical intervention will minimize long-term complications. Three methods are currently used, separately or in combination, to effect closure. Initial medical management consists of providing adequate respiratory support, maintaining a relatively high hematocrit (greater than 40%), restricting fluids, and using diuretics (to decrease pulmonary edema) and perhaps digoxin while waiting for spontaneous closure of the ductus to occur. The administration of prostaglandin synthetase inhibitors, such as indomethacin, impairs synthesis of the E series prostaglandins responsible for dilatation of the ductus and can cause ductal closure. Indomethacin is effective, but it is not without side effects and must be used cautiously. If medical management is unsuccessful or contraindicated, then the ductus may be surgically ligated. Patent ductus arteriosus will often prolong the course of illness in a preterm newborn and lead to chronic pulmonary dysfunction.

CLINICAL TIP

When using Indocin to treat a PDA in conjunction with an aminoglycoside (ie, Gentamicin), the aminoglycoside should either be changed to another broad-spectrum antibiotic that is not nephrotoxic or be placed on hold and a trough checked before dosing. The rationale is that Indocin can decrease renal function and cause a decrease in excretion of the Gentamicin.

Apnea

Apnea of prematurity refers to cessation of breathing for 20 seconds or longer or for less than 20 seconds when associated with cyanosis and bradycardia. Apnea is a common problem in the preterm infant (of less than 37 weeks' gestation) and is thought to be primarily a result of neuronal immaturity, a factor that contributes to the preterm infant's irregular breathing patterns. Factors that adversely affect brain nerve cells include hypoxia, acidosis, edema, intracranial bleeding, anemia, hyperbilirubinemia, hypoglycemia, hypocalcemia, and sepsis. Gastroesophageal reflux (GER) has also been implicated in the production of apnea, although with much controversy. It is believed that GER causes laryngospasm, which leads to bradycardia and apnea.

Apneic onset is often insidious; cardiorespiratory monitoring allows for early recognition and intervention, thus decreasing the need for resuscitative efforts. Apnea may occur during feeding, suctioning, or stooling. However, there may be no observable activity related to apnea. All episodes of apnea are documented. The documentation includes activity at the time of apnea, length of episode, along with any bradycardia, color change, or desaturation on pulse-oximeter associated with apneic episodes, and treatment required to bring the baby out of the apneic spell. These data are useful in determining etiology and possible treatment.

The nurse makes careful observations, quickly assessing the need for intervention or ascertaining that the infant is having periodic breathing. The intervention required depends on the severity of the apneic episode and the baby's response. Gentle stimulation of the infant may be sufficient. Respiratory support is provided if needed, and methylxanthine drugs (aminophylline, theophylline, or caffeine) are often used to treat apnea of prematurity. Reflux precautions should be initiated. The infant is placed in 30-degree prone position 1 hour after feeding. Feedings are thickened with rice cereal. Metoclopramide (Cisapride) is used to increase tone of the lower esophageal sphincter as well as increase peristalsis of the duodenum (Premji, Wilson, Paes, & Gray, 1997).

Intraventricular Hemorrhage

Intraventricular hemorrhage (IVH) is the most common type of intracranial hemorrhage in the small preterm infant, especially those weighing less than 1500 g or of less than 34 weeks' gestation.

The most common site of hemorrhage is the periventricular subependymal germinal matrix, where there is a rich blood supply and the capillary walls are thin and fragile. The matrix provides little supportive tissue for the fragile blood vessels. Before 32 weeks' gestation, an infant is much more susceptible to hemorrhage of these tiny vessels because they are vulnerable to hypoxic events (such as respiratory distress, birth trauma, birth asphyxia) that damage and rupture vessel walls.

Prenatal interventions include preventing premature birth and transporting the mother to a tertiary care center. Administration of phenobarbital and vitamin K to the mother is being studied for their preventive effect. Postnatal preventive interventions include careful resuscitation, correction or prevention of major hemodynamic disturbances, and correction of coagulation abnormalities. Potential postnatal preventive pharmacologic interventions include phenobarbital to control seizures, narcotics for sedation, and vitamin E for its antioxidant abilities (Volpe, 1995).

The outcome for the infant depends on the size of the intracerebral bleed and the gestational age of the infant. The most severe hemorrhages may cause motor deficits, posthemorrhagic hydrocephalus, hearing loss, and blindness. Less severe bleeds may have no observable effects. In caring for the infant with an IVH, the nurse provides continuing support for the parents, identifying their level of understanding and facilitating interdisciplinary communication with them.

Long-Term Needs and Outcome

The care of the preterm infant and the family does not stop on discharge from the nursery. Follow-up care is extremely important because many developmental problems are not noted until the infant is older and begins to demonstrate motor delays or sensory disability. Within the first year of life, low-birth-weight preterm infants face higher mortality than term infants. Causes of death include sudden infant death syndrome (SIDS)—which occurs about five times more frequently in the preterm infant—respiratory infections, and neurologic defects. Morbidity is also much higher among preterm infants, with those weighing less than 1500 g at highest risk for long-term complications.

The most common long-term problems observed in preterm infants include retinopathy of prematurity, speech defects, neurologic defects, and auditory defects.

Retinopathy of Prematurity Premature newborns are particularly susceptible to characteristic retinal changes known as retinopathy of prematurity (ROP). Until recently, ROP was thought to be exclusively the result of excessive use of oxygen in the treatment of premature infants. However, ROP has also occurred in premature infants who never received oxygen, in full-term infants with cyanotic congenital heart disease, and in certain other congenital anomalies. The disease is now viewed as multifactorial in origin. Increased survival of very-low-birth-weight (VLBW) infants may be the most important factor in the increased incidence of ROP.

Treatment of the acute stages of ROP with laser or cryotherapy is an option. Because most acute cases of ROP regress spontaneously with no long-term visual impairment, the possibility of regression must be weighed against the risk of an unfavorable outcome. For infants with bilateral traction and retinal detachment, surgical vitrectomy and scleral buckling have been used experimentally. Because they are experimental, further follow-up is required for evaluation.

Nursing care for the visually impaired infant must concentrate on parental support and education. When the crisis of premature birth is quickly followed by the devastating news of suspected visual impairment or blindness, the parents will need extensive support by all members of the interdisciplinary health team. The parents again experience overwhelming anxiety and uncertainty about their infant's future abilities. Premature infants with blindness due to ROP may be at increased risk of cognitive and emotional problems. The evidence suggests that this increased risk may be due to environmental factors rather than to inherent intellectual or neurologic factors.

Speech Defects The most frequently observed speech defects involve delayed development of receptive and expressive ability that may persist into the school-age years.

Neurologic Defects The most common neurologic defects include cerebral palsy, hydrocephalus, seizure disorders, lower IQ scores, and learning disabilities. However, the socioeconomic climate and family support systems have been shown to be important factors influencing the child's ultimate school performance in the absence of major neurologic defects. Families can be reminded that risk does not equal injury, injury does not equal damage, and description of damage does not allow a precise prediction about recovery or outcome.

Auditory Defects Preterm infants have a 1% to 4% incidence of moderate to profound hearing loss and should have a formal audiologic examination prior to discharge and at 3 to 6 months (corrected age). The test currently used to measure hearing functions of the newborn is the evoked otoacoustic emissions (EOAE) test. Earphones are used on each ear and independently measure sounds produced in the inner ear in response to acoustic stimuli. Any infant with repeated, abnormal results should be referred to speech-and-language specialists. Infants at increased risk include those with congenital viral infections, hyperbilirubinemia, perinatal asphyxia, and birth trauma. Damage from ototoxic drugs such as gentamicin and furosemide (Lasix) is variable and related to multiple factors, including renal function, age, duration of treatment, and concomitant administration of other ototoxic agents.

When evaluating an infant's abilities and disabilities, parents must understand that the developmental progress must be evaluated based on chronologic age from the expected date of birth, not from the actual date of birth (corrected age). In addition, the parents need the consistent support of health care professionals in the long-term management of their infant. Many new and ongoing concerns arise as the high-risk infant grows and develops; the goal is to promote the highest quality of life possible.

NURSING CARE MANAGEMENT

Nursing Assessment and Diagnosis

Accurate assessment of the physical characteristics and gestational age of the preterm newborn is imperative to anticipate the special needs and problems of this baby. Physical characteristics vary greatly, depending on the gestational age, but the following characteristics are frequently present:

- *Color.* Usually pink or ruddy but may be acrocyanotic (Cyanosis, jaundice, or pallor are abnormal and should be noted.)
- *Skin.* Reddened, translucent, blood vessels readily apparent, lack of subcutaneous fat
- *Lanugo.* Plentiful, widely distributed
- *Head size.* Appears large in relation to body
- *Skull.* Bones pliable, fontanelle smooth and flat
- *Ears.* Minimal cartilage, pliable, folded over
- *Nails.* Soft, short
- *Genitals.* Small; testes may not be descended
- *Resting position.* Flaccid, froglike
- *Cry.* Weak, feeble
- *Reflexes.* Poor suck, swallow, and gag
- *Activity.* Jerky, generalized movements (Seizure activity is abnormal.)

Determining gestational age in preterm newborns requires knowledge and experience in administering gestational assessment tools. The tool used should be specific, reliable, and valid. For a discussion of gestational age assessment tools, see Chapter 25. Nursing diagnoses that may apply to the preterm newborn include:

- ***Impaired Gas Exchange*** related to immature pulmonary vasculature and inadequate surfactant production
- ***Ineffective Breathing Pattern*** related to immature central nervous system
- ***Alteration in Cardiovascular Status*** related to hypotension related to decreased tissue perfusion secondary to PDA
- ***Ineffective Thermoregulation*** related to hypothermia secondary to decreased glycogen and brown fat stores
- ***Potential Hyperbilirubinemia*** secondary to immature liver to conjugate bilirubin
- ***Altered Nutrition: Less than Body Requirements*** related to weak suck and swallow reflexes and decreased ability to absorb nutrients
- ***Fluid Volume Deficit*** related to high insensible water losses and inability of kidneys to concentrate urine
- ***High Risk for Intraventricular Hemorrhage*** related to fragile capillary network in the germinal matrix
- ***Ineffective Family Coping*** related to anger/guilt at having delivered a premature baby
- ***Dysfunctional Grieving*** related to actual or perceived loss of a normal newborn

Nursing Plan and Implementation

Maintenance of Respiratory Function

There is increased danger of respiratory obstruction in preterm newborns because their bronchi and trachea are so narrow that mucus can obstruct the airway. The nurse must maintain patency through judiciously suctioning, but only on an as-needed basis.

Positioning of the newborn can also affect respiratory function. If the baby is in the supine position, the nurse should slightly elevate the infant's head to maintain the airway, being careful not to hyperextend the neck because the trachea will collapse. Also, because the newborn has weak neck muscles and cannot control head movement, the nurse should ensure that this head position is maintained by using a small roll under the shoulders. The prone position splints the chest wall and decreases the amount of respiratory effort used to move the chest wall. The prone position therefore facilitates chest expansion and improves air entry and oxygenation. Weak or absent cough or gag reflexes increase the chance of aspiration in the premature newborn. The nurse should ensure that the infant's position facilitates drainage of mucus or regurgitated formula.

The nurse monitors heart and respiratory rates with cardiorespiratory monitors as well as through physical assessments to identify alterations in the newborn's cardiopulmonary status. Signs of respiratory distress include the following:

- Cyanosis (serious sign when generalized)
- Tachypnea (sustained respiratory rate greater than 60/minute after first 4 hours of life)
- Retractions
- Expiratory grunting
- Nasal flaring
- Apneic episodes
- Presence of rales or rhonchi on auscultation
- Diminished air entry

The nurse who observes any of these alterations records and reports them for further evaluation. If respiratory distress occurs, the nurse administers oxygen per physician/nurse practitioner order to relieve hypoxemia. If hypoxemia is not treated immediately, it may result in patent ductus arteriosus or metabolic acidosis. If oxygen is administered to the newborn, the nurse monitors the oxygen concentration with devices such as the transcutaneous oxygen monitor ($tcPO_2$)or the pulse oximeter. Monitoring of oxygen concentration in the baby's blood is essential because hyperoxemia may lead to ROP.

The nurse also needs to consider respiratory function during feeding. To prevent aspiration, increased energy expenditure, and increased oxygen consumption, the nurse needs to ensure that the infant's gag and suck reflexes are intact before initiating oral feedings.

Maintenance of Neutral Thermal Environment

Providing a neutral thermal environment minimizes the oxygen consumption required to maintain a normal core temperature; it also prevents cold stress and facilitates growth by decreasing the calories needed to maintain body temperature. The preterm infant's immature central nervous system, as well as small brown fat stores, provides poor temperature control. A small infant (<1200 g) can lose 80 kcal/kg/day through radiation of body heat. The nurse should implement all the usual thermoregulation measures discussed in Chapter 26. In addition, to minimize heat loss and the effects of temperature instability for preterm and low-birth-weight newborns, the nurse should do the following:

1. Warm and humidify oxygen to minimize evaporative heat loss and decrease oxygen consumption.
2. Place the baby in a double-walled incubator, or use a plexiglass heat shield over small preterm infants in single-walled incubators to avoid radiative heat losses. Some institutions use radiant warmers and plastic wrap over the baby and pipe in humidity

(swamping). Do not use plexiglass shields on radiant warmer beds because it blocks the infrared heat.

3. Avoid placing the baby on cold surfaces, such as metal treatment tables and cold x-ray plates; pad cold surfaces with diapers and use radiant warmers during procedures; place the preterm infant on prewarmed mattresses; and warm hands before handling the baby to prevent heat transfer via conduction.
4. Use warmed ambient humidity. The use of humidity and its role in decreasing insensible water loss remains controversial ("Neonatal Thermoregulation," 1997).
5. Keep the skin dry, and place a cap on the baby's head to prevent heat loss via evaporation. (The head makes up 25% of the total body size.)
6. Keep radiant warmers, incubators, and cribs away from windows and cold external walls and out of drafts to prevent heat loss by radiation.
7. Open incubator portholes and doors only when necessary, and use plastic sleeves on portholes to decrease convective heat loss.
8. Use a skin probe to monitor the baby's skin temperature. Correlate ambient temperatures with the skin probe in the incubator using the servocontrol rather than the manual mode. The temperature should be 36C to 37C (96.8F to 97.7F). Temperature fluctuations indicate hypothermia or hyperthermia. Be careful not to place skin temperature probes over bony prominences; areas of brown fat; poorly vasoreactive areas, such as extremities; or excoriated areas ("Neonatal Thermoregulation," 1997).
9. Warm formula or stored breast milk before feeding.
10. Use reflector patch over the skin temperature probe when using a radiant warmer bed so that the probe does not sense the higher infrared temperature as the baby's skin temperature and therefore decreases the heater output.

Once preterm infants are medically stable, they should be clothed with a double-thickness cap, cotton shirt and diaper and, if possible, swaddled in a blanket. The nurse begins the process of weaning to a crib when the premature infant is medically stable, doesn't require assisted ventilation, weighs approximately 1500 g, has 5 days of consistent weight gain, and is taking oral feedings and when apnea and bradycardia episodes have stabilized. The nurse should be familiar with the individual institution's protocol for weaning to crib for preterm infants.

Maintenance of Fluid and Electrolyte Status

Hydration is maintained by providing adequate intake based on the newborn's weight, gestational age, chronologic age, and volume of sensible and insensible water losses. Adequate fluid intake should provide sufficient water to compensate for increased insensible losses and to provide the amount needed for renal excretion of metabolic products. Insensible water losses can be minimized by providing a high ambient humidity, humidifying oxygen, using heat shields, covering the skin with plastic wrap, and placing the infant in a double-walled incubator. Some units use zero humidity and adjust their intravenous fluid support accordingly to control insensible water losses.

The nurse evaluates the baby's hydration status by assessing and recording signs of dehydration. Signs of dehydration include the following:

- Sunken fontanelle
- Loss of weight
- Poor skin turgor (skin returns to position slowly when squeezed gently)
- Dry oral mucous membranes
- Decreased urine output
- Increased urine specific gravity (>1.013)

The nurse must also identify signs of overhydration by observing the newborn for edema or excessive weight gain and by comparing urine output with fluid intake.

The preterm infant should be weighed at least once daily at the same time each day. Weight change is the most sensitive indicator of fluid balance. Weighing diapers is also important for accurate input and output measurement (1 mL = 1 g). A comparison of intake and output measurements over an 8-hour or 24-hour period provides important information about renal function and fluid balance. Assessment of patterns—in particular, whether they show a net gain or loss over several days—is also essential to fluid management. Monitor blood serum levels and pH to evaluate for electrolyte imbalances.

Accurate hourly intake calculations should be maintained when administering intravenous fluids. Because the preterm infant is unable to excrete excess fluid, it is important that the nurse maintain the correct amount of intravenous fluid to prevent fluid overload. This can be accomplished by using neonatal or pediatric infusion pumps. To prevent electrolyte imbalance, overhydration and dehydration, the nurse must take care to give the correct intravenous solutions and volumes and concentrations of formulas. Urine specific gravity and pH are obtained periodically. Urine osmolality provides an indication of hydration, although this factor must be correlated with other assessments (for example, serum sodium). Hydration is considered adequate when the urine output is 1 to 3 mL/kg/hour.

Provision of Adequate Nutrition and Prevention of Fatigue during Feeding

The feeding method depends on the preterm newborn's feeding abilities and health status (see Methods of Feeding, earlier in this chapter). Both nipple and gavage methods are initially supplemented with intravenous therapy until oral intake is sufficient to support growth (110 to

130 kcal/kg/day). Early, small-volume enteral feedings (0.1 mL to 0.5 mL per hour), called hypocaloric or trophic feedings, have proved to be of benefit to the very-low-birth-weight infant. Gastrointestinal priming with these small-volume enteral feedings are not intended to contribute to the total nutritional intake but rather to enhance gut metabolism. Trophic feedings may also help to encourage earlier advancement to full feedings, thereby decreasing the development of necrotizing enterocolitis (NEC) and the complications of parenteral nutrition (cholestatic jaundice, metabolic bone disease, glucose intolerance). In addition, there is an increase in serum gastrin levels, a gastrointestinal hormone that is thought to play a role in improved tolerance of feedings. Formula or breast milk (with or without fortifiers to increase caloric content) is incorporated into the feedings slowly; initially, it may be at quarter-strength, then half-strength, and so on. This is done to avoid overtaxing the digestive capacity of the preterm newborn. The nurse should carefully watch for any signs of feeding intolerance, including:

- Increasing gastric residuals
- Abdominal distention (measured routinely before feedings) with visible bowel loops
- Guaiac-positive stools (occult blood in stools)
- Lactose in stools (reducing substance in the stools)
- Vomiting
- Diarrhea

Before each feeding, the nurse measures abdominal girth and auscultates the abdomen to determine the presence and quality of bowel sounds. Such assessments permit early detection of abdominal distention and decreased peristaltic activity, which may indicate NEC or paralytic ileus. The nurse also checks for residual formula in the stomach prior to feeding. This is done when the newborn is fed by gavage method. This procedure also can be performed when the nipple-fed newborn presents with abdominal distention. The presence of residual formula may indicate intolerance to the type or amount of feeding. Residual formula is usually readministered because digestive processes have already been initiated and subtracted from the amount to be given at that feeding.

Preterm newborns who are ill or fatigue easily with nipple feedings are usually fed by gavage or transpyloric feeding. The infant is essentially passive with these methods, thus conserving energy and calories. As the baby matures, gavage feedings are replaced with breast- or bottle-feedings to assist in strengthening the sucking reflex and meeting oral and emotional needs. Factors used to indicate readiness are a strong gag reflex, presence of nonnutritive sucking, rooting behavior, gestational age of 34 weeks or more, and weight over 1500 g. Both low-birth-weight and preterm infants nipple-feed more effectively in a quiet state (Kinneer & Beachy, 1994). The nurse establishes a nipple-feeding program that progresses slowly, such as one nipple feeding per day, then one nipple feeding per shift, and then a nipple feeding every other feeding. Daily weights are monitored because often there is a small weight loss when nipple feedings are started. After feedings, the baby is placed on the right side (with support to maintain this position) or on the abdomen. These positions enhance gastric emptying and decrease the chance of aspiration if regurgitation occurs. Gastroesophageal reflux is not uncommon in preterm newborns.

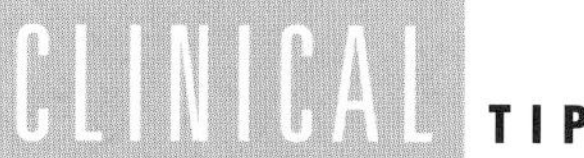

TIP

For an otherwise healthy, growing premature infant who is receiving total enteral intake and has started to experience apnea and bradycardia, one differential diagnosis to think about is reflux rather than sepsis, although sepsis may need to be ruled out.

The nurse involves the parents in feeding their preterm baby. This is essential to the development of attachment between parents and infant. In addition, such involvement increases parental knowledge about the care of their infant and helps them cope with the situation.

Prevention of Infection

The nurse is responsible for minimizing the preterm newborn's exposure to pathogenic organisms. The preterm newborn is susceptible to infection because of an immature immune system and thin, permeable skin. Invasive procedures, techniques such as umbilical catheterization and mechanical ventilation, and prolonged hospitalization place the infant at greater risk for infection.

Strict hand washing and the use of separate equipment for each infant help minimize exposure of the preterm newborn to infectious agents. In addition, most nurseries around the country have adopted the CDC's standard precautions whereby every baby is isolated. Staff members are required to scrub 2 to 3 minutes using iodine-containing antibacterial solutions, which inhibit the growth of gram-positive cocci and gram-negative rod organisms. Other nursing interventions include limiting visitors; requiring visitors to wash their hands; and maintaining strict aseptic practices when changing intravenous tubing and solutions (IV solutions and tubing should be changed every 24 hours), administering parenteral fluids, and assisting with sterile procedures. Incubators and radiant warmers should be changed weekly. Pressure area breakdown is prevented by changing the baby's position, doing range-of-motion exercises, using a sheepskin (cover sheepskin with blanket, or diaper portion of sheepskin beneath infant's head) or a water bed. To avoid skin tears, a protective transparent covering can be applied over vulnerable joints but use very sparingly ("Neonatal Skin Care," 1997). Chemical skin preps and tape may cause skin trauma and should be avoided as much as possible.

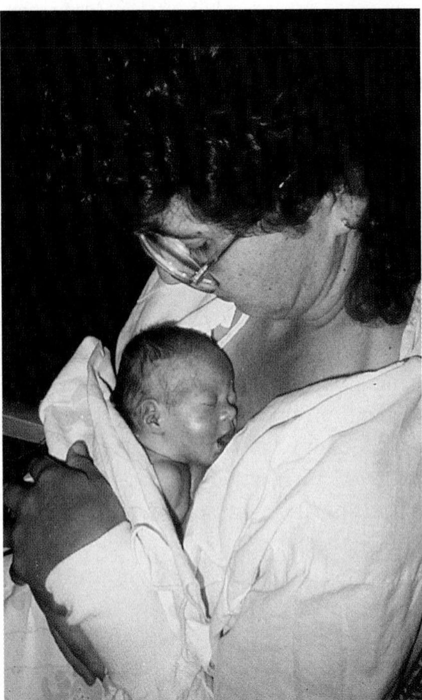

FIGURE 28–10 Kangaroo (skin-to-skin) care facilitates a closeness and attachment between parents and their premature infant. SOURCE: Courtesy of Kadlac Medical Center Kangaroo Care Study and Carol Thompson, RNC, MSN, NNP.

If infection (sepsis) occurs in the preterm newborn, the nurse may be the first to identify the associated subtle clinical signs. The nurse informs the clinician of the findings immediately and implements the treatment plan per clinician orders in the presence of infection. For specific nursing care required for the newborn with an infection, see Chapter 29.

Promotion of Parent-Infant Attachment

Preterm newborns can be separated from their parents for prolonged periods after illness or complications that are detected in the first few hours or days following birth. The resultant interruption in parent-newborn bonding necessitates intervention to ensure successful attachment of parent and infant.

Nurses should take measures to promote positive parental feelings toward the newborn. Photographs of the baby are given to parents to have at home or to the mother if she is in a different hospital or too ill to come to the nursery and visit. The infant's first name is placed on the incubator as soon as it is known to help the parents feel that their infant is a unique and special person. A weekly card with the baby's footprint, weight, and length is also sent to promote bonding. The nurse provides the parents with the telephone number of the nursery or intensive care unit and names of staff members so that they have access to information about their baby at any time of the day or night.

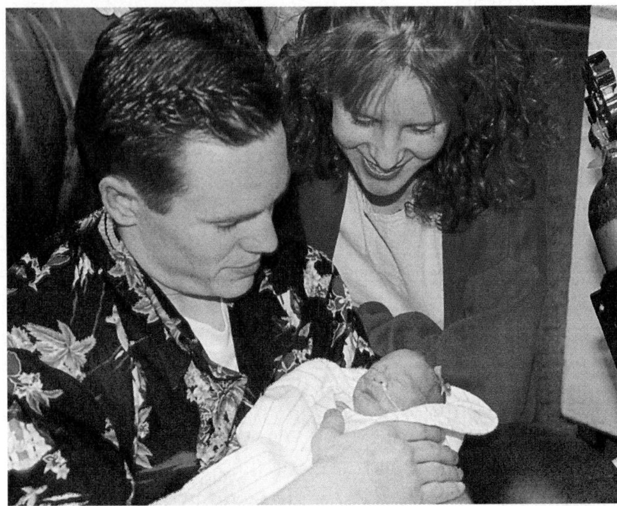

FIGURE 28–11 Family bonding occurs when parents have oppurtunities to spend time with their infant. SOURCE: Courtesy of Carol Harrigan, RNC, MSN, NNP.

The nurse includes the parents in determining the baby's plan of care. Early involvement in the care and decisions regarding their baby provides parents with realistic expectations for their baby. The individual personality characteristics of the infant and the parents influence bonding and contribute to the interactive process. Information is another important variable. Parents need education to develop caregiving skills and to understand the premature infant's behavioral characteristics. Their daily participation (if possible) is encouraged, as are early and frequent visits. The nurse provides opportunities for the parents to touch, hold, talk to, and care for the baby. Skin-to-skin (kangaroo care) helps parents feel close to their small infants. Kangaroo care has been shown to improve sleep periods and parents' perception of their caregiving ability (Messmer et al, 1997) (Figure 28–10).

Some parents may progress easily to touching and cuddling their infant; others will not (Figure 28–11). Parents need to know that their apprehension is normal and the progression of acquaintanceship is slow. Rooming-in can provide another opportunity for the stable preterm infant and family to get acquainted. It offers an environment that is more private but where help is readily available.

Promotion of Developmentally Supportive Care

Prolonged separation and the neonatal intensive care unit (NICU) environment necessitate individualized sensory stimulation programs for the baby. The nurse plays a key role in determining the appropriate type and amount of visual, tactile, and auditory stimulation (Horns, 1998).

Research has shown that some preterm infants are not developmentally able to deal with more than one sensory input at a time. The assessment of preterm infant behavior (APIB) scale identifies the individual preterm newborn behaviors according to five areas of development (Als, Lester, Tronick, & Brazelton, 1982). The infant's physiologic and behavioral subsystems are autonomic, motor control, state differentiation, attention maintenance and social interaction, and finally overall system regulation or self-regulation. Integration of these subsystems improves with increasing gestational and postconceptual age. If the premature infant's self-regulatory capacity is exceeded and the infant is not able to return to previously integrated subsystem functioning, maladaptive behaviors may result when the infant is confronted with environmental demands. The nurse observes the baby's behavioral reactions to stimulation and then bases developmental interventions on reducing detrimental environmental stimuli to the lowest possible level and providing appropriate opportunities for development (Als et al, 1998).

The NICU environment contains many detrimental stimuli that the nurse can help reduce. Noise levels can be lowered by replacing alarms with lights or silencing alarms quickly and keeping conversations away from the baby's bedside. Dimmer switches should be used to shield the baby's eyes from bright lights with blankets over the top portion of the incubator. Dimming the lights may encourage infants to open their eyes and be more responsive to their parents (Cusson & Lee, 1994). Nursing care should be planned to decrease the number of times the baby is disturbed. Signs (ie, "Quiet Please") can be placed near the bedside to allow the baby some periods of uninterrupted sleep (National Association of Neonatal Nurses [NANN] Practice Committee, 1993; Modrein-McCarthy, McCue & Walker, 1997). Some other suggested developmentally supportive interventions include:

- Facilitate handling by using containment measures when turning or moving the infant or doing procedures such as suctioning. Use the hands to hold the infant's arms and legs, flexed, close to the midline of the body. This helps stabilize the infant's motor and physiologic subsystems during stressful activities.
- Touch the infant gently, and avoid sudden postural changes.
- Promote self-consoling or soothing activities, such as placing blanket rolls or approved manufactured devices next to the infant's sides and against the feet, to provide "nesting." Swaddle the infant to maintain extremities in a flexed position while ensuring that the hands can reach the face. This permits the infant to do hand-to-mouth activities, which can be consoling (Figure 28–12).
- Simulate the kinesthetic advantages of the intrauterine environment by using sheepskin and approved water beds. Water bed use has been reported to improve sleep and decrease motor activity as well as lead to more mature motor behavior, fewer state changes, and a decreased heart rate.

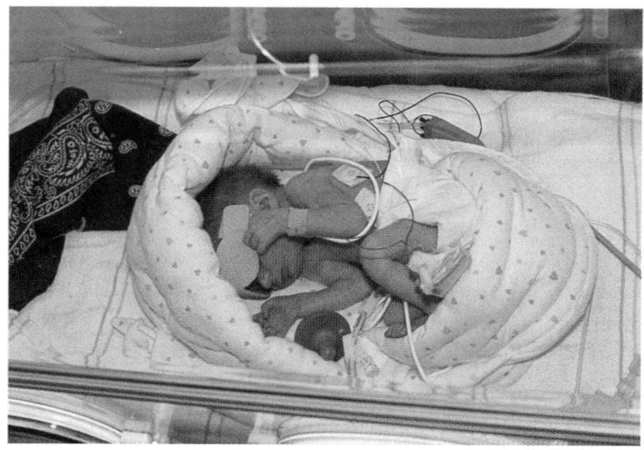

FIGURE 28–12 Infant is "nested." Hand-to-face behavior facilitates self-consoling and soothing activities. SOURCE: Courtesy of Theresa Kledzik, RN, Developmental Nurse, Memorial Hospital, Colorado Springs, Colorado.

- Provide opportunities for nonnutritive sucking with a pacifier. This improves transcutaneous oxygen saturation; decreases body movement; improves sleep, especially after feedings; and increases weight gain (Engebretson & Wardell, 1997).
- Provide objects for the infant to grasp (eg, a piece of blanket, oxygen tubing, or a finger) during caregiving. Grasping may comfort the baby.

Teaching the parents to read behavioral cues will help them move at their infant's pace when providing stimulation. Parents are ideally equipped to meet the baby's need for stimulation. Stroking, rocking, cuddling, quiet singing, and talking to the baby can all be an integral part of the baby's care. Visual stimulation in the form of en face interaction with the caregivers and mobiles is also important.

Preparation for Home Care

Parents are often anxious when their premature infant is transferred out of the NICU or is discharged home. Parents of preterm babies should receive the same postpartal teaching as any parent taking a new infant home. In preparing for discharge, the nurse encourages the parents to spend time caring directly for their baby. This familiarizes them with their baby's behavior patterns and helps them establish realistic expectations about the infant. Some hospitals have a special room near the nursery where a mother can spend the night with her baby prior to discharge.

Discharge instruction includes breastfeeding and bottle-feeding techniques, formula preparation, and vitamin administration. If the mother wishes to breastfeed, the nurse teaches her to pump her breasts to keep the milk flowing and provide milk even before discharge. The nurse gives information on bathing, diapering, hygiene, and normal elimination patterns and prepares the parents to expect changes in the color of the baby's stool, number of bowel movements, and timing of elimination when the infant is switched from bottle-feeding to breastfeeding. This information can prevent unnecessary concern by the parents. The nurse also discusses normal growth and development patterns, reflexes, and activity for preterm infants. In these discussions, the nurse should emphasize ways to promote bonding behaviors and deal with newborn crying. Care of the preterm infant with complications, preventing infections, recognizing signs of a sick baby, and the need for continued medical follow-up are other key issues.

Families with preterm infants usually do not need to be referred to community agencies, such as visiting nurse assistance. Referral may be necessary if the infant has severe congenital abnormalities, feeding problems, or complications with infections or respiratory problems or if the parents seem unable to cope with an at-risk baby. Parents of preterm infants can benefit from meeting with others in a similar situation to share common experiences and concerns. Nurses should refer parents to support groups sponsored by the hospital or by others in the community and make connection for parents with early education intervention centers.

Evaluation

Expected outcomes of nursing care include the following:

- The preterm newborn is free of respiratory distress and establishes effective respiratory function.
- The preterm newborn gains weight and shows no signs of fatigue or aspiration during feedings.
- The parents are able to verbalize their anger, anxieties, and guilt feelings about the birth of a preterm baby and show attachment behavior such as frequent visits and growing confidence in their participatory care activities.
- The preterm newborn demonstrates a serial head circumference growth rate of 1 cm/week.

CRITICAL THINKING QUESTION

What ethical issues arise from the birth and survival of increasing numbers of very-low-birth-weight infants?

Care of the Infant of a Substance-Abusing Mother

An infant of a substance-abusing mother (ISAM) was formerly called an infant of an addicted mother. The newborn of an alcoholic or drug-addicted woman may also be alcohol or drug dependent. After birth, when an infant's connection with the maternal blood supply is severed, the baby may suffer withdrawal. In addition, the drugs the mother ingested may be teratogenic, resulting in congenital anomalies.

Alcohol Dependence

The **fetal alcohol syndrome (FAS)** includes a series of malformations frequently found in infants exposed to alcohol in utero. It has been estimated that complete FAS syndrome occurs in 1 to 2 live births per 1000 (Kenner & D'Apolito, 1997). FAS rates among Native Americans and Alaska natives are estimated at 1.3 to 10.3 per 1000 live births in the groups studied. If infants with fetal alcohol effects are included, the incidence may more approximate 4 in 1000 live births (Kenner & D'Apolito, 1997).

Fetal alcohol effects (FAE), or alcohol-related birth defects (ARBD), are usually determined only by a positive maternal drinking history and cognitive difficulties (Institute of Medicine [IOM], 1996). The new diagnostic categories for FAS take into consideration the various clinical manifestations of FAS, the social and family environment, and, if available, the maternal alcohol history (Hess & Kenner, 1998).

Although it is known that ethanol freely crosses the placenta to the fetus, it is still not known whether the alcohol alone or the breakdown products of alcohol cause the damage. For in-depth discussion of alcohol abuse in pregnancy, see Chapter 15. The effects of other substances that are often combined with alcohol, such as nicotine, diazepam (Valium), marijuana, and caffeine, as well as poor diet, enhance the likelihood of FAS.

Long-Term Complications for the Infant with FAS

The long-term prognosis for the FAS newborn is less than favorable. Many FAS infants are evaluated for organic and inorganic failure to thrive.

Feeding problems are frequently present during infancy and preschool years. These infants have a delay in the normal progression of oral feeding because of weak suck development. Many FAS infants nurse poorly and have persistent vomiting until 6 to 7 months of age.

Central nervous system dysfunctions are the most common and serious problems associated with FAS. Hypotonicity and increased placidity is seen in these infants. They also have a decreased ability to habituate repetitive stimuli. Children exhibiting FAS can be severely mentally retarded or have normal intelligence. The more abnormal the facial features, the lower the IQ scores. Often there is little improvement in intelligence (as measured by IQ) despite positive environmental and educational factors (Hess & Kenner, 1998). These children show impulsivity, cognitive impairment, speech and language abnormalities, and learning disabilities indicative of CNS involvement (Church & Abel, 1998).

NURSING CARE MANAGEMENT

Nursing Assessment and Diagnosis

Newborns with FAS show the following characteristics:

- *Abnormal structural development and CNS dysfunction,* including mental retardation, microcephaly, and hyperactivity.
- *Growth deficiencies.* Infants with FAS are often growth retarded with weight, length, and head circumference being affected. These infants continue to show a persistent postnatal growth deficiency with head circumference and linear growth most affected.
- *Distinctive facial abnormalities.* These include short palebral fissures, epicanthal folds, broad nasal bridge, flattened midfacies, short upturned or beaklike nose, micrognathia (abnormally small lower jaw), hypoplastic maxilla, thin upper lip or vermilion border, and smooth philtrum (groove on upper lip). Facial dysmorphology can change with age (Kenner & D'Apolito, 1997).
- *Associated anomalies.* Abnormalities affecting the heart (primarily septal and valvular defects), eyes, kidneys, and skeletal system (especially those involving joints, such as congenital dislocated hips) are often noted.

Alcohol-exposed infants in the first week of life may show symptoms that include sleeplessness, excessive arousal states, inconsolable crying, abnormal reflexes, hyperactivity with little ability to maintain alertness and attentiveness to environment, jitteriness, abdominal distention, and exaggerated mouthing behaviors such as hyperactive rooting and increased nonnutritive sucking. These symptoms commonly persist throughout the first month of life but may continue longer (Gardner, 1997). Alcohol dependence in the infant is physiologic, not psychologic.

Nursing diagnoses that may apply to the FAS newborn include the following:

- ***Altered Nutrition: Less than Body Requirements*** related to decreased food intake and hyperirritability
- ***Alteration in Neurodevelopmental Status*** related to central nervous system involvement secondary to maternal alcohol use
- ***Ineffective Family Coping*** related to dysfunctional family dynamics and substance-dependent mother

Nursing Plan and Implementation

Hospital-Based Nursing Care

The nurse's awareness of the signs and symptoms of fetal alcohol syndrome is important in structuring and guiding nursing care. Nursing care of the FAS newborn is aimed at avoiding heat loss, providing adequate nutrition, and reducing environmental stimuli. The FAS baby is most comfortable in a quiet, dimly lighted environment. Because of feeding problems, these infants require extra time and patience during feedings. Its important to provide consistency in the staff working with the baby and parents and to keep personnel and visitors to a minimum at any one time (Gardner, 1997).

The nurse should inform the alcohol-dependent mother that breastfeeding is not contraindicated but that excessive alcohol consumption may intoxicate the newborn and inhibit the let-down reflex. The nurse should monitor the newborn's vital signs closely and observe for evidence of seizure activity and respiratory distress.

Community-Based Nursing Care

Infants affected by maternal alcohol abuse are also at risk psychologically. Restlessness, sleeplessness, agitation, resistance to cuddling or holding, and frequent crying can be frustrating to parents as their efforts to relieve the distress are unrewarded. Feeding dysfunction can also result in frustrations for the caregiver and digestive upsets for the infant. Frustration may cause the parents to punish the baby or result in the unconscious desire to stay away from the infant. Either outcome may create an unstable family environment and result in the infant's failure to thrive.

The nurse should focus on providing support for the parents and reinforcing positive parenting activity. Prior to discharge, parents should be given opportunities to provide baby care so that they can feel confident in their interpretations of their baby's cues and their ability to meet the baby's needs. Referring the family to social services and visiting nurse or public health nurse associations is essential for the well-being of the infant. Follow-up care and teaching can strengthen the parents' skills and coping abilities and help them create a stable, healthy environment for their family. The infant with FAS/ARBD should be involved in intervention programs that monitor the child's developmental progress, health, and home environment.

Evaluation

Expected outcomes of nursing care include the following:

- The FAS newborn is able to tolerate feedings and gain weight.
- The FAS infant's hyperirritability are controlled, and the baby has suffered no physical injuries.
- The parents are able to identify and meet the special needs of their newborn and accept outside assistance as needed.

Drug Dependence

Drugs of abuse by the pregnant woman can include the following singularly or in combination: tobacco, cocaine, phencyclidine (PCP), methamphetamines, inhalants, marijuana, heroin, and methadone.

Drug-dependent infants are predisposed to a number of problems. Almost all narcotic drugs cross the placenta and enter the fetal circulation, so the fetus can develop problems in utero or soon after birth. The effects of polydrug use on the newborn must be taken into consideration.

The greatest risks to the fetus of the drug-dependent mother are listed below:

- *Intrauterine asphyxia.* Often a direct result of fetal withdrawal secondary to maternal withdrawal, fetal withdrawal is accompanied by hyperactivity with increased oxygen consumption. If not adequately compensated, this can lead to fetal asphyxia. Moreover, narcotic-addicted women tend to have a higher incidence of pregnancy-induced hypertension (PIH), abruptio placentae, and placenta previa, resulting in placental insufficiency and fetal asphyxia.
- *Intrauterine infection.* Sexually transmitted infections, HIV infection, and hepatitis are often connected with the pregnant addict's lifestyle. Such infections can involve the fetus.
- *Alterations in birth weight.* These may depend on the type of drug the mother uses. Women using predominantly heroin or cocaine have infants of lower birth weight who are SGA. Women maintained on methadone have higher-birth-weight infants, some of whom are LGA.
- *Low Apgar scores.* These may be related to the intrauterine asphyxia or the medication the woman received during labor. The use of a narcotic antagonist (nalorphine or naloxone) to reverse respiratory depression is contraindicated because it may precipitate acute withdrawal in the infant.

Patterns of abuse of alcohol, marijuana, and heroin in childbearing women have changed very little in the past few years, but the incidence of cocaine (especially "crack") use has recently risen dramatically. (See Chapter 15 for more discussion of maternal substance abuse.) Marijuana, alcohol, and nicotine are often used in conjunction with cocaine.

Common Complications of the Drug-Dependent Newborn

The newborn of a woman who abused drugs during her pregnancy is predisposed to the following problems:

- *Respiratory distress.* The heroin-addicted newborn frequently suffers respiratory stress, mainly meconium-aspiration pneumonia and transient tachypnea. Meconium aspiration is usually secondary to increased oxygen consumption and activity experienced by the fetus during intrauterine withdrawal. Transient tachypnea may develop secondary to the inhibitory effects of narcotics on the reflex responsible for clearing the lungs. Respiratory distress syndrome, however, occurs less often in heroin-addicted newborns, even in those who are premature, because they have tissue-oxygen unloading capabilities comparable to those of a 6-week-old term infant. In addition, heroin stimulates production of glucocorticoids via the anterior pituitary gland.
- *Jaundice.* Newborns of methadone-addicted women may develop jaundice due to prematurity. By contrast, infants of mothers addicted to heroin or cocaine have a lower incidence of hyperbilirubinemia because these substances contribute to early maturity of the liver.
- *Congenital anomalies and growth retardation.* The incidence of anomalies of the genitourinary and cardiovascular systems is slightly increased in infants of heroin- and cocaine-addicted mothers. Infants of cocaine-addicted mothers exhibit congenital malformations involving bony skull defects, such as microencephaly, and symmetric intrauterine growth retardation, cardiac defects, and genitourinary defects. Congenital anomalies, however, are rare (Frank, Bresnahan, & Zuckerman, 1996; Kenner & D'Apolito, 1997).
- *Behavioral abnormalities.* Babies exposed to cocaine have poor state organization. They exhibit decreased interactive behaviors when tested with the Brazelton Neonatal Behavioral Assessment Scale (Wagner, Katikaneni, Cox, & Ryan, 1998). These infants also have difficulty moving through the various sleep and awake states and have problems attending to and actively engaging in auditory and visual stimuli.
- *Withdrawal.* The most significant postnatal problem of the drug-addicted newborn is narcotic withdrawal (usually from heroin or methadone). The onset of the withdrawal manifestations often occurs after discharge, especially with short birthing unit stays. See Table 28–2 on page 836 in Nursing Assessment for a discussion of withdrawal symptoms.

Long-Term Effects

During the first 2 years of life, many cocaine-exposed infants demonstrate susceptibility to behavior lability and the inability to express strong feelings such as pleasure, anger, or distress, or even a strong reaction to being separated from their parents. Cocaine-exposed infants are at higher risk for motor development problems, delays in expressive language skills, and feeding difficulties due to swallowing problems (Kenner & D'Apolito, 1997).

Infants of drug-addicted mothers often demonstrate a higher incidence of gastrointestinal and respiratory illnesses; it is believed these are related not to drug exposure but to the mothers' lack of education regarding proper infant care, feeding, and hygiene.

Another important long-term complication is the high rate (15 to 20 per 1000 births) of sudden infant death syndrome (SIDS) for heroin- or methadone-exposed infants in comparison to those in the general infant population (Kenner & D'Apolito, 1997). After birth the infant born to a drug-dependent mother may also be subject to neglect, abuse, or both (Kenner & D'Apolito, 1997).

Clinical Therapy

The goal of clinical therapy is to prevent complications through prenatal management (see Chapter 15) and pharmacologic management of newborn narcotic withdrawal. For optimal fetal and newborn outcome, the narcotic-addicted woman should receive complete prenatal care as early as possible. She should be started on a methadone program with a reduction in dosage to 20 mg or less, if possible (Buchi, 1998). The aim of methadone maintenance during pregnancy is to prevent heroin use. The dose of methadone used for maintenance should be sufficient to ensure this goal even if the dose is greater than 20 mg. It is not recommended that the woman be withdrawn completely from narcotics while pregnant because this induces fetal withdrawal with poor newborn outcomes.

Newborn treatment may include management of complications; serologic tests for syphilis, HIV, and hepatitis B; urine drug screen and meconium analysis; and social service referral. About 50% of newborns of addicted mothers experience withdrawal symptoms severe enough to require pharmacologic intervention. The choice of pharmacologic intervention should be based not only on the drug of exposure, but also on the origin of the presenting withdrawal symptoms—for example, gastrointestinal or central nervous system. Drugs used to control withdrawal symptoms vary and may be regionally based. They include phenobarbital, paregoric, oral morphine sulfate solution, Donnatal elixir, and simethicone (Mylicon) drops. Nutritional support is important in light of the increase in energy expenditure that withdrawal may entail.

NURSING CARE MANAGEMENT

Nursing Assessment and Diagnosis

Early identification of the newborn needing clinical or pharmacologic interventions decreases the incidence of mortality and morbidity. During the newborn period, nursing assessment focuses on the following:

- Discovering the mother's last drug intake and dosage level. This is accomplished through the prenatal history and laboratory tests. Women may be reluctant to disclose this information; therefore, a nonjudgmental interview technique is essential.
- Assessing for congenital malformations and the complications related to intrauterine withdrawal, such as SGA, intrauterine asphyxia, meconium aspiration, and prematurity.
- Identifying the signs and symptoms of newborn withdrawal or newborn abstinence syndrome. Signs and symptoms of newborn withdrawal can be classified in five groups:

1. Central nervous system signs
   a. Hyperactivity
   b. Hyperirritability (incessant shrill cry)
   c. Increased muscle tone
   d. Exaggerated reflexes (myoclonic jerks)
   e. Tremors, seizures
   f. Sneezing, hiccups, yawning
   g. Short, unquiet sleep
   h. Fever
2. Respiratory signs
   a. Tachypnea (> 60 breaths/min when quiet)
   b. Excessive secretions
3. Gastrointestinal signs
   a. Disorganized, vigorous suck
   b. Vomiting
   c. Drooling
   d. Sensitive gag reflex
   e. Hyperphagia
   f. Diarrhea
   g. Abdominal cramping
   h. Poor feeding (<15 mL on first day of life; takes longer than 30 min per feeding)
4. Vasomotor signs
   a. Stuffy nose, yawning, sneezing
   b. Flushing
   c. Sweating
   d. Sudden, circumoral pallor
5. Cutaneous signs
   a. Excoriated buttocks, knees, elbows
   b. Facial scratches
   c. Pressure point abrasions

Although many of the signs and symptoms of narcotic withdrawal are similar to those seen with hypoglycemia and hypocalcemia, glucose and calcium values are reported to be within normal limits for this group of infants.

The severity of withdrawal can be assessed by a scoring system based on clinical manifestations. It evaluates the infant on potentially life-threatening signs, such as vomiting, diarrhea, weight loss, irritability, tremors, and tachypnea (Table 28–2).

Nursing diagnoses that may apply to drug-dependent newborns include the following:

TABLE 28–2 Assessment of the Clinical Severity of Neonatal Narcotic Withdrawal

Symptom	Mild	Moderate	Severe
Vomiting	Spitting up	Extensive vomiting for three successive feedings	Vomiting associated with imbalance of serum electrolytes
Diarrhea	Watery stools < four times per day	Watery stools five to six times per day for 3 days; no electrolyte imbalance	Diarrhea associated with imbalance of serum electrolytes
Weight loss	<10% of birth weight	10%–15% of birth weight	>15%
Irritability	Minimal	Marked but relieved by cuddling or feeding	Unrelieved by cuddling or feeding
Tremors or twitching	Mild tremors when stimulated	Marked tremors or twitching when stimulated	Convulsions
Tachypnea	60–80 breaths/minute	80–100 breaths/minute	>100 breaths/minute; associated with respiratory alkalosis

SOURCE: Ostrea EM, Chavez CJ, Stryker JS: *The Care of the Drug Dependent Woman and Her Infant.* Lansing, MI: Michigan Department of Public Health, 1978, p 33.

- ***Altered Nutrition: Less than Body Requirements*** related to vomiting and diarrhea, uncoordinated suck and swallow reflex, hypertonia secondary to withdrawal
- ***Impaired Skin Integrity*** related to constant activity
- ***Altered Parenting*** related to hyperirritable behavior of the infant
- ***Ineffective Family Coping: Disabling*** related to drug abuse, poverty, and lack of education
- ***Sleep Pattern Disturbance*** related to CNS excitation secondary to drug withdrawal

Nursing Plan and Implementation

Hospital-Based Nursing Care

Care of the drug-dependent newborn is based on reducing withdrawal symptoms and promoting adequate respiration, temperature, and nutrition. See the Critical Pathway for Newborn of a Substance-Abusing Mother on the facing page for specific nursing care measures. Some general nursing care measures include the following:

- Temperature regulation
- Careful monitoring of pulse and respirations every 15 minutes until stable; stimulation if apnea occurs
- Small, frequent feedings, especially in the presence of vomiting, regurgitation, and diarrhea
- Intravenous therapy as needed
- Medications as ordered, such as phenobarbital and paregoric. Methadone should not be given because of possible newborn addiction to it. There is controversy about the use of paregoric because it contains alcohol and camphor (American Academy of Pediatrics Committee on Drugs, 1998).
- Proper positioning on the right side to avoid possible aspirations of vomitus or secretions
- Monitoring frequency of diarrhea and vomiting, and weighing infant every 8 hours during withdrawal
- Observation for problems of SGA or LGA newborns
- Swaddling with hands near mouth to minimize injury and achieve more organized behavioral state. Gentle, vertical rocking can be successful in calming an infant who is out of control (Gardner-Cole, 1996)
- Placing newborn in quiet, dimly lighted area of nursery

CRITICAL THINKING QUESTION

What issues need to be addressed to meet the needs of babies of substance-abusing mothers?

Community-Based Nursing Care

Parents need assistance to prepare for what they can expect for the first few months at home. At the time of discharge, the mother should be instructed to anticipate mild jitteriness and irritability in the newborn, which may persist from 8 to 16 weeks, depending on the initial severity of the withdrawal. The nurse should demonstrate and help the mother learn feeding techniques, comforting measures, how to recognize newborn cues, and appropriate parenting responses (French, Pituch, Brandt, & Pohorecki, 1998). Parents are to be counseled regarding available resources, such as support groups, and signs and symptoms that indicate the need for further care. Ongoing evaluation is necessary because of the potential for long-term problems. Follow-up on missed appointments can bring parents back into the health care system, thereby improving parent and infant outcomes and promoting a positive, interactive environment after delivery.

Evaluation

Expected outcomes of nursing care include the following:

- The newborn tolerates feedings, gains weight, and has a decreased number of stools.

Text continues on page 840.

CRITICAL PATHWAY FOR NEWBORN OF A SUBSTANCE-ABUSING MOTHER

Category	Day of Birth—First 4 Hours	Remainder of Birth Day
Referral	Report from L&D, neonatal nurse practitioner Check ID bands High-risk peds/neonatology consults prn	Check ID bands q shift As parents request, obtain circumcision permit after their discussion with MD
Assessments	Complete set of VS Admission wt, length, HC Assess skin color, skin integrity for rashes, breakdown Gestational age assessment Monitor activity (lethargy, character of cry, exaggerated startle responses) Maternal hx of drugs consumed during each month of pregnancy Obtain prior hx of addiction and treatment Withdrawl s/s: hyperactivity, jitteriness, irritability, shrill high-pitched cry, vomiting, diarrhea, weak suck, stuffy nose, frequent sneezing, yawning, tachycardia, hypertension, apnea, seizure activity Cocaine withdrawal pattern may be unpredictable or may be asymptomatic with only subtle behavioral state organization problems	Vital signs: T/P/R q4h and prn, BP prn Newborn assessment q shift Assess for hypothermia Assess mother/baby interaction
Teaching/ psychosocial	(See Newborn Critical Pathway, pp. 754 to 755) Admission activities performed at mother's bedside if possible; orient parents to NSY, handwashing; assess teaching needs and readiness for learning Evaluate additional psychosocial needs (provide time for verbalizing concerns, determine parental understanding of substance abuse) Provide information including: • s/s of baby's withdrawal, current condition, and rationale of treatment • Newborn capabilities and developmental behaviors, cues • Newborn's need for appropriate stimulation as well as rest, depending on cues • Physical care needs (feeding, bathing, clothing, holding) • Safety-bulb syringe, choking, positioning	Reinforce previous teaching Discuss/teach infant security, identification Discuss/teach temperature maintenance with clothing/blankets Teach parents/guardian feeding methods, burping, diapering, and elimination norms Teach parents calming techniques, s/s of stress and infant cues to stress
Nursing care management and reports	• Serum electrolytes to detect losses from vomiting/diarrhea • Blood type, Rh, Coombs' on cord blood when applicable • Chemstrip prn; BP prn • Baer hearing test • Maintain Universal Precautions • Bathe ASAP if foul smelling amniotic fluid/cord care per policy • Hep B form reviewed and/or signed by parent, administer if ordered after bath • Peripheral hematocrit per protocol • Toxicology screen to identify drugs and drug levels in infant • CBC and blood cultures to detect sepsis • Intavenous access for meds, hydration, nutritional support	• Check for Baer hearing test results • Femoral pulse or BP all 4 extremities if early DC • Vital signs: q4h, T/P/R • Daily wt • Assess color q shift and prn • Cord care per policy (alcohol to cord stump q diaper change) • Monitor for s/s of substance withdrawal, seizure activity; notify NP/MD prn, offer supportive care • Maintain intravenous access prn
Activity and comfort	• Adjust and monitor radiant warmer to maintain skin temp until stable • Provide calming techniques: Swaddling infant tightly in side-lying or prone position with blanket roll to back, nest Provide quiet, dim environment for rest Hold, rock, and cuddle infant. Use touching, petting, smiling, talking. Use infant snuggly for closeness, carrying infant. Provide pacifier or swaddle to allow infant's hands to mouth.	Leave in radiant warmer until stable, then swaddle in open crib Continue calming/soothing techniques prn Cluster care, provide care on infant's schedule Avoid overstimulation

➤

CRITICAL PATHWAY FOR NEWBORN OF A SUBSTANCE-ABUSING MOTHER *CONTINUED*

Category	Day of Birth—First 4 Hours	Remainder of Birth Day
Nutrition	Initiate bottle-feeding Initiate breastfeeding as soon as mother/baby condition allows lavage and gavage prn Supplement breast only when medically indicated or ordered by MD per protocol Assess for increased nutritional needs because of gestational age, weight, uncoordinated suck and swallow, vomiting, diarrhea, and regurgitation	Continue feeding schedule Encourage frequent feedings at least q3–4h during day Feed on demand breast or bottle Consider breast milk evaluation to r/o active or residual drug presence
Elimination	Note first void and stool color Urine specific gravity to detect dehydration	Monitor stools for amount, type, consistency and pattern changes Monitor all voids q shift
Medication	Administer medications for withdrawal as ordered, such as paregoric, chlorpromazine, Valium, phenobarbital, tincture of opium, observe for effectiveness and side effects Aquamephyton IM, dosage according to infant wt and protocol after bath Ilotycin ophth ointment OU—after bath	Continue medications as ordered and necessary to alleviate s/s substance withdrawal, to allow newborn rest and ability to suck/maintain nutritional status
Discharge planning/ home care	Evaluate for social services, visiting nurses service, and DC planning needs Plan DC with parent/guardian in 1–3 days	Present birth certificate instructions/worksheet Car seat available for DC Newborn photographs
Family involvement	Evaluate parent teaching Access community resources prn, ie, Teen "Healthy Starts" Encourage/support positive mothering/parenting behaviors with infant	Evaluate parent teaching Assess parents' knowledge of newborn behavior and reflexes Encourage family involvement in infant's care as soon as possible and as infant tolerates
Date		
Category	**Day 1**	**Day 2/3 (if applicable)**
Referral	Check ID bands when baby leaves nursery Lactation consult prn	Check ID bands q shift **Expected Outcomes** Mother/baby ID bands correlate at time of DC Consults completed prn
Assessments	Assess mother/baby interaction Continue newborn assessments q shift Assess thermoregulation/VS q shift and prn Assess abdominal distension, gastric residuals Assess altered sleep-wake cycle and rhythm at 24–48h	Assess mother/baby interaction Assess abdominal distension, gastric residuals, wt gain, s/s drug withdrawal and complications **Expected Outcomes** Physical assessments, VS WNL; no complications of newborn of substance-abusing mother noted
Teaching/ psychosocial	(See Newborn Critical Pathway, pp. 754 to 755) Reinforce previous teaching Parental Teaching: bathing, cord care, skin/nail care, use of thermometer, activity, sleep patterns, calming activities, reflexes, s/s jaundice, growth/feeding patterns, special nutritional needs, report feeding intolerance, circumcision care Evaluate mother/parent teaching; provide information about HIV s/s, group support and community resources for persons with substance abuse issues	Final Discharge Teaching: (See Newborn Critical Pathway, pp. 754 to 755) Review with parents/guardian infant safety, s/s illness and when to call health care provider **Expected Outcomes** Mother verbalizes comprehension of instructions, demonstrates care capabilities

Category	Day 1	Day 2/3 (if applicable)
Nursing care management and reports	Newborn assessment q shift Daily wt Circumcision care q diaper change Femoral pulse or BP all 4 extremities before DC or first 48h Unclamp cord clamp, alcohol to cord q diaper change HSV culture per parental hx of HSV Maintain NTE Newborn screen Continue to monitor for s/s of drug withdrawal, seizure activity Administer meds for withdrawal s/s as ordered; monitor infant response, report to NP/MD prn	Newborn assessment and VS q shift Daily wt Cord care per policy Note Baer hearing test results Cord care, circumcision care q diaper change **Expected Outcomes** Physical assessments WNL; cord unclamped and dry without s/s infection; circ site unremarkable; gaining wt or stabilized to not >10% loss; labs WNL; without s/s of substance withdrawal or infection; infant not requiring medication for relief of s/s of drug withdrawal
Activity and comfort	Swaddled in open crib Incubator if temp instability; adjust incubator for infant size, gestation, layers of clothing to maintain NTE	Swaddle to allow movement of hands to face **Expected Outcomes** Maintains temp WNL swaddled in open crib
Nutrition	• Supplement oral or gavage feedings with intravenous intake per orders; evaluate necessity prn • Give small, frequent feedings q3–4h breast milk or formula as ordered, increasing strength of feeding as tolerated and as ordered (may start with half-strength breast milk/formula) • Feed calorically enhanced breast milk/formula as ordered; monitor infant's tolerance to feedings • Check for gastric residuals before q feeding; adjust volume of feeding prn with high or increasing residuals. Notify NP/MD of increasing residuals • Increase feeding volume as tolerated and as hyperactivity decreases • Supplement breast only when medically indicated and ordered by NP/MD • Feed on demand, minimally q3–4h	Feed on demand, minimally q3–4h Gavage feed prn, as ordered to maintain nutrition Supplement breast only when medically indicated and ordered by NP/MD Encourage frequent feedings during day Monitor infant for s/s of active or residual presence of drugs with breastmilk feedings versus normal satiation after feeding. Consider toxicology screen of breast milk, fresh or frozen, prn **Expected Outcomes** Infant tolerates feedings, feeds on demand; breastfeeds without supplement, nipples without problems; regaining lost wt or wt stabilized
Elimination	Monitor stools for amount, consistency, pattern changes, occult blood, reducing substances Monitor voids q8h	Continue monitoring of all voids and stools q shift, noting changes **Expected Outcomes** Voids qs; stools without difficulty qs with stool character WNL; diaper area without s/s breakdown
Medication	Hep B vaccine before DC Administer meds for withdrawal or seizure activity prn as ordered; observe for s/s of effectiveness and side effects	**Expected Outcomes** Infant has received ophth ointment OU and Aquamephyton injection; received first Hep B vaccine if ordered and parental consent received; infant not requiring meds for s/s withdrawal or seizure activity
Discharge planning/ home care	Newborn photographs Complete birth certificate packet If vag birth, complete DC teaching Access community referrals, support groups for mother/family prn, ie, drug rehab, developmental, occupational and physical therapy, WIC, financial resources, public health nursing for home visits	If cesarean birth, complete DC teaching Complete DC summary (See Newborn Critical Pathway, pp. 754 to 755) **Expected Outcomes** Infant DC home with mother; mother verbalizes follow-up appointment times, dates, referral sources
Family involvement	Bath, newborn care, and feeding class Newborn channel as available Assess mother/baby bonding/interaction Incorporate significant other/siblings in infant care Support positive parenting behaviors Evaluate mother/parent teaching	Assess mother/baby interaction Identify community referral needs and refer to community agencies Evaluate mother/parent teaching Encourage questions **Expected Outcomes** Mother/family demonstrates caring and family incorporation of infant
Date		

- The parents learn ways to comfort their newborn.
- The parents are able to cope with their frustrations and begin to use outside resources as needed.

Care of the Newborn Exposed to HIV/AIDS

Increasing numbers of newborns are born infected with HIV or at risk for acquiring it in the newborn period or early infancy. Transmission during the perinatal and newborn periods can occur across the placenta or through breast milk or contaminated blood. Ongoing prospective studies indicate maternal to newborn vertical transmission rates of about 20% to 30%; the majority of infants who are born to an infected mother ultimately remain uninfected (Committee on Pediatric AIDS, 1997). Vertical transmission can be decreased by two-thirds in mothers taking azidothymidine (AZT) during gestation. For further discussion of maternal and fetal HIV/AIDS, see Chapter 15.

Early identification of babies with or at risk for HIV/AIDS is essential during the newborn period. The currently available HIV serologic tests (ELISA and Western blot test) cannot distinguish between maternal and infant antibodies; therefore, they are inappropriate for infants up to 15 months of age. It may take up to 15 months for infected infants to form their own antibodies to HIV (Committee on Pediatric AIDS, 1997). Testing by HIV DNA polymerase chain reaction (PCR) or viral culture should be performed at birth and again at 1 to 2 months of age (Committee on Pediatric AIDS, 1997). Umbilical cord blood should not be used for HIV testing. If PCR and viral culture are unavailable, the p24 antigen may be used to assess HIV infection status in infants older than 1 month, but the sensitivity of p24 antigen testing is substantially less than the other tests. Opportunistic diseases such as gram-negative sepsis and problems associated with prematurity are the primary causes of mortality in HIV-infected babies. Some infants infected by maternal-fetal transmission suffer from severe immunodeficiency, with HIV disease progressing more rapidly during the first year of life (Rodriguez, Diaz & Fowler, 1997). For infants who have two or more negative HIV antibody tests, the National Pediatric HIV Resource Center recommends a final HIV antibody test at 24 months of age for HIV-exposed infants whose previous testings have been negative.

NURSING CARE MANAGEMENT

Nursing Assessment and Diagnosis

Many newborns exposed to HIV/AIDS are premature, SGA, or both and show failure to thrive during the newborn and infant periods. They can show signs and symptoms of disease within days of birth. Signs that may be seen in the early infancy period include enlarged spleen and liver, swollen glands, recurrent respiratory infections, rhinorrhea, interstitial pneumonia (rarely seen in adults), recurrent gastrointestinal problems (diarrhea and weight loss), organic failure to thrive, urinary system infections, persistent or recurrent oral and genital candidiasis infections, and loss of developmental milestones (Gray, 1997). Some cranial and facial stigmas have been associated with AIDS contracted in utero. However, these findings do not establish a diagnosis of HIV infection at birth. Nursing diagnoses that may apply to the infant exposed to HIV/AIDS include the following:

- ***Altered Nutrition: Less than Body Requirements*** related to formula intolerance and inadequate intake
- ***Risk for Impaired Skin Integrity*** related to chronic diarrhea
- ***Risk for Infection*** related to perinatal exposure and immunoregulation suppression secondary to HIV/AIDS
- ***Impaired Physical Mobility*** related to decreased neuromuscular development
- ***Altered Growth and Development*** related to lack of attachment and stimulation
- ***Altered Parenting*** related to diagnosis of HIV/AIDS and fear of future outcome

Nursing Plan and Implementation

Hospital-Based Nursing Care

Nursing care of the newborn exposed to HIV/AIDS calls for all the normal care required for any newborn in a nursery. See the Critical Pathway for Newborn at Risk for HIV/AIDS on pages 842 to 844. In addition, the nurse must include care for a newborn suspected of having a blood-borne infection, as with hepatitis B. Standard (universal) precautions should be used when caring for the newborn immediately after birth and when obtaining blood samples via vein puncture or heel stick. (The blood of all newborns must be considered potentially infectious because the status of the infant's blood is often not known until after the infant is discharged. There is also a window of time before seroconversion occurs, during which the baby is still considered infectious.) Nursing care involves providing for comfort; keeping the newborn well nourished and protected from opportunistic infections; and facilitating growth, development, and attachment. Most institutions recommend that their caregivers wear gloves during all diaper changes and examination of babies. Disposable gloves are worn when changing diapers or cleaning the diaper area, especially in the presence of diarrhea, because blood may be in the stool. Good skin care is essential to prevent skin rashes.

CRITICAL THINKING IN PRACTICE

Mrs Jean Corrigan, a 23-year old G1P1, positive for HIV, has just given birth to a 7 lb 1 oz baby girl. As she watches you assessing her daughter in the birthing room, she asks why you are wearing gloves and whether her daughter will have to be in isolation. How do you respond?

Answers can be found in Appendix I.

Community-Based Nursing Care

Hand washing is crucial when caring for newborns at risk for AIDS. Parents should be taught proper hand-washing technique. Nutrition is essential because failure to thrive and weight loss are common. Small, frequent feedings and food supplementation are helpful. The nurse should discuss with the parents sanitary techniques for preparing formula. The nurse should also inform parents that the baby should not be put to bed with juice or formula because of potential bacteria growth. Parents need to be alert to the signs of feeding intolerance, such as increasing regurgitation, abdominal distention, and loose stools. The newborn should be weighed three times a week.

The baby should have his or her own skin care items, towels, and washcloths. Most clothing and linens can be washed with other household laundry. Linen that is visibly soiled with blood or body fluids should be kept separate and washed separately in hot, sudsy water with household bleach. Prompt diaper changing and perineal care can prevent or minimize diaper rash and promote comfort. The diaper-changing area in the home should be separate from the food preparation and serving areas. The diapers are to be placed in plastic bags, sealed, and disposed of daily. Diaper-changing areas should be cleaned with a 1:10 dilution of household bleach after each diaper change. Toys should be kept as clean as possible, and they should not be shared with other children. Toys should be checked for sharp edges to prevent scratches.

The nurse should instruct parents in what signs of infection to be alert for and when to call their health care provider. The inability to feed without pain may indicate esophageal yeast infection. Topical mycostatin or Desitin ointment is used for diaper rashes and oral mycostatin for oral thrush. If diarrhea occurs, the baby requires frequent perineal care and fluid replacements. Antidiarrheal medications are often ineffective. Irritability may be the first sign of fever. Taking rectal temperatures should be avoided, as it may stimulate diarrhea. Fluids, antipyretics, and sponging with tepid water are of use in managing fever.

Parents and family members need to be reassured that there are no documented cases of people contracting HIV/AIDS from routine care of infected babies. Emotional support for the family is essential because of the stress and social isolation they may face. Because of these stresses, parents may not bond with the baby or fail to provide the baby with enough sensory and tactile stimulation. The nurse should instruct the parents to hold the baby during feedings because the infant will benefit from frequent, gentle touch. Auditory stimulation may also be provided using music or tapes of parents' voices. The nurse should offer information to families about support groups, available counseling, and information resources. Current therapeutic information regarding HIV disease is available to both health care providers and families through the AIDS Clinical Trials Information Service (1-800-TRIALS-A). The CDC recommends that HIV-infected women in developed countries not breastfeed because HIV has been found to be transmitted via breast milk. Therefore, if there is a viable alternative feeding method, it should be used (Committee on Pediatric AIDS, 1997).

All infants born to HIV-positive mothers require regular clinical, immunologic, and virologic monitoring. Preventive care for exposed infants is the same as for other infants and includes routine immunizations, except that the live polio vaccine should be avoided. At 1 month of age, the baby's physical examination should include a developmental assessment; complete blood count, including differential blood count, CD4+ count, and platelet count. Prophylaxis for *pneumocystis carinii* pneumonia (PCP) for all infants born to HIV-infected women should be initiated at 4 to 6 weeks of age, regardless of the infant's CD4+ lymphocyte count (Committee on Pediatric AIDS, 1997). Pediatric HIV disease raises many health care issues for the family. The parents, depending on their health status, may or may not be able to care for their infant, and they must deal with many psychosocial and economic issues.

Evaluation

Expected outcomes of nursing care include the following:

- The parents are able to bond with their infant and have realistic expectations about the baby.
- Potential opportunistic infections are identified early and treated promptly.
- The parents verbalize their concerns surrounding their baby's existing and potential health problems and accept outside assistance as needed.

Care of the Newborn with Congenital Anomalies

The birth of a baby with a congenital defect places both newborn and family at risk. Many congenital anomalies can be life-threatening if not corrected within hours after

Text continues on page 844.

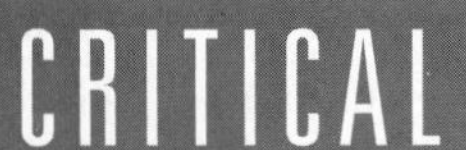

PATHWAY FOR NEWBORN AT RISK FOR HIV/AIDS

Category	Day of Birth—1st 4 Hours	Remainder of Birth Day
Referral	Report from L&D, neonatal nurse practitioner Check ID bands High-risk peds/neonatology/infectious disease consults	Check ID bands q shift As parents desire, obtain circumcision permit after their discussion with physician Lactation consult
Assessments	(See Newborn Critical Pathway, pp. 754 to 755) • Complete set of VS • Admission wt, length, HC • Assess skin color, skin integrity for rashes or skin breakdown • Gestational age assessment • Monitor activity • Maternal hx of drug abuse or needle sharing • Check hx of mother's sexual partner(s) for HIV status as available	Newborn assessment q shift (See Newborn Critical Pathway, pp. 754 to 755) VS: T/P/R q4h and prn, BP prn Assess mother/baby interaction
Teaching/ psychosocial	(See Newborn Critical Pathway, pp. 754 to 755) Admission activities performed at mother's bedside if possible, orient to nursery, handwashing, assess teaching needs Teach mother/parents rationale for Universal Precautions	(See Newborn Critical Pathway, pp. 754 to 755) Reinforce previous teaching Discuss infant security Teach parent/guardian bottle-feeding method, burping, diapering, calming techniques, s/s stress, elimination norms
Nursing care management and reports	Diagnostic Tests: blood type, Rh, Coombs on cord blood when applicable; chemstrip within 1h of birth and per protocol for infant size Baer hearing test Maintain Universal Precautions Bathe ASAP per policy; cord care per policy Hep B form reviewed and/or signed by parent, administer if ordered after bath Peripheral hematocrit per protocol	Check for Baer hearing test results Femoral pulses or BP all 4 extremities if early discharge VS: q4h T/P/R Daily weight Cord care q diaper change (alcohol to cord stump) Assess color q shift and prn
Activity and comfort	Adjust and monitor radiant warmer to maintain skin temp until stable Provide calming techniques: nesting, touch, talking, holding, pacifier	Leave in radiant warmer until stable, then swaddle in open crib Continue calming techniques prn
Nutrition	Initiate bottle-feeding Lavage and gavage prn only Educate mother on rationale for formula feeds to avoid HIV in BM	Continue feeding schedule Evaluate tolerance of formula feedings Encourage demand feedings, minimally q3–4h during day
Elimination	Note first void and stool color	Note all voids, amount and color of stools with diaper changes or q4h
Medication	After initial bath: administer Aquamephyton dosage according to infant weight per MD/NP orders, Ilotycin ophth ointment OU Initiate retroviral prophylaxis per MD/NP orders, ie, Zidovudine	Hep B vaccine after initial bath as ordered by MD/NP and after consent reviewed and signed by parents
Discharge planning/ home care	Evaluate for social services, visiting nurse services, and DC planning needs Plan DC with parent/guardian in 1–3 days	Present birth certificate instructions/worksheet Car seat available for DC Newborn photographs as desired by family
Family involvement	Evaluate parent teaching Access community resources prn, ie, Teen "Healthy Starts" program Encourage/support positive mothering/parenting behaviors with infant	
Date		

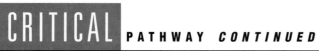

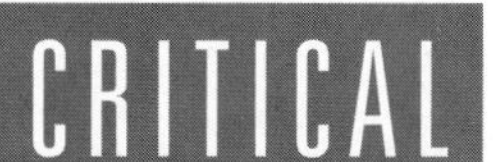 PATHWAY *CONTINUED*

Category	Day 1	Day 2/3 (if applicable)
Referral	Check ID bands when baby leaves nursery	Check ID bands q shift **Expected Outcomes** Mother/baby ID bands correlate at time of DC Consults completed prn
Assessments	Continue newborn assessments q shift: suck, color, resp. status Assess mother/baby interaction VS: q shift and prn, monitor thermoregulation Assess for abdominal distension, gastric residuals	Assess mother/baby interaction Continue newborn assessments, feeding tolerance, wt gain **Expected Outcomes** Physical assessments, VS WNL
Teaching/ psychosocial	Reinforce previous teaching Parental teaching: bathing, cord care, skin/nail care, use of thermometer, activity/sleep patterns, calming activities, reflexes, s/s of jaundice, growth/feeding patterns, circ/uncirc penis care, special nutritional needs, report feeding intolerance Evaluate parental teaching; provide information on cause of AIDS, s/s of HIV in infants, support groups and community resources Provide information on preventing HIV infection	Final Discharge Teaching: (See Newborn Critical Pathway, pp. 754 to 755) Review with parents/guardian infant safety, s/s illness and when to call health care provider **Expected Outcomes** Mother/parents verbalizes comprehension of instructions, demonstrates care capabilities
Nursing care management and reports	Newborn assessment q shift, vital signs q shift and prn Daily wt Circumcision care q diaper change DC cord clamp, alcohol to cord q diaper change HSV culture per parental hx of HSV Femoral pulse or BP all 4 extremities before DC or first 48h Newborn screen Maintain NTE Continue Universal Precautions	Newborn assessment and vital signs q shift Daily wt Cord care, circumcision care q diaper change Note Baer hearing test results **Expected Outcomes** Physical assessments WNL; cord unclamped and dry without s/s infection; circ site unremarkable; gaining wt or stabilized to not >10% loss; labs WNL; no s/s HIV or immune system alteration
Activity and comfort	Swaddled in open crib Incubator if temp instability; adjust incubator for infant size, gestation, layers of clothing to maintain NTE	Swaddle to allow movement of hands to face Hold, talk to infant, rock, provide short periods soft music **Expected Outcomes** Maintains temp WNL swaddled in open crib; attempts self-calming
Nutrition	Encourage small, frequent feedings q3–4h Demand feeding Formula feeding per parent preference or MD/NP orders Gavage feed only as necessary and per MD/NP orders	Continue on demand formula feeding, minimally q3–4h during day Teach mother how to mix/store formula for proper cal/oz **Expected Outcomes** Infant tolerates formula feedings; feeds on demand; nipples without problems; regaining lost wt or wt stabilized before DC
Elimination	Monitor stools for amount, consistency, pattern changes, occult blood, reducing substances Monitor voids q shift	Continue monitoring of all voids and stools q shift, noting changes **Expected Outcomes** Voids qs; stools without difficulty qs; stool character WNL; skin intact at diaper area without s/s rash or breakdown
Medication	Hep B vaccine before DC Continue retroviral prophylaxis; instruct mother/parent on retroviral medication dosing and emphasize importance of continuity	**Expected Outcomes** Infant has received ophth ointment OU, Aquamephyton IM and first Hep B injection if ordered and parental consent received; retroviral prophylactic medication continues; mother/parents verbalize retroviral medication dosing schedule and rationale for medication, can demonstrate ability to dose infant
Discharge planning/ home care	Complete birth certificate packet If vag birth, complete DC teaching Access community referrals, support groups for people who are HIV positive and their families; financial assistance, ie, WIC, public health nursing prn	If cesarean birth, complete DC teaching Complete DC summary (See Newborn Critical Pathway, pp. 754 to 755) **Expected Outcomes** Infant DC home with mother; mother verbalizes follow-up appointment times, dates, referral resources, support resources

➤

CRITICAL PATHWAY FOR NEWBORN AT RISK FOR HIV/AIDS *CONTINUED*

Category	Day 1	Day 2/3 (if applicable)
Family Involvement	Bath and feeding class Newborn channel as available Incorporate significant other/siblings in infant care Support positive parenting behaviors Evaluate mother/parent teaching Teach family essentials of universal precautions; how HIV is contracted	Identify community referral needs and refer to community agencies Evaluate mother/parent teaching Encourage questions **Expected Outcomes** Mother/family demonstrates caring and family incorporation of infant
Date		

birth; others are very visible and cause the families emotional distress. When one congenital anomaly is found, health care providers should look for other ones, particularly in body systems that develop at the same time during gestation. Table 28–3 identifies some of the more common anomalies and their early management and nursing care in the newborn period.

Care of the Newborn with Congenital Heart Defect

The incidence of congenital heart defects is 4 to 5 per 1000 live births. They account for one-third of the deaths caused by congenital defects in the first year of life. Because accurate diagnosis and surgical treatment are now available, many such deaths can be prevented. It is now possible to perform corrective surgery at an earlier age; for example, more than one-half of children undergoing surgery are less than 1 year of age, and one-fourth are less than 1 month old. It is crucial for the nurse to have comprehensive knowledge of congenital heart disease to detect deviations from normal and to initiate interventions.

Overview of Congenital Heart Defects

Factors that might influence development of congenital heart malformations can be classified as environmental or genetic. Infections of the pregnant woman, such as rubella, cytomegalovirus, coxsackie B, and influenza, have been implicated. Thalidomide, steroids, alcohol, lithium, and some anticonvulsants have been shown to cause malformations of the heart. Seasonal spraying of pesticides has also been linked to an increase in congenital heart defects. Clinicians are also beginning to see cardiac defects in infants of mothers with phenylketonuria (PKU) who do not follow their diets. Infants with Down syndrome and trisomy 13/15 and 16/18 frequently have heart lesions. Increased incidence and risk of recurrence of specific defects occur in families.

It is customary to describe congenital malformations of the heart as either *acyanotic* (those that do not present with cyanosis) or *cyanotic* (those that do present with cyanosis). If an opening exists between the right and left sides of the heart, blood will normally flow from the area of greater pressure (left side) to the area of lesser pressure (right side). This process is referred to as left-to-right shunt and does not produce cyanosis because oxygenated blood is being pumped out to the systemic circulation. If pressure in the right side of the heart, due to obstruction of normal flow, exceeds that in the left side, unoxygenated blood will flow from the right side to the left side of the heart and out into the system. This right-to-left shunt causes cyanosis. If the opening is large, there may be a bidirectional shunt with mixing of blood in both sides of the heart, which also produces cyanosis.

The common cardiac defects seen in the first 6 days of life are left ventricular outflow obstructions (mitral stenosis, aortic stenosis, or atresia), hypoplastic left heart, coarctation of the aorta, patent ductus arteriosus (PDA, the most common defect), transposition of the great vessels, tetralogy of Fallot, and large ventricular septal defect or atrial septal defects. Many cardiac defects may not clearly manifest themselves until after discharge from the birthing unit.

NURSING CARE MANAGEMENT

The primary goals of the neonatal nurse are early identification of cardiac defects and initiation of referral to the physician. The three most common manifestations of cardiac defect are cyanosis, detectable heart murmur, and signs of congestive heart failure (tachycardia, tachypnea, diaphoresis, hepatomegaly, and cardiomegaly). Table 28–4 on page 848 presents the clinical manifestations and medical/surgical management of these cardiac defects. Initial repair of heart defects in the newborn period is becoming more commonplace. The staff of NICUs are now more involved in both the preoperative and postoperative care of cardiac newborns. The benefits for the cardiac infant

Text continues on page 847.

TABLE 28–3 Congenital Anomalies: Identification and Care in Newborn Period

Congenital Anomaly	Nursing Assessments	Nursing Goals and Interventions
Congenital hydrocephalus	Enlarged head Enlarged or full fontanelles Split or widened sutures "Setting sun" eyes Head circumference > 90% on growth chart	Assess presence of hydrocephalus: Measure and plot occipital-frontal baseline measurements; then measure head circumference once a day. Check fontanelles for bulging and sutures for widening. Assist with head ultrasound and transillumination. Maintain skin integrity: Change position frequently. Clean skin creases after feeding or vomiting. Use sheepskin pillow under head. Postoperatively, position head off operative site. Watch for signs of infection.
Choanal atresia	Occlusion of posterior nares Cyanosis and retractions at rest Snorting respirations Difficulty breathing during feeding Obstruction by thick mucus	Assess patency of nares: Listen for breath sounds while holding baby's mouth closed and alternately compressing each nostril. Assist with passing feeding tube to confirm diagnosis. Maintain respiratory function: Assist with taping airway in mouth to prevent respiratory distress. Position with head elevated to improve air exchange.
Cleft lip	Unilateral or bilateral visible defect May involve external nares, nasal cartilage, nasal septum, and alveolar process Flattening or depression of midfacial contour 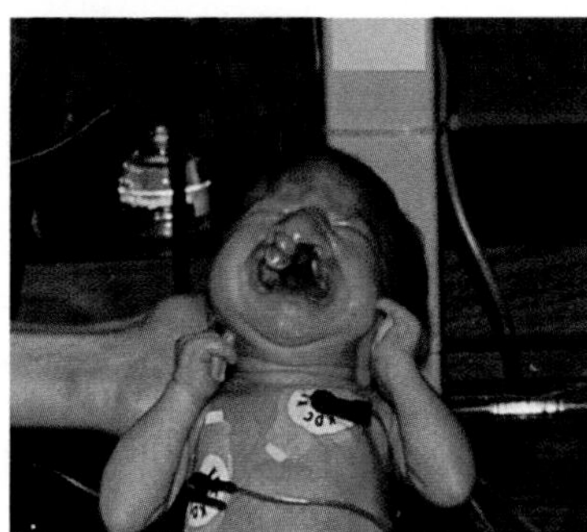	Provide nutrition: Feed with special nipple. Burp frequently (increased tendency to swallow air and reflex vomiting). Clean cleft with sterile water (to prevent crusting on cleft prior to repair). Support parental coping: Assist parents with grief over loss of idealized baby. Encourage verbalization of their feelings about visible defect. Provide role model in interacting with infant. (Parents internalize others' responses to their newborn.) (At left) Unilateral cleft lip with cleft abnormality involving both hard and soft palates.
Cleft palate	Fissure connecting oral and nasal cavity May involve uvula and soft palate May extend forward to nostril involving hard palate and maxillary alveolar ridge Difficulty in sucking Expulsion of formula through nose	Prevent aspiration/infection: Place prone or in side-lying position to facilitate drainage. Suction nasopharyngeal cavity (to prevent aspiration or airway obstruction) During newborn period feed in upright position with head and chest tilted slightly backward (to aid swallowing and discourage aspiration). Provide nutrition: Feed with special nipple that fills cleft and allows sucking. Also decreases chance of aspiration through nasal cavity. Clean mouth with water after feedings. Burp after each ounce (tend to swallow large amounts of air). Thicken formula to provide extra calories. Plot weight gain patterns to assess adequacy of diet. Provide parental support: Refer parents to community agencies and support groups. Encourage verbalization of frustrations because feeding process is long and frustrating. Praise all parental efforts. Encourage parents to seek prompt treatment for upper respiratory infection (URI) and teach them ways to decrease URI.
Tracheoesophageal fistula (type 3)	History of maternal hydramnios Excessive mucous secretions Constant drooling Abdominal distention beginning soon after birth Periodic choking and cyanotic episodes Immediate regurgitation of feeding Clinical symptoms of aspiration pneumonia (tachypnea, retractions, rhonchi, decreased breath sounds, cyanotic spells) Failure to pass nasogastric tube	Maintain respiratory status and prevent aspiration: Withhold feeding until esophageal patency is determined. Quickly assess patency before putting to breast in birth area. Place on low intermittent suction to control saliva and mucus (to prevent aspiration pneumonia). Place in warmed, humidified incubator (liquefies secretions, facilitating removal). Elevate head of bed 20–40 degrees (to prevent reflux of gastric juices). Keep quiet (crying causes air to pass through fistula and to distend intestines, causing respiratory embarrassment). Maintain fluid and electrolyte balance: Give fluids to replace esophageal drainage and maintain hydration. Provide parent education: Explain staged repair—provision of gastrostomy and ligation of fistula, then repair of atresia. Keep parents informed; clarify and reinforce physician's explanations regarding malformation, surgical repair, preoperative and postoperative care, and prognosis (knowledge enhances feelings of self-worth).

➤

Congenital Anomaly	Nursing Assessments	Nursing Goals and Interventions
Tracheoesophageal fistula (type 3) *continued*		Involve parents in care of infant and in planning for future; facilitate touch and eye contact (to dispel feelings of inadequacy, increase self-esteem and self-worth, and promote incorporation of infant into family).
Diaphragmatic hernia	Difficulty initiating respirations Gasping respirations with nasal flaring and chest retraction Barrel chest and scaphoid abdomen Asymmetric chest expansion Breath sounds may be absent Usually on left side Heart sounds displaced to right Spasmodic attacks of cyanosis and difficulty in feeding Bowel sounds may be heard in thoracic cavity	Nurse should never ventilate with bag and mask O_2 because the stomach will inflate, further compressing the lungs. Maintain respiratory status: Immediately administer oxygen. Initiate gastric decompression. Place in high semi-Fowler's position (to use gravity to keep abdominal organs' pressure off diaphragm). Turn to affected side to allow unaffected lung expansion. Carry out interventions to alleviate respiratory and metabolic acidosis. Assess for increased secretions around suction tube (denotes possible obstruction). Aspirate and irrigate tube with air or sterile water.

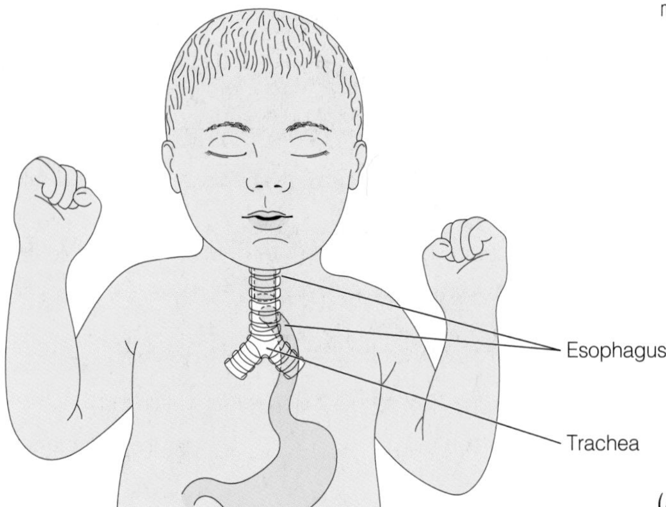

(At left) The most frequently seen type of congenital tracheoesophageal fistula and esophageal atresia.

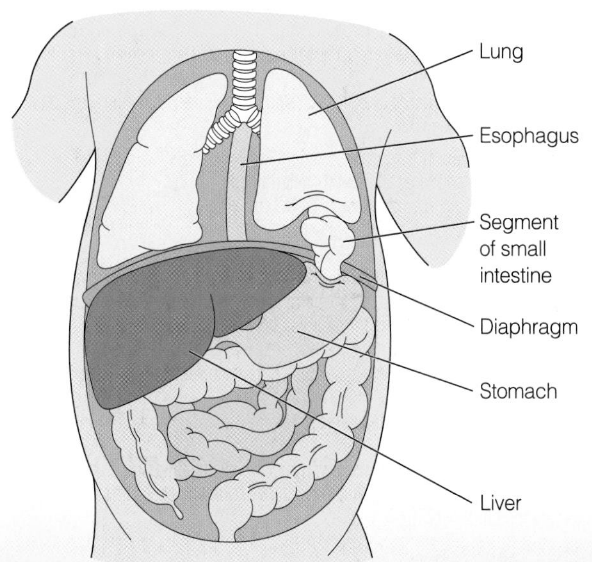

(At left) Diaphragmatic hernia. Note compression of the lung by the intestine on the affected side.

Congenital Anomaly	Nursing Assessments	Nursing Goals and Interventions
Myelomeningocele	Saclike cyst containing meninges, spinal cord, and nerve roots in thoracic and/or lumbar area Myelomeningocele directly connects to subarachnoid space so hydrocephalus often associated No response or varying response to sensation below level of sac May have constant dribbling of urine Incontinence or retention of stool Anal opening may be flaccid	Prevent trauma and infection. Position on abdomen or on side and restrain (to prevent pressure and trauma to sac). Meticulously clean buttocks and genitals after each voiding and defecation (to prevent contamination of sac and decrease possibility of infection). May put protective covering over sac (to prevent rupture and drying). Observe sac for oozing of fluid or pus. Credé bladder (apply downward pressure on bladder with thumbs, moving urine toward the urethra) as ordered to prevent urinary stasis. Assess amount of sensation and movement below defect. Observe for complications: Obtain occipital-frontal circumference baseline measurements; then measure head circumference once a day (to detect hydrocephalus). Check fontanelle for bulging.
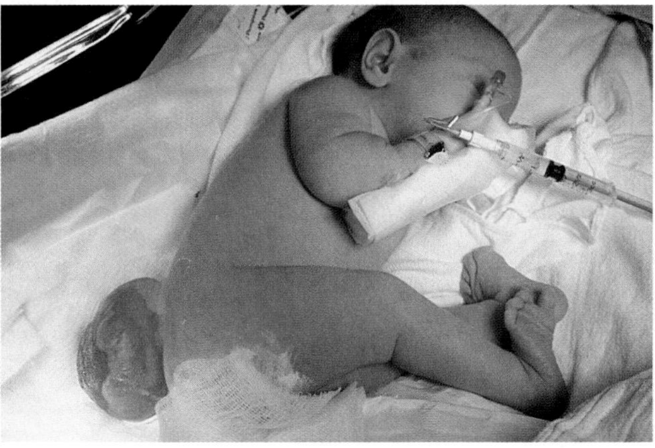		(At left) Newborn with lumbar myelomeningocele. SOURCE: Courtesy Dr Paul Winchester.
Omphalocele	Herniation of abdominal contents into base of umbilical cord May have an enclosed transparent sac covering	Maintain hydration and temperature: Provide D_5LR and albumin for hypovolemia. Place infant in sterile bag up to and covering defect. Cover sac with moistened sterile gauze, and place plastic wrap over dressing (to prevent rupture of sac and infection). Initiate gastric decompression by insertion of nasogastric tube attached to low suction (to prevent distention of lower bowel and impairment of blood flow). Prevent infection and trauma to defect. Position to prevent trauma to defect. Administer broad-spectrum antibiotics.
Gastroschisis	Lateral defect in abdominal wall allowing viscera outside the body to the left of an intact umbilical cord. No sac covering. Associated with intestinal atresia, malrotation	Maintain hydration and temperature. Prevent trauma and infection to defect. Provide D_5LR and albumin for hypovolemia. Place infant in sterile bag up to cord and covering defect. Initiate gastric decompression by insertion of nasogastric tube attached to low suction. Administer broad-spectrum antibiotics.
Imperforate anus, congenital dislocated hip, and clubfoot	See discussion in Chapter 25, Anus and Extremities	Identify defect and initiate appropriate referral early.

of being cared for by NICU staff include the staff's knowledge of neonatal anatomy and physiology, experience in supporting the family, and an awareness of the developmental needs of the newborn (Buckley & Friend, 1997).

After the baby is stabilized, decisions are made about the special ongoing care needs. The parents need careful and complete explanations and the opportunity to take part in decision making. They also require ongoing emotional support. Families of any baby born with a congenital abnormality need genetic counseling regarding future conception. Parents need opportunities to verbalize their concern about their baby's health maintenance and understand the rationale for follow-up care.

Care of the Newborn with Inborn Errors of Metabolism

Inborn errors of metabolism are a group of hereditary disorders that are transmitted by mutant genes. Each

Text continues on page 850.

TABLE 28–4 Cardiac Defects of the Early Newborn Period

Congenital Heart Defect	Clinical Findings	Medical/Surgical Management
Acyanotic		
Patent ductus arteriosus (PDA) ↑ in females, maternal rubella, RDS, <1500 g preterm newborns, high-altitude births 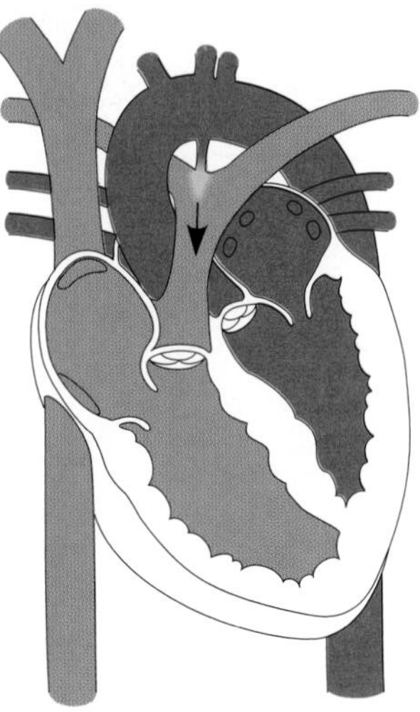	Harsh grade 2–3 machinery murmur upper left sternal border (LSB) just beneath clavicle ↑ difference between systolic and diastolic pulse pressure Can lead to right heart failure and pulmonary congestion ↑ left atrial (LA) and left ventricular (LV) enlargement, dilated ascending aorta ↑ pulmonary vascularity The patent ductus arteriosus is a vascular connection that, during fetal life, short-circuits the pulmonary vascular bed and directs blood from the pulmonary artery to the aorta. Postnatally, blood shunts through the ductus from the aorta to the pulmonary artery.	Indomethacin—0.2 mg/kg orally (prostaglandin inhibitor) Surgical ligation Use of O_2 therapy and blood transfusion to improve tissue oxygenation and perfusion Fluid restriction and diuretics
Atrial septal defect (ASD) ↑ in females and Down syndrome	Initially frequently asymptomatic Systolic murmur second left intercostal space (LICS) With large ASD, diastolic rumbling murmur lower left sternal (LLS) border Failure to thrive, upper respiratory infection (URI), poor exercise tolerance	Surgical closure with patch or suture
Ventricular septal defect (VSD) ↑ in males	Initially asymptomatic until end of first month or large enough to cause pulmonary edema Loud, blowing systolic murmur between the third and fourth intercostal space (ICS) pulmonary blood flow Right ventricular hypertrophy Rapid respirations, growth failure, feeding difficulties Congestive right heart failure at 6 weeks–2 months of age	Follow medically—some spontaneously close Use of lanoxin and diuretics in congestive heart failure (CHF) Surgical closure with Dacron patch
Coarctation of aorta Can be preductal or postductal 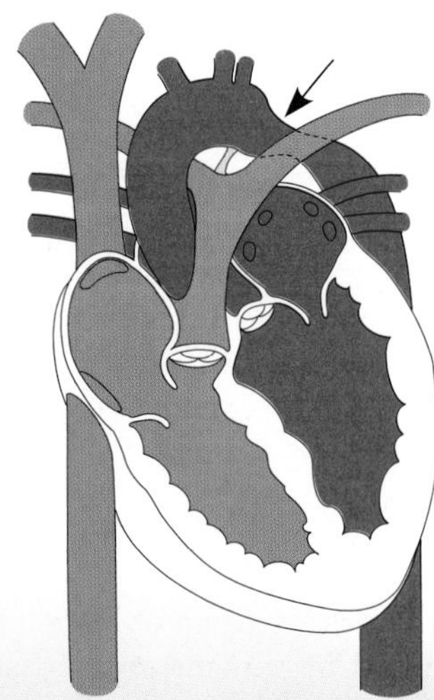	Absent or diminished femoral pulses Increased brachial pulses Late systolic murmur left intrascapular area Systolic BP in lower extremities Enlarged left ventricle Can present in CHF at 7–21 days of life Coarctation of the aorta is characterized by a narrowed aortic lumen. The lesion produces an obstruction to the flow of blood through the aorta, causing an increased left ventricular pressure and work load.	Surgical resection of narrowed portion of aorta

Congenital Heart Defect	Clinical Findings	Medical/Surgical Management
Hypoplastic left heart syndrome	Normal at birth—cyanosis and shocklike congestive heart failure develop within a few hours to days Soft systolic murmur just left of the sternum Diminished pulses Aortic and/or mitral atresia Tiny, thick-walled left ventricle Large, dilated, hypertrophied right ventricle X-ray examination: cardiac enlargement and pulmonary venous congestion	Currently no effective corrective treatment
Cyanotic		
Tetralogy of Fallot (Most common cyanotic heart defect) Pulmonary stenosis Ventricular septal defect (VSD) Overriding aorta Right ventricular hypertrophy	May be cyanotic at birth or within first few months of life Harsh systolic murmur LSB Crying or feeding increases cyanosis and respiratory distress X-ray: boot-shaped appearance secondary to small pulmonary artery Right ventricular enlargement	Prevention of dehydration, intercurrent infections Alleviation of paroxysmal dyspneic attacks Palliative surgery to increase blood flow to the lungs Corrective surgery—resection of pulmonic stenosis, closure of VSD with Dacron patch

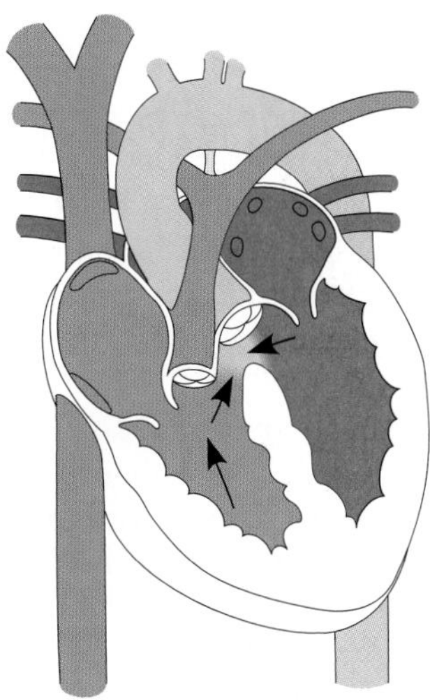

In tetralogy of Fallot, the severity of symptoms depends on the degree of pulmonary stenosis, the size of the ventricular septal defect, and the degree to which the aorta overrides the septal defect.

Congenital Heart Defect	Clinical Findings	Medical/Surgical Management
Transposition of great vessels (TGA) (↑ females, IDMs, LGAs)	Cyanosis at birth or within 3 days Possible pulmonic stenosis murmur Right ventricular hypertrophy Polycythemia "Egg on its side" x-ray finding	Prostaglandin E to vasodilate ductus to keep it open Initial surgery to create opening between right and left side of heart if none exists Total surgical repair—usually the arterial switch procedure

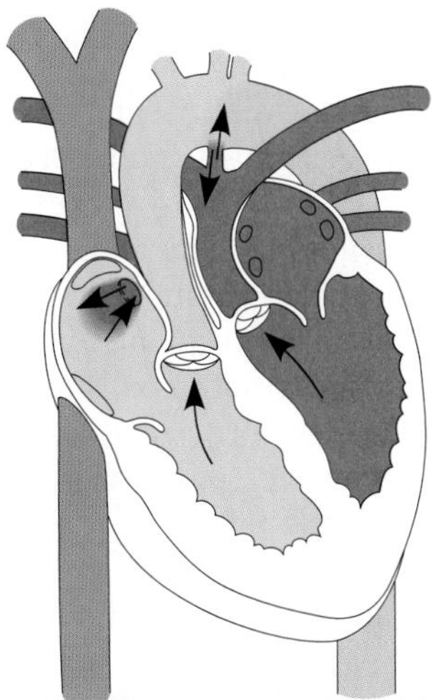

Complete transposition of great vessels is an embryologic defect caused by a straight division of the bulbar trunk without normal spiraling. As a result, the aorta originates from the right ventricle, and the pulmonary artery from the left ventricle. An abnormal communication between the two circulations must be present to sustain life.

SOURCE: All illustrations from *Congenital Heart Abnormalities.* Clinical Education Aid no 7, Ross Laboratories, Columbus, OH.

causes an enzyme defect that blocks a metabolic pathway and leads to an accumulation of toxic metabolites. Most of the disorders are transmitted by an autosomal recessive gene, requiring two heterozygous parents to produce a homozygous infant with the disorder. Heterozygous parents carrying some inborn errors of metabolism disorders can be identified by special tests, and some inborn errors of metabolism can be detected and treated in utero.

Many inborn errors of metabolism are now detected neonatally through newborn screening programs. These programs test principally for disorders associated with mental retardation.

Phenylketonuria (PKU) is the most common of the group of metabolic errors known as amino acid disorders. Newborn screenings have set its incidence at about 1 in 12,000 live births worldwide and 1 in 10,000 to 25,000 live births in the United States; however, the incidence varies considerably among ethnic groups (American Academy of Pediatrics Committee on Genetics, 1996). The highest incidence is noted in white populations from northern Europe and the United States. It is rarely observed in people of African, Jewish, or Japanese descent.

Phenylalanine is an essential amino acid used by the body for growth, and in the normal individual any excess is converted to tyrosine. The newborn with PKU lacks this converting ability, which results in an accumulation of phenylalanine in the blood. Phenylalanine produces two abnormal metabolites, phenylpyruvic acid and phenylacetic acid, which are eliminated in the urine, producing a musty odor. Excessive accumulation of phenylalanine and its abnormal metabolites in the brain tissue leads to progressive mental retardation.

Maple syrup urine disease (MSUD) is an inborn error of metabolism that, when untreated, is a rapidly progressing and often fatal disease caused by an enzymatic defect in the metabolism of the branched chain amino acids leucine, isoleucine, and valine.

Homocystinuria is a disorder caused by a deficiency of the enzyme cystathionine B synthase, which blocks the normal conversion of methionine to cystine.

Galactosemia is an inborn error of carbohydrate metabolism in which the body is unable to use the sugars galactose and lactose. Enzyme pathways in liver cells normally convert galactose and lactose to glucose. In galactosemia, one step in that conversion pathway is absent, either because of the lack of the enzyme galactose 1-phosphate uridyl transferase or because of the lack of the enzyme galactokinase. High levels of unusable galactose circulate in the blood, causing cataracts, brain damage, and liver damage (American Academy of Pediatrics Committee on Genetics, 1996).

Another disorder frequently included in mandatory newborn blood screening tests is *congenital hypothyroidism.* An inborn enzymatic defect, lack of maternal dietary iodine, or maternal ingestion of drugs that depress or destroy thyroid tissue can cause congenital hypothyroidism.

The incidence of metabolic errors is relatively low, but for affected infants and their families these disorders pose a threat to survival and frequently require lifelong treatment.

NURSING CARE MANAGEMENT

Nursing Assessment and Diagnosis

The clinical picture of a PKU baby involves a normal-appearing newborn, most often with blond hair, blue eyes, and fair complexion. Decreased pigmentation may be related to the competition between phenylalanine and tyrosine for the available enzyme tyrosinase. Tyrosine is needed for the formation of melanin pigment and the hormones epinephrine and thyroxin. Without treatment, the infant fails to thrive and develops vomiting and eczematous rashes. By about 6 months of age, the infant exhibits behavior indicative of mental retardation and other CNS involvement, including seizures and abnormal electroencephalogram (EEG) patterns.

Newborns with MSUD have feeding problems and neurologic signs (seizures, spasticity, opisthotonos) during the first week of life. A maple syrup odor of the urine is noted, and when ferric chloride is added to the urine, its color changes to gray-green.

Homocystinuria varies in its presentation, but the more common characteristics are skeletal abnormalities, dislocation of ocular lenses, intravascular thromboses, and mental retardation. Abnormalities occur because of the toxic effects of the accumulation of methionine and the metabolite homocystine in the blood.

Clinical manifestations of galactosemia include vomiting soon after ingestion of milk-based formula or breast milk, diarrhea, failure to thrive (Chung, 1997), hepatosplenomegaly, jaundice, and mental retardation. The condition is frequently associated with anemia, sepsis, and cataracts in the newborn period. Except for cataracts and mental retardation, those findings are reversible when galactose is excluded from the diet. Mental retardation can be prevented by early diagnosis and careful dietary management.

A large tongue, umbilical hernia, cool and mottled skin, low hairline, hypotonia, and large fontanelles (especially the posterior fontanelle in term infants) are frequently associated with congenital hypothyroidism. Early symptoms include prolonged newborn jaundice, poor feeding, constipation, low-pitched cry, poor weight gain, inactivity, and delayed motor development.

Nursing diagnoses that may apply to the newborn with an inborn error of metabolism include the following:

- ***Knowledge Deficit*** related to parental lack of information about appropriate weight gain and nutritional status due to need for special dietary management required for inborn errors of metabolism

- ***Ineffective Family Coping: Compromised*** related to parental guilt secondary to hereditary nature of disease

Nursing Plan and Implementation

Hospital-Based Nursing Care

All states have universal screening of newborns for phenylketonuria (PKU) and congenital hypothyroidism (CH) (Stoddard & Farrell, 1997). Mandatory newborn screening for other inborn errors of metabolism varies among states. Some states simultaneously test all hospitalized newborns for MSUB, homocystinuria, and PKU during the first 3 to 4 days of life. Identification via newborn screening and early clinical intervention for inborn errors of metabolism have become more difficult with the advent of early discharge of newborns. If the initial specimen is obtained before 24 hours of age, then a second specimen should be obtained at 1 to 2 weeks of age (American Academy of Pediatrics [AAP] and American College of Obstetricians and Gynecologists [ACOG], 1997). It is important to recognize that newborns in NICU who required interhospital transfers and early discharged healthy newborns are at risk for nonscreening (Gray, Sorrentino, Matheson, Wise, & McCormick, 1997). The first filter paper test screens for PKU, homocystinuria, MSUD, galactosemia, and sickle cell anemia. A second blood specimen is often required, but the nurse must remember that this second blood specimen tests only for PKU.

In most states, the Guthrie blood test for PKU is required for all newborns before discharge. The Guthrie test uses a drop of blood collected from a heel stick and placed on filter paper. The Guthrie test should be done at least 24 hours, but preferably 72 hours, after the initiation of feedings containing the usual amounts of breast milk or formula. Phenylalanine is found in milk, so its metabolites begin to build up in the baby with PKU once milk feedings are initiated. Because it is possible to do the testing on an infant with PKU before the phenylalanine concentration rises and thus miss the diagnosis, some states routinely request a repeat test at 10 to 14 days (Sinai, Kim, Casey, & Pinto-Martin, 1995). When the Guthrie blood test is performed early, during the first 3 to 4 days of life, a phenylalanine blood level of about 4 to 6 mg/dL is considered a presumptive positive; but only 1 in 20 to 30 infants with this level is a true positive (Seashore & Rinaldo, 1993).

High-risk newborns should be receiving a 60% milk intake, with no more than 40% of their total intake coming from nonprotein intravenous fluids. The PKU testing of high-risk newborns should be deferred for at least 48 hours after hyperalimentation is initiated. It is vital that the parents understand the need for the screening procedure, and a follow-up check is necessary to confirm that the test was done.

Community-Based Nursing Care

Some clinicians have the parents perform a diaper test for PKU. At about 6 weeks of age, the parent takes a freshly wet diaper and presses the prepared test stick against the wet area. The parent notes the color of the test stick, records the color on the prepared sheet, and mails the form back to the physician. A green color reaction is positive and indicates probable PKU.

Treatment involves stringent restrictions of phenylalanine intake. Once identified, an afflicted PKU infant can be treated by a special diet that limits ingestion of phenylalanine. Special formulas low in phenylalanine, such as Lofenalac, Phenyl-Free, PKU1, and PKU2 are available. Special food lists are helpful for parents of a PKU child (Bowe, 1995). If treatment is begun before 3 months of age, CNS damage can be minimized. Most centers now recommend keeping blood phenylalanine levels below 15 mg/dL, or even 10mg/dL, for life. There is a 95% risk of producing a child with mental retardation if the mother with PKU is not on a low-phenylalanine diet during pregnancy. It is recommended that the woman reinstate her low-phenylalanine diet a few months before becoming pregnant (Acosta, 1995).

Diagnosis of MSUD is made by analyzing blood levels of leucine, isoleucine, and valine. Confirmation of the diagnosis depends on blood assay for the enzyme oxidative decarboxylase. Dietary management of MSUD must be initiated immediately with a formula that is low in the branched-chain amino acids leucine, isoleucine, and valine and must be continued indefinitely. Dietary treatment prior to 12 days of life has been reported to result in normal intelligence (American Academy of Pediatrics Committee on Genetics, 1996).

In several states, newborn screening includes an enzyme assay for galactose 1-phosphate uridyl transferase; this test, however, does not detect galactosemia if it is caused by a deficiency of the enzyme galactokinase. There appear to be ethnic differences in age of onset of symptoms and in severity of course. Caucasians have more severe symptoms and earlier onset (3 to 14 days) than people of African descent (14 to 28 days) (Wright, Brown, & Davidson-Mundt, 1992). Treatment involves a galactose-free diet. Galactose-free formulas include Nutramigen (a protein hydrolysate process formula), meat-based formulas, or soybean formulas. As the infant grows, parents must be educated not only to avoid giving their child milk and milk products but also to read all labels carefully and avoid any foods containing dry milk products. Even with early treatment, children may have learning disabilities, speech problems, and female ovarian failure (Chung, 1997).

For hypothyroidism, immediate and appropriate thyroid replacement therapy is established based on newborn screening and laboratory data. Frequently, premature infants of less than 30 weeks' gestation have low T_4 or thyroid-stimulating hormone (TSH) values when compared with normal values of term infants. This may

RESEARCH IN PRACTICE

What is the study about? Transition and progression of the premature infant to full nipple feedings is often used as a criterion of the infant's readiness for discharge. For the preterm infant to establish full nipple feedings to maintain nutritional needs requires learning on the infant's part. The length of transition also has social and economic implications for the family. The purpose of this descriptive study was to: (1) explore the contribution of history, environment, and infant factors on the initiation and achievement of full nipple feedings (transition time) for premature infants with a history of lung disease; (2) examine historical difference (from 1983–1995) in care and their contribution to environmental and infant factors that affect transition time; and (3) compare transition times and their relationship to infant and environmental factors of infants with respiratory distress syndrome (RDS) and bronchopulmonary dysplasia (BPD).

How was the study done? A retrospective chart review of all hospital records of infants ≤32 weeks and appropriate for gestational age was conducted. Ninety-two infant charts (46 infants with BPD and 36 infants with RDS) served as the sample. Data were collected on three factors: (1) infant (birthweight, gender, type length of experience being breastfed or nasogastric or orogastric fed, indices of maturity [apnea of prematurity, weight on the first day of nipple feeding, estimation of postconceptual age (PCA) at initiation of nipple feeding], and severity of lung disease), (2) environmental (the type of NICU caring for the infant), and (3) historical (years between 1983 and 1995 and the onset of use of surfactant for treatment of severe lung disease).

What were the results of the study? All three variables—infant, environment, and history—contributed significantly to shortening or lengthening transition time to full nippling. The number of days on tube feedings significantly lengthened transition time, the order of the PCA at the time of initiation of nipple feeds shortened the transition time, and the diagnosis of BPD over the early 1980s and late 1990s eras significantly lengthened and shortened transition time respectively.

What additional questions might I have? (1) What contribution might the type of caregiver (nurse versus parent) have on transition time to full nippling and (2) Why do many units still use weight as the ultimate criteria for initiation of nipple feedings of infants?

How can I use this study? This study reveals the importance of environmental and historical variables on the transition time of infants with lung disease to full nipple feedings. The infant factors of PCA, apnea incidents, birthweight, and days of tube feeding also play a role in the transition time. Nurses play a significant role in assessing the readiness of infants to begin nipple feedings and this study provides some interesting variables that may decrease the transition time for infants with lung disease.

SOURCE: Pridham, K., Brown, R., Sondel, S., Green, C., Wedel, N., & Lai, H-C (1998). Transition time to full nipple feeding for premature infants with a history of lung disease. *JOGNN, 27*(5), 533–545.

reflect the premature infant's inability to bind thyroid. Management includes frequent laboratory monitoring and adjustment of thyroid medication to accommodate growth and development of the infant. With adequate treatment, children remain free of symptoms, but if the condition is untreated, stunted growth and mental retardation occur.

Infants with homocystinuria are managed on a diet that is low in methionine but supplemented with cystine and pyridoxine (vitamin B_6). Early diagnosis and careful management may prevent mental retardation.

Parents of affected newborns should be referred to support groups. The nurse should also ensure that parents are informed about centers that can provide them with information about biochemical genetics and dietary management.

Evaluation

Expected outcomes of nursing care include the following:

- The risk of inborn errors of metabolism is promptly identified, and early intervention is initiated.
- The parents verbalize their concerns about their baby's nutritional status, health problems, long-term care needs, and potential outcomes.
- The parents are aware of available community health resources and use them as indicated.

Care of the Family of the At-Risk Newborn

The birth of a preterm or ill infant or an infant with a congenital anomaly is a serious crisis situation for a family. Acute grief reactions follow the loss of the perfect baby they have fantasized. In the case of a preterm birth, the mother is denied the last few weeks of pregnancy that seem to prepare her psychologically for the stress of birth and the attachment process. Attachment at this time is fragile, and interruption of the process by separation can affect the future mother-child relationship.

Feelings of guilt and failure often plague mothers of preterm newborns. They may ask themselves, "Why did labor start? What did I do (or not do)?" A woman may have guilt fantasies and wonder what they may have done to cause the early labor: "Was it because I carried three loads of wash up from the basement?" "Am I being punished for something I did in the past—even in childhood?"

The birth of the newborn with an illness or congenital abnormalities also engenders feelings of guilt and failure. As in the birth of a preterm infant, the woman may entertain ideas of personal guilt: "What did I do (or not do) to cause this?" "Am I being punished for something?"

Parental reactions and steps of attachment are altered by the birth of a preterm infant or one with an illness or a congenital anomaly. A variety of new feelings, reactions, and stresses must be recognized and dealt with before the family can work toward establishing a healthy parent-infant relationship.

Although reactions and steps of attachment are altered by the birth of these infants, a healthy parent-child relationship can occur. Kaplan and Mason (1974) have identified four psychologic tasks as essential for coping with the stress of an at-risk newborn and for providing a basis for the maternal-infant relationship:

1. Anticipatory grief as a psychologic preparation for possible loss of the child while still hoping for his or her survival.
2. Acknowledgement of maternal failure to produce a term or perfect newborn expressed as anticipatory grief and depression and lasting until the chances of survival seem secure.
3. Resumption of the process of relating to the infant, which was interrupted by the threat of nonsurvival. This task may be impaired by a continuous threat of death or abnormality, and the mother may be slow in her response of hope for the infant's survival.
4. Understanding of the special needs and growth patterns of the at-risk newborn, which are temporary and yield to normal patterns.

Most authorities agree that the birth of a preterm infant or a less-than-perfect infant does require major adjustments as the parents are forced to surrender the image of the ideal child they had nurtured for so long.

Solnit and Stark (1961) postulate that grief and mourning of the loss of the loved object—the idealized child—mark parental reactions to an infant with abnormalities. The parents must grieve the loss of the valued object—their wished-for perfect child. Simultaneously, they must adopt the imperfect child as the new love object. Parental responses to an infant with health problems may also be viewed as a five-stage process (Klaus & Kennell, 1982):

1. *Shock* is felt at the reality of the birth of this baby. This stage may be characterized by forgetfulness, amnesia of the situation, and a feeling of desperation.
2. There is *denial* (disbelief) of the reality that the child is defective. This stage is exemplified by assertions such as, "It didn't really happen!" "There has been a mistake; it's someone else's baby."
3. *Depression* over the reality of the situation and a corresponding grief reaction follows acceptance of the situation. This stage is characterized by much crying and sadness. Anger about the reality of the situation may also occur at this stage. A projection of blame on others or on self and feelings of "why me?" are characteristic of this stage.
4. *Equilibrium and acceptance* are characteristic of a decrease in the emotional reactions of the parents. This stage is variable and may be prolonged because of continuing threat to the infant's survival. Some parents experience chronic sorrow in relation to their child.
5. *Reorganization* of the family is necessary to deal with the child's problems. Mutual support of the parents facilitates this process, but the crisis of the situation may precipitate alienation between the mother and father.

In the birth of an infant with an anomaly or illness or a preterm infant, the mourning process is necessary for attachment to the less-than-perfect baby. **Grief work,** the emotional reaction to significant loss, must occur before adequate attachment to the actual baby is possible. Parental detachment precedes parental attachment.

NURSING CARE MANAGEMENT

Nursing Assessment and Diagnosis

Development of a nurse-family relationship facilitates information gathering in areas of concern. A concurrent illness of the mother or other family members or other concurrent stress (lack of hospitalization insurance, loss of job, age of parents) may alter the family response to the baby. Feelings of apprehension, guilt, failure, and grief that are verbally or nonverbally expressed are important aspects of the nursing history. These observations enable all professionals to be aware of the parental state, coping behaviors, and readiness for attachment, bonding, and caretaking. Appropriate nursing observations while interviewing and relating to the family may include:

1. *Level of understanding.* Observations concerning the family's ability to assimilate information given and to ask appropriate questions; the need for constant repetition of "the same" information
2. *Behavioral responses.* Appropriateness of behavior in relation to information given; lack of response; "flat" affect
3. *Difficulties with communication.* Deafness (reads lips only); blindness; dysphasia; understanding only a foreign language
4. *Paternal and maternal education level.* For example: parents unable to read or write; only eighth grade completed; mother an MD, RN, or PhD; and so on

Documentation of such information, obtained by the nurse through continuing contact and development of a therapeutic family relationship, enables all professionals to understand and use the nursing history in providing continuous individual care.

Visiting and caregiving patterns indicate the level or lack of parental attachment. A record of visits, caretaking procedures, affect (in relating to the newborn), and telephone calls from parents is essential. Serial observations, rather than just isolated instances of concern, must be obtained. Grant (1978) has developed a conceptual framework depicting adaptive and maladaptive responses to parenting of a preterm or less-than-perfect infant (Figure 28–13).

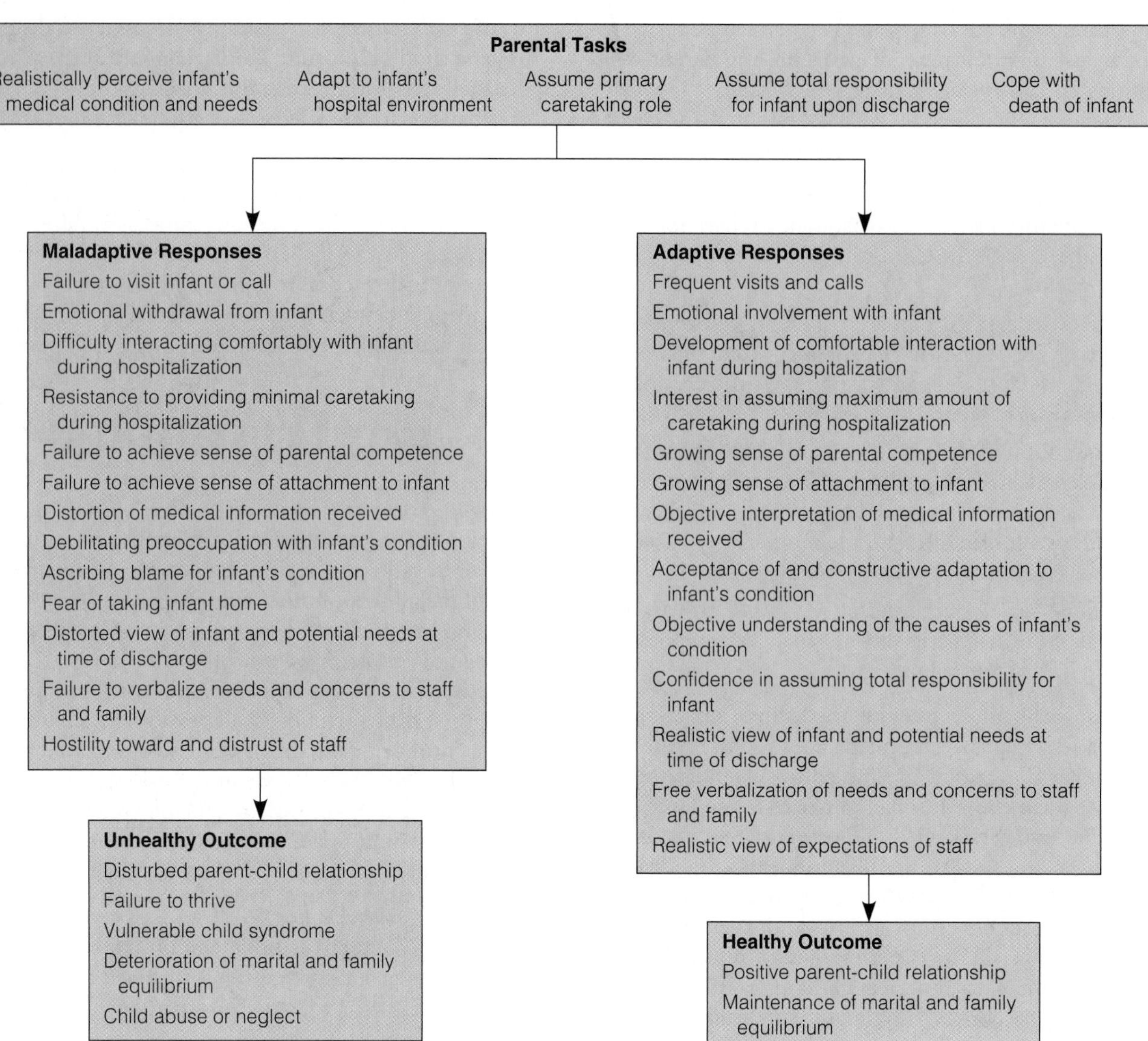

Parental Tasks
Realistically perceive infant's medical condition and needs
Adapt to infant's hospital environment
Assume primary caretaking role
Assume total responsibility for infant upon discharge
Cope with death of infant
Maladaptive Responses
Failure to visit infant or call
Emotional withdrawal from infant
Difficulty interacting comfortably with infant during hospitalization
Resistance to providing minimal caretaking during hospitalization
Failure to achieve sense of parental competence
Failure to achieve sense of attachment to infant
Distortion of medical information received
Debilitating preoccupation with infant's condition
Ascribing blame for infant's condition
Fear of taking infant home
Distorted view of infant and potential needs at time of discharge
Failure to verbalize needs and concerns to staff and family
Hostility toward and distrust of staff
Unhealthy Outcome
Disturbed parent-child relationship
Failure to thrive
Vulnerable child syndrome
Deterioration of marital and family equilibrium
Child abuse or neglect
Adaptive Responses
Frequent visits and calls
Emotional involvement with infant
Development of comfortable interaction with infant during hospitalization
Interest in assuming maximum amount of caretaking during hospitalization
Growing sense of parental competence
Growing sense of attachment to infant
Objective interpretation of medical information received
Acceptance of and constructive adaptation to infant's condition
Objective understanding of the causes of infant's condition
Confidence in assuming total responsibility for infant
Realistic view of infant and potential needs at time of discharge
Free verbalization of needs and concerns to staff and family
Realistic view of expectations of staff
Healthy Outcome
Positive parent-child relationship
Maintenance of marital and family equilibrium

FIGURE 28–13 Maladaptive and adaptive parental responses during crisis period, showing unhealthy and healthy outcomes. SOURCE: Grant P: Psychological needs of families of high-risk infants. *Fam Commun Health* 1978; 11:93. By permission of Aspen Systems Corporation.

If a pattern of distancing behaviors evolves, the nurse should institute appropriate intervention. Follow-up studies have found that a statistically significant number of preterm, sick, and congenitally defective infants suffers from failure to thrive, battering, or other disorders of parenting. Early detection and intervention may prevent these aberrations in parenting behaviors from leading to irreparable damage or death.

Nursing diagnoses that may apply to the family of a newborn at risk include the following:

- ***Dysfunctional Grieving*** related to loss of idealized newborn
- ***Fear*** related to emotional involvement with an at-risk newborn
- ***Altered Parenting*** related to impaired bonding secondary to feelings of inadequacy about caretaking activities

Nursing Plan and Implementation

Hospital-Based Nursing Care

Support of Parents in Initial Viewing of the Newborn Before parents see their child, the nurse must prepare them for the visit. It is important that a positive, realistic attitude regarding the infant, rather than a pessimistic one, be presented to the parents. An overly negative, fatalistic attitude further alienates the parents from their infant and retards attachment behaviors. In this case, instead of allowing attachment and bonding to develop, the mother will begin the process of grieving for the loss of her infant. Once started, this process is very difficult to reverse.

In preparing parents for the first view of their infant, the professional should have already looked at the baby. The nurse should prepare the parents to see both the deviations and the normal aspects of their infant. All infants exhibit strengths as well as deficiencies. The nurse may say, "Your baby is small, about the length of my two hands. She weighs 2 lb 3 oz but is very active and cries when we disturb her. She is having some difficulty breathing but is breathing without assistance and on only 35% oxygen."

The equipment being used for the at-risk newborn and its purpose should be described before the parents enter the intensive care unit. Many NICUs have booklets for parents to read before entering the unit. Through explanations and pictures, the parents can be better prepared to deal with the feelings they may experience when they see their infant for the first time.

On entering the unit, parents may be overwhelmed by the sounds of monitors, alarms, and respirators, as well as by the unfamiliar language and "foreign" atmosphere. Preparing the parents by having the same health care professional(s) accompany them to the unit can be reassuring. The primary nurse and physician caring for the newborn should be with the parents when they first visit the baby. Parental reactions vary, but there is usually an element of initial shock. Providing them with chairs and time to regain composure will assist the parents. Slow, complete, and simple explanations—first about the infant and then about the equipment—allay fear and anxiety.

As parents attempt to deal with the initial stages of shock and grief, they may fail to grasp new information. The parents may need repeated explanations in order to accept the reality of the situation, procedures, equipment, and the infant's condition on subsequent visits.

Concern about the infant's physical appearance is common yet may remain unvoiced. Parents may express such concerns as, "He looks so small and red—like a drowned rat." "Why do her genitals look so abnormal?" "Will that awful looking mouth [cleft lip and palate] ever be normal?" Such questions need to be anticipated by the nurse and addressed. Use of pictures, such as of an infant after cleft lip repair, may be reassuring to doubting parents. Knowledge of the development of a "normal" preterm infant will allow the nurse to make reassuring statements such as "The baby's skin may look very red and transparent with lots of visible veins, but it is normal for her maturity. As she grows, subcutaneous fat will be laid down, and these superficial veins will begin to disappear. Your baby's normal for her level of maturity."

The tone of the neonatal intensive care unit is set by the nursing staff. Development of a safe, trusting environment depends on viewing the parents as essential caregivers, not as visitors or nuisances in the unit. Providing parents privacy when needed and easy access to staff and facilities are important in developing an open, comfortable environment. An uncrowded and welcoming atmosphere lets parents know, "You are welcome here." However, even in crowded physical surroundings an attitude of openness and trust can be conveyed by the nursing staff.

A trusting relationship is essential for collaborative efforts in caring for the infant. Nurses must therapeutically use their own responses to relate on a one-to-one basis with the parents. Each individual has different needs, different ways of adapting to crisis, and different means of support. Professionals must use techniques that are real and spontaneous to them and avoid adopting words or actions that are foreign to them. Nurses must also gauge their interventions to match the parents' pace and needs.

Facilitation of Attachment If Neonatal Transport Occurs In the event that a small hospital may not be able to care for a sick infant, transport to a regional referral center may be necessary. These centers may be as far as 500 miles from the parents' community; it is therefore essential that the mother see and touch her infant before the infant is transported.

Bringing the mother to the nursery or taking the infant in a warmed transport incubator to the mother's bedside will allow her to see the infant before transportation to the center. When the infant reaches the referral center, a staff member should call the parents with information about the infant's condition during transport, safe arrival at the center, and present condition.

Support of parents, with explanations from the professional staff, is crucial. Occasionally, the mother may be unable to see the infant prior to transport, for example, if she is still under general anesthesia or experiencing postpartum complications. In these cases, the infant should be photographed before transport. The picture should be given to the mother, along with an explanation of the infant's condition, present problems, and a detailed description of the infant's characteristics, to facilitate the attachment process until the mother can visit. An additional photograph is also helpful for the father to share with siblings or the extended family. With the increased attention to improved fetal outcome, prenatal maternal transports, rather than neonatal transports, are occurring more frequently. This practice gives the mother of an at-risk infant the opportunity to visit and care for her infant during the early postpartal period.

Promotion of Touching and Parental Caretaking Parents visiting a small or sick infant may need several visits to become comfortable and confident in their abilities to touch the infant without injuring her or him. Barriers such as incubators, incisions, monitor electrodes, and tubes may delay the mother's confidence. Knowledge of this "normal" delay in touching behavior will enable the nurse to understand parental behavior.

Klaus and Kennell (1982) found a significant difference in the amount of eye contact and touching behaviors

STAGE I: Touching
Uses fingertips
Uses whole hand
Strokes child
Holds and studies child "en face"
Spontaneously lowers crib rails to fondle, hold, or talk to child

↓

STAGE II: Caretaking
Provides clean clothing, toys, grooming aids
Performs activities of daily living (bathing, diapering, feeding, dressing)
Performs caretaking tasks with proficiency and expresses pleasure in meeting infant's needs
Able to comfort child when distressed or crying
Able to meet child's special health needs (suctioning, cleaning stoma sites, treatments)

↓

STAGE III: Identity
Brings linens from home
Takes photographs
Brings individualized toys
Can make personalized observations about child
Offers suggestions and makes demands for personalized care
Demonstrates "advocacy" behavior
Feels he or she can care for child better than anyone else
Demonstrates consistent visiting and/or calling pattern
Questions focus on total child, not only physiologic parameters

FIGURE 28–14 Stages of parenting behavior toward an infant in intensive care. SOURCE: Schraeder BD: Attachment and parenting despite lengthy intensive care. *MCN* January/February 1980; 5:38. Reprinted with permission of the American Journal of Nursing Company.

of mothers of normal newborns and mothers of preterm infants. Whereas mothers of normal newborns progress within minutes to palm contact of the infant's trunk, the mother of a preterm infant is slower to progress from fingertip to palm contact and from the extremities to the trunk. The progression to palm contact with the infant's trunk may take several visits to the nursery.

Through support, reassurance, and encouragement, the nurse can facilitate the mother's positive feelings about her ability and her importance to her infant. Touching facilitates "getting to know" the infant and thus establishes a bond with the infant. Touching as well as seeing the infant helps the mother to realize the "normals" and potentials of her baby (Figure 28–14).

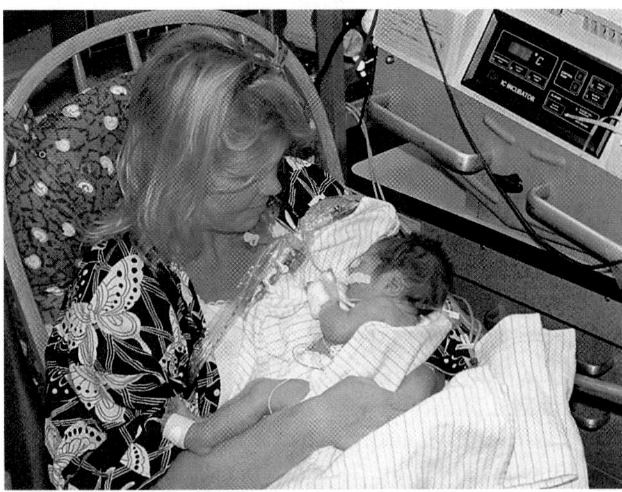

FIGURE 28–15 This mother of a 35 week gestational age infant with respiratory distress syndrome is getting acquainted with her infant. Physical contact is vital to the bonding process and should be encouraged whenever possible. SOURCE: Courtesy of Carol Harrigan, RNC, MSN, NNP.

The nurse can also encourage parents to meet their newborn's need for stimulation. Stroking, rocking, cuddling, singing, and talking should be an integral part of the parents' caretaking responsibilities. Bonding can be facilitated by encouraging parents to visit and become involved in their baby's care (Figure 28–15). When visiting is impossible, the parents should feel free to phone whenever they wish to receive information about their baby. A warm receptive attitude on the part of the nurse is very supportive. Nurses can also facilitate parenting by personalizing a baby to the parents, by referring to the infant by name, or by relating personal behavioral characteristics to the parents. Remarks such as, "Jenny loves her pacifier" help make the infant more individual and unique.

Caretaking may be delayed for the mother of a preterm or sick infant. The variety of equipment needed for life support is hardly conducive to anxiety-free caretaking by the parents. However, even the sickest infant may be cared for, if only in a small way, by the parents. As a facilitator of parental caretaking, the nurse should promote the parents' success. Demonstration and explanation, followed by support of the parents in initial caretaking behaviors, positively reinforce this behavior. Changing the infant's diaper, giving their infant skin care or oral care, or helping the nurse turn the infant may at first be anxiety provoking for the parents, but they will become more comfortable and confident in caretaking and receive satisfaction from the baby's reactions and their ability "to do something." Complimenting the parent's competence in caretaking also increases their self-esteem, which has received recent "blows" of guilt and failure. It is vitally important that the parents never be given a task if there is any possibility they will not be able to accomplish it.

Often mothers of high-risk infants have ambivalent feelings toward the nurse. As the mother watches the nurse competently perform the caretaking tasks, she feels both grateful for the nurse's abilities and expertise and jealous of the nurse's ability to care for her infant. These feelings may be acted out in criticism of the care being received by the infant, manipulation of staff, or personal guilt. Instead of fostering (by silence) these inferiority feelings within mothers, nurses should recognize such feelings and intervene appropriately to enhance mother-infant attachment. The nurse needs to deal with ambivalent feelings that contribute to a competitive atmosphere. For example, the nurse should avoid making unfavorable comparisons between the baby's response to parental caretaking and the child's responses to the nurses. During a quiet time, it may help for the nurse to encourage the parents to talk about their hopes and fears and to facilitate their involvement in parent groups (Raines, 1998).

Nurses who are understanding and secure will be able to support the parents' egos instead of collecting rewards for themselves. To reinforce positive parenting behaviors, professionals must first believe in the importance of the parents. The nurse can hardly convince doubting parents of their importance to the infant unless the nurse really believes it. Both attitudes and words must say: "You are a good mother/father. You have an important contribution to make to the care of your infant." Unless as much care is taken in facilitating parental attachment as in providing physiologic care, the outcome will not be a healthy family.

Verbalizations by the nurse that improve parental self-esteem are essential and easily shared. The nurse can point out that, in addition to physiologic use, breast milk is important because of the emotional investment of the mother. Pumping, storing, labeling, and delivering quantities of breast milk is time-consuming and a "labor of love" for mothers. Positive remarks regarding breast milk reinforce the maternal behavior of caretaking and providing for her infant: "Breast milk is something that only you can give your baby" or "You really have brought a lot of milk today" or "Even small amounts of milk are important, and look how rich it is."

If the infant begins to gain weight while being fed breast milk, it is important to point this out to the mother. Parents should also be advised that initial weight loss with beginning nipple feedings is common because of the increased energy expended when the infant begins active rather than passive nutritional intake.

Provision of care by the parents is appropriate even for a very sick infant who is likely to die. It has been found that detachment is easier after attachment because the parents are comforted by the knowledge that they did all they could for their child while he or she was alive.

Facilitation of Family Adjustment During crisis, maintaining interpersonal relationships is difficult. Yet in a newborn intensive care area, the parents are expected to relate to many different care providers. It is important that parents have as few professionals as possible relaying information to them. A primary nurse should coordinate and provide continuity in information giving to parents. Care providers are individuals and thus will use different terms, inflections, and attitudes. These subtle differences are monumental to parents and only confuse, confound, and produce anxiety. The transfer of the baby from NICU to a step-down unit or back transport to home hospital is very anxiety producing for the parents because they must now deal with new health care professionals. The nurse not only functions as a liaison between the parents and the wide variety of professionals interacting with the infant and parents, but also offers clarification, explanation, interpretation of information, and support to the parents.

The nurse should encourage the parents to deal with the crisis with help from their support system. The support system attempts to meet the emotional needs and provide support for the family members in crisis and stress situations. Biologic kinship is not the only valid criterion for a support system; an emotional kinship is the most important factor. In our mobile society of isolated nuclear families, the support system may be a next-door neighbor, a best friend, or perhaps a schoolmate. The nurse must search out the significant others in the lives of the parents and help them understand the problems so that they can be a constant parental support.

The impact of the crisis on the family is individual and varied. The nurse obtains information about the family's ability to adapt to the situation through the relationship with the family. To institute appropriate interventions, the nurse should view the birth of the infant (normal newborn, preterm infant, infant with illness or congenital anomaly) as it is defined by the family.

Because the family is a unit composed of individuals who must deal with the situation, it is important to encourage open intrafamily communication. The nurse should discourage the family from keeping secrets from one another, especially between spouses, because secrets undermine the trust of their relationship. Well-meaning rationales such as, "I want to protect her," "I don't want him to worry about it," and so on, can be destructive to open communication and to the basic element of a relationship—trust.

The nurse should encourage open communication among family members, particularly between spouses. Open communication is especially important when the mother is hospitalized apart from the infant. The first person to visit the infant relays information regarding the infant's care and condition to the mother and family. In this situation, the mother has had minimal contact, if any, with her infant. Because of her anxiety and isolation, she may mistrust all those who provide information (the nurse, physician, or extended family) until she can see the infant for herself. This can put tremendous stress on the relationship between family members. The parents (and family) should be given information together. This practice helps overcome misunderstandings and misinterpretations and promotes mutual "working through" of problems.

The nurse should encourage the entire family—siblings as well as extended relatives—to visit and receive information about the baby. Methods of intervention in assisting the family to cope with the situation include providing support, confronting the crisis, and helping the family understand the reality. Support, explanations, and the helping role must extend to the kin network, as well as to the nuclear family, to aid them in communication and support ties with the nuclear family.

The needs of siblings should not be overlooked. They have been looking forward to the new baby, and they too suffer a degree of loss. Young children may react with hostility and older ones with shame at the birth of an infant with an anomaly. Both reactions make them feel guilty. Parents, preoccupied with working through their own feelings, often cannot give the other children the attention and support they need. Sometimes another child becomes the focus of family tension. Anxiety thus directed can take the form of finding fault or of overconcern. This is a form of denial; the parents cannot face the real worry—the infant at risk. After assessing the situation, the observant nurse could see to it that another family member or friend step in and give the needed support to the siblings of the affected baby.

The nurse must respect and facilitate the desires and needs of the individuals involved; differences are tolerable and should be able to exist side by side. The nurse can easily elicit the parents' feelings and the meaning of this experience to them by asking, "How are you doing?" The emphasis is on "you," and the interest must be sincere.

Families with children in the newborn intensive care unit become friends and support one another. To encourage the development of these friendships and to provide support, many units have established parent groups. The core of the groups consists of parents who previously have had an infant in the intensive care unit. Most groups make contact with families within a day or two of the infant's admission to the unit, either through phone calls or visits to the hospital. Early one-on-one parent contacts help families work through their feelings better than discussion groups. This personalized method gives the grieving parents an opportunity to express personal feelings about the pregnancy, labor, and birth and their "different from expected" infant with others who have experienced the same feelings and with whom they can identify.

Community-Based Nursing Care

Predischarge planning begins once the infant's condition becomes stable and indications suggest the newborn will survive (American Academy of Pediatrics, Hospital Discharge of the High Risk Neonate, 1998). Adequate predischarge teaching will help the parents transform their feelings of inadequacy and competition with the nurse into feelings of self-assurance and attachment. From the beginning, the parents should be taught about their infant's special needs and growth patterns (Bracht, Ardal, Bot, & Cheng, 1998). This teaching and involvement are best facilitated by a nurse who has been familiar with the infant and family over a period of time and who has developed a comfortable and supportive relationship with them.

The nurse's responsibility is to provide home care instructions in an optimal environment for parental learning. Learning should take place over time, to avoid the necessity of bombarding the parents with instructions in the day or hour before discharge. Parents often enjoy doing minimal caretaking tasks with gradual expansion of their role.

Many intensive care units provide facilities for parents to room in with their infants for a few days before discharge. This allows parents a degree of independence in the care of their infant with the security of nursing help nearby. This practice is particularly helpful for anxious parents, parents who have not had the opportunity to spend extended time with their infant, or parents who will be giving complex physical care at home, such as tracheostomy care (Costello & Chapman, 1998; Dracup, Doering, Moser, & Evangelista, 1998).

The basic elements of home care instruction are as follows:

1. Teaching parents routine well-baby care, such as bathing, temperature taking, formula preparation, and breastfeeding.
2. Training parents to do special procedures as needed by the newborn, such as gavage or gastrostomy feedings, tracheostomy or enterostomy care, medication administration, cardiopulmonary resuscitation (CPR), and operation of an apnea monitor. Before discharge, the parents should be as comfortable as possible with these tasks and should demonstrate independence. Written tools and instructions are useful for parents to refer to once they are home with the infant, but these should not replace participation in the infant's care.
3. Referring parents to community health and support organizations. The visiting nurses association, public health nurses, or social services can assist the parents in the stressful transition from hospital to home by providing the necessary home teaching and support. Some intensive care nurseries have their own parent support groups to help bridge the gap between hospital and home care. Parents can also find support from a variety of community support organizations, such as mothers of twins groups, March of Dimes Birth Defects Foundation,

handicapped children services, and teen mother and child programs. Each community has numerous agencies capable of assisting the family in adapting emotionally, physically, and financially to the chronically ill infant. The nurse should be familiar with community resources and help the parents identify which agencies may benefit them.

4. Helping parents recognize the growth and development needs of their infant. A developmental care program begun in the hospital can be continued at home, or parents may be referred to an infant development program in the community.
5. Arranging medical follow-up care before discharge. The infant will need to be followed up by a family pediatrician, a well-baby clinic, or a specialty clinic. The first appointment should be made before the infant is discharged from the hospital (Hussey-Gardner, Wachtel, & Viscardi, 1998).
6. Evaluating the need for special equipment for infant care (such as a respirator, oxygen, apnea monitor, feeding pump) in the home. Any extra equipment or supplies should be placed in the home before the infant's discharge.

Further evaluation after the infant has gone home is useful in determining whether the crisis has been resolved satisfactorily. The parents are usually given the intensive care nursery's telephone number to call for support and advice. The staff can follow up each family with visits or telephone calls at intervals for several weeks to assess and evaluate the infant's (and parents') progress.

Evaluation

Expected outcomes of nursing care include the following:

- The parents are able to verbalize their feelings of grief and loss.
- The parents verbalize their concerns about their baby's health problems, care needs, and potential outcome.
- The parents are able to participate in their infant's care and show attachment behaviors.

Considerations for the Nurse Who Works with At-Risk Newborns

Support cannot be given unless it can be received. Working in an emotional environment of "lots of living and lots of dying" takes its toll on staff. Neonatal intensive care units are among the most stressful areas in health care for patients, families, and nurses. Nurses bear most of the stress and largely determine the atmosphere of the NICU. The nurse's ability to cope with stress is the key to creating an emotionally healthy environment and a positive working atmosphere. The emotional needs and feelings of the staff must be recognized and dealt with in order to enable them to support the parents. An environment of openness to feelings and support in dealing with their own human needs and emotions is essential for staff. As caregivers, nurses may be unaware of their need to grieve for their own losses in the NICU. Nurses must also go through the grief work that parents experience. Techniques such as group meetings, individual support, and primary care nursing may assist in maintaining staff mental health.

The staff NICU nurses may never see the long-term results of the specialized, sensitive care they give to parents and their newborns. Their only immediate evidence of effective care may be the beginning of resolution of parental grief, discharge of a recovered thriving infant to the care of happy parents, and the beginning of reintegration of family life.

FOCUS YOUR STUDY

- Early identification of potential high-risk fetuses through assessment of preconception, prenatal, and intrapartal factors facilitates strategically timed nursing observations and interventions.
- High-risk newborns, whether they are premature, SGA, LGA, postterm, or infants of a diabetic or substance-abusing mother, have many similar problems, although their problems are based on different physiologic processes.
- Small-for-gestational-age newborns are associated with perinatal asphyxia and resulting aspiration syndrome, hypothermia, hypoglycemia, hypocalcemia, polycythemia, congenital anomalies, and intrauterine infections. Long-term problems include continued difficulties with growth and learning.
- Large-for-gestational-age newborns are at risk for birth trauma as a result of cephalopelvic disproportion, hypoglycemia, polycythemia, and hyperviscosity.
- Infants of diabetic mothers are at risk for hypoglycemia, hypocalcemia, hyperbilirubinemia, polycythemia, and respiratory distress due to delayed maturation of their lungs.
- Postterm newborns often encounter intrapartal problems such as CPD (shoulder dystocia) and birth traumas, hypoglycemia, polycythemia, meconium aspiration, cold stress, and possible seizure activity. Long-term complications may involve poor weight gain and low IQ scores.
- The common problems of the preterm newborn are results of the baby's immature body systems. Potential problem areas include respiratory distress (respiratory distress syndrome), patent ductus arteriosus, hypothermia and cold stress, feeding difficulties and necrotizing enterocolitis, marked insensible water loss and loss of buffering agents through the kidneys, infection, anemia of prematurity, apnea and intraventricular hemorrhage, retinopathy of prematurity, and behavioral state disorganization. Long-term needs and problems include bronchopulmonary dysplasia, speech defects, sensorineural hearing loss, and neurologic defects.
- Newborns of alcohol-dependent mothers are at risk for alterations in physical characteristics and the long-term complications of feeding problems; CNS dysfunction, including lower IQ, hyperactivity, and language abnormalities; and congenital anomalies.
- Newborns born to drug-dependent mothers experience drug withdrawal as well as respiratory distress, jaundice, congenital anomalies, and behavioral abnormalities. With early

recognition and intervention, the potential long-term physiologic and emotional consequences of these difficulties can be avoided or at least lessened in severity.

- Newborns born to mothers with AIDS require early recognition and treatment so that the physiologic and emotional consequences may be lessened in severity and CDC guidelines implemented.
- Cardiac defects are a significant cause of morbidity and mortality in the newborn period. Early identification and nursing and medical care of newborns with cardiac defects are essential to the improved outcome of these infants. Care is directed toward lessening the workload of the heart and decreasing oxygen and energy consumption.
- Inborn errors of metabolism such as galactosemia, PKU, homocystinuria, and maple syrup urine disease are usually included in a newborn screening program designed to prevent mental retardation through dietary management and medication.
- The nursing care of the newborn with special problems involves understanding normal physiology, the pathophysiology of the disease process, clinical manifestations, and supportive or corrective therapies. Only with this theoretical background can the nurse make appropriate observations concerning responses to therapy and development of complications.
- Newborns communicate needs only by their behavior; the nurse caring for newborns, through objective observations and evaluations, interprets this behavior to obtain meaningful information about the infant's condition.
- The nurse is the facilitator of interdisciplinary communication with the parents, identifying their understanding of their infant's care and their needs for emotional support.
- Parents of at-risk newborns need support from nurses and health care providers to understand the special needs of their baby and to feel comfortable in an overwhelmingly strange environment.

REFERENCES

Acosta, P. B. (1995). Nutrition support of maternal phenylketonuria. *Seminars in Perinatology, 19*(3), 182–190.

Als, H. (1998). Developmental care in the newborn intensive care unit. *Current Opinion in Pediatrics, 10*, 138–142.

Als, H., Lester, B. M., Tronick, E., & Brazelton, T. B. (1982). Assessment of preterm infant behavior (APIB). In B. M. Fitzgerald Lester & M. W. Yogman (Eds.), *Theory and research in behavioral pediatrics* (Vol. 1). New York: Plenum.

American Academy of Pediatrics Committee on Drugs. (1998). Neonatal drug withdrawal. *Pediatrics, 101*(6), 1079–1088.

American Academy of Pediatrics (AAP) and American College of Obstetricians and Gynecologists (ACOG). (1997). *Guidelines for perinatal care* (4th ed.). Elk Grove Village, IL: Author.

American Academy of Pediatrics Committee on Fetus and Newborn. (1998). Hospital discharge of the high-risk neonate—Proposed guidelines. *Pediatrics, 102*,(2), 411–417.

American Academy of Pediatrics Committee on Genetics. (1996). Newborn screening fact sheets. *Pediatrics, 98*(3), 473–501.

American College of Obstetricians and Gynecologists. (1992). ACOG Technical Bulletin No. 159: Fetal macrosomia—September, 1991. *International Journal of Gynecological and Obstetrics 39*(4), 341–345.

Bakketeig, L. S. (1998). Current growth standards, definitions, diagnosis and classification of fetal growth retardation. *European Journal of Clinical Nutrition 52*(S1), S1–S4.

Bowe, K. (1995). Phenylketonuria: An update for pediatric community health nurses. *Pediatric Nursing, 21*(2), 191–194.

Bracht, M., Ardal, F., Bot, A., & Cheng, C. M. (1998). Initiation and maintenance of a hospital-based parent group for parents of premature infants: Key factors for success. *Neonatal Network 17*,(3), 33–37.

Buchi, K. F. (1998). The drug-exposed infant in the well-baby nursery. *Clinics in Perinatology, 25*(2), 335–350.

Buckley, T. P., & Friend, C. (1997). Recovery of the neonate after open heart surgery: Strategies for preparing the NICU. *Neonatal Network, 16*(8), 27–33.

Chung, M. A. (1997). Galactosemia in infancy: Diagnosis, management, and prognosis. *Pediatric Nursing, 23*(6), 563–569.

Church, M. W., & Abel, E. L. (1998). Fetal alcohol syndrome: Hearing, speech, language, and vestibular disorders. *Obstetrics and Gynecology of North America, 25*(1), 85–97.

Committee on Pediatric AIDS (1997). Evaluation and medical treatment of the HIV-exposed infant. *Pediatrics 99*(6), 909–917.

Costello, A., & Chapman, J. (1998). Mothers' perceptions of the care-by-parent program prior to hospital discharge of their preterm infants. *Neonatal Network, 17*(4), 37–42.

Cusson, R. M., & Lee, A. L. (1994). Parental interventions and the development of the preterm infant. *Journal of Obstetric, Gynecologic, and Neonatal Nursing, 23*(1), 60–68.

Dracup, K., Doering, L. V., Moser, D. K., & Evangelista, L. (1998). Retention and use of cardiopulmonary resuscitation skills in parents of infants at risk for cardiopulmonary arrest. *Pediatric Nursing, 24*(3), 219–225.

Doshier, S. (1995). What happens to the offspring of diabetic pregnancies? *American Journal of Maternal Child Nursing, 20*(1), 25–28.

Engebretson, J. C., & Wardell, D. W. (1997). Development of a pacifier for low-birth-weight infants' nonnutritive sucking. *Journal of Obstetric, Gynecologic, and Neonatal Nursing 26*(6), 660–664.

Frank, D. A., Bresnahan, K., & Zuckerman, B. S. (1996, Feb.). Maternal cocaine use: Impact on child health and development. *Current Problems in Pediatrics*, 52–70.

French, E. D., Pituch, M., Brandt, J., & Pohorecki, S. (1998). Improving interactions between substance-abusing mothers and their substance-exposed newborns. *Journal of Obstetric, Gynecologic, and Neonatal Nursing, 27*(3), 262–269.

Gardner, J. (1997). Fetal alcohol syndrome: Recognition and intervention. *American Journal of Maternal Child Nursing, 22*(6), 318–322.

Gardner-Cole, J. G. (1996). Intervention strategies for infants with prenatal drug exposure. *Infants and Young Children, 8*(3), 35.

Grant, P. (1978). Psychological needs of families of high risk infants. *Family and Community Health, 1*(3), 91–102.

Gray, J. (1997). HIV in the neonate. *Journal of Hospital Infection, 37*, 181–198.

Gray, J. E., Sorrentino, J. E., Matheson, G. A., Wise, P., & McCormick, M. C. (1997). Failure to screen newborns for inborn disorders: A potential consequence of changes in newborn care. *Early Human Development, 48*, 277–285.

Harrington, K., & Campbell, S. (1993). Fetal size and growth. *Current Opinion in Obstetrics & Gynecology, 5*(2), 186–194.

Hess, D. J., & Kenner, C. (1998). Families caring for children with fetal alcohol syndrome: The nurse's role in early identification and intervention. *Holistic Nursing Practice, 12*(3), 47–54.

Homko, C. J., Sivan, E., Nyirjesy, P., & Reece, E. A. (1995). The interrelationship between ethnicity and gestational diabetes in fetal macrosomia. *Diabetes Care, 18*(11), 1442–1445.

Horns, K. M. (1998). Being-in-tune caregiving. *Journal of Perinatal Neonatal Nursing, 12*(3), 38–49.

Hurst, N. M., Valentine, C. J., Renfro, L., Burns, P., & Ferlic, L. (1997). Skin-to-skin holding in the neonatal intensive care unit influences maternal milk volume. *Journal of Perinatology, 17*(3), 213–217.

Hussey-Gardner, B. T., Wachtel, R. C., & Viscardi, R. M. (1998). Parent perceptions of an NICU follow-up clinic. *Neonatal Network, 17*(1), 33–39.

Institute of Medicine (IOM). (1996). *Fetal alcohol syndrome: Diagnosis, epidemiology, prevention and treatment.* Washington, DC: National Academy Press.

Jaeger, M. C., Lawson, M., & Filteau, S. (1997). The impact of prematurity and neonatal illness on the decision to breast-feed. *Journal of Advanced Nursing 25*, 729–737.

Kaplan, D. M., & Mason, E. A. (1974). Maternal reactions to premature birth viewed as an acute emotional disorder. In H. J. Parad (Ed.), *Crisis intervention.* New York: Family Services Association of America.

Kenner, C., & D'Apolito, K. (1997). Outcomes for children exposed to drugs in utero. *Journal of Obstetric, Gynecologic, and Neonatal Nursing, 26*(5), 595–603.

Kinneer, M. D., & Beachy, P. (1994). Nipple feeding premature infants in the neonatal intensive-care unit: Factors and decisions. *Journal of Obstetric, Gynecologic, and Neonatal Nursing, 23*(2), 105–112.

Klaus, M. H., & Kennell, J. H. (1982). *Maternal-infant bonding* (2nd ed.). St. Louis: Mosby.

Kliegman, R. M. (1997). Intrauterine growth retardation. In A. A. Fanaroff & R. J. Martin (Eds.), *Neonatal-perinatal medicine: Diseases of the fetus and infant* (6th ed.). St. Louis: Mosby.

Kochenour, N. K. (1997). Postterm pregnancy. In A. A. Fanaroff & R. J. Martin (Eds.), *Neonatal-perinatal medicine: Diseases of the fetus and infant* (6th ed.). St. Louis: Mosby.

McMahon, M. J., Kuller, J. A., & Yankowitz, J. (1996). Assessment of the post-term pregnancy. *American Family Physician, 54*(2), 631–636, 641–642.

Merenstein, G. B., & Gardner, S. L. (1998). *Handbook of neonatal intensive care* (4th. ed.). St. Louis: Mosby.

Messmer, P. R., Rodriguez, S., Adams, J., Wells-Gentry, J., Washburn, K., Zabaleta, I., & Abreu, S. (1997). Effects of kangaroo care on sleep time for neonates. *Pediatric Nursing 23*(4), 408–414.

Modrein-McCarthy, M. A., McCue, S., & Walker, J. (1997). Preterm infants and stress: A tool for the neonatal nurse. *Journal of Perinatal Neonatal Nursing 10*(4), 62–71.

Nagey, V. A., & Viscardi, R. M. (1993). Retarded intrauterine growth. In J. J. Pomerance & C. J. Richardson (Eds.), *Neonatology for the clinician.* Norwalk, CT: Appleton & Lange.

National Association of Neonatal Nurses (NANN) Practice Committee. (1993). *Infant development care guidelines.* Petaluma, CA: NANN.

Neonatal skin care. (1997). In *NANN guidelines for practice.* Petaluma, CA: National Association of Neonatal Nurses.

Neonatal thermoregulation. (1997). In *NANN Guidelines for Practice.* Petaluma, CA: National Association of Neonatal Nurses.

Ogata, E. S. (1994). Carbohydrate homeostasis. In G. B. Avery, M. A. Fletcher, & M. G. MacDonald (Eds.), *Neonatology: Pathophysiology and management of the newborn* (4th ed.). Philadelphia: Lippincott.

Pickler, R. H., Mauck, A. G., & Geldmaker, B. (1997). Bottle-feeding histories of preterm infants. *Journal of Obstetric, Gynecologic, and Neonatal Nursing, 26*(4), 414–420.

Premji, S. S., Wilson, J., Paes, B., & Gray, S. (1997). Cisapride: A review of the evidence supporting its use in premature infants with feeding intolerance. *Neonatal Network, 16*(7), 17–21.

Pressler, J. L., & Hepworth, J. T. (1997). Behavior of macrosomic and appropriate-for-gestational-age newborns. *Journal of Obstetric, Gynecologic, and Neonatal Nursing, 26*(2), 198–205.

Raines, D. A. (1998). Values of mothers of low birth weight infants in the NICU. *Neonatal Network, 17*(4), 41–46.

Rodriguez, E. M., Diaz, C., & Fowler, M. G. (1997). The clinical management of children perinatally exposed to HIV. *HIV/AIDS Management in Office Practice, 24*(3), 643–666.

Seashore, M. R., & Rinaldo, P. (1993). Metabolic disease of the neonate and young infant. *Seminars in Perinatology, 17*(5), 318–329.

Seppänen, M. P., Ojanperä, O. S., Kääpä, O., & Kero, P. O. (1997). Delayed postnatal adaptation of pulmonary hemodynamics in infants of diabetic mothers. *Journal of Pediatrics, 131*(4), 545–548.

Sinai, L. N., Kim, S. C., Casey, R., & Pinto-Martin, J. A. (1995). Phenylketonuria screening: Effect of early newborn discharge. *Pediatrics, 96*(4 Pt. 1), 605–608.

Sohl, B., & Moore, T. R. (1998). Abnormalities of fetal growth. In H. W. Taeusch & R. A. Ballard (Eds.), *Avery's diseases of the Newborn* (7th ed.). Philadelphia: Saunders.

Solnit, A., & Stark, M. (1961). Mourning and the birth of a defective child. *Psychoanalytic Study of the Child, 16*, 505.

Stoddard, J. J., & Farrell, P. M. (1997). State-to-state variations in newborn screening policies. *Archives of Pediatric and Adolescent Medicine, 151*(6), 561–564.

Strauss, R. S., & Dietz, W. H. (1997). Effects of intrauterine growth retardation in premature infants on early childhood growth. *Journal of Pediatrics, 130*(1), 95–102.

Taeusch, H. W., & Sniderman, S. (1998). History and physical examination of the newborn. In H. W. Taeusch & R. A. Ballard (Eds.), *Avery's diseases of the newborn.* (7th ed.). Philadelphia: Saunders.

Theis, J. G. W., Selby, P., Ikizler, Y., & Koren, G. (1997). Current management of the neonatal abstinence syndrome: A critical analysis of the evidence. *Biology of the Neonate, 71*, 345–356.

Tyrala, E. E. (1996). The infant of the diabetic mother. *Obstetrics and Gynecology Clinics of North America, 23*(1), 221–241.

Volpe, J. J. (1995). *Neurology of the newborn.* Philadelphia: Saunders.

Wagner, C. L., Katikaneni, L. D., Cox, T. H., & Ryan, R. M. (1998). The impact of prenatal drug exposure on the neonate. *Obstetrics and Gynecology Clinics of North America, 25*(1), 169–194.

Wright, L., Brown, A., & Davidson-Mundt, A. (1992). Newborn screening: The miracle and the challenge. *Journal of Pediatric Nursing, 17*(1), 26.

29 The Newborn at Risk: Birth-Related Stressors

Key Terms

Bronchopulmonary dysplasia (BPD)
Cold stress
Erythroblastosis fetalis
Hemolytic disease of the newborn
Hydrops fetalis
Hyperbilirubinemia
Hypoglycemia
Jaundice
Kernicterus
Meconium aspiration syndrome (MAS)
Persistent pulmonary hypertension of the newborn (PPHN)
Phototherapy
Physiologic anemia
Polycythemia
Respiratory distress syndrome (RDS)
Sepsis neonatorum

I WATCHED HER BREATHE EVERY PRECIOUS BREATH on the respirator. I saw her covered with wires and tubes. I kept watch. She was special to me and I would tell her over and over, "Daddy is here. Daddy loves you." The three days she lived were hell—not knowing if she would make it, uncertain about what plans we should make. Somehow I thought she would live; I was hopeful. When she died, at least I was there with her. The grief was unbearable. But there was also a sense of relief. The uncertainty, the waiting were finally over.
~ *When Pregnancy Fails* ~

Objectives

- Discuss how to identify infants in need of resuscitation and the appropriate method of resuscitation based on the labor record and observable physiologic indicators.
- Based on clinical manifestation, differentiate among the various types of respiratory distress (respiratory distress syndrome, transient tachypnea of the newborn, and meconium aspiration syndrome).
- Identify the components of nursing care for a newborn with respiratory distress syndrome.
- Discuss selected metabolic abnormalities (including cold stress and hypoglycemia), their effects on the newborn, and their nursing implications.
- Differentiate between physiologic and pathologic jaundice according to onset, cause, possible sequelae, and specific management.
- Explain the circumstances that must be present for the development of erythroblastosis and ABO incompatibility.
- Identify the nurse's role in the care of an infant with hemolytic disease.
- Identify the nursing responsibilities in caring for the newborn receiving phototherapy.
- Discuss selected hematologic problems such as anemia and polycythemia and the nursing implications associated with each one.
- Describe the nursing assessment that would lead the nurse to suspect newborn sepsis.
- Relate the consequences of selected maternally transmitted infections, such as maternal syphilis, gonorrhea, herpesvirus, or chlamydia, to the management of the infant in the neonatal period.
- Identify the special initial and long-term needs of parents of at-risk infants.

MARKED HOMEOSTATIC CHANGES OCCUR during the transition from fetal to newborn life. The most rapid anatomic and physiologic changes of this period occur in the cardiopulmonary system. Thus the major problems of the newborn are usually related to this system. These problems include asphyxia, respiratory distress syndrome, cold stress, jaundice, hemolytic disease, and anemia. Ideally, problems are anticipated and identified prenatally, and appropriate intervention measures are begun at or immediately after birth. See Essential Precautions in Practice: At-Risk Newborns.

ESSENTIAL PRECAUTIONS IN PRACTICE

At-Risk Newborns

Examples of times when disposable gloves should be worn include the following:

- Handling baby prior to first bath, before all blood and amniotic fluid have been removed
- Suctioning oral and nasal secretions
- During resuscitation, with use of bag and mask ventilation
- Administering vitamin K injection, eye prophylaxis, and cord care
- Carrying out routine heel stick blood work (ie, glucose, hematocrit)
- Inserting umbilical catheter lines—umbilical artery (UAC) and umbilical vein (UVC)—and any other invasive lines
- Flushing and blood drawing from umbilical catheter lines (UAC, UVC)

All invasive procedures require sterile gloves and should be carried out over thoroughly cleansed areas of skin. At times, goggles and protective gowns or aprons may be required.

REMEMBER to wash your hands before putting on the disposable gloves and AGAIN immediately after you remove the gloves.

For further information, consult OSHA and CDC guidelines.

Care of the Newborn at Risk Due to Asphyxia

Newborn asphyxia results from circulatory, respiratory, and biochemical factors. Circulatory patterns that accompany asphyxia indicate an inability to make the transition to extrauterine circulation—in effect, a return to fetal circulatory patterns. Failure of lung expansion and establishment of respiration rapidly produces hypoxia (decreased PaO_2), acidosis (decreased pH), and hypercarbia (increased PCO_2). These biochemical changes result in pulmonary vasoconstriction and high pulmonary vascular resistance, hypoperfusion of the lungs, and a large right-to-left shunt through the ductus arteriosus. As right atrial pressure exceeds left atrial pressure, the foramen ovale reopens, and blood flows from right to left. See Chapter 25 for review of normal newborn cardiopulmonary adaptation.

Biochemical changes that occur in asphyxia contribute to these circulatory changes. The most serious biochemical abnormality is a change from aerobic to anaerobic metabolism due to hypoxia. This change results in the accumulation of lactate and the development of metabolic acidosis. Simultaneously, respiratory acidosis may also occur due to a rapid increase in PCO_2 during asphyxia. In response to hypoxia and anaerobic metabolism, the amounts of free fatty acids (FFA) and glycerol in the blood increase. Glycogen stores are mobilized to provide a continuous glucose source for the brain. Hepatic and cardiac stores of glycogen may be used up rapidly during an asphyxial attack.

The newborn is supplied with protective mechanisms against hypoxic insults. These include a relatively immature brain and a resting metabolic rate lower than that observed in the adult; an ability to mobilize substances within the body for anaerobic metabolism and to use the energy more efficiently; and an intact circulatory system able to redistribute lactate and hydrogen ions in tissues still being perfused. Unfortunately, severe prolonged hypoxia will overcome these protective mechanisms, resulting in brain damage or death of the newborn.

The newborn who is apneic at birth requires immediate resuscitative efforts. The need for resuscitation can be anticipated if specific risk factors are present during the pregnancy or labor and birth period.

Risk Factors Predisposing to Asphyxia

The need for resuscitation may be anticipated if the mother demonstrates the antepartal and intrapartal risk factors described in Tables 11–1 and 19–1. Neonatal risk factors for resuscitation are as follows:

- Nonreassuring fetal heart rate pattern
- Difficult birth
- Fetal blood loss
- Apneic episode that is unresponsive to tactile stimulation
- Inadequate ventilation
- Prematurity
- Structural lung abnormality (congenital diaphragmatic hernia, lung hypoplasia)
- Cardiac arrest

At times, no risk factors may be apparent prenatally. Particular attention must be paid to all at-risk pregnancies during the intrapartal period. Certain aspects of labor and birth challenge the oxygen supply to the fetus, and often the at-risk fetus has less tolerance to the stress of labor and birth.

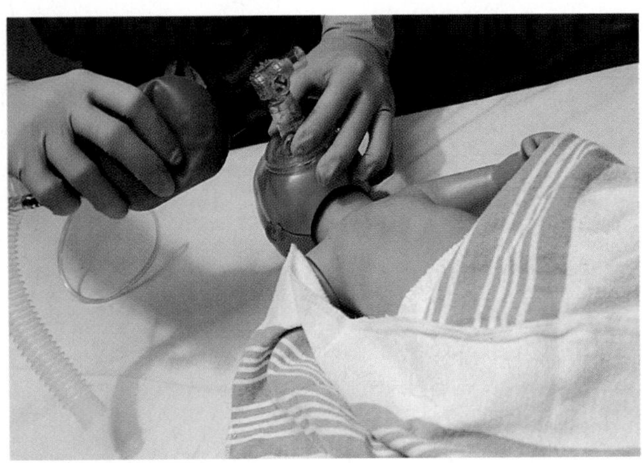

FIGURE 29–1 Demonstration of resuscitation of an infant with bag and mask. Note that the mask covers the nose and mouth and that the head is in a neutral position. The resuscitation bag is placed to the side of the baby so that chest movement can be seen.

Clinical Therapy

The initial goal of clinical management is to identify the fetus at risk for asphyxia so that resuscitative efforts can begin at birth.

Fetal biophysical assessment (see Chapter 17) and monitoring of fetal and maternal pH, blood gases, and fetal heart rates during the intrapartal period may help identify fetal distress. If fetal distress is present, appropriate measures can be taken to deliver the fetus immediately, before major damage occurs, and to treat the asphyxiated newborn.

The fetal biophysical profile enhances the ability to predict an abnormal perinatal outcome. In addition, fetal scalp blood sampling may indicate asphyxic insult and the degree of fetal acidosis, when considered in relation to the stage of labor, uterine contractions, and nonreassuring fetal heart rate (FHR) patterns. During labor, a fetal pH of 7.25 or higher is considered normal. A pH value of 7.20 or less is considered an ominous sign of fetal asphyxia (Jepson, Talashek, & Tichy, 1991). However, low fetal pH without associated hypoxia can be caused by maternal acidosis resulting from prolonged labor, dehydration, and maternal lactate production.

The treatment of fetal or newborn asphyxia is resuscitation. The goal of resuscitation is to provide an adequate airway with expansion of the lungs, to decrease the PCO_2 and increase the PO_2, to support adequate cardiac output, and to minimize oxygen consumption by reducing heat loss.

Initial resuscitative management of a compromised newborn is extremely important. Caregivers should keep the newborn in a head-down position before the first gasp to avoid aspiration of the oropharynx secretions and must suction the oropharynx and nasopharynx immediately. Clearing the nasal and oral passages of fluid that may obstruct the airway establishes a patent airway. Suction is always performed before resuscitation so that mucus, blood, or meconium is not aspirated into the lungs.

After the first few breaths, the nurse places the newborn in a level position under a radiant heat source and dries the baby quickly with warm blankets to maintain skin temperature at about 36.5C (97.7F). Drying is also a good stimulation to breathing. Heat loss through evaporation is tremendous during the first few minutes of life. The temperature of a wet 1500 g baby in a cold room (16C [62F]) drops 1C every 3 minutes. Hypothermia increases oxygen consumption. In an asphyxiated infant, it increases the hypoxic insult and may lead to severe acidosis and development of respiratory distress.

Assessment of the newborn's need for resuscitation begins at the time of birth. The time of the first gasp, first cry, and onset of sustained respirations should be noted in order of occurrence. The Apgar score (see Chapter 20) may be helpful in determining the severity of neonatal depression but should not be used to determine the need for resuscitation of the newborn (Letko, 1996).

Breathing is established by employing the simplest form of resuscitative measures initially, with progression to more complicated methods as required, for example:

1. Simple stimulation is provided by rubbing the back.
2. If respirations have not been initiated or are inadequate (gasping or occasional respirations), the lungs must be inflated with positive pressure. The mask is positioned securely on the face (over nose and mouth, avoiding the eyes) with the head in "sniffing" or neutral position (Figure 29–1). Hyperextension of the infant's neck will obstruct the trachea. An airtight connection is made between the baby's face and the mask (thus allowing the bag to inflate). The lungs are inflated rhythmically by squeezing the bag. Oxygen can be delivered at 100% with an anesthesia or Laerdal bag and adequate liter flow. The self-inflating bag delivers only 40% oxygen unless it has been adapted. In addition, it may not be possible to maintain adequate inspiratory pressure with Ambu or Hope bags. In a crisis situation, it is crucial that 100% O_2 be delivered with adequate pressure.
3. The rise and fall of the chest are observed for proper ventilation. Air entry and heart rate are checked by auscultation. Manual resuscitation is coordinated with any voluntary efforts. The rate of ventilation should be between 40 and 60 breaths per minute. Pressure should be adequate to move the chest wall. The pressure gauge (manometer) must be in place to avoid overdistention of the newborn's lungs and other problems such as pneumothorax or abdominal distension. In newborns with normal lungs, 15 to 25 cm H_2O may be adequate. If the newborn has lung disease, 20 to 40 cm H_2O may be necessary. If the newborn has not taken a first breath after birth, pressures of 30 to 40 cm H_2O may be transiently required to expand collapsed alveoli. If ventilation

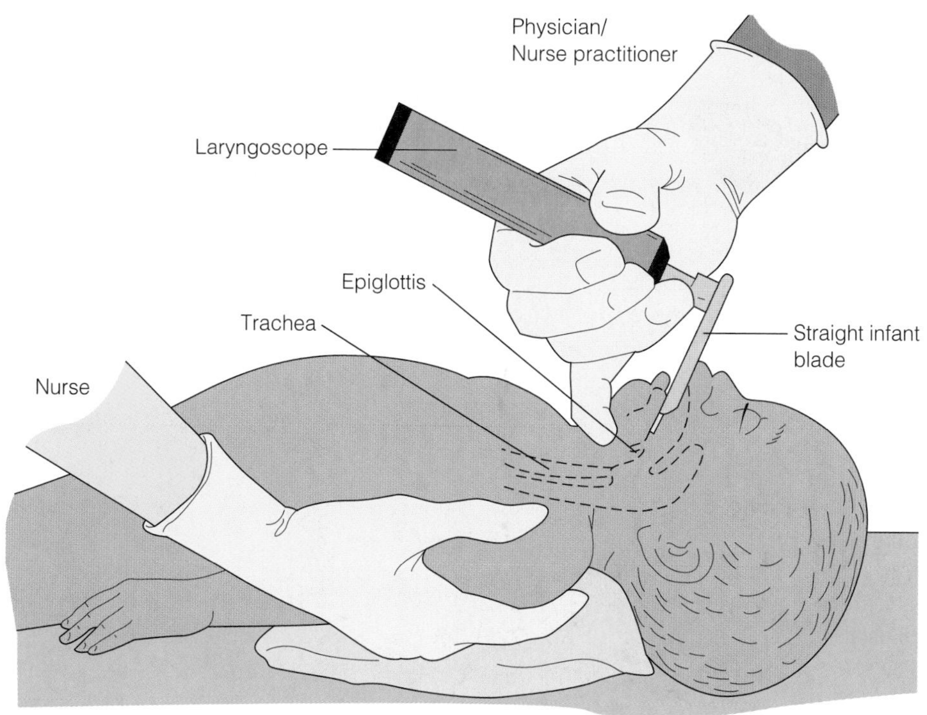

FIGURE 29–2 Endotracheal intubation is accomplished with the infant's head in the "sniffing" position. The clinician places the fifth finger under the chin to hold the tongue forward and inserts the laryngoscope blade. Once the blade is in position as shown, an endotracheal tube is inserted through the groove in the laryngoscope blade. The endotracheal tube is not seen in this illustration.

is adequate, the chest moves with each inspiration, bilateral breath sounds are audible, and the lips and mucous membranes become pink. If color and heart rate fail to respond to ventilatory efforts, poor or improper placement of an endotracheal tube may be the cause. If the baby is intubated properly, pneumothorax, diaphragmatic hernia, or hypoplastic lungs (Potter's association) may exist. Distention of the stomach is controlled by inserting a nasogastric tube for decompression.

4. Endotracheal intubation (Figure 29–2) may be needed. However, most newborns, except for very-low-birth-weight (VLBW) infants, can be resuscitated by bag and mask ventilation.

Once breathing has been established, the heart rate should increase to over 100 beats per minute. If the heart rate is less than 60 beats per minute or between 60 and 80 beats per minute and is not increasing despite 15 to 30 seconds of ventilation with 100% oxygen, external cardiac massage (chest compression) is begun. Chest compressions are started immediately if there is no detectable heartbeat.

1. The infant is positioned properly on a firm surface.
2. The resuscitator uses the two-fingers method (Figure 29–3) or may stand at the foot of the infant and place both thumbs over the lower third of the sternum (just below an imaginary line drawn between the nipples) with the fingers wrapped around and supporting the back.
3. The sternum is depressed approximately two-thirds of the distance to the vertebral column (1 to 2 cm or ½ to ¾ in) at a rate of 90 beats per minute (Bloom & Cropley, 1994).
4. A 3:1 ratio of heartbeat to assisted ventilation is used.

Drugs that should be available in the birthing area include those needed in the treatment of shock, cardiac arrest, and narcosis. Oxygen, because of its effective use in ventilation, is the drug most often used.

If after 30 seconds of ventilation and cardiac compression, the newborn has not responded with spontaneous respirations and a heart rate above 80 beats per minute, it is necessary to administer resuscitative medications. The most accessible route for administering medications is the umbilical vein. If bradycardia is present, epinephrine (0.1 to 0.3 mL/kg of a 1:10,000 solution) is given through the umbilical vein catheter, the peripheral IV setup, or the endotracheal tube (if an IV setup has not yet been started). When epinephrine is administered by endotracheal tube, two to three times the IV dose of epinephrine is given followed immediately by 1 mL of normal saline (Young & Mangum, 1997). In a severely asphyxiated newborn, sodium bicarbonate (2 mEq/kg of 4.2% solution) is given slowly, at a rate of 1 mEq/kg/minute to correct metabolic acidosis, but only after adequate ventilation is established. Dextrose is given to prevent progression of hypoglycemia. A 10% dextrose in water intravenous solution is usually sufficient to prevent or treat hypoglycemia in the birthing area. Naloxone hydrochloride (0.1 mg/kg), a narcotic antagonist, is used to reverse narcotic depression (Young & Mangum, 1997). See Drug Guide: Naloxone Hydrochloride (Narcan).

If shock develops (eg, low blood pressure or poor peripheral perfusion), the baby may be given a volume

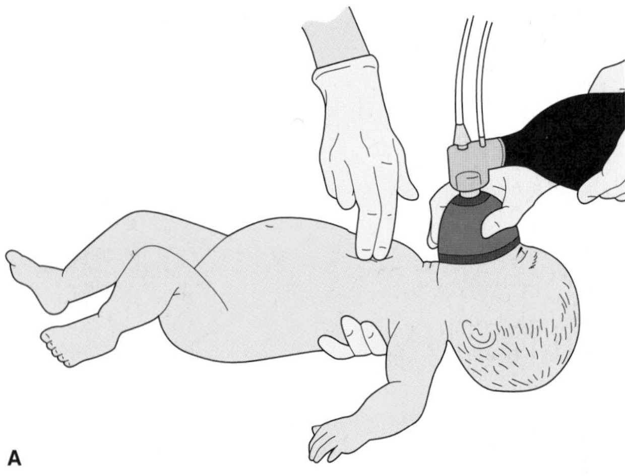

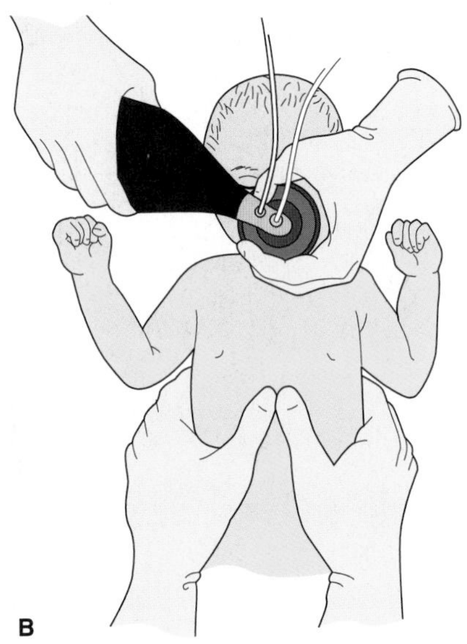

FIGURE 29–3 External cardiac massage. The lower third of the sternum is compressed with two fingertips or thumbs at a rate of 90 beats/minute. ***A,*** In the two-fingers method, the tips of two fingers of one hand compress the sternum, and the other hand or a firm surface supports the infant's back. ***B,*** In the thumb method, the fingers support the infant's back, and both thumbs compress the sternum.

expander such as 5% albumin or lactated Ringer's in a dose of 10 mL/kg. Whole blood, fresh-frozen plasma, plasminate, and packed red blood cells can also be used for volume expansion and treatment of shock. In some instances of prolonged resuscitation associated with shock and poor response to resuscitation, dopamine (5 μg/kg/minute) may be necessary.

NURSING CARE MANAGEMENT

Nursing Assessment and Diagnosis

Communication between the obstetric office or clinic and the birthing area nurse facilitates the identification of newborns who may be in need of resuscitation. When the woman arrives in the birthing area, the nurse should have the antepartal record and should note any contributory prenatal history factors and assess present fetal status. As labor progresses, nursing assessments include ongoing monitoring of fetal heartbeat and its response to contractions, assisting with fetal scalp blood sampling, and observing the presence of meconium in the amniotic fluid to identify fetal asphyxia. In addition, the nurse should alert the resuscitation team and the practitioner responsible for the care of the newborn of any potential high-risk laboring woman.

Nursing diagnoses that may apply to the newborn with asphyxia and the newborn's parents include:

- ***Ineffective Breathing Pattern*** related to lack of spontaneous respirations at birth secondary to in utero asphyxia
- ***Decreased Cardiac Output*** related to impaired oxygenation
- ***Ineffective Family Coping: Compromised*** related to baby's lack of spontaneous respirations at birth and fear of losing their newborn

Nursing Plan and Implementation

Hospital-Based Nursing Care

Following identification of possible high-risk situations, the next step in effective resuscitation is assembling the necessary equipment and ensuring proper functioning. It is desirable to provide for pH and blood gas determinations as well. Necessary equipment includes a radiant warmer that provides an overhead radiant heat source (a thermostatic mechanism that is taped to the infant's abdomen triggers the radiant warmer to turn on or off in order to maintain a level of thermoneutrality) and an open bed for easy access to the newborn. It is essential that the nurse keep the infant warm. To do so, the nurse dries the newborn quickly with warmed towels or blankets to prevent evaporative heat loss and places the baby under a prewarmed radiant warmer with servocontrol set at 36.5C.

Resuscitative equipment in the birthing room must be sterilized after each use. In the high-risk nursery, the need for resuscitation may occur at any time. The reliability of the equipment must be maintained before an emergency arises, and the equipment must be restocked immediately after use. The nurse inspects all equipment—bag and mask, pressure manometer, oxygen and flow meter, laryngoscope, and suction machine—for damaged or nonfunctioning parts before a birth or when setting up an admission bed. A systematic check of the emergency cart and equipment is a routine responsibility of each shift.

Training and knowledge about resuscitation are vital to personnel in the birth setting for both normal and high-risk births. Resuscitation is at least a two-person effort, and the nurse should call for additional support as needed. The resuscitative efforts are recorded on the newborn's chart so that all members of the health care team will have access to this information.

Parent Teaching

Birthing room resuscitation is particularly distressing for the parents. If the need for resuscitation is anticipated, the parents should be assured that a team will be present at the birth to care specifically for their newborn. As soon as stabilization is accomplished, a member of the interdisciplinary team needs to discuss the baby's condition with the parents. The parents may have many fears about the reasons for resuscitation and the condition of their baby following the resuscitation.

Evaluation

Expected outcomes of nursing care include the following:

- The risk of asphyxia is promptly identified, and intervention is started early.
- The newborn's metabolic and physiologic processes are stabilized, and recovery proceeds without complications.
- The parents can describe the reason for resuscitation and what was done to resuscitate their newborn.
- The parents can verbalize their fears about the resuscitation process and potential implications for their baby's future. ●

Care of the Newborn with Respiratory Distress

One of the severest conditions to which the newborn may fall victim is respiratory distress—an inappropriate respiratory adaptation to extrauterine life. The nursing care of a baby with respiratory distress requires understanding of the normal pulmonary and circulatory physiology (Chapter 24), the pathophysiology of the disease process, clinical manifestations, and supportive and corrective therapies. Only with this knowledge can the nurse make appropriate observations concerning responses to therapy and development of complications. Unlike the verbalizing adult client, the newborn communicates needs only by behavior. The neonatal nurse interprets this behavior as clues about the individual baby's condition.

Respiratory distress syndrome (RDS), also referred to as *hyaline membrane disease (HMD)*, is the result of a primary absence, deficiency, or alteration in the production of pulmonary surfactant. It is a complex disease

DRUG GUIDE

Naloxone Hydrochloride (Narcan)

Overview of Neonatal Action

Naloxone hydrochloride (Narcan) is used to reverse respiratory depression due to acute narcotic toxicity. It displaces morphinelike drugs from receptor sites on the neurons; therefore the narcotics can no longer exert their depressive effects. Naloxone reverses narcotic-induced respiratory depression, analgesia, sedation, hypotension, and pupillary constriction.

Route, Dosage, Frequency

Intravenous dose is 0.1 to 0.2 mg/kg (0.25 to 0.5 mL/kg of 0.4 mg/mL preparation) concentration at birth, including premature infants. This drug is usually given through the umbilical vein or endotracheal tube, although naloxone can be given intramuscularly or subcutaneously. The use of neonatal naloxone (Narcan 0.02 mg/mL) is no longer recommended by the American Academy of Pediatrics Committee on Drugs because of the extremely large fluid volumes that are required.

Reversal of drug depression occurs within 1 to 2 minutes after IV administration. The duration of action is variable (minutes to hours) and depends on the amount of the drug present and the rate of excretion. Dose may be repeated in 3–5 minutes. If there is no improvement after two or three doses, discontinue naloxone administration. If initial reversal occurs, repeat dose as needed.

Neonatal Contraindications

Naloxone should not be administered to infants of narcotic-addicted mothers because it may precipitate acute withdrawal syndrome (increased HR and BP, vomiting, tremors).

Respiratory depression may result from nonmorphine drugs, such as sedatives, hypnotics, anesthetics, or other nonnarcotic CNS depressants.

Neonatal Side Effects

Excessive doses may result in irritability, increased crying, and possible prolongation of partial thromboplastin time (PTT).
Tachycardia may occur.

Nursing Considerations

- Monitor respirations closely—rate and depth.
- Assess for return of respiratory depression when naloxone effects wear off and effects of longer-acting narcotics reappear.
- Have resuscitative equipment, O_2, and ventilatory equipment available.
- Monitor bleeding studies.
- Note that naloxone is incompatible with alkaline solutions.
- Store at room temperature and protect from light.
- Compatible with heparin.

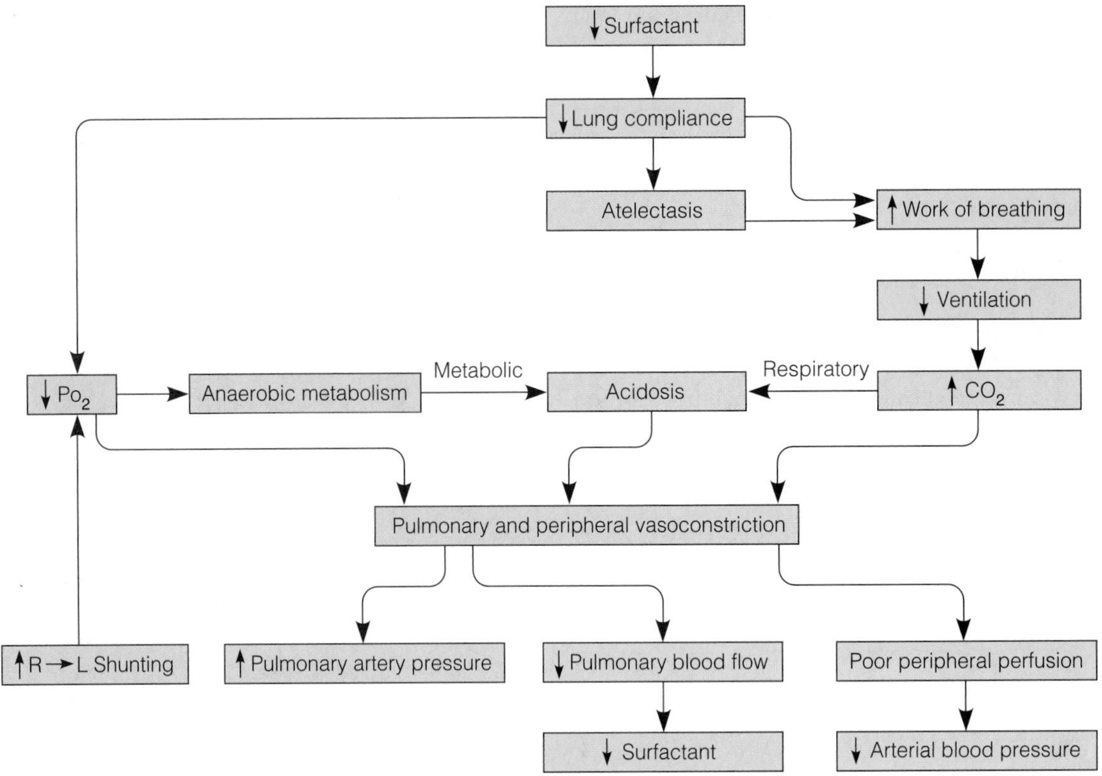

FIGURE 29–4 Cycle of events of RDS leading to eventual respiratory failure. SOURCE: Modified from Gluck L, Kulovich MV: Fetal lung development. *Pediatr Clin North Am* 1973; 20:375.

that affects approximately 40,000 infants a year in the United States, most of whom are preterm infants. Nearly 65% of these infants are born at gestational ages of 30 weeks or less (Askin, 1997). The syndrome occurs more frequently in premature Caucasian infants than in infants of African descent and almost twice as often in males as in females.

All the factors precipitating the pathologic changes of RDS have not been determined, but the main factors associated with its development are as follows:

1. *Prematurity.* All preterm newborns—whether AGA, SGA, or LGA—and especially IDMs are at risk for RDS. The incidence of RDS increases with the degree of prematurity, with most deaths occurring in newborns weighing less than 1500 g. The maternal and fetal factors resulting in preterm labor and birth, complications of pregnancy, indications for cesarean birth, and familial tendency are all associated with RDS.
2. *Surfactant deficiency disease.* Normal pulmonary adaptation requires adequate surfactant, a lipoprotein that coats the inner surface of the alveoli. Surfactant provides alveolar stability by decreasing the alveoli's surface tension and tendency for collapse. Surfactant is produced by type II alveolar cells starting at about 24 weeks' gestation. In the normal or mature newborn lung, it is continuously synthesized, oxidized during breathing, and replenished. Adequate surfactant levels lead to better lung compliance and permit breathing with less work. Respiratory distress syndrome is due to alterations in surfactant quantity, composition, function, or production (Askin, 1997).

Development of RDS indicates a failure to synthesize surfactant, which is required to maintain alveolar stability (see Chapter 24). Upon expiration, the instability increases atelectasis, which causes hypoxia and acidosis because of the lack of gas exchange. These conditions further inhibit surfactant production and cause pulmonary vasoconstriction. The resulting lung instability causes the biochemical problems of hypoxemia (decreased Po_2), hypercarbia (increased PCo_2), and acidemia (decreased pH), which further increases pulmonary vasoconstriction and hypoperfusion. The cycle of events of RDS leading to eventual respiratory failure is diagrammed in Figure 29–4.

Because of these pathophysiologic conditions, the newborn must expend increasing amounts of energy to reopen the collapsed alveoli with every breath, so that each breath becomes more difficult than the last. The progressive expiratory atelectasis upsets the physiologic homeostasis of the pulmonary and cardiovascular systems and prevents adequate gas exchange. Lung compliance decreases, which accounts for the difficulty of inflation, labored respirations, and the increased work of breathing.

The physiologic alterations of RDS produce the following complications:

1. *Hypoxia.* As a result of hypoxia, the pulmonary vasculature constricts, pulmonary vascular resistance increases, and pulmonary blood flow is reduced. Increased pulmonary vascular resistance may precipitate a return to fetal circulation as the ductus arteriosus opens and blood flow is shunted around the lungs. This increases the hypoxia and further decreases pulmonary perfusion. Hypoxia also causes impairment or absence of metabolic response to cold; reversion to anaerobic metabolism, resulting in lactate accumulation (acidosis); and impaired cardiac output, which decreases perfusion to vital organs.
2. *Respiratory acidosis.* Increased PCO_2 and decreased pH are results of alveolar hypoventilation. A persistent rise in PCO_2 is a poor prognostic sign of pulmonary function and adequacy.
3. *Metabolic acidosis.* Because of the lack of oxygen at the cellular level, the newborn begins an anaerobic pathway of metabolism, with an increase in lactate levels and a resultant base deficit (loss of bicarbonate). As the lactate levels increase, the pH decreases, and the buffer base decreases in an attempt to maintain acid-base homeostasis.

The classic radiologic picture of RDS is diffuse reticulogranular density that occurs bilaterally, with portions of the air-filled tracheobronchial tree (air bronchogram) outlined by the opaque ("white-out") lungs with widespread atelectasis (Hansen, Cooper, & Weisman, 1998) (Figure 29–5). Opacification of the lungs on x-ray image may be due to massive atelectasis, diffuse alveolar infiltrate, or pulmonary edema. The progression of x-ray findings parallels the pattern of resolution, which usually occurs in 4 to 7 days, and the time of surfactant reappearance, unless surfactant replacement therapy has been used. Echocardiography is a valuable tool in diagnosing vascular shunts that shunt blood either away from or toward the lungs.

Clinical Therapy

The primary goal of prenatal management is to prevent preterm birth through aggressive treatment of preterm labor and administration of glucorticoids to enhance fetal lung development (see Chapter 16). Clinical trials have shown antenatal steriod and possibly β-adrenergic agonist (ritodrine) therapy reduce neonatal mortality and incidence of RDS in preterm infants (Askin, 1997; Jobe, Newnham, Willet, Sly, & Ikegami, 1998). The goals of postnatal therapy are to maintain adequate oxygenation and ventilation, to correct acid-base abnormalities, and to provide the supportive care required to maintain homeostasis.

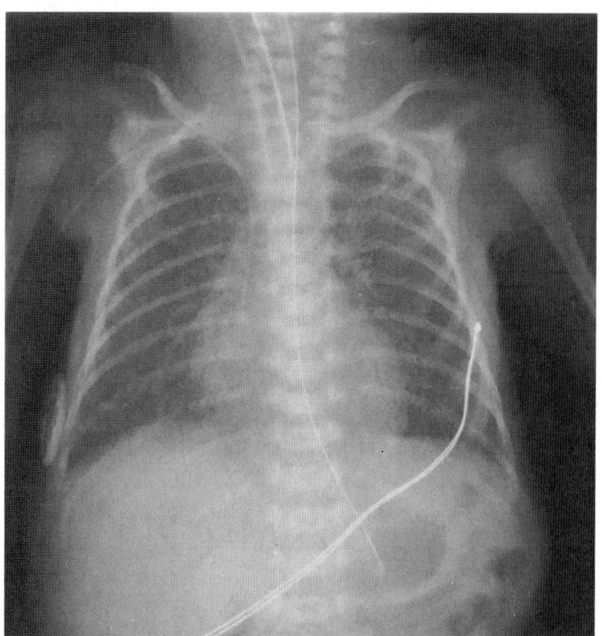

FIGURE 29–5 RDS chest x-ray. Chest radiograph of respiratory distress syndrome characterized by a reticulogranular pattern with areas of microatelectasis of uniform opacity and air bronchograms. SOURCE: Courtesy of Carol Harrigan, RNC, MSN, NNP.

Supportive medical management consists of oxygenation, ventilatory therapy, transcutaneous oxygen and carbon dioxide monitoring, blood gas monitoring, correction of acid-base imbalance, environmental temperature regulation, adequate nutrition, and protection from infection. Ventilatory therapy is directed toward preventing hypoventilation and hypoxia. Mild cases of RDS may require only increased humidified oxygen concentrations. Use of continuous positive airway pressure (CPAP) may be required in moderately afflicted infants. Babies with severe cases of RDS require mechanical ventilatory assistance from a respirator (Figure 29–6). Surfactant replacement therapy is now available for infants to decrease the severity of RDS in low-birth-weight newborns. Surfactant replacement therapy is delivered through an endotracheal tube, and it may be given either in the delivery room or in the nursery after hospitalization and as indicated by the severity of respiratory distress syndrome. Repeat doses are often required. The most generally reported response to treatment is rapidly improved oxygenation and decreased need of ventilatory support.

High-frequency ventilation and extracorporeal membrane oxygenation (ECMO) have been tried when conventional ventilator therapy has not been successful (Askin, 1997). Both of these have specific protocols for eligibility for use and require specially trained nurses and respiratory therapists. Nitric oxide inhalation therapy may also be a useful adjunctive therapy for infants with RDS (Gomez, Hansen, & Corbet, 1998). In some institutions, morphine or fentanyl is used for its analgesic and

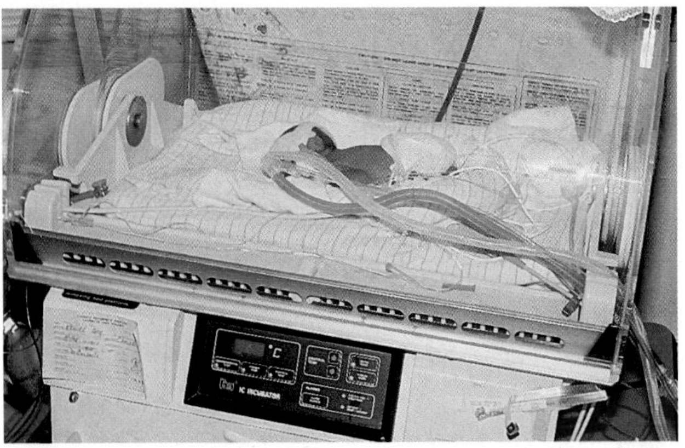

FIGURE 29–6 One day old, 29 weeks gestational age, 1450 gram baby on respirator and in isolette. SOURCE: Carol Harrigan RNC, MSN, NNP.

sedative effects. Sedation may be indicated for infants most likely to have air leak respiratory problems. Use of pancuronium for muscle relaxation in infants with RDS is controversial.

NURSING CARE MANAGEMENT

Nursing Assessment and Diagnosis

Characteristics of RDS the nurse should look for are increasing cyanosis, tachypnea, grunting respirations, nasal flaring, significant retractions, and apnea. Table 29–1 reviews clinical findings associated with respiratory distress in general. The Silverman-Andersen index (Figure 29–7) may be helpful in evaluating the signs of respiratory distress and can be done in the birthing area.

Nursing diagnoses that may apply to the newborn with respiratory distress syndrome include the following:

- ***Impaired Gas Exchange*** related to inadequate lung surfactant
- ***Altered Nutrition: Less than Body Requirements*** related to increased metabolic needs of stressed infants
- ***Risk for Infection*** related to invasive procedures

Nursing Plan and Implementation

Hospital-Based Nursing Care

Based on clinical parameters, the neonatal nurse implements therapeutic approaches to maintain physiologic homeostasis and provides supportive care to the newborn with RDS. See Critical Pathway for the Care of Newborn with Respiratory Distress on pages 874 to 877.

Nursing interventions and criteria for instituting mechanical ventilatory assistance are done per institutional protocol. Methods of noninvasive oxygen monitoring and nursing interventions are described in Table 29–2 on page 875. (The nursing care of infants on ventilators or with umbilical artery catheters is not discussed here.

CLINICAL TIP

In babies with respiratory distress syndrome who are on ventilators, increased urination (determined by weighing diapers) may be an early clue that the baby's condition is improving. As fluid moves out of the lungs into the bloodstream, alveoli open, and kidney perfusion increases, which results in increased voiding. At this point, the nurse must monitor chest expansion closely. If chest expansion is increasing, ventilator settings may have to be decreased. Too high a ventilator setting may "blow the lungs," resulting in pneumothorax.

These infants have severe respiratory distress and are cared for in intensive care nurseries by nurses with advanced knowledge and training.) Ventilatory assistance with high-frequency ventilators has shown positive results. The parents of a baby born having respiratory distress should be provided with a very supportive environment (see Chapter 28).

Evaluation

Expected outcomes of nursing care include the following:

- The risk of RDS is promptly identified, and early intervention is initiated.
- The newborn is free of respiratory distress and metabolic alterations.
- The parents verbalize their concerns about their baby's health problem and survival and understand the rationale behind management of their newborn. ●

Transient Tachypnea of the Newborn

Some newborns, primarily AGA and near-term infants, may develop progressive respiratory distress that clinically can resemble RDS. They may have had intrauterine or intrapartal asphyxia due to maternal oversedation, maternal bleeding, prolapsed cord, breech birth, or maternal diabetes. The resultant effect on the newborn is failure to clear the airway of lung fluid, mucus, and other debris, or an excess of fluid in the lungs due to aspiration of amniotic or tracheal fluid. It is also more prevalent in cesarean born newborns who have not had the thoracic squeeze that occurs during vaginal birth and removes some of the lung fluid.

Usually the newborn experiences little or no difficulty at the onset of breathing. However, shortly after birth, expiratory grunting, flaring of the nares, and mild cyanosis may be noted in the newborn breathing room air. Tachypnea is usually present by 6 hours of age, with respiratory rates as high as 100 to 140 breaths per minute.

Clinical Therapy

Initial x-ray findings may be identical to those showing RDS within the first 3 hours. However, radiographs of

TABLE 29–1 Clinical Assessments Associated with Respiratory Distress

Clinical Picture	Significance
Skin Color	
Pallor or mottling	These represent poor peripheral circulation due to systemic hypotension and vasoconstriction and pooling of independent areas (usually in conjunction with severe hypoxia).
Cyanosis (bluish tint)	Depending on hemoglobin concentration, peripheral circulation, intensity and quality of viewing light, and acuity of observer's color vision, this is frankly visible in advanced hypoxia. Central cyanosis is most easily detected by examination of mucous membranes and tongue.
Jaundice (yellow discoloration of skin and mucous membranes due to presence of unconjugated [indirect] bilirubin)	Metabolic alterations (acidosis, hypercarbia, asphyxia) of respiratory distress predispose to dissociation of bilirubin from albumin-binding sites and deposition in the skin and central nervous system.
Edema (presents as slick, shiny skin)	This is characteristic of preterm infants because of low total protein concentration with decrease in colloidal osmotic pressure and transudation of fluid. Edema of hands and feet is frequently seen within first 24 hours and resolved by fifth day in infants with severe RDS.
Respiratory System	
Tachypnea (normal respiratory rate 30–60/minute, elevated respiratory rate 60+/minute)	Increased respiratory rate is the most frequent and easily detectable sign of respiratory distress after birth. This compensatory mechanism attempts to increase respiratory dead space to maintain alveolar ventilation and gas exchange in the face of an increase in mechanical resistance. As a decompensatory mechanism it increases work load and energy output by increasing respiratory rate, which causes increased metabolic demand for oxygen and thus increases alveolar ventilation of an already overstressed system. During shallow, rapid respirations, there is an increase in dead space ventilation, thus decreasing alveolar ventilation.
Apnea (episode of nonbreathing for more than 20 seconds; periodic breathing, a common "normal" occurrence in preterm infants, is defined as apnea of 5–10 seconds alternating with 10–15 seconds of ventilation)	This poor prognostic sign indicates cardiorespiratory disease, CNS disease, metabolic alterations, intracranial hemorrhage, sepsis, or immaturity. Physiologic alterations include decreased oxygen saturation, respiratory acidosis, and bradycardia.
Chest	Inspection of the thoracic cage includes shape, size, and symmetry of movement. Respiratory movements should be symmetrical and diaphragmatic; asymmetry reflects pathology (pneumothorax, diaphragmatic hernia). Increased anteroposterior diameter indicates air trapping (meconium aspiration syndrome).
Labored respirations (Silverman-Anderson chart in Figure 29–7 indicates severity of retractions, grunting, and nasal flaring, which are signs of labored respirations)	Indicates marked increase in the work of breathing.
Retractions (inward pulling of soft parts of the chest cage—suprasternal, substernal, intercostal, subcostal—at inspiration)	These reflect the significant increase in negative intrathoracic pressure necessary to inflate stiff, noncompliant lungs. Infants attempt to increase lung compliance by using accessory muscles. Lung expansion markedly decreases. Seesaw respirations are seen when the chest flattens with inspiration and the abdomen bulges. Retractions increase the work of breathing and O_2 need so that assisted ventilation may be necessary due to exhaustion.
Flaring nares (inspiratory dilation of nostrils)	This compensatory mechanism attempts to lessen the resistance of the narrow nasal passage.
Expiratory grunt (Valsalva maneuver in which the infant exhales against a closed glottis, thus producing an audible moan)	This increases transpulmonary pressure, which decreases or prevents atelectasis, thus improving oxygenation and alveolar ventilation. Intubation should not be attempted unless the infant's condition is rapidly deteriorating, because it prevents this maneuver and allows the alveoli to collapse.
Rhythmic body movement with labored respirations (chin tug, head bobbing, retractions of anal area)	This is a result of using abdominal and other respiratory accessory muscles during prolonged forced respirations.
Auscultation of chest reveals decreased air exchange with harsh breath sounds or fine inspiratory rales; rhonchi may be present	Decrease in breath sounds and distant quality may indicate interstitial or intrapleural air or fluid.
Cardiovascular System	
Continuous systolic murmur may be audible	Patent ductus arteriosus is a common occurrence with hypoxia, pulmonary vasoconstriction, right-to-left shunting, and congestive heart failure.
Heart rate usually within normal limits (fixed heart rate may occur with a rate of 110–120/minute)	A fixed heart rate indicates a decrease in vagal control.
Point of maximal impulse usually located at fourth to fifth intercostal space, left sternal border	Displacement may reflect dextrocardia, pneumothorax, or diaphragmatic hernia.
Hypothermia	This is inadequate functioning of metabolic processes that require oxygen to produce necessary body heat.
Muscle Tone	
Flaccid, hypotonic, unresponsive to stimuli	These may indicate deterioration in the newborn's condition and possible CNS damage due to hypoxia, acidemia, or hemorrhage.
Hypertonia and/or seizure activity	

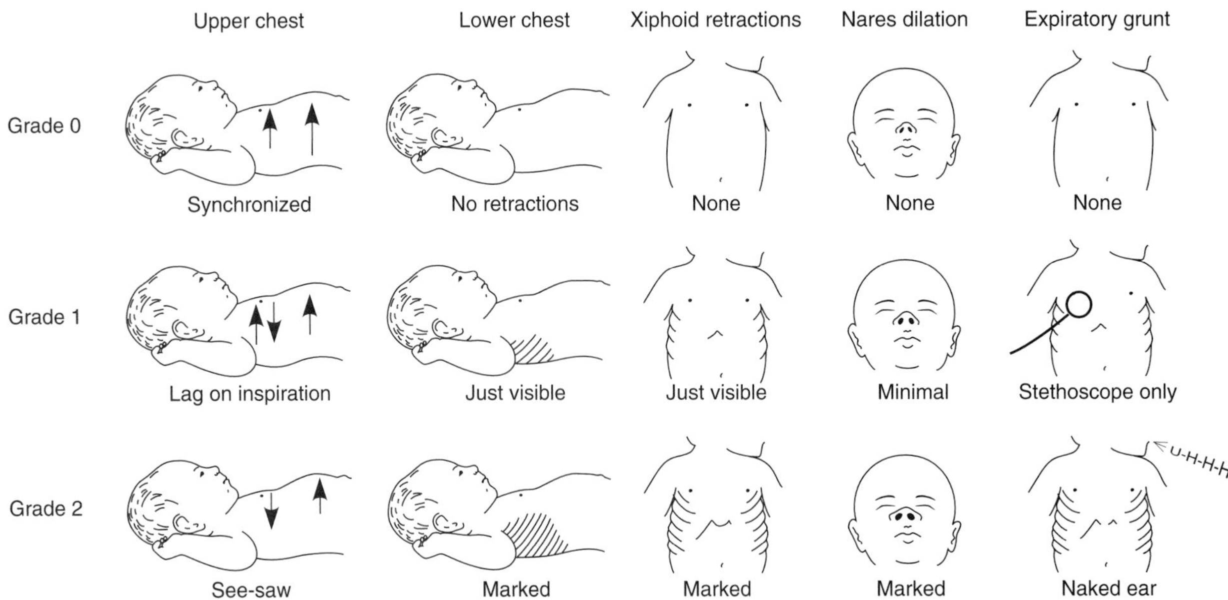

FIGURE 29–7 Evaluating respiratory status using the Silverman-Andersen index. The baby's respiratory status is assessed. A grade of 0, 1, or 2 is determined for each area, and a total score is charted in the baby's record or on a copy of this tool and placed in the chart.

SOURCES: Ross Laboratories, Nursing Inservice Aid No. 2, Columbus, OH; Silverman WA, Andersen DH: *Pediatrics* 1956; 17:1. Copyright 1956, American Academy of Pediatrics.

infants with transient tachypnea usually reveal a generalized overexpansion of the lungs (hyperaeration of alveoli), which is identifiable principally by flattened contours of the diaphragm. Dense streaks (increased vascularity) radiate from the hilar region and represent engorgement of the lymphatic vessels, which clear alveolar fluid on initiation of air breathing. Within 48 to 72 hours, the chest x-ray examination is normal (Hansen, Cooper, & Weisman, 1998).

Ambient oxygen concentrations of 30% to 50%, usually under an oxyhood, may be required to correct the hypoxemia (Figure 29–8). Fluid and electrolyte requirements should be met with intravenous fluids during acute phase of the disease. Oral feedings are contraindicated because of rapid respiratory rates. The infant should be improving by 8 to 24 hours. The duration of the clinical course of transient tachypnea is approximately 72 hours. Mild respiratory and metabolic acidosis may be present at 2 to 6 hours.

When hypoxemia is severe and tachypnea continues, persistent pulmonary hypertension must be considered and treatment measures initiated. If pneumonia is suspected initially, antibiotics may be administered prophylactically.

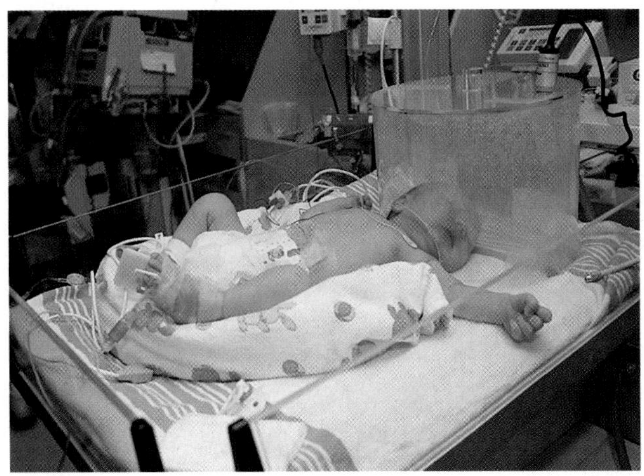

FIGURE 29–8 Infant in oxygen hood.

CRITICAL THINKING IN PRACTICE

You are caring for baby girl Linn, who is a 39-week, AGA female born by repeat cesarean birth to a 34-year-old G3 now P3 mother. Baby Linn's Apgar scores were 7 and 9 at 1 and 5 minutes. At 2 hours of age, an elevated respiratory rate of 70 to 80 and mild cyanosis were noted. She is now receiving 30% oxygen and has a respiratory rate of 100 to 120. The baby's clinical course, chest x-ray examination, and lab work are all consistent with transient tachypnea of the newborn. Her mother calls you to ask about her baby. She tells you that her last child was born at 30 weeks' gestation, had respiratory distress syndrome requiring ventilator support, and was hospitalized for 6 weeks. She asks you, "Is this the same respiratory distress?" What will you tell her?

Answers can be found in Appendix I.

TABLE 29–2 Oxygen Monitors

Type	Function and Rationale	Nursing Interventions
Pulse Oximetry—Spo_2		
Estimates beat-to-beat arterial oxygen saturation.	Calibration is automatic.	Understand and use oxyhemoglobin dissociation curve.
Microprocessor measures saturation by the absorption of red and infrared light as it passes through tissue.	Less dependent on perfusion than $TcPo_2$ and $TcPco_2$; however, functions poorly if peripheral perfusion is decreased due to low cardiac output.	Monitor trends over time and correlate with arterial blood gases (Merenstein & Gardner, 1998). Check disposable sensor at least q8h.
Changes in absorption related to blood pulsation through vessel determine saturation and pulse rate (Merenstein & Gardner, 1998).	Much more rapid response time than $TcPo_2$—offers "real-time" readings.	Use disposable cuffs (reusable cuffs allow too much ambient light to enter, and readings may be inaccurate).
	Can be located on extremity, digit, or palm of hand, leaving chest free; not affected by skin characteristics.	
	Requires understanding of oxyhemoglobin dissociation curve.	
	Pulse oximeter reading of 85% to 95% reflects clinically safe range of saturation.	
	Extreme sensitivity to movement; decreases if average of 7th or 14th beat is selected rather than beat to beat.	
	Poor correlation with extreme hyperoxia.	
Transcutaneous Oxygen Monitor—$TcPo_2$		
Measures oxygen diffusion across the skin	When transcutaneous monitors are properly calibrated and electrodes are appropriately positioned, they will provide reliable, continuous, noninvasive measurements of Po_2, Pco_2, and oxygen saturation.	Use $TcPo_2$ to monitor trends of oxygenation with routine nursing care procedures. Clean electrode surface to remove electrolyte deposits; change solution and membrane once a week.
Clark electrode is heated to 43C (preterm) or 44C (term) to warm the skin beneath the electrode and promote diffusion of oxygen across the skin surface. Po_2 is measured when oxygen diffuses across the capillary membrane, skin, and electrode membrane (Merenstein & Gardner, 1998).	Readings vary when skin perfusion is decreased. Reliable as trend monitor.	Allow machine to stabilize before drawing arterial gases; note reading when gases are drawn, and use values to correlate.
	Frequent calibration necessary to overcome mechanical drift.	Ensure airtight seal between skin surface and electrode; place electrodes on clean, dry skin on upper chest, abdomen, or inner aspect of thigh; avoid bony prominences.
	Following membrane change, machine must "warm up" 1 hour prior to initial calibration; otherwise, after turning it on, it must equilibrate for 30 minutes prior to calibration.	
	When placed on infant, values will be low until skin is heated; approximately 15 minutes required to stabilize.	
	Second-degree burns are rare but can occur if electrodes remain in place too long.	Change skin site and recalibrate at least every 4 hours; inspect skin for burns; if burns occur, use lowest temperature setting and change position of electrode more frequently.
	Decreased correlations noted with older infants (related to skin thickness); with infants with low cardiac output (decreased skin perfusion); and with hyperoxic infants.	
	The adhesive that attaches the electrode may abrade the fragile skin of the preterm infant.	Adhesive disks may be cut to a smaller size, or skin prep may be used under the adhesive circle only; allow membrane to touch skin surface at center.
	May be used for both preductal and postductal monitoring of oxygenation for observations of shunting.	

NURSING CARE MANAGEMENT

For nursing actions, see the Critical Pathway for Care of the Newborn with Respiratory Distress on page 874 to 877.

Care of Newborn with Meconium Aspiration Syndrome

The presence of meconium in amniotic fluid indicates an asphyxial insult to the fetus before or during labor unless the baby is in breech position. The physiologic response to asphyxia is increased intestinal peristalsis, relaxation of the anal sphincter, and passage of meconium into the amniotic fluid.

Among all pregnancies, 8% to 29% will manifest meconium-stained fluid (Askin, 1997). This fluid may be aspirated into the tracheobronchial tree by the fetus in utero or during the first few breaths taken by the newborn. This aspiration is called **meconium aspiration syndrome (MAS).** This syndrome primarily affects term, SGA, and postterm newborns and those who have experienced a long labor.

Presence of meconium in the lungs produces a ball-valve action (air is allowed in but not exhaled), so that alveoli overdistend; rupture with pneumomediastinum or pneumothorax is a common occurrence. The meconium

Text continues on page 877.

CRITICAL PATHWAY FOR CARE OF A NEWBORN WITH RESPIRATORY DISTRESS

Category	Day of Birth—1st 4 Hours	Remainder of Birth Day
Referral	Report from L&D, Neonatal Nurse Practitioner Check ID bands Consults prn: High-risk peds, neonatology	Check ID bands q shift Lactation consult prn
Assessments	Assess development of s/s respiratory distress: • Tachypnea (>60 respirations/min) • Expiratory grunting (audible), subcostal/intercostal/suprasternal retractions, nasal flaring on inspiration • Cyanosis and pallor • Signs of increased air hunger (apnea, hypotonus), labored respirations • Arterial blood gases (indicating respiratory failure): Pa_{O_2} less than 50 mm Hg, and Pc_{O_2} above 60 mm Hg Auscultation: • Initially breath sounds may be normal, then decreased air exchange occurs with harsh breath sounds and, upon deep inspiration, rales • Later, a low-pitched systolic murmur indicates patent ductus arteriosus Determine baseline of respiratory effort and ventilatory adequacy: • Observe chest wall movement • Assess skin, mucous membranes color, capillary refill • Auscultate quality of air entry bilaterally • Assess arterial blood gases and pH Increasing oxygen concentration requirements to maintain adequate P_{O_2} levels VS: temp (ax), pulse, respirations, BP Admission wt, length, HC, peripheral pulses × 4 Monitor pulse oximeter Gestational age assessment (only as tolerated without increasing infant's work of breathing, or defer) Gestational history: recent episodes of fetal or intrapartal stress (maternal hypotension, bleeding, maternal and resultant fetal oversedation), fetal lung circulation compromise Lung maturity assessment: amniotic, tracheal and/or gastric aspirates as available for PG Newborn Hx: birth asphyxia resulting in acute hypoxia, hypothermia, low Apgar scores, bag/mask resuscitation Monitor activity (increasing lethargy, s/s seizure activity)	Continue previous assessments q2–4h and prn Assess color, respiratory status Assess mother/baby interaction as appropriate Observe infant for temperature instability, signs of increased oxygen consumption and metabolic acidosis Observe infant for s/s sepsis: apnea, lethargy, cyanosis, temp instability
Teaching/ psychosocial	Admission activities performed at mother's bedside as possible; orient parents to nursery, handwashing; assess teaching needs and readiness for learning Provide parents information on infant's condition, minimal handling rationale, equipment and monitoring devices prn	Reinforce previous teaching; keep parents apprised of infant's status Discuss/teach infant security, identification Teach parents s/s respiratory distress, calming techniques, bulb syringe, positioning, when to call for assistance
Nursing care management and reports	Admit directly to special care nursery prn Labs as ordered: blood type, Rh, Coombs' on cord blood prn, tracheal or gastric aspirate for PG, chemstrip, peripheral hct, blood cultures, CBC, electrolytes, arterial or capillary blood gas Administer IV antibiotics as ordered Intravenous access for meds, hydration, nutritional support Assist MD/NP with placement of umbilical or arterial lines prn Attach servo probe to infant's skin, radiant warmer bed on servo control Attach 3-lead EKG for continuous cardiac, resp monitoring prn Attach pulse oximeter to infant extremity Set up, monitor oxygen administration prn (or assist respiratory therapist prn), nasal cannula, oxygen hood	Vital signs: q4h and prn, use monitoring devices to decrease infant stimulation; daily wt using bedscale as necessary Monitor antibiotic drug levels Continue assessments q4h and prn Cord care per policy (alcohol to cord q diaper change after infant stable and possibility of placing umbilical lines remote) Rotate pulse oximetry sites q8h and prn; TCOM sites q4h and prn depending on infant's skin integrity
Activity and comfort	Adjust and monitor radiant warmer to maintain skin temp and NTE Provide calming techniques Cluster cares (allow recovery time between procedures), nest Minimal stimulation, quiet and dim environment Provide pacifier for nonnutritive sucking	Leave in radiant warmer until stable, then swaddle and move to isolette or open crib as condition allows Encourage parent interaction/holding as soon as infant tolerates Avoid overstimulation, cluster cares, assess on infant's schedule Reposition for comfort q4h, prn; position on surfboard while prone

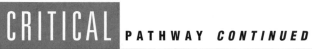

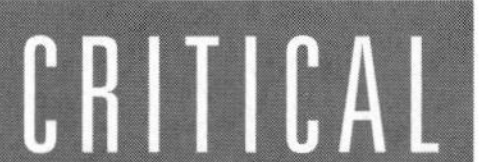

PATHWAY *CONTINUED*

Category	Day of Birth—1st 4 Hours	Remainder of Birth Day
Nutrition	Provide total parenteral nutrition (TPN) as ordered and indicated Provide adequate caloric intake: consider amount of intake, route of administration, need for supplementation of intake by other routes, type of feeding breast/formula Gavage feeding prn Maintain IV rate via infusion pump (usually 60–80 ml/kg/day dependent on gestational age, and organ efficiency) • Record intake hourly (oral, parenteral type and amount) • Monitor vital signs, lung auscultation, heart sounds for s/s fluid overload	Advance intake as tolerated from parenteral to gastrointestinal. Gavage or nipple feed, supplementing with IV prn, discontinue IV when oral intake sufficient Initiate breastfeeding as soon as mother/baby condition allows Supplement breastfeeding only when medically indicated and ordered by MD/NP Initiate bottle feeding as applicable
Elimination	Note first void and stool Record hourly output Monitor urine specific gravity	Continue accurate hourly output monitoring (1–3 ml/kg/h) Monitor stools for amt, type, pattern changes Continue specific gravity monitoring
Medication	Aquamephyton IM, dosage according to infant wt per MD order Ilotycin ophth ointment OU after retinal assessment by MD/NP Antibiotic therapy as ordered	Continue antibiotic therapy as ordered
Discharge planning/ home care	Plan DC with parent/guardian Evaluate for Social Services/home care/DC planning needs	Birth certificate instructions/worksheet Car seat available for DC
Family involvement	Evaluate psychosocial needs: provide time for expressions of concerns, determine parents' understanding of respiratory distress syndrome (RDS) Evaluate parent teaching	Encourage family involvement in infant's care as possible and as infant tolerates Keep family apprised of infant's progress and current status Evaluate parent teaching
Date		
Category	**Day 1 after Birth**	**Day 2/3 (as applicable) after Birth**
Referral	Check ID bands q shift	Check ID bands q shift **Expected Outcomes** Mother/baby ID bands correlate at time of DC Consults completed prn
Assessments	Continue high risk assessment for RDS q4h Assess respiratory effort and ventilatory adequacy Assess mother/baby interaction Assess thermoregulation Assess abdominal distention, gastric residuals Monitor blood gases, capillary refill, O_2 saturation, pulses all 4 extremities	Assess respiratory effort and level of distress Continue high risk assessment for resp distress q4h as needed Assess mother/baby interaction Continue monitoring blood gases, capillary refill, O_2 saturation, pulses all 4 extremities q4h prn, wean to q8h as infant recovers **Expected Outcomes** Physical assessments, VS WNL; no complications or residual respiratory distress noted
Teaching/ psychosocial	(See Newborn Critical Pathway, pp. 754 to 755) Reinforce previous teaching Parental teaching: bathing, cord care, skin/nail care, use of thermometer, activity, sleep patterns, calming methods, reflexes, jaundice, growth/feeding patterns, burping, diapering, elimination norms Provide information including: • Newborn capabilities and developmental behaviors, cues • Temperature maintenance with clothing and blankets • Safety (choking, positioning, use of bulb syringe)	Final discharge teaching: (See Newborn Critical Pathway, pp. 754 to 755) Review infant safety, s/s illness and when to call health care provider with parents **Expected Outcomes** Mother verbalizes comprehension of instructions, demonstrates care capabilities

CRITICAL PATHWAY FOR CARE OF A NEWBORN WITH RESPIRATORY DISTRESS *CONTINUED*

Category	Day 1 after Birth	Day 2/3 (as applicable) after Birth
Nursing care management and reports	Maintain on respiratory and cardiac monitors: • Check and calibrate all monitoring and measuring devices q8h • Calibrate oxygen devices to 21% and 100% O_2 concentrations Provide warmed air and humidified oxygen Monitor oxygen concentrations at least q1h Femoral pulses or BPs all 4 extremities before DC or at 48h VS q4h Daily wt Continue high risk assessments for resp distress q4h, wean to q8h as infant stabilizes and recovers Isolette if temp instability • Adjust and monitor to maintain skin temp and NTE Use servo control to maintain constant temp regulation Monitor activity Administer meds as ordered Newborn screen, monitor therapeutic drug levels, blood gases prn	Newborn/high-risk assessment q8h if resp status WNL and stable Baer hearing test Daily wt VS q8h and prn Continue oxygen administration as warranted (oxyhood, nasal cannula) Monitor O_2 concentrations q1–2h Prepare infant for/assist with circumcision as applicable Cord care per policy (alcohol to cord q diaper change) Administer antibiotics/monitor levels as ordered Continue Universal Precautions HSV culture per parental hx HSV Wean from radiant warmer or isolette to open crib if VS WNL, stable **Expected Outcomes** Physical assessments WNL; cord unclamped and dry without s/s infection; circ site unremarkable; no s/s respiratory distress; labs WNL; wt stabilized to not >10% loss
Activity and comfort	Change position q4h and prn Swaddled in open crib as condition permits Isolette if temp instability; adjust temp for infant size, gestation layers of clothing to maintain NTE	Swaddled in open crib as condition permits Allow movement of hands to face **Expected Outcomes** Maintains temp WNL swaddled in open crib
Nutrition	Supplement breast only when medically indicated/ordered Gavage feed prn Encourage on demand feedings as tolerated, minimally q3–4h Bottle feed q3–4h on demand Decrease parenteral support as oral feedings increase	Continue feeding schedule Feed on demand breast or bottle Supplement breast only when medically indicated/ordered **Expected Outcomes** Infant tolerates feedings, feeds on demand; breastfeeds without supplement, nipples without problems or s/s increased WOB; regaining lost wt or wt stabilized after birth
Elimination	Monitor stools for amount, consistency, pattern changes, occult blood, reducing substances Monitor voids q8h Continue accurate intake and output as warranted	Continue monitoring of all voids and stools q shift, noting changes. Accurate intake and output as warranted **Expected Outcomes** Voids qs, stools without difficulty qs, stool character WNL
Medication	Hep B vaccine as ordered by MD/NP after consent signed by parent	Hep B vaccine before DC **Expected Outcomes** Infant has received ophthalmic ointment OU and Aquamephyton injection; received first Hep B vaccine if ordered and parental consent given; antibiotics regimen completed with resolution RDS
Discharge planning/ home care	Newborn photographs Complete birth certificate packet Continue DC teaching Access community referrals, support groups for mother/family prn, ie, WIC, financial resources, public health nursing	Complete DC teaching Complete DC summary, give written copy DC instructions (See Newborn Critical Pathway, pp. 754 to 755) Set up appointment for follow-up newborn screening blood test All discharge referrals made, follow-up appointments scheduled **Expected Outcomes** Infant discharged home with family; mother verbalizes f/u appointments times and dates; mother verbalizes comprehension of DC instructions and available resources, ie, lactation, new parents support groups

Category	Day 1 after Birth	Day 2/3 (as applicable) after Birth
Family involvement	Bath and feeding class Newborn channel as available Assess mother/baby bonding/interaction Incorporate significant other/siblings in care Support positive parenting behaviors Evaluate mother/parent teaching Encourage significant other's presence during MD visits with mother on infant's progress, current status, and plan formation	Assess mother/baby bonding/interaction Identify community referral needs and refer to community agencies **Expected Outcomes** Demonstrates caring and family incorporation of infant
Date		

also initiates a chemical pneumonitis in the lung with oxygen and carbon dioxide trapping and hyperinflation. Secondary bacterial pneumonias can occur.

Clinical manifestations of MAS include (1) fetal hypoxia in utero a few days or a few minutes prior to birth, indicated by a sudden increase in fetal activity followed by diminished activity, slowing of fetal heart rate or weak and irregular heartbeat, loss of beat-to-beat variability, and meconium staining of amniotic fluid; and (2) presence of signs of distress at birth, such as pallor, cyanosis, apnea, slow heartbeat, and low Apgar scores (below 6) at 1 and 5 minutes. As victims of intrauterine asphyxia, meconium-stained newborns or newborns who have aspirated meconium often have respiratory depression at birth and require resuscitation to establish adequate respiratory effort.

After the initial resuscitation, the severity of clinical symptoms correlates with the extent of aspiration. Many infants require mechanical ventilation at birth due to immediate signs of distress (generalized cyanosis, tachypnea, and severe retractions). An overdistended, barrel-shaped chest with increased anteroposterior diameter is common. Auscultation reveals diminished air movement with prominent rales and rhonchi. Abdominal palpation may reveal a displaced liver caused by diaphragmatic depression resulting from the overexpansion of the lungs. Yellowish staining of the skin, nails, and umbilical cord is usually present.

The chest x-ray film for newborns with MAS reveals nonuniform, coarse, patchy densities and hyperinflation (9- to 11-rib expansion). Evidence of pulmonary air leak is frequently present. These infants have serious biochemical alterations, which include (1) extreme metabolic acidosis resulting from the cardiopulmonary shunting and hypoperfusion; (2) extreme respiratory acidosis due to shunting and alveolar hypoventilation; and (3) extreme hypoxia, even in 100% O_2 concentrations and with ventilatory assistance. The extreme hypoxia is also caused by the cardiopulmonary shunting and resultant failure to oxygenate and can lead to *persistent pulmonary hypertension of the newborn (PPHN).*

Clinical Therapy

The combined efforts of the obstetric and pediatric teams are needed to prevent MAS. The most effective form of preventive management is outlined as follows:

1. After the head of the newborn is born and the shoulders and chest are still in the birth canal, the baby's oropharynx and then the nasopharynx are suctioned. (The same procedure is followed with a cesarean birth.) To decrease the possibility of HIV transmission, low-pressure wall suction is used.
2. If the infant is vigorous and there is thick meconium in the amniotic fluid, the glottis is visualized, and meconium is suctioned from the trachea.
3. If the infant is vigorous and there is only thin meconium in the amniotic fluid, no subsequent special resuscitation is indicated.
4. For any depressed infant (heart rate less than 100 beats per minute or poor respiratory effort with meconium staining), the glottis is visualized and the trachea suctioned (Greenough, 1995).

If the newborn's head is not adequately suctioned on the perineum (at the time the head is born but the shoulder and chest are still in the vagina), respiratory or resuscitative efforts will push meconium into the airway and into the lungs. Stimulation of the newborn should be avoided to minimize respiratory movements. Further resuscitative efforts are undertaken as indicated, following the same principles mentioned in clinical/medical therapy for asphyxia earlier in this chapter. Resuscitated newborns should be immediately transferred to the nursery for closer observation. An umbilical arterial line may be used for direct monitoring of arterial blood pressures; blood sampling for pH and blood gases; and infusion of intravenous fluids, blood, or medications.

Treatment usually involves delivery of high ambient oxygen concentrations and controlled ventilation. Low positive end-expiratory pressures (PEEP) are preferred to avoid air leaks. Unfortunately, high pressures may be needed to cause sufficient expiratory expansion of the obstructed terminal airways or to stabilize airways that are weakened by inflammation so that the most distal atelectatic alveoli are ventilated.

Surfactant replacement therapy is most effective when given as a prophylactic measure. It improves oxygenation and decreases the incidence of air leaks (Findlay, Taeusch, & Walther, 1996). Systemic blood pressure and pulmonary blood flow must be maintained. Dopamine or dobutamine and/or volume expanders may be used to maintain systemic blood pressure.

Full-term newborns over 3.17 kg (7 lb) with respiratory failure who are not responding to conventional ventilator therapy may require treatment with high-frequency ventilation and/or nitric oxide therapy or extracorporeal membrane oxygenation (ECMO). ECMO treatment, a form of heart-lung bypass, has proven successful for newborns with meconium aspiration, pneumonia, and PPHN who are not responding to traditional treatment modalities (Findlay et al, 1996).

Treatment also includes chest physiotherapy (chest percussion, vibration, and drainage) to remove the debris. Prophylactic antibiotics are frequently given. Bicarbonate may be necessary for several days for severely ill newborns. Mortality in term or postterm infants is very high because the cycle of hypoxemia and acidemia is difficult to break.

NURSING CARE MANAGEMENT

Nursing Assessment and Diagnosis

During the intrapartal period, the nurse should observe for signs of fetal hypoxia and meconium staining of amniotic fluid. At birth, the nurse assesses the newborn for signs of distress. During the ongoing assessment of the newborn, the nurse carefully observes for complications such as pulmonary air leaks; anoxic cerebral injury manifested by cerebral edema and/or convulsions; anoxic myocardial injury evidenced by congestive heart failure or cardiomegaly; disseminated intravascular coagulation (DIC) resulting from hypoxic hepatic damage with depression of liver-dependent clotting factors; anoxic renal damage demonstrated by hematuria, oliguria, or anuria; fluid overload; sepsis secondary to bacterial pneumonia; and any signs of intestinal necrosis from ischemia, including gastrointestinal obstruction or hemorrhage.

Nursing diagnoses that may apply to the newborn with meconium aspiration syndrome and the infants' parents include the following:

- ***Ineffective Gas Exchange*** related to aspiration of meconium and amniotic fluid during birth
- ***Altered Nutrition: Less than Body Requirements*** related to respiratory distress and increased energy requirements
- ***Ineffective Family Coping: Compromised*** related to life-threatening illness in a term newborn

Nursing Plan and Implementation

Hospital-Based Nursing Care

Initial interventions are aimed primarily at preventing the aspiration by assisting with the removal of the meconium from the infant's oropharynx and nasopharynx prior to the first extrauterine breath.

When significant aspiration occurs, therapy is supportive with the primary goals of maintaining appropriate gas exchange and minimizing complications. Nursing interventions after resuscitation should include maintaining adequate oxygenation and ventilation, regulating temperature, performing glucose testing by glucometer at 2 hours of age to check for hypoglycemia, observing intravenous fluids, calculating necessary fluids (which may be restricted in the first 48 to 72 hours because of cerebral edema), providing caloric requirements, and monitoring intravenous antibiotic administration.

Evaluation

Expected outcomes of nursing care include the following:

- The risk of MAS is promptly identified, and early intervention is initiated.
- The newborn is free of respiratory distress and metabolic alterations.
- The parents verbalize their concerns about their baby's health problem and survival and understand the rationale behind management of their newborn.

Care of the Newborn with Persistent Pulmonary Hypertension

Persistent pulmonary hypertension of the newborn (PPHN) is a serious disorder that may affect near-term, term, or postterm newborns. It has been called persistent fetal circulation (PFC) because the problems that occur are a result of right-to-left (R-L) shunting of blood away from the lungs and through the fetal ductus arteriosus and patent foramen ovale.

PPHN has been associated with several events causing hypoxemia and acidosis: postmaturity syndrome, RDS, MAS, intrapartal asphyxia, pneumonia, group B streptococcal sepsis, and diaphragmatic hernia. Many fetuses have problems that compromise fetal oxygenation prior to the onset of labor.

Depending on the cause, PPHN is classified as primary or secondary. Primary disease results from pulmonary vascular changes prior to birth, which cause abnormally high pulmonary vascular resistance (PVR). Secondary PPHN occurs when the initial sequences of respiration and change in circulation after birth are interrupted by events that increase the PVR. Hypoxemia and acidosis are the most potent stimulants of pulmonary vasoconstriction. The increased vascular resistance increases pulmonary artery pressure, hypoxemia, and R-L shunting of pulmonary blood across fetal shunts. Once this process has begun, it is self-perpetuating and difficult to interrupt. Clinical deterioration is rapid (DeBoer & Stephens, 1997).

Clinical Therapy

The first goal of medical management is early diagnosis of this disorder to halt the progressive worsening of the R-L shunt. Certain diagnostic tests are often used to evaluate the increased PVR and shunting. Simultaneous preductal and postductal blood gases or pulse oximetry and/or transcutaneous monitoring can be used to demonstrate ductal shunting. The hyperoxia-hyperventilation test is the most definitive test for PPHN. A positive indication of PPHN is when the prehypertension PaO_2 is less than 50 mm Hg and rises to greater than 100 mm Hg with hyperoxia and hyperventilation. The improved oxygenation can be noted clinically if the infant's mucous membranes turn pink. Echocardiography (bubble echo) can demonstrate R-L shunting and a prolonged ratio of right ventricular ejection period to right ventricular ejection time in infants with PPHN.

The goal of therapeutic intervention is to lower the PVR and reverse the process of shunting. Maintaining tissue oxygenation in the presence of R-L shunting presents the greatest therapeutic challenge but is essential to minimize complications.

Ventilatory management is undertaken to decrease the PVR and increase oxygenation. Hyperventilation to achieve respiratory alkalosis (pH >7.55) will cause pulmonary vasodilatation, which increases oxygenation. To prevent respiratory interference and achieve hypocarbia, most infants require paralysis with a neuromuscular blocking agent such as fentanyl. Either respiratory or metabolic alkalosis may decrease pulmonary vascular resistance.

If alkalosis alone does not lead to a decrease in the PVR, pharmacologic vasodilators may be given to decrease pulmonary vascular resistance. In the presence of systemic hypotension, volume expanders such as isotonic crystalloids, albumin, plasma, or packed red cells should be administered. Infusion of vasopressors (such as dopamine, dobutamine, or isoproterenol) and/or afterload reducers (nitroprusside) are also advocated. Vasopressors increase the systemic vascular resistance, thereby decreasing the amount of right-to-left shunting, which increases cardiac output (DeBoer & Stephens, 1997; Merenstein & Gardner, 1998).

Oxygenation, ventilation, and drug therapy efforts continue until the PaO_2 can be consistently maintained greater than 100 mm Hg. Alkalosis and hyperoxia may have to be maintained for several days to avoid a sudden return of hypoxemia and increased PVR. Inhaled nitric oxide and high frequency or oscillatory jet ventilation are also used.

NURSING CARE MANAGEMENT

The nurse assesses for the onset of symptoms, which usually occur in the first 12 to 24 hours of life. Affected newborns exhibit signs of respiratory distress (grunting, nasal flaring, tachypnea), with increased anteroposterior diameter and cyanosis. They typically fail to respond to conventional methods of oxygenation and ventilation. Significant unexplained hypoxemia exists in the absence of congenital heart disease. The chest radiograph might show no evidence of pulmonary parenchymal disease (depending on the underlying disease). The hypoxemia and cyanosis associated with PPHN are characteristic of extreme changeability. Marked, rapid changes in PaO_2 and color are seen with agitation, stimulation, or therapeutic intervention (suctioning).

Infants with PPHN are critically ill and require experienced, highly skilled nurses to provide optimal care with minimal manipulation. Any disturbance may cause agitation, which leads to hypoxemia. If a paralyzing agent is used, nursing care includes monitoring the newborn's response to artificial oxygenation and mechanical ventilation. The nurse ensures that the oxygen is delivered in correct amounts and route and records the percentage of oxygen flow. The ventilator settings are checked frequently and recorded every 2 hours. The nurse carefully suctions the endotracheal tube as necessary while assessing the effect of the procedure on the baby's oxygenation and perfusion. The amount and type of secretions are noted. The nurse carefully assesses arterial blood gases and notifies the clinician if the results are out of the acceptable range. Oxygen monitoring is essential for identifying activities that may compromise the infant's status. (Nursing interventions required for noninvasive oxygen monitoring is discussed in Table 29–2.) Continuous monitoring of vital signs and blood pressure is required, and careful inspection of the skin during positioning is necessary to avoid pressure necrosis.

Pharmacologic vasodilation may lead to precipitous central hypotension, which must be quickly identified and corrected. If tolazoline therapy is used, the infant is monitored for other side effects, such as increased gastric secretion, gastrointestinal bleeding, and oliguria.

Aggressive ventilation poses a potential risk for pneumothorax. The nurse can best prevent complications by advanced preparation and close monitoring for signs of compromise. (See Pneumothorax later in this chapter for appropriate nursing interventions.)

Parent Teaching

Many infants suffering PPHN are born at or near term at a time when parents least expect problems—especially life-threatening problems—to occur. The magnitude of the infant's illness and the rapid deterioration may be overwhelming to parents. The nurse should assess their level of understanding and assist them by providing information about their baby's condition and therapies in easily understandable terms.

Attachment becomes difficult when the infant responds poorly to touching (as seen by decreased PaO_2). Instead, the nurse can encourage parents to talk very softly to their infant because this will usually not compromise the baby's condition. Continuity of nursing care is helpful because it will be less threatening for the parents to relate to a smaller group of nurses.

Evaluation

Expected outcomes of nursing care include the following:

- The risks for development of persistent pulmonary hypertension of the newborn (PPHN) are identified early, and immediate action is taken to minimize the development of sudden, severe illness.
- The newborn is free of respiratory distress and establishes effective respiratory function.
- The parents verbalize their concerns about their baby's illness and understand the rationale behind the management of their newborn. ●

Care of the Newborn with Complications Due to Respiratory Therapy

Oxygen and mechanical ventilation, although required as therapeutic interventions to reduce hypoxia, hypercarbia, ischemia, and infarction to vital organs, may also have harmful effects. The concentrations of ambient oxygen administered to the newborn must be titrated according to oxygen tension within arterial blood in order to avoid development of retinopathy of prematurity. In addition, pulmonary air leaks occur in approximately 15% of mechanically ventilated newborns. But air leaks can be a consequence of injury due to the disease rather than the mechanical ventilation.

Pulmonary Interstitial Emphysema

Pulmonary interstitial emphysema (PIE) is the accumulation of air in lung tissues. Extra-alveolar air collections are most common with use of positive pressure ventilation. Air collections outside the lung are a function of lung compliance and use of increased pressures to ventilate. Overdistention of alveoli may progress to PIE when rupture occurs and air escapes into the interstitial spaces. Air moves along perivascular spaces but not into the pleural space or mediastinum. As the air collections increase, blood vessels are constricted, and blood gas exchange is impaired. This condition is highly associated with subsequent bronchopulmonary dysplasia (BPD). It may also precede pneumothorax or pneumomediastinum.

Pneumothorax

Pneumothorax, a common complication of respiratory therapy, is an accumulation of air in the thoracic cavity between the parietal and visceral pleura. Pneumothorax occurs when alveoli are overdistended, usually by excessive intra-alveolar pressure and rupture; air then leaks into the thoracic cavity.

Pneumothorax in the newborn causes several physiologic changes: collapse of the lung, compression of the heart and lungs, compromise of venous return to the right heart with mediastinal air, and development of tension in the pleural space. Symptoms of pneumothorax include a sudden, unexplained deterioration in the newborn's condition; decreased breath sounds; apnea; bradycardia; cyanosis; increased oxygen requirements; higher PCO_2; decrease in pH; mottled, asymmetric chest expansion; decreased arterial blood pressure; shocklike appearance; and a shift in the apical cardiac impulses to the side opposite the pneumothorax.

Transillumination of the chest is used for rapid evaluation of pneumothorax. Transillumination is the visualization of light through the air in the affected side (or sides, for bilateral pneumothorax) of the baby's chest. However, x-ray examination is the main method of diagnosing this complication (Figure 29–9).

Pneumothorax is a life-threatening situation for the neonate and demands immediate removal of the accumulated air. The thoracentesis procedure is done only as an emergency measure and carries a risk of damaging the lung pleura with needle tracks as the air is evacuated and the collapsed lung reexpands. Only skilled and specifically trained personnel should perform this procedure. For complete resolution of the pneumothorax, a chest tube may be inserted.

Bronchopulmonary Dysplasia

Bronchopulmonary dysplasia (BPD), also called *chronic lung disease of prematurity (CLD),* most commonly occurs in very compromised low-birth-weight (LBW) infants who require oxygen therapy and assisted mechanical ventilation for the treatment of respiratory distress syndrome (Verklan, 1997). It has also been associated with neonatal pneumonia, MAS, PPHN, congenital heart disease (PDA), other congenital anomalies requiring high levels of ventilatory support, and low-grade or asymptomatic pulmonary infection with *Ureaplasma urealyticum.* The cause is multifactorial. The process of BPD is one of continuous lung tissue injury and repair, delaying both lung and body growth.

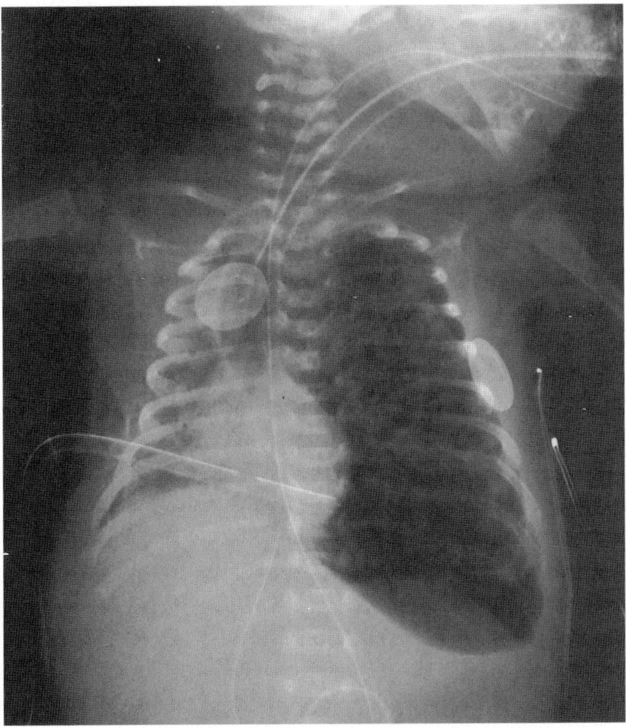

FIGURE 29–9 Chest x-ray of a left-sided pneumothorax. A rupture of the alveolic sacs allows air to leak through the pleura forming collections of air outside the lung (air shows on x-ray as dark area over lung). SOURCE: Courtesy of Carol Harrigan RNC, MSN, NNP.

Clinical Therapy

The goals of therapeutic intervention for the newborn with BPD are to provide adequate oxygenation and ventilation, prevent further lung damage, promote optimal nutrition, and give supportive care to ensure adequate rates of growth and development. New therapies, such as exogenous surfactant administration, high-frequency ventilation, and steroids (prenatal and postnatal) have altered the severity of BPD, but chronic lung disease remains a major clinical problem. Because of the chronic nature of this disease, therapeutic intervention must be individualized to meet the specific needs of the infant. Diuretics and fluid restriction are frequently used to control pulmonary fluid retention and to improve lung function; electrolyte supplements are necessary to offset the results of chronic diuretic therapy (Verklan, 1997). In addition, bronchodilators are indicated to decrease airway resistance and to control bronchospasm. The infant with chronic lung disease is often on long-term steroids. Serial echocardiography is used to monitor cardiac response to the chronic pulmonary disease.

NURSING CARE MANAGEMENT

Hospital-Based Nursing Care

The nurse observes carefully any changes in the newborn's oxygenation, giving special attention to maintaining the prescribed oxygen concentration during all activities, especially during periods of stress, such as when the infant is crying; when blood is drawn; while starting an IV infusion; and during a lumbar puncture (LP), suctioning, chest physiotherapy (CPT), and feeding (Figure 29–10).

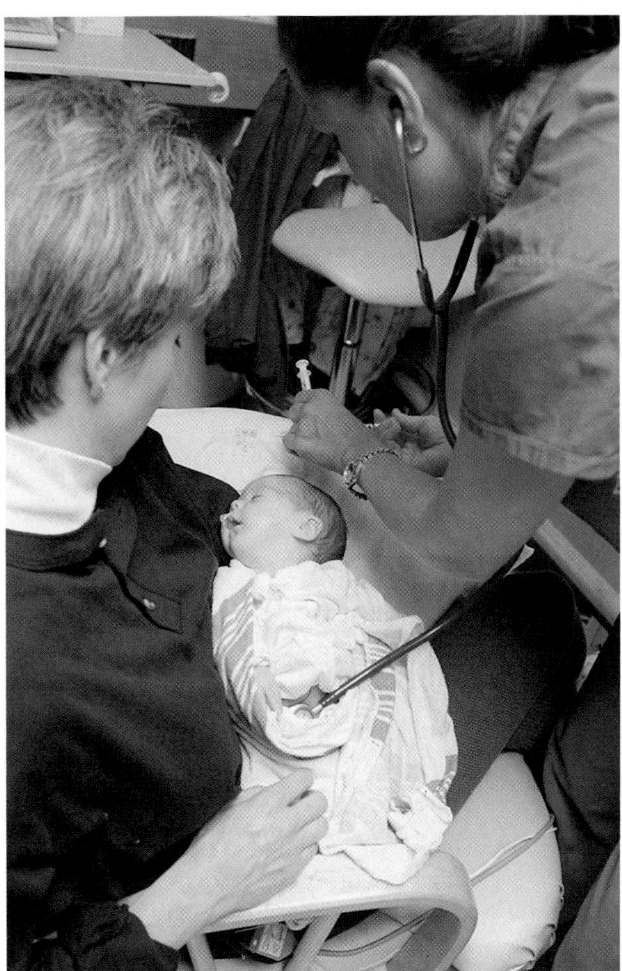

FIGURE 29–10 The baby with BPD has ongoing oxygen and nutritional needs as well as the need for gentle individualized care.

The current goal is to adjust the level of supplemental oxygen to consistently keep O_2 saturations between 92% and 96%, depending on the presence of associated clinical problems such as poor growth, recurrent bradycardia, and pulmonary hypertension (Verklan, 1997). The nurse obtains blood gases based on the institution's chronic blood gas protocol—for example, every 3 days, 20 minutes after a permanent change in ambient oxygen concentration (FiO_2), or more frequently if the infant experiences increasing respiratory distress or increasing lethargy.

Postural drainage, chest physiotherapy (CPT), and vibration followed by suctioning are carried out with close attention to the baby's tolerance. It is essential to time the care activities with rest periods to avoid fatiguing the infant. The nurse maintains the infant's body temperature because hypothermia or hyperthermia will increase oxygen consumption and may increase oxygen requirements. Positioning on the abdomen helps the baby maintain higher transcutaneous oxygen saturation ($TcPo_2$) and improved ventilation.

Bronchodilators such as theophylline, albuterol, and terbutaline; diuretics; steroids; and electrolyte supplements may be used in the clinical management of the BPD infant (Bancalari, 1998). Appropriate timing of administration is essential to maintain adequate blood levels. Many of the electrolyte (hypokalemia) and mineral (fractures) side effects can be avoided by giving the diuretics every other day.

CRITICAL THINKING QUESTION

Why is nutrition a critical therapy in BPD?

Providing for adequate nutrition enhances formation of new alveoli and enlargement of the airway diameter. The nurse helps provide adequate nutrition and monitors the newborn's caloric intake and the energy expended during the feeding process. The more severely ill the baby, the higher the caloric need to meet the greater expenditure of energy for survival and healing. As soon as tolerated, a 24 kcal/oz formula for preterm infants is started, especially if the baby is on fluid restriction. More oxygen may be required during feeding, and the least energy-consuming feeding method should be used. If the feeding schedule is too stressful, smaller, more frequent feedings may be initiated.

Infants with BPD frequently experience negative oral sensations due to suctioning and intubation. These can adversely affect their transition to nipple or spoon feeding. Positioning is often the key to adequate intake and decreasing gastroesophogeal reflux (GER) (Ryan, 1998). In addition, most infants receive numerous, possibly unpalatable, medications with meals. Attempts must be made to include pleasurable activities such as cuddling at mealtime to develop positive associations with appropriate feeding behaviors. Premature infants with BPD frequently require some type of feeding therapy to help them eat successfully.

Infants with BPD are very susceptible to infection, especially if they are on long-term steriods; therefore, it is important to discourage anyone with early signs of infectious disease from having contact with them. The infant's behavior and vital signs should be monitored for changes that might indicate early developing infection. Changes in color, quantity, or quality of pulmonary secretions are noted and reported. The frequency of CPT and suctioning may need to be increased.

Because BPD infants require prolonged hospitalization and/or home care, the nurse should give special attention to formulating a program of early stimulation activities. Psychomotor delays are seen frequently in these infants and are most likely due in part to prolonged exposure to the hospital environment. Because their tolerance level for activity is limited because of their illness, activities must be individualized for each baby. Families need to be included in the plans for their baby.

Community-Based Nursing Care

When the infant develops BPD and the family becomes aware of the implications of chronic illness and prolonged hospitalization, they may experience despair and find it difficult to cope with this added burden. The nurse can help the family cope by encouraging them to take an active role in their infant's daily activities. Their involvement will help dispel feelings of inadequacy and prepare them to perform the unique tasks necessary to meet their infant's needs.

Parents need to be able to demonstrate their ability to provide all the care their child will require at home before leaving the hospital. This may include feeding, adjusting O_2 support, O_2 saturation monitoring, suctioning and airway management, CPT, bathing, and giving medications. They also need to know when to call the home health nurse who is providing care. Parents should be taught how to assess the infant's respiratory condition and understand the BPD baseline respiratory pattern (frequency of respiration, rhythm, degree of retractions, and color of skin and mucous membranes) (Mitchell, 1996). Finally, parents must be taught to evaluate their infant's tolerance of activities and to recognize signs of distress due to poor oxygenation, inadequate ventilation, infection, fluid retention, and bronchospasm.

Care of the Newborn with Cold Stress

Cold stress is excessive heat loss resulting in the use of compensatory mechanisms (such as increased respirations and nonshivering thermogenesis) to maintain core body temperature. Heat loss that results in cold stress occurs in the newborn through the mechanisms of evaporation, convection, conduction, and radiation. (See Chapter 24 for a detailed discussion of thermoregulation.) Heat loss at birth that leads to cold stress can play a significant role in the severity of RDS and the ultimate outcome for the infant.

The amount of heat lost by an infant depends to a large extent on the actions of the nurse or caregiver. Both preterm and SGA newborns are at risk for cold stress because they have decreased adipose tissue, brown fat stores, and glycogen available for metabolism.

As discussed in Chapter 24, the newborn infant's major source of heat production in nonshivering thermogenesis (NST) is brown fat metabolism. The ability of an infant to respond to cold stress by NST is impaired in the presence of several conditions:

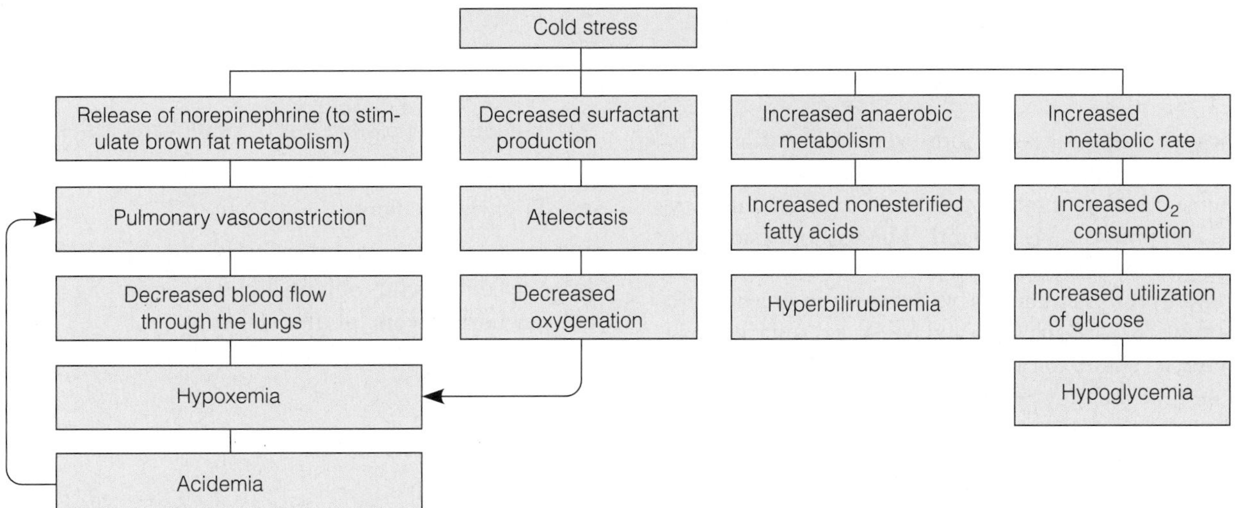

FIGURE 29–11 Cold stress chain of events. The hypothermic, or cold-stressed, newborn attempts to compensate by conserving heat and increasing heat production. These physiologic compensatory mechanisms initiate a series of metabolic events that result in hypoxemia and altered surfactant production, metabolic acidosis, hypoglycemia, and hyperbilirubinemia.

- Hypoxemia (PO_2 less than 50 torr)
- Intracranial hemorrhage or any CNS abnormality
- Hypoglycemia (blood glucose < 40 mg/dL)

When these conditions occur, the infant's temperature should be monitored more closely and the neutral thermal environment conscientiously maintained. It is important for the nurse to recognize these conditions and treat them as soon as possible. The metabolic consequences of cold stress can be devastating and potentially fatal to an infant. Oxygen requirements increase, glucose use increases, acids are released into the bloodstream, and surfactant production decreases. The effects are graphically depicted in Figure 29–11.

CRITICAL THINKING QUESTION

Why are the physiologic alterations associated with cold stress potentially fatal for an infant?

NURSING CARE MANAGEMENT

The nurse observes the baby for signs of cold stress. These include increased movements and respirations, decreased skin temperature and peripheral perfusion, development of hypoglycemia, and possibly development of metabolic acidosis.

Skin temperature assessments are used because initial response to cold stress is vasoconstriction, resulting in a decrease in skin temperature. Therefore, monitoring rectal temperature is not satisfactory. A decrease in rectal temperature means that the infant has long-standing cold stress with decompensation in the newborn's ability to maintain core body temperature.

If a decrease in skin temperature is noted, the nurse determines whether hypoglycemia is present. Hypoglycemia is a result of the metabolic effects of cold stress and is suggested by glucose strip values below 45 mg/mL, tremors, irritability or lethargy, apnea, or seizure activity.

If hypothermia occurs, the following nursing interventions should be initiated ("Neonatal Thermoregulation," 1997):

- Keep the ambient air temperature 1C to 1.5C higher than the infant's temperature.
- Warm the newborn slowly, because rapid temperature elevation may cause hypotension and apnea.
- Increase the air temperature in hourly increments of 1C until infant's temperature is stable.
- Monitor skin temperature every 15 to 30 minutes to determine whether the newborn's temperature is increasing.
- Remove plastic wrap, caps, and heat shields while rewarming the infant so that cool air as well as warm air is not trapped.
- Warm intravenous fluids prior to infusion.
- Initiate efforts to block heat loss by evaporation, radiation, convection, conduction, and maintain the newborn in a neutral thermal environment.

The presence of anaerobic metabolism is assessed and interventions initiated for the resulting metabolic acidosis. Attempts to burn brown fat increase oxygen consumption, lactic acid levels, and metabolic acidosis. Hypoglycemia may be reversed by adequate glucose intake, as described in the following section.

Care of the Newborn with Hypoglycemia

Hypoglycemia in the newborn occurs when their blood glucose level is less than 40 mg/dL (Brooks, 1997). It is the most common metabolic disorder occurring in IDM, SGA, and preterm AGA infants. The pathophysiology of hypoglycemia differs for each classification.

AGA preterm infants have not been in utero a sufficient time to store glycogen and fat. As a result, they have a decreased ability to carry out gluconeogenesis. This situation is further aggravated by increased use of glucose by the tissues (especially the brain and heart) during stress and illness (chilling, asphyxia, sepsis, and RDS).

Infants of White's class A through C or type I diabetic mothers (women with diagnosed or gestational diabetes) have increased stores of glycogen and fat (Chapter 28). Circulating insulin and insulin responsiveness are also higher when compared with other newborns. Because the high glucose loads present in utero stop at birth, the newborn experiences rapid and profound hypoglycemia (Halamek, Benaron, & Stevenson, 1997; Williams, 1997). The SGA infant has used up glycogen and fat stores because of intrauterine malnutrition and has a blunted hepatic enzymatic response with which to produce and use glucose. Any newborn who is stressed at birth (from asphyxia or cold) also quickly uses up available glucose stores and becomes hypoglycemic. Also epidural anesthesia may alter maternal-fetal glucose homeostasis, resulting in hypoglycemia.

Hypoglycemia may also be defined as a glucose oxidase reagent strip below 45 mg/dL, but only when corroborated with laboratory blood glucose (see Procedure 29–1: Performing a Heelstick on a Newborn). Glucose reagent strips should not be used by themselves to screen and diagnose hypoglycemia because their results depend on the baby's hematocrit, and there is a wide variance (5 to 15 mg/dL) when compared to laboratory determinations, especially with blood glucose values of less than 40 to 50 mg/dL (Brooks, 1997). Newer techniques, such as using a glucose oxidase analyzer or an optical bedside glucose analyzer, are more reliable for bedside screening but must also be validated with laboratory chemical analysis. A definitive diagnosis of hypoglycemia is made based on at least two successive values that are significantly low.

Clinical Therapy

The goal of medical management includes early identification of hypoglycemia through observation and screening of newborns at risk. The baby may be asymptomatic, or any of the following may occur:

- Lethargy, jitteriness
- Poor feeding
- Vomiting
- Pallor
- Apnea, irregular respirations, respiratory distress, cyanosis
- Hypotonia, possible loss of swallowing reflex
- Tremors, jerkiness, seizure activity
- High-pitched cry

Differential diagnosis of a newborn with nonspecific hypoglycemic symptoms includes determining whether the newborn has any of the following:

- CNS disease
- Sepsis
- Metabolic aberrations
- Polycythemia
- Congenital heart disease
- Drug withdrawal
- Temperature instability
- Hypocalcemia

Aggressive treatment is recommended after a single low blood glucose value if the infant shows any of these symptoms. In high-risk infants, routine screening should be carried out at 2, 4, 6, 12, 24, and 48 hours of age or whenever any of the noted clinical manifestations appear. Blood glucose sampling techniques and analysis methods can significantly affect the accuracy of the blood glucose value. For example, whole blood glucose concentrations are 15% lower than plasma glucose. The higher the hematocrit, the greater the difference between whole blood and plasma values. Also, venous blood glucose concentrations are approximately 10% to 15% lower than arterial blood glucose concentrations because the glucose has been extracted by the tissues prior to entering the venous system ("Neonatal Hyperglycemia," 1996).

Adequate caloric intake is important. Early breastfeeding or formula feeding is one of the major preventive approaches. If early feeding or intravenous glucose is started to meet the recommended fluid and caloric needs, the blood glucose is likely to remain above the hypoglycemic level. During the first hours after birth, asymptomatic newborns may be given oral glucose, and then another plasma glucose measurement is obtained within 30 to 60 minutes after feeding. Intravenous infusions of a dextrose solution (5% to 10%) begun immediately after birth should prevent hypoglycemia. Plasma glucose levels are obtained when the parenteral infusion is started. However, in the very small AGA infant, infusions of 10% dextrose solution may cause *hyperglycemia* to develop, requiring an alteration in the glucose concentration (Schwartz, 1997). Infants require 6 to 8 mg/kg/minute of glucose to maintain normal glucose concentrations. Therefore an intravenous glucose solution should be calculated based on body weight of the infant and fluid requirements and correlated with blood glucose tests to determine adequacy of the infusion treatment.

PROCEDURE 29–1 PERFORMING A HEELSTICK ON A NEWBORN

Nursing Action	*Rationale*
Objective: Assemble the equipment.	*Equipment organization facilitates the procedure.*
• Microlancet (do not use a needle)	*A needle may nick the periosteum.*
• Alcohol swabs	
• 2 × 2 sterile gauze squares	
• Small bandage	
• Transfer pipette	
• Glucose reagent strips or reflectance meters	
• Gloves	*Gloves are used to implement universal precautions and prevent nosocomial infections.*
Objective: Prepare the infant's heel for the procedure.	
• Use a warm wet wrap or specially designed chemical heat pad to warm the infant's heel for 5–10 seconds to facilitate blood flow.	
• Select a clear, previously unpunctured site.	*The selection of a previously unpunctured site minimizes the risk of infection and excessive scar formation.*
• Clean the site by rubbing vigorously with 70% isopropyl alcohol swab, followed by a dry gauze square.	*Friction produces local heat, which aids vasodilation.*
• Blot the site dry completely before lancing.	*Alcohol is irritating to injured tissue and it may also produce hemolysis.*
Objective: Lance the infant's heel and ensure accurate blood sampling. See the step-by-step instructions below.	
Objective: Prevent excessive bleeding.	
• Apply a folded gauze square to the puncture site and secure it firmly with a bandage.	
• Check the puncture site frequently for the first hour after sampling.	
Objective: Record the findings on the infant's chart.	
Report immediately any results under 45 mg/dL or over 175 mg/dL for glucose.	*Recording the results helps identify possible complications.*

Performing the Heelstick

The infant's lateral heel is the site of choice because it precludes damaging the posterior tibial nerve and artery, plantar artery, and the important longitudinally oriented fat pad of the heel, which in later years could impede walking (Figure 29–12). This is especially important for infants undergoing multiple heel stick procedures. Toes are acceptable sites if necessary.

Lancing the Heel

- Grasp the infant's lower leg and foot so as to impede venous return slightly. This will facilitate extraction of the blood sample.
- With a quick, piercing motion, puncture the lateral heel with a microlancet. Be careful not to puncture too deeply. Optimal penetration is 4 mm (Figure 29–13).

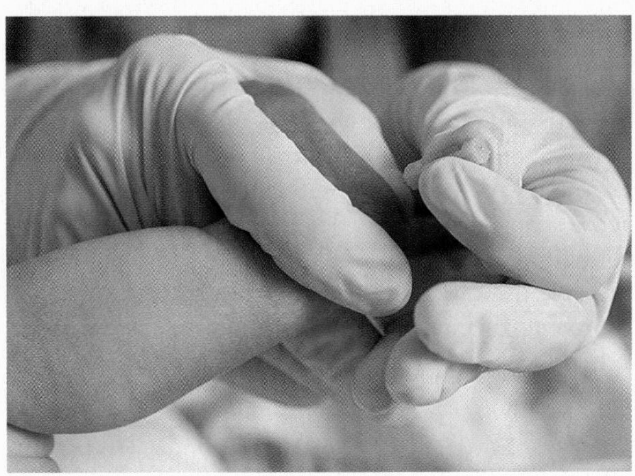

FIGURE 29–12 Heel stick.

Collecting the Blood Sample

- Use transfer pipette to place drop of blood on glucose reflectance meter.
- Use capillary tube for hematocrit testing.

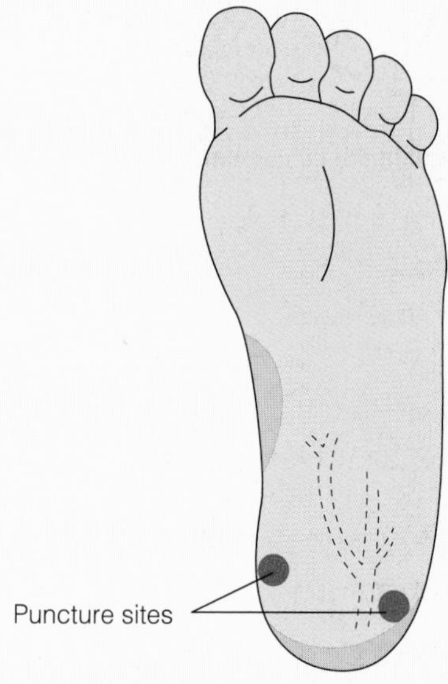

FIGURE 29–13 Potential sites for heel sticks. Avoid shaded areas in order to avoid injury to arteries and nerves in the foot.

A rapid infusion of 25% to 50% dextrose is contraindicated because it may lead to profound rebound hypoglycemia following an initial brief increase. In more severe cases of hypoglycemia, corticosteroids may be administered. It is thought that steroids enhance gluconeogenesis from noncarbohydrate protein sources (Brooks, 1997).

The prognosis for untreated hypoglycemia is poor. It may result in permanent, untreatable CNS damage or death.

NURSING CARE MANAGEMENT

Nursing Assessment and Diagnosis

The objective of nursing assessment is to identify newborns at risk and to screen symptomatic infants. For newborns who are diagnosed with hypoglycemia, assessment is ongoing with careful monitoring of glucose values. Glucose strips, urine dipsticks, and urine volume (monitor only if above 1 to 3 mL/kg/hour) are evaluated frequently for osmotic diuresis and glycosuria.

Nursing diagnoses that may apply to the newborn with hypoglycemia include the following:

- ***Altered Nutrition: Less than Body Requirements*** related to increased glucose use secondary to physiologic stress
- ***Ineffective Breathing Pattern*** related to tachypnea and apnea
- ***Pain*** related to frequent heel sticks for glucose monitoring

Nursing Plan and Implementation

When caring for a preterm AGA infant, the nurse should monitor blood glucose levels using glucose strips or laboratory determinations every 4 to 8 hours for the first day of life and daily or as necessary thereafter. The IDM should be monitored hourly for the first several hours after birth because it is at this time that precipitous falls in glucose are most likely. In the SGA newborn, symptoms usually appear between 24 and 72 hours of age; occasionally, they may begin as early as 3 hours of age. Infants who are below the 10th percentile on the intrauterine growth curve should have blood sugar assessments at least every 8 hours until 4 days of age or more frequently if any symptoms develop. Once an infant's blood sugar is stable, glucose testing every 2 to 4 hours, or prior to feedings, adequately monitors glucose levels (Brooks, 1997).

Calculating glucose requirements and maintaining intravenous glucose will be necessary for any symptomatic infant with low serum glucose levels. Careful attention to glucose monitoring is again required when the transition from intravenous to oral feedings is attempted. Titration of intravenous glucose may be required until the infant is able to take adequate amounts of formula or breast milk to maintain a normal blood sugar level. This titration is accomplished by decreasing the concentration of parenteral glucose gradually to 5%, then reducing the rate of infusion to 6 mg/kg/minute, then to 4 mg/kg/minute, and slowly discontinuing it over 4 to 6 hours.

The method of feeding greatly influences glucose and energy requirements. In addition, the therapeutic nursing measure of nonnutritive sucking during gavage feedings has been reported to increase the baby's daily weight gain and lead to earlier bottle-feeding or breast-feeding and discharge. Nonnutritive sucking may also lower activity levels, which allows newborns to conserve their energy stores. Activity can increase energy requirements; crying alone can double the baby's metabolic rate. Establishment and maintenance of a neutral thermal environment has a potent influence on the newborn's metabolism. The nurse pays careful attention to environmental conditions, physical activity, and organization of care and integrates these factors into delivery of nursing care. The nurse identifies any discrepancies between the baby's caloric requirements and received calories and weighs the newborn daily at consistent times, preferably before a feeding. Only then can findings of unusual weight losses or gains, as well as the pattern of weight gain, be considered reliable.

Evaluation

Expected outcomes of nursing care include the following:

- The risk of hypoglycemia is promptly identified, and intervention is started early.
- The newborn's metabolic and physiologic processes are stabilized; recovery proceeds without sequelae.

RESEARCH IN PRACTICE

What is this study about? Interpretations of pain in newborns, especially those in NICUs, is different because evidence of pain is often assessed based on the patient's ability to verbalize the degree of pain. Compounding this problem of pain assessment in the newborn is the lack of valid and reliable pain assessment tools for the preterm and term newborn. The purpose of this descriptive study was to identify the indicators used by neonatal nurses in interpreting the pain experienced by newborns in the NICU.

How was this study done? Neonatal nurses were recruited and asked to complete a structured questionnaire that identified the physiologic and behavioral indicators used by them to interpret the pain experience of their infants. A sample of 72 NICU nurses completed the questionnaire.

What were the results of the study? Ten pain indicators were used by more than 50% of the neonatal nurses in this study. These indicators included in decreasing order of frequency: (1) fussiness, (2) restlessness, (3) grimacing, (4) crying, (5) increasing heart rate, (6) increasing respirations, (7) wiggling, (8) rapid state change, (9) wrinkling of forehead, and (10) clenching of fists.

What additional questions might I have? (1) How are these physiologic and behavioral indicators used to determine the management of the newborn's pain and (2) Does a pain instrument exist for neonates that includes these physiologic and behavioral indicators?

How can I use this study? Recognition and interpretation of neonatal pain indicators is dependent on the caretaker's sensitivity to the behavioral and physiologic cues of the newborn. This study suggests that neonatal nurses interpret newborn pain using behavioral and physiologic cues. Establishing an increased awareness of newborn pain during daily care is critical. This study provides some important clues used by nurses to assess pain in newborns.

SOURCE: Howard, V. & Thurber, F. (1998). The interpretation of infant pain: Physiological and behavioral indicators used by NICU nurses. **Journal of Pediatric Nursing, 13(3), 164–174.**

Care of the Newborn with Jaundice

The most common abnormal physical finding in newborns is **jaundice** (icterus neonatorium). Jaundice develops from the deposit of yellow pigment *bilirubin* in lipid tissues, as described in Chapter 24. Fetal unconjugated bilirubin is normally cleared by the placenta in utero, so total bilirubin at birth is usually less than 3 mg/dL unless an abnormal hemolytic process has been present. Postnatally, the infant must conjugate bilirubin (convert a lipid-soluble pigment into a water-soluble pigment) in the liver.

The rate and amount of conjugation of bilirubin depend on the rate of hemolysis, the bilirubin load, the maturity of the liver, and the presence of albumin-binding sites. See Chapter 24 for discussion of conjugation of bilirubin. A normal, healthy, full-term infant's liver is usually mature enough and producing enough glucuronyl transferase that the total serum bilirubin concentration does not reach a pathologic level. However, physiologic jaundice remains a common problem for the term newborn and may require treatment with phototherapy. Physiologic jaundice is due to the newborn's shorter red cell life span, slower uptake by the liver, lack of intestinal bacteria, and poorly established hydration.

Pathophysiology

Serum albumin-binding sites are usually sufficient to meet the normal demands. However, certain conditions tend to decrease the sites available. Fetal or neonatal asphyxia decreases the binding affinity of bilirubin to albumin, as acidosis impairs the capacity of albumin to hold bilirubin. Hypothermia and hypoglycemia release free fatty acids that dislocate bilirubin from albumin. Also, premature infants have less albumin available for binding with bilirubin.

Although the exact mechanism of bilirubin-produced neuronal injury is uncertain, it is known that high concentrations of unconjugated bilirubin can be neurotoxic. Unconjugated bilirubin has a high affinity for extravascular tissue, such as fatty tissue (subcutaneous tissue) and the brain. Various conditions decrease albumin binding, including hypothermia, hypoglycemia, asphyxia, and neonatal medications such as indomethacin. Maternal use of sulfa drugs or salicylates interferes with conjugation or with serum albumin binding sites by competing with bilirubin for these sites. Bilirubin not bound to albumin then can cross the blood-brain barrier, damage cells of the CNS, and produce kernicterus or bilirubin encephalopathy (Bratlid, 1996). **Kernicterus** (meaning "yellow nucleus") usually refers to the deposition of unconjugated bilirubin in the basal ganglia of the brain and to permanent neurologic sequelae of untreated hyperbilirubinemia. The classic bilirubin encephalopathy of kernicterus most commonly found with Rh and ABO blood group incompatibility is less common today because of aggressive treatment with phototherapy and exchange transfusions. But cases of kernicterus are reappearing as a result of early discharge and the increase incidence of dehydration (a result of discharge before mother's milk is established). Current therapy can reduce the incidence of kernicterus encephalopathy but cannot distinguish all infants who are at risk.

Causes of Hyperbilirubinemia

A primary cause of **hyperbilirubinemia** is **hemolytic disease of the newborn** secondary to Rh incompatibility. All pregnant women who are Rh negative or who have blood type O (possible ABO incompatibility) should be asked about outcomes of any previous pregnancies, including abortions, and their history of blood transfusion. Prenatal amniocentesis with spectrophotographic examination may be indicated in some cases. Cord blood from newborns is evaluated for bilirubin level, which normally does not exceed 5 mg/dL. Newborns of Rh negative and O blood type mothers are carefully assessed for blood type status, appearance of jaundice, and levels of serum bilirubin.

Isoimmune hemolytic disease, also known as **erythroblastosis fetalis,** occurs when an Rh negative mother is pregnant with an Rh positive fetus and transplacental passage of maternal antibodies takes place. Maternal antibodies enter the fetal circulation, then attach to and destroy the fetal RBCs. The fetal system responds by increasing red blood cell production. Jaundice, anemia, and compensatory erythropoiesis result. A marked increase in immature red blood cells (erythroblasts) also occurs, hence the designation erythroblastosis fetalis.

Hydrops fetalis, the most severe form of erythroblastosis fetalis, occurs when maternal antibodies attach to the Rh site on the fetal red blood cells, making them susceptible to destruction. The fetal system responds by increased production of immature red blood cells that do not have the functional capabilities of mature cells and cause multiple organ system failure.

If anemia is severe, as seen in hydrops fetalis, cardiomegaly with severe cardiac decompensation and hepatosplenomegaly occur. Severe generalized massive edema (anasarca) and generalized fluid effusion into the pleural cavity (hydrothorax), pericardial sac, and peritoneal cavity (ascites) develop. Jaundice is not present until the newborn period because the bilirubin pigments for the fetus are being excreted through the placenta into the maternal circulation. The hydropic hemolytic disease process is also characterized by hyperplasia of the adrenal cortex and pancreatic islets, which predisposes the infant to neonatal hypoglycemia similar to that of IDMs. These infants also have increased bleeding tendencies due to associated thrombocytopenia and hypoxic damage to the capillaries. Hydrops is a frequent cause of intrauterine death among infants with Rh disease.

ABO incompatibility (the mother is blood type O and the baby is blood type A or B) may result in jaundice, although it rarely results in hemolytic disease severe enough to be clinically diagnosed and treated. Hepatosplenomegaly may be found occasionally in newborns with ABO incompatibility, but hydrops fetalis and stillbirth are rare.

Certain prenatal and perinatal factors predispose the newborn to hyperbilirubinemia. During pregnancy, maternal conditions that predispose to neonatal hyperbilirubinemia include hereditary spherocytosis, diabetes, intrauterine infections, gram-negative bacilli infections that stimulate production of maternal isoimmune antibodies, drug ingestion (such as sulfas, salicylates, novobiocin, and diazepam), and oxytocin.

In addition to Rh or ABO incompatibility, other newborn conditions predispose to hyperbilirubinemia: polycythemia (central hematocrit 65% or more), pyloric stenosis, obstruction or atresia of the biliary duct or of the lower bowel, low-grade urinary tract infection, sepsis, hypothyroidism, enclosed hemorrhage (cephalhematoma, extensive bruising), asphyxia neonatorum, hypothermia, acidemia, and hypoglycemia. Neonatal hepatitis, atresia of the bile ducts, and gastrointestinal atresia all can alter bilirubin metabolism and excretion.

Abnormal red cell shape is another hemolytic cause of hyperbilirubinemia because these cells may have abnormal, less deformable cell membranes and a shorter than normal life span. Other factors such as enzyme deficiency and drug effects may also produce hemolysis. Newborns with congenital biliary duct atresia have a poor prognosis; for some, a liver transplant is now an option.

The prognosis for a newborn with hyperbilirubinemia depends on the extent of the hemolytic process and the underlying cause. Severe hemolytic disease may result in fetal or early neonatal death from the effects of anemia—cardiac decompensation, edema, ascites, and hydrothorax. Hyperbilirubinemia may lead to kernicterus. The resultant neurologic damage may be responsible for cerebral palsy, mental retardation, sensory difficulties, or, to a lesser degree, perceptual impairment, delayed speech development, hyperactivity, muscle incoordination, or learning difficulties.

Clinical Therapy

The best treatment for hemolytic disease is prevention. Prenatal identification of the fetus at risk for Rh or ABO incompatibility will allow prompt treatment. See Chapter 16 for discussion of in utero management of this condition.

When one or more of the predisposing factors are present, the maternal and neonatal blood types should be tested in the laboratory for Rh or ABO incompatibility. Other necessary laboratory evaluations include Coombs' test, serum bilirubin levels (direct and total), hemoglobin, reticulocyte percentage, white blood cell count, and positive smear for cellular morphology.

Neonatal hyperbilirubinemia must be considered pathologic if any of the following criteria are met (Bland, 1996):

1. Clinically evident jaundice in the first 24 hours of life, or after the fourth day of life, unless infant is a premature infant
2. Serum bilirubin concentration rising by more than 5 mg/dL per day
3. Total serum bilirubin concentrations exceeding 12.9 mg/dL in term infants or 15 mg/dL in preterm babies (because preterm newborns have less subcutaneous fat, bilirubin may reach higher levels before it is visible)
4. Conjugated bilirubin concentrations greater than 2 mg/dL
5. Persistence of clinical jaundice beyond 7 days in term infants or beyond 14 days in preterm infants

Initial diagnostic procedures are aimed at differentiating jaundice resulting from increased bilirubin production, impaired conjugation or excretion, increased intestinal reabsorption, or a combination of these factors. Coombs' test is performed to determine whether jaundice is due to Rh or ABO incompatibility.

If the hemolytic process is due to Rh sensitization, laboratory findings reveal the following: (1) an Rh positive newborn with a positive Coombs' test, (2) increased erythropoiesis with many immature circulating red blood cells (nucleated blastocysts), (3) anemia, in most cases, (4) elevated levels (5 mg/dL or more) of bilirubin in cord blood, and (5) a reduction in albumin-binding capacity. Maternal data may include an elevated anti-Rh titer and spectrophotometric evidence of fetal hemolytic process.

The indirect Coombs' test measures the amount of Rh positive antibodies in the mother's blood. Rh positive red blood cells are added to the maternal blood sample. If the mother's serum contains antibodies, the Rh positive red blood cells will agglutinate (clump) when rabbit immune antiglobulin is added, and the test results are labeled positive.

The direct Coombs' test reveals the presence of antibody-coated (sensitized) Rh positive red blood cells in the newborn. Rabbit immune antiglobulin is added to the specimen of neonatal blood cells. If the neonatal red blood cells agglutinate, they have been coated with maternal antibodies, a positive result.

If the hemolytic process is due to ABO incompatibility, laboratory findings reveal an increase in recticulocytes. The resulting anemia is usually not significant during the newborn period and is rare later on. The direct Coombs' test may be negative or mildly positive; the indirect Coombs' test may be strongly positive. Infants with a positive direct Coombs' test have increased incidence of jaundice with bilirubin levels in excess of 10 mg/dL. Increased numbers of spherocytes (spherical, plump, mature erythrocytes) are seen on a peripheral blood smear. Increased numbers of spherocytes are not seen on smears from Rh disease infants.

Regardless of the cause of hyperbilirubinemia, management of these infants is directed toward alleviating anemia, removing maternal antibodies and sensitized erythrocytes, increasing serum albumin levels, reducing serum bilirubin levels, and minimizing the consequences of hyperbilirubinemia.

Early discharge of newborns from birthing centers has significantly influenced the diagnosis and management of neonatal jaundice, increasing the emphasis on outpatient and home care management.

Therapeutic methods of management of hyperbilirubinemia include phototherapy, exchange transfusion, infusion of albumin, and drug therapy. If hemolytic disease is present, it may be treated by phototherapy, exchange transfusion, and drug therapy. When determining the appropriate management of hyperbilirubinemia due to hemolytic disease, the three variables that must be taken into account are the newborn's (1) serum bilirubin level, (2) birth weight, and (3) age in hours. If a newborn has hemolysis with an unconjugated bilirubin level of 14 mg/dL, weighs less than 2500 g (birth weight), and is 24 hours old or less, an exchange transfusion may be the best management. However, if that same newborn is over 24 hours old, which is past the time where an increase in bilirubin would occur due to pathologic causes, phototherapy may be the treatment of choice to prevent the possible complications of kernicterus.

Phototherapy

Phototherapy is the exposure of the newborn to high-intensity light. It may be used alone or in conjunction with exchange transfusion to reduce serum bilirubin levels. Exposure of the newborn to high-intensity light (fluorescent light bulbs or bulbs in the blue-light spectrum) decreases serum bilirubin levels in the skin by facilitating

TABLE 29–3 American Academy of Pediatrics Guidelines for the Management of Hyperbilirubinemia in the Healthy Term Newborn

	Total Serum Bilirubin Level, mg/dL (μmol/L)			
Age (hours)	**Consider Phototherapy°**	**Phototherapy**	**Exchange Transfusion if Intensive Phototherapy Fails†**	**Exchange Transfusion and Intensive Phototherapy**
25–48‡	≥12 (170)	≥15 (260)	≥20 (340)	≥25 (430)
49–72	≥15 (260)	≥18 (310)	≥25 (430)	≥30 (510)
>72	≥17 (290)	≥20 (340)	≥25 (430)	≥30 (510)

°Phototherapy at these total serum bilirubin (TSB) levels is a clinical option, meaning that the intervention is available and may be used on the basis of individual clinical judgment.

†Intensive phototherapy should produce a decline of TSB of 1 to 2 mg/dL within 4 to 6 hours, and the TSB level should continue to decline and remain below the threshold level for exchange transfusion. If this does not occur, phototherapy has failed. Intensive phototherapy includes the use of more than one bank of lamps containing "special blue" bulbs, maximizing the surface area illuminated by using a phototherapy blanket or other means, and providing phototherapy on a continuous, noninterrupted schedule.

‡Term infants who are clinically jaundiced at ≤24 hours old are not considered healthy and require further evaluation.

SOURCE: Used with permission of the American Academy of Pediatrics: Practice parameter: Management of hyperbilirubinemia in the healthy term newborn. **Pediatrics** 94:560, 1994.

biliary excretion of unconjugated bilirubin. This occurs when light absorbed by the tissue converts unconjugated bilirubin into two isomers called photobilirubin. The photobilirubin moves from the tissues to the blood by a diffusion mechanism. In the blood it is bound to albumin and transported to the liver. It moves into the bile and is excreted into the duodenum for removal with feces without requiring conjugation by the liver. In addition, the photodegradation products formed when light oxidizes bilirubin can be excreted in the urine.

Phototherapy plays an important role in preventing a rise in bilirubin levels but does not alter the underlying cause of jaundice, and hemolysis may continue to produce anemia. Currently, there is no evidence that healthy term infants without a pathologic cause for the jaundice are at risk for brain damage, even at levels in the 20 to 24 mg/dL range (Newman & Maisels, 1992).

It is generally accepted that phototherapy should be started at 4 to 5 mg/dL below the calculated exchange level for each infant. Sick newborns of less than 1000 g should have phototherapy instituted at a bilirubin concentration of 5 mg/dL. Many authors have recommended initiating phototherapy "prophylactically" in the first 24 hours of life in high-risk, very-low-birth-weight infants (Dennery, Rhine, & Stevenson, 1995). Sick preterm infants who are at least 1500 g should have phototherapy instituted when the bilirubin level is 10 mg/dL. Any newborn with a bilirubin level of 20 mg/dL or above may need an exchange transfusion if illness or associated conditions are present (Dennery et al, 1995) (Table 29–3).

Phototherapy can be provided through conventional banks of phototherapy lights or by a fiber-optic blanket attached to a halogen light source around the trunk of the newborn or a combination of both delivery methods (American Academy of Pediatrics [AAP], 1994). With the fiber-optic blanket, the light stays on at all times, and the newborn is accessible for care, feeding, and diaper changes. The eyes are not covered. Fluid and weight loss are not complications of this system. Furthermore, it makes the infant accessible to the parents and is less alarming to parents than standard phototherapy (Thureen, Deacon, O'Neill, & Hernandez, 1999). Many institutions and pediatricians use fiber-optic blankets for home care. A combination of a fiber-optic light source in the mattress under the baby and a standard light source above has been recommended (MacMahon, Stevenson, & Oski, 1998).

Exchange Transfusion

Exchange transfusion is the withdrawal and replacement of the newborn's blood with donor blood. It is used to treat anemia with red blood cells that are not susceptible to maternal antibodies, remove sensitized red blood cells that would be lysed soon, remove serum bilirubin, and provide bilirubin-free albumin and increase the binding sites for bilirubin. Concerns over doing an exchange transfusion are related to the use of blood products and associated potential for HIV infection and hepatitis.

NURSING CARE MANAGEMENT

Nursing Assessment and Diagnosis

Assessment is aimed at identifying prenatal and perinatal factors that predispose to development of jaundice and identifying jaundice as soon as it is apparent. Clinically, ABO incompatibility presents as jaundice and occasionally as hepatosplenomegaly. Fetal hydrops or erythoblastosis fetalis is rare (see Chapter 16). Hemolytic disease of the newborn is suspected if the placenta is enlarged, if the newborn is edematous with pleural and pericardial effusion plus ascites, if pallor or jaundice is noted during the first 24 to 36 hours, if hemolytic anemia is diagnosed, or if the spleen and liver are enlarged. The nurse carefully notes changes in behavior and observes for evidence of bleeding. If laboratory tests indicate elevated bilirubin levels, the nurse checks the newborn for jaundice about every 2 hours and records observations.

To check for jaundice in lighter-skinned babies, the nurse should blanch the skin over a bony prominence (forehead, nose, or sternum) by pressing firmly with the thumb. After pressure is released, if jaundice is present, the area appears yellow before normal color returns. The nurse should check oral mucosa and the posterior portion of the hard palate and conjunctival sacs for yellow pigmentation in darker-skinned babies. Assessment in daylight gives best results, because pink walls and surroundings may mask yellowish tints and yellow light makes differentiation of jaundice difficult. The time of onset of jaundice is recorded and reported. If jaundice appears, careful observation of the increase in depth of color and the infant's behavior is mandatory.

The newborn's behavior is assessed for neurologic signs associated with hyperbilirubinemia, which are rare but may include hypotonia, diminished reflexes, lethargy, seizures, or opisthotonic posturing.

Nursing diagnoses that may apply to a newborn with jaundice include the following:

- ***Fluid Volume Deficit*** related to increased insensible water loss and frequent loose stools
- ***Risk for Injury*** related to use of phototherapy
- ***Sensory/Perceptual Alterations*** related to neurologic damage secondary to kernicterus
- ***Risk for Altered Parenting*** related to parenting a newborn with jaundice

Nursing Plan and Implementation

Hospital-Based Nursing Care

Hospital-based care is described in the Critical Pathway for Care of a Newborn with Hyperbilirubinemia on page 892. Ideally, the entire skin surface of the newborn is exposed to the light. Minimal covering may be applied over the genitals and buttocks to expose maximum skin surface while still protecting the bedding from soiling. Phototherapy success is measured every 12 hours or daily by serum bilirubin levels. The lights must be turned off while drawing blood for serum bilirubin levels. Because it is not known whether phototherapy injures the delicate eye structures, particularly the retina, the nurse applies eye patches over the newborn's closed eyes during exposure to banks of phototherapy lights (Figure 29–14). Phototherapy is discontinued and the eye patches are removed at least once per shift to assess the eyes for the presence of conjunctivitis. Patches are also removed to allow eye contact during feeding (for social stimulation) or when parents are visiting (to promote parental attachment).

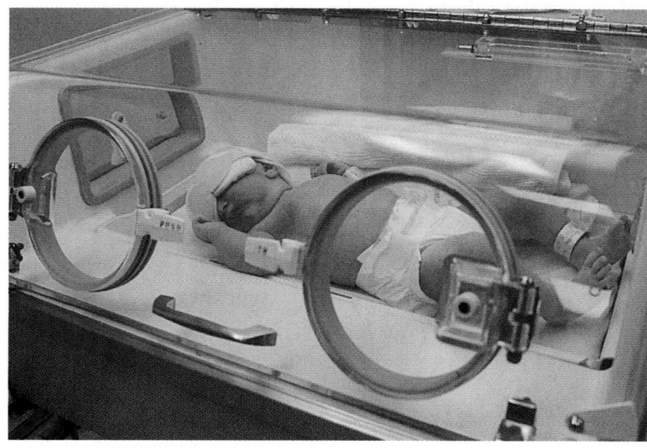

FIGURE 29–14 Infant receiving phototherapy. The phototherapy light is positioned over the incubator. Bilateral eye patches are always used during phototherapy to protect the baby's eyes.

The irradiance level at the skin determines the effectiveness of the phototherapy. The standard desired level of irradiance is 5 to 6 microwatts per square centimeter per nanometer, whereas superphoto therapy delivers 50 to 60 microwatts. Most phototherapy units will provide this level of irradiance 42 to 45 cm below the lamps. Irradiance levels can be increased slightly as indicated. The nurse can use a photometer to measure and maintain desired levels.

The newborn's temperature is monitored to prevent hyperthermia or hypothermia. The newborn will require additional fluids to compensate for the increased water loss through the skin and loose stools. Loose stools and increased urine output are the results of increased bilirubin excretion. The infant is observed for signs of dehydration and perianal excoriation.

A benign transient bronze discoloration of the skin may occur with phototherapy when the infant has elevated direct serum bilirubin levels or liver disease. As a side effect of phototherapy, some newborns develop a maculopapular rash. In addition to assessing the newborn's skin color for jaundice and bronzing, the nurse examines the skin for developing pressure areas. The newborn should be repositioned at least every 2 hours to permit the light to reach all skin surfaces, to prevent pressure areas, and to vary the stimulation to the infant. The nurse keeps track of the number of hours each lamp is used so that each can be replaced before its effectiveness is lost. The nurse must be careful about using ointment under bilirubin lights because they may cause burns.

The terms *jaundice*, *hyperbilirubinemia*, *exchange transfusion*, and *phototherapy* may sound frightening and threatening. Some parents may feel guilty about their baby's condition and think they have caused the problem. Under stress, parents may not be able to understand the physician/nurse practitioner's first explanations. The

CRITICAL PATHWAY FOR CARE OF A NEWBORN WITH HYPERBILIRUBINEMIA

Category	Day 1	Day 2/Discharge
Referral	Refer to lactation consultant	**Expected Outcomes** Consults completed
Assessments	Lab work (CBC, Rh, Coombs'-direct, retic count, bilirubin level, both direct and indirect) Baer hearing test if bilirubin > 18 Obtain maternal/paternal history Obtain birth and newborn history Assess sclera and skin color for jaundice; assess mucous membranes for jaundice with dark pigmented skin Continue routine newborn assessments (See Newborn Critical Pathway pp. 754 to 755)	Bilirubin levels as ordered BID Assess for s/s of dehydration Assess sclera and skin color for progression of jaundice **Expected Outcomes** Physical assessments, VS WNL; skin/mucous membranes pink, sclera clear of jaundice color; laboratory work WNL, total bilirubin level stabilized or decreasing
Teaching/ psychosocial	Evaluate additional psychosocial needs of parents/family Orient family to nursery, equipment, patient room if rooming-in Instruct parents on s/s of hyperbilirubinemia (slight lethargy, irritability) Discuss possible side effects of phototherapy (stool character changes, increased fluid loss, temp changes, rash, altered sleep/wake patterns) Instruct parents on care and treatment of hyperbilirubinemia: • Phototherapy rationale, indications and precautions • Placement of bili mask over closed eyes • Lab draws; rationale, frequency • Accurate intake and output to monitor for s/s dehydration Review cord care, skin care, care of genitalia (circumcision care as applicable) Review role of pumping breasts if necessary and offering formula for limited period of time	Teach/encourage parents to provide cuddling, tactile stimulation and eye contact during diaper changes and feedings, talk to baby frequently Reinforce previous teaching; evaluate parental comprehension Provide opportunities for parents to express concerns/feelings **Expected Outcomes** Parents verbalize comprehension of care of infant with hyperbilirubinemia and potential sequelae of no treatment; parents verbalize comprehension of the risks/benefits of phototherapy as treatment; parents demonstrate developmentally appropriate care for infant during diaper changes and feedings; parents verbalize concerns, ask appropriate questions prn
Nursing care management and reports	Vital signs q4h with axillary temps Monitor thermoregulation Daily wt Initiate phototherapy as indicated and ordered • Maintain bili mask over eyes • Keep genitalia covered per policy • Check eyes for discharge, excessive pressure, corneal abrasions • Expose as much skin surface as possible to bili lights • Bilimeter reading q shift • No lotion or ointment on infant skin • Turn bili lights off during lab draws Continue infant assessments including: • Note and document skin color q shift • Thorough skin care with diaper changes; note s/s breakdown, rash • Assess neuro status for s/s abnormality q interaction (hypotonia, lethargy, poor sucking reflex)	VS q4h with axillary temps Monitor thermoregulation, maintain NTE Daily wt Continue phototherapy as indicated • Maintain bili mask over eyes • Cover genitalia per policy • Check eyes for discharge, conjunctivitis, corneal abrasions • Expose as much skin surface as possible to bili lights • Bilimeter reading q shift • No lotion or ointment on infant skin • Turn bili lights off during lab draws Continue infant assessments as per Day 1 **Expected Outcomes** VS WNL; wt stabilized or gaining wt; no s/s kernicterus; skin integrity intact; skin and mucous membranes pink; eyes without drainage, sclera clear; labs WNL with stabilized or decreasing bilirubin level

nurse must expect that the parents will need explanations repeated and clarified and that they may need help voicing their questions and fears. Eye and tactile contact with the infant is encouraged. The nurse can coach parents when they visit with the baby. After the mother's discharge, parents are kept informed of their infant's condition and are encouraged to return to the hospital or telephone at any time so that they can be fully involved in the care of their infant.

While the mother is still hospitalized, phototherapy can also be carried out in the mother's room if the only problem is hyperbilirubinemia. The mother must be willing to keep the baby in the room for 24 hours a day, be able to take emergency action, as for choking, if necessary, and complete instruction checklists. Some institutions require that parents sign a consent form. The nurse gives the instructions to the parents but also continues to monitor the infant's temperature, activity, intake and out-

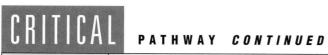

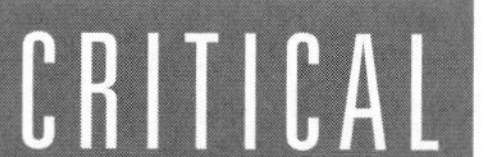

PATHWAY *CONTINUED*

Category	Day 1	Day 2/Discharge
Activity and comfort	Nest in open crib if infant able to maintain temp beneath bili lights Isolette if infant unable to maintain temp beneath bili lights Reposition q2–4h Remove bili mask, swaddle and cuddle during feedings Cluster cares, remove from lights for feedings	Nest in open crib if infant's temp stable beneath bili lights Isolette if infant unable to maintain temp beneath bili lights **Expected Outcomes** Infant's temp WNL; infant able to rest with nested boundaries; infant cuddled, has eye contact with caregiver during cares and feedings
Nutrition	Breast or bottle feed q2–4h Monitor for dehydration, supplement with oral/IV fluid as indicated Remove newborn from bili lights, remove mask for feedings	Continue to feed q2–4h, monitor for dehydration, cuddle for feeding **Expected Outcomes** Infant tolerating feedings q2–4 without sequelae
Elimination	Record urine color and frequency Specific gravity each void Record quantity and characteristics each stool Strict intake and output (weigh diapers before discarding)	Continue noting urine and stool quantity and characteristics **Expected Outcomes** Voids qs, stools qs without difficulty, stool characteristics WNL for resolving hyperbilirubinemia; specific gravity WNL, no s/s dehydration
Medication	Evaluate routine meds Evaluate need for IV fluids	**Expected Outcomes** Routine meds given; IV fluids administered prn, IV fluids tapered as oral intake adequate to prevent dehydration
Discharge planning/ home care	Evaluate social services/visiting nurse/DC planning needs Possible home phototherapy Schedule follow-up bili levels as outpatient; follow-up with MD/NP	Offer info on CPR classes and/or film, give CPR booklet **Expected Outcomes** Infant DC home with parent(s); mother verbalizes follow-up appointments
Family involvement	Evaluate additional psychosocial needs Orient family to NSY, equipment, room Discuss rationale for treatment and possible side effects of phototherapy with family (stool changes, increased fluid loss, possible temp instability, slight lethargy, rash, altered sleep/wake patterns) Instruct family on infant's care while undergoing phototherapy: • Safety precautions—bili mask, isolette door closed and latched, covering genitalia per policy • Skin care, cord care, circ care as appropriate • Lab draws, rationale for intake and output As necessary, review role of pumping breasts and offering formula for limited time Encourage parents/significant others/sibling involvement in infant care as possible Evaluate family's understanding of information	Encourage parents to provide tactile stimulation during feeding and diaper changes Encourage cuddling and eye contact during feedings Offer suggestions to comfort restless infant: • Nesting beneath bili lights • Talking softly/singing quietly to infant • Taped music or tape recording of evening activities from home • Rhythmic patting of infant's buttocks • Firm, nonstroking touch, assisting with control of extremities • Pacifier for nonnutritive sucking Encourage family/friend support of mother/parents, ie, meals, rest, child care for siblings, allow expression of concerns/feelings **Expected Outcomes** Parents verbalize understanding of rationale and possible side effects of phototherapy; parents/family demonstrate safety precautions when caring for infant; parents getting meals, rest, verbalize support given
Date		

put, and positioning of eye patches (if conventional light banks are used) at regular intervals (Table 29–4).

Community-Based Nursing Care

If the baby is to receive phototherapy at home, parents are taught to record the infant's temperature, weight, fluid intake and output, stools, and feedings and to use the phototherapy equipment. In addition, if phototherapy lights are being used, parents must agree that the baby will be exposed to the lights for long periods of time; that they will hold the baby for only short periods for feedings, comforting, and cleansing of the perineal area; and that the room temperature will be regulated to minimize heat loss. Fiber-optic phototherapy blankets eliminate the need for eye patches, decrease heat loss because the baby is clothed, and provide more opportunities for interaction between the baby and parents. The best method of home phototherapy depends on the cause of the hyperbilirubinemia and the rate of progression of the jaundice.

Evaluation

Expected outcomes of nursing care include the following:

- The risks for development of hyperbilirubinemia are identified, and action is taken to minimize the potential impact of hyperbilirubinemia.
- The baby will not have any corneal irritation or drainage, skin breakdown, or major fluctuations in temperature.
- Parents will understand the rationale for, goal of, and expected outcome of therapy. Parents verbalize their concerns about their baby's condition and identify how they can facilitate their baby's improvement.

TABLE 29–4 Instructional Checklist for In-Room Phototherapy

Explain and demonstrate the placement of eye patches and explain that they must be in place when the infant is under the lights.
Explain the clothing to be worn (diaper under lights, dress and wrap when away from the lights).
Explain the importance of taking the infant's temperature regularly.
Explain the importance of adequate fluid intake.
Explain the charting flow sheet (intake, output, eyes covered).
Explain how to position the lights at a proper distance.
Explain the need to keep the infant under phototherapy except during feeding and diaper changes.

Care of the Newborn with Anemia

Neonatal anemia is often difficult to recognize by clinical evaluation alone. The hemoglobin concentration in a full-term newborn is 15 to 20 g/dL, slightly higher than in premature infants, in whom the mean hemoglobin is 14 to 18 g/dL. Infants with hemoglobin values of less than 14 mg/dL (term) and 13 g/dL (preterm) are usually considered anemic. The most common causes of neonatal anemia are blood loss, hemolysis, and impaired red blood cell production.

Blood loss (hypovolemia) occurs in utero from placental bleeding (placenta previa or abruptio placentae). Intrapartal blood loss may be fetomaternal, fetofetal, or the result of umbilical cord bleeding. Birth trauma to abdominal organs or the cranium may produce significant blood loss, and cerebral bleeding may occur because of hypoxia.

Excessive hemolysis of red cells is usually a result of blood group incompatibilities but may be due to infections. The most common cause of impaired red cell production is a deficiency in G-6-PD, which is genetically transmitted. Anemia and jaundice are the presenting signs.

A condition known as **physiologic anemia** exists as a result of the normal gradual drop in hemoglobin for the first 6 to 12 weeks of life. Theoretically, the bone marrow stops production of red blood cells in response to the elevated oxygenation of extrauterine respirations. When the amount of hemoglobin decreases, reaching levels of 10 to 11 g/dL at about 6 to 12 weeks of age, the bone marrow begins production of RBCs again, and the anemia disappears.

Anemia in preterm newborns occurs earlier, and reversal by bone marrow is initiated at lower levels of hemoglobin (7 to 9 g/dL). The preterm baby's hemoglobin reaches a low sooner (4 to 8 weeks after birth) than does a term newborn's (6 to 12 weeks) because preterm red blood cell survival time is shorter than in the term newborn (Mentzer & Glader, 1998). This is due to two factors: The preterm infant's growth rate is relatively rapid, and a vitamin E deficiency is common in small preterm newborns.

Clinical Therapy

Hematologic problems can be anticipated based on the pregnancy history and clinical manifestations. The age at which anemia is first noted is also of diagnostic value.

Clinically, light-skinned anemic infants are very pale in the absence of other symptoms of shock and usually have abnormally low red blood cell counts. In acute blood loss, symptoms of shock may be present, such as pallor, low arterial blood pressure, and a decreasing hematocrit value. The initial laboratory workup should include hemoglobin and hematocrit measurements, reticulocyte count, examination of peripheral blood smear, bilirubin determinations, direct Coombs' test of infant's blood, and examination of maternal blood smear for fetal erythrocytes (Kleihauer-Betke test). Clinical management depends on the severity of the anemia and whether blood loss is acute or chronic. The baby should be placed on constant cardiac and respiratory monitoring. Mild or chronic anemia in an infant may be treated adequately with iron supplements alone or with iron-fortified formulas. Frequent determinations of hemoglobin, hematocrit, and bilirubin levels (in hemolytic disease) are essential. In severe cases of anemia, transfusions are the preferred method of treatment. Management of anemia of prematurity includes recombinant human erythropoietin and supplemental iron. Blood transfusions are kept to a minimum (Downey, 1997).

NURSING CARE MANAGEMENT

The nurse assesses the newborn for symptoms of anemia (pallor). If the blood loss is acute, the baby may exhibit signs of shock (a capillary filling time greater than 3 seconds, decreased pulses, tachycardia, and low blood pressure). Continued observations will be necessary to identify physiologic anemia as the preterm newborn grows. Signs of compromise include poor weight gain, tachycardia, tachypnea, and apneic episodes. The nurse promptly reports any symptoms indicating anemia or shock. The amount of blood drawn for all laboratory tests is recorded so that total blood removed can be assessed and replaced by transfusion when necessary. If the newborn exhibits signs of shock, the nurse may need to initiate interventions.

Care of the Newborn with Polycythemia

Polycythemia, a condition in which blood volume and hematocrit values are increased, is observed more commonly in small-for-gestational age (SGA) and full-term infants with delayed cord clamping, maternal-fetal and twin-to-twin transfusions, or chronic intrauterine hypoxia (Werner, 1995). An infant is considered polycythemic when the central venous hematocrit value is greater than 65% to 70% or the venous hemoglobin level is greater than 22 g/dL during the first week of life. Other conditions that present with polycythemia are chromosomal anomalies such as trisomy 21, 18, and 13; endocrine disorders such as hypoglycemia and hypocalcemia; and births at altitudes over 5000 feet.

Clinical Therapy

The goal of therapy is to reduce the central venous hematocrit to a range of 50% to 55% in symptomatic infants. Treatment of asymptomatic infants is more controversial, but many authorities agree that these newborns benefit from prophylactic exchanges (Werner, 1995). To decrease the red cell mass, the symptomatic infant receives a partial exchange transfusion in which blood is removed from the infant and replaced milliliter for milliliter with fresh plasma, plasmanate, or 5% albumin. Supportive treatment of presenting symptoms is required until resolution, which usually occurs spontaneously following the partial exchange transfusion.

NURSING CARE MANAGEMENT

The nurse assesses, records, and reports symptoms of polycythemia. The nurse also does an initial screening of the newborn's hematocrit on admission to the nursery. If a capillary hematocrit is done, warming the heel prior to obtaining the blood helps to decrease falsely high values (Procedure 29–1: Heelstick in Newborn). Peripheral venous hematocrit samples are usually obtained from the antecubital fossa.

Many infants are asymptomatic, but as symptoms develop, they are related to the increased blood volume, hyperviscocity (thickness) of the blood, and decreased deformability of red blood cells, all of which result in poor perfusion of tissues. The infants have a characteristic plethoric (ruddy) appearance. The most common symptoms observed include the following:

- Tachycardia and congestive heart failure due to the increased blood volume
- Respiratory distress with grunting, tachypnea, and cyanosis; increased oxygen need; or hemorrhage in respiratory system due to pulmonary venous congestion, edema, and hypoxemia
- Hyperbilirubinemia due to increased numbers of red blood cells breaking down
- Decrease in peripheral pulses, discoloration of extremities, renal vein thrombosis with decreased urine output, hematuria, or proteinuria due to thromboembolism
- Jitteriness, decreased activity and tone, seizures due to decreased perfusion of the brain and increased vascular resistance secondary to sluggish blood flow (This can result in neurologic or developmental problems.)

The nurse observes closely for signs of distress or change in vital signs during the partial exchange. The nurse assesses carefully for potential complications resulting from the exchange such as transfusion overload (which can result in congestive heart failure), irregular cardiac rhythm, bacterial infection, hypovolemia (because of decreased plasma volume), and anemia. Parents need specific explanations about polycythemia and its treatment. The newborn needs to be reunited with the parents as soon after the exchange as the baby's status permits.

Care of the Newborn with Infection

Newborns up to 1 month of age are particularly susceptible to infection, referred to as **sepsis neonatorum,** caused by organisms that do not cause significant disease in older children. Once any infection occurs in the newborn, it can spread rapidly through the bloodstream, regardless of its primary site. The incidence of primary neonatal sepsis is 1 to 10 per 1000 live births (0.1% to 1%) (Wolach, 1997). Nosocomial infection frequency ranges from 0.6% to 1.7% in normal newborn infants and from 0.9% to 18.2% in infants in the NICU (Payne, Schilling, & Steinberg, 1994).

One factor predisposing the newborn to infection is prematurity. Prematurity and low birth weight are associated with nosocomial infection rates up to 15 times higher than average (Payne et al, 1994). The general debilitation and underlying illness often associated with prematurity necessitates invasive procedures such as umbilical catheterization, intubation, resuscitation, ventilatory support, monitoring, and parenteral alimentation (especially lipid emulsions); and prior broad-spectrum antibiotic therapy. However, even full-term infants are susceptible because their immunologic systems are immature. They lack the complex factors involved in effective phagocytosis and the ability to localize infection or to respond with a well-defined recognizable inflammatory response. In addition, newborns lack IgM immunoglobin, which is necessary to protect against bacteria, because it does not cross the placenta (refer to Chapter 24 for immunologic adaptations in newborn period).

Most nosocomial infections in the NICU present as bacteremia/sepsis, urinary tract infections, meningitis, or pneumonia. Maternal antepartal infections such as rubella, toxoplasmosis, cytomegalic inclusion disease, and herpes may cause congenital infections and resulting disorders in the newborn. Intrapartal maternal infections, such as amnionitis and those resulting from premature rupture of membranes and precipitous birth, are sources of neonatal infection. (See Chapter 16 for more detailed information.) Passage through the birth canal and contact with the vaginal flora (β-hemolytic streptococci, herpes, *Listeria*, and gonococci) expose the infant to infection (Table 29–5). With infection anywhere in the fetus or newborn, the adjacent tissues or organs are very easily penetrated, and the blood-brain barrier is ineffective. Septicemia is more common in males, except for those infections caused by group B β-hemolytic streptococcus.

At present gram-negative organisms (especially *E coli*, *Enterobacter*, *Proteus*, and *Klebsiella*) and the gram-positive organism β-hemolytic streptococcus are the most common causative agents. *Pseudomonas* is a common fomite contaminant of ventilatory support and oxygen therapy equipment. Gram-positive bacteria, especially coagulase-negative staphylococci, are common pathogens in nosocomial bacteremias, pneumonias, and urinary tract infections. Other gram-positive bacteria frequently isolated are enterococci and *Staphylococcus aureus* (Gaynes, Edwards, Jarvis, Culver, Tolson, & Martone, 1996).

Protection of the newborn from infections starts prenatally and continues throughout pregnancy and birth. Prenatal prevention should include maternal screening for sexually transmitted infection and monitoring of rubella titers in women who test negative. Intrapartally, sterile technique is essential. Smears from genital lesions are taken, and placenta and amniotic fluid cultures are obtained if amnionitis is suspected. If genital herpes is present toward term, cesarean birth may be indicated. Local eye treatment with silver nitrate or an antibiotic ophthalmic ointment is given to all newborns to prevent damage from gonococcal infections. Prophylactic antibiotic therapy, for asymptomatic GBS-culture-positive women during the intrapartum period, has been shown to be beneficial in preventing early-onset sepsis (Schuchat, 1998).

Clinical Therapy

Infants with a history of possible exposure to infection in utero (for example, premature rupture of membranes [PROM] more than 24 hours before birth or questionable maternal history of infection) should have cultures taken as soon after birth as possible. Cultures are obtained before antibiotic therapy is begun.

1. Two blood cultures are obtained from different peripheral sites. They are taken from a peripheral rather than an umbilical vessel because catheters have yielded false-positive results due to contamination. The skin is prepared by cleaning with an antiseptic solution, such as one containing iodine, and allowed to dry; the specimen is obtained with a sterile needle/syringe.
2. Spinal fluid culture is done following a spinal tap.
3. The specimen for urine culture is best obtained by a suprapubic bladder aspiration.
4. Skin cultures are taken of any lesions or drainage from lesions or reddened areas.
5. Nasopharyngeal, rectal, ear canal, and gastric aspirate cultures may be obtained.

Other laboratory investigations include a complete blood count, chest x-ray examination, serology, and Gram stains of cerebrospinal fluid, urine, skin exudate, and umbilicus. White blood cell (WBC) count with differential may indicate the presence or absence of sepsis. A level of 30,000 WBC may be normal in the first 24 hours of life, whereas low WBC may be indicative of sepsis. A low neutrophil count and high band (immature white cells) count indicate that an infection is present. Stomach aspirate should be sent for culture and smear if a gonococcal infection or amnionitis is suspected. C-reactive protein may or may not be elevated. Serum IgM levels are elevated (normal level less than 20 mg/dL) in response to

TABLE 29–5 Maternally Transmitted Newborn Infections

Infection	Nursing Assessment	Nursing Plan and Implementation
Group B Streptococcus 1% to 2% colonized with one in ten developing disease. Early onset—usually within hours of birth or within first week. Late onset—1 week to 3 months.	Severe respiratory distress (grunting and cyanosis). May become apneic or demonstrate symptoms of shock. Meconium-stained amniotic fluid seen at birth.	Early assessment of clinical signs necessary. Assist with x-ray examination—shows aspiration pneumonia or hyaline membrane disease. Immediately obtain blood, gastric aspirate, external ear canal and nasopharynx cultures. Administer antibiotics, usually aqueous penicillin or ampicillin combined with gentamicin, as soon as cultures are obtained. Early assessment and intervention are essential to survival. Initiate referral to evaluate for blindness, deafness, learning or behavioral problems.
Syphilis Spirochetes cross placenta after 16th–18th week of gestation.	Check perinatal history for positive maternal serology. Assess infant for Elevated cord serum IgM and FTA-ABS IgM Rhinitis (snuffles) Fissures on mouth corners and excoriated upper lip Red rash around mouth and anus Copper-colored rash over face, palms, and soles Irritability Generalized edema, particularly over joints; bone lesions; painful extremities Hepatosplenomegaly, jaundice Congenital cataracts SGA and failure to thrive	Initiate isolation techniques until infants have been on antibiotics for 48 hours. Administer penicillin. Provide emotional support for parents because of their feelings about mode of transmission and potential long-term sequelae.
Gonorrhea Approximately 30%–35% of newborns born vaginally to infected mothers acquire the infection.	Assess for Ophthalmia neonatorum (conjunctivitis) Purulent discharge and corneal ulcerations Neonatal sepsis with temperature instability, poor feeding response, and/or hypotonia, jaundice	Administer 1% silver nitrate solution or ophthalmic antibiotic ointment (see Drug Guide: Erythromycin [Ilotycin] Ophthalmic Ointment in Chapter 26) or, in lieu of silver nitrate, penicillin. Initiate follow-up referral to evaluate any loss of vision.
Herpes Type 2 1 in 7500 births. Usually transmitted during vaginal birth; a few cases of in utero transmission have been reported.	Small cluster vesicular skin lesions over all the body. Check perinatal history for active herpes genital lesions. Disseminated form—DIC, pneumonia, hepatitis with jaundice, hepatosplenomegaly, and neurologic abnormalities. Without skin lesions, assess for fever or subnormal temperature, respiratory congestion, tachypnea, and tachycardia.	Carry out careful hand washing and gown and glove isolation with linen precautions. Administer intravenous vidarabine (Vira A) or acyclovir (Zovirax). Initiate follow-up referral to evaluate potential sequelae of microcephaly, spasticity, seizures, deafness, or blindness. Encourage parental rooming-in and touching of their newborn. Show parents appropriate hand-washing procedures and precautions to be used at home if mother's lesions are active. Obtain throat, conjunctiva, cerebral spinal fluid (CSF), blood, urine, and lesion cultures to identify herpesvirus type 2 antibiotics in serum IgM fraction. Cultures positive in 24–48 hours.
Oral Candidal Infection (Thrush) Acquired during passage through birth canal.	Assess newborn's buccal mucosa, tongue, gums, and inside the cheeks for white plaques (seen 5 to 7 days of age). Check diaper area for bright red, well-demarcated eruptions. Assess for thrush periodically when newborn is on long-term antibiotic therapy.	Differentiate white plaque areas from milk curds by using cotton tip applicator (if it is thrush, removal of white areas causes raw, bleeding areas). Maintain cleanliness of hands, linen, clothing, diapers, and feeding apparatus. Instruct breastfeeding mothers on treating their nipples with nystatin. Administer gentian violet (1% to 2%) swabbed on oral lesions 1 hour after feeding or nystatin instilled in baby's oral cavity and on mucosa. Swab skin lesions with topical nystatin. Discuss with parents that gentian violet stains mouth and clothing. Avoid placing gentian violet on normal mucosa; it causes irritation.
Chlamydia Trachomatis Acquired during passage through birth canal.	Assess for perinatal history of preterm birth. Symptomatic newborns present with pneumonia—conjunctivitis after 3–4 days. Chronic follicular conjunctivitis (corneal neovascularization and conjunctival scarring).	Instill ophthalmic erythromycin (see Drug Guide: Erythromycin [Ilotycin] Ophthalmic Ointment in Chapter 26). Initiate follow-up referral for eye complications and late development of pneumonia at 4–11 weeks postnatally.

transplacental infections. If available, counterimmunoelectrophoresis tests for specific bacterial antigens are performed.

Evidence of congenital infections may be seen on skull x-rays for cerebral calcifications (cytomegalovirus, toxoplasmosis), on bone x-rays (syphilis, cytomegalovirus), and in serum-specific IgM levels (rubella). Cytomegalovirus infection is best diagnosed by urine culture.

Because neonatal infection causes high mortality, therapy is instituted before results of the sepsis workup are obtained. A combination of two broad-spectrum antibiotics, such as ampicillin and gentamicin, is given in large doses until a culture with sensitivities results are obtained.

After the pathogen and its sensitivities are determined, appropriate specific antibiotic therapy is begun.

TABLE 29–6 Neonatal Sepsis Antibiotic Therapy

Drug	Dose (mg/kg) Total Daily Dose	Schedule for Divided Doses	Route	Comments
Ampicillin	50–100 mg/kg	Every 12 hours* Every 8 hours†	IM or IV	Effective against gram-positive microorganisms, *Haemophilus influenzae,* and majority of *E coli* strains. Higher doses indicated for meningitis. Used with aminoglycoside for synergy.
Cefotaxime	50 mg/kg 100–150 mg/kg/day	Every 12 hours* Every 8 hours†	IM or IV	Active against most major pathogens in infants; effective against aminoglycoside-resistant organisms; achieves CSF bactericidal activity; lack of ototoxicity and nephrotoxicity; wide therapeutic index (levels not required); resistant organisms can develop rapidly if used extensively; ineffective against pseudomonas, listeria.
Gentamicin	2.5–3 mg/kg 5.0–7.5 mg/kg/day	Every 12–24 hours*‡ Every 8–24 hours†	IM or IV	Effective against gram-negative rods and staphylococci; may be used instead of kanamycin against penicillin-resistant staphylococci and *E coli* strains and *Pseudomonas aeruginosa.* May cause ototoxicity and nephrotoxicity. Need to follow serum levels. Must never be given as IV push. Must be given over at least 30–60 minutes. In presence of oliguria or anuria, dose must be decreased or discontinued. In infants less than 1000 g or 29 weeks, lower dosage 2.5–3.0 mg/kg/day. Monitor serum levels before administration of second dose. Peak 5–10 μg/mL Trough 1–2 μg/mL
Methicillin	25–50 mg/dose 50–100 mg/kg/day	Every 12 hours* Every 6–8 hours†	IM or IV	Effective against penicillinase-resistant staphylococci. Monitor CBC and UA. Slow IV push.
Nafcillin	25–50 mg/kg 50–100 mg/kg/day	Every 8–12 hours* Every 6–8 hours†	IM or IV	Effective against penicillinase-resistant staphylococci. Caution in presence of jaundice.
Penicillin G (aqueous crystalline)	25,000–50,000 IU/kg 50,000–125,000 IU/kg/day	Every 12 hours* Every 8 hours†	IM or IV	Initial sepsis therapy effective against most gram-positive microorganisms except resistant staphylococci; can cause heart block in infants.
Vancomycin	10–20 mg/kg 30 mg/kg/day	Every 12–24 hours*‡ Every 8 hours†	IV	Effective for methicillin-resistant strains (*S epidermidis*); must be administered by slow intravenous infusion to avoid prolonged cutaneous eruption. For smaller infants <1200 g; <29 weeks, smaller dosages and longer intervals between doses. Nephrotoxic, especially when given in combination with aminoglycosides. Slow IV infusion over 60 minutes. Peak 25–40 μg/mL Trough 5–10 μg/mL

*Up to seven days of age.

†Greater than seven days of age.

‡Dependent on GA.

Combinations of penicillin or ampicillin and kanamycin have been used in the past, but new kanamycin-resistant enterobacteria and penicillin-resistant staphylococcus necessitate increasing use of gentamicin.

Rotating aminoglycosides has been suggested to prevent development of resistance. Use of cephalosporins and, in particular, cefotaxime has emerged as an alternative to aminoglycoside therapy in the treatment of neonatal infections. Duration of therapy varies from 7 to 14 days (Table 29–6). However, if cultures are negative and symptoms subside, antibiotics may be discontinued after 3 days. Supportive physiologic care may be required to maintain respiratory, hemodynamic, nutritional, and metabolic homeostasis.

CRITICAL THINKING QUESTION

What is the danger in early or aggressive use of antibiotics to treat neonatal sepsis?

NURSING CARE MANAGEMENT

Nursing Assessment and Diagnosis

Symptoms of infection are most often noticed by the nurse during daily care of the newborn. The infant may deteriorate rapidly in the first 12 to 24 hours after birth if β-hemolytic streptococcal infection is present, with signs and symptoms mimicking RDS. In other cases, the onset of sepsis may be gradual, with more subtle signs and symptoms. The most common symptoms include the following:

- Subtle behavioral changes—the infant "isn't doing well" and is often lethargic or irritable (especially after first 24 hours), hypotonic, and hypotensive. Color changes may include pallor, duskiness, cyanosis, or a "shocky" appearance. Skin is cool and clammy.
- Temperature instability, manifested most commonly by hypothermia (recognized by a decrease in skin temperature) or, rarely in newborns, hyperthermia

(elevation of skin temperature) necessitates a corresponding increase or decrease in incubator temperature to maintain a neutral thermal environment.

- Feeding intolerance is evidenced by a decrease in total intake, abdominal distention, vomiting, poor sucking, lack of interest in feeding, and diarrhea.
- Hyperbilirubinemia.
- Tachycardia initially, followed by spells of apnea/bradycardia.

Signs and symptoms may suggest CNS disease (jitteriness, tremors, seizure activity), respiratory system disease (tachypnea, labored respirations, apnea, cyanosis), hematologic disease (jaundice, petechial hemorrhages, hepatosplenomegaly), or gastrointestinal disease (diarrhea, vomiting, bile-stained aspirate, hepatomegaly). A differential diagnosis is necessary because of the similarity of symptoms to other more specific conditions.

Nursing diagnoses that may apply to the infant with sepsis neonatorum and the family include the following:

- ***Risk for Infection*** related to immature immunologic system
- ***Fluid Volume Deficit*** related to feeding intolerance
- ***Ineffective Family Coping: Compromised*** related to present illness resulting in prolonged hospital stay for the newborn

Nursing Plan and Implementation

In the nursery, controlling the environment and preventing acquired infection are the responsibilities of the neonatal nurse. The nurse must promote strict handwashing technique for all who enter the nursery, including nursing colleagues; physicians; laboratory, x-ray, and inhalation technicians; and parents. The nurse must be prepared to assist in the aseptic collection of specimens for laboratory investigations. Scrupulous care of equipment—changing and cleaning incubators at least every 7 days, removing and sterilizing wet equipment every 24 hours, preventing cross-use of linen and other equipment, cleaning sinkside equipment such as soap containers periodically, and taking special care with the open radiant warmers (access without prior hand washing is much more likely than with the closed incubator)—will prevent fomite contamination or contamination through improper hand washing. An infected newborn can be effectively isolated in an incubator and receive close observation. Visits to the nursery area by unnecessary personnel should be discouraged.

Antibiotic Therapy Provision

The nurse administers antibiotics as ordered by the nurse practitioner/physician. It is the nurse's responsibility to be knowledgeable about the following:

- The proper dose to be administered, based on the weight of the newborn and desired peak and trough levels
- The appropriate route of administration, because some antibiotics cannot be given intravenously
- The appropriate rate of administration
- Admixture incompatibilities because some antibiotics are precipitated by intravenous solutions or by other antibiotics
- Side effects and toxicity

In the case of term infants who are being treated for infections, neonatal home infusion of antibiotics should be considered as a viable alternative to continued hospitalization. The infusion of antibiotics at home by skilled RNs facilitates parent-infant bonding while meeting the ongoing health care needs of the infant (Anastasi, 1998).

Provision of Supportive Care

In addition to antibiotic therapy, physiologic supportive care is essential in caring for a septic infant (Askin, 1995). The nurse should carry out the following:

- Observe for resolution of symptoms or development of other symptoms of sepsis.
- Maintain a neutral thermal environment with accurate regulation of humidity and oxygen administration.
- Provide respiratory support: Administer oxygen and observe and monitor respiratory effort.
- Provide cardiovascular support: Observe and monitor pulse and blood pressure; observe for hyperbilirubinemia, anemia, and hemorrhagic symptoms.
- Provide adequate calories, because oral feedings may be discontinued due to increased mucus, abdominal distention, vomiting, or aspiration.
- Provide fluids and electrolytes to maintain homeostasis. Monitor weight changes, urine output, and urine specific gravity.
- Observe for the development of hypoglycemia, hyperglycemia, acidosis, hyponatremia, and hypocalcemia.

Restricting parental visits has not been shown to have any effect on the rate of infection and may be harmful to the newborn's psychologic development. With instruction and guidance from the nurse, both parents should be allowed to handle the baby and participate in daily care. Support to the parents is crucial. They need to be informed of the newborn's prognosis as treatment continues and to be involved in care as much as possible. They also need to understand how infection is transmitted.

Evaluation

Expected outcomes of nursing care include the following:

- The risks for development of sepsis are identified early, and immediate action is taken to minimize the development of the illness.

- Appropriate use of aseptic technique protects the newborn from further exposure to illness.
- The baby's symptoms are relieved, and the infection is treated.
- The parents verbalize their concerns about their baby's illness and understand the rationale behind the management of their newborn.

Care of the Family of a Newborn with a Complication

Adaptation of the Family

The birth of a baby with a problem or disorder is a traumatic event with the potential for either total disruption or growth of the involved family. Throughout the pregnancy, both parents, together and separately, have felt excitement, experienced thoughts of acceptance, and pictured what their baby would look like. Both parents have wished for a perfect baby and feared a damaged, unhealthy one. Each parent and family member must accept and adjust when the fantasized fears become reality.

Grieving for the loss of the hoped-for perfect child is necessary before the development of a positive relationship to the existing child can begin. Parents express grief as shock and disbelief, denial of reality, anger toward self and others, guilt, blame, and concern for the future. Self-esteem and feelings of self-worth are jeopardized.

In some cases fear, separation, and grief begin during the birth, when the newborn requires immediate resuscitation or special treatment. Instead of being handed to its mother, the baby is given to a nurse or a pediatrician, who rushes it to a special care area. The joyful cries of "It's a boy!" or "It's a girl!" are absent; there is only the mother's pleading question, "What's wrong with my baby?" If no answer is given to the mother, she frequently fantasizes the worst and assumes that the baby is dead. It is extremely important for the mother's health and the mother-infant relationship that some immediate answer be given to the parents. Honest, simple, and positive facts can be shared: "Your baby is alive"; "Your baby is a girl"; "Your baby has a strong heartbeat but needs some help with breathing"; "Your baby is alive but needs some special care right now"; "The pediatrician/nurse practitioner is helping your baby now and will talk with you soon." The information that nurses share with parents must always be honest data that nurses can observe and document. Nurses should not make promises that they cannot fulfill and should refrain from offering empty reassurances that everything will be all right.

The period of waiting between suspicion and confirmation of abnormality or dysfunction is a very anxious one for parents because it is difficult, if not impossible, to begin attachment to the infant if the newborn's future is questionable. During the "not knowing period," parents need support and acknowledgment that this is an anxious time and must be kept informed about efforts to gather additional data and maintain the infant's livelihood. It is helpful to tell both parents about the problem at the same time with the baby present. An honest discussion of the problem and anticipatory management at the earliest possible time by health professionals help the parents (1) maintain trust in the physician and nurse, (2) appreciate the reality of the situation by dispelling fantasy and misconception, (3) begin the grieving process, and (4) mobilize internal and external support.

Nurses need to be aware that anger is a universal response and that it is best directed outward because holding it in check requires great energy, which is diverted away from grieving and physical recovery from pregnancy and giving birth. Anger may be directed unjustifiably at the physician and/or nurse, at the food, at nursing care, or at hospital regulations and routines. Parents rarely show anger with the baby and such responses can precipitate guilt feelings.

A heightened concern for self may be misinterpreted by health professionals as rejection of the newborn. Both parents need time and understanding to deal with their own feelings before they can direct concern toward the baby. In a short span of time, the parent is confronted with the loss of the idealized child, the need to accept a child who deviates from normal, and a sense of personal failure. In addition, the new mother may be suffering from fatigue and sleep deprivation from her pregnancy and labor and from discomforts arising from cesarean birth, episiotomy, inability to void, hemorrhoids, and afterpains. In the postpartal period, concern for self and dependence are normal events.

In their sensitive and vulnerable state, parents are acutely perceptive about others' responses and reactions (particularly nonverbal) to the child. Parents can be expected to identify with the responses of others. Therefore it is imperative that medical and nursing staff be fully aware of their feelings and come to terms with those feelings so that they are comfortable and at ease with the baby and the grieving family.

Nurses may feel uncomfortable not knowing what to say to parents or may fear confronting their own feelings as well as those of the parents. Each nurse must work out personal reactions with instructors, peers, clergy, parents, or significant others. It is helpful to have a stockpile of therapeutic questions and statements to initiate meaningful dialogue with parents. Opening statements can be as follows: "You must be wondering what could have caused this"; "Are you thinking that you (or someone else) may have done something?"; "How can I help?"; "Go ahead and cry. It's worth crying about"; or "Are you wondering how you are going to manage?" Avoid statements such as, "It could have been worse"; "It's God's will"; "You have other children"; "You are still young and can have more"; and "I understand how you feel." This child is important now.

Some nurses find relief for themselves or a means of escape from painful circumstances by overzealous and unrealistic reassurance that "everything will be all right" and by avoiding the newborn and family. Other medical and nursing staff take refuge in technical jargon and involvement in the technical aspects of the mother's care rather than taking time to talk about the situation. These approaches confuse the parents at a time when they need most to be understood and to understand.

Nurses show concern and support by planning time to spend with the parents, by being psychologically as well as physically present, by encouraging open discussion and grieving, by repetitious explanations (as necessary), by providing privacy as needed, and by encouraging contact with the newborn. Identifying and clarifying feelings and fears decrease distortions in perception, thinking, and feeling. Nurses invest the baby with value in the eyes of the parents when they provide meticulous care to the newborn, talk and coo (especially in the face-to-face position) while holding or providing care to the newborn, refer to the child by gender or name, and relate the newborn's activities ("He took a whole ounce of formula"; "She burped so loudly that . . . "; "He took hold of the blanket and just wouldn't let go"; "He voided all over the doctor"). Nurses should note the "normal" characteristics and capabilities of each newborn as well as the newborn's needs. The nurse should also learn the baby's name and refer to him or her by name.

Many physicians show parents "before" and "after" photographs of conditions requiring surgical intervention. Parents also may benefit from meeting other parents who have faced the same problem through a parental support group or organization that is specific to that problem. Specialists (plastic surgeons, perinatal clinic nurse specialists, neurosurgeons, orthopedists, oral surgeons, dentists, and rehabilitation therapists) can be reassuring and supportive of parents in their short- and long-term goals. However, these types of interventions must be carefully timed to the readiness of the parents.

Cues that the parents are ready to become involved with the child's care or planning for the future include their reference to the baby as "she" or "he" or by name and their questioning as to amount of feeding taken, appearance today, and the like.

Mothers may feel inadequate or guilty when they do not feel motherly toward their baby. One mother, for example, looking at her child born with a severe cleft lip and palate, said, "God help me. I can't stand looking at her. I wish she weren't mine. What a horrid thing to say, but I can't . . . I just can't." She could not bring herself to hold or touch the infant prior to cleft lip repair. She needed considerable assistance to talk of these feelings in a nonjudgmental and accepting atmosphere before she was able to hold the infant after surgery. She proceeded to learn to feed her daughter (whose cleft palate was not yet repaired) and become very "motherly" before the infant was discharged. Her husband, fortunately, facilitated the whole process by his continued love for and acceptance of his wife throughout the experience.

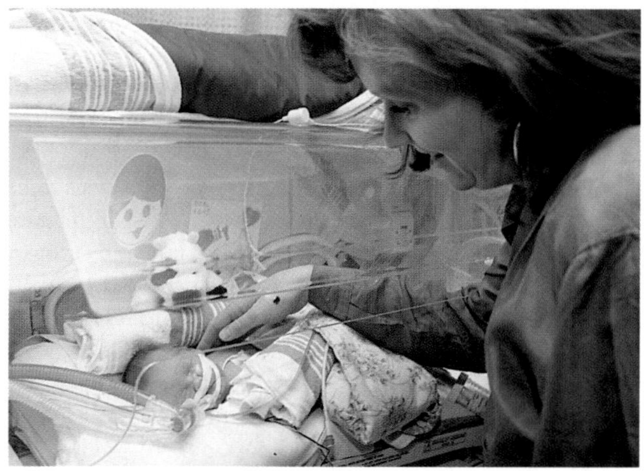

FIGURE 29–15 When parents participate in their baby's care, they tend to have realistic expectations of the child's long-term developmental needs.

Occasionally, a mother may become overprotective and overoptimistic shortly after the baby's birth. The nurse should accept her behavior but continue to remind her that it is okay and natural to feel disappointment, a sense of failure, helplessness, or anger. The overprotectiveness and overoptimism are defense mechanisms. To deny the negative feelings only entrenches them further, delays their resolution, and delays realistic planning.

Developmental Consequences

The baby who is born prematurely, is ill, or has a malformation or disorder is at risk in emotional and intellectual, as well as physical, development. The risk is directly proportional to the seriousness of the problem and the length of treatment.

Medical, surgical, and technical advances in recent years have been responsible for salvaging increasing numbers of preterm and ill newborns. However, the necessary physical separation of family and infant and the tremendous emotional and financial burdens adversely affect the parent-child relationship. A considerable percentage of these children have been rescued only to be emotionally or physically battered by the parents. The most recent trend in many hospitals is to involve the parents with the neonate early, repeatedly, and over protracted periods of time. Early and continued involvement may only mean opportunities to look at or stroke the baby (Figure 29–15). Later, when the mother's and baby's conditions warrant it, the mother should participate in her baby's care (to the extent she is willing) and in planning for the future. This type of involvement facilitates early bonding, attachment, and emotional investment. The parents need a sense of personal success, self-worth, self-esteem, and confidence from the knowledge that they can cope with the situation. This atmosphere aids the baby, as well—the child may escape abuse and may instead be assisted toward self-actualization.

Mothers of newborns who are gravely ill are often unable to chance an emotional investment in their child. When their baby stabilizes, these mothers need assistance in perceiving the cues and hearing the words that indicate the baby is going to survive. They need time and support to establish a positive relationship with the newborn. A mother who is unable to develop maternal feelings may reject the baby or overcompensate because of underlying guilt feelings; in either case an unproductive relationship may develop. The child may then be further handicapped by inability to relate well to others and by seeing the world as unsatisfying and painful.

The parents must have a clear picture of the reality of the handicap and the types of developmental hurdles ahead. Unexpected behaviors and responses from the baby due to his or her defect or disorder can be upsetting and frightening. For example, parents find it difficult to cope with a baby's lack of motor or social responsiveness and tend to interpret the lack as a form of rejection. The parents may in return respond with rejection, and an unfortunate cycle is begun.

The demands of care of the child and disputes regarding management or behavior stress family relationships. A variety of behavioral patterns may occur. For example, one or more members of the family may make a scapegoat of the child. Another may become the youngster's champion to the exclusion of others. One or the other spouse may feel pushed aside or denied attention and thus may withdraw or leave the family unit. Parents or siblings may feel that their own needs (schooling, material goods, freedom of movement) are being set aside while all assets (financial and other) go to support the one child's needs.

The entire multidisciplinary team may need to pool their resources and expertise to help parents of children born with problems or disorders so that both parents and children can thrive.

FOCUS YOUR STUDY

- The sick newborn—whether preterm, term, or postterm—must be managed within narrow physiologic parameters.
- These parameters (respiratory, cardiovascular, and thermal regulation) will maintain physiologic homeostasis and prevent introduction of iatrogenic stress to the already stressed infant.
- The nursing care of the newborn with special problems involves understanding normal physiology, the pathophysiology of the disease process, clinical manifestations, and supportive or corrective therapies. Only with this theoretical background can the newborn nurse make appropriate observations concerning responses to therapy and development of complications.
- Asphyxia results in significant circulatory, respiratory, and biochemical changes in the newborn that make the successful transition to extrauterine life difficult. Asphyxia requires early identification and resuscitative management.
- Newborn conditions that commonly present with respiratory distress and require oxygen and ventilatory assistance are respiratory distress syndrome, transient tachypnea of the newborn, meconium aspiration syndrome, and persistent pulmonary hypertension.
- Cold stress sets up the chain of physiologic events of hypoglycemia, pulmonary vasoconstriction, hyperbilirubinemia, respiratory distress, and metabolic acidosis.
- Nurses are responsible for early detection and initiation of treatment for hypoglycemia.
- Differentiation between pathologic and physiologic jaundice is the key to early and successful intervention.
- Anemia (decreased amount of red blood cell volume) or polycythemia (excess amount) place the newborn at risk for alterations in blood flow and the oxygen-carrying capacity of the blood.
- Nursing assessment of the septic newborn involves identifying very subtle clinical signs that are also seen in other clinical disease states.
- The nurse is the facilitator for interdisciplinary communication with the parents, identifying their understanding of their infant's care and their needs for emotional support.
- Parents of at-risk newborns need support from nurses and health care providers to understand the special needs of their baby and to feel comfortable in an overwhelmingly strange environment.

REFERENCES

American Academy of Pediatrics Provisional Committee for Quality Improvement and Subcommittee on Hyperbilirubinemia. (1994). Practice parameter: Management of hyperbilirubinemia in the healthy term newborn [published erratum appears in *Pediatrics, 95*(3), 458–461. (1995).] *Pediatrics, 94*(4 Pt. 1), 558–665.

Anastasi, J. M. (1998). Innovations in care: Neonatal home antibiotic infusion therapy. *Neonatal Network, 17*(4), 33–38.

Askin, D. F. (1995). Bacterial and fungal infections in the neonate. *Journal of Obstetric, Gynecologic, and Neonatal Nursing, 24*(7), 635–643.

Askin, D. F. (1997). *Acute respiratory care of the neonate* (2nd ed.). Petaluma, CA: NICU INK.

Bancalari, E. (1998). Corticosteriods and neonatal chronic lung disease. *European Journal of Pediatrics, 157 Suppl 1*, S31–S37.

Bland, H. E. (1996, Nov./Dec.). Jaundice in the healthy term neonate: When is treatment indicated? *Current Problems in Pediatrics*, 355–362.

Bloom, R. S., & Cropley, C. (1994). *Textbook of neonatal resuscitation.* Elk Grove Village, IL: American Heart Association and American Academy of Pediatrics.

Bratlid, D. (1996). Criteria for treatment of neonatal jaundice. *Journal of Perinatology, 16*(3), Pt 2, 583–588.

Brooks, C. (1997). Neonatal hypoglycemia. *Neonatal Network, 16*(2), 15–21.

DeBoer, S. L., & Stephens, D. (1997). Persistent pulmonary hypertension of the newborn: Case study and pathophysiology review. *Neonatal Network, 16*(1), 7–13.

Dennery, P. A., Rhine, W. D., & Stevenson, D. K. (1995). Neonatal jaundice: What now? *Clinical Pediatrics, 34*(2), 103–107.

Downey, P. (1997). Recombinant human erythropoietin as a treatment for anemia of prematurity. *Journal of Perinatal and Neonatal Nursing, 11*(3), 57–68.

Findlay, R. D., Taeusch, H. W., & Walther, F. J. (1996). Surfactant replacement therapy for meconium aspiration syndrome. *Pediatrics, 97*(1), 48–52.

Gaynes, R. P., Edwards, J. R., Jarvis, W. R., Culver, D. H., Tolson, J. S., & Martone, W. J. (1996). Nosocomial infections among neonates in high-risk nurseries in the United States. National Nosocomial Infections Surveillance System. *Pediatrics, 98*(3 Pt. 1), 357–361.

Gomez, M., Hansen, T., & Corbet, A. (1998). Therapies for intractable respiratory failure. In H. W. Taeusch & R. A. Ballard (Eds.), *Avery's diseases of the newborn* (7th ed.). Philadelphia: Saunders.

Greenough, A. (1995, April 28). Meconium aspiration syndrome: Prevention and treatment. *Early Human Development, 41*(3), 183–192.

Halamek, L. P., Benaron, D. A., Stevenson, D. K. (1997, Dec.). Neonatal hypoglycemia, Part I: Background and definition. *Clinical Pediatrics*, 675–680.

Hansen, T. N., Cooper, T. R., & Weisman, L. E. (1998). *Contemporary diagnosis and management of neonatal respiratory diseases* (2nd ed.). Newtown, PA: Handbooks in Health Care.

Jepson, H. A., Talashek, M. L., & Tichy, A. M. (1991). The Apgar score: Evolution, limitations, and scoring guidelines. *Birth, 18*(2), 83–92.

Jobe, A. H., Newnham, J., Willet, K., Sly, P., & Ikegami, M. (1998). Fetal versus maternal and gestational age effects of repetitive antenatal gluco corticoids. *Pediatrics, 102*(5), 116–1125.

Kerem, E., Dollberg, S., Paz, I., Armon, Y., Seidman, D. S., Stevenson, D. K., & Gale, R. (1997). Prenatal ritodrine administration and the incidence of respiratory distress syndrome in premature infants. *Journal of Perinatology, 17*(2), 101–106.

Letko, M. D. (1996). Understanding the Apgar score. *Journal of Obstetric, Gynecologic, and Neonatal Nursing, 25*(4) 299–303.

MacMahon, J. R., Stevenson, D. K., & Oski, F. A. (1998). Management of neonatal hyperbilirubinemia. In H. W. Taeusch & R. A. Ballard (Eds.), *Avery's diseases of the newborn* (7th ed.). Philadelphia: Saunders.

Mentzer, W. C., & Glader, B. E. (1998). Erythrocyte disorders of infancy. In H. W. Taeusch & R. A. Ballard (Eds.), *Avery's diseases of the newborn* (7th ed.). Philadelphia: Saunders.

Merenstein, G. B., & Gardner, S. L. (1998). *Handbook of neonatal intensive care* (4th ed.). St. Louis: Mosby.

Mitchell, S. H. (1996). Infants with bronchopulmonary dysplasia: A developmental perspective. *Journal of Pediatric Nursing, 11*(3), 145–151.

Neonatal hyperglycemia. (1996). In *NANN guidelines for practice* (pp 1–7). Petaluma, CA: NICU INK. NANN.

Neonatal thermoregulation. (1997). In *NANN guidelines for practice* (pp 1–15). Petaluma, CA: NICU INK. NANN.

Newman, T. B., & Maisels, M. J. (1992). Evaluation and treatment of jaundice in the term newborn: A kinder, gentler approach. *Pediatrics, 89*(5 Pt. 1), 809–818.

Payne, N. R., Schilling, C. G., & Steinberg, S. (1994). Selecting antibiotics for nosocomial bacterial infections in patients requiring neonatal intensive care. *Neonatal Network, 13*(3), 41–51.

Ryan, S. (1998). Nutrition in neonatal chronic lung disease. *European Journal of Pediatrics, 157*(Suppl 1), S19–S22.

Schwartz, R. P. (1997). Neonatal hypoglycemia: How low is too low? *Journal of Pediatrics, 131*(2), 171–173.

Schuchat, A. (1998). Epidemiology of group B streptococcal disease in the United States: Shifting paradigms. *Clinical Microbiology Reviews, 11* (3), 497–513.

Thureen, P. J., Deacon, J., O'Neill, P., & Hernandez, J. (1999). *Assessment and care of the well newborn.* Philadelphia: Saunders.

Verklan, M. T. (1997). Bronchopulmonary dysplasia: Its effects upon the heart and lungs. *Neonatal Network, 16*(8), 5–12.

Werner, E. J. (1995). Neonatal polycythemia and hyperviscosity. *Clinics in Perinatology, 22*(3), 693–710.

Williams, A. F. (1997). Hypoglycemia of the newborn: A review. *Bulletin of the World Health Organization, 75*(3), 261–290.

Wolach, B. (1997). Neonatal sepsis: Pathogenesis and supportive therapy. *Seminars in Perinatology, 21*(1), 28–38.

Young, T. E., & Mangum, O. B. (1997). *Neofax: A manual of drugs used in neonatal care* (10th ed.). Raleigh, NC: Acorn Publishing.

Postpartum

seven

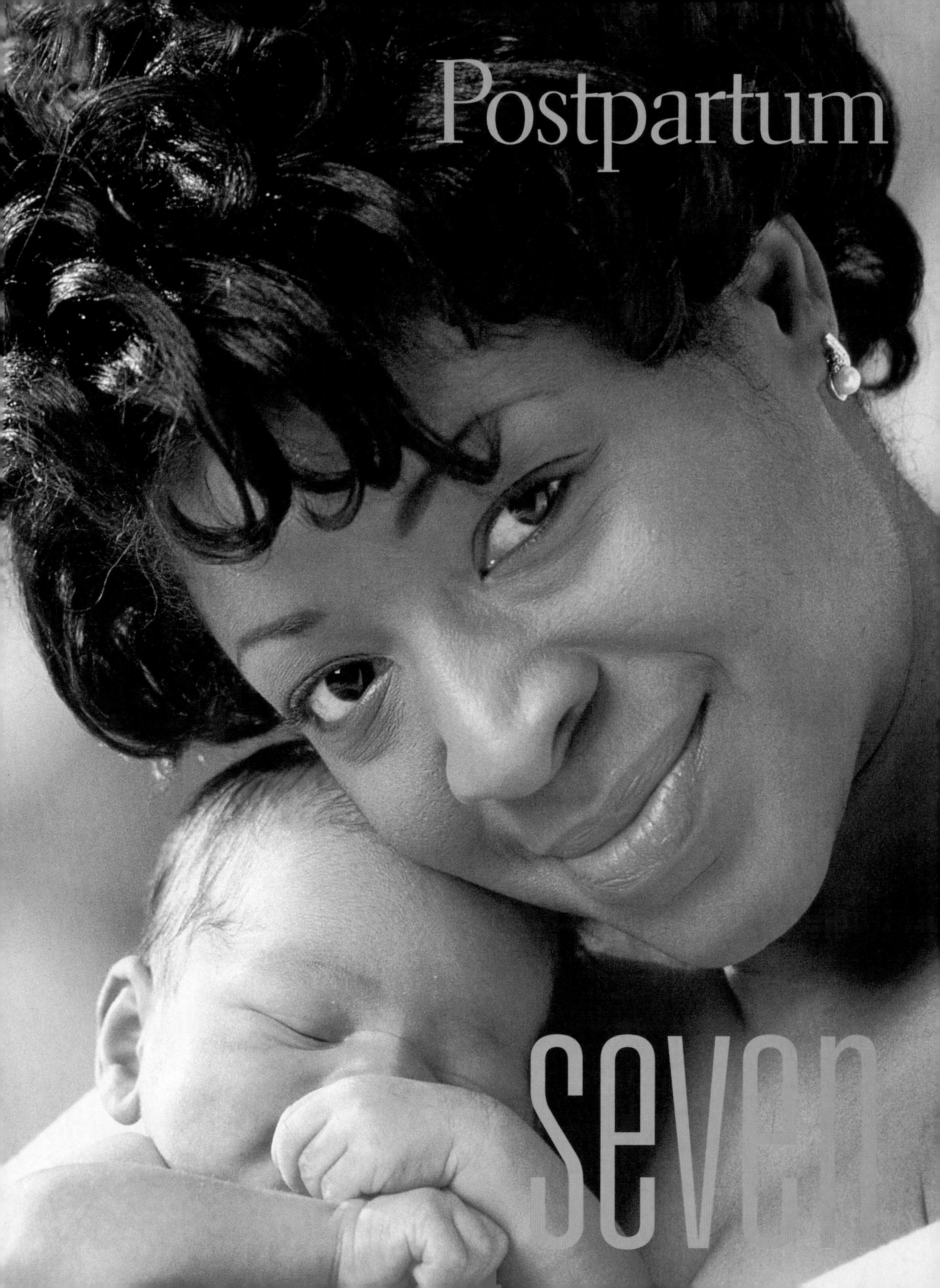

30

Postpartal Adaptation and Nursing Assessment

Key Terms

Afterpains
Boggy uterus
Diastasis recti abdominis
En face
Engrossment
Fundus
Involution
Lochia
Lochia alba
Lochia rubra
Lochia serosa
Maternal role attainment
Postpartum blues
Puerperium
Reciprocity
Subinvolution

I HAD HEARD ABOUT THE NEGATIVES—THE FATIGUE, the loneliness, loss of self. But nobody told me about the wonderful parts: holding my baby close to me, seeing her first smile, watching her grow and become more responsive day by day. How can I describe the way I felt when she stroked my breast while nursing, or looked into my eyes or arched her eyebrows like an opera singer? This was the deepest connection I'd felt to anybody. Sometimes the intensity almost frightened me. For the first time I cared about somebody else more than myself, and I would do anything to nurture and protect her.
~ *The New Our Bodies, Ourselves* ~

Objectives

- Describe the basic physiologic changes that occur in the postpartal period as a woman's body returns to its prepregnant state.
- Discuss the psychologic adjustments that normally occur during the postpartal period.
- Identify those organs that will not return completely to a prepregnant state following childbirth.
- Delineate the physiologic and psychosocial components of a normal postpartal assessment.
- Summarize the physical and developmental tasks that the mother must accomplish during the postpartal period.

The puerperium, or postpartal period, is the period during which the woman adjusts, physically and psychologically, to pregnancy and birth. It begins immediately after birth and continues for approximately 6 weeks or until the body has returned to a near prepregnant state.

This chapter describes the physiologic and psychologic changes and adaptations that occur postpartally and the basic aspects of a thorough postpartal assessment.

Postpartal Physical Adaptations

Comprehensive nursing assessment is based on a sound understanding of the normal anatomic and physiologic processes of the puerperium. These processes involve the reproductive organs and other major body systems.

Reproductive System

Involution of the Uterus

The term **involution** is used to describe the rapid reduction in size of the uterus and its return to a condition similar to its prepregnant state, although it remains slightly larger than it was before the first pregnancy.

Following separation of the placenta, the decidua of the uterus is irregular, jagged, and varied in thickness. With the dramatic decrease in the levels of circulating estrogen and progesterone following placental separation, the uterine cells atrophy, and the hyperplasia of pregnancy begins to reverse. The process is one in which the size of the cells decreases markedly; the number of cells does not decrease (Cunningham et al, 1997). Proteolytic enzymes are released, and macrophages migrate to the uterus to promote autolysis (self-digestion). Protein material in the uterine wall is broken down and absorbed. The spongy layer of the decidua is cast off as lochia, and the basal layer of the decidua remains in the uterus to become differentiated into two layers within the first 48 to 72 hours after birth. The outermost layer becomes necrotic and is sloughed off in the lochia. The layer closest to the myometrium contains the fundi of the uterine endometrial glands, and these glands lay the foundation for the new endometrium. Except at the placental site, this process is completed in approximately 3 weeks.

Involution of the placental site is a similar process but takes up to 6 to 7 weeks for completion. Following separation, the placental site contracts to an area about 8 to 10 cm in diameter that appears raised, irregular, and 4 to 10 cm above the surface of the uterus. Bleeding from the larger uterine vessels of the placental site is controlled by compression of the retracted uterine muscle fibers. The clotted blood is gradually absorbed by the body. Some of these vessels are eventually obliterated and replaced by new vessels with smaller lumens.

TABLE 30–1 Factors That Retard Uterine Involution

Factor	Rationale
Prolonged labor	Muscles relax because of prolonged time of contraction during labor.
Anesthesia	Muscles relax.
Difficult birth	The uterus is manipulated excessively.
Grandmultiparity	Repeated distention of uterus during pregnancy and labor leads to muscle stretching, diminished tone, and muscle relaxation.
Full bladder	As the uterus is pushed up and usually to the right, pressure on it interferes with effective uterine contraction.
Incomplete expulsion of placenta or membranes	The presence of even small amounts of tissue interferes with ability of uterus to remain firmly contracted.
Infection	Inflammation interferes with uterine muscle's ability to contract effectively.
Overdistention of uterus	Overstretching of uterine muscles with conditions such as multiple gestation, hydramnios, or a very large baby may set the stage for slower uterine involution.

Rather than forming a fibrous scar in the decidua, the placental site heals by a process of exfoliation. The placental site is undermined by the growth of the endometrial tissue, both from the margins of the site and from the fundi of the endometrial glands left in the basal layer of the site. The infarcted superficial tissue then becomes necrotic and is sloughed off. *Exfoliation* is one of the most important aspects of involution. If the healing of the placental site left a fibrous scar, the area available for further implantation would be limited, as would the number of possible pregnancies.

Factors that enhance involution include an uncomplicated labor and birth, complete expulsion of the amniotic membranes and the placenta, breastfeeding, and early ambulation. Factors that slow uterine involution and the rationale for each factor are listed in Table 30–1.

Changes in Fundal Position

Immediately following the expulsion of the placenta, the uterus contracts firmly to the size of a large grapefruit. The **fundus** (top portion of the uterus) is situated in the midline of the abdomen, one-half to two-thirds of the way between the symphysis pubis and the umbilicus (Figure 30–1). The walls of the contracted uterus, each about 4 to 5 cm thick, are close together, and the uterine blood vessels are firmly compressed by the myometrium. Within 6 to 12 hours after birth, the fundus of the uterus rises to the level of the umbilicus because of blood and clots that remain within the uterus and changes in support of the uterus by the ligaments (Zlatnik, 1994). A fundus that is above the umbilicus and boggy (feels soft and spongy rather than firm and well contracted) is associated with excessive uterine bleeding. As blood collects and forms clots within the uterus, the fundus rises; firm con-

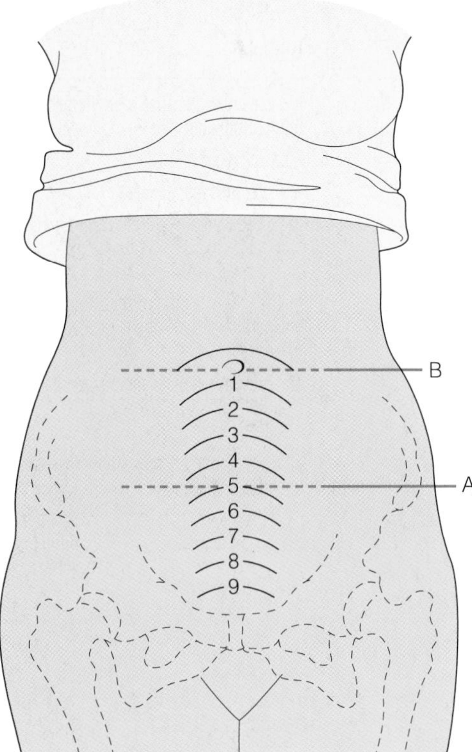

FIGURE 30–1 Involution of the uterus. Immediately after delivery of the placenta, the top of the fundus is in the midline and approximately halfway between the symphysis pubis and the umbilicus (A). About 6 to 12 hours after birth, the fundus is at the level of the umbilicus (B). The height of the fundus then decreases about one fingerbreadth (approximately 1 cm) each day.

tractions of the uterine muscle are interrupted, causing a **boggy uterus.** When the fundus is higher than expected and deviated from the midline (usually to the right), bladder distention should be suspected. Because the uterine ligaments are still stretched, a full bladder can move the uterus.

After birth, the top of the fundus remains at the level of the umbilicus for about half a day. On the first postpartum day (first day following birth), the top of the fundus is located about 1 cm below the umbilicus. The top of the fundus descends approximately one fingerbreadth (width of index, second, or third finger), or 1 cm, per day until it descends into the pelvis on about the tenth day (Cunningham et al, 1997).

If the mother is breastfeeding, the release of endogenous oxytocin from the posterior pituitary in response to suckling hastens this process. Barring complications, such as infection or retained placental fragments, the uterus approaches its prepregnant size and location by 5 to 6 weeks (Cunningham et al, 1997). In women who had an oversized uterus during the pregnancy (hydramnios, birth of a large-for-gestational-age [LGA] infant, or multiple gestation), the time frame for immediate uterine involution process is lengthened. If intrauterine infection is present, the uterine fundus descends much more slowly. This slowing of descent is called **subinvolution** (for further discussion of subinvolution, see Chapter 33).

Lochia

One of the unique capabilities of the uterus is its ability to rid itself of the debris remaining after birth. This discharge, termed **lochia,** is classified according to its appearance and contents. **Lochia rubra** is dark red in color. It is present for the first 2 to 3 days postpartum and contains epithelial cells, erythrocytes, leukocytes, bacteria, shreds of the decidua, and occasionally fetal meconium, lanugo, and vernix caseosa. Lochia should not contain large clots; if it does, the cause should be investigated without delay. A few small clots (no larger than a nickel) are considered normal. **Lochia serosa** is a pinkish to brownish color. It follows from about the third to the tenth day. Lochia serosa is composed of serous exudate (hence the name), shreds of degenerating decidua, erythrocytes, leukocytes, cervical mucus, and numerous microorganisms.

The blood cell component decreases gradually, and a creamy or yellowish discharge persists for an additional week or two. This final discharge, termed **lochia alba,** is composed primarily of leukocytes, decidual cells, epithelial cells, fat, cervical mucus, cholesterol crystals, and bacteria. In breastfeeding women, lochia may continue beyond 6 weeks postpartum. It is believed that the flow is associated with the exfoliation process of the placental site, which does not terminate until after this time (Visness, Kennedy, & Ramos, 1997). When the lochia stops, the cervix is considered closed, and chances of infection ascending from the vagina to the uterus decrease.

Like menstrual discharge, lochia has a musty, stale odor that is not offensive. Microorganisms are always present in the vaginal lochia, and by the second day following birth the uterus is contaminated with the vaginal bacteria. Researchers speculate that infection does not develop because the organisms involved are relatively nonvirulent. In addition, by the time the bacteria reach the raw, exposed surface of the uterus, the process of granulation has begun, forming a protective barrier. Any foul smell to the lochia or used peri-pad suggests infection and the need for prompt additional assessment, such as white blood cell count and differential and assessment for uterine tenderness and fever.

The total volume of lochia is approximately 240 to 270 mL (8 to 9 oz), and the daily volume decreases gradually. Discharge is greater in the morning because of pooling in the vagina and uterus while the mother lies sleeping. The amount of lochia may also be increased by exertion or breastfeeding.

Evaluation of lochia is necessary not only to determine the presence of hemorrhage but also to assess uterine involution. The type, amount, and consistency of lochia determine the state of healing of the placental site, and a progressive change from bright red at birth to dark red to pink to white or clear discharge should be observed. Persistent discharge of lochia rubra or a return to lochia rubra indicates subinvolution or late postpartal hemorrhage (see Chapter 33).

The nurse should exercise caution in evaluating bleeding immediately after birth. The continuous seepage of blood is more consistent with cervical or vaginal lacerations and may be effectively diagnosed when the bleeding is evaluated in conjunction with the consistency of the uterus. Lacerations should be suspected if the uterus is firm and of expected size and if no clots can be expressed.

Cervical Changes

Following birth, the cervix is spongy, flabby, and formless and may appear bruised. The lateral aspects of the external os are frequently lacerated during the birth process (Cunningham et al, 1997). However, the original form of the cervix is regained within a few hours (Resnik, 1999). The external os is markedly irregular and closes slowly. It admits two fingers for a few days following birth, but by the end of the first week it will admit only a fingertip.

The shape of the external os is permanently changed by the first childbearing. The characteristic dimplelike os of the nullipara changes to the lateral slit (fish-mouth) os of the multipara. After significant cervical laceration or several lacerations, the cervix may appear lopsided. Because of the slight change in the size of the cervix, a diaphragm or cervical cap will need to be refitted if the woman is using one of these methods of contraception.

Vaginal Changes

Following birth, the vagina appears edematous and may be bruised. Small superficial lacerations may be evident, and the rugae have been obliterated. The apparent bruising of the vagina is due to pelvic congestion and will quickly disappear. The hymen, torn and jagged, heals irregularly, leaving small tags called the *carunculae myrtiformes.*

The size of the vagina decreases and rugae return within 3 weeks. This facilitates the gradual return to smaller, although not to nulliparous, dimensions. By 6 weeks, the nonlactating woman's vagina usually appears normal. The lactating woman is in a hypoestrogenic state because of ovarian suppression, and her vaginal mucosa may be pale and without rugae. This may lead to dyspareunia (painful intercourse) (Cunningham et al, 1997). Tone and contractibility of the vaginal opening may be improved by perineal tightening exercises (Kegel's exercises, discussed in Chapter 12), which may begin soon after birth. The labia majora and labia minora are looser in the woman who has borne a child than in the nullipara.

Perineal Changes

During the early postpartal period, the soft tissue in and around the perineum may appear edematous with some bruising (Figure 30–2). If an episiotomy or laceration is present, the edges should be approximated. Occasionally, ecchymosis occurs, and this may delay healing.

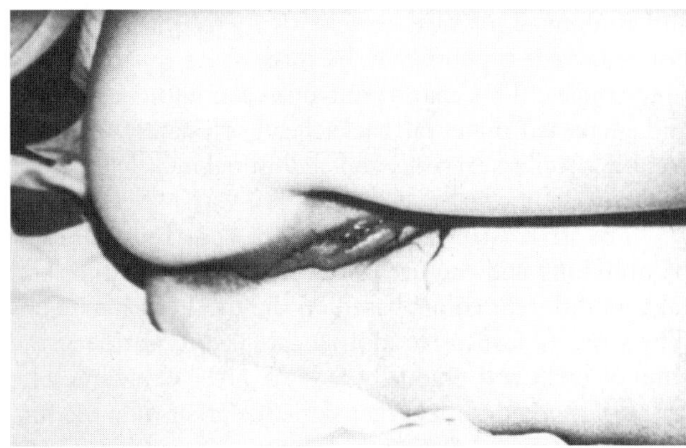

FIGURE 30–2 Bruising and edema of the vulva and perineum in a primipara 3 days after a forceps delivery. SOURCE: Bennett VR, Brown LK: *Myles Textbook for Midwives,* 11th ed. Edinburgh, Scotland: Churchill Livingstone, 1989, p 235.

Recurrence of Ovulation and Menstruation

The return of menstruation and ovulation varies for each postpartal woman. Menstruation generally returns in nonnursing mothers between 7 and 9 weeks after birth, and the first cycle is anovulatory (Resnik, 1999). Overall, 90% of nonnursing mothers resume menstruation by 12 weeks after birth.

The return of menstruation and ovulation in nursing mothers is usually prolonged and is associated with the length of time the woman breastfeeds and whether formula supplements are used. If a nursing mother breastfeeds for less than 1 month, the return of menstruation and ovulation is similar to the nonnursing mother. In women who continue to breastfeed, the return of menstruation may occur as early as the second or as late as the 18th month after delivery (Cunningham et al, 1997).

Abdomen

The uterine ligaments (notably the round and broad ligaments) are stretched and require time to recover. The stretched abdominal wall appears loose and flabby, but it will respond to exercise within 2 to 3 months. In the grandmultipara, in the woman whose abdomen is overdistended, or in the woman whose muscle tone was poor before pregnancy, the abdomen may fail to regain good tone and will remain flabby. **Diastasis recti abdominis,** a separation of the rectus abdominis muscles, may occur with pregnancy, especially in women with poor abdominal muscle tone. If diastasis occurs, part of the abdominal wall has no muscular support but is formed only by skin, subcutaneous fat, fascia, and peritoneum. Improvement depends on the physical condition of the mother, the total number of pregnancies, and the type and amount of physical exercise. If rectus muscle tone is not regained, support may be inadequate during future pregnancies. This may result in a pendulous abdomen and increased maternal backache. Fortunately, diastasis responds well to exercise, and abdominal muscle tone can improve significantly.

The striae (stretch marks), which occurred as a result of stretching and rupture of the elastic fibers of the skin, take on different colors based on the mother's skin color. The striae of Caucasian mothers are red to purple at the time of birth and gradually fade to silver or white. The striae of mothers with darker skin are darker than the surrounding skin and remain darker.

Lactation

During pregnancy, the breasts develop in preparation for lactation as a result of the influence of both estrogen and progesterone. After birth, the interplay of maternal hormones leads to the establishment of milk production (see Chapter 27).

Gastrointestinal System

Hunger following birth is common, and the mother may enjoy a light meal. Frequently, she is quite thirsty and will drink large amounts of fluid. Drinking fluids helps replace fluid lost during labor, in the urine, and through perspiration.

The bowels tend to be sluggish after birth because of the lingering effects of progesterone and decreased abdominal muscle tone. Women who have had an episiotomy may tend to delay elimination for fear of increasing their pain or in the belief that their stitches will be torn if they bear down. In most instances the initial bowel movement is not uncomfortable. However, refusing or delaying the bowel movement may cause constipation and more discomfort when elimination finally occurs.

The woman with a cesarean birth may receive clear liquids shortly after surgery, and once bowel sounds are present the diet is quickly advanced to solid food. The woman may experience some initial discomfort from flatulence. This is relieved by early ambulation and use of antiflatulent medications. It may take a few days for the bowel to regain its tone. The woman who has had a cesarean or a difficult birth may benefit from stool softeners. In some cases it may be necessary to administer an enema or suppository to promote elimination.

Urinary Tract

The postpartal woman has an increased bladder capacity, swelling and bruising of the tissues around the urethra, decreased sensitivity to fluid pressure, and decreased sensation of bladder filling. Consequently, she is at risk for overdistention, incomplete emptying, and buildup of residual urine. Women who have had an anesthetic block have inhibited neural functioning of the bladder and are more susceptible to bladder distention, difficulty voiding, and bladder retention.

Urinary output increases during the early postpartal period (first 12 to 24 hours) due to *puerperal diuresis*. The kidneys must eliminate an estimated 2000 to 3000 mL of extracellular fluid with a normal pregnancy, which causes rapid filling of the bladder. Thus adequate bladder elimination is an immediate concern. Women with pregnancy-induced hypertension (PIH), chronic hypertension, and diabetes experience even greater fluid retention, and postpartal diuresis is increased accordingly.

Bladder elimination presents an immediate problem. If stasis exists, chances increase for urinary tract infection because of bacteriuria and the presence of dilated ureters and renal pelves, which persist for about 6 weeks after birth. A full bladder may also increase the tendency of the uterus to relax by displacing the uterus and interfering with its contractility, leading to hemorrhage.

Hematuria, resulting from bladder trauma, may occasionally occur after birth, but the presence of lochia may mask this sign. If hematuria occurs in the second or third postpartal week, there may be a bladder infection. Acetone may be present in the urine of women with diabetes or of women with prolonged labor and dehydration. Slight (1+) proteinuria may occur during the first week following birth. However, proteinuria may be associated with an infectious process (cystitis, pyelitis), so it should be evaluated further. A urine specimen contaminated with lochia may falsely indicate proteinuria, so any specimen should be obtained as a midstream or a catheterized specimen.

Vital Signs

During the postpartal period, with the exception of the first 24 hours, the woman should be afebrile. A temperature of up to 38C (100.4F) may occur up to 24 hours after birth as a result of the exertion and dehydration of labor. Infection must be considered in the woman with a temperature of 38C or above after the first 24 hours (see Chapter 33).

Blood pressure readings should remain stable and within normal range following the birth. A decrease may indicate physiologic readjustment to decreased intrapelvic pressure, or it may be related to uterine hemorrhage. Blood pressure elevations, especially when they are accompanied by headache (nondependent edema or proteinuria) suggest PIH, and the woman should be evaluated further.

Puerperal bradycardia with rates of 50 to 70 beats per minute commonly occurs during the first 6 to 10 days of the postpartal period. It may be related to decreased cardiac strain, the decreased blood volume following placental separation, contraction of the uterus, and increased stroke volume. Tachycardia occurs less frequently and is related to increased blood loss or difficult, prolonged labor and birth.

Blood Values

Blood values should return to the prepregnant state by the end of the postpartal period. Pregnancy-associated activation of coagulation factors may continue for variable amounts of time. This condition, in conjunction with trauma, immobility, or sepsis, predisposes the woman to development of thromboembolism. Plasma fibrinogen is maintained at pregnancy levels for a week following childbirth, accounting for the higher sedimentation rate observed in the early postpartum period.

Leukocytosis with white blood cell (WBC) counts up to 30,000 per mL persists in the early postpartal days (Cunningham et al, 1997). The leukocytosis does not necessarily indicate infection. An increase of greater than 30% in 6 hours is an indication of pathology. Other clinical signs of infection (elevation of temperature, redness, swelling, and pain) must be evaluated.

Blood loss averages 200 to 500 mL with a vaginal birth and 700 to 1000 mL with a cesarean birth. Hemoglobin and erythrocyte values vary during the early puerperium, but they should approximate or exceed prelabor values within 2 to 6 weeks. As extracellular fluid is excreted, hemoconcentration occurs, with a concomitant rise in hematocrit. A drop in values indicates an abnormal blood loss. The following is a convenient rule of thumb: a 2-point drop in hematocrit equals a blood loss of 500 mL (Varney, 1997).

Weight Loss

An initial weight loss of 10 to 12 lb occurs as a result of the birth of infant, placenta, and amniotic fluid. Puerperal diuresis accounts for the loss of an additional 5 lb during the early puerperium. By the sixth to eighth week after birth, many women have returned to approximately prepregnant weight if they gained the average 25 to 30 lb. For others, a return to prepregnant weight takes longer or does not occur.

Postpartal Chill

Most mothers experience a shaking chill immediately after birth, which may be related to a neurologic response or to vasomotor changes. Covering the woman with warmed bath blankets will help alleviate the chill and increase her comfort. The mother may also find a warm beverage helpful. Chills and fever later in the puerperium indicate infection and require further evaluation.

Postpartal Diaphoresis

The elimination of excess fluid and waste products via the skin during the puerperium greatly increases perspiration. Diaphoretic episodes frequently occur at night, and the woman may awaken drenched with perspiration. This perspiration is not significant clinically, but the mother should be protected from chilling.

Afterpains

Afterpains occur more commonly in multiparas than in primiparas and are caused by intermittent uterine contractions. Although the uterus of the primipara usually remains consistently contracted, the lost tone of the uterus of the multipara results in alternate contraction and relaxation. This phenomenon also occurs if the uterus has been markedly distended, as with multiple pregnancies or hydramnios, or if clots or placental fragments were retained. These afterpains may cause the mother severe discomfort for 2 to 3 days following birth. The administration of oxytocic agents (intravenous infusion with Pitocin or oral administration of Methergine) stimulates uterine contraction and increases the discomfort of the afterpains. Because oxytocin is released when the infant suckles, breastfeeding also increases the severity of the afterpains. The nursing mother may find it helpful to take a mild analgesic agent approximately 1 hour before feeding her infant. The nurse can assure the nursing mother that the prescribed analgesic agents are not harmful to the newborn and help improve the quality of the breastfeeding experience. An analgesic agent is also helpful at bedtime if the afterpains interfere with the mother's rest.

Postpartal Psychologic Adaptations

Maternal Role

The postpartal period is a time of readjustment and adaptation for the entire childbearing family, but especially for the mother. The woman experiences a variety of responses as she adjusts to a new family member, postpartal discomforts, changes in her body image, and the reality that she is no longer pregnant. One young mother described her responses well:

> *I feel like it's the day after Christmas. I'm relieved that everything went well and I have a fine baby, but I feel so let down. I had an image of what childbirth would be like, but everything was a little different. I figured that as soon as I gave birth, I would feel fine. Why didn't someone tell me I would still be sore; the pain didn't magically disappear! When I was pregnant, everyone treated me as though I was a little fragile. Now when people call or visit, all they talk about is the baby. I don't think I'm really jealous, but I do miss the attention. During this past day I've started to realize that my life will never, ever be the same again. I've always wanted to be a mother, but I'm not really sure how to do it. Isn't that strange?*

During the first day or two following birth, the woman tends to be passive and somewhat dependent. The new mother follows suggestions, is hesitant about making decisions, and is still rather preoccupied with her needs. She may have a great need to talk about her perceptions of her labor and birth. This helps her work through the process, sort out the reality from her fantasized experience, and clarify anything that she did not understand. Food and sleep are major focuses. The woman is talkative but passive. In her early work, Rubin (1961) labeled this the *taking-in* period.

By the second or third day after birth, the new mother is then ready to resume control of her life. She may be concerned about controlling bodily functions, such as elimination. If she is breastfeeding, she may worry about the quality of her milk and her ability to nurse her baby. She requires assurance that she is doing well as a mother. If her baby spits up following feeding, she may view it as a personal failure. She may also feel demoralized by the fact that the nurse handles her baby proficiently while she feels unsure and tentative. Rubin (1961) labeled this phase as *taking-hold.*

Today's environment and birthing care has changed drastically from the time of Rubin's research. Mothers are more independent and adjust more rapidly. Ament (1990) found that women did exhibit behavior characteristics of "taking-in" and "taking-hold" but found that the time frames were shorter than those cited by Rubin. Martell (1996) discovered that aspects of "taking-in" and "taking-hold" surfaced during the first 12 hours postpartally. Examples cited by study participants of "taking-in" were inactivity, tiredness, and a desire to converse regarding the labor and birth process. Plans for discharge, proactive personal control, and requests for needs were aspects of the "taking-hold" phase recounted by participants. These behaviors were found to be elements of the original concepts described by Rubin; however, because of the prevailing changes in postpartal women, the paradigm first described by Rubin (1961) is no longer relevant as originally stated. More research and the development of a new theory directed at contemporary postpartal clients is vital. It will be interesting to see what further study brings to this subject.

Postpartally, the woman must adjust to a changed body image. Often women, especially primiparas, are surprised and rather dismayed to discover that they do not return to their prepregnant weight and shape as soon as the baby is born. Women often express dissatisfaction about their appearance and concern about the return of their weight and figure to normal. Multiparas tend to be more positive about their appearance postpartally than primiparas. This may be because the multipara's previous experience has prepared her for the fact that the body does not immediately return to a prepregnant state.

The psychologic outcomes of the postpartal period are far more positive when the parents have access to a support network. Women and their partners may find that family relationships become increasingly important, and the attention that their infant receives from family members is a source of satisfaction to the new parents. In many cases, the ties to the woman's family become especially good. Fathers may report that their relationships with their in-laws become far more positive and supportive. But the increased family interaction can be a source of stress, especially for the new mother, who tends to have more contact with the families.

Childbearing couples often change their social network somewhat following the birth of their child. Once the new parents have made the transition to parenthood, they both tend to have more contact with other parents of small children. For the woman, interaction with coworkers often declines postpartally, but contact with friends increases. Thus the woman maintains the size of her support group but alters it to meet the changes that have occurred in her lifestyle.

Perhaps the greatest concern involves women and their partners who have no family available and no friends to form a social network. Isolation during a time in which the woman feels an increased need for support can result in tremendous stress and is often a contributing factor in situations of child neglect or abuse.

A prime focus of research in recent years has been maternal role attainment. **Maternal role attainment** is the process by which a woman learns mothering behaviors and becomes comfortable with her identity as a mother. The formation of a maternal identity indicates that the woman has attained the maternal role. Formation of a maternal identity occurs with each child a woman bears. As the mother grows to know this child and forms a relationship with her or him, the mother's maternal identity gradually, systematically evolves, and she "binds in" to the infant (Rubin, 1984).

Maternal role attainment occurs in four stages (Mercer, 1995):

1. The *anticipatory stage* occurs during pregnancy. The woman looks to role models, especially her own mother, for examples of how to mother.
2. The *formal stage* begins when the child is born. The woman is still influenced by the guidance of others and tries to act as she believes others expect her to act.
3. The *informal stage* begins when the mother begins to make her own choices about mothering. The woman begins to develop her own style of mothering and finds ways of functioning that work well for her.
4. The *personal stage* is the final stage of maternal role attainment. When the woman reaches this stage, she is comfortable with the notion of herself as "mother."

The formal and informal stages of maternal role attainment correspond with the taking-in and taking-hold stages previously identified by Rubin (1961).

In most cases, maternal role attainment occurs within 3 to 10 months following birth. Social support, the woman's age and personality traits, the temperament of her infant, and the family's socioeconomic status all influence the woman's success in attaining the maternal role. Research by Sethi (1995) suggests that the process of becoming a mother requires a minimum of 3 months. Following the birth, the woman initially experiences sensations that are profoundly opposite in meaning, such as devotion/sacrifice or happiness/frustration. The woman gives unselfishly of herself while establishing a new role. Following that phase, women go through a metamorphosis in which they finally evolve as a mother of a young infant. This changes other facets of their life, such as professional goals or personal relationships (McVeigh, 1998).

The postpartal woman faces a number of challenges as she adjusts to her new role (Mercer, 1995):

- For many women, finding time for themselves is one of the greatest challenges. It is often difficult for the new mother to find time to read a book, talk to her partner, or even eat a meal without interruption.
- Women also report feelings of incompetence because they have not mastered all aspects of the mothering role. Often they are unsure of what to do in a given situation.
- The next greatest challenge involves fatigue resulting from sleep deprivation. The demands of nighttime care are tremendously draining, especially if the woman has other children.
- One challenge the new mother faces involves the feeling of responsibility that having a child brings. Women experience a sense of lost freedom, an awareness that they will never again be quite as carefree as they were before becoming mothers. Mothers sometimes cite the infant's behavior as a problem, especially when the child is about 8 months old. Stranger anxiety develops, the infant begins crawling and getting into things, teething may cause fussiness, and the baby's tendency to put everything in his or her mouth requires constant vigilance by the parent.

Mothers, whether primiparas or multiparas, have a variety of concerns following childbirth related to their own physiologic changes, newborn care, and methods to manage recovery from childbirth. The Maternal Concerns Questionnaire developed by Sheil and colleagues (1995) is a useful tool for nurses. It helps the mother identify the degree of concern she has regarding her own and the baby's needs, concerns related to her partner and family, and concerns related to the community. For each area, the mother can note specific needs and rate each as of no concern, little concern, moderate concern, or much concern. After the mother completes the questionnaire, the nurse can identify the woman's concerns and informational needs and address each one. Postpartum nurses must be aware of the long-term adjustments and stresses that the childbearing family faces as its members adjust to new and different roles. Nurses can help by providing anticipatory guidance about the realities of being a mother. Agencies should have literature available for reference at home. Ongoing parenting groups give parents an opportunity to discuss problems and become comfortable in new roles.

Postpartum Blues

The term **postpartum blues** describes a transient period of depression that occurs in most women during the first week or two after birth. It may be manifested by mood swings, anger, weepiness, anorexia, difficulty sleeping, and a feeling of letdown. Because of the practice of early postpartum discharge, the depression often occurs at home. Psychologic adjustments and hormonal changes are thought to be the main causes, although fatigue, discomfort, and overstimulation may play a part. The postpartum blues usually resolve naturally, especially if the woman receives understanding and support. If symptoms persist or intensify, the woman may need evaluation for postpartum depression (see Chapter 33).

Development of Parent-Infant Attachment

A mother's first interaction with her infant is influenced by many factors, including her family of origin, her relationships, the stability of her home environment, the communication patterns she has developed, and the degree of nurturing she received as a child. Certain characteristics of that self are also important:

- *Level of trust.* What level of trust has this mother developed in response to her life experiences? What is her philosophy of childrearing? Will she be able to treat her infant as a unique individual with changing needs that should be met as much as possible?
- *Level of self-esteem.* How much does she value herself as a woman and as a mother? Does she feel generally able to cope with the adjustments of life?
- *Capacity for enjoying herself.* Is the mother able to find pleasure in everyday activities and human relationships?
- *Interest in and adequacy of knowledge about childbearing and childrearing.* What beliefs about the course of pregnancy, the capacities of newborns, and the nature of her emotions may influence her behavior at first contact with her infant and later?
- *Her prevailing mood or usual feeling tone.* Is the woman predominantly content, angry, depressed, or anxious? Is she sensitive to her own feelings and those of others? Will she be able to accept her own needs and to obtain support in meeting them?
- *Reactions to the present pregnancy.* Was the pregnancy planned? Did it go smoothly? Were there ongoing life events that enhanced her pregnancy or depleted her reserves of energy?

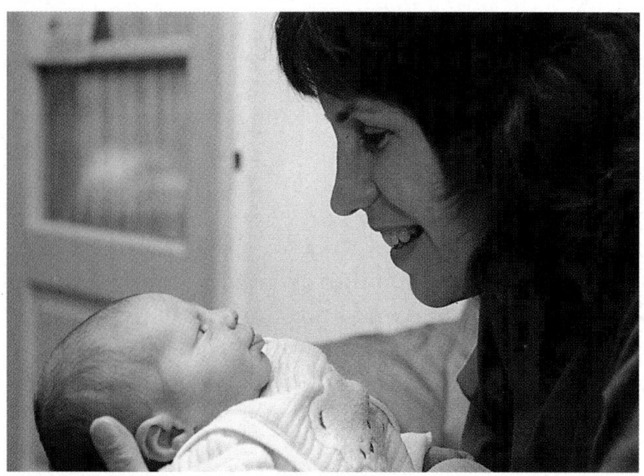

FIGURE 30–3 The mother has direct face-to-face and eye-to-eye contact in the *en face* position.

By the time of birth, each mother has developed an emotional orientation of some kind to the baby based on these factors, as well as a physical awareness of the fetus within her and her fantasy images and perceptions.

Initial Attachment Behavior

New mothers demonstrate a fairly regular pattern of maternal behaviors at first contact with a normal newborn. In a progression of touching activities, the mother proceeds from fingertip exploration of the newborn's extremities toward palmar contact with larger body areas and finally to enfolding the infant with the whole hand and arms. The time taken to accomplish these steps varies from minutes to days, depending, it appears, on the timing of the first contact, the clothing barriers present, and the physical condition of the baby. Maternal excitement and elation tend to increase during the time of the initial meeting. The mother also increases the proportion of time spent in the **en face** position (Figure 30–3). She arranges herself or the newborn so that she has direct face-to-face and eye-to-eye contact. There is an intense interest in having the infant's eyes open. When the eyes are open, the mother characteristically greets the newborn and talks in high-pitched tones to him or her.

In most instances the mother relies heavily on her senses of sight, touch, and hearing in getting to know what her baby is really like. She tends also to respond verbally to any sounds emitted by the newborn, such as cries, coughs, sneezes, and grunts. The sense of smell may also be involved, although this possibility has not yet been adequately studied.

In addition to interacting with the newborn, the mother is undergoing her own emotional reactions to the birth and, more specifically, to the baby as she perceives him or her. The frequency of the "I can't believe" reaction leads to speculation that human beings meet gains as well as losses with a degree of shock, disbelief, and denial. Among mothers, a feeling of emotional distance from the newborn is quite common: "I felt he was a stranger." However, the mother may express feelings of connectedness between the newborn and the rest of the family, either in positive or in negative terms: "She's got your cute nose, Daddy,"or "Oh, no! He looks just like the first one, and he was an impossible baby." A mother's facial expression or the frequency and content of her questions may demonstrate concerns about the infant's general condition or normality, especially if her pregnancy was complicated or if a previously delivered baby was not normal.

What are the characteristic behaviors of a newborn? Unless care is taken to effect a gentle birth, many harsh stimuli assault the senses of the newborn at birth. The newborn is probably suctioned, held with head down somewhat, exposed to bright lights and cool air, and in some way cleansed. The infant usually responds by crying. In fact, caregivers typically stimulate the newborn to cry to reassure themselves that the baby is well and normal. When newborns no longer need to concentrate most of their energy on physical and physiologic responses to the immediate crisis of birth, they are able to lie quietly with eyes open, looking about, moving their limbs occasionally, making sucking motions, possibly attempting to get hand to mouth. Placed in appropriate proximity to the mother, the newborn appears to focus briefly on her face and attend to her voice in the first moment of life.

During the first few days after her child's birth, the new mother applies herself to the task of getting to know her baby. This is termed the *acquaintance phase*. If the infant gives clear behavioral cues about needs, the infant's responses to mothering will be predictable, which will make the mother feel effective and competent. Other behaviors that make an infant more attractive to caretakers are smiling, grasping a finger, nursing eagerly, cuddling, and being easy to console.

During this time the newborn is also becoming acquainted. Within a few days after birth, infants show signs of recognizing recurrent situations and responding to changes in routine. To the extent that their mother is their world, it can be said that they are actively acquainting themselves with her.

During the *phase of mutual regulation*, mother and infant seek to deal with the issue of the degree of control to be exerted by each in their relationship. In this phase of adjustment, a balance is sought between the needs of the mother and the needs of the infant. The most important consideration is that each should obtain a good measure of enjoyment from the interaction. During the mutual adjustment phase, negative maternal feelings are likely to surface or intensify. Because they feel that they are expected to love their babies, mothers often fail to express these negative feelings, which often then build up. If the mother does express these feelings, friends, relatives, or health care personnel often respond by denying them: "You don't mean that." Some negative feelings are normal in the first few days after birth, and the nurse should be supportive when the mother vocalizes these feelings.

When mutual regulation arrives at the point where both mother and infant primarily enjoy each other's company, reciprocity has been achieved. **Reciprocity** is an interactional cycle that occurs simultaneously between mother and infant. It involves mutual cuing behaviors, expectancy, rhythmicity, and synchrony. The mother develops a new relationship with an individual who has a unique character and evokes a response entirely different from the fantasy response of pregnancy. When reciprocity is synchronous, the interaction between mother and infant is mutually gratifying and is sought and initiated by both partners. They find pleasure and delight in each other's company and grow in mutual love.

Father-Infant Interactions

Traditionally in Western cultures, the primary role of the expectant father has been one of support for the pregnant woman. Commitment to family-centered maternity care, however, has fostered interest in understanding the feelings and experiences of the new father. Evidence suggests that the father has a strong attraction to his newborn and that the feelings he experiences are similar to the mother's feelings of attachment (Figure 30–4). The characteristic sense of absorption, preoccupation, and interest in the infant demonstrated by fathers during early contact has been termed **engrossment.**

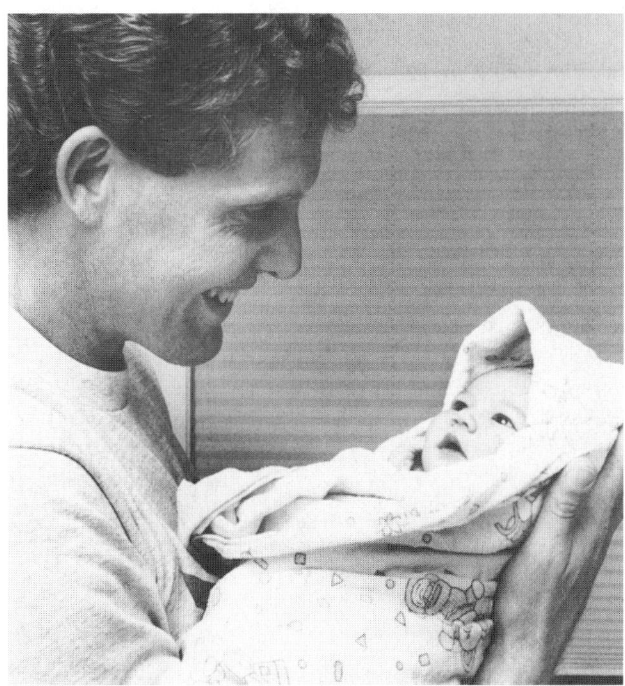

FIGURE 30–4 The father experiences strong feelings of attraction during engrossment.

CRITICAL THINKING QUESTION

At times men may feel funny talking to their newborns. How can the nurse encourage the father to vocalize with his baby?

Siblings and Others

Infants are also capable of maintaining a number of strong attachments without loss of quality. These attachments may include siblings, grandparents, aunts, and uncles. The social setting and personality of the individual seem to be significant factors in the development of multiple attachments. The advent of open visiting hours and rooming-in permits siblings and grandparents to participate in the attachment process.

Cultural Influences in the Postpartal Period

The new mother's beliefs about her postpartal care are influenced by her culture and personal values. Her expectations regarding food, fluids, rest, hygiene, medications and relief measures, support and counsel—as well as other aspects of her life—will be influenced by the beliefs and values of her family and cultural group. Sometimes a new mother's wishes will differ from the expectations of the CNM/physician or nurse.

Nurses also belong to a particular culture, as well as to the health care cultural group. As a part of the health care cultural group, nurses implement practices that support their general beliefs, such as offering food in the recovery period following birth, providing iced fluids, expecting the woman to ambulate as soon as possible, and assuming the woman will want to shower and perhaps wash her hair soon after birth. However, these practices may be in opposition to the woman's beliefs and expectations. To individualize care for each mother, the nurse needs to assess the woman's preferences, have her exercise her choices when possible, and support those choices, with the help of cultural awareness and a sound knowledge base (Pope-Davis, Eliason, & Ottavi, 1994).

Although describing the practices of different cultural groups always involves some generalization, it is helpful for nurses to understand some of the possible differences in beliefs and practices that they may encounter. For example, a woman of European heritage may expect to eat a full meal and have a large amount of iced fluids following the birth, in the belief that the food restores energy and the fluids help replace fluid lost during the labor. She may want to ambulate shortly after the birth and shower, wash her hair, and put on a fresh gown. She may expect a relatively short stay in the hospital and may or may not be interested in educational classes. Women of the Islamic faith have specific modesty requirements; the woman must be completely covered, with only her feet and hands exposed. A man, other than the husband or family member, may not be alone with the woman (Hutchinson & Baqi-Aziz, 1994).

Many cultures emphasize certain postpartal routines or rituals for mother and baby, which are designed to restore the harmony, or the hot-cold balance, of the body.

TABLE 30–2 Postpartal High-Risk Factors

Factor	Maternal Implication
PIH	↑ Blood pressure ↑ CNS irritability ↑ Need for bed rest → ↑ risk thrombophlebitis
Diabetes	Need for insulin regulation Episodes of hypoglycemia or hyperglycemia ↓ Healing
Cardiac disease	↑ Maternal exhaustion
Cesarean birth	↑ Healing needs ↑ Pain from incision ↑ Risk of infection ↑ Length of hospitalization
Overdistention of uterus (multiple gestation, hydramnios)	↑ Risk of hemorrhage ↑ Risk of anemia ↑ Stretching of abdominal muscles ↑ Incidence and severity of afterpains
Abruptio placentae, placenta previa	Hemorrhage → anemia ↓ Uterine contractility after birth → ↑ infection risk
Precipitous labor (<3 hours)	↑ Risk of lacerations to birth canal → hemorrhage
Prolonged labor (>24 hours)	Exhaustion ↑ Risk of hemorrhage Nutritional and fluid depletion ↑ Bladder atony and/or trauma
Difficult birth	Exhaustion ↑ Risk of perineal lacerations ↑ Risk of hematomas ↑ Risk of hemorrhage → anemia
Extended period of time in stirrups at birth	↑ Risk of thrombophlebitis
Retained placenta	↑ Risk of hemorrhage ↑ Risk of infection

For example, some women of India, Mexican, African, and Asian cultures may avoid cold after birth. This prohibition includes cold air, wind, and all water (even if heated). Dietary changes also reflect the need to avoid cold foods and restore the balance between hot and cold (Howard & Berbiglia, 1997; Andrew & Boyle, 1995; Jambunathan, 1995; Hutchinson & Baqi-Aziz, 1994). For instance, a traditional Mexican woman may avoid eating "hot" foods, such as pork, just after the birth of her baby. It is important to note that each individual or cultural group may define hot and cold conditions as well as hot and cold foods differently. Therefore, the nurse should ask each woman what she can eat and what foods she thinks would be helpful for healing (Choudhry, 1997; Andrew & Boyle, 1995). The nurse may encourage family members to bring preferred food and drink for the mother.

In many cultures, the extended family plays an essential role during the puerperium. The grandmother is often the primary helper to the mother and newborn (Choudhry, 1997). She brings wisdom and experience, allowing the new mother time to rest as well as giving her ready access to someone who can help with problems and concerns as they arise. It is important to ensure access of all family members during the postpartal period. Visiting rules may be waived to allow family members or authority figures access to the mother and newborn. These practices show respect and foster a blending of old and new behaviors to meet the goals of all concerned.

CRITICAL THINKING QUESTION

How can you use your knowledge of cultural beliefs to influence delivery of postpartum care?

Postpartal Nursing Assessment

Comprehensive care is based on a thorough assessment, with identification of individual needs or potential problems. (See the accompanying Assessment Guide: Postpartal—First 24 Hours After Birth.)

Risk Factors

The emphasis on ongoing assessment and education during the puerperium is designed to meet the needs of the childbearing family and to detect and treat possible complications. Table 30–2 identifies factors that may place the new mother at risk during the postpartal period. The nurse uses this knowledge during the assessment and is particularly alert for possible complications that may occur in an individual because of identified risk factors.

CRITICAL THINKING QUESTION

Using your knowledge of general physical assessment, how would you alter your approach to doing a postpartal physical assessment?

Physical Assessment

The nurse should use the following principles in preparing for and completing an assessment of the postpartal woman:

- Select the time that will provide the most accurate data. Palpating the fundus when the woman has a full bladder, for example, may give false information about the progress of involution.
- Provide an explanation of the purposes of regular assessment to the woman.
- Ensure that the woman is relaxed before starting; perform the procedures as gently as possible to avoid unnecessary discomfort.
- Record and report the results as clearly as possible.

Text continues on page 920.

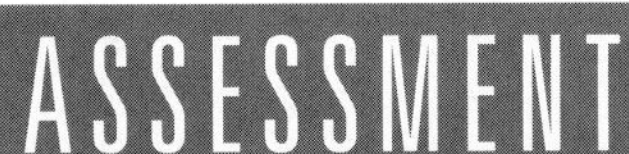 GUIDE: POSTPARTAL—FIRST 24 HOURS AFTER BIRTH

Physical Assessment/ Normal Findings	Alterations and Possible Causes*	Nursing Responses to Data†
Vital Signs		
Blood pressure (BP): Should remain consistent with baseline BP during pregnancy.	High BP (PIH, essential hypertension, renal disease, anxiety). Drop in BP (may be normal; uterine hemorrhage).	Evaluate history of preexisting disorders and check for other signs of PIH (edema, proteinuria). Assess for other signs of hemorrhage (↑ pulse, cool clammy skin).
Pulse: 50–90 beats/minute. May be bradycardia of 50–70 beats/minute.	Tachycardia (difficult labor and birth, hemorrhage).	Evaluate for other signs of hemorrhage (↓ BP, cool clammy skin).
Respirations: 16–24/minute.	Marked tachypnea (respiratory disease).	Assess for other signs of respiratory disease.
Temperature: 36.2–38C (98–100.4F).	After first 24 hours temperature of 38C (100.4F) or above suggests infection.	Assess for other signs of infection; notify physician/certified nurse-midwife.
Breasts		
General appearance: Smooth, even pigmentation, changes of pregnancy still apparent; one may appear larger.	Reddened area (mastitis).	Assess further for signs of infection.
Palpation: Depending on postpartal day, may be soft, filling, full, or engorged.	Palpable mass (caked breast, mastitis). Engorgement (venous stasis). Tenderness, heat, edema (engorgement, caked breast, mastitis).	Assess for other signs of infection: If blocked duct, consider heat, massage, position change for breastfeeding. Assess for further signs. Report mastitis to physician/certified nurse-midwife.
Nipples: Supple, pigmented, intact; become erect when stimulated.	Fissures, cracks, soreness (problems with breastfeeding), not erectile with stimulation (inverted nipples).	Reassess technique; recommend appropriate interventions.
Abdomen		
Musculature: Abdomen may be soft, have a "doughy" texture; rectus muscle intact.	Separation in musculature (diastasis recti abdominis).	Evaluate size of diastasis; teach appropriate exercises for decreasing the separation.
Fundus: Firm, midline; following expected process of involution.	Boggy (full bladder, uterine bleeding).	Massage until firm; assess bladder and have woman void if needed; attempt to express clots when firm. If bogginess remains or recurs, report to physician/certified nurse-midwife.
May be tender when palpated.	Constant tenderness (infection).	Assess for evidence of endometritis.
Lochia		
Scant to moderate amount, earthy odor; no clots.	Large amount, clots (hemorrhage). Foul-smelling lochia (infection).	Assess for firmness, express additional clots; begin peri-pad count. Assess for other signs of infection; report to physician/certified nurse-midwife.

*Possible causes of alterations are placed in parentheses.

†This column provides guidelines for further assessment and initial nursing actions.

Physical Assessment/ Normal Findings	Alterations and Possible Causes*	Nursing Responses to Data†
Normal progression: First 1–3 days: rubra. Following rubra Days 3–10: serosa (alba seldom seen in hospital).	Failure to progress normally or return to rubra from serosa (subinvolution).	Report to physician/certified nurse-midwife.
Perineum		
Slight edema and bruising in intact perineum.	Marked fullness, bruising, pain (vulvar hematoma).	Assess size; apply ice glove or ice pack; report to physician/certified nurse-midwife.
Episiotomy: No redness, edema, ecchymosis, or discharge; edges well approximated.	Redness, edema, ecchymosis, discharge, or gaping stitches (infection).	Encourage sitz baths; review perineal care, appropriate wiping techniques.
Hemorrhoids: None present; if present, should be small and nontender.	Full, tender, inflamed hemorrhoids.	Encourage sitz baths, side-lying position; tucks pads, anesthetic ointments, manual replacement of hemorrhoids, stool softeners, increased fluid intake.
Costo-Vertebral Angle (CVA) Tenderness		
None.	Present (kidney infection).	Assess for other symptoms of urinary tract infection (UTI); obtain clean-catch urine; report to physician/certified nurse-midwife.
Lower Extremities		
No pain with palpation; negative Homans' sign.	Positive findings (thrombophlebitis).	Report to physician/certified nurse-midwife.
Elimination		
Urinary output: Voiding in sufficient quantities at least every 4–6 hours; bladder not palpable.	Inability to void (urinary retention). Symptoms of urgency, frequency, dysuria (UTI).	Employ nursing interventions to promote voiding; if not successful, obtain order for catheterization. Report symptoms of UTI to physician/certified nurse-midwife.
Bowel elimination: Should have normal bowel movement by second or third day after birth.	Inability to pass feces (constipation due to fear of pain from episiotomy, hemorrhoids, perineal trauma).	Encourage fluids, ambulation, roughage in diet; sitz baths to promote healing of perineum; obtain order for stool softener.

Cultural Assessment‡	Variations to Consider	Nursing Responses to Data†
Determine customs and practices regarding postpartum care. Ask the mother whether she would like fluids, and ask what temperature she prefers.	Individual preference may include • Room-temperature or warmed fluids rather than iced drinks.	Provide for specific request if possible. If woman is unable to provide specific information, the nurse may draw from general information regarding cultural variation.

‡These are only a few suggestions. It is not our intent to imply this is a comprehensive cultural assessment.

*Possible causes of alterations are placed in parentheses.

†This column provides guidelines for further assessment and initial nursing actions.

Cultural Assessment[‡]	Variations to Consider	Nursing Responses to Data[†]
Ask the mother what foods or fluids she would like.	• Special foods or fluids to hasten healing after childbirth.	Mexican women may want food and fluids that restore hot-cold balance to the body. Women of European background may ask for iced fluids.
Ask the mother whether she would prefer to be alone during breastfeeding.	Some women may be hesitant to have someone with them when their breast is exposed.	Provide privacy as desired by mother.
Psychosocial Assessment/ Normal Findings	**Variations to Consider**	**Nursing Responses to Data**
Psychologic Adaptation		
During first 24 hours: Passive; preoccupied with own needs; may talk about her labor and birth experience; may be talkative, elated, or very quiet.	Very quiet and passive; sleeps frequently (fatigue from long labor; feelings of disappointment about some aspect of the experience; may be following cultural expectation).	Provide opportunities for adequate rest; provide nutritious meals and snacks that are consistent with what the woman desires to eat and drink; provide opportunities to discuss birth experience in nonjudgmental atmosphere if the woman desires to do so.
By 12 hours: Beginning to assume responsibility; some women eager to learn; easily feels overwhelmed.	Excessive weepiness, mood swings, pronounced irritability (postpartum blues; feelings of inadequacy; culturally prescribed behavior).	Explain postpartum blues; provide supportive atmosphere; determine support available for mother; consider referral for evidence of profound depression.
Attachment		
En face position; holds baby close; cuddles and soothes; calls by name; identifies characteristics of family members in infant; may be awkward in providing care.	Continued expressions of disappointment in sex, appearance of infant; refusal to care for infant; derogatory comments; lack of bonding behaviors (difficulty in attachment, following expectations of cultural/ethnic group).	Provide reinforcement and support for infant caretaking behaviors; maintain nonjudgmental approach and gather more information if caretaking behaviors are not evident.
Initially may express disappointment over sex or appearance of infant but within 1–2 days demonstrates attachment behaviors.		
Client Education		
Has basic understanding of self-care activities and infant care needs; can identify signs of complications that should be reported.	Unable to demonstrate basic self-care and infant care activities (knowledge deficit; postpartum blues; following prescribed cultural behavior and will be cared for by grandmother or other family member).	Determine whether woman understands English and provide interpreter if needed; provide reinforcement of information through conversation and through written material (remember that some women and their families may not be able to understand written materials because of language difficulties or inability to read); provide information regarding infant care skills that are culturally consistent; give woman opportunity to express her feelings; consider social service home referral for women who have no family or other support, are unable to take in information about self-care and infant care, and demonstrate no caretaking activities.

[‡]These are only a few suggestions. It is not our intent to imply this is a comprehensive cultural assessment.

[†]This column provides guidelines for further assessment and initial nursing actions.

ESSENTIAL PRECAUTIONS IN PRACTICE

During Postpartal Assessment

Examples of times when disposable gloves should be worn include the following:

- Assessing the breast if there is leakage of colostrum or milk
- Assessing the perineum and lochia
- Changing or handling perineal pads
- Handling clothing, perineal pads, and/or bedding contaminated with lochia
- Handling used breast pads

REMEMBER to wash your hands prior to putting the disposable gloves on and AGAIN immediately after you remove the gloves.

For further information, consult OSHA and CDC guidelines.

TABLE 30–3 Common Postpartal Concerns

Source of Concern	Explanation
Gush of blood that sometimes occurs when she first arises	Due to normal pooling of blood in vagina when the woman lies down to rest or sleep. Gravity causes blood to flow out when she stands.
Night sweats	Normal physiologic occurrence that results as body attempts to eliminate excess fluids that were present during pregnancy. May be aggravated by plastic mattress pad.
Afterpains	More common in multiparas. Due to contraction and relaxation of uterus. Increased by oxytocin, breastfeeding. Relieved with mild analgesics and time.
"Large stomach" after birth and failure to lose all weight gained during pregnancy	The baby, amniotic fluid, and placenta account for only a portion of the weight gained during pregnancy. The remainder takes approximately 6 weeks to lose. Abdomen also appears large due to ↓ muscle tone. Postpartal exercises will help.

- Take appropriate precautions to prevent exposure to body fluids. (See Essential Precautions in Practice: During Postpartal Assessment.)

While completing the physical assessment, the nurse should also teach the woman. For example, when assessing the breasts of a nursing woman, the nurse can discuss breast milk production, the let-down reflex, and breast self-examination. Mothers may be very receptive to instruction on postpartal abdominal tightening exercises when the nurse assesses the woman's fundal height and diastasis. The assessment also provides an excellent time to provide information about the body's postpartal physical and anatomic changes as well as danger signs to report (Table 30–3). Because the time the woman spends in the postpartum unit is limited, nurses should use every available opportunity for client teaching regarding self-care. To assist nurses in recognizing these opportunities, examples of client teaching during the assessment have been provided throughout the following discussion.

Vital Signs

The nurse may organize the physical assessment in a variety of ways. Many nurses choose to begin by assessing vital signs because the findings are more accurate when they are obtained with the woman at rest. In addition, establishing whether the vital signs are within the expected normal range will assist the nurse in determining other assessments that might be needed. For instance, if the temperature is elevated, the nurse considers the time since birth and begins to gather information to determine whether the woman is dehydrated or whether an infection is developing.

Alterations in vital signs may indicate complications, so they are assessed at regular intervals. The blood pressure should remain stable. The pulse often shows a characteristic slowness that is no cause for alarm. Pulse rates return to prepregnant norms very quickly unless complications arise.

Temperature elevations (up to 38C [100.4F]) due to normal processes should last for only a few days and should not be associated with other clinical signs of infection. The nurse should evaluate any temperature elevation in light of other signs and symptoms and should carefully review the woman's history to identify other factors, such as premature rupture of membranes (PROM) or prolonged labor, that might increase the incidence of infection in the genital tract.

The nurse informs the woman of the results of the vital signs assessment, providing information regarding the normal changes in blood pressure and pulse. This may also be an opportunity to assess whether the mother knows how to take her own and her infant's temperatures, how to read a thermometer, and how to select a thermometer from the wide variety now available.

Auscultation of Lungs

The breath sounds should be clear. Women who have been treated for preterm labor or PIH are especially at risk for pulmonary edema (see Chapter 15).

Breasts

A properly fitting bra provides support to the breasts and helps maintain breast shape by limiting stretching of supporting ligaments and connective tissue. The nurse can first assess the fit and support provided by the woman's bra. The nurse provides information about how to select a bra. If the mother is breastfeeding, the straps of the bra should be cloth, not elastic (because cloth has less stretch and provides more support) and easily adjustable. The back should be wide and have at least three rows of hooks

CLINICAL TIP

During the first few hours after birth, the woman may have some orthostatic hypotension. This will cause her to have a lower blood pressure reading in a sitting position. For the most accurate reading, measure her BP with her in the same position each time, preferably lying on her back with her arm at her side.

to adjust for fit. Traditional nursing bras have a fixed inner cup and a separate half-cup that can be unhooked for breastfeeding while continuing to support the breast. Purchasing a nursing bra one size too large during pregnancy will usually result in a good fit because the breasts increase in size with milk production.

The bra is then removed so the breasts can be examined. The nurse notes the size and shape of the breasts and any abnormalities, reddened areas, or engorgement. The nurse also palpates the breasts lightly for softness, slight firmness associated with filling, or firmness associated with engorgement, warmth, or tenderness. The nipples are assessed for fissures, cracks, soreness, or inversion. The nurse teaches the woman the characteristics of the breast and explains how to recognize problems such as fissures or cracks in the nipples.

The nurse assesses the nonnursing mother for evidence of breast discomfort and provides relief measures if necessary. (See discussion of lactation suppression in the nonnursing mother in Chapter 31.) Breast assessment findings for a nonnursing woman may be recorded as follows: "Breasts soft, filling, no evidence of nipple tenderness or cracking."

Abdomen and Fundus

The woman should void before her abdomen is examined. This practice ensures that a full bladder is not causing displacement of the uterus or any uterine atony; if atony is present, other causes (such as uterine relaxation associated with a regional block, overstretched uterus, or distended bladder) must be investigated.

The nurse determines the relationship of the fundus to the umbilicus and also assesses the firmness of the fundus. The nurse notes whether the fundus is in the midline or displaced to either side of the abdomen. The most common cause of displacement is a full bladder; thus this finding requires further assessment. If the fundus is in the midline but higher than expected, it is usually associated with clots within the uterus. The results of the assessment should then be recorded. (See Procedure 30–1 on page 922.)

While completing the assessment, the nurse teaches the woman about fundal position and how to determine firmness. The mother can be taught to massage her fundus gently if it is not firm.

CLINICAL TIP

During postpartal assessment, a firm uterus typically feels like a grapefruit because the muscles are well contracted. If the uterus loses its ability to contract and begins to relax, it is called boggy. A boggy uterus feels softer, like a sponge, or may become so relaxed that you can't feel it at all. If the uterus is boggy but you can still feel it, massage it until it becomes firm. If you can't feel it at all, place the side of one hand just above the woman's symphysis pubis to provide stability. Then place the other hand at the level of the umbilicus. (The fundus may have risen to this level because it is relaxed and filling with blood.) Press deeply into the abdomen and massage in a circular motion. You will usually feel the uterus begin to firm up under your hand. If you don't, move your hand slightly lower on the abdomen, and repeat the process.

A well-contracted uterus feels as firm as the uterus does during a strong labor contraction. If handled gently, the uterus should not be overly tender. Excessive pain in the uterus during postpartal examination should alert the nurse to possible uterine infection. If the uterus is not firm, the nurse should gently massage the fundus with the fingertips of the examining hand, then assess the results. If the uterus becomes firm, the chart should read: "Uterus: boggy → firm c̄ light massage." A good habit for the nurse to develop during the postpartal examination is to have the woman lie flat on her back with her head on a pillow and legs flexed. Then the nurse can release the perineal pad to observe the results of uterine massage based on the amount of expelled blood. Occasionally, oxytocic agents, such as an intravenous Pitocin infusion or methylergonovine maleate (Methergine), need to be administered postpartally to maintain uterine contraction and prevent or treat hemorrhage (see Drug Guide: Methylergonovine Maleate [Methergine] in Chapter 31).

A boggy uterus that does not contract with light, gentle massage may need more vigorous massage. The nurse assesses the amount and character of any expelled blood obtained while massaging the fundus. When a woman has postpartal uterine atony (the uterus does not remain firm), the nurse should do the following:

1. Reevaluate for full bladder; if the bladder is full, have the woman void.
2. Question the woman on her bleeding history since the birth or last examination. How heavy does her flow seem? Has she passed any clots? How frequently has she changed pads? Were the pads saturated? Look at the discarded pads.
3. For the nursing mother, put the newborn to the mother's breast for feeding to stimulate oxytocin production.
4. Assess maternal blood pressure and pulse to identify hypotension.

PROCEDURE 30–1 ASSESSING THE FUNDUS FOLLOWING VAGINAL BIRTH

Nursing Action	*Rationale*
Objective: Prepare the woman.	
• Explain the procedure.	*Explanation decreases anxiety and increases cooperation.*
• Ask the woman to void.	*A full bladder will cause uterine atony.*
• Position the woman flat in bed with her head comfortable on a pillow. If the procedure is uncomfortable, the woman may flex her legs.	*The supine position prevents falsely high assessment of fundal height. Flexing the legs relaxes the abdominal muscles.*
Objective: Determine uterine firmness.	
• Gently place one hand on the lower segment of the uterus. Using the side of the other hand, palpate the abdomen until you locate the top of the fundus.	*This position provides support for the uterus and a larger surface for palpation.*
• Determine whether the fundus is firm. If it is not firm, massage the abdomen lightly until the fundus is firm.	*A firm fundus indicates that the muscles are contracted and bleeding will not occur.*
Objective: Determine the height of the fundus.	
Measure the top of the fundus in fingerbreadths above, below, or at the umbilicus (Figure 30–5).	*Fundal height gives information about the progress of involution.*

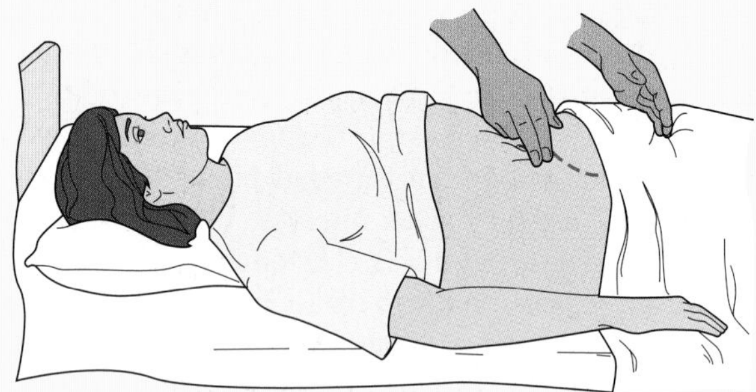

FIGURE 30–5 Measuring the descent of the fundus. The fundus is located two fingerbreadths below the umbilicus.

Nursing Action	*Rationale*
Objective: Ascertain the position of the fundus.	
• Determine whether the fundus has deviated from the midline. If it is not in the midline, locate the position. Evaluate the bladder for distention.	*The fundus may be deviated when the bladder is full.*
• Measure urine output for the next few hours until normal elimination status is established.	
Objective: Correlate the uterine status with lochia.	
Observe the amount, color, and odor of the lochia and the presence of clots.	*As normal involution occurs, the lochia decreases and changes from rubra to serosa. Increased amounts of lochia may be associated with uterine relaxation; failure to progress to the next type of lochia may indicate uterine relaxation or infection.*

PROCEDURE 30–1 *CONTINUED*

Nursing Action	*Rationale*
Objective: Record the findings. • Fundal height is recorded in fingerbreadths; for example, "2 FB ↓ U; 1 FB ↑ U." • If massage was necessary: "Uterus: Boggy → firm c̄ light massage."	*Provides a permanent record.*

5. Reassess the fundus; if the fundus is still boggy, alert the certified nurse-midwife or physician immediately, because further intervention, such as intravenous fluids and an oxytocic medication, are needed.

In the woman who has had a cesarean birth, the nurse should inspect the abdominal incision for signs of healing, such as approximation and minimal redness, and for any signs of infection, including drainage, foul odor, or redness. During the assessment, the nurse teaches the woman about her incision. The nurse can also review characteristics of normal healing and discuss signs of infection.

Lochia

Lochia is then assessed for character, amount, odor, and the presence of clots. The nurse must wear disposable gloves when assessing the perineum and lochia. Nurses may put on the gloves before beginning the assessment, just before assessing the abdomen and fundus, or when they are ready to assess the perineum and lochia. (See Essential Precautions in Practice: During Postpartal Assessment on page 920.) During the first 1 to 3 days, the lochia should be rubra. A few small clots are normal and occur as a result of blood pooling in the vagina. However, the passage of numerous or large clots is abnormal, and the cause should be investigated immediately. After 2 to 3 days, the lochia becomes serosa.

Lochia should never exceed a moderate amount, such as that needed to partially saturate four to eight peri-pads daily, with an average of six. However, the number of pads alone is not the sole indicator; the nurse must also consider two other factors. First, some birth facilities use peri-pads that are super absorbent; a saturated pad of this type would contain a greater amount of lochia than a regular pad. The nurse needs to assess the volume absorbed in the pad. The other factor is the individual woman's pad-changing practices. The nurse should ask the mother how long the current pad has been in use, and whether any clots were passed prior to this examination, such as during voiding. If heavy bleeding is reported but not seen, the nurse asks the woman to put on a clean perineal pad and reassesses the discharge in 1 hour (Figure 30–6).

Research suggests that visual estimations of blood loss are influenced by the brand of peri-pad used (Luegenbiehl, Brophy, Artigue, Phillips, & Flak, 1990). Consequently, the clinical facility's standards for estimating blood loss should be brand specific and need to be reassessed whenever brands are changed. When a more accurate assessment of blood loss is needed, the perineal pads can be weighed, with 1 g considered equivalent to 1 mL blood.

Clots and heavy bleeding may be caused by uterine relaxation (atony) or retained placental fragments, and they require further assessment. Because of the evacuation of the uterine cavity during cesarean birth, women with such surgery usually have less lochia after the first 24 hours than mothers who give birth vaginally. Therefore, amounts of lochia that would be normal in women who had vaginal births are suspect in women who have undergone cesarean birth.

If the woman is at increased risk for bleeding or is actually experiencing heavy flow of lochia rubra, her blood pressure, pulse, and uterus need to be assessed frequently, and the physician may prescribe methylergonovine maleate (Methergine). The odor of the lochia is nonoffensive and never foul. If foul odor is present, so is an infection. When using narrative nursing notes, the amount of lochia is charted first, followed by character, for example, "Lochia: moderate rubra" or "Lochia: small rubra/serosa."

CRITICAL THINKING IN PRACTICE

You have completed your assessment of Patty Clark, a 24-year-old G2P2 woman who is 24 hours past birth. The fundus is just above the umbilicus and slightly to the right. Lochia rubra is present, and a pad is soaked every 2 hours. What would you do?

Answers can be found in Appendix I.

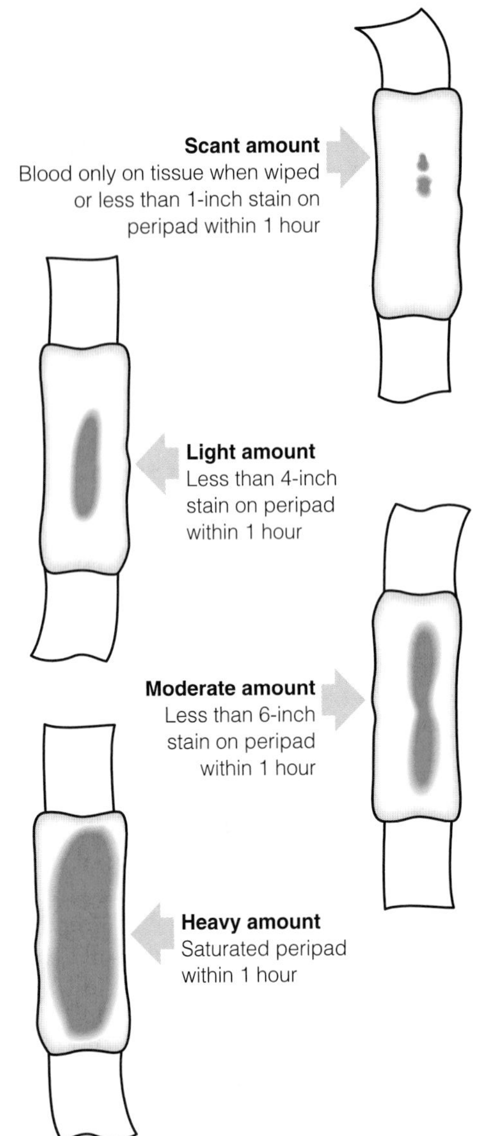

FIGURE 30–6 Suggested guidelines for assessing lochia volume. SOURCE: Jacobson H: A standard for assessing lochia volume. *Am J Mat Child Nurs* May/June 1985; 10:175.

Client teaching that the nurse may address during assessment of the lochia may center on normal changes that can be expected in the amount and color of the flow. Hygienic measures, such as wiping the perineum from front to back and washing her hands after toileting and changing pads, may be reviewed if appropriate. The nurse should approach the timing of teaching hygienic practices delicately, along with the content to be included. By establishing positive goals for the teaching—promoting comfort, enhancing tissue healing, and preventing infection—the nurse can avoid value-laden statements regarding personal beliefs about the need for cleanliness or control of body odor.

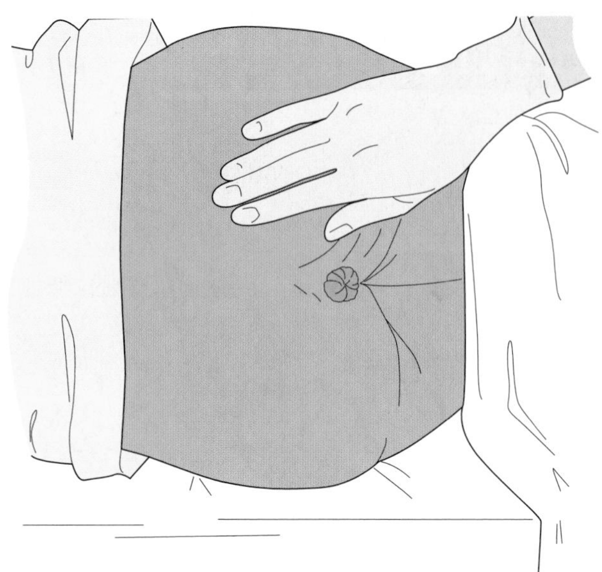

FIGURE 30–7 Intact perineum with hemorrhoids. Note how the examiner's hand raises the upper buttocks to fully expose the anal area.

Perineum

The perineum is inspected with the woman lying in Sims' position. The buttock is lifted to expose the perineum and anus.

If an episiotomy was performed or a laceration required suturing, the nurse assesses the wound. To evaluate the state of healing, the nurse inspects the wound for redness, edema, ecchymosis, discharge, and approximation. After 24 hours, some edema may still be present, but the skin edges should be "glued" together (well approximated) so that gentle pressure does not separate them. Gentle palpation should elicit minimal tenderness, and there should be no hardened areas suggesting infection. Ecchymosis interferes with normal healing, as does infection. Foul odors associated with drainage indicate infection.

The nurse next assesses whether hemorrhoids are present around the anus. If present, they are assessed for size, number, and pain or tenderness (Figure 30–7).

During the assessment, the nurse talks with the woman to determine the effectiveness of comfort measures that have been used. The nurse provides teaching about the episiotomy. Some women do not thoroughly understand what an episiotomy is and where it is and may believe that the stitches must be removed, as with other types of surgery. Frequently, when women fear that the stitches must be removed manually, they are afraid to ask about them. While explaining the findings of the assessment, the nurse can provide information about the episiotomy, its location, and signs that are being assessed. In addition, the nurse can casually add that the sutures dissolve slowly over the next few weeks as the tissues heal. By the time the sutures are dissolved, the tissues are strong, and the incision edges will not separate. This is also an opportunity to teach comfort measures that may be used (see Chapter 31).

An example of charting a perineal assessment might read: "Midline episiotomy; no edema, tenderness, or ecchymosis present. Skin edges well approximated. Woman reports sitz bath and pain relief measures are controlling discomfort."

Lower Extremities

If thrombophlebitis occurs, the most likely site will be the woman's legs. To assess for this condition, the nurse should have the woman stretch her legs out, with the knees slightly flexed, and the legs relaxed. The nurse then grasps the foot and dorsiflexes it sharply. No discomfort or pain should be present. If pain is elicited, the nurse notifies the certified nurse-midwife or physician that the woman has a positive Homans' sign (see Figure 33–3). The pain is caused by inflammation of a vessel. The nurse also evaluates the legs for edema, noting any areas of redness, tenderness, and increased skin temperature.

Early ambulation is an important aspect of preventing thrombophlebitis. Most women are able to get up shortly after birth or once they have fully recovered from the effects of the regional anesthetic agent, if one has been used. The cesarean birth client requires passive range-of-motion exercises until she is ambulating more freely.

Client teaching associated with assessment of the lower extremities focuses on the signs and symptoms of thrombophlebitis. In addition, the nurse may review self-care measures to promote circulation and prevent thrombophlebitis, such as leg exercises that may be performed in bed, dorsiflexion on an hourly basis while on bed rest, ambulation, avoiding pressure behind the knees, avoiding use of the knee gatch on the bed, and avoiding crossing the legs.

Usually, the nurse records the results of the assessment on a flowsheet or a summary nursing note. If tenderness and warmth have been noted, they might be recorded as follows: "Tenderness, warmth, slight edema, and slight redness noted on posterior aspect of left calf—positive Homans'. Woman advised to avoid pressure to this area; lower leg elevated and moist heat applied per agency protocol. Call placed to Dr Garcia to report findings."

Elimination

During the hours after birth, the nurse carefully monitors a new mother's bladder status. A displaced uterus, palpable bladder, or boggy uterus is a sign of bladder distention and requires nursing intervention.

The postpartal woman should be encouraged to void at least every 4 to 6 hours. The nurse should assess the bladder for distention until the woman is able to completely empty her bladder with each voiding. The nurse may employ techniques to assist voiding, such as helping the woman out of bed to void, pouring warm water on the vulva, and running water in the sink, and encouraging the woman to relax and take deep breaths. Catheterization is required when the bladder is distended and the woman cannot void or when she is voiding small amounts (<100 mL) frequently. Although many physicians/CNMs write orders stating that the woman can be catheterized in 8 hours if she has not voided, the nurse needs to assess the bladder and any voiding pattern frequently prior to the end of the 8-hour period. Some women may require catheterization sooner. The cesarean birth mother may have an indwelling catheter inserted prophylactically. The nurse should perform the same assessments in evaluating bladder emptying once the catheter is removed.

During the physical assessment, the nurse elicits information from the woman regarding the adequacy of her fluid intake, whether she feels she is emptying her bladder completely when she voids, and any signs of urinary tract infection (UTI) she may be experiencing.

In the same way, the nurse obtains information about the new mother's intestinal elimination and any concerns she may have about it. Many mothers fear that the first bowel movement will be painful and possibly even damaging if an episiotomy has been performed. Stool softeners may be ordered to increase bulk and moisture in the fecal material and to allow more comfortable and complete evacuation. Constipation may cause pressure on sutures and increase discomfort and therefore should be prevented. Encouraging ambulation, forcing fluids (up to 2000 mL/day or more), and providing fresh fruits and roughage in the diet enhance bowel elimination and help the woman reestablish her normal bowel pattern.

During the assessment, the nurse may provide information regarding postpartum diuresis, explaining why the woman may be emptying her bladder so frequently. Information about the need for additional fluid intake, with suggestions of specific amounts, may be helpful. The woman should drink at least eight 8-oz glasses of water or juice in addition to other fluids. The nurse discusses signs of retention and overflow voiding and reviews symptoms of UTI with the mother at this time if it seems an appropriate moment for teaching. The nurse can also review methods of assisting bowel elimination and provide opportunities for the woman to ask questions.

Rest and Sleep Status

As part of the postpartal assessment, the nurse evaluates the amount of rest the new mother is getting. If the woman reports difficulty sleeping at night, the nurse should try to determine the cause. If it is simply the strange environment, a warm drink, back rub, or mild sedative may prove helpful. Appropriate nursing measures are indicated if the woman is bothered by normal postpartal discomforts such as afterpains, diaphoresis, or episiotomy or hemorrhoidal pain.

TABLE 30–4 Daily Eating to Encourage Healthful Nutrition During the Postpartal Period

2–3 servings of milk, yogurt, and cheese group
2–3 servings of meat or protein group
3–5 servings of vegetable group
4 servings of whole grain
2–4 servings of fruit group
6–11 servings of bread, cereal, rice, and pasta group
Fats, oils, and sweets sparingly

A daily rest period should be encouraged, and hospital activities should be scheduled to allow time for napping. The nurse can also provide information about the fatigue a new mother experiences and the impact it can have on her emotions and sense of well-being.

Nutritional Status

The nurse determines postpartal nutritional status by evaluating information provided by the mother and by direct assessment. During pregnancy, the daily recommended dietary allowances call for increases in calories, proteins, and most vitamins and minerals. After birth, the nonnursing mother's dietary requirements return to prepregnancy levels.

Visiting mothers during mealtime provides an opportunity for unobtrusive nutritional assessment and counseling. The nonnursing mother should be advised about the need to reduce her caloric intake by about 300 kcal and to return to prepregnancy levels for other nutrients. The nursing mother should increase her caloric intake by about 200 kcal over the pregnancy requirements, or a total of 500 kcal over the nonpregnant requirement. Basic discussion will usually prove helpful, followed by referral as needed. In all cases, the nurse should provide literature on nutrition so that the woman will have a source of information following discharge.

The dietitian should be informed of any mother who is a vegetarian or whose cultural or religious beliefs require specific foods. Appropriate meals can then be prepared for her. Many women, especially those who gained more than the recommended number of pounds, are interested in losing weight after birth. The dietitian can design weight-reduction diets to meet nutritional needs and food preferences. The nurse may also refer women with unusual eating habits or numerous questions about good nutrition to the dietitian.

New mothers are also advised that it is common practice to prescribe iron supplements for 4 to 6 weeks after birth. Hemoglobin and hematocrit values are assessed at a postpartal visit to detect any anemia.

As a part of the nutritional assessment, the nurse can provide teaching about the nutritional needs of the woman during the postpartal period. See Table 30–4 as well as the discussion in Chapter 14.

CRITICAL THINKING QUESTION

What techniques might you use to accurately assess the new mother's psychologic status?

Psychologic Assessment

Adequate assessment of the mother's psychologic adjustment is an integral part of postpartal evaluation. This assessment focuses on the mother's general attitude, feelings of competence, available support systems, and caregiving skills. It also evaluates her fatigue level, sense of satisfaction, and ability to accomplish her developmental tasks.

The concepts of postpartal/childbearing fatigue and tiredness are not synonymous. During the initial hospitalization following childbirth, the woman typically suffers from tiredness, which is less severe and more easily relieved; fatigue, by contrast, tends to be more severe and lasts longer, with both physiologic and psychologic aspects (Milligan, Lenz, Parks, Pugh, & Kitzman, 1996). Frequently, the woman is so tired from a long labor and birth that everything seems to be an effort. To avoid inadvertently classifying a very tired mother as one with a potential attachment problem, the nurse should perform the psychologic assessment on more than one occasion. After a nap, the new mother is often far more receptive to her baby and her surroundings.

Some new mothers have little or no experience with newborns and may feel totally overwhelmed. They may show these feelings by asking questions and reading all available material or by becoming passive and quiet because they simply cannot deal with their feelings of inadequacy. Unless a nurse questions the woman about her plans and previous experience in a supportive, nonjudgmental way, the nurse might conclude that the woman is uninterested, withdrawn, or depressed. Clues that may indicate a problem include excessive, continued fatigue; marked depression; excessive preoccupation with physical status or discomfort; evidence of low self-esteem; lack of support systems; marital problems; inability to care for or nurture the newborn; and current family crises (such as illness or unemployment). These characteristics frequently indicate a potential for maladaptive parenting, which may lead to child abuse or neglect (physical, emotional, intellectual) and cannot be ignored. Referrals to public health nurses or other available community resources may provide greatly needed assistance and alleviate potentially dangerous situations.

Assessment of Early Attachment

Attachment is a desired outcome of maternal-newborn interactions during the postpartal period. The nurse in the postpartum setting can periodically observe and note the mother's progress toward attachment. The following questions can be addressed in the course of nurse-client interaction:

1. Is the mother attracted to her newborn? To what extent does she seek face-to-face contact and eye contact? Has she progressed from fingertip touch to palmar contact, to enfolding the infant close to her own body? Is attraction increasing or decreasing? If the mother does not exhibit increasing attraction, why not? Do the reasons lie primarily within her, in the baby, or in the environment?
2. Is the mother inclined to nurture her infant? Is she progressing in her interactions with her infant?
3. Does the mother act consistently? If not, is the source of unpredictability within her or her infant?
4. Is her mothering consistently carried out? Does she seek information and evaluate it objectively? Does she develop solutions based on adequate knowledge of valid data? Does she evaluate the effectiveness of her maternal care and make appropriate adjustments?
5. Is she sensitive to the newborn's needs as they arise? How quickly does she interpret her infant's behavior and react to cues? Does she seem happy and satisfied with the infant's responses to her efforts? Is she pleased with feeding behaviors? How much of this ability and willingness to respond is related to the baby's nature, and how much to her own?
6. Does she seem pleased with her baby's appearance and sex? Is she experiencing pleasure in interaction with her infant? What interferes with the enjoyment? Does she speak to the baby frequently and affectionately? Does she call him or her by name? Does she point out family traits or characteristics she sees in the newborn?
7. Are there any cultural factors that might modify the mother's response? For instance, is it customary for the grandmother to assume most of the child care responsibilities while the mother recovers from childbirth?

When the nurse has addressed these questions and assembled the facts, the nurse's intuition and formal background of knowledge combine to answer three more questions: Is there a problem in attachment? What is the problem? What is its source? The nurse can then devise a creative approach to the problem as it presents itself in the context of a unique, developing mother-infant relationship.

CRITICAL THINKING QUESTION

How can the nurse positively influence the bonding or attachment process in this era of short birthing stays?

Assessment of Physical and Developmental Tasks

During the first several weeks postpartum, the woman must accomplish certain physical and developmental tasks. These include the following:

- Restoring physical condition
- Developing competence in caring for and meeting the needs of her infant
- Establishing a relationship with her new child
- Adapting to altered lifestyles and family structure resulting from the addition of a new member

The new mother and her family may have an inadequate or incorrect understanding of what to expect during the early postpartal weeks. She may be concerned with restoring her figure and surprised because of continuing physical discomfort from sore breasts, episiotomy, or hemorrhoids (Fishbein & Burggraf, 1998). Fatigue is perhaps her greatest, yet most underestimated, problem during the early weeks. This may be aggravated if she has no extended family support or if there are other young children at home. Smith-Hanrahan and Deblois (1995) studied fatigue and functional ability in women following discharge. In their study, 95% of the women were found to suffer from some degree of fatigue at the end of the first week, and one-third of these mothers described their fatigue as severe. After 6 weeks, 50% of mothers continued to experience moderate to severe levels of fatigue.

Developing skill and confidence in caring for an infant may provoke extreme anxiety in a new mother. As she struggles to establish a mutually acceptable pattern with her baby, small unanticipated concerns may seem monumental. The woman may begin to feel inadequate and, if she lacks support systems, isolated.

Nurses have been in the forefront of health care providers attempting to improve the care given during the postpartal period. Many obstetricians, certified nurse-midwives, and nurse practitioners now routinely see all postpartal women 1 to 2 weeks after birth in addition to the routine 6-week checkup. These visits provide opportunities for physical assessment as well as assessment of the mother's psychologic and informational needs and needs of the family. Glazener, Abdalla, Stroud, Naji, Templeton, and Russell (1995) discovered that 87% of the women they studied suffered from self-described health problems during the first 8 weeks postpartum. Seventy-six percent of the study population continued to suffer from at least one health problem at 18 months following birth. The surprising results of this study indicate that health care professionals need to have a greater awareness of the needs and potential problems the postpartal woman may experience.

COMMUNITY IN FOCUS

Midwifery Services in Rural New York

Mary Imogene Bassett Hospital (MIBH) in Cooperstown serves ten rural counties in upstate New York. For many years the hospital served as a clinical site for obstetrical residents from Columbia University in New York City. However, census declines in the mid-1980s led to the elimination of the residency program. Without program services, the community was faced with the problem of how best to meet the needs of childbearing women in the counties MIBH served.

The chief of obstetrics and the hospital administration recognized that certified mid-wives (CNMs) could provide needed services, and in 1986 the first CNM was hired. Currently the nurse-midwifery service is staffed by seven CNM's. Of the 592 babies born in the Bassett Birthing Center at MIBH in 1998, 510 births were attended by nurse-midwives. This figure is especially impressive because it represents 86% of the nonsurgical births at Bassett.

The organizational model employed by the nurse-midwifery service represents a truly collaborative approach. The service is housed within the Department of Obstetrics and Gynecology; however the director of nurse-midwifery services reports directly to both the head of the ob/gyn department and the vice-president for nursing and patient care services. Moreover, the director is a member of the nursing administration council, and several staff CNMs serve on various hospital committees.

When a woman first seeks prenatal care services, she is encouraged to attend the 2-hour orientation program, New Beginnings, taught by maternity nurse educators. The program covers a variety of topics related to pregnancy and explains the Bassett system. Following the program, the woman and a staff member complete a health history and routine lab tests. An appointment is then scheduled with one of the CNMs for a physical examination. CNMs complete the initial risk assessment and examination of all pregnant women except those specifically requesting a physician. Based on the results, three methods of client management are available: (1) exclusive CNM management for women with low-risk status; (2) collaborative management by CNMs and physician for women who are considered high risk; and (3) exclusive physician care for women who request it. Four of the fourteen satellite clinics are managed by CNMs. For women seeking prenatal care at one of the remaining clinics, the initial plan of care is developed by the nurse-midwife; a nurse practitioner then provides ongoing management. If questions arise, CNM and physician coverage is available at Bassett around the clock.

For women who are considered high risk, the physician generally addresses the medical issues (eg, insulin requirements), whereas the CNM addresses issues related to support and the birth process. Careful collaboration between physician and certified nurse-midwife is essential. Often the CNM attends the birth, with the physician immediately available to lend assistance if necessary. No woman who wishes to have a midwife with her during labor is excluded from the midwifery service.

This collaborative model has resulted in favorable outcomes. The number of women who have given birth at Bassett has increased significantly since the program began. More importantly, the cesarean birth rate has declined from 26.2% to 12.8%, with a concurrent increase in the number of VBACs (vaginal birth after cesarean). The incidence of episiotomies and lacerations has also decreased.

Although the obstetricians with whom the CNM practice remain committed to the collaborative model, the nurse-midwifery service is feeling the effects of budget cuts as well as a concerted effort on the part of some administrators to retain or increase physician positions despite funding restrictions related to managed care. Specifically, the number of funded CNM positions decreased from 9 in 1996 to 6.5 in 1999 even though the nurse-midwives provide extremely cost-effective care. During the same period, the number of funded physician positions increased from 5 to 6. Hopefully, senior management will recognize the value of this innovative approach to maternity care, both in terms of client outcomes and satisfaction and in terms of cost effectiveness, and continue to support this high-quality program.

SOURCE: Personal communication with M. Patricia Brown, RN, MS, CNM, Director of Nurse-Midwifery Services at Bassett Healthcare.

Early Discharge Postpartal Care

The Centers for Disease Control and Prevention (1995) note that the postpartal woman's length of hospitalization decreased from 4.1 days in 1970 to 2.6 days in 1992. The disclosure of this fact fueled continuing interest in researching the implications of early discharge on the mother/newborn dyad. For the low-risk postpartal client, the advantages of early discharge are early promotion of the bonding process, facilitation of early return to family life, decreased length of pathogenic exposure, and reduction of health-care costs (Havens & Hannan, 1996).

Goals of postpartal nursing care include promoting physical stability for both mother and baby, ensuring the mother's ability to care for the infant, and providing follow-up care (Margolis, Kotelchuck, & Chang, 1997). Nurses must be flexible in their delivery of care (McGregor, 1996). Many interventions must be organized and performed simultaneously to provide expedient, thorough nursing care. Some research suggests that during the first 24 hours following birth of a baby, a woman experiences a memory deficit; therefore, this time frame is not optimal for client teaching (Brown, Towne, & York, 1996). Stover and Marnejon (1995) recommended that nurses provide all educational information in a written format and establish a specific plan of care for the follow-up period.

CRITICAL THINKING IN PRACTICE

You walk in and find Dana Sullivan, a 29-year-old G2P2 at 48 hours post repeat c-section, crying. She states, "I'm not ready to go home. With my first baby they made me go home after 2 days. Can they make me again?"

Answers can be found in Appendix I.

Postpartal Home Care

Nurses may provide postdischarge care for the postpartal woman by home visits, follow-up phone calls, or both. A home visit 1 to 3 days after discharge provides opportunities for further assessment and teaching. The follow-up phone call is usually initiated by a nurse from the postpartal unit of the agency where the mother gave birth. It is made soon after discharge (within 24 to 48 hours) and is designed to provide assessment and, if necessary, care; to reinforce knowledge and provide additional teaching; and to make referrals if indicated (Gagnon, Edgar, Kramer, Papageorgiou, Wagner, & Klein, 1997).

The routine physical assessment, which can be made rapidly, focuses on the woman's general appearance, breasts, reproductive tract, bladder and bowel elimination, and any specific problems or complaints. (See the postpartal Assessment Guide: First Home Visit and Anticipated Progress at 6 Weeks, in Chapter 32.) In addition, the nurse should talk with the mother about her diet, fatigue level, family adjustment, and psychologic status. The nurse explores any problems with child care and refers the mother to a pediatric nurse practitioner or pediatrician if needed. Available community resources, including public health department follow-up visits, are mentioned when appropriate. If not already discussed, teaching about family planning is appropriate at this time, and the nurse provides information regarding birth control methods.

In ideal situations, a family approach involving the father, newborn, and other siblings permits a total evaluation and provides an opportunity for all family members to ask questions and express concerns. In addition, a family approach can sometimes enable the nurse to identify disturbed family patterns more readily and suggest, or even institute, therapeutic measures to prevent future problems of neglect or abuse.

FOCUS YOUR STUDY

- The uterus involutes rapidly, primarily through a reduction in cell size.
- Involution is assessed by measuring fundal height. The fundus is at the level of the umbilicus within a few hours after birth and should decrease by approximately 1 fingerbreadth per day.
- The placental site heals by a process of exfoliation, so no scar formation occurs.
- Lochia progresses from rubra to serosa to alba and is assessed in terms of type, quantity, and characteristics.
- The abdomen may have decreased muscle tone (flabby consistency) initially. Diastasis recti abdominis, separation of the rectus abdominus muscles, should be assessed for.
- Constipation may develop postpartally because of decreased tone in the abdominal muscles, limited diet, and denial of the urge to defecate due to fear of pain.
- Decreased bladder sensitivity, increased capacity, and postpartal diuresis may lead to problems with bladder elimination. Frequent assessment and prompt intervention are indicated. A fundus that is boggy but does not respond to massage, is higher than expected, or deviates to the side usually indicates a full bladder.
- Postpartally, a healthy woman should be normotensive and afebrile. Bradycardia is common.
- Postpartally the WBC count is often elevated. Activation of clotting factors predisposes the woman to thrombus formation.
- Psychologic adaptations of the postpartal woman are traditionally described as "taking-in" and "taking-hold."
- In consideration of the client's background, the nurse should recognize and respect cultural variations and individual preferences.
- Postpartal assessment should be completed in a systematic way, usually head to toe. The assessment provides opportunities for informal client teaching.
- In the weeks following birth, the woman's physical condition returns to a nonpregnant state, and she gains competence in caregiving and confidence in herself as a parent.

REFERENCES

Ament, L. A. (1990). Maternal tasks of the puerperium reidentified. *Journal of Obstetric, Gynecologic, and Neonatal Nursing, 19*(4), 330–335.

Andrew, M. M., & Boyle, J. S. (1995). *Transcultural concepts in nursing care.* Glenview, IL: Scott, Foresman/Little, Brown.

Brown, L. P., Towne, S. A., & York, R. (1996). Controversial issues surrounding early postpartum discharge. *Nursing Clinics of North America, 31*(2), 333–339.

Centers for Disease Control. (1995, May 5). Trends in length of stay for hospital deliveries—United States, 1970–1992. *Morbidity and Mortality Weekly Report, 44*(17), 335–337.

Choudhry, U. K. (1997). Traditional practices of women from India: Pregnancy, childbirth, and newborn care. *Journal of Obstetric, Gynecologic, and Neonatal Nursing, 26*(5), 533–539.

Cunningham, F. G., MacDonald, P. C., Gant, N. F., Leveno, K. J., Gilstrap, L. C., III, Hankins, G. D. V., & Clark, S. L. (1997). The puerperium. In F. G. Cunningham, P. C. MacDonald, N. F. Gant, K. J. Leveno, L. C. Gilstrap, III, G. D. V. Hankins, & S. L. Clark (Eds.), *Williams obstetrics* (20th ed.). Stamford, CT: Appleton & Lange.

Fishbein, E. G. & Burggraf, E. (1998). Early postpartum discharge: How are mothers managing? *Journal of Obstetric, Gynecologic, and Neonatal Nursing, 27*(2), 142–148.

Gagnon, A. J., Edgar, L., Kramer, M. S., Papageorgiou, A., Waghorn, K., & Klein, M. C. (1997). A randomized trial of a program of early postpartum discharge with nurse visitation. *American Journal of Obstetrics and Gynecology, 176*(1 Pt. 1), 205–211.

Gennaro, S., Fehder, W. P., York, R., & Douglas, S. D. (1997). Weight, nutrition, and immune status in postpartal women. *Nursing Research, 46*(1), 20–25.

Glazener, C. M., Abdalla, M., Stroud, P., Naji, S., Templeton, A., & Russell, I. T. (1995). Postnatal maternal morbidity: Extent, causes, prevention and treatment. *British Journal of Obstetrics and Gynaecology, 102*(4), 282–287.

Havens, D. M., & Hannan, C. (1996). Legislation to mandate maternal and newborn length of stay. *Journal of Pediatric Health Care, 10*(3), 141–144.

Howard, J. Y., & Berbiglia, V. A. (1997). Caring for childbearing Korean women. *Journal of Obstetric, Gynecologic, and Neonatal Nursing, 26*(6), 665–671.

Hutchinson, M. K., & Baqi-Aziz, M. (1994). Nursing care of the childbearing Muslim family. *Journal of Obstetric, Gynecologic, and Neonatal Nursing, 23*(9), 767–771.

Jacobson, H. (1985). A standard for assessing lochia volume. *American Journal of Maternal Child Nursing, 10*(3), 174–175.

Jambunathan, J. (1995). Hmong cultural practices and beliefs: The postpartum period. *Clinical Nursing Research, 4*(3), 335–345.

Luegenbiehl, D. L., Brophy, G. H., Artigue, G. S., Phillips, K. E., & Flak, R. J. (1990). Standardized assessment of blood loss. *American Journal of Maternal Child Nursing, 15*(4), 241–244.

Margolis, L. H., Kotelchuck, M., & Chang, H. Y. (1997). Factors associated with early maternal postpartum discharge from the hospital. *Archives of Pediatrics and Adolescent Medicine, 151*(5), 466–472.

Martell, L. K. (1996). Is Rubin's "taking-in" and "taking-hold" a useful paradigm? *Health Care for Women International, 17*(1), 1–13.

McGregor, L. A. (1996). Short, shorter, shortest: Continuing to improve the hospital stay for mothers and newborns. *American Journal of Maternal Child Nursing, 21*(4), 191–196.

McVeigh, C. (1998). Functional status after childbirth in an Australian sample. *Journal of Obstetric, Gynecologic, and Neonatal Nursing, 27*(4), 402–409.

Mercer, R. T. (1985). The process of maternal role attainment over the first year. *Nursing Research, 34*(4), 198–204.

Mercer R. T. (1995). *Becoming a mother.* New York: Springer.

Milligan, R., Lenz, E. R., Parks, P. L., Pugh, L. C., & Kitzman, H. (1996, Fall). Postpartum fatigue: Clarifying a concept. *Scholarly Inquiry for Nursing Practice, 10*(3), 279–291.

Pope-Davis, D. B., Eliason, M. J., & Ottavi, T. M. (1994). Are nursing students multiculturally competent? An exploratory investigation. *Journal of Nursing Education, 33*(1), 31–33.

Resnik, R. (1999). The puerperium. In R. K. Creasy & R. Resnik (Eds.), *Maternal-fetal medicine* (4th ed.). Philadelphia: Saunders.

Rubin, R. (1961). Puerperal change. *Nursing Outlook, 9*, 753.

Rubin, R. (1984). *Maternal identity and the maternal experience.* New York: Springer.

Sethi, S. (1995). The dialectic in becoming a mother: Experiencing a postpartum phenomenon. *Scandinavian Journal of Caring Sciences, 9*(4), 235–244.

Sheil, E. P., Bull, M. J., Moxon, B. E., Muehl, P. A., Kroening, K. L., Peterson-Palmberg, G., & Kelber, S. (1995). Concerns of childbearing women: A Maternal Concerns Questionnaire as an assessment tool. *Journal of Obstetric, Gynecologic, and Neonatal Nursing, 24*(2), 149–155.

Smith-Hanrahan, C., & Deblois, D. (1995). Postpartum early discharge: Impact on maternal fatigue and functional ability. *Clinical Nursing Research, 4*(1), 50–66.

Stover, A. M., & Marnejon, J. G. (1995). Postpartum care. *American Family Physician, 52*(5), 1465–1472.

Varney, H. (1997). *Nurse midwifery* (3rd ed.). Sudbury, MA: Jones and Bartlett.

Visness, C. M., Kennedy, K. I., & Ramos, R. (1997). The duration and character of postpartum bleeding among breast-feeding women. *Obstetrics and Gynecology, 89*(2), 159–163.

Zlatnik, F. J. (1994). The normal and abnormal puerperium. In J. R. Scott, P. J. DiSaia, C. B. Hammond, & W. N. Spellacy (Eds.), *Danforth's obstetrics and gynecology* (7th ed.). Philadelphia: Lippincott.

A Day in the Life of a Nurse-Midwife

TO ME, PREGNANCY IS A WONDERFUL, normal experience—part of the cycle of life. That's why I love the fact that I can participate in all aspects of it, from pregnancy through birth and into the postpartal period. My practice enables me to ensure that a family's childbirth experience incorporates their personal beliefs and meets their expectations as much as possible. Come along with me for a day.

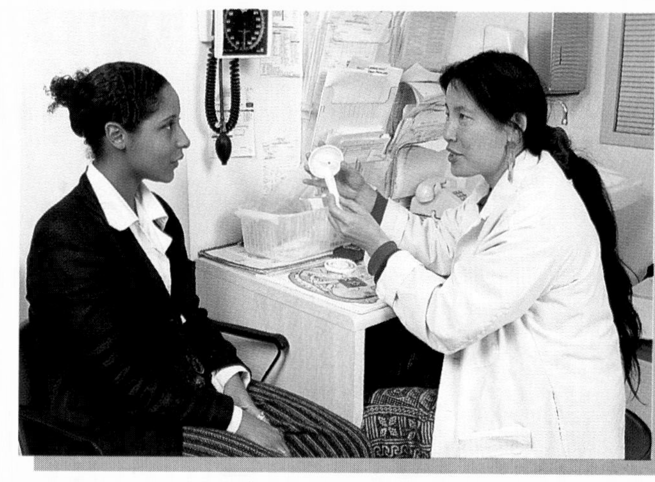

Cherrene has come for contraceptive information. I find it helpful to use models and examples during the discussion.

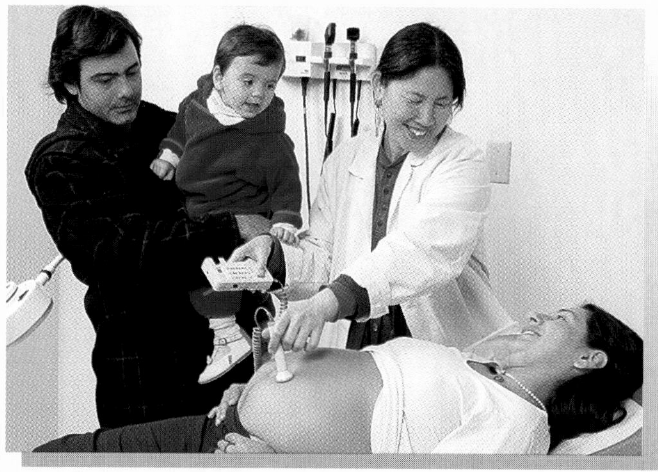

Dianne and her family come together for every appointment. We all enjoy listening to the fetal heartbeat.

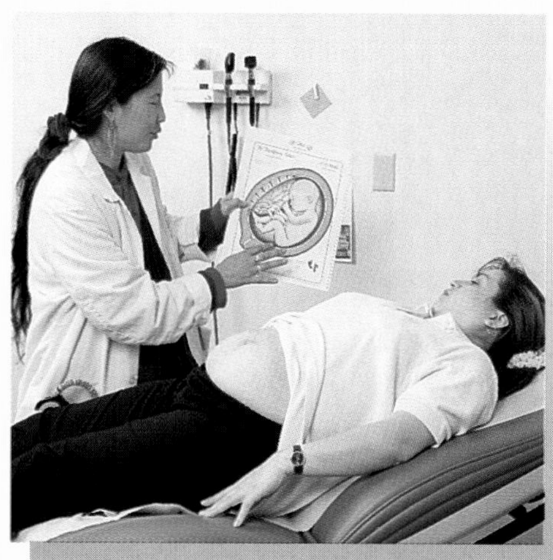

Gretchen's pregnancy is progressing well. She asks what her baby looks like now. I like to use a visual device as I talk with her about her baby's development.

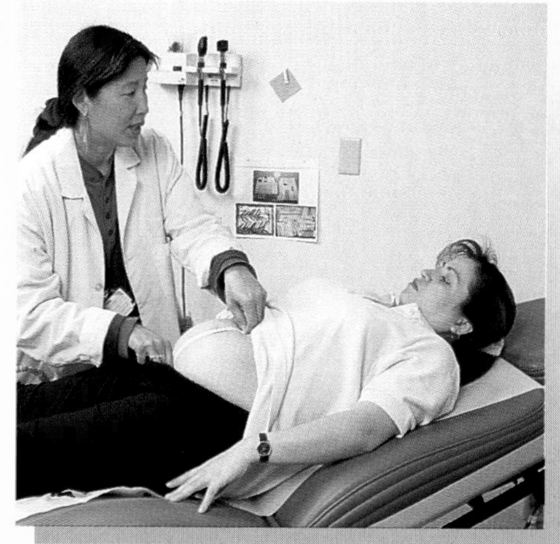

I measure the height of the fundus to determine if the baby is growing as expected. Gretchen and I talk about the impact of her nutrition, exercise, and healthy lifestyle habits on her baby and the outcome of her pregnancy.

8 WEEKS

Development is rapid; heart begins to pump blood; limb buds are well developed. Facial features and major divisions of the brain are discernible. Ears develop from skin folds; tiny bones and muscles are formed beneath the thin skin.

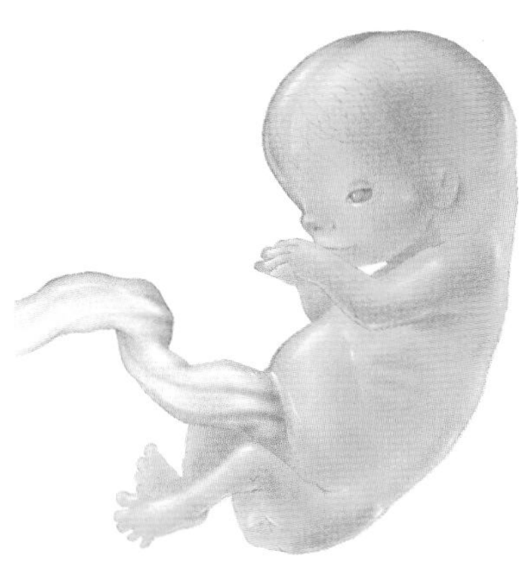

Morning sickness, may persist to 12 weeks. Uterus changes from pear to globular shape. Hegar's, Goodell's and Piskacek's signs appear. Cervix flexes; leukorrhea increases. Surprise and ambivalence about pregnancy may occur. No noticeable weight gain.

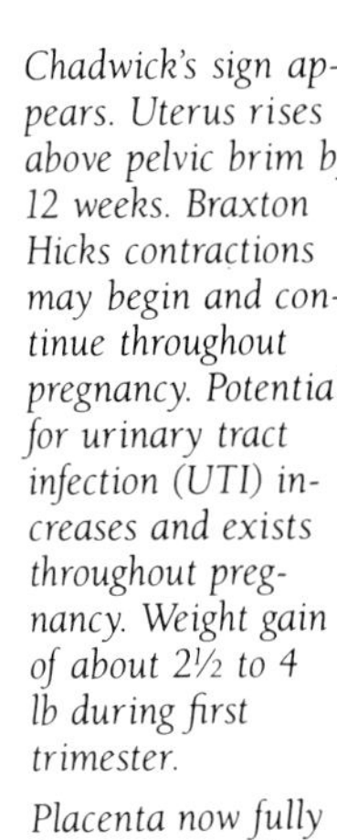

Eat dry crackers before arising; try frequent small, dry, low-fat meals with fluids taken between meals. Avoid use of hot tubs, saunas, and steam rooms throughout pregnancy.

Discuss attitudes toward pregnancy. Discuss value of early pregnancy classes that focus on what to expect during pregnancy. Provide information about childbirth preparation classes.

12 WEEKS

Embryo becomes a fetus, its beating heart discernible by ultrasound. Assumes a more human shape as lower body develops. At week 12, first movements begin. Sex is determinable. Kidneys produce urine.

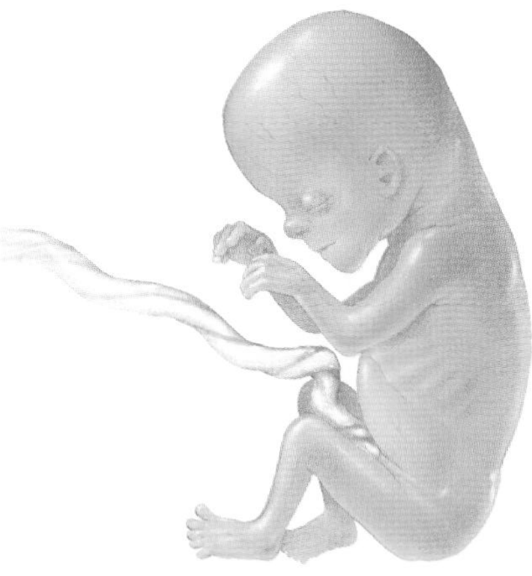

Chadwick's sign appears. Uterus rises above pelvic brim by 12 weeks. Braxton Hicks contractions may begin and continue throughout pregnancy. Potential for urinary tract infection (UTI) increases and exists throughout pregnancy. Weight gain of about 2½ to 4 lb during first trimester.

Placenta now fully functioning and producing hormones.

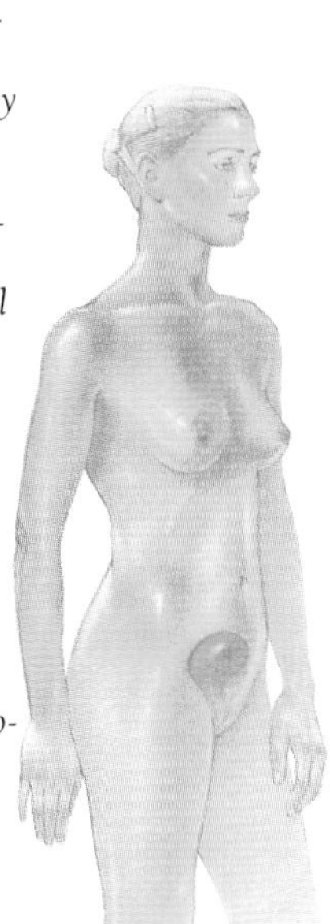

Adequate fluid intake and frequent voiding (every 2 hr while awake) help prevent UTI. Also helpful to void following intercourse. Wipe from front to rear.

Discuss nutrition and appropriate weight gain. Stress value of regular physical exercise, especially nonweightbearing activities or walking. Discuss possible effects of pregnancy on sexual relationship.

16 WEEKS

Musculoskeletal system has matured; nervous system begins to exert control. Blood vessels rapidly develop. Fetal hands can grasp; legs kick actively. All organs begin to mature and grow. Fetus weighs about 7 oz (½ lb). FHT discernible with Doppler. Pancreas produces insulin.

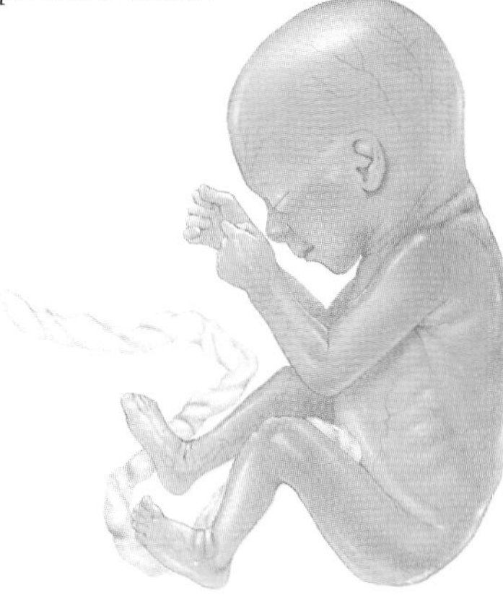

Fundus halfway between symphysis and umbilicus. Woman gains slightly less than 1 lb per wk for remainder of pregnancy. May feel more energetic. BPD measurement on ultrasound. Vaginal secretions increase. Itching, irritation, malodor suggest infection. Woman may begin wearing maternity clothes. Pressure on bladder lessens and urinary frequency decreases.

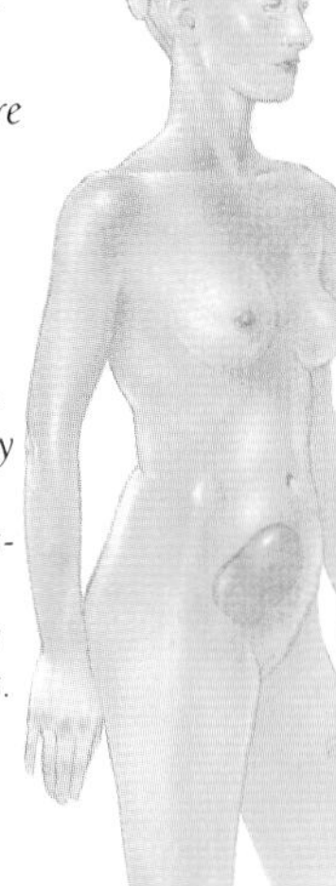

Daily shower or bath and thorough drying of vulva helpful; avoid douching during pregnancy. Consult caregiver if infection suspected; use only prescribed medications.

Review danger signs of pregnancy. Discuss infant feeding options; provide information on the value of breastfeeding. Provide information about clothing, shoes.

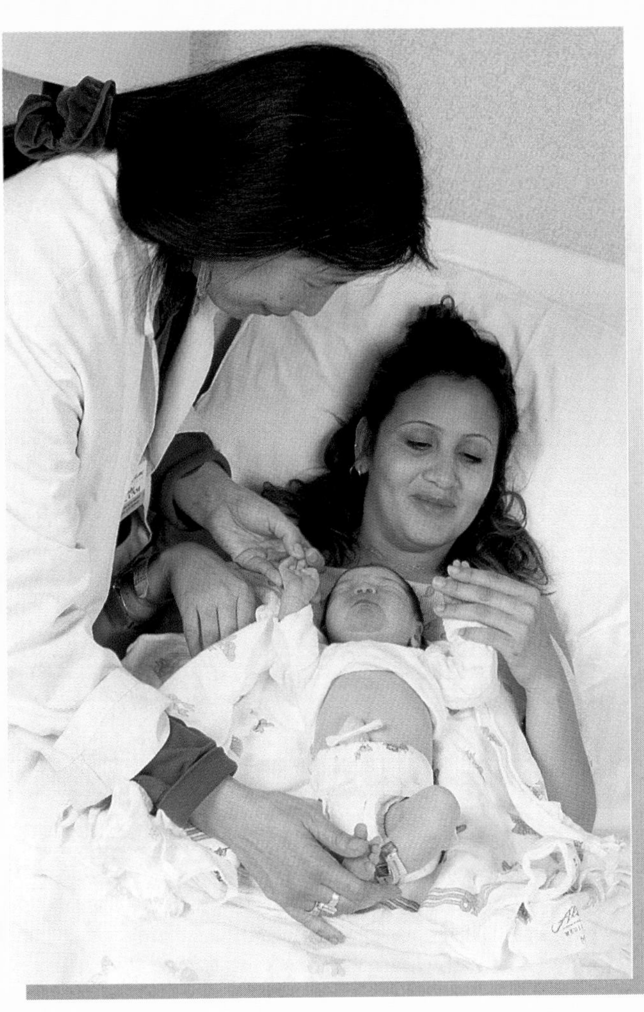

Alisa is fascinated with baby Lydia's tiny fingers and toes. I love being with parents as they explore their baby. Each new baby is such a wonder. . . such a miracle.

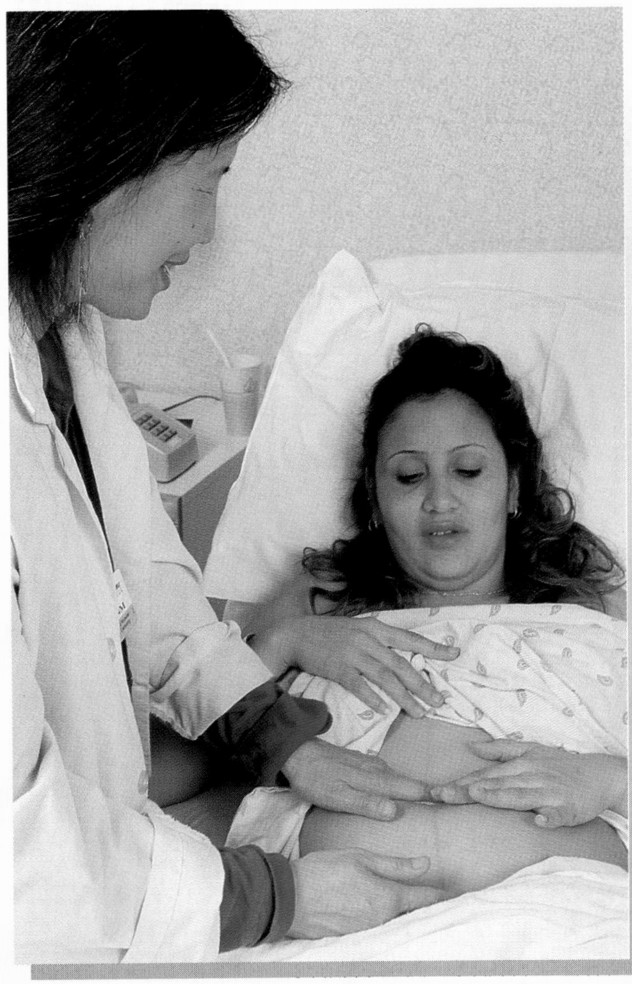

Now my attention turns to Alisa. As part of my assessment, I check the position and tone of her fundus. All is well. I head home after a busy, but rewarding, day.

5 — 20 WEEKS

/ernix protects the body; fine hair
(lanugo) covers the body and keeps the
oil on the skin. Eyebrows, eyelashes,
and head hair develop. Fetus develops
a regular schedule of sleeping, sucking
and kicking.

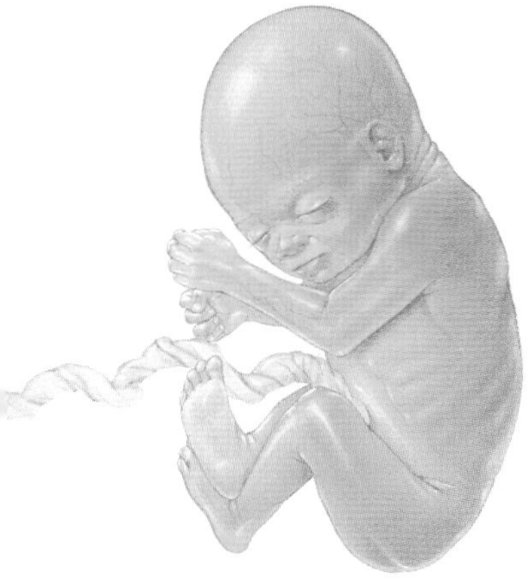

Fundus reaches level
of umbilicus. Breasts
begin secreting co-
lostrum. Amniotic
sac holds about
400mL fluid.
Faintness and diz-
ziness may occur,
especially with sud-
den position changes.
Varicose veins may
begin to develop.
Woman experiences
fetal movement, and
pregnancy may sud-
denly seem more
"real." Areola
darken. Nasal stuff-
iness may develop.
Leg cramps may
begin to occur. Con-
stipation may
develop.

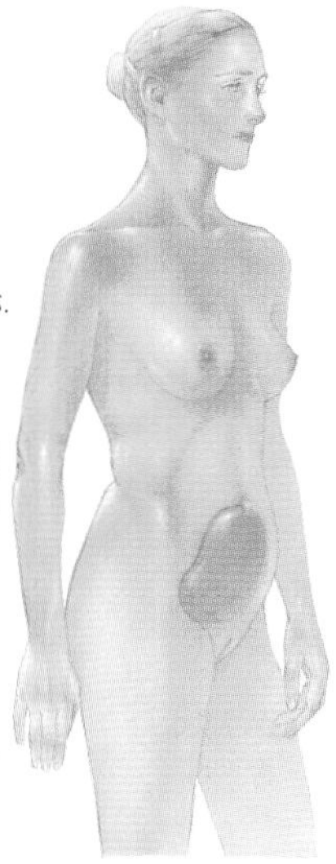

Sit with feet elevated when possible; rise slowly and carefully. Avoid pressure on lower thighs. Support stockings may be helpful. Cool-air vaporizer may help. Eat foods containing fiber, such as raw fruits, vegetables, cereals with bran; drink liquids and exercise frequently.

Discuss breast care. Discuss dorsiflexion of foot to relieve cramps; heat to affected muscle.

6 — 24 WEEKS

Skeleton develops rapidly as bone-forming cells increase activity. Respiratory movements begin. Fetus weighs about 1 lb, 10 oz.

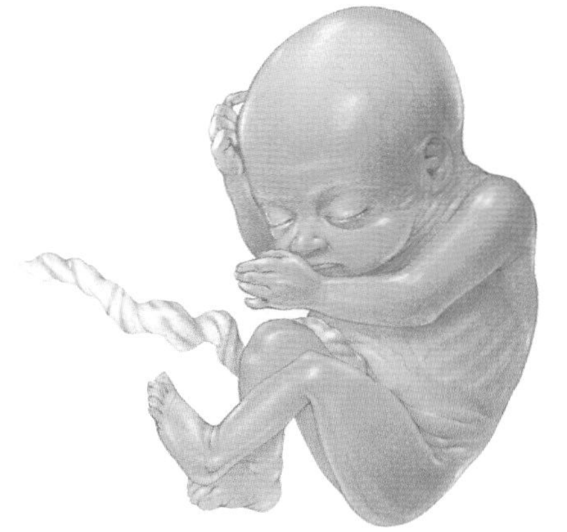

Fundus above umbilicus. Backache and leg cramps may begin. Skin changes can include striae gravidarum, chloasma, linea negra, acne, redness on palms of hands and soles of feet. Nosebleeds can occur. May experience abdominal itching as uterus enlarges; will continue until end of pregnancy.

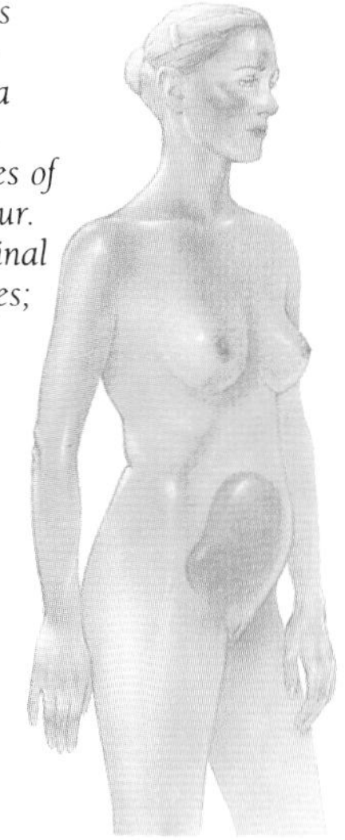

Assure woman that skin changes generally subside soon after birth. Discuss specific exercises such as pelvic tilt to help strengthen back and abdominal muscles, and stress importance of good body mechanics. Reiterate importance of avoiding medications, caffeine, alcohol and smoking.

Woman may choose to apply petroleum jelly in nostrils to relieve nosebleeds. Cool vaporizer may also help. Lanolin-based cream can relieve itching. Mild soap can remove excess oil associated with acne.

7 — 28 WEEKS

Fetus can breathe, swallow, regulate temperature. Surfactant forms in lungs. Eyes begin to open and close. Baby is $\frac{2}{3}$ the size it will be at birth.

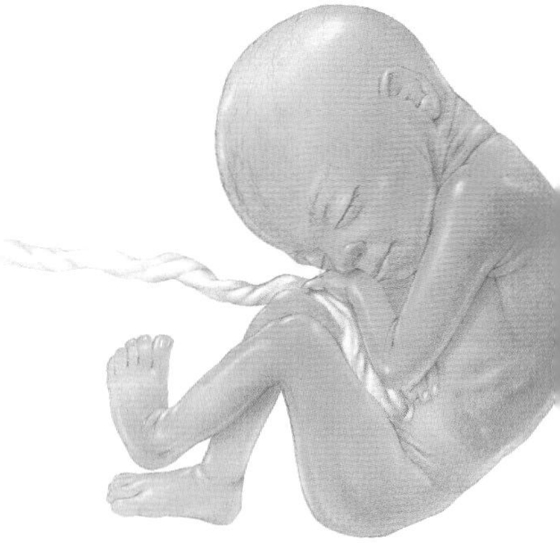

Fundus halfway between umbilicus and xyphoid process. May develop hemorrhoids. Thoracic breathing replaces abdominal breathing. Fetal outline palpable. May be tired of pregnancy and eager for the mothering role. Heartburn may begin to occur. May begin taking childbirth preparation classes with partner or support person.

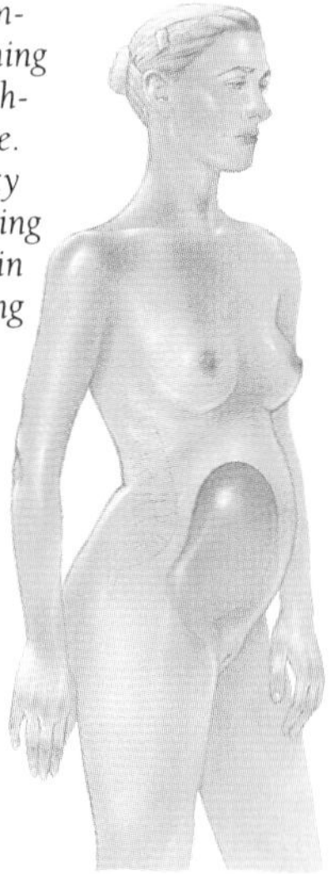

Avoid constipation; use sitz baths, gentle reinsertion of hemorrhoids with a fingertip as necessary. Topical anesthetic agents may offer relief of hemorrhoids. Stool softeners may be prescribed by caregiver. Elevate legs and assume sidelying position when resting. Eat small, more frequent meals; avoid fatty foods, lying down after eating. Maalox or mylanta may be helpful; Avoid sodium bicarbonate. Discuss expectations about labor and delivery, caring for an infant.

32 WEEKS

Brown fat deposits are developing beneath the skin to insulate the baby following birth. Baby has grown to about 15–17 in. Begins storing iron, calcium, and phosphorus.

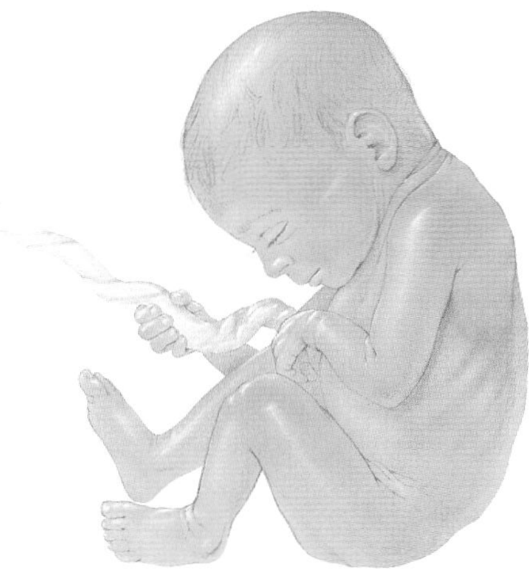

Fundus reaches xyphoid process; breasts full and tender. Urinary frequency may return. Swollen ankles and sleeping problems may develop. Dyspnea may develop.

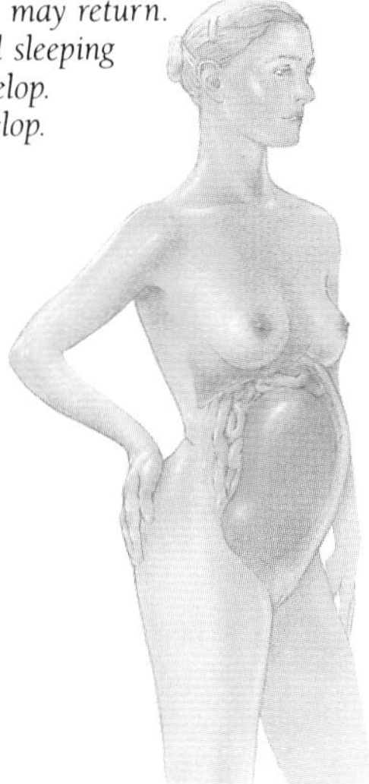

Wear well-fitting supportive bra. Elevate legs once or twice daily for an hour or so. Sleep on left side if possible. Use naturally occurring diuretics such as 2 tbsp lemon juice in 1 cup water or a generous serving of watermelon if available. Avoid most diuretics unless specifically prescribed. Maintain proper posture; use extra pillows at night for severe dyspnea. Following culture and personal preference, may begin preparing nursery now.

Review signs of labor. Discuss plans for other children (if any), transportation to agency.

38 WEEKS

The entire uterus is occupied by the baby, thus restricting its activity. Maternal antibodies are transferred to the baby. This provides immunity for about 6 months until the infant's own immune system can take over.

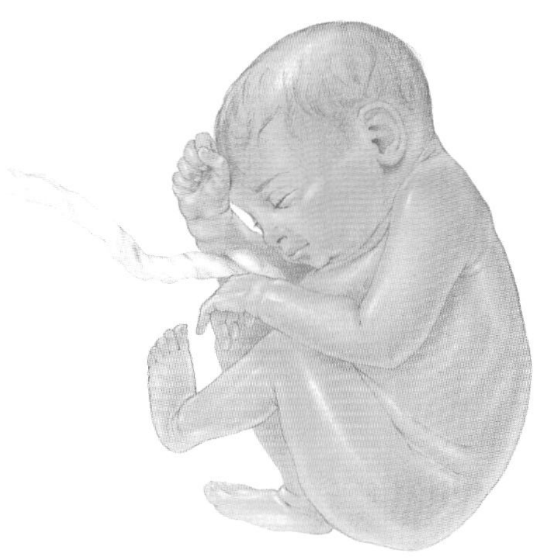

The fetus descends deeper into the mother's pelvis (lightening). The placenta is nearly 4 times as thick as it was 20 weeks ago, weighing nearly 20 oz. Mother is eager for birth, may have final burst of energy. Backaches, urinary frequency increase. Braxton Hicks contractions intensify as cervix and lower uterine segment prepare for labor. Couple may tour labor and delivery area.

Continue pelvic tilt exercises. Wear low-heeled shoes or flats. Avoid heavy lifting. Sleep on side to relieve bladder pressure. Urinate frequently. Avoid all analgesics except acetominophen. Pack suitcase for delivery.

Discuss postpartum period including decisions such as circumcision, rooming-in. Discuss common postpartum discomforts; mention postpartum blues. Discuss family planning methods, infant care. Stress need for adequate rest postpartally. Provide support, especially if baby is overdue.

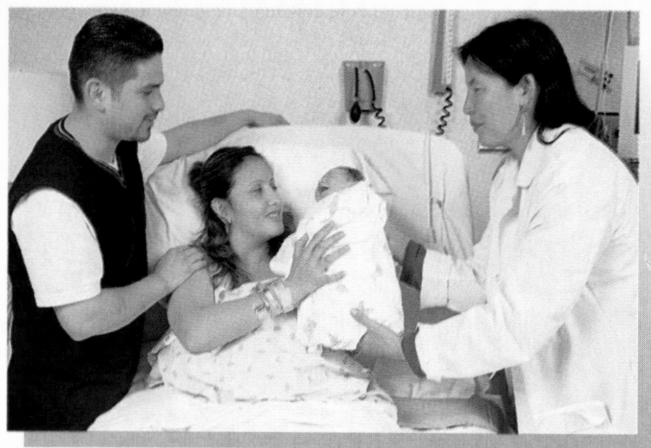

While I'm at the birth center, I check in on Alisa and Richard. Their baby, Lydia Rose, was born 6 hours ago. Alisa has asked for help with breastfeeding. Baby Lydia is a sleepy little one and needs encouragement to latch on and begin feeding.

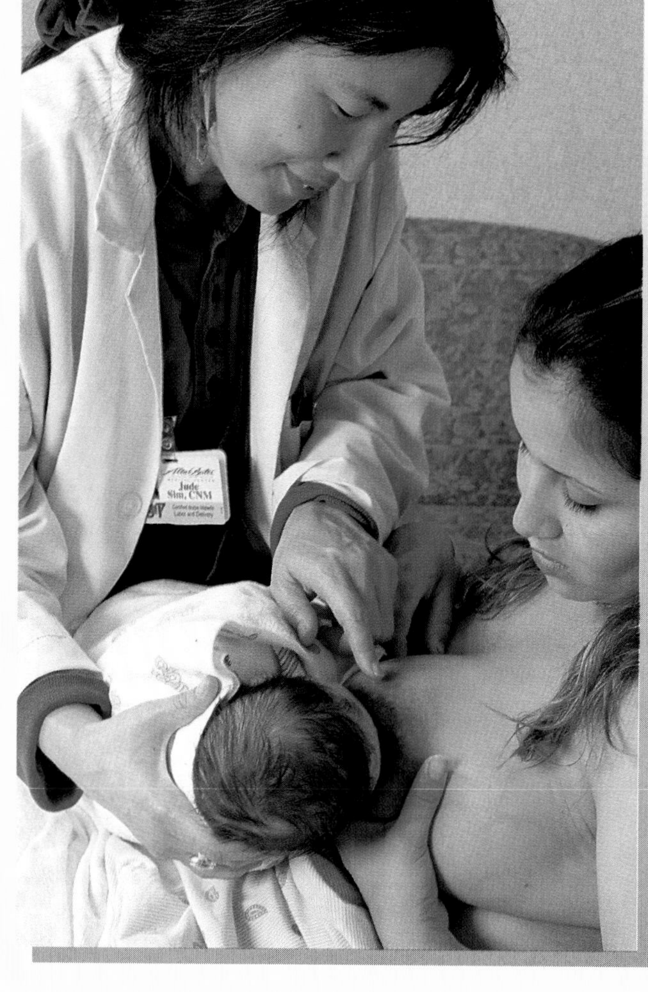

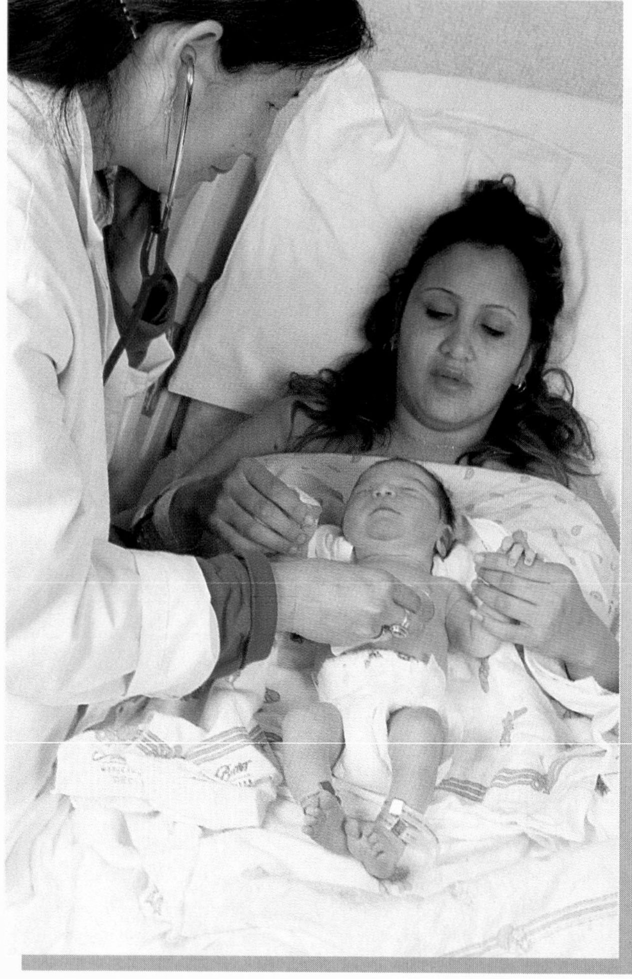

After baby Lydia has finished nursing, I do a physical assessment. I prefer to do an assessment in the room with the parents. It is such a wonderful opportunity for them to learn about their baby.

TEACHING ABOUT METHODS OF CONTRACEPTION

Factors to Consider in Choosing a Method of Contraception Effectiveness • Safety • Age and future childbearing plans • Contraindications in health history • Religious or moral factors • Personal preferences, biases • Lifestyle: frequency of intercourse, number of partners, cost factors, access to medical care • Partner's support and willingness to cooperate

Fertility Awareness or Natural Family Planning Methods Include basal body temperature (BBT), calendar (rhythm), cervical mucus (ovulation or Billings), and symptothermal methods • Require periodic abstinence • Generally require no artificial devices or substances • Readily reversible • 20% failure rate

Mechanical Contraceptives Include male condome (12% failure rate), female condom (21% failure), diaphragm (18% failure), cervical cap (nulliparous → 18% failure), intrauterine device (IUD) (1% failure) • Condoms available over-the-counter • All barrier methods readily reversible and generally free of side effects in appropriate clients • IUDs recommended only to women in monogamous relationships who have already had at least one child

(continued)

TEACHING HOME CARE OF THE POSTPARTAL FAMILY

When possible the nurse prepares for the home visit by establishing contact and a beginning relationship with the family while they are still in the birthing center or hospital setting • Purpose of the home visit is to assess maternal, neonatal, and family status and to provide teaching and make referrals as needed

Fostering a Caring Relationship with the Family Introduce yourself to the family • Address family members by their surnames until invited to use the given name • Ask to be introduced to other family members • Ask for permission before sitting • Be genuine; make sure your verbal and nonverbal messages are congruent, don't make assumptions, demonstrate caring behaviors, answer questions honestly and thoroughly, provide opportunity for family members to ask further questions for clarification, provide opportunity for return demonstration if needed • Demonstrate empathy; listen to the family without judgement, be attentive, listen to their perspective • Establish trust; do what you say you will do, be on time, be prepared for the visit, provide any follow-up as needed, provide information about community resources

(continued)

TEACHING ABOUT SEXUAL ACTIVITY DURING PREGNANCY

During Pregnancy the Woman May Experience Sexual desire may change or may remain unchanged • First trimester: possible changed sexual desire due to discomforts such as breast tenderness, nausea, fatigue • Second trimester: woman tends to feel at her best; sexual desire may increase • Third trimester: possible decreased sexual desire due to discomfort and fatigue • More intense orgasms followed by cramping possible in last weeks of pregnancy

During Pregnancy the Partner May Experience Sexual desire may change or may remain unchanged • Possible changed desire due to feelings about partner's changing appearance, beliefs about sexual activity with a pregnant woman, concern about hurting the woman or fetus, personal view of pregnancy as erotic or not, response to the notion of partner as a mother

Sexual Activities Suggest positions such as side-lying, female superior, or vaginal rear entry for more comfortable intercourse in later pregnancy • If male superior position is used, woman should place pillow under right hip to displace uterus and avoid venal caval syndrome • Encourage sexual activities enjoyed by both partners (generally not

(continued)

TEACHING ABOUT EXERCISE DURING PREGNANCY

Value of Regular Exercise During Pregnancy Improves maternal fitness and muscle tone • Relieves stress, improves sleep • Helps control weight gain • Promotes more rapid recovery following birth • Promotes sense of well-being

Choosing the Best Exercise In general, continue any exercise at which woman is proficient • Avoid learning new, strenuous sports • Avoid high-risk activities or sports that require good balance and coordination • Non-weight bearing activities (swimming, cycling) may be more comfortable as pregnancy progresses • When in doubt, contact caregiver

Basic Guidelines for Exercise During Pregnancy Exercise regularly, at least three times/week if possible • Avoid exercising while lying supine • Decrease intensity of exercise as pregnancy progresses and stop when fatigued • Avoid high-risk activities or activities that require good balance and coordination • Avoid prolonged overheating • Warm up before and cool down after exercising • Wear supportive shoes and supportive bra • Stop exercising if the following signs/symptoms develop: extreme fatigue, dizziness or faintness, sudden sharp pain, difficulty in breathing, nausea and vomiting,

(continued)

Teaching in the Home The home provides an excellent setting as the family is in their own territory and may feel more in control of the visit; the nurse is a visitor • During the introduction, observe family relationships and communication style; who is the greeter, who makes the decisions, who asks the questions and how is information shared, who is the primary caretaker of the infant, how are siblings incorporated into care of the new baby • During the assessment of the mother and newborn, continue to provide information regarding findings of each assessment and encourage mother to ask questions • Ask for return demonstrations when appropriate and maintain a supportive environment in which they may occur • Make referrals to appropriate health care professionals, agencies as needed • Carry a listing of resources within your community so information can be easily shared • Assist the family in problem solving and locating special resources or in meeting health care needs • Act as an advocate for health care that meets the needs of the mother, child, and new family

Oral Contraceptives and Other Methods Combination birth control pills (3% failure) have rare but serious medical complications and may have annoying side effects • Spermicides such as jellies, creams, foam, film, and vaginal suppositories (21% failure) minimally effective if used alone • Operative sterilization (vasectomy [0.15% failure] and tubal ligation [0.4% failure]) theoretically reversible, but 30–85% reversible in men and 40–75% reversible in women

Correct Procedure for Using Method Identify supplies or equipment needed • Provide details of how method is used • Discuss what to do if unusual circumstances arise (missed pill, missed AM temperature, second episode of intercourse with diaphragm)

Warning Signs Requiring Immediate Action For oral contraceptive pill users: shortness of breath or chest pain; severe headaches; severe abdominal pain; visual disturbances such as double vision, reduced visual fields, blindness; severe leg pain or swelling • For IUD users: severe or persistent abdominal pain, late or missed periods, fever, chills, noticeable or foul discharge, spotting, bleeding, heavy periods, clots

pain, vaginal bleeding, excessive muscle soreness; contact caregiver if symptoms persist

Basic Body Conditioning Exercises Pelvic tilt to reduce back strain and strengthen abdominal muscles (may be done standing, on hands and knees, or lying down) • Exercises to strengthen abdominal tone: abdominal muscle tightening, partial sit-ups (kness must be flexed and feet flat on the floor) • Kegel exercises to improve perineal muscle tone • Tailor sitting to prepare inner thigh muscles for birth

contraindicated medically) • To avoid introducing *E coli* into the vagina, the couple should *not* go from anal to vaginal penetration without thoroughly washing the penis • Encourage the exploration of other methods of expressing affection such as hugging, cuddling, and stroking each other to increase feelings of closeness • Suggest masturbation, either privately or as a shared experience, to provide release • Woman's orgasmic contractions from masturbation may be unusually intense in later pregnancy • Encourage openly expressing feelings, preferences, and concerns to partner

Contraindications to Sexual Intercourse Ruptured membranes • Presence of bleeding • Woman with history of preterm labor due to release of oxytocin with orgasm (breast stimulation also triggers the release of oxytocin and should therefore be avoided)

after eating, and sodium bicarbonate • *Ankle edema:* elevate legs frequently; dorsiflex feet when standing; avoid tight garters or constricting bands • *Varicose veins:* elevate legs; wear support hose; don't cross legs, wear tight garters, or stand for long periods • *Hemorrhoids*: gently reinsert into rectum as necessary; avoid constipation; use ice packs, topical ointments, anesthetic agents, warm soaks, or sitz baths • *Constipation:* increase fluid intake; eat high fiber diet; get regular exercise; develop regular bowel habits; use stool softeners as recommended by caregiver • *Backache:* perform good body mechanics; do pelvic tilt exercise; avoid uncomfortable working heights, high heel shoes, heavy lifting, and fatigue • *Leg cramps:* dorsiflex foot to stretch affected muscle; apply heat to affected muscle; evaluate diet • *Faintness*: arise slowly from resting position; avoid prolonged standing in warm or stuffy environments • *Dyspnea* (shortness of breath): maintain proper posture when sitting and standing; sleep propped up on pillows if dyspnea occurs at night • *Flatulence:* avoid gas-forming foods; chew food thoroughly; get regular daily exercise; maintain normal bowel habits • *Carpal tunnel syndrome:* avoid aggravating hand movements; use splint as prescribed; elevate affected arm

Additional Considerations Consider calories in making choices (not all nutritionally equivalent foods have same number of calories) • Eat foods with low nutrient value (sometimes called empty calories) sparingly (cakes, doughnuts, potato chips, butter, mayonnaise) • Combine foods to enhance nutrition (for example, 1 c spaghetti with a 2 oz meatball and ¼ c tomato sauce = 1 serving of meat, 1⅓ servings of grain, and ½ serving of vegetable)

that you can make a phone call from a pay phone if necessary • Carry needed phone numbers with you in an easily accessible place • If you are very uncomfortable with the location of the home or have concerns for your safety, pay attention to your feelings and leave, contact the family immediately and arrange another appointment at a time when another nurse can accompany you • It is important to follow your intuition

Pushing Breaths Begin with a cleansing breath • Breathe in 2 additional breaths and, holding them, push down on the perineum • Visualize pushing down through the vagina • Exhale during the pushing effort or hold breath whichever is more comfortable

heart rate) • Explain assessments and the results (prior to vaginal examinations, explain what will be done and validate the woman's discomfort during the examination) • Assist the woman in pushing when the first stage is completed and the woman has a natural urge to push

Essential Points Remember that the woman (couple) has the right to determine what happens, and the nurse acts as an advocate when needed • The nurse should be prepared to act as an advocate for analgesia and anesthesia if the woman requests it, regardless of her social status • Insist that a nurse is available to the couple during labor and birth, and that the nurse be supportive • Request privacy during the labor and birth if desired

left side • The right side may also be used • Monitoring may continue while the woman ambulates by using a mobile unit

Normal Findings with Electric Fetal Monitoring Normal fetal heart rate baseline between 120 and 160 beats per minute • Short-term variability is present, and long term variability is average (accurate assessment of variability is accomplished only by an internal fetal scalp electrode, not by external means) • Accelerations of FHR occur with fetal movement • Early decelerations may be present (indicate pressure of fetal head on the cervix) • Absence of late and/or variable decelerations

Indications of Fetal Stress Fetal heart rate baseline below 120 bpm (bradycardia) or above 160 bpm (tachycardia) • Decreased variability (short-term variability absent and/or long-term variability decreased or absent) • Development of periodic decelerations (late or variable) • Meconium stained amniotic fluid • Signs of fetal distress not always clear

Interventions that May Be Used when There Is Possible Fetal Stress As a result of changes in the FHR pattern, the maternal position may be changed from one side to the other, oxygen administered by face mask • An IV may be started or, if one is in place, the rate may be increased • Blood pressure is checked more frequently to identify hypotension

TEACHING INITIAL POSTPARTUM CARE

Checking the Uterine Fundus Determine location of the fundus (normally at umbilicus or one finger breadth above within hours of birth; descends at rate of about one finger breadth per day for first 10–14 days) • Assess position and consistency (affected by distention of bladder, presence of infection, breastfeeding, ambulation, and retention of products of conception) • Gently massage the fundus to alleviate atonic (boggy) uterus • Report recurrence of bogginess to the caregiver immediately

How to Apply Perineal Pads Apply from front to back • Change after voiding or whenever they are soiled

Caring for the Perineum Use perineal spray, rinse bottle, or cleansing pads, and pat dry with toilet paper • Always clean from front (at the symphysis pubis) to back (around the anus)

Beginning Ambulation Call for assistance the first time • Anticipate some dizziness

Changes in the Lochia Lochia dark red (lochia rubra) for first 1–3 days (similar to menstrual flow) • Lochia pinkish-brownish or serous (lochia serosa) after 2–3 days

(continued)

TEACHING POSTPARTUM COMFORT MEASURES

Relief of Breast Discomfort for Nonnursing Mothers Wear supportive, well-fitting bra • Apply ice packs for 20 minutes, 4 times a day • Avoid breast stimulation

Relief of Uterine Cramping (Afterpains) Lie on abdomen with a small pillow placed under it to apply pressure • Apply heat • Walk (obtain assistance for first ambulation) • Take analgesic medication (if breastfeeding, take mild analgesic about one hour before nursing)

Relief of Episiotomy Discomfort Apply ice packs to the perineum during the first few hours after delivery • Take 20-minute sitz baths 3–4 times a day • Shine a heat lamp on the cleaned perineum for 20 minutes, 2–3 times a day • Use perineal analgesic/anesthetics sprays • Keep perineum clean and free from dried discharge • Use gentle spray of warm water on perineum after voiding to provide cleansing; then pat dry, front to back • Take analgesic medication

Relief of Hemorrhoidal Discomfort Take 20-minute sitz baths 3–4 times a day • Apply anesthetic ointments or witch hazel pads • Maintain side-lying or prone position when

(continued)

TEACHING POSTPARTUM WARNING SIGNS

Warning Signs: Possible Causes *Alterations in pattern of lochia* (increased amount, change from lochia alba to serosa or from lochia serosa ro rubra, and/or presence of clots): possible uterine infection or uterine relaxation • *Development of foul smelling lochia:* uterine infection • *Maternal temperature elevation above 38C (100.4F):* infection • *Constant uterine tenderness:* infection • *Failure of fundus to descend as expected:* uterine infection or subinvolution • *Continued or increased discomfort in the episiotomy site* (separation of the suture line, development of swelling, increased tenderness, or presence of whitish or gray-green discharge at the site of episiotomy): infection • *Tenderness, swelling, and warmth in any area of the legs:* thrombophlebitis • *Swelling, warmth, and tenderness in any area of the breast:* mastitis

If a Warning Sign Develops Call caregiver immediately • Note specific information about the sign: length of time it has been present, related problems or activites, and specific characteristics of the problem

POSTPARTUM DISCHARGE TEACHING

Review Important Self-Care Measures Care of breasts • Expected positional changes in the uterus, and continued comfort measures for decreasing uterine cramping (afterpains) • Care of the episiotomy and hemorrhoids if present • Expected changes in lochia • Need for adequate nutrition and fluid intake • Measures to promote bowel elimination • Strategies to promote rest and relaxation • Postpartum exercises • Resumption of sexual activity • Warning signs of possible problems

Review Important Infant Care Measures Information and support regarding feeding techniques • Bathing and diaper changes • Umbilical cord care • Care of the uncircumcised and circumcised penis • Recognizing normal characteristics of the newborn • Maintaining safety • Soothing techniques • Recognizing illness or problems in the newborn in bed • Avoid prolonged sitting • Maintain adequate fluid intake • Take stool softener if needed to avoid constipation

• Moderate flow (use of 4–8 perineal pads per day) and small clots normal • *Signs of possible problems:* increase in amount, change from serosa back to rubra, presence of larger clots, change in odor drop of blood may be present when cord falls off • Never pull on cord or attempt to loosen it

Circumcision Care Squeeze soapy water over circumcision site once a day • Rinse area off with warm water and pat dry • Apply small amount of petroleum jelly (unless a Plastibell is in place) with each diaper change • Fasten diaper loosely over penis • Since the glans is sensitive, avoid placing baby on his stomach • Check for any foul smelling drainage or bleeding at least once a day • Let Plastibell fall off by itself (about 8 days after circumcision), Plastibell should not be pulled off • Light, sticky, yellow drainage (part of healing process) may form over head of penis

Uncircumcision Care Clean uncircumcised penis with water during diaper changes and with bath • Do not force foreskin back over the penis; foreskin will retract normally over time (may take 3–5 years)

menstruation by the 6th week after birth, and 45% of *lactating* mothers resume menstruation by the 12th week after birth • Breastfeeding does not provide adequate protection against pregnancy

"defrost" setting on microwave oven and carefully check temperature of formula before feeding

Positioning the Baby for Feeding Hold baby close, establishing eye contact as in breastfeeding • Hold baby's bottom or foot firmly, keeping his or her back straight to aid digestion and provide a sense of security • Quiet baby before feeding • Alternate the side baby is fed from to give baby two-sided stimulation • Avoid feeding while baby is on his or her back • Don't prop the bottle

Procedure for Feeding Nipple hole should allow only drops of milk to flow • Keep nipple full with milk to decrease air ingestion

How to Burp a Baby Position baby so his or her head rests on mother's shoulder or face down on lap, or sit baby on lap with baby's chin and chest supported • Gently pat or stroke baby's back • Burp baby halfway through feeding and at end of feeding • Learn baby's preferred burping position and whether baby is a slow or quick burper • Regurgitation of small amounts of formula is common • Have "burp cloth" available

Helpful Hints Be certain baby is well awake before attempting feeding • Alternate breast at which baby begins feeding (use safety pin as reminder) • Lift breast slightly or press lightly on breast above nares if mother's large breast occludes infant's nares • Avoid using nipple shields • Rotate baby's position at breast to avoid undue trauma to nipples and improve emptying of ducts • Avoid supplementary formula feedings until lactation is established • Check with caregiver before taking any medication while breastfeeding (because medications may cross into breast milk)

• Ineffective Management of Therapeutic Regimen: Individuals • Noncompliance (Specify) • Ineffective Management of Therapeutic Regimen: Families • Ineffective Management of Therapeutic Regimen: Individual • Decisional Conflict (Specify) • Health-Seeking Behaviors (Specify)
Pattern 6: Moving Impaired Physical Mobility • Risk for Peripheral Neurovascular Dysfunction • Risk for Perioperative Positioning Injury • Impaired Walking • Impaired Wheelchair Mobility • Impaired Transfer Ability • Impaired Bed Mobility • Activity Tolerance • Fatigue • Risk for Activity Intolerance • Sleep Pattern Disturbance • Sleep Deprivation • Diversional Activity Deficit • Impaired Home Maintenance Management • Altered Health Maintenance • Delayed Surgical Recovery • Adult Failure to Thrive • Feeding Self-Care Deficit • Impaired Swallowing • Ineffective Breastfeeding • Interrupted Breastfeeding • Effective Breastfeeding • Ineffective Infant Feeding Pattern • Bathing/Hygiene Self-Care Deficit • Dressing/Grooming Self-Care Deficit • Toileting Self-Care Deficit • Altered Growth and Development • Risk for Altered Development • Risk for Altered Growth • Relocation Stress Syndrome • Risk for Disorganized Infant Behavior • Disorganized Infant Behavior • Potential for Enhanced Organized Infant Behavior
Pattern 7: Perceiving Body Image Disturbance • Self-Esteem Disturbance • Chronic Low Self-Esteem • Situational Low Self-Esteem • Personal Identity Disturbance • Sensory/Perceptual Alterations (Specify: Visual, Auditory, Kinesthetic, Gustatory, Tactile, Olfactory) • Unilateral Neglect • Hopelessness • Powerlessness
Pattern 8: Knowing Knowledge Deficit (Specify) • Impaired Environmental Interpretation Syndrome • Acute Confusion • Chronic Confusion • Altered Thought Processes • Impaired Memory
Pattern 9: Feeling Pain • Chronic Pain • Nausea • Dysfunctional Grieving • Anticipatory Grieving • Chronic Sorrow • Risk for Violence: Directed at Others • Risk for Self-Mutilation • Risk for Violence: Self-Directed • Post-Trauma Syndrome • Rape-Trauma Syndrome • Rape-Trauma Syndrome: Compound Reaction • Rape-Trauma Syndrome: Silent Reaction • Risk for Post-Trauma Syndrome • Anxiety • Death Anxiety • Fear

Used by permission of NANDA.

General Considerations Bathe baby in warm, draft-free room ● Collect all supplies before starting the bath so baby is never unattended ● Use only tepid water (warm to inner wrist) ● Test water each time before putting baby in ● Bathe baby every day in warm, humid weather; give full body bath twice a week in dry weather ● Keep one hand on baby at all times during bath, cradling baby's head and back with arm while securely holding onto thigh ● Ointments are better than lotions for dry cracked hands and feet ● Lotion or talc-free powder may be used, but controversy exists over their use (do not let baby inhale powder) ● Don't immerse baby in bath water until umbilical cord falls off ● Choose a convenient bath time that allows parents and baby to enjoy the experience ● Baths may be useful in soothing a fussy baby

How to Obtain Baby's Temperature Shake thermometer down until end of the mercury line is below 94F ● Never leave baby unattended, no matter which method is used ● After taking baby's temperature, find and note the end of the mercury line ● Rectal temperatures are not recommended

Taking Axillary Temperature Place bulb of thermometer underneath baby's armpit ● Hold outer aspect of baby's arm next to his or her body ● Hold thermometer securely in place for 3–4 minutes

Taking Rectal Temperature Lubricate end of rectal thermometer bulb ● Place baby on his or her back ● Hold baby's legs up with one hand, exposing the anus ● Insert thermometer's silver bulb only until about ½ inch of it is covered ● Hold thermometer in place for 5 minutes

Helpful temperature ranges (Centigrade and Fahrenheit values)

Temperatures: 36.5C (97.7F), 37.0C (98.6F), 37.8C (100.0F), 38.3C (101.0F), 38.9C (102.0F), 39.4C (103.0F), or 40.0C (104.0F)

The Postpartal Family: Needs and Care

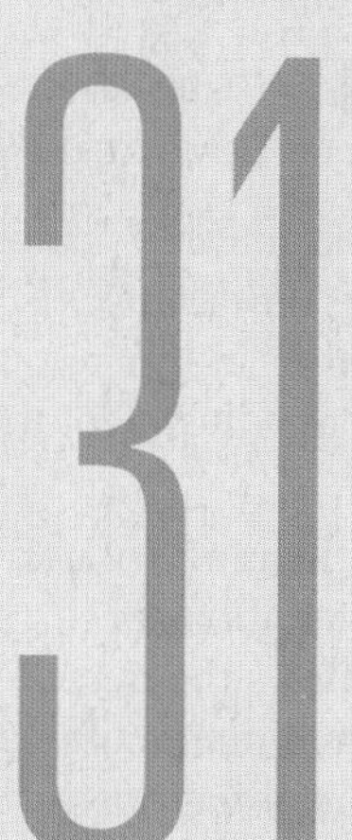

THE WORD "FAMILY" TO ME HAS ALWAYS HAD VERY meaningful and positive thoughts and experiences associated with it. I vividly remember growing up being the oldest of six children. With constant love, affection, and support from my parents, I always thought, "How can they do it? How can they nurture and raise so many kids and yet still make every one of us feel so special and important?" I truly believed that I would never be able to accomplish the successful parenting they so consistently provided to all of us, and I was actually scared and fearful to begin a family of my own. My husband and I now laugh about these thoughts I shared with him 4 1/2 years ago, as our family continues to grow quite rapidly. Trying to raise a 4-year-old, a 2-year-old, and a 10-week-old is extremely challenging, but it is the most rewarding experience in my life.

In addition to parenting three very small children I have balanced a full-time position as a nurse manager, and I completed my master's degree this spring. All of this has demanded an enormous amount of energy, motivation, and self-control. I realize now that my uneasiness and hesitation to begin our family was merely a time in my life in which I lacked the self-esteem and self-confidence to be a successful parent.

Key Terms

Bogginess
Couplet care
Mother-baby care
Patient-controlled analgesia (PCA)

Objectives

- Delineate nursing responsibilities for client teaching during the early postpartum period.
- Discuss appropriate nursing interventions to meet identified nursing goals for the childbearing family.
- Compare the nursing needs of a woman who experienced a cesarean birth with the needs of a woman who gave birth vaginally.
- Summarize the nursing needs of the childbearing adolescent during the postpartal period.
- Describe possible approaches to follow-up nursing care for the childbearing family.
- Determine the nurse's responsibilities related to early postpartum discharge.

Certain premises form the basis of effective nursing care during the postpartal period.

- The best postpartal care is family centered and disrupts the family unit as little as possible. This approach uses the family's resources to support an early and smooth adjustment to the newborn by all family members.
- Knowledge of the range of normal physiologic and psychologic adaptations occurring during the postpartal period allows the nurse to recognize alterations and initiate interventions early. Communicating information about postpartal adaptations to the family facilitates their adjustment to their situation.
- Nursing care is aimed at accomplishing specific goals that ultimately meet individual needs. These goals are formulated after careful assessment and consideration of factors that could influence the outcome of care.

Chapter 30 provided a thorough discussion of postpartal assessment. This chapter describes how the nurse can plan and implement nursing care management strategies. Specific nursing responses to the mother's physical needs and the family's psychosocial needs are described at length. See also the Critical Pathway for the Postpartal Period.

Community-Based Nursing Care

Various services are available to meet the needs of the childbearing family during the postpartal period and beyond. These services range from educational opportunities, such as classes on nutrition, exercise, infant care, parenting and the like, to specific health care programs, such as well-baby checkups, immunization clinics, and family planning services. Some are offered by private caregivers, some are provided by volunteer and charitable organizations, and some are the domain of city, state, or federal agencies. In all cases, the goal is consistent: to help ensure that the mother, the father (if he is involved), siblings, and the newborn have the opportunity to meet specific health care needs regardless of their personal resources.

Home Care

Home care is one of the most important forms of community-based nursing care offered to postpartal families. Home care visits and phone contacts (telephone follow-up) help ensure that families have the necessary skills and resources to care for an infant and to meet their own health needs. Because of its importance today in caring for childbearing families, home care is discussed in depth in Chapter 32.

Nursing Care Management during the Early Postpartal Period

Nursing Diagnosis

For most postpartal women, physical recovery proceeds smoothly and is considered a healthy process. Because of this perception, it is all too common for caregivers to think that the woman and her family have no "real" needs and thus that no care plan is needed. Nothing could be further from the truth. Every member of the family has needs, although they may not be obvious, especially if they are psychologic or educational.

The postpartal family's needs, which should be identified during assessment, are the basis for developing nursing diagnoses. Once a nursing diagnosis is made and recorded, systematic action, as delineated in a nursing care plan, can be taken to meet the identified need.

Many nurses have suggested that nursing diagnoses are difficult to make in a wellness setting because of their emphasis on "problems." Nurses involved in the effort to formulate standardized diagnoses recognize this difficulty and are working to develop diagnoses that are more useful in wellness settings.

Often agencies that use nursing diagnoses prefer to use only the NANDA list. Consequently, physiologic alterations form the basis of many postpartal diagnoses. Examples of such diagnoses include the following:

- ***Altered Patterns of Urinary Elimination*** related to dysuria or urinary retention
- ***Constipation*** related to fear of tearing stitches or pain
- ***Pain*** related to perineal edema from birth, episiotomy, and generalized muscular discomfort
- ***Sleep Pattern Disturbance*** related to frequent interruption of rest for newborn care

Diagnoses related to family coping or instructional needs are also used frequently. Examples of these diagnoses include the following:

- ***Knowledge Deficit*** related to lack of knowledge regarding newborn care, self-care, infant feeding, and infant growth and development
- ***Family Coping: Potential for Growth*** related to successful adjustment to new baby

After completing the assessment and diagnosis steps of the nursing process, the nurse identifies expected outcomes and selects nursing interventions that will effect the expected outcomes.

Nursing Plan and Implementation

Nursing care management is individualized to meet the needs of each postpartal woman and her newborn The plan of care needs to consider the newborn's schedule of activities during the day, such as feeding times, because they frequently determine the mother's schedule.

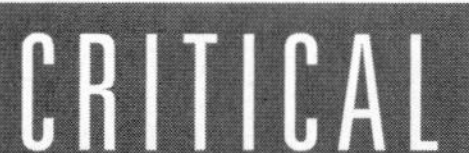

PATHWAY FOR THE POSTPARTAL PERIOD

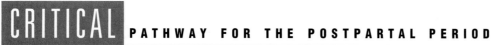

Category	First 4 Hours	4–8 Hours Past Birth	8–24 Hours Past Birth
Referral	Report from labor nurse if not continuing in an LDR room	Lactation consultation as needed	Home nursing, WIC referral if indicated **Expected Outcomes** Referrals made
Assessments	Postpartum assessments q30min × 2, q1h × 2, then q4h. Includes: • Fundus firm, midline, at or below umbilicus • Lochia rubra < 1 pad/h; no free flow or passage of clots with massage • Bladder: voids large amounts of urine spontaneously; bladder not palpable following voiding • Perineum: sutures intact; no bulging or marked swelling; no c/o severe pain. Minimal bruising may be present. If hemorrhoids present, no tenseness or marked engorgement; < 2 cm diameter • Breasts: soft, colostrum present Vital Signs: • BP WNL; no hypotension; not > 30 mm systolic or 15 mm diastolic over baseline • Temperature: < 38C (100.4F) • Pulse: bradycardia normal, consistent with baseline • Respirations: 12–20/min; quiet, easy Comfort level: < 3 on scale of 1–10	Continue postpartum assessment q4h × 2, then q8h Breast: evaluate nipple status; should be no evidence of cracks or bruising Observe feeding technique with newborn Vital signs assessment q8h; all WNL; report temperature > 38C (100.4F) Assess Homan's sign q8h Continue assessment of comfort level	Continue postpartum assessment q8h Breasts: nipples should remain free of cracks, fissures, bruising Feeding technique with newborn: should be good or improving Vital signs assessment q8h; all WNL; report temperature > 38 C (100.4 F) Continue assessment of comfort level **Expected Outcomes** Vital signs medically acceptable, voids qs, postpartum assessment WNL; comfort level < 3 on 1–10 scale, involution of uterus in process, demonstrates and verbalizes appropriate newborn feeding techniques
Teaching/ psychosocial	Explain postpartum assessments Teach self-massage of fundus and expected findings; rationale for fundal massage Instruct to call for assistance first time OOB and PRN Demonstrate peri-care, surgigator, sitz bath prn Explain comfort measures Begin newborn teaching; bulb suctioning, positioning, feeding, diaper change, cord care Orient to room if transferred from LDR room Provide information on early postpartal period Assess mother/infant attachment	Discuss psychologic changes of postpartum period; facilitate transition through tasks of taking on maternal role Discuss peri care/hygiene; encourage use of supportive brassiere for breast- or bottle-feeding Stress need for frequent rest periods Continue newborn teaching: soothing/comforting techniques, swaddling; return demonstrations indicate woman's understanding Provide opportunities for questions and review; reinforce previous teaching Breastfeeding: nipple care: air-drying, lanolin; proper latch-on technique; tea bags Bottle-feeding; supportive bra, ice bags, breast binder Assess mother/infant attachment	Reinforce previous teaching, complete teaching evaluation Discuss involution; anticipated physical changes in first 2 weeks postpartum; postpartal exercises; need to limit visitors Discuss postpartal nutrition; balanced diet Breastfeeding: • Increase calories by 500 kcal over nonpregnant state (200 kcal over pregnant intake) • Explain milk production, let-down reflex, use of supplements, breast pumping, and milk storage Bottle-feeding: • Return to nonpregnant caloric intake • Explain formula preparation and storage Discuss birth control options, sexuality Discuss sibling rivalry and plan for supporting siblings at home Discuss pets; suggestions for improving acceptance of infant by pets **Expected Outcomes** Mother verbalizes teaching comprehension. Positive bonding and emotional behaviors observed.
Nursing care management and reports	Ice pack to perineum to decrease swelling and increase comfort Straight catheter prn × 1 if distended or voiding small amounts If continues unable to void or voiding small amounts, insert Foley catheter and notify CNM/physician	Sitz baths prn If woman Rh− and infant Rh+, RhoGAM work up; obtain consent; complete teaching Determine rubella status Obtain consent for rubella vaccine if indicated; explain purpose, procedure, implications of vaccine Obtain hematocrit	Continue sitz baths prn May shower if ambulating without difficulty DC buffalo cap (heplock) if present Administer rubella vaccine as indicated **Expected Outcomes** Using sitz bath; voids qs; lab work WNL; performs ADL without sequelae

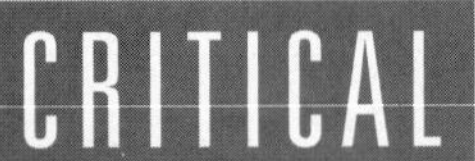

CRITICAL PATHWAY FOR THE POSTPARTAL PERIOD *CONTINUED*

Category	First 4 Hours	4–8 Hours Past Birth	8–24 Hours Past Birth
Activity	Assistance when OOB first time, then prn Ambulate ad lib Rests comfortably between assessments	Encourage rest periods Ambulate ad lib; may leave birthing unit after notifying staff of plan to ambulate off unit	Up ad lib **Expected Outcomes** Ambulates ad lib
Comfort	Institute comfort measures: • Perineal discomfort: peri-care; sitz baths, topical analgesics • Hemorrhoids: sitz baths, topical analgesics, digital replacement of external hemorrhoids; side-lying or prone position • Afterpains: prone with small pillow under abdomen; warm shower or sitz baths; ambulation • Administer pain medication ________	Continue with pain management techniques Offer alternative pain management options: distraction with music, television, visitors; massage; warmed blankets or towels to affected area; using breathing techniques when infant latches on to breast and/or during cramping until medication's action is felt	Continue with pain management techniques **Expected Outcomes** Comfort level < 3 on 1–10 scale Verbalizes alternative pain management options
Nutrition	Regular diet Fluid $\geqq$ 2000 mL/day	Continue diet and fluids	Continue diet and fluids **Expected Outcomes** Regular diet/fluids tolerated
Elimination	Voiding large amounts straw-colored urine	Voiding large quantities May have bowel movement	Same **Expected Outcomes** Voiding qs; passing flatus or bowel movement
Medications	Pain medications as ordered Methergine 0.2 mg q4h po if ordered Stool softener ________________ Tucks pad prn, perineal analgesic spray	Continue meds Lanolin to nipples PRN; tea bags to nipples if tender; heparin flush to buffalo cap/heplock (if present) q8h or as ordered May take own prenatal vitamins	Continue medications RhoGAM and rubella vaccine administered if indicated **Expected Outcomes** Vaccines administered; pain controlled
Discharge planning/home care	Evaluate knowledge of normal postpartum and newborn care Evaluate support systems	Discuss typical newborn schedule; plan for periods of rest Birth certificate paperwork completed Evaluate plans for transporting newborn; car seat available	Review discharge instruction sheet/checklist Describe postpartum warning signs and when to call CNM/physician Provide prescriptions. Gift packs given appropriate for bottle- or breastfeeding Arrangements for baby pictures as desired Postpartum and newborn visits scheduled **Expected Outcomes** Discharged home; mother verbalizes postpartum warning s/s, follow-up appointment times/dates
Family involvement	Identify available support persons Assess family perceptions of birth experience Parenting: demonstrates culturally expected early parenting behaviors	Involve support persons in care, teaching; answer questions Evidence of parental bonding behaviors present	Continue to involve support persons in teaching, involve siblings as appropriate. Plans made for providing support to mother following discharge **Expected Outcomes** Evidence of parental bonding behavior; support persons verbalize understanding of woman's need for rest, good nutrition, fluids and emotional support
Date			

An important component of nursing care is client teaching, which is designed to help the woman and her family become self-sufficient and effective in dealing with changes postpartum and in providing effective newborn care. Sophisticated, detailed forms and guidelines are often available to assist in health teaching. Such tools are a useful adjunct but cannot take the place of the nurse's client-specific plan. As part of client teaching, the nurse should discuss desired client outcomes or goals with the mother as soon as possible on her arrival in the postpartum unit. Examples of these desired client outcomes (adapted from the Rose Women's Center, Denver, Colorado) include the following:

- Maintains health for self and baby
- Reviews educational resources for self and baby care
- Demonstrates care for self and baby
- Displays appropriate interaction between parent and baby
- Practices principles of infant safety
- Demonstrates proper breastfeeding and breast care or describes formula preparation for bottle-feeding, feeding techniques, and breast care

Additional outcomes for the cesarean birth mother include the following:

- States in own words the reason for the cesarean birth
- Maintains desired pain control
- Maintains moderate mobility level

In summary, all components of nursing care management are designed to achieve the desired outcomes identified for the woman and her family.

Promotion of Maternal Physical Well-Being

The nurse promotes and restores maternal physical well-being by monitoring the status of the uterus, vital signs, cardiovascular status, elimination, nutritional needs, sleep and rest, and support and educational needs. In addition, medications may be needed to promote comfort, treat anemia, provide immunity to rubella, and prevent development of antibodies in the nonsensitized Rh negative woman.

TABLE 31–1 Key Facts To Remember About Monitoring Postpartal Uterine Status

Position of the Uterine Fundus Following Birth

Immediately after birth: The top of the fundus is in the midline about midway between the symphysis pubis and umbilicus.

Six to 12 hours after birth: The top of the fundus is in the midline and at the level of the umbilicus.

One day after birth: The top of the fundus is in the midline and one finger-breadth below the umbilicus.

Second day after birth and thereafter: The top of the fundus remains in the midline and descends about one fingerbreadth per day.

Normal Characteristics of Lochia

Lochia rubra is red and is present for the first 2–3 days.

Lochia serosa is pinkish red and is present from day 3 to day 10.

Lochia alba is creamy white and is present from day 11 to about day 21.

Monitoring Uterine Status

The nurse completes an assessment of the uterus as discussed in Chapter 30. The assessment interval is every 15 minutes for the first hour after childbirth, every 30 minutes for the next hour, and then hourly for approximately 2 hours. Thereafter, the nurse monitors uterine status every 8 hours or more frequently if problems, such as **bogginess** (softening of the uterus due to inadequate contraction of the muscle tissue), positioning out of midline, heavy lochia flow, or the presence of clots, arise (Table 31–1).

The amount, consistency, color, and odor of the lochia are monitored on an ongoing basis. Changes in lochia that need to be assessed further, documented, and reported to the physician/certified nurse-midwife are presented in Table 31–2.

CRITICAL THINKING QUESTION

The postpartum unit you work on as a staff nurse is changing the type of perineal pads (peri-pads) that will be used. You volunteer to assist with the change. How will you establish an accurate visual method of assessing the amount of lochia on the pad?

Occasionally a medication such as methylergonovine maleate (Methergine) is prescribed to promote uterine

TABLE 31–2 Changes in Lochia That Cause Concern

Change	Possible Problem	Nursing Action
Presence of clots	Inadequate uterine contractions that allow bleeding from vessels at the placental site.	Assess location and firmness of fundus. Assess voiding pattern. Record and report findings.
Persistent lochia rubra	Inadequate uterine contractions; retained placental fragments; infection	Assess location and firmness of fundus. Assess activity pattern. Assess for signs of infection. Record and report findings.

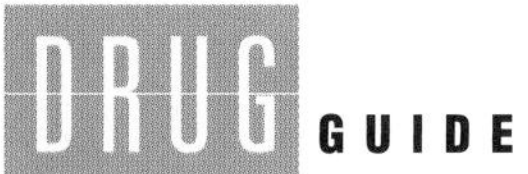

Methylergonovine Maleate (Methergine)

Overview of Action

Methylergonovine maleate (Methergine) is an ergot alkaloid that stimulates smooth muscle tissue. Because the smooth muscle of the uterus is especially sensitive to this drug, it is used postpartally to stimulate the uterus to contract in order to decrease blood loss by clamping off uterine blood vessels and to promote the involution process. In addition, the drug has a vasoconstrictive effect on all blood vessels, especially the larger arteries. This may result in hypertension, particularly in a woman whose blood pressure is already elevated.

Route, Dosage, and Frequency

Methergine has a rapid onset of action and may be given orally or intramuscularly.
Usual IM dose: 0.2 mg following delivery of the placenta. The dose may be repeated every 2–4 hours if necessary.
Usual oral dose: 0.2 mg every 4 hours (six doses).

Maternal Contraindications

Pregnancy, hepatic or renal disease, cardiac disease, hypertension or pregnancy induced hypertension contraindicate this drug's use. Methylergonovine maleate must be used with caution during lactation (PDR Nurse's Handbook, 1999).

Maternal Side Effects

Hypertension, nausea, vomiting, headache, bradycardia, dizziness, tinnitus, abdominal cramps, palpitations, dyspnea, chest pain, and allergic reactions may be noted.

Effects on Fetus or Neonate

Because Methergine has a long duration (3 hours [Karch, 1999]) and action and can thus produce tetanic contractions, it **should never be used during pregnancy or in labor,** when it may result in a sustained uterine contraction that may cause amniotic fluid embolism (increased pressure in uterus may allow entry of amniotic fluid under the edge of the placenta and thus entry into the maternal venous system), uterine rupture, cervical and perineal lacerations (resulting from tetanic contractions and rapid birth of the baby), and hypoxia and intracranial hemorrhage in the baby (because of tetanic contractions, which severely decrease the maternal-placental-fetal blood flow, or uterine rupture, which causes cessation of blood flow to the unborn baby) (PDR Nurse's Handbook, 1999).

Nursing Considerations

- Monitor fundal height and consistency and the amount and character of the lochia.
- Assess the blood pressure before and routinely throughout drug administration.
- Observe for adverse effects or symptoms of ergot toxicity (ergotism) such as nausea and vomiting, headache, muscle pain, cold or numb fingers and toes, chest pain, and general weakness (PDR Nurse's Handbook, 1999).
- Provide client/family teaching regarding importance of not smoking during methergine administration (nicotine from cigarettes leads to constricted vessels and may lead to hypertension), signs of toxicity.

contractions. In some cases an intravenous infusion of oxytocin (Pitocin) may be necessary if the uterus does not remain firm and uterine bleeding is excessive. See Drug Guide: Methylergonovine Maleate (Methergine) in this chapter and Drug Guide: Pitocin in Chapter 23.

Teaching for Self-Care The nurse teaches the woman to assess her fundus for firmness and position and to massage the fundus gently to promote uterine muscle contraction. In addition, the nurse instructs her to monitor the amount and color of the lochia flow to determine whether normal progression is occurring. Being aware of normal involutional changes will help the woman identify problems and know when to contact her health care provider once she is discharged.

Promotion of Comfort and Relief of Pain

Discomfort may be present to varying degrees in the postpartal woman. Potential sources of discomfort include an edematous perineum; a distended bladder; an episiotomy, perineal laceration, or extension; a vaginal hematoma; engorged hemorrhoids; engorged breasts; or sore nipples.

Relief of Perineal Discomfort

Many nursing interventions are available for relieving perineal discomfort. Before selecting a method, the nurse needs to have assessed the perineum to determine the degree of edema and other problems. It is also important to ask the woman whether there are special measures that she feels will be particularly effective and to offer her choices when possible. The nurse uses disposable gloves while applying all relief measures and washes hands before and after using the gloves. (See Essential Precautions in Practice: During Postpartal Care.)

At all times it is necessary to use basic hygienic practices, such as moving from the front (area of the symphysis pubis) to the back (area around the anus) of the perineum. The nurse should follow this principle when

ESSENTIAL PRECAUTIONS IN PRACTICE

During Postpartal Care

Examples of times when disposable gloves should be worn include

- Assessing the perineum and lochia
- Changing perineal pads and chux
- Assessing the breast if there is leakage of colostrum or milk
- Handling used breast pads
- Handling used clothing, chux, perineal pads, and/or bedding contaminated with lochia
- Applying ice packs or topical anesthetic sprays to the perineum. (Although an ice pack or anesthetic spray could be applied in such a manner that contact with the perineum and a perineal pad is avoided, it is best to have gloves on so that you can assist with removal of the pad if needed.)

REMEMBER to wash your hands before putting on the disposable gloves and again immediately after you remove them.

For further information, consult OSHA and CDC guidelines.

CLINICAL TIP

You may be surprised by how quickly the postpartal woman shows signs of bladder distention, possibly as soon as 1 to 2 hours after childbirth. This is because of normal postpartal diuresis. You can help prevent overdistention by palpating the woman's bladder frequently and encouraging her to void. When urinating the first time after vaginal birth, some mothers may feel the urge to urinate but are unable to begin the flow of urine. Possible interventions include: let her hear running water by turning water on in the sink; run warm water in the sink and have her place one hand in the water; place her feet in a basin of warm water; and place a few drops of peppermint oil in the urine collection device ("hat"). Be sure to measure the first few voidings. The amount should be at least 150cc. If she is still unable to void and catheterization becomes necessary, be prepared for difficulty in visualizing the urethra because of localized swelling and discomfort and tenderness in the area.

placing ice packs, placing perineal pads, and applying topical anesthetic agents or pain relief products. Avoiding contamination between the anal area and the urethral-vaginal area is essential to prevent infection.

Ice Pack If an episiotomy is performed at the time of birth, an ice pack is generally applied to reduce edema and numb the tissues, which promotes comfort. In some agencies chemical ice bags are used. These are usually activated by folding both ends toward the middle. Inexpensive ice bags can be made by filling a disposable glove with ice chips or crushed ice and then taping the top of the glove. To protect the perineum from burns caused by contact with the ice pack, the disposable glove is first rinsed under running water to remove any powder that may be present and then wrapped in an absorbent towel or washcloth before it is placed against the perineum. To attain the maximum effect of this cold treatment, the ice pack should remain in place approximately 20 minutes and then be removed for about 10 minutes before it is replaced. Ice packs may be continued for as long as necessary. Usually, they are needed for the first 24 hours.

Teaching for Self-Care The nurse provides information regarding the purpose of the ice pack, anticipated effects, benefits, and possible problems and how to prepare an ice pack for home use if edema is present and early discharge is planned.

Sitz Bath The warmth of the water in the sitz bath provides comfort, decreases pain, and increases circulation to the tissues, which promotes healing and reduces the incidence of infection. Sitz baths may be ordered three times daily (TID) and as needed (PRN). The nurse prepares the sitz bath by cleansing the portable sitz and then fills it with water at 102F to 105F. The nurse instructs the woman to remain in the sitz for 20 minutes. Care needs to be taken during the first sitz bath because the warm, moist heat may cause the woman to faint. The nurse should place a call bell well within reach and check on the woman at frequent intervals to ensure her safety, observing for signs that she may faint, such as pallor or complaints of dizziness, a floating or spacy feeling, or difficulty hearing. It is important for the woman to have a clean unused towel to pat dry her perineum after the sitz bath and to have a clean perineal pad ready to apply.

Recently, cool sitz baths have gained popularity because they are effective in reducing perineal edema. Until definite research supports one temperature (warm or cold) as more effective, it may be best to offer the woman a choice.

Teaching for Self-Care The nurse provides information about the purpose and use of the sitz bath, anticipated effects, benefits, possible problems, and safety measures to prevent injury from fainting, slipping, or excessive water temperature. Home use of sitz baths may be recommended for the woman with an extensive episiotomy; the woman may use a portable sitz or her bathtub. It is important for the nurse to emphasize that in using a bathtub, the woman draws only 4 to 6 inches of water, assesses the temperature of the water, and uses the water only for the sitz, not for bathing. If the woman takes a tub bath, she should release the water, clean the tub, and draw new water prior to the sitz to prevent infection.

Topical Agents Topical anesthetic agents, such as Dermoplast aerosol spray or Americain spray, may be used to relieve perineal discomfort. The woman is advised to apply the anesthetic agent after a sitz bath or perineal care. Because of the danger of tissue burns, she must be cautioned not to apply the anesthetic agent before using a heat lamp.

Witch hazel compresses may be used to relieve perineal discomfort and edema. Nupercainal ointment or Tucks may be ordered for relief of hemorrhoidal pain. It is important for the nurse to emphasize the need for the woman to wash her hands before and after using the topical treatments.

Teaching for Self-Care The nurse provides information regarding the anesthetic spray or topical agent. The woman needs to understand the purpose, use, anticipated effects, benefits, and possible problems associated with the product. Demonstration of application by the nurse can be combined with explanation. A return demonstration is a useful method of evaluating the woman's understanding.

Perineal Care Perineal care after each elimination cleanses the perineum and helps promote comfort. Many agencies provide "peri bottles" that the woman can use to squirt warm tap water over her perineum following elimination. To cleanse her perineum, the woman may use a Surgigator, moist antiseptic towelettes, or toilet paper in a blotting (patting) motion and should be taught to start at the front (area just under the symphysis pubis) and proceed toward the back (area around the anus) to prevent contamination from the anal area. In addition, to prevent contamination, the perineal pad should be applied from front to back, placing the front portion against the perineum first.

Teaching for Self-Care The nurse demonstrates how to cleanse the perineum and assists the woman as necessary, for example, by offering additional information regarding the use of perineal pads. The pad needs to be placed snugly against the perineum but should not produce pressure. If the pad is worn too loosely, it may rub back and forth, irritating perineal tissues and causing contamination between the anal and vaginal areas. Many women have never used a perineal pad or belt and will need additional assistance in using them during the postpartal period. (See Teaching Guide: Episiotomy Care.)

Relief of Hemorrhoidal Discomfort

Some mothers experience hemorrhoidal pain after giving birth. Relief measures include the use of sitz baths, anesthetic ointments, rectal suppositories, or witch hazel pads applied directly to the anal area. The woman can be taught to digitally replace external hemorrhoids in her rectum. She may also find it helpful to maintain a side-lying position when possible or to tighten her buttocks when sitting down to reduce contact of the perineum with the seat and to avoid prolonged sitting. The mother is encouraged to maintain an adequate fluid intake, and is given stool softeners to ensure greater comfort with bowel movements. The hemorrhoids usually disappear a few weeks after birth if the woman did not have them prior to her pregnancy.

Relief of Afterpains

Afterpains are the result of intermittent uterine contractions. A primipara may not notice afterpains because her uterus is able to maintain a contracted state. Multiparous women and those who have had an overdistended uterus (due to multiple gestation or hydramnios) frequently experience discomfort from afterpains as the uterus intermittently contracts more vigorously. Breastfeeding women are also more likely to experience afterpains than bottle-feeding women because of the release of oxytocin when the infant suckles. The nurse can suggest the woman lie prone with a small pillow under the lower abdomen, explaining that the discomfort may be intensified for about 5 minutes but then will diminish greatly, if not completely. The prone position applies pressure to the uterus and therefore stimulates contractions. When the uterus maintains a constant contraction, the afterpains cease. Additional nursing interventions include a sitz bath (for warmth), positioning, ambulation, or administration of an analgesic agent, such as Motrin, Tylenol, or Percoset. When administering an analgesic agent, the nurse must make a clinical judgment about the type, dosage, and frequency based on the medications ordered. The mother's description of the type and severity of her pain is usually the most reliable method of determining which analgesic agent would provide her the comfort she desires. Many women who are breastfeeding have concerns about the effects of medications on the infant. For breastfeeding mothers, a mild analgesic agent administered an hour before feeding will promote comfort and enhance maternal-infant interactions.

Teaching for Self-Care The nurse provides information about the cause of afterpains and methods to decrease discomfort. The nurse also explains any medications that are ordered, expected effect, benefits, possible side effects, and any special considerations such as the possibility of dizziness or sleepiness with particular medications.

Relief of Discomfort from Immobility

Discomfort may also be caused by immobility. The woman who pushed for a long time during labor may experience muscular aches. It is not unusual for women to experience joint pains and discomfort in both arms and legs, depending on the effort they exerted during the second stage of labor. Early ambulation is encouraged to help reduce the incidence of complications such as constipation and thrombophlebitis. It also helps promote a general feeling of well-being.

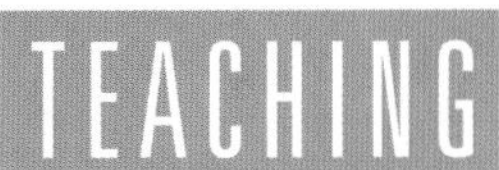 GUIDE: EPISIOTOMY CARE

Assessment During the time following labor and birth, assess the woman's understanding of the purpose of the episiotomy, the factors that contribute to wound healing, and the comfort measures available if needed. The woman's level of knowledge may be influenced by several factors, including, for example, childbirth preparation activities and previous childbirth experience.

Nursing Diagnosis The key nursing diagnosis will probably be ***Knowledge Deficit*** related to lack of information about self-care measures to promote episiotomy healing and personal comfort.

Nursing Plan and Implementation The teaching will focus on the process of healing, factors that increase the risk of infection, and steps the woman can take to promote healing and increase her personal comfort.

Client Goals At the completion of teaching, the woman will be able to:

- Identify the factors that both promote and interfere with wound healing.
- Summarize self-care activities to promote healing and increase personal comfort.
- Demonstrate the correct procedure for taking a sitz bath.
- Discuss the judicious use of prescribed analgesics as needed.

Teaching Plan

Content	*Teaching Method*
• Describe the process of wound healing, including the value of healing by first intention as opposed to a jagged tear. Discuss the risk of contamination of the episiotomy by bacteria from the anal area.	*Many women do not consider the episiotomy a surgical incision. Discussion helps them understand the importance of good wound care.*
• Explain techniques that are used to keep the episiotomy clean and promote healing such as: • Sitz bath • Use of peribottle following each voiding or defecation • Pad change following each elimination and at regular intervals	*Focus on open discussion. Demonstrate the peri bottle or sitz bath if necessary.*
• Describe comfort measures: • Ice pack or glove immediately following birth • Sitz bath • Judicious use of analgesics or topical anesthetics • Tightening buttocks before sitting	*Focus on discussion and provide an opportunity for questions.*
• Identify signs of episiotomy infection. Advise the woman to contact her caregiver if infection develops.	*Encourage discussion and provide printed handouts. Some of this content may also be covered during a small postpartum class.*

Evaluation At the end of the teaching session the woman will be able to verbalize the principles of wound healing and episiotomy care. She will also be able to demonstrate self-care measures such as peri-care and taking a sitz bath.

CLINICAL TIP

It is not unusual for the postpartum mother to feel faint the first few times she gets up. Be alert for signs of faintness, such as loss of color in her lips or face; complaints of feeling warm, dizzy, or having buzzing in her ears; and difficulty hearing. If any of these signs are noted, immediately support her body so she doesn't fall. Then help her sit with her head between her knees or lie down.

I'd like to tell you about a memorable moment that occurred in my nursing practice with a new postpartum mother. I was walking a new mother from the bathroom back to bed. The mother and I were quite unequal in size. As I felt her body begin to slump, I realized I could not gently let her slide down to the floor. I quickly looked around, saw a big upholstered chair behind me and sat down, pulling her with me. I maintained safety for her; however, she was lying on top of me. I could not move, could not reach the call button, and had shut the door to the room. I began to call out "yoo-hoo . . . I need help in here." I did not call out loudly because I would have been yelling in her ear. When assistance came, the mother was still unconscious and my colleagues could not refrain from smiling and rolling their eyes at our predicament. I usually share this story with beginning nursing students as they learn how to ambulate patients. The students smile and laugh with me and I think it helps them know that all of us will have some unusual experiences.

The nurse assists the woman the first few times she gets up during the postpartal period. Fatigue, effects of medications, loss of blood, and possibly even lack of food may cause feelings of dizziness or faintness when the woman stands up. Because this may be a problem during the woman's first shower, the nurse should remain in the room, check the woman frequently, and have a chair close by in case she becomes faint. Dizziness may be aggravated by standing still and by the warmth of the water, so it is best to keep the first shower somewhat brief. On many postpartal units, ammonia inhalants (referred to as "smelling salts") are taped to the bathroom door for use in case of fainting. During this first shower the nurse instructs the woman in the use of the emergency call button in the bathroom; if she becomes faint during a future shower, she can call for assistance.

Teaching for Self-Care The nurse provides information about ambulation and the importance of monitoring any signs of dizziness or weakness. If she becomes dizzy, the woman should sit down and call for assistance.

Relief of Discomfort from Excessive Perspiration

Postpartal diaphoresis (excessive perspiration) may cause discomfort for new mothers. The nurse can offer a fresh dry gown and bed linens to enhance comfort.

CLINICAL TIP

The woman who has had an epidural during labor may not have full control of her legs for a while after birth. Before getting her up to the bathroom for the first time, assess for orthostatic hypotension. Obtain her blood pressure lying down, wait 2 minutes, assist her into a sitting position with her legs over the side of the bed and take her blood pressure. If her blood pressure drops more than 20 points systolic, or she feels dizzy, assist her back to a supine position. If the blood pressure remains fairly stable, wait 2 minutes, have her stand beside the bed, and reassess the blood pressure. If orthostatic hypotension is present, assist her to a sitting and then a supine position. If the blood pressure is stable, you can assist her to the bathroom. You will need to stay with her in case she needs further assistance.

Some women may feel refreshed by a shower. It is important to consider cultural practices and realize that some women of Mexican or Asian cultural background may prefer not to shower in the first few days following birth. Women from India may take a warm bath, but they, too, are often reluctant to shower (Choudhry, 1997). Because diaphoresis also may lead to increased thirst, the nurse can offer fluids as the woman desires. Again, cultural practices are important to consider. Women of western European background may prefer iced water; Asian women may prefer water at room temperature. It is essential that the nurse ascertains the woman's wishes rather than operate solely from the nurse's own values or cultural belief system.

Teaching for Self-Care The nurse provides information about the normal physiologic changes that cause diaphoresis and methods to increase comfort.

Suppression of Lactation in the Non-nursing Mother

For the woman who chooses not to breastfeed, lactation may be suppressed by mechanical inhibition. Although signs of engorgement do not usually occur until the second or third day postpartum, engorgement is best prevented by beginning mechanical methods of lactation suppression as soon as possible after birth. Ideally, this involves having the woman begin wearing a supportive, well-fitting bra within 6 hours after birth. The bra is worn continuously until lactation is suppressed (usually about 5 days) and is removed only for showers. The bra provides support and eases the discomfort that can occur with tension on the breasts because of fullness. A snug breast binder may be used if the woman does not have a bra available or if she finds the binder more comfortable. Ice packs should be applied over the axillary area of each breast for 20 minutes four times daily. This, too, should be begun soon after birth. Ice is also useful in relieving discomfort if engorgement occurs.

CLINICAL TIP

Each episode of diaphoresis may result in a fluid loss of more than 1000 mL. The woman who wakes up soaked may be very worried that something is wrong. It is important for her to understand what is happening and that it is normal. It is also very important to assist her in washing herself if she desires, and then into dry clothing and bedding.

I bottle-fed my baby. It worked very well and my baby and I enjoyed the special closeness of cuddling during feeding. With the bottle, my husband was also able to share the feeding experience. He felt very involved as such an integral member of our new family. The only problem I had was getting through breast engorgement in the first 2 or so weeks after our baby was born. My breasts became so hard, tender, and painful, and nothing brought relief. I was so surprised when the breast tissue all the way under my arms became sore and I had to hold my arms away from my body. The breast discomfort affected how I held our baby, positions for sleep, and even getting a hug from my husband. I guess one of the most important realizations was that not one of my nurses ever mentioned to me what engorgement really meant and how to deal with it. I'd like to encourage all nurses to ask postpartum mothers what their experience is or was, and to share realistic and practical information with all new mothers. Even with excellent teaching, there are so many questions for new parents.

Teaching for Self-Care The mother is advised to avoid any stimulation of her breasts by her baby, herself, breast pumps, or her sexual partner until the sensation of fullness has passed (usually about 5 to 7 days). Such stimulation will increase milk production and delay the suppression process. Heat is avoided for the same reason, and the mother is encouraged to let shower water flow over her back rather than her breasts. Suppression takes only a few days in most cases, but small amounts of milk may be produced up to a month after birth.

Promotion of Rest and Graded Activity

Following birth, some women feel exhausted and in need of rest. Other women are euphoric and full of psychic energy, ready to retell their experience of birth repeatedly. The nurse evaluates individual needs, always with the goal of providing opportunities for rest. The nurse can provide time for the excited, euphoric woman to air her feelings and then can encourage a period of rest. The nurse may also help the family limit visitors and provide a comfortable sleep chair or bed for the father.

Physical fatigue often affects other adjustments and functions of the new mother. For example, fatigue may reduce milk flow, thereby increasing problems with establishing breastfeeding. The mother requires energy to make the psychologic adjustments to a new infant and to assume new roles. She makes these adjustments more smoothly when she gets adequate rest. The nurse can encourage rest by organizing activities to avoid frequent interruptions for the woman. If the new mother chooses, rest times may be arranged by having the newborn remain in the holding nursery for a period of time, or the mother can rest or sleep when the baby is sleeping in her room. It is important for the new mother to know that physical fatigue may persist for a number of months. Persistent fatigue is affected by physiologic, psychologic, situational, and environmental factors (Parks, Lenz, Milligan & Han, 1999).

Although most mothers feel fatigued, they tend to view themselves as healthy and well if they perceive pregnancy and birth as natural processes. Some mothers, however, view the postpartal period as a time of sickness. For instance, some Korean women and their families view the new mother as sick and in need of care by the mother-in-law and the father. A Korean mother may take on some activities, but for the most part they will be directed to the baby, such as picking up the baby from the nursery, rather than to herself (Schneiderman, 1996).

Ambulation and activity may gradually increase after discharge. The new mother should avoid heavy lifting, excessive stair climbing, and strenuous activity. One or two daily naps are essential and are most easily achieved if the mother sleeps when her baby does.

By the second week at home, the new mother may resume light housekeeping activities. Although it is customary to delay returning to work for 6 weeks, most women are physically able to resume practically all activities by 4 to 5 weeks. Delaying returning to work until after the final postpartal examination will minimize the possibility of problems.

Postpartal Exercises

The nurse should encourage the woman to begin simple exercises while in the birthing unit and continue them at home, advising her that increased lochia or pain means she should reevaluate her activity and make necessary alterations. Most agencies provide a booklet describing suggested postpartal activities. (Exercise routines vary for women undergoing tubal ligation following birth or for cesarean birth clients.) See Figure 31–1 on page 942 for a description of some commonly used exercises. Sampselle, Seng, Yeo, Killion, and Oakley (1999) report that exercise during the prenatal period is associated with positive views of the childbirth experience. The postpartal woman is more likely to have positive views of her own well-being and less fatigue if she continues to do stretching and/or her own programmed pattern of exercise.

Pharmacologic Interventions

Rubella Vaccine

Women who have a rubella titer of less than 1:10 or are ELISA antibody negative are usually given rubella vaccine in the postpartal period (Cunningham et al, 1997).

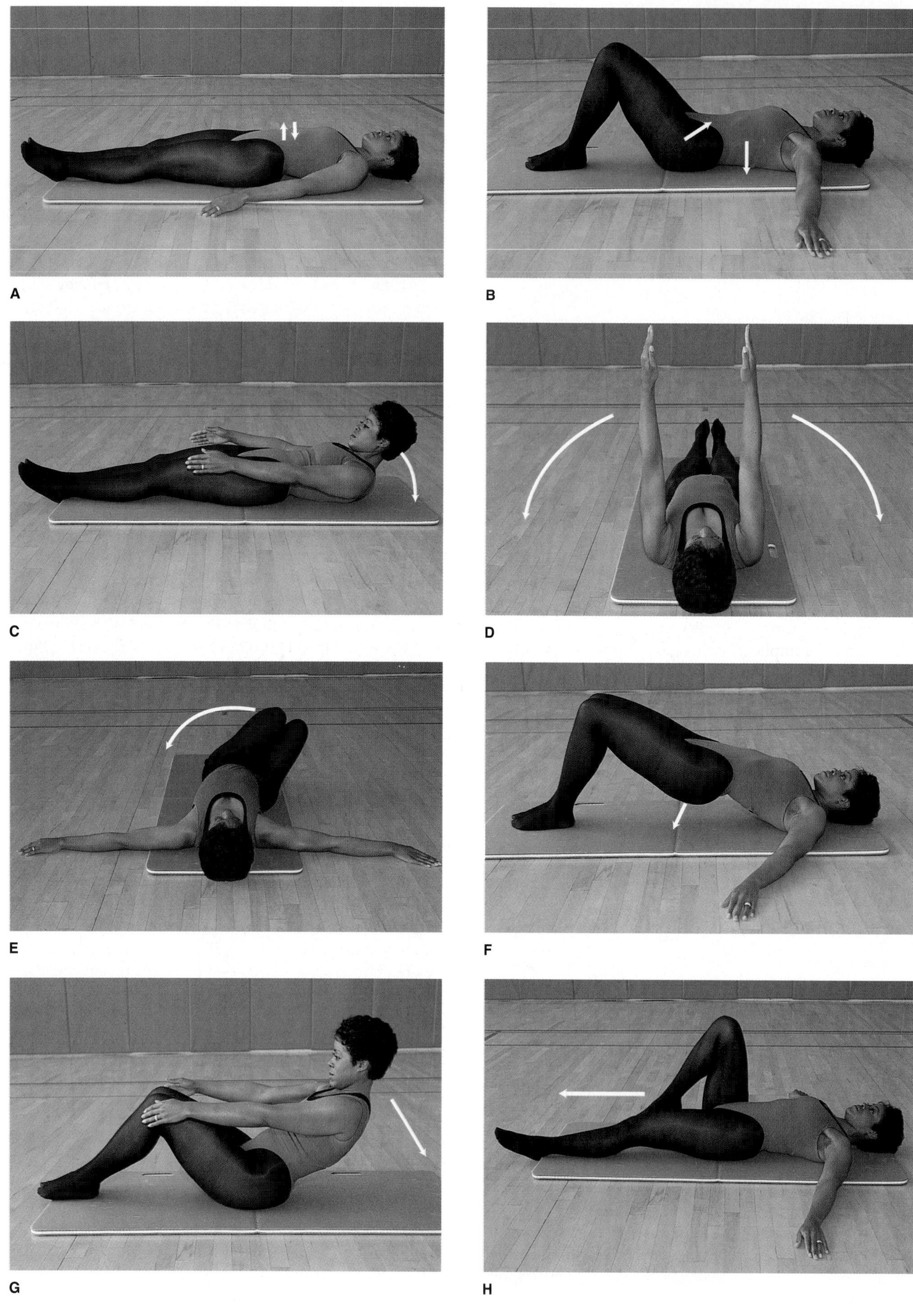

A

B

C

D

E

F

G

H

Because the vaccine needs to be given when the woman is not pregnant, administering the injection just after childbirth has the advantage of targeting a time period when the woman is definitely not pregnant and in most cases does not want another pregnancy in the next 3 months. If the woman is not rubella immune and is also Rh negative and receives RhoGAM, the RhoGAM may interfere with the production of antibodies to rubella. In this case, most physicians/certified nurse-midwives continue to order rubella vaccine and repeat the rubella titer in a few weeks to determine immunity (Varney, 1997). See Table 31–3.

Teaching for Self-Care The nurse needs to ensure that the woman understands the purpose of the vaccine and that she must avoid becoming pregnant in the next 3 months. To ensure that the woman understands, an informed consent is usually signed prior to administration. Because avoiding pregnancy is so important, counseling regarding contraception is suggested.

RhIgG (RhoGAM)

All Rh negative women who meet specific criteria should receive RhIgG (RhoGAM) within 72 hours after childbirth to prevent sensitization from a fetomaternal transfusion of Rh positive fetal red blood cells. See discussion of criteria in Procedure 16–2.

Teaching for Self-Care The Rh negative woman needs to understand the implications of her Rh negative status in future pregnancies. (See Chapter 15 for a detailed discussion.) The nurse provides opportunities for questions during teaching.

Promotion of Maternal Psychologic Well-Being

The birth of a child, with the role changes and increased responsibilities it produces, is a time of emotional stress for the new mother. This stress is increased by the tremendous physiologic changes that occur as her body adjusts to a nonpregnant state. During the early postpartal days, mood swings and tearfulness are common.

At first the mother may repeatedly discuss her experiences in labor and birth and how it compared with her fantasized picture. This storytelling allows her to reexperience and integrate her experiences (Banks-Wallace, 1999). If she feels that she did not cope well with labor, she may have feelings of inadequacy and may benefit from reassurance that she did well. Open discussion of feelings is possible only if the postpartum nurse has established a warm, supportive relationship with the woman. Follow-up visits from the nurse who assisted her in labor and birth provide additional opportunities for the mother to relive her experiences and come to terms with them.

During the postpartal period, the mother must also adjust to the loss of her fantasized child and accept the child she has borne. This may be more difficult if the child is not of the desired sex or has birth defects.

Immediately following the birth (the taking-in period), the mother is dependent and focused inward on bodily concerns. During this time, teaching other than for self-care may not be totally effective. Because early discharge has become so common, however, the nurse should offer classes and information and provide printed handouts for reference as questions arise at home.

Following the initial dependent period, the mother becomes very concerned about her ability to be a successful parent (the taking-hold period). Skillful intervention by the nurse, with continual reassurance that the woman is a successful mother, is vital. During this time the mother is most receptive to teaching, and tactful instruction and demonstration assist her in developing mothering skills. The nurse must carefully avoid "taking over" the infant. By functioning as an adviser and allowing the mother to perform the actual care, the nurse demonstrates confidence in the mother's skill and ability, which in turn increases the mother's self-confidence about her effectiveness as a parent. Recognition and praise of her

FIGURE 31–1 Postpartal exercises. Begin with five repetitions two or three times daily, and gradually increase to ten repetitions. First day: ***A,*** Abdominal breathing. Lying supine, inhale deeply, using the abdominal muscles. The abdomen should expand. Then exhale slowly through pursed lips, tightening the abdominal muscles. ***B,*** Pelvic rocking. Lying supine with arms at sides, knees bent, and feet flat, tighten abdomen and buttocks, and attempt to flatten back on floor. Hold for a count of ten; then arch the back, causing the pelvis to "rock." On the second day, add ***C,*** Chin to chest. Lying supine with legs straight, raise head and attempt to touch chin to chest. Slowly lower head. ***D,*** Arm raises. Lying supine, arms extended at a 90-degree angle from body, raise arms so that they are perpendicular and hands touch. Lower slowly. On fourth day, add ***E,*** Knee rolls. Lying supine with knees bent, feet flat, arms extended to the side, roll knees slowly to one side, keeping shoulders flat. Return to original position, and roll to opposite side. ***F,*** Buttocks lift. Lying supine, arms at sides, knees bent, feet flat, slowly raise the buttocks, and arch the back. Return slowly to starting position. On sixth day, add ***G,*** Abdominal tighteners. Lying supine, knees bent, feet flat, slowly raise head toward knees. Arms should extend along either side of legs. Return slowly to original position. ***H,*** Knee to abdomen. Lying supine, arms at sides, bend one knee and thigh until foot touches buttocks. Straighten leg and lower it slowly. Repeat with other leg. After 2–3 weeks, more strenuous exercises, such as sit-ups and side leg raises, may be added as tolerated. Kegel exercises, begun antepartally, should be done many times daily during postpartum to restore vaginal and perineal tone.

TABLE 31–3 Essential Information for Common Postpartum Drugs

EMPIRIN #3 (325 mg aspirin and 30 mg codeine)

Drug class: Narcotic analgesic.

Dose/Route: Usual adult dose: 1–2 tablets PO every 4 hours PRN.

Indication: For relief of mild to moderate pain.

Adverse Effects: Aspirin: Nausea, dyspepsia, epigastric discomfort, dizziness. Codeine: Respiratory depression, apnea, light-headedness, dizziness, nausea, sweating, dry mouth, constipation, facial flushing, suppression of cough reflex, ureteral spasm, urinary retention, pruritus.

Nursing Implications: Determine whether woman is sensitive to aspirin or codeine; has history of impaired hepatic or renal function.
Monitor bowel sounds, respirations, urine output.
Administer with food or after meals if GI upset occurs; encourage woman to drink one full glass (240 mL) with the tablet to reduce the risk of the tablet lodging in the esophagus.

Client Teaching: Inform client about name of drug, expected action, possible side effects, that it is secreted in breast milk (Note: Some physicians/certified nurse-midwives may avoid ordering this medication for nursing mothers), and review safety measures (assess for dizziness, use side rails, call for assistance when getting out of bed and ambulating, report to nurse any signs of adverse effects); ask if she has any questions.

Nursing Diagnoses Related to Drug Therapy: ***Knowledge Deficit*** related to lack of information regarding the drug therapy.
Risk for injury related to dizziness secondary to effect of drug.

PERCOSET (325 mg acetaminophen and 5 mg oxycodone)

Drug Class: Narcotic analgesic.

Dose/Route: 1–2 tablets PO every 4 hours PRN.

Indication: For moderate to moderately severe pain. Can be used in aspirin-sensitive women.

Adverse Effects: Acetaminophen: Hepatotoxicity, headache, rash, hypoglycemia. Oxycodone: Respiratory depression, apnea, circulatory depression, euphoria, facial flushing, constipation, suppression of cough reflex, ureteral spasm, urinary retention.

Nursing Implications: Determine whether woman is sensitive to acetaminophen or codeine; has bronchial asthma, respiratory depression, convulsive disorder.
Observe woman carefully for respiratory depression if given with barbiturates or sedative/hypnotics. Consider that postcesarean-birth woman may have depressed cough reflex, so teaching and encouragement to deep breathe and cough is needed.
Monitor bowel sounds, urine and bowel elimination.

Client Teaching: Teaching should include name of drug, expected effect, possible adverse effects, that drug is secreted in the breast milk, encouragement to report any signs of adverse effects immediately.

Nursing Diagnoses Related to Drug Therapy: ***Ineffective Breathing Pattern*** related to depression.
Constipation related to slowed gastrointestinal activity.

RUBELLA VIRUS VACCINE, LIVE (Meruvax 2)

Dose/Route: Single dose vial, inject subcutaneously in outer aspect of the upper arm.

Indication: Stimulate active immunity against rubella virus.

Adverse Effects: Burning or stinging at the injection site; about 2–4 weeks later may have rash, malaise, sore throat, or headache.

Nursing Implications: Determine whether woman has sensitivity to neomycin (vaccine contains neomycin); is immunosuppressed, or has received blood transfusions (not to be administered within 3 months of blood transfusion, plasma transfusion, or serum immune globulin).
Note: If a woman is to receive both RhoGAM and rubella, there is a possibility that the formation of antibodies to rubella may be suppressed by the RhoGAM injection. Most physicians will go ahead and order both injections and retest for maternal rubella immune status in about 3 months (Varney, 1997).

Client Teaching: Name of drug, expected effect, possible adverse effects, possible comfort measures to use if adverse effects occur; rubella titer will be assessed in about 3 months. Instruct woman to AVOID PREGNANCY FOR 3 MONTHS following vaccination. Provide information regarding contraceptives and their use.

Nursing Diagnoses Related to Drug Therapy: ***Knowledge Deficit*** regarding drug therapy. ***Knowledge Deficit*** regarding types and use of contraceptives.
Pain related to rash and malaise.

RhoGAM (Rh immune globulin specific for D antigen)

Dose/Route: Postpartum: One vial IM within 72 hours of birth. Antepartal: One vial microdose RhoGAM IM at 28 weeks in Rh negative women; after amniocentesis, spontaneous or therapeutic abortion, or ectopic pregnancy.

Indication: Prevention of sensitization to the Rh factor in Rh negative women and to prevent hemolytic disease in the newborn in subsequent pregnancies. Mother must be Rh negative, not previously sensitized to Rh factor. Infant must be Rh positive, direct antiglobulin negative.

Adverse Effects: Soreness at injection site.

Nursing Implications: Confirm criteria for administration are present. Assure correct vial is used for the client (each vial is cross-matched to the specific woman and must be carefully checked).
Inject entire contents of vial.

Client Teaching: Name of drug, expected action, possible side effects; report soreness at injection site to nurse; woman should carry information regarding Rh status and dates of RhoGAM injections with her at all times; explain use of RhoGAM with subsequent pregnancies.

Nursing Diagnoses Related to Drug Therapy: ***Knowledge Deficit*** related to the need for RhoGAM and future implications.
Pain related to soreness at injection site.

TABLE 31–3 *continued*

SECONAL SODIUM (secobarbital sodium)

Drug Class: Sedative, short-acting barbiturate.

Dose/Route: 100 mg PO at bedtime.

Indication: Promote sleep.

Adverse Effects: Somnolence, confusion, ataxia, vertigo, nightmares, hypoventilation, bradycardia, hypotension, nausea, vomiting, rashes.

Nursing Implications: Determine whether woman has sensitivity to barbiturates, or respiratory distress. Monitor respirations, blood pressure, pulse. Modify environment to increase relaxation and promote sleep.
Monitor for drug interaction if woman also is taking tranquilizers or TACE.

Client Teaching: Name of drug, expected effect, possible adverse effects, safety measures (siderails, use call bell, ask for assistance when out of bed); medication is secreted in breast milk.

Nursing Diagnoses Related to Drug Therapy: ***Risk for Injury*** related to possible ataxia or vertigo.
Altered Thought Processes related to drug-induced confusion.
Knowledge Deficit related to lack of information regarding drug therapy.

success helps the mother develop feelings of competence in caring for her baby.

The depression, weepiness, and "let down feeling" that characterize the postpartum blues are often a surprise for the new mother. She and her family may require reassurance that these feelings are normal and an explanation about why they occur. It is vital to provide a supportive environment that permits the mother to cry without feeling guilty.

I was amazed by how awkward I felt at first taking care of my new son. Nothing was easy—the day he was born he sprayed my mother-in-law when I took off his diaper and didn't know enough to cover him quickly. Now it is a family joke, but I remember feeling mortified—as though he had done it on purpose! I felt like a total incompetent and ended up in tears more than once. A wonderful student nurse helped me get through that early time. He taught me all kinds of little tricks and told funny stories about problems he had had with the babies. He helped me understand that my feelings of uncertainty were normal and gave me confidence that I could be the mother I wanted to be. I hope he knows what a difference he made.

Promotion of Effective Parent Teaching

Meeting the educational needs of the new mother and her family is one of the primary challenges facing the postpartum nurse. Each woman's educational needs vary according to age, background, experience, and expectations. However, because the mother spends only a brief period of time in the postpartal area, identifying and addressing individual instructional needs can be difficult. Effective education provides the childbearing family with sufficient knowledge to meet many of their own health needs and to seek assistance if necessary.

The nurse assesses the learning needs of the new mother through observation, sensitivity to nonverbal clues, and tactfully phrased questions. For example, "What plans have you made for handling things when you get home?" will elicit a more detailed response than, "Will someone be available to help you at home?" To assess learning needs, some agencies provide a client handout listing the most frequently identified areas of concern for new mothers. The mother checks those that apply to her or writes in concerns not included.

The nurse should plan and implement learning experiences in a logical, nonthreatening way based on knowledge of and respect for the family's cultural values and beliefs. For example, some Korean women look to their mother-in-law for information regarding all aspects of self-care and infant care (Schneiderman, 1996). The nurse needs to recognize this and honor the role the mother-in-law plays in the family. Unless there is a culturally-related activity the nurse believes would be harmful, most cultural customs can be supported and encouraged.

The educational method the nurse chooses varies. Agencies with many clients and limited staff may rely heavily on structured classes. Smaller units may provide individualized instruction through the use of one-on-one teaching or prepared videotapes. Some agencies use a television channel to show instructional videotapes at scheduled times during the day. Women should have pencil and paper to jot down questions that arise as they view the material. Afterward nurses need to be available to clarify material or answer any questions about the content. Because more effective learning occurs when there is sensory involvement and active participation, videotapes (sight and hearing) are more helpful than lecture (hearing only), and demonstration–return demonstration (sight, touch, hearing, and possibly smell and taste) is even more effective.

Timing is important in implementing educational activities. The new mother is more receptive to teaching after the first 24 to 48 hours, when she is ready to assume responsibility for her own care and that of her newborn (Lamp & Howard, 1999). However, many women are discharged in the early, dependent phase. Because of this, the nurse needs to provide whatever teaching the woman is ready for, with written handouts for future reference.

Research suggests that following discharge, many primiparas want additional information on self-care topics such as diet, exercise, nutrition, resuming normal activities, and feelings of fatigue. They also desire more information on baby care topics (Moran, Holt, & Martin,

1997). These needs may be addressed through home visits and postpartum educational programs.

Timing is also important for new fathers, who are more likely to attend sessions planned for them if they are scheduled in the evening after visiting hours. If material is planned for siblings, late afternoon teaching after school or naps might be most effective.

Teaching should not be limited to "how to" activities, however. Anticipatory guidance is essential in assisting the family to cope with role changes and the realities of a new baby. Small group discussions provide a chance for the new parents to talk about fears and expectations. Questions may arise about sexuality, contraception, child care, and even the grief associated with giving up the fantasized infant in order to accept the actual one.

Information is also essential for individuals with special educational needs—the mother who had a cesarean birth, the adolescent mother, the parents of an infant with congenital anomalies, and so on (Koniak-Griffin, Mathenge, Anderson, & Verzemnieks, 1999). They may feel overwhelmed, have difficult feelings to work through, and not even realize what it is they need to know. Nurses who are attuned to these individual problems can begin providing guidance as soon as possible.

Methods for evaluating learning vary according to the objectives and teaching methods. Return demonstrations, question-and-answer sessions, and even programmed instruction are opportunities for evaluating learning, as are formal evaluation tools.

Evaluation of attitudinal or less concrete learning is more difficult. For example, a mother's ability to express her frustrations over an unanticipated cesarean birth or a new mother's decision to delay for several weeks a family dinner originally scheduled for the first weekend after she arrives home may be the nurse's only clues that learning has occurred. Follow-up phone calls after discharge may provide additional evaluative information and continue the helping process as the nurse assesses the family's current educational needs and begins planning accordingly.

Promotion of Family Wellness

A satisfactory maternity experience may have a positive impact on the entire family. The new or expanding family that receives appropriate information and has adequate time to interact with its newest member in a supportive environment will feel more comfortable and secure at home.

In the past, newborns were typically separated from their parents immediately after birth. Today most facilities support family-centered care, which is focused on keeping the mother and baby together as much as the mother desires. **Mother-baby care,** or **couplet care** (care of both the mother and her baby), is an important part of the family-centered approach, in which the infant remains at the mother's bedside and both are cared for by the same nurse. Couplet care allows the nurse to teach and role model and to integrate the entire family into the care of the woman and her infant. It also enables the mother to have time to bond with her baby and learn to care for him or her in a supportive environment (Association of Women's Health, Obstetric, and Neonatal Nursing [AWHONN], 1998).

In a mother-baby unit, the newborn's crib is placed near the mother's bed, where she can see her baby easily. The crib should be a self-contained unit stocked with items the mother might require in providing care. A bulb syringe for suctioning the mouth or nares should always be accessible, and the mother and father/partner should be familiar with its use. The mother-baby unit is conducive to a self-demand feeding schedule for both breastfeeding and bottle-feeding infants.

Mothers are frequently very tired after birth, so the responsibility for providing total infant care could be overwhelming. The mother-baby policy must be flexible enough to permit the mother to return the baby to the nursery if she finds it necessary because of fatigue or physical discomfort. Some mother-baby units also return the newborns to a central nursery at night so the mothers can get more rest.

Many agencies have unlimited visiting hours for the father or significant others of the mother's choice. These opportunities to hold and care for the child promote paternal self-confidence and foster paternal attachment.

Reactions of Siblings

Sibling visitation helps meet the needs of both the siblings and their mother. A visit to the hospital reassures children that their mother is well and still loves them. It also provides an opportunity for the children to become familiar with the new baby. For the mother, the pangs of separation are lessened as she interacts with her children and introduces them to the newest family member.

Most agencies now recognize the importance of providing siblings with opportunities to see their mother and meet the infant during the early postpartal period (Figure 31–2). Approaches to this issue vary from specified visiting hours for siblings to unlimited visiting privileges.

Teaching for Self-Care Although the parents have prepared the child for the presence of a new brother or sister, the actual arrival of the infant requires some adjustments. If the woman gives birth in a birthing center, her children may be present for the birth. They then have an opportunity to spend time with their new sibling and their parents. They may even remain throughout the woman's hospitalization, especially if it is brief, and all go home as a family.

For the mother who is returning home to small children, it is often helpful to have the father carry the new baby inside. This practice keeps the mother's arms free to hug and hold her older children. She thereby reaffirms her love for them before introducing them to their new sibling. Many mothers have found that bringing a doll home with them for the older child is helpful. The child cares for the doll alongside his or her parents, thereby identifying with the parent. This identification helps decrease anger and the need to regress to get attention.

Often older children enjoy working with the parents to care for the newborn. Involvement in care helps the older child develop a sense of closeness to the baby. It also helps the child learn acceptable behavior toward the newborn, feel a sense of accomplishment, and develop tenderness and caring. With constant supervision and assistance as necessary, even very young children can hold the baby or a bottle during feeding. Breastfeeding mothers may allow siblings to help give the new infant an occasional bottle of water.

Regression is a common occurrence even when siblings have been well prepared. The nurse can provide anticipatory guidance so that parents do not become overly upset if their previously toilet-trained child begins to have accidents or requests a bottle.

Regardless of age, an older sibling needs reassurance that he or she is still special to the parents, a truly loved and valued family member. Words of love and praise coupled with hugs and kisses are very important. So, too, is special parent-child time. Both parents should spend quality time in a one-to-one experience with each of their older children. This may require some careful planning, but its worth cannot be overestimated. It confirms the parents' love for the child and often helps the child accept the new baby.

The child, especially one of the opposite sex from the newborn, may raise queries about the appearance of the genitals as compared to his or her own. A simple explanation, such as, "That's what little girls (boys) look like," is often sufficient.

Resumption of Sexual Activity

Nursing interventions in the postpartal period acknowledge that the parent is also a sexual being. Couples were formerly discouraged from engaging in sexual intercourse until 6 weeks postpartum. Currently, the couple is advised to abstain from intercourse until the episiotomy is healed and the lochial flow has stopped (usually by the end of the third week). During this period, couples can be encouraged to express their affection and love through kissing, holding, and talking. Because the vaginal vault is still "dry" (hormone-poor), some form of lubrication, such as K-Y jelly, may be necessary initially during intercourse. The female-superior or side-by-side positions for coitus may be preferable because they enable the woman to control the depth of penile penetration.

Breastfeeding couples should be forewarned that during orgasm, milk may spout from the nipples because of the release of oxytocin. Some couples find this pleasurable or amusing; other couples choose to have the woman wear a bra during sexual activity. Nursing the baby prior to lovemaking may reduce the chance of milk release.

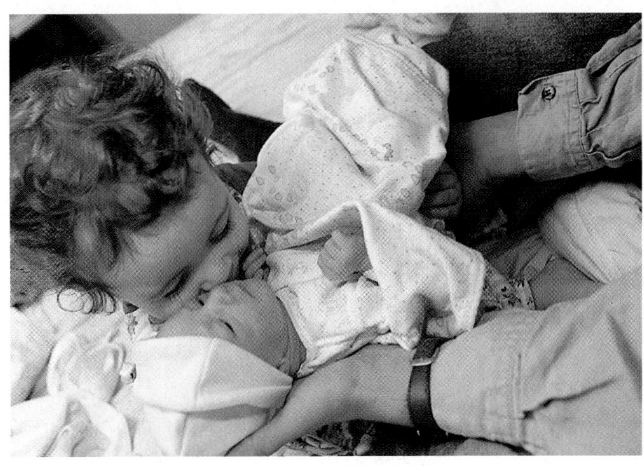

FIGURE 31–2 The sister of this newborn becomes acquainted with the new family member while the nurse performs a nursing assessment.

Other factors may inhibit satisfactory sexual experience. The baby's crying may "spoil the mood"; the woman's changed body may be unattractive to her or to her partner; and maternal sleep deprivation may interfere with a mutually satisfying experience. Couples may also be frustrated if there is decreased libido or other changes in the woman's physiologic response to sexual stimulation. These changes are due to hormonal changes and may persist for several months.

Maternal fatigue is often a significant factor limiting the resumption of sexual intercourse. Consequently, couples should be encouraged to find a time for lovemaking when both are interested and awake. By 3 months postpartum, sexual interest and activity are generally regular in frequency. However, a return to prepregnant levels of sexual activity varies by couple and may take from a few weeks to a year after childbirth to occur (Alteneder & Hartzell, 1997).

Anticipatory guidance during the prenatal and postnatal periods can forewarn the couple of these eventualities and of their temporary nature. See Teaching Guide: Resuming Sexual Activity after Childbirth.

Contraception

Because many couples resume sexual activity before the postpartal examination, family-planning information should be made available before discharge. A couple's decision to use a contraceptive is often motivated by a desire to gain control over the number of children they will conceive or to determine the spacing of future children. In choosing a specific method, consistency of use outweighs the absolute reliability of a given method. The nurse must identify risk factors and contraindications of the various methods to help the couple select a contraceptive method that has practical application and is compatible with the couple's health and physical needs.

TEACHING GUIDE: RESUMING SEXUAL ACTIVITY AFTER CHILDBIRTH

Assessment Recognize that couples, especially if they have become parents for the first time, may have questions about resuming sexual activity. Although the woman may initiate this discussion, you can often best assess the woman's (and her partner's) understanding by providing general information followed by some tactful questions.

Nursing Diagnosis The key nursing diagnosis will probably be ***Knowledge Deficit*** related to lack of information about changes in sexual activity that commonly occur postpartally.

Nursing Plan and Implementation First establish rapport with the couple and promote an environment that is conducive to teaching and discussion. It is helpful to provide privacy during the session so that the couple feels free to ask questions without fear of interruption. The format is generally a question-and-answer or discussion approach.

Client Goals At the completion of teaching, the couple will be able to:

- Discuss the changes in the woman's body that affect sexual activity.
- Formulate alternative approaches to sexual activity based on an understanding of these changes.
- Identify the length of time it is advisable to wait before resuming sexual activity.
- Discuss information needed to make contraceptive choices.

Teaching Plan

Content	*Teaching Method*
• Present information about changes that may affect sexual activity, including the following: • Tenderness of the vagina and perineum • Presence of lochia and the healing process • Dryness of the vagina • Breast engorgement and tenderness • Escape of milk during sexual activity	*Discussion is a logical approach. It may be useful to make a universal statement and link it with a question to determine a couple's initial level of knowledge. For example, "Many women experience vaginal dryness when they resume intercourse for the first several weeks after childbirth. Are you familiar with this change and the cause for it?" Use the information gained during this discussion to determine the depth to which to cover the material.*
• Discuss healing at the placental site and stress that the presence of lochia indicates that healing is not yet complete. Point out that because the vagina is "hormone-poor" postpartally, vaginal dryness may pose a problem. This can be avoided by using a water-soluble lubricant. Explain that escape of milk during sexual activity can be minimized by nursing the baby immediately beforehand.	*Provide printed information to clarify content and serve as a resource for the couple following discharge. See the Self-Care Guide, "Guidelines for Resuming Sexual Activity after Childbirth," in the perforated section at the end of the book.*
• Discuss the importance of contraception during the early postpartal period. Provide information on the advantages and disadvantages of different methods. The woman's body needs adequate time to heal and recover from the stress of pregnancy and childbirth. Couples who are opposed to contraception may choose abstinence at this time.	*Provide samples of different types of contraceptives.* *Provide literature on specific contraceptive methods. See the Self-Care Guide, "Summary of Contraceptive Methods," in the perforated section at the end of the book.*
• Discuss the impact of fatigue and the new baby's schedule on the woman's feelings of desire. Refer the couple to a physician or certified nurse-midwife for additional information if needed.	*Many couples are unprepared for the impact of fatigue and the baby's schedule on lovemaking. Information enables the couple to anticipate this impact.*

Evaluation Determine the couple's learning by providing time for discussion and questions. If the couple indicates that they plan to use a particular contraceptive method, you may ask them about aspects of the method to ascertain that they have correct and complete information.

TABLE 31–4 Parent Attachment Behaviors

Assessment Area	Attachment	Behavior Requiring Assessment and Information
Caretaking	Talks with baby. Demonstrates and seeks eye-to-eye contact. Touches and holds baby. Changes diapers when needed. Baby is clean. Clothing is appropriate for room temperature. Feeds baby as needed and baby is gaining weight. Positions baby comfortably and checks on baby.	Does not refer to baby. Completes activities without addressing the baby or looking at the baby. Lack of interaction. Does not recognize need for or demonstrate concern for baby's comfort or needs. Feeding occurs intermittently. Baby does not gain weight. Waits for baby to cry and then hesitates to respond.
Perception of the baby	Has knowledge of expected child development. Understands that the baby is dependent and cannot meet parent's needs. Accepts sex of child and characteristics.	Has unrealistic expectations of the baby's abilities and behaviors. Expects love and interaction from the baby. Believes that the baby will fulfill parent's needs. Is strongly distressed over sex of baby or feels that some aspect of the baby is unacceptable.
Support	Has friends who are available for support. Seems to be comfortable with being a parent. Has realistic beliefs of parenting role.	Is alone or isolated. Is on edge, tense, anxious, and hesitant with the baby. Demonstrates difficulty incorporating parenting with own wants and needs.

Please note: These are a few of the behaviors that may be associated with attachment. It is vitally important for the nurse to observe the parents on more than one occasion and to take into consideration individual characteristics, values, beliefs, and customs.

Often different methods of contraception are appropriate at different times in the couple's life. Thus they should have a clear understanding of all of the methods available to them so that they can make an appropriate choice. The currently available contraceptive methods are discussed in detail in Chapter 3.

Promotion of Parent-Infant Attachment

Nursing interventions to enhance the quality of parent-infant attachment should be designed to promote feelings of well-being, comfort, and satisfaction. Table 31–4 describes parental attachment behaviors and those that require further assessment. Following are some suggestions for ways of achieving this.

- Determine the childbearing and childrearing goals of the infant's mother and father, and adapt them wherever possible in planning nursing care for the family. This includes giving the parents choices about their labor and birth experience and their initial time with their new infant.
- Postpone eye prophylaxis for 1 hour after birth to facilitate eye contact between parents and their newborn (eye ointment further clouds the newborn's vision and makes eye contact difficult for the baby).
- Provide time in the first hour after birth for the new family to become acquainted, with as much privacy as possible.
- Arrange the health care setting so that the individual nurse-client relationship can be developed and maintained. A primary nurse can develop rapport and assess the mother's strengths and needs.
- Encourage the parents to involve the siblings in integrating the infant into the family by bringing them to the birthing center for sibling visits.
- Use anticipatory guidance from conception through the postpartal period to prepare the parents for expected problems of adjustment.
- Include parents in any nursing intervention, planning, and evaluation. Give choices whenever possible.
- Initiate and support measures to alleviate fatigue in the parents.
- Help parents identify, understand, and accept both positive and negative feelings related to the overall parenting experience.
- Support and assist parents in determining the personality and unique needs of their infant.

Whenever possible, the mother should be allowed to care for her baby. This practice gives the mother a chance to learn her newborn's normal patterns and develop confidence in caring for him or her. It also allows the father more uninterrupted time with his infant in the first days of life. If mother and baby are doing well, help is available for the mother at home and the family and certified nurse-midwife/physician agree, early discharge may be advantageous.

The nurse may observe beginnings of parent-newborn attachment in the first few hours after birth, continuing assessments in home visits after discharge. As the nurse assesses attachment, it is important to remember that cultural values, beliefs, and practices will direct child-care activities and self-care practices. For example, some Mexican American women treat the umbilical stump by placing a coin or belly band over it. Some Mexican American women and Hmong women may not want the baby to receive compliments or any attention, because they believe that this may bring on unwanted attention of bad spirits (AWHONN, 1998; Fadiman, 1997).

RESEARCH IN PRACTICE

What is this study about? Although a woman may achieve physiologic recovery within 6 weeks postpartum her return to functional status may take considerably longer. In Australia, Carol McVeigh designed a prospective longitudinal study to examine the changes in functional status from 6 weeks to 6 months after delivery.

How was the study done? The investigator recruited a random sample of 200 culturally diverse women to participate in the study. Selection criteria included normal pregnancy and delivery, 20 to 35 years of age, and a healthy newborn born between 37 and 42 weeks gestation. Data were collected at 6 weeks, 3 months, and 6 months postpartum. Study tools, mailed to the participants, included printed information and questionnaires about maternal-infant attributes and about functional status. Functional status was evaluated through the use of the Inventory of Functional Status After Childbirth (IFSAC) which includes subscales for infant care, self-care, household activities, social and community activities, and occupational activities.

What were the results of the study? Of the original sample of 200 women, 173 returned data at 6 weeks, 154 at 3 months, and 142 completed all three surveys. At 6 weeks the respondents reported the highest mean score in infant care (3.79 of a possible 4) or that they had achieved the higher level of functional status in this area. The lowest mean score for this time period was in social activities (2.79). The means for both household responsibilities and social activities increased significantly from 6 weeks to 3 months ($p = 0.0001$) and again between 3 months and 6 months ($p = 0.02$). Functional status in the area of self-care increased significantly from 6 weeks to 3 months ($p = 0.0001$) but not from 3 to 6 months. The IFSAC grand mean increased significantly from 3 to 6 months ($p = 0.02$) but not for the first measurement period. None of the Australian women reported returning to full functional status within 6 months in all areas. In the highest subscale area of infant care only 64% felt they had achieved full functional status, and in the area of self-care only 0.7% related return to a fully functional status.

What additional questions might I have? Although the author describes the sample as culturally diverse, very little description is given related to racial or ethnic characteristics. How was the author defining culturally diverse?

How can I use this study? As noted by the author, in order to design individualized care, nurses should ask the new mother how she feels about the changes that have occurred since childbirth. Also the nurses can help new mothers have more realistic goals by sharing the results of studies such as this one which demonstrate a much longer period than 6 weeks for the achievement of full functional status.

SOURCE: McVeigh, C. (1998). Functional status after childbirth in an Australian sample. *JOGNN, 27*(4), 402–409.

Nursing Care Management after Cesarean Birth

After a cesarean birth, the new mother has postpartal needs similar to those of women who gave birth vaginally. Because she has undergone major abdominal surgery, however, the woman who has had a cesarean also has nursing care needs similar to those of other surgical clients.

Promotion of Maternal Physical Well-Being

Immobility after the use of narcotic and sedative agents and alterations in the immune response of postoperative clients increase the chances of pulmonary infection. For this reason, the woman is encouraged to cough and deep breathe and to use incentive spirometry every 2 to 4 hours while awake for the first few days following cesarean birth.

The nurse continues to assess the woman's pain level and provide relief measures as needed. Sources of pain include incisional pain, gas pain, referred shoulder pain, periodic uterine contractions (afterbirth pains), and pain from voiding, defecation, or constipation.

Nursing interventions are oriented toward preventing or alleviating pain or helping the woman cope with pain. The nurse should undertake the following measures:

- Administer analgesic medications as needed, especially during the first 24 to 72 hours. Their use will relieve the woman's pain and enable her to be more mobile and active.
- Promote comfort through proper positioning, back rubs, oral care, and the reduction of noxious stimuli, such as noise and unpleasant odors.
- Encourage the presence of significant others, including the newborn. This provides distraction from the painful sensations and helps reduce the woman's fear and anxiety.
- Encourage the use of breathing, relaxation, and distraction techniques (for example, stimulation of cutaneous tissue) taught in childbirth preparation class.

Epidural analgesia administered just after the cesarean birth is an effective method of pain relief for most women in the first 24 hours following birth (see Drug Guide: Postpartum Epidural Morphine).

The physician may prescribe **patient-controlled analgesia (PCA).** With this approach, the woman is given a bolus of analgesia, usually morphine or meperidine, at the beginning of therapy. Using a special IV pump system, the woman presses a button to self-administer small doses of the medication as needed. For safety, the pump is preset with a time lockout so that the pump

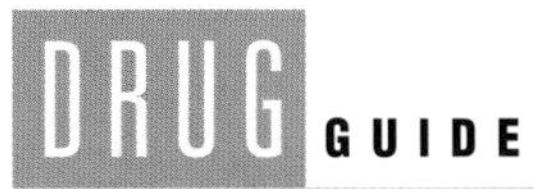

Postpartum Epidural Morphine

Overview of Obstetric Action

Epidural morphine is used to provide relief of pain associated with cesarean birth, extensive episiotomies (mediolaterals), or third- and fourth-degree lacerations. Epidural morphine pain relief results directly from its effect on the opiate receptors in the spinal cord (it depresses pain impulse transmission). Morphine binds opiate receptors, thereby altering both the perception of and emotional response to pain. Women experience little or no discomfort or pain during recovery and for up to 24 hours afterward. There is no motor or sympathetic block or associated hypotension. Onset of analgesia is slower, but duration is longer.

Route, Dosage, and Frequency

Five to seven and one-half mg of morphine is injected through a catheter into the epidural space, providing pain relief for about 24 hours (Datta, 1995).

Maternal Contraindications

Allergy to morphine, narcotic addition, chronic debilitating respiratory disease, infection at the injection site, or administration of parenteral corticosteriods in past 14 days (PDR Nurse's Handbook, 1999).

Maternal Side Effects

Late-onset respiratory depression (rare but may occur 8–12 hours after administration), nausea and vomiting (occurring between 4 and 7 hours after injection), itching (begins within 3 hours and lasts up to 10 hours), urinary retention, and, rarely, somnolence. Side effects can be managed with naloxone.

Neonatal Effects

No adverse effects since medication is injected after birth of baby.

Nursing Considerations

- Obtain history: sensitivity (allergy) to morphine, presence of any contraindications (PDR Nurse's Handbook, 1999).
- Assess orientation, reflexes, skin color, texture, breath sounds, presence of lesions or infection over area of lumbar spine, voiding pattern, urinary output within normal limits (Karch, 1999).
- Monitor and evaluate analgesic effect. Ask client about comfort level and notify anesthesiologist of inadequate pain relief.
- Check catheter for obvious knots, breaks, and leakage at insertion site and catheter hub.
- Assess for pruritus (scratching and rubbing, especially around face and neck).
- Administer comfort measures for narcotic-induced pruritus, such as: lotion, back rubs, cool/warm packs, or diversional activities. If the itching can be tolerated, naloxone should be avoided, especially since it counteracts the pain relief.
- If allergic reaction (urticaria, edema, or respiratory difficulties) occurs, administer naloxone or diphenhydramine per physician order.
- Provide comfort measures for nausea/vomiting, such as frequent oral hygiene or gradual increase of activity; administer naloxone, trimethobenzamide (Tigan), or metoclopramide HCl per physician order.
- Assess postural blood pressure and heart rate before ambulation.
- Assist client with her first ambulation and then as needed.
- Assess respiratory function every hour for 24 hours, then q2–8 hrs as needed. Also assess level of consciousness and mucous membrane color. May need to monitor client via apnea monitor for 24 hours.
- Monitor urinary output and assess bladder for distention. Assist client to void.

cannot deliver another dose until a specified time has elapsed. Women using PCA feel less anxious and have a greater sense of control with less dependence on the nursing staff. The frequent smaller doses help the woman experience rapid pain relief without grogginess and also eleminates the discomfort of injections.

CRITICAL THINKING QUESTION

The postpartal woman you are caring for is on a PCA pump. She tells you she cannot let herself fall asleep because she wakes up in terrible pain and it takes an hour for the pain medication to catch up. What is happening? What will you do?

If general anesthesia was used, abdominal distention from the accumulation of gas in the intestines may produce discomfort for the woman during the first postpartal days. Measures to prevent or minimize gas pains include leg exercises, abdominal tightening, ambulation, avoiding carbonated or very hot or cold beverages, avoiding the use of straws, and providing a high-protein liquid diet for the first 24 to 48 hours until bowel sounds return. The woman may find it helpful to lie prone or on her left side. Lying on the left side allows gas to rise from the descending colon to the sigmoid colon so that it can be expelled more readily. Other women report that a rocking chair helps them obtain relief. Medical interventions for gas pain include the use of antiflatulents (such as Mylicon), suppositories, and enemas.

The nurse can minimize discomfort and promote satisfaction as the mother assumes the activities of her new role. Instruction and assistance in assuming comfortable positions when holding or breastfeeding the infant will do much to increase the mother's sense of competence and comfort. Sitting in a chair or tailor fashion in bed, leaning slightly forward with the infant propped on a pillow in her lap, will prevent irritation to the incision. Another preferred position for breastfeeding during the first postoperative days is lying on the side with the newborn positioned along the mother's body.

By the first or second day after the cesarean birth, the mother is usually receptive to learning how to care for herself and her infant. Demonstration of proper body mechanics in getting out of bed without the use of a side rail and ways of caring for the infant that prevent strain and torsion on the incision are also indicated. The nurse needs to place special emphasis on home management, encouraging the woman to let others assume responsibility for housekeeping and cooking. Fatigue not only prolongs recovery but also interferes with breastfeeding and mother-infant interaction.

The woman usually does extremely well postoperatively. If spinal anesthesia was used, the side effects of general anesthesia are absent. Even after general anesthesia, however, most women are ambulating by the day after the surgery. Usually by the second postpartal day, the incision can be covered with plastic wrap so the woman can shower, which seems to provide a mental as well as physical lift. If staples have been used, the incision is sometimes left open to the air, and showering is permitted without covering it. Most women are discharged on the third postoperative day.

Research suggests that women with cesarean births have several special needs following discharge: increased need for rest and sleep; incisional care; assistance with household chores, infant care, and self-care; and relief of pain and discomfort. In addition, women with planned cesarean births expressed a need for socialization or help with depression and improved family closeness (Eakes & Brown, 1998). Nurses need to address these areas during hospitalization and discharge planning. Perhaps one of the most important considerations for cesarean birth mothers is the need to plan for additional assistance at home to enable the new mother to rest and heal.

Promotion of Parent-Infant Interaction after Cesarean Birth

Many factors associated with cesarean birth may hinder successful and frequent maternal-infant interaction. These include the physical condition of the mother and newborn and maternal reactions to stress, anesthesia, and medications. The mother and her infant may be separated after birth because of hospital routines, prematurity, or neonatal complications. A healthy infant born by an uncomplicated cesarean birth is no more fragile than an infant born vaginally. Many agencies are beginning to provide time for the family together in the operating room if the mother's and infant's conditions permit, but some agencies still automatically place cesarean birth newborns in a high-risk nursery for a time.

Signs of depression, anger, or withdrawal in the cesarean birth mother may indicate a grief response to the loss of the fantasized vaginal birth experience. Fathers as well as mothers may experience feelings of "missing out," guilt that the surgery was the result of something they did "wrong," and even jealousy toward another couple who had a vaginal birth. The cesarean birth couple may also feel guilty that they are considering their personal needs and not simply the welfare of the infant.

The nurse can support the parents in a variety of ways. Initially, nurses must work through their own feelings about cesarean birth. The nurse who considers a vaginal birth "normal" and refers to it as such indicates that a cesarean birth is "abnormal," rather than simply an alternative method. Thus language and terminology, though seemingly insignificant, can convey to the couple negative messages about their cesarean birth experience.

The nurse should offer positive support to the couple. The cesarean birth couple may need the opportunity to tell their story repeatedly to work through their feelings. The nurse can provide factual information about their situation and support the couple's effective coping behaviors. The nurse should provide the parents with choices by allowing them to participate in decision making about the options available to them.

The presence of the father or significant other during the birth process positively influences the woman's perception of the birth event. His or her presence not only reduces the woman's fears but also enhances her sense of control and enables the couple to share feelings and respond to one another with touch and eye contact. Later they have the opportunity to relive the experience and fill in any gaps or missing pieces. This is especially valuable if the mother has had general anesthesia. The father or significant other can take pictures, hold the baby, and foster the discovery process by directing the mother's attention to details about her newborn.

The perception of and reactions to a cesarean birth experience depend on how the woman defines that experience. Her reality is what she perceives it to be. If the woman's attitude is more positive than negative, successful resolution of subsequent stressful events is more likely. Because the definition of events is transitory in nature, the possibility of change and growth is present. Often the mothering role is perceived as an extension of the childbearing role, and inability to fulfill expected childbearing behavior (vaginal birth) may lead to parental feelings of role failure and frustration. The nurse can help families alter their negative definitions of cesarean birth and bolster and encourage positive perceptions.

COMMUNITY IN FOCUS

Tot and Teen Clinic: Shreveport, Louisiana

Until the mid-1980s, follow-up care for adolescent mothers and their children was only available through the parish (Louisiana equivalent of a county) public health unit. This approach was not as successful as desired because it involved a great deal more time for these young mothers, who had to have separate appointments for themselves and their children. To address the problem and ensure greater continuity of care, two pediatricians established the Tot and Teen Clinic in 1986 at the Louisiana State University Medical Center (LSUMC) in Shreveport.

In 1989 the Tot and Teen Clinic obtained formal funding through a grant awarded by the Louisiana Maternal Child Health Department. The grant provided funding for a full-time nurse, social worker, and clerical person. The pediatric nurse practitioners and pediatricians who provided direct patient care were on the faculty at LSUMC and their salaries were provided by that organization.

The program has several goals: (1) to promote regular prenatal care and thereby help ensure the birth of a healthy baby; (2) to provide well-baby immunizations; (3) to role model effective child care skills and provide information about good parenting; (4) to provide primary medical care for the mother and baby; (5) to offer family planning options and thereby prevent another pregnancy; and (6) to promote physical, mental, and social development in the baby. In addition to the primary care and educational benefits the clinic provides, young mothers who are eligible can also receive WIC vouchers there.

To use the Tot and Teen Clinic, the mother must be 17 years of age or under at the time of childbirth and she must reside in Shreveport or its sister city, Bossier City. The mother may stay in the program until she is 20 years of age or her child is 5 years of age. According to Yvonne Mitchell, RN, MS, one of the two nurse coordinators of the clinic, the goal is to provide a "one stop" approach to health care for the teen mother and child. Prospective clients are located during their pregnancy by the nurse practitioners and physicians of the OB department or by the Tot and Teen nurses while they are in the hospital following the birth of the baby.

The children are evaluated using the DDST II. Language delays are the most prevalent problem detected. To address this problem, the clinic has added a new offering—the federally funded, "Reach Out and Read" program. This program encourages parents to read to children by having people "role model" (read) to the children in the waiting room. In addition the nurse practitioner or primary care physician provides a book to the child following the visit. This program is designed for children from 6 months until 5 years of age.

Currently about 350 new mothers make use of the clinic services each year. The Tot and Teen Clinic is a wonderful example of a long-lasting program that is meeting a major community need.

SOURCE: Information provided by Lisa A. Smith-Pedersen, RN, MSN, faculty member, Northwestern State University of Louisiana and Yvonne Mitchell, RN, MS, Clinic Coordinator.

Nursing Care Management of the Postpartal Adolescent

Over half the teens who become pregnant give birth and keep their babies. Very few adolescents give up their babies for adoption (National Campaign to Prevent Teen Pregnancy, 1997). Consequently, the adolescent mother's ability to relate to her infant is important. Earlier studies demonstrated that teenage mothers interact less positively with their babies than older mothers do. However, recent research suggests that this is related more to lower levels of maternal education than to age (Diehl, 1997) and to the amount of support an adolescent receives in the prenatal period (Koniak-Griffin et al, 1999).

During the postpartal period, the adolescent may have special needs, depending on her level of maturity, support systems, and cultural background. The nurse should assess maternal-infant interaction, roles of support people, plans for discharge, knowledge of childrearing, and plans for follow-up care. It is imperative to have a community health service be in touch with the young woman shortly after discharge.

Contraception counseling is an important part of teaching. Often the young woman tells the nurse that she does not plan on engaging in sex again. This denial mechanism is unrealistic, and the nurse must help the young woman realize this. The nurse should make sure that the woman has some method of birth control available to her and that she understands ovulation and fertility in relation to her menstrual cycle. This is an excellent opportunity for sex education.

The nurse has many opportunities for teaching the adolescent about the newborn in the postpartal unit. Because the nurse serves as a role model, the manner in which she handles the baby greatly influences the young mother. The father should be included in as much of the teaching as possible.

A newborn physical examination performed at the bedside gives the adolescent immediate feedback about the newborn's health and shows her methods of handling an infant. The nurse can teach as the examination progresses, giving the new mother information about the fontanelles, cradle cap, shampooing the newborn's hair, and so on. The nurse might also use this time to teach the young mother about infant stimulation techniques. Because adolescent mothers tend to concentrate their interactions in the physical domain, they need to comprehend the importance of verbal, visual, and auditory stimulation for newborns as well.

Performing an examination at the bedside also gives the adolescent permission to explore her baby, which she may have been hesitant to do. A Brazelton neonatal assessment (Chapter 26) will help the mother understand the newborn's response to stimuli, a key factor in the adolescent's response to the individuality of her newborn once she goes home. Parents who have some idea of what to expect from their infants will be less frustrated with the newborn's behavior.

The adolescent mother appreciates positive feedback about her fine newborn and her developing maternal responses. This praise and encouragement will increase her confidence and self-esteem.

Group classes for adolescent mothers should include infant care skills, information about growth and development, infant feeding, well-baby care, and danger signals in the ill newborn. If classes are offered in the hospital during the postpartum stay, the adolescent mother should be strongly encouraged to attend. If the child's father is involved, he should also be encouraged to attend and participate. The nurse can correct misconceptions and unrealistic expectations about growth and development. The nurse should also make a thorough assessment of the support systems and resources already in place for the mother and additional resources from the hospital or the community that may be appropriate for the situation.

Ideally, teenage mothers should visit adolescent clinics where mother and baby are assessed for several years after birth. In this way, classes on parenting, vocational guidance, and school attendance can be followed closely. School systems' classes for young mothers are an excellent way of helping adolescents finish school and learn how to parent at the same time.

Nursing Care Management for the Woman with an Unwanted Pregnancy

Sometimes a pregnancy is unwanted. The woman may be single, an adolescent, or economically restricted, or the pregnancy may be the result of incest or rape. She may dislike children or the idea of being a mother. She may feel that she is not emotionally ready for the responsibilities of parenthood. Her partner may disapprove of the pregnancy. These and many other reasons may cause the woman to continue to reject the idea of her pregnancy. An emotional crisis arises as she attempts to resolve the problem. She may choose to have an abortion, to carry the fetus to term and keep the baby, or to have the baby and relinquish it for adoption. Regardless of her decision, she needs nonjudgmental, supportive nursing care. The nurse can ensure that she has opportunities to discuss her feelings and carefully consider the decisions she must make.

In the event that a woman decides to keep an unwanted child, the nurse should be aware of the potential for parenting problems. Families with unwanted children are more prone to crisis than others, although in many cases parents grow to love their child after attachment occurs. The nurse should be ready to initiate crisis management strategies or make appropriate referrals as the need arises.

Denial of Pregnancy

Initial denial of pregnancy by women usually progresses to acceptance of the pregnant state. Occasionally, however, a nurse may encounter a woman who denies she is pregnant even as she is admitted to the maternity unit. This may be an unconscious reaction to an unwanted pregnancy. It may seem impossible to the nurse that a woman who is so obviously pregnant could maintain this delusion. Because of this denial, the woman has not sought prenatal care. Preparation for the birth experience may be incomplete, and the mother and infant may be at risk.

The nurse must establish a trusting relationship with this woman. While building rapport with the woman, the nurse should gently guide her to accept reality. If the woman remains in denial, a psychiatric referral may be indicated.

Nursing Care Management for the Woman Who Relinquishes Her Infant

Often mothers who choose to give their infants up for adoption are young, unmarried, or both. A mother's decision to relinquish her infant is an extremely difficult one, especially because there are social pressures against giving up one's child even though relinquishment may be in the child's best interest.

The mother who chooses to let her child be adopted often experiences intense ambivalence about her decision. She usually has made considerable adjustments in her lifestyle to give birth to this child. She may not have told friends and relatives about the pregnancy and so lacks an extended support system. During the prenatal period, the nurse can help her by encouraging her to express her grief, loneliness, guilt, and other feelings. It is often helpful to encourage the mother to visit the hospital prior to birth. She may be given a tour of the birthing area as well as the postpartum area.

When the relinquishing mother is admitted to the birthing unit, the staff should be informed about the mother's decision to relinquish the infant. Any special requests regarding the birth should be respected, and the woman should be encouraged to express her emotions.

Her feelings of ambivalence may heighten just before birth. If the woman is accompanied by family members or a significant other, the nurse provides support to them throughout the labor and birth. If no support person is present, the nurse acts as the primary support person and ensures that the woman has a clear understanding of all that occurs.

After the birth, the mother should be able to decide whether she wants to see the newborn. Seeing the newborn often facilitates the grieving process. When the mother sees her baby, she may feel strong attachment and love, and her ambivalence may be especially pronounced. The nurse needs to assure the woman that these feelings do not mean that her decision to relinquish the child is a wrong one; relinquishment is often a painful act of love (Arms, 1990).

The well-being of the baby is one of the relinquishing mother's greatest concerns, and research indicates that relinquishing mothers often report great feelings of pride, satisfaction, and relief when they give birth to a healthy child. This heightened response may be a reflection of the compressed time period during which the woman is able to demonstrate maternal behaviors (Keen-Payne & Bond, 1997).

After the birth, relinquishing mothers frequently feel tremendous fatigue. Consequently they may focus on pain relief, rest, and sleep. They often feel both excitement and anxiety about returning home and adjusting to life following pregnancy. Thus postpartum is a time of both physical and emotional recovery (Keen-Payne & Bond, 1997). During the postpartum period, the mother needs to complete a grieving process to work through her loss.

Discharge Information

The postpartum stay allowed by most third-party payors has decreased dramatically in recent years. Hospital stays that were measured in weeks in the 1940s are now measured in hours. Postpartum nursing care that has traditionally included a strong focus on the adjustments of the mother, newborn, and family is very difficult to accomplish because of the brief length of stay. Mothers and newborns are being discharged before many of their important postbirth health care needs can be addressed. These include establishing breastfeeding, ruling out infections, supporting infant-family bonding, and client teaching. Home health services are increasingly being recognized as a cost-effective means of meeting the postbirth needs of mothers and newborns.

Ideally, preparation for discharge begins the moment a woman enters the birthing unit to give birth. Nursing efforts should be directed toward assessing the couple's knowledge, expectations, and beliefs and then providing anticipatory guidance and teaching accordingly (Table 31–5). Because teaching is one of the primary responsibilities of the postpartum nurse, many agencies have elaborate teaching programs and classes. Before the actual discharge, however, the nurse should spend time with the couple to determine whether they have any last-minute questions. In general, discharge teaching should include at least the following.

1. The woman should contact her caregiver if she develops any of the signs of possible complications:
   a. Sudden persistent or spiking fever
   b. Change in the character of the lochia—foul smell, return to bright red bleeding, excessive amount
   c. Evidence of mastitis, such as breast tenderness, reddened areas, malaise
   d. Evidence of thrombophlebitis, such as calf pain, tenderness, redness
   e. Evidence of urinary tract infection, such as urgency, frequency, burning on urination
   f. Evidence of infection in an incision (either episiotomy or cesarean), such as redness, edema, bruising, discharge, or lack of approximation
   g. Continued severe or incapacitating postpartal depression
2. The woman should review the literature she has received that explains recommended postpartum exercises, the need for adequate rest, the need to avoid overexertion initially, and the recommendation to abstain from sexual intercourse until lochia has ceased. The woman may take a shower and may continue sitz baths at home if she desires.
3. The woman should be given the phone numbers of the postpartum unit and nursery and be encouraged to call if she has any questions, no matter how simple.
4. The woman should receive information on local agencies or support groups, such as La Leche League and Mothers of Twins, that might be of particular assistance to her.
5. Both breastfeeding and bottle-feeding mothers should receive information geared to their specific nutritional needs. They should also be told to continue their vitamin and iron supplements until their postpartal examination.
6. The woman should have a scheduled appointment for her postpartal examination and for her infant's first well-baby examination before they are discharged.
7. The mother should clearly understand the correct procedure for obtaining copies of her infant's birth certificate.
8. The new parents should be able to provide home care for their infants and should know when to

Text continues on page 958.

TABLE 31–5 Areas to Include in Postpartal Teaching

Knowledge and Skills To Be Taught	Teaching Method: Video	Verbal Only	Verbally Reinforced	Demonstration
Care of the Mother				
Breast care Breast feeding or lactation suppression				
Possible problems and care				
Involutional changes Position of fundus				
Aftercontractions				
Changes in lochia				
Signs of possible problems				
Bladder function Fluid needs				
Signs of possible problems				
Bowel function Normal patterns				
Dietary assistance				
Perineal care Expected healing changes in episiotomy				
Comfort measures (rinsing with warm water, use of analgesic/anesthetic spray, sitz bath), home care				
Signs of possible problems				
Rest and activity Scheduling rest periods, handling fatigue				
Ambulation				
Watching for circulatory problems in legs				
Emotional changes Changes in mood, crying, depression				
Care of the Father/Partner				
Emotional changes Emotional changes and challenges that may occur				
Encouragement to seek support as needed				
Physiologic and psychologic changes that may occur in the mother and newborn				
Infant care concerns Possible supportive measures for the new family				
Care of the Baby				
Observing the baby General appearance				
Senses Visual				
Hearing				
Touch				
Smell				
Taste				
Vital signs Normal parameters				
How to take a temperature				
Skin Coloring				
Normal sign rashes				
Diaper care				
Stool cycle Normal characteristics				
Signs of diarrhea and treatment				
Signs of constipation and treatment				

TABLE 31–5 *continued*

Knowledge and Skills To Be Taught	Teaching Method			
	Video	Verbal Only	Verbally Reinforced	Demonstration
Care of the Baby *continued* Observing the baby *continued* Emotional and comforting needs				
Protective reflexes Blinking				
Sneezing				
Swallowing				
Normal reflexes Moro				
Fencing				
Head lag				
Stepping				
Feeding the baby Schedule				
Breastfeeding				
Positioning, initiating and ending feeding				
Infant cues for feeding				
Identifying problem areas and possible solutions				
Breast care				
Bottle-feeding Positioning				
Preparation of bottles and formula				
Burping or bubbling the baby				
Holding, wrapping and diapering the baby Various holds (cradle, football)				
Securing baby in blanket to provide warmth				
Diapering Comparison of reusable (cloth) and single use (paper)				
Methods of diapering and care of soiled diapers				
Perineal skin care				
Positioning the baby for sleep				
Bathing the baby Supplies				
Method				
Safety Use of bulb syringe and care if choking				
Positioning				
Car seat				
Health promotion When to call health care provider				
Temp				
Diarrhea				
Eating problems				
Malaise				
Protecting baby from infections				
Immunization schedule				
Aspects of Parenting				
Interaction with newborn Newborn cues and capacity for interaction				
Parenting needs				
Acquaintance with individual characteristics of their newborn and possible techniques to use				
Resources available				

anticipate that the cord will fall off, when the infant can have a tub bath, when the infant will need his or her first immunizations, and so on. They should also be comfortable feeding and handling the baby and should be aware of basic safety considerations, including the need to use a car seat whenever the infant is in a car.

9. The parents should be aware of signs and symptoms in the infant that indicate possible problems and whom they should contact about them.

The nurse can also use this final period to reassure the couple of their ability to be successful parents, stressing the infant's need to feel loved and secure. The nurse can also urge parents to talk to each other and work together to solve any problems that may arise.

The nurse addresses follow-up visits when appropriate. If not already discussed, teaching about family planning is appropriate at this time, and the nurse can provide information regarding birth control methods.

In ideal situations, a family approach involving the father, infant, and possibly other siblings would permit a total evaluation and provide an opportunity for all family members to ask questions and express concerns. In addition, a family approach can enable the nurse to identify disturbed family patterns more readily and initiate interventions to prevent future problems of neglect or abuse.

FOCUS YOUR STUDY

- Nursing diagnoses can be used effectively in planning care for the postpartal woman.
- Postpartum discomfort may be due to a variety of factors, including engorged breasts, an edematous perineum, an episiotomy or extension, engorged hemorrhoids, or hematoma formation. Various self-care approaches are helpful in promoting comfort.
- Lactation may be suppressed by mechanical techniques or by administering medication.
- The new mother requires opportunities to discuss her childbirth experience with an empathetic listener.
- The first day or two following birth are marked by maternal behaviors that are more dependent and oriented to the woman's comfort. Thereafter the woman becomes more independent and ready to assume responsibility.
- Rooming-in provides the childbearing family with opportunities to interact with their new member during the first hours and days of life. This enables the family to develop some confidence and skill in a "safe" environment.
- Sexual intercourse may resume once the episiotomy has healed and lochia has stopped. Couples should be forewarned of possible changes; for example, the vagina may be "dry," fatigue may inhibit the level of desire, or the woman's breasts may leak milk during orgasm.
- Following cesarean birth, a woman has the nursing care needs of a surgical client in addition to her needs as a postpartum client. She may also require assistance in working through her feelings if the cesarean birth was unexpected.
- Postpartally, the nurse evaluates the adolescent mother in terms of her level of maturity, available support systems, cultural background, and existing knowledge and then plans care accordingly.
- The mother who decides to relinquish her baby needs emotional support. She should be able to decide whether to see and hold her baby and should have any special requests regarding the birth honored.
- Prior to discharge, the nurse should give the couple any information necessary for the woman to provide appropriate self-care. They should have a beginning skill in caring for their newborn and should be familiar with warning signs of possible complications for mother or baby. Printed information is valuable in helping couples deal with questions that may arise at home.
- Because of the trend toward early discharge, follow-up care is more important than ever. Many approaches are used, especially home visits.

REFERENCES

Alteneder, R. R., & Hartzell, D. (1997). Addressing couples' sexuality concerns during the childbearing period: Use of the PLISSIT model. *Journal of Obstetric, Gynecologic, and Neonatal Nursing, 26*(6), 651–658.

Arms, S. (1990). *Adoption: A handful of hope.* Berkeley, CA: Celestial Arts.

Association of Women's Health, Obstetric, and Neonatal Nursing (AWHONN). (1998). Guidelines for planning family-centered care to meet the needs of the mother and baby. *Standards and guidelines for professional nursing practice in the care of women and newborns* (5th ed.). Washington, DC: Author.

Banks-Wallace, J. (1999). Storytelling as a tool for providing holistic care to women. *American Journal of Maternal Child Nursing, 24,* 20–24.

Bucknell, S., & Sikorski, K. (1989). Putting patient-controlled analgesia to the test. *American Journal of Maternal Child Nursing, 14*(1), 37–40.

Choudhry, U. K. (1997). Traditional practices of women from India: Pregnancy, childbirth, and newborn care. *Journal of Obstetric, Gynecologic, and Neonatal Nursing, 26*(5), 533–539.

Cunningham, F. G., MacDonald, P. C., Gant, N. F., Leveno, K. J., Gilstrap, L. C., III, Hankins, G. D. V., & Clark, S. L. (Eds.). (1997). *Williams obstetrics* (20th ed.). Stamford, CT: Appleton & Lange.

Datta, S. (1995). *The obstetric anesthesia handbook* (2nd ed.). St. Louis: Mosby.

Diehl, K. (1997). Adolescent mothers: What produces positive mother-infant interaction? *American Journal of Maternal Child Nursing, 22*(2), 89–95.

Eakes, M., & Brown, H. (1998). Home alone: Meeting the needs of mothers after cesarean birth. *AWHONN Lifelines, 2*(1), 36–40.

Fadiman, A. (1997). *The spirit catches you and you fall down: A Hmong child, her American doctors, and the collision of two cultures.* The Noonday Press: New York.

Gosha, J., & Brucker, M. C. (1986). A self-help group for new mothers: An evaluation. *American Journal of Maternal Child Nursing, 11*(1), 20–23.

Harrison, L. L. (1990). Patient education in early postpartum discharge programs. *American Journal of Maternal Child Nursing, 15*(1), 39.

Inturrisi, M., Camenga, C. F., & Rosen, M. (1988). Epidural morphine for relief of postpartum, postsurgical pain. *Journal of Obstetric, Gynecologic, and Neonatal Nursing, 17*(4), 238–243.

Jansson, P. (1985). Early postpartum discharge. *American Journal of Nursing, 85*(5), 547–550.

Karch, A. M. (1999). *1999 Lippincott's nursing drug guide.* Pp. 773–774, 815–818. Philadelphia: Lippincott.

Keen-Payne, R., & Bond, M. L. (1997). Voices of clients and caregivers in a maternity home. *Western Journal of Nursing Research, 19*(2), 190–204.

Koniak-Griffin, D., Mathenge, C., Anderson, N. L. R., & Verzemnieks, I. (1999). An early intervention program for adolescent mothers: A nursing demonstration project. *Journal of Obstetric, Gynecologic, and Neonatal Nursing, 28,* 51–59.

Lamp, J. M., & Howard, P. A. (1999). Guiding parents' use of the internet for newborn education. *American Journal of Maternal Child Nursing, 24,* 33–36.

Moran, C. F., Holt, V. L., & Martin, D. P. (1997). What do women want to know after childbirth? *Birth, 24,* 27–34.

National Campaign to prevent teen pregnancy. (1997). Whatever happened to childhood? The problem of teen pregnancy in the United States. Washington, D.C.: Author.

Nursing '99. (1999). *Drug handbook.* Springhouse, PA: Springhouse Corp.

Parks, P. L., Lenz, E. R., Milligan, R. A., & Han, H-R. (1999). What happens when fatigue lingers for 18 months after delivery? *Journal of Obstetric, Gynecologic, and Neonatal Nursing, 28,* 87–93.

PDR Nurse's Handbook. Pp. 869–870, 911–912. Montvale, NJ: Medical Economics Co.

Rhode, M. A., & Barger, M. K. (1990). Perineal care: Then and now. *Journal of Nurse-Midwifery, 35*(4), 220–230.

Sampselle, C. M., Seng, J., Yeo, S., Killion, C., & Oakley, D. (1999). Physical activity and postpartum well-being. *Journal of Obstetric, Gynecologic, and Neonatal Nursing, 28,* 41–49.

Schneiderman, J. U. (1996). Postpartum nursing for Korean mothers. *MCN; American Journal of Maternal Child Nursing, 21*(3), 155–158.

Scott, J. R., DiSaia, P. J., Hammond, C. B., & Spellacy, W. N. (1994). *Danforth's obstetrics and gynecology* (7th ed.). Philadelphia: Lippincott.

Sheil, E. P., Bull, M. J., Moxon, B. E., Muehl, P. A., Kroening, K. L., Peterson-Palmberg, G., & Kelber, S. (1995). Concerns of childbearing women: A maternal concerns questionnaire as an assessment tool. *Journal of Obstetric, Gynecologic, and Neonatal Nursing, 24*(2), 149–155.

Varney, H. (1997). *Varney's midwifery* (3rd ed.). Sudbury, MA: Jones and Bartlett.

Williams, L. R., & Cooper, M. K. (1993). Nurse-managed postpartum home care. *Journal of Obstetric, Gynecologic, and Neonatal Nursing, 22*(1), 25–31.

32

Home Care of the Postpartal Family

Key Terms

Active awake state

Crying state

Quiet alert state

Quiet sleep

I AM AMAZED BY THE FACT THAT I LOVE MAKING home visits. I always thought that nothing could be more satisfying than hospital nursing, but when I go into a home and help a family with a teaching need or work out a problem using my knowledge, common sense, and the resources available in the community, I know I am making an incredible difference in the lives of a new family.

Objectives

- Discuss the components of postpartal home care.
- Identify the main purposes of home visits during the postpartum period.
- Summarize actions the nurse should take to ensure personal safety during a home visit.
- Delineate aspects of fostering a caring relationship in the home.
- Describe assessment, care of the newborn, and reinforcement of parent teaching in the home.
- Discuss maternal and family assessment and anticipated progress after birth.

HOME CARE HAS BECOME ESSENTIAL because the length of stay in the birth setting has decreased steadily over the past few years. The length of time the woman and newborn spend in the hospital or birthing center after birth has been referred to as *short stay;* however, there is no agreement about how long this period should be. The trend toward short stay has been fueled by efforts to contain health care costs rather than by well-developed research studies that validate the efficacy and safety of this practice (Braveman, Egerter, Pearl, Marchi, & Miller, 1995) or cooperative decision making between health care professionals and families (American Academy of Pediatrics (AAP) Committee on Fetus and Newborn, 1995).

As the length of stay has declined, a number of new issues have been identified. Fishbein and Burggraf (1998) suggest that new mothers who are discharged in 48 hours or less following childbirth must adjust to motherhood without the benefit of the assessment and teaching that are possible with a longer stay. In addition, the shortened stay (less than 48 hours) has implications for the newborn because many conditions, such as jaundice, ductal dependent cardiac lesions, and gastrointestinal obstructions, often develop several days after birth and can be identified only by a skilled, experienced professional (AAP Committee on Fetus and Newborn, 1995; Soskolne, Schumacher, Fyock, Young, & Schork, 1996). Catz, Hanson, Simpson, and Yaffe (1995) found that in one year, 1% to 4% of term newborns (up to 110,000 newborns) with less than a 48-hour stay were readmitted, and in 85% of the cases the reason was jaundice.

Many educated, well-prepared women with strong support systems are eager to return home and often press for early discharge. However, the shortened stay has implications for the new mother who is less prepared. The stability of her health, availability of support systems, and opportunities to become comfortable with her new baby may be compromised; moreover, a period of fewer than 48 hours is too little time to establish breastfeeding (AAP Committee on Fetus and Newborn, 1995). In addition, the first 24 hours after birth is the taking-in phase for the mother, which is not conducive to learning (Soskolne et al, 1996). The AAP Committee on Fetus and Newborn (1995) has developed minimum criteria to guide the timing of early discharge in order to enhance excellence in maternal-newborn care (Table 32–1).

TABLE 32–1 Minimal Criteria for Discharge of Newborns

1. Uncomplicated prenatal, intrapartal, and postpartal course and vaginal birth.
2. A single baby who is term, 38–42 weeks, and AGA (average weight for gestational age).
3. The newborn's vital signs are within normal limits and have been stable for the 12 hours preceding discharge. (Respirations < 60/min; apical pulse 100–160 beats per minute; axillary temperature of 36.1C–37C in an open crib with appropriate clothing)
4. The newborn has passed at least one stool and has urinated.
5. At least two feedings have been successfully completed, and the baby's ability to coordinate sucking, swallowing, and breathing has been observed and documented.
6. No physical abnormalities have been found that require continued hospitalization.
7. If a circumcision has been done, no excessive bleeding has been evident for at least two hours before discharge.
8. There has been no significant jaundice in the first 24 hours of life.
9. The mother has received education about breastfeeding or bottle-feeding; the newborn's expected stool and urinary patterns; care of circumcision; cord, skin, and genital care; ways to recognize signs of illness or distress and common infant problems; signs of jaundice and who to contact if it develops; infant safety, including positioning of baby after feeding and for sleep; and use of a car seat.
10. Review of pertinent laboratory data including maternal syphilis and hepatitis B surface antigen status; cord or infant blood type.
11. Completion of screening tests (eg, phenylketonuria [PKU]).
12. First hepatitis B vaccine has been administered or appointment for administration has been scheduled within the first week.
13. Method and schedule for continuing care has been ascertained and planned, and the family is aware of the plan.
14. Family assessment has been completed for social and environmental risk factors such as history of previous child abuse or neglect; spousal or partner abuse either preceding or beginning during the pregnancy; parental substance abuse; lack of support within the family or community; lack of funds, shelter, or food; mental illness of one of the parents that impairs ability to care for self and newborn; single first-time mother without social support.

SOURCE: Committee on Fetus and Newborn: Hospital stay for healthy term newborns. *Pediatrics* 1995; 96(4):788.

In January 1998, the Newborns' and Mothers' Health Protection Act of 1996, which was signed into law in 1997, took effect. The bill provides for a guaranteed minimum stay of up to 48 hours following vaginal birth and 96 hours following cesarean birth at the discretion of the new mother and her health care provider. It does not, however, require follow-up home visits for women who leave earlier than the mandated time. Currently over half the states have passed legislation strengthening the federal legislation by mandating coverage for home care follow-up (Carpenter, 1998). Locklin and Johnson (1999) describe additional aspects of the Newborns' and Mothers' Health Protection Act that went into effect January 1, 1998. The purpose of the bill is multifaceted: insurance-driven early discharge from the birthing center or hospital is discouraged for mothers and their newborns after a normal vaginal birth; and insurance payment for physician directed home visits by skilled nurses for the mother and newborn who are discharged in less than 48 hours (Locklin & Johnson, 1999).

Because of the short length of stay, nursing professionals in birthing centers are pressed to complete essential assessments, ensure holistic care (physiologic, psychologic, and spiritual) and provide opportunities for education about maternal self-care and newborn care. The new family, eager to learn about important aspects of care, also need to rest and spend time with their newborn. The needs of the family and the goals of the health care provider can be addressed through the development of postpartal home care.

Home care for the postpartal family is focused more on assessment, teaching, and counseling than on physical care. *Postpartal home care* provides opportunities for expanding information and reinforcing self- and infant care techniques initially presented in the birth setting. In addition, the home setting provides an opportunity for the nurse and family to interact in a more relaxed environment, one in which the family has control of the setting. In some instances, a home provides unique challenges in assessing and enhancing the woman's self-care and infant care, and the nurse has many opportunities to exercise critical thinking and develop creative options with the family. Most important perhaps, initial research suggests that there are no significant differences in perceived maternal competence, identification of neonatal jaundice, infant weight gain, infant use of health care services, or predominant breastfeeding in women who remain in the birth setting for 48 hours or more with standard postpartum follow-up and women discharged 6 to 36 hours postpartum who receive follow-up home visits (Gagnon, Edgar, Kramer, Papageorgiou, Waghorn, & Klein, 1997). Furthermore, there is no increase in the incidence of neonatal readmission when early discharge is combined with a structured program of postpartum home visits (Bragg, Rosenn, Khoury, Miodovnik, & Siddiqi, 1997).

Considerations for the Home Visit

In planning a home visit, the nurse should clearly understand the purpose of the visit and identify the maximum amount of content to be addressed. Other important considerations include ways of creating and fostering relationships with families, techniques for preplanning and executing the visit while maintaining safety, documentation of the visit, and telephone follow-up.

The postpartal home visit differs from community health visits in that only one or two postpartal visits are typically planned, and long-term follow-up by the postpartal nurse is not anticipated. Although the postpartal home visit is comprehensive, it is more specifically focused on postpartal family needs and care.

Because of the established guidelines for early discharge of the mother and baby (refer to Table 32–1), the nurse can logically expect to find certain levels of health and wellness. However, because the status of the mother and newborn can change, the nurse should stay alert for deviations from the norm.

Purpose and Timing of the Home Visit

The postpartal home visit has many purposes. It provides an opportunity to assess the mother's and infant's status after birth for signs of any complications and to complete follow-up blood work if needed. The nurse also assesses current needs for information and provides additional information as needed. The home visit also provides time to cover additional information in a more relaxed setting. In addition, the nurse assesses adaptation of the family to the new baby and adjustment of any siblings, answers questions about breastfeeding, provides support and encouragement, and addresses the need for referrals (Lowdermilk, 1995).

The postpartal home visit usually occurs within 24 to 48 hours of discharge and is conducted by a registered nurse who is experienced in postpartal maternal and newborn care. This timing is designed to provide assistance to the family as they deal with questions or concerns that may have arisen as they begin caring for their new infant. Because the visit typically occurs on about the infant's third day of life, it generally occurs when the breastfeeding mother's milk volume has increased significantly and provides an opportunity for her to ask questions about infant feeding, nipple care, and the like. At this point, too, the infant's bilirubin levels are peaking and the nurse can assess for jaundice (Carpenter, 1998).

Fostering a Caring Relationship with the Family

Although the nurse in the birthing center strives to enhance family autonomy and control, the inherent atmosphere of the institutional environment may cause the new mother and family to feel unempowered. It is important for the professional nurse to recognize that the parameters of the home visit are different in many ways from those of the hospital or birthing center environment. In the home, the family has control of their environment and the nurse is an invited visitor. The nurse can rely on the same characteristics of a caring relationship that have been integral to hospital-based practice—regard for clients, genuineness, empathy, and establishment of trust and rapport—but the relationship may take on new elements as the nurse moves into the home setting for the first time (Table 32–2).

Planning the Home Visit

Prior to the home visit, the nurse prepares by identifying the purpose of the home visit and gathering anticipated materials and equipment. A personal contact while the woman is still in the birth setting or a previsit telephone call is used to arrange the appointment with the woman and her family. During the previsit contact, it is important for the nurse to identify clearly the purpose and goals of the visit and to begin establishing rapport.

Maintaining Safety

In the past, nurses were viewed as a mainstay of communities and could move in most settings without fear or concern for safety. However, in current times some communities are not safe for visiting nurses. Thus it is important for the nurse to follow some basic safety rules when conducting a home visit. Specifically, the nurse should:

TABLE 32–2 Fostering a Caring Relationship

Demonstrated Goal	Approaches to Achieve Goal
Regard	Introduce yourself to the family. Call the family members by their surnames until you have been invited to use the given or a less formal name. Ask to be introduced to other members of the family who are present. Allow the mother or spokesperson to assume this role. Use active listening. Maintain objectiveness. Ask permission before sitting.
Genuineness	Mean what you say. Make sure that your verbal and nonverbal messages are congruent. Be nonjudgmental. Don't make assumptions about individuals or settings. Always strive to demonstrate caring behaviors. Be prepared for the visit, honestly answer questions and provide information, and be truthful. If you don't know the answer to a question, tell the client you will find the information and report back.
Empathy	Listen to the mother and family without judgment, trying to view events and circumstances from their point of view. Be attentive to what the birthing experience means to them so that you will understand their concerns from their perspective.Remember empathy denotes understanding, not sympathy.
Trust and rapport	Do what you say you will do. Be prepared for the visit and be on time. Follow-up on any areas that are needed.

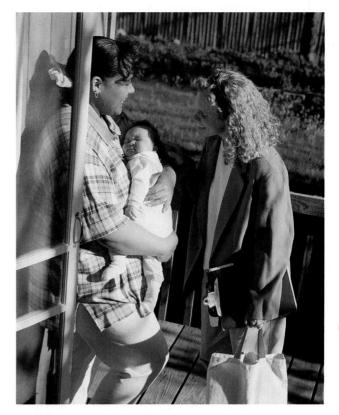

FIGURE 32–1 Nurse arriving for a home visit.

- Know the specific address, and ask for directions during the previsit contact.
- Trace out the route to the client's home on a map before leaving for the visit and take the map along.
- Notify an instructor or supervisor when leaving for a visit and check in as soon as the visit is completed.
- Carry a cellular phone or another method of communication.
- Carry enough change to make a call from a pay phone if needed.
- Wear a name tag.
- Avoid wearing expensive jewelry.
- Terminate the visit if a situation arises that feels unsafe.
- Avoid entering areas where violence is in progress. In such cases, return to the car and make appropriate contacts, such as calling 911. If the visit is in an area that seems very unsafe, it may be wise for two nurses to go together.

Most people are more comfortable in familiar settings and have some hesitation in entering other residential areas. It is always important for nurses to be aware of their surroundings and the people who are nearby. First home visits may feel uncomfortable because they are unfamiliar, but with experience the nurse's comfort increases (Figure 32–1).

Carrying Out the Home Visit

When the door is answered, the nurse should introduce herself or himself and confirm that the location is correct. If a place to sit is not indicated, the nurse may inquire, "Where is the best place to sit so that we can talk for a while?" In some homes, the mother or family may offer refreshments, and this may be an important aspect of welcoming a visitor. In this case, it is beneficial to the relationship to accept the refreshment graciously.

Many agencies have developed a uniform assessment tool to be used during postpartum home visits. This ensures that the nurse completes a physical assessment of both the mother and the newborn; assesses infant feeding and weight gain; evaluates maternal psychosocial adjustment, parental bonding, parenting behaviors, family adaptation, and coping skills; and determines environmental strengths and risk factors. Based on these assessments the nurse may do any of the following:

- Provide direct physical care (assessments, interventions, consultation and referrals).
- Carry out client and family teaching.

COMMUNITY IN FOCUS

Postpartum Home Care Program

The Maternity and Newborn Home Visit Program, a joint effort of Professional Nurse Associates, Inc (PNA) and Kaiser Permanente of Ohio, is designed to address the needs of childbearing families following their hospital stay. The program, which has been in effect since 1989, is an example of an effective partnership between a private nursing practice and a managed care organization.

The program consists of three phases: the prenatal phase, referral process, and home visit program. The prenatal phase is educationally focused and includes waiting room videotapes, childbirth classes, and educational mailings. The mailings provide information on a variety of topics including the short length of stay and the home follow-up visit program.

The referral process begins about one month before the woman's expected date of birth when her prenatal history and demographic information is sent to PNA. PNA in turn assigns a nurse case manager who will complete the postpartum home visit. The actual home visit is initiated by a hospital nurse or discharge planner who completes a summary of the woman's hospital stay and forwards it to PNA.

As initially designed, the postpartum home visit program, implemented by registered nurses, was provided for women discharged on the first postpartum day following vaginal birth or the third postpartum day following cesarean birth. Because of the positive outcomes demonstrated by the program, a home visit is currently provided to all postpartum families regardless of length of stay. The home visit program includes a previsit phone call to the family, case management from PNA, and a home visit within 72 hours of discharge if a problem that requires immediate attention (such as poor infant feeding) is identified. Additional home visits may also be scheduled if a need is identified by the home visit nurse or medical providers. PNA nurses make necessary referrals to a variety of community resources such as WIC, parent support groups, domestic violence prevention programs. In addition, a 24-hour PNA help line, staffed by clinical nurse specialists, is also available for families with questions, concerns, or problems. Over half the families served make use of it.

On the average, home visits last approximately 97 minutes; the average number of phone contacts per family is 2.4. Despite the shortened length of stay, the readmission rate for both mothers and newborns is less than 1 percent. Client satisfaction is measured via a survey mailed with a stamped self-addressed envelope after the case is closed. Response rates approach 75 percent and reflect an impressive 99 percent satisfaction rate. Equally impressive is the cost benefit, which is estimated at one million dollars each year since 1991.

This program is a wonderful example of innovative approaches to limited resources. It also exemplifies the best of entrepreneurial nursing practice.

SOURCES: Personal communication with Lenore R. Williams, Director, Professional Nurse Associates, Inc; Williams LR, Cooper MK.

- Consult with the physician or a specialist, such as a lactation consultant.
- Refer the woman or family to appropriate community agencies.
- Schedule additional home visits or telephone follow-up.

The nurse should report significant medical concerns to the certified nurse-midwife or physician immediately and plan for appropriate follow-up (Carpenter, 1998).

The remainder of the chapter focuses on specific aspects of newborn and maternal care that are assessed, addressed, and evaluated during the home visit.

Home Care: The Newborn

Positioning and Handling

The nurse demonstrates methods of positioning and handling the newborn as needed. When the family provides care for their newborn, the nurse can instill confidence by giving them positive feedback. If the family encounters problems, the nurse can suggest alternatives and serve as a role model.

When the newborn is out of the crib, one of the following holds can be used (Figure 32–2). The *cradle hold* is frequently used during feeding. It provides a sense of warmth and closeness, permits eye contact, frees one of the adult's hands, and provides security because the cradling protects the newborn's body. Extra security is provided by gripping the thigh with the hand while the arm supports the newborn's body. The *upright position* provides security and a sense of closeness and is ideal for burping. One hand should support the neck and shoulders while the other hand holds the buttocks or is placed between the newborn's legs. The newborn may also be held upright in a cloth sling carrier that gently holds the baby against the mother or father's chest and frees the hands for other tasks. The *football hold* frees one of the caregiver's hands and permits eye contact. This hold is ideal for shampooing, carrying, or breastfeeding. It frees the caregiver to talk on the telephone, answer the door, or do the myriad tasks that await attention at this busy time.

The newborn is most frequently positioned on her or his side with a rolled blanket or diaper behind the back to provide support and to prevent rolling (Figure 32–3). The side-lying position aids drainage of mucus and allows air to circulate around the cord. It is also more comfortable for the newly circumcised male. After feeding, the newborn is placed on the right side to aid digestion

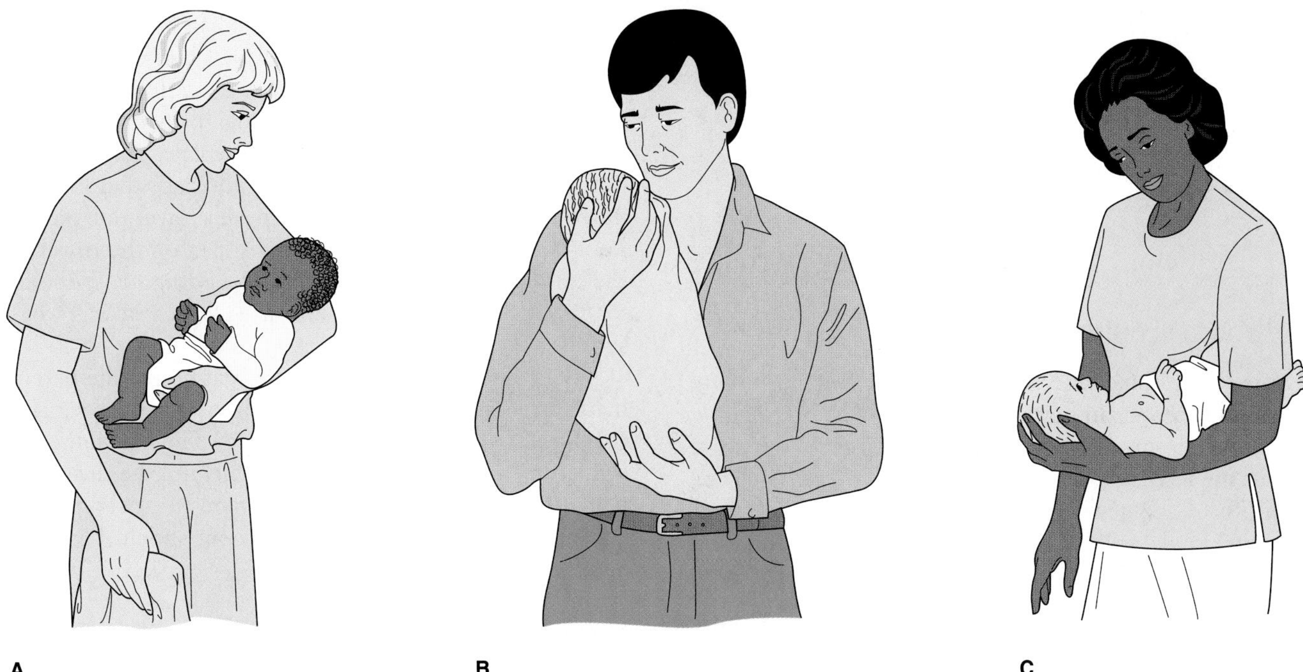

FIGURE 32–2 Various positions for holding an infant. ***A,*** Cradle hold. ***B,*** Upright position. ***C,*** Football hold.

and to prevent aspiration of regurgitated feedings; this position also makes it easier to expel air bubbles from the stomach.

A firm, flat mattress without pillows should be provided for the newborn. Recent studies have shown an increased incidence of sudden infant death syndrome (SIDS) in infants who sleep on their stomachs. There is no evidence that sleeping on the back or side is harmful to healthy infants. Certain infants may need to be placed on their stomachs, including premature infants with respiratory distress (severe breathing problems); infants with symptoms of gastroesophageal reflux (severe spitting up); and infants with certain upper airway abnormalities. There may be other valid reasons for infants to be placed on their stomachs for sleep. Parents should discuss their individual circumstances with their care provider. Although the risk of SIDS for infants who sleep on their stomachs may be higher than for those who sleep on their sides or backs, the actual risk of SIDS for infants placed on their stomachs is still extremely low (*Infant Sleep Position and SIDS Position Statement*, 1992).

The infant's position should be changed periodically during the early months of life, because skull bones are soft and permanently flattened areas may develop if the newborn consistently lies in one position. A newborn in the first days of life should not be left in a supine position when unattended, because of the danger of aspiration.

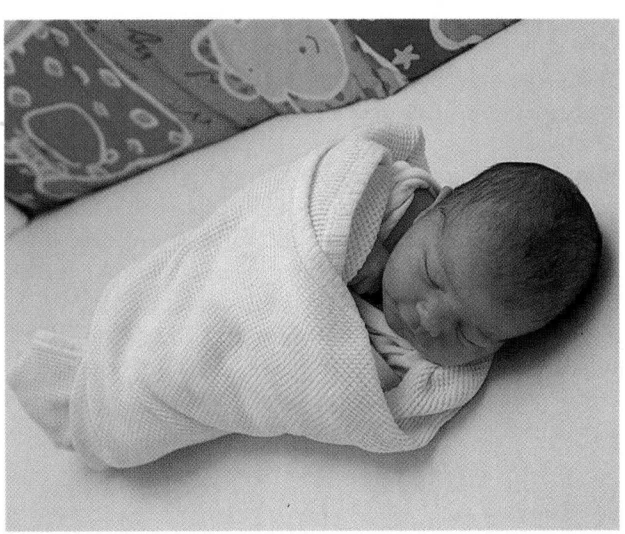

FIGURE 32–3 The most common sleeping position of the newborn is on the side. A rolled blanket may be placed behind the back to provide additional support.

TABLE 32–3 Bath Supplies

Washcloths (2)	Petroleum jelly or A and D ointment
Towels (2)	Rubbing alcohol
Blankets (2)	Cotton balls
Unperfumed mild soap (eg, Castile, Neutrogena)	Diapers
	Clean clothes
Shampoo	

Newborn Feeding

On the first home visit, the nurse can anticipate finding that the parents and newborn have established a feeding pattern. The nurse will take this opportunity to inquire about the feedings and determine if the parents have any questions. The newborn's status regarding fluid and nutritional intake will be assessed by obtaining information regarding a number of factors (Locklin & Jansson, 1999):

- The physical assessment to establish if normal findings are present
- The newborn's nude weight is determined. If the weight loss has been 10% since birth, signs of dehydration may be present (loose skin with decreased skin turgor, dry mucous membranes, sunken anterior fontanelle, decreased number and frequency of voidings and stooling).

If the mother is breastfeeding, continued support by the nurse and a lactation consultant is advised. Information regarding the breastfeeding experience may be obtained by: observation of a feeding for positioning; evaluation of newborn feeding behaviors and satiation; assessment of the mother's breasts for engorgement, pain during nursing and/or reddened nipples; and gathering information about the newborn's sleep and crying patterns. Locklin and Jansson (1999) report that mothers who are at particularly high risk for breastfeeding difficulties are those who are greater than 35 years of age, had an operative birth (low forceps or vacuum extractor assisted birth), and isolation from the mother's immediate family. Newborn factors include small for gestational age, being post-term, and being one of a multiple gestation (Locklin & Jansson, 1999).

Bathing

An actual bath demonstration is the best way for the nurse to provide information to parents. Because excess bathing and use of soap removes natural skin oils and dries out the newborn's sensitive skin, bathing should be done every other day or twice a week. Sponge baths are recommended for the first 2 weeks or until the umbilical cord completely falls off and the umbilicus has healed. Some agencies use a tub bath for the bath demonstration and apply alcohol to the cord after the bath to facilitate drying.

Supplies can be kept in a plastic bag or some type of container to eliminate the necessity of hunting for them each time (Table 32–3). At home, the family may want to use a small plastic tub, a clean kitchen or bathroom sink, or a large bowl as the baby's tub. Expensive baby tubs are not necessary, but some prefer to purchase them. Some nurses recommend spreading a beach towel out on the floor and placing a small plastic dishpan on the towel. If the mother or father is comfortable sitting on the floor for the bath, this arrangement provides a spacious work surface.

Before starting, if no one else is at home, the parent may want to take the phone off the hook and put a sign on the door to avoid being disturbed. Having someone home during the first few baths is helpful, because that person can get forgotten items, attend to interruptions, and provide moral support. The room should be warm and free of drafts.

Sponge Bath

After the supplies are gathered, the tub (or any of the containers mentioned) is filled with water that is warm to the touch. Even though the newborn won't be placed in the tub, the bath giver carefully tests the water temperature with an elbow or forearm. Families may also choose to purchase a thermometer to help them determine when the bath water is at approximately 37.8C (100F) and safe to use. Soap should not be added to the water. The newborn should be wrapped in a blanket, with a T-shirt and diaper on, to keep her or him warm and secure.

To start the bath, the adult wraps a washcloth around the index finger once. Each eye is gently wiped from inner to outer corner. This direction prevents the potential for clogging the tear duct at the inner corner, where the eye naturally drains. A different portion of the washcloth is used for each eye to prevent cross-contamination. Cotton balls can also be used for this purpose, using a new one for each eye. Some eye swelling and drainage may be present the first few days after birth as a result of the eye prophylaxis.

The bath giver washes the ears next by wrapping the washcloth once around an index finger and gently cleaning the external ear and behind the ear. Cotton swabs are never used in the ear canal because it is possible to put the swab too far into the ear and damage the ear drum. In addition, the swab may back any discharge farther down into the ear canal.

The caregiver then wipes the remainder of the baby's face with the soap-free washcloth. Many babies start to cry at this point. The face should be washed every day and the mouth and chin wiped off after each feeding.

The neck is washed carefully but thoroughly with the washcloth. Soap may now be used. Formula or breast milk and lint collect in the skinfolds of the neck, so it may be helpful to sit the newborn up, supporting the neck and shoulders with one hand while washing the neck with the other hand.

The bath giver now unwraps the blanket, removes the T-shirt, and wets the chest, back, and arms with the washcloth. The bath giver may then lather the hands with soap and wash the baby's chest, back, and arms. Wetting the cord is avoided, if possible, because it delays drying. Soap is rinsed off with the wet washcloth, and the upper part of the body is dried with a towel or blanket. The newborn's upper body is then wrapped with a clean, dry blanket to prevent chill.

Next the bath giver unwraps the newborn's legs, wets them with the washcloth, and lathers, rinses, and dries them well. If the newborn has dry skin, a small amount of unscented lotion or ointment (petroleum jelly or A and D ointment) may be used. Ointments are thought to be better than lotions for dry, cracked feet and hands. Baby oil is not recommended because it clogs skin pores. Powders are not currently recommended. Some believe they aggravate dry skin, and others avoid powders because of the possible danger of inhalation.

Families should be warned that baby powder can cause serious respiratory problems for the baby if it is inhaled. If parents want to use powder, they should be advised to use one that is talc free. Parents should avoid shaking powder directly onto the baby. Rather they can shake the powder into their hands and then rub it on the newborn.

The genital area is cleansed daily with soap and water, and with water after each wet or dirty diaper. Females are washed from the front of the genital area toward the rectum to avoid fecal contamination of the urethra and thus the bladder. Newborn females often have a thick, white mucous discharge or a slight bloody discharge from the vaginal area. This discharge is normal for the first 1 to 2 weeks of age and should be wiped off with a damp cloth during diaper changes.

Parents of uncircumcised males should cleanse the penis daily. Even minimal retraction of the foreskin is not advised (see in-depth discussion of care of uncircumcised male babies in Chapter 23). Males who have been circumcised also need their penis cleansed daily. A very wet washcloth is rubbed over a bar of soap. The washcloth is squeezed above the baby's penis, letting the soapy water run over the circumcision site. The area is rinsed off with plain warm water and lightly patted dry. A small amount of petroleum jelly, A and D, or bactericidal ointment may be put on the circumcised area, but excessive amounts may block the urinary meatus and should be avoided. It is important to avoid using ointments if a Plastibell is in place because ointments may cause the Plastibell ring to slip off the penis too early. The Plastibell usually falls off within 5 to 8 days. If it doesn't, the family needs to call the health care provider.

The diaper area should be cleansed with each diaper change to prevent diaper rash. Even when this cleansing is done regularly, a diaper rash may occasionally occur. Baby powder (or cornstarch) is not recommended for diaper rash. Baby powder may cake with urine and irritate the perineal area. Cornstarch may promote fungal infection. Ointments that provide a barrier, such as zinc oxide, A and D ointment, or petroleum jelly are more effective for diaper rash. If the ointment does not help the rash, families using single-use (disposable) diapers should try another brand. If they use cloth diapers, a different detergent or fabric softener, more thorough rinsing, and hanging them in the sun to dry may alleviate the problem. If the rash persists, parents should discuss the problem with their nurse practitioner or physician, because it may be due to a yeast or fungal infection.

The umbilical cord should be kept clean and dry. The close proximity of the umbilical vessels makes the cord a common entry area for infection. At discharge, most parents are advised to cleanse the area around the cord with a cotton ball and alcohol (70% isopropyl) two to three times a day until the cord falls off and the umbilicus is healed. The cord stump generally falls off in 7 to 14 days. The diaper should be folded down to allow air to circulate around the cord. The parents should consult their health care provider if redness, bright red bleeding, or puslike drainage with foul odor appears around the umbilicus, or if the area remains unhealed 2 to 3 days after the cord stump has sloughed off.

The last step in bathing is washing the hair (some prefer to do this step first). The newborn is swaddled in a dry blanket, leaving only the head exposed, and held in the football hold with the head tilted slightly downward to prevent water running in the eyes. Water should be brought to the head by a cupped hand. The hair is moistened and lathered with a small amount of shampoo. A very soft brush may be used to massage the shampoo over the entire head, including the fontanelles, which families often call the "soft spots." The hair is then rinsed and toweled dry. Oils or lotions are not used on the newborn's head unless there is evidence of cradle cap. Moistening the scaly area with lotion or mineral oil a half an hour or more before shampooing softens the crusts or scales and makes it easier to remove them with a soft brush during the shampoo.

Tub Baths

The baby may be put in a small tub after the cord has fallen off and the circumcision site is healed (approximately 2 weeks) (Figure 32–4). Newborns usually enjoy a tub bath more than a sponge bath, although some cry during either one.

The tub is filled with 3 to 5 inches of water. To prevent slipping, a washcloth is placed in the bottom of the tub or sink. Some parents choose to bring the newborn into the tub with them.

The baby's face is washed in the same manner as for a sponge bath. The parent then places the newborn in the tub using the cradle hold and grasping the distal thigh. The neck is supported by the parent's elbow in the cradle position. An alternative hold is to support the newborn's

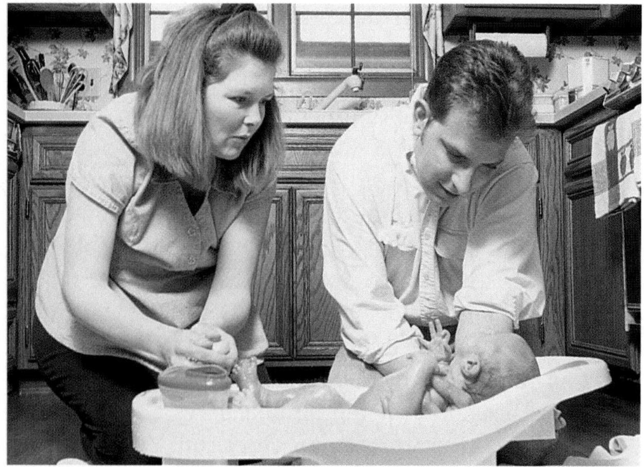

FIGURE 32–4 When bathing the newborn, the caregiver must support the head. Wet babies are very slippery.

head and neck with the forearm while grasping the distal shoulder and arm.

Because wet newborns are slippery, some parents pull a cotton sock (with the holes cut out for the fingers) over the supporting arm to provide a "nonskid" surface. The newborn's body is washed with a soapy washcloth or hand. To wash the back, the bath giver places the noncradling hand on the newborn's chest with the thumb under the newborn's arm closest to the adult. Gently tipping the newborn forward onto the supporting hand frees the cradling arm to wash the back. After the bath, the newborn is lifted out of the tub in the cradle position, dried well, and wrapped in a dry blanket. The hair is then washed in the same way as for a sponge bath.

Nail Care

The nails of the newborn are seldom cut in the birthing center. During the first days of life, the nails may adhere to the skin of the fingers, and cutting is contraindicated. Within a week the nails separate from the skin and frequently break off. If the nails are long or if the newborn is scratching his or her face, the nails may be trimmed. This is most easily done while the infant is asleep. Nails should be cut straight across using adult cuticle scissors or blunt-ended infant cuticle scissors.

Dressing the Newborn

Newborns need to wear a T-shirt, diaper (diaper cover or plastic pants if using cloth diapers), and a sleeper. On a fairly cool day, they should be wrapped in a light blanket while being fed. Newborns should be covered with a blanket in air-conditioned buildings. The blanket can be unwrapped or removed when inside a warm building.

At home, the amount of clothing the newborn wears is determined by the temperature. Families who maintain their home at 60F to 65F should dress the infant more warmly than those who maintain a temperature of 70F to 75F.

CLINICAL TIP

Dressing a newborn baby with a T-shirt may be quite a challenge. The T-shirt is first pulled over the baby's head. The next challenge is getting the arms in the sleeves, because the newborn grasps at the fabric of the T-shirt as you try to pull it over the hands and arms. It will help, if you put your hand through the right sleeve of the T-shirt and hold the baby's right hand. Then pull the sleeve over your hand. Repeat the same movements for the left sleeve.

Newborns should wear a head covering outdoors to protect their sensitive ears from drafts. A blanket can also be wrapped around the baby, leaving one corner free to place over the head for added protection while outdoors or in crowds. The nurse must advise families about the ease with which a newborn's skin can burn when exposed to the sun. To prevent sunburn, the newborn should remain shaded, wear a light layer of clothing, or be protected with sunscreen.

Diaper shapes vary and are subject to personal preference (Figure 32–5). Prefolded and disposable diapers are usually rectangular. Cloth diapers may also be triangular or kite-folded. Extra material is placed in front for males and toward the back for females to increase absorbency.

Baby clothing should be laundered separately with a mild soap or detergent. Diapers are generally presoaked before washing. All clothing should be rinsed twice to remove soap and residue and to decrease the possibility of rash. Some newborns may not tolerate clothing treated with fabric softeners added to the washer or dryer.

Temperature Assessment

As the nurse prepares to teach parents about taking their baby's temperature, it is important to provide opportunities for discussion and demonstration. Bordman and Holzman (1996) found that even with individual teaching in the hospital setting, more than half the mothers in their study were unsure how to take their baby's temperature, and almost half of them were unsure when to call their primary health care provider. The study encourages nurses to create opportunities for questions and to pose questions to the parents about what they would do in different situations. This can be accomplished only after a supportive relationship has been established.

The nurse shows the family how to take an axillary temperature and discusses the different types of thermometers. It is important that parents understand the differences and how to select the appropriate one. If the parents are planning to use a glass thermometer, they need information about shaking the mercury down (the mercury needs to be below 94F on the thermometer), reading the thermometer, and making sure that the thermometer bulb is underneath the armpit. To take an axil-

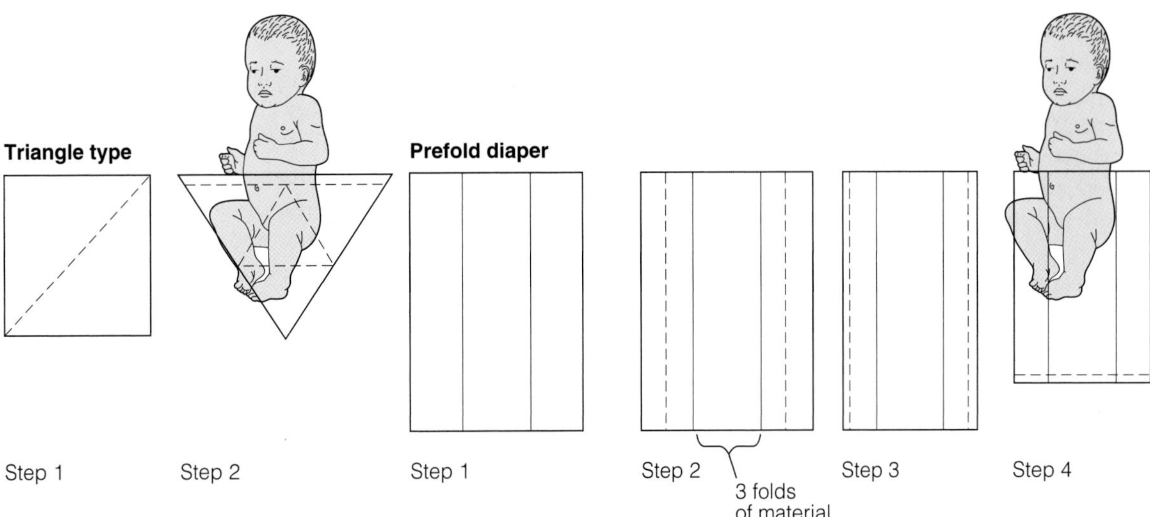

FIGURE 32–5 Two basic cloth diaper shapes. Dotted lines indicate folds.

lary temperature, the thermometer is placed under one of the newborn's arms and held in place 3 to 4 minutes. It is important to hold the baby's arm still, because friction between the arm and chest creates heat and can make the thermometer record an inaccurate temperature. Parents should not take the temperature rectally because this method can be both irritating and unsafe for the baby. When taken properly, the axillary method is an accurate way to measure the baby's temperature.

CRITICAL THINKING QUESTION

Parents may purchase a variety of thermometers. For example, there are inexpensive digital models and pacifier devices, as well as thermometer strips that can be placed on the baby's forehead. What differences are there between thermometers? How do the current methods compare in accuracy? If a parent does decide to use a mercury thermometer, what teaching is needed regarding what to do if the thermometer breaks? What precautions are needed for the mercury?

Parents need to take the newborn's temperature only when signs of illness are present. They should call their physician or pediatric nurse practitioner immediately if any signs of illness are present. Parents should also check with their clinician for advice about over-the-counter medications to keep in the medicine cabinet.

When parents find that their newborn has a fever, they may expect to give an antipyretic medication, such as Tylenol (acetaminophen). They should not give any form of aspirin for an illness that may be viral; use of aspirin in viral illnesses has been linked to Reye's syndrome in children. They should discuss management of flu, colds, teething, constipation, diarrhea, and other common ailments with their clinician before they occur. When analgesic or antipyretic medication is needed, clinicians frequently recommend acetaminophen drops.

Stools and Urine

The appearance and frequency of a newborn's stools can cause concern for parents. The nurse prepares them by discussing and showing pictures of meconium stools and transitional stools and by describing the difference between breast milk and formula stools. Although each baby develops his or her own stooling patterns, parents can get an idea what to expect (see Figure 24–12).

- Breastfed newborns may have 6 to 10 small, semiliquid, yellow stools per day by the third or fourth day after milk production is established, unless the mother is having problems with her milk supply. Once breastfeeding is well established, usually by 1 month, the newborn may have only 1 stool every few days because of the increased digestibility of breast milk, or the newborn may still have several daily. Constipation is unlikely to occur in newborns receiving only breast milk. Infrequent stooling in the first few weeks may indicate inadequate milk intake.
- Formula-fed babies may have only 1 or 2 stools a day; they are more formed and yellow or yellow-brown.

The parents may also be shown pictures of a constipated stool (small, pelletlike) and diarrhea (loose, green, or perhaps blood-tinged). Families should understand that a green color is common in transitional stools so that they do not mistake transitional stools for diarrhea during the first week of a newborn's life. Constipation may indicate that the newborn needs additional fluid intake. Parents may try offering water in an attempt to reverse the constipation.

Babies normally void (urinate) five to eight times per day. Fewer than six to eight wet diapers a day may indicate the newborn needs more fluids. Frequency of voiding is easy to assess with cloth diapers. Parents who use super-absorbent single-use disposable diapers may have difficulty determining voiding patterns because the surface of the diaper feels dry. The liquid pools inside the filling of the diaper.

Sleep and Activity

The newborn demonstrates several different sleep-wake states after the initial periods of reactivity described in Chapter 24. It is not uncommon for a newborn to sleep almost continuously for the first 2 to 3 days following birth, awakening only for feedings every 3 to 4 hours. Some newborns bypass this stage of deep sleep and require only 12 to 16 hours of sleep. The parents need to know that this is normal.

Quiet sleep is characterized by regular breathing and no movement except for sudden body jerks. During this sleep state, normal household noise will not awaken the infant. In the active sleep state, the newborn has irregular breathing and fine muscular twitching. The newborn may cry out during sleep, but this does not mean he or she is uncomfortable or awake. Unusual household noise may awaken the newborn more easily in this state; however, he or she will quickly go back to sleep.

Quiet alert state is a state in which newborns are quietly involved with the environment. They watch a moving mobile, smile, and, as they become older, discover and play with their hands and feet. When newborns become uncomfortable due to wet diapers, hunger, or cold, they enter the **active awake state** and **crying state.** In these states, parents should identify and eliminate the cause of the crying. Sometimes families are frustrated as they try to identify the external or internal stimuli that are causing the angry, hurt crying. Parents need to be told that they may change the state from crying to quiet alert by moving the newborn toward an upright position, where scanning and exploration are possible (Klaus & Klaus, 1985). See Table 32–4 for the characteristics of the various states.

It was so exciting to go home with our new baby. The rest of that first day went quite well and Joe and I felt that we were on our way as new parents. Our son had been fed and diapered a number of times and it was now time for bed. When we snuggled him in his bed, he lay quietly and didn't cry. Then we looked at each other, and at the same time said "What if we don't hear him in the middle of the night?" We went on to bed but with much trepidation. Our baby's first cry in the night woke us immediately. We both sat up and simultaneously said "There he is!"

After a few weeks, we could laugh at the anxiety we had during those first few days. I'm sure all new parents must have had similar experiences.

Crying

For the newborn, crying is the only means of expressing needs vocally. Families learn to distinguish different tones and qualities of the newborn's cry. The amount of crying is highly individual. Some will cry as little as 15 to 30 minutes in 24 hours, or as long as 2 hours every 24 hours. When crying continues after such causes as discomfort or hunger are eliminated, the newborn may be comforted by swaddling or by rocking and other reassuring activities. There is some indication that newborns who are held more tend to be calmer and cry less when not being held. Some parents may be afraid that holding may "spoil" the newborn and will need reassurance that that is not the case. Picking babies up when they cry teaches them that adults try to meet their needs and are responsive to them. This helps build a sense of trust in humankind. Caregivers should note and assess excessive crying, taking other factors into consideration. After the first 2 or 3 days, newborns settle into individual patterns.

Safety Considerations

Newborns should not have pillows or stuffed animals in the crib while they sleep; these items could cause suffocation. Mattresses should fit snugly in a crib to prevent entrapment and suffocation, and the crib should be inspected regularly to determine whether it is in safe working order. Crib slats should be no more than 2⅜ inches apart. Parents can be encouraged to attend infant cardiopulmonary resuscitation (CPR) classes, especially if there is a family history of SIDS or if the infant requires special care.

During the home visit, the nurse also discusses signs of infection in the newborn as well as other possible indications of developing complications. Table 26–4 identifies findings in the newborn that the parents should report to the baby's health care provider.

Newborn Screening and Immunization Program

Before the newborn and mother are discharged from the hospital, the nurse informs parents about the normal screening tests for newborns and tells them when to return for further tests if needed. Newborn screening tests detect disorders that cause mental retardation, physical handicaps, or death if left undiscovered. Inborn errors of metabolism that can usually be detected from a drop of blood obtained by a heel stick on the second or third day include galactosemia, homocystinuria, hypothyroidism, maple syrup urine disease, phenylketonuria (PKU), and sickle cell anemia. Parents should be instructed that a second blood specimen will be required from the newborn after 7 to 14 days. In some states, the second blood specimen is not recommended if the first specimen is obtained after 48 hours of age. However, it must be clarified that an abnormal test result is not diagnostic. More defin-

TABLE 32–4 Infant State* Chart (Sleep and Awake States)

Sleep States	Body Activity	Eye Movement	Facial Movement	Breathing Pattern	Level of Response	Implications for Caregiving
	Characteristics of State					
Deep sleep	Nearly still except for occasional startle or twitch	None	Without facial movements, except for occasional sucking movement at regular intervals	Smooth and regular	Only very intense and disturbing stimuli will arouse infants.	Caregivers trying to feed infant in deep sleep will probably find the experience frustrating. Infants will be unresponsive, even if caregivers use disturbing stimuli (flicking feet) to arouse infants. Infants may arouse only briefly and then become unresponsive as they return to deep sleep. If caregivers wait until infants move to a higher, more responsive state, feeding or caregiving will be much more pleasant.
Light sleep	Some body movements	Rapid eye movement (REM): fluttering of eyes beneath closed eyelids	May smile and make brief fussy or crying sounds	Irregular	Infants are more responsive to internal and external stimuli. When these stimuli occur, infants may remain in light sleep or move to drowsy state.	Light sleep makes up the highest proportion of newborn sleep and usually precedes awakening. Caregivers who are not aware that the brief fussy or crying sounds made during this state occur normally may think it is time for feeding and may try to feed infants before they are ready to eat.
Drowsy	Activity level variable, with mild startles interspersed from time to time; movements usually smooth	Eyes open and close occasionally; are heavy-lidded with dull, glazed appearance	May have some facial movements; often are none and the face appears still	Irregular	Infants react to sensory stimuli although responses are delayed. State change after stimulation frequently noted.	From the drowsy state infants may return to sleep or awaken further. In order to wake them, caregivers can provide something for infants to see, hear, or suck. This may arouse them to a quiet alert state, a more responsive state. Infants left alone without stimuli may return to a sleep state.
Quiet alert	Minimal	Brightening and widening of eyes	Faces have bright, shining, sparkling looks	Regular	Infants attend most to environment, focusing attention on any stimuli that are present.	Infants in this state provide much pleasure and positive feedback for caregivers. Providing something for infants to see, hear, or suck will often maintain a quiet alert state in the first few hours after birth. Most newborns commonly experience a period of intense alertness before going into a long sleeping period.
Active alert	Much body activity; may have periods of fussiness	Eyes open with less brightening	Much facial movement; faces not as bright as in alert state	Irregular	Infants are increasingly sensitive to disturbing stimuli (hunger, fatigue, noise, excessive handling).	Caregivers may intervene at this stage to console and to bring infants to a lower state.
Crying	Increased motor activity with color changes	Eyes may be tightly closed or open	Grimaces	More irregular	Infants are extremely responsive to unpleasant external or internal stimuli.	Crying is the infant's communication signal. It is a response to unpleasant stimuli from the environment or from within infants (fatigue, hunger, discomfort). Crying tells us infants have been reached. Sometimes infants can console themselves and return to lower states. At other times they need help from caregivers.

**State* is a group of characteristics that regularly occur together: body activity, eye movements, facial movements, breathing pattern, and level of response to external stimuli (eg, handling) and internal stimuli (eg, hunger).

SOURCE: Blackburn S, Kang R; Early Parent-Infant Relationships, 2nd edition, module 3, series 1. *The First Six Hours after Birth.* White Plains, NY: March of Dimes Birth Defects Foundation, 1991. Reprinted with permission of the copyright holder.

itive tests must be performed to verify the results. It is important to follow protocols that incorporate state laws about newborn testing.

If additional tests are positive, treatment is initiated. These conditions may be treated by dietary means or by administering missing hormones. The inborn conditions cannot be cured, but they can be treated. They are not contagious, but they may be inherited (Chapter 28).

Follow-Up Care

Each newborn has variations in normal physiologic responses and growth-and-development patterns. Parents need to learn to interpret these changes in their child. To help parents care for their newborn at home, some physicians encourage prenatal pediatric visits to establish contact before the birth. Public health nurses have long been involved as guides in newborn care and parent education.

Many birthing units are now expanding their primary care functions to the new family to include one home visit by the nurse who cared for the family in the birthing unit. The birthing unit nursery staff may also make themselves available as a 24-hour telephone resource for the new family that needs additional support and consultation during the first few days at home with their newborn.

Routine well-baby visits should be scheduled with the clinic, pediatric nurse practitioner, or physician.

The family should have been taught all necessary caregiving methods before discharge. However, during the home visit the nurse may use a checklist to determine that the family clearly understands material. If not, the nurse should complete pertinent teaching. The nurse needs to review with the couple all areas for understanding and answer any questions they may have, making sure that the mother has the phone number and address of, and any specific instructions from, the certified nurse-midwife/nurse practitioner/physician and lactation consultant. Having the nursery phone number is also reassuring to a new family. The nurse encourages them to call with questions.

RESEARCH IN PRACTICE

What is this study about? Due to the effort to control health care costs through early discharge, many mothers undergo the intense experience of giving birth and are also expected to learn to care for their newborn within 24 hours or less. The information obtained needs to enable the mother to function effectively at home without further health care interaction until the 6-week checkup. Sandra Brown and Bonne Johnson developed a pilot project whereby two nurses, one having expertise in postpartum or labor and delivery and the other in newborn care, provided home visits to mother-infant dyads.

How was the study done? Twenty-nine of the beginning 41 dyads concluded the project. Eligibility criteria included being 18 years or older, residing within 20 miles of the hospital, and having no identified problems during the perinatal period. The nurses conducted a telephone assessment within 24 hours of discharge, paid a home visit within 72 hours, followed up with another telephone assessment at one week and a second home visit in the third postpartum week if needed. A randomly selected group of 29 mother-infant dyads who met the same eligibility criteria as the intervention group served as the control group.

What were the results of the study? When contacted 6 to 8 weeks post delivery by the project director, 79% of the mothers in the treatment group and 100% of the infants had received scheduled routine follow-up care. Only 55% of the mothers and 90% of the infants in the control group had received this care. Ten percent of the mothers and 43% of the infants in the control group required non-routine care with 2 of the mothers and 13 infants needing hospitalization. Only 3% of the mothers and 28% of the infants in the treatment group received non-routine care with 8 infants requiring hospitalization. Costs for the control group were $6,631 for non-routine care while treatment group costs only reached $646.

Interestingly, the initial assumption that first-time mothers with limited education were more in need of the program and were likely to obtain more benefit from the program did not hold true. Types of questions and information sought did not relate to either parity or educational level. Younger mothers appeared to have stronger support systems and need the project less.

What additional questions might I have? Were the demographic data statistically the same for both treatment and control group? Was the control group selected during the same time period as the treatment group or afterwards?

How can I use this study? This study originated because a faculty member responsible for baccalaureate nursing students making postpartum home visits identified the need for follow-up home visits with mothers and babies. All students can help identify research needs based on clinical problems observed in their practice.

SOURCE: Brown, S.G. & Johnson, B.T. (1998). Enhancing early discharge with home follow-up: A pilot project. *JOGNN, 27*(1), 33–38.

Home Care: The Mother and Family

During the first few postpartal weeks, many changes occur. The family adjusts to incorporating a new family member, and siblings become familiar with new roles and responsibilities. During this period, the woman must accomplish a variety of physical and developmental tasks:

- Restoring physical condition
- Developing competence in caring for and meeting the needs of her infant
- Establishing a relationship with her new child
- Adapting to altered lifestyles and family structure resulting from the addition of a new member

Assessment and Care of the Mother and Family

The nurse can complete ongoing postpartum assessment following discharge by telephone follow-up, home visit, or a combination. The approach used depends on the mother's needs and preferences and established practices in the community.

Telephone Follow-Up

Telephone follow-up option is offered to families prior to discharge, and a mutually agreeable time is set for the call, usually within 3 days after discharge or earlier if desired. Calls typically last about 20 minutes and are preplanned and goal directed. The initial goal is to assess the woman's perceptions of her current circumstances, her recovery from childbirth, her adjustment and that of her partner to parenthood, the newborn's condition, family-newborn bonding, and any problems or concerns the woman may have. The nurse asks specifically about the following areas: (1) progression of lochia (color, amount of flow, presence of foul odor or clots; (2) fever or malaise; (3) dysuria or difficulty voiding; (4) pain in the pelvis or perineum; (5) painful, reddened hot spots or shooting pains in the breasts during or between feedings; (6) areas of redness, edema, tenderness, or warmth in the legs. The nurse also inquires about the woman's emotional status, comfort level, fatigue, any problems sleeping, reactions to the baby, appetite, and adaptation to her new role.

To perform an effective telephone assessment, the nurse must be able to listen skillfully, use open-ended questions and wait for answers, projecting a warm, caring attitude so that the mother feels comfortable talking to a faceless caller.

The plan of care developed and implemented during a telephone conversation is limited to supportive counseling, teaching, and referral. The new mother may have many questions, especially about newborn care, and is generally at a high level of learning readiness. The nurse can answer the woman's questions and use the questions as a "stepping stone" for further teaching. When nursing assessment reveals signs of an initial or recurring postpartum complication, the nurse should refer the woman to her primary care provider for further evaluation.

Home Visit

During the home visit, the nurse completes a physical and psychologic assessment. The physical assessment focuses on maternal physical adaptation, which is assessed by evaluating vital signs, breasts, abdominal musculature, elimination patterns, reproductive tract, and laboratory values. The nurse should also talk with the mother about her diet, fatigue level, ability to rest and sleep, pain management, and signs of postpartal complications. Prior to completing the assessment, the nurse should ensure privacy.

If not addressed previously, the nurse provides information about family planning options at this time (see Chapter 3) and answers any questions the woman or her partner may have about methods of birth control.

The psychologic assessment focuses on attachment, adjustment to the parental role, sibling adjustment, and educational needs. When appropriate, the nurse mentions available community resources, including public health department follow-up visits. In ideal situations, a family approach involving the presence of the father and any siblings provides an opportunity to observe family interactions and opportunities for all family members to ask questions and express concerns. In addition, this approach may surface any questionable family interaction pattern, such as one suggestive of abuse or neglect; the nurse can consider further referral if needed. See Postpartal Assessment Guide: First Home Visit and Anticipated Progress at 6 Weeks.

During the home visit, the nurse continues to provide teaching to the mother and her family as needed and describes self-care measures when needed. The nurse also reviews the signs of developing illness with the woman and her partner. If signs of potential complications are present, the nurse completes a more in-depth evaluation and determines whether it is necessary for the woman to see her primary care provider or whether therapy can be initiated immediately following phone consultation. For example, if the woman is febrile and shows signs of developing mastitis, the nurse can contact the certified nurse-midwife or physician and obtain a prescription for an antibiotic for the woman and a follow-up appointment. For more severe problems, for example, signs of developing pyelonephritis in the woman, the nurse can refer her immediately to her primary care provider.

The nurse usually makes a follow-up telephone call a few days after the home visit. During the call, the nurse can provide additional information, address questions or areas of confusion, and make referrals if indicated.

Return Visits

If the mother and family and physician/certified nurse-midwife have chosen discharge earlier than 48 hours after vaginal birth, the mother may, in some states, request a total of three visits. In such cases, the nurse would schedule the first visit about 24 hours after discharge and then space out the other two visits over the next week. In other instances, the nurse may schedule additional home visits based on the findings of the first home visit and the follow-up phone call.

Help Lines for Parents

Many communities have established 24-hour help lines for new parents to call when they have questions or need support. In areas where help lines are not available, parents may be directed to call the birthing center. In either case, the nurse may provide the number so that it is readily accessible for the family.

Postpartal Classes and Support Groups

Postpartal classes are becoming more common as caregivers recognize the continuing needs of the childbearing family. In many instances, classes are prepared to meet the specific needs of a variety of families so that, for example, single mothers and adolescent mothers can attend class with peers. A series of structured classes may focus on topics such as parenting, postpartal exercise, or nutrition, or there may be loosely structured group sessions that address mothers' concerns as they arise. Such classes offer chances for the new mother to socialize, share her

Text continues on page 978.

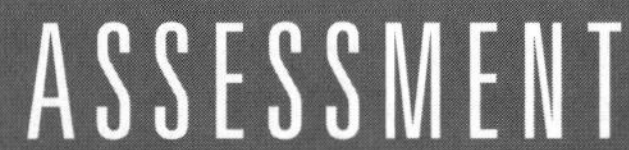

ASSESSMENT GUIDE: POSTPARTAL—FIRST HOME VISIT AND ANTICIPATED PROGRESS AT SIX WEEKS

Physical Assessment/ Normal Findings	Alterations and Possible Causes*	Nursing Responses to Data†
Vital Signs		
Blood pressure: Return to normal prepregnant level.	Elevated blood pressure (anxiety, essential hypertension, renal disease).	Review history, evaluate normal baseline; refer to physician/CNM if necessary.
Pulse: 60–90 beats/minute (or prepregnant normal rate).	Increased pulse rate (excitement, anxiety, cardiac disorders).	Count pulse for full minute, note irregularities; marked tachycardia or beat irregularities require additional assessment and possible physician/CNM referral.
Respirations: 16–24/minute.	Marked tachypnea or abnormal patterns (respiratory disorders).	Evaluate for respiratory disease; refer to physician/CNM if necessary.
Temperature: 36.2C–37.6C (98F–99.6F).	Increased temperature (infection).	Assess for signs and symptoms of infection or disease state.
Weight		
2 days: Possible weight loss of 12–20+ lb.	Minimal weight loss (fluid retention, pregnancy-induced hypertension [PIH]).	Evaluate for fluid retention, edema, deep tendon reflexes and blood pressure elevation.
6 weeks: Returning to normal prepregnant weight.	Retained weight (excessive caloric intake).	Determine amount of daily exercise. Provide dietary teaching. Refer to dietitian if necessary for additional dietary counseling.
	Extreme weight loss (excessive dieting, inadequate caloric intake).	Discuss appropriate diets; refer to dietitian for additional counseling if necessary.
Breasts		
Nonnursing 2 days: May have mild tenderness; small amount of milk may be expressed. 6 weeks: Soft, with no tenderness; return to prepregnant size.	Some engorgement (incomplete suppression of lactation). Redness; marked tenderness (mastitis). Palpable mass (tumor).	Engorgement may be seen in nonnursing mothers. Advise client to wear a supportive, well-fitted bra, avoid very warm showers, use ice packs for comfort; evaluate for signs and symptoms of mastitis (rare in nonnursing mothers).
Nursing Full, with prominent nipples; lactation established.	Cracked, fissured nipples (feeding problems). Redness, marked tenderness, or even abscess formation (mastitis). Palpable mass (full milk duct, tumor).	Counsel about nipple care. Evaluate client condition, evidence of fever; refer to physician/certified nurse-midwife for initiation of antibiotic therapy, if indicated. Opinion varies as to value of breast examination for nursing mothers; some feel a nursing mother should examine her breasts monthly, after feeding, when breasts are empty; if palpable mass is felt, refer to physician for further evaluation.

*Possible causes of alterations are placed in parentheses.

†This column provides guidelines for further assessment and initial nursing intervention.

Physical Assessment/ Normal Findings	Alterations and Possible Causes*	Nursing Responses to Data[†]
Breasts ***continued***		For breast inflammation instruct the mother to **1.** Keep breast empty by frequent feeding. **2.** Rest when possible. **3.** Take prescribed pain relief med. **4.** Force fluids. If symptoms persist for more than 24 hours, instruct her to call her physician/CNM.
Abdominal Musculature		
2 days: Improved firmness, although "bread dough" consistency is not unusual, especially in multipara. Striae pink and obvious.	Marked relaxation of muscles.	Evaluate exercise level; provide information on appropriate exercise program.
Cesarean incision healing.	Drainage, redness, tenderness, pain, edema (infection).	Evaluate for infection; refer to physician/ CNM if necessary.
6 weeks: Muscle tone continues to improve; striae may be beginning to fade, may not achieve a silvery appearance for several more weeks; linea nigra fading.		
Elimination Pattern		
Urinary Tract		
Return to prepregnant urinary elimination routine.	Urinary incontinence, especially when lifting, coughing, laughing, and so on (urethral trauma, cystocele).	Assess for cystocele; instruct in appropriate muscle tightening exercises; refer to physician/CNM.
	Pain or burning when voiding, urgency and/or frequency, pus or white blood cells (WBC) in urine, pathogenic organisms in culture (urinary tract infection).	Evaluate for urinary tract infection; obtain clean-catch urine; refer to physician/certified nurse-midwife for treatment if indicated.
Routine urinalysis within normal limits (proteinuria disappeared).	Sugar or ketone in urine—may be some lactose present in urine of breastfeeding mothers (diabetes).	Evaluate diet; assess for signs and symptoms of diabetes; refer to physician/CNM.
Bowel Habits		
2 days: May be some discomfort with defecation, especially if client had severe hemorrhoids or third- or fourth-degree extension.	Severe constipation or pain when defecating (trauma or hemorrhoids).	Discuss dietary patterns; encourage fluid, adequate roughage. Continue use of stool softener if necessary to prevent pain associated with straining; continue sitz baths, periods of rest for severe hemorrhoids; assess healing of episiotomy and/or lacerations; severe constipation may require administration of laxatives, stool softeners, and an enema.

*Possible causes of alterations are placed in parentheses.

[†]This column provides guidelines for further assessment and initial nursing intervention.

Physical Assessment/ Normal Findings	Alterations and Possible Causes*	Nursing Responses to Data[†]
Bowel Habits continued		
6 weeks: Return to normal prepregnancy bowel elimination.	Marked constipation.	See above.
	Fecal incontinence or constipation (rectocele).	Assess for evidence of rectocele; instruct in muscle tightening exercises; refer to physician/CNM.
Reproductive Tract		
Lochia		
2 days: Lochia rubra or lochia serosa, scant amounts, fleshy odor.	Excessive amounts (nonfirm uterus), foul odor (infection).	Assess for evidence of infection and/or failure of the uterus to decrease in size; refer to physician/CNM.
6 weeks: No lochia, or return to normal menstruation pattern.	See above.	See above.
Fundus and Perineum		
2 days: Fundus is at least two fingerbreadths below the umbilicus; uterine muscles still somewhat lax; introitus of vagina lacks tone—gapes when intra-abdominal pressure is increased by coughing or straining.	Uterus not decreasing in size appropriately (infection).	Assess fundus for firmness and/or signs of infection; refer to physician/CNM if indicated.
Episiotomy and/or lacerations healing; no signs of infection.	Evidence of redness, tenderness, poor tissue approximation in episiotomy and/or laceration (wound infection).	
6 weeks: Uterus almost returned to prepregnant size with almost completely restored muscle tone.	Continued flow of lochia, failure to decrease appropriately in size (subinvolution).	Assess for evidence of subinvolution and/or infection; refer to physician for further evaluation and for dilatation and curettage if necessary.
Hemoglobin and Hematocrit Levels		
6 weeks: Hb 12 g/dL. Hct 37% $\pm$ 5%.	Hb $<$ 12 g/dL. Hct 32% (anemia).	Assess nutritional status, begin (or continue) supplemental iron; for marked anemia (Hb $\leq$ 9 g/dL) additional assessment and/or physician/CNM referral may be necessary.
Attachment		
Bonding process demonstrated by soothing, cuddling, and talking to infant; appropriate feeding techniques; eye-to-eye contact; calling infant by name.	Failure to bond demonstrated by lack of behaviors associated with bonding process, calling infant by nickname that promotes ridicule, inadequate infant weight gain, infant is dirty, hygienic measures are not being maintained, severe diaper rash, failure to obtain adequate supplies to provide infant care (malattachment).	Provide counseling; talk with the woman about her feelings regarding the infant; provide support for the caretaking activities that are being performed; refer to public health nurse for continued home visits.

*Possible causes of alterations are placed in parentheses.

[†]This column provides guidelines for further assessment and initial nursing intervention.

Psychosocial Assessment/ Normal Findings	Alterations and Possible Causes*	Nursing Responses to Data†
Attachment *continued*		
Parent interacts with infant and provides soothing, caretaking activities.	Parent is unable to respond to infant needs (inability to recognize needs, inadequate education and support, fear, family stress).	Provide support for caretaking activities observed; provide information regarding caretaking activities, such as responding to infant cry; methods of wrapping infant; methods of soothing the infant such as swaddling, rocking, increasing stimuli by singing to the infant or decreasing stimuli by putting infant to rest in quiet room; methods of holding the infant; differences in the cry. Identify support system such as friends, neighbors; provide information regarding community resources and support groups.
Parents express feelings of comfort and success with the parent role.	Evidence of stress and anxiety (difficulty moving into or dealing with the parent role).	Provide support and encouragement; provide information regarding progression into parent role and assist parents in talking through their feelings; refer to community resources and support groups.
Woman is in the informal or personal stage of maternal role attainment.	Woman is still greatly influenced by others, has not developed an image or style of her own (woman remains in the anticipatory stage).	Provide role modeling for the woman in working through problem solving with the infant; provide encouragement as she thinks through decisions and develops her sense of problem solving; encourage her to make decisions regarding infant care.
Adjustment to Parental Role		
Parents are coping with new roles in terms of division of labor, financial status, communication, readjustment of sexual relations, and adjusting to new daily tasks.	Inability to adjust to new roles (immaturity, inadequate education and preparation, ineffective communication patterns, inadequate support, current family crisis).	Provide counseling; refer to parent groups.
Education		
Mother understands self-care measures.	Inadequate knowledge of self-care (inadequate education).	Provide education and counseling.
Parents are knowledgeable regarding infant care.	Inadequate knowledge of infant care (inadequate education).	
Siblings are adjusting to new baby.	Excessive sibling rivalry.	
Parents have a method of contraception.	Birth control method not chosen.	

*Possible causes of alterations are placed in parentheses.

†This column provides guidelines for further assessment and initial nursing intervention.

concerns, and receive encouragement. Because baby-sitting arrangements may be difficult or expensive, it is desirable to provide child care for newborns and siblings; in some instances infants may remain with mothers in the class.

Some cities offer support groups through birthing centers or hospitals or as a community effort. Once again, the support group provides an opportunity for parents to interact with one another and to share information and experiences.

Many parents look to Internet resources for additional information on parenting and newborn care. Internet sites can be devised by anyone, so the quality, usefulness, and accuracy of the information may vary. Nurses have an opportunity to assist parents in evaluating the reliability of the information they find. Criteria that suggests Internet information is reliable and high in quality include: affiliation with a university medical or nursing school; inclusion of the authors' credentials, education, board certification, and affiliations; referencing of information; currency of information; similarity of information when compared with other sources and easy accessibility (Lamp & Howard, 1999).

FOCUS YOUR STUDY

- The overall goal of postpartal home visits is to enhance opportunities for smooth transition of the new family. The home visit provides opportunities for assessment, teaching, and fostering a caring relationship with new families.
- Professional nurses play an important role in establishing and maintaining excellence in care for the new family after discharge from the birthing center.
- Nursing goals during home visits include reinforcing daily newborn care, maintaining neutral thermal environment, promoting adequate hydration and nutrition, preventing complications, promoting safety, and enhancing attachment and family knowledge of child care.
- Essential care during a home visit includes assessments of the vital signs, weight, overall color, intake/output, umbilical cord and circumcision, newborn nutrition, parent education, and attachment.
- The physician or pediatric nurse practitioner should be notified if there is evidence of redness around the newborn's umbilicus or bright red bleeding or puslike drainage near the cord stump or if the umbilicus remains unhealed.
- Following a circumcision, the newborn must be observed closely for inability to void and signs of infection.
- Newborn screening for galactosemia, hemocystinuria, hypothyroidism, maple syrup urine disease, phenylketonuria, and sickle cell anemia is performed on all newborns in the first 1 to 3 days, with a second blood specimen drawn after 7 to 14 days.
- Signs of illness in mothers include mastitis, excessive or foul-smelling lochia, failure of fundus to descend at anticipated rate; temperature of 101.4F or above, elevation of blood pressure, and tenderness, redness, or pain in the legs.

REFERENCES

American Academy of Pediatrics (AAP) Committee on Fetus and Newborn. (1995). Hospital stay for healthy term newborns. *Pediatrics, 96*(4 Pt. 1), 788–790.

Barnes, L. P. (1996). Meeting the challenge of early postpartum discharge. *MCN; American Journal of Maternal Child Nursing, 21*(3), 129.

Bordman, H. B., & Holzman, I. R. (1996). Infant care knowledge of primiparous urban mothers. *Journal of Perinatology, 16*(2 Pt. 1), 107–110.

Bowers, S. (1995). Legislative action. *Perinatal Home Care News, 1*(1), 1.

Bragg, E. J., Rosenn, B. M., Khoury, J. C., Miodovnik, M., & Siddiqi, T. A. (1997). The effect of early discharge after vaginal delivery on neonatal readmission rates. *Obstetrics & Gynecology, 89*(6), 930–933.

Braveman, P., Egerter, S., Pearl, M., Marchi, K., & Miller, C. (1995). Problems associated with early discharge of newborn infants. Early discharge of newborns and mothers: A critical review of the literature. *Pediatrics, 96*(4 Pt. 1), 716–726.

Brown, L. P., Towne, S. A., & York, R. (1996). Controversial issues surrounding early postpartum discharge. *Nursing Clinics of North America, 31*(2), 333–339.

Carpenter, J. A. (1998). Shortening the short stay. *AWHONN Lifelines, 2*(1), 29–34.

Catz, C., Hanson, J. W., Simpson, L., & Yaffe, S. J. (1995). Summary of workshop: Early discharge and neonatal hyperbilirubinemia. *Pediatrics, 96*(4 Pt. 1), 743–745.

Fishbein, E. G., & Burggraf, E. (1998). Early postpartum discharge: How are mothers managing? *Journal of Obstetric, Gynecologic, and Neonatal Nursing, 27*(2), 142–150.

Gagnon, A. J., Edgar, L., Kramer, M. S., Papageorgiou, A., Waghorn, K., & Klein, M. C. (1997). A randomized trial of a program of early postpartum discharge with nurse visitation. *American Journal of Obstetrics and Gynecology, 176*(1 Pt. 1), 205–211.

Infant sleep positioning and SIDS position statement. (1992). Evanston, IL: American Academy of Pediatrics.

Klaus, M., & Klaus, P. (1985). *The amazing newborn.* Menlo Park, CA: Addison-Wesley.

Lamp, J. M., & Howard, P. A. (1999). Guiding parents' use of the internet for newborn education. *American Journal of Maternal-Child Nursing, 24,* 33–36.

Locklin, M. P., & Jansson, M. J. (1999). Home visits: Strategies to protect the breastfeeding newborn at risk. *Journal of Obstetric, Gynecologic, and Neonatal Nursing, 28,* 33–40.

Lowdermilk, D. (1995, Dec. 14–15). *AWHONN perinatal home care guidelines: An overview.* Perinatal home care conference. New Orleans, LA: AWHONN and Mosby.

Lynch, A. M. (1996a). Controversies in practice: Discharge decisions and dollars. *House Calls, 1*(1), 12.

Lynch, A. M. (1996b). Postpartum home care. *House Calls, 1*(1), 1.

Soskolne, E. I., Schumacher, R., Fyock, C., Young, M. L., & Schork, A. (1996). The effect of early discharge and other factors on readmission rates of newborns. *Archives of Pediatric and Adolescent Medicine, 150,* 373.

The Postpartal Family at Risk

33

WE ARE SURVIVING. JUST. WHY DON'T THEY GIVE the Croix de Guerre to people who can go without more than two hours total daily sleep for five weeks? I thought babies ate at six-ten-two-six-ten-two—mine does. He also eats at five-seven-nine-eleven and four-eight-twelve. I am getting rather used to going around with my breasts hanging out. They are either drying from the last feed or getting ready for the next one. But the love—I never knew, never imagined that I would love him like this. This incredible feeling of boundless, endless love—a wish to protect his innocence from ever being hurt or wounded or scratched. And that awful, horrible, mad feeling in the first week that you'll never be able to keep anything so precious and so vulnerable alive.
~ *The New Our Bodies, Ourselves* ~

Key Terms

Early postpartal hemorrhage
Endrometritis/metritis
Late postpartal hemorrhage
Mastitis
Pelvic cellulitis (parametritis)
Peritonitis
Puerperal morbidity
Subinvolution
Thrombophlebitis
Uterine atony
Warm lines

Objectives

- Describe assessment of the woman for predisposing factors, signs, and symptoms of various postpartum complications to facilitate early and effective management of complications.
- Incorporate preventive measures for various complications of the postpartal period into nursing care of the postpartum woman.
- List the causes of and appropriate nursing interventions for hemorrhage during the postpartal period.
- Develop a nursing care plan that reflects a knowledge of etiology, pathophysiology, and current clinical management for the woman experiencing postpartal hemorrhage, reproductive tract infection, thromboembolic disease, urinary tract infection, mastitis, or a postpartal psychiatric disorder.
- Evaluate the mother's knowledge of self-care measures, signs of complications to be reported to the primary care provider, and measures to prevent recurrence of complications.
- Describe the role of telephone follow-up and home care in the extended care of postpartal families at risk.

THE POSTPARTAL PERIOD IS TYPICALLY seen as a smooth, uneventful time that follows the anticipation of pregnancy and the excitement and work of labor and birth—and often it is. However, it is important for the nurse to be aware of problems that may develop postpartally and their implications for the childbearing family. This chapter discusses several serious complications of the postpartal period and describes hospital-based and community-based care that may apply.

Hospital-Based Care of At-Risk Women

When providing care to the childbearing woman during the postpartal period, the nurse continues to apply the nursing process to make ongoing assessments, institute preventive measures, and detect, as early as possible, the development of any complications. If a complication does develop, assessment remains important to determine the effectiveness of therapy and to detect any signs that the problem is worsening.

Comprehensive nursing assessment of postpartal clients is an important aspect of care. Systematic data collection allows the nurse to note the normality of findings and to identify early signs of complications that would necessitate a longer hospital stay. Data collected prior to hospital discharge represent baseline findings against which subsequent data, collected by telephone or home visits, may be judged.

Signs and symptoms of many postpartal complications (late hemorrhage, mastitis, thromboembolic disease, and major depression) typically occur only after the woman has returned home. Consequently, it is critical that predischarge teaching for the woman and her partner (or her identified others) include signs of postpartal complications; findings to report to her physician or certified nurse-midwife; and preventive measures, if available. Written instructions to supplement any discussion will be of great value in the early weeks at home with a newborn, when life can be chaotic and instructions may be forgotten. The family should have telephone numbers for postpartum follow-up services and other resources for getting answers to questions. By communicating an attitude of willingness to answer questions and listen to concerns, the nurse enhances the family's comfort in making calls later for what they might otherwise perceive as "too trivial to bother someone about." Knowing the difficult schedules of obstetricians and certified nurse-midwives, many women are hesitant to "bother them" for what might be interpreted as a nonurgent concern. However, if an atmosphere of accessibility has been created by hospital-based nurses and community resources have been identified, families are more likely to feel empowered to seek assistance from one of those sources or feel legitimized in calling their obstetrician or CNM.

Community-Based Care of At-Risk Women

Telephone or home-visit follow-up may allow early recognition of postpartal complications and helps the mother get earlier intervention from her primary provider than might otherwise be available. Prior to the telephone call or visit, the nurse reviews the antepartal record and summary documents from the hospital stay to conduct a risk assessment. When either telephone follow-up or an examination at the home visit provides evidence of a developing complication, the nurse shares these findings or impressions with the woman, and they mutually plan an appropriate next step. In the case of telephone follow-up, the nurse usually counsels the woman to notify her physician or certified nurse-midwife, being prepared to schedule an appointment immediately if risk assessment indicates.

The nurse who identifies a complication at the home visit will need to communicate the clinical findings to the primary health provider and document them and any interventions for the permanent record. Complications, by their very nature, suggest the need for collaborative management with the physician and/or certified nurse-midwife. Moreover, they demand immediate communication rather than a follow-up letter or copy of the record. When nurses telephone the office of a physician or certified nurse-midwife to report the clinical findings, they should identify themselves and their employing agency; identify the client and specify that she was assessed at home; clearly and concisely provide a logical, systematic summary of clinical findings and any intervention provided on site; and elicit orders for management. Once this is done, the nurse carefully and clearly interprets the information with the woman and her family (if available) and supports them in working out any details of the management plan. Occasionally, the primary provider will order specimen collection for a diagnostic test, such as wound culture, or specify a particular treatment to be provided on site.

More hospitals and communities are addressing the issue of continuity of care for postpartal women and their families with unique follow-up services and resources. Being at "home alone" with a newborn and the inherent, seemingly neverending role demands is difficult enough when postpartal recovery is proceeding normally. If complications arise, it can seem overwhelming. It is not surprising that couples welcome the continuity of care offered by postpartal follow-up telephone calls, home visits, and resources for advice, such as warm lines. Postpartum **warm lines** are telephone services designated for questions and concerns of new parents. These 24-hour-per-day services, usually staffed by perinatal nurses, are available for the myriad questions that arise in the early weeks of parenthood. That warm lines are not substitutes for 911 emergency calls must be clear to prospective users.

While most calls relate to newborn care and questions about breastfeeding, occasionally advice is given that prevents complications (Seigel, 1992). At times, callers seek validation of the appropriateness of their reasoned solutions to problems. For example, consider the case of a woman who experienced a sudden increase in vaginal bleeding. She thought it might be related to increasing her activity. At the insistence of her husband, however, she called the community warm line, where a nurse quickly assessed the amount of bleeding occurring, the absence of other related symptoms, and the comparative difference in activity level. The telephone nurse agreed with the woman's assessment of increased activity as a likely cause of an increase in flow. This led to a mutually developed plan for the woman to lie down for 1 to 2 hours, recheck the extent of her bleeding, and report back to the nurse. Receiving positive feedback from the warm line nurse about the practical wisdom of her problem solving increased the esteem of the caller while averting a potential problem. Obviously, if the caller's bleeding had not lessened after the 1 to 2 hours of bed rest, the nurse would have referred the woman to the physician or certified nurse-midwife for follow-up.

Telephone or home visit follow-up care by a professional nurse may also be initiated or extended in response to referral from a physician who has diagnosed a postpartal complication. In either event, the nurse will continue systematic assessment and will plan and implement strategies in collaboration with the physician and family, assuring ongoing communication with the primary provider.

Care of the Woman with Postpartal Hemorrhage

Hemorrhage in the postpartum period is described as either early (immediate) or late (delayed) postpartal hemorrhage. **Early postpartal hemorrhage** occurs in the first 24 hours after childbirth. **Late postpartal hemorrhage** occurs from 24 hours to 6 weeks after birth. Statistically, postpartal hemorrhage (PPH) occurs in 5% to 8% of vaginal births and continues to be a cause of significant maternal mortality and morbidity (Druelinger, 1994).

The traditional definition of postpartal hemorrhage has been a blood loss of greater than 500 mL following childbirth. This definition is being questioned, because careful quantification indicates that the average blood loss in a vaginal birth is actually greater than 500 mL, and the average blood loss after cesarean childbirth exceeds 1000 mL. Some clinicians believe that postpartal hemorrhage can be objectively and reliably defined as a decrease in the hematocrit of 10 points between the time of admission and the time postbirth, or the need for fluid replacement following childbirth (Norris, 1997). Clinical estimation of blood loss at childbirth may be difficult to estimate because blood mixes with amniotic fluid and is obscured as it oozes onto sterile drapes or is sponged away; without vigilance, it may be difficult over the next hours to appreciate the significance of slow, steady blood loss. As the amount of blood loss increases, as in the case of hemorrhage, estimates are likely to be even less accurate. Moreover, postpartal hemorrhage may occur intra-abdominally, into the broad ligament, or into hematomas arising from genital tract trauma, wherein the blood loss is concealed. Given the increased blood volume of pregnancy, the clinical signs of hemorrhage, such as decreased blood pressure, increasing pulse, and decreasing urinary output do not appear until as much as 1000 mL has been lost, shortly before the woman becomes hemodynamically unstable (Norris, 1997).

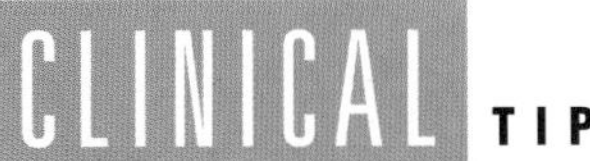

TIP

Women who are natural redheads tend to experience heavier bleeding after childbirth.

Early Postpartal Hemorrhage

At term, blood volume and cardiac output have increased so that 20% of cardiac output, or 600 mL/minute, perfuses the pregnant uterus, supporting the developing fetus. When the placenta separates from the uterine wall, the many uterine vessels that have carried blood to and from the placenta are severed abruptly. The normal mechanisms for hemostasis after birth of the placenta is contraction of the interlacing uterine muscles to occlude the open sinuses that previously brought blood into the placenta. Absence of prompt and sustained uterine contraction (uterine atony) can cause significant blood loss (Roberts, 1995). Other causes of postpartal hemorrhage include laceration of the genital tract: episiotomy; retained placental fragments; vulvar, vaginal, or subperitoneal hematomas; uterine inversion; uterine rupture; problems of placental implantation; and coagulation disorders.

Uterine Atony

Uterine atony (relaxation of the uterus) accounts for 80% to 90% of early postpartal hemorrhage (Norris, 1997). Although uterine atony can occur after any childbirth, its contributing factors include the following:

- Overdistention of the uterus due to multiple gestation, hydramnios, or a large infant (macrosomia)
- Dysfunctional or prolonged labor, which indicates that the uterus is contracting abnormally
- Oxytocin augmentation or induction of labor

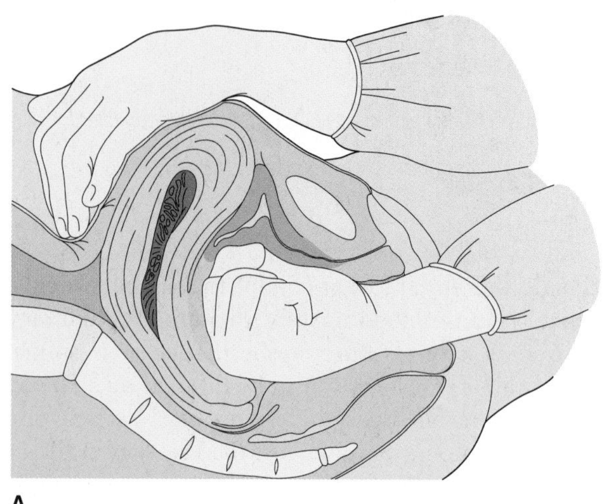

A

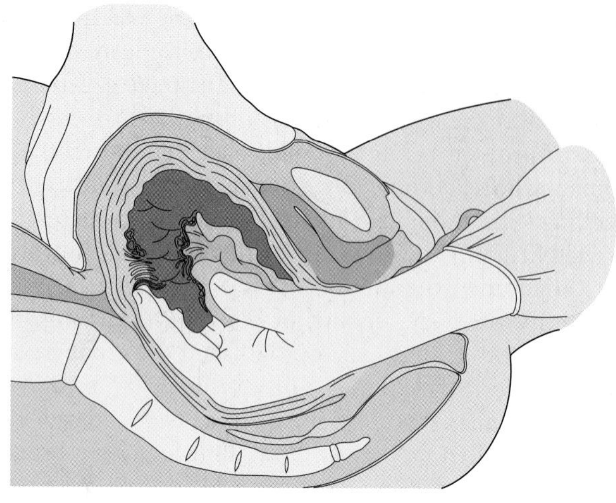

B

FIGURE 33–1 ***A,*** Manual compression of the uterus and massage with the abdominal hand usually will effectively control hemorrhage from uterine atony. ***B,*** Manual removal of placenta. The fingers are alternately abducted, adducted, and advanced until the placenta is completely detached. Both procedures are performed only by the medical clinician. SOURCE: Adapted from Cunningham FG, MacDonald PC, Gant NF [editors]: *Williams Obstetrics,* 18th ed. Norwalk, CT: Appleton & Lange, 1989, pp 417–418.

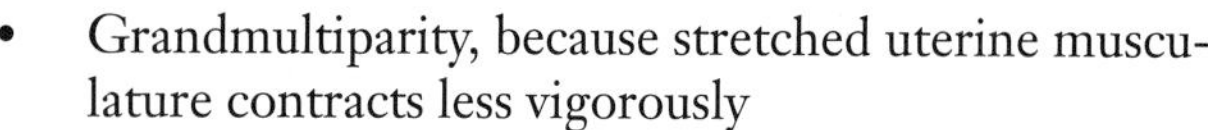

- Grandmultiparity, because stretched uterine musculature contracts less vigorously
- Use of anesthesia (especially halothane) or other drugs such as magnesium sulfate, which cause the uterus to relax
- Prolonged third stage of labor—more than 30 minutes
- Pregnancy-induced hypertension (PIH)
- Asian or Hispanic heritage

Hemorrhage from uterine atony may be slow and steady or sudden and massive. The blood may escape vaginally or collect in the uterus, evident as large clots. The uterine cavity may distend with up to 1000 mL or more of blood while the perineal pad and linen protectors remain suspiciously dry. A treacherous feature of postpartal hemorrhage is that maternal blood pressure and pulse may not change until significant blood loss has occurred because of the increased blood volume associated with pregnancy. The woman with PIH is an exception to this finding because she does not have the normal hypervolemia of pregnancy and cannot tolerate even normal postchildbirth blood loss (Cunningham et al, 1997).

Ideally, postpartal hemorrhage is prevented, beginning with adequate prenatal care, good nutrition, avoidance of traumatic procedures, risk assessment, early recognition, and management of complications as they arise. Any woman at risk should be typed and crossmatched for blood and have intravenous lines in place with needles suitable for blood transfusion (18-gauge minimum). Excellent labor management and childbirth techniques are imperative.

After expulsion of the placenta, the fundus is palpated to ensure that it is firmly contracted. If it is not firm, fundal massage is performed until the uterus contracts. Fundal massage is painful for the woman who has not received regional anesthesia; she will need explanations for why this uncomfortable procedure is necessary and support as massage is initiated. If bleeding is excessive, the clinician will likely order intravenous oxytocin at a rapid infusion rate and may elect to do a bimanual massage (Figure 33–1). Other uterine stimulants may be necessary to manage postpartal uterine atony. Table 33–1 summarizes critical nursing information about the use of uterine stimulants. The need for intravenous fluid replacement and blood transfusion is determined on the basis of hemoglobin and hematocrit results.

In addition to the previously described measures, severe uncontrolled hemorrhage may require radiographic embolization of the pelvic vessels using Gelfoam. Ligation of the uterine artery or internal iliac (hypogastric) artery may be used to slow blood loss and allow normal clotting mechanisms to occur (Chin, 1997). Hysterectomy may be necessary to control hemorrhage but is usually reserved for women of high parity or those in whom excessive bleeding has become life threatening (Craigo & Kapernick, 1994).

Lacerations of the Genital Tract

Some investigators associate 20% of early postpartum hemorrhage with lacerations of the perineum, vagina, or cervix (Craigo & Kapernick, 1994). Several factors predispose women to higher risk of reproductive tract lacerations:

- Nulliparity
- Epidural anesthesia
- Precipitous childbirth
- Macrosomia
- Forceps- or vacuum-assisted birth

TABLE 33–1 Uterine Stimulants Used to Prevent and Manage Uterine Atony

Drug	Dosing Information	Contraindications	Expected Effects	Side Effects
Oxytocin (Pitocin, Syntocinon)	IV use: 10–40 units in 500–1000 mL crystalloid fluid @ 50m U/min administration rate. Onset: immediate. Duration: 1 h. **IV bolus administration not recommended.** IM use: 10–20 units. Onset: 3–5 min. Duration: 2–3 h.		Rhythmic uterine contractions that help to prevent or reverse postpartal hemorrhage caused by uterine atony.	Uterine hyperstimulation, mild transient hypertension, water intoxication rare in postpartum use.
Methylergonovine Malaeate (Methergine)	IM use: 0.2 mg q2–4h. Onset: 2–5 min. Duration: 3 h (× 5 dose maximum). PO use: 0.2 mg q6–12h. Onset: 7–15 min. Duration: 3 h (× 1 week). **IV administration not recommended.**	Women with labile or high blood pressure or known sensitivity to drug.	Sustained uterine contractions that help to prevent or reverse postpartal hemorrhage caused by uterine atony; management of postpartal subinvolution.	Hypertension, dizziness, headache, flushing/hot flashes, tinnitus, nausea and vomiting, palpitations, chest pain. Overdose or hypersensitivity is recognized by seizures; tingling and numbness of fingers and toes from vasoconstrictive effect, leading rarely to gangrene; hypertension; weak pulse; chest pain.
Ergonovine Maleate (Ergotrate Maleate)	IM use: 0.2 mg q2–4h. Onset 7 min. Duration: 3 h (5 dose maximum). PO use: 0.2 mg q6–12h. Onset: 15 min. Duration: 3 h (× 2–7 days). **IV administration not recommended.**	Women with labile or high blood pressure or known sensitivity to drug.	Sustained uterine contractions that help to prevent or reverse postpartal hemorrhage caused by uterine atony; management of postpartal subinvolution.	Hypertension, dizziness, headache, nausea and vomiting, chest pain. Hypersensitivity is noted by systemic vasoconstrictive effects: seizure, chest pain, and tingling and numbness of fingers and toes that leads rarely to gangrene.
Prostaglandin (PGF_{2a}, Hemabate, Prostin/15M)	IM use: 0.25 mg repeated up to maximum 5 doses; may be repeated q15–90min. Physician may elect to administer by direct intramyometrial injection.	Women with active cardiovascular, renal, liver disease, or asthma or with known hypersensitivity to drug.	Control of refractory cases of postpartal hemorrhage caused by uterine atony; generally used after failed attempts at control of hemorrhage with oxytoxic agents.	Nausea, vomiting, diarrhea, headache, flushing, bradycardia, bronchospasm, wheezing, cough, chills, fever.

Implications for Nursing Management of the Postpartal Woman Receiving Uterine Stimulants

- Assess fundus for evidence of contraction and amount of uterine bleeding at least q10–15min × 1–2 h after administration, then q30–60min until stable. **More frequent assessments are determined by the woman's condition or by orders of the physician or certified nurse-midwife.**
- Weigh pads to estimate blood loss.
- Monitor blood pressure and pulse q15min for at least 1 h after administration, then q30–60min until stable.
- Note expected duration of action of drug being administered, and take care to recheck fundus at that time.
- When the drug is ineffective, the fundus remains atonic (boggy or uncontracted) and bleeding continues, massage the fundus. If massage fails to cause sustained contraction, notify the physician or certified nurse-midwife immediately.
- Monitor woman for signs of known side effects of the drug; report to physician or certified nurse-midwife if side effects occur.
- Remind the woman and her support person that uterine cramping is an expected result of these drugs and that medication is available for discomfort. Administer analgesic medications as needed for pain relief. Provide nonpharmacologic comfort measures. If analgesic medication ordered is insufficient for pain relief, notify the physician or certified nurse-midwife.

When Prostaglandin Is Used

- Check temperature q1–2h and/or after chill. Administer antipyretic medication as ordered for prostaglandin-induced fever.
- Auscultate breath sounds frequently for signs of adverse respiratory effects.
- Assess for nausea, vomiting, and diarrhea. Administer antiemetic and antidiarrheal medications as ordered. (In some settings, women are premedicated with these drugs).

Thorough inspection of the genital tract by the birth attendant allows recognition and timely repair of most lacerations. Genital tract lacerations should be suspected when vaginal bleeding persists in the presence of a firmly contracted uterus. The nurse who suspects a laceration should notify the clinician so that the laceration can be immediately sutured to control hemorrhage and repair the integrity of the reproductive tract.

Episiotomies can be a source of postpartal blood loss. Episiotomy is an often underappreciated source because of slow, steady bleeding. The risk for bleeding is increased with mediolateral episiotomies.

Retained Placental Fragments

Retained placental fragments may be a cause of immediate postpartal hemorrhage and are the most common cause of delayed hemorrhage. The most common cause of partial separation of the placenta with retention of fragments is massage of the fundus *prior* to placental separation, so this practice should be avoided.

Following birth, the placenta should always be inspected for intactness and evidence of missing fragments or cotyledons on the maternal side and for vessels that transverse to the edge of the placenta outward along the membranes of the fetal side, which may indicate succenturiate placenta and a retained lobe. Uterine exploration may be required at that time to remove missing fragments. This cause should be immediately suspected if bleeding persists and no lacerations are noted. Sonography may be used to diagnose retained placental fragments. Curettage, formerly standard treatment, is now thought by some to traumatize the implantation site, thereby increasing bleeding and the potential for uterine adhesions. It may be necessitated by the degree of hemorrhage, however (Cunningham et al, 1997).

Vulvar, Vaginal, and Pelvic Hematomas

Hematomas occur as a result of injury to a blood vessel from birth trauma, often without noticeable trauma to the superficial tissue or from inadequate hemostasis at the site of repair of an incision or laceration. The soft tissue in the area offers little resistance, and hematomas containing 250 to 500 mL of blood may develop rapidly. Hematomas may be vulvar (involving branches of the pudendal artery), vaginal (especially in the area of the ischial spines), vulvovaginal, or subperitoneal. The latter are rare but most dangerous because of the large amount of blood loss that can occur without clinical symptoms until the woman becomes hemodynamically unstable. Subperitoneal hematomas involve the uterine artery branches or vessels in the broad ligaments.

Risk factors for hematomas include the following: PIH, use of pudendal anesthesia, first full-term birth, precipitous labor, prolonged second stage of labor, macrosomia, forceps- or vacuum-assisted births, and history of vulvar varicosities. Frequent assessment of the perineum of the woman under the effects of regional anesthesia is important. Once the effects of anesthesia have subsided, vaginal and vulvar hematomas are generally associated with perineal pain, often intense and out of proportion to what seems apparent in the area. If the hematoma is localized in the posterior vaginal area, rectal pressure may also be a presenting complaint. Hematomas that develop in the upper vagina may cause difficulty voiding because of pressure against the urinary meatus or urethra. Rather than automatically attributing complaints of perineal pain to the presence of an episiotomy, the nurse should examine the perineal area for signs of hematomas: ecchymosis, edema, tenseness of tissue overlying the hematoma, a fluctuant mass bulging at the introitus, and extreme tenderness to palpation. Estimating the size on first assessment of the perineum enables the nurse to better identify increases in size and the potential blood loss. The nurse notifies the physician or certified nurse-midwife if a hematoma is suspected.

Hematomas less than 5 cm in size and nonexpanding are managed expectantly with ice packs and analgesia. They usually resolve over several days. For larger hematomas and those that expand, surgical management is usually required: the hematoma is evacuated, the bleeding vessel ligated, and the wound closed, with or without a vaginal packing. An indwelling urinary catheter may be necessary for 24 hours because voiding may be impossible with a vaginal pack in place (Cunningham et al, 1997).

The initial sign of subperitoneal hematoma may be hypovolemic shock; however, the woman may also complain of severe pelvic pain, flank pain, or abdominal distention. A parametrial mass may be identified on bimanual examination. Expectant management with serial ultrasonography and hematocrit may be possible. In rare cases, angiographic embolization or ligation of the hypogastric vessels may be required to manage the hemorrhage associated with postpartal hematomas.

The hematoma site is an ideal medium for proliferation of flora normally present in the genital tract. Consequently, broad-spectrum antibiotics are usually ordered to prevent infection or abscess.

The nurse can decrease the risk of vulvar or vaginal hematoma by applying an ice pack to the woman's perineum during the first hour after birth and intermittently thereafter for the next 8 to 12 hours. If a hematoma develops despite preventive measures, a sitz bath after the first 12 hours will aid fluid absorption once bleeding has stopped and will promote comfort, as will the judicious use of analgesic agents.

Uterine Inversion

Uterine inversion, a prolapse of the uterine fundus to or through the cervix so that the uterus is, in effect, turned inside-out after birth, is a rare (the incidence is 1 in 20,000 or more) but life-threatening cause of postpartal hemorrhage (Craigo & Kapernick, 1994). Although not always preventable, uterine inversion is often associated with these factors: fundal implantation or abnormal adherence of the placenta, weakness of the uterine musculature or other uterine abnormalities, protracted labor, uterine relaxation secondary to anesthesia or drugs such as magnesium sulfate, and excess traction on the umbilical cord or vigorous manual removal of the placenta.

Uterine Rupture

Spontaneous rupture of the uterus is rare in the United States but continues to be seen in developing countries where emergency surgery for obstructed labors may be less immediately accessible (Roberts, 1995). The woman with a ruptured uterus will have acute, severe abdominal pain, with minimal to diffuse external bleeding. Concealed hemorrhage may occur in the abdominal cavity or broad ligaments, undetected until the woman becomes symptomatic from hypovolemic shock. Risk factors for uterine rupture include prior uterine surgery, including cesarean birth; fetal malpresentation; grandmultiparity; operative vaginal birth; and oxytocic induction of labor. With uterine rupture, immediate surgery is required with fluid and blood replacement as needed (Norris, 1997).

Abnormal Placental Implantation

Normally, a layer of decidual tissue separates the proliferating placental villi from the myometrium at the site of placental implantation. A defect in the formation of this decidual layer, possibly related to a poorer blood supply, can contribute to a placenta that directly adheres to the myometrium (placenta accreta) or penetrates deeply into the myometrium (placenta increta). See Chapter 23. Abnormally adherent placentas are rare in normal pregnancies but occur in 5% of women with placenta previa, especially those with cesarean births (Roberts, 1995). Uncontrollable hemorrhage is possible; as a result, this complication is associated with emergency hysterectomy.

Coagulation Disorders (Coagulopathies)

Coagulopathies should be suspected when postpartal bleeding persists with no identifiable cause (Norris, 1997). Preexisting coagulation defects, such as von Willebrand's disease and idiopathic thrombocytopenia purpura, should have been identified prenatally and managed in consultation with a hematologist. A consumptive coagulopathy such as disseminated intravascular coagulation (DIC) may occur during pregnancy as a result of pregnancy-induced hypertension, amniotic fluid embolism, sepsis, abruptio placentae, or prolonged intrauterine fetal demise syndrome. Coagulopathy can also result from excessive blood loss (Roberts, 1995). Oozing from a puncture site or development of petechiae may be initial clues of coagulopathy. Coagulation studies (prothrombin time, partial thromboplastin time, platelet count, fibrinogen level, and fibrin degradation products) should be assessed immediately.

Late Postpartal Hemorrhage

Although early postpartal hemorrhage most often occurs within hours of birth, delayed hemorrhage occurs most often within 1 to 2 weeks after childbirth, most frequently as a result of subinvolution of the placental site due to retention of placental tissue. Blood loss at this time may be excessive but rarely poses the same risk as that from immediate postpartal hemorrhage.

The site of placental implantation is always the last area of the uterus to regenerate after childbirth. In the case of subinvolution, adjacent endometrium and the decidua basalis fail to regenerate to cover the placental site. Deficiency of immunologic factors has been implicated as a cause. Faulty implantation in the less vascular lower uterine segment, retention of placental tissue, or infection may contribute to subinvolution (Craigo & Kapernick, 1994). With **subinvolution,** the postpartum fundal height is greater than expected. In addition, lochia often fails to progress from rubra to serosa to alba normally. Lochia rubra that persists longer than 2 weeks postpartum is highly suggestive of subinvolution (Cunningham et al, 1997). Some women report scant brown lochia or irregular heavy bleeding. Leukorrhea, backache, and foul lochia may occur if infection is a cause. There may be a history of heavy early postpartal bleeding or difficulty in delivery of the placenta (Chin, 1997).

When portions of the placenta have been retained in the uterus, bleeding continues because normal uterine contraction that constricts the bleeding site is prohibited. Presence of placental tissue within the uterus can be confirmed by pelvic ultrasonography. Occasionally the placental fragment becomes necrotic over time and, when it separates from the uterus, hemorrhage occurs suddenly.

Subinvolution is most commonly diagnosed during the routine postpartal examination at 4 to 6 weeks. The woman may relate a history of irregular or excessive bleeding or describe the symptoms listed previously. An enlarged, softer than normal uterus, palpated bimanually, is an objective indication of subinvolution. Treatment includes oral administration of methylergonovine maleate (Methergine) 0.2 mg orally every 3 to 4 hours for 24 to 48 hours (see Drug Guide: Methergine, in Chapter 31, page 936). When uterine infection is present, antibiotics are also administered. The woman is reevaluated in 2 weeks. If retained placenta is suspected or other treatment is ineffective, curettage may be indicated (Cunningham et al, 1997).

NURSING CARE MANAGEMENT

Nursing Assessment and Diagnosis

Careful and ongoing assessment of the woman during labor and birth and evaluation of her prenatal history will help identify factors that put her at risk for postpartal hemorrhage. Following birth, periodic assessment for evidence of bleeding is a major nursing responsibility. Regular and frequent assessment of fundal height and evidence of uterine tone or contractility will alert the nurse to the possible development or recurrence of hemorrhage. Careful observation and documentation of vaginal

ESSENTIAL PRECAUTIONS IN PRACTICE

During Postpartal Hemorrhage

The same basic precautions that apply in caring for any woman during the postpartal period apply when caring for a woman experiencing postpartal hemorrhage. In addition, remember the following specifics:

- Wear gloves when assessing the perineum and when changing or disposing of peri-pads, chux, or linens soiled with blood or body fluids.
- Place blood-soaked disposable material in appropriate waste containers. Store blood-soaked bedding in an appropriate receptacle for the laundry according to agency procedure.
- Wear a splash apron when changing very soiled bedding or helping a clinician control severe hemorrhage.

For further information, consult OSHA and CDC guidelines.

CLINICAL TIP

As you know, bogginess indicates that the uterus is not contracting well, which results in increased uterine bleeding. This blood may remain in the uterus and form clots or may result in increased flow. In assessing the amount of blood loss, you must first massage the uterus until it is firm and then express clots. Don't be misled by the fact that a woman has a firm uterus. Significant bleeding can occur from causes other than uterine atony. To accurately determine the amount of blood loss, it is not sufficient to assess only the peri-pad. You should also ask the woman to turn on her side so you can assess underneath her for pooling of blood.

bleeding are important to determine whether further medical intervention is needed. This assessment can be done visually, by pad counts, or by weighing the perineal pads. See Essential Precautions in Practice: During Postpartal Hemorrhage.

Nursing diagnoses that may apply when a woman experiences postpartal hemorrhage include the following:

- ***Knowledge Deficit*** related to lack of information about signs of delayed postpartal hemorrhage
- ***Fluid Volume Deficit*** related to blood loss secondary to uterine atony, lacerations, hematomas, coagulation disorders, or retained placental fragments

Nursing Plan and Implementation

If the nurse detects a soft, boggy uterus, it is massaged until firm. If the uterus is not contracting well and appears larger than anticipated, the nurse may express clots during fundal massage. Once clots are removed, the uterus tends to contract more effectively.

If the woman seems to have a slow, steady, free flow of blood, the nurse begins weighing the perineal pads (1mL = 1g) and monitors the woman's vital signs at least every 15 minutes—more frequently if indicated. If the fundus is displaced upward or to one side because of a full bladder, the nurse encourages the woman to empty her bladder—or catheterizes her if she is unable to void—to allow for efficient uterine contractions.

When there are risk factors for postpartal hemorrhage or frequent fundal massage has been necessary to sustain uterine contractions, the nurse should maintain the vascular access (IV) initiated during labor in case additional fluid or blood becomes necessary. Sometimes physicians and certified nurse-midwives write orders that specify "discontinue IV after present bottle." The astute postpartum nurse will assess the consistency of the fundus and the presence of normal versus excessive lochia prior to discontinuing the infusion. If the assessments are not reassuring, the nurse continues the IV and notifies the physician or certified nurse-midwife.

In most settings, postpartum collection of blood for hemoglobin and hematocrit determination is routine. The nurse reviews these findings when available, compares them to the admission baseline, and notifies the physician or certified nurse-midwife if the hematocrit has decreased by 10 points or more. In cases where there is risk of postpartal hemorrhage and blood has been crossmatched earlier, the nurse checks that blood is available in the blood bank.

The nurse evaluates the woman for signs of anemia, such as fatigue, pallor, headache, thirst, and orthostatic changes in pulse or blood pressure, and reviews the results of all hematocrit determinations. All medical interventions, intravenous infusions, blood transfusions, oxygen therapy, and medications such as uterine stimulants are monitored as necessary and evaluated for effectiveness. Urinary output should be monitored to determine adequacy of fluid replacement and renal perfusion, with amounts less than 30 mL per hour reported to the physician. The nurse also helps the woman plan activities so that adequate rest is possible.

The woman who is experiencing anemia and fatigue related to hemorrhage may need assistance with self-care and progressive ambulation for several days. When she is able to be out of bed to shower, use of a shower chair permits independence while providing a measure of safety should the woman experience weakness or dizziness. The emergency call light should be easily accessible.

The mother may find it difficult to care for her baby because of the fatigue associated with blood loss. The nurse can often find ways to promote attachment while still recognizing the health needs of the mother. The mother may require additional assistance in caring for her infant. If she has intravenous lines in place, even carrying the newborn may be awkward. For the mother who feels compelled to do as much as possible, the nurse may also need to "give permission" to the mother to return her infant to the nursery so she can have adequate periods of uninterrupted rest.

If the father of the child is involved in the birth experience, including him in the plan of care is a productive strategy. He supports the mother's recovery by helping to meet her physical needs while encouraging her to rest. The mother is likely to feel less concern over her limited opportunities for newborn care if she can witness the father's interactions with and care for the newborn. The couple may wish for arrangements to be made for the father to stay in the hospital room, sleeping on a cot and eating with the mother so that limited rooming-in with the newborn is still an option. In that way, even if the mother is too fatigued to care for the infant, she can enjoy the infant's presence and bond with the baby. The extent to which the father becomes involved with the care of the mother and baby must be carefully balanced with his need to be rested for the extra responsibilities he will assume when his partner and newborn child are discharged from the hospital.

Teaching for Self-Care

The woman and her family or other support persons should receive clear, preferably written, explanations of the normal postpartal course, including changes in the lochia and fundus and signs of abnormal bleeding. Instructions for the prevention of bleeding should include fundal massage, ways to assess the fundal height and consistency, and inspection of the episiotomy and lacerations, if present. The woman should receive instruction in perineal care. The woman and her family are advised to contact their caregiver if any of the following occur: excessive or bright red bleeding (saturation of more than one pad per hour), a boggy fundus that does not respond to massage, abnormal clots, leukorrhea, high temperature, or any unusual pelvic or rectal discomfort or backache. See Table 33–2. If iron supplementation is ordered, instructions for proper dosage should be provided in order to enhance absorption and avoid constipation and stomach upset.

Community-Based Nursing Care

For most postpartal women, routine discharge instructions include advice such as: "You take care of the baby, and let someone else care for you, the family, and the household." Because of her fatigue and weakened condition, the woman who experienced postpartal hemorrhage may be unable even to care for her newborn unassisted. The caregivers at home need clear, concise explanations of her condition and needs for recovery. For example, all should understand the woman's need to rest and to be given extra time to rest after any necessary activity.

To ensure her safety, the woman should be advised to rise slowly to minimize the likelihood of orthostatic hypotension. Until she regains strength, the mother should be seated when holding the newborn.

TABLE 33–2 Signs of Postpartal Hemorrhage

Excessive or bright red bleeding
A boggy fundus that does not respond to massage
Abnormal clots
Any unusual pelvic discomfort or backache
Persistent bleeding in the presence of a firmly contracted uterus
Rise in the level of the fundus of the uterus
Increased pulse or decreased BP
Hematoma formation or bulging/shiny skin in the perineal area
Decreased level of consciousness

The person who assumes responsibility for grocery shopping and meal preparation will need advice about the importance of including foods high in iron in the daily menus. Having the woman indicate her preferences from a list of such foods will promote cooperation with the diet. The nurse also explains the rationale for continuing medications containing iron.

The woman should continue to count perineal pads for several days so she can recognize any recurring problem with excessive blood loss. The debilitated condition and anemia associated with hemorrhage increase the woman's risk of puerperal infection. She and her caregivers should use good hand-washing technique and minimize exposure to infection in the home. They should be given a list of signs of infection and should understand the importance of alerting the physician immediately should signs occur.

A sense of emergency often exists in the event of late postpartal hemorrhage. Because it commonly occurs 1 to 2 weeks after birth, the couple is generally at home, involved in the day-to-day activities demanded by their new roles, when the unexpected, excessive bleeding begins. Quick decisions about child care arrangements must often be made so that the mother can return to the hospital. Both mother and father are likely to be alarmed by the excessive bleeding and concerned about her prognosis. There will be additional worries about separation from the newborn, especially when the mother is breastfeeding. The father may find himself torn between the needs of the mother and those of the newborn. Ideally, arrangements can be made to minimize separation of the family members.

In addition to meeting the woman's physical needs, which may include those related to recovery from emergency dilation and curettage (D & C), the nurse will assess the couple for impending crisis by addressing these factors: (1) What is their perception of the current situation? Is the perception realistic? (2) What coping strategies have been helpful in previous difficult circumstances? Are they in use at this time, and are they effective? (3) What degree of support do they have from significant others? Do they have necessary resources? Providing realistic information, offering to call those in their support network, and exploring effective coping strategies can be of immeasurable value as they try to maintain a sense of balance in this difficult situation.

Evaluation

Expected outcomes of nursing care include:

- Signs of postpartal hemorrhage are detected quickly and managed effectively.
- Maternal-infant attachment is maintained successfully.
- The woman is able to identify abnormal changes that might occur following discharge and understands the importance of notifying her caregiver if they develop. ●

CRITICAL THINKING QUESTION

If hypovolemic shock is present, what signs might you see?

Care of the Woman with a Reproductive Tract Infection or Wound

Because shortened inpatient stays are the norm in maternity care, women will be discharged following childbirth before clinical signs of puerperal infection are evident. Consequently, hospital-based nurses are challenged to analyze the woman's history and clinical course for risk assessment and to recognize the sometimes early subtle signs of infection so that discharge may be delayed as needed. Prior to discharge, the nurse advises the postpartal woman about preventive measures and signs of infection. Community and home care nurses review the prenatal and birth record for continuity of risk assessment, conduct physical assessment for objective findings of infection, collect specimens as ordered for diagnosing infection, and collaborate with the primary caregiver in managing infection.

Obviously, postpartal women are at risk for both genital and other sources of infection. A thorough history, including antepartal and intrapartal risk assessments, help differentiate the site of infection, including the possibility of exposure to illness prior to admission in labor. When fever occurs, the physical examination should include the pharynx, neck, lungs, costovertebral angle (CVA) region, breasts, abdomen, extremities, IV sites, and incisions. Timing of fever also helps in differentiating the source of infection: atelectasis generally occurs within the first 48 hours; pneumonia or urinary tract infection usually occurs within 72 hours after childbirth; and wound infections and septic thrombophlebitis are likely to occur at 3 to 7 days postpartum, with wound abscess formation at 7 to 14 days. Although mastitis may occur as early as 3 to 7 days, it usually presents at 2 weeks postpartum, as does pulmonary embolism (Calhoun & Brost, 1995).

Puerperal infection is an infection of the reproductive tract associated with childbirth that occurs at any time up to 6 weeks postpartum. The most common postpartal infection is metritis (endometritis), which is limited to the uterus. However, infection can spread by way of the lymphatic system and circulatory system to become a progressive disease resulting in parametrial cellulitis and peritonitis. The woman's prognosis is directly related to the stage of the disease at the time of diagnosis, the causative organism, and the state of her health and immune system.

The standard definition of **puerperal morbidity** established in the 1930s by the Joint Committee on Maternal Welfare is a temperature of 38C (100.4F) or higher, with the temperature occurring on any 2 of the first 10 days postpartum, exclusive of the first 24 hours, and when taken by mouth by a standard technique at least four times a day. However, serious infections can occur in the first 24 hours or may cause only persistent low-grade temperatures. Therefore, careful assessment of all postpartal women with elevated temperatures is essential.

Antibiotic therapy alone has not caused the decrease in postpartal morbidity and mortality that is seen today. Aseptic technique, fewer traumatic operative births, a better understanding of labor dystocia, improved surgical intervention, and a population that is generally at less risk from malnutrition and chronic debilitative disease have also contributed to this reduction.

The vagina and cervix of approximately 70% of all healthy pregnant women contain pathogenic bacteria that, alone or in combination, are sufficiently virulent to cause extensive infections. Why the organisms do not cause infection during pregnancy is not altogether clear; however, recent studies indicate that more than the presence of a pathogen in the woman's reproductive tract is necessary for infection to begin.

Although the uterus is considered a sterile cavity prior to rupture of the fetal membranes, bacterial contamination of amniotic fluid with the membranes still intact at term is more common than previously believed and may contribute to premature labor. Following rupture of the membranes and during labor, contamination of the uterine cavity by vaginal or cervical bacteria can easily occur. Despite that finding, uterine infections are relatively uncommon following uncomplicated vaginal births. They continue to be a major source of morbidity for women who deliver by cesarean, occurring in 12% to 51% of cases (Gibbs & Sweet, 1999).

Postpartal Uterine Infection

Postpartal uterine infection is known variously as metritis, endometritis, endomymetritis, and endoparametritis. Because the infection involves the decidual lining of the uterus, the myometrium, and parametrial tissue, some authorities are proposing the terminology *metritis with parametrial cellulitis* (Cunningham et al, 1997). Risk factors for postpartal uterine infection include the following:

- Cesarean birth is the single most significant risk
- Prolonged rupture of the amniotic membranes (PROM)
- Multiple vaginal examinations during labor
- Compromised health status (low socioeconomic status, anemia, obesity, smoker, user of illicit drugs or alcohol)
- Use of fetal scalp electrode or intrauterine pressure catheter for internal monitoring during labor
- Obstetric trauma—episiotomy, laceration of perineum, vagina, or cervix
- Chorioamnionitis
- Preexisting bacterial vaginosis or *Chlamydia trachomatis* infection
- Instrument-assisted childbirth—vacuum or forceps
- Manual removal of the placenta
- Lapses in aseptic technique by surgical staff

Endometritis (Metritis)

Endometritis, or **metritis,** an inflammation of the endometrium, may occur postpartally. After expulsion of the placenta, the placental site provides an excellent culture medium for bacterial growth. The site in the contracted uterus is a round, dark red, elevated area of 4 cm, with a nodular surface composed of numerous veins, many of which may become occluded because of clot formation. The remaining portion of the decidua is also susceptible to infection because of its thinness (approximately 2 mm) and its large blood supply. The cervix presents a bacterial breeding ground because of multiple small lacerations attending normal labor and spontaneous birth. Pathogenic bacteria deposited at the cervix during vaginal examinations and those that are already present infect the decidua and eventually involve the entire mucosa. If the infection is confined to this region, the area will be necrotic and will be sloughed off within 3 to 5 days. With the extra surgical trauma associated with cesarean birth, more tissue is devitalized and there are more foreign bodies (eg, sutures) and blood, which can act as a medium for bacterial proliferation, making infection more probable. Both aerobic and anaerobic organisms cause postpartal uterine infections. Late-onset postpartal endometritis/metritis is most commonly associated with genital mycoplasmas and *Chlamydia trachomatis.* Chlamydia trachomatis has a longer replication time and latency period than other bacteria and is not consistently eradicated by antibiotics used for early postpartal infections.

In mild cases of endometritis, the woman generally has vaginal discharge that may be scant or profuse, bloody, and foul smelling. In more severe cases, she also has uterine tenderness; saw-tooth temperature spikes, usually between 38.3C (101F) and 40C (104F); tachycardia; and chills. Foul-smelling lochia is cited as a classic sign of endometritis, but in the case of infection with β-hemolytic streptococcus, the lochia may be scant and odorless (Cunningham et al, 1997).

Pelvic Cellulitis (Parametritis)

Pelvic cellulitis (parametritis) is infection involving the connective tissue of the broad ligament or, in more severe forms, the connective tissue of all the pelvic structures. The infection generally ascends upward in the pelvis by way of the lymphatic vessels in the uterine wall but may also occur if pathogenic organisms invade a cervical laceration that extends upward into the connective tissue of the broad ligament—a direct pathway into the pelvis.

A pelvic abscess may form in the case of postpartal peritonitis and most commonly is found in the uterine ligaments, cul-de-sac of Douglas, and the subdiaphragmatic space. Pelvic cellulitis may be a secondary result of pelvic vein thrombophlebitis. This condition occurs when the clot, usually in the right ovarian vein, becomes infected, and the wall of the vein breaks down from necrosis, spilling the infection into the connective tissues of the pelvis.

As the course of pelvic cellulitis advances, a mass of exudate develops along the base of the broad ligament that may push the uterus toward the opposite wall (if the infection is unilateral), where it will become fixed. If the exudate spreads into the rectocervical septum, a firm mass develops behind the cervix instead. The abscess that results should be drained or resolved through appropriate antibiotic therapy to avoid rupture of the abscess into the peritoneal cavity and development of a possibly fatal peritonitis.

A woman suffering from parametritis may demonstrate a variety of symptoms, including marked high temperature (38.9C to 40C or 102F to 104F), chills, malaise, lethargy, abdominal pain, subinvolution of the uterus, tachycardia, and local and referred rebound tenderness. If peritonitis develops, the woman will be acutely ill with severe pain; marked anxiety; high fever; rapid, shallow respirations; pronounced tachycardia; excessive thirst; abdominal distention; nausea; and vomiting. Infection involving the peritoneal cavity is **peritonitis.**

Perineal Wound Infections

Given the degree of bacterial contamination that occurs with normal vaginal birth, it is surprising that more women do not have infections of the episiotomy or repaired lacerations of perineum, vagina, or vulva. When perineal wound infection does occur, it is recognized by the classic signs: redness, warmth, edema, purulent drainage, and later, gaping of the wound that has previously been well approximated. Local pain may be severe. Infected perineal wounds, like other infected wounds, are treated by draining purulent material. Sutures are removed, and the wound is left open. A regimen of broad-spectrum antibiotics is used. When the surface of the wound is free of infectious exudate and tissue granulation is evident, the mother returns for secondary closure of the wound under regional anesthesia (Cunningham et al, 1997).

Cesarean Wound Infections

The infection rate following cesarean births is 4% to 12%, with the highest rate occurring after emergency cesarean because there is more traumatization of the tissue. Predisposing factors include obesity, diabetes mellitus, prolonged postpartal hospitalization, PROM, metritis, prolonged labor, anemia, steroid therapy, and immunosuppression (Gibbs & Sweet, 1999). Signs of an abdominal wound infection, which may not be evident until after discharge, include erythema; warmth; skin discoloration; edema; tenderness; purulent drainage, sometimes mixed with serosanguineous fluid; or gaping of the wound edges. Fever, pain, malodorous lochia, and other systemic signs of infection are also common. Abdominal distention and decreased bowel sounds may be noted. Culture of wound drainage commonly reveals mixed pathogens.

Postpartal wound dehiscence (opening of wound edges) is uncommon because pregnant women are usually a healthy population and because lower uterine/skin (Pfannensteil) incisions rarely dehisce. An infected open wound may be left open for delayed closure after the debridement.

Clinical Therapy

The infection site and causative organism are diagnosed by careful history and complete physical examination, blood tests, aerobic and anaerobic endometrial cultures (although this may be of limited value, because multiple organisms are usually present), and urinalysis to rule out urinary tract infection. When a localized infection develops, it is treated with antibiotics, sitz baths, and analgesics as necessary for pain relief. If an abscess has developed or a stitch site is infected, the suture is removed, and the area is allowed to drain. Packing the wound with saline gauze twice to three times daily, using aseptic technique, allows removal of necrotic debris when packing is removed. Broad-spectrum antibiotic coverage is used to treat postpartal wound infections. Cephalosporins, penicillinase-resistant penicillin, and vancomycin are commonly used with anaerobic coverage by clindamycin or ampicillin/sulbactam (Gibbs & Sweet, 1999).

Endometritis (metritis) is treated by the administration of antibiotics. With appropriate antibiotic coverage, improvement should occur within a few days. Antibiotics are generally continued until the woman is afebrile for 24 to 48 hours. If the clinical manifestations show no response to the drugs, the clinician should consider the possibility of nonpelvic causes of infection, septic thrombophlebitis, or pelvic abscess. The route and dosage are determined by the severity of the infection. Careful monitoring is also necessary to prevent the development of a more serious infection.

Parametritis and peritonitis are treated with intravenous antibiotics. Broad-spectrum antibiotics effective against the most common causative organisms are chosen initially until the results of culture and sensitivity reports are available. If multiple organisms are present, the approach to antibiotic therapy is continued unless no improvement is observed; then the antibiotic is changed.

An abscess is frequently manifested by the development of a palpable mass and may be confirmed with ultrasound. An abscess usually requires incision and drainage to avoid rupture into the peritoneal cavity and the possible development of peritonitis. After drainage of the abscess, the cavity may be packed with iodoform gauze to promote drainage and facilitate healing.

The woman with a severe systemic infection is acutely ill and may require care in an intensive care unit. Supportive therapy includes maintenance of adequate hydration with intravenous fluids, analgesic medications, ongoing assessment of the infection, and possibly continuous nasogastric suctioning if paralytic ileus develops.

Standard antibiotic coverage has been provided by clindamycin and gentamicin, broad-spectrum antibiotics with nearly 90% effectiveness. Single-agent therapy with effectiveness against aerobic and anaerobic organisms is slightly less effective. Third-generation cephalosporins, such as cefoxitin, have also been of value in cases of metritis. Antibiotics are generally continued until the woman has been afebrile for 48 hours. Oral antibiotics are rarely needed on discharge.

NURSING CARE MANAGEMENT

Nursing Assessment and Diagnosis

The nurse should inspect the woman's perineum every 8 to 12 hours for signs of early infection. The REEDA scale helps the nurse remember to consider *r*edness, *e*dema, *e*cchymosis, *d*ischarge, and *a*pproximation. Any degree of induration (hardening) should be immediately reported to the clinician.

Fever, malaise, abdominal pain, foul-smelling lochia, larger than expected uterus, tachycardia, and other signs of infection should be noted and reported immediately so that treatment can begin. The WBC count, a usual objective measure of infection, cannot be used reliably because of the normal increase in white blood cells during the postpartum period; a WBC of 14,000 to 16,000 mm is not an unusual finding. Some clinicians believe that WBC counts of 20,000 plus are not abnormal at this time, likely resulting from the physiologic stress response of labor and also cite a primary increase in neutrophils. An increase in WBC level of more than 30% in a 6-hour period, however, is indicative of infection.

Nursing diagnoses that may apply to the women with a puerperal infection include the following:

- ***Risk for Injury*** related to the spread of infection
- ***Pain*** related to the presence of infection
- ***Knowledge Deficit*** related to lack of information about condition and its treatment
- ***Risk for Altered Parenting*** related to delayed parent-infant attachment secondary to woman's malaise and other symptoms of infection

Nursing Plan and Implementation

Hospital-Based Nursing Care

Careful attention to aseptic technique during labor, birth, and postpartum is essential.

The nurse caring for a woman during the postpartal period is responsible for teaching the woman self-care measures that are helpful in preventing infection. The woman should understand the importance of good perineal care, hygiene practices to prevent contamination of the perineum (such as wiping from front to back, changing the perineal pad after voiding), and thorough hand washing. Once edema and perineal pain are under control, the nurse can also encourage sitz baths, which are cleansing and promote healing. Adequate fluid intake, coupled with a diet high in protein and vitamin C, which are necessary to promote wound healing, also helps prevent infection.

If the woman has a draining wound or purulent lochia, it is especially important that those in contact with soiled items and linens practice good hand washing. Clear, concise instructions about wound care and how to discard soiled dressings appropriately must be provided to safeguard the woman and her caregivers.

If the woman is seriously ill, ongoing assessment of urine specific gravity and intake and output is necessary. The nurse also carefully administers antibiotics as ordered and regulates the intravenous fluids. Ongoing assessment of the woman's condition is vital to detect subtle changes in her health status. The nurse also recognizes the woman's comfort needs related to hygiene, positioning, oral hygiene, and pain relief.

Promoting maternal-infant attachment can be difficult with the acutely ill woman. The nurse may provide pictures of the infant and keep the mother informed of the infant's well-being. If she feels up to it, the new mother will also benefit from brief visits with her newborn.

The woman who wishes to breastfeed when her condition allows can maintain lactation by pumping her breasts regularly. The mother needs to know that this special mothering opportunity is simply delayed, not eliminated, by the infectious process and may improve the woman's morale.

The partner of a seriously ill woman has particular needs. He will be concerned about her condition and torn about spending time with her and with their newborn. Because maternal-infant bonding may be compromised, father-newborn bonding can be especially important. Mementos, such as a footprint, a note "written" by the baby to the mother, or a videotape of the baby can be comforting to the mother during their separation. See the Critical Pathway for the Woman with a Puerperal Infection on pages 992 to 994 for specific nursing measures.

Community-Based Nursing Care

The woman with a puerperal infection needs assistance when she is discharged from the hospital. If the family cannot provide this home assistance, a referral to home care services is needed. Home care services should be contacted as soon as puerperal infection is diagnosed so that the nurse can meet with the woman for a family and home assessment and development of a home care plan.

The family needs instruction in the care of a newborn, including feeding, bathing, cord care, immunizations, and significant observations that should be reported. A well-baby appointment should be scheduled. Breastfeeding mothers receiving antibiotics should be instructed to inspect the infant's mouth for signs of thrush and to report the finding to their physician.

The mother should be instructed regarding activity, rest, medications, diet, and signs and symptoms of complications, and she should be scheduled for a return medical visit. She needs to know the importance of taking the entire course of prescribed antibiotics even though she may begin to feel better before the bottle is empty. She also needs to be informed about the importance of pelvic rest; that is, she should not use tampons or douches nor have intercourse until she has been examined by the physician and told it is safe to resume those activities.

Evaluation

Expected outcomes of nursing care include:

- The infection is quickly assessed, and treatment is instituted successfully without further complications.
- The woman understands the nature of the infection and the purpose of therapy; she carries out any ongoing antibiotic therapy necessary after discharge.
- Maternal-infant attachment is maintained. ●

Care of the Woman with a Urinary Tract Infection (UTI)

Urinary tract infection occurs in 2% to 4% of postpartal women (Clark, 1995) and represents the second most common postpartal infection. The postpartal woman is at increased risk of developing urinary tract problems because of the normal postpartal diuresis, increased bladder capacity, decreased bladder sensitivity from stretching or

Text continues on page 994.

CRITICAL PATHWAY FOR THE WOMAN WITH A PUERPERAL INFECTION

Category	1–4 Hours Postpartum	4–8 Hours Postpartum	8–24 Hours Postpartum
Referral	Report from labor nurse if not continuing in an LDR room	Lactation consultation if needed	Home nursing referral if indicated **Expected Outcomes** Appropriate resources identified and utilized
Assessment	Postpartum assessments q$\frac{1}{2}$h ×2, q1h ×2, then q4h. Includes: • Fundus firm, in midline, at or below umbilicus • Lochia rubra <1 pad/h; no free flow or passage of clots with massage • Bladder: voids large amounts of urine spontaneously; bladder not palpable following voiding • Perineum: sutures intact; no bulging or marked swelling; no c/o severe pain. Minimal bruising may be present. If hemorrhoids present, no tenseness or marked engorgement; <2 cm diameter. • Breasts: soft, colostrum present Vital signs: • BP WNL; no hypotension; not >30 mm systolic or 15 mm diastolic over baseline • Temperature: <38C (100.4F) • Pulse: Bradycardia normal; consistent with baseline • Respirations: 12–20/min; quiet; easy Comfort level: <3 on scale of 1 to 10	Continue postpartum assessment q4h ×2, then q8h • Assess for bowel sounds • Assess lochia for color, odor, amount Breasts: evaluate nipple status; should be no evidence of cracks or bruising Observe feeding technique with newborn Assess VS q8h; all WNL; report temp >38C (100.4F) Continue assessment of comfort level q3–4h	Continue postpartum assessment q8h Breasts: nipples should remain free of cracks, fissures, bruising Feeding technique with newborn should be good or improving Assess VS q4h; report temp >38C (100.4F) Continue assessment of comfort level q3–4h Continue s/sx of infection (ie, episiotomy, endometritis, pelvic cellulitis, or puerperal peritonitis) Inspect incision/episiotomy for redness, approximation, and drainage Assess for signs of progressive infection (ie, uterine subinvolution, foul-smelling lochia, uterine tenderness, severe lower abdominal pain, fever, elevated WBC, malaise, chills, lethargy, tachycardia, nausea and vomiting, abdominal rigidity) **Expected Outcomes** Findings indicate infection identified, treated and reduced or eliminated in timely manner No additional complications found
Comfort	Institute comfort measures: • Perineal discomfort: peri-care, sitz baths, topical analgesics • Hemorrhoids: sitz baths, topical analgesics, digital replacement of external hemorrhoids, side-lying or prone position • Afterpains: prone with small pillow under abdomen; warm shower or sitz baths; ambulation Administer pain medication__________	Continue with pain management techniques	Continue with pain management techniques Promote comfort by: • Ensuring adequate periods of rest • Minimizing disturbing environmental stimuli • Judicious use of analgesics and antipyretics • Providing emotional support • Using supportive nursing measures (ie, back rubs, instruction in relaxation techniques, maintenance of cleanliness, provision of diversional activities)
Teaching/ psychosocial	Explain postpartum assessments Teach self-massage of fundus and expected findings Instruct to call for assistance first time OOB and prn Demonstrate peri-care, surgigator, sitz baths prn Explain comfort measures Begin newborn teaching (bulb suctioning, positioning, feeding, diaper change, cord care) Orient to room if transferred from LDR room Provide information on early postpartum period If breastfeeding mother is unable to nurse, assist her in pumping her breasts to maintain adequate milk supply	Discuss psychologic changes of postpartum period Stress need for frequent rest periods Continue newborn teaching: soothing/comforting techniques, swaddling; return demonstrations indicate woman's understanding Provide opportunities for questions and review; reinforce previous teaching Breastfeeding: nipple care; air-drying, lanolin; tea bags; proper latch-on technique Bottle-feeding: supportive bra; ice bags, breast binder **Expected Outcomes** Client verbalizes/demonstrates understanding of teaching and related plan of care Client incorporates teaching into self-care	Reinforce previous teaching: answer questions Discuss need to take antibiotics until course completed Discuss involution; anticipated physical changes in first 2 weeks postpartum; postpartum exercises; need to limit visitors Breastfeeding/bottle-feeding: • Explain milk production, let-down reflex, use of supplements, breast pumping, and milk storage • If cannot breastfeed, assist mother with pumping her breasts • Explain formula preparation and storage Discuss sibling rivalry; mother should have plan for supporting siblings at home Teaching evaluation completed

Category	1–4 Hours Postpartum	4–8 Hours Postpartum	8–24 Hours Postpartum
Therapeutic nursing interventions and reports	Ice pack to perineum to decrease swelling and increase comfort Straight cath prn × 1 if distended or voiding small amounts If continues unable to void or voiding small amounts, insert Foley catheter and notify CNM/physician	Sitz baths prn If woman Rh− and infant Rh+, RhoGAM work up; obtain consent; complete teaching Obtain consent for rubella vaccine if indicated; explain purpose, procedure, implications Obtain hematocrit Determine rubella status **Expected Outcomes** Labs and cultures indicate infection reduced/resolved Complications have been minimized	Continue sitz baths 2–3 times/day or surgigator May shower if ambulating without difficulty Obtain blood cultures per dr order if temp elevated Obtain wound culture and assist with wound drainage and packing Use principles of medical asepsis in handwashing and disposal of contaminated material by client and caregiver Promote normal wound healing by peri-care, wiping front to back after each voiding, frequent changing of pads
Activity	Assistance when OOB first time, then prn Ambulate ad lib Rests comfortably between checks	Encourage rest periods Ambulate ad lib; may leave birthing unit	Up ad lib **Expected Outcomes** Optimal comfort and activity maintained
Nutrition	Regular diet, high in vit C and protein Fluid intake ≥2000 mL/day	Continue diet and fluids **Expected Outcomes** Nutritional needs met with emphasis on calories needed for healing	Continue diet and fluids Increase calories by 500 kcal over nonpregnant state (200 kcal over pregnant intake) if breast-feeding Return to normal caloric intake for nonpregnant state if bottle feeding
Elimination	Voiding large amounts straw-colored urine	Voiding large quantities May have bowel movement, assess bowel sounds	Monitor I/O, urine specific gravity, and level of hydration **Expected Outcomes** Intake and output WNL
Medications	Methergine 0.2 mg q4h prn if ordered Stool softener___________ Tucks pads prn	Continue meds Lanolin to nipples prn; tea bags to nipples if tender; heparin flush to buffalo cap (if present) q8h or as ordered	IV antibiotics Continue meds May take own prenatal vitamins RhoGAM administered if indicated Rubella vaccine administered if indicated **Expected Outcomes** Infection successfully treated Medications utilized to further support health
Discharge planning/ home care	Evaluate knowledge of normal postpartum, newborn care Evaluate support systems	Discuss typical newborn schedule; plan for periods of rest Birth certificate paperwork completed Evaluate plans for transporting newborn; car seat used	Provide information regarding predisposing factors, s/sx, and treatment Discuss the value of a nutritious diet in promoting healing Review hygiene practice (ie, correct wiping after voiding, and hand washing, to prevent the spread of infection) Discuss home care routines to be used following postpartal infection Review discharge instruction sheet and check-list Describe postpartum and infection warning signs and when to call CNM/physician Provide prescriptions; gift pack given to woman Arrangements made for baby pictures if desired Postpartum visit scheduled Newborn check scheduled **Expected Outcomes** Woman participates in self-care and continued medication therapy Discharge teaching complete with emphasis on follow-up care, adequate rest and infant attachment

Category	1–4 Hours Postpartum	4–8 Hours Postpartum	8–24 Hours Postpartum
Family involvement	Identify available support persons Assess family perceptions of birth experience Parenting: demonstrates culturally expected early parenting behaviors	Involve support persons in care, teaching; answer questions Evidence of parental bonding behaviors apparent Provide and maintain mother-infant interaction: • Provide opportunities for the mother to see and hold her infant • Encourage partner or support person to discuss infant with woman and to become involved in infant's care if the woman is not able to do so	Continue to involve support persons in teaching Evidence of parental bonding behaviors continued Plans made for providing support to mother following discharge. Support persons verbalize understanding of need for woman to rest, eat nutritionally, recover **Expected Outcomes** Family demonstrates understanding of resources Support network identified Family development unimpaired
Date			

trauma, and possible inhibited neural control of the bladder following the use of general or regional anesthesia and contamination from catheterization.

Emptying the bladder is vital. Women who have not sufficiently recovered from the effects of anesthesia cannot void spontaneously, and catheterization is necessary.

Retention of residual urine, bacteria introduced at the time of catheterization, and a bladder traumatized by childbirth combine to provide an excellent environment for the development of cystitis. As many as 5% of women who have one catheterization, and 50% of those with intermittent catheterization develop bacteriuria (Clark, 1995).

Overdistention of the Bladder

Overdistention occurs postpartally when the woman is unable to empty her bladder as a result of the predisposing factors previously identified. After the effects of regional anesthesia have worn off, postpartal urinary retention is highly indicative of urinary tract infection.

Clinical Therapy

Overdistention in the early postpartal period is often managed by draining the bladder with a straight catheter as a one-time measure. If the overdistention recurs or is diagnosed later in the postpartal period, an indwelling catheter is generally ordered for 24 hours.

NURSING CARE MANAGEMENT

Nursing Assessment and Diagnosis

The overdistended bladder appears as a large mass, reaching sometimes to the umbilicus and displacing the uterine fundus upward. There is increased vaginal bleeding, the fundus is boggy, and the woman may complain of cramping as the uterus attempts to contract. Some women also experience backache and restlessness.

Nursing diagnoses that may apply when a woman has difficulties due to overdistention include the following:

- ***Risk for Infection*** related to urinary stasis secondary to overdistention
- ***Urinary Retention*** related to decreased bladder sensitivity and normal postpartal diuresis

Nursing Plan and Implementation

Diligent monitoring of the bladder during the recovery period and preventive health measures greatly reduce the chance for overdistention of the bladder. Encouraging the mother to void spontaneously and helping her use the toilet, if possible, or the bedpan if she has received conductive anesthesia, prevents overdistention in most cases. The nurse assists the woman to a normal position for voiding (ie, sitting with the legs and feet lower than the trunk) and provides privacy to encourage voiding. The woman should be medicated for whatever pain she may be having before attempting to void because pain may cause a reflex spasm of the urethra. Perineal ice packs applied after birth will minimize any edema, which may interfere with voiding. Pouring warm water over the perineum or having the woman void in a sitz bath may also be effective.

If catheterization becomes necessary, careful, meticulous, aseptic technique should be employed during catheter insertion. The vagina and vulva are traumatized to some degree by vaginal birth, and edema is common. This edema may obscure the urinary meatus; therefore the nurse needs to be extremely careful in cleansing the vulva and inserting the catheter. It is imperative to discard a catheter that has inadvertently been introduced into the vagina and thus contaminated. Because catheterization is an uncomfortable procedure due to the postpartal trauma and edema of the tissue, the nurse should be careful and gentle not only in inserting the catheter but also in handling and cleaning the perineal area.

If the amount of urine drained from the bladder reaches 900 to 1000 mL, the catheter should be clamped and taped firmly to the woman's leg. The nurse should carefully document the procedure, including taking the woman's vital signs before and after the procedure and noting her responses. After an hour, the catheter may be unclamped and removed or, in the case of an indwelling catheter, placed on gravity drainage. This technique protects the bladder and avoids rapid intra-abdominal decompression. When the indwelling catheter is removed, a urine specimen is often sent to the laboratory. The tip of the catheter may also be removed and sent for culture.

Evaluation

Expected outcomes of nursing care include:

- The woman voids adequately to meet the demands of the increased fluid shifts during the postpartal period.
- The woman doesn't develop infection due to stasis of urine.
- The woman actively incorporates self-care measures to decrease bladder overdistention. ●

Cystitis (Lower Urinary Tract Infection)

Escherichia coli has been demonstrated to be the causative agent in most cases of postpartal cystitis and pyelonephritis (in both lower and upper UTI). In most cases, the infection ascends the urinary tract from the urethra to the bladder and then to the kidneys because vesiculoureteral reflux forces contaminated urine into the renal pelvis.

Clinical Therapy

When cystitis is suspected, a clean-catch midstream urine sample is obtained for microscopic examination, culture, and sensitivity tests. The specimen may require collection by the nurse with the woman on a bedpan because few postpartal women can collect a true midstream, clean-catch specimen without contaminating the specimen with lochia. A catheterized specimen is avoided when possible because of the increased risk of infection. When the bacterial concentration is greater than 100,000 colonies of the same organism per milliliter of fresh urine, infection is generally present. Counts between 10,000 and 100,000 suggest infection, particularly if clinical symptoms are noted.

Treatment is theoretically delayed until urine culture and sensitivity reports are available. In the clinical setting, however, antibiotic therapy is often initiated using trimethoprim-sulfamethoxazole (Bactrim, Septra), one of the short-acting sulfonamides, nitrofurantoin (Macrodantin), or, in the case of sulfa allergy, ampicillin. The antibiotic is begun immediately and then can be changed if indicated by the results of the sensitivity report (Cunningham et al, 1997). Antispasmodic or urinary analgesic agents, such as Pyridium, may be given to relieve discomfort.

Pyelonephritis (Upper Urinary Tract Infection)

Pyelonephritis is an infection of the upper urinary tract. In most cases, the infection has ascended from the lower urinary tract. It occurs more commonly on the right, although both kidneys may be affected. If untreated, the renal cortex may be damaged and kidney function impaired.

Clinical Therapy

When pyelonephritis is diagnosed, intravenous antibiotic therapy is begun immediately. If sensitivity reports so indicate, the antibiotic can be changed later. Bed rest and careful monitoring of intake and output are necessary to detect the development of bacterial shock. Fluids are encouraged. Antispasmodic, analgesic, and antipyretic medications are given to relieve discomfort. The woman usually continues to take antibiotics for 2 to 4 weeks after clinical and bacteriologic response. A clean-catch urine culture should be obtained 2 weeks after completion of therapy and then periodically for the next 2 years. An intravenous pyelogram may be ordered in 2 to 4 months to identify any residual renal damage.

Continuation of breastfeeding during therapy is limited only by the degree of the mother's malaise and clinical discomfort. For the breastfeeding mother, the antibiotic should be selected carefully to avoid problems for the infant via the milk.

NURSING CARE MANAGEMENT

Nursing Assessment and Diagnosis

Symptoms of cystitis often appear 2 to 3 days after birth. The initial symptoms of cystitis may include frequency, urgency, dysuria, and nocturia. Hematuria and suprapubic pain may also be present. A slightly elevated temperature may occur, but systemic symptoms are often absent.

When a urinary tract infection progresses to pyelonephritis, systemic symptoms usually occur, and the woman becomes acutely ill. Symptoms include chills, high fever, flank pain (unilateral or bilateral), nausea, and vomiting, in addition to all the signs of lower UTI. Costovertebralangle tenderness on palpation and pain also may or may not be present. The nurse obtains a urine culture so that sensitivity tests can identify the causative organism.

Nursing diagnoses that may apply if a woman develops a UTI postpartally include the following:

- ***Pain*** with voiding related to dysuria secondary to infection
- ***Knowledge Deficit*** related to lack of information about self-care measures to prevent UTI

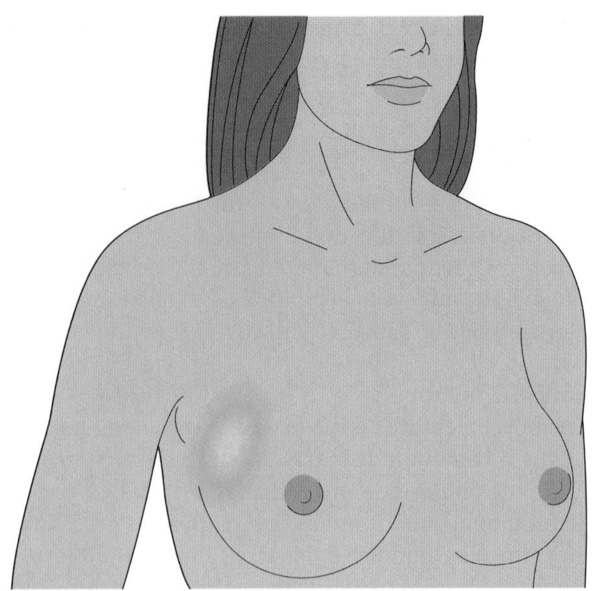

FIGURE 33–2 Mastitis. Erythema and swelling are present in the upper outer quadrant of the breast. Axillary lymph nodes are enlarged and tender.

Nursing Plan and Implementation

Screening for asymptomatic bacteriuria in pregnancy should be routine. Frequent emptying of the bladder during labor and postpartum should be encouraged to prevent overdistention and trauma to the bladder. Catheterization technique and nursing actions to prevent overdistention (previously discussed) also apply. The woman with pyelonephritis must understand the importance of follow-up care after discharge to prevent recurrence or further complications.

Teaching for Self-Care

The nurse should advise the postpartal woman to continue good perineal hygiene following discharge. The nurse also advises her to maintain a good fluid intake, especially of water, and to empty her bladder whenever she feels the urge to void, but at least every 2 to 4 hours while awake. Once sexual intercourse is resumed, the new mother should void before (to prevent bladder trauma) and following intercourse (to wash contaminants from the vicinity of the urinary meatus). Wearing cotton-crotch underwear to facilitate air circulation also reduces the risk of urinary tract infection.

Acidification of the urine is thought to aid in preventing and managing urinary tract infection. The nurse thus advises the woman to avoid carbonated beverages, which increase alkalinity of urine, and to drink cranberry, plum, apricot, and prune juices, which increase the acidity of urine.

Evaluation

Expected outcomes of nursing care include:

- Signs of urinary tract infection are detected quickly, and the condition is treated successfully.
- The woman incorporates self-care measures to prevent the recurrence of UTI as part of her personal hygiene routine.
- The woman continues with any long-term therapy or follow-up.
- Maternal-infant attachment is maintained; the woman is able to care for her newborn effectively. ●

Care of the Woman with Mastitis

Mastitis is an infection of the breast connective tissue, primarily occurring in women who are lactating. The usual causative organisms are *Staphylococcus aureus*, *Escherichia coli*, and *Streptococcus* species (Appling, 1998). Because symptoms seldom occur before the second to fourth week postpartum, birthing unit nurses often are not fully aware of how uncomfortable and acutely ill the woman may be. No definitive data exist that allow caregivers to predict which woman will experience mastitis, so all breastfeeding women need to be taught preventive techniques and ways of recognizing this condition should it develop. The infection usually begins when bacteria invade the breast tissue. Often the tissue has been traumatized in some way (fissured or cracked nipples, overdistention, manipulation, or milk stasis) and is especially susceptible to pathogenic invasion. The most common sources of these organisms are the infant's nasopharynx, although other sources include the hands of the mother or birthing unit personnel or the woman's circulating blood.

Poor drainage of milk, lowered maternal defenses due to fatigue or stress, and poor hygiene practices make the woman susceptible to mastitis. Tight clothing, missed feedings, poor support of pendulous breasts, lack of regular breast pumping when away from the baby, or a baby who suddenly begins to sleep through the night can all result in milk stasis, which is a milder inflammatory condition.

Infectious mastitis is a more serious infection with fever, headache, flulike symptoms, and a warm, reddened, painful area of the breast, often wedge shaped because of septal distribution of connective tissue (Figure 33–2).

In other cases, *Candida albicans* is the causative organism of mastitis, entering the breast through a small fissure or abrasion on the nipple. Signs include late-onset nipple pain, followed by shooting pain during and between feedings. Eventually, the skin of the affected breast will become pink, flaking, and pruritic.

Clinical Therapy

Diagnosis is usually based on history and physical examination; culture and sensitivity may be done (Appling, 1998). A culture of breast milk allows susceptibility-directed antibiotic therapy; a leukocyte count of 1 million/mL and bacterial colony count of greater than 1000/mL is diagnostic (Chin, 1997). Treatment involves bed rest (may be needed for the first several days), increased fluid intake (at least 2 to 3 liters per day), a supportive bra, frequent breastfeeding, local application of heat, and cold compresses and analgesics (such as acetaminophen) as needed for discomfort. Nonsteroidal anti-inflammatory agents are also recommended to treat both fever and inflammation. Early treatment may prevent the progression of milk stasis and noninfectious inflammation to mastitis. Treatment of mastitis includes all of the measures mentioned previously, plus a 10-day course of antibiotics, usually a penicillinase-resistant penicillin or cephalosporin (Appling, 1998). Improved outcome, a decreased duration of symptoms, and decreased incidence of breast abscess result if the breasts continue to be emptied by either nursing or pumping. Thus continued breastfeeding is recommended in the presence of mastitis. The woman should be contacted within 24 hours of initiation of treatment to ensure that symptoms are subsiding (Wheeler, 1997). Ten percent of all cases will result in abscess formation requiring aspiration (if small) or, more commonly, incision and drainage (Appling, 1998).

Occasionally, the process of mastitis continues, and a frank abscess develops. The mother's milk and any drainage from the nipple should be cultured and antibiotic therapy instituted. Breast abscess requiring operative drainage is rare (Stover & Marnejon, 1995).

NURSING CARE MANAGEMENT

Nursing Assessment and Diagnosis

Daily assessment of breast consistency, skin color, surface temperature, nipple condition, and presence of pain is essential to detect early signs of problems that may predispose to mastitis. The mother should be observed breastfeeding her baby to ensure use of proper technique.

If an infection has developed, the nurse should assess for contributing factors such as cracked nipples, poor hygiene, engorgement, supplemental feedings, change in routine or infant feeding pattern, abrupt weaning, or lack of proper breast support so that these factors may be corrected as part of the treatment plan.

Nursing diagnoses that may apply to the woman with mastitis include the following:

- ***Knowledge Deficit*** related to lack of information about appropriate breastfeeding practices
- ***Ineffective Breastfeeding*** related to pain secondary to development of mastitis

Nursing Plan and Implementation

Preventing mastitis is far simpler than treating it. Ideally, mothers should be instructed in proper breastfeeding technique prenatally. The nurse should help the mother breastfeed soon after birth and should review correct technique. Co-management of breastfeeding between the nurse and a certified lactation specialist is often possible. All women, even those not breastfeeding, are encouraged to wear a good supportive bra at all times to avoid milk stasis, especially in the lower lobes.

Meticulous hand washing by the breastfeeding mother and all personnel is the primary measure for preventing epidemic nursery infections and subsequent maternal mastitis. Prompt attention to mothers who have blocked milk ducts eliminates stagnant milk as a growth medium for bacteria. If the mother finds that one area of her breast feels distended, she can rotate the position of her infant for nursing, manually express milk remaining in the breast after nursing (usually only necessary if the infant is not sucking well), or massage the caked area toward the nipple as the infant nurses. Mothers who have developed mastitis can apply warm, moist compresses to the affected area before breastfeeding. The nurse encourages the mother to breastfeed frequently, starting with the unaffected breast until let-down occurs in the affected breast, then encourages feeding from the affected breast until it is emptied completely (Appling, 1998). After nursing, the mother can leave a small amount of milk on each nipple to prevent cracking and allow nipples to air dry. Early identification of and intervention for sore nipples are also essential, as is prompt assessment of the nursing mother's breasts when thrush is discovered in her newborn's mouth.

Teaching for Self-Care

The nurse stresses to the breastfeeding woman the importance of adequate breast and nipple care to prevent the development of cracks and fissures, a common portal for bacterial entry. For a detailed discussion of breastfeeding, see Chapter 27.

The woman should be aware of the importance of regular, complete emptying of the breasts to prevent engorgement and stasis. She should also understand the role of let-down in successful breastfeeding, correct positioning of the infant on the nipple, proper latch-on, and the principles of supply and demand. Breastfeeding mothers who will be returning to work outside the home need information on how to do so successfully. Because mastitis tends to develop following discharge, it is important to include information about signs and symptoms in the discharge teaching (Table 33–3). All flulike symptoms should be considered a sign of mastitis until proved otherwise. If symptoms develop, the woman should contact her caregiver immediately, because prompt treatment helps to avoid abscess formation.

Community-Based Nursing Care

The home care nurse who suspects mastitis on the basis of assessment findings refers the woman to the physician. The nurse may be asked to obtain a sample of breast milk to be cultured for the causative organism.

If the mother feels too ill to breastfeed or develops an abscess that prevents nursing, the home care nurse can

TABLE 33–3 Comparison of Findings of Engorgement, Plugged Duct, and Mastitis

Characteristics	Engorgement	Plugged Duct	Mastitis
Onset	Gradual, immediately postpartum	Gradual, after feedings	Sudden, after 10 days
Site	Bilateral	Unilateral	Usually unilateral
Swelling and heat	Generalized	May shift, little or no heat	Localized, red, hot, and swollen
Pain	Generalized	Mild but localized	Intense but localized
Body temperature	<38.4C	<38.4C	>38.4C
Systemic symptoms	Feels well	Feels well	Flulike symptoms

SOURCE: Lawrence RA: *Breastfeeding—A Guide for the Medical Profession.* St Louis: Mosby, 1994, p 261.

help the mother obtain an appropriate breast pump to help her maintain lactation and can provide opportunities for demonstration and return demonstration of pumping. The nurse can assist the mother to deal with her feelings about temporarily being unable to breastfeed. Referral to a lactation consultant or to La Leche League can be invaluable to the woman's physical and emotional adjustment to mastitis.

Evaluation

Expected outcomes of nursing care include:

- The woman is aware of the signs and symptoms of mastitis.
- The woman's mastitis is detected early and treated successfully.
- The woman continues breastfeeding if she chooses.
- The woman understands self-care measures she can use to prevent recurrence of mastitis. ●

Care of the Woman with Thromboembolic Disease

Thromboembolic disease may occur antepartally, but it is generally considered a postpartal complication. Venous thrombosis refers to thrombus formation in a superficial or deep vein with the accompanying risk that a portion of the clot might break off and result in pulmonary embolism. When the thrombus is formed in response to inflammation in the vein wall, it is termed **thrombophlebitis.** In this type of thrombosis, the clot tends to be more firmly attached and therefore is less likely to result in embolism. In noninflammatory venous thrombosis (also called phlebothrombosis), the clot tends to be more loosely attached, and the risk of embolism is greater. The primary factor responsible for noninflammatory deep vein thrombosis is venous stasis (Cunningham et al, 1997).

Factors contributing directly to the development of thromboembolic disease postpartally include (1) increased amounts of certain blood clotting factors; (2) postpartal thrombocytosis (increased quantity of circulating platelets and their increased adhesiveness); (3) release of thromboplastin substances from the tissue of the decidua, placenta, and fetal membranes; and (4) increased amounts of fibrinolysis inhibitors. Predisposing factors are (1) obesity, increased maternal age, and high parity; (2) anesthesia and surgery, with possible vessel trauma and venous stasis due to prolonged inactivity; (3) previous history of venous thrombosis; (4) maternal anemia, hypothermia, or heart disease; (5) endometritis (metritis); (6) varicosities. Thromboembolic disease is more likely to occur after cesarean birth (Laros, 1999).

Superficial Leg Vein Disease

Superficial thrombophlebitis is far more common postpartally than during pregnancy. Often the clot involves the saphenous veins. This disorder is more common in women with preexisting varices (enlarged veins), although it is not limited to these women. Symptoms usually become apparent about the third or fourth postpartal day: tenderness in a portion of the vein, some local heat and redness, absent or low-grade fever, and occasionally slight elevation of the pulse. Treatment involves application of local heat, elevation of the affected limb, bed rest and analgesic agents, and the use of elastic support hose. Anticoagulants are usually not necessary unless complications develop. Pulmonary embolism is extremely rare. Occasionally, the involved veins have incompetent valves, and as a result the problem may spread to the deeper leg veins, such as the femoral vein.

Deep Vein Thrombosis (DVT)

Deep venous thrombosis or thrombophlebitis is more frequently seen in women with a history of thrombosis. Certain obstetric complications such as hydramnios, PIH, and operative birth are associated with an increased incidence.

Clinical manifestations may include edema of the ankle and leg and an initial low-grade fever often followed by high temperature and chills. Depending on the vein involved, the woman may complain of pain in the

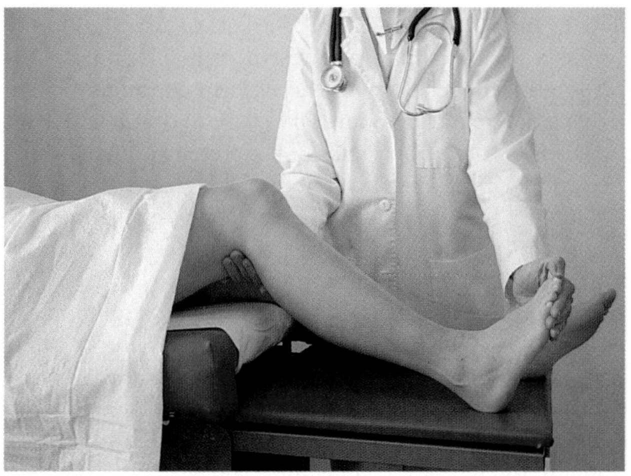

FIGURE 33–3 Homans' sign. With the client's knee flexed to decrease the risk of embolization, the nurse dorsiflexes the client's foot. Pain in the foot or leg is a positive Homans' sign.

popliteal and lateral tibial areas (popliteal vein), entire lower leg and foot (anterior and posterior tibial veins), inguinal tenderness (femoral vein), or pain in the lower abdomen (iliofemoral vein). Homans' sign (Figure 33–3) may or may not be positive, but pain often results from calf pressure. Because of reflex arterial spasm, sometimes the limb is cool to the touch—the so-called milk leg or phlegmasia alba dolens—and peripheral pulses may be decreased.

Septic Pelvic Thrombophlebitis

Septic pelvic thrombophlebitis is a complication that develops in conjunction with infections of the reproductive tract and is more common in women who have had a cesarean birth. Infection ascends upward along the venous system, and thrombophlebitis develops in the uterine, ovarian, or hypogastric veins (Cunningham et al, 1997). This diagnosis is suspected when infection is unresponsive to antibiotics. Abdominal or flank pain, or both, sometimes accompanied by guarding, occurs on the second or third day postpartum with fever and tachycardia. Bimanual exam may reveal a parametrial mass. On occasion, paralytic ileus develops. A complete blood count (CBC), blood chemistry, coagulation profile, chest x-ray examination, computed tomography, and magnetic resonance imaging are useful for diagnosis. Treatment consists of anticoagulation and antibiotic therapy. Although most women show significant clinical improvement with antibiotics, a saw-tooth fever spike and chills may persist (Laros, 1999).

Clinical Therapy

Because cases of thromboembolic disease are seldom clear-cut, diagnosis involves a variety of approaches, such as client history and physical examination, occlusive cuff impedence plethysmography (IPG), Doppler ultrasonography, and contrast venography. In questionable cases, contrast venography provides the most accurate diagnosis of deep vein thrombosis. Unfortunately, venography is not practical for multiple examinations or prospective screening and may itself induce phlebitis.

Treatment involves the administration of intravenous heparin, using an infusion pump to permit continuous, accurate infusion of medication. Strict bed rest and elevation of the legs are required, and analgesics are given as necessary to relieve discomfort. If fever is present, deep thrombophlebitis is suspected, and the woman is also given antibiotic therapy. In most cases thrombectomy is not necessary.

Once the symptoms have subsided (usually in several days), the woman may begin walking while wearing elastic support stockings. Intravenous heparin is continued, and treatment with sodium warfarin (Coumadin) is begun. When prothrombin time reaches 1.5 to 1.7, the heparin is discontinued. The woman will continue on Coumadin for 2 to 6 months at home. While the woman is on warfarin, prothrombin times are assessed periodically to maintain correct dosage levels.

CRITICAL THINKING IN PRACTICE

Lei Chang, G1P1, had a cesarean birth after a prolonged labor and failure to progress. As she is walking in the hallway with her husband, you notice that Lei is limping slightly, and you comment on that observation. Lei responds that she is having pain in her right lower leg. She says, "Maybe I pulled a muscle during labor." What would you do?

Answers can be found in Appendix I.

NURSING CARE MANAGEMENT

Nursing Assessment and Diagnosis

The nurse carefully assesses the woman's history for factors predisposing to development of thrombosis or thrombophlebitis. In addition, as part of regular postpartal assessment, the nurse is alert to any client complaints of pain in the leg, inguinal area, or lower abdomen because such pain may indicate deep venous thrombosis. The nurse also assesses the woman's legs for evidence of edema, temperature change, or pain with palpation.

Nursing diagnoses that may apply to a postpartal woman with thromboembolic disease include the following:

- ***Altered Tissue Perfusion*** in periphery related to obstructed venous return
- ***Pain*** related to tissue hypoxia and edema secondary to vascular obstruction

- ***Risk for Altered Parenting*** related to decreased maternal-infant interaction secondary to bed rest and intravenous lines
- ***Altered Family Processes*** related to illness of family member
- ***Knowledge Deficit*** related to lack of information about the DVT/thrombophlebitis, its treatment, preventive measures, and the medication (warfarin)

Nursing Plan and Implementation

Women with varicosities should be evaluated for the need for support hose during labor and postpartum. Adequate fluid intake is necessary during labor to avoid dehydration. Because trauma is often a factor in the development of thrombophlebitis, the nurse avoids keeping the woman's legs elevated in stirrups for prolonged periods. If stirrups are used, they should be comfortably padded and adjusted to provide correct support and prevent pressure on popliteal vessels. In addition, early ambulation is encouraged following birth, and the use of the knee gatch on the bed should be avoided. Women confined to bed following a cesarean birth are encouraged to perform regular leg exercises to promote venous return.

Once the diagnosis of deep venous thrombosis is made, the nurse maintains the heparin therapy, provides for appropriate comfort measures, and monitors the woman closely for signs of pulmonary embolism. The nurse also assesses for evidence of bleeding related to heparin and keeps the antagonist for heparin, protamine sulfate, readily available.

The nurse instructs the woman to avoid prolonged standing or sitting, because these positions contribute to venous stasis. She is also instructed to avoid crossing her legs because of the pressure it causes. The nurse also advises her to take frequent breaks, such as when taking car trips or at a job where she sits most of the day. Walking is acceptable because it promotes venous return. The woman is reminded to identify her history of thrombosis or thrombophlebitis to her physician during subsequent pregnancies so that preventive measures may be instituted early.

Women who are discharged on warfarin must understand the purpose of the medication and be alert to signs of hemorrhage, such as bleeding gums, epistaxis, petechiae or ecchymosis, or evidence of blood in the urine or stool. Because careful monitoring is important, the woman should clearly understand the need to keep scheduled appointments for prothrombin time assessment. Certain medications, such as aspirin and other nonsteroidal anti-inflammatory drugs, increase anticoagulant activity, so they should be avoided. In fact, while she is taking warfin the woman should check for possible medication interaction before taking *any* other medication. The nurse should encourage the woman to carry a MedicAlert card in case of emergency and to inform all medical care providers, including dentists, that she is taking anticoagulants. She should also have vitamin K available in case bleeding occurs. Warfarin is excreted in the breast milk and thus may present problems for breastfeeding mothers. Women who wish to continue nursing may be maintained at home on low doses of subcutaneous heparin, because heparin is not excreted in breast milk. See the Critical Pathway for the Woman with Thromboembolic Disease for specific nursing care measures.

Community-Based Nursing Care

Because the mother with postpartal thromboembolic disease will depend on others for much of her initial home care, it is helpful for the father to be involved in preparations for discharge. The nurse should provide ample opportunities to answer questions and clarify instructions, verbally and in writing. The nurse will evaluate the extent to which both mother and father have understood instructions regarding the plan of care. It is especially important before discharge to assess the couple's plans in order to ensure complete bed rest for the mother. They might explore ways for her to maintain bed rest and still spend quality time with her newborn and any other children. For example, young children can sit on the bed for storytelling or play quiet games, and the newborn's crib can be placed adjacent to the mother's bed.

Many concerns will not surface until the couple actually returns home and fully comprehends the reality of their situation. For that reason, it is valuable to provide them with an accessible resource person and to plan telephone or home visit follow-up care.

The father may be assuming multiple roles in the circumstances—household manager, parent, worker, and caregiver. Fatigue is inevitable. There may be financial concerns as a result of prolonged health care or his extended time away from work to care for the family. The couple must keep their communication lines open and spend quality time together. Referral to social services and assessment of the presence and use of a continued support system and coping strategies are necessary to avert potential crises.

Signs of postpartum thrombophlebitis may not occur until after discharge from the hospital. Consequently, all couples must be taught about the signs and symptoms and to appreciate the importance of reporting them immediately and of not massaging the affected leg. Should signs and symptoms occur after discharge from the postpartum unit, a short readmission might be required. Every effort is made in that case to allow mother, father, and newborn to remain together.

Evaluation

Expected outcomes of nursing care include:

- If thrombosis or thrombophlebitis develops, it is detected quickly and managed successfully without further complications.
- At discharge, the woman is able to explain the purpose, dosage regimen, and necessary precautions

Text continues on page 1004.

CRITICAL PATHWAY FOR THE WOMAN WITH THROMBOEMBOLIC DISEASE*

Category	Antepartal Management	Intrapartal Management	Postpartal Management
Referral	Perinatologist Internist Social worker Psychiatric clinical nurse practitioner Dietary/nutrionist Infectious disease consult	Obtain prenatal record	Home nursing referral if indicated **Expected Outcomes** Appropriate resources identified and utilized
Assessment	Obtain hx of present pregnancy Assess estimated gestational age Assess any sensitivity to medications Obtain complete physical examination to include: • Fetal size, fetal status (FHR), and fetal maturity • Signs of fatigue, weakness, recurrent diarrhea, pallor, night sweats • Present weight and amount of weight gain or weight loss Obtain diagnostics studies: • Ultrasound • Fetal maturity studies (L/S ratio, PG, creatinine) • Hemoglobin, hematocrit, platelet count • WBC and differential • HIV-I • CD4+ T lymphocyte count • ESR		Monitor daily Hct Continue normal postpartum assessment q8h Feeding technique with newborn: should be good or improving TPR assessment: q8h; all WNL; report temperature >38C (100.4F) Continue assessment of comfort level Assess for superficial thrombophlebitis: • Tenderness along involved vein • Areas of palpable thrombosis • Warmth and redness in the involved area Deep venous thrombosis (DVT): • Positive Homans' sign (pain occurs when foot is dorsiflexed while leg is extended) • Tenderness and pain in affected area • Fever (initially low, followed by high fever and chills) • Edema in affected extremity • Pallor and coolness in affected limb • Diminished peripheral pulses • Increased potential for pulmonary embolus Immediately report the development of any signs of pulmonary embolism, including the following: • Sudden onset of severe chest pain, often located substernally • Apprehension and sense of impending catastrophe • Cough (may be accompanied by hemoptysis) • Tachycardia • Fever • Hypotension • Diaphoresis, pallor, weakness • Shortness of breath • Neck engorgement • Friction rub and evidence of atelectasis upon auscultation **Expected Outcomes** Findings indicate complications of thrombosis minimized, and condition stable/improved
Comfort			Continue with pain management techniques. No aspirin or ibuprofen. Acetaminophen may be ordered. Provide supportive nursing comfort measures such as back rubs, provision of quiet time for sleep, diversional activities Maintain warm moist soaks as ordered with legs elevated

*All of the interventions for a normal labor and birth and postpartal client may be found in those appropriate critical pathways.

CRITICAL PATHWAY FOR THE WOMAN WITH THROMBOEMBOLIC DISEASE *CONTINUED*

Category	Antepartal Management	Intrapartal Management	Postpartal Management
Teaching/ psychosocial	Room orientation Explain s/sx of labor Increase client awareness of fetal monitoring Evaluation of client teaching	Tour of ICN Discuss with woman: • Mode of childbirth • Postpartum expectation	Implement normal postpartum teaching and psychosocial support (see Chapter 31) Maintain mother/infant attachment; when mother is on bed rest provide frequent contacts for mother and infant; modified rooming-in is possible if the crib is placed close to the mother's bed and nurse checks often to help mother lift or move infant **Expected Outcomes** Woman demonstrates/verbalizes understanding of plan of care and teaching Infant/maternal bonding unimpaired
Nursing care management and reports	Assess emotional response so that support and teaching can be planned accordingly Weigh woman Obtain food history Establish rapport Provide opportunities to talk without interruption Monitor for signs of infection Maintain appropriate isolation precautions	Ongoing monitoring of blood pressure Electronic fetal monitoring in place Try to have same nurses caring for woman during her hospitalization Monitor for signs of infection **Expected Outcomes** Maternal/fetal circulation optimized	Continue sitz baths prn May shower if ambulating without difficulty DC buffalo cap (heparin lock) if present Monitor for signs of infection For DVT obtain prothrombin time (PT) and review prior to beginning warfarin. Repeat periodically per physician order **Expected Outcomes** Thromoembolic disease treated successfully, without related complications
Activity and comfort	Decreased stimulation in room including visitors		Maintain bed rest and limb in elevated position Initiate progressive ambulation following the acute phase; provide properly fitting elastic stockings prior to ambulation for management of superficial thrombophlebitis and DVT **Expected Outcomes** Activity initiated as appropriate Optimal comfort maintained
Nutrition	Plan high-protein, high-calorie diet		Continue diet and fluids **Expected Outcomes** Nutritional needs met
Elimination			
Medications		Continuous IV infusion	May take own prenatal vitamins RhoGAM administered if indicated Rubella vaccine administered if indicated For DVT administer intravenous heparin as ordered by continuous intravenous drip, heparin lock, or subcutaneously, including : • Monitor IV or heparin lock site for signs of infiltration • Obtain Lee-White clotting times or partial thromboplastin time (PTT) per physician order, and review prior to administering heparin • Observe for signs of anticoagulant overdose with resultant bleeding, including the following: hematuria, epistaxis, ecchymosis, and bleeding gums • Provide protamine sulfate per physician order to combat bleeding problems related to heparin overdosage **Expected Outcomes** Thrombosis resolved and control of related bleeding problems achieved Minimized complications and side effects

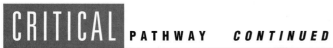

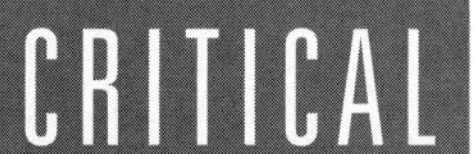 PATHWAY *CONTINUED*

Category	Antepartal Management	Intrapartal Management	Postpartal Management
Discharge planning/ home care	Assess home care needs Provide support and counseling		Discuss ways of avoiding circulatory stasis such as avoiding prolonged standing, sitting, and crossing legs Review need to wear support stockings and to plan for rest periods with legs elevated In the presence of DVT, discuss the following: • The use of warfarin, its side effects, possible interactions with other medications, and need to have dosage assessed through periodic checks of the prothrombin time • Signs of bleeding, which may be associated with warfarin sodium and which need to be reported immediately, including the following: hematuria, epislaxis, ecchymosis, bleeding gums, and rectal bleeding • Monitor menstrual flow: bleeding may be heavier • Review need for woman to eat a consistent amount of leafy green vegetables (lettuce, cabbage, brussels sprouts, broccoli) every day (high in vit K so affects dose of warfarin and PT balance) • Instruct the woman to report any bleeding that continues more than 10 minutes • Instruct the woman to do the following: • Routinely inspect the body for bruising • Carry MedicAlert card indicating she is on anticoagulant therapy • Use electric razor to avoid scratching skin • Use soft bristle toothbrush • Avoid alcohol intake or keep intake at minimum • Avoid taking any other drugs without checking with the physician • Note that stools may change color to pink, red, or black as a result of anticoagulant use • Advise all health providers, including dentists, that she is taking anticoagulants Review discharge instructions and checklist Provide list or make appropriate referrals to available community resources Describe postpartum warning signs and when to call CNM/physician Provide prescriptions: Gift pack given to woman Arrangements made for baby pictures if desired Postpartum visit scheduled Newborn check scheduled **Expected Outcome** Client discharge teaching done with emphasis on follow-up care, continued therapy needs and precautions Support network identified

CRITICAL PATHWAY FOR THE WOMAN WITH THROMBOEMBOLIC DISEASE *CONTINUED*

Category	Antepartal Management	Intrapartal Management	Postpartal Management
Family involvement	Assess support systems	Encourage family member to stay with the woman as long as possible throughout labor and childbirth	Involve support persons in teaching Plans made for providing support to mother following discharge. Support persons verbalize understanding of need for woman to rest, eat nutritionally, recover Encourage woman to express her concerns to her partner. Assist couple in planning ways to manage while woman is hospitalized and after her discharge Encourage partner or support person to bring other children to hospital to visit mother and meet new sibling Encourage partner or support person to bring in family pictures. Encourage phone calls Contact social services if indicated to obtain additional assistance for family if needed **Expected Outcomes** Family demonstrates resource availability and utilization Family bonding and development unimpaired
Date			

associated with any prescribed medications, such as anticoagulants.

- The woman can discuss self-care measures and ongoing therapies (such as the use of elastic stockings) that are indicated.
- The woman has bonded successfully with her newborn and is able to care for the baby effectively. ●

Care of the Woman with a Postpartum Psychiatric Disorder

Many types of psychiatric problems may occur in postpartum. The classification of postpartum psychiatric disorders is a subject of some controversy. The *Diagnostic and Statistical Manual of Mental Disorders*, 4th edition (DSM-IV), has added a postpartum onset specifier to the mood disorder diagnostic category of psychiatric disorders. It is proposed that postpartum psychiatric disorders be considered one diagnosable syndrome with three subclasses: (1) adjustment reaction with depressed mood, (2) postpartum psychosis, and (3) postpartum major mood disorder. The incidence, etiology, symptoms, treatment, and prognosis vary with each subclass.

Adjustment reaction with depressed mood is also known as postpartum, maternal, or "baby" blues. It occurs in as many as 50% to 80% of mothers and is characterized by mild depression interspersed with happier feelings. Postpartum blues typically occur within a few days after the baby's birth and are self-limiting, lasting from a few hours to 10 days or longer (Beck, 1998). It is more severe in primiparas and seems related to the rapid alteration of estrogen, progesterone, and prolactin levels after birth. New mothers experiencing postpartum blues commonly report feeling overwhelmed, unable to cope, fatigued, anxious, irritable, and oversensitive. A key feature is episodic tearfulness, often without an identifiable reason.

Validating the existence of this phenomenon, labeling it as a real but normal adjustment reaction, and providing reassurance can offer a measure of relief. Assistance with self and infant care, information, and family support is helpful to recovery. The partner should be encouraged to watch for and report signs that the new mother is not returning to a more normal mood but is instead slipping into a deeper depression.

Postpartum psychosis, which has an incidence of 1 to 2 per 1000, usually becomes evident within the first 3 months postpartum. Symptoms include agitation, hyperactivity, insomnia, mood lability, confusion, irrationality, difficulty remembering or concentrating, poor judgment, delusions, and hallucinations. Improvement is seen in 95% of women in 2 to 3 months (Wood, Thomas, Droppleman, & Meighan, 1997). There is a 10% to 25% recurrence rate in subsequent pregnancies. Risk factors include (1) previous puerperal psychosis; (2) history of bipolar (manic-depressive) disorder; (3) prenatal stressors, such as lack of social support, lack of a partner, and low socioeconomic status; (4) obsessive personality; and

(5) a family history of a mood disorder. Treatment may include hospitalization, antipsychotic medications, sedatives, electroconvulsive therapy, removal of the infant, social support, and psychotherapy.

Postpartum major mood disorder, also known as *postpartum depression*, develops in about 8% to 26% of all postpartal women (Beck, 1998). Although it may occur at any time during the first year postpartum, the greatest risks occur around the fourth week, just prior to the initiation of menses, and upon weaning. Surprisingly, it is not associated with depression during pregnancy.

Many of the symptoms of this major depression are indistinguishable from serious depression at other times: sadness, frequent crying, insomnia, appetite change, difficulty concentrating and making decisions, feelings of worthlessness, obsessive thoughts of inadequacy as a person and parent, lack of interest in usual activities (including sexual relations), and lack of concern about personal appearance. Persistent anxiety further contributes to the woman's feeling out of control. Irritability and hostility toward others, including the newborn, may be evident. Beck (1993) describes these debilitating symptoms as "teetering on the edge" between sanity and insanity. Women participating in Beck's qualitative research on postpartum depression described a sense of living their daily life in a sort of fog, from which they believed they would never emerge. Once they improved, they often grieved over the time lost with their newborns while in this "fog."

Risk factors for postpartum depression include the following:

- Primiparity
- Ambivalence about maintaining the pregnancy
- History of postpartum depression or bipolar illness
- Lack of social support
- Lack of a stable relationship with parents or partner
- The woman's dissatisfaction with herself, including body image problems and eating disorders
- Lack of a supportive relationship with her parents, especially her father, as a child

Certain other factors that have been highly correlated with postpartum depression may be assessed via screening questions for the disorder: (1) history of infertility, (2) early menarche (before age 11), (3) unrealistic expectations of parenthood, and (4) adverse emotional reactions (irritability or depression) resulting from earlier use of oral contraceptives (Horowitz, Damato, Solon, & von Metzech, 1995).

Clinical Therapy

Medication, individual or group psychotherapy, and practical assistance with child care and other demands of daily life are common treatment measures. Treatment of postpartum depression is not unlike treatment of any significant depression: psychotherapy and antidepression medications, usually the selective serotonin reuptake inhibitors such as sertraline (Zoloft), paroxetine (Paxil), and fluoxetine (Prozac) or tricyclic agents, such as amitriptyline (Elavil) or imipramine (Tofranil). Support groups have proved to be successful adjuncts to such treatment. Within a support group of postpartal women and their partners, a couple may feel consolation that they are not alone in their experience. Moreover, the support group provides a forum for gaining information about postpartum depression, learning stress reduction measures, and experiencing renewed self-esteem and support. If a support group is not available locally, the woman and her family may be encouraged to contact Depression After Delivery (DAD), a national support network that provides literature and volunteers, at PO Box 1282, Morrisville, PA 19067, or 800-944-4773.

In about 10% of cases, symptoms of postpartum depression occur secondary to postpartum thyroiditis. Laboratory studies of TSH (thyroid-stimulating hormone) and T_4 levels should be ordered to rule out a transient thyroid disorder as a cause of depression. Treatment of the disorder may be necessary (Wheeler, 1997). There is some indication that prophylactic antidepressants begun within 24 hours of subsequent childbirth may prevent recurrence of postpartum depression (Wisner & Wheeler, 1994).

Women with a history of depression or postpartum psychosis should be referred to a mental health professional for counseling and biweekly visits between the second and sixth week postpartum for evaluation of depression.

Treatment of postpartum psychosis is directed at the specific type of psychotic symptoms displayed. Emergency hospitalization in an inpatient psychiatric unit is usually indicated. Treatment may include lithium; antipsychotic medications, such as chlorpromazine (Thorazine) or haloperidol (Haldol); or electroconvulsive therapy in combination with psychotherapy. It is important for the nurse to realize that many of the drugs used in treating postpartum psychiatric conditions are contraindicated in breastfeeding women.

NURSING CARE MANAGEMENT

Nursing Assessment and Diagnosis

Assessment for factors predisposing a client to postpartum depression or psychosis should begin prenatally (Beck, 1998). Questions designed to detect problems can be included as part of the routine prenatal history interview or questionnaire. Women with a personal or family history of psychiatric disease, particularly postpartum depression or psychosis, need prenatal instructions on the signs and symptoms of depression and may need additional emotional support. If not done previously, the nurse assesses the woman for predisposing factors during her labor and postpartum stay.

TABLE 33–4 Suggested Questions to Elicit Responses from the Postpartum Depression Checklist (PDC)*

Lack of Concentration

Are you experiencing difficulty concentrating?
Does your mind seem to be filled with cobwebs?
Does it seem at times like fogginess sets in?

Loss of Interests

Do you feel your life is empty of your previous interests and goals?
Have you lost interest in your hobbies that used to bring you pleasure and enjoyment?

Loneliness

Are you experiencing feelings of loneliness?
Do you feel as though no one really understands what you are experiencing?
Do you feel uncomfortable around other people?
Have you been isolating yourself from other people?

Insecurity

Have you been feeling insecure, fragile, or vulnerable?
Does the responsibility of motherhood seem overwhelming?

Obsessive Thinking

Is your mind constantly filled with obsessive thinking such as, "What's wrong with me?" "Am I going crazy?" "Why can't I enjoy being with my baby?"
When trying to fall asleep at night, is your mind still racing with repetitive thoughts?

Lack of Positive Emotions

Are you experiencing feelings of emptiness?
Do you feel like a robot just going through the motions?
When caring for your infant/child, do you feel any joy or love?

Loss of Self

Do you feel as though you are not the same person you used to be?
Are you afraid that your life will never be normal again?

Anxiety Attacks

Are you experiencing uncontrollable anxiety attacks?
Are you experiencing periods of palpitations, chest pains, sweating, or tingling hands?
When going through an anxiety attack, do you feel as though you're losing your mind?

Loss of Control

Do you feel you are in control of your emotions and thoughts?
Are you experiencing loss of control in any aspects of your life?

Guilt

Are you feeling guilty because you believe you are not giving your infant/child the love and attention he/she needs?
Are you experiencing guilt over thoughts of harming your infant/child?
Do you feel you are a good mother?

Contemplating Death

Have you experienced thoughts of harming yourself?
Have you been feeling so low that the thought of leaving this world was appealing to you?

*Bold print reflects areas of concern expressed by depressed women in Beck's qualitative studies. Questions answered "Yes" by women during screening with this checklist can be followed with further dialogue between nurse and client. SOURCE: Beck CT: Screening methods for postpartum depression. *JOGNN 1995; 24*(4): 113. Used with permission of Lippincott-Raven Publishers.

Becoming a mother is idealized by most societies as a joyful event. Consequently, the woman who experiences depression, instead of joy, often suffers silently because she feels guilty and hesitant to disclose her honest feelings with family and caregivers. Some women believe that admission of emotional difficulty and mothering inadequacy will be used against them. Prior to assessment for evidence of depression, the nurse can give voice to this societal myth of joyful motherhood, giving the woman permission to share negative feelings and thoughts she might be feeling (Beck, 1995). Several depression scales are available for assessing postpartum depression; one of the most widely used is a self-report, the Edinburgh Postnatal Depression Scale, which consists of ten brief statements of symptoms commonly associated with depression. There are four responses for each statement; the woman selects the response most descriptive of how she has felt in the previous week. For example, to the symptom statement, "I have felt sad or miserable," the woman would select one of these responses: "Yes, most of the time"; "Yes, quite often"; "Not very often"; or "No, not at all." Each of the 10 items is scored 0, 1, 2, or 3, according to severity. Mothers who score above 12 are likely to be suffering from postpartum depression (Fowles, 1998).

Beck (1995) developed a practical and simple screening checklist for use during routine care with all postpartal women to identify those who might be experiencing postpartum depression so that early management might be initiated. There are 11 symptoms on the Postpartum Depression Checklist (PDC). Questions are asked to elicit yes/no answers about each symptom; when a "yes" answer is elicited, the nurse provides opportunities for additional exploration, using open-ended questions (Table 33–4). Willingness to listen as the mother shares her experience of postpartum depression not only enables the nurse to recognize symptoms and initiate timely management, but also is commonly perceived by the mother as caring (Beck, 1996).

In providing daily care, the nurse observes the woman for objective signs of depression—anxiety, irritability, poor concentration, forgetfulness, sleeping difficulties, appetite change, fatigue and tearfulness—and listens for statements indicating feelings of failure and self-accusation. Severity and duration of symptoms should be noted. Behavior and verbalization that are bizarre or seem to indicate a potential for violence against herself or others, including the infant, are reported as soon as possible for further evaluation.

The nurse needs to be aware that many normal physiologic changes of the puerperium are similar to symptoms of depression (lack of sexual interest, appetite change, and fatigue). It is essential that observations be as specific and as objective as possible and that they be carefully documented.

Possible nursing diagnoses that may apply to a woman with a postpartum psychiatric disorder include the following:

- ***Ineffective Individual Coping*** related to postpartum depression
- ***Risk for Altered Parenting*** related to postpartal mental illness

Nursing Plan and Implementation

Nurses working in antepartal settings or teaching childbirth classes play indispensable roles in helping prospective parents appreciate the lifestyle changes and role demands associated with parenthood. Offering realistic information and anticipatory guidance and debunking myths about the perfect mother or perfect newborn may help prevent postpartum depression.

The nurse should alert the mother, partner, and other family members to the possibility of postpartum blues in the early days after birth and reassure them of the short-term nature of the condition. Symptoms of postpartum depression should be described and the mother encouraged to call her health care provider if symptoms become severe, if they fail to subside quickly, or if at any time she feels she is unable to function. Encouraging the mother to plan how she will manage at home and providing concrete suggestions on how to cope will aid in her adjustment to motherhood.

Community-Based Nursing Care

Home visits, especially for early discharge families, are essential to fostering positive adjustments for the new family constellation. Telephone follow-up at 3 weeks postpartum to ask whether the mother is experiencing difficulties is also helpful.

In all women, the presence of three symptoms on one day or one symptom for 3 days may signal serious depression and requires immediate referral to a mental health professional. Immediate referral should also be made if rejection of the infant or threatened or actual aggression against the infant has occurred. In such cases, the newborn is never left unattended with the mother.

Depression does appear to interfere with optimal mothering; there is less interaction between mother and child, more mood and cognitive development problems, and more visits to the doctor in these children (Beck, 1998).

A diagnosis of postpartum depression or other psychiatric disorder will pose major problems for the family, especially the father. The symptoms of these disorders are difficult to witness and may be harder to understand than physical problems such as hemorrhage or infection. The father may feel hurt by his partner's hostility and may worry that she is becoming insane, or be baffled by her mood swings and lack of concern about herself, the newborn, or household responsibilities. He may be troubled by their lack of intimacy or deteriorating communication. Certainly, he has cause for concern about how the newborn and any other children are being affected. There may be very real practical matters to handle—running the household; managing the children, including the totally dependent newborn; and caring for the mother—added to his usual routines and work responsibilities. It is not surprising that even in the most supportive families relationships may suffer in response to these circumstances. It is often a family member who in desperation makes contact with the health care agency. This is especially difficult when the mother is reluctant to admit she is suffering emotional difficulty or is too ill to recognize her own needs.

RESEARCH IN PRACTICE

What is this study about? The quality of the interactions between a mother and her infant may depend on the mother's response to cues provided by her infant. The interactions between a substance-abusing mother and her substance-exposed infant can be hampered by emotional instability of the mother and irritability of the newborn. Impaired interactions may lead to neglect or even abuse. Evelyn French, Martha Pituch, Jean Brandt, and Sharon Pohorecki developed a study to determine whether teaching interaction and comforting techniques to substance-abusing mothers would improve the mother-infant interaction after discharge.

How was the study done? The researchers randomly assigned 40 women with drug-positive prenatal urine tests to either the control or intervention group. Since the Nursing Child Assessment Feeding Scale (NCAFS) tool had previously been validated with 1- to 3-month-old infants, and not with newborns less than one week old, the investigators included 20 women with negative prenatal urine results as a comparison group. The comparison group was matched in age, race, marital status, and education to the women in the control and intervention groups. Each of the 3 groups comprised of 10 first-time mothers and 10 mothers with more than one child. Trained observers evaluated each mother feeding her child after delivery. The observers were not informed of the mothers' drug history, and to evaluate mother-child interaction, used the NCAFS. The NCAFS assesses sensitivity to cues, response to distress, social-emotional and cognitive growth fostering of the parent, as well as clarity of cues and responsiveness of the infant. Mothers in the intervention group were shown a culturally sensitive video, received a booklet, and received instruction on interaction techniques and comforting a newborn. Within 48 to 72 hours after discharge, observers again used the NCAFS to evaluate each mother's interaction while feeding her infant. Control and comparison groups received the booklet after the home visit.

What were the results of the study? Using one-way analysis of variance the investigators found equivalence among the groups at the beginning of the study. Total home scores for the intervention and comparison groups were significantly different ($p = 0.05$) from the control group. Further analysis showed the total parent subscale for the control group to be significantly different from the other two groups with no difference found on the child subscale.

What additional questions might I have? How did the investigators determine that the video was culturally sensitive? What was the attrition rate? Statistical tables denote an n of 20 per group yet the article text discusses an anticipated 28% attrition rate.

How can I use this study? Nurses can help new mothers recognize and respond to cues from their newborn and enhance mother-infant interactions.

SOURCE: French, E. D., Pituch, M., Brandt, J. & Pohorecki, S. (1998). Improving interactions between substance-abusing mothers and their substance-exposed newborns. *JOGNN, 27*(3), 262–269.

Information, emotional support, and assistance in providing or obtaining care for the infant may be needed. The nurse can assist family members by identifying community resources and making referrals to public health nursing services and social services. Postpartum follow-up is especially important, as well as visits from a psychiatric home health nurse.

Evaluation

Expected outcomes of nursing care include:

- Signs of potential postpartal disorders are detected quickly, and therapy is implemented.
- The newborn is cared for effectively by the father or another support person until the mother is able to do so. ●

FOCUS YOUR STUDY

- Nursing assessment and intervention play a large role in preventing postpartum complications.
- The main causes of early postpartal hemorrhage are uterine atony, lacerations of the vagina and cervix, and retained placental fragments.
- The most common postpartal infection is endometritis, which is limited to the uterine cavity.
- Thromboembolic disease originating in the veins of the leg, thigh, or pelvis may occur antepartally or postpartally and carries with it the potential for creating a pulmonary embolus.
- A postpartal woman is at increased risk for developing urinary tract problems because of normal postpartal diuresis, increased bladder capacity, decreased bladder sensitivity from stretching or trauma, and, possibly, inhibited neural control of the bladder following the use of anesthetic agents.
- Mastitis is an inflammation of the breast often caused by *Staphylococcus aureus*, *Escherichia coli*, and *Streptococcus* species. Mastitis is seen primarily in breastfeeding women. Symptoms seldom occur before the second to fourth postpartal week.
- Although many different types of psychiatric problems may be encountered in the postpartal period, depression is the most common. Episodes occur frequently in the week after birth and are typically transient.
- Telephone calls and home visits are effective measures for extending comprehensive care into the home setting of the postpartal family at risk.

REFERENCES

American Psychiatric Association (APA). (1994). *Diagnostic and statistical manual of mental disorders: DSM-IV* (4th ed.). Washington, DC: Author.

Appling, S. E. (1998). Mastitis. *Lippincott's primary care practice—Breast conditions, 2*(2), 184–188.

Beck, C. T. (1993). Teetering on the edge: A substantive theory of postpartum depression. *Nursing Research, 42*(1), 42–48.

Beck, C. T. (1995). Perceptions of nurses' caring by mothers experiencing postpartum depression. *Journal of Obstetric, Gynecologic, and Neonatal Nursing, 24*(9), 819–825.

Beck, C. T. (1996). Postpartum depressed mothers' experiences interacting with their children. *Nursing Research, 45*(2), 98–104.

Beck, C. T. (1998). A checklist to identify women at risk for developing postpartum depression. *Journal of Obstetric, Gynecologic, and Neonatal Nursing, 27*, (1), 39–46.

Calhoun, B. C., & Brost, B. (1995). Emergency management of sudden puerperal fever. *Obstetrics & Gynecology Clinics of North America, 22*(2), 357–367.

Chin, H. G. (1997). *On call obstetrics and gynecology*. Philadelphia: Saunders.

Clark, R. A. (1995). Infections during the postpartum period. *Journal of Obstetric, Gynecologic, and Neonatal Nursing, 24*(6), 542–548.

Craigo, S. D., & Kapernick, P. S. (1994). Postpartum hemorrhage and the abnormal puerperium. In A. H. DeCherney & M. L. Pernoll (Eds.), *Current obstetrics and gynecologic diagnosis and treatment.* Norwalk, CT: Appleton & Lange.

Cunningham, F. G., McDonald, P. C., Gant, N. F., Leveno, K. J., Gilstrap, L. C., III, Hankins, G. D. V., & Clark, S. L. (1997). *Williams obstetrics* (20th ed.). Stamford, CT: Appleton & Lange.

Druelinger, L. (1994). Postpartum emergencies. *Emergency Medicine Clinics of North America, 12*(1), 219–237.

Fowles, E. R. (1998). The relationship between maternal role attainment and postpartum depression. *Health Care for Women International 19*, 83–94.

Gibbs, R. S., & Sweet, R. L. (1999). Maternal and fetal infectious disorders. In R. K. Creasy & R. Resnik (Eds.), *Maternal-fetal medicine* (4th ed.). Philadelphia: Saunders.

Horowitz, J. A., Damato, E., Solon, L., & von Metzech, G. (1995). Identification of symptoms of postpartum depression: Linking research to practice. *Journal of Perinatology, 16*(5), 360–365.

Laros, R. K. (1999). Thromboembolic disease. In R. K. Creasy & R. Resnik (Eds.), *Maternal-fetal medicine* (4th ed.). Philadelphia: Saunders.

Norris, T. C. (1997, Feb. 1). Management of postpartum hemorrhage. *American Family Physician, 55*(2), 635–640.

Roberts, W. E. (1995). Emergent obstetric management of postpartum hemorrhage. *Obstetrics & Gynecology Clinics of North America, 22*(2), 283–302.

Seigel, S. B. (1992). Telephone follow-up programs as creative nursing interventions. *Pediatric Nursing, 18*(1), 86–89.

Stover, A. M., & Marnejon, J. G. (1995). Postpartum care. *American Family Physician, 52*(5), 1465–1472.

Wheeler, L. (1997). *Nurse-midwifery handbook: A practical guide to prenatal and postpartal care.* Philadelphia: Lippincott-Raven.

Wisner, K. L., & Wheeler, S. B. (1994). Prevention of recurrent postpartum major depression. *Hospital & Community Psychiatry, 45*(12), 1191–1196.

Wood, A. F., Thomas, S. P., Droppleman, P. G., & Meighan, M. (1997). The downward spiral of postpartum depression. *American Journal of Maternal Child Nursing, 22*(6), 308–318.

Appendices

Appendix A

Common Abbreviations in Maternal-Newborn and Women's Health Nursing

accel	Acceleration of fetal heart rate
AC	Abdominal circumference
AFAFP	Amniotic fluid α-fetoprotein
AFP	α-fetoprotein
AFV	Amniotic fluid volume
AGA	Average for gestational age
AID or AIH	Artificial insemination donor (H designates mate is donor)
ARBOW	Artificial rupture of bag of waters
AROM	Artificial rupture of membranes
BAT	Brown adipose tissue (brown fat)
BBT	Basal body temperature
BL	Baseline (fetal heart rate baseline)
BOW	Bag of waters
BPD	Biparietal diameter *or* Bronchopulmonary dysplasia
BPP	Biophysical profile
BSE	Breast self-examination
BSST	Breast self-stimulation test
CC	Chest circumference *or* Cord compression
C–H	Crown-to-heel length
CID	Cytomegalic inclusion disease
CMV	Cytomegalovirus
CNM	Certified nurse-midwife
CNS	Clinical nurse specialist
CPAP	Continuous positive airway pressure
CPD	Cephalopelvic disproportion *or* Citrate-phosphate-dextrose
CRL	Crown-rump length
C/S	Cesarean section (or C-section)
CST	Contraction stress test
CVA	Costovertebral angle
CVS	Chorionic villus sampling
D&C	Dilatation and curettage
decels	Deceleration of fetal heart rate
DFMR	Daily fetal movement response
dil	Dilatation
DRG	Diagnostic related groups
DTR	Deep tendon reflexes
ECMO	Extracorporal membrane oxygenator
EDB	Estimated date of birth
EDC	Estimated date of confinement
EDD	Estimated date of delivery
EFM	Electronic fetal monitoring
EFW	Estimated fetal weight
EIA	Enzyme immunoassay
ELF	Elective low forceps
ELISA	Enzyme-linked immunosorbent assay
epis	Episiotomy
ERT	Estrogen replacement therapy
FAD	Fetal activity diary
FAE	Fetal alcohol effects
FAS	Fetal alcohol syndrome
FBD	Fibrocystic breast disease
FBM	Fetal breathing movements
FBS	Fetal blood sample *or* Fasting blood sugar test
FECG	Fetal electrocardiogram
FHR	Fetal heart rate
FHT	Fetal heart tones
FL	Femur length
FM	Fetal movement
FPG	Fasting plasma glucose test
FSH	Follicle-stimulating hormone
FSHRH	Follicle-stimulating hormone–releasing hormone
G or grav	Gravida
GDM	Gestational diabetes mellitus
GIFT	Gamete intrafallopian transfer
GnRF	Gonadotropin-releasing factor
GnRH	Gonadotropin-releasing hormone
GTD	Gestational trophoblastic disease
GTPAL	Gravida, term, preterm, abortion, living children; a system of recording maternity history
HA	Head-abdominal ratio
HAI	Hemagglutination-inhibition test
HC	Head compression
hCG	Human chorionic gonadotropin
hCS	Human chorionic somatomammotropin (same as hPL)
HMD	Hyaline membrane disease

hMG	Human menopausal gonadotropin
hPL	Human placental lactogen
HPV	Human papilloma virus
HVH	Herpesvirus hominis
IDM	Infant of a diabetic mother
IPG	Impedance phlebography
IU	International units
IUD	Intrauterine device
IUFD	Intrauterine fetal death
IUGR	Intrauterine growth restriction
IVF	In vitro fertilization
LADA	Left-acromion-dorsal-anterior
LADP	Left-acromion-dorsal-posterior
LBW	Low birth weight
LDR	Labor, delivery, and recovery room
LGA	Large for gestational age
LH	Luteinizing hormone
LHRH	Luteinizing hormone–releasing hormone
LMA	Left-mentum-anterior
LML	Left mediolateral (episiotomy)
LMP	Last menstrual period *or* Left-mentum-posterior
LMT	Left-mentum-transverse
LOA	Left-occiput-anterior
LOF	Low outlet forceps
LOP	Left-occiput-posterior
LOT	Left-occiput-transverse
L/S	Lecithin/sphingomyelin ratio
LSA	Left-sacrum-anterior
LSP	Left-sacrum-posterior
LST	Left-sacrum-transverse
MAS	Meconium aspiration syndrome
mec	Meconium
mec st	Meconium stain
ML	Midline (episiotomy)
MSAFP	Maternal serum α-fetoprotein
MUGB	4-methylumbelliferyl quanidinobenzoate
multip	Multipara
NEC	Necrotizing enterocolitis
NGU	Nongonococcal urethritis
NP	Nurse practitioner
NSCST	Nipple stimulation contraction stress test
NST	Nonstress test *or* Nonshivering thermogenesis
NSVD	Normal sterile vaginal delivery
NTD	Neural tube defects
OA	Occiput anterior
OC	Oral contraceptives
OCT	Oxytocin challenge test
OF	Occipito-frontal diameter of fetal head
OFC	Occipito-frontal circumference
OGTT	Oral glucose tolerance test
OM	Occipitomental (diameter)
OP	Occiput posterior
p	Para
Pap smear	Papanicolaou smear
PDA	Patent ductus arteriosus
PEEP	Positive end-expiratory pressure
PG	Phosphatidylglycerol *or* Prostaglandin
PI	Phosphatidylinositol
PID	Pelvic inflammatory disease
PIH	Pregnancy-induced hypertension
Pit	Pitocin
PKU	Phenylketonuria
PMS	Premenstrual syndrome
PPHN	Persistent pulmonary hypertension
Premie	Premature infant
primip	Primipara
PROM	Premature rupture of membranes
PSI	Prostaglandin synthesis inhibitor
PUBS	Percutaneous umbilical blood sampling
RADA	Right-acromion-dorsal-anterior
RADP	Right-acromion-dorsal-posterior
RDS	Respiratory distress syndrome
REM	Rapid eye movements
RIA	Radioimmunoassay
RLF	Retrolental fibroplasia
RMA	Right-mentum-anterior
RMP	Right-mentum-posterior
RMT	Right-mentum-transverse
ROA	Right-occiput-anterior
ROM	Rupture of membranes
ROP	Right-occiput-posterior *or* Retinopathy of prematurity
ROT	Right-occiput-transverse
RRA	Radioreceptor assay
RSA	Right-sacrum-anterior
RSP	Right-sacrum-posterior
RST	Right-sacrum-transverse
SET	Surrogate embryo transfer
SFD	Small for dates
SGA	Small for gestational age
SIDS	Sudden infant death syndrome
SMB	Submentobregmatic diameter
SOB	Suboccipitobregmatic diameter
SPA	Sperm penetration assay
SRBOW	Spontaneous rupture of the bag of waters
SROM	Spontaneous rupture of membranes
STI	Sexually transmitted infection
STH	Somatotropic hormone
STS	Serologic test for syphilis
SVE	Sterile vaginal exam
TC	Thoracic circumference
TCM	Transcutaneous monitoring
TDI	Therapeutic Donor Insemination
TNZ	Thermal neutral zone
TOL	Trail of labor
TORCH	Toxoplasmosis, rubella, cytomegalovirus, herpesvirus hominis type 2
TSS	Toxic shock syndrome
ū	Umbilicus
UA	Uterine activity

UAC	Umbilical artery catheter
UAU	Uterine activity units
UC	Uterine contraction
UPI	Uteroplacental insufficiency
US	Ultrasound
VBAC	Vaginal birth after cesarean
VDRL	Venereal Disease Research Laboratories
VLBW	Very low birth weight
WIC	Supplemental food program for Women, Infants, and Children
ZIFT	Zygote intrafallopian transfer

Appendix B

Conversions and Equivalents

TEMPERATURE CONVERSION

(Fahrenheit temperature – 32) x $\frac{5}{9}$ = Celsius temperature
(Celsius temperature – $\frac{9}{5}$) + 32 = Fahrenheit temperature

SELECTED CONVERSIONS TO METRIC MEASURES

Known value	Multiply by	To find
inches	2.54	centimeters
ounces	28	grams
pounds	454	grams
pounds	0.45	kilogram

SELECTED CONVERSIONS FROM METRIC MEASURES

Known value	Multiply by	To find
centimeters	0.4	inches
grams	0.035	ounces
grams	0.0022	pounds
kilograms	2.2	pounds

CONVERSION OF POUNDS AND OUNCES TO GRAMS

	Ounces															
S	0	1	2	3	4	5	6	7	8	9	10	11	12	13	14	15
0	—	28	57	85	113	142	170	198	227	255	283	312	340	369	397	425
1	454	482	510	539	567	595	624	652	680	709	737	765	794	822	850	879
2	907	936	964	992	1021	1049	1077	1106	1134	1162	1191	1219	1247	1276	1304	1332
3	1361	1389	1417	1446	1474	1503	1531	1559	1588	1616	1644	1673	1701	1729	1758	1786
4	1814	1843	1871	1899	1928	1956	1984	2013	2041	2070	2098	2126	2155	2183	2211	2240
5	2268	2296	2325	2353	2381	2410	2438	2466	2495	2523	2551	2580	2608	2637	2665	2693
6	2722	2750	2778	2807	2835	2863	2892	2920	2948	2977	3005	3033	3062	3090	3118	3147
7	3175	3203	3232	3260	3289	3317	3345	3374	3402	3430	3459	3487	3515	3544	3572	3600
8	3629	3657	3685	3714	3742	3770	3799	3827	3856	3884	3912	3941	3969	3997	4026	4054
9	4082	4111	4139	4167	4196	4224	4252	4281	4309	4337	4366	4394	4423	4451	4479	4508
10	4536	4564	4593	4621	4649	4678	4706	4734	4763	4791	4819	4848	4876	4904	4933	4961
Pounds 11	4990	5018	5046	5075	5103	5131	5160	5188	5216	5245	5273	5301	5330	5358	5386	5415
12	5443	5471	5500	5528	5557	5585	5613	5642	5670	5698	5727	5755	5783	5812	5840	5868
13	5897	5925	5953	5982	6010	6038	6067	6095	6123	6152	6180	6209	6237	6265	6294	6322
14	6350	6379	6407	6435	6464	6492	6520	6549	6577	6605	6634	6662	6690	6719	6747	6776
15	6804	6832	6860	6889	6917	6945	6973	7002	7030	7059	7087	7115	7144	7172	7201	7228
16	7257	7286	7313	7342	7371	7399	7427	7456	7484	7512	7541	7569	7597	7626	7654	7682
17	7711	7739	7768	7796	7824	7853	7881	7909	7938	7966	7994	8023	8051	8079	8108	8136
18	8165	8192	8221	8249	8278	8306	8335	8363	8391	8420	8448	8476	8504	8533	8561	8590
19	8618	8646	8675	8703	8731	8760	8788	8816	8845	8873	8902	8930	8958	8987	9015	9043
20	9072	9100	9128	9157	9185	9213	9242	9270	9298	9327	9355	9383	9412	9440	9469	9497
21	9525	9554	9582	9610	9639	9667	9695	9724	9752	9780	9809	9837	9865	9894	9922	9950
22	9979	10007	10036	10064	10092	10120	10149	10177	10206	10234	10262	10291	10319	10347	10376	10404

Appendix C

Spanish Translations of English Phrases[1]

This Appendix includes phrases you might find helpful in working with families during pregnancy, labor and birth, and after the birth. There are many ways to phrase questions. We have chosen some statements we consider essential and have tried to phrase them in a straightforward way. The phrases are designed to help you in situations in which translation is not possible at the moment.

This list begins with introductory statements, which are presented in a logical conversational flow. The remaining phrases are arranged according to the phases of pregnancy and birth during which they are most applicable.

Essential Introductory Phrases	**Frases Introductoras Esenciales**
Hello.	Hola.
I am a nurse.	Soy enferera (enfermero).[2]
I am a student nurse.	Soy estudiante de enfermería.
My name is ________________	Mi nombre es ________________
	Me llamo ________________
What is your name?	¿Cuál es su nombre?
	¿Cómo se llama?
What name should I call you?	¿Cómo quiere que la llamemos?
	¿Cómo quiere ser llamada?
Thank you.	Gracias.
Please.	Por favor.
Is someone here with you?	¿Hay alquien aquí con usted?
Does he (she) speak English?	¿Habla él (ella) English?
Goodbye.	Adiós.
Phrases for the Antepartal Period	**Frases para el Periodo Prenatal**
Are you taking any medications now?	¿Está tomando algunas medicinas ahora?
Show me the medicine bottles please.	Por favor, muéstreme los frascos.
Have you ever had trouble with your blood pressure?	¿Ha tenido problemas alguna vez con la presión arterial?
When was the first day of your last period?	¿Cuál fue el primer día de su última regla?
	¿Cuál fue el primer día de su última menstruación?
Have you had any spotting or bleeding since your last period?	¿Ha sangrado o ha tenido manchas de sangre desde su última regla?
Have you been on birth control pills?	¿Ha estado tomando píldoras anticonceptivas?
When did you stop taking them?	¿Cuándo dejó de tomarlas?

1. Prepared by Elizabeth Medina, PhD. Associate Professor of Spanish, Regis University, Denver, Colorado

2. In Spanish, nouns that end in *a* indicate female gender. Nouns that end in *o* indicate male gender.

Phrases for the Antepartal Period	Frases para el Periodo Prenatal
Do you have an intrauterine device (IUD)?	¿Usa un aparato intrauterino?
How many times have you been pregnant?	¿Cuántas veces ha estado usted embarazada?
Are you having any problems with your pregnancy?	¿Tiene problemas con us embarazo?
Is there anything that is worrying you?	¿Hay algo o alguna cosa que la preocupe?
I would like to take your blood pressure.	Quisiera tomarle la presió arterial.
I would like to take your pulse.	Quisiera tomarle el pulso.
I would like to take your temperature.	Quisiera tomarle la temperatura.
I would like to listen to your heart and lungs.	Quisiera escucharle el corazon y los pulmones.
I would like to check your uterus.	Quisiera examinarle el útero.
Would you please urinate in this cup and leave it in the bathroom.	Puede orinar en este vaso y dejarlo en el baño.
Please stand up.	Por favor, levántese.
Please sit down.	Por favor, siéntense.
Please lie down.	Por favor, acuéstese.

Phrases Related to Client Safety	Frases Relacionadas con la Seguridad del Cliente
I would like to talk to you alone.	Quisiera hablar a solas con usted.
Are you safe at home?	¿Sufre de peligros en case?
Are you afraid of your partner?	¿Le tiene miedo a su compañero?
During your pregnancy has your partner hit, slapped, kicked, or punched you?	Durante su embarazo, ¿la ha golpeado? ¿la ha abofeteado? ¿la ha pateado? o ¿le ha dado puñetazos?
How many times?	¿Cuántas veces?
Do you have someone for support?	¿Cuénta con alguien que la pueda ayudar?

Questions the Mother or Father May Ask	Posibles Preguntas que Madres y Padres Hacen
How big is my baby?	¿De qué tamaño es el (la) bebé ahora?
How much does the baby weigh now?	¿Cuánto pesa el bebé ahora?
When will I feel my baby move?	¿Cuándo lo (la) voy a sentir moverse?

Phrases for the Intrapartal Period	Frases Durante el Parto
Note: Review the Essential Introductory Phrases for beginning conversation.	Nota: Repase las frases introductoras para comenzar una conversación.
Are you having labor pains?	¿Tiene dolores de parto?
Are you having contractions?	¿Tiene contracciones?
Are you having pain?	¿Tiene dolores?
Do you need medicine for pain?	¿Necesita medicina para el dolor?
Do you need to urinate?	¿Necisita orinar?
This is a bedpan to urinate in.	Aquí tiene el bacín (la chata) (el pato) para orinar.
Can I help you to the bathroom?	¿La ayudo a ir al baño?
Do you need to have a bowel movement?	¿Necisita mover el vientre (obrar)? Necesita "Hacer caca"—coloquial
Has your bag of water broken?	¿Se le ha roto la bolsa de agua(s)?
Have you had any bright red bleeding during your pregnancy?	¿Ha tenido algún sangramiento de color rojo durante su embarazo?

Phrases for the Intrapartal Period

How many births have you had?

I need to do a vaginal examination.

I will help you.

I will stay with you.

Please pant. I will show you how.

Please do not push.

Push now.

Stop pushing.

The doctor needs to do a cesarean birth.

This is medicine for your pain. You will feel better soon.

When is your baby supposed to be born?

January	February
March	April
May	June
July	August
September	October
November	December

What is your doctor's name?

What is your midwife's name?

Your baby is having a little trouble now.

El bebé está sufriendo algunas dificultades.

I need to put this oxygen mask on you. It will help your baby. It may smell funny, but it is ok.

Please turn on your left side.

Please turn on your right side

Your baby is ok.

Phrases for the Postpartal Period and the Newborn Area

Note: Review the Essential Introductory Phrases for beginning conversation.

Are you hungry?

Are your thirsty?

Are you cold?

Are you tired?

I am going to put antibiotic ointment in the baby's eyes. It will help protect your baby from some infections.

I am going to take some blood from your baby's foot to check the blood sugar and hemocrit.

If your baby begins to spit up, please turn him (her) on his (her) side.

It may help to position your baby like this.

I would like to suggest that you clean your nipples this way before your breastfeed your baby.

Frases Durante el Parto

¿Cuántos niños le han nacido?

Necesito hacerle un exaen vaginal.

La voy a ayudar.

Me quedaré con usted.

Por favor, jadee. Le voy a mostrar cómo.

No puje ahora.

Puje ahora.

Pare de pujar.

No puje más.

El doctor le va a hacer una operación cesárea.

Esta medicina es para el dolor. Va a sentirse mejor pronto.

¿Cuando está supuesto a nacer el bebé?

enero	febrero
marzo	abril
mayo	junio
julio	agosto
septiembre	octubre
noviembre	diciembre

¿Cuál es el nombre de su doctor?

¿Cuál is el nombre de su comadrona (partera)?

El bebé está pasando por algunos problemas.

Le voy a poner esta máscara de oxígeno. Va a ayudar al bebé. Huele extraño, pero no hay problemas.

Por favor voltéese al lado izquierdo.

Por favor voltéese al lado derecho.

El bebé está bien.

Frases para el Periodo Despues del Parto y el Area del Recien Nacido

Nota: Repase las frases introductoras para comenzar una conversación.

¿Tiene hambre?

¿Tiene sed?

¿Tiene frío?

¿Está cansada?

Le voy a poner al bebé un ungüento antibiótico alrededor de los ojos. Lo (la) va a proteger contra infecciones.

Le voy a sacar sangre del pie al bebé para determinar el azúcar del la sangre ye el hematocrítico.

Si el bebé comienza a vomitar, colóquelo (colóquela) de costado.

Lo (la) ayudará—si lo coloca así.

Lo (la) ayudaría—si lo colocara así.

Es bueno que se lave los pezones de esta manera antes de darle el pecho al bebé.

Phrases for the Postpartal Period and the Newborn Area	**Frases para el Periodo Despues del Parto y el Area del Recien Nacido**
I would like to suggest that you clean your baby's cord this way.	Es mejor para el bebé que le lave el ombligo de esta man era.
I would like to suggest that you bathe your baby this way.	Es mejor que lo (la) bañe de esta manera.
I would like to suggest that you clean your baby's penis this way.	Es mejor que le limpie el pene así.
I would like you to fold the diaper this way.	Le sugiero que doble el pañal así.
I would like to suggest that you fasten the diaper this way.	Le sugiero que asegure el pañal así.
I would like to suggest that you take the baby's temperature this way.	Tómele la temperature así.
I need to check your breasts, your uterus, your flow, your stitches, your legs and feet.	Necesito examinarle los pechos, el útero, el flujo, los puntos, las pierns y los pies.
I need to feel your uterus.	Necesito examinarle el útero.
I need to massage your uterus.	Necesito darle un masaje en la región del útero.
Place your baby on its side.	Coloque al bebé de costado.
Place the baby's used diaper here.	Coloque aquí los pañales usados.
Please rub your uterus every half hour to keep it firm. I will show you how.	Necesita darse un masaje en la región del útero cada me dia hora para mantenerlo firme. Le voy a mostrar cómo.
Would you like to see your baby now?	¿Quiere ver a su bebé ahora?
Would you like me to help you feed your baby?	¿Quiere que le ayude a alimentarlo (la)?
Your baby needs a car seat to go home in.	El (la) bebé necesita un asiento para bebé en el automóvil.

Special Neonatal Needs	**Necesidades del Recien Nacido**
We are giving your baby oxygen.	Le vamos a dar oxígeno al (a la) bebé.
Your baby is having some problems breathing.	El (la) bebé tiene problemas al respirar.
Your baby needs extra help.	El (la) bebé necesita ayuda especial.
Your baby needs to go to a special care nursery.	El (la) bebé necesita ir a la sala de cuidados especiales para bebés.

Appendix D

Guidelines for Working with Deaf Clients and Interpreters

1. First, remember that it requires trust on the part of the client to allow non-signing caregivers and an interpreter into their life.
2. It is important to use a registered interpreter. Medical interpreters are registered with the Registry of Interpreters for the Deaf. Although family members and friends may offer to interpret, it is best to use a registered medical interpreter because they are required to translate the clients and nurses words accurately without adding in any other opinion.
3. Greet the client and family with a handshake and body posture that indicates welcome. You may point to your name tag and use the American Sign Language (ASL) alphabet cards to spell out your name. The client may wish to select cards to indicate their name. It is especially important as you work together to make the effort to provide a greeting as you would with speaking clients, this will help develop rapport.
4. Once the interpreter is present, continue to look at the client and speak directly to her. There will be a temptation to look at the interpreter and it will help to remember that you are speaking to the client.
5. Avoid phrasing your words as if you are talking to the interpreter. For example, "Can you tell her . . . . ". Instead phrase your questions as you do with speaking clients. For example, "I'm going to ask you some questions now."
6. Depend on the deaf client to ask questions.
7. Look at the client's face for signs of difficulty in understanding. Deaf clients have a behavior of "gesturing" which involves shaking their head as if to indicate "yes" even when they do not understand. If the client is nodding "yes", ask her to repeat the directions you have just given.
8. Be as direct as possible. Keep to what you want to know or what you want to convey. Speak in short sentences using nontechnical words. Avoid colloquial or slang words. Be sure to explain what you want to do, before you do it. For instance, tell her you want to start an IV and explain the equipment. Then with her permission, start the IV.
9. Be aware that deaf clients may have difficulty understanding when to take medications. It will be helpful to associate taking medications or completing some treatment/activity with meals. (For instance, while showing her the two capsules she is to take when she goes home, tell her to take the two capsules at breakfast and another two capsules at bedtime). Avoid saying "take two capsules at 8:00 AM, 2:00 PM and 12:00 AM."
10. The difference in interpreting time may also effect obtaining a history. It is best to begin with a specific event in the past and work forward.

What to Do Until the Interpreter Arrives

1. Role play as much as possible.
2. Demonstrate what you want the client to do or what you want to do.
3. Be resourceful.
4. Remember that some deaf clients can read lips. Some may read written language, but use care in assuming the client understands.

What to Do to Prepare for Working with a Deaf Client

1. Contact local agencies that work with deaf clients to see what resources are available. Ask about classes in ASL. Learning some basic signs will be very helpful until an interpreter arrives.
2. Read to learn more about the deaf culture. Contact your local agency or the National Information Center on Deafness, Silver Springs, Maryland to suggest books you might read.
3. Investigate your health facility. What is available to assist you? Look for videos used for teaching in the maternal-child unit and note if they have captions. Remember that many deaf clients do not read written language, so it will be important to review the content of the video with an interpreter present.

Prepared with the kind assistance of Mr. Gerald Dement, Interpreter Coordinator, Pikes Peak Center on Deafness, Colorado Springs, Colorado.

Appendix E

Sign Language for Health Care Professionals

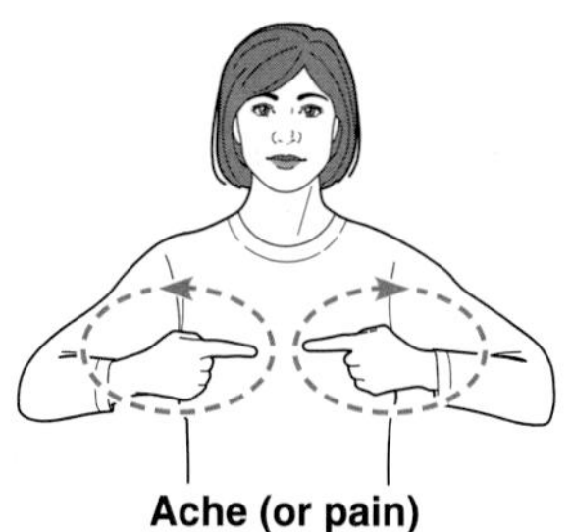
Ache (or pain)

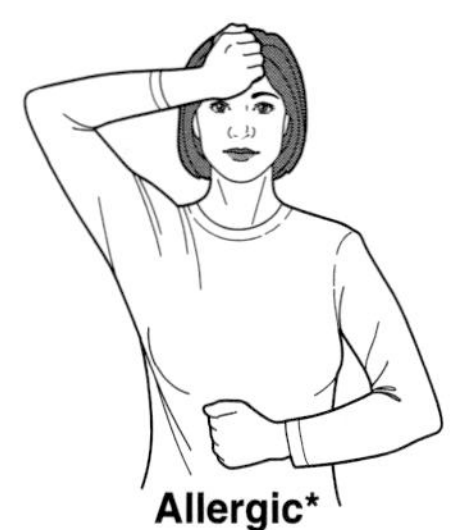
Allergic*

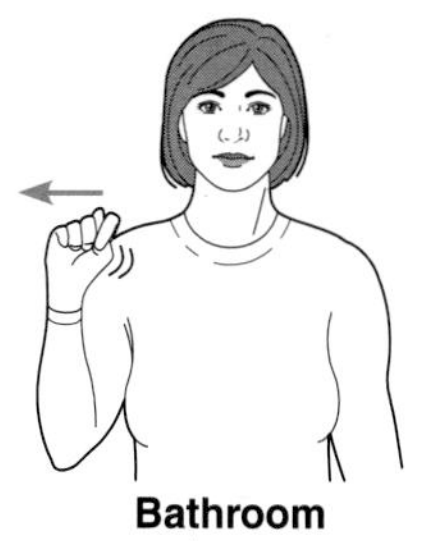
Bathroom

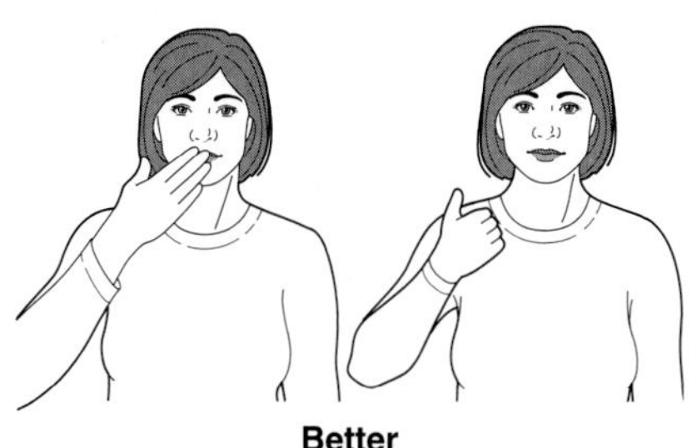
Better

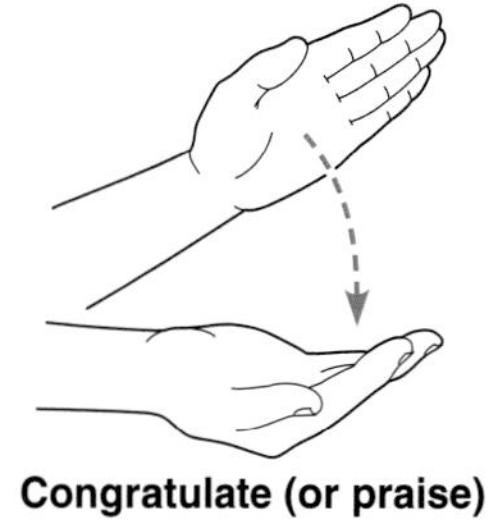
Congratulate (or praise)

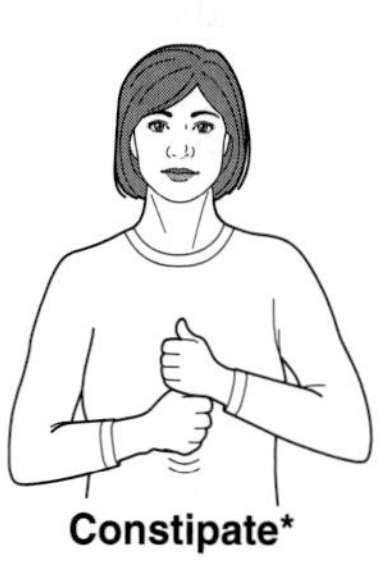
Constipate*

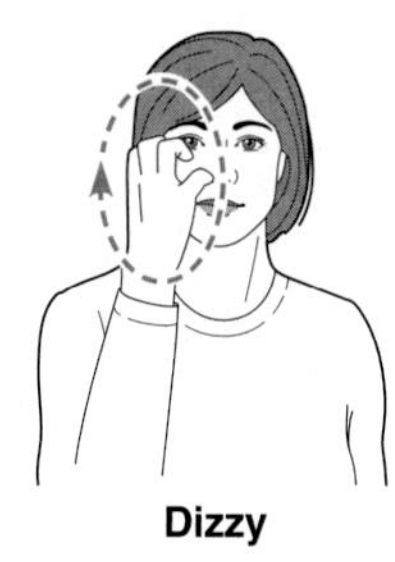
Dizzy

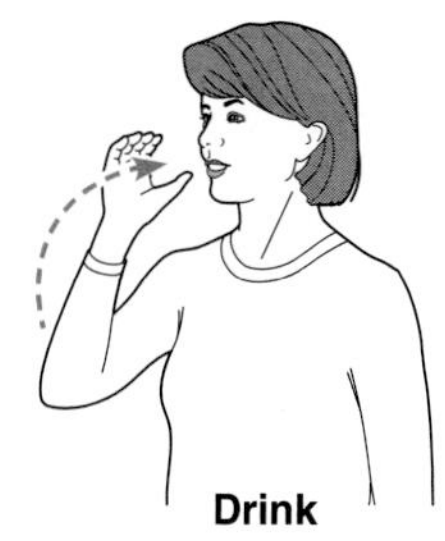
Drink

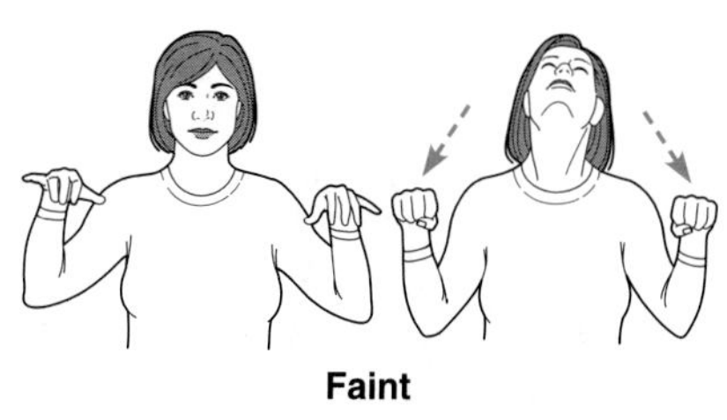
Faint

*Indicates signs that are in manually signed English. Those without an asterisk are in American Sign Language.

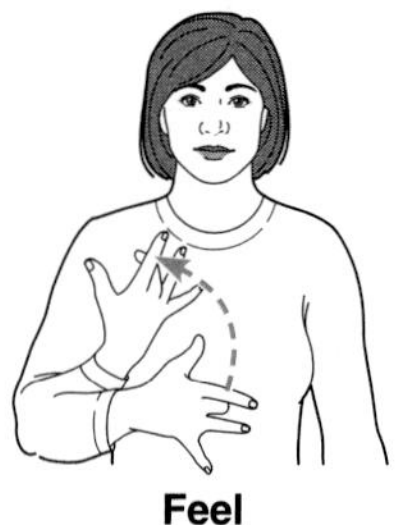
Feel

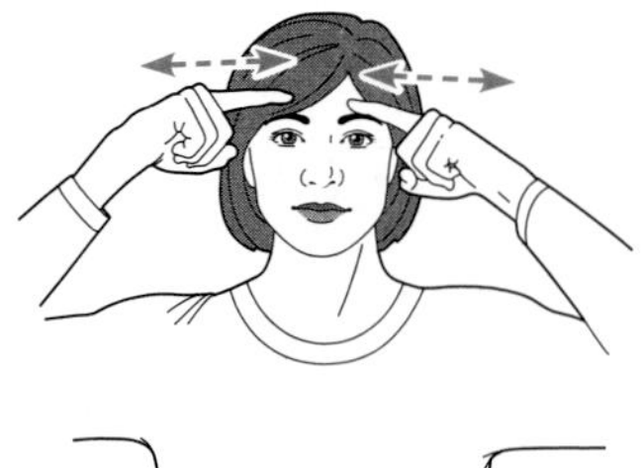
Headache

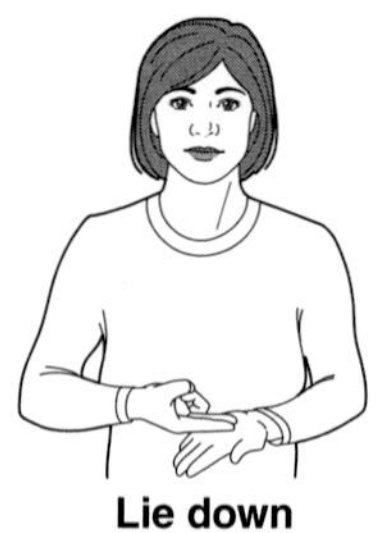
Lie down

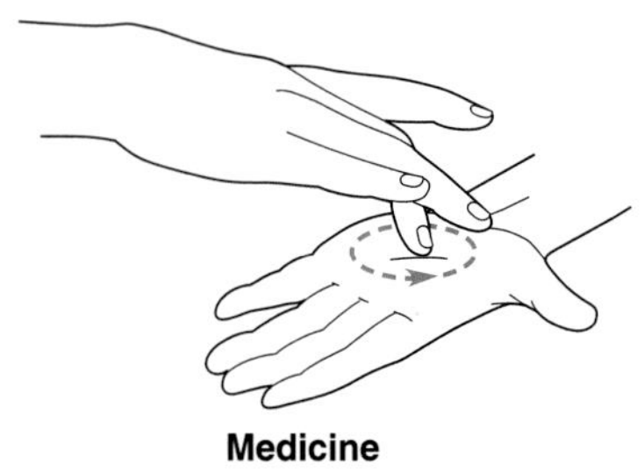
Medicine

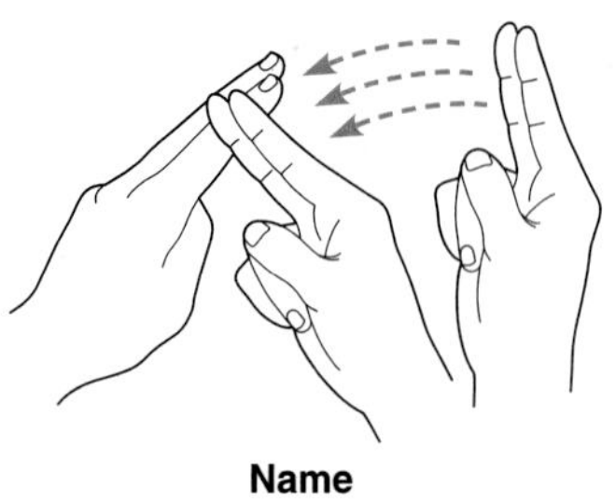
Name

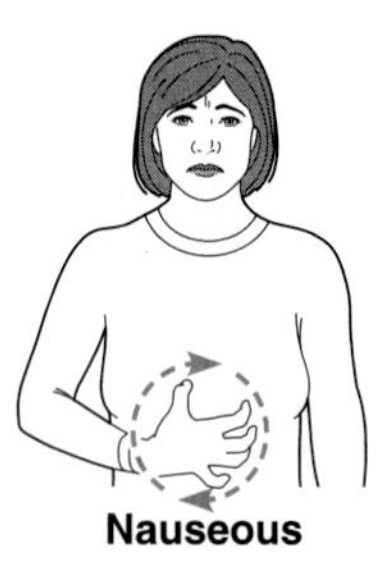
Nauseous

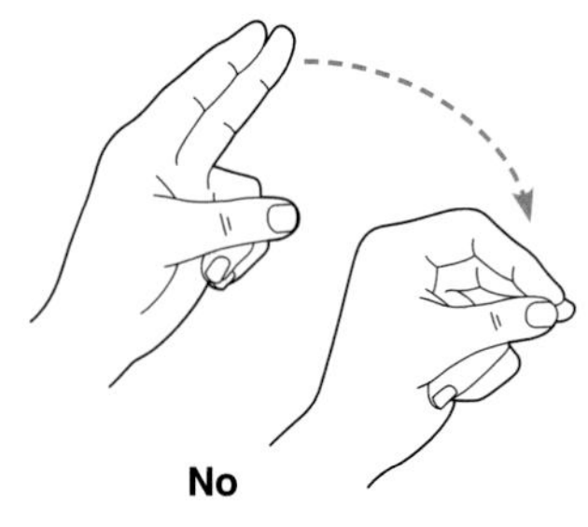
No

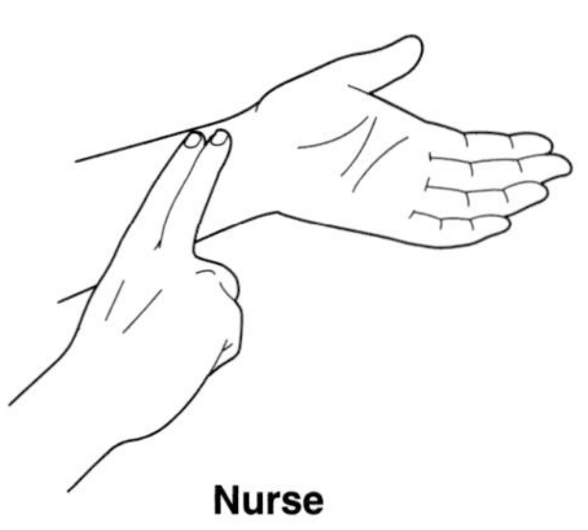
Nurse

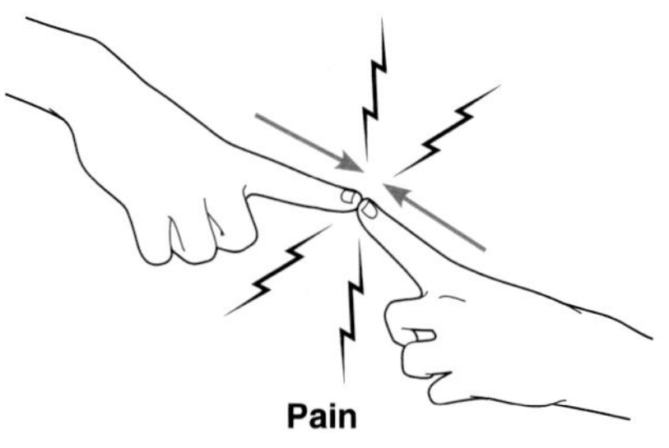
Pain

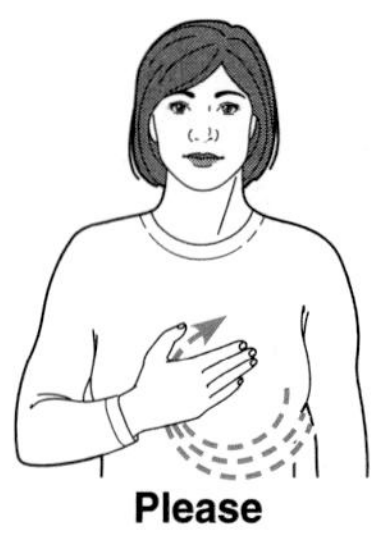
Please

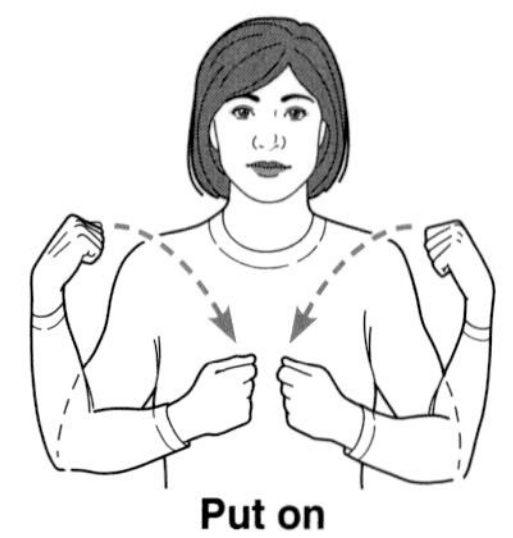
Put on

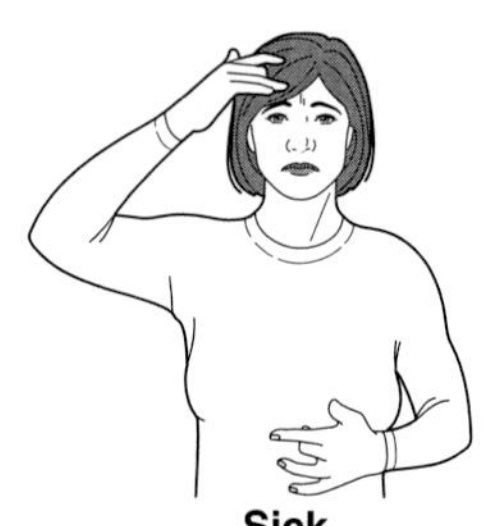
Sick

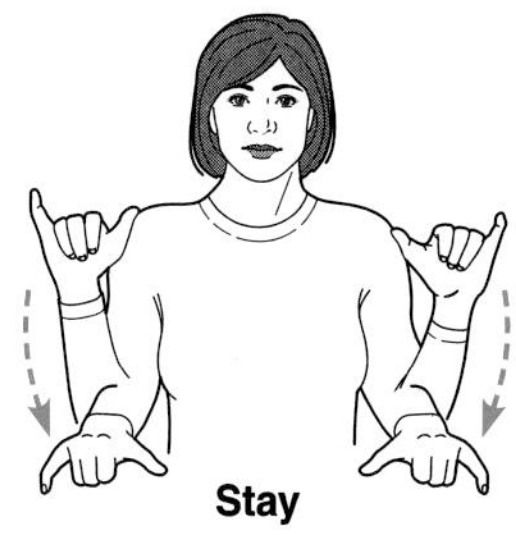
Stay

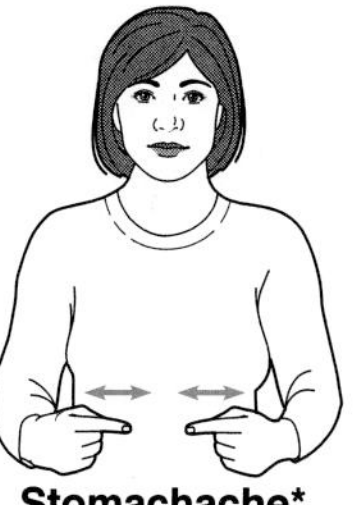
Stomachache*

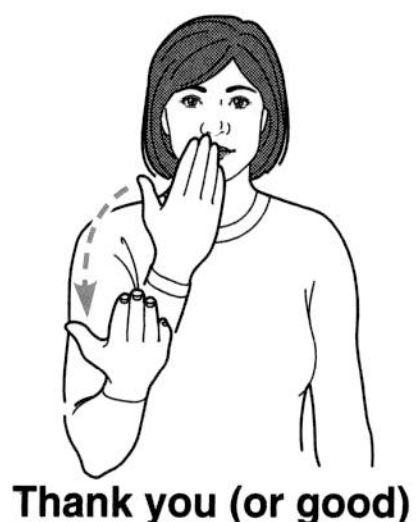
Thank you (or good)

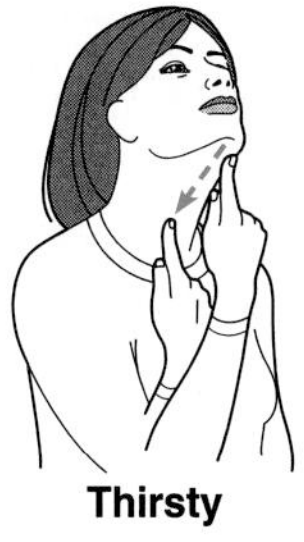
Thirsty

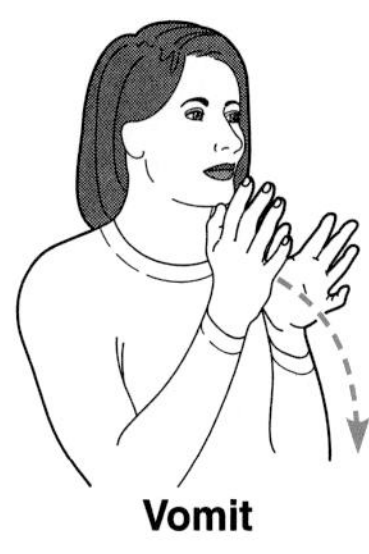
Vomit

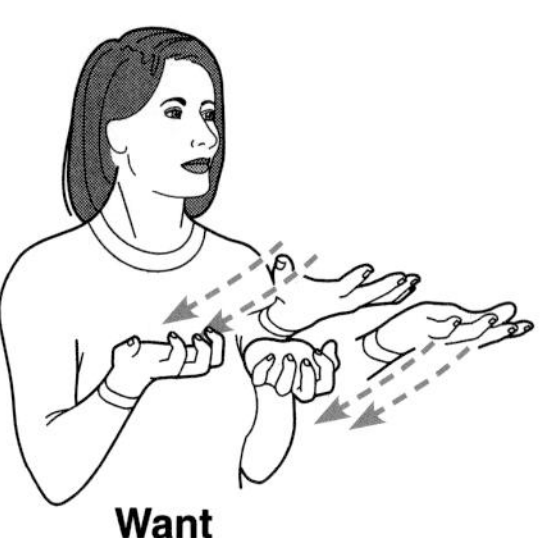
Want

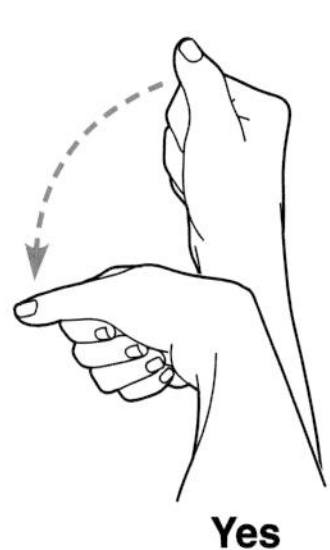
Yes

*Indicates signs that are in manually signed English. Those without an asterisk are in American Sign Language.

Appendix F

Clinical Estimation of Gestational Age

Examination First Hours

CLINICAL ESTIMATION OF GESTATIONAL AGE

An Approximation Based on Published Data*

PHYSICAL FINDINGS		WEEKS GESTATION																												
		20	21	22	23	24	25	26	27	28	29	30	31	32	33	34	35	36	37	38	39	40	41	42	43	44	45	46	47	48
VERNIX		APPEARS				COVERS BODY, THICK LAYER														ON BACK, SCALP, IN CREASES		SCANT, IN CREASES		NO VERNIX						
BREAST TISSUE AND AREOLA		AREOLA & NIPPLE BARELY VISIBLE NO PALPABLE BREAST TISSUE														AREOLA RAISED		1-2 MM NODULE		3-5 MM	5-6 MM	7-10 MM				?12 MM				
EAR	FORM	FLAT, SHAPELESS														BEGINNING INCURVING SUPERIOR		INCURVING UPPER 2/3 PINNAE			WELL-DEFINED INCURVING TO LOBE									
	CARTILAGE	PINNA SOFT, STAYS FOLDED												CARTILAGE SCANT RETURNS SLOWLY FROM FOLDING				THIN CARTILAGE SPRINGS BACK FROM FOLDING				PINNA FIRM, REMAINS ERECT FROM HEAD								
SOLE CREASES		SMOOTH SOLES T̄ CREASES												1-2 ANTERIOR CREASES			2-3 ANTERIOR CREASES	CREASES ANTERIOR 2/3 SOLE		CREASES INVOLVING HEEL				DEEPER CREASES OVER ENTIRE SOLE						
SKIN	THICKNESS & APPEARANCE	THIN, TRANSLUCENT SKIN, PLETHORIC, VENULES OVER ABDOMEN EDEMA												SMOOTH THICKER NO EDEMA				PINK		FEW VESSELS		SOME DESQUAMATION PALE PINK		THICK, PALE, DESQUAMATION OVER ENTIRE BODY						
	NAIL PLATES	APPEAR	NAILS TO FINGER TIPS																					NAILS EXTEND WELL BEYOND FINGER TIPS						
HAIR		APPEARS ON HEAD			EYE BROWS & LASHES					FINE, WOOLLY, BUNCHES OUT FROM HEAD									SILKY, SINGLE STRANDS LAYS FLAT					?RECEDING HAIRLINE OR LOSS OF BABY HAIR SHORT, FINE UNDERNEATH						
LANUGO		APPEARS	COVERS ENTIRE BODY												VANISHES FROM FACE					PRESENT ON SHOULDERS				NO LANUGO						
GENITALIA	TESTES									TESTES PALPABLE IN INGUINAL CANAL								IN UPPER SCROTUM						IN LOWER SCROTUM						
	SCROTUM									FEW RUGAE								RUGAE, ANTERIOR PORTION				RUGAE COVER		PENDULOUS						
	LABIA & CLITORIS											PROMINENT CLITORIS LABIA MAJORA SMALL WIDELY SEPARATED						LABIA MAJORA LARGER NEARLY COVERED CLITORIS				LABIA MINORA & CLITORIS COVERED								
SKULL FIRMNESS		BONES ARE SOFT								SOFT TO 1" FROM ANTERIOR FONTANELLE							SPONGY AT EDGES OF FONTANELLE CENTER FIRM			BONES HARD SUTURES EASILY DISPLACED				BONES HARD, CANNOT BE DISPLACED						
POSTURE	RESTING	HYPOTONIC LATERAL DECUBITUS						HYPOTONIC				BEGINNING FLEXION THIGH		STRONGER HIP FLEXION		FROG-LIKE		FLEXION ALL LIMBS		HYPERTONIC				VERY HYPERTONIC						
	RECOIL - LEG	NO RECOIL												PARTIAL RECOIL						PROMPT RECOIL										
	ARM	NO RECOIL														BEGIN FLEXION NO RECOIL		PROMPT RECOIL MAY BE INHIBITED				PROMPT RECOIL AFTER 30" INHIBITION								
		20	21	22	23	24	25	26	27	28	29	30	31	32	33	34	35	36	37	38	39	40	41	42	43	44	45	46	47	48

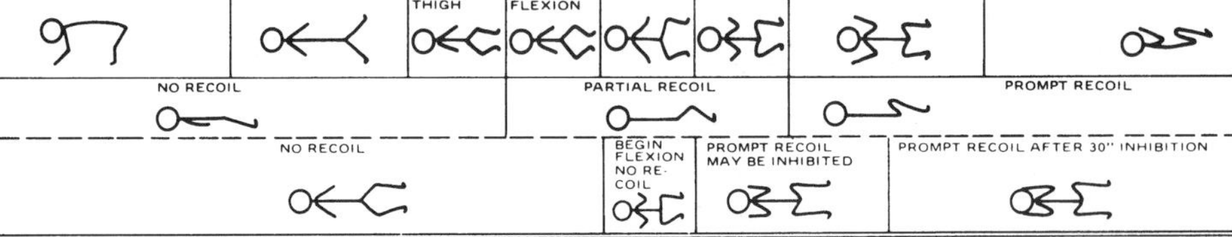

*Brazie JV and Lubchenco LO. The estimation of gestational age chart. In Kempe, Silver and O'Brien, *Current Pediatric Diagnosis and Treatment*, ed 3. Los Altos, Calif. Lange Medical Publications, 1974, ch 4.
Form courtesy of Mead Johnson Laboratories, Evansville, IN.

Appendix G

Actions and Effects of Selected Drugs During Breastfeeding*

Anticoagulants
Coumarin derivatives (Warfarin Dicumarol): Only small amount in breast milk; check PTT
Heparin: Relatively safe to use; check PTT
Phenindione (Hedulin): Not used in USA, Passes easily into breast milk; neonate may have increased prothrombin time and PTT

Anticonvulsants
Phenytoin (Dilantin), phenobarbital: Generally considered safe; if high doses of phenobarbital are ingested, may cause drowsiness; short-acting phenobarbiturates (secobarbital) preferred, as they appear in lower concentration in milk

Antihistamines
Diphenhydramine (Benadryl), pheniramine (Dimetane), Coricidin, Drixoral: May cause decreased milk supply; infant may become drowsy, irritable, or have tachycardia

Antimetabolites Unknown, probably long-term anti-DNA effect on the infant; potentially very toxic

Antimicrobials
Aminoglycosides: May cause ototoxicity or nephrotoxicity if given for more than 2 weeks
Ampicillin: Skin rash, candidiasis; diarrhea
Chloramphenicol: Possible bone marrow suppression; too low a dose for Gray syndrome; refusal of breast
Methacycline: Possible inhibition of bone growth; may cause discoloration of the teeth; use should be avoided
Metronidazole (Flagyl): Possible neurologic disorders or blood dyscrasias; delay breastfeeding for 12 hours after dose
Penicillin: Possible allergic response; candidiasis
Quinolones (synthetic antibiotics): Can cause arthropathies
Sulfonamides: May cause hyperbilirubinemia; use contraindicated until infant over 1 week old
Tetracycline: Long-term use and large doses should be avoided; may cause tooth staining or inhibition of bone growth

Antithyroids
Thiouracil: Contraindicated during lactation; may cause goiter or agranulocytosis

Barbiturates
Propylthiouracil: safe-monitor infamthroid function
Phenothiazines: May produce sedation

Bronchodilators
Aminophylline: May cause insomnia or irritability in the infant
Ephedrine, cromolyn (Intal): Relatively safe

Caffeine Excessive consumption may cause jitteriness or wakefulness

Cardiovascular
Methyldopa: Increase in milk volume
Propranolol (Inderal): May cause hypoglycemia; possibility of other blocking effects, especially if infant has renal or liver dysfunction
Quinidine: May cause arrhythmias in infant
Reserpine (Serpasil): Nasal stuffiness, lethargy, or diarrhea in infant

Corticosteroids Adrenal suppression may occur with long-term administration of doses greater than 10 mg/day

Diuretics
Furosemide (Lasix): Not excreted in breast milk
Thiazide diuretics (Œsidrix, Hydrodiuril, Oretic): Safe but can cause dehydration, reduce milk production

Heavy metals
Gold: Potentially toxic; Gold salts-compatible with nursing
Mercury: Excreted in the milk and hazardous to infant

Hormones
Androgens: Suppress lactation
Thyroid hormones: May mask hypothyroidism

Laxatives
Cascara: May cause diarrhea in infant
Milk of magnesia: Relatively safe

Narcotic analgesics
Codeine: Accumulation may lead to neonatal depression
Meperidine: May lead to neonatal depression
Morphine: Long-term use may cause newborn addiction

*Based on data from Riordan J, Auerbach KG: *Breastfeeding and Human Lactation.* Boston: Jones and Bartlett, 1993, pp 135–166. Fanaroff, AA, Martin RJ: *Neonatal-Perinatal Medicine: Diseases of the Fetus and Infant.* 6th ed. Vol 1, 1997 p 148–152. St. Louis: Mosby. Briggs GG, Freeman RK, Yaffe SJ: *Drugs in Pregnancy and Lactation* 5th ed. 1998, Baltimore: Williams & Wilkins Committee on Drugs, American Academy of Pediatrics. The transfer of drugs and other chemicals into human milk. *Pediatrics* 1994; 93:137–50. Taeusch, H and Ballard, RA (1998): *Avery's Diseases of the Newborn* 7th ed. Philadelphia: W. B. Saunders. p 1348–1352.

Nonnarcotic analgesics, NSAIDs
Acetaminophen (Tylenol): Relatively safe for short-term analgesia
Ibuprofen (Motrin): Safe
Propoxyphene (Darvon): May cause sleepiness and poor nursing in infant
Salicylates (aspirin): Safe after first week of life; monitor protime

Oral contraceptives
Combined estrogen/progestin pills: Significantly decrease milk supply; may alter milk composition; may cause gynecomastia in male infants
Progestin only: Safe if started after lactation is established

Radioactive materials for testing
Gallium citrate (^{67}G): Insignificant amount excreted in breast milk; no nursing for 2 weeks
Iodine: Contraindicated; may affect infant's thyroid gland
^{125}I: Discontinue nursing for 48 hours
^{131}I: Nursing should be discontinued until excretion is no longer significant; nursing may be resumed after 10 days
Technetium-99m: Discontinue nursing for 3 days (half-life = 6 hours)

Sedatives/Tranquilizers
Diazepam (Valium): May accumulate to high levels; may increase neonatal jaundice; may cause lethargy and weight loss
Lithium carbonate: Contraindicated; may cause neonatal flaccidity and hypotonia

Substance Abuse
Alcohol: Potential motor developmental delay; mild sedative effect
Amphetamines: Controversial; may cause irritability, poor sleeping pattern
Cocaine, crack: Extreme irritability, tachycardia, vomiting, apnea
Marijuana: Drowsiness
Heroin: Tremors, restlessness, vomiting, poor feeding
Nicotine (smoking): Shock, vomiting, diarrhea, decreased milk production

Appendix H

Selected Maternal-Newborn Laboratory Values

Normal Maternal Laboratory Values

Test	Non-Pregnant Values	Pregnant Values
Hematocrit	37%–47%	32%–42%
Hemoglobin	12–16 g/dL*	10–14 g/dL*
Platelets	150,000–350,000/mm^3	Significant increase 3–5 days after birth (predisposes to thrombosis)
Partial thromboplastin time (PTT)	12–14 seconds	Slight decrease in pregnancy and again in labor (placental site clotting)
Fibrinogen	250 mg/dL	400 mg/dL
Serum Glucose:		
Fasting	70–80 mg/dL	65 mg/dL
2-hour postprandial	60–110 mg/dL	Less than 140 mg/dL
Total protein	6.7–8.3 g/dL	5.5–7.5 g/dL
White blood cell total	4500–10,000/mm^3	5000–15,000/mm^3
Polymorphonuclear cells	54%–62%	60%–85%
Lymphocytes	38%–46%	15%–40%

Normal Neonatal Laboratory Values

Test	Normal Values
Hematocrit	51%–56%
Hemoglobin	16.5 g/dL (cord blood)
Platelets	150,000–400,000/mm^3
White blood cell total	18,000/mm^3
White blood cell differential:	
Bands	1600/mm^3 (9%)
Polymorphonuclear (segs)	9400/mm^3 (52%)
Eosinophils	400/mm^3 (2.2%)
Basophils	100/mm^3 (0.6%)
Lymphocytes	5500/mm^3 (31%)
Monocytes	1050/mm^3 (5.8%)
Serum glucose	40–80 mg/dL
Serum electrolytes:	
Sodium	135–147 mEq/L
Potassium	4–6 mEq/L
Chloride	90–114 mEq/L
Carbon dioxide	15–25 mEq/L
Bicarbonate	18–23 mEq/L
Calcium	7–10 mg/dL

*at sea level

Appendix I

Suggested Answers to Critical Thinking in Practice Questions

Chapter 3

Rita has described a normal menstrual cycle. While it is variable in frequency, it is not outside the range of what is acceptable in a teenager. The flow that she thinks is heavy is really quite normal and the fact that she has cramps indicates that she is having ovulatory cycles.

It is important to reassure Rita that there is nothing wrong with her menstrual cycle. It would be appropriate to suggest an anti-prostaglandin such as ibuprofen for the relief of dysmenorrhea. Of utmost importance is to follow up on her request for birth control pills. It may be that she is considering becoming sexually active and needs contraception. Sometimes teenagers have a difficult time asking for what they really want and this is an ideal situation in which to bring up issues of sexuality with a young woman.

Chapter 3

The use of feminine hygiene products can result in vaginitis and actually promote sexually transmitted diseases, especially PID. Feminine hygiene products, especially douches, alter the acid-base balance of the vagina, allowing opportunistic organisms to replicate. Also, douching washes out the protective normal flora of the vagina, and the altered acid-base vaginal environment prevents the protective bacteria from growing. The action of douching can propel pathogenic organisms upward and promote an ascending infection such as PID. CW should be told that douching is seldom necessary, and that cleansing daily with soap and water are adequate hygienic measures (Rosenberg and Phillips, 1992).

CW should be told that she is at increased risk for PID because she has multiple sexual partners, uses an IUD, and douches. She should be counseled to consider other forms of contraceptives that are more protective against STDs and to consider limiting her sexual activity to a monogamous relationship.

Chapter 5

Marsha's story of how she got her injury is not consistent with the type of injury she has. Injuries that are accidental are usually to the extremities and not the trunk. Also, the bruising and edema suggest that the injury happened several hours ago. You should suspect that Marsha received her injuries from physical abuse, probably by Fred. The type of injury and the delay in coming for treatment are possible indicators of abuse. Also the fact that she looks to Fred to agree with her statements is suspicious. You should make every attempt to separate Marsha from Fred, so that she can speak more openly if she chooses. It is likely that if Fred is in the room she will deny the abuse for fear of further abuse. You do not want to put her in danger. You may need to be creative in separating Fred from Marsha, since often the abuser does not want to leave.

Chapter 10

Elena's height and prepregnancy weight are normal. Her weight gain during pregnancy has been appropriate but not excessive. Research indicates that assessment of fundal height is more accurate between 22–24 and 34 weeks' gestation. At 33 weeks Elena's baby was growing normally. Thus this finding is not abnormal by itself and may simply be a reflection of decreased accuracy of the procedure late in pregnancy. It may also reflect variations in growth of the baby. To make your best assessment you need further information about the results of this week's examination. If during her examination there are no indicators of problems such as decreased fetal activity, maternal urinary tract infection, maternal hypertension, and so forth, you can reassure Elena that this finding is probably a normal variation.

Chapter 11

At this point it would be important to realize that this is this couple's first exposure to the health care system of the United States and that the goal should be to make their first experience a positive one, as this may greatly influence their utilization of the system in the future. Take a moment to critically examine your own cultural values. Perhaps reflect upon your value of the importance of seeking early prenatal care and realize that for the Southeast Asian individual, seeking health care is usually related to a crisis and relief of symptoms. Pregnancy is not viewed as an illness, and therefore this couple would not usually be entering the health care system. What has brought them here today? Is Mrs Nguyen experiencing any problems with her pregnancy?

While reflecting upon questions such as these, one of the first things you can do to make this a positive experience for them is to immediately arrange for an interpreter. Once the interpreter is available, you will be able to obtain a more thorough history of Mrs Nguyen's pregnancy. Include a cultural assessment as part of your history. What are their expectations of the health care system? Are they using any traditional healing practices? Based upon the information provided, you will be able to provide prenatal education and care with consideration for their cultural values and beliefs.

Chapter 12

Competing in the marathon is not recommended. Even though Constance is in excellent shape, we do not know what impact prolonged participation in such a strenuous event might have on her fetus. Uterine blood flow is decreased during exercise as blood is shunted to the muscles, and the normal fetus seems able to withstand this. We don't know, however, whether this decreased blood flow to the fetus interferes with the fetus's ability to dissipate heat, especially since the fetus is not able to decrease temperature via perspiration or respiration (Fishbein & Phillips, 1990). With this in mind, ACOG guidelines recommend that, during pregnancy, competitive athletes avoid competition, and all women exercise for shorter intervals (no longer than 15 minutes at a time).

Chapter 13

Cindy has only recently turned 15. She may not be aware of good nutrition, and probably has minimal knowledge about how her nutritional habits impact the growing fetus. The nurse can begin by showing Cindy and her boyfriend pictures of the uterus, placenta, and umbilical cord, and discussing how the fetus is nourished. She then needs to help Cindy understand good nutritional habits and which of her favorite foods in the different food groups will also be healthy for her fetus. The use of audiovisual aids is important in teaching young teenagers. The nurse needs to determine food practices in Cindy's home. Who is cooking and preparing the food? How much control does Cindy have? If the mother prepares the food, the nurse and Cindy can discuss ways of sharing information about good nutrition with Cindy's mother. Evaluation of nutritional habits and reinforcement for positive changes throughout her pregnancy will be important. Since this was a planned pregnancy with a supportive boyfriend, compliance in health behaviors to produce a healthy baby is likely.

Expected weight gain in pregnancy also needs to be discussed. Body image is a concern in the teen years. Knowing a specific amount of weight that needs to be gained each trimester for normal growth of a healthy fetus, and that this weight will be lost after pregnancy, will be important for both Cindy and her boyfriend.

Chapter 14

Although Jane's intake is supporting an appropriate weight gain, her diet is not nutritionally adequate. Comparing her diet to the Food Guide Pyramid shows that she lacks servings from the grain and dairy groups and that she has a high intake from the meat group.

Grain group	Jane should not restrict her intake from this group. Breads, pasta, and other grain products will not cause weight gain unless they are prepared with large amounts of fat or eaten in excessive quantities.
Meat group	The number of servings from this group exceeds the recommended intake. This contributes to Jane's fat and calorie intake even though she may be selecting lean cuts of meat. The number of servings should be decreased and each portion size should be about 2–3 ounces.
Dairy group	A restricted dairy intake has decreased Jane's calcium intake. The items she does consume from this group tend to have a high fat content. She could use dairy products that have a reduced fat content in order to limit her calorie intake but maintain the calcium level in her diet.
Vegetable group	Broccoli and green leafy vegetables such as beet greens, collards, and kale will provide calcium to the diet but must be consumed in amounts greater than usual serving sizes in order to obtain adequate calcium (Table 14–5). Most salad greens contain very little calcium.
Beverages	The total amount of fluid consumed is adequate. The consumption of soda should be limited because it would increase the calorie intake without contributing to the nutrient content of the diet.

Chapter 15

It is not unusual for women to be upset and frustrated with news that they may have newly diagnosed glucose intolerance during pregnancy. It has been described that women with gestational diabetes approach the new diagnosis as a crisis or anxiety-provoking situation. These women may experience more difficulty with coping and learning than do women with chronic diabetes who become pregnant (Keohane 1991).

It is important for the nurse to first assess the woman's knowledge about gestational diabetes before attempting to provide any teaching. The woman will benefit most from discussions that build on her current knowledge level. It will usually take several sessions to ensure that the new information is accurately understood and retained.

The nurse can reassure Mrs Chang that the baby should be fine, and can stress the importance of keeping her glucose levels in a normal range. Women with gestational diabetes usually require treatment with diet therapy alone, but occasionally may need insulin administration to control hyperglycemia.

It is felt that gestational diabetes does not cause birth defects because it occurs later in pregnancy, after the baby's organs are formed. The two most common risks to the baby are macrosomia, potentially causing a problem in labor and birth, and hypoglycemia.

Chapter 16

This approach is not appropriate for Rachel. While it is unusual for a nonpregnant woman to develop pyelonephritis from a bladder infection, 25% to 65% of pregnant women with bacteriuria develop pyelonephritis unless their bladder infection is treated (Shortliffe 1992). This is related to the anatomic and physiologic changes of pregnancy, including decreased ureteral peristalsis, ureteral dilation, and increased bladder capacity. Since Rachel is 6 months pregnant, she is probably being seen monthly for prenatal care. Because prompt treatment is essential, you should urge her to call her care giver and discuss her symptoms.

Chapter 21

We hope you would encourage her to take medication if she felt she needed it. There are many types of analgesic agents and many types of regional blocks that can help her if she decides she needs them. Sometimes, giving permission for someone to ask relieves her anxiety and decreases the need for intervention.

Chapter 22

The pattern described is within normal limits. No further action is needed because the pattern is reassuring.

Chapter 23

Once uterine contractions reach the desired characteristics (frequency of every 2–3 minutes, duration of 40–60 seconds, and moderate to strong intensity), and cervical dilitation is 5–6 cm, the infusion rate can be decreased by increments similar to those by which it was increased. In this case you should decrease the rate to the step it was just prior to 6 mU/min (36 mL/hr).

Chapter 24

The twin at greatest risk of developing tissue hypoxia is David. Hypoxia develops when there is inadequate delivery of oxygen to the tissues. This occurs when there is inadequate circulation to the tissues or, as in this case, the blood delivered to the tissues has a decreased oxygen-carrying capacity. The oxygen-carrying capacity of blood is calculated as: 1.26 mL O_2/gram of hemoglobin (the O_2-carrying capacity of fetal hemoglobin) multiplied by the grams of hemoglobin in the sample. Thus, the oxygen vols% and the oxygen-carrying capacity of David's blood is $1.26 \times 11 = 13.86$ vols%. Therefore, David is at greater risk of developing tissue hypoxia than is his brother.

Caution should be exercised when using oxygen saturation monitors to assess hypoxia. The monitors determine the amount of oxygenated versus deoxygenated hemoglobin in the blood and report this value as a percentage; for example, "94% saturated" means 94 percent of the hemoglobin has bound to oxygen molecules. The monitors do not evaluate the amount of hemoglobin present in the blood, nor the actual oxygen-carrying capacity. In this case, David is at greater risk of developing tissue hypoxia despite his oxygen saturation of 100% because he has a lower oxygen-carrying capacity and his tissues are receiving less oxygen per volume of blood.

Chapter 25

The unique behavioral and temperament characteristics of newborn infants should be discussed. Additionally, aspects of the Brazelton exam may be helpful to show Mrs Reyes how her infant changes state with different stimuli and intervention. Teaching her how to console her newborn may also be helpful.

Chapter 26

Reassure mother that you will help her baby as you carry out the following activities:

- Position the infant with her head lowered and to the side.
- Bulb suction the nares and mouth repeatedly until the airway is cleared.
- Hold and comfort the infant when normal respirations are restored.
- Reassure the mother, and review this procedure with her.

Note: If bulb suctioning alone does not clear the airway, use DeLee wall suction and administer oxygen as needed to restore normal respirations.

Chapter 27

Acknowledge Ann's frustration and pain. Tell her you are glad she called and ask how you may be of help. Let her ventilate about how she feels. Explain that her breasts are engorged, which is a problem that many women encounter. It is not unusual for infants to refuse to nurse when the breast is hard and the nipple difficult to grasp.

Identify methods to relieve the engorgement.

a. Warm or cool soaks, whichever she prefers, for comfort and to stimulate let-down.
b. Express a small amount of milk.
c. Put the baby to breast after stimulating let-down and expressing a little milk. (The breast will be softer and it will be easier to grasp the nipple.)
d. Use analgesics. (If taken immediately before nursing, less medication will go to the baby.)

Explain to Ann that her emotional upheaval is probably the "baby blues" or "postpartum blues" and that they usually subside in 24–72 hours. Instruct her to call her physician if the blues do not subside, or if she develops symptoms of depression.

Ask why she started supplemental feedings. Upon questioning, Ann tells you that she had started supplementing her baby with formula after each feeding because her mother-in-law told her that the baby was nursing too frequently (every 1–3 hours, sometimes clustering 3–4 feedings in one 2–3 hour period). She told Ann that the baby was obviously not getting enough breast milk. After receiving supplemental feedings, the baby began feeding once every 3–5 hours.

Tactfully explain that although Ann's mother-in-law meant well, her comments indicate a lack of information about breastfeeding; that is,

a. Breast milk digests faster than formula, so breastfeeding babies feed more frequently.
b. On average, babies nurse 8–12 times in 24 hours.
c. After lactation is well established, the baby will nurse less frequently. During growth spurts, however, all babies nurse more frequently for a few days.

Explain that Ann may still breastfeed successfully, and if she desires to continue breastfeeding, she should stop supplementing with formula.

Chapter 28

We hope that you would tell her that nurses always wear gloves during the initial assessment of a newborn, during all admission procedures until the newborn has its first bath, and sometimes during diaper changes. You should also tell her that her baby will not be isolated from the other babies when in the nursery, and that her baby can remain with her if she wishes. It is important to recognize the concern that Mrs Corrigan may have about people knowing that her baby may have HIV, and to assess her own feelings of social isolation.

Chapter 29

It is important to give this mother clear, factual information regarding the type, cause, and usual course of the baby's respiratory problem. You see that Linn's laboratory tests, chest x-ray, and clinical course so far are indicative of transient tachypnea of the newborn. Respiratory distress syndrome is probably not the problem since Linn is not premature and didn't have any asphyxia at birth. You recognize that prior experience with a premature newborn with respiratory distress and prolonged hospitalization will add to this mother's fear and anxiety regarding her new baby. Therefore, in addition to giving factual information regarding the baby's condition, it is important for you to see whether the mother can be brought to the nursery to see her baby, or to have the mother receive a picture of the baby for reassurance. Before the mother visits the baby, clearly describe the oxygen and monitoring equipment that is helping Linn so that the mother will not be alarmed upon seeing her daughter.

Chapter 30

These findings are not within the normal range. At 24 hours past birth the fundus should be approximately one finger-breadth below the umbilicus and located in the midline. A uterus that is deviated to the right may indicate that the bladder is full and the woman needs to urinate. You should determine whether she is having difficulty urinating and emptying her bladder; if so, you can try some nursing measures to help her void. The lochia will still be rubra, but the amount is excessive and may be related to a boggy uterus.

Chapter 30

Your best response would be, "You can only be discharged if both you and your physician feel you are ready. Federal law now states that you can stay in the hospital for up to 4 days (96 hours) when you have had a c-section."

Chapter 33

You should have Lei return to her room via wheelchair. Assess her leg for warmth, edema, redness, tenderness, and Homan's sign. Discuss with Lei that she should not massage her leg or get out of bed until you consult with the primary provider concerning your findings. Notify her primary health care provider and document your assessment findings.

Appendix J

Resource Directory

General Information Resources

National Center for Health Statistics (NCHS)
Hyattsville, MD
301-436-8500
www.cdc.gov/nchswww

National Health Information Center
Washington DC
800-336-4797
www.nhic-nt.heath.org

National Institute of Child Health and Human Development (NICHD)
Bethesda, MD
301-496-5133
www.nih.gov/nichd

National Maternal and Child Health Clearinghouse
Vienna, VA
703-625-8410
www.circsol.com/mch

National Technical Information Service (NTIS)
Springfield, VA
800-553-6847
www.ntis.gov

Office of Research for Women's Health
Bethesda, MD
800-994-WOMAN
www.4woman.gov or
www.aamc.org/research/adhocgp/women.html

Dialogue Corporation (formerly Knight-Ridder Information, Inc.)
Mountain View, CA
800-334-2564
www.dialogue.com

National Library of Medicine
800-272-4787
www.nlm.nih.gov

Ovid Technologies
Murray, Utah
800-289-4277
www.ovid.com

Resources By Topic

Abortion

National Abortion Federation
Washington DC
800-772-9100
www.prochoice.org

National Abortion Rights Action League (NARAL)
Washington DC
www.naral.org

National Right to Life Committee
www.nrlc.org

Planned Parenthood Federation of America
New York, NY
800-829-7732
www.plannedparenthood.org

Abuse

Incest Survivors Anonymous (ISA)
Box 5613
Long Beach, CA 90805

National Coalition Against Domestic Violence
800-333-SAFE

National Council on Child Abuse and Family Violence
Washington DC
800-222-2000

Adoption

AASK (Adopt a Special Kid)
Oakland, CA
510-451-1748
www.aask.org

Adoptees' Liberty Movement Association (ALMA) Society
New York, NY
212-581-1568
www.almanet.com

Child Welfare Administration
New York, NY
718-291-1900
www.ci.nyc.ny.us/html/acs/html/acscms1t.html

Child Welfare League of America
Washington DC
202-638-2952
www.cwla.org

AIDS (Acquired Immune Deficiency Syndrome)

American Foundation for AIDS Research (AmFar)
New York, NY
800-39-AMFAR
www.amfar.org

American Social Health Association
RTP, NC
www.ashastd.org

AIDS Information Hotline
800-342-AIDS
www.ashastd.org

AIDS Research Information Center, Inc.
Baltimore, MD
www.critpath.org/aric

SIDA Hotline
(provides AIDS information in Spanish)
800-344-7432

TTY/TTD Hotline
(provides AIDS information for the deaf)
800-243-7889

Community Health Education Core
New York, NY
212-740-7292
cpmcnet.columbia.edu/dept/sph

National AIDS Hotline
800-HIV-0440 AIDS Treatment Information
800-TRIALS-A AIDS Clinical Trials Information
800-843-9388 AZT Information Hotline
800-458-5231 Center for Disease Control's National AIDS Clearinghouse
www.cdcnpin.org

CDC National Prevention Information Network
www.cdcnac.org

Shanti Project
San Francisco, CA
415-864-2273
www.emf.net/%7Echeetham/gshpct-1.html

Alcohol Abuse

Al-Anon/Alateen
New York, NY
800-344-2666
www.al-anon-alateen.org

Alcoholics Anonymous
New York, NY
212-870-3400
www.alcoholics-anonymous.org

National Clearinghouse for Alcohol and Drug Information
Rockville, MD
800-729-6686
www.health.org

Victim Outreach Program
Mothers Against Drunk Driving (MADD)
Dallas, TX
214-744-6233
www.madd.org

Women for Sobriety, Inc.
Quakertown, PA
800-333-1606
www.mediapulse.com/wfs/

Birth Control

See Family Planning

Birth Defects

See also Down Syndrome; Genetic Disorders; Sickle Cell Anemia

American Cleft Palate Association
Pittsburgh, PA
800-24-CLEFT
www.cleft.com/index.htm

Cystic Fibrosis Foundation
Atlanta, GA
800-476-4483
www.cff.org

Institutes for the Achievement Human Potential
Philadelphia, PA
215-233-2050
www.iahp.org

March of Dimes Birth Defects Foundation
White Plains, NY
888-MODBABY
www.modimes.org

Spina Bifida Association of America
Washington DC
800-621-3141
www.sbaa.org

Breast Cancer

Reach to Recovery
New York, NY
800-ACS-2345
www.cancer.org

Breastfeeding

Human Lactation Center
Westport, CT
203-259-5995

Lactation and Related Resources
www.telcomplus.net/kga/lactation.htm

La Leche League International
Chalmburg, IL
800-525-3243
www.lalecheleague.org

Lact-Aid
Athens, TN
615-744-9090
www.lact-aid.com

Lactation Consultants Association, Ltd. (ILCA)
Charlottesville, VA
919-787-5181
www.ilca.org

Cancer

American Cancer Society National Office
Atlanta, GA
800-ACS-2345
www.cancer.org

Cancer Information Service, Cancer Inquiries
Bethesda, MD
800-4-CANCER
www.nci.nih.gov

Cesarean Birth

C/SEC, Inc. (Cesarean/Support Education and Concern)
Farmingham, MA
508-877-8266

International Cesarean Awareness Network's Homepage
www.childbirth.org/section/ICAN.html

VBAC (Vaginal Birth After Cesarean)
Needham, MA
www.midwife.org/prof/vbac.htm

Child Abuse

C. Henry Kempe National Center for Prevention and Treatment of Child Abuse and Neglect
Denver, CO
303-864-5252
www.kempecenter.org

Clearinghouse on Child Abuse and Neglect Information
Washington DC
800-FYI-3666
www.calib.com/nccanch

National Committee for Prevention of Child Abuse (NCPCA)
Chicago, IL
312-663-3520
www.childabuse.org

Child Health and Development

Canadian Institute of Child Health
Ottawa, Canada
613-224-4144
www.cich.ca

National Center for Education in Maternal and Child Health
Washington DC
202-625-8400
www.circsol.com/mch

National Institute of Child Health and Human Development (NICHD)
Bethesda, MD
301-496-4000
www.nih.gov/nichd

4 Parents Hotline
Denver, CO
303-620-4444
www.unitedwaydenver.org

Childbirth

Alliance for the Improvement of Maternity Services
aimsusa.org

Birth: Issues in Prenatal Care and Education
Cambridge, MA
888-661-5800

International Childbirth Education Association
Minneapolis, MN
612-854-8660
www.icea.org

Maternity Center Association
New York, NY
212-369-7300

National Association of Childbearing Centers
Perkiomenville, PA
215-234-8068
www.birthcenters.org

Childbirth Education/Preparation

American Academy of Husband-Coached Childbirth
Sherman Oaks, CA
818-788-6662
www.bradleybirth.com

Childbirth Graphics, Ltd.
Rochester, NY
716-272-0300
www.acegraphics.com

Lamaze International
Washington DC
800-368-4404
www.lamaze-childbirth.com

The Natural Family Web Site: Natural Childbirth
www.bygpub.com/natural/natural-childbirth.htm

Circumcision

American Academy of Pediatrics
Elk Grove, IL
800-433-9016
www.aap.org

Circumcision Resource List
www.cirp.org/pages/general/resource-list

Circumcision Publications—Fathering Magazine
www.fathermag.com/health/circ

National Organization of Circumcision
Information Resource Center (No-Circ)
San Anselmo, CA
415-488-9883
www.nocirc.org

Congenital Disorders/Defects

See Birth Defects; Genetic Disorders

Contraception

See Family Planning

Counseling Services

Alliance For Children and Families
www.alliance1.org

Women in Transition (WIT)
Philadelphia, PA
215-751-1111
www.libertynet.org/wit

DES (Diethylstilbestrol) Exposure

Cancer Information Service, Cancer Inquiries
Bethesda, MD
301-496-5583
www.nci.nih.gov

DES Action
Oakland, CA
1-800-DES-9288
www.desaction.org

Down Syndrome

National Association for Down Syndrome (NADS)
Atlanta, GA
800-232-6372
www.nads.org

National Down Syndrome Society Hotline
New York, NY
800-221-4602
www.ndss.org

Family

Displaced Homemakers Network
Washington DC
202-467-6346
www.womenwork.org

Extended Family
www.kidscampaigns.org/start/101extended.html

Fathers for Equal Rights
Miami, FL
305-895-6351
www.merchantfind.com/fathers.htm

Family Service America
Milwaukee, WI
414-359-1040
www.nahsc.org

Parents Without Partners
Silver Springs, MD
800-637-7974
www.parentswithoutpartners.org

Step Family Foundation
New York, NY
212-877-3244
www.stepfamily.org

Family Planning

Association of Voluntary Sterilization, Inc.
New York, NY
212-561-8000

Couple to Couple League International, Inc. (CCL)
Cincinnati, OH 45211
513-471-2000
www.ccli.org

Family Life Information Exchange
Bethesda, MD
301-654-6190
www.dhhs.gov/progorg/opa

Planned Parenthood Federation of America
New York, NY
800-829-7732
www.plannedparenthood.org

Vasectomy
www.gynpages.com/ultimate/vasectomy.html

Food and Nutrition

See Nutrition

Genetic Disorders

National Center for Education in Maternal and Child Health
Washington DC
202-625-8100
www.circsol.com/mch

Hearing Impaired Children

Alexander Graham Bell Association for the Deaf
Washington DC
202-337-5220
www.agbell.org

American Society for Deaf Children
Sacramento, CA
800-942-ASDC
www.deafchildren.org

International Organization for the Education of the Hearing Impaired
Washington, DC
202-337-5220
www.agbell.org

Infant Death

Compassionate Friends
Oak Brook, IL
708-990-0010
www.compassionatefriends.org

SHARE (Source of Help in Airing and Resolving Experiences)
Springfield, IL
800-821-6819
www.nationalshareoffice.com

Infant Health

American Foundation for Maternal and Child Health
New York, NY
212-759-5510
aimsusa.org

American Red Cross
Washington DC
800-234-5272
www.redcross.org

Infertility

Fertility Research Foundation (FRF)
New York, NY
212-744-5500

Resolve, Inc.
Somerville, MA
617-643-2424
www.resolve.org

Test-Tube Fertilization
Norfolk, VA
804-446-8948
www.jonesinstitute.org

Intrauterine Procedures

National Institute for Child Health and Human Development (NICHD)
Bethesda, MD
301-496-4000
www.nih.gov/science/campus

Legal Concerns

Reproductive Freedom Project (ACLU)
New York, NY
212-944-9800
www.aclu.org

Medical Organizations

American Academy of Family Physicians
Kansas City, MO
816-333-9700
www.aafp.org

American Academy of Pediatrics
Elk Grove, IL
800-433-9016
www.aap.org

American College of Obstetricians and Gynecologists
Chicago, IL
202-638-5577
www.acog.org

American Medical Association
Chicago, IL
312-464-5000
www.ama-assn.org

Society of Obstetricians and Gynecologists of Canada
Ottawa, Canada
613-730-4192
sogc.medical.org

Medications (Prescriptions and Over-the-Counter)

Gold Standard Multimedia-Clinical Pharmacology On-line
ww.gsm.cponline.com

Midwifery

Ask the Midwife
www.parentsplace.com/genobject.cgi/readroom/midwife/mi

Multiple Birth

Center for the Study of Multiple Birth
Chicago, IL
312-266-9093

National Organization of Mothers of Twins Club
Albuquerque, NM
505-275-0955
www.nomotc.org

Nurse-Midwifery

American College of Nurse Midwives
Washington DC
www.acnm.org

Journal of Nurse-Midwifery
New York, NY
212-989-5800

Nursing Organizations

American Association of Nurse Anesthetists (AANA)
Park Ridge, IL
708-692-7050
www.aana.com/information/contact.htm

American Nurses Association and Foundation
Washington DC
202-651-7000
www.nursingworld.org

Canadian Nurses Association
Ottwawa, Canada
613-237-2133
www.cna-nurses.ca

Association of Women's Health, Obstetric and Neonatal Nurses (AWHONN)
Washington DC
202-662-1600
www.awhonn.org

National League for Nursing (NLN)
New York, NY
212-363-5555
www.nln.org

Nutrition

American Institute of Nutrition
Bethesda, MD
301-530-7050
www.nutrition.org

Food and Drug Administration (FDA)
Rockville, MD
888-INFO-FDA
www.fda.gov

Obesity

See Nutrition; Weight Control

Occupational Health

Clearinghouse for Occupational Safety and Health Information
Cincinnati, OH
800-356-4674
www.cdc.gov/niosh

Premenstrual Syndrome

See Women's Health

Rape

See your telephone directory for local Rape Centers.

Sex Education

Advocacy for Youth
Washington DC
202-347-5700
www.advocatesforyouth.org

Planned Parenthood Federation of America
New York, NY
800-829-7732
www.plannedparenthood.org

Sexual Abuse and Assault

National Committee for Prevention of Child Abuse
Chicago, IL
800-556-2722
www.childabuse.org

Voices in Action, Inc.
Chicago, IL
800-7-VOICE-8
www.voices-action.org

Sexually Transmitted Infections

See also AIDS; Sex Education

American Social Health Association
Atlanta, GA
800-227-8922
www.ashastd.org

V.D. National Hotline
800-227-8922

Sickle Cell Anemia

Center for Sickle Cell Disease
Washington DC
202-806-7930
www.jericho.org

Smoking

The following organizations provide information about the effects of smoking as well as how to quit smoking. See the white pages of your telephone directory for local chapters.

American Cancer Society
New York, NY
800-ACS-2345
www.cancer.org

American Heart Association
Dallas, TX
800-AHA-USA1
www.americanheart.org

American Lung Association
New York, NY
800-586-4872
www.lungusa.org

Sudden Infant Death Syndrome

Loyola University
Maywood, IL
708-216-9000
www.lumc.edu

National Sudden Infant Death Syndrome Clearinghouse (NSIDSC)
McLean, VA
703-821-8955 ext. 249
www.circol.com/SIDS

Weight Control

The following groups provide information about weight control and support for their members. See the white pages of your telephone directory for local chapters.

Overeaters Anonymous
Rio Rancho, NM
505-891-2664
www.overeatersanonymous.org

TOPS (Take Off Pounds Sensibly)
Milwaukee, WI
414-482-4620
www.tops.org

Weight Watchers International, Inc.
Jericho, NY
800-651-6000
www.weightwatchers.com

Women's Health

Boston Women's Health Book Collective
(*publishes* Our Bodies, Ourselves, *a well-known book on women's health*)
Summerville, MA
617-625-0271
www.feminist.com/ourbodies.htm

National Coalition for Homelessness
San Francisco, CA
415-346-3740
www.sfo.com/~coh

Community Health Education Core
New York, NY
212-740-7292
http://cpmcnet.columbia.edu

National Women's Health Network
Washington DC
202-347-1140
www.aoa.dhhs.gov/aoa/dir

Office of Minority Health Resource Center
www.os.dhhs.gov/progort/ophs/omh/omhrs.htm

Women's Sports Foundation
East Meadow, NY
800-2227-3988
www.lifetimetv.com/WoSport

Glossary

Abdominal effleurage Gentle stroking used in massage.

Abortion Loss of pregnancy before the fetus is viable outside the uterus; miscarriage.

Abruptio placentae (ab-rŭp'shē-ō pla-sen'tē) Partial or total premature separation of a normally implanted placenta.

Abstinence Refraining voluntarily, especially from indulgence in food, alcoholic beverages, or sexual intercourse.

Acceleration Periodic increase in the baseline fetal heart rate.

Acini cells Secretory cells in the human breast that create milk from nutrients in the bloodstream.

Acme Peak or highest point; time of greatest intensity (of a uterine contraction).

Acrocyanosis Cyanosis of the extremities.

Acrosomal reaction Breakdown of the hyaluronic acid in the corona radiata by enzymes from the heads of sperm; allows one spermatozoon to penetrate the ovum zona pellucida.

Active acquired immunity Formation of antibodies by the pregnant woman in response to illness or immunization.

Adnexa Adjoining or accessory parts of a structure, such as the uterine adnexa: the ovaries and fallopian tubes.

Adolescence Period of human development initiated by puberty and ending with the attainment of young adulthood.

Afterbirth Placenta and membranes expelled after the birth of the infant, during the third stage of labor. Also called secundines.

Afterpains Cramplike pains due to contractions of the uterus that occur after childbirth. They are more common in multiparas, tend to be most severe during nursing, and last 2 to 3 days.

AIDS (Acquired immune deficiency syndrome) A sexually transmitted viral disease that so far has proved fatal in 100% of cases.

Allele One of a series of alternative genes at the same locus; one form of a gene.

Alveoli Small units of the breast tissue in which milk is synthesized by the alveolar secretory epithelium.

Amenorrhea Suppression or absence of menstruation.

Amniocentesis Removal of amniotic fluid by insertion of a needle into the amniotic sac; amniotic fluid is used to assess fetal health or maturity.

Amnion The inner of the two membranes that form the sac containing the fetus and the amniotic fluid.

Amnionitis Infection of the amniotic fluid.

Amniotic fluid The liquid surrounding the fetus in utero. It absorbs shocks, permits fetal movement, and prevents heat loss.

Amniotic fluid embolism Amniotic fluid that has leaked into the chorionic plate and entered the maternal circulation.

Amniotomy (am-nē-ot'ō-mē) The artificial rupturing of the amniotic membrane.

Ampulla The outer two-thirds of the fallopian tube; fertilization of the ovum by a spermatozoon usually occurs here.

Androgen Substance producing male characteristics, such as the male hormone testosterone.

Android pelvis Male-type pelvis.

Antepartum Time between conception and the onset of labor; usually used to describe the period during which a woman is pregnant.

Anterior fontanelle Diamond-shaped area between the two frontal and two parietal bones just above the newborn's forehead.

Anthropoid pelvis Pelvis in which the anteroposterior diameter is equal to or greater than the transverse diameter.

Apgar score A scoring system used to evaluate newborns at 1 minute and 5 minutes after birth. The total score is achieved by assessing five signs: heart rate, respiratory effort, muscle tone, reflex irritability, and color. Each of the signs is assigned a score of 0, 1, or 2. The highest possible score is 10.

Apnea A condition that occurs when respirations cease for more than 20 seconds, with generalized cyanosis.

Areola Pigmented ring surrounding the nipple of the breast.

Artificial rupture of membranes (AROM) Use of a device such as an amnihook or allis forceps to rupture the amniotic membranes.

Artificial insemination Introduction of viable semen into the vagina by artificial means for the purpose of impregnation.

Assisted reproductive technology (ART) Term used to describe the highly technologic approaches used to produce pregnancy.

Attachment Enduring bonds or relationship of affection between persons.

Attitude Attitude of the fetus refers to the relationship of the fetal parts to each other.

Autosome A chromosome that is not a sex chromosome.

Babinski reflex Reflex found normally in infants under 6 months of age in which the great toe dorsiflexes when the sole of the foot is stimulated.

Bacterial vaginosis A bacterial infection of the vagina, formerly called *Gardnerella vaginalis* or *Hemophilus vaginalis*, characterized by a foul-smelling, grayish vaginal discharge that exhibits a characteristic fishy odor when 10% potassium hydroxide (KOH) is added. Microscopic examination of a vaginal wet prep reveals the presence of "clue cells" (vaginal epithelial cells coated with gram-negative organisms).

Bag of waters (BOW) The membrane containing the amniotic fluid and the fetus.

Ballottement (bal-ot-maw′) A technique of palpation to detect or examine a floating object in the body. In obstetrics, the fetus, when pushed, floats away and then returns to touch the examiner's fingers.

Barr body Deeply staining chromatin mass located against the inner surface of the cell nucleus. It is found only in normal females. Also called sex chromatin.

Basal body temperature (BBT) The lowest waking temperature.

Baseline rate The average fetal heart rate observed during a 10-minute period of monitoring.

Baseline variability Changes in the fetal heart rate that result from the interplay between the sympathetic and the parasympathetic nervous systems.

Battledore placenta Placenta in which the umbilical cord is inserted on the periphery rather than centrally.

Bimanual palpation Examination of the pelvic organs by placing one hand on the abdomen and one or two fingers of the other hand into the vagina.

Biophysical profile Assessment of five variables in the fetus that help to evaluate fetal risk: breathing movement, body movement, tone, amniotic fluid volume, and fetal heart rate reactivity.

Birth center A setting for labor and birth that emphasizes a family-centered approach rather than obstetric technology and treatment.

Birth plan Decisions made by the expectant couple about aspects of the childbearing experience that are most important to them.

Birth rate Number of live births per 1000 population.

Birthing room A room for labor and birth with a relaxed atmosphere.

Bishop score A prelabor scoring system to assist in predicting whether an induction of labor may be successful. The total score is achieved by assessing five components: cervical dilatation, cervical effacement, cervical consistency, cervical position, and fetal station. Each of the components is assigned a score of 0 to 3, and the highest possible score is 13.

Blastocyst The inner solid mass of cells within the morula.

Blended family Families established through remarriage; may include children from previous marriages of each spouse as well as children of the current marriage.

Bloody show Pink-tinged mucous secretions resulting from rupture of small capillaries as the cervix effaces and dilates.

Body stalk Future umbilical cord; structure that attaches the embryo to the yolk sac and contains blood vessels that extend into the chorionic villi.

Boggy uterus A term used to describe the uterine fundus when it is not firmly contracted after the birth of the baby and in the early postpartum period; excessive bleeding occurs from the placental site and maternal hemorrhage may occur.

Bonding Process of parent-infant attachment occurring at or soon after birth.

Brachial palsy Partial or complete paralysis of portions of the arm resulting from trauma to the brachial plexus during a difficult birth.

Bradley method Partner-coached natural childbirth.

Braxton Hicks contractions Intermittent painless contractions of the uterus that may occur every 10 to 20 minutes. They occur more frequently toward the end of pregnancy and are sometimes mistaken for true labor signs.

Brazleton's neonatal behavioral assessment A brief examination used to identify the infant's behavioral states and responses.

Breasts Mammary glands.

Breast self-examination Recommended monthly procedure by which women may detect changes or abnormalities in their breasts.

Breech presentation A birth in which the buttocks and/or feet are presented instead of the head.

Broad ligament The ligament extending from the lateral margins of the uterus to the pelvic wall; keeps the uterus centrally placed and provides stability within the pelvic cavity.

Bronchopulmonary dysplasia (BPD) Chronic pulmonary disease of multifactorial etiology characterized initially by alveolar and bronchial necrosis, which results in bronchial metaplasia and interstitial fibrosis. Appears in x-ray films as generalized small, radiolucent cysts within the lungs.

Brown adipose tissue (BAT) Fat deposits in neonates that provide greater heat-generating activity than ordinary fat. Found around the kidneys, adrenals, and neck; between the scapulas; and behind the sternum. Also called brown fat.

Calorie Amount of heat required to raise the temperature of 1 kg of water 1 degree Celsius.

Capacitation Removal of the plasma membrane overlying the spermatozoa's acrosomal area with the loss of seminal plasma proteins and the glycoprotein coat. If the glycoprotein coat is not removed, the sperm will not be able to penetrate the ovum.

Caput succedaneum (kap′ut)/(suk″sĕ-da′ne-um) Swelling or edema occurring in or under the fetal scalp during labor.

Cardinal ligaments The chief uterine supports, suspending the uterus from the side walls of the true pelvis.

Cardinal movements of labor The positional changes of the fetus as it moves through the birth canal during labor and birth. The positional changes are descent, flexion, internal rotation, extension, restitution, and external rotation.

Cardiopulmonary adaptation Adaptation of the neonate's cardiovascular and respiratory systems to life outside the womb.

Cephalhematoma (sef′ăl-hē-mă-tō′mă) Subcutaneous swelling containing blood found on the head of an infant several days after birth, which usually disappears within a few weeks to 2 months.

Cephalic presentation Birth in which the fetal head is presenting against the cervix.

Cephalopelvic disproportion (CPD) A condition in which the fetal head is of such a shape or size, or in such a position, that it cannot pass through the maternal pelvis.

Certified nurse-midwife (CNM) An RN who has received special training and education in the care of the family during childbearing and the prenatal, labor and birth, and postpartal periods. After a period of formal education, the nurse-midwife takes a certification test to become a CNM.

Cervical cap A cup-shaped device placed over the cervix to prevent pregnancy.

Cervical dilatation Process in which the cervical os and the cervical canal widen from less than a centimeter to approximately 10 cm, allowing birth of the fetus.

Cervix The "neck" between the external os and the body of the uterus. The lower end of the cervix extends into the vagina.

Cesarean birth Birth of the fetus by means of an incision into the abdominal wall and the uterus.

Chadwick's sign Violet bluish color of the vaginal mucous membrane caused by increased vascularity; visible from about the fourth week of pregnancy.

Chemical conjunctivitis Irritation of the mucus membrane lining of the eyelid; may be due to instillation of silver nitrate ophthalmic drops.

Child abuse Nonaccidental physical or threatened harm, including mental or emotional injury, sexual abuse, and sexual exploitation.

Child neglect Failure by parents or other custodians to meet the medical, emotional, physical, or supervisory needs of a child.

Chloasma (klō-az′mă) Brownish pigmentation over the bridge of the nose and the cheeks during pregnancy and in some women who are taking oral contraceptives. Also called mask of pregnancy.

Chorioamnionitis (kō′rē-ō-am′nē-ō-nī′tis) An inflammation of the amniotic membranes stimulated by organisms in the amniotic fluid, which then becomes infiltrated with polymorphonuclear leukocytes.

Chorion The fetal membrane closest to the intrauterine wall that gives rise to the placenta and continues as the outer membrane surrounding the amnion.

Chorionic villus sampling Procedure in which a specimen of the chorionic villi is obtained from the edge of the developing placenta at about 8 weeks' gestation. The sample can be used for chromosomal, enzyme, and DNA tests.

Chromosomes The threadlike structures within the nucleus of a cell that carry the genes.

Chronic grief Grief response involving a denial of the reality of the loss, which prevents any resolution.

Circumcision Surgical removal of the prepuce (foreskin) of the penis.

Circumoral cyanosis Bluish appearance around the mouth.

Circumvallate (ser-kŭm-val′āt) **placenta** A placenta with a thick white fibrous ring around the edge.

Cleavage Rapid mitotic division of the zygote; cells produced are called blastomeres.

Client advocacy An approach to client care in which the nurse educates and supports the client and protects the client's rights.

Climacteric The period of time that marks the cessation of a woman's reproductive function; the "change of life" or menopause.

Clitoris Female organ homologous to the male penis; a small oval body of erectile tissue situated at the anterior junction of the vulva.

Coitus Sexual intercourse between a male and female.

Coitus interruptus Method of contraception in which the male withdraws his penis from the vagina prior to ejaculation.

Cold stress Excessive heat loss resulting in compensatory mechanisms (increased respirations and nonshivering thermogenesis) to maintain core body temperature.

Colostrum (kō-los′trŭm) Secretion from the breast before the onset of true lactation; contains mainly serum and white blood corpuscles. It has a high protein content, provides some immune properties, and cleanses the neonate's intestinal tract of mucus and meconium.

Colposcopy The use of an instrument inserted into the vagina to examine the cervical and vaginal tissues by means of a magnifying lens.

Conception Union of male sperm and female ovum; fertilization.

Conceptional age The number of complete weeks since the moment of conception. Because the moment of conception is almost impossible to determine, conceptional age is estimated at 2 weeks less than gestational age.

Condom A rubber sheath that covers the penis to prevent conception or disease.

Conduction Loss of heat to a cooler surface by direct skin contact.

Condyloma (kon-di-lō′mă) Wartlike growth of skin, usually seen on the external genitals or anus. There are two types, a pointed variety and a broad, flat form usually found with syphilis.

Conjugate Important diameter of the pelvis, measured from the center of the promontory of the sacrum to the back of the symphysis pubis. The diagonal conjugate is measured and the true conjugate is estimated.

Conjugate vera The true conjugate, which extends from the middle of the sacral promontory to the middle of the pubic crest.

Contraception The prevention of conception or impregnation.

Contraction Tightening and shortening of the uterine muscles during labor, causing effacement and dilatation of the cervix; contributes to the downward and outward descent of the fetus.

Contraction stress test A method of assessing the reaction of the fetus to the stress of uterine contractions. This test may be utilized when contractions are occurring spontaneously or when contractions are artificially induced by OCT (oxytocin challenge test) or BSST (breast self-stimulation test).

Convection Loss of heat from the warm body surface to cooler air currents.

Coombs' test (kōōmz) A test for antiglobulins in the red cells. The indirect test determines the presence of Rh-positive antibodies in maternal blood; the direct test determines the presence of maternal Rh-positive antibodies in fetal cord blood.

Cornua The elongated portions of the uterus where the fallopian tubes open.

Corpus The upper two-thirds of the uterus.

Corpus luteum A small yellow body that develops within a ruptured ovarian follicle; it secretes progesterone in the second half of the menstrual cycle and atrophies about 3 days before the beginning of menstrual flow. If pregnancy occurs, the corpus luteum continues to produce progesterone until the placenta takes over this function.

Cotyledon (kot-i-lē′don) One of the rounded portions into which the placenta's uterine surface is divided, consisting of a mass of villi, fetal vessels, and an intervillous space.

Couvade (kū-vahd′) In some cultures, the male's observance of certain rituals and taboos to signify the transition to fatherhood.

Crack A form of free base cocaine that is smoked.

Crisis intervention Actions taken by the nurse to help the client deal with an impending, potentially overwhelming crisis, regain his or her equilibrium, grow from the experience, and improve coping skills.

Critical thinking Intellectual processes that include separating fact from opinion, identifying prejudices and stereotypes that may influence interpretation of information, exploring differing ideas and views, and arriving at conclusions or insights.

Crowning Appearance of the presenting fetal part at the vaginal orifice during labor.

Deceleration Periodic decrease in the baseline fetal heart rate.

Decidua (dē-sid′yū-ă) Endometrium or mucous membrane lining of the uterus in pregnancy that is shed after childbirth.

Decidua basalis The part of the decidua that unites with the chorion to form the placenta. It is shed in lochial discharge after childbirth.

Decidua capsularis The part of the decidua surrounding the chorionic sac.

Decidua vera (parietalis) Nonplacental decidua lining the uterus.

Decrement Decrease or stage of decline, as of a contraction.

Depo-Provera A long acting, injectable progestin contraceptive.

Descriptive statistics Statistics that describe or summarize a set of data.

Desquamation (des-kwă-mā′shŭn) Shedding of the epithelial cells of the epidermis.

Diagonal conjugate Distance from the lower posterior border of the symphysis pubis to the sacral promontory; may be obtained by manual measurement.

Diaphragm A flexible disk that covers the cervix to prevent pregnancy.

Diastasis (dī-as′tă-sis) **recti** (rek-ti′tis) **abdominis** Separation of the recti abdominis muscles along the median line. In women, it is seen with repeated childbirths or multiple gestations. In the newborn, it is usually caused by incomplete development.

Dilatation and curettage (D and C) Stretching of the cervical canal to permit passage of a curette, which is used to scrape the endometrium to empty the uterine contents or to obtain tissue for examination.

Dilatation of the cervix Expansion of the external os from an opening a few millimeters in size to an opening large enough to allow the passage of the infant.

Diploid number of chromosomes Containing a set of maternal and a set of paternal chromosomes; in humans, the diploid number of chromosomes is 46.

Dissociation relaxation A pattern of active relaxation in which the woman learns to tighten one area of the body and then relax other areas simultaneously. This relaxation pattern is very effective for some women during labor.

Doula A supportive companion who accompanies a laboring woman to provide emotional, physical, and informational support and acts as an advocate for the woman and her family.

Down syndrome An abnormality resulting from the presence of an extra chromosome number 21 (trisomy 21); characteristics include mental retardation and altered physical appearance. Formerly called mongolism.

Drug-dependent infant The newborn of an alcoholic or drug-addicted woman.

Ductus arteriosus A communication channel between the main pulmonary artery and the aorta of the fetus. It is obliterated after birth by rising Po_2 and changes in intravascular pressure in the presence of normal pulmonary functioning. It normally becomes a ligament after birth but sometimes remains patent (patent ductus arteriosus, a treatable condition).

Ductus venosus A fetal blood vessel that carries oxygenated blood between the umbilical vein and the inferior vena cava, bypassing the liver; it becomes a ligament after birth.

Duncan's mechanism Occurs when the maternal surface of the placenta presents upon delivery rather than the shiny fetal surface.

Duration The time length of each contraction, measured from the beginning of the increment to the completion of the decrement.

Dysmenorrhea Painful menstruation.

Dyspareunia Painful intercourse.

Dystocia (dis-tō'sē-ă) Difficult labor due to mechanical factors produced by the fetus or the maternal pelvis, or due to inadequate uterine or other muscular activity.

Early decelerations Periodic change in fetal heart rate pattern caused by head compression; deceleration has a uniform appearance and early onset in relation to maternal contraction.

Early postpartal hemorrhage See *Postpartal hemorrhage.*

Eclampsia (ek-lamp'sē-ă) A major complication of pregnancy. Its cause is unknown; it occurs more often in the primigravida and is accompanied by elevated blood pressure, albuminuria, oliguria, tonic and clonic convulsions, and coma. It may occur during pregnancy (usually after the 20th week of gestation) or within 48 hours after childbirth.

Ectoderm Outer layer of cells in the developing embryo that gives rise to the skin, nails, and hair.

Ectopic pregnancy Implantation of the fertilized ovum outside the uterine cavity; common sites are the abdomen, fallopian tubes, and ovaries. Also called oocyesis.

Effacement Thinning and shortening of the cervix that occurs late in pregnancy or during labor.

Effleurage (e-fler-ahz') A light stroking movement of the fingertips over the abdominal area during labor; used to provide distraction during labor contractions.

Ejaculation Expulsion of the seminal fluids from the penis.

Embryo The early stage of development of the young of any organism. In humans the embryonic period is from about 2 to 8 weeks of gestation, and is characterized by cellular differentiation and predominantly hyperplastic growth.

Embryonic membranes The amnion and chorion.

Endoderm The inner layer of cells in the developing embryo that give rise to internal organs such as the intestines.

Endometriosis Ectopic endometrium located outside the uterus in the pelvic cavity. Symptoms may include pelvic pain or pressure, dysmenorrhea, dispareunia, abnormal bleeding from the uterus or rectum, and sterility.

Endometritis Infection of the endometrium.

Endometrium (en'dō-mē'trē-ŭm) The mucous membrane that lines the inner surface of the uterus.

En face An assumed position in which one person looks at another and maintains his or her face in the same vertical plane as that of the other.

Engagement The entrance of the fetal presenting part into the superior pelvic strait and the beginning of the descent through the pelvic canal.

Engorgement Vascular congestion or distention. In obstetrics, the swelling of breast tissue brought about by an increase in blood and lymph supply to the breast, preceding true lactation.

Engrossment Characteristic sense of absorption, preoccupation, and interest in the infant demonstrated by fathers during early contact with their infants.

Entrainment Phenomenon in which a newborn moves in rhythm to adult speech.

Epidural block Regional anesthesia effective through the first and second stages of labor.

Episiotomy (ĕ-piz″e-ot'o-me) Incision of the perineum to facilitate birth and to avoid laceration of the perineum.

Epstein's (ep'stīnz) **pearls** Small, white blebs found along the gum margins and at the junction of the hard and soft palates; commonly seen in the newborn as a normal manifestation.

Erb-Duchenne palsy Paralysis of the arm and chest wall as a result of a birth injury to the brachial plexus or a subsequent injury to the fifth and sixth cervical nerves.

Erythema toxicum Innocuous pink papular rash of unknown cause with superimposed vesicles; it appears within 24 to 48 hours after birth and resolves spontaneously within a few days.

Erythroblastosis fetalis Hemolytic disease of the newborn characterized by anemia, jaundice, enlargement of the liver and spleen, and generalized edema. Caused by isoimmunization due to Rh incompatibility or ABO incompatibility.

Estimated date of birth (EDB) During a pregnancy, the approximate date when childbirth will occur; the "due date."

Estrogen replacement therapy (ERT) Use of estrogen and a progestin to decrease the symptoms of menopause and to help prevent osteoporosis.

Estrogens The hormones estradiol and estrone, produced by the ovary.

Ethnocentrism An individual's belief that the values and practices of his or her own culture are the best ones.

Evaporation Loss of heat incurred when water on the skin surface is converted to a vapor.

Exchange transfusion The replacement of 70% to 80% of circulating blood by withdrawing the recipient's blood and injecting a donor's blood in equal amounts, for the purpose of preventing the accumulation of bilirubin or other by-products of hemolysis in the blood.

External os The opening between the cervix and the vagina.

External (cephalic) version Procedure involving external manipulation of the maternal abdomen to change the presentation of the fetus from breech to cephalic.

Fallopian tubes Tubes that extend from the lateral angle of the uterus and terminate near the ovary; they serve as a passageway for the ovum from the ovary to the uterus and for the spermatozoa from the uterus toward the ovary. Also called oviducts and uterine tubes.

False labor Contractions of the uterus, regular or irregular, that may be strong enough to be interpreted as true labor but that do not dilate the cervix.

False pelvis The portion of the pelvis above the linea terminalis; its primary function is to support the weight of the enlarged pregnant uterus.

Family-centered care An approach to health care based on the concept that a hospital can provide professional services to mothers, fathers, and infants in a homelike environment that would enhance the integrity of the family unit.

Female condom A thin, disposable polyurethane sheath with a flexible ring at each end which is placed inside the vagina and serves to prevent sperm from entering the cervix, thus preventing conception.

Female reproductive cycle (FRC) The monthly rhythmic changes in sexually mature women.

Ferning Formation of a palm-leaf pattern by the crystallization of cervical mucus as it dries at mid-menstrual cycle. Helpful in determining time of ovulation. Observed via microscopic examination of a thin layer of cervical mucus on a glass slide. This pattern is also observed when amniotic fluid is allowed to air dry on a slide and is a useful and quick test to determine whether amniotic membranes have ruptured.

Fertility awareness methods Natural family planning.

Fertility rate Number of births per 1000 women aged 15 to 44 in a given population per year.

Fertilization Impregnation of an ovum by a spermatozoon; conception.

Fetal acoustic stimulation test (FAST) A fetal assessment test that uses sound from a speaker, bell, or artificial larynx to stimulate acceleration of the fetal heart; may be used in conjunction with the nonstress test.

Fetal activity diary (FAD) A method for tracking fetal activity taught to pregnant women.

Fetal alcohol effects (FAE) The less severe fetal manifestations of maternal alcohol ingestion, including mild to moderate cognitive problems and physical growth retardation.

Fetal alcohol syndrome (FAS) Syndrome caused by maternal alcohol ingestion and characterized by microcephaly, intrauterine growth retardation, short palpebral fissures, and maxillary hypoplasia.

Fetal attitude Relationship of the fetal parts to one another. Normal fetal attitude is one of moderate flexion of the arms onto the chest and flexion of the legs onto the abdomen.

Fetal blood sampling Blood sample drawn from the fetal scalp (or from the fetus in breech position) to evaluate the acid-base status of the fetus.

Fetal bradycardia A fetal heart rate less than 120 beats per minute during a 10-minute period of continuous monitoring.

Fetal death Death of the developing fetus after 20 weeks' gestation. Also called fetal demise.

Fetal distress Evidence that the fetus is in jeopardy, such as a change in fetal activity or heart rate.

Fetal heart rate (FHR) The number of times the fetal heart beats per minute; normal range is 120 to 160.

Fetal lie Relationship of the cephalocaudal axis (spinal column) of the fetus to the cephalocaudal axis (spinal column) of the woman. The fetus may be in a longitudinal or transverse lie.

Fetal movement record See *Fetal activity diary.*

Fetal position Relationship of the landmark on the presenting fetal part to the front, sides, or back of the maternal pelvis.

Fetal presentation The fetal body part that enters the maternal pelvis first. The three possible presentations are cephalic, shoulder, or breech.

Fetal tachycardia A fetal heart rate of 160 beats per minute or more during a 10-minute period of continuous monitoring.

Fetoscope An adaptation of a stethoscope that facilitates auscultation of the fetal heart rate.

Fetoscopy A technique for directly observing the fetus and obtaining a sample of fetal blood or skin.

Fetus The child in utero from about the seventh to ninth week of gestation until birth.

Fibrocystic breast disease Benign breast disorder characterized by a thickening of normal breast tissue and the formation of cysts.

Fimbria Any structure resembling a fringe; the fringelike extremity of the fallopian tubes.

Folic acid An important vitamin directly related to the outcome of pregnancy and to maternal and fetal health.

Follicle-stimulating hormone (FSH) Hormone produced by the anterior pituitary during the first half of the menstrual cycle, stimulating development of the graafian follicle.

Fontanelle (fon′tă-nel′) In the fetus, an unossified space or soft spot consisting of a strong band of connective tissue lying between the cranial bones of the skull.

Foramen ovale Special opening between the atria of the fetal heart. Normally, the opening closes shortly after birth; if it remains open, it can be repaired surgically.

Forceps Obstetric instrument occasionally used to aid in childbirth.

Foremilk Breast milk obtained at the beginning of the breastfeeding episode.

Fourth trimester First several postpartal weeks during which the woman returns to an essentially prepregnant state and becomes competent in caring for her newborn.

Frequency The time between the beginning of one contraction and the beginning of the next contraction.

Fundus The upper portion of the uterus between the fallopian tubes.

Galactorrhea Nipple discharge.

Gamete (gam′ēt) Female or male germ cell; contains a haploid number of chromosomes.

Gamete intrafallopian transfer (GIFT) Retrieval of oocytes by laparoscopy; immediately combining oocytes with washed, motile sperm in a catheter; and placement of the gametes into the fimbriated end of the fallopian tube.

Gametogenesis The process by which germ cells are produced.

Genotype The genetic composition of an individual.

Gestation (jes-tā′shŭn) Period of intrauterine development from conception through birth; pregnancy.

Gestational age The number of complete weeks of fetal development, calculated from the first day of the last normal menstrual cycle.

Gestational age assessment tools Systems used to evaluate the newborn's external physical characteristics and neurologic and/or neuromuscular development to accurately determine gestational age. These replace or supplement the traditional calculation from the woman's last menstrual period.

Gestational diabetes mellitus A form of diabetes of variable severity with onset or first recognition during pregnancy.

Gestational trophoblastic disease (GTD) Disorder classified into two types: benign (hydatidiform mole) and malignant.

Gonadotropin-releasing hormone (GnRH) A hormone secreted by the hypothalamus that stimulates the anterior pituitary to secrete FSH and LH.

Goodell's sign Softening of the cervix that occurs during the second month of pregnancy.

Graafian follicle The ovarian cyst containing the ripe ovum; it secretes estrogens.

Grasping reflex Normal newborn reflex elicited by stimulating the palm with a finger or object, resulting in newborn firmly holding on to the finger or object.

Gravida (grav′i-dă) A pregnant woman.

Grief work The inner process of working through or managing the bereavement.

Gynecoid pelvis Typical female pelvis in which the inlet is round instead of oval.

Habituation (ha-bit-chū-ā′shŭn) Infant's ability to diminish innate responses to specific repeated stimuli.

Haploid number of chromosomes Half the diploid number of chromosomes. In humans there are 23 chromosomes, the haploid number, in each germ cell.

Harlequin sign A rare color change that occurs between the longitudinal halves of the newborn's body, such that the dependent half is noticeably pinker than the superior half when the newborn is placed on one side; it is of no pathologic significance.

Hegar's sign A softening of the lower uterine segment found upon palpation in the second or third month of pregnancy.

HELLP syndrome A cluster of changes including *h*emolysis, *el*evated *l*iver enzymes, and *l*ow *p*latelet count; sometimes associated with severe preeclampsia.

Hemolytic disease of the newborn *Hyperbilirubinemia* secondary to Rh incompatibility.

Heterozygous A genotypic situation in which two different alleles occur at a given locus on a pair of homologous chromosomes.

Hindmilk Breast milk released after initial letdown reflex; high in fat content.

Homozygous A genotypic situation in which two similar genes occur at a given locus on homologous chromosomes.

Hormone replacement therapy (HRT) Administration of hormones, usually estrogen and a progestin, to alleviate the symptoms of menopause.

Huhner test Postcoital examination to evaluate sperm and cervical mucus.

Human chorionic gonadotropin (hCG) A hormone produced by the chorionic villi and found in the urine of pregnant women. Also called prolan.

Human placental lactogen (hPL) A hormone synthesized by the syncytiotrophoblast that functions as an insulin antagonist and promotes lipolysis to increase the amounts of circulating free fatty acids available for maternal metabolic use.

Hydatidiform (hī-da-tid'i-form) **mole** Degenerative process in chorionic villi, giving rise to multiple cysts and rapid growth of the uterus with hemorrhage.

Hydramnios (hī-dram'-nē-os) An excess of amniotic fluid, leading to overdistention of the uterus. Frequently seen in diabetic pregnant women, even if there is no coexisting fetal anomaly. Also called polyhydramnios.

Hydrops fetalis See *Erythroblastosis fetalis.*

Hyperbilirubinemia (hī'per-bil'i-rū-bi-nē'mē-ă) Excessive amount of bilirubin in the blood; indicative of hemolytic processes due to blood incompatibility, intrauterine infection, septicemia, neonatal renal infection, and other disorders.

Hyperemesis gravidarum Excessive vomiting during pregnancy, leading to dehydration and starvation.

Hypnoreflexogenous method A combination of hypnosis and conditioned reflexes used during childbirth.

Hypoglycemia Abnormally low level of sugar in the blood.

Hysterectomy Surgical removal of the uterus.

Hysterosalpingogram Result of testing by instillation of radiopaque substance into the uterine cavity to visualize the uterus and fallopian tubes.

Hysteroscopy Use of a special endoscope to examine the uterus.

In vitro fertilization (IVF) Procedure during which oocytes are removed from the ovary, mixed with spermatozoa, fertilized, and incubated in a glass petri dish; then up to four viable embryos are placed in the woman's uterus.

Inborn error of metabolism A hereditary deficiency of a specific enzyme needed for normal metabolism of specific chemicals.

Incompetent (dysfunctional) cervix The premature dilatation of the cervix, usually in the second trimester of pregnancy.

Increment Increase or addition; to build up, as of a contraction.

Induction of labor The process of causing or initiating labor by use of medication or surgical rupture of membranes.

Infant A child under 1 year of age.

Infant mortality rate Number of deaths of infants under 1 year of age per 1000 live births in a given population per year.

Infant of a diabetic mother (IDM) At-risk infant born to a woman previously diagnosed as diabetic, or who develops symptoms of diabetes during pregnancy.

Inferential statistics Statistics that allow an investigator to draw conclusions about what is happening between two or more variables in a population and to suggest or refute casual relationships between them.

Infertility Diminished ability to conceive.

Informed consent A legal concept that protects a person's rights to autonomy and self-determination by specifying that no action may be taken without that person's prior understanding and freely given consent.

Infundibulopelvic ligament Ligament that suspends and supports the ovaries.

Innominate bone The hip bone, ilium, ischium, and pubis.

Intensity The strength of a uterine contraction during acme.

Internal os An inside mouth or opening; the opening between the cervix and the uterus.

Internal version Procedure used to vaginally deliver a second twin. The obstetrician inserts a hand into the uterus, grasps the feet of the fetus, and changes the fetus from a transverse to a breech presentation.

Intrapartum The time from the onset of true labor until the birth of the infant and delivery of the placenta.

Intrauterine catheter A catheter that can be placed through the cervix into the uterus to measure uterine pressure during labor. Some types of catheters may be inserted for the purpose of infusing warmed saline to add additional intrauterine fluid when oligohydramnios is present.

Intrauterine device (IUD) Small metal or plastic form that is placed in the uterus to prevent implantation of a fertilized ovum.

Intrauterine fetal surgery Surgery performed on a fetus to correct anatomic lesions that are not compatible with life if left untreated.

Intrauterine growth restriction (IUGR) Fetal undergrowth due to any etiology, such as intrauterine infection, deficient nutrient supply, or congenital malformation. Formerly called intrauterine growth retardation.

Introitus Opening or entrance into a cavity or canal such as the vagina.

Involution Rolling or turning inward; the reduction in size of the uterus following childbirth.

Ischial spines Prominences that arise near the junction of the ilium and ischium and jut into the pelvic cavity; used as a reference point during labor to evaluate the descent of the fetal head into the birth canal.

Isthmus The straight, narrow part of the fallopian tube with a thick muscular wall and an opening (lumen) 2–3 mm in diameter; the site of tubal ligation. Also a constriction in the uterus that is located above the cervix and below the corpus.

Jaundice Yellow pigmentation of body tissues caused by the presence of bile pigments. See also *Physiologic jaundice*.

Karyotype The set of chromosomes arranged in a standard order.

Kegel's exercises Perineal muscle tightening that strengthens the pubococcygeus muscle and increases its tone.

Kernicterus (ker-nik′ter-ŭs) An encephalopathy caused by deposition of unconjugated bilirubin in brain cells; may result in impaired brain function or death.

Kilocalorie (kcal) Equivalent to 1000 calories, it is the unit used to express the energy value of food.

Klinefelter syndrome A chromosomal abnormality caused by the presence of an extra X chromosome in the male; characteristics include tall stature, sparse pubic and facial hair, gynecomastia, small firm testes, and absence of spermatogenesis.

Labor The process by which the fetus is expelled from the maternal uterus. Also called childbirth, confinement, or parturition.

Lactation The process of producing and supplying breast milk.

Lacto-ovovegetarians Vegetarians who include milk, dairy products, and eggs in their diets, and occasionally fish, poultry, and liver.

Lactose intolerance A condition in which an individual has difficulty digesting milk and milk products.

Lactovegetarians Vegetarians who include dairy products but no eggs in their diets.

La Leche League Organization that provides information on and assistance with breastfeeding.

Lamaze method A method of childbirth preparation. See also *Psychoprophylaxis*.

Lanugo (lă-nū′gō) Fine, downy hair found on all body parts of the fetus, with the exception of the palms of the hands and the soles of the feet, after 20 weeks' gestation.

Laparoscopy Procedure that enables direct visualization of pelvic organs.

Large for gestational age (LGA) Excessive growth of a fetus in relation to the gestational time period.

Last menstrual period (LMP) The last normal menstrual period experienced by the woman prior to pregnancy; sometimes used to calculate the infant's gestational age.

Late decelerations Periodic change in fetal heart rate pattern caused by uteroplacental insufficiency; deceleration has a uniform shape and late onset in relation to maternal contraction.

Late postpartal hemorrhage See *Postpartal hemorrhage*.

Lecithin/sphingomyelin (les′i-thin sfing′gō-mī′ĕ-lin) **(L/S) ratio** Lecithin and sphingomyelin are phospholipid components of surfactant; their ratio changes during gestation. When the L/S ratio reaches 2:1, the fetal lungs are thought to be mature and the fetus will have a low risk of respiratory distress syndrome if born at that time.

Leiomyoma A benign tumor of the uterus, composed primarily of smooth muscle and connective tissue. Also referred to as a myoma or a fibroid.

Leopold's maneuvers A series of four maneuvers designed to provide a systematic approach whereby the examiner may determine fetal presentation and position.

Letdown reflex Pattern of stimulation, hormone release, and resulting muscle contraction that forces milk into the lactiferous ducts, making it available to the infant. Also called milk ejection reflex.

Leukorrhea Mucous discharge from the vagina or cervical canal that may be normal or pathologic, as in the presence of infection.

Lie Relationship of the long axis of the fetus and the long axis of the pregnant woman. The fetal lie may be longitudinal, transverse, or oblique.

Lightening Moving of the fetus and uterus downward into the pelvic cavity.

Linea (lin′ē-ă) **nigra** (ni′gră) The line of darker pigmentation extending from the umbilicus to the pubis noted in some women during the later months of pregnancy.

Local anesthesia Injection of an anesthetic agent into the subcutaneous tissue in a fanlike pattern.

Lochia (lō′kē-ă) Maternal discharge of blood, mucus, and tissue from the uterus; may last for several weeks after birth.

Lochia alba White vaginal discharge that follows lochia serosa and that lasts from about the 10th to the 21st day after birth.

Lochia rubra Red, blood-tinged vaginal discharge that occurs following birth and lasts 2 to 4 days.

Lochia serosa Pink, serous, and blood-tinged vaginal discharge that follows lochia rubra and lasts until the seventh to tenth day after birth.

Long-term variability (LTV) Large rhythmic fluctuations of the FHR that occur from two to six times per minute.

Luteinizing hormone (LH) Anterior pituitary hormone responsible for stimulating ovulation and for development of the corpus luteum.

Macrosomia (mak-rō-sō′mē-ă) A condition seen in neonates of large body size and high birth weight, as those born of prediabetic and diabetic mothers.

Malposition An abnormal position of the fetus in the birth canal.

Malpresentation A presentation of the fetus into the birth canal that is not "normal," that is, brow, face, shoulder, or breech presentation.

Mammogram A soft tissue radiograph of the breast without the injection of a contrast medium.

Mastitis Inflammation of the breast.

Maternal mortality The number of maternal deaths from any cause during the pregnancy cycle per 100,000 live births.

Mature milk Breast milk that contains 10% solids for energy and growth.

McDonald's sign A probable sign of pregnancy characterized by an ease in flexing the body of the uterus against the cervix.

Meconium Dark green or black material present in the large intestine of a full-term infant; the first stools passed by the newborn.

Meconium aspiration syndrome (MAS) Respiratory disease of term, postterm, and SGA newborns caused by inhalation of meconium or meconium-stained amniotic fluid into the lungs; characterized by mild to severe respiratory distress, hyperexpansion of the chest, hyperinflated alveoli, and secondary atelectasis.

Meiosis The process of cell division that occurs in the maturation of sperm and ova that decreases their number of chromosomes by one-half.

Menarche (me-nar′kē) Beginning of menstrual and reproductive function in the female.

Mendelian inheritance A major category of inheritance whereby a trait is determined by a pair of genes on homologous chromosomes. Also called single gene inheritance.

Menopause The permanent cessation of menses.

Menorrhagia Excessive or profuse menstrual flow.

Menstrual cycle Cyclic buildup of the uterine lining, ovulation, and sloughing of the lining occurring approximately every 28 days in nonpregnant females.

Mentum The chin.

Mesoderm The intermediate layer of germ cells in the embryo that gives rise to connective tissue, bone marrow, muscles, blood, lymphoid tissue, and epithelial tissue.

Metrorrhagia Abnormal uterine bleeding occurring at irregular intervals.

Mifepristone (RU 486) Experimental postcoital contraceptive.

Milia (mil′ē-ă) Tiny white papules appearing on the face of a neonate as a result of unopened sebaceous glands; they disappear spontaneously within a few weeks.

Milk/plasma ratio Comparison of the concentration of substances in the breast milk and the maternal blood serum.

Miscarriage See *Spontaneous abortion.*

Mitosis Process of cell division whereby both daughter cells have the same number and pattern of chromosomes as the original cell.

Molding Shaping of the fetal head by overlapping of the cranial bones to facilitate movement through the birth canal during labor.

Mongolian spot Dark, flat pigmentation of the lower back and buttocks noted at birth in some infants; usually disappears by the time the child reaches school age.

Moniliasis Yeastlike fungal infection caused by *Candida albicans.*

Mons (monz) **pubis** (pu′bis) Mound of subcutaneous fatty tissue covering the anterior portion of the symphysis pubis.

Moro reflex Flexion of the newborn's thighs and knees accompanied by fingers that fan, then clench, as the arms are simultaneously thrown out and then brought together, as though embracing something. This reflex can be elicited by startling the newborn with a sudden noise or movement. Also called the startle reflex.

Morula Developmental stage of the fertilized ovum in which there is a solid mass of cells.

Mosaicism Condition of an individual who has at least two cell lines with differing karotypes.

Mottling (mot′ling) Discoloration of the skin in irregular areas; may be seen with chilling, poor perfusion, or hypoxia.

Mucous plug A collection of thick mucus that blocks the cervical canal during pregnancy. Also called operculum.

Multigravida (mŭl-tē-grav′i-dă)Woman who has been pregnant more than once.

Multipara (mŭl-tip′ă-ră) Woman who has had more than one pregnancy in which the fetus was viable.

Multiple pregnancy More than one fetus in the uterus at the same time.

Myometrium Uterine muscular structure.

Nägele's rule A method of determining the estimated date of birth (EDB): after obtaining the first day of the last menstrual period, subtract 3 months and add 7 days.

Natural childbirth Prepared childbirth, in which the couple attends a prenatal education program and learns exercises and breathing patterns that are used during labor and childbirth.

Neonatal mortality rate Number of deaths of infants in the first 28 days of life per 1000 live births.

Neonatal mortality risk The chance of death within the newborn period.

Neonatal transition The first few hours of life in which the newborn stabilizes its respiratory and circulatory functions.

Neonate Infant from birth through the first 28 days of life.

Neonatology The specialty that focuses on the management of high-risk conditions of the newborn.

Nevus (nē′vŭs) **flammeus** Large port-wine stain.

Nevus vasculosus "Strawberry mark": raised, clearly delineated, dark red, rough-surfaced birthmark commonly found in the head region.

Newborn screening tests Tests that detect inborn errors of metabolism that, if left untreated, cause mental retardation and physical handicaps.

Nidation Implantation of a fertilized ovum in the endometrium.

Nipple A protrusion about 0.5 to 1.3 cm in diameter in the center of each mature breast.

Nipple preparation Prenatal activities designed to toughen the nipple in preparation for breastfeeding.

Non-Mendelian (multifactorial) inheritance The occurrence of congenital disorders that result from an interaction of multiple genetic and environmental factors.

Nonstress test (NST) An assessment method by which the reaction (or response) of the fetal heart rate to fetal movement is evaluated.

Norplant A subdermal progestin contraceptive which is implanted in a woman's arm and provides contraceptive protection for up to 5 years.

Nuchal cord Term used to describe the umbilical cord when it is wrapped around the neck of the fetus.

Nulligravida (nŭl-i-grav′i-dă) A woman who has never been pregnant.

Nullipara A woman who has not delivered a viable fetus.

Obstetric conjugate Distance from the middle of the sacral promontory to an area approximately 1 cm below the pubic crest.

Oligohydramnios (ol′i-gō-hī-dram′nē-os) Decreased amount of amniotic fluid, which may indicate a fetal urinary tract defect.

Oocyte Early primitive ovum before it has completely developed.

Oogenesis Process during fetal life whereby the ovary produces oogenia, cells that become primitive ovarian eggs.

Oophoritis Infection of the ovaries.

Ophthalmia (of-thal′mē-ă) **neonatorum** Purulent infection of the eyes or conjunctiva of the newborn, usually caused by gonococci.

Oral contraceptives "Birth control pills" that work by inhibiting the release of an ovum and by maintaining a type of mucus that is hostile to sperm.

Orgasm Climax of the sexual experience.

Orientation Infant's ability to respond to auditory and visual stimuli in the environment.

Ortolani's maneuver A manual procedure performed to rule out the possibility of congenital hip dysplasia.

Ovarian ligaments Ligaments that anchor the lower pole of the ovary to the cornua of the uterus.

Ovary Female sex gland in which the ova are formed and in which estrogen and progesterone are produced. Normally there are two ovaries, located in the lower abdomen on each side of uterus.

Ovulation Normal process of discharging a mature ovum from an ovary approximately 14 days prior to the onset of menses.

Ovum Female reproductive cell; egg.

Oxygen toxicity Excessive levels of oxygen therapy that result in pathologic changes in tissue.

Oxytocin Hormone normally produced by the posterior pituitary, responsible for stimulation of uterine contractions and the release of milk into the lactiferous ducts.

Oxytocin challenge test (OCT) See *Contraction stress test (CST)*.

Papanicolaou (Pap) smear Procedure to detect the presence of cancer of the uterus by microscopic examination of cells gently scraped from the cervix.

Para (par′ă) A woman who has borne offspring who reached the age of viability.

Parametritis Inflammation of the parametrial layer of the uterus.

Parent-newborn attachment Close affectional ties that develop between parent and child. See also *Attachment.*

Passive acquired immunity Transfer of antibodies (IgG) from the mother to the fetus in utero.

Pedigree Graphic representation of a family tree.

Pelvic cavity Bony portion of the birth passages; a curved canal with a longer posterior than anterior wall.

Pelvic cellulitis Infection involving the connective tissue of the broad ligament or, in severe cases, the connective tissue of all the pelvic structures.

Pelvic diaphragm Part of the pelvic floor composed of deep fascia and the levator ani and the coccygeal muscles.

Pelvic floor Muscles and tissue that act as a buttress to the pelvic outlet.

Pelvic inflammatory disease (PID) An infection of the fallopian tubes that may or may not be accompanied by a pelvic abscess; may cause infertility secondary to tubal damage.

Pelvic inlet Upper border of the true pelvis.

Pelvic outlet Lower border of the true pelvis.

Pelvic tilt Also called pelvic rocking; exercise designed to reduce back strain and strengthen abdominal muscle tone.

Penis The male organ of copulation and reproduction.

Percutaneous umbilical blood sampling (PUBS) A technique used to obtain pure fetal blood from the umbilical cord while the fetus is in utero. Also called cordocentesis.

Perimetrium The outermost layer of the corpus of the uterus. Also known as the serosal layer.

Perinatal mortality rate The number of neonatal and fetal deaths per 1000 live births.

Perinatology The medical specialty concerned with the diagnosis and treatment of high-risk conditions of the pregnant woman and her fetus.

Perineal (per′i-nē′ăl) **body** Wedge-shaped mass of fibromuscular tissue found between the lower part of the vagina and the anal canal.

Perineum (per′i-nē′ŭm) The area of tissue between the anus and scrotum in a man or between the anus and vagina in a woman.

Periodic breathing Sporadic episodes of apnea, not associated with cyanosis, that last for about 10 seconds and commonly occur in preterm infants.

Periods of reactivity Predictable patterns of neonate behavior during the first several hours after birth.

Persistant occiput posterior position Malposition of the fetus in which the fetal occiput is posterior in the maternal pelvis.

Persistent pulmonary hypertension of the newborn (PPHN) Respiratory disease resulting from right-to-left shunting of blood away from the lungs and through the ductus arteriosus and patent foramen ovale.

Phenotype The whole physical, biochemical, and physiologic makeup of an individual as determined both genetically and environmentally.

Phenylketonuria (fen′il-kē′tō-nū′rē-ă) A common metabolic disease caused by an inborn error in the metabolism of the amino acid phenylalanine.

Phosphatidylglycerol (PG) (fos-fă-tī′dĭl-glis′er-ol) A phospholipid present in fetal surfactant after about 35 weeks' gestation.

Phototherapy The treatment of jaundice by exposure to light.

Physiologic anemia of infancy A harmless condition in which the hemoglobin level drops in the first 6 to 12 weeks after birth, then reverts to normal levels.

Physiologic anemia of pregnancy Apparent anemia that results because during pregnancy the plasma volume increases more than the erythrocytes increase.

Physiologic jaundice A harmless condition caused by the normal reduction of red blood cells, occurring 48 or more hours after birth, peaking at the fifth to seventh day, and disappearing between the seventh to tenth day.

Pica The eating of substances not ordinarily considered edible or to have nutritive value.

Placenta (plă-sen′tă) Specialized disk-shaped organ that connects the fetus to the uterine wall for gas and nutrient exchange. Also called afterbirth.

Placenta accreta Partial or complete absence of the decidua basalis and abnormal adherence of the placenta to the uterine wall.

Placenta previa Abnormal implantation of the placenta in the lower uterine segment. Classification of type is based on proximity to the cervical os: *total*—completely covers the os; *partial*—covers a portion of the os; *marginal*—is in close proximity to the os.

Platypelloid pelvis An unusually wide pelvis, having a flattened oval transverse shape and a shortened anteroposterior diameter.

Polar body A small cell resulting from the meiotic division of the mature oocyte.

Polycythemia An abnormal increase in the number of total red blood cells in the body's circulation.

Polydactyly (pol-ē-dak′ti-lē) A developmental anomaly characterized by more than five digits on the hands or feet.

Positive signs of pregnancy Indications that confirm the presence of pregnancy.

Postconception age periods Period of time in embryonic/fetal development calculated from the time of fertilization of the ovum.

Postmature newborn See *Postterm newborn.*

Postpartal hemorrhage A loss of blood of greater than 500 mL following birth. The hemorrhage is classified as *early* or *immediate* if it occurs within the first 24 hours and *late* or *delayed* after the first 24 hours.

Postpartum After childbirth or delivery.

Postpartum blues A maternal adjustment reaction occurring in the first few postpartal days, characterized by mild depression, tearfulness, anxiety, headache, and irritability.

Postterm newborn Any infant born after 42 weeks' gestation.

Postterm labor Labor that occurs after 42 weeks of gestation.

Postterm pregnancy Pregnancy that lasts beyond 42 weeks' gestation.

Precipitous birth (1) Unduly rapid progression of labor. (2) A birth in which no physician is in attendance.

Precipitous labor Labor lasting less than 3 hours.

Preeclampsia (prē-ē-klamp′sē-ă) Toxemia of pregnancy, characterized by hypertension, albuminuria, and edema. See also *Eclampsia.*

Pregnancy-induced hypertension (PIH) A hypertensive disorder including preeclampsia and eclampsia as conditions, characterized by the three cardinal signs of hypertension, edema, and proteinuria.

Premature infant See *Preterm infant.*

Premature rupture of the membranes (PROM) See *Rupture of membranes.*

Premenstrual syndrome (PMS) Cluster of symptoms experienced by some women, typically occurring from a few days up to 2 weeks prior to the onset of menses.

Prenatal education Programs offered to expectant families, adolescents, women, or partners to provide education regarding the pregnancy, labor, and birth experience.

Prep Shaving of the pubic area.

Presentation The fetal body part that enters the maternal pelvis first. The three possible presentations are cephalic, shoulder, or breech.

Presenting part The fetal part present in or on the cervical os.

Presumptive signs of pregnancy Symptoms that suggest but do not confirm pregnancy, such as cessation of menses, quickening, Chadwick's sign, and morning sickness.

Preterm infant Any infant born before 38 weeks' gestation.

Preterm labor Labor occurring between 20 and 38 weeks of pregnancy. Also called premature labor.

Primigravida (prī-mi-grav′i-dă) A woman who is pregnant for the first time.

Primipara (prī-mip′ă-ră) A woman who has given birth to her first child (past the point of viability), whether or not that child is living or was alive at birth.

Probable signs of pregnancy Manifestations that strongly suggest the likelihood of pregnancy, such as a positive pregnancy test, enlarging abdomen, and positive Goodell's, Hegar's, and Braxton Hicks signs.

Progesterone A hormone produced by the corpus luteum, adrenal cortex, and placenta whose function is to stimulate proliferation of the endometrium to facilitate growth of the embryo.

Progressive relaxation A relaxation technique that involves relaxing first one portion of the body and then another portion, until total body relaxation is achieved; may be used during labor.

Prolactin A hormone secreted by the anterior pituitary that stimulates and sustains lactation in mammals.

Prolapsed cord Umbilical cord that becomes trapped in the vagina before the fetus is born.

Prolonged labor Labor lasting more than 24 hours.

Prostaglandins Complex lipid compounds synthesized by many cells in the body.

Pseudomenstruation Blood-tinged mucus from the vagina in the newborn female infant; caused by withdrawal of maternal hormones that were present during pregnancy.

Psychoprophylaxis (Lamaze) Psychophysical training aimed at preparing the expectant parents to cope with the processes of labor and to avoid concentration on the discomforts associated with childbirth.

Ptyalism Excessive salivation.

Pubic Pertaining to the pubes or pubis.

Pudendal (pyū-den′dăl) **block** Injection of an anesthetizing agent at the pudendal nerve to produce numbness of the external genitals and the lower one third of the vagina, to facilitate childbirth and permit episiotomy if necessary.

Puerperal morbidity A maternal temperature of 38C (100.4F) or higher on any 2 of the first 10 postpartal days, excluding the first 24 hours. The temperature is to be taken by mouth at least 4 times per day.

Puerperium (pyū-er-pēr′ē-ŭm)The period after completion of the third stage of labor until involution of the uterus is complete, usually 6 weeks.

Quickening The first fetal movements felt by the pregnant woman, usually between 16 to 18 weeks' gestation.

Radiation Heat loss incurred when heat transfers to cooler surfaces and objects not in direct contact with the body.

Rape Sexual activity, often intercourse, against the will of the victim.

Read method Natural childbirth preparation centered on eliminating the fear-tension-pain syndrome.

Reciprocal inhibition The principle that it is impossible to feel relaxed and tense at the same time; the basis for relaxation techniques.

Recommended dietary allowances (RDA) Government-recommended allowances of various vitamins, minerals, and other nutrients.

Regional anesthesia Injection of local anesthetic agents so that they come into direct contact with nervous tissue.

Relaxin A water-soluble protein secreted by the corpus luteum that causes relaxation of the symphysis and cervical dilatation.

Respiratory distress syndrome (RDS) Respiratory disease of the newborn characterized by interference with ventilation at the alveolar level, thought to be caused by the presence of fibrinoid deposits lining the alveolar ducts. Formerly called hyaline membrane disease.

Retinopathy (ret-i-nop′ă-thē) **of prematurity** Formation of fibrotic tissue behind the lens; associated with retinal detachment and arrested eye growth, seen with hypoxemia in preterm infants.

Rh factor Antigens present on the surface of blood cells that make the blood cell incompatible with blood cells that do not have the antigen.

RhoGAM An anti-Rh (D) gamma-globulin given after delivery to an Rh-negative mother of an Rh-positive fetus or child. Prevents the development of permanent active immunity to the Rh antigen.

Rhythm method The timing of sexual intercourse to avoid the fertile time associated with ovulation.

Risk factors Any findings that suggest the pregnancy may have a negative outcome, either for the woman or her unborn child.

Rooting reflex An infant's tendency to turn the head and open the lips to suck when one side of the mouth or cheek is touched.

Round ligaments Ligaments that arise from the side of the uterus near the fallopian tube insertion to help the broad ligament keep the uterus in place.

Rugae (rū'gē) Transverse ridges of mucous membranes lining the vagina, which allow the vagina to stretch during the descent of the fetal head.

Rupture of membranes (ROM) Rupture may be PROM (premature), SROM (spontaneous), or AROM (artificial). Some clinicians may use the abbreviation RBOW (rupture of bag of waters).

Sacral promontory A projection into the pelvic cavity on the anterior upper portion of the sacrum; serves as an obstetric guide in determining pelvic measurements.

Salpingitis Infection of the fallopian tubes.

Saltatory pattern A fetal heart rate pattern of marked or excessive variability.

Scalp stimulation test (SST) A test used during labor to assess fetal well-being by pressing a fingertip on the fetal scalp. A fetus not under excessive stress will respond to the digital stimulation with heart rate accelerations.

Scarf sign The position of the elbow when the hand of a supine infant is drawn across to the other shoulder until it meets resistance.

Schultze's mechanism Delivery of the placenta with the shiny or fetal surface presenting first.

Self-quieting activity Infant's ability to use personal resources to quiet and console him- or herself.

Semen Thick whitish fluid ejaculated by the male during orgasm and containing the spermatozoa and their nutrients.

Sepsis neonatorum Infections experienced by a neonate during the first month of life.

Sex chromosomes The X and Y chromosomes, which are responsible for sex determination.

Sexually transmitted infection (STI) Refers to infections ordinarily transmitted by direct sexual contact with an infected individual. Also called sexually transmitted disease.

Short-term variability (STV) Refers to the differences between successive heart beats as measured by the R—R wave interval of the QRS cardiac cycle. Measured only by internal electronic fetal monitoring.

Show A pinkish mucous discharge from the vagina that may occur a few hours to a few days prior to the onset of labor.

Simian line A single palmar crease frequently found in children with Down syndrome.

Sinusoidal pattern A wave form of fetal heart rate where long-term variability is present but there is no short-term variability.

Situational contraceptives Contraceptive methods that involve no prior preparation, for instance, abstinence or coitus interruptus.

Skin turgor Elasticity of skin; provides information on hydration status.

Small for gestational age (SGA) Inadequate weight or growth for gestational age; birth weight below the tenth percentile.

Spermatogenesis The process by which mature spermatozoa are formed, during which the number of chromosomes is halved.

Spermatozoa Mature sperm cells of the male animal, produced by the testes.

Spermicides A variety of creams, foams, jellies, and suppositories that, when inserted into the vagina prior to intercourse, destroy sperm or neutralize any vaginal secretions and thereby immobilize sperm.

Spinal block Injection of a local anesthetic agent directly into the spinal fluid in the spinal canal to provide anesthesia for vaginal and cesarean births.

Spinnbarkeit The elasticity of the cervical mucus that is present at ovulation.

Spontaneous abortion Abortion that occurs naturally. Also called miscarriage.

Station Relationship of the presenting fetal part to an imaginary line drawn between the pelvic ischial spines.

Sterility Inability to conceive or to produce offspring.

Stillbirth The delivery of a dead infant.

Striae (strī'ă) **gravidarum** Stretch marks; shiny reddish lines that appear on the abdomen, breasts, thighs, and buttocks of pregnant women as a result of stretching the skin.

Structural-functional framework Defines the family as a social system.

Subconjunctival (sŭb'kon-jŭnk-tī'văl) **hemorrhage** (hem'ŏ-rij) Hemorrhage on the sclera of a newborn's eye usually caused by changes in vascular tension during birth.

Subdermal implants (Norplant) Silastic capsules containing levonorgestrel; when 6 are implanted in a woman's upper arm, they act as a contraceptive for up to 5 years.

Subinvolution (sŭb-in-vō-lū'shŭn) Failure of a part to return to its normal size after functional enlargement, such as failure of the uterus to return to normal size after pregnancy.

Sucking reflex Normal newborn reflex elicited by inserting a finger or nipple in the newborn's mouth, resulting in forceful, rhythmic sucking.

Surfactant (ser-fak'tănt) A surface-active mixture of lipoproteins secreted in the alveoli and air passages that reduces surface tension of pulmonary fluids and contributes to the elasticity of pulmonary tissue.

Suture Fibrous connection of opposed joint surfaces, as in the skull.

Symphysis pubis Fibrocartilaginous joint between the pelvic bones in the midline.

Syndactyly (sin-dak′ti-lē) Malformation of the fingers or toes in which there may be webbing or complete fusion of two or more digits.

Telangiectatic (tel-an′jē-ek-tat′ik) **nevi** (nē′vī) **(stork bites)** Small clusters of pink-red spots appearing on the nape of the neck and around the eyes of infants; localized areas of capillary dilatation.

Teratogens Nongenetic factors that can produce malformations of the fetus.

Term The normal duration of pregnancy.

Testes The male gonads, in which sperm and testosterone are produced.

Testosterone The male hormone; responsible for the development of secondary male characteristics.

Therapeutic abortion Medically induced termination of pregnancy when a malformed fetus is suspected or when the woman's health is in jeopardy.

Thermal neutral zone (TNZ) An environment that provides for minimal heat loss or expenditure.

Thrombophlebitis Inflammation of a vein wall resulting in thrombus.

Thrush A fungal infection of the oral mucous membranes caused by *Candida albicans.* Most often seen in infants; characterized by white plaques in the mouth.

Tocolysis Use of medications to arrest preterm labor.

Tonic neck reflex Postural reflex seen in the newborn. When the supine infant's head is turned to one side, the arm and leg on that side extend while the extremities on the opposite side flex. Also called the fencing position.

TORCH An acronym used to describe a group of infections that represent potentially severe problems during pregnancy. TO 5 toxoplasmosis, R 5 rubella, C 5 cytomegalovirus, H 5 herpesvirus.

Total serum bilirubin Sum of conjugated (direct) and unconjugated (indirect) bilirubin.

Touch relaxation A relaxation technique that involves relaxing an area of one's body as another person provides a "touch" cue to that specific area. Touch relaxation is very effective during labor contractions.

Toxic shock syndrome Infection caused by *Staphylococcus aureaus,* found primarily in women of reproductive age.

Transitional milk Breast milk produced from the end of colostrum production until about 2 weeks postpartum.

Transverse diameter The largest diameter of the pelvic inlet; helps determine the shape of the inlet.

Transverse lie A lie in which the fetus is positioned crosswise in the uterus.

Trichomonas vaginalis A parasitic protozoan that may cause inflammation of the vagina, characterized by itching and burning of vulvar tissue and by white, frothy discharge.

Trimester Three months, or one-third of the gestational time for pregnancy.

Trisomy The presence of three homologous chromosomes rather than the normal two.

Trophoblast The outer layer of the blastoderm that will eventually establish the nutrient relationship with the uterine endometrium.

True pelvis The portion that lies below the linea terminalis, made up of the inlet, cavity, and outlet.

Tubal ligation Sterilization of a woman accomplished by transecting or occluding the fallopian tubes.

Turner syndrome A number of anomalies that occur when a woman has only one X chromosome; characteristics include short stature, little sexual differentiation, webbing of the neck with a low posterior hairline, and congenital cardiac anomalies.

Ultrasound High-frequency sound waves that may be directed, through the use of a transducer, into the maternal abdomen. The ultrasonic sound waves reflected by the underlying structures of varying densities allow various maternal and fetal tissues, bones, and fluids to be identified.

Umbilical (ŭm-bil′i-kăl) **cord** (kōrd) The structure connecting the placenta to the umbilicus of the fetus and through which nutrients from the woman are exchanged for wastes from the fetus.

Uterine atony Relaxation of uterine muscle tone following birth.

Uterine inversion Prolapse of the uterine fundus through the cervix into the vagina; may occur just prior to or during delivery of the placenta; associated with massive hemorrhage requiring emergency treatment.

Uterosacral ligaments Ligaments that provide support for the uterus and cervix at the level of the ischial spines.

Uterus The hollow muscular organ in which the fertilized ovum is implanted and in which the developing fetus is nourished until birth.

Vagina The musculomembranous tube or passageway located between the external genitals and the uterus of a woman.

Vaginal birth after cesarean (VBAC) Practice of permitting a trial of labor and possible vaginal birth for women following a previous cesarean birth for nonrecurring causes such as fetal distress or placenta previa.

Variable deceleration Periodic change in fetal heart rate caused by umbilical cord compression; decelerations vary in onset, occurrence, and waveform.

Vasectomy Surgical removal of a portion of the vas deferens (ductus deferens) to produce infertility.

Vegan A "pure" vegetarian; one who consumes no food from animal sources.

Vena caval syndrome Symptoms of dizziness, pallor, and clamminess that result from lowered blood pressure when a pregnant woman lies supine and the enlarged uterus presses on the vena cava. Also known as supine hypotensive syndrome.

Vernix (ver′niks) **caseosa** (kā′sē-ōs) A protective cheese-like whitish substance made up of sebum and desquamated epithelial cells that is present on the fetal skin.

Version Turning of the fetus in utero.

Vertex The top or crown of the head.

Vulva The external structure of the female genitals, lying below the mons veneris.

Weaning The process of discontinuing breastfeeding and accustoming an infant to another feeding method.

Wharton's (hwar'tunz) **jelly** Yellow-white gelatinous material surrounding the vessels of the umbilical cord.

Zona pellucida Transparent inner layer surrounding an ovum.

Zygote A fertilized egg.

Zygote intrafallopian transfer (ZIFT) Retrieval of oocytes under ultrasound guidance followed by in vitro fertilization and laparoscopic replacement of fertilized eggs into fimbriated end of the fallopian tube.

Art and Photography Credits

Art Credits

Chapter 3
3-1: Nea Hanscomb. 3-2B: Precision Graphics. 3-3B–D: Precision Graphics. 3-4A–D: Precision Graphics. 3-6: Nea Hanscomb. 3-8: Precision Graphics. 3-9A–D: Precision Graphics.

Chapter 6
6-1: Kristin Mount. 6-2: Nea Hanscomb. 6-3: Barbara Cousins. 6-4: Wendy Hiller Gee/Biomed Arts Associates. 6-5: Wendy Hiller Gee/Biomed Arts Associates. 6-6A: Kristin Mount. 6-6B: Kristin Mount. 6-7A: Precision Graphics. 6-7B: Precision Graphics. 6-8A–C: Precision Graphics. 6-9: Wendy Hiller Gee/Biomed Arts Associates. 6-10: Wendy Hiller Gee/Biomed Arts Associates. 6-11A: Kristin Mount. 6-11B: Kristin Mount. 6-12: Kristin Mount. 6-13A: Precision Graphics. 6-13B: Precision Graphics. 6-14: Precision Graphics. 6-15: Kristin Mount. 6-16: Wendy Hiller Gee/Biomed Arts Associates. 6-17: Kristin Mount. 6-18: Nea Hanscomb. 6-19: Kristin Mount. 6-20A: Nea Hanscomb. 6-20B: Nea Hanscomb. 6-23: Barbara Cousins. 6-24A: Wendy Hiller Gee/Biomed Arts Associates. 6-24B: Wendy Hiller Gee/Biomed Arts Associates. 6-25: Kristin Mount.

Chapter 7
7-1: Nea Hanscomb. 7-2: Nea Hanscomb. 7-3: Nea Hanscomb. 7-4: Nea Hanscomb. 7-5A: Kristin Mount. 7-6A: Precision Graphics. 7-6B: Precision Graphics. 7-7: Kristin Mount. 7-8A–C: Kristin Mount. 7-9: Kristin Mount. 7-10: Kristin Mount. 7-11: Precision Graphics. 7-14: Nea Hanscomb. 7-15: Kristin Mount. 7-16: Kristin Mount. 7-17: Precision Graphics.

Chapter 8
8-1: Nea Hanscomb. 8-2: Nea Hanscomb. 8-3: The Left Coast Group. 8-4A: Precision Graphics. 8-5: Nea Hanscomb. 8-12: Nea Hanscomb. 8-15: Precision Graphics. 8-16: Precision Graphics. 8-17: Precision Graphics. 8-18A: Kristin Mount. B: Kristin Mount. 8-19A: Precision Graphics. 8-19B: Precision Graphics. 8-20: Precision Graphics.

Chapter 9
9-1: Nea Hanscomb. 9-2: The Left Coast Group. 9-6A: Precision Graphics. 9-6B: Precision Graphics.

Chapter 10
10-1: Kristin Mount. 10-3: Kristin Mount. 10-4: Kristin Mount. 10-5A–C: Precision Graphics. 10-6: Kristin Mount.

Chapter 11
11-1: Nea Hanscomb. 11-2: The Left Coast Group. 11-4: Kristin Mount. 11-6: Kristin Mount. 11-7A–D: Kristin Mount. 11-8: Kristin Mount. 11-9A–D: Kristin Mount.

Chapter 12
12-4: The Left Coast Group. 12-5A–C: Nea Hanscomb. 12-6: Kristin Mount. 12-11: Kristin Mount.

Chapter 13
13-1: Shirley Bortoli.

Chapter 14
14-1: Robert Voights/Nea Hanscomb. 14-2: Shirley Bortoli. 14-4: The Left Coast Group.

Chapter 16
16-1A–C: Precision Graphics. 16-2: Kristin Mount. 16-3: Precision Graphics. 16-4: Nea Hanscomb. 16-5A: Precision Graphics. 16-5B: Precision Graphics. 16-8A–E: Kristin Mount

Chapter 17
17-11A–D: Nea Hanscomb. 17-14: Nea Hanscomb. 17-15: Nea Hanscomb. 17-17: Nea Hanscomb. 17-18: Nea Hanscomb. 17-19: Kristin Mount.

Chapter 18
18-1: Kristin Mount. 18-2: Kristin Mount. 18-3A: Kristin Mount. 18-3B: Kristin Mount. 18-4A: Precision Graphics. 18-4B: Precision Graphics. 18-5A–D: Precision Graphics. 18-6A–C: Precision Graphics. 18-7: Precision Graphics. 18-8: Precision Graphics. 18-9: Nea Hanscomb. 18-10A–D: Precision Graphics. 18-12: Kristin Mount. 18-13A: Kristin Mount. 18-13B: Kristin Mount. 18-14: Precision Graphics. 18-15: Precision Graphics. 18-16: Precision Graphics. 18-17: Precision Graphics.

Chapter 19
19-1: Kristin Mount. 19-2A–D: Precision Graphics. 19-3: Precision Graphics. 19-6: Precision Graphics. 19-8: Kristin Mount. 19-10: Precision Graphics. 19-11: Precision Graphics. 19-12A–C: Precision Graphics. 19-13: Nea Hanscomb. 19-14A–D: Nea Hanscomb. 19-15: Nea Hanscomb. 19-16: Nea Hanscomb. 19-17A: Nea Hanscomb. 19-17B: Nea Hanscomb. 19-18: Nea Hanscomb. 19-19: Nea Hanscomb. 19-20: Nea Hanscomb. 19-21: Nea Hanscomb. 19-22: Nea Hanscomb. 19-23: Nea Hanscomb. 19-24: Nea Hanscomb. 19-25: Nea Hanscomb. 19-26: Nea Hanscomb. 19-27: Precision Graphics.

Chapter 20
20-10A: Precision Graphics. 20-10B: Precision Graphics. 20-10C: Precision Graphics. 20-11: Precision Graphics. Table 20-4: Nea Hanscomb.

Chapter 21
21-1A–C: Precision Graphics. 21-2: Kristin Mount. 21-3A: Precision Graphics. 21-3B: Kristin Mount. 21-3C: Precision Graphics. 21-3D: Kristin Mount. 21-4A–D: Kristin Mount. 21-5: Kristin Mount. 21-6A: Kristin Mount. 21-6B: Kristin Mount. 21-7A: Kristin Mount. 21-7B: Kristin Mount. 21-8A: Kristin Mount. 21-8B: Kristin Mount. 21-9: Kristin Mount.

Chapter 22
22-1: Nea Hanscomb. 22-2A: The Left Coast Group. 22-2B: The Left Coast Group. 22-3A: Precision Graphics. 22-3B: Precision Graphics. 22-4A–D: Precision Graphics. 22-5A–E: Precision Graphics. 22-6A–D: Nea Hanscomb. 22-7A: Precision Graphics. 22-7B: Precision Graphics. 22-8A: Precision Graphics. 22-8B: Precision Graphics. 22-9: Precision Graphics. 22-10A: Precision Graphics. 22-10B: Precision Graphics. 22-11A–D: Precision Graphics. 22-12A: Precision Graphics. 22-12B: Precision Graphics. 22-13A–C: Precision Graphics. 22-14: Precision Graphics. 22-15: Kristin Mount. 22-16: Nea Hanscomb. 22-17A–C: Precision Graphics. 22-18A–C: Precision Graphics. 22-20: Nea Hanscomb. 22-21: Precision Graphics. Table 22-4: Nea Hanscomb.

Chapter 23
23-1: Precision Graphics. 23-2A–D: Precision Graphics. 23-3: Wendy Hiller Gee/Biomed Arts Associates/Biomed Arts Associates. 23-4: Nea Hanscomb. 23-5A–C: Precision Graphics. 23-6A–C: Precision Graphics. 23-7A–C: Nea Hanscomb.

Chapter 24
24-1: Nea Hanscomb. 24-2A–D: Kristin Mount. 24-3: Nea Hanscomb. 24-4: Nea Hanscomb. 24-5: Kristin Mount. 24-6A–C: Kristin Mount. 24-7: Nea Hanscomb. 24-8: Kristin Mount. 24-9A–D: Precision Graphics. 24-10: Precision Graphics. 24-11: Nea Hanscomb.

Chapter 25
25-1: The Left Coast Group. 25-11: Nea Hanscomb. 25-12: The Left Coast Group. 25-14A: Precision Graphics. 25-14B: Precision Graphics. 25-15: Precision Graphics. 25-24-1: Kristin Mount. 25-25: Kristin Mount. 25-34A–C: Kristin Mount.

Chapter 26
26-3: Kristin Mount. 26-5A: Precision Graphics. 26-5B: Precision Graphics. 26-6: Precision Graphics. 26-7: The Left Coast Group. 26-10: Precision Graphics. 26-11: Precision Graphics. 26-12: Shirley Bortoli.

Chapter 27
27-2A–D: Precision Graphics. 27-3: Nea Hanscomb. 27-5A: Precision Graphics. 27-6: Precision Graphics. 27-7: Precision Graphics. 27-8: Shirley Bortoli. 27-12: Precision Graphics.

Chapter 28
28-1: Nea Hanscomb. 28-2: Nea Hanscomb. 28-8: Precision Graphics. 28-9: Precision Graphics. 28-13: Nea Hanscomb. 28-14: Nea Hanscomb. Table 28-3: Kristin Mount.

Chapter 29
29-2: Precision Graphics. 29-3A: Precision Graphics. 29-3B: Precision Graphics. 29-4: Nea Hanscomb. 29-7: Nea Hanscomb. 29-11: Nea Hanscomb. 29-13: Nea Hanscomb.

Chapter 30
30-1: Kristin Mount. 30-5: Precision Graphics. 30-6: Nea Hanscomb. 30-7: Precision Graphics.

Chapter 32
32-2A–C: Precision Graphics. 32-5: Precision Graphics.

Chapter 33
33-1A: Kristin Mount. 33-1B: Kristin Mount. 33-2: Kristin Mount.

Appendix E: Kristin Mount.

Photography Credits

Chapter 1
1-1: © Richard Tauber/Addison Wesley Longman. 1-2: © Jenny Thomas Photography/Addison Wesley Longman. 1-3: © Elena Dorfman/Addison Wesley Longman.

Chapter 2
2-1: © Elena Dorfman/Addison Wesley Longman.

Chapter 3
3-2A: © Kathleen Cameron/Addison Wesley Longman. 3-3A: © Kathleen Cameron/Addison Wesley Longman. 3-5: © Kathleen Cameron/Addison Wesley Longman. 3-7 (left): © Kathleen Cameron/Addison Wesley Longman. 3-7 (right): © Alain McLaughlin/Addison Wesley Longman. 3-10: Courtesy of Centers for Disease Control and Prevention. 3-11: Courtesy of Centers for Disease Control and Prevention. 3-12: © D.M. Phillips/Visuals Unlimited. 3-13: © Kenneth Greer/Visuals Unlimited.

Chapter 4
4-1: © Elena Dorfman/Addison Wesley Longman. 4-2: Courtesy of Edward Zieserl, MD.

Chapter 6
6-21A and B: Courtesy of Dr. E. S. E. Hafez, Wayne State University. 6-22: Courtesy of Dr. E. S. E. Hafez, Wayne State University.

Chapter 7
7-5B: © Lennart Nilsson/*A Child is Born*, Dell. 7-12: Courtesy of Marcia London, RNC, MSN, NNP. 7-13: Courtesy of Marcia London, RNC, MSN, NNP. 7-18: © Petit Format/Nestle/Science Source/Photo. 7-19: © Petit Format/Nestle/Science Source/Photo. 7-20: © Petit Format/Nestle/Science Source/Photo. 7-21: © Petit Format/Nestle/Science Source/Photo. 7-22: © Lennart Nilsson/*A Child is Born*, Dell. 7-23: © Lennart Nilsson/*A Child is Born*, Dell. 7-24: © Lennart Nilsson/*A Child is Born*, Dell.

Chapter 8
8-4B: Courtesy of Lovena L. Porter. 8-4C: From Speroff et al.: *Clinical Gynecologic Endocrinology and Infertility*, 5th ed. 8-6: Courtesy of David Peakman, Reproductive Genetics Center, Denver, Colorado. 8-7: Courtesy of David Peakman, Reproductive Genetics Center, Denver, CO. 8-8: Courtesy of Dr. Arthur Robinson, National Jewish Hospital and Research Center, Denver, CO. 8-9: From *Smith's Recognizable Patterns of Human Malformations*, 4th ed. Philadelphia: Saunders 1988. 8-10: From *Smith's Recognizable Patterns of Human Malformations*, 4th ed. Philadelphia: Saunders 1988. 8-11: From *Smith's Recognizable Patterns of Human Malformations*, 4th ed. Philadelphia: Saunders 1988. 8-13: From Thompson JS, Thompson MW: *Genetics in Medicine*, 5th ed. Philadelphia: Saunders, 1991. 8-14: From Lemli L, Smith DW: *The XO Syndrome: A Study of the differential phenotype in 25 patients.* J Pediatr 1963; 63:577.

Chapter 9
9-3: © Elena Dorfman/Addison Wesley Longman. 9-4: © Anne Dowie/Addison Wesley Longman. 9-5: © Richard Tauber/Addison Wesley Longman.

Chapter 10
10-2: Unknown.

Chapter 11
11-3: © Elena Dorfman/Addison Wesley Longman. 11-5: © Elena Dorfman/Addison Wesley Longman.

Chapter 12
12-1: © Richard Tauber/Addison Wesley Longman. 12-2: © Richard Tauber/Addison Wesley Longman. 12-3: © Jenny Thomas Photography/Addison Wesley Longman. 12-7: © Elena Dorfman/Addison Wesley Longman. 12-8: © Elena Dorfman/Addison Wesley Longman. 12-9: © Elena Dorfman/Addison Wesley Longman. 12-10: © Elena Dorfman/Addison Wesley Longman. 12-12: © Elena Dorfman/Addison Wesley Longman.

Chapter 13
13-2: © Elena Dorfman/Addison Wesley Longman. 13-3: © Jenny Thomas Photography/Addison Wesley Longman.

Chapter 14
14-3: © Elena Dorfman/Addison Wesley Longman.

Chapter 15
15-1: © Jenny Thomas Photography/Addison Wesley Longman.

Chapter 16
16-6: © Elena Dorfman/Addison Wesley Longman. 16-7: © Elena Dorfman/Addison Wesley Longman.

Chapter 17
17-1: © Elena Dorfman/Addison Wesley Longman. 17-2: © Elena Dorfman/Addison Wesley Longman. 17-3: Courtesy of Diane Roth. 17-4: From Callen: *Ultrasonography and Obstetrics and Gynecology*, 2nd ed. Philadelphia: WB Saunders, 1988 17-5A and B: From Callen: *Ultrasonography and Obstetrics and Gynecology*, 2nd ed. Philadelphia: WB Saunders, 1988 17-6A and B: From Callen: *Ultrasonography and Obstetrics and Gynecology*, 2nd ed. Philadelphia: WB Saunders, 1988 17-7A and B: From Callen: *Ultrasonography and Obstetrics and Gynecology*, 2nd ed. Philadelphia: WB Saunders, 1988 17-8A and B: From Callen: *Ultrasonography and Obstetrics and Gynecology*, 2nd ed. Philadelphia: WB Saunders, 1988 17-9A–C: From Callen: *Ultrasonography and Obstetrics and Gynecology*, 2nd ed. Philadelphia: WB Saunders, 1988 17-10: From Callen: *Ultrasonography and Obstetrics and Gynecology*, 2nd ed. Philadelphia: WB Saunders, 1988 17-12: From Cundiff, J.L., Haybrich, K.L., Hinzman, N.G.: *Umbilical artery Doppler flow studies during pregnancy.* JOGNN November/December 1990; 19(6):475, fig 3. 17-13: From Cundiff, J.L., Haybrich, K.L., Hinzman, N.G.: *Umbilical artery Doppler flow studies during pregnancy.* JOGNN November/December 1990; 19(6):475, fig 4. 17-16: © Elena Dorfman/Addison Wesley Longman. 17-20: © John Watney/Photo Researchers, Inc.

Chapter 18
18-11: © Stella Johnson/Addison Wesley Longman.

Chapter 19
19-4: © Stella Johnson/Addison Wesley Longman. 19-5: Courtesy of Hewlett-Packard Company. 19-7: © Elena Dorfman/Addison Wesley Longman. 19-9A and B: © Elena Dorfman/Addison Wesley Longman. 19-9C: © Stella Johnson/Addison Wesley Longman.

Chapter 20
20-1: © Elena Dorfman/Addison Wesley Longman. 20-2: © Elena Dorfman/Addison Wesley Longman. 20-3: © Elena Dorfman/Addison Wesley Longman. 20-4: © Suzanne Arms/Addison Wesley Longman. 20-5: © Elena Dorfman/Addison Wesley Longman. 20-6A: © Elena Dorfman/Addison Wesley Longman. 20-7: © Elena Dorfman/Addison Wesley Longman. 20-8: © Stella Johnson/Addison Wesley Longman. 20-9: © Elena Dorfman/Addison Wesley Longman. 20-3: © Elena Dorfman/Addison Wesley Longman. 20-6B: © Stella Johnson/Addison Wesley Longman. 20-8: © Stella Johnson/Addison Wesley Longman.

Chapter 22
22-19: Courtesy of Dr. Dan Farine, University of Toronto.

Chapter 24
24-13: © Beth Elkin/Addison Wesley Longman. 24-14: © Elena Dorfman/Addison Wesley Longman.

Chapter 25
25-2A–C: Reprinted by permission of V. Dubowitz, M.D., Hammersmith Hospital, London, England. 25-3A: Courtesy of Barbara Carey, RNC, MSN, NNP. 25-3B and C: Reprinted by permission of V. Dubowitz, M.D., Hammersmith Hospital, London, England. 25-4A and B: Reprinted by permission of V. Dubowitz, M.D., Hammersmith Hospital, London, England. 25-4C: © Suzanne Arms/Addison Wesley Longman. 25-5A and B: Reprinted by permission of V. Dubowitz, M.D., Hammersmith Hospital, London, England. 25-5C: © Suzanne Arms/Addison Wesley Longman. 25-6A and C: Reprinted by permission of V. Dubowitz, M.D., Hammersmith Hospital, London, England. 25-6B: © Suzanne Arms/Addison Wesley Longman. 25-7A–C: Reprinted by permission of V. Dubowitz, M.D., Hammersmith Hospital, London, England. 25-8A–C: Reprinted by permission of V. Dubowitz, M.D., Hammersmith Hospital, London, England. 25-9A–C: Reprinted by permission of V. Dubowitz, M.D., Hammersmith Hospital, London, England. 25-10A and B: Reprinted by permission of V. Dubowitz, M.D., Hammersmith Hospital, London, England. 25-13: © Elena Dorfman/Addison Wesley Longman. 25-16: © Elena Dorfman/Addison Wesley Longman. 25-23: From Korones, S.B.: High Risk Newborn Infants 4th ed. St. Louis: Mosby, 1986- 25-24: Reproduced with permission from Potter, E.L., Craig, J.M.: *Pathology of the Fetus and Infant*, 3rd ed. ©1975 by Year Book Medical Publishers, Chicago. 25-25: Courtesy of Mead Johnson & Company, Evansville, IN. 25-26: Courtesy of Dr. Ralph Platow from Potter, E.L., Craig, J.M.: *Pathology of the Fetus and Infant*, 3rd ed. © 1975 by Year Book Medical Publishers, Chicago. 25-27: Courtesy of Mead Johnson & Company, Evansville, IN. 25-28: © Stella Johnson/Addison Wesley Longman. 25-29A and B: Courtesy of Mead Johnson & Company, Evansville, IN. 25-30: From Korones, S.B.: *High Risk Newborn Infants*, 4th ed. St. Louis: Mosby, 1986- 25-31A and B: © Elena Dorfman/Addison Wesley Longman. 25-32: © Elena Dorfman/Addison Wesley Longman. 25-33: Reproduced with permission from Potter, E.L., Craig, J.M.: *Pathology of the Fetus and Infant*, 3rd ed. © 1975 by Year Book Medical Publishers, Chicago. 25-35A: Courtesy of Mead Johnson & Company, Evansville, IN. 25-35B: © Stella Johnson/Addison Wesley Longman. 25-36: © Stella Johnson/Addison Wesley Longman. 25-37: © Stella Johnson/Addison Wesley Longman. 25-38: © Stella Johnson/Addison Wesley Longman. 25-39: © Stella Johnson/Addison Wesley Longman. 25-40: © Elena Dorfman/Addison Wesley Longman.

Chapter 26
26-1: © Stella Johnson/Addison Wesley Longman. 26-2: © Elena Dorfman/Addison Wesley Longman. 26-4: Courtesy of Ruth Likler, RNC, BSN. 26-8: © Stella Johnson/Addison Wesley Longman. 26-9: © Stella Johnson/Addison Wesley Longman.

Chapter 27
27-1: © Stella Johnson/Addison Wesley Longman. 27-4: © Stella Johnson/Addison Wesley Longman. 27-5B: © Stella Johnson/Addison Wesley Longman. 27-9: © Elena Dorfman/Addison Wesley Longman. 27-10: © Stella Johnson/Addison Wesley Longman. 27-11: © Stella Johnson/Addison Wesley Longman. 27-13: © Jenny Thomas Photography/Addison Wesley Longman.

Chapter 28
28-3: Courtesy of Carol Harrigan, RNC, MSN, NNP. 28-4: © Stella Johnson/Addison Wesley Longman. 28-5: From Dubowitz, L., Dubowitz, V.: *Gestational Age of the Newborn.* Menlo Park, CA: Addison-Wesley. 28-6: Courtesy of Carol Harrigan, RNC, MSN, NNP. 28-7: © Stella Johnson/Addison Wesley Longman. 28-10: Courtesy of Kadlac Medical Center/Carol Thompson, MSN, NNP. 28-11: Courtesy of Theresa Kledzik. 28-12: Courtesy of Theresa Kledzik, RN. 28-15: Courtesy of Carol Harrigan, RNC, MSN, NNP. Table 28-1: Courtesy of Marcia London, RNC, MSN, NNP.

Chapter 29
29-1: © Stella Johnson/Addison Wesley Longman. 29-5: Courtesy of Marcia London, RNC, MSN, NNP. 29-6: © Stella Johnson/Addison Wesley Longman. 29-8: ©Stella Johnson/Addison Wesley Longman. 29-9: Courtesy of Marcia London, RNC, MSN, NNP. 29-10: © Stella Johnson/Addison Wesley Longman. 29-12: © Elena Dorfman/Addison Wesley Longman. 29-14: © Stella Johnson/Addison Wesley Longman. 29-15: © Stella Johnson/Addison Wesley Longman.

Chapter 30
30-2: From Myles *Textbook for Midwives*, 11th ed. by Bennett and Brown. Churchill Livingstone, 1989. 30-3: © Stella Johnson/Addison Wesley Longman. 30-4: ©Beth Elkin/Addison Wesley Longman.

Chapter 31
31-1A–H: © Anne Dowie/Addison Wesley Longman. 31-2: © Stella Johnson/Addison Wesley Longman.

Chapter 32
32-1: © Kathy Kieliszewski/Addison Wesley Longman. 32-3: © Stella Johnson/Addison Wesley Longman. 32-4: © Kathy Kieliszewski/Addison Wesley Longman.

Chapter 33
33-3: © Elena Dorfman/Addison Wesley Longman.

Part Openers
1: © Ed Eckstein/Phototake. 2: © Jim Cummins/FPG. 3: Philip Matson/Tony Stone Images, Inc. 4: © V. Clement/Jerrican/Photo Researchers. 5: © Yoav Levy/ Phototake. 6: © Mitch Diamond/Uniphoto/Pictor. 7: © Bruce Ayres/Tony Stone Images, Inc.

Insert, *A Day in the Life of a Nurse-Midwife:* © Jenny Thomas Photography/Addison Wesley Longman.

Index

NOTE: An *f* following a page number indicates a figure and a *t* following a page number indicates a table.

continued

continued

continued

continued

continued

continued

continued

continued

continued

continued

Fertility Awareness (also called Natural Family Planning)	***Basal Body Temperature (BBT)*** Methodology: The woman measures and records BBT until ovulation can be predicted according to BBT. Action: Abstain from intercourse for several days before the anticipated time of ovulation and for 3 days after ovulation. ***Rhythm Method (also called Calendar Method)*** Methodology: The woman uses a calendar to calculate the fertile and infertile phases of her menstrual cycle. Action: Abstain from intercourse during the fertile period. ***Cervical Mucus Method (also called Ovulation Method or Billings Method)*** Methodology: The woman assesses cervical mucus for changes in wetness, color, and clearness throughout the menstrual cycle until ovulation can be predicted by the condition of the mucus. Action: Abstain from intercourse when the mucus is wet, clear, and stretchable. ***Symptothermal Method*** Methodology: The woman assesses and records information about primary signs (eg, cycle days, cervical mucus changes) and secondary signs (eg, increased libido, abdominal bloating) until ovulation can be predicted according to the signs. Action: Abstain from intercourse for several days before the anticipated time of ovulation and for 3 days after ovulation.
Situational Contraceptives	***Abstinence*** ***Coitus Interruptus (Withdrawal)*** Methodology/Action: The man withdraws from the vagina when he feels that ejaculation is impending and then ejaculates away from the woman's external genitalia. NOTE: This is one of the least reliable methods of contraception. ***Douching*** Methodology/Action: The woman douches with a saline solution directly after intercourse. NOTE: This is an ineffective method and is not recommended. It may actually facilitate conception by pushing sperm farther up the birth canal.
Spermicides	***Creams, Jellies, Foams, Vaginal Film, Suppositories*** Methodology: The substances destroy or immobilize sperm. Action: The woman inserts one of the substances into the vagina before intercourse. NOTE: Spermicides are minimally effective when used alone, but effectiveness increases when used with a diaphragm, cervical cap, or condom.
Mechanical Contraceptives	***Male Condom*** Methodology: The condom covers the penis and prevents sperm from entering the birth canal. Action: The man applies the condom to the erect penis before vulvar or vaginal contact. ***Female Condom*** Methodology: The condom, which fits over the cervix and also covers a portion of the woman's external genitalia and the base of the man's penis, prevents sperm from entering the birth canal. Action: The woman inserts the condom prior to intercourse. ***Diaphragm*** Methodology: The spermicide-filled diaphragm covers the cervix, preventing sperm from entering the birth canal. Action: The woman fills the diaphragm with spermicidal cream and inserts it into the vagina prior to intercourse. NOTE: The diaphragm must be left in place for 6 hours following intercourse.

SUMMARY OF CONTRACEPTIVE METHODS *CONTINUED*

Mechanical Contraceptives *continued*	***Cervical Cap*** Methodology: This cup-shaped device filled with spermicidal cream fits snugly over the cervix and is held in place by suction. It prevents sperm from entering the birth canal. Action: Insertion is similar to the diaphragm, but the cap may be left in place for up to 48 hours. It should be inserted at least 20 minutes before intercourse and not more than 4 hours before intercourse. ***Intrauterine Device (IUD)*** Methodology: The IUD immobilizes sperm and impedes their progress from the cervix through the uterus to the fallopian tubes. It also causes a sterile inflammatory response of the endometrium that is spermicidal. Action: The IUD is inserted by a physician into the uterus with its string or tail protruding through the cervix into the vagina. The woman must check for the string after each menses.
Oral Contraceptives	Methodology: Oral contraceptives inhibit the release of an ovum and maintain cervical mucus that is hostile to sperm. Action: The woman takes the pill for 21 days, waits 7 days, then restarts the next cycle of pills.
Long-Acting Progestin Contraceptives	***Subdermal Implants (Norplant)*** Methodology: The progestin implant prevents ovulation in most women, and it stimulates the production of thick cervical mucus, which inhibits sperm penetration. ***Depo-Provera*** Methodology: The 150 mg injection interacts with hormones to suppress ovulation, and it thickens the cervical mucus to block sperm penetration. Action: The injection is effective for 3 months; however, return of fertility may be delayed for an average of 9 months.
Operative Sterilization	***Vasectomy*** Methodology/Action: The vas deferens on both sides of the scrotum is surgically severed, interrupting the flow of sperm from the epididymis. ***Tubal Ligation*** Methodology/Action: The fallopian tubes are clipped or plugged, preventing the ovum and the sperm from meeting.

SELF-CARE GUIDE: HOW TO PERFORM BREAST SELF-EXAMINATION (BSE)

1. Stand or sit in front of a mirror to inspect your breasts in three positions.

With both arms relaxed at your side

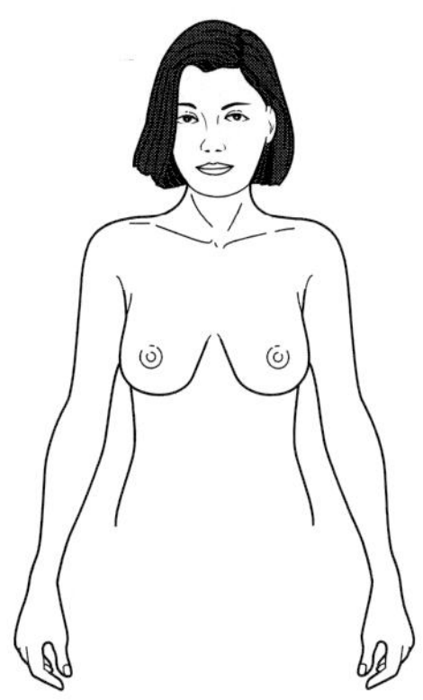

With both arms stretched straight over your head

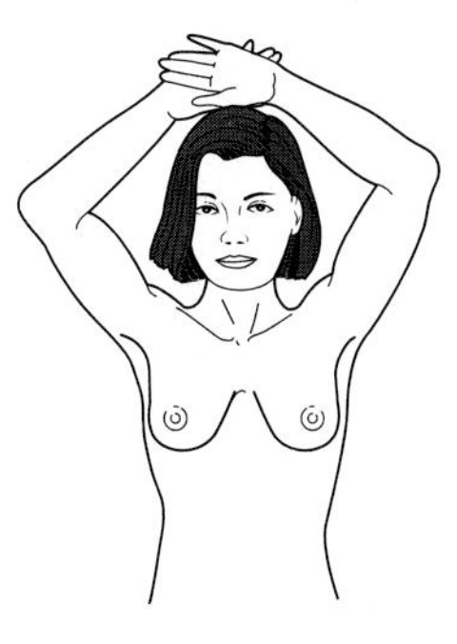

With both hands on your hips while leaning forward

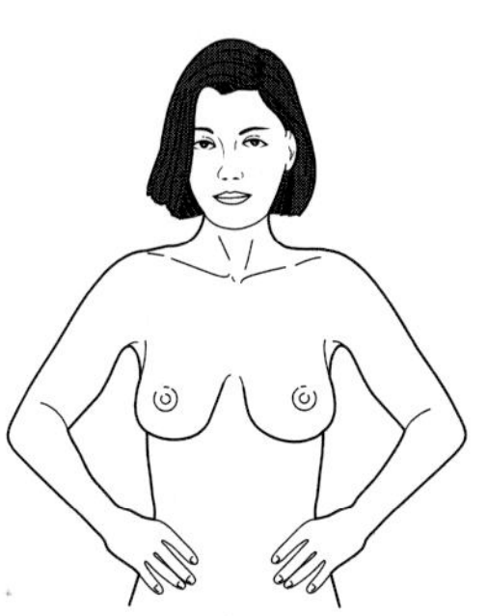

2. Look at your breasts individually and in comparison with one another. Note the following characteristics for each position.

Size and Symmetry of the Breasts

1. Breasts may vary, but the variations should remain constant during rest or movement—note abnormal contours.
2. Some size difference between the breasts is normal.

Shape and Direction of the Breasts

1. The shape of the breasts can be rounded or pendulous with some variation between breasts.
2. The breasts should be pointing slightly laterally.

Surface of the Breasts

1. Skin dimpling, puckering, or retraction (pulling) when the woman presses her hands together or against her hips suggest malignancy.
2. Striae (stretch marks) red at onset and whitish with age are normal.

Color, Thickening, Edema, and Venous Patterns

1. Check for redness or inflammation.
2. A blue hue with a marked venous pattern that is focal or unilateral may indicate an area of increased blood supply due to tumor. Symmetric venous patterns are normal.
3. Skin edema observed as thickened skin with enlarged pores ("orange peel") may indicate blocked lymphatic drainage due to tumor.

Nipple Size and Shape, Direction, Rashes, Ulcerations, and Discharge

1. Long-standing nipple inversion is normal, but an inverted nipple previously capable of erection is suspicious. Note any deviation, flattening, or broadening of the nipples.
2. Check for rashes, ulcerations, or discharge.

➤

3. Palpate (feel) your breasts as follows:

- Lie down, with one hand behind your head. Flatten your fingers and press lightly on your breast, feeling gently for a lump or thickening.

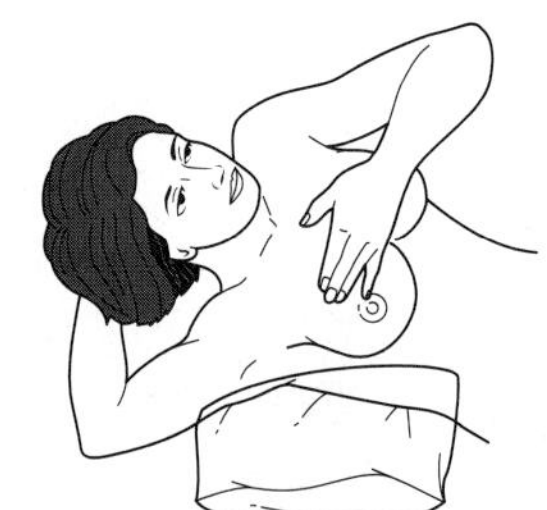

- Check each breast in a circular fashion. Remember to feel all parts of each breast.

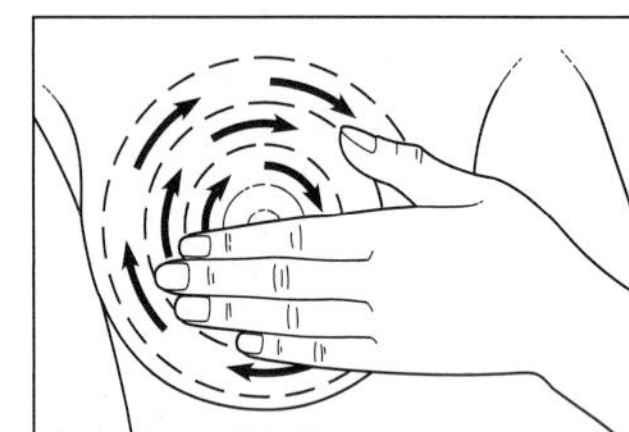

- Repeat the same procedure sitting up, with your hand still behind your head.

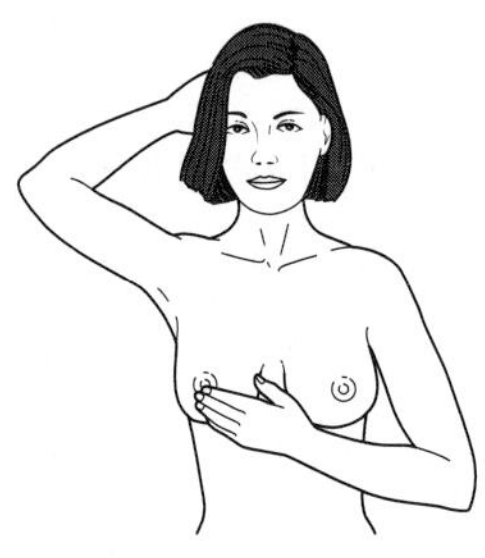

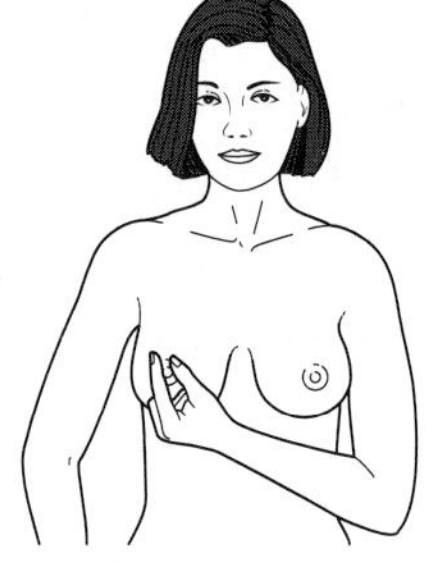

- Squeeze your nipple between your thumb and forefinger. Look for any clear or bloody discharge.

The Warning Signs of Breast Cancer

- Breast mass or thickening
- Unusual lump in the underarm or above the collarbone
- Persistent skin rash near the nipple area
- Flaking or eruption near the nipple
- Dimpling, pulling, or retraction in an area of the breast
- Nipple discharge
- Change in nipple position
- Burning, stinging, or pricking sensation

If you have any of the above signs, see your health care professional immediately.

SELF-CARE GUIDE: HOW TO DETERMINE OVULATION

You can perform two noninvasive tests to help pinpoint your ovulation.

Basal Body Temperature (BBT) Method

By charting your BBT, you can predict when you will ovulate by the rise and fall of your temperature (see chart below). You will need to take your BBT for 3 to 4 months to determine a pattern. For accurate results, take your temperature using a BBT thermometer for 5 minutes every morning before you get out of bed and before you begin any activity. Choose one site (oral, vaginal, rectal or tympanic) and use the same site each time.

Procedure

- Insert the BBT thermometer and after 5 minutes record your temperature on a special BBT chart (with 0.1 [tenths of a degree] markings).
- Connect the temperature dots for each day to see baseline temperature readings.
- Shake down the thermometer to prepare for the next day.

BBT Measurements and Indications

- Right before ovulation, BBT drops.
- Ovulation has occurred when there is a 0.3 to 0.6 degree rise in BBT for 3 consecutive days.
- BBT is elevated 12–14 days prior to menstruation.

Cervical Mucus Method

Your mucus is normally yellow, thick, and dry; absent or white and cloudy. Close to or during ovulation, mucus is clear, slippery, and elastic. Ovulation most likely occurs about 24 hours after the last day of abundant, slippery discharge. Four days after peak mucus or when it is again dry, thick and cloudy, you have passed your fertile time and may resume intercourse.

Procedure

- Check your vagina every day when you use the bathroom, either by dabbing the vaginal opening with toilet paper or by putting a finger inside the opening.
- Note the wetness, collect mucus, and look at its color and consistency.

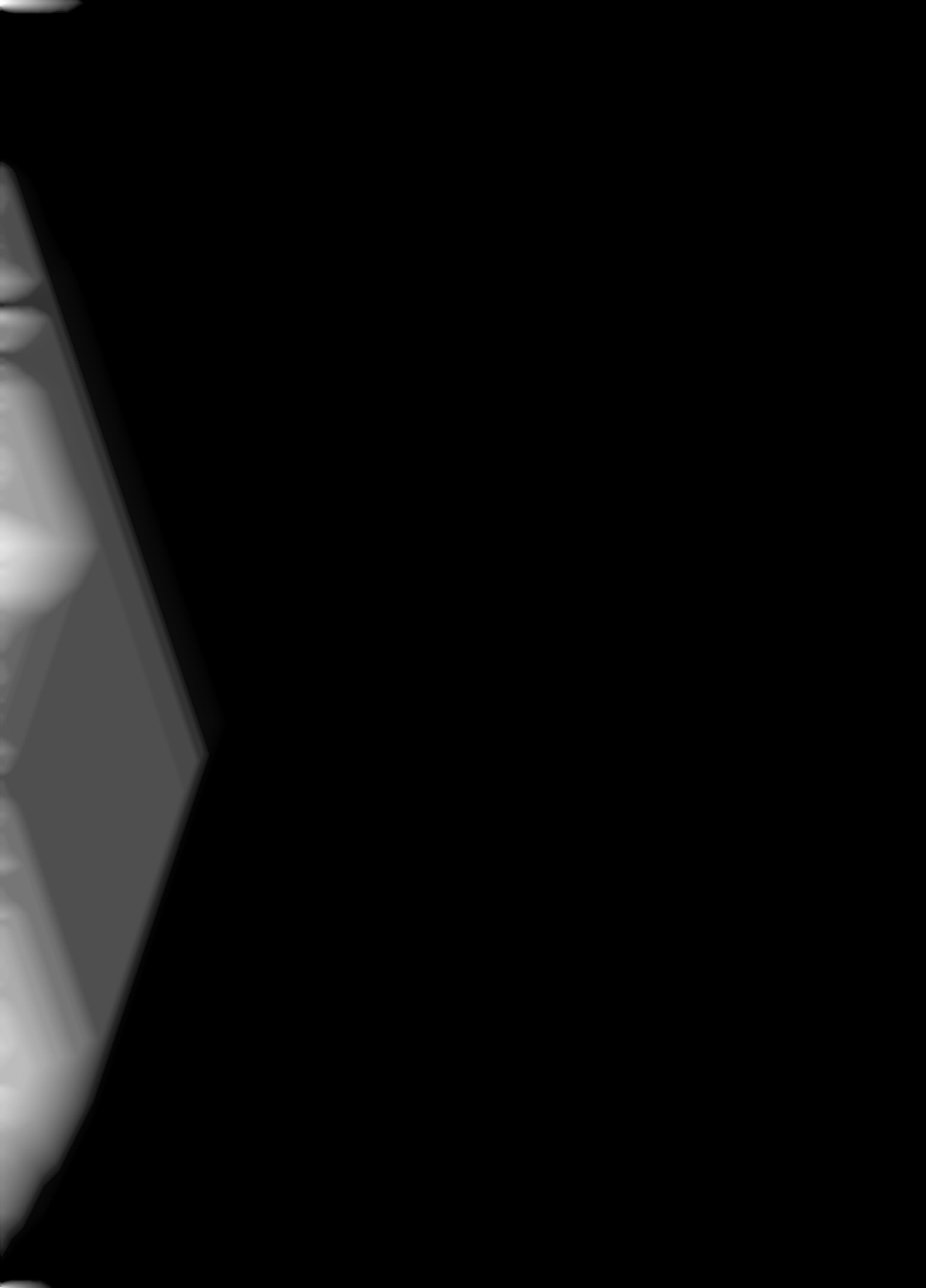

SELF-CARE GUIDE: HOW TO ASSESS FETAL ACTIVITY

Your fetus will begin to move enough for you to feel it when it is about 18 weeks old, and the movements will be stronger and easier to detect as your pregnancy progresses. The normal amount of movement varies considerably; however, most expectant women feel fetal movement at least 10 times in 3 hours.

You can use the **Cardiff Count-to-Ten method** or the **Daily Fetal Monitor Record (DFMR)** to keep a record of your fetus' activity, beginning in the 27th week of gestation. You may choose what time you start each day, but once you choose a time, try to begin counting at the same time every day. If possible, schedule the counting periods about 1 hour after you eat.

Cardiff Count-to-Ten Method

- Begin by photocopying the Cardiff Count-to-Ten scoring card on the other side of this page.
- Lie quietly on your side.
- Begin counting at the hour you have chosen and count up to 10 fetal movements. Place an X on the chart for each movement.

Daily Fetal Movement Record (DFMR)

- Photocopy the DFMR scoring card on the other side of this page.
- Count 3 times a day for 20–30 minutes each session.
- If there are fewer than 3 movements per session, count for 1 hour or more.

When To Contact Your Health Care Provider

- If there are fewer than 10 movements in 3 hours.
- If overall the fetus's movements are slowing, and it takes much longer each day to note 10 movements.
- If there are no movements in the morning.
- If there are fewer than 3 movements in 8 hours.

➤

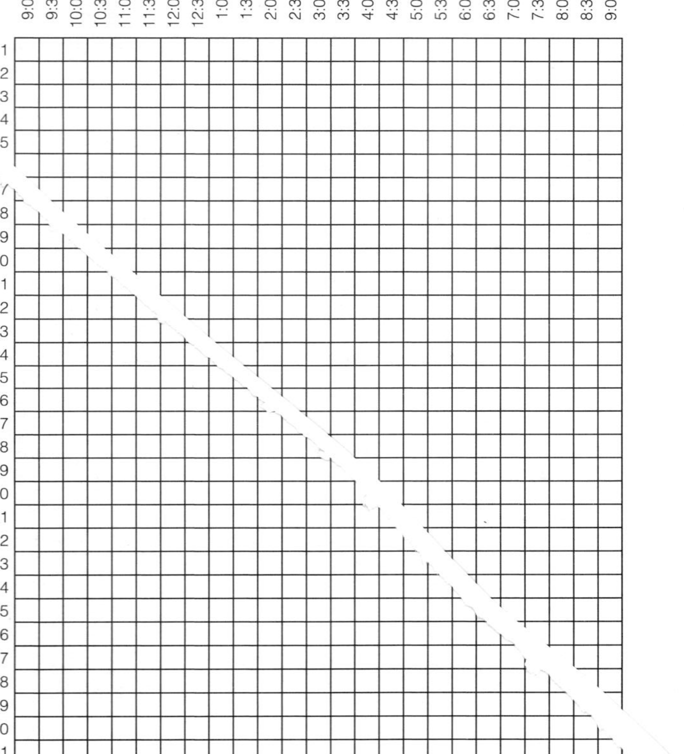

Cardiff Count–to–Ten Scoring Card

Month: ________

Week of gestation at beginning of month: ________

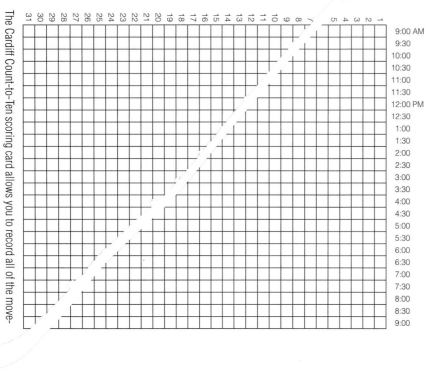

	9:00 AM	9:30	10:00	10:30	11:00	11:30	12:00 PM	12:30	1:00	1:30	2:00	2:30	3:00	3:30	4:00	4:30	5:00	5:30	6:00	6:30	7:00	7:30	8:00	8:30	9:00
1																									
2																									
3																									
4																									
5																									
7																									
8																									
9																									
10																									
11																									
12																									
13																									
14																									
15																									
16																									
17																									
18																									
19																									
20																									
21																									
22																									
23																									
24																									
25																									
26																									
27																									
28																									
29																									
30																									
31																									

The Cardiff Count-to-Ten scoring card allows you to record all of the movements for the month.

DFMR Scoring Card

Month: _______ Week of gestation at beginning of month: _______

	1st Counting Period (number of movements)	2nd Counting Period (number of movements)	3rd Counting Period (number of movements)
1			
2			
3			
4			
5			
6			
7			
8			
9			
10			
11			
12			
13			
14			
15			
16			
17			
18			
19			
20			
21			
22			
23			
24			
25			
26			
27			
28			
29			
30			
31			

The DFMR scoring card allows for three counting periods per day.

SELF-CARE GUIDE: HOW TO ADD 300KCAL TO YOUR DIET

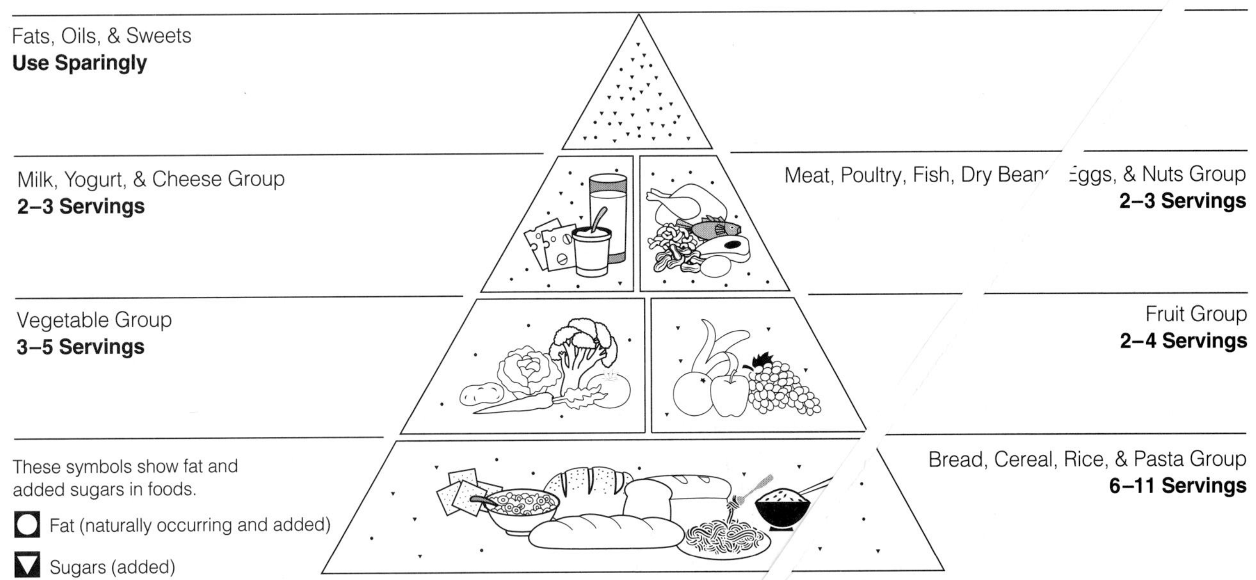

1. Familiarize yourself with the **Food Guide Pyramid.** The grain, fruit, and vegetable groups at the base of the pyramid should account for the majority of your food selections.
2. Use the information about basic food groups below to plan your diet. It is important to consider that not all foods that are nutritionally equivalent have the same number of calories when making food choices.
3. To add 300 Kcals per day, add two milk servings and one meat or alternative serving. Consider using low-fat milk and lean cuts of meat to minimize fat consumption.

About the Food Groups

Grains: 6–11 servings
One serving = 1 slice bread, ½ hamburger roll, 1 oz dry cereal, 1 tortilla, ½ cup pasta, rice, or grits

Fruits: 2–4 servings
One serving = 1 medium-sized piece of fruit, ½ cup of juice

Vegetables: 3–5 servings
One serving = 1 cup raw vegetable, 1 cup green leafy vegetable, ½ cup cooked vegetable

Dairy: 2–3 servings
One serving = 1 cup milk or yogurt, 1.5 oz hard cheese, 2 cups cottage cheese, 1 cup pudding made with milk

Meats and Alternatives: 2–3 servings
One serving = 2 oz lean cooked meat, poultry, or fish; 2 eggs; ½ cup cottage cheese; 1 cup cooked legumes (kidney, lima, garbanzo, or soy beans, split peas); 6 oz tofu; 2 oz nuts or seeds; 4 tsp peanut butter

Combining Foods
Spaghetti and meatball:
2 oz meatball = 1 serving meat
¾ cup spaghetti = 1 grain
¼ cup tomato sauce = ½ cup vegetable

Safety Measures

- Watch for excessive mucus; use a bulb syringe to remove if necessary.
- Keep your baby in a crib or in your arms.
- Avoid leaving your baby unattended on your bed.
- Always wash your hands before handling the baby.

Waking and Quieting Your Baby

Waking Techniques

- Loosen clothing, change diaper.
- Hand express milk onto baby's lips.
- Talk with your baby while making eye contact.
- Hold the baby in upright position (sitting or standing).
- Gently and rhythmically bend your baby back and forth while grasping under knees and supporting head and back with your other hand.
- Play patty-cake with the baby.
- Brush one cheek with your hand or nipple to stimulate the baby's rooting reflex.
- Gently rub the baby's hands and feet.

Quieting Techniques

- Check for a soiled diaper.
- Swaddle or bundle the baby to increase sense of security.
- Use slow, calming movements.
- Softly talk, sing, or hum.

When Your Baby Is Ill

- Call your primary caregiver.
- Be prepared to tell care giver length of time since onset, related activities or problems, specific characteristics of the problem, and the baby's temperature.

Signs of Possible Illness

- Rectal temperature above 38.4C (101F) or above 38C (100.4F) axillary and less than 36.6C (97.8F) axillary.
- More than one episode of forceful vomiting or frequent vomiting (over 6 hours).
- Refusal of two feedings in a row.
- Lethargy (listlessness), difficulty in waking.
- Inconsolable or uses continuous high-pitched cry.
- Cyanosis (bluish discoloration of skin) with or without a feeding.
- Absence of breathing longer than 15 seconds.
- Abdominal distention, crying when trying to pass stools, or absence of stools after stool pattern is established.
- Two consecutive green or black, watery stools or increased frequency of stooling.
- No wet diapers for 18–24 hours or less than 6 wet diapers per day after 4 days of age.
- Increasing jaundice (yellow tone) of the skin.
- Reddened umbilical cord.
- Pustules, rashes, or blisters other than normal newborn rash.

SELF-CARE GUIDE: HOW TO CARE FOR YOUR BABY'S UMBILICAL CORD

Your baby's umbilical cord will fall off within 7 to 14 days after birth. While it is still attached, you will need to perform cord care at least two to three times a day, or you may wish to do it with each diaper change.

Be sure to check the cord every day for odor, oozing of yellow drainage, or reddened, tender areas around the cord. Report any signs of infection to your health care provider.

Follow this procedure to clean your baby's umbilical cord:

1. Lift the cord stump.

2. Using a cotton ball or a cotton-tipped swab moistened with 70% isopropyl alcohol, start at the top and wipe halfway around the cord. Rotate the cotton ball and wipe around the other half of the cord.

3. Swab around the base of the cord to clean away any drainage.

4. Fold the diaper below the umbilical cord to expose it to air.

Helpful Hints

- It is normal for the cord to look dark and to dry up before it falls off. A little drop of blood may appear on the diaper as the cord is about to fall off.
- Your baby may cry when the cold alcohol touches the abdomen, but cord care is not painful because there are no nerve endings in the cord.
- Do not give your baby a tub bath until the cord falls off.
- Never pull the cord or attempt to loosen it.

SELF-CARE GUIDE: RESUMING SEXUAL ACTIVITY AFTER BIRTH

Your ability and willingness to resume sexual activity may depend on a variety of physical factors, such as vaginal tenderness, vaginal dryness, breast tenderness, and the presence of vaginal discharge, among others. The following guidelines will help you and your partner when you are ready to resume lovemaking.

What You May Experience

For the first few weeks after childbirth, the following situations may affect your desire for sexual activity. They are all normal postpartal responses and should disappear within a few weeks or months.

- vaginal dryness and/or tenderness
- difficulty feeling excitement because of fatigue due to the demands of newborn care and recovery from childbirth
- awkwardness if there is leakage of breast milk during sexual activity
- fear of pain during intercourse
- fear of another pregnancy

Your partner may experience:

- fear that you will be uncomfortable during intercourse
- disruption of the established sexual pattern
- fear of another pregnancy
- reduced interest in sex because of fatigue associated with newborn care

When You May Resume Activity

It is best to abstain from intercourse until the episiotomy is healed, if applicable, and the flow of vaginal discharge (lochia) has stopped (usually by the end of the third week following birth).

In the Meantime

- Try expressing your affection and love through kissing, holding, and talking.
- When you do have intercourse, use some form of lubrication, such as K-Y jelly, and use female-superior or side-by-side positions for greater comfort.

A Word About Contraception

Forty percent of nonlactating mothers resume menstruation by the 6th week after birth, and 45% of lactating mothers resume menstruation by the 12th week after birth. Breastfeeding does not provide adequate protection against pregnancy, so be prepared to use contraception if desired.

CERVICAL DILATATION ASSESSMENT AID

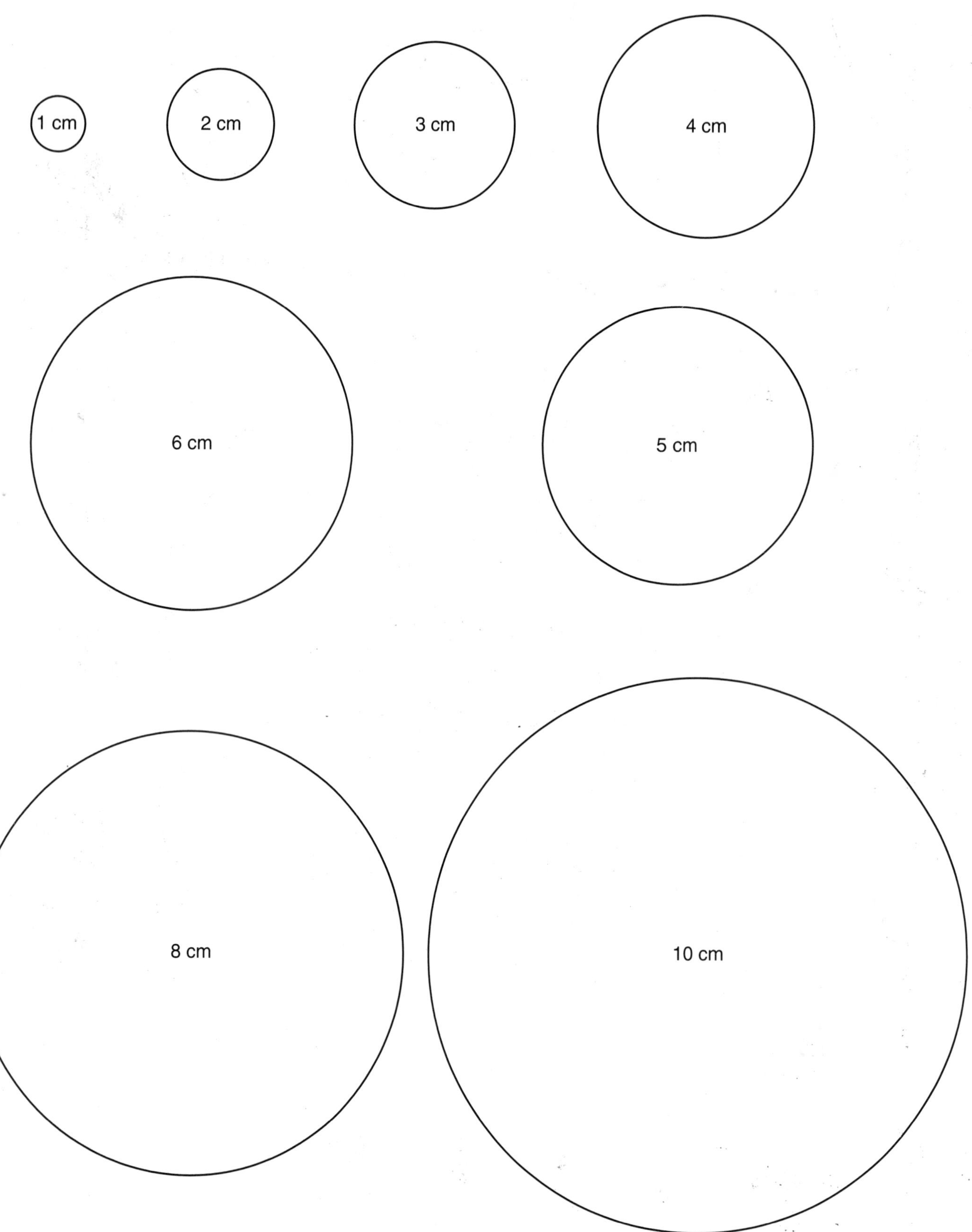